D1074714

Diagnostic Abdominal Imaging

Diagnostic Abdominal Imaging

Wallace T. Miller Jr., MD

Associate Professor of Radiology and Medicine
University of Pennsylvania School of Medicine
Philadelphia, Pennsylvania

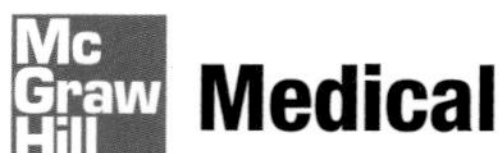

New York Chicago San Francisco Lisbon London Madrid Mexico City
Milan New Delhi San Juan Seoul Singapore Sydney Toronto

Diagnostic Abdominal Imaging

1 2 3 4 5 6 7 8 9 0 CTP/CTP 18 17 16 15 14 13

ISBN 978-0-07-162353-7
MHID 0-07-162353-1

This book was set in Scala Pro by Thomson Digital.
The editors were Michael Weitz and Cindy Yoo.
The production supervisor was Sherri Souffrance.
Project management was provided by Asheesh Ratra, Thomson Digital.
The designer was Eve Siegel; the cover designer was The Gazillion Group.
China Translation & Printing Services, Ltd., was printer and binder.

Library of Congress Cataloging-in-Publication Data

Miller, Wallace T., 1958-
Diagnostic abdominal imaging / Wallace Miller.
p. ; cm.
ISBN 978-0-07-162353-7 (hardcover : alk. paper)
ISBN 0-07-162353-1 (hardcover : alk. paper)
I. Title.
[DNLM: 1. Digestive System Diseases—diagnosis. 2. Abdomen—pathology. 3. Diagnostic Imaging. 4. Urologic Diseases—diagnosis. WI 141]
616.3'075—dc23

2012020791

Dedication

To my Mom, my first teacher.

Contents

Contributors

Skip M. Alderson, MD
Staff Radiologist
Department of Radiology
Radiology Affiliates Imaging
Hamilton, New Jersey

Stanley Chan, MD
Associate Radiology Residency Program Director
Director of Body Imaging
Mercy Catholic Medical Center
Darby, Pennsylvania

Lauren Ehrlich, MD
Assistant Professor of Radiology
Department of Diagnostic Radiology
Yale-New Haven Hospital
New Haven, Connecticut

Naraínder K. Gupta, MD, DRM, MSc, FRCR
Associate Professor of Clinical Radiology
Department of Radiology
The Perelman School of Medicine at the University of Pennsylvania
Philadelphia, Pennsylvania

Susan Hilton, MD
Co-Chief and Modality Chief, CT Section
Professor of Clinical Radiology
Department of Radiology
The Perelman School of Medicine at the University of Pennsylvania
Philadelphia, Pennsylvania

Jason N. Itri, MD, PhD
Assistant Professor
Director of Quality and Safety
Department of Radiology, University of Pittsburgh Medical Center
Pittsburgh, Pennsylvania

Saurabh Jha, MBBS, MRCS
Assistant Professor
Department of Radiology
The Perelman School of Medicine at the University of Pennsylvania
Philadelphia, Pennsylvania

Lisa P. Jones, MD, PhD
Assistant Professor of Clinical Radiology
Department of Radiology
The Perelman School of Medicine at the University of Pennsylvania
Philadelphia, Pennsylvania

Sharyn I. Katz, MD, MTR
Assistant Professor of Radiology
Department of Radiology
The Perelman School of Medicine at the University of Pennsylvania
Philadelphia, Pennsylvania

Stephanie Carruth Kurita, MD
Assistant Professor of Radiology
Department of Radiology and Radiological Sciences
Vanderbilt University Medical Center
Nashville, Tennessee

Jill Langer, MD
Associate Professor of Radiology
Department of Radiology
The Perelman School of Medicine at the University of Pennsylvania
Philadelphia, Pennsylvania

Wallace T. Miller Jr., MD
Associate Professor of Radiology and Medicine
Department of Radiology
The Perelman School of Medicine at the University of Pennsylvania
Philadelphia, Pennsylvania

Edward R. Oliver, MD, PhD
Assistant Professor of Radiology
Department of Radiology
The Perelman School of Medicine at the University of Pennsylvania
Philadelphia, Pennsylvania

Nicholas Papanicolaou, MD, FACR
Co-Chief, Body CT Section
Professor of Radiology
The Perelman School of Medicine at the University of Pennsylvania
Philadelphia, Pennsylvania

Parvati Ramchandani, MD
Section Chief, Genitourinary Radiology
Professor of Radiology and Surgery
The Perelman School of Medicine at the University of Pennsylvania
Philadelphia, Pennsylvania

Mark Alan Rosen, MD, PhD
Associate Professor of Radiology
Department of Radiology
The Perelman School of Medicine at the University of Pennsylvania
Philadelphia, Pennsylvania

Drew A. Torigian, MD, MA
Associate Professor of Radiology
Department of Radiology
The Perelman School of Medicine at the University of Pennsylvania
Philadelphia, Pennsylvania

Hanna M. Zafar, MD, MHS
Assistant Professor of Radiology
Department of Radiology
The Perelman School of Medicine at the University of Pennsylvania
Philadelphia, Pennsylvania

Preface

It is the intention of this book to provide a comprehensive review of pattern recognition in abdominal imaging. At some level, diagnostic imaging is primarily an exercise in predicting disease states based on gross pathology. The underlying pathology of disease is constant and so the imaging characteristics of diseases are essentially the same regardless of imaging modality. Thus, it is the intent of this text to unify abdominal x-ray, ultrasonography, CT, MRI, and nuclear radiology interpretations of these underlying disease states, emphasizing when individual modalities have characteristics that can also provide unique insight into disease diagnosis. Furthermore, it is my belief that accurate imaging diagnosis of abdominal diseases can only be performed with the addition of appropriate clinical history. Therefore, the characteristic clinical presentations of the various diseases will be discussed in conjunction with the imaging findings. The book will be divided into chapters based the organ of interest. Chapters will be organized to stress differentiation of diseases based on imaging patterns. In general this pattern based approach will follow a similar format emphasizing differentiation of disease based on "focal," "multifocal," and "diffuse," abnormalities within the organ in interest followed by a discussion of diseases causing unique imaging features. Each section will follow a similar format. The most salient pathologic, histologic, and clinical features of the disorder will be reviewed, followed by a discussion of imaging characteristics. When possible, differentiating features, both clinical and radiographic, between etiologies producing similar imaging patterns will be emphasized. Many diseases have a variety of imaging features. When this occurs, they will be discussed under each pattern but the most comprehensive review of the subject will occur under the pattern that is most characteristic of the disease.

Acknowledgments

I would like to begin by thanking the many residents and fellows I have had the good fortune to work with. Through their many questions and input, they constantly refine my understanding of human illness and the imaging manifestations of disease.

I could not have completed a textbook on Abdominal Imaging of this magnitude without the excellent help of the many chapter authors. They are my coworkers in the Department of Radiology at the University of Pennsylvania's Perelman School of Medicine and I am very proud that this work represents a collective effort of our department. They worked tirelessly on the manuscript and graciously accepted the editing necessary to maintain a uniform format throughout the text.

There would be no book if I didn't have clinical colleagues. The many cases illustrating this text often have detailed clinical histories as well as final answers thanks to the feedback we have received from the many clinicians who consult with us. Since the completion of my residency, I am sure that I have learned more from my many friends in clinical medicine than from any other source.

I would also like to thank my secretary Tisha Grant for her help in preparing the manuscript.

Lastly, I would like to thank Cristina for her patience, understanding, and support.

CHAPTER 1

Fluid, Fat, Blood, Calcium, and Contrast: General Imaging Features

Wallace T. Miller Jr., MD
Sharyn I. Katz, MD, MTR

Certain abnormalities can be seen in different organs but have a common imaging feature regardless of the organ involved. Before discussing abnormalities of specific organs, we will note some of these common features.

IMAGING FEATURES OF FLUID

Simple serous fluid has characteristic features on computed tomography (CT), ultrasonography (US), and magnetic resonance imaging (MRI). This fluid can exist freely in various potential anatomical spaces, for example, ascites, pleural effusion, and pericardial effusion, or can be loculated in cysts within solid organs. On CT images, simple physiologic fluid has an attenuation of 0 to 20 Hounsfield units (HUs). This measurement can be made during evaluation of the computer data at the imaging workstation. A visual estimate can also be made by comparing the abnormality to known structures. Simple fluid will usually have an attenuation between that of skeletal muscle and fat (see Figure 1-1). When the accumulated fluid is not a simple transudate of blood but rather becomes "complex," admixed with proteinaceous material such as that derived from infection or hemorrhage, the attenuation will increase to greater than 20 HU (see Figure 1-2). One potential caveat that must be considered is that volume averaging within a reconstructed slice can confound Hounsfield unit density measurements and so it should be confirmed that the measurement of the tissue in question be made in a slice that has tissue in the slice above and below it so that volume averaging with adjacent distinct tissues does not occur.

Simple fluid in US examinations is uniformly anechoic because there are no interfaces to reflect the sound, and therefore it appears uniformly black (see Figure 1-1B). Fluid-containing structures will also demonstrate increased through transmission of sound, which appears as a band of bright echoes behind the fluid structure (see Figure 1-1B). Simple fluid has no structures to reflect sound, and therefore more sound passes through to the tissues deep to a fluid-containing structure. Therefore, compared to an ultrasound wave that passes through solid tissue, there is more sound to reflect back when it strikes an interface in the tissues deep to the fluid-containing structure. The US computer records this increased sound as brighter lines. So, the tissues deep to the fluid-containing structure appear brighter than adjacent tissues that are not deep to the fluid-containing structure. This artifact is known as "increased through transmission" of sound and is characteristic of any structure that contains fluid: cysts, gallbladder, urinary bladder, and pleural effusions.

Complex fluid, which contains internal debris, can be observed in a number of scenarios such as hemorrhagic collections, abscesses, or central necrosis within a malignancy. US of these processes will often demonstrate multiple internal bright floating specks or "echoes." These echoes represent the reflection of sound from floating particulate debris within the fluid. If plentiful in debris or clot and relatively low in water content, complex fluid can actually

Imaging Notes 1-1. Imaging Characteristics of Simple Fluid

CT	Attenuation between 0 and 20 HU
	Nonenhancing
US	Anechoic
	Increased through transmission
MRI	High signal T2W images
	Intermediate signal T1W images
	Nonenhancing

Imaging Notes 1-2. Imaging Features of Nonsimple Fluid

Internal septations
Internal debris • Echogenic foci and increased through transmission on US • Attenuation >20 HU and nonenhancing on CT • Decreased T2 signal on MRI
Fluid-debris levels

have a similar appearance to solid tissues on US. In these cases, the inherently higher than normal fluid content usually preserves the enhanced through transmission typical of fluid on US, a property characteristic of fluid structures (see Figure 1-3). In some cases, further imaging with MRI or CT will be necessary to confirm a diagnosis of a fluid-containing structure.

In some instances, there will be septations within the fluid. These will appear as fine lines of increased echogenicity within the fluid-filled structure. US is often the most sensitive imaging test for the presence of septations. However, MRI can have an advantage in evaluating fluid-filled structures where US is limited because of large body habitus. For example, evaluation of complex renal cysts in an obese patient can be impaired by poor sound transmission through excess adipose tissue. MRI, on the other hand, is not limited in the setting of obesity and will accurately characterize the internal architecture of the cystic structure. CT is the least sensitive cross-sectional modality for detection of internal septations. Occasionally, CT can detect septations when there is enhancement of the septa by intravenous (IV) contrast, thereby increasing tissue contrast. Otherwise, septations will typically remain unrecognized by CT studies (see Figure 1-4).

Fluid on an MRI examination appears uniformly high intensity (bright white) on T2-weighted images and appears a uniform intermediate intensity (gray) on T1-weighted images (see Figures 1-1 and 1-4). The bright signal intensity typical of fluid on T2-weighted images is a result of

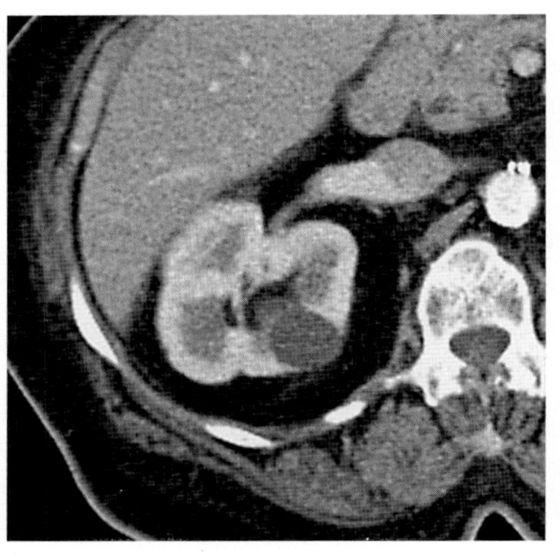

A

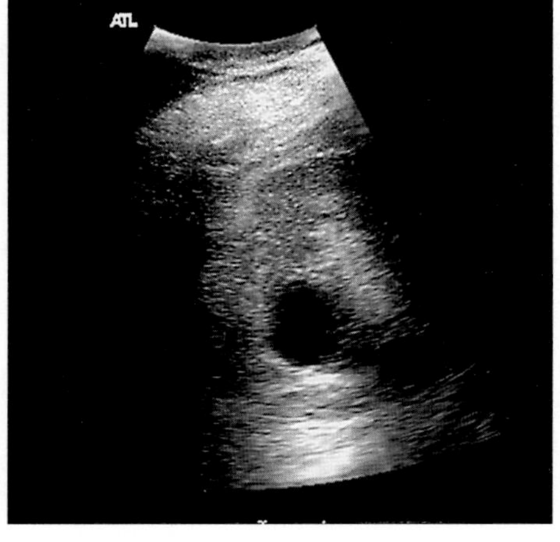

B

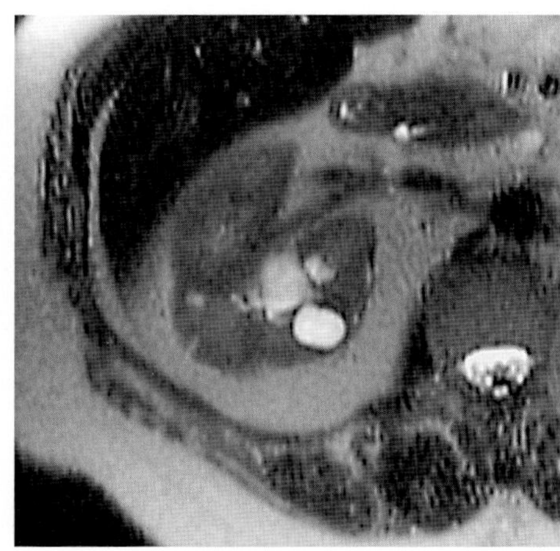

C

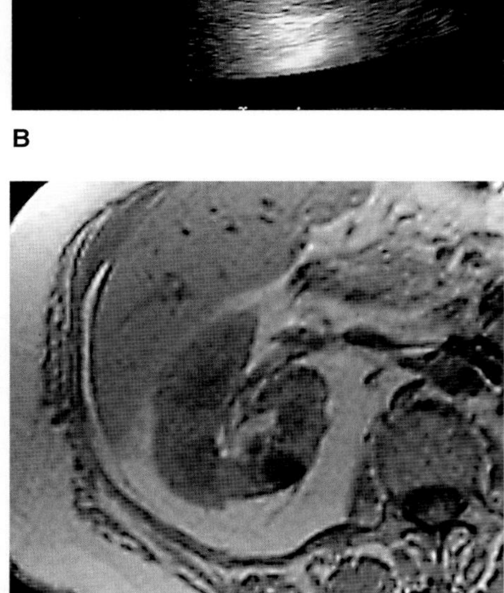

D

Figure 1-1 Simple Cyst of the Kidney This 72-year-old woman had undergone a left nephrectomy for renal cell carcinoma. **A.** CT image through the right kidney demonstrates a small, round, uniform, nonenhancing lesion in the upper pole of the kidney. This region measured 13 HU. **B.** US of the same lesion shows it to be round and anechoic. The tissue below the lesion appears brighter than the adjacent tissues, representing increased through transmission of sound. **C.** MRI images through the lesion show it to be uniformly high signal on T2-weighted images. **D.** Low to intermediate signal on T1-weighted sequences. These findings are all characteristic of a simple cyst.

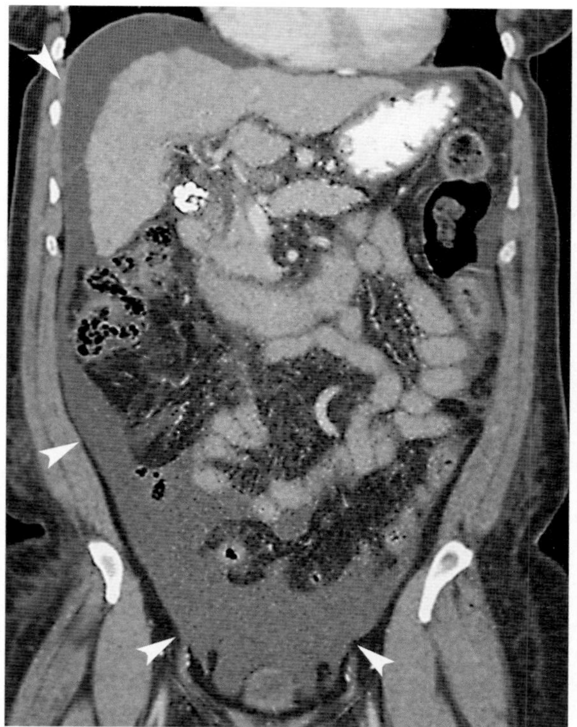

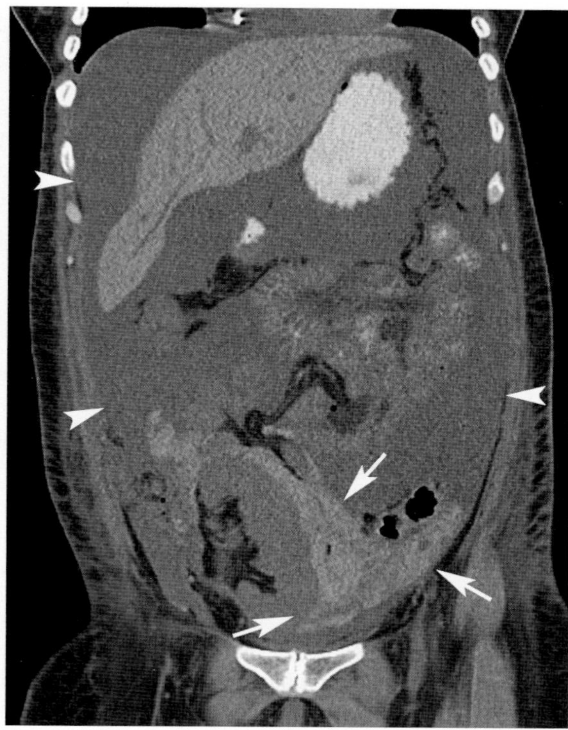

Figure 1-2 Ascites versus Hemoperitoneum
A. Contrast-enhanced coronal CT image from a 58-year-old man with cirrhosis shows a large amount of low attenuation acites (*arrowheads*) surrounding the liver and small bowel mesentery and filling the pelvis. Note how the attenuation of the fluid is less than the attenuation of muscle and liver but is greater than fat. **B.** Unenhanced coronal CT image from a 51-year-old woman with abdominal pain status post renal transplantation shows similar low attenuation fluid (*arrowheads*); however, there is also an amorphous region of higher attenuation in the pelvis and lower abdomen. This represents acute clotted blood within the peritoneum. Notice how it is slightly higher attenuation than the attenuation of unenhanced muscle.

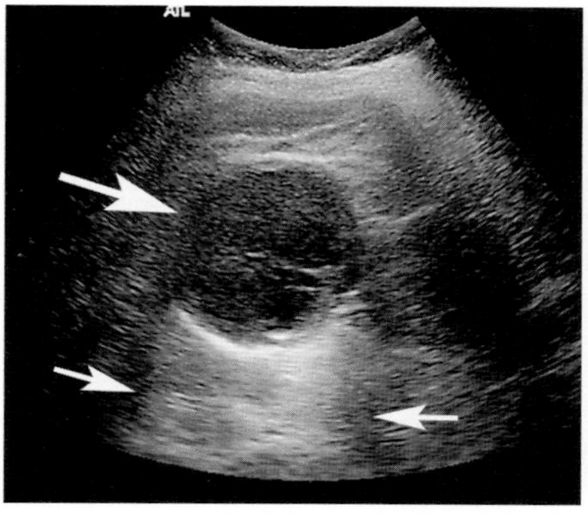

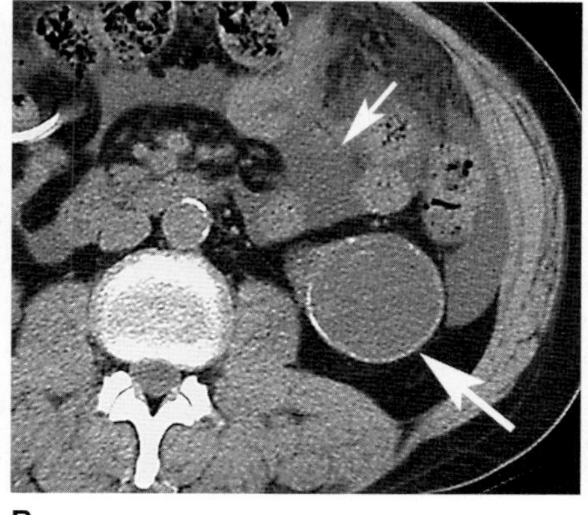

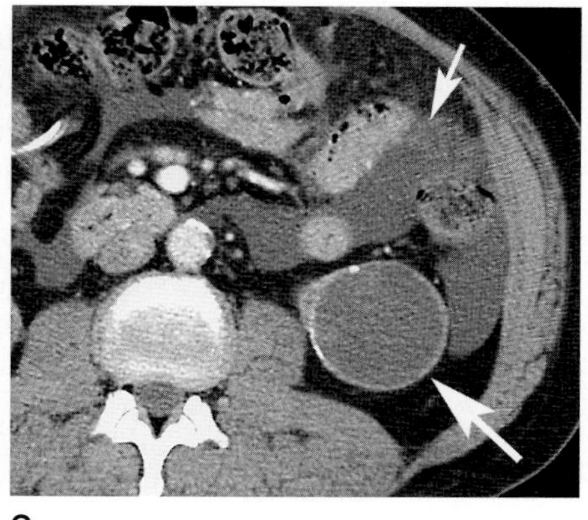

Figure 1-3 Complicated Cyst
This 68-year-old woman was being evaluated for voiding dysfunction. **A.** US of the lower pole of the right kidney reveals a round hypoechoic structure (*large arrow*) in the lower pole with faint internal echoes. These internal echoes could indicate either a solid lesion or a cyst with internal debris. However, in the tissues deep to the lesion, there is a band of increased echogenicity (*small arrows*), an artifact called increased through transmission that indicates that this lesion is a cyst. Unenhanced (**B**) and enhanced (**C**) CT images through the cyst show the cyst (*large arrows*) to be faintly higher attenuation than some adjacent ascites (*small arrows*). The cyst measured 28 HU on the unenhanced image and 25 HU on the enhanced image. This indicates the lesion is nonenhancing and is consistent with a "hyperdense" cyst. Note also the faint rim calcification in the cyst on CT seen as thin foci of high attenuation in the medial rim of the cyst.

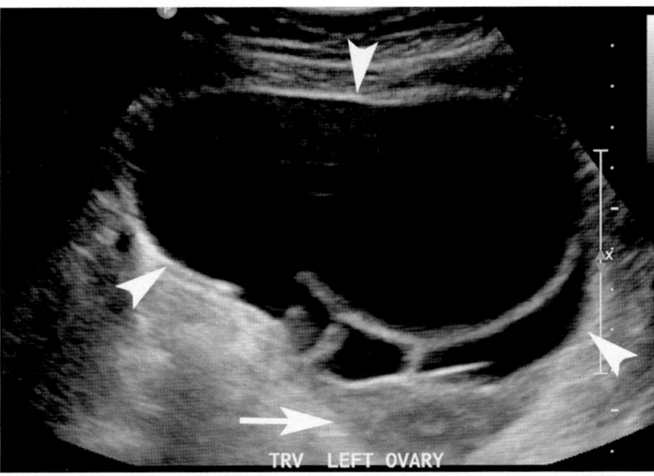

A

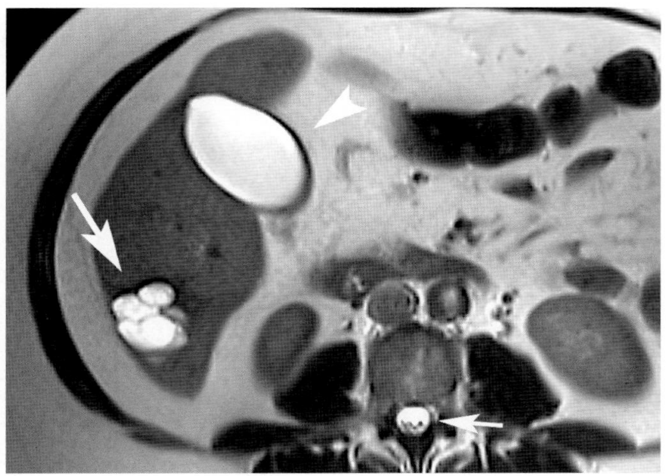

B

Figure 1-4 Complicated Cysts with Internal Septations in 2 Patients
A. This 26-year-old woman had a palpable adnexal lesion. Transvaginal ultrasound shows a large anechoic structure with several echogenic septations projecting from the left ovary. These are features of a cyst with internal septations. Surgical resection demonstrated a mucinous cystadenocarcinoma.

B. This 49-year-old woman was being evaluated for carcinoid tumor. T2-weighted MRI sequence shows a multiloculated hyperintense lesion (*large arrow*) in the liver. High intensity on T2-weighted sequences will usually indicate the presence of fluid. The internal septations indicate that this represents a complex cyst. Note the high signal fluid in the gallbladder (*arrowhead*) and cerebrospinal fluid (*small arrow*).

the slower loss of phase coherence of the proton nuclei in the transverse plane immediately following the imaging radiofrequency pulse. Interactions between adjacent proton nuclei results in loss of spin synchrony and causes measured MR signal in the horizontal plane. This process requires dissipation of energy, which is not efficient within water, thus leading to a prolonged or "brighter" T2 signal. As with other imaging modalities, an estimate of the composition of the structure of interest can be inferred from comparison to normal structures of known composition. For example, when considering the fluid nature of a cyst, the T2-weighted signal may be compared to the spinal fluid within the spinal canal, which is mostly composed of water.

If the fluid being studied is "complex," T2-weighted images may reveal low T2-weighted signal intensity debris or septae within otherwise high T2-weighted signal intensity water (see Figure 1-4). Cysts containing hemorrhage can have a variety of imaging appearances based on the MR signal characteristics of various phases of hemoglobin. However, in general, hemorrhagic cysts will be hyperdense on T1-weighted imaging. This phenomenon is discussed later in the section Imaging Characteristics of Hemorrhage.

Simple fluid can collect as cysts in many organs. Besides the various characteristics of fluid in different modalities, there are several common characteristics of simple cysts: (1) smooth, thin, well-defined walls; (2) round or oval shape; and (3) internal characteristics of simple fluid within the cyst: attenuation between 0 and 20 HU on CT, anechoic, increased through transmission on US, and high T2-weighted signal on MRI (see Figure 1-1). Furthermore, if IV contrast is administered, there is no enhancement of the structure.

IMAGING FEATURES OF FAT AND OTHER LIPIDS

Like fluid, fat has a unique appearance on cross-sectional imaging studies. Fat is less dense than other soft tissues, and because density is the major determinant of x-ray attenuation, pure fat will have a lower attenuation than other soft tissues on unenhanced CT exams. Moreover, because fat is also relatively hypovascular compared with other soft tissues, it will remain low attenuation on

Imaging Notes 1-3. Imaging Features of Macroscopic Fat

CT	Attenuation between −40 and −120 HU
US	Hyperechoic
MRI	High signal T1W images
	Intermediate-high signal T2W images
	Etching artifact on opposed-phase T1W images

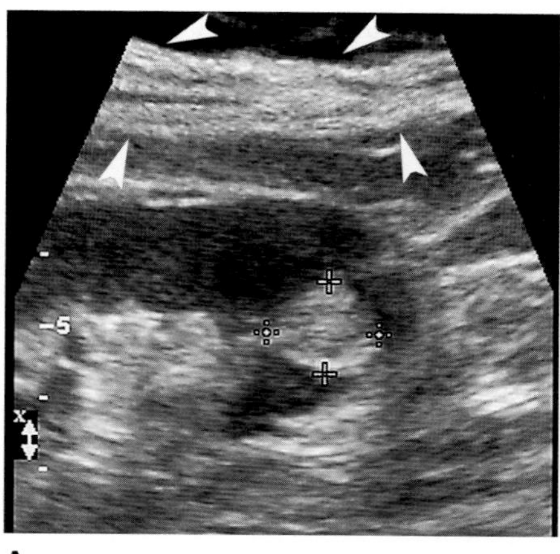

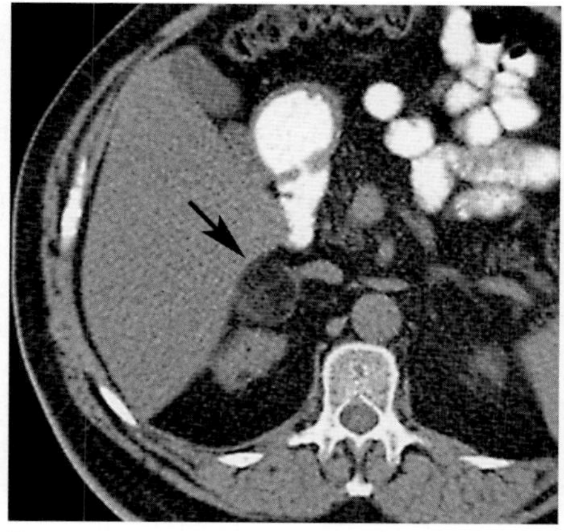

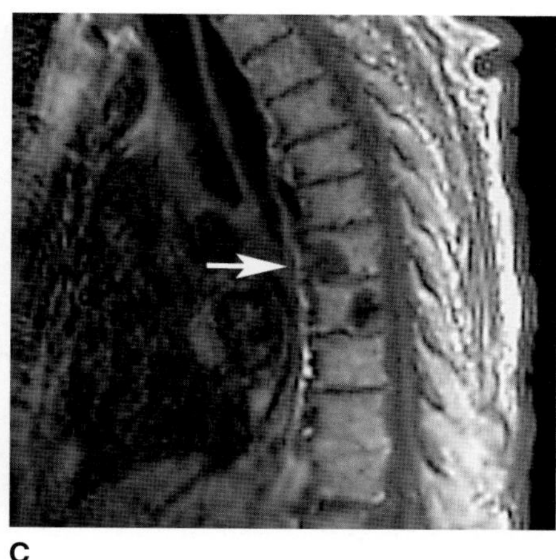

Figure 1-5 Imaging Characteristics of Fat
A. This ultrasonographic image shows a brightly echogenic nodule (*cursors*) in the lower pole of the kidney. Note how the echogenicity of the nodule is similar to the subcutaneous fat (*arrow*). This represents a small angiomyolipoma, a fatty tumor of the kidney. A metastasis or second renal cell carcinoma would usually be less echogenic. **B.** This 63-year-old woman had a lung mass discovered on chest x-ray. This unenhanced CT image at the level of the adrenals shows a normal left adrenal and a 2.5 cm right adrenal mass (*arrow*). The mass has a thin rim of tissue resembling muscle, but the majority of the mass is low attenuation, resembling retroperitoneal fat. Mature fat within an adrenal mass is diagnostic of an adrenal myelolipoma, a benign adrenal tumor. **C.** This 75-year-old woman had back pain and a history of breast cancer. Sagittal T1-weighted MRI image through the thoracic spine shows the normal vertebral bodies to have a relatively high signal because of the intramedullary fat. In the central thoracic spine are 2 spherical areas of decreased signal representing bone metastasis. The breast cancer is very conspicuous on these T1-weighted sequences because of the relative differences in intensity of the fatty marrow and the nonfatty metastasis.

contrast-enhanced CT images. It has been shown that mature fat has an attenuation between −40 and −120 HU. The attenuation can be measured directly at the PACS workstation, but most often it is easiest to compare the attenuation of the structure in question with the attenuation of subcutaneous fat. If the attenuations are similar, then the structure contains macroscopic fat (see Figure 1-5).

On US examinations, fat appears as regions of densely increased echogenicity. The numerous small fibrous septae that surround small fat globules act as innumerable specular reflectors, resulting in fine even echoes throughout the fat (see Figure 1-5). The appearance of densely increased echogenicity is not unique to fat and can be seen with structures that contain psammomatous (numerous fine punctate) calcifications or with structures that are composed of a complex network of interfaces, such as hepatic hemangiomas (see Figure 1-6).

On MRI, the majority of tissue contrast is derived from the intrinsic T1 time or spin-lattice relaxation time of a tissue. This T1 time refers to the time required for the radiofrequency energy of magnetization from the imaging pulse to dissipate through the infrastructure of the tissue, allowing the proton nuclear spin to return—or "relax"—to its original orientation within the magnetic field. This T1 time is a result of proton–proton nuclear interactions of different molecules within the tissue being imaged and generates relatively unique T1 times for different tissue compositions. By exploiting the relative tissue properties of T1 imaging, not only can the presence of fat be detected but also macroscopic fat can be differentiated from microscopic fat (ie, microscopic lipid admixed with fluid). These additional fatty characteristics can provide further information as to the nature of the tissue being studied.

Macroscopic fat typically appears uniformly bright on T1-weighted sequences and intermediate to high signal intensity on T2-weighted sequences although typically not as bright as fluid. The bright T1-weighted signal of fat is a result of the fast dissipation of radiofrequency energy of magnetization within the tissue structure, resulting in a short T1 time leading to bright T1-weighted signal because the protons have relaxed, are synchronized, and are now generating signal in the plane of imaging signal acquisition (see Figure 1-5). As with CT, the easiest method of identifying fat in a structure is to compare the intensity of the structure in question with the intensity of subcutaneous fat. If the signal pattern on *all* sequences parallels that of subcutaneous fat, then the structure contains macroscopic fat. Note that it is important to compare all sequences. Some other substances, for example blood, can be very bright on T1-weighted sequences but will not follow subcutaneous fat on all sequences and are generally low in T2-weighted signal, with some exceptions. Macroscopic fat will also produce an artifact on opposed-phase images called the etching artifact. With this pulse

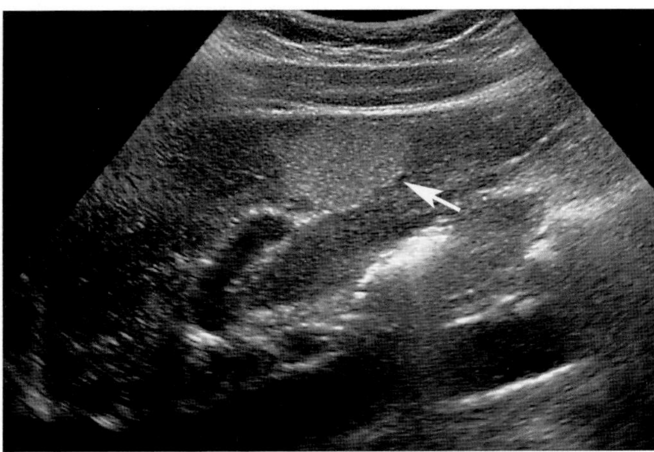

Figure 1-6 Hemangioma
This 17-year-old woman was being evaluated for abdominal pain. Longitudinal US of the liver shows an echogenic mass (*arrow*) in the left lobe of the liver. This is a typical appearance of a hepatic hemangioma. The multiple vascular channels of the tumor serve as specular reflectors, resulting in the increased echogenicity of the mass.

sequence, voxels containing both lipid and water molecules will lose signal. At places where macroscopic fat is adjacent to nonfatty soft tissue, voxels will contain both lipid and water molecules, and a thin black line will be artifactually produced that appears to outline the abdominal organs (see Figure 1-7).

Microscopic fat—lipid molecules admixed with water molecules—yields a signal intensity that is generally intermediate on T1- and T2-weighted imaging. However, microscopic lipid can be identified with the use of T1-weighted in-phase and opposed-phase imaging. As mentioned earlier, proton nuclei of lipids dissipate energy more efficiently and hence have a shorter T1 relaxation time than proton nuclei in water. In fact, the T1 time for water is approximately twice that of lipid. Therefore, in a voxel with approximately 50% lipid and 50% water, if the time-to-echo is timed at multiples of the T1 time of lipid, the signals between lipid and water will be opposed, termed *opposed-phase*, and thus cancel out at the odd multiples and be additive, termed *in-phase*, at even multiples of the lipid T1 time. When compared to in-phase T1-weighted images, the signal generated by a tissue where water and lipid are mixed within a voxel will result in a drop in signal in out-of-phase T1-weighted images, and the drop in signal will be maximal when the mix of molecules within that voxel is close to 50% water and 50% lipid. For this reason, macroscopic fat tissue, which has proportionally much more fat than water in any given voxel, will not exhibit a drop in signal from in- to out-of-phase T1-weighted imaging. This phenomenon is primarily used to identify the presence of cholesterol in adrenal adenomas but occasionally can be used for other purposes such as the detection of microscopic lipid in tumors of hepatic origin and in the differentiation

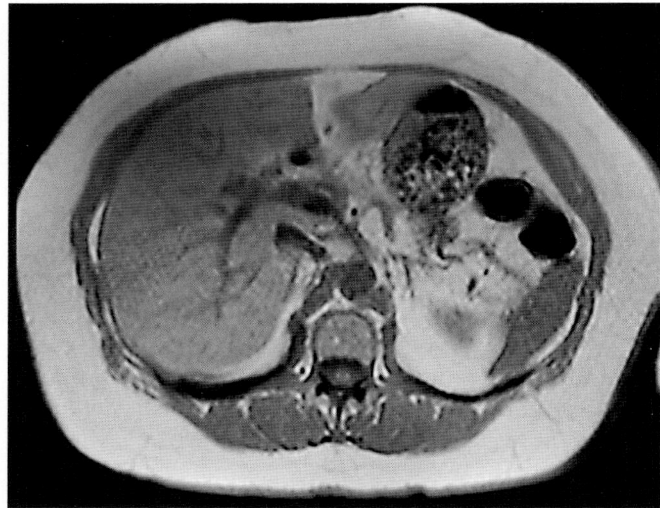

A

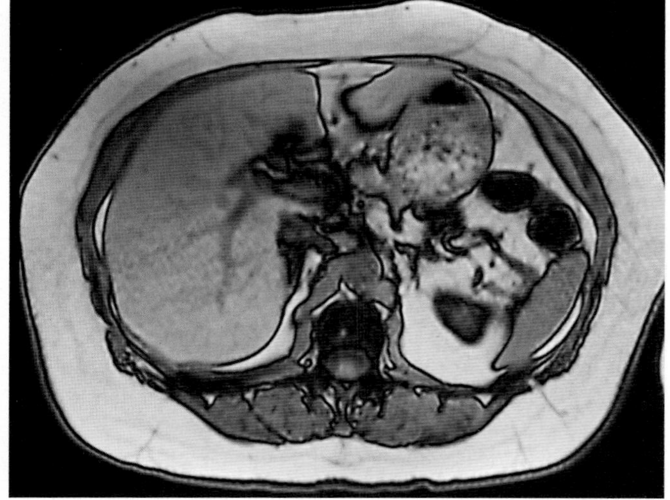

B

Figure 1-7 Etching Artifact on Opposed-Phase Images
This 66-year-old woman was being evaluated for an adrenal mass. In-phase (**A**) and opposed-phase (**B**) T1-weighted MRI images through the upper abdomen show thin black lines that outline the liver, spleen, stomach, psoas muscles, and erector spinae muscles on the opposed-phase images but are not present on the in-phase images. This is an artifact of the way the image is created. There is fat surrounding the surface of each of these organs and therefore the voxels present at the margins of the organs contain both fat and water protons. In the in-phase image, the signal from these protons is added; however, in the opposed-phase image, the fat signal and the water signal is subtracted, resulting in the thin black lines. Thus, this technique can be used to identify the presence of microscopic or macroscopic lipid within tissues.

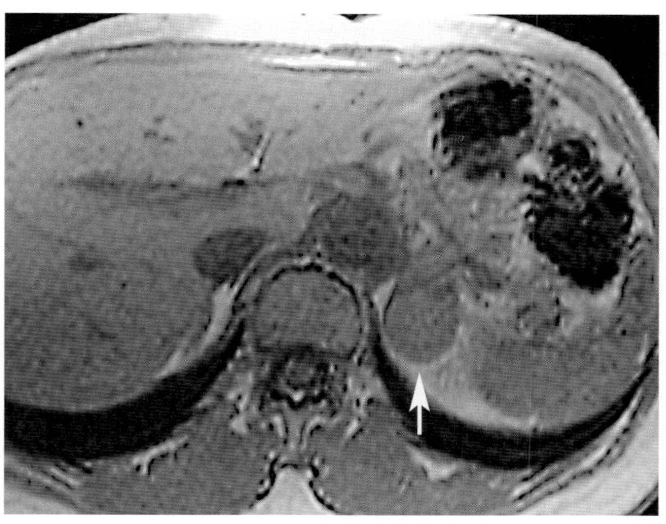

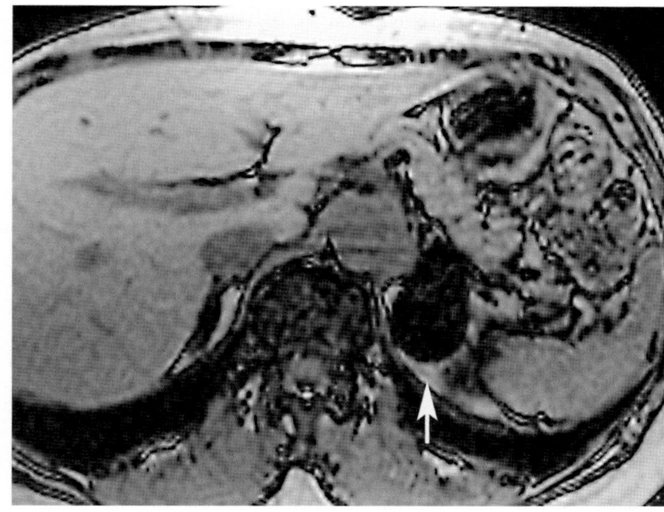

Figure 1-8 Subtraction Images in Adrenal Adenomas
This 73-year-old man had lung cancer. In-phase (**A**) T1-weighted and out-of-phase (**B**) T1-weighed images show a 2.5-cm nodule in the left adrenal gland that loses signal in the out-of-phase images. This is indicative of the presence of microscopic lipid within the lesion and is diagnostic of an adrenal adenoma.

of thymic hyperplasia, which normally contains diffuse microscopic lipid, from thymomas (see Figure 1-8).

IMAGING CHARACTERISTICS OF HEMORRHAGE

A hematoma undergoes various stages of evolution. Initially, extravasated blood forms a dense coagulated mass. With time, the hematoma undergoes degradation via the action of extracellular proteases and macrophage phagocytosis leading to liquification of the clot. Coincident with this process, hemoglobin undergoes a transition from oxygenated (oxyhemoglobin) to deoxygenated (deoxyhemoglobin) to methylated hemoglobin (methemoglobin). Various characteristics of this transition process can be identified by imaging exams and can suggest the presence of extravasated blood.

Computed tomographic examinations will often show acute hemorrhage as a high attenuation region relative to unenhanced tissues (see Figure 1-2). This high attenuation is a direct result of increased density of acute iron-containing clot relative to soft tissues. Although initially characterized for evaluating subarachnoid, subdural, epidural, intraparenchymal, and intraventricular hemorrhage in the brain, this phenomenon is now routinely used to identify acute hemorrhage throughout the body. It is important to note that extravasated blood is only high attenuation relative to surrounding vascularized tissues when those tissues are *unenhanced* with IV contrast. Use of IV contrast increases the CT attenuation of vascularized soft tissues such that acute hemorrhage will be relatively lower in attenuation. However, acute hemorrhage will always remain higher in CT attenuation than simple fluid.

As a clot ages, it begins to degrade and becomes progressively less dense, and so the attenuation falls until it approaches or equals simple fluid attenuation (0-20 HU). In an intermediate phase, hemorrhage can equal the attenuation of unenhanced tissues and as a consequence can be difficult to identify. In many cases, an old liquefied hematoma will contain simple fluid in the nondependent portion of the hematoma and debris will settle by gravity into the dependent portion of the hematoma, generating a "fluid-debris level." The presence of debris within a fluid collection will often indicate the presence of prior hemorrhage but can also be seen in abscesses and some neoplasms.

On US examinations, acute hematoma will appear as an echogenic mass within the tissues. It is believed that the multiple fibrin strands act as specular reflectors and lead to many small echogenic foci. This can be confused with other echogenic masses such as fat-containing lesions or hemangiomas. As the hematoma liquefies, debris from within the clot will cause internal echoes within the fluid collection. This will appear as an echogenic cyst with increased through transmission. Similar to CT, the debris will often settle dependently within the collection, leading to a fluid-debris level. The complex cyst of a liquefying hematoma cannot be distinguished from other debris-filled cysts that can be seen with abscesses and some neoplasms.

The imaging properties of blood products on MRI is dependent on location of the hemorrhage within the body, and hence surrounding tissues, and timing of imaging relative to time of hemorrhage. In the brain, the MRI appearance of a hemorrhage has been extensively studied and can yield very specific information on the age of the hemorrhagic products. In the hyperacute phase of intracranial

Imaging Notes 1-4. MRI Characteristics of Evolving Brain Hemorrhage

Phase of Hemorrhage	Hemoglobin State	T1W	T2W
Hyperacute (<12 h)	oxy-Hg	iso	hyper
Acute (12-72 h)	deoxy-Hg	iso	hypo
Early subacute (4-7 d)	met-Hg (intracellular)	hyper	hypo
Late subacute (1-4 wk)	met-Hg (extracellular)	hyper	hyper
Chronic (mo)	hemosiderin	hypo	hypo

hemorrhage (less than 12 hours from the hemorrhagic event), the predominant form of hemoglobin within the blood clot is oxyhemoglobin, which is isointense to brain parenchyma on T1-weighted signal and high intensity on T2-weighted signal. Over the initial 12 hours, the predominant blood product is oxyhemoglobin, but during the acute stage (12-72 hours posthemorrhage), the hemoglobin within the hematoma becomes increasingly deoxygenated and results in deoxyhemoglobin, which is a paramagnetic substance and leads to marked shortening (darkening) of the T2-weighted MR signal within the hematoma. During the early subacute phase of hemorrhage (3-7 d posthemorrhage), failure of extravasated red blood cells to maintain an intracellular functional reductase enzyme system results in oxidation of deoxyhemoglobin to methemoglobin, which is a strongly paramagnetic substance resulting in marked shortening of T1-weighted signal (signal brightening), the most dominant effect, and further shortening of T2-weighted signal (signal darkening) (see Figure 1-9). This is followed by release of methemoglobin into the extracellular environment, as the red blood cells subsequently degenerate and lyse, resulting in further T1-weighted signal shortening (brightening). In the chronic phase, which begins in the weeks following the hemorrhagic event, ongoing macrophage activity along the periphery of the evolving chronic intracranial hemorrhage will result in steady conversion of methemoglobin to hemosiderin, which results in marked T2 shortening (darkening) because of the strongly ferromagnetic properties of hemosiderin. This hemosiderin ring of markedly low T2-weighted signal around the intracranial hematoma increases in thickness with time, whereas the central scar contracts and ultimately collapses, usually resulting in a band-like hypointense ferromagnetic scar that sometimes persists indefinitely.

Another location in the body where the MR signal characteristic of hemorrhage is studied, temporally, is the aorta. Similar to the brain, in the setting of an acute intramural

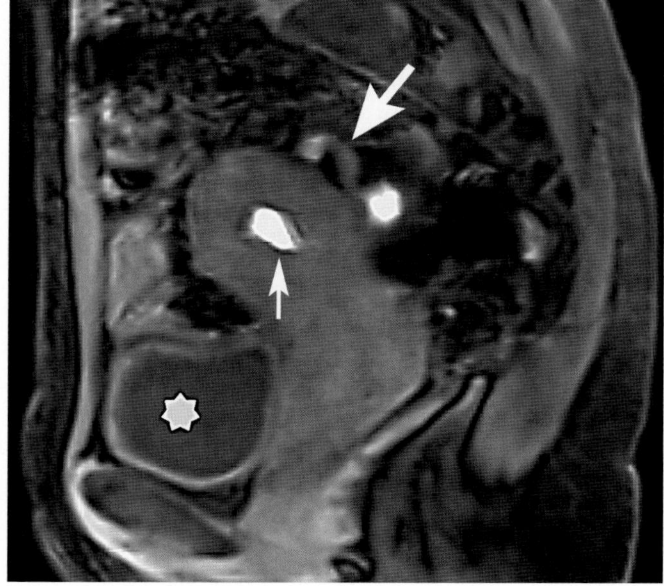

A

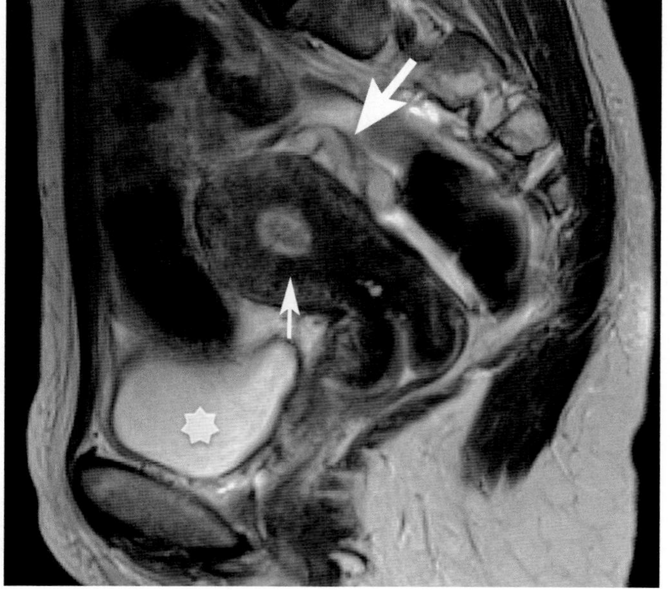

B

Figure 1-9 Differentiation Between Fluid and Hemorrhage on MRI Sagittal T1-weighted (**A**) and T2-weighted (**B**) MRI images through the pelvis reveal a dilated tubular structure posterior to the uterine fundus in keeping with the Fallopian tube (*thick white arrow*). There is also a small amount of fluid (*thin white arrow*) in the endometrial canal. The fluid in these structures is high signal on T1-weighted sequence (A) and intermediate signal on the T2-weighted sequence (B) typical of early subacute hemorrhage related to menses. By contrast, the predominately water-filled bladder (*star*) exhibits the typical MRI appearance of simple fluid, that is, low in signal intensity on T1-weighted images and high in signal intensity on T2-weighted images.

hematoma, the formation of a hematoma within the aortic wall results in an isointense T1-weighted signal and high T2-weighted signal because of the presence of oxyhemoglobin. With increasing age and conversion first to deoxyhemoglobin then methemoglobin, seen after 7 days from hemorrhage, the T2-weighted signal decreases and the T1-weighted signal increases. In this case, as in the brain, the changing MR signal generated by evolving hemorrhagic blood products results in an imaging signature providing information not only on the nature of the tissue composition but timing of pathophysiology.

The specific timing of conversion from oxyhemoglobin, to deoxyhemoglobin, to intracellular and extracellular methemoglobin in tissues other than the brain and aorta is not well defined. Hemorrhage will typically pass through the same sequence of stages of hemoglobin degradation; however, regional tissue characteristics can influence differentially the imaging appearance of an evolving hemorrhage. Examples of these regional tissue influences include the local tissue partial pressure of oxygen, pH, glucose concentration, hemoglobin concentration, and vascularity of the tissue. Other factors that can affect the MR signal of hemorrhage, or MR signal in general, include the patient's temperature and hematocrit, specific imaging parameters selected for the scanning sequences, and field strength of the MRI magnet. In most cases, acute or subacute hemorrhage within the abdomen will appear as homogeneously or heterogeneously high signal on T1-weighted sequences. T2-weighted sequences can be high attenuation or intermediate attenuation. The mass does not enhance following contrast administration. Chronic hematoma will typically appear as high attenuation on T1-weighted sequences and low attenuation on T2-weighted sequences (see Figure 1-10).

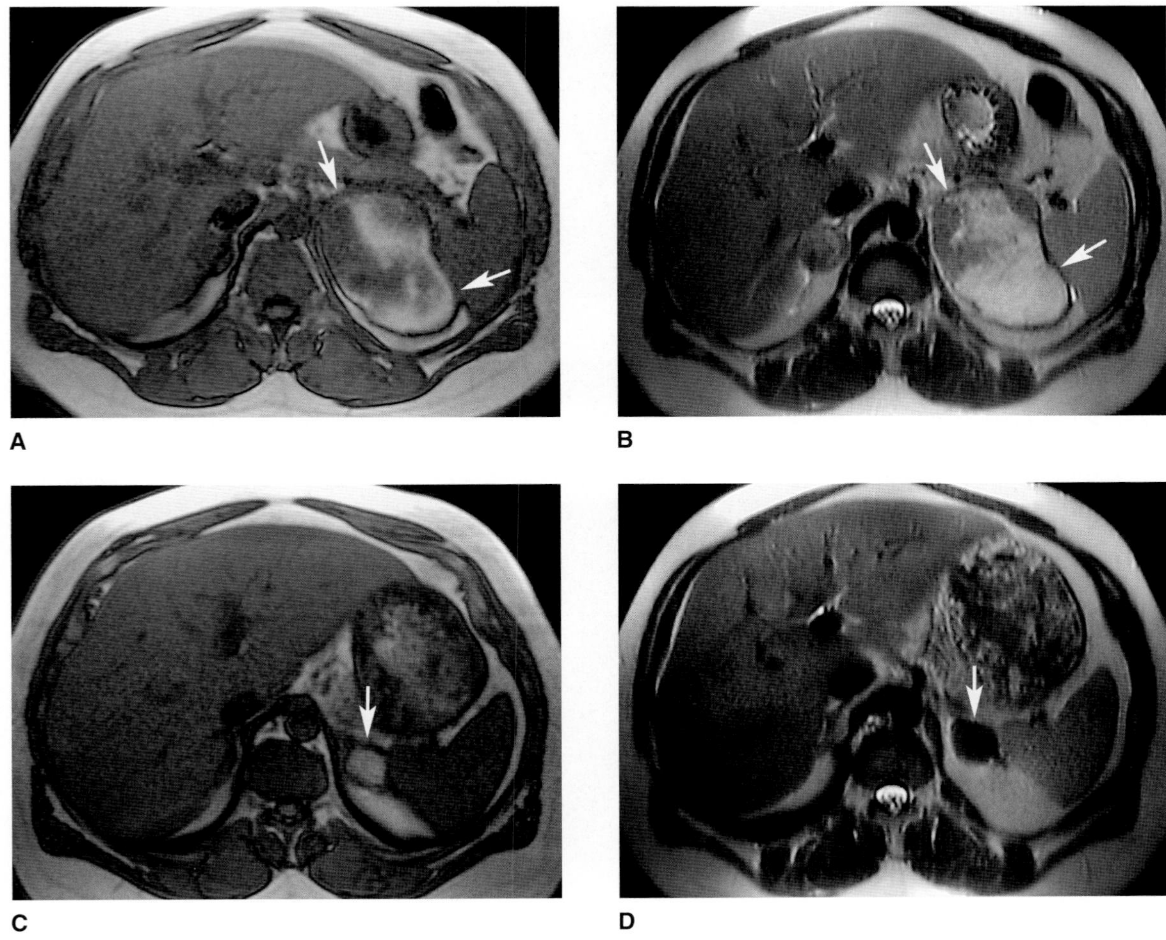

Figure 1-10 MRI Features of Hemorrhage
This 49-year-old man had an adrenal mass discovered on outside imaging exams. T1-weighted (**A**) and T2-weighted (**B**) MRI sequences show a mixed high and intermediate signal mass (*arrows*) in the left adrenal. This is a typical appearance of a subacute hematoma containing admixtures of various stages of hemoglobin degradation, primarily intracellular and extracellular methemoglobin. T1-weighted (**C**) and T2-weighted (**D**) MRI images obtained 9 months later shows decrease in size of the mass (*arrows*), which is now high signal on T1-weighted and very low signal on T2-weighted sequences. This is a typical appearance of chronic hematomas in the abdomen.

IMAGING CHARACTERISTICS OF CALCIFICATION

Calcification is a common feature of many abnormalities of the body. Microscopic calcifications are not identifiable by any imaging method; however, macroscopic calcifications often have characteristic features. Calcium is of higher density and higher atomic number than soft tissues and as a consequence it appears as a high attenuation (bright white) structure with values often greater than 200 or 300 HU on CT exams. Calcified structures will appear to have a similar attenuation to cortical bone (see Figures 1-3 and 1-11).

As a result of its dense structure, calcification will usually reflect the entire sound beam in a US examination. The result is a uniformly bright echogenic stripe. Beneath the echogenic stripe will be an anechoic band extending from the stripe to the deepest aspect of the image. This band is known as "shadowing" and is an artifact created by the absence of sound waves passing through the calcification

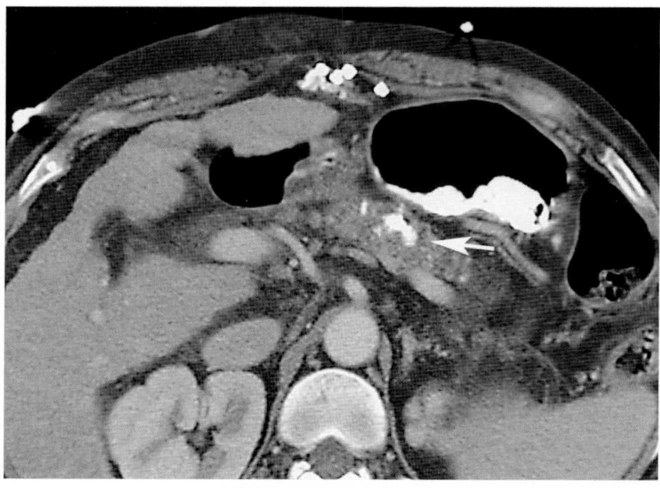
A

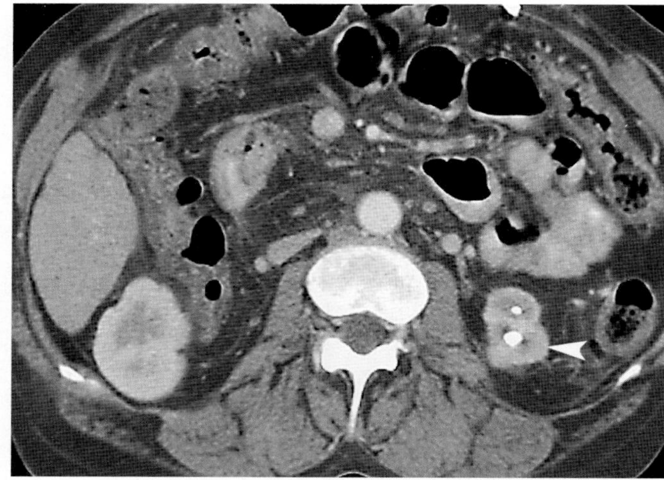
B

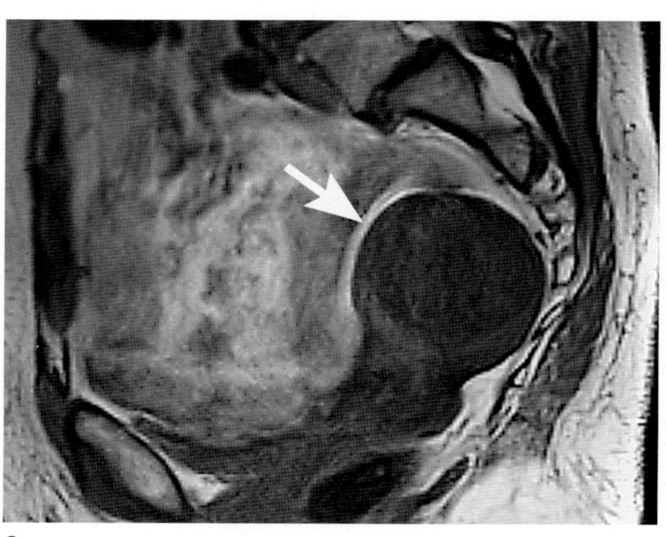
C

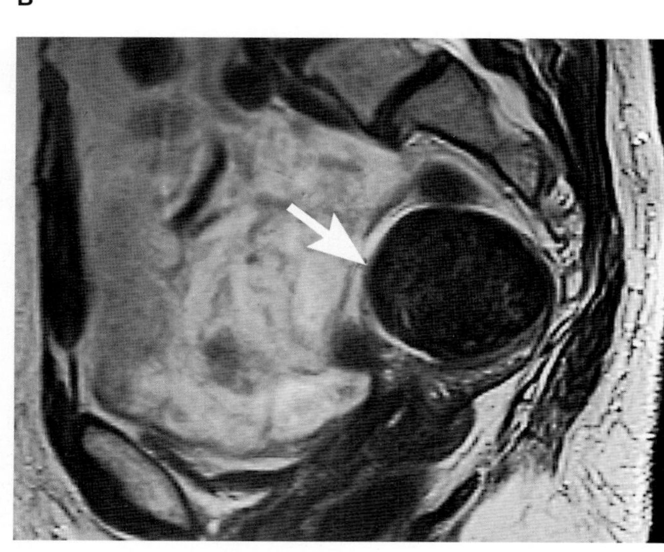
D

Figure 1-11 Calcification in 2 Patients
A and **B.** This 51-year-old woman was found unconscious. Contrast-enhanced image through the pancreas shows an irregular area of calcification (*arrow*) seen as a very bright white structure and indicates the presence of chronic pancreatitis (A). Contrast-enhanced image shows 2 bright white structures (*arrowhead*) in the lower pole of the left kidney, indicating the presence of renal calculi (B). **C** and **D.** This 53-year-old woman had menometrorrhagia. Sagittal T1-weighted (C) and T2-weighted (D) images through the pelvis depict a large densely calcified uterine leiomyoma (*white arrows*). The calcification provides very little signal, making the mass hypointense on both T1-weighted and T2-weighted images.

because all sound waves are reflected by the surface of the calcification (see Figure 1-12).

MRI examinations are created by the recognition of signals produced from spinning hydrogen protons. Because there are little or no hydrogen protons in regions of dense calcification, little or no signal is typically derived from calcified tissue and signal recognition is dependent on the amount and density of calcium in the deposit. In general, a calcified lesion will appear low/black signal intensity on T1-weighted and low/black to intermediate signal intensity on T2-weighted sequences (see Figure 1-11). Pure calcium will appear as a focus of absent signal both on T1-weighted and T2-weighted signal. On gradient echo sequences, the paramagnetic effects of a heavy calcium deposit can induce a local degradation of the MR signal by inducing inhomogeneities in the local magnetic field. This can result in an exaggerated "signal void" or area of absent MR signal in and immediately around the paramagnetic substance. This artifact is termed *susceptibility artifact* and is typically modest for calcium but can become quite pronounced for certain materials most commonly manifested in clinical MRI by metallic joint prostheses and metallic surgical clips (see Figure 1-13).

CONTRAST ENHANCEMENT

IV contrast is a marker for where blood travels in tissues. Because disease states will frequently alter blood flow to affected tissues, alterations in contrast enhancement can be used to detect the presence of disease and, in some cases, to more precisely identify the cause of the disorder. The precise alteration in blood flow will depend on the character of the disease and the character of the underlying organ.

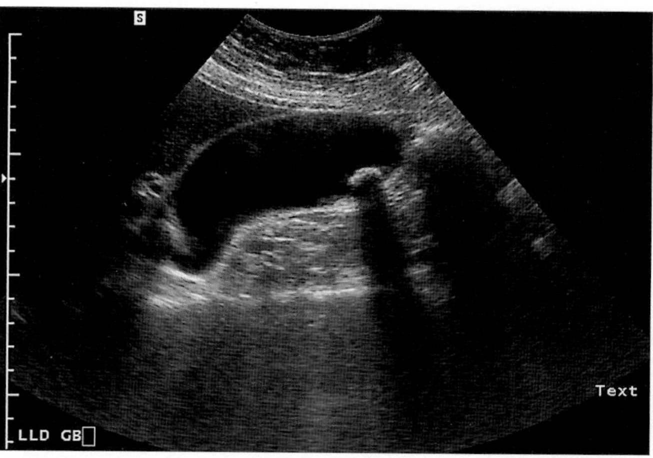

Figure 1-12 Gallstones
This longitudinal view of the gallbladder shows a predominantly anechoic lumen, typical of bile. However, within the gallbladder fundus is a brightly echogenic curved line, typical of a gallstone. The brightness is because the gallstone reflects the entire ultrasound signal. The tissues deep to the gallstone are uniformly anechoic, a finding which is an artifact of the gallstone. Because no sound reaches this portion of the body, no signals can be returned to the ultrasound transducer and it appears anechoic, a phenomenon called "acoustic shadowing." Just inferior (to the right of) to the gallbladder fundus is a second brightly echogenic region, which also produces posterior acoustic shadowing. This is a loop of bowel filled with air. Air is a poor conductor of sound, and so the majority of the sound wave is reflected at the air surface, causing acoustic shadowing.

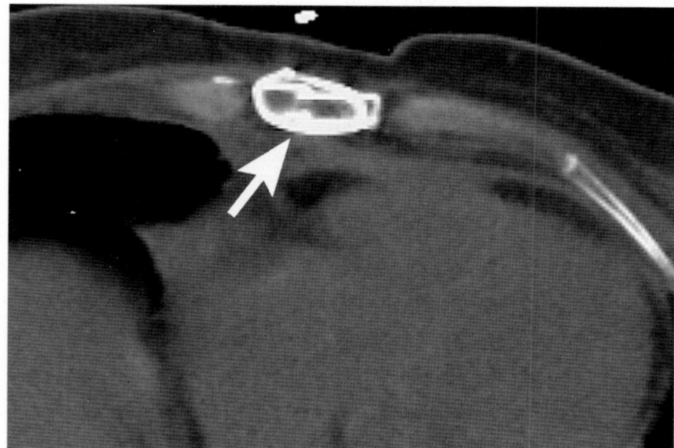

A

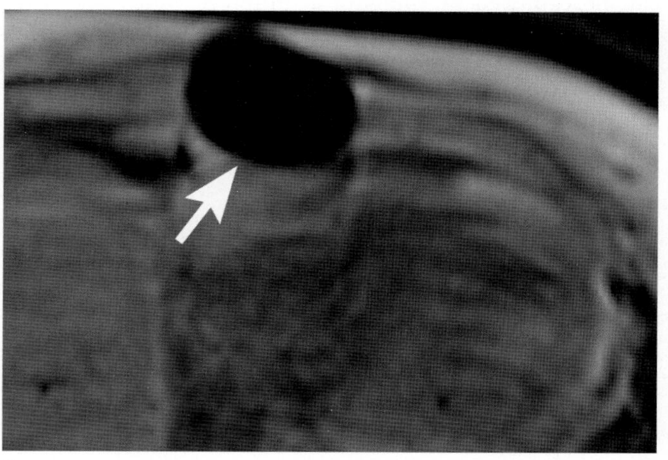

B

Figure 1-13 Susceptibility Artifact Due to Metallic Wires
A. Unenhanced CT shows the typical appearance of metal wires on CT in this patient who had received a median sternotomy.

B. T1-weighted MRI sequence shows a signal void in the area of the sternal wires. This is an artifact due to the paramagnetic properties of ferromagnetic metals termed *susceptibility artifact*.

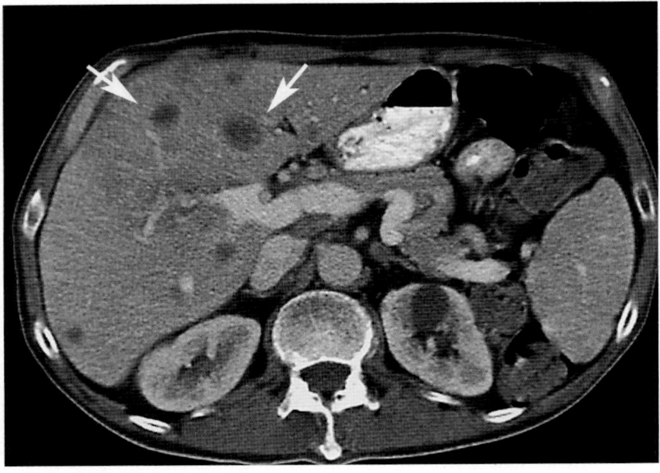

A

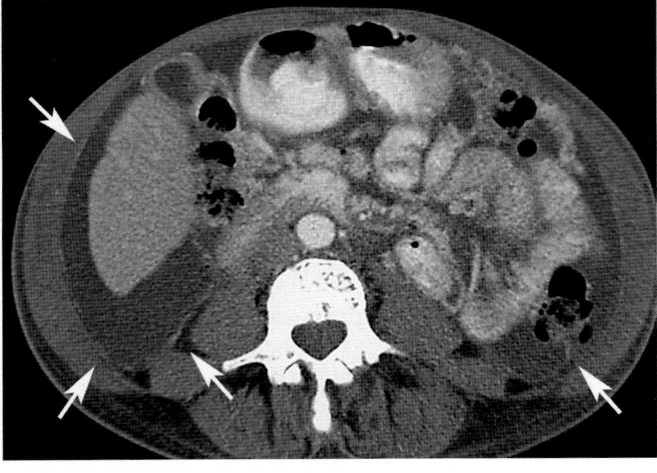

B

Figure 1-14 Affects of Contrast Enhancement
A. This 57-year-old man had gastric cancer. Contrast-enhanced CT shows multiple lesions that are lower attenuation than the very brightly enhancing liver. These were consistent with metastasis. **B.** This 58-year-old woman had breast cancer. Along the surface of the peritoneum are small foci of increased attenuation relative to the adjacent ascites and psoas muscles indicating contrast-enhancing peritoneal nodules, which represented peritoneal metastasis.

For example, the liver is among the most highly vascularized organs and, therefore, in the majority of disease states there will be less blood flow than that in a healthy liver. Thus, most metastases, infections, traumas, and other hepatic lesions appear less attenuating and of lower signal on contrast-enhanced CT and MRI exams. Whereas normal blood flow to the peritoneum is relatively small, nearly all disease states of the peritoneum, such as peritonitis and peritoneal metastasis, will appear as increased attenuation/signal than the normal peritoneum after contrast administration (see Figure 1-14).

In some cases, alterations in blood flow characteristics can be captured by imaging at different times following contrast administration. The most notable example of this relates to the dual blood supply of the liver. Following IV injection of a bolus of contrast, the contrast travels throughout the body as a column of high attenuation blood. This column of blood reaches the hepatic artery (approximately 15-30 seconds after IV injection) prior to the portal vein (approximately 45-75 seconds after IV injection), because the contrast reaching the portal vein must first pass through the mesenteric arteries and return via the mesenteric veins to the portal vein. As a consequence, structures that are primarily supplied by the hepatic artery will preferentially enhance in the "arterial phase" of liver enhancement compared with other structures that are primarily supplied by the portal vein, which enhance greatest during the "portal venous phase" of contrast enhancement. Arterial phase enhancement is characteristic of lesions derived from hepatocytes, including regenerative nodules, hepatic adenoma, focal nodular hyperplasia, and hepatocellular carcinoma. Therefore, these lesions will typically appear to intensely enhance during the arterial phase of contrast enhancement and relatively less enhancement on portal venous phases of imaging (see Figure 1-15).

Another tissue where blood flow mechanics can be used to identify the underlying abnormality is scar tissue. Scar tissue will characteristically have a relatively less robust venous drainage and a larger extracellular space than normal tissues. As a consequence, scar tissue will typically retain contrast longer than the normal surrounding tissues. Delayed imaging, several minutes following IV contrast injection, will typically show persistent enhancement of scar tissue and little enhancement of the surrounding normal tissues. This property of scar tissue has been employed in cardiac MRI to demonstrate nonviable myocardium in patients being considered for revascularization. In the abdomen, this property of scar tissue primarily is used to identify characteristic scars in some types of liver neoplasms, for example, focal nodular hyperplasia, which characteristically has a well-defined late-enhancing central scar (see Figure 1-15).

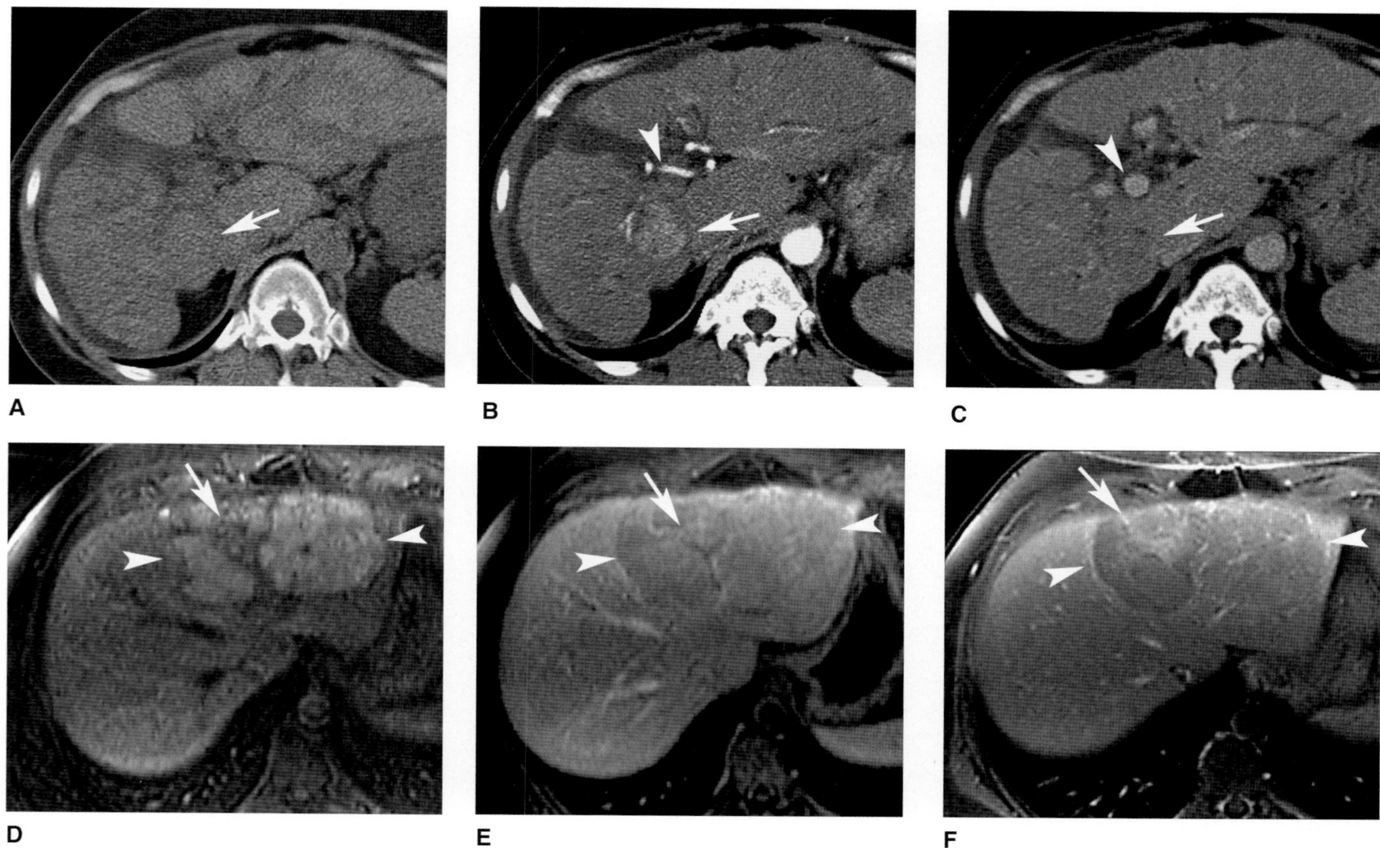

Figure 1-15 Timing Effects With Contrast Enhancement
A-C. This 53-year-old man with autoimmune hepatitis. Unenhanced (A), hepatic arterial phase (B), and portal venous phase (C) CT images demonstrate an enhancing nodule (*arrow*) that is only seen on the arterial phase image. This is a characteristic feature of hepatocyte-derived lesions of the liver, in this case a small hepatocellular carcinoma. Note the dense enhancement of the hepatic arteries (*arrowhead* in B), which is best seen on the arterial phase image, and the moderate enhancement of the portal veins (*arrowhead* in C), which is best seen on the portal venous phase image. **D-F.** This 28-year-old woman was being evaluated for complications of gastric bypass when a liver lesion was detected. Hepatic arterial phase (D), portal venous phase (E), and delayed enhancement phase (F) gadolinium-enhanced T1-weighted MRI sequences show a large lobulated mass (*arrowheads*) that enhances briskly on the arterial phase, is nearly isoenhancing in the venous phase and hypoenhancing in the delayed phase. There is also a small Y-shaped area (*arrow*) in the center of the mass that is hypoenhancing on the arterial and venous phases but brightly enhances on the delayed phase. This delayed enhancement is typical of scar tissue, in this case within a large hepatic adenoma.

CHAPTER

Imaging of the Bowel

Hanna M. Zafar, MD, MHS
Wallace T. Miller Jr., MD

ANATOMY OF THE BOWEL

The abdominal portion of the gastrointestinal (GI) tract consists of the stomach, small and large intestines, rectum, and anal canal. It is a muscular tube, approximately 9 m in length, and it is controlled by the autonomic nervous system.

The stomach is a curved sacklike structure in the left upper quadrant of the abdomen and is divided into 3 portions, the capacious fundus, and progressively smaller body and antrum. There are thick longitudinal folds called rugae that run from the fundus to antrum. The stomach terminates in a thick muscular sphincter, the pylorus, that regulates the passage of gastric contents into the small bowel.

The small intestine begins at the pyloric sphincter, joins the colon at the ileocecal valve, and is divided into 3 separate segments: the duodenum, jejunum, and ileum. It has a diameter of approximately 2.5 cm and is approximately 6.5 m in length. The surface area of the small intestine is increased by the presence of circular folds approximately 10 mm high called valvulae conniventes.

The duodenum is divided into 4 segments, the bulb, descending, transverse, and ascending portions and forms a U-shaped structure that surrounds the head of the pancreas. With the exception of the bulb, the duodenum is entirely retroperitoneal in position and remains fixed. The common bile duct and pancreatic duct join at the sphincter of Oddi and enter the lower portion of the descending duodenum along the medial wall. The minor papilla enters the duodenum approximately 1 to 2 cm proximal to the major papilla. The jejunum begins at the ligament of Treitz, then winds through the left upper quadrant and then the right upper quadrant and midabdomen. There is no precise juncture between the jejunum and ileum, which represents the small bowel that occupies the pelvis and then passes into the right lower quadrant, terminating at the illeocecal valve.

The large intestine is approximately 1.5 m in length and is divided into 4 segments: the ascending, transverse, descending, and sigmoid colons. Its size decreases gradually from the cecum, where it is approximately 7 cm in diameter, to the sigmoid, where it is approximately 2.5 cm in diameter. The majority of the ascending and descending colons are retroperitoneal in location and are therefore fixed in position, with the exception of the cecum, which can have a mesentery that allows for movement. The transverse and sigmoid colons are introperitoneal in location and are suspended on mesenteries. The ileocecal valve represents a fold of mucous membrane that allows the passage of material from the small intestine into the large intestine and prevents the reflux of contents from the colon back into the ileum.

The vermiform appendix is attached to the cecal tip and is typically 8 to 13 cm in length but can vary from 2.5 to 23 cm in length.

The rectum is approximately 13 cm in length and begins where the colon loses its mesentery—at about the level of the third sacral vertebra. It lies in the posterior aspect of the pelvis and ends 2 to 3 cm anteroinferiorly to the tip of the coccyx, where it bends downwards to form the anal canal. The anal canal is the terminal segment of the large intestine and is approximately 4 cm in length, opening to the exterior as the anus.

The stomach is supplied by all 3 branches of the celiac axis, including the left gastric artery; the gastroduodenal artery, which arises from the hepatic artery; and the short gastric arteries, which arise from the splenic artery. The superior mesenteric artery (SMA) supplies the whole of the small intestine and the proximal colon to the level of the splenic flexure. These regions of the bowel are drained by the superior mesenteric vein (SMV), which meets the splenic vein to form the portal vein. The descending and sigmoid colon are supplied by the inferior mesenteric artery (IMA) and drained by the inferior mesenteric vein (IMV). The internal iliac arteries supply the distal sigmoid, rectum, and anus, and venous drainage is primarily by the SMV and IMV.

IMAGING OF THE BOWEL

Computed tomographic (CT) examinations of the abdomen with oral and intravenous (IV) contrast is currently the most commonly employed examination of the GI tract. However, diseases of the bowel can be identified through many different imaging examinations, including abdominal plain films, contrast upper GI tract examinations, contrast enemas, sonography, magnetic resonance imaging (MRI) and specialized CT examinations such as CT colonography (CTC) and CT enterography.

Abdominal Plain Films

A single abdominal radiograph without IV or oral contrast is variously called "abdominal plain films" or "KUB" for kidney-ureter-bladder. When both supine and horizontal beam films are obtained, they are called an "obstruction series" (see Figure 2-1). The abdominal plain film is a very poor means of evaluating the abdominal contents. Contrast between the non-air-containing and noncalcified soft tissues is poor and, therefore, the evaluation of the solid abdominal viscera is limited. However, because bowel contains air, some information can be inferred about the GI tract, predominantly information about obstruction and paralytic ileus. Abdominal plain films can also detect calcified stones and calcified abdominal masses.

Contrast Examinations of the Bowel

Contrast examinations with water-soluble contrast and barium suspensions were the first means of directly evaluating the bowel with imaging. Ingestion or instillation of these contrast agents opacify the lumen of the bowel and are called "single contrast" examinations (see Figure 2-2). These studies allow for identification of lesions, such as polyps or carcinomas, protruding into the lumen of the bowel or outpouchings, such as diverticula or ulcers, extending from the lumen of the bowel. "Double contrast" examinations are performed with both high-density barium and air or CO_2 gas. The patient is asked to roll backwards and forwards on the examining table, causing the barium to coat the surface of the bowel mucosa. The air or gas distends the lumen of the bowel and the combination of these actions results in imaging that can detect fine mucosal changes, including small ulcerations, irregular mucosal thickening called "cobblestoning," and thin plaquelike elevations. Historically, these examinations were an important part of the evaluation of GI diseases. However, the combination of CT imaging, which is readily available and can be performed in a single breath-hold, and evaluation with endoscopy and colonoscopy has reduced the uses for contrast examinations of the bowel, except in special circumstances.

Abdominal CT

Abdominal CT allows the reader to directly observe the macroscopic anatomy of the abdominal organs, including the stomach, small bowel, and colon (see Figure 2-3). Unlike plain films and contrast examinations, CT directly visualizes the bowel wall and will directly show intrinsic and extrinsic masses of the bowel and focal, segmental, or diffuse thickening of bowel wall. In the standard examination, the bowel lumen is opacified with positive contrast (the lumen appears whiter than soft tissues) with gastrographin or barium sulfate. This has the advantage of rapidly distinguishing bowel from peritoneal fluid collections; however, positive contrast will obscure small polyps and fine details of the mucosa. CT enterography and CTC fill the bowel lumen with negative oral contrast (the lumen appears darker than soft tissues) and CO_2, respectively, both of which allow for evaluation of more subtle mucosal lesions.

CT Enterography

Although routine CT is excellent at evaluation of most routine causes of abdominal pain, CT enterography and enteroclysis are believed to be more sensitive for subtle mucosal diseases of the small bowel and colon, especially Crohn disease. Because of the superior distension achieved with CT enteroclysis, this study is more sensitive for suspected partial small-bowel obstruction (SBO) than routine abdominal CT.[1,2] There are no formal studies on the performance of these methods in the evaluation of ulcerative colitis, small-bowel tumors, and celiac disease although they have been used in these indications.

CT enterography is performed following the ingestion of a large volume of low-concentration barium with sorbitol, a nonabsorbable sugar alcohol that promotes luminal distention and limits resorption of water. In CT enteroclysis, a nasojejunal tube is placed prior to the examination terminating in the distal duodenum under fluoroscopy. Oral contrast is injected through the nasojejunal tube at a rapid rate, approximately 100 mL/min. When Crohn disease or a small-bowel mass is suspected, water is the preferred oral agent, whereas when partial bowel obstruction is suspected, positive oral contrast is preferred. Bowel distension achieved with both CT enterography and CT enteroclysis permits visualization of luminal narrowing with prestenotic dilation and pseudodiverticulum.

Similar to routine CT, both of these examinations utilize IV contrast. However, they differ from routine CT in that they typically utilize negative rather than positive oral contrast, as above, and they are acquired using thin-section collimation that allows for near-isotropic resolution. The

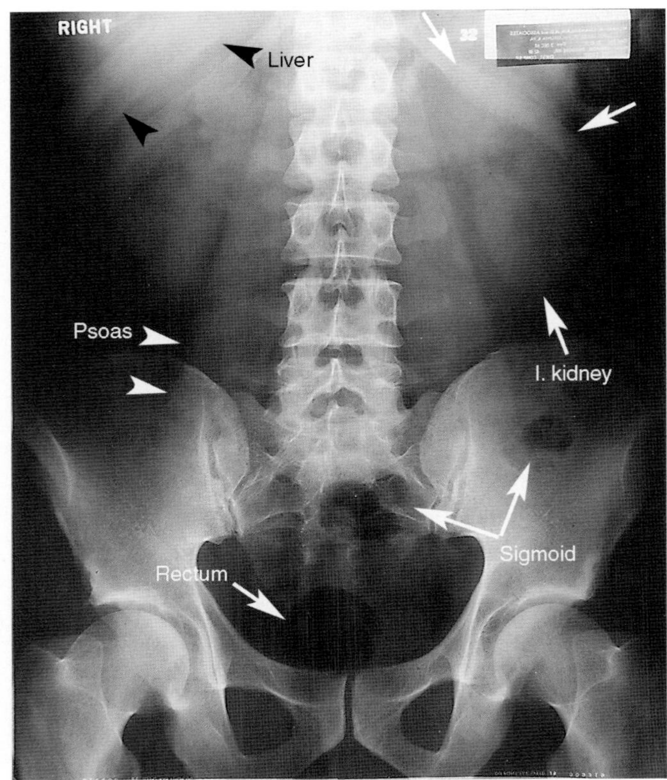

A

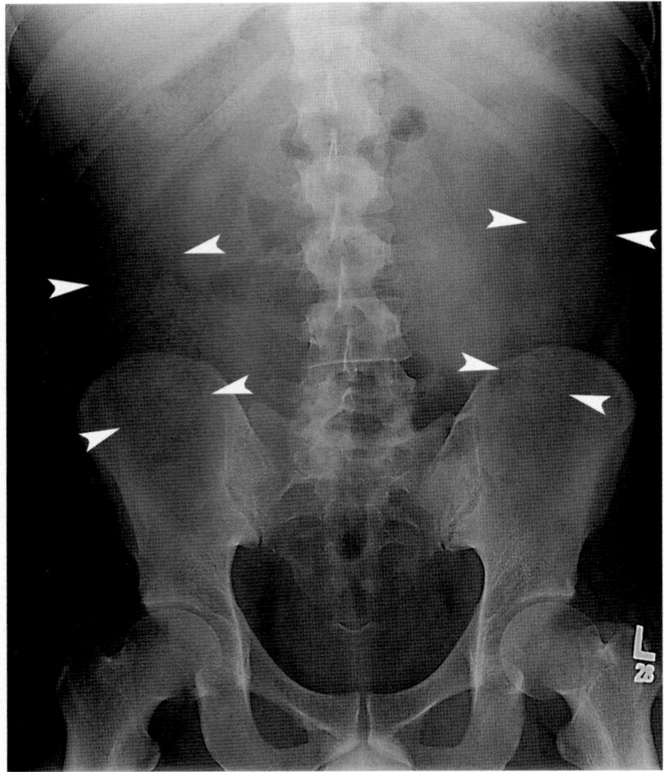

B

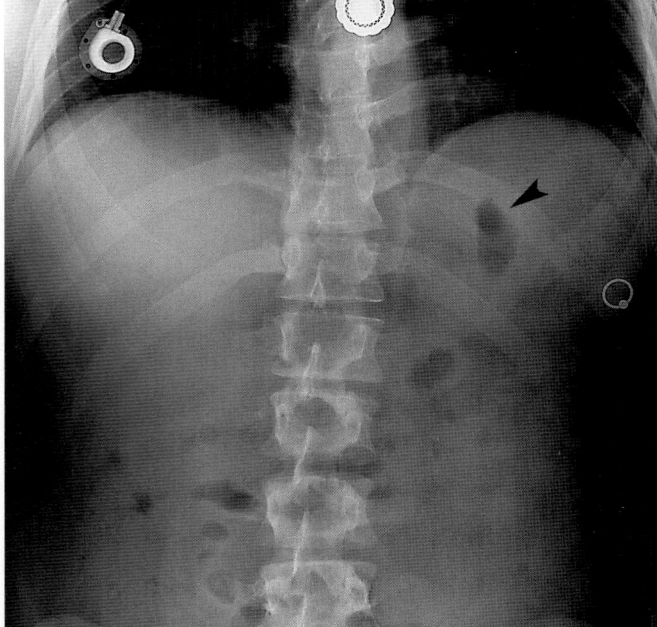

C

Figure 2-1 Normal Abdominal X-ray
A. This supine view of the abdomen is taken after a colonic cleansing regimen. The kidneys, psoas muscles, and liver edge can be identified because the surrounding retroperitoneal and peritoneal fat is more radiolucent than nonfatty soft tissues. Supine (**B**) erect (**C**) radiographs in a patient without a colonic cleansing regimen. Small bubbles of air and soft tissue (*white arrowheads*) represent feces in the ascending and descending colon. Small collections of gas are seen in other bowel loops including air in the stomach (*black arrowhead*). See if you can identify the liver edge, kidney, and psoas shadows in B. They are difficult to see because of the overlying feces.

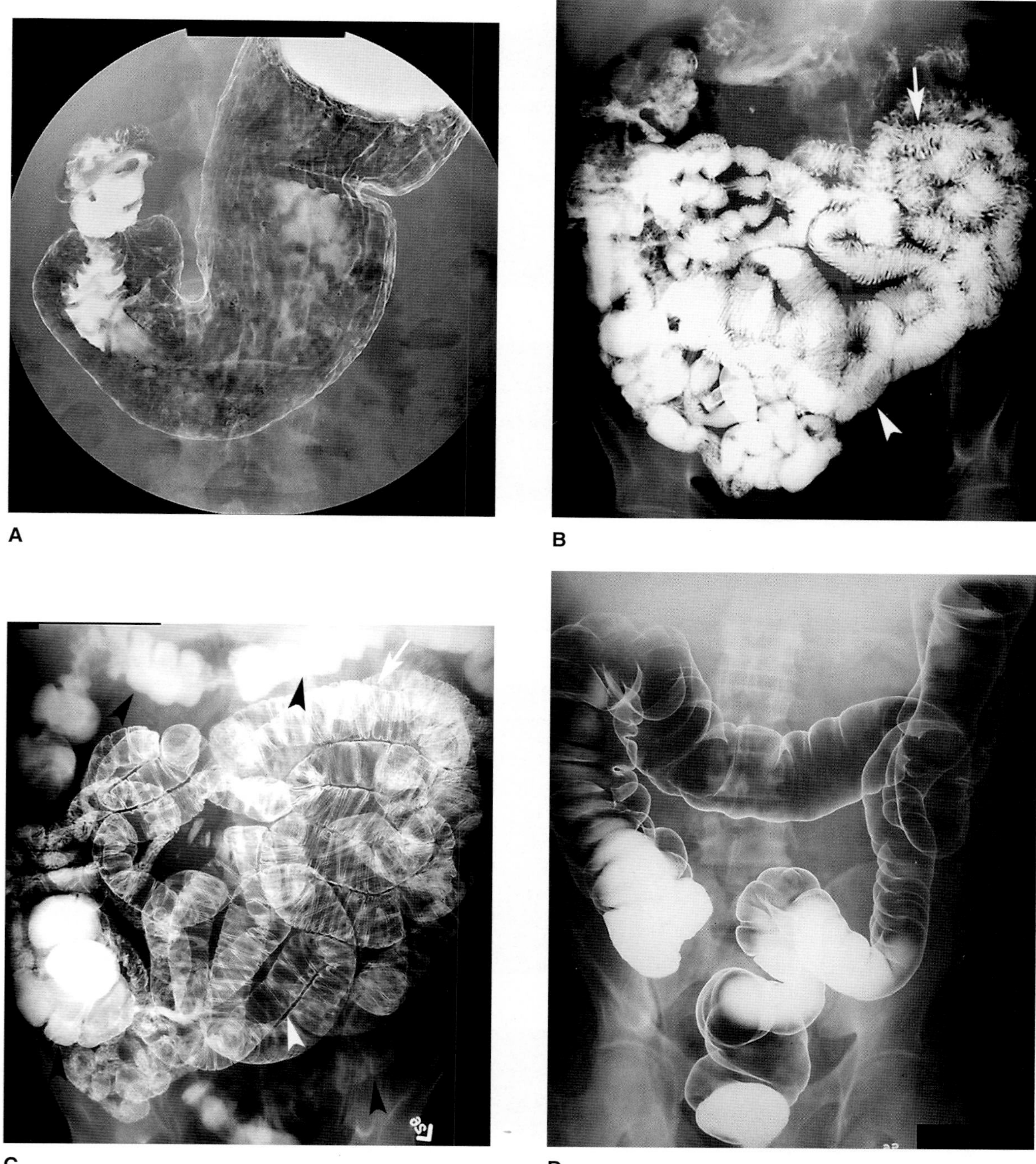

Figure 2-2 Normal-Contrast GI Examinations
A. This is a double-contrast examination of the stomach. The patient swallows small granules that convert to CO_2 gas on dissolving in water in the stomach. High-density barium is then ingested and coats the surface of the stomach. **B.** This is a small-bowel follow-through examination. The patient drinks a barium solution and images are taken as the contrast passes through the small bowel into the colon. **C.** This is a small-bowel enema. In this examination, a tube is passed from the mouth into the proximal jejunum. Barium is first injected into the tube followed by a solution of methylcellulose. The barium adheres to the small-bowel wall and the methylcellulose fills the lumen producing a "double-contrast" examination. Note how there are more folds (plica circularis) in the proximal small bowel (*white arrows*) than there are in the distal small bowel (*white arrowheads*). Note also the relative positions of the centrally placed small bowel (*white arrows and arrowheads*) compared with the colon (*black arrowheads*). **D.** This is a normal double-contrast barium enema. In this examination, a large-bore tube is inserted into the rectum and barium is administered by gravity. Then air is insufflated through the tube to distend the lumen of the colon. The barium adheres to the surface of the colon and the air distends the lumen. This provides fine detail of the mucosa of the colon. Single-contrast barium enema can also be performed and shows a cast of the outline of the lumen of the colon.

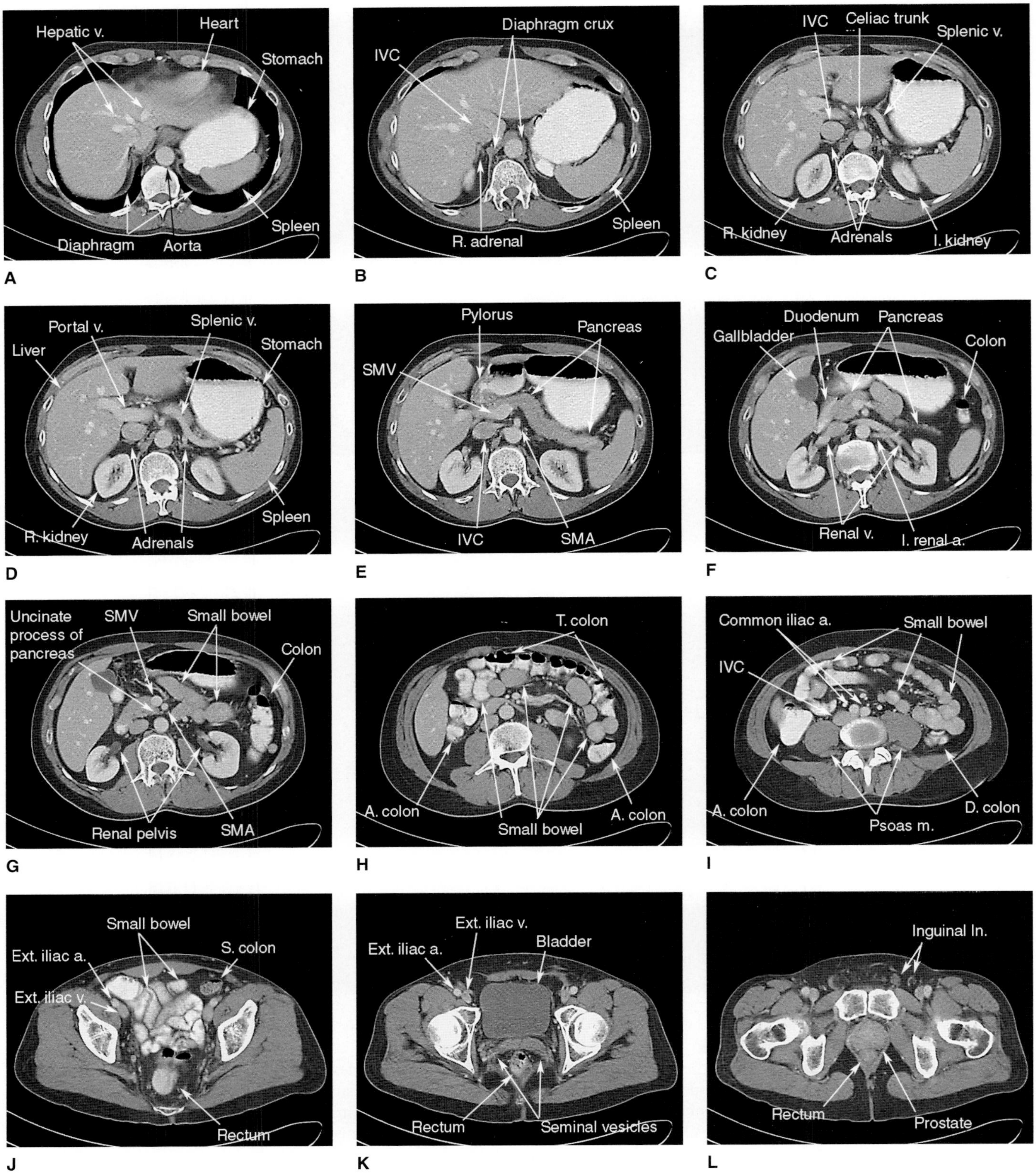

Figure 2-3 Normal Male Abdominal CT
Review the normal cross-sectional anatomy depicted in these CT images.

low attenuation of negative oral contrast enables the viewer to evaluate the degree of mucosal enhancement and the presence of subtle intraluminal masses, which are not possible with the positive oral contrast used in standard CT. When findings at fluoroscopic examination are used as a reference, CT enterography has a sensitivity of more than 85% in the detection of active inflammatory Crohn disease, compared with 78% for convential enteroclysis.[3,4] When endoscopic or surgical findings are used as a reference standard, CT enterography has a sensitivity of 77% in the detection of active inflammatory Crohn disease.[5]

CT Colonography

CTC is a noninvasive method of evaluating the colon for neoplasia that has been in practice since the mid-1990s. This technology utilizes thin section CT imaging of the insufflated colon with evaluation of that data using both 2D axial and 3D endoluminal images (see Figure 2-4). Two of the largest national trials comparing same-day CTC and optical colonoscopy demonstrated that the sensitivity of CTC in the detection of polyps ≥10 mm ranged from 90% to 94.0% and of polyps at least 6 mm was 80% to 89%.[6,7]

The success of CTC relies on 3 factors: (1) bowel preparation, (2) fecal tagging, and (3) colonic distension. Bowel preparation is key to the successful visualization of colonic polyps or masses and their differentiation from stool.[8] Utilization of a bowel preparation that leaves behind the least amount of fluid is desirable to ensure that the maximal mucosal surface is visualized. Although IV contrast can be administered in order to demonstrate polyp enhancement, it is not administered at the majority of institutions as it is not necessary when adequate bowel preparation is achieved. Fecal tagging is accomplished by providing a barium tagging agent to food that is ingested on the last day of solid meals, usually 2 days before the CTC. Fecal tagging facilitates improved differentiation of stool from polyps by making the stool high attenuation.[9,10] Colonic distension is achieved by placing a rectal catheter and administering air or continuous CO_2 during scanning. Because CO_2 is resorbed by the colon, continuous CO_2 has the advantage of less delayed cramping relative to insufflated air. However, if CO_2 is not administered continuously, it will be resorbed, causing colonic collapse.

Dual positioning, in the supine and prone positions, is necessary in order to optimally distend different portions of the bowel, to redistribute fluid and to distinguish mobile stool from fixed polyps. At times, additional views in the right or left lateral decubitus views may also be needed depending on the amount of fluid or collapse of different portions of the colon. Typically 8- and 16-multidetector CT scanning factors include 1.25-mm collimation, 1.0- to 1.25-mm reconstruction interval, and 120 kVp.[2] Because of the high degree of contrast between the gas-filled colonic lumen and soft-tissue polyps, significant dose reduction can be achieved relative to diagnostic CT examinations. Specifically, the dose can be reduced either automatically through Multidetector computed tomography (MDCT) scanner tube current modulation system, or through a tube current-time product in the range of 50 to 75 mAs that produced diagnostic images, excepting morbidly obese patients.[11]

Data interpretation is accomplished using both 2-dimensional (2D) and 3-dimensional (3D) images, although the choice of whether to perform a primary 2D or 3D interpretation lies with the reader. The primary 2D read utilizes serial thin-section axial images to track the colon from the rectum to the cecum using a "polyp" window, which lies between a lung and bone window.[12-16] In this approach, each colonic segment is evaluated from the "floor" to the "ceiling," and any questionable lesions detected and characterized on the 2D images can be further evaluated on the 3D images. The primary 3D read utilizes the virtual colonoscopy or endoluminal view of the colon. This approach requires both anterograde and retrograde interrogation of the colon in order to see abnormalities on the back of a fold.[16] Any questionable lesions detected on the 3D images must then be further characterized using the 2D images as there are a host of polypoid-appearing entities that mimic polyps on the 3D images, including tagged stool, bulbous folds, and fecoliths within diverticula.[17] The merits of the primary 2D and 3D read with regards to polyp sensitivity and time efficiency remain a subject of debate.[17-19] The 2D method is more intuitive to radiologists because of the similarity to reading CT and permits characterizion of abnormalities at the time of detection. The primary 3D read is limited by the inability to view the mucosal surface with colonic collapse or large amounts of fluid.[8,20] However, a primary 3D read can identify smaller polyps (<5 mm) with greater ease than a 2D read and is generally faster than primary 2D reads.[17]

Three criteria are used to distinguish stool from polyp: (1) attenuation, (2) morphology, and (3) mobility. When stool is tagged with high-attenuation barium, discrimination between stool and polyps can be made quickly and confidently. However, in those cases where stool is poorly tagged or untagged, discrimination from polyps rests on characterization of morphology and mobility. Characteristic features of stool include geographic or angulated borders and heterogenous attenuation often with foci of gas.[15,21] In contrast, polyps or small cancers typically demonstrate smooth, rounded, or lobulated borders and homogenous soft-tissue attenuation. Changes in lesion position between supine and prone images also favor a diagnosis of stool.[21,22] However, pedunculated polyps and polyps located within colonic segments attached to a mesentery can also move with changes in position.[23]

Currently accepted indications for performing CTC include (1) failed or incomplete optical colonoscopy,[24-26] in which the examination can be performed the same day with the use of oral iodinated contrast; (2) to evaluate the colon proximal to an obstructing mass or stricture; (3) patients on chronic anticoagulation; and (4) those at risk for receiving sedation.

Imaging Notes 2-1. Criteria Distinguishing Stool From Polyps on CT Colonoscopy

Characteristic	Stool	Polyp
Attenuation	Heterogenous Hyperattenuating internal gas	Homogenous Soft-tissue attenuation
Morphology	Angulated, irregular borders	Smooth, lobulated borders
Mobility	Location mobile	Location fixed

Sonography of the Bowel

Ultrasonography (US) is often the first imaging modality used for evaluation of abdominal pain. Normal bowel is poorly evaluated by US because of interference of bowel gas and peristalsis. However, in the setting of bowel pathology, US can visualize wall thickening, luminal narrowing or dilation, and inflammation of the adjacent fat if the lumen is filled with fluid and contains no air. Despite the limitations of US in evaluating gas-filled bowel, the 1 situation it has been frequently employed is in the evaluation of appendicitis. These examinations can be especially useful in pregnant patients and in other situations where ionizing radiation is relatively contraindicated.

In contrast to CT and MRI, US permits both targeted evaluation of the exact point of discomfort, and dynamic evaluation of bowel peristalsis.[27] When evaluating the area of discomfort, it is necessary to perform graded compression in order to minimize patient pain and avoid pushing the bowel entirely out of the field of view while decreasing the distance between the probe and the bowel, particularly for heavy patients.[28]

The large intestine is characterized by the fixed position of the ascending and descending colon. Colonic haustra and small-bowel valvulae conniventes can be visualized when the bowel is distended with fluid. When attempting to find the appendix, the cecum should initially be identified as a blind-ending loop of large intestine arising from the fixed ascending colon. Subsequently, the terminal ileum should be visualized, and tracing inferiorly along the same side of the cecal wall, the region of the appendix can be evaluated.[27]

The normal wall thickness of the colon on US is 4 mm or less and thinner for the small intestine.[29] Normal bowel on US demonstrates a layered appearance, is compressible, and shows intermittent peristalsis.[27] Abnormal intestine can demonstrate increased wall thickness, loss of the normal layered appearance, and lack of compressibility.[30] When determining the underlying cause, evaluation of the degree and distribution of wall thickening is important. When a focal mass is noted, its location relative to the bowel wall can be classified into intraluminal, mural, or exophytic. Finally, color Doppler is of value in inflammatory conditions such as appendicitis or bowel inflammation in demonstrating wall hyperemia.

Imaging Notes 2-2. Indications for CT Colonoscopy

1. Failed or incomplete optical colonoscopy
2. Evaluation of the colon proximal to an obstructing mass or stricture
3. Chronic anticoagulation
4. Patients at risk for receiving sedation.

MRI of the Bowel

MRI is not routinely used in the evaluation of bowel diseases. However, over the past decade, MRI enterography and enteroclysis have had an increasing impact in the diagnosis and management of patients with Crohn disease. The benefits of these modalities compared to fluoroscopy and CT include high soft-tissue contrast, static and dynamic imaging capabilities, direct multiplanar imaging capabilities, and the use of nonionizing radiation.[31,32]

Magnetic resonance (MR) is more reliable than fluoroscopic enteroclysis in the correct identification of affected regions of Crohn disease involvement but less reliable in detection of mucosal abnormalities.[32,33] Despite higher image quality with CT enterography, studies have demonstrated equivalent results using either MR or CT enterography in the detection of active disease and the demonstration of extraenteric complications.[31,34-37] Because Crohn disease typically affects young patients who are most vulnerable to radiation exposure, MRI has emerged as the preferable method of follow-up in this patient population.[31] Although MR enterography and enteroclysis have been used in other small-bowel disease such as lymphoma and celiac disease, their role in these diseases are yet to be determined.[31]

MR enterography and MR enteroclysis differ in technique from one another and also from CT enterography and CT enteroclysis. Similar to CT enterography, MR enterography involves the ingestion of a large volume of oral contrast incrementally over 1 hour preceding the examination. This oral contrast is composed of dilute barium and sorbitol and superparamagnetic iron oxide, which is used to increase the contrast between the lumen and bowel wall in postcontrast and T2-weighted images. The result is that bowel contents are high in T2 but low in T1 signal.

Similar to CT enteroclysis, the major drawback of MR enteroclysis is that it requires intubation of the patient and positioning of an intestinal tube within the duodenum. Also similar to CT enteroclysis, the major benefit of MR

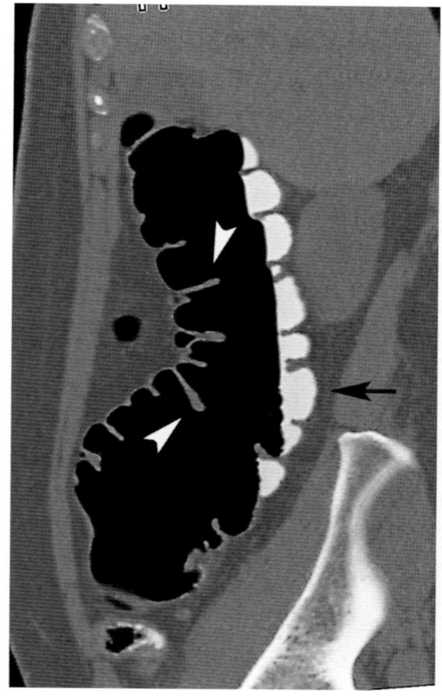
A

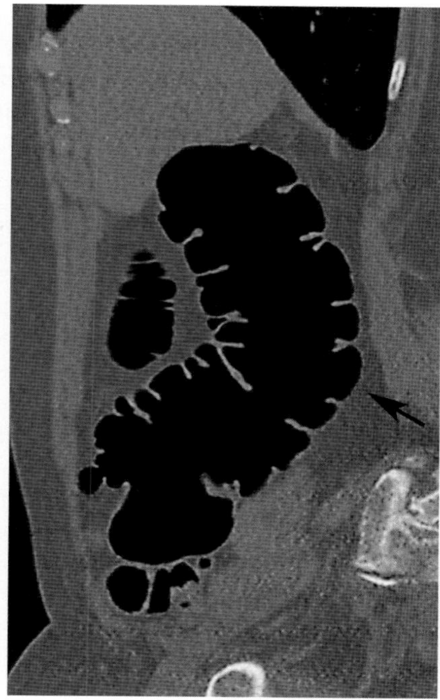
B

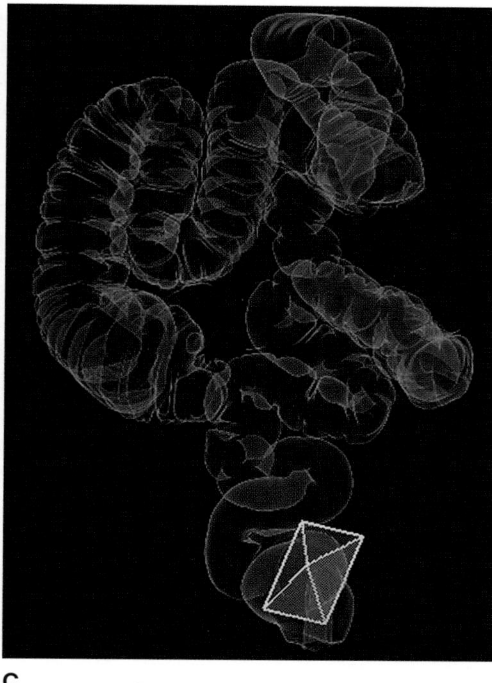
C

Figure 2-4 Normal CTC
Sixty-two-year-old woman referred for CTC following incomplete optical colonoscopy. **A.** Sagittal image of the normal ascending colon in the supine plane using polyp windows demonstrates colonic distension with CO_2 and thin, almost imperceptible walls. Multiple colonic haustra project within the colonic lumen (*white arrowheads*). Note the presence of a small amount of homogenously tagged fluid from Gastroview ingestion along the posterior (dependent) wall (*black arrow*). **B.** Corresponding image of the proximal colon at the same level with the patient in the left lateral decubitus view illustrates that the fluid has shifted, now with clear visualization of the posterior wall (*black arrow*). **C.** Overhead view demonstrates gaseous distension from the rectum to the cecum.

enteroclysis is the ability to control the administration of oral contrast into the small bowel allowing for optimal distension of all bowel segments. However, this improved distention does not necessarily translate into a clinically significant improvement in diagnostic effectiveness between MR enterography and MR enteroclysis.[38,39] Comparison of these 2 techniques demonstrate equivalent diagnostic performances in the identification of stenoses and fistulas, although MR enteroclysis may be superior to MR enterography in demonstrating mucosal abnormalities.[32]

FOCAL DISORDERS OF THE STOMACH

Cross-sectional imaging is generally insensitive for the detection of gastric abnormalities and double-contrast upper GI tract contrast examinations are the most sensitive imaging examination for subtle mucosal lesions. Regardless of the imaging modality, distension of the stomach improves the detection of gastric lesions.[40-43] With collapse of the stomach, the gastric wall becomes thickened, a phenomenon that can hide abnormal wall thickening. Gastric distension will stretch the normal gastric wall and unmask the abnormal wall thickening or depict protruding lesions that hide within collapsed gastric folds. Double-contrast upper GI examinations use CO_2 gas to distend the stomach. In CT examinations, the use of water as a negative oral contrast agent in conjunction with IV contrast will improve detection of gastric lesions because an enhancing mucosal mass will appear more conspicuous against the low attenuation water compared with traditional positive contrast agents.[40-43] Dual-phase dynamic contrast-enhanced CT can also be helpful in visualizing subtle lesions.[44] Specifically, arterial-phase imaging can highlight differences between the normal gastric wall and neoplasms.[40]

Focal lesions of the bowel can either present as soft-tissue masses or as lesions that protrude (ulcers and diverticula) outward from the bowel lumen. The term *polyp* is a descriptive term meaning a growth of tissue that projects from a mucous membrane into the hollow cavity of a tubular structure. If the polyp is connected to the mucosal surface by an elongated stalk, it is said to be "pedunculated." As mass lesions grow, they become progressively larger polyps, then form eccentric masses filling 1 side of the lumen of the bowel and finally progress to circumferential or "annular" masses that focally thicken the wall and narrow the lumen of the GI tract. In general, the differential diagnosis for polyps and masses will be similar, with the exception that some nonneoplastic lesions will always remain small, that is, polypoid. The differential diagnosis of focal GI lesions is dependent on the appearance of the lesion and the organ of origin.

Polyps and Masses of the Stomach

When evaluating sessile polys, it is useful to try to determine whether the mass is epithelial or submucosal in origin. If accurately recognized, this distinction allows for narrowing of the differential diagnosis. On barium examination, submucosal masses are characterized by their smooth well-circumscribed borders and obtuse angles with the bowel wall, similar to the extrapleural sign of pleural and chest wall lesions on chest radiographs. CT and MRI will demonstrate a focal, smoothly marginated nodule or mass within the wall of the GI tract structure that, when viewed in profile, will demonstrate obtuse angles with the bowel wall as seen on barium (see Figure 2-5). However, regardless of the modality used, it is not always possible to reliably distinguish submucosal from epithelial lesions (Table 2-1).

Hyperplastic polyps

Hyperplastic polyps are the most common cause of small gastric polyps, accounting for 75% to 90% of all gastric polyps.[45] They range from a few millimeters to a few centimeters in diameter and have been reported to be associated with various types of chronic gastritis, particularly autoimmune gastritis, *Helicobacter pylori* gastritis, and the postantrectomy stomach.[46,47] Histopathologically, they represent proliferations of the gastric mucosa characterized by prominent foveolar hyperplasia, tortuosity, and edema and inflammation of the intervening lamina propria.[47] Similar to hyperplastic polyps of the colon, they

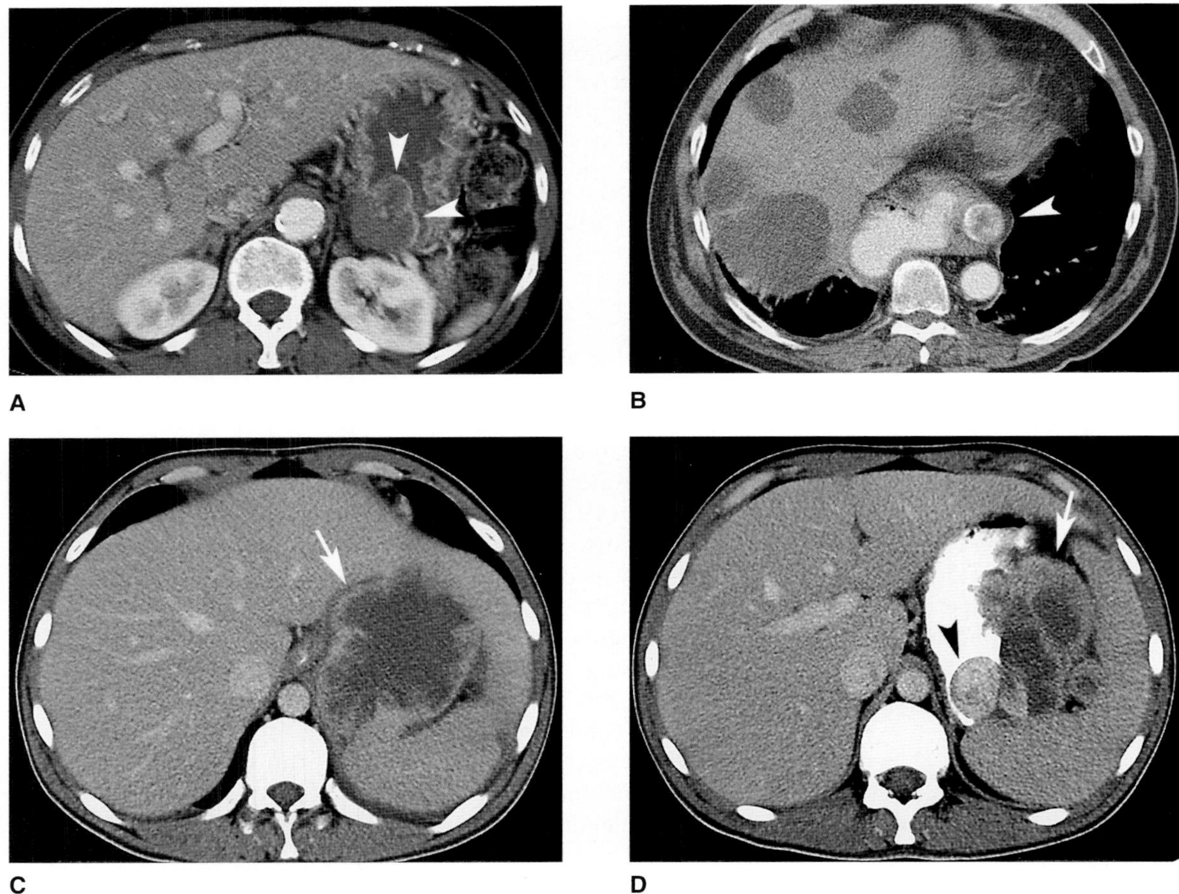

Figure 2-5 Gastrointestinal Stromal Tumor in 3 Patients
A and **B.** In these 2 cases, a lobulated submucosal mass (*white arrowheads*) was incidentally found in the fundus of the stomach. Note the enhancing mucosa on the surface of the mass in **A** indicating the intramural location of the mass. **C** and **D.** This man presented with weight loss. Contrast-enhanced axial CT shows a large, lobulated multicavitary mass (*white arrow*) with a small intensely enhancing nodule (*black arrowhead*). All 3 were proven to represent GISTs.

Table 2-1. Polyps and Masses of the Stomach

1. Epithelial lesions
a. Benign polyps
i. Hyperplastic polyps
ii. Fundic gland polyps
iii. Juvenile (Peutz-Jeghers) polyp
b. Adenoma/adenocarcinoma
c. Carcinoid tumor
2. Submucosal lesions
a. Gastrointestinal stromal tumor (GIST)
b. Lipoma
c. Other stromal tumors
i. Leiomyoma
ii. Neurofibroma
iii. Schwannoma

rarely undergo malignant degeneration.[47] However, studies have shown that 8% to 28% of patients with hyperplastic polyps will have a synchronous gastric carcinoma.[48,49] This association is believed to be due to the association of hyperplastic polyps with underlying atrophic gastritis that predisposes patients to the development of both polyps and cancer.[50]

Most patients with hyperplastic polyps are clinically asymptomatic and are discovered incidentally on radiologic or endoscopic examinations.[50] Rarely, they can present with low-grade GI bleeding or symptoms of gastric outlet obstruction as a result of the prolapse of a polyp through the pylorus.

On barium examinations, they typically appear as multiple, small, smooth, sessile, round, or oval polyps projecting into the gastric lumen, typical of polyps of any cause (see Figure 2-6).[51,52] Most hyperplastic polyps are less than 1 cm but can rarely be as large as 6 cm in diameter.[51,52] Because of their small size, hyperplastic polyps are rarely discovered on cross-sectional imaging but can occasionally be seen as polypoid protrusions from the gastric wall into the gastric lumen.

Fundic gland polyps

Fundic gland polyps arise from the epithelium of the small glands that line the lumen of the stomach.[53] Histologically, they appear as cystically dilated, hyperplastic fundic glands. In the majority of cases, multiple polyps, as many as 50 in number, will occur synchronously. Fundic gland polyps are typically discovered in middle-aged women and can occur sporadically or as part of the inherited syndrome: familial adenomatous polyposis (FAP).[54,55] These polyps are usually benign; however, those arising in patients with FAP have an increased risk of developing colon cancer. Like hyperplastic polyps, fundic gland polyps are typically asymptomatic and their imaging appearance is indistinguishable from polyps due to other causes, although they predominantly occur in the fundus and body of the stomach (see Figure 2-7).[54,56]

Imaging Notes 2-3. Gastric Polyps

Most gastric polyps are of either hyperplastic or adenomatous histology

Polyposis syndromes

There are a variety of predominantly inherited disorders that lead to multiple GI polyps, including familial adenomatous polyposis, Gardner syndrome, Turcot syndrome, Peutz-Jeghers syndrome, juvenile polyposis syndrome, Cronkhite-Canada syndrome, and PTEN hamartoma tumor syndrome. With the exception of Peutz-Jeghers syndrome, which has its most important manifestations in the small bowel and is discussed most completely under the heading **Focal Polyps or Masses of the Small Bowel** later in this chapter, these disorders have their most important manifestations in the colon and are discussed most completely under the heading **Focal Polyps or Masses of the Colon**, later in this chapter. However, we will briefly outline their gastric manifestations here.

Familial adenomatous polyposis and gardner syndrome: Familial adenomatous polyposis (FAP) is an autosomal dominant inherited syndrome causing the development of hundreds to thousands of adenomatous polyps of the colon but is also associated with the formation of polyps in the stomach and small bowel. Unlike colon polyps that have adenomatous histology, most gastric polyps are fundic gland polyps and, therefore, not predisposed to malignancy.[57] These polyps are typically confined to the fundus of the stomach. Uncommonly, gastric polyps associated with familial adenomatous polyposis will have adenomatous histology and have the potential for malignant transformation.

Gardner syndrome was once thought to be a separate syndrome but is now known to result from mutations of the FAP gene and is considered a variant of FAP. It is distinct from FAP; in that, the multiple GI manifestations are also associated with the presence of multiple osteomas (especially of the jaw and skull), desmoid tumors, fibromas, dental abnormalities, and congenital hypertrophy of the retinal epithelial pigment.

Upper GI examinations will demonstrate multiple small, 1- to 5-mm, sessile polyps clustered in the gastric fundus.[58]

Peutz-Jeghers syndrome: Peutz-Jeghers syndrome is an inherited, autosomal dominant disorder characterized by the Peutz-Jeghers type of juvenile polyp. Patients have multiple small skin and GI hamartomas.[59] Imaging

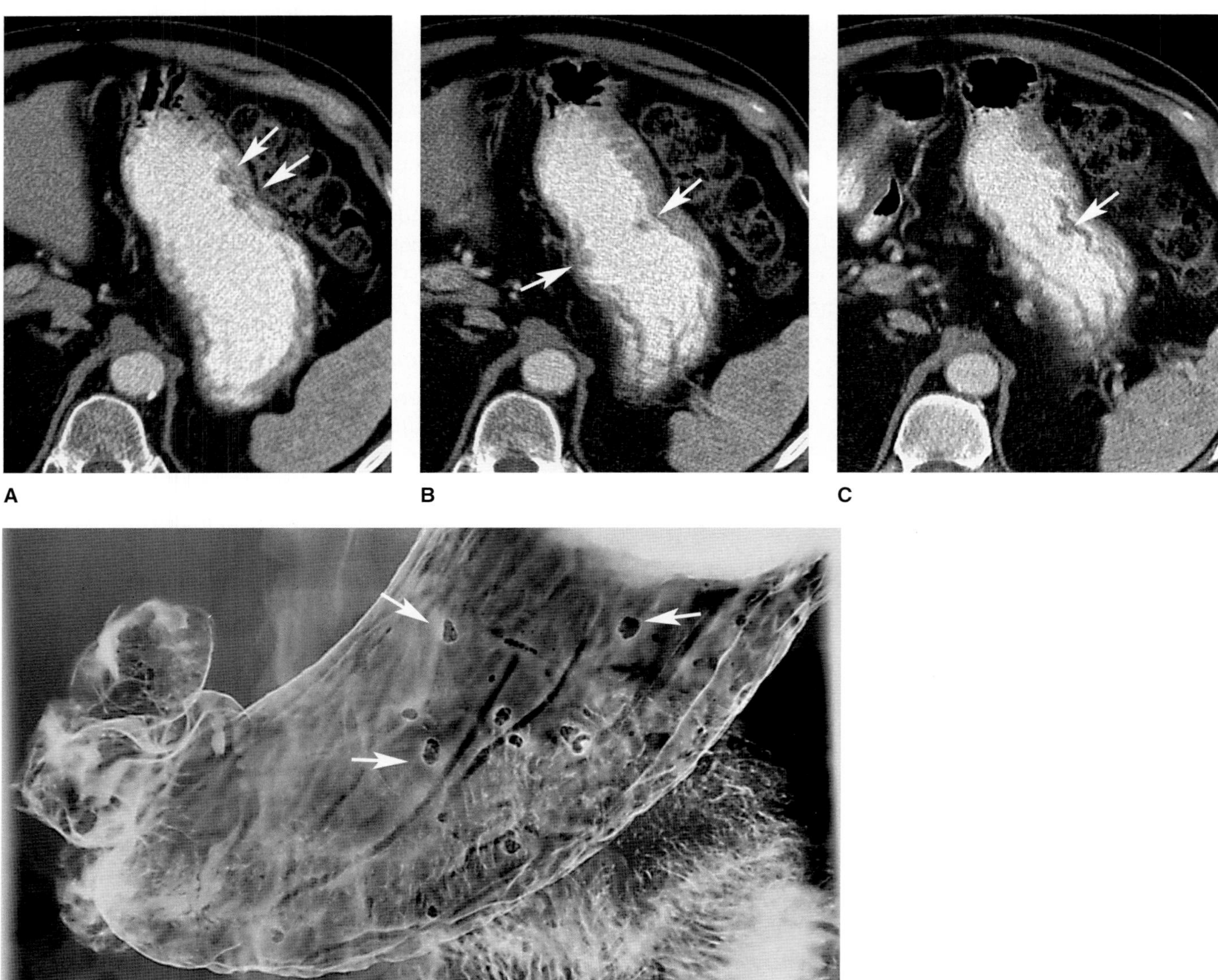

Figure 2-6 Hyperplastic Polyps of the Stomach in 2 Patients This 75-year-old man was being evaluated for non-Hodgkin lymphoma. **A-C.** Axial CT images through the stomach demonstrate multiple small polyps (*arrows*) within the gastric lumen. **D.** Double-contrast upper gastrointestinal examination (UGI) in a second 49-year-old woman with anemia also shows multiple small gastric polyps (*arrows*). There is no histologic proof in these 2 cases; however, these polyps are most likely to be hyperplastic in etiology.

examinations will demonstrate multiple polyps within the small bowel, stomach, and colon but most commonly in the small bowel.[59]

Juvenile polyps and juvenile polyposis syndrome: Juvenile polyps are a form of hamartomatous polyp that can occur sporadically or as part of juvenile polyposis syndrome. Juvenile polyps are found most commonly in the colon but can also occur in the small bowel and stomach.[60]

Adenoma and adenocarcinoma

Adenocarcinoma is the most common gastric malignancy representing more than 95% of malignant tumors of the stomach.[16,40] The peak prevalence of adenocarcinoma is between 50 and 70 years of age.[61] There is wide geographic variation in the incidence of this disease, with the highest incidence of gastric carcinoma occurring in Japan (62.1 cases per 100 000) compared to Western Europe (12.8 cases per 100 000).[62] Prognosis depends on the stage at presentation and early gastric cancers are usually curable lesions, with 5-year survival rates of more than 90%.[63]

Histologically, gastric adenocarcinomas are subdivided into papillary, tubular, mucinous, and signet-ring cell histologies.[64] Most will form fungating masses within the stomach. However, the signet-ring cell histology is associated with submucosal spread of tumor that often

Imaging Notes 2-4. Distinguishing Features of Gastric Polyps

Type	Number	Location	Other
Hyperplastic	Multiple Rarely solitary	Any	Most common Associated with gastritis
Fundic gland	Multiple	Fundus	Middle-aged women Sporadic or associated with familial adenomatous polyposis
Juvenile	Multiple	Any	Associated with Peutz-Jeghers syndrome
Adenoma/ Carcinoma	Solitary	Any	
Carcinoid	Solitary (sporadic) Multiple	Body and fundus Submucosal	Multiple, associated with chronic atrophic gastritis and Zollinger-Ellison syndrome
GIST	Solitary	Body and fundus Submucosal	
Lipoma	Solitary	Submucosal	
Metastasis	Solitary or multiple	Any	

causes a severe desmoplastic response in the gastric wall leading to the features of scirrhous carcinoma, also called "linitis plastica."[65] Classically, linitis plastica involves the distal half of the stomach, arising in the pyloric region and extending toward the body and fundus. However, it can also be seen as a localized lesion involving the gastric fundus or body.[66] In advanced cases, the entire stomach is infiltrated by the tumor.

Unfortunately, gastric carcinoma is generally an aggressive tumor that typically presents late in the course of disease with overall 5-year survival rates of less than 20% in the United States.[40] However, in some Asian countries, especially Japan, aggressive screening for gastric cancer with endoscopy and double-contrast upper GI examinations can lead to detection of early-stage disease with an improved prognosis.[67]

Multiple risk factors for the formation of gastric adenocarcinoma have been described, including salt-rich diets, smoked or poorly preserved foods, nitrates, nitrites, secondary amines, *H pylori* infection, chronic atrophic gastritis, pernicious anemia, partial gastrectomy, smoking, obesity, Ménétrier disease, and gastric polyps.[68,69]

Roughly 30% of cancers are located in the antrum, the body, and the fundus or cardia, respectively. The remaining 10% are scirrhous carcinomas, which are diffusely infiltrating lesions that involve the entire stomach.[68,69]

More than 75% of patients will present with lymphatic spread of tumor,[70] typically to the perigastric lymph nodes. The frequency of lymphatic metastases is correlated with

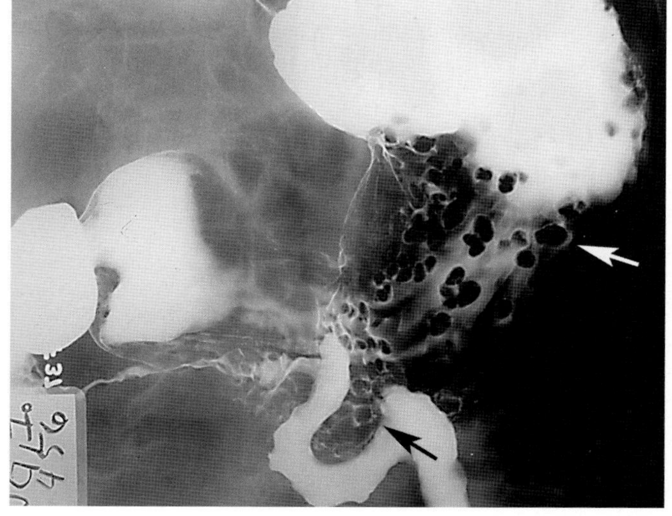

Figure 2-7 Fundic Gland Polyps
This 80-year-old woman complained of weight loss, malaise, and anorexia. Double-contrast barium enema demonstrates multiple polyps in the fundus and body of the stomach, which are seen as filling defects in the barium pool (*white arrow*) or etched in white as small circles (*black arrow*). The distribution of disease is typical of fundic gland polyps. Differential diagnosis could include multiple gastric carcinoids in a patient with chronic atrophic gastritis or Zollinger-Ellison syndrome. Multiple gastric polyps can also be seen in patients with FAP syndrome and Peutz-Jeghers syndrome.

the size and depth of penetration of the tumor. Abnormal nodes, as elsewhere in the abdomen, are classified based on size as well as morphologic and enhancement criteria. Of note, lymph node involvement outside the perigastric location is considered metastatic (M1 disease).

Metastases from gastric carcinoma spread hematogenously and most often involve the liver because the stomach is drained by the portal vein (see Figure 2-8). However, other sites of spread include the lungs, adrenal glands, kidneys, bones, and brain. Peritoneal carcinomatosis can be seen with advanced cancer. Rarely, patients with gastric carcinomas can metastasize to the ovaries, a phenomenon known as Krukenberg tumors.[63] This occurs most frequently in patients with signet-ring cell histology.

Presenting symptoms include vague abdominal pain, evidence of GI bleeding such as hematemesis, melena, hematochezia, or evidence of bowel obstruction such as nausea, vomiting, or early satiety. Some patients will be discovered while still asymptomatic either on screening examinations intended to detect unsuspected GI malignancies or accidentally on examinations performed for reasons unrelated to the presence of the cancer.

On contrast upper GI examinations, early gastric cancers typically take 1 of 2 appearances: (1) small superficial plaquelike lesions or (2) as small irregular ulcers.[71,72] In some cases, there will be associated mucosal nodularity and/or amputation of radiating folds. Advanced carcinomas typically present as polypoid, plaquelike, ulcerated, infiltrating lesions, or as thickened irregular folds (see Figure 2-9). Double-contrast barium evaluation is superior to single-contrast technique for the detection of these tumors.[73,74]

On CT and MRI, early gastric cancers will appear as small to large polypoid or plaquelike projections into the gastric lumen. Protruded lesions are easier to detect on CT than are flat or ulcerated lesions.[63] Advanced gastric cancer can present with a diversity of imaging appearances, including focal eccentric or concentric masses with or without central ulceration, or as segmental or diffuse wall thickening with irregular lobulation (see Figures 2-8 and 2-9).[63,73-75] Carcinomas of the cardia can be difficult to differentiate from the normal soft-tissue thickening that occurs at the gastroesophageal junction.

On CT and MRI, transmural extension of gastric cancer is characterized by haziness of the serosal margin with strandlike areas of increased soft-tissue attenuation or increased T2 signal extending into the perigastric fat (see Figures 2-9 and 2-10). Cancer will often spread through ligamentous and peritoneal reflections to adjacent organs, including the liver, via the gastrohepatic ligament; the pancreas, via the lesser sac; and the transverse colon, via the gastrocolic ligament. Carcinoma of the cardia will involve the distal esophagus in approximately 60% of patients, whereas carcinoma of the antrum will involve the duodenum in 13% to 18% of patients.[63]

Detection of a gastric cancer should lead to a careful review of the perigastric and retroperitoneal lymph nodes for evidence of metastasis (see Figures 2-10 and 13-34). The liver and other visualized organs should be carefully evaluated for evidence of metastasis.

The clinical value of ^{18}F-fludeoxyglucose positron emission tomography (FDG-PET) in gastric cancer is not as well established as that of other GI tumors and is currently not reimbursed by Medicare.[76] The sensitivity

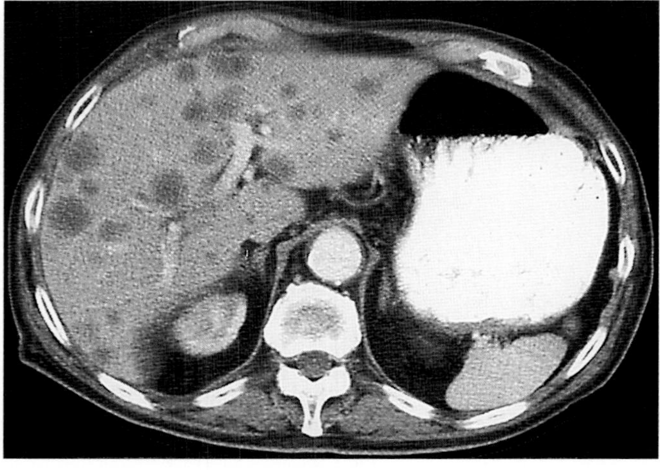

A

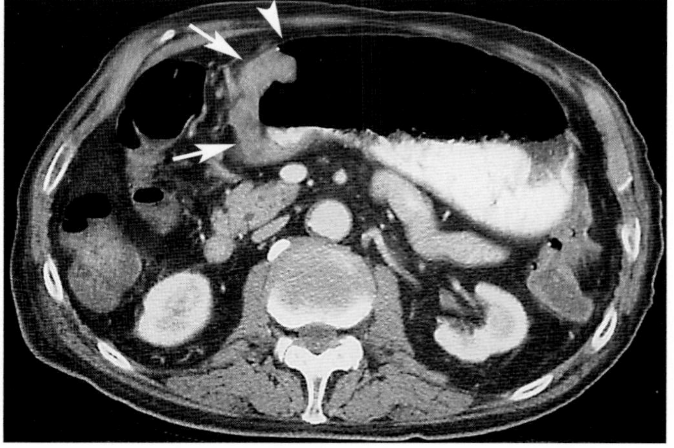

B

Figure 2-8 Gastric Carcinoma
This 85-year-old man presented with heme-positive stool. **A.** CT image through the liver demonstrates multiple low attenuation nodules, most likely due to hepatic metastasis. **B.** CT image through the antrum and body of the stomach shows a focal lobulated area of wall thickening (*arrows*) in the antrum. The sharp division between abnormal gastric wall and normal gastric wall (*arrowhead*) indicates that this abnormality represents an eccentric gastric mass, most likely a gastric carcinoma. Endoscopic biopsy confirmed a diagnosis of adenocarcinoma of the stomach.

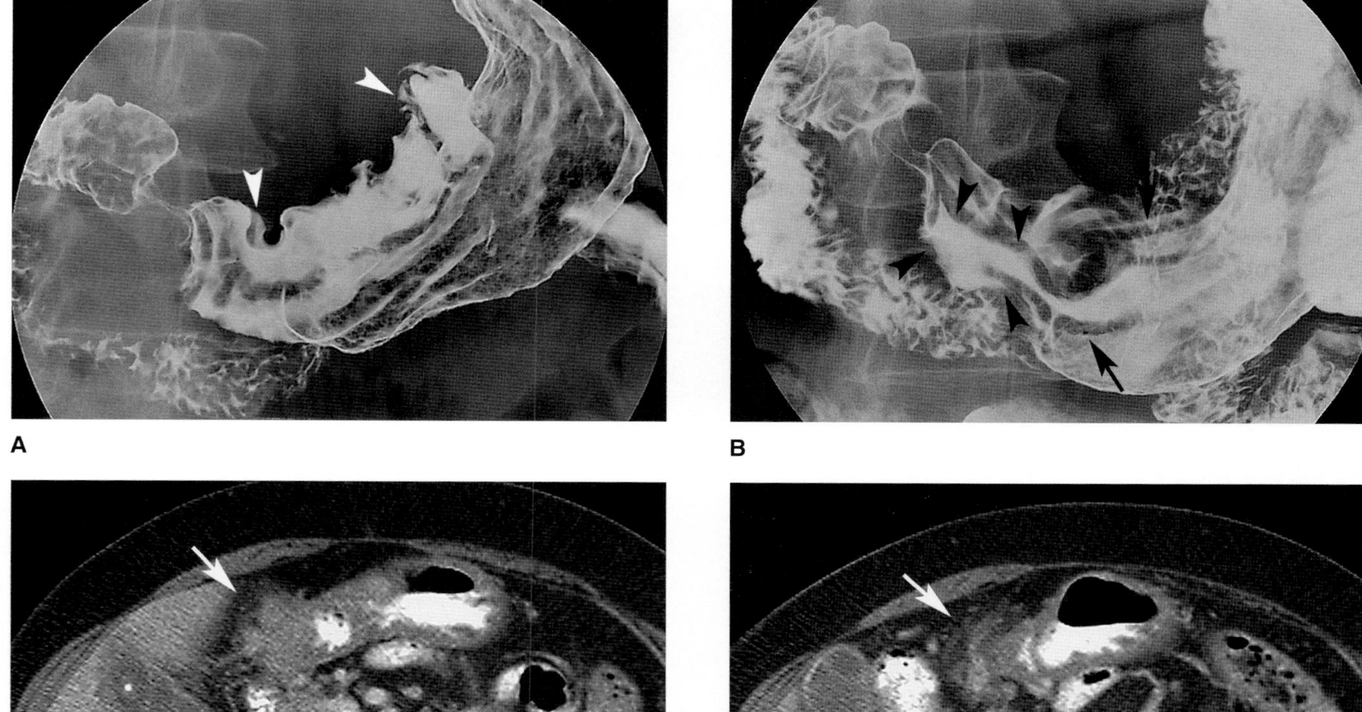

Figure 2-9 Ulcerated Gastric Carcinoma
A. Double-contrast UGI in this 79-year-old woman shows a large mass in profile, seen as a raised plaquelike lesion projecting into the lumen of the stomach along the lesser curvature between the 2 white arrowheads. The central region of the mass is depressed indicating a central ulcer. Note how the ulcer does not project beyond the lumen of the stomach, a feature usually indicating the presence of a malignancy. **B.** In this view, the mass is seen as an irregularly shaped ulcer (*black arrowheads*) in the antrum. Note how the gastric folds (*black arrows*) stop at the margins of the mass. **C** and **D.** Contrast-enhanced CT in the same patient shows a soft-tissue mass in the antrum of the stomach. Note how the margins between the mass and the gastric fat are indistinct, indicating invasion of the perigastric fat. The anterior wall of the stomach proximal to the mass also appears thickened in C, indicating extension of the cancer into the more proximal stomach.

of PET in T-staging ranges from 60% to 80%.[77-79] PET is similarly insensitive for detecting nodal involvement, distant metastases,[79-81] and detection of recurrent disease. One promising area for FDG-PET is in evaluating tumor response to chemotherapy,[78] although this indication requires further validation.

Carcinoid tumor

Gastric carcinoids are uncommon gastric neoplasms, most of which arise from oxyntic mucosa in the gastric body and fundus.[82,83] These tumors arise from enterochromaffin-like cells (Kulchitsky cells) within the gastric mucosa.[39] Approximately three-fourths of gastric carcinoids are associated with autoimmune chronic atrophic gastritis, slightly greater than 5% are associated with Zollinger-Ellison (ZE) syndrome, and the remainder occur sporadically without associated atrophic gastritis or hypergastrinemia.[85]

Chronic atrophic gastritis results in the loss of acid-secreting parietal cells in the body and fundus of the stomach, causing permanent reduction of gastric acid secretion.[41] As a result, antral G cells are hyperstimulated to produce gastrin. Hypergastrinemia causes hyperplasia of the enterochromaffin-like cells. In some cases, enterochromaffin-like hyperplasia goes on to develop carcinoid tumors. As a consequence of this process, carcinoid tumors associated with chronic atrophic gastritis

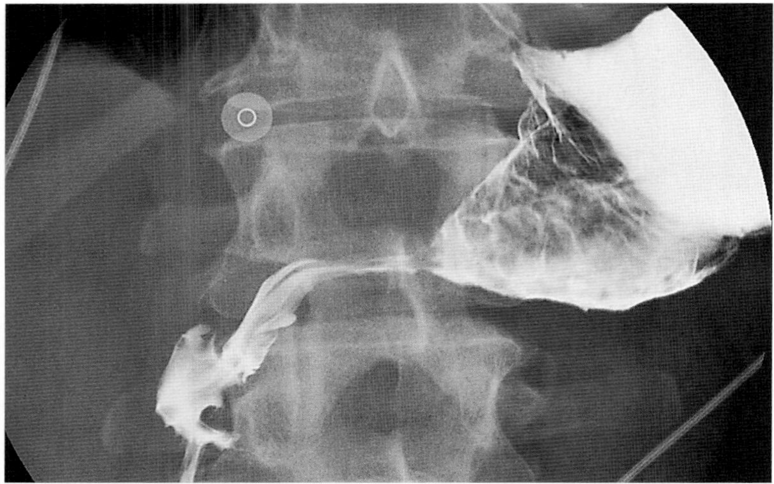

A

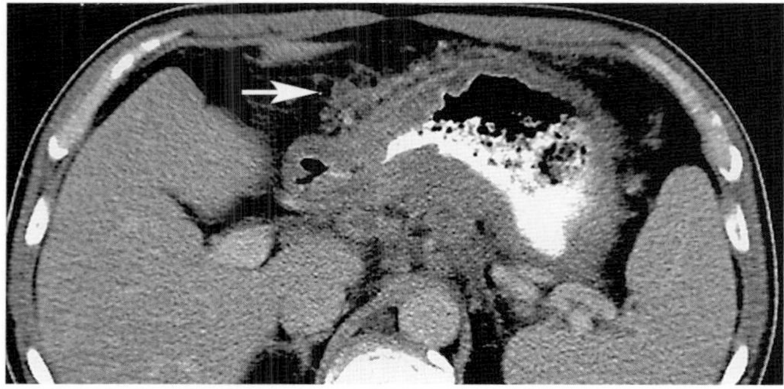

B

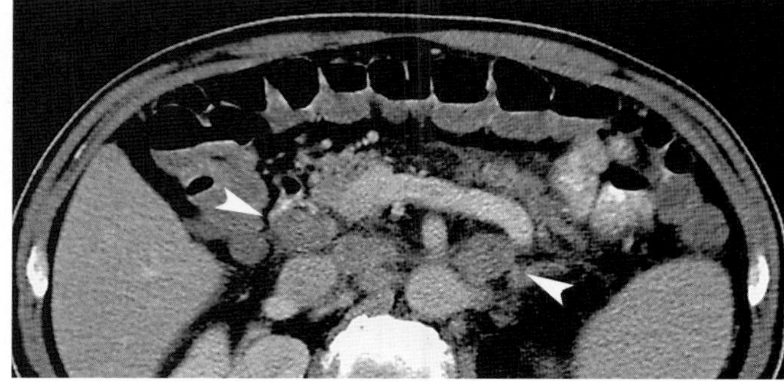

C

Figure 2-10 Scirrhous Gastric Carcinoma
This 58-year-old man complained of nausea and vomiting. **A.** Double-contrast upper GI tract examination shows circumferential narrowing of the gastric antrum. Although this could be due to a severe benign stricture, it is most likely due to a diffusely infiltrating carcinoma. **B** and **C.** Contrast-enhanced CT images show concentric thickening of the wall of the antrum. Note the indistinctness of the perigastric fat (*arrow*) indicating invasion beyond the wall of the stomach. There are also multiple enlarged celiac axis lymph nodes (*arrowheads*).

and ZE syndrome are typically numerous and low-grade.[86] Lymph node and hepatic metastasis are rare, occurring in approximately 2% of patients with chronic atrophic gastritis and a slightly higher percentage in those with ZE syndrome.[86-88]

Sporadic carcinoids are distinctly different from those that occur in association with hypergastrinemia.[86,87] They are seen predominantly in men (89%), are typically larger and solitary, and carry a greater malignant potential. The risk of metastasis correlates with the size of the tumor. The risk of metastases is 10% among patients with tumors less than 1 cm in diameter as opposed to 66% among patients with tumors greater than 3 cm in diameter.

When they metastasize, gastric carcinoids typically involve the regional lymph nodes draining the stomach, involving first the gastrohepatic and gastrosplenic ligament and then the celiac axis and paraaortic lymph nodes.[41] Hematogenous metastasis will most often occur in the liver.

Carcinoid tumors will usually be found in patients older than age 40 years. Patients are typically asymptomatic but can present with abdominal pain, nausea, vomiting, or weight loss or with symptoms of GI bleeding.[89] The overwhelming majority of gastric carcinoids are nonsecretory and, therefore, do not present with carcinoid syndrome.

As above, carcinoid tumors associated with hypergastrinemia will typically appear as multiple small smoothly marginated, 1- to 2-cm polypoid, mucosal, or submucosal masses located in the gastric body and fundus (see Figure 2-11).[90] In comparison, sporadic carcinoids will typically appear as single large mucosal or submucosal masses in the stomach (see Figure 2-12). Larger carcinoids can demonstrate mucosal ulcerations along the surface of the mass, which are readily identified at double-contrast upper GI radiography or CT as focal, irregular collections of barium, contrast material, or air on the surface of the

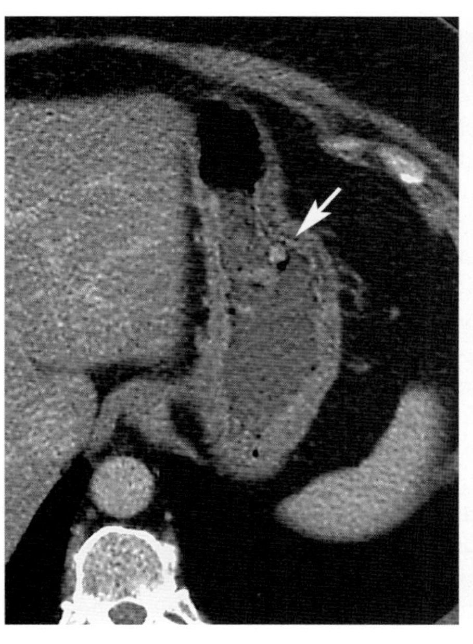

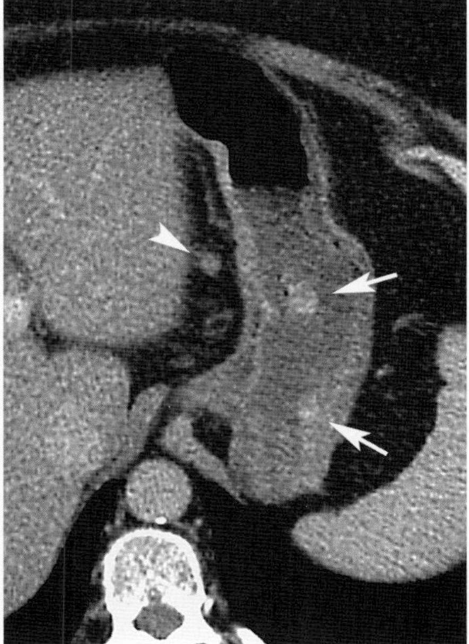

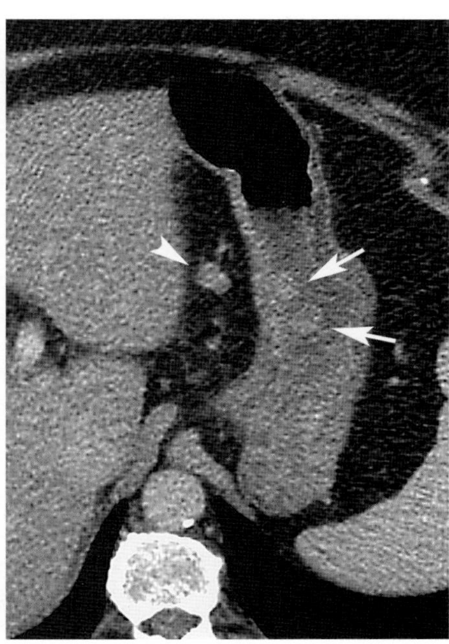

A B C

Figure 2-11 Multiple Gastric Carcinoid Tumors
This 64-year-old man had multiple polyps identified on endoscopy. **A-C.** Narrow windows on a contrast-enhanced CT can also demonstrate multiple intensely enhancing gastric polyps predominantly involving the gastric body and fundus. There are also mildly enlarged gastrohepatic ligament lymph nodes. Causes of multiple gastric polyps include hyperplastic polyps, fundic gland polyps, and multiple carcinoid tumors. The dense enhancement and enlarged lymph nodes would favor gastric carcinoid tumors. Histologic samples confirmed a diagnosis of multiple carcinoid tumors in a background of chronic atrophic gastritis.

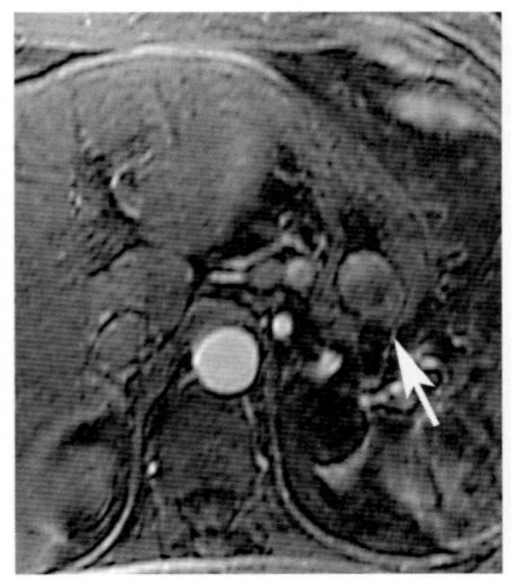

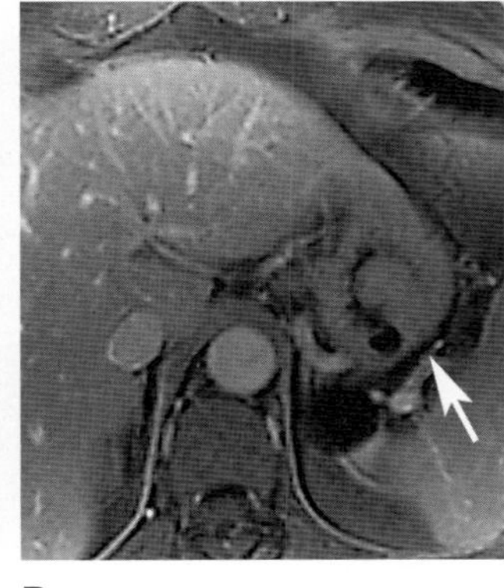

A B

Figure 2-12 Solitary Gastric Carcinoid
This 55-year-old man had a mass noted on endoscopy. T1-weighted post-gadolinium MRI images performed in the (**A**) arterial and (**B**) venous phases of imaging show a smoothly marginated oval polypoid mass (*arrows*) projecting into the lumen of the gastric fundus. Note the brisk enhancement of the mass in A prior to enhancement of the gastric wall in A, indicating the presence of a hypervascular mass, most likely to indicate a neuroendocrine tumor. Biopsy was diagnostic of a gastric carcinoid.

mass. When larger than 1 cm in diameter, gastric carcinoids can be seen on contrast-enhanced CT as 1 or multiple mural masses with arterial enhancement (see Figures 2-11 and 2-12).[85] Gastrointestinal carcinoids are discussed most completely under the subsequent heading **Focal Polyps and Masses of the Small Bowel**.

Lymphoma

Primary gastric lymphoma accounts for 1% to 5% of all gastric malignancies overall, and for 50% to 70% of all primary GI lymphomas.[91] It is believed that most primary gastric lymphomas often originate as a low-grade mucosa-associated lymphoid tissue (MALT) lymphoma, which transforms into intermediate or high-grade large cell lymphoma if not diagnosed or treated in time.[92] Although the stomach contains a paucity of lymphoid tissue, chronic infection with *H pylori* is thought to lead to a proliferation of lymphoid tissue that can result in the development of low-grade MALT lymphoma. It has been estimated that chronic *H pylori* gastritis accounts for 50% to 72% of all primary gastric lymphomas.[92]

Both primary and secondary GI lymphoma can involve any portion of the GI tract. However, secondary GI lymphoma usually involves multiple sites, whereas primary GI lymphoma usually involves only 1 site.[93] The stomach is the most common site of involvement in primary GI lymphoma, followed by the small bowel, large intestine, and esophagus.[93-96]

Clinical symptoms can include abdominal pain, early satiety, weight loss, nausea, and vomiting.[97] Overall, 20% to 30% of patients will present with hematemesis or melena.

On upper GI examinations, gastric lymphoma will typically appear as a large irregularly marginated mass projecting into the lumen of the stomach—an appearance that can be indistinguishable from gastric adenocarcinoma. In some cases, gastric lymphoma will present as multiple rounded and confluent nodules within the stomach. When visualized, this appearance can be a clue that the gastric mass represents lymphoma rather than carcinoma. Unfortunately, this nodularity is difficult to distinguish from enlarged area gastricae, which are also seen in *H pylori* gastritis. Similar to other large gastric tumors, large lymphomas can develop central ulceration.[94,98-100] In some cases, the central necrosis can be so severe that it leads to gastric perforation. Occasionally, gastric lymphoma can present as extensive infiltration of the gastric wall, with gastric fold thickening producing a linitis plastica appearance.[92,101]

On CT and MRI examinations, the most common manifestation of lymphoma is as segmental or diffuse wall thickening, measuring up to 4.0 cm in diameter.[40,102] However, lymphoma can also appear as a large exophytic mass with or without ulceration (see Figure 2-13). Wall thickening can be difficult to appreciate without distention of the stomach. Subtle thickening is more common with MALT lymphoma than other gastric lymphomas.

Several imaging features are helpful to distinguish lymphoma from adenocarcinoma in the stomach. On CT, both adenocarcinoma and lymphoma present with gastric wall thickening. However, lymphoma is favored when there is preservation of the perigastric fat planes[103] and/or involvement of more than 1 region of the stomach.[40] Adenocarcinoma will usually cause the wall to become rigid and narrows the lumen of the stomach, increasing the likelihood of gastric outlet obstruction. Lymphoma, on the other hand, retains the pliability of the gastric wall without luminal narrowing, making gastric outlet obstruction rare.[104] Finally, extension of adenopathy below the renal hila or visualization of bulky nodes also favors lymphoma over adenocarcinoma.[102,103] Both the primary disease and

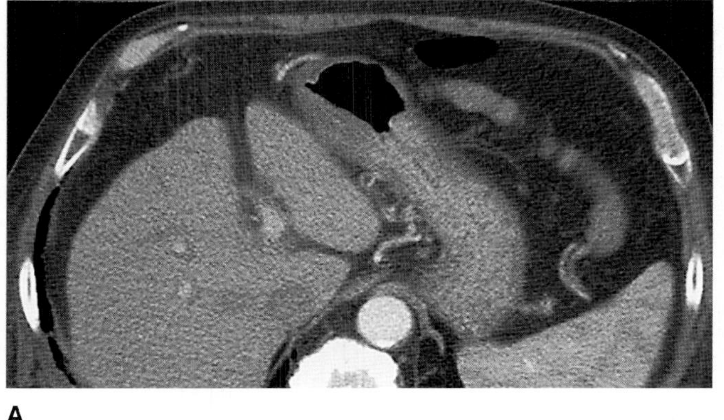

A

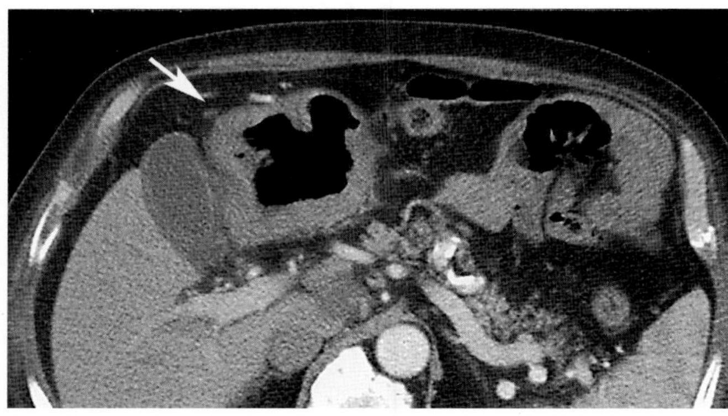

B

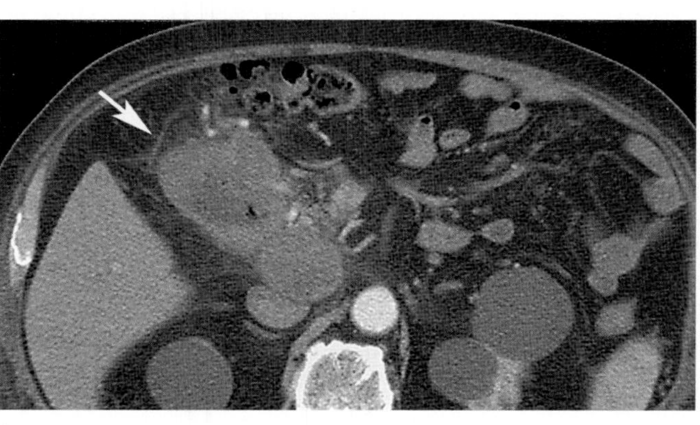

C

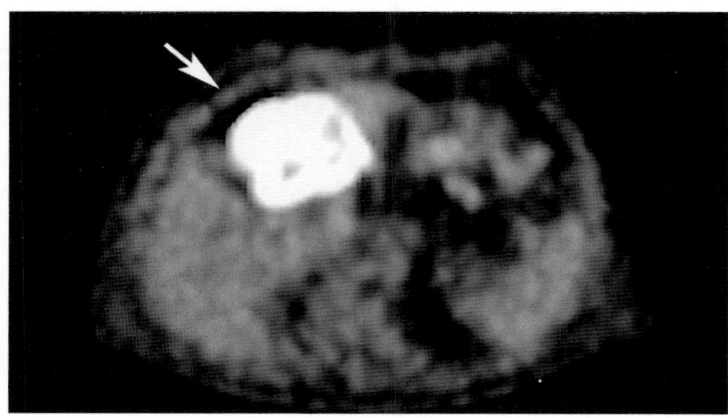

D

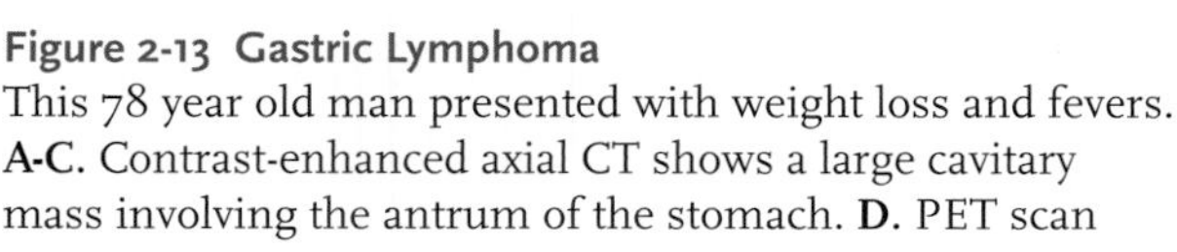

Figure 2-13 Gastric Lymphoma
This 78 year old man presented with weight loss and fevers. **A-C.** Contrast-enhanced axial CT shows a large cavitary mass involving the antrum of the stomach. **D.** PET scan shows increased metabolic activity in the mass without other abnormality demonstrated. Differential diagnosis would include adenocarcinoma, lymphoma, and malignant GIST. Biopsy was diagnostic of B-cell lymphoma.

Imaging Notes 2-5. Imaging Features Distinguishing Gastric Lymphoma From Carcinoma

Characteristic	Adenocarcinoma	Lymphoma
Plasticity	Rigid	Distensible
Lumen	Narrowed	Little or no narrowing
Adjacent fat	Infiltrated	Not infiltrated
Regional involvement	Single region	Multiple regions
Adenopathy	Only drainage Region of stomach	Involvement of lymph nodes outside of gastric drainage

the treatment of lymphoma can result in a number of complications, including obstruction, perforation, or fistulization. These complications can be detected with CT and barium studies.[93]

Gastrointestinal stromal tumor

Gastrointestinal stromal tumors (GISTs) are a group of tumors that are distinct from smooth muscle and neural tumors and are the most common mesenchymal tumor of the GI tract.[85] These tumors are defined by the expression of KIT (CD117), a tyrosine kinase growth factor receptor.[85] Approximately 45% to 70% of these tumors are found in the stomach, followed by the small bowel (20%-30%) and the anorectal region (9%), but they can be located anywhere from the esophagus to the rectum.[85,105] These tumors are usually found in patients older than age 50 years,[106] and can be associated with neurofibromatosis type I.

These tumors arise from the muscularis propria of the stomach and intestinal wall. When large, they have a predilection to present as an exophytic mass projecting outside the organ of origin.[85,107] They present as well-circumscribed masses that range in size from several millimeters to more than 30 cm.[107] As they enlarge, focal regions of hemorrhage, necrosis, and cystic degeneration are common, which can result in cavity formation connecting the necrotic center of the mass with the bowel lumen.[85] Unlike lymphoma and adenocarcinoma, lymphatic metastases are rare. Instead, most malignant GISTs will spread by local invasion or hematogenous dissemination to the liver or peritoneum.

On upper GI examinations, GISTs will appear as submucosal mass characterized by smooth margins and obtuse angles with the gastric wall when viewed in profile.[108] In smaller tumors, the mucosa is usually intact; however, large tumors demonstrate central mucosal ulceration in more than half of cases thought to reflect outgrowth of tumor blood supply.[108,109] As a result, these lesions demonstrate a characteristic “bull’s eye” or “target” appearance on barium, which can also be seen in metastatic disease, particularly melanoma and Kaposi sarcoma.[110-113] Approximately 90% of malignant GISTs occur in the fundus or body of the stomach.[16]

On CT and MRI examinations, GISTs will typically appear as a large, sharply defined, soft-tissue mass involving the fundus or body of the stomach but projecting esophytically into the surrounding perigastric fat. An intramural component can be visualized on CT and MRI in almost all cases, but when these tumors become large (>5 cm), they often appear as an exophytic mass. Larger tumors will often present with central necrosis and calcification.[109,114] More than 80% of these large tumors will demonstrate extragastric extension to the gastrohepatic or gastrosplenic ligament or the lesser sac.[85] Because the bulk of the tumor is usually located outside of the stomach, it can be difficult to visualize the thin pedicle connecting this mass to the stomach. In this situation, careful evaluation of the stomach for subtle wall thickening can be a clue to the site of origin (see Figure 2-5).[85]

Following the administration of contrast, greater than 90% of tumors demonstrate peripheral enhancement corresponding to viable tumor, with central regions of low attenuation corresponding to hemorrhage, necrosis, or cyst formation.[115] Cavitation of extensive hemorrhagic or necrotic components with resultant communication between the mass and the gastric lumen can be seen on CT.[116] The imaging appearance on MRI varies with the degree of necrosis. However, in general, the solid portions of GIST on MRI usually demonstrate low T1 and high T2 signal.[117]

Lymphadenopathy is rarely seen in GISTs. In some cases, this can be an important distinguishing feature between GISTs and some gastric carcinomas and lymphomas.[85] Malignant GISTs can both invade adjacent organs and metastasize hematogenously, usually to the lung or liver.[40] In the absence of these findings, imaging cannot usually help differentiate between malignant and benign gastric stromal tumors, although small tumors (less than 4-5 cm) are usually benign.[40]

Imaging Notes 2-6. Large Masses of the Stomach

Type	Location	Ulceration
Adenocarcinoma	Any	+++
Lymphoma	Any	++
GIST	Body or fundus Submucosal	+++
Carcinoid	Body and fundus Submucosal	++
Lipoma	Submucosal	rare

Kaposi sarcoma

Kaposi sarcoma is a rare malignancy of vascular origin that was an important opportunistic malignancy found in HIV-positive homosexual men. With recent advances in the control of HIV infection and increased awareness of the risks of unprotected sex in the gay community, the incidence of Kaposi sarcoma has fallen precipitously. Although primarily a skin disease, rarely, this malignancy can involve the GI tract, primarily the stomach and small bowel.[118,119]

In most cases, gastric lesions are clinically asymptomatic and are discovered on endoscopic and barium examinations performed for other reasons.[120] These lesions are submucosal in location and are visualized on barium as 1 or several raised lesions that form obtuse angles with the gastric mucosa when viewed in profile.[119,120] These lesions range from 0.5 to 3.0 cm in diameter, and larger lesions will often demonstrate central ulceration along the submucosal surface because of outgrowth of their blood supply. This central ulceration produces a bull's-eye or target appearance on barium. That can also be seen in metastatic disease, particularly melanoma, and lymphoma discussed above.[110-113] Rarely, Kaposi sarcoma can cause thickened nodular folds or a linitis plastica appearance.[119,121,122]

Lipoma

Lipomas are uncommon, slow-growing submucosal tumors that can be found throughout the GI tract.[123,124] The colon is the most common site of lipoma in the GI tract, followed by the small bowel and stomach.[123,125] In most cases, they will appear as smooth, sharply marginated ovoid masses on barium studies, CT, and MRI.

Other mesenchymal tumors of the stomach

The vast majority of mesenchymal tumors of the stomach will represent GISTs or lipomas. However, rarely true leiomyomas, leiomyosarcomas, schwannomas, and neurofibromas occur within in the stomach. These tumors will typically have an appearance that is similar to that of GISTs.

Gastric metastasis

Metastasis to the stomach are rare and found in only 2% of autopsies of patients who die of carcinoma.[126] Most metastases occur as a result of hematogenous spread but can rarely be due to direct extension of an adjacent cancer. Melanoma, breast, and lung cancers are the most common primary sites for gastric metastasis. Most gastric metastases are asymptomatic, but rarely they can present with evidence of GI bleeding, nausea, vomiting, early satiety, epigastric pain, or weight loss.[127,128]

Hematogenous metastasis will most often appear as 1 or several submucosal masses of the stomach. These will appear as smoothly marginated masses projecting into the lumen of the stomach on upper GI studies of the stomach. As these lesions outgrow their blood supply, they may develop central ulceration along their submucosal surface presenting with a bull's-eye or target appearance that can also be seen in lymphoma and Kaposi sarcoma.[110-113] Occasionally, lesions can achieve such a large size that they may be confused with primary lesions of the gastric wall such as GISTs.[129-131] On CT, hematogenous metastasis can appear as a discrete enhancing mass within the wall of the stomach or as focal wall thickening.[132,133]

Rarely, hematogenous metastasis will infiltrate the wall of the stomach, reducing the distensibility of the stomach and causing the linitis plastica appearance.[54,55] On CT scans, this will appear as diffuse thickening of the wall of the stomach.[132,133]

Ulcers and Diverticula of the Stomach

Gastric ulcers can be divided into benign inflammatory causes and malignant causes. Epiphrenic diverticula are common incidental findings in the fundus of the stomach.

Gastritis and peptic ulcer disease

Gastritis is among the most common causes of epigastric pain and is a frequent cause of emergency room admissions. It can be an acute or chronic phenomenon. Causes of acute gastritis include alcohol consumption, aspirin or other nonsteroidal anti-inflammatory drugs (NSAIDs), stress, trauma, burns, Crohn disease, and viral or fungal infections.[73,134-139] In approximately one-half of patients with acute gastritis, no predisposing factor will be identified.

The most common causes of chronic gastritis are *H pylori* infection. *Helicobacter pylori* is a microaerophilic bacterium, which has evolved to live in the highly acidic environment of the stomach and can be found in more than half of Americans older than age 60.[140] The organism induces a low-grade chronic inflammation of the gastric mucosa that can lead to chronic gastritis.

Many patients with gastritis are asymptomatic. Those with symptoms will typically present with dyspepsia and epigastric pain. Other symptoms can include nausea, vomiting, belching, bloating, hematemesis, melena, and unexplained weight loss.

Histopathologically, gastritis causes inflammation and edema of the mucosa and submucosal tissues of the stomach. The inflammation can also cause gastric erosions, which are small epithelial defects that do not project beyond the muscularis mucosa.[134] With greater severity of disease, there is destruction of the muscularis mucosa and deeper submucosal tissues resulting in the formation of a gastric ulcer. *Helicobacter pylori* is thought to be the major factor in the development of gastric ulcers.[73] Approximately 60% to 80% of patients with gastric ulcer disease test positive for *H pylori*.[141] Treatment of *H pylori* with antibiotics and antisecretory agents leads to both, more rapid healing of gastric ulcers and also to lower rates of recurrence.[142,143] Edema of the submucosal tissues of the stomach results in enlargement or apparent thickening of the gastric folds.

There are 2 characteristic features of gastritis on imaging examinations: (1) defects in the mucosa (erosions and ulcers) and (2) wall or fold thickening. On double-contrast upper GI examinations, 0.5% to 20% of patients with gastritis will demonstrate erosions of 2 types.[73,144-148] The most common is the complete or "varioliform" erosion, which is characterized by a punctate or slitlike collection of barium surrounded by a radiolucent halo of edematous, raised mucosa (see Figure 2-14). These are usually located in the gastric antrum and are often aligned on folds. Five percent of erosions will be incomplete or "flat" and appear

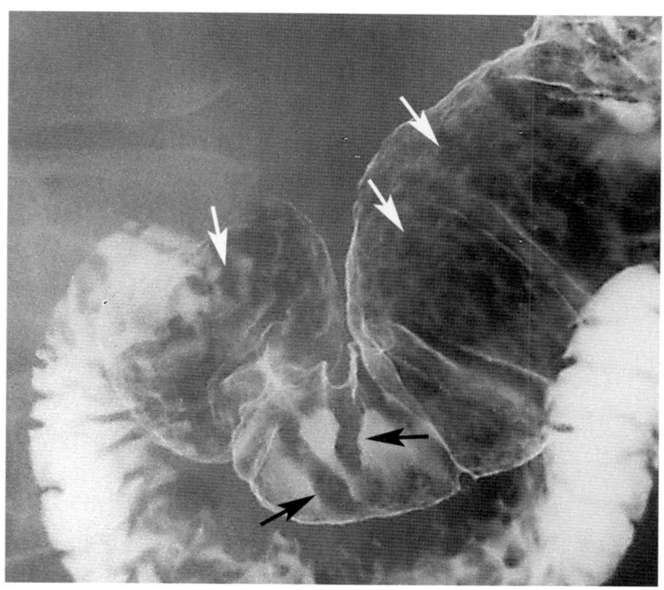

A

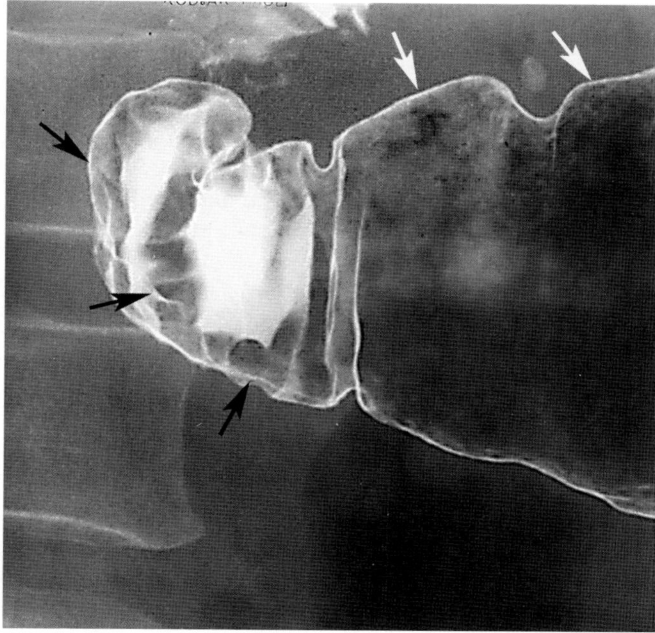

B

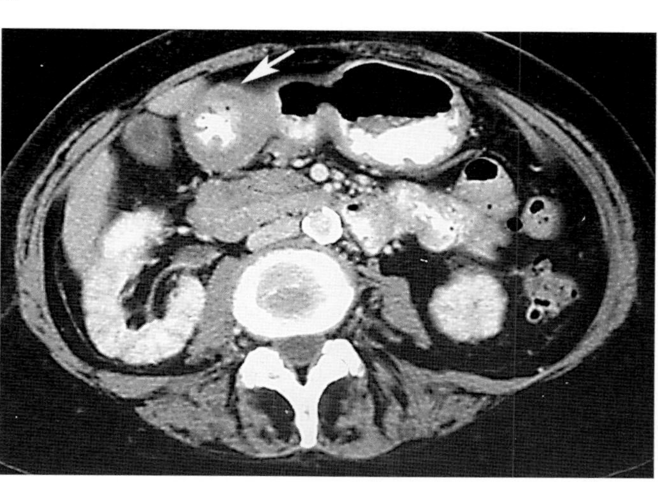

C

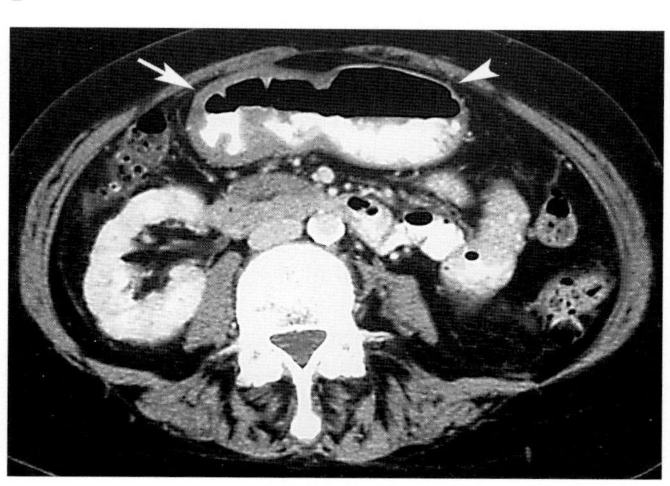

D

Figure 2-14 Gastritis in 2 Patients
A. This 67-year-old man had epigastric pain and heme-positive stool. The examination demonstrates multiple radiolucent mounds of edema with small dotlike collections of barium typical of varioloform ulcerations. There are also mildly thickened antral folds with small dotlike ulcers. **B-D.** This 75-year-old man had epigastric pain and burning. B. Double-contrast barium examination of the stomach shows slight stippling of the mucosa of the body of the stomach suggesting small incomplete erosions (*white arrow*). There are also several thickened folds in the gastric antrum (*black arrows*). C and D. CT images of the same patient as B confirm focal thickening of the antrum of the stomach (*arrows*). Compare the thickness of the antrum, with the normal wall thickness of the gastric body (*arrowhead*). Although this could be caused by an infiltrative tumor, this finding most likely represents antral gastritis. Endoscopy confirmed a diagnosis of *Helicobacter pylori* gastritis.

as small collections of barium without elevation of the surrounding mucosa. They are visualized as linear streaks or dots of barium and are more difficult to detect than varioliform erosions.[148,149]

In most cases, the imaging features of erosions do not allow differentiation of the underlying cause. However, erosions associated with NSAID use often have a distinct configuration and location, appearing as a cluster of linear or serpiginous erosions on or near the greater curvature of the stomach.[150] This location of erosions is thought to be due to accumulation of pill fragments along the greater curvature as a result of gravity. Stasis of the highly acidic NSAIDs in this location results in local mucosal injury. Other patterns associated with NSAID use include linear erosions in the antrum or body away from the greater curvature or flattening, straightening, or retraction of the greater curvature of the distal antrum likely reflecting scarring from multiple cycles of recurrent erosion formation and healing.[151]

With progressive destruction, erosions can deepen to form small or large ulcers in the wall of the stomach. Most gastric ulcers are a result of severe gastritis, however, some gastric ulcers will indicate the presence of a necrotic gastric neoplasm and it is important to differentiate between benign gastric ulcers and those that represent ulcerated neoplasm.

Most benign ulcers are located on the lesser curvature, the posterior wall of the antrum, or body of the stomach.[152-155] The size of the ulcer is not related to the presence of carcinoma.[73] Age affects the distribution of ulcers such that younger patients present with ulcers in the distal stomach, whereas older patients present with ulcers in the proximal stomach along the lesser curvature.[156,157]

Peptic ulcers represent small to large craters within the wall of the stomach or duodenum and will have a variable appearance on double-contrast upper GI examinations depending on the location of the ulcer within the stomach and on patient position. In profile, peptic ulcers are seen as outpouchings from the mucosal surface on barium studies (see Figure 2-15). When seen "en face," an ulcer on the dependent wall of the stomach will usually appear as a circular or oval pool of barium, but can occasionally appear as a thin ring of barium ("ring shadow") if there is not enough barium trapped within the ulcer crater (see Figure 2-15).[158] If the ulcer is located on the nondependent wall, it will also appear as a ring shadow because of barium coating the rim of the crater. Turning the patient 180 degrees will fill the ulcer crater with barium.[73] Ulcers can assume a variety of shapes, including oval, linear, rectangular, serpiginous, or flame-shaped lesions (see Figure 2-15).[73] The linear shape is thought to represent the healing phase of larger ulcers.[152]

Most gastric erosions and ulcers are not visible on routine CT and MRI examinations because they involve only the superficial layers of the gastric mucosa.[40,159] As a consequence, these examinations are less sensitive for the diagnosis of gastritis than a high-quality double-contrast upper GI examination. However, on occasion, an ulcer will be sufficiently deep to be detected by CT or MRI.[160]

Perforation of gastric ulcers is an important complication, which can be detected as pneumoperitoneum on abdominal x-rays and CT scan. Contrast upper GI examinations can show extravasation of contrast, and CT scans can show extraluminal gas or contrast in the tissues centered near the site of the perforated ulcer (see Figure 2-16).[40]

In many cases, patients with gastritis will also have thickened folds. Fold thickening is usually most severe in the antrum followed by the body, with the fundus usually having the least severe involvement. This manifestation of gastritis is discussed and illustrated in the subsequent section titled **Diffuse Diseases of the Stomach.**

Crohn disease

Crohn disease is a common autoimmune disorder primarily involving the GI tract, especially the small bowel and colon. Gastric involvement is uncommon but can be discovered incidentally during evaluation for disease in the more distal bowel or can present with abdominal pain, vomiting, weight loss, or signs and symptoms of GI bleeding.[161]

Upper GI examinations will typically demonstrate disease in the antrum and body of the stomach and the proximal duodenum.[162] Fundal involvement is rare. Aphthoid ulcers can be seen as punctate or slitlike collections of barium surrounded by radiolucent mounds of edema similar to erosions from other causes of gastritis.[163] In more advanced disease, 1 or more ulcers can be found, associated with diffusely thickened gastric folds.[162] Chronic scarring can result in an irregular, narrowed, funnel-shaped antrum and/or proximal duodenum with a resultant appearance that has been likened to a ram's horn (see Figure 2-17). Crohn disease is covered most completely later in this chapter under the heading **Long-Segment Wall Thickening of the Small Bowel and Colon**.

Malignant gastric ulcers

More than 95% of gastric ulcers diagnosed in the United States are benign and related to peptic ulcer disease.[164] However, a small number of gastric ulcers will represent necrotic neoplasms.[73] These most often represent adenocarcinomas but can occasionally be due to lymphomas, GISTs, and rarely other neoplasms.

Features of a benign ulcer on upper GI examinations include projection of the ulcer beyond the expected luminal contour when viewed in profile and visualization of a discrete crater ulcer surrounded by a smooth rim of edema when demonstrated en face. Radiating folds or area gastricae can be seen up to the edge of the ulcer crater, and the surrounding mucosa is intact (see Figure 2-15).[152,154,165]

Features of a malignant ulcer on double-contrast barium examination include absence of projection beyond the expected luminal contour when viewed in profile and

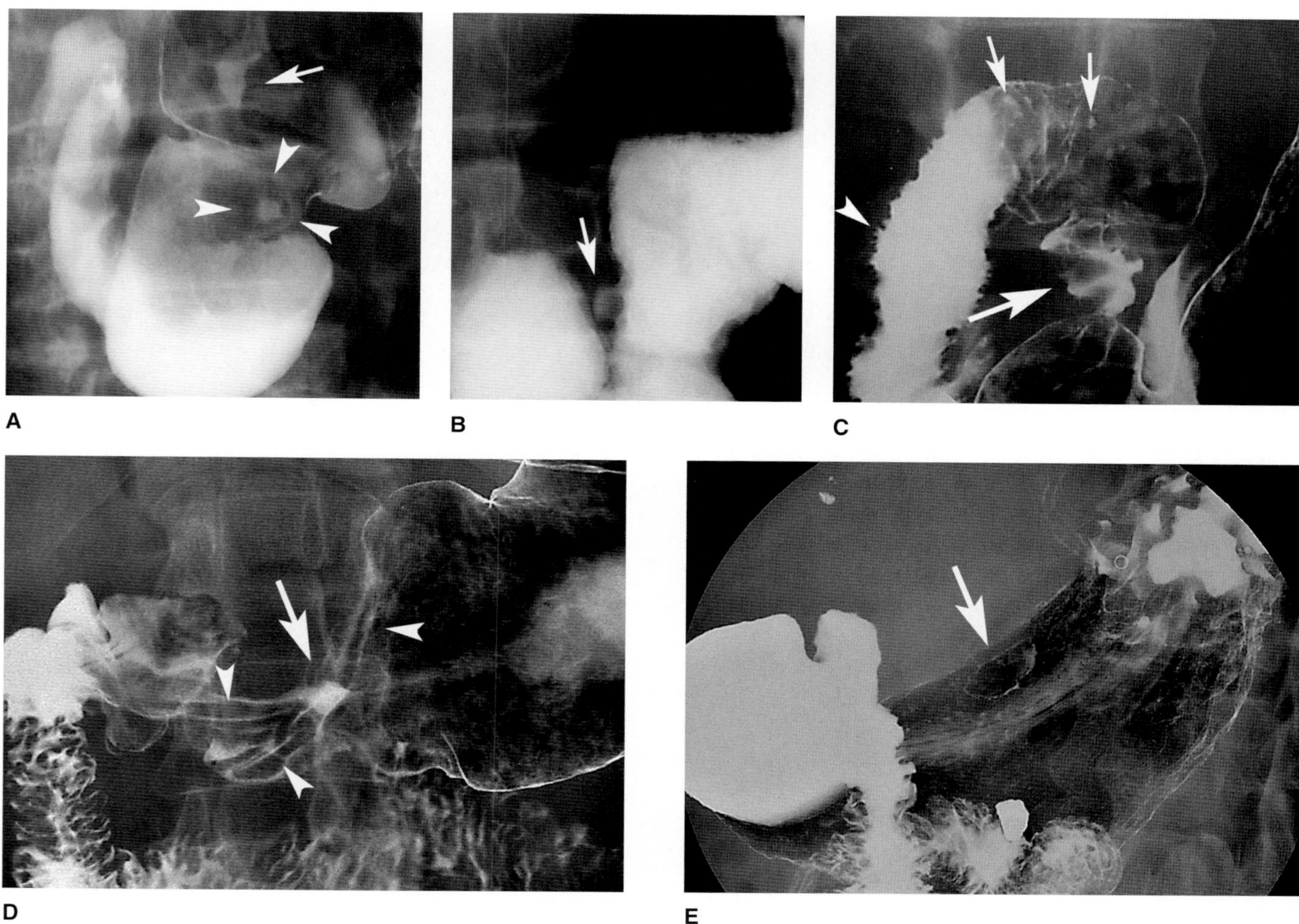

Figure 2-15 Peptic Ulcers in 4 Patients
A and **B.** This 76-year-old man had heme-positive stool. A. Single-contrast UGI demonstrates 2 ulcers, 1 as a small pool of barium (*arrow*) and the other as a small pool of barium with a faint hallow of edema (*arrowheads*). B. The larger ulcer is seen as a projection from the contour of the lesser curvature of the stomach. **C.** This 57-year-old man had received radiation therapy for pharyngeal cancer and developed heme-positive stool. Double-contrast UGI shows many small barium pools (*small arrows*) in the duodenal bulb typical of small erosions. These erosions are seen as small spikes (*arrowhead*) projecting from the surface of the duodenum in profile. There is also a large cross-shaped ulcer in the pyloric channel (*large arrow*). **D.** This 62-year-old man complained of epigastric pain. Double-contrast UGI shows a barium-filled ulcer (*arrow*) with thin radiating folds (*arrowheads*) typical of a peptic ulcer on the dependent surface (in this case the posterior wall). **E.** This 60-year-old man had nausea and abdominal pain. Double-contrast UGI shows a thin ring shadow (*arrow*) near the lesser curvature of the stomach. This is the typical appearance of an ulcer on the nondependent surface, in this case the anterior wall.

visualization of an irregular ulcer crater located eccentrically within an irregular mass when viewed en face. (see Figure 2-9).[152] Radiating folds may be present; however, they are nodular or clubbed and stop short of the ulcer crater. These findings are best visualized on a double-contrast upper GI examination. Ulcers located along the proximal half of the greater curvature are almost always malignant.[152]

On CT and MRI examinations, virtually all malignant gastric ulcers will also show a large mass involving the wall of the stomach (see Figure 2-13).

Gastric diverticulum

Gastric diverticulum is an uncommon outpouching of the stomach, found in 0.1% to 2.6% of autopsy series in the general population.[166] These diverticulum are usually detected near the gastric cardia and it is unclear whether they are congenital or acquired. Some gastric diverticula have been noted in embryo, suggesting that they may be congenital.[167] One theory suggests that during embryogenesis, failure of fusion of the dorsal mesentery with the posterior body wall could result in a focal constriction of the gastric fundus, with creation of a diverticulum that extends

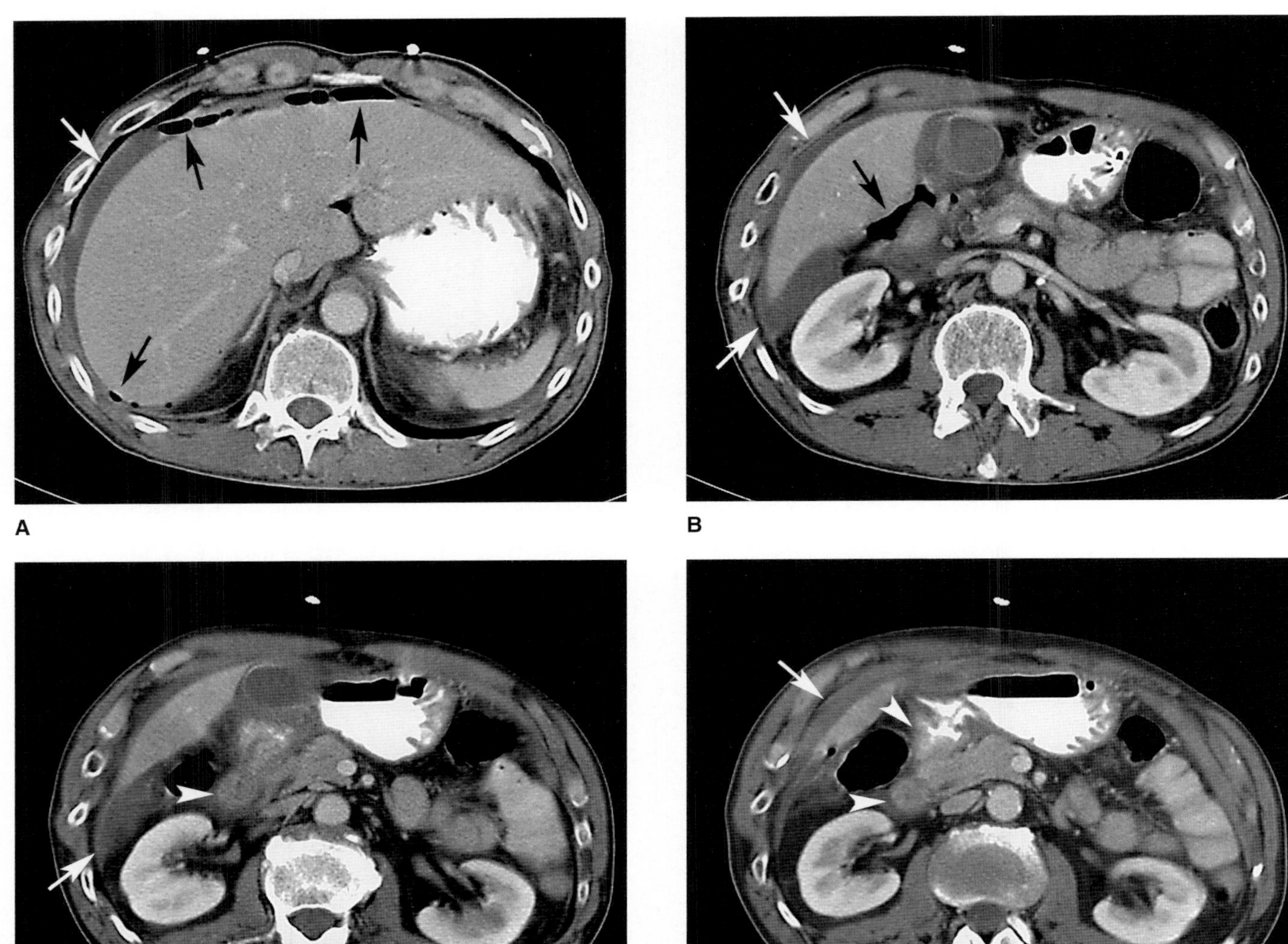

Figure 2-16 Pneumoperitoneum due to a Perforated Duodenal Ulcer This 55-year-old man presented with abdominal pain and rebound tenderness. **A-D.** CT images through the abdomen demonstrate small bubbles of pneumoperitoneum (*black arrows*), which was not seen on an abdominal radiograph and ascites (*white arrows*). The presence of air in the lesser sack (*black arrow* in B) suggests a perforation in the stomach or duodenum. There is also thickening of the proximal duodenum (*white arrowheads*). These findings suggest a perforated duodenal ulcer that was confirmed by surgical exploration and repair.

into the retroperitoneum near the adrenal gland and superior pole of the kidney.[168] Other authors have speculated that gastric diverticula are the result of 1 or several factors including focal weakness of the longitudinal muscle fibers, perforating arterioles, and absence of the visceral peritoneum in this region.[169] Most cases of gastric diverticulum are clinically silent and discovered incidentally by imaging examinations or endoscopy.[61] However, patients can occasionally present with dyspepsia, vomiting, abdominal pain, or hemorrhage.[169]

Barium examinations will show a small smoothly marginated outpouching from the gastric mucosa of the posterior wall of the gastric fundus, near the cardia (see Figure 2-18).[62] The presentation of these diverticulum on CT or MRI will vary depending on whether they are filled with gas and fluid or collapsed. When they are filled with air or fluid, they are seen as oval structures adjacent and attached to the posterior aspect of the stomach near the gastric cardia (see Figure 2-18).[168] However, if they are collapsed, they may simulate a small soft-tissue mass adjacent to the gastric fundus (see Figure 2-19). Specifically, because they often project medially into the region of the adrenal gland, they can be confused with an adrenal mass.[168]

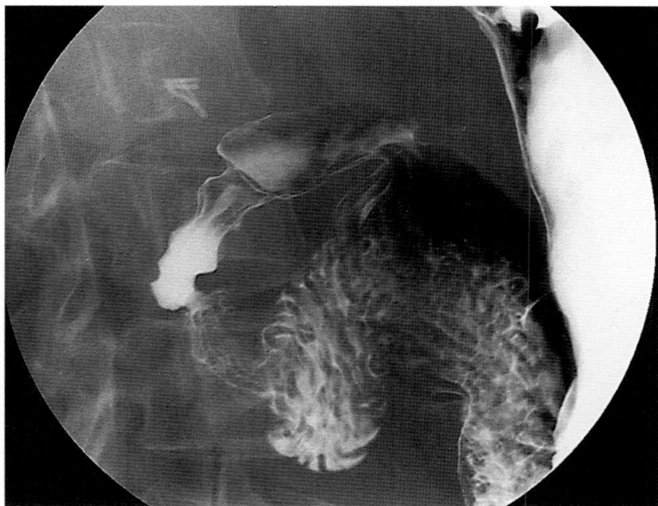

Figure 2-17 Ram's Horn Appearance of Duodenal Crohn Disease This 57-year-old man had Crohn disease. Anteroposterior (AP) view from an UGI exam shows a patulous pylorus and a gentle tapered stricture of the descending duodenum causing the descending duodenum to resemble a ram's horn. This is a typical appearance of Crohn disease of the duodenum.

DIFFUSE DISEASES OF THE STOMACH

The only diffuse abnormality of the stomach is widespread mucosal fold or wall thickening with or without associated narrowing of the gastric lumen. Diffuse gastric fold or wall thickening can be caused by mucosal edema or by submucosal neoplasms. A study of giant gastric fold thickening on CT suggests that this finding is most often due to scirrhous gastric cancer (30/64, 47%) (mean thickness: 15.8 mm), followed by large B cell lymphoma (15/64, 23%) (mean thickness: 26.6 mm), acute gastritis (14/64, 22%) (mean thickness: 4.4 mm), and Ménétrier disease (5/64, 8%) (mean thickness: 11.2 mm), in decreasing order.[171] Of these causes, lymphoma results in the greatest degree of wall thickening (Table 2-2).

Malignant Wall/Fold Thickening

Malignancies causing diffuse wall thickening include primary adenocarcinoma, lymphoma, and metastasis.

Scirrhous adenocarcinoma ("Linitis plastica")

Gastric adenocarcinoma can loosely be subdivided into (1) discrete mass-like tumors that arise from the wall of the stomach and grow in a fungating manner and (2) scirrhous tumors that infiltrate and thicken the gastric wall without causing a discrete mass.[172] Scirrhous tumors incite an inflammatory reaction within the wall of the stomach, resulting in fibrosis and fixed narrowing of the gastric lumen. In the majority of cases, scirrhous gastric cancers will have signet-ring histology.[65] *Linitis plastica* is an old term that denotes a diffuse, intramurally infiltrating carcinoma in a hollow structure resulting in a shrunken organ with thickened walls.[173]

On upper GI examinations, scirrhous carcinoma appears as irregular narrowing and rigidity of the gastric wall (see Figure 2-10). On CT and MRI examinations, it is characterized by loss of the normal gastric folds and diffuse thickening of the gastric wall (see Figure 2-10).[63] Loss of mucosal striation on enhanced CT is also associated with the presence of an infiltrative malignancy, rather than an inflammatory cause of thickening.[171] Classically, linitis plastica involves the distal half of the stomach, arising in the pyloric region and extending toward the body and fundus. However, it can also be seen as a localized lesion involving the gastric fundus or body (see Figure 2-20).[66] In advanced cases, the entire stomach is infiltrated by tumor.

Gastric carcinoma is discussed most completely under the heading **Focal Polyps and Masses of the Stomach**.

Lymphoma

Lymphoma is among the most common gastric malignancies. In most cases, it will present as a large focal mass, with or without ulceration, and with or without thickening of the stomach wall. However, occasionally, gastric lymphoma can present as extensive infiltration of the gastric wall with widespread gastric fold thickening that can be visualized on upper GI examinations[92,101] as well as CT and MRI examinations.[40,102,171] This finding can occasionally be confused with the various causes of severe gastritis, especially Ménétrier disease and ZE syndrome. The more massive the fold thickening and the more irregular the wall thickening, the more likely the disease is to represent lymphoma. Loss of mucosal striation on enhanced CT is also associated with the presence of an infiltrative malignancy, rather than an inflammatory cause of thickening.[171] However, in some cases, these causes of diffuse wall thickening cannot be differentiated (see Figure 2-21).

Gastric metastasis causing diffuse gastric narrowing

Scirrhous carcinoma of the stomach can be a result of a primary carcinoma of the stomach or due to metastasis to the wall of the stomach. Secondary scirrhous carcinoma is most often due to breast cancer (see Figure 2-22).

Gastric metastases are discussed more completely under the heading **Focal Polyps and Masses of the Stomach**.

Inflammatory Wall/Fold Thickening

Inflammatory wall or fold thickening can be due to gastritis, ZE syndrome, Ménétrier disease, eosinophilic gastroenteritis, and Crohn disease.

Gastritis

Gastritis is a common disorder due to a variety of causes that have been discussed in detail under the previous

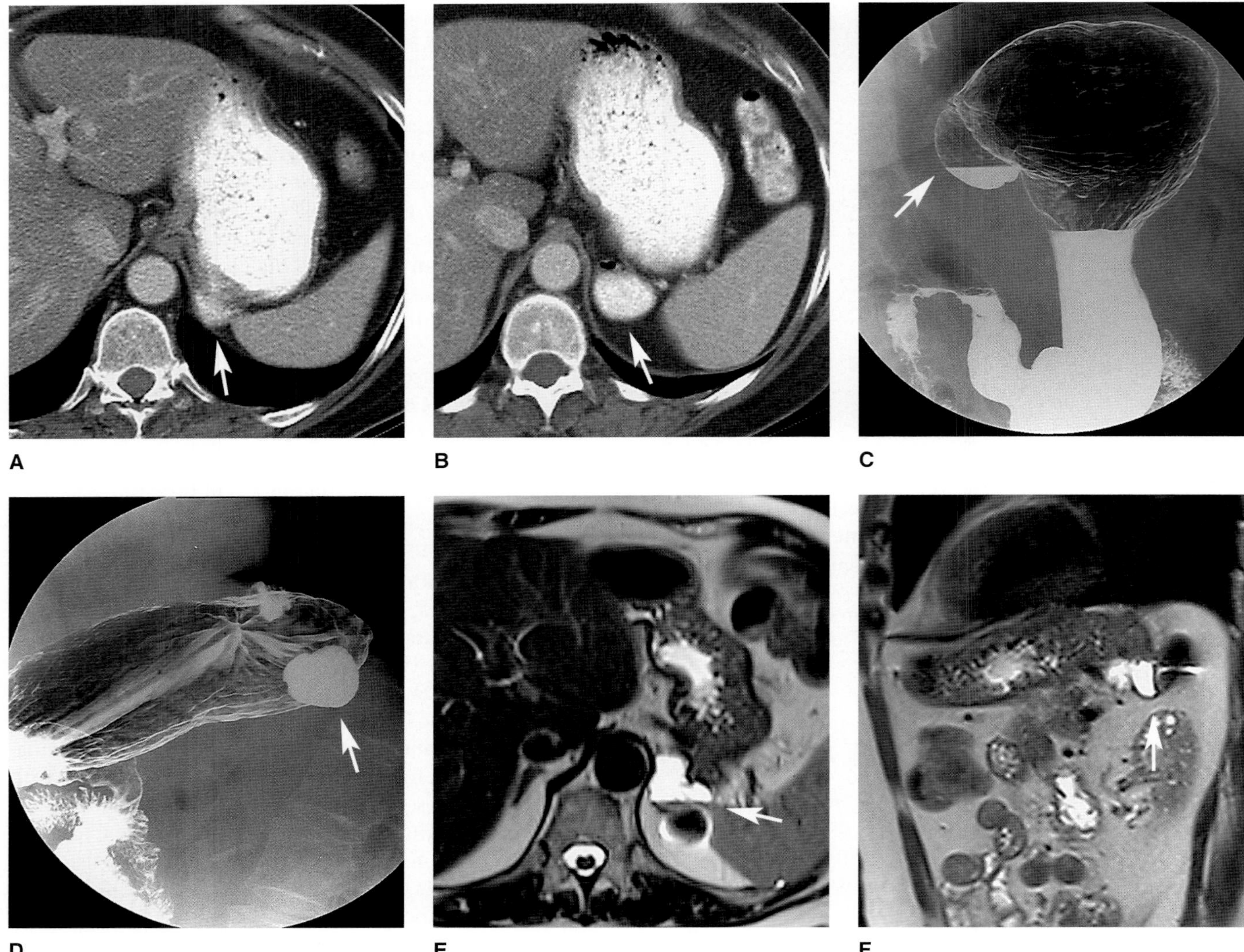

Figure 2-18 Gastric Diverticulum in 2 Patients
This 63-year-old woman complained of epigastric pain. **A** and **B**. Axial CT images show a contrast- and air-filled structure (*arrows*) projecting from the posterior wall of the gastric fundus. Double-contrast UGI in the (**C**) AP projection and in the (**D**) lateral projection show a saccular collection of barium and air (*arrows*) projecting from the posterior medial wall of the fundus of the stomach. T2-weighted MRI sequences in a second patient with a history of carcinoid tumor from the (**E**) axial and (**F**) sagittal projection show a fluid- and debris-filled structure (*arrows*) projecting from the posterior medial wall of the gastric fundus. These are typical appearances of a gastric diverticulum.

heading: **Ulcers and Diverticula of the Stomach**. In addition to mucosal ulceration, gastritis causes edema and inflammation of the wall of the stomach. Wall edema can be seen as thickened gastric folds on upper GI examinations and as wall thickening on CT and MRI.

On upper GI contrast examinations, thickened folds will appear as linear and serpiginous filling defects within pools of contrast on either single- or double-contrast examinations.[141,174] On double-contrast examinations, there will also be visualization of parallel linear or curvilinear lines outlining the edges of the folds (see Figure 2-14). In some double-contrast examinations, gastritis will also lead to prominent area gastricae.

Double-contrast upper GI examination is the preferred imaging method of diagnosing suspected peptic ulcer disease. However, because CT is usually the first imaging test in patients with nonspecific abdominal complaints, it may be the first study to suggest a diagnosis of gastritis.[40] Thickening of the gastric folds and wall is the most common finding of gastritis on CT (see Figure 2-14). Wall thickening can be focal, segmental, or diffuse in distribution. On upper GI examinations, the stomach is purposefully distended with contrast or air. In CT and MRI examinations, however, the degree of gastric distention is variable. When the stomach is collapsed on these modalities, recognition of mild wall thickening is impaired.

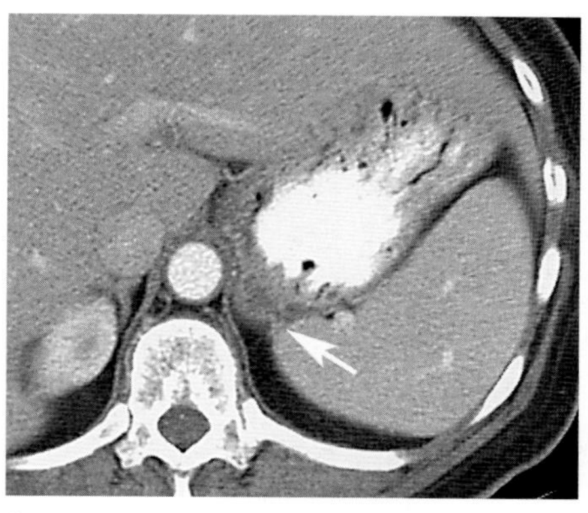
A

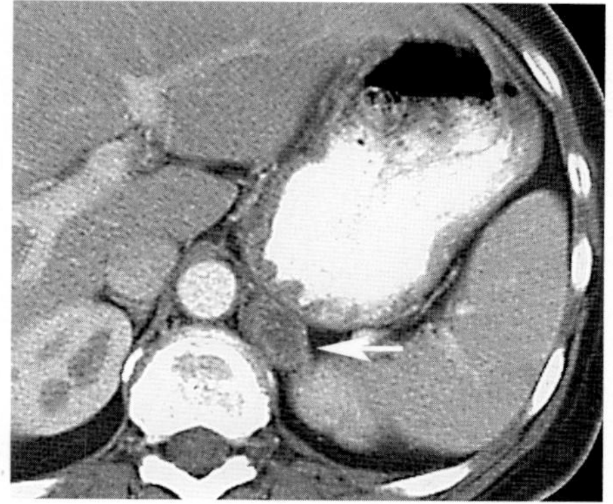
B

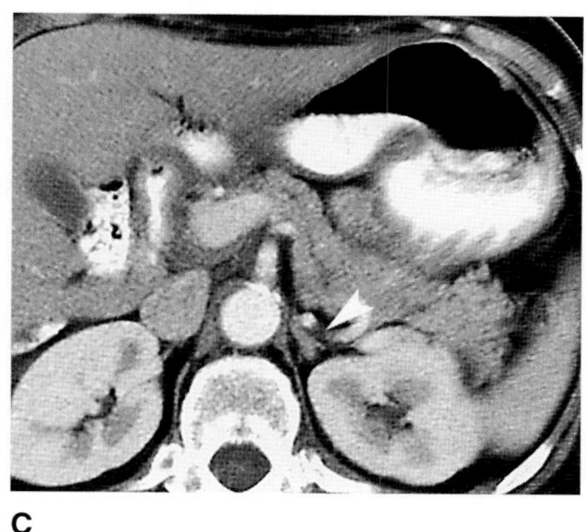
C

Figure 2-19 Gastric Diverticulum Appearing as a Retroperitoneal Mass
This 70-year-old woman had endometrial carcinoma. **A-C.** Axial CT images show a low attenuation mass (*arrows*) posterior to the stomach and inferior to the kidney. This can be confused with an adrenal mass; however, the normal adrenal (*arrowhead*) is seen in a more caudad image. This appearance is typical of a gastric diverticulum.

In severe gastritis, the gastric wall will in some cases demonstrate low attenuation on CT as a result of submucosal edema with simultaneous mucosal hyperemia, which is best seen on arterial phase imaging (see Figure 2-23).[40,175] However, the CT appearance of gastritis can overlap with that of malignancy, and further evaluation with barium evaluation or with endoscopic visualization and biopsy may be necessary.

Zollinger-Ellison syndrome

Zollinger-Ellison syndrome is the uncommon clinical triad of gastric acid hypersecretion, severe peptic ulceration, and gastrinoma.[176] Gastrinomas are neuroendocrine cancers, which were initially found primarily in the pancreas. However, recent studies indicate that slightly greater than 50% of gastrinomas are found outside the pancreas, most commonly in the duodenum, but also within abdominal lymph nodes, ovaries, liver, bile ducts, and a variety of other intraabdominal and extraabdominal sites.[176] Approximately 90% of gastrinomas are located in the "gastrinoma triangle" formed by the junction between the neck and body of the pancreas medially, the second and third parts of the duodenum inferiorly, and the junction of the cystic and common ducts superiorly.[177] These tumors secrete the hormone gastrin, which causes the parietal cells of the stomach to hypersecrete hydrogen ions into the stomach, resulting in the excessive production of hydrochloric acid. Gastrin also causes hyperplasia of parietal cells, further increasing acid production. The hyperacidity of gastric contents results in inflammation and ultimately ulceration of the gastric and duodenal mucosa. Gastrinomas can be single or multiple small lesions, and in approximately one-half to two-thirds of cases they will be malignant. Approximately 25% of cases of ZE syndrome will be associated with multiple endocrine neoplasia type 1 (MEN 1).[176] The presence of multiple gastrinomas should raise the possibility of underlying MEN 1.

The mean age of onset of symptoms is approximately 41 years but final diagnosis will often be delayed by 5 to 6 years from the onset of symptoms.[176] Patients will typically present with abdominal pain and diarrhea but can also complain of nausea, vomiting, GI bleeding, and heartburn. A helpful clue to the diagnosis of ZE syndrome is the presence of diarrhea with peptic ulcer disease or *H pylori* infection because diarrhea is less common in patients with isolated peptic disease or *H pylori* infection without ZE syndrome.[176,178] The failure of known peptic ulcers to respond to conventional treatment can be another clue to the diagnosis of ZE syndrome. The diagnosis is established by measuring fasting gastrin levels.

The diagnostic imaging test of choice for ZE syndrome is somatostatin receptor scintigraphy. However, ZE syndrome can also be visualized on barium, CT, and MRI. There are a variety of characteristic imaging features of ZE syndrome on upper GI.[179-181] Hypersecretion of acid can

Table 2-2. Causes of Diffuse Gastric Fold/Wall Thickening

1. Submucosal neoplasm a. Primary adenocarcinoma b. Lymphoma c. Metastasis
2. Mucosal edema a. Gastritis b. Zollinger-Ellison syndrome c. Ménétrier disease d. Eosinophilic gastroenteritis e. Crohn disease

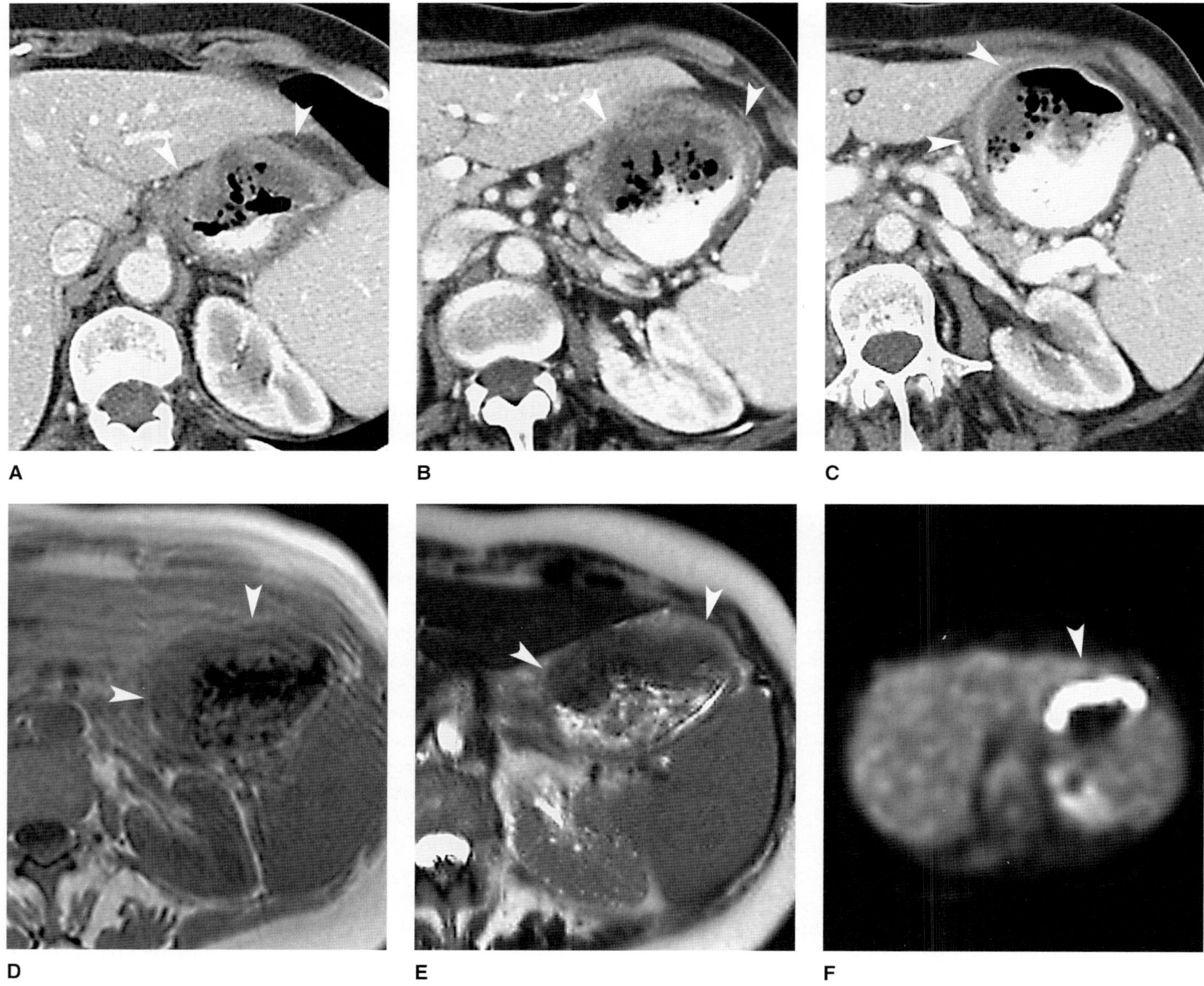

Figure 2-20 Scirrhous Carcinoma of the stomach
A-C. Axial CT in this 71-year-old woman shows segmental thickening of the gastric fundus and anterior wall of the stomach. Similar gastric thickening is seen on this (**D**) T1-weighted and (**E**) T2-weighted MRI sequences. **F.** PET scan shows segmental increased metabolic activity in the region of the gastric wall thickening. Biopsy was diagnostic of a poorly differentiated adenocarcinoma.

result in a large volume of gastric fluid that impairs barium coating of the gastric and duodenal mucosa. Patients will demonstrate severely thickened gastric and duodenal folds because of a combination of acid-related edema and gastrin-induced parietal cell hyperplasia. Gastric fold thickening is especially pronounced in the body and fundus of the stomach, which are unusual locations for fold thickening in standard peptic disease (see Figure 2-24). Ulcers in the stomach and duodenum are also a common finding. These are indistinguishable from the more common peptic ulcer. However, the possibility of ZE syndrome should be considered in patients with multiple ulcers in unusual locations.[178]

The role of CT and MRI in ZE syndrome is typically to locate the primary tumor and to evaluate for metastatic lymph nodes or liver metastases for surgical planning.[182] Optimal CT technique for the detection of gastrinomas includes a triple-phase protocol, use of water to distend the stomach and duodenum, and the administration of an antiperistaltic agent.[183] Gastrinomas are usually hypervascular on both CT and MRI, best seen on the arterial-phase images, although they can enhance variably. On MRI, they typically demonstrate increased T2 signal, best seen on fat-saturated images. Tumor size and location are highly correlated with visualization on CT and MRI. Because most gastrinomas in ZE syndrome are less than 1 cm in size and multiple in number discrimination of these lesions is challenging with both CT and MRI.[69] The sensitivity of CT ranges from 30% to 50%

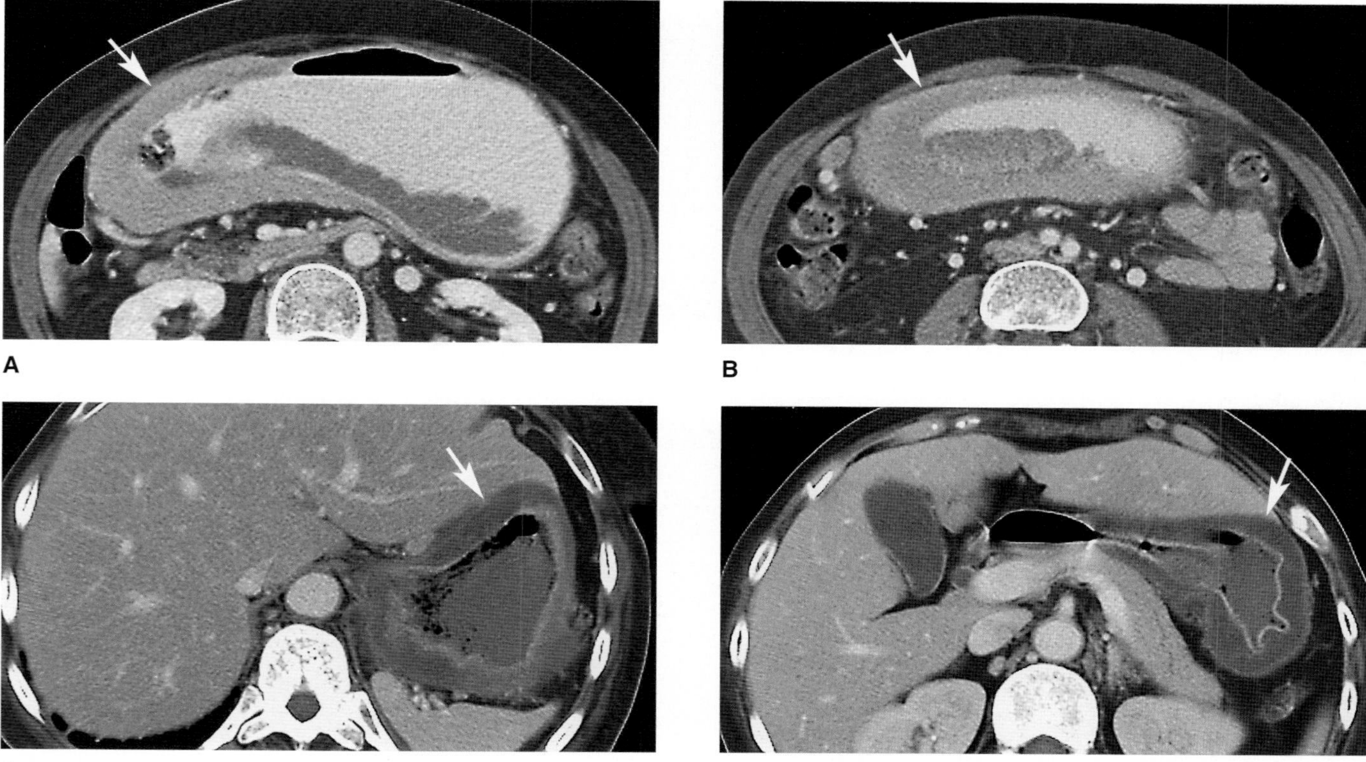

Figure 2-21 Thickened Gastric Wall due to Lymphoma
These 2 women both complained of weight loss, dysphagia and abdominal pain. **A** and **B.** Contrast-enhanced axial CT demonstrates extensive thickening of the gastric antrum (*arrows*) and body with sparing of the fundus. Biopsies were diagnostic of a marginal zone lymphoma. **C** and **D.** Contrast-enhanced axial CT images shows extensive low attenuation thickening of the gastric body and fundus (*arrows*) with sparing of the antrum. The low attenuation of the wall will, in most, cases indicate edema and a benign diagnosis. However, biopsies were diagnostic of a diffuse large B-cell lymphoma.

in the detection of extrahepatic and extrapancreatic gastrinomas.[184-186] MRI is comparable if not better than CT in the detection of primary tumors.[187-189] Both CT and MRI are highly sensitive (>94%) in the detection of liver metastases.[182]

There are no published series of the gastric findings of ZE syndrome as detected by CT or MRI. However, ZE syndrome would be expected to demonstrate diffuse gastric wall thickening and hyperemia by CT and MRI examinations (see Figure 2-24).

Ménétrier disease

Ménétrier disease, also called hyperplastic, hypersecretory gastropathy, is a rare disorder of the stomach resulting in dramatic thickening of the gastric rugae such that they resemble the gyri of the brain. It is now thought to be due to overexpression of transforming growth factor-α (TGF-α) that results in the selective expansion of surface mucous cells in the body and fundus of the stomach.[190] The expansion of these surface mucous cells is at the expense of parietal and chief cells that, when reduced, result in decreased output or absence of gastric acid (achlorhydria). Ménétrier disease is histologically characterized by thickening and hyperplasia of the gastric mucosa with cystic dilation and elongation of the gastric mucous glands and deepening of the foveolar pits.[191] Ménétrier disease also often leads to a protein loosing enteropathy that results in hypoalbuminemia and soft-tissue edema.

There are 2 forms of disease, 1 seen in childhood and the second in adulthood. The adult form of the disease is progressive, whereas the childhood form has been associated with cytomegalovirus (CMV) infection and resolves spontaneously.[190,192]

The mean age of presentation is approximately 55 years and patients typically present with abdominal pain, nausea, vomiting, anemia (due to gastric blood loss), hypochlorhydria, and peripheral edema.[190] There is an increased incidence of thrombotic events throughout the body, possibly due to a decrease in intravascular volume. Ménétrier disease is believed to carry an increased risk of gastric malignancy; however, the magnitude is not known.

Upper GI examinations will demonstrate massively thickened, lobulated rugal folds, which are most pronounced in the gastric fundus and body along the greater curvature.[193] Although the antrum was initially thought to

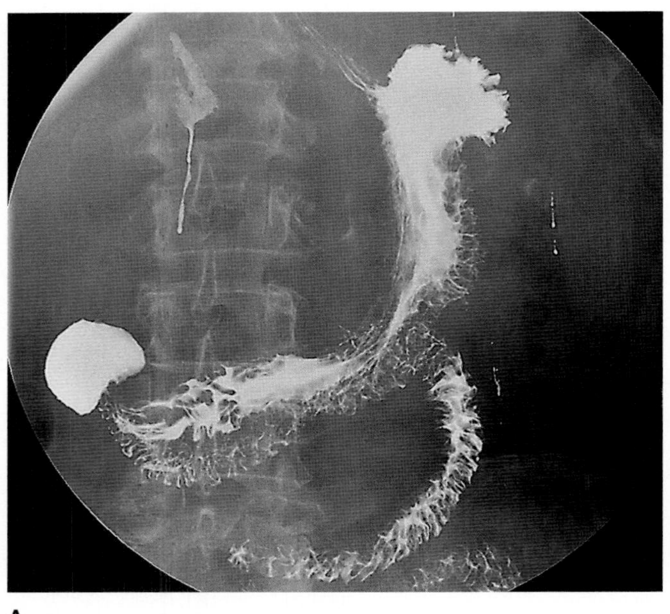

A

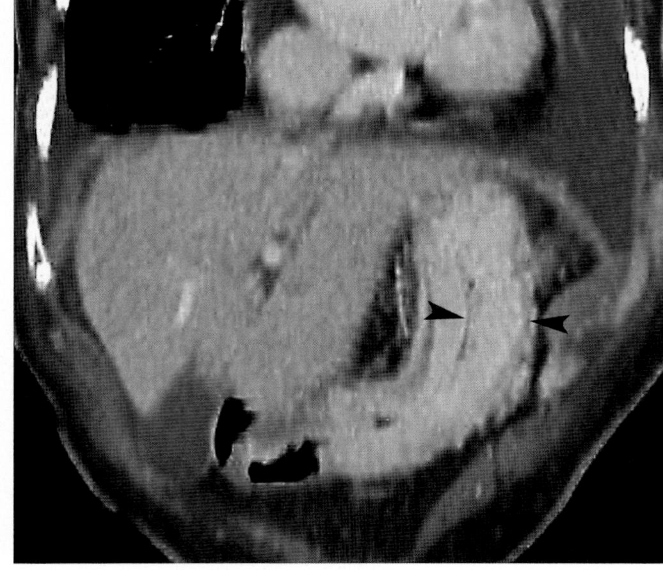

B

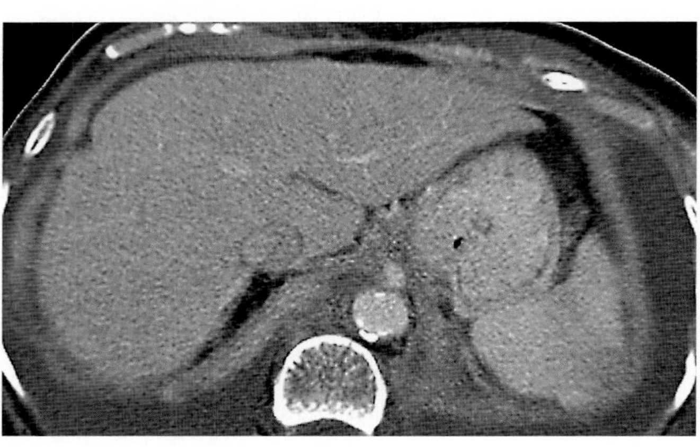

C

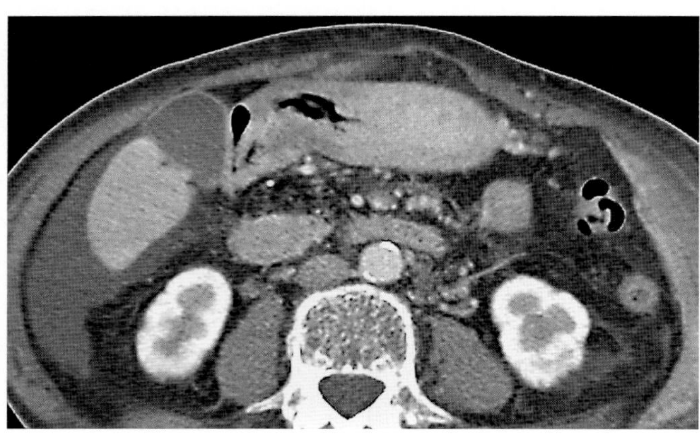

D

Figure 2-22 Scirrhous Metastasis to the Stomach
This 92-year-old woman with breast carcinoma complained of dysphagia. **A.** Single-contrast UGI examination shows diffuse narrowing of the body of the stomach that could not be distended despite repeated swallows of barium. This appearance is indicative of rigidity of the stomach and suggests the presence of scirrhous metastasis to the stomach. Coronal oblique reconstruction (**B**) and axial contrast-enhanced CT images (**C** and **D**) show diffuse thickening of the gastric wall (*arrowheads*). On CT examinations, it is difficult to determine whether this is due to inadequate distension or wall thickening. Endoscopic biopsy confirmed a diagnosis of breast cancer metastasis.

be spared, some studies have shown antral fold thickening in Ménétrier disease in nearly 50% of patients.[194] Rarely, the disease results in focal fold thickening that can be confused with lymphoma or infiltrating forms of carcinoma. Similar to ZE syndrome, there is an excess of gastric fluid that can cause poor coating of the mucosa by high-density barium.

Cross-sectional imaging will demonstrate massive thickening of the gastric wall, which enhances avidly following contrast administration.[171,195] In some cases, rugal fold hypertrophy can appear as a mass lesion that can mimic the appearance of a gastric lymphoma or carcinoma.[196]

Eosinophilic gastroenteritis

Eosinophilic gastroenteritis is a rare, poorly defined condition characterized by eosinophilic infiltration of the wall of the GI tract that can variably involve the mucosal, muscularis, or serosal portions of the intestines.[197] It most often involves the stomach, followed by the small bowel and colon.[198] The pathogenesis of this disease is not certain, but because of the association of eosinophilic gastroenteritis with a variety of allergic conditions, including seasonal allergies, food sensitivity, eczema, and asthma, it is believed that hypersensitivity likely plays a role.[199] Some

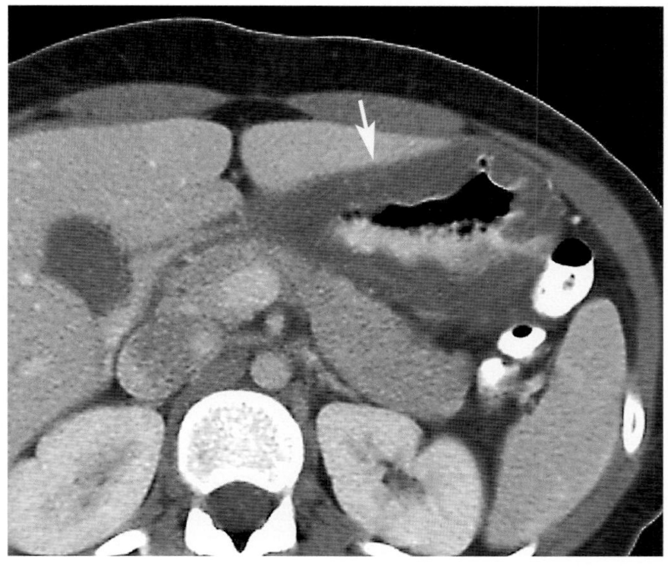

A

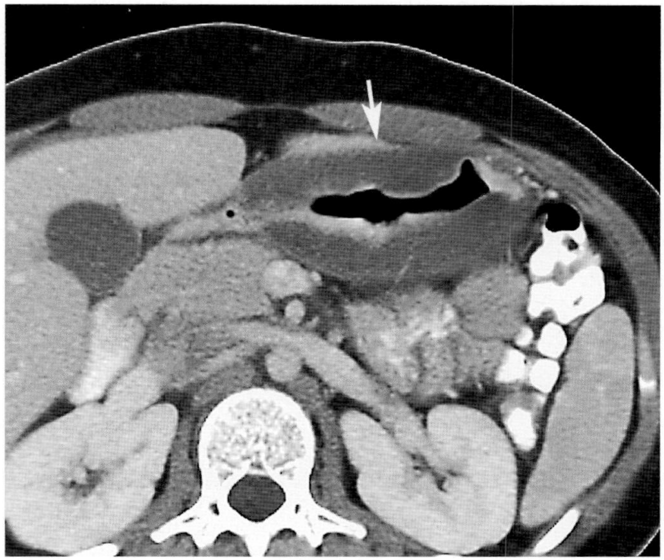

B

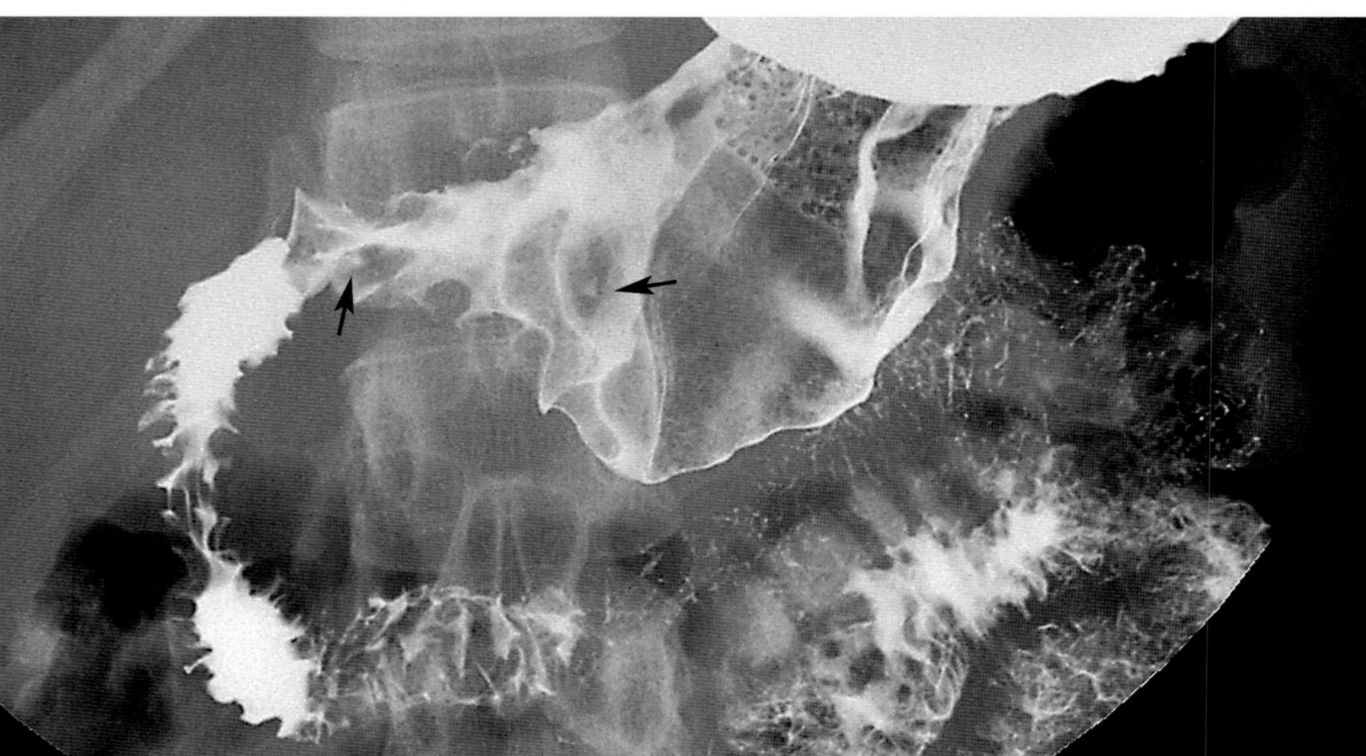

C

Figure 2-23 Severe Acute Gastritis
This 19-year-old woman complained of several weeks of severe epigastric pain, nausea, and vomiting. **A** and **B.** A contrast-enhanced CT was ordered and demonstrated severe, low-attenuation thickening (*white arrows*) of the antral wall. Note the mucosal enhancement on the nondependent wall. This low attenuation thickening usually indicates wall edema. **C.** Upper GI examination confirms the presence of multiple thickened antral folds and also shows punctate collections of barium (*black arrows*), indicating the presence of small ulcerations on the surface of the thickened folds. Note the thickened duodenal folds suggesting duodenitis. Gastric biopsy demonstrated acute and chronic gastritis and duodenitis.

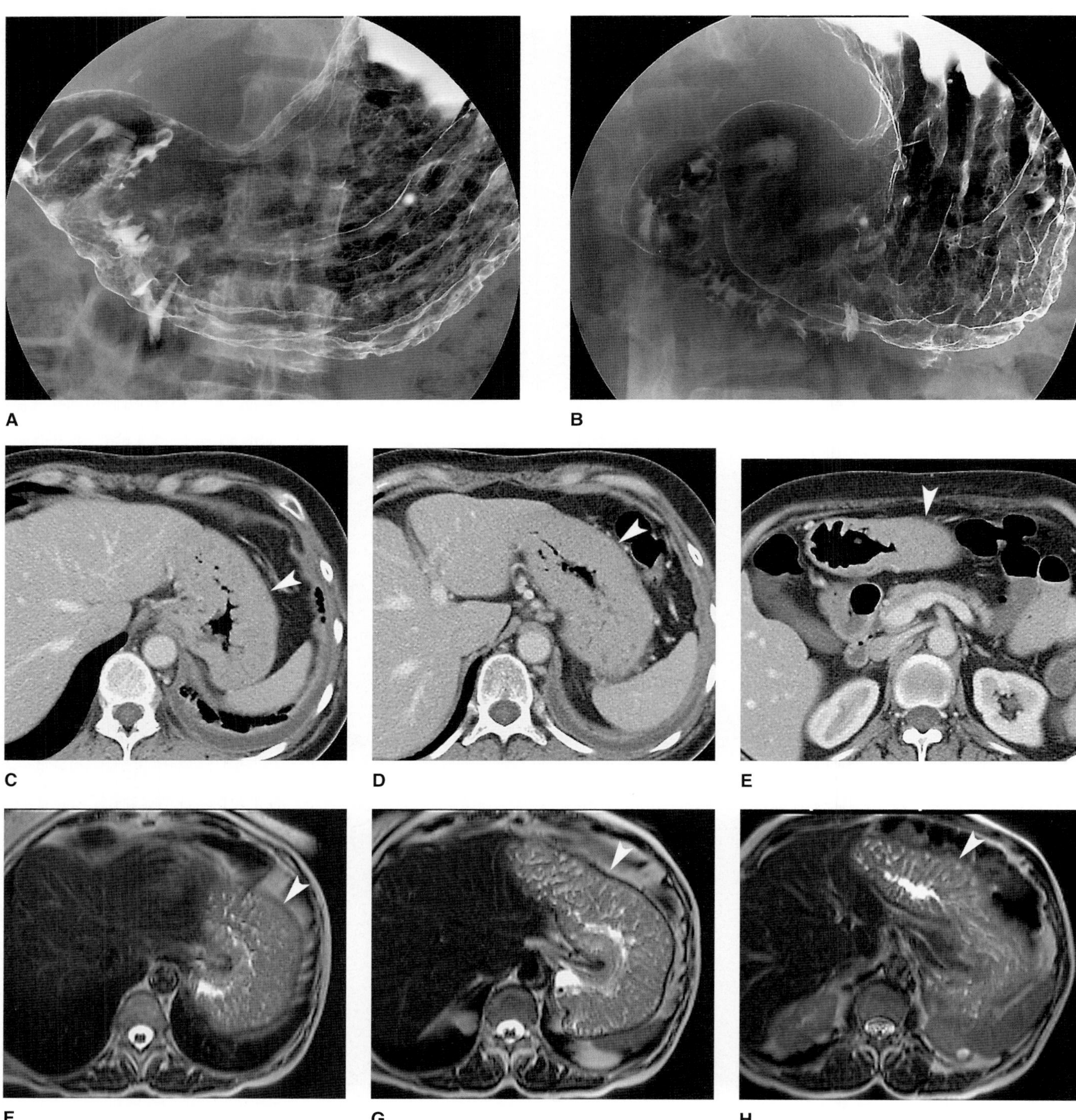

Figure 2-24 Zollinger-Ellison Syndrome in 3 Patients
A and **B.** This 37-year-old man had severe abdominal pain. AP (A) and lateral (B) projections from a double-contrast barium enema show increased number and thickness of rugal folds in the body and fundus of the stomach. Gastrin levels were elevated and a diagnosis of Zollinger-Ellison syndrome was made. **C-E.** This 49-year-old woman complained of abdominal pain. Enhanced CT shows apparent thickening of the wall of the stomach (*arrowheads*). Careful observation suggests that this is due to apposition of multiple enlarged rugal folds. When the stomach is collapsed, the wall can appear thickened and so a normal variation cannot be excluded as a cause for this apparent thickening. **F-H.** Axial T2-weighted MRI sequences in a third patient show similar findings but more easily demonstrate the increased number of rugal folds. Both of these patients were diagnosed with Zollinger-Ellison syndrome.

studies suggest that degranulation of eosinophils in the tissues of the GI tract leads to damage and subsequent symptoms.

Patients typically present with nonspecific GI symptoms, including abdominal pain, nausea, vomiting, diarrhea, weight loss, and/or abdominal distension. Patients will often have peripheral eosinophilia and elevated IgA. The site of involvement can influence clinical symptoms. Mucosal involvement will characteristically present with features of malabsorption and protein-losing enteropathy. Muscular involvement is more likely to present with mass lesions that can occasionally lead to obstructive symptomatology, whereas serosal involvement is associated with ascites.

Upper GI examinations will typically demonstrate thickened mucosal folds, mucosal nodularity, and luminal narrowing, which predominantly involves the distal half of the stomach.[200,201] In approximately 50% of patients, there is associated thickening and nodularity of small-bowel folds. Occasionally, eosinophilic gastroenteritis can present with luminal narrowing and obstruction of either the stomach or small bowel.[202]

There are no studies that have directly evaluated the cross-sectional imaging manifestations of eosinophilic gastroenteritis. However, there are scattered case reports of eosinophilic gastroenteritis that include descriptions of CT findings. In many cases, CT failed to detect the presence of disease.[202] However, in 1 case, focal wall thickening of the stomach was noted on enhanced CT scans.[203]

Crohn disease

Crohn disease is a common autoimmune disorder primarily involving the small bowel and colon. Gastric involvement is uncommon. Upper GI examinations will typically demonstrate aphthoid ulcers. In more advanced disease, 1 or more ulcers can be found, associated with diffusely thickened gastric folds.[162] The cross-sectional imaging features of gastric involvement by Crohn disease have not been systematically evaluated. Similar to other causes of gastritis, however, it is expected that Crohn involvement of the stomach is likely to cause thickening of the gastric wall. Given the predilection of Crohn disease to involve the gastric body and antrum, this fold thickening will predominantly involve the distal stomach. Crohn disease has been more completely covered later in this chapter under the heading: **Long-Segment Wall Thickening of the Small Bowel and Colon**.

FOCAL DISORDERS OF THE SMALL BOWEL

Focal Polyps and Masses of the Small Bowel

The majority of focal mass lesions of the small bowel represent either benign or malignant neoplasms. The most common neoplasms of the small bowel are adenocarcinoma and carcinoid tumor. Other neoplasms include lymphoma, GISTs, lipomas, and hamartomatous polyps (Table 2-3).

Table 2-3. Polyps and Masses of the Small Bowel

1. Epithelial lesions
   a. Adenoma/adenocarcinoma
   b. Carcinoid tumor
2. Submucosal lesions
   a. Lymphoma
   b. Gastrointestinal stromal tumor (GIST)
   c. Lipoma
   d. Hamartomatous polyps
      i. Peutz-Jeghers
      ii. Juvenile
   e. Kaposi sarcoma
   f. Other mesenchymal tumors
      i. Leiomyoma/leiomyosarcoma
      ii. Neurofibroma
      iii. Schwannoma

Adenoma and adenocarcinoma

Adenocarcinoma is the most common tumor of the small bowel but is still only half as common as colonic adenocarcinoma.[204-206] Among small-bowel adenocarcinomas, 50% are found in the duodenum, mainly near the ampulla of Vater, or in the proximal jejunum within 30 cm of the ligament of Treitz.[204,207] Risk factors for the development of adenocarcinoma of the small bowel include a history of Crohn disease, celiac sprue, Peutz-Jeghers syndrome, Lynch syndrome II, congenital bowel duplication, ileostomy, and duodenal or jejunal bypass surgery.[205]

Patient symptoms vary with tumor size, location, blood supply, and the presence of ulceration.[208] Smaller lesions are typically asymptomatic. Annular lesions eventually produce obstruction[209] and, rarely, polypoid lesions can result in bowel obstruction due to intussusception. Duodenal adenocarcinomas can also present with obstructive jaundice, because of biliary obstruction of the tumor, or pancreatitis, because of pancreatic duct obstruction of the tumor.[207]

Unlike adenocarcinoma of the colon and rectum, the size of small-bowel adenocarcinoma is not correlated with its tendency to spread. Small tumors can manifest with distant metastases.[210] Unlike the remainder of the small bowel, the duodenum is retroperitoneal in location, and direct spread into the retroperitoneum is an important additional mode of spread that often leads to unresectability. Approximately half of small-bowel adenocarcinomas are unresectable, and the 5-year survival of these tumors is approximately 20%.[208]

The imaging appearance of a small-bowel adenocarcinoma varies. Typically, it will involve a short segment of bowel and will appear as one of the following: (1) an annular region of luminal narrowing with abrupt "shelf-like" margins or "overhanging edges," (2) as a discrete tumor mass, or (3) as an ulcerative lesion (see Figure 2-25).[205] Distal small-bowel adenocarcinomas are usually annular,

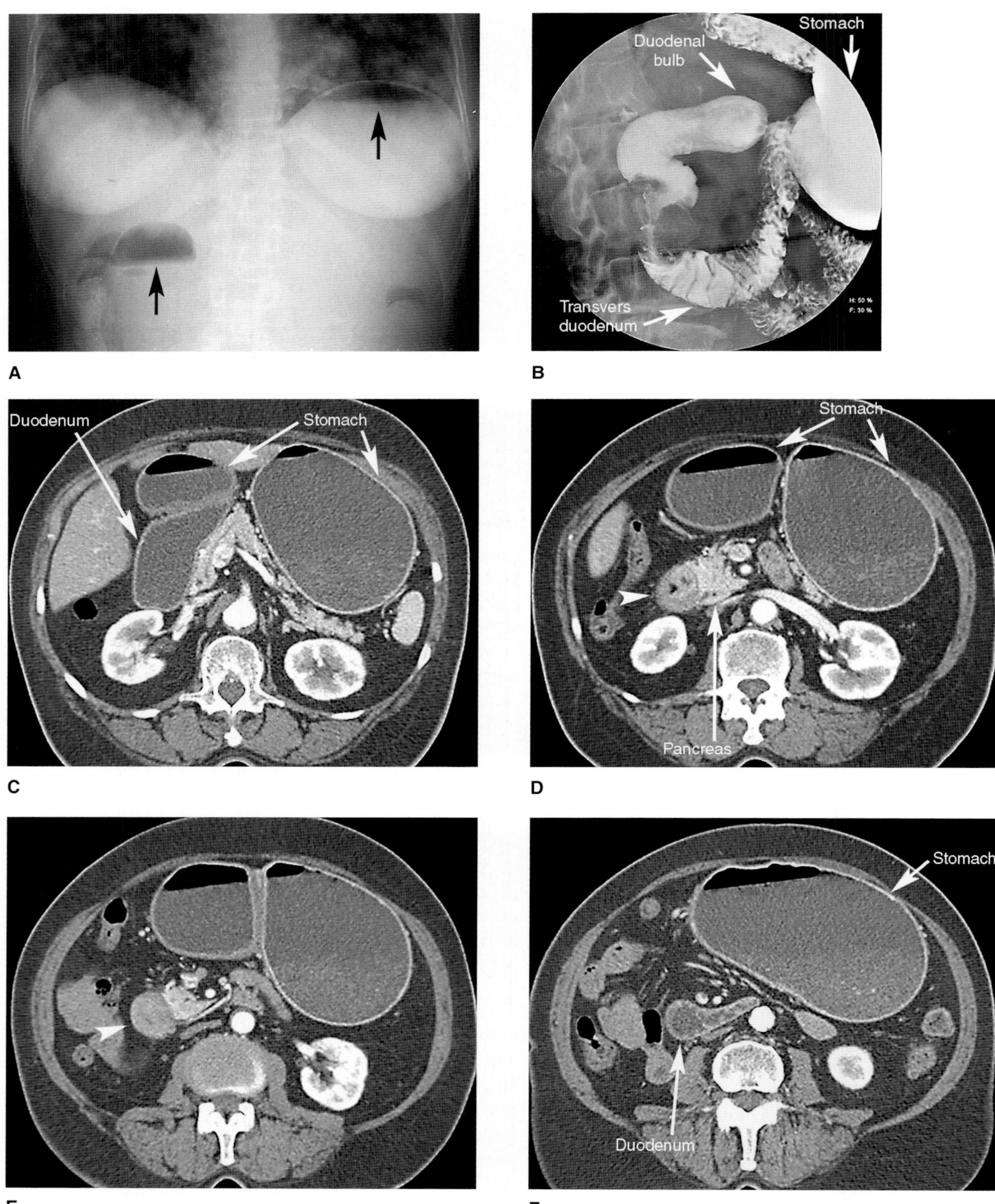

Figure 2-25 Duodenal Obstruction due to Adenocarcinoma

This 75-year-old woman complained of melena and vomiting. **A.** Examination of the upper abdomen shows 2 air-fluid levels (*arrows*), 1 underneath the left hemidiaphragm and the other in the right upper quadrant. This is the characteristic appearance of the double bubble sign and indicates a duodenal obstruction. **B.** Barium swallow confirms the presence of focal narrowing of the descending duodenum with a shelflike shoulder between the narrowed and normal segments of the bowel. This appearance is typical of an annular carcinoma. **C-F.** CT images of the upper abdomen show a distended stomach and proximal duodenum with a normal-caliber distal duodenum. Images D and E show a concentric mass involving the descending biopsy that was diagnostic of adenocarcinoma of the duodenum.

constricting, and partially ulcerated, whereas duodenal adenocarcinomas are typically polypoid with little ulceration or infiltration.[208,211] On barium examination, these tumors will be seen as an annular lesion with shelflike overhanging margins or a polypoid mass within the lumen of the bowel. Because barium coats the mucosa of these lesions, ulceration of these tumors is more readily demonstrated on barium compared to CT.

On CT, these tumors will present as heterogeneously attenuating soft-tissue masses with moderate levels of enhancement.[16] They can appear as small polypoid lesions, larger eccentric masses, or annular masses of the wall of the small bowel. Although a large, aggressive, ulcerated adenocarcinoma can be mistaken for lymphoma, the presence of bulky metastatic lymphadenopathy favors lymphoma rather than adenocarcinoma.[212] Metastatic lymphadenopathy typically occurs in the root of the mesentery and in the pyloric, hepatic, peripancreatic, cecal, and ileocolic regions.[213] CT can also detect hematogenous metastasis to the liver and other abdominal organs. Both barium examinations and CT can also demonstrate complications of the tumor such as obstruction and intussusception.[214-216]

Carcinoid tumor

Gastrointestinal carcinoid tumors are relatively uncommon, although their incidence has increased over the past 30 years. Approximately two-thirds of carcinoid tumors in the body are located in the GI tract, with most of the remaining one-third located in the tracheobronchial system.[217] Within the GI tract, these tumors are located most frequently in the small intestine (41.8%), followed by the rectum (27.4%), appendix (24.1%), and stomach (8.7%).[85,217]

Carcinoid tumors are a diverse group of typically low-grade, slow-growing malignancies that arise from specialized endocrine cells populating the GI mucosa and submucosa.[85,213] The wide variety of hormones produced by these tumors can produce multiple syndromes, including carcinoid syndrome and ZE syndrome. Alternatively, carcinoid tumors can be a manifestation of the inherited syndromes: multiple endocrine neoplasia (MEN) type 1 and neurofibromatosis (NF) type 1.[85]

Approximately 90% of carcinoid tumors arise in the ileum.[213] Primary carcinoid tumors of the small intestine are typically small, rarely exceeding 3.5 cm.[85] At the time of diagnosis, almost two-thirds of patients with small intestinal carcinoid tumors have disease that has spread beyond the intestine to regional lymph nodes or the liver.[217] Unlike the primary tumor, metastasis to the lymph nodes, mesentery, and liver often attain large sizes, overshadowing the primary tumor. Involvement of the subserosa and adjacent mesentery stimulates a desmoplastic reaction that results in kinking, retraction, and angulation of the bowel, a finding that is characteristic of carcinoid and can suggest the correct diagnosis.[85]

Complications of carcinoid tumors include hormonal syndromes (listed above), intestinal ischemia, and intestinal obstruction. The classic carcinoid syndrome consists of cutaneous flushing, sweating, bronchospasm, colicky abdominal pain, diarrhea, and right-sided cardiac valvular fibrosis.[85] Approximately 10% of patients who do develop carcinoid syndrome will have a primary tumor of the small bowel. Carcinoid syndrome develops when vasoactive substances produced by the tumor, including serotonin, gastrin, somatostatin, cholecystokinin, and secretin enter systemic circulation without undergoing metabolic degeneration.[85] These substances are cleared from the circulation by the liver and, therefore, only 10% of patients with bowel carcinoid tumors develop carcinoid syndrome.[218] Unsurprisingly, most patients with a GI carcinoid who develop carcinoid syndrome have extensive hepatic metastasis such that the vasoactive secretions of the metastasis do not undergo degradation by liver enzymes and instead enter the systemic circulation. Although duodenal carcinoids are rare, approximately 62% will secrete gastrin, one-third of which have sufficient hormone production to cause ZE syndrome.[82,219]

Secretion of serotonin and other vasoactives substances can produce thickening, multifocal stenoses, or occlusion of mesenteric arteries and veins with resultant local, regional, or diffuse intestinal ischemia.[220] Both the primary tumor and associated desmoplastic reaction can result in partial or complete SBO.

The imaging appearance of jejunal and ileal carcinoids varies by tumor size, extent of mesenteric involvement, and presence or absence of lymph node or liver metastases.[85] Enteroclysis is the most sensitive test for the detection of small primary lesions, although these lesions may be seen on routine small-bowel follow-through (SBFT). When visualized, these tumors typically present as small (<2 cm), solitary or multifocal, polypoid lesion of the distal ileum.[84,85] Carcinoids are submucosal in location, resulting in lesions with smooth, sharply defined borders. However, occasionally the mucosa overlying the nodule of carcinoid can ulcerate, producing a barium-filled crater on the surface of the lesion.[85]

Small primary carcinoid tumors often go undetected on CT and MRI examinations. However, larger polypoid lesions can be visualized within the lumen of the bowel on CT and MRI. The lesions typically enhance intensely during arterial-phase images and are best appreciated on multiplanar reformatted CT using water for oral contrast[222] or on fat-suppressed postgadolinium MRI images.[223] Larger tumors will appear as asymmetric or concentric mural thickening of the small-bowel wall (see Figure 2-26).

In many cases, the secondary findings of carcinoid tumor are initially detected, which then leads to recognition of the small primary lesion. Secondary findings include (1) mesenteric fibrosis, (2) kinking of the bowel, (3) intussusception, (4) bowel ischemia, and (5) SBO.

The mesenteric desmoplastic response to carcinoid tumors typically appears as a soft-tissue attenuation mesenteric mass with spiculated margins and radiating soft-tissue

Imaging Notes 2-7. Imaging Features of Small-Bowel Carcinoid Tumors

Primary tumor	Undetected; or Small polyp (often dense enhancement); or Asymmetric or concentric mass
Secondary features	Mesenteric fibrosis (calcified soft-tissue mass/radiating strands) Kinking of bowel Intussusception
Distant disease	Mesenteric adenopathy (70% calcified) Hepatic metastasis (hyperenhancing)

strands. These mesenteric masses are usually easier to identify than the primary carcinoid tumor and are highly suggestive but not specific for this disease.[16,213] Interestingly, the degree of spiculation manifest by these masses correlates with the degree of mesenteric retraction and fibrosis from the local effects of vasoactive substances rather than tumor infiltration.[220] Enhancement of these masses varies depending on the degree of fibrosis and necrosis. Approximately 70% of these metastatic masses and nodes contain calcification (see Figures 2-26 and 2-27).[220]

In contrast to the spiculation of mesenteric masses, kinking of the small-bowel wall is thought to be the result of tumor infiltration and fibrosis of both the small-bowel wall and the adjacent mesentery, causing a tight "hairpin turn." These hairpin turns are visualized as rigid, curved segments

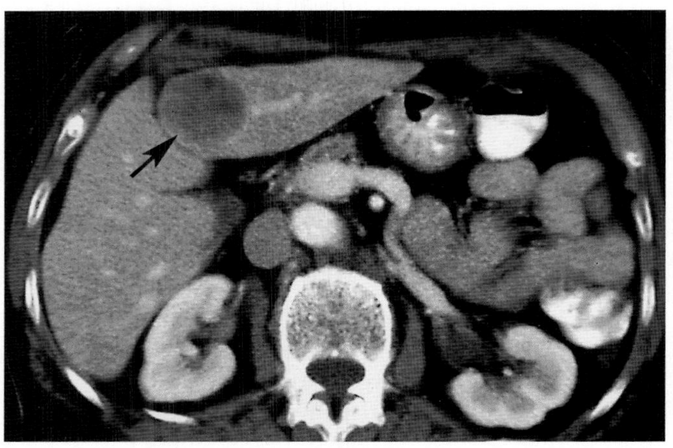

A

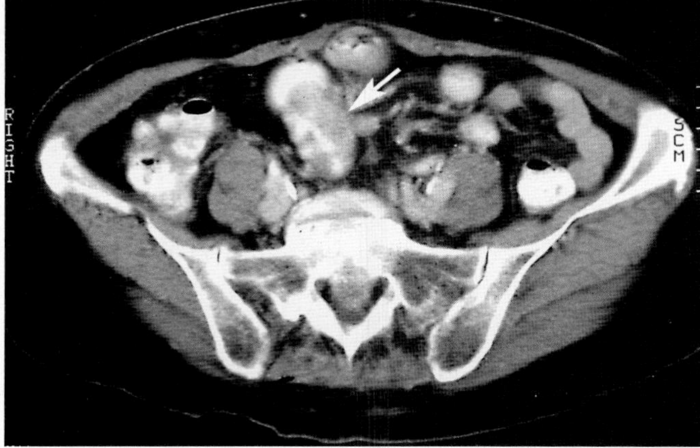

B

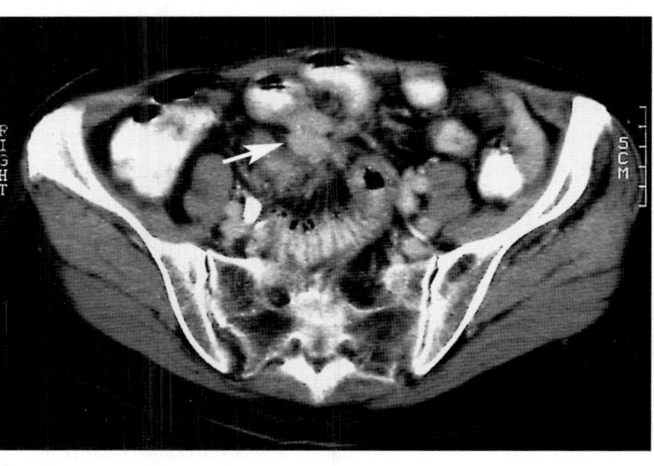

C

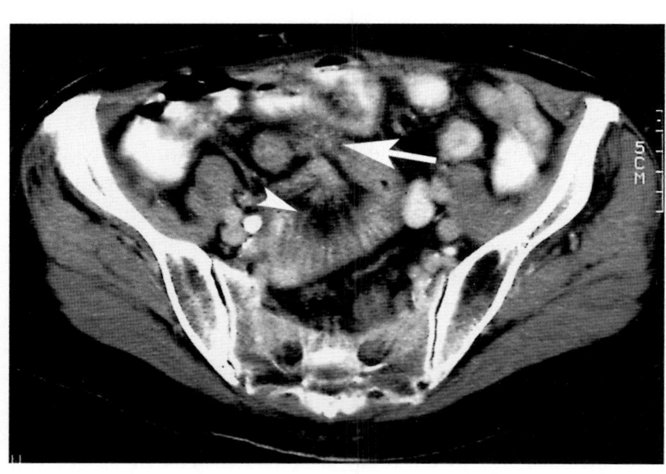

D

Figure 2-26 Carcinoid Tumor of the Small Bowel
This 82-year-old man presented with intermittent abdominal pain. **A-D.** CT images through the abdomen demonstrate an eccentric mass involving the left lateral and inferior walls of a loop of ilium (*small white arrows*). This is associated with a spiculated appearance of the mesentery (*large white arrow*) and tethering of an adjacent bowel loop (*white arrowhead*). These findings are typical of a small-bowel carcinoid. A solitary hepatic metastasis is also seen (*black arrow*).

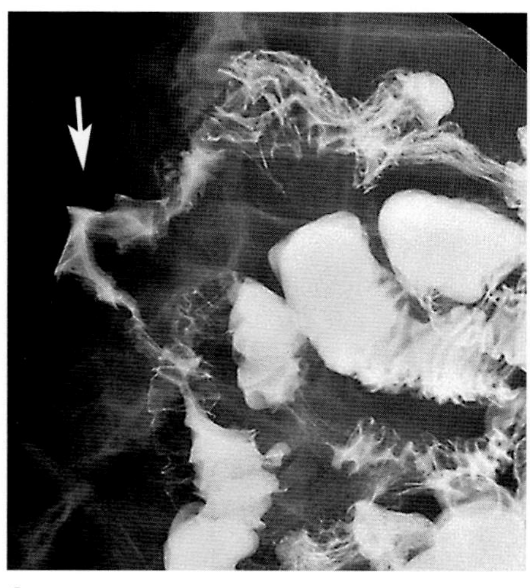
A

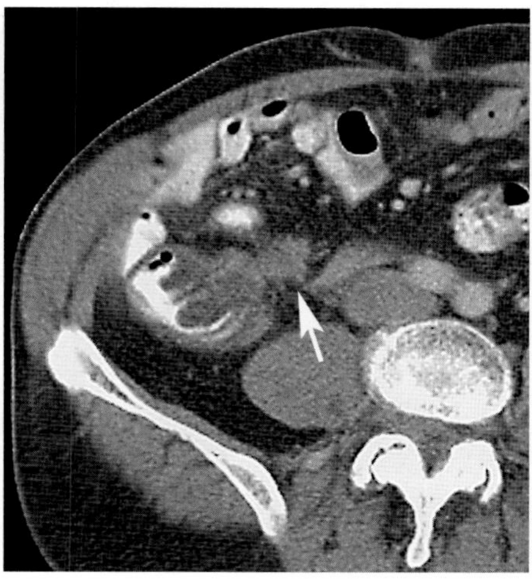
B

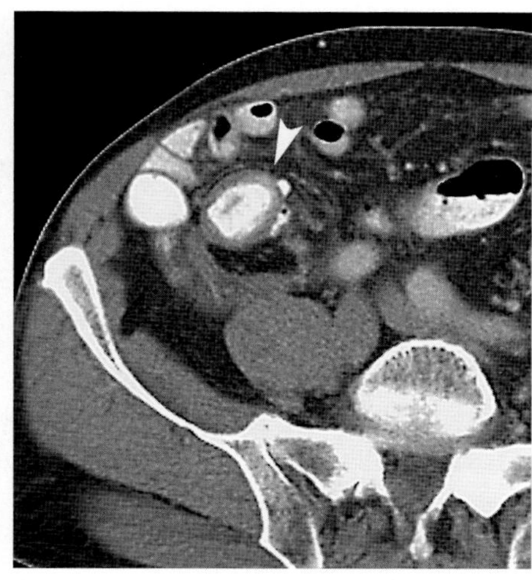
C

Figure 2-27 Small-bowel Tethering due to Carcinoid
A. Small-bowel follow-through in this 83-year-old man demonstrates distortion and angulation of a small-bowel loop (*arrow*) in the right side of the abdomen. This appearance is most often due to adhesions but can be a result of mesenteric scarring of any cause including carcinoid tumor. **B** and **C.** Contrast-enhanced images through the right side of the abdomen demonstrates a small speculated mesenteric mass with radiating strands in the mesenteric fat. Although this can be due to a variety of desmoplastic masses, this is most typical of carcinoid tumor. There is thickening of a loop of small bowel fed by the portion of mesentery with the desmoplastic mass. This probably indicates small-bowel ischemia due to vascular compromise by the mesenteric fibrotic mass.

of the small intestine that are easily appreciated on enteroclysis and SBFT examinations. On CT, they manifest as a thickened, distorted segment of small intestine. Although the curvature or kinking of the small bowel may be present on axial images, multiplanar reformatting will illustrate the hairpin turn to the best advantage (see Figure 2-27).[85]

The liver and mesenteric nodes are the most common sites of metastasis from midgut carcinoid tumors, defined as the small bowel and proximal colon. Metastases to the pancreas, bone, and peritoneum are uncommon, and metastases to the soft tissue, breast, and orbit are rare.[224-226] Ovarian metastases can be found in up to 2% of GI carcinoid tumors.[227] Metastases from small-bowel carcinoids are usually hypervascular and often best seen during the arterial phase of IV contrast material administration on CT and MR images.[223,228]

Small-bowel lymphoma

Lymphoma of the small bowel accounts for 20% to 30% of all primary GI lymphomas.[93] The distal ileum is the most common location, particularly near the ileocecal valve, because of the higher concentration of lymphoid tissue in this region.[229] Most small-bowel lymphomas are of the B-cell type.[93,230] T-cell lymphomas are uncommon and usually occur in the setting of celiac disease.[93]

B-cell lymphoma of the small bowel can assume a number of imaging appearances on double-contrast barium enema (DCBE) examination and CT.[93]. Small-bowel lymphomas most commonly appear as single or multiple segments of symmetric and marked bowel wall thickening. Wall thickness ranges from 1.5 to 7 cm and the mass is typically homogenous in attenuation, with uniform enhancement following IV contrast (see Figure 2-28).[213,231,232] Small-bowel lymphoma can also appear as an exocentric or circumferential mass that extends into the small-bowel mesentery (see Figure 2-29). In some cases, usually when the tumor reaches a large size, it will undergo central necrosis leading to a large central ulcer that communicates with the bowel lumen.[93,229] Occasionally, small-bowel lymphoma will appear as a long distensible infiltrating lesion with or without aneurysmal dilation of the lumen of the bowel (see Figure 2-28). This distention is a result of denervation of the muscularis propria by the infiltrating malignancy. Rarely, small-bowel lymphoma can appear as a focal polypoid intraluminal mass without wall thickening or lymphadenopathy that can serve as a lead point for intussusception.[93,232]

T-cell lymphoma in the small bowel has a higher incidence of multifocal involvement. Usually it presents with mild to moderate wall thickening relative to the marked degree of wall thickening manifest by B-cell lymphoma, and has a predilection for perforation.[233]

Gastrointestinal stromal tumor

The small bowel is the second most common location of GISTs after the stomach. Although benign GISTs can occur anywhere in the small bowel, malignant GISTs tend to arise in the distal small bowel.[213]

On barium examination, these tumors will be visualized as an intraluminal or submucosal mass with sharply

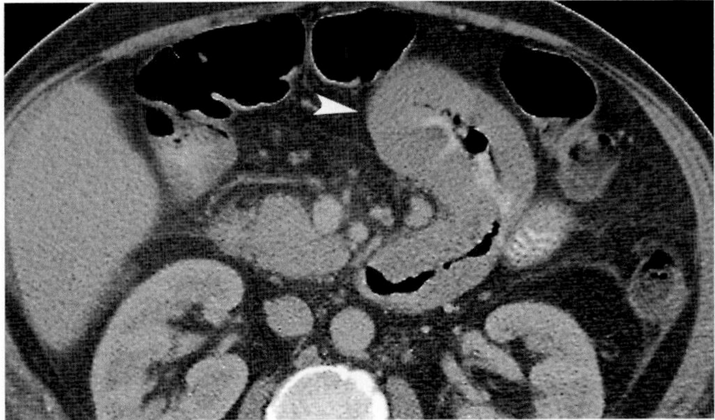

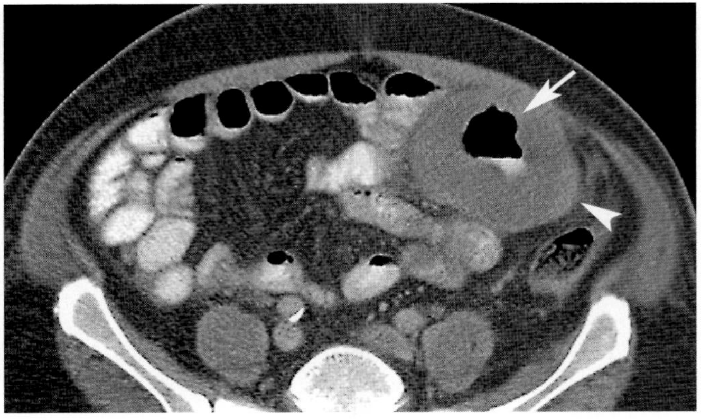

Figure 2-28 Luminal Distension in Small-bowel Lymphoma This 54-year-old man with AIDS complained of abdominal pain and nausea. **A** and **B.** Contrast-enhanced CT shows a loop of small bowel with massive wall thickening (*arrowheads*) and a focally dilated lumen. These are characteristic features of small-bowel lymphoma.

defined margins. Similar to GISTs in the stomach, the mucosal surface can show focal ulceration, especially in large tumors, and usually demonstrate an extraserosal component.

On CT and MRI examinations, most GISTs will appear as a smoothly marginated intramural mass of the wall of the small bowel that projects either intraluminally or extraserosally.[213] Rarely, GISTs can appear as an intraluminal polyp.[213] Smaller tumors are typically uniform in attenuation on CT and signal intensity on MRI; however, larger tumors will often demonstrate heterogenous enhancement with areas of low attenuation corresponding to hemorrhage, central necrosis, or cyst formation.[234] In some cases, this central necrosis will cavitate, resulting in communication between the tumor and the lumen of the small bowel that presents as a large central wall ulcer.[234] When large, GISTs can exert significant mass effect on the small bowel segment of origin as well as adjacent segments, making it challenging to determine the exact origin of the tumor. Lymphadenopathy is rare in patients with small-bowel GISTs, a finding that can help differentiate GISTs from lymphoma (see Figure 2-30). GISTs are discussed most completely earlier in this chapter under the heading **Polyps and Masses of the Stomach**.

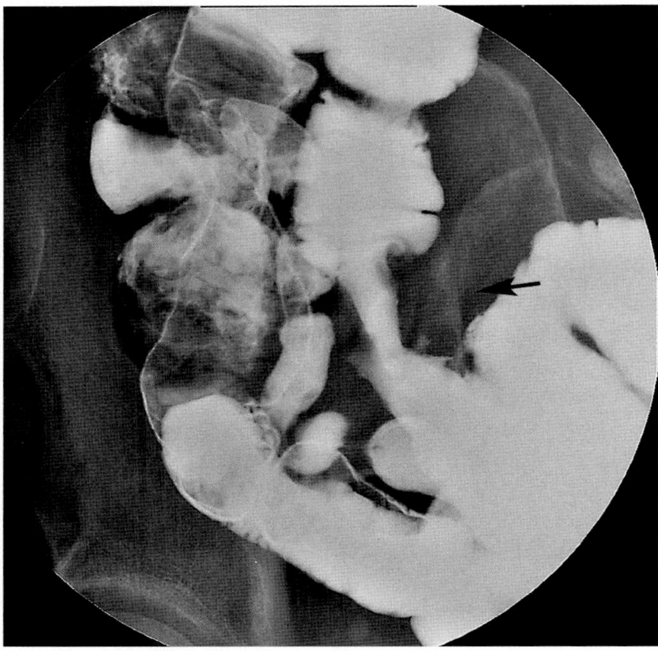

Figure 2-29 Follicular Lymphoma of the Small Bowel This 71-year-old man has a focal moderately sharply marginated stricture (*arrow*) of the distal small bowel. This would most often be due to a small-bowel carcinoma or carcinoid but in this case was proven to represent a follicular lymphoma.

Lipoma

Lipomas are uncommon, slow-growing submucosal tumors that can be found throughout the GI tract.[123,124] The colon is the most common site of lipoma in the GI tract, followed by the small bowel and stomach.[123,125] In most cases, they will appear as a smooth, sharply marginated ovoid mass on barium studies, CT, and MRI. However, because they are located superficial to the muscularis propria, regular peristaltic contractions of the bowel may propel this lesion into the bowel lumen, resulting in the appearance of a polyp on a pseudopedicle.[124] CT and MRI will reveal the fatty nature of the mass (see Figure 2-31).

Familial adenomatous polyposis and gardner syndrome

FAP is an autosomal dominant, inherited disorder resulting in hundreds of GI polyps.[235,236] Polyps are commonly

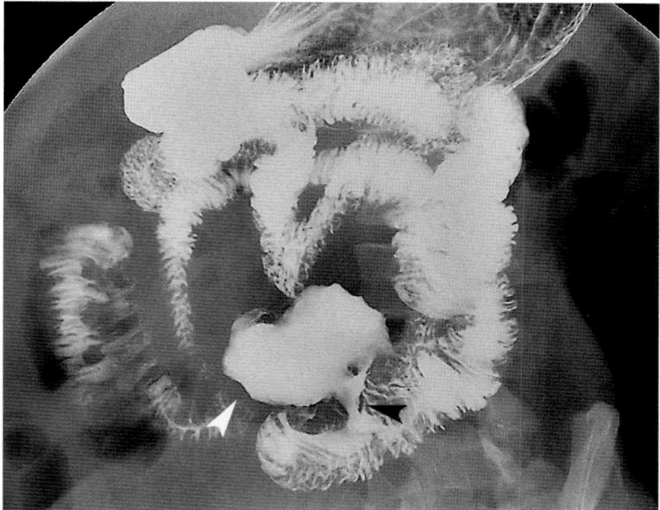

A

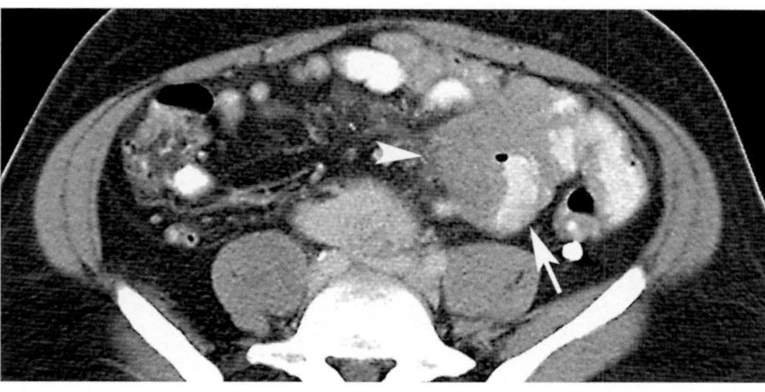

B

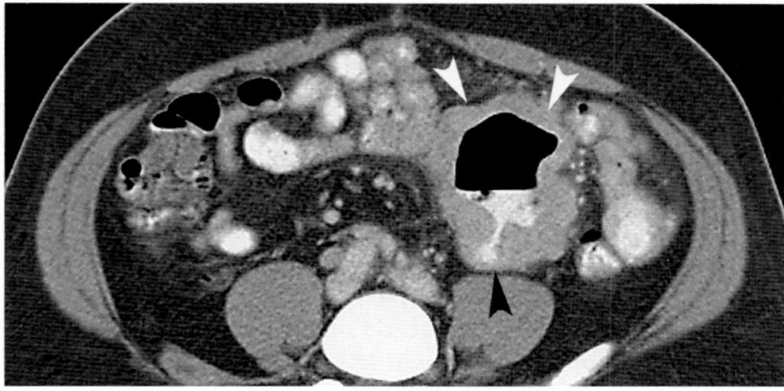

C

Figure 2-30 Cavitary Small-Bowel Gastrointestinal Stromal Tumor This 49-year-old man complained of abdominal pain and weight loss. **A.** Double-contrast upper GI tract examination shows an amorphous collection of barium (*white arrowhead*), which communicates with the adjacent small bowel by a narrow neck (*black arrowhead*). Notice how the region around the collection is devoid of most bowel loops. The bowel is being displaced by a large mass with a central cavity that communicates with the lumen of the small bowel. **B** and **C.** CT images confirm the presence of a thick-walled cavitary mass (*white arrowheads*) that communicates with the small bowel (*small white arrow*) via a narrow neck (*black arrowhead*). Both the UGI and CT appearance is typical of a cavitary mass of the wall of the small bowel, usually a lymphoma or GIST. Surgical biopsy was diagnostic of a GIST.

found in the stomach and colon but can also be seen in the small bowel. When they occur, small bowel polyps are most often located in the duodenum, are of adenomatous histology, and have the potential for malignant transformation (see Figure 2-32).[52] Gardner syndrome, once thought to be a related but separate syndrome, is now known to result from mutations of the FAP gene and is considered a variant of that syndrome. It is distinct from FAP; in that, the multiple GI manifestations are also associated with the presence of multiple osteomas, especially of the jaw and skull, desmoid tumors, fibromas, dental abnormalities, and congenital hypertrophy of the retinal epithelial pigment. Upper GI examinations can demonstrate small, <5-mm polyps in the duodenum, and more distal small bowel. FAP and Gardner syndromes are discussed most completely under the heading **Focal Polyps or Masses of the Colon** later in this chapter.

Hamartomatous polyps

Hamartomas are nonneoplastic, tumorlike lesions composed of an excess or abnormal arrangement of tissues normally found in the region where they are discovered.[59] There are 2 main types of hamartomatous polyps, Peutz-Jeghers polyps, and juvenile polyps, which are associated with a few polyposis syndromes, including Peutz-Jeghers syndrome, juvenile polyposis syndrome, Cronkhite-Canada syndrome, and PTEN hamartoma tumor syndrome.

Peutz-Jeghers syndrome: Peutz-Jeghers syndrome is an inherited, autosomal dominant disorder characterized by the presence of unique GI hamartomatous polyps and mucocutaneous pigmentation.

Peutz-Jeghers polyps are characterized by a core of smooth muscle contiguous with the muscularis mucosa and is surrounded by fronds of mature epithelium.[59] The core has a central trunk with branchlike projections that extend into the surrounding fronds. When viewed in cross section, the trunk and fronds resemble the trunk, branches, and needles of a Christmas tree. The polyps are most commonly found in the small bowel followed by the colon and then the stomach. These polyps are benign. However, the syndrome is associated with the development of a variety of malignancies, most commonly of the GI, breast, pancreas, and the reproductive organs.[59] Of 31 patients with Peutz-Jeghers syndrome in the Johns Hopkins Polyposis registry over 12 years, 15 patients developed cancer.[237]

Although autosomally dominantly inherited, Peutz-Jeghers syndrome has variable penetrance. Therefore, a negative family history does not exclude the diagnosis. Patients will have multiple flat, pigmented lesions that most prominently involve the face, especially the perioral region, and resemble freckles that, with time, will increase in size, number, and depth.[59] These represent small skin hamartomas. Patients typically present in childhood with intermittent episodes of abdominal pain as a result of intermittent

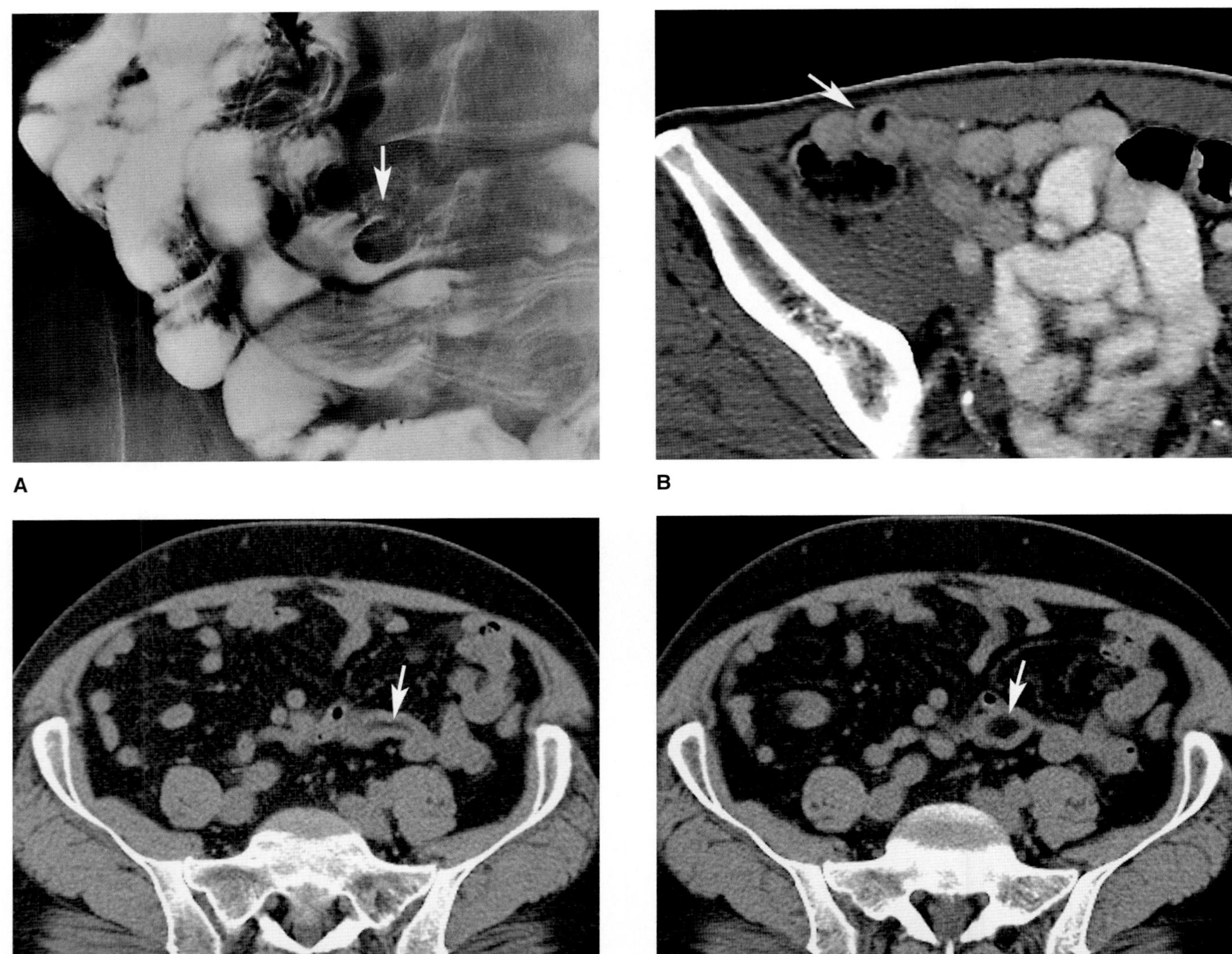

Figure 2-31 Jejunal Lipoma in 2 Patients
A and **B.** This 58-year-old man complained of nausea and vomiting. A. Film from a small-bowel follow-through shows a smoothly marginated filling defect (*arrow*) within a loop of ilum consistent with a polyp. B. Axial CT shows the polyp to be a small lipoma (*arrow*). **C** and **D.** This 69-year-old man was being evaluated for kidney stones. C and D. CT images without oral contrast show a thin fatty stalk (*arrow* in C) and a polypoid fatty nodule (*arrow* in D) within the lumen of a loop of distal jejunum. This is diagnostic of a pedunculated, submucosal jejunal lipoma.

intussusception.[59] In most cases, the intussusception will spontaneously reduce, but occasionally, patients will present with SBO. Rarely, patients will present with symptoms of GI bleeding.

Imaging examinations will demonstrate multiple polyps within the small bowel, stomach, and colon.[59] Polyps can be sessile or pedunculated and can range from a few millimeters to several centimeters in diameter. In most patients there are multiple polyps, which are widely scattered over areas of normal mucosa but can occasionally carpet the surface of the stomach or small bowel.[59] In most cases, these lesions are detected by barium examinations but can occasionally be detected by CT or US examinations.[238]

Juvenile polyps and juvenile polyposis syndrome: Juvenile polyps are a form of hamartomatous polyp that can occur sporadically or as part of juvenile polyposis syndrome. Juvenile polyps are found most commonly in the colon but can also occur in the small bowel and stomach.[60]

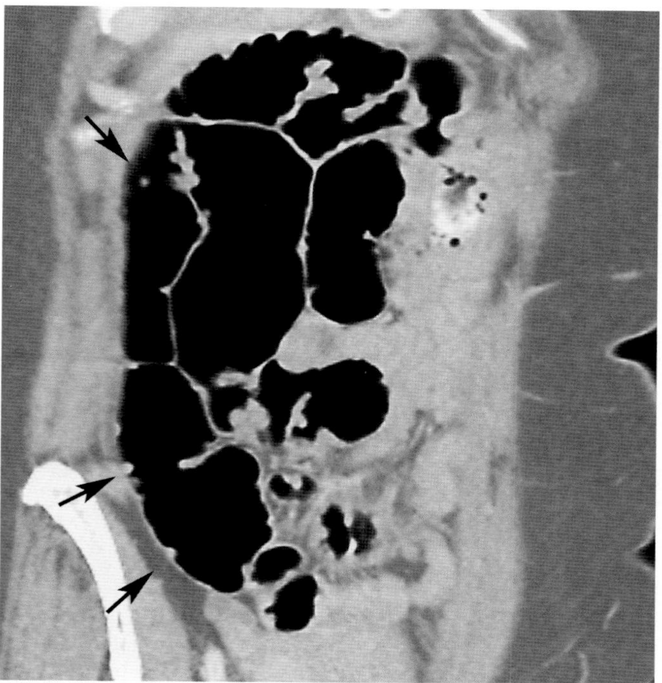

A

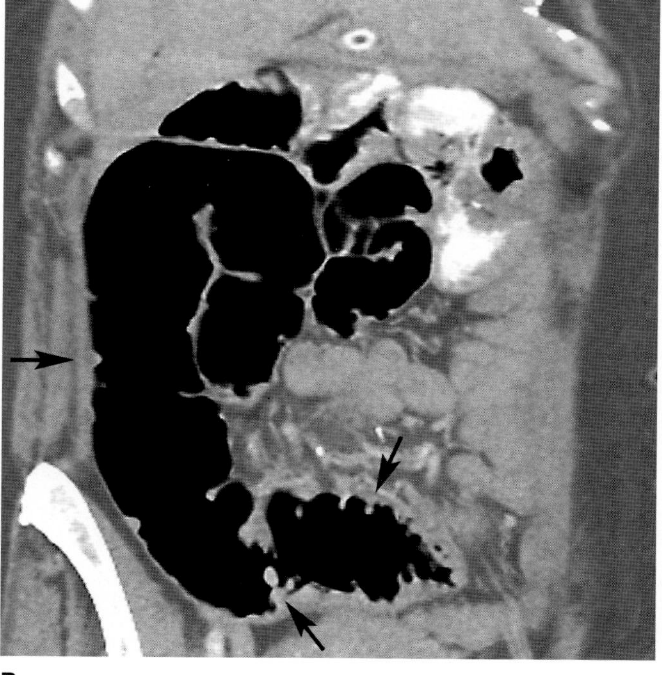

B

Figure 2-32 FAP
This 46-year-old man had had a total colectomy for FAP. **A** and **B.** Coronal reconstructions from a CT of the abdomen demonstrate multiple small polyps projecting from the lumen of the small bowel.

Juvenile polyps and juvenile polyposis syndrome are discussed more completely under the heading **Focal Polyps or Masses of the Colon** later in this chapter.

Kaposi sarcoma in HIV

During the initial AIDS epidemic in the 1980s, 40% of patients with HIV had Kaposi sarcoma involving the GI tract. These tumors are now rare in HIV-infected patients. Kaposi sarcoma in HIV patients typically presents with multiple small elevated submucosal lesions in the jejunum or ilium that can mimic multiple small GISTs or lymphoma.[239,240] On barium evaluation, these submucosal lesions demonstrate a characteristic central umbilication that produces a bull's-eye or target appearance.[241] These lesions can then coalesce to form diffusely thickened small-bowel folds, resembling small-bowel lymphoma. Retroperitoneal and mesenteric adenopathy is seen in about 50% of cases of Kaposi sarcoma on CT or MRI examinations, making this diagnosis additionally difficult to distinguish from lymphoma.[85,239]

Small-bowel metastasis

Metastases to the small bowel are uncommon. Imaging can show lesions from small submucosal lesions to larger cavitary masses (see Figure 2-33). Occasionally, small-bowel metastasis can act as a lead point for intussusception.

Ulcers and Diverticula of the Small Bowel

Ulcers of the small bowel occur in the setting of peptic ulcer disease and are found in the duodenum or in the setting of a necrotic tumor. Diverticula of the small bowel are due to congenital malformation of the bowel during fetal development.

Duodenal ulcers

Unlike gastric ulcers, duodenal ulcers are almost always a result of peptic ulcer disease.[73] Approximately 90% to 100% of patients with duodenal ulcers are infected with *H pylori*.[141] These ulcers demonstrate gastric metaplasia along their borders with *H pylori* infection of the metaplastic epithelium; a finding that may explain why the infected mucosa is more susceptible to ulceration.[242] Treatment of *H pylori* in these patients both accelerates the healing of ulcers and also decreases the rate of ulcer recurrence.[143]

Approximately 95% of duodenal ulcers are located in the bulb,[243] usually on the anterior wall.[157] These ulcers are typically <1 cm in diameter and appear as an ovoid or round barium collection surrounded by a smooth radiolucent mound of edematous mucosa with radiating folds that converge centrally to the edge of the crater.[73] Similar to gastric ulcers, duodenal ulcers can occasionally have unusual, linear flamelike or other shapes (see Figure 3-28).

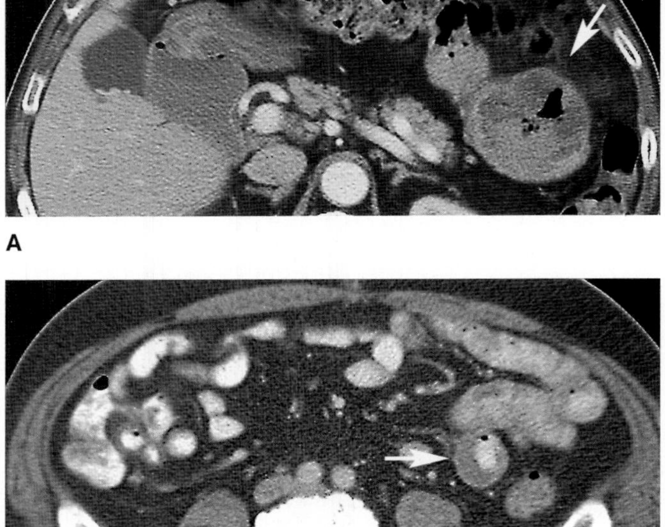

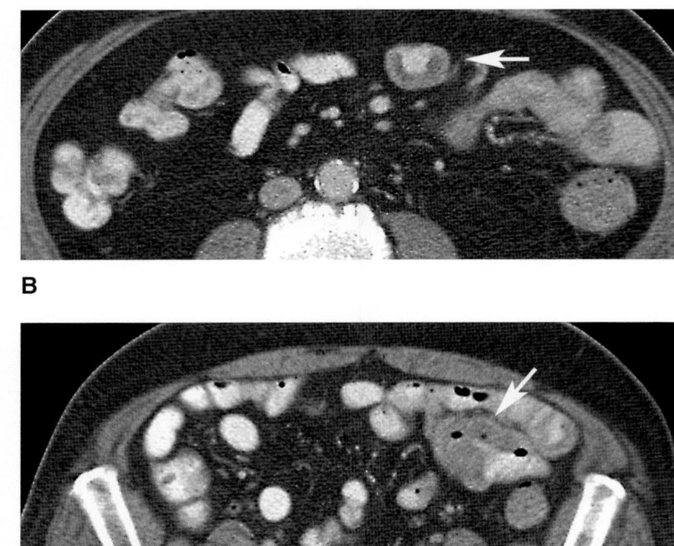

Figure 2-33 Small-Bowel Metastasis in 2 Patients
Both of these patients were being evaluated for malignant melanoma. **A.** Axial CT image shows a large cavitary mass in the proximal jejunum. **B-D.** Axial CT images show several annular and semiannular lesions (*arrows*) in the small bowel. Surgical biopsies were diagnostic of metastatic melanoma in both patients.

CT and MRI do not play a role in the primary detection of duodenal ulcers. CT is useful in the detection of perforated duodenal ulcers characterized by the presence of the following: (1) wall thickening, (2) periduodenal fluid, (3) retroperitoneal air, or (4) free intraperitoneal air.[244]

Malignant ulcers of the small bowel

Malignant ulcers of the small bowel are usually a manifestation of central necrosis of a bowel malignancy that communicates with the lumen of the bowel. This is most frequently found in patients with GISTs and lymphomas but can occasionally occur with adenocarcinoma and some other malignancies (see Figure 2-30). In most cases, imaging will show a large mass with central ulceration. Ulceration without evidence of a mass lesion is uncommon.

Diverticula of the small bowel

Virtually all diverticula of the small bowel are congenital in origin. Congenital diverticula can be found from the esophagus to the rectum but are most commonly found in the small bowel. Most congenital diverticula are discovered incidentally. Occasionally, individuals will present with symptoms of malabsorption, such as weight loss and diarrhea, as a result of bacterial overgrowth within the diverticulum. Other patients can present with abdominal pain, fever, and/or leucocytosis as a result of diverituculitis.[73,245] Rarely, congenital diverticula can be a cause for intussusception whereby patients will present with symptoms of bowel obstruction. In addition to the more common sporadic congenital diverticula, there are 2 specific types of congenital diverticula in the small bowel: jejunal diverticulosis and Meckel diverticulum.

Sporadic congenital diverticula are most commonly found in the duodenum, often near the third portion. They appear as air-, fluid-, or contrast-filled round or oval fluid collections along the antimesenteric border of the bowel.

Jejunal diverticulosis occurs along the mesenteric border of the small bowel. Their incidence ranges between 0.06% and 1.3% on autopsy and 0.02% to 0.04% on imaging examinations.[73,245] On imaging, they are visualized as air-, fluid-, and/or contrast-filled sacculations with narrow necks and no normal small-bowel mucosal features (see Figure 2-34).

Meckel diverticula are the most common congenital abnormality of the small bowel with an incidence of between 1% and 4%.[246] These are true diverticula, composed of all layers of the intestinal wall,[247,248] and are usually found within 100 cm of the ileocecal valve.[246] They occur because of a failure of the omphalomesenteric duct to involute completely, with fibrous obliteration of the umbilical end and patency of the ileal end of the duct.[249] Potential complications of Meckel diverticulum include GI bleeding, intussusception, obstruction, perforation, strangulation, diverticulitis, volvulus, hernia, and neoplasm in decreasing order of frequency. The lifetime risk for developing a complication is 4.2% to 6.4%,[250] with the highest risk occurring in the pediatric age group. Bleeding is due

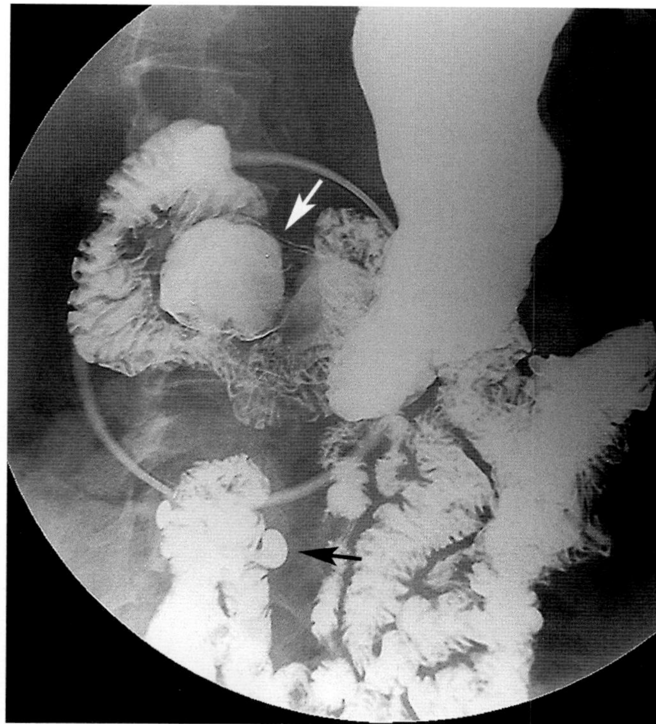

A

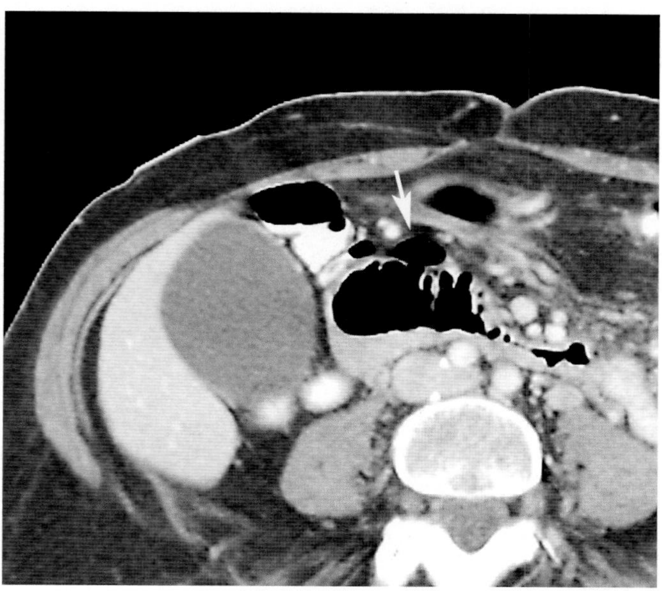

B

Figure 2-34 Jejunal Diverticulosis
A. Barium upper GI examination of this 75-year-old woman demonstrates 2 outpouchings of barium, 1 in the duodenum (*white arrow*) and 1 in the jejunum (*black arrow*) consistent with small-bowel diverticula. Despite the woman's age, these are most likely to be congenital diverticula. **B.** CT examination shows a small diverticula projecting off a loop of small bowel (*white arrow*).

to ectopic gastric, pancreatic, or duodenal mucosa, which occurs in 15% to 50% of Meckel diverticula.

On barium studies, Meckel diverticula are visualized as a smooth-walled diverticulum arising from the antimesenteric border of the distal ileum or, if it is inverted, as a filling defect within the lumen of the ileum. This is in contrast to duplication cysts or acquired diverticula, both of which arise from the mesenteric border of the ileum.[246] Small filling defects or mucosal irregularity within the diverticulum can be seen, representing ectopic gastric mucosa[251] or blood clots in cases where the patient has presented with hemorrhage.[252]

It is often difficult to recognize an uncomplicated Meckel diverticulum on CT examinations because it appears similar to normal segments of the small bowel. In the setting of Meckel diverticulitis, however, there will be visualization of a thick-walled loop of bowel in the region of the terminal ileum with associated inflammatory change in the surrounding mesentry located separate from the appendix (see Figure 2-35).[253] When present, CT is more sensitive than plain films both in detecting the presence of and the localization of enteroliths in relation to the ileum.[254]

FOCAL DISEASES OF THE COLON

Similar to the stomach and small bowel, focal colonic lesions can be due to polypoid or masslike lesions that protrude into or narrow the lumen of the colon or due to lesions that protrude outward from the colonic epithelium and represent ulcers or diverticula.

Focal Polyps or Masses of the Colon

Focal mass lesions of the colon include the non-neoplastic lesions: hyperplastic and inflammatory polyps, and the neoplastic lesions: adenoma, adenocarcinoma, carcinoid tumor, lymphoma, GIST, lipoma, and some other rare lesions. Colon-related infections, including diverticulitis, appendicitis, and abscesses related to inflammatory bowel disease (IBD), can also appear as colonic mass lesions (Table 2-4).

Hyperplastic polyps

The majority of colonic polyps measuring 5 mm or less represent hyperplastic polyps or normal mucosal tags.[10,12,255] The prevalence of hyperplastic polyps ranges from 25% to 80% in the general population.[97,256,257] They appear as smooth, round, and sessile lesions that increase in frequency with increasing age and are primarily found in patients older than age 40.[258-260] Histopathologically, hyperplastic polyps appear as protrusions of the colonic mucosa characterized by elongated serrated crypts lined by proliferative epithelium and enlarged goblet cells with a saw-toothed outline.[261] These polyps almost never undergo malignant degeneration, so there is minimal or no risk of cancer developing in these lesions.

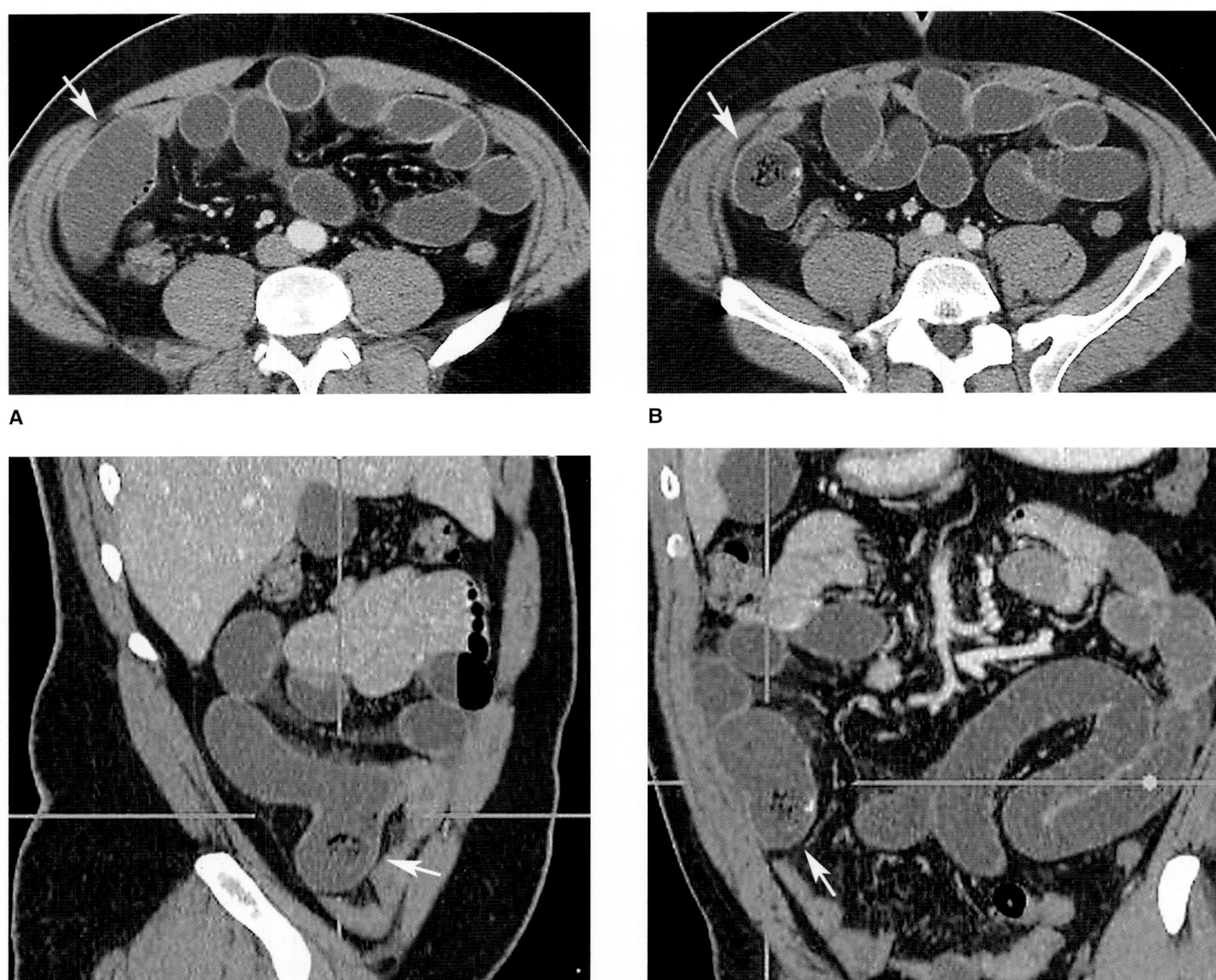

Figure 2-35 Meckel Diverticulitis by CT
This 46-year-old man had periumbilical pain, nausea, and vomiting. **A** and **B**. Axial images demonstrate dilated small-bowel loops and a small-bowel feces sign (*arrows*). This was initially interpreted as representing a small-bowel obstruction. **C** and **D**. Sagittal and coronal reconstructions show the small-bowel feces sign to be in a wide mouth diverticulum (*arrows*) extending form the distal small bowel. Surgical resection demonstrated a Meckel diverticulitis with gastric mucosa. The bowel dilation represented an adynamic ileus due to the diverticulitis rather than a small-bowel obstruction.

The vast majority of hyperplastic polyps are clinically asymptomatic and do not affect the health and well-being of the patient. Their significance is that they have imaging and colonoscopic appearance identical to adenomatous polyps that do have the potential to harbor malignancy. From an imaging perspective, the size of a polyp is the most important determinant of malignant potential. Most polyps less than or equal to 5 mm in diameter will represent hyperplastic

Imaging Notes 2-8. Importance of Polyp Size

Most colonic polyps are of either hyperplastic or adenomatous histology. The size of colonic polyps is of considerable importance because of the risk of carcinoma increases with increasing polyp size[21-23]

Table 2-4. Polyps and Masses of the Colon

A. Inflammatory lesions
 1. Hyperplastic polyps
 2. Inflammatory polyps

B. Neoplasms
 1. Epithelial lesions
  a. Adenoma/adenocarcinoma
  b. Carcinoid tumor
 2. Submucosal lesions
  a. Lymphoma
  b. Gastrointestinal stromal tumor (GIST)
  c. Lipoma
  d. Melanoma
  e. Other mesenchymal tumors
   i. Leiomyoma/leiomyosarcoma
   ii. Neurofibroma
   iii. Schwannoma

C. Hamartomatous polyps
 1. Peutz-Jeghers polyp
 2. Juvenile polyp

D. Focal infections
 1. Diverticulitis
 2. Appendicitis

polyps. With increasing polyp size, however, there is an increased risk of adenomatous polyps. Polyps larger than 1 cm in diameter are more likely to harbor adenocarcinoma, in particular if they have a lobulated contour or have a basal indentation.[258,262] A pedunculated polyp with a stalk longer than 2 cm is rarely associated with invasive carcinoma.[263]

On barium examination, sessile polyps appear as filling defects in the barium pool if they are located on the dependent wall, and as ring shadows etched in white due to barium coating along the rim of the polyp if they are located on the nondependent wall.[264] When viewed in obliquity, sessile polyps may appear as "bowler hats," where the brim of the hat represents the base of the polyp and the dome of the hat represents the head of the polyp.[265] Although both polyps and diverticula can present as bowler hats on double-contrast images,[266,267] the dome of the hat points toward the lumen of the bowel for polyps and away from the lumen for diverticula.[258,268]

Pedunculated polyps are identified by the presence of a discrete stalk. When the patient is in the supine or prone position, a polyp on the nondependent wall may appear as a "Mexican hat." This refers to presence of a pair of concentric rings, where the outer ring represents the head of a polyp and the inner ring represents the stalk seen through the head.[264] When this finding is identified, the stalk can be visualized simply by rotating the patient 180° or moving the patient into the erect position.

On cross-sectional imaging, including CT, CTC, US, and MRI examinations, sessile and pedunculated polyps are characterized by homogenous soft-tissue attenuation, echogenicity or signal intensity, by smooth, rounded, or lobulated borders and by a fixed relationship to the bowel wall with patient repositioning.[21] Villous adenomas can also be characterized on CTC, much as on barium examinations, by visualization of a lobulated mass that contains barium within the interstices.

Polyposis syndromes

There are a variety of predominantly inherited disorders that lead to multiple GI polyps. They can lead to either multiple adenomatous polyps or multiple hamartomatous polyps.

Adenomatous polyposis syndromes

Familial adenomatous polyposis is the most common polyposis syndrome and results in innumerable GI adenomatous polyps. Gardner syndrome and Turcot syndrome are 2 other adenomatous polyposis syndromes (Table 2-5).

Familial adenomatous polyposis and gardner syndrome: FAP is an autosomal dominant inherited syndrome diagnosed by the presence of more than 100 adenomatous

Table 2-5. Polyposis Syndromes

Syndrome	Inheritance	Colon Polyp	Gastric Polyp	Major Disease Site
Familial adenomatous polyposis	Autosomal dominant	Adenoma	Hyperplastic	Colon
Gardner syndrome	Autosomal dominant	Adenoma	Hyperplastic	Colon, bone, small bowel mesentery
Peutz-Jeghers	Autosomal dominant	Hamartoma	Hamartoma	Small bowel
Juvenile polyposis	Autosomal dominant	Hamartoma	Hamartoma	Colon
PTEN hamartoma tumor	Autosomal dominant	Hamartoma	Hamartoma	Brain and skin
Cronkhite-Canada syndrome	None	Hamartoma	Hamartoma	Skin, colon, stomach

colorectal polyps. In most cases, however, patients will present with hundreds to thousands of polyps.[235,236] The disease is caused by mutations in the FAP gene, a tumor suppressor gene on chromosome 5, and has a prevalence of approximately 1 in 10 000 births. Approximately 30% of patients will have spontaneous mutation of the gene and will, therefore, not have a family history of the disease.[269] Nearly all patients with the FAP gene will develop polyps by the age of 35 years, and approximately 7% of patients will develop colon cancer by the age of 21 years.[235,236]

FAP is associated with the formation of polyps in the stomach, small bowel, and colon. Colon polyps of FAP are adenomatous, typically of tubular or tubulovillous histology but can occasionally be of villous adenoma histology.[235,236] Unlike colon polyps of FAP, which are adenomatous, most gastric polyps of FAP are fundic gland polyps and, therefore, not predisposed to malignancy. Small-bowel polyps of FAP most often occur in the duodenum and are usually of adenomatous histology with corresponding malignant potential (see Figure 2-32). In addition to the increased risk of colon cancer, patients with FAP are at increased risk of cholangiocarcinoma, hepatoblastoma, and cancers of the thyroid gland, adrenal gland, and pancreas.[236]

Gardner syndrome, once thought to be a related but separate syndrome, is now known to result from mutations of the FAP gene and considered a variant of familial adenomatous polyposis. It is distinct from FAP; in that, the multiple GI manifestations are also associated with the presence of multiple osteomas, especially of the jaw and skull, desmoid tumors, fibromas, dental abnormalities, and congenital hypertrophy of the retinal epithelial pigment.

Patients with FAP typically present with either symptoms of rectal bleeding or diarrhea, but some will be asymptomatic until a colon cancer develops.[235,236,270] Some patients' polyps will become large enough to ulcerate and cause rectal bleeding or cause obstructive symptoms. Virtually 100% of patients will ultimately develop colon cancer, usually at a younger age than typically seen with sporadic colon cancer. As a result, prophylactic total colectomy is recommended for these patients in their late teenage years.[271]

Contrast enema will typically demonstrate innumerable small or moderate filling defects within the colon.[236] Although these patients typically have as many as several thousand <5-mm polyps, contrast studies will typically underestimate the total number of polyps because of their small size.[235,236] In most cases, the polyps will be relatively uniformly distributed across the colon but can occasionally be predominant in 1 region of the colon.

Upper GI examination will demonstrate multiple small, 1- to 5-mm, sessile polyps clustered in the gastric fundus. Small, <5-mm polyps can also be found in the duodenum and distal small bowel.

CT and MRI examinations have not been used in the evaluation of colonic polyps but have been used to monitor duodenal polyps and desmoid tumors.[272-274]

Turcot syndrome: Turcot syndrome is a hereditary disease in which multiple GI polyps are associated with primary brain tumors, especially gliomas, glioblastomas, and astrocytomas. Patients typically present in the first or second decades of life with symptoms related to the brain tumor.

Hamartomatous (juvenile) polyps and polyposis syndromes

Hamartomas are nonneoplastic, tumorlike lesion composed of an excess or abnormal arrangement of tissues normally found in the region where they are discovered.[59] There are 2 main types of hamartomatous polyps, including Peutz-Jeghers polyps and juvenile polyps, which are associated with several polyposis syndromes: Peutz-Jeghers syndrome, juvenile polyposis syndrome, Cronkhite-Canada syndrome, and PTEN hamartoma tumor syndrome.

Peutz-Jeghers syndrome: Peutz-Jeghers syndrome is an inherited, autosomal dominant disorder characterized by the Peutz-Jeghers polyp. Patients have multiple small skin and GI hamartomas.[59] Imaging examinations will demonstrate multiple polyps within the small bowel, stomach, and colon but most commonly in the small bowel.[59] Peutz-Jeghers syndrome is discussed most completely under the heading **Focal Polyps or Masses of the Small Bowel** earlier in this chapter.

Juvenile polyps and juvenile polyposis syndrome: Juvenile polyps are a form of hamartomatous polyp that is characterized by cystically dilated GI glands with expanded lamina propria. Juvenile polyps are the most common GI polyps in children and may have as high as a 2% prevalence in preschool children.[60] The majority occur sporadically and are found in the rectosigmoid colon. Uncommonly, they can occur as part of juvenile polyposis syndrome.

Juvenile polyposis syndrome is a rare autosomally dominantly inherited syndrome of multiple GI polyps. Three genes have been associated with juvenile polyposis syndrome: *SMAD4*, *BMPR1A*, and *ENG*.[60] The World Health Organization defines juvenile polyposis syndrome as any of 3 conditions:

1. more than 3 to 10 juvenile polyps in the colon or rectum,
2. juvenile polyps outside of the colon, or
3. any number of juvenile polyps in a person with a family history of juvenile polyposis syndrome.[60]

Twenty percent to 50% of patients with juvenile polyposis syndrome will have a family history of the disease with a mean age at presentation of 18.5 years.[60] Many patients will by asymptomatic but others will present with symptoms, including rectal bleeding, anemia, abdominal pain, diarrhea, intussusception, obstruction, and polyp prolapse through the anus.[60] Patients with the syndrome are at increased risk of developing colorectal, gastric, small intestinal, and pancreatic carcinoma. However, the juvenile polyp does not appear to be a premalignant lesion but is rather a marker for the development of adenomatous and carcinomatous change in the GI epithelium.[60] One group has reported a 38% risk of colorectal cancer risk and a 55% cumulative risk of GI cancer in patients with juvenile polyposis syndrome, with a mean age of 43 years (age range, 17-68 years).[275] In patients with gastric polyps, the incidence of gastric carcinoma is more than 20%.[276]

Polyp size can range from several millimeters to at least 3 cm in diameter and are found predominantly in the colon but can also be discovered in the stomach and small bowel.[27] Their imaging appearance on oral contrast examinations, CT, and MRI is similar to that of other causes of GI polyps.

PTEN hamartoma tumor syndrome: PTEN hamartoma tumor syndrome is a new term to describe 2 disorders, Cowden syndrome and Banya-Riley-Ruvalcaba syndrome that are now known to be a result of mutations in the PTEN gene, a tumor suppressor gene.[60] Both Cowden syndrome and Banya-Riley-Ruvalcaba syndrome are rare, autosomally dominantly inherited disorders characterized by multiple GI juvenile polyps and a variety of extraintestinal manifestations. In both cases, the extraintestinal manifestations are the dominant clinical finding. Cowden syndrome is characterized by macrocephaly, mucocutaneous lesions (especially trichilemmoma), acral keratosis, papillomatous papules, and glycogenic acanthosis of the esophagus. Neoplasms and other disorders of the thyroid gland, breast, and endometrium are also seen in Cowden syndrome. Banya-Riley-Ruvalcaba syndrome is characterized by macrocephaly, developmental delays, pigmented speckling of the penis, and lipomas and hamartomatous polyps of the intestine.

Cronkhite-Canada syndrome: Cronkhite-Canada syndrome is a rare systemic disease characterized by diffuse GI hamartomatous polyps, dystrophic changes in the fingernails, alopecia, cutaneous hyperpigmentation, diarrhea, weight loss, and hyperpigmentation.[277] Unlike most other polyposis syndromes, it is not inherited and occurs primarily in older adults with a mean age of onset in the fifth to sixth decade. To date, approximately 400 cases have been reported worldwide—approximately 75% from Japan. There is evidence, such as elevated ANA and IG4 levels, to suggest that it is an autoimmune disorder of unknown cause. Morbidity and mortality is primarily related to chronic diarrhea and protein-losing enteropathy; however, some individuals can develop associated malignancies. The incidence of secondary malignancy may be as high as 15%, primarily tumor of the colon and stomach. Polyps are most commonly found in the colon and stomach but can occasionally be found in the small intestine.

Inflammatory polyps

Inflammatory polyps are a result of the healing process of ulcerative colitis and Crohn disease. Widespread mucosal ulceration from either Crohn disease or ulcerative colitis sometimes leaves linear zones of surviving tissue separated by denuded mucosa. With healing, the regions of spared mucosa form multiple linear tendrils of tissue projecting into the lumen of the colon. These lesions have been termed inflammatory pseudopolyps and demonstrate a characteristic "filiform" appearance (see Figure 2-36).[16,278-282] Inflammatory bowel disease is discussed most completely later in this chapter under the heading **Long-Segment Wall Thickening of the Small Bowel and Colon**.

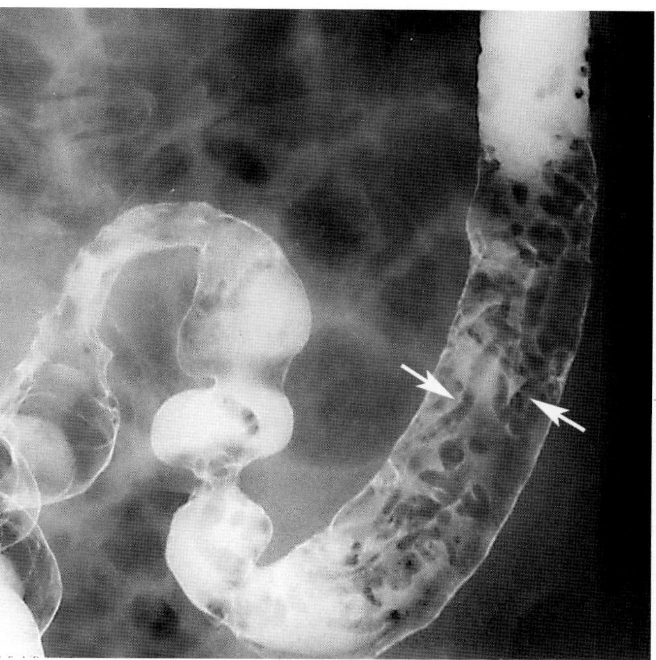

Figure 2-36 Filiform Polyps due to Crohn Colitis
This 45-year-old man had a long history of poorly controlled ulcerative colitis. This image from a double-contrast barium enema shows multiple wormlike or "filiform" filling defects within the descending and sigmoid colon. These represent multiple inflammatory polyps as a result of his ulcerative colitis.

Adenoma and adenocarcinoma

Colorectal adenocarcinoma is the third most commonly diagnosed malignancy among both men and women, and the second leading cause of cancer-related death in the United States. Although improved screening has led to a slow decline in the incidence and mortality of colorectal cancer, approximately 40% of the eligible US population do not receive screening.[283]

Pathophysiology of colon cancer and screening strategies: The adenoma-carcinoma sequence refers to a series of genetic mutations whereby small adenomatous colon polyps (<5 mm) transform into large adenomatous polyps (>1 cm), noninvasive carcinomas, and then invasive carcinomas. This sequence takes an average of 10 years to evolve.[284] It is believed that up to 90% of colorectal carcinomas develop through the adenoma-carcinoma sequence.[285,286]

Adenomatous lesions of the colon typically have a tubular histology but in some cases will have a villous histology. Villous adenomas carry a higher risk of malignant degeneration than tubular adenomas or tubulovillous adenomas.

Given that colon cancer develops through the adenoma-carcinoma sequence, this disease is virtually preventable through regular screening. The American Cancer Society colorectal cancer screening guidelines include optical colonoscopy every 10 years or DCBE and CTC at 5-year intervals.[287] Regardless of the methodology utilized to perform screening, the importance of visualizing the entire colon cannot be underscored. Approximately 5% of patients with colorectal cancers have synchronous colonic carcinomas, and more than one-third of these patients have other adenomatous polyps in the colon.[288-290] In addition, half of colon cancers are located proximal to the descending colon.[291] Therefore, CTC or barium enema for patients with failed incomplete optical colonoscopy is imperative to ensure proper screening. Once the diagnosis of colorectal cancer is made, careful follow-up is merited, as approximately 5% of patients will develop metachronous carcinomas at a later point in time.[288]

Risk factors for colon cancer: Age is the biggest risk factor for both diagnosis and mortality due to colorectal cancer. More than 90% of new cases and 94% of deaths attributable to colorectal cancer occur in individuals 50 and older, which has led to the recommendation that screening for colorectal carcinoma begin at the age of 50.[292] Other risk factors in the general population include diets high in fat or low in fiber and calcium, obesity, low levels of physical activity, tobacco smoking, and high alcohol intake (see Table 2-6).[293] The lifetime risk of colorectal cancer doubles among patients with 1 first-degree relative with colorectal cancer and quadruples among patients with more than 1 first-degree relative with colorectal cancer or a first-degree relative who was diagnosed below the age of 45.[294,295] Hereditary syndromes such as familial adenomatous polyposis, hereditary nonpolyposis colorectal cancer syndrome, and MutY homolog polyposis account for 6% of colorectal carcinoma.[263] In addition, patients with IBD, including chronic ulcerative colitis and Crohn colitis, also have at least double the risk of developing colorectal cancer.[296]

Table 2-6. Risk Factors for Colorectal Carcinoma

1. Age >50
2. High-fat, low-fiber, low-calcium diet
3. Obesity
4. Low levels of physical activity
5. Tobacco smoking
6. High alcohol consumption

Imaging Notes 2-9. Polyp Size and Risk of Colon Carcinoma

<5 mm	66% nonadenomas/34% adenomas
5-10 mm	<1% risk of carcinoma
10-20 mm	10%-20% risk of carcinoma
>20 mm	40%-50% risk of carcinoma

Size is the most important imaging feature, indicating the risk that a polyp contains malignancy. Approximately 34% of polyps measuring ≤5 mm and 60% of polyps ≥6 mm represent adenomas.[297] Among these, the number of adenomatous polyps that will undergo malignant transformation into colorectal cancer is roughly 3%.[298] Therefore, short of direct sampling, size is the most important determinant of malignancy potential. Specifically, fewer than 1% of adenomas less than 1 cm harbor adenocarcinoma, 10% to 20% of adenomas 1 to 2 cm in diameter harbor adenocarcinoma and 40% to 50% of those greater than 2 cm in diameter harbor adenocarcinoma.[284-286] As adenomatous polyps grow, they will cause eccentric thickening of the bowel wall, producing a semiannular carcinoma, which, over time, will progress to a circumferential or annular carcinoma (see Figure 2-37).

Clinical features of colon cancer: Presenting symptoms include vague abdominal pain, evidence of GI bleeding such as melena or hematochezia, or evidence of bowel obstruction such as nausea, vomiting, early satiety, or colicky abdominal pain. Some patients will be discovered while still asymptomatic either on screening examinations or accidentally on examinations performed for reasons unrelated to the presence of the cancer.

Metastatic disease is detected on initial presentation, in less than 15% of cases, and is usually suggested by symptoms, including right upper quadrant pain, abnormality on physical examination, such as hepatomegaly, or abnormal laboratory tests, especially elevations in liver function tests and carcinoembryonic antigen levels.[299-301] The liver is the most common site of colorectal cancer metastases because the portal vein receives the majority of colonic venous drainage. Other common sites of metastasis include the lungs, adrenal glands, and bones. Because the rectum has dual venous drainage via the superior hemorrhoidal vein into the portal venous system and the middle and inferior hemorrhoidal veins, which drain into the inferior vena cava, rectal cancer has a predilection to cause lung metastasis directly without the presence of liver metastasis.

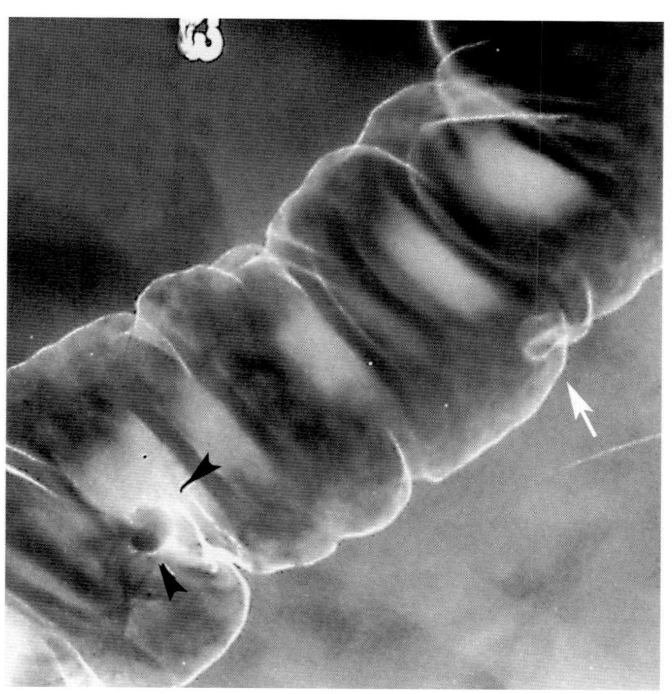

A

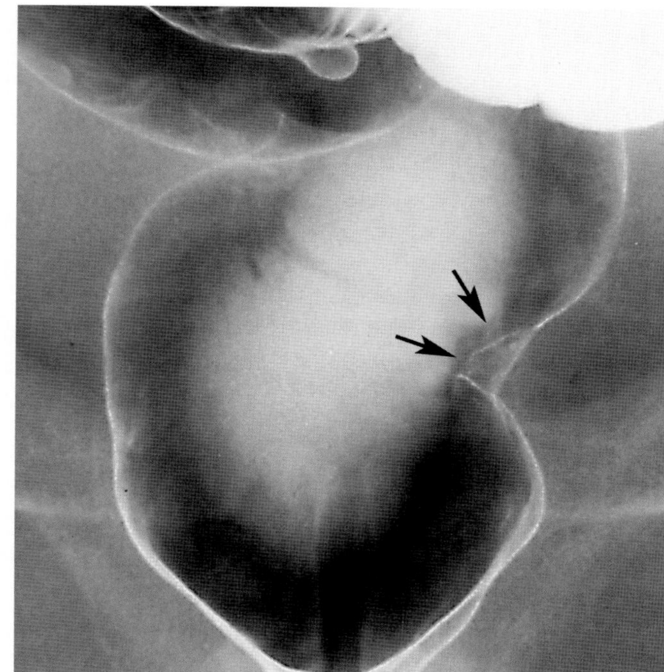

B

C

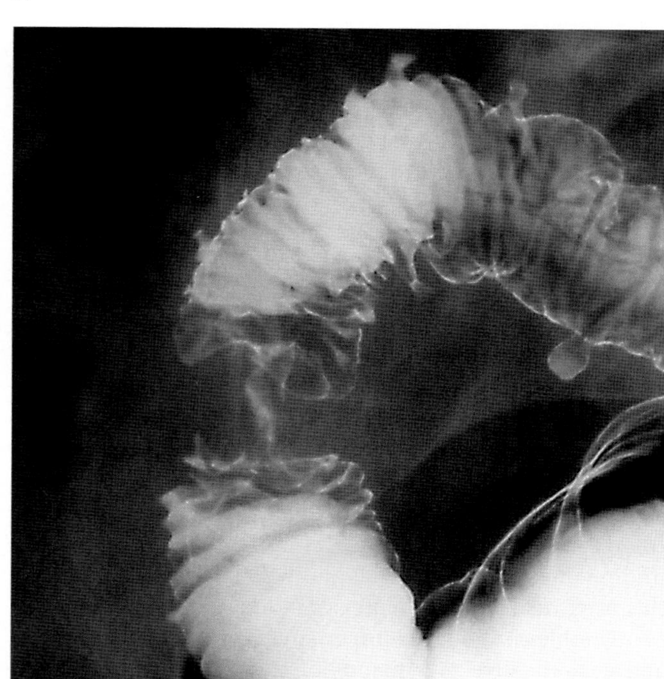

D

Figure 2-37 Barium Enema Features of Adenomas and Adenocarcinomas in 4 Patients
A. Screening barium enema shows a small bowler hat polyp (*white arrow*) and a small polyp as a filling defect in the barium pool (*black arrowheads*). Both represented small adenomas. **B.** This 64-year-old man had hematochezia. Double-contrast barium enema shows a thin curvilinear line along the left lateral wall of the rectum suggesting a small flat lesion. This appearance could have represented adherent feces, but biopsy was diagnostic of an adenoma. **C.** Screening barium enema in a third patient shows a large polyp of the cecum (*black arrowheads*), which was biopsied and shown to represent an adenocarcinoma. **D.** This 55-year-old man had melena. Double-contrast barium enema shows a short-length, abruptly shouldered stricture of the sigmoid colon. This resembles an apple core and is the typical appearance of an annular carcinoma of the colon. Biopsy was diagnostic of an adenocarcinoma.

Recurrent disease occurs in 37% to 44% of patients[302-304] within 2 years of surgical resection.[299] Up to half of recurrent disease (19%-48%) will occur locally at the surgical site, with the remaining disease (25%-44%) occurring distant to the primary disease.[299] Hematogenous metastasis involves primarily the liver in 20% of all patients, followed by the peritoneum, and then the lungs.[76] In general, multiple sites of recurrence are more common than a single site of disease. Fewer than 20% of patients with recurrent colon cancer are eligible for repeat surgical resection with curative intent. Of those patients who undergo repeat resection, long-term survival is demonstrated in only 30% of cases.[263,305,306]

Currently, CT remains the standard of care in detecting colorectal recurrence. However, recent studies have shown that PET-CT adds clinical value over routine enhanced CT in the detection of recurrent intrahepatic metastatic disease, extrahepatic metastases, and local recurrence at the initial surgical site.[307] FDG-PET has demonstrated a sensitivity (93%) for colorectal metastasis that is comparable to intraoperative ultrasound (89%) and higher than CT or MRI (78%).[306,308] FDG-PET has also demonstrated value in the monitoring of chemotherapy response for advanced colorectal cancer and multimodality treatment response for rectal cancer.[309]

Although a number of combined clinical and imaging surveillance strategies following resection of colon cancer have been reported, there is little consensus on what constitutes the optimal surveillance strategy. In part, this lack of consensus stems from studies showing that although intense follow-up, including routine imaging, leads to a higher proportion of resectable tumor recurrence,[310] there is no significant difference in survival between those patients with resected disease versus those who were unresectable.[71,72] In addition, the costs associated with this intense follow-up are high.[311,312]

Imaging features of colon cancer: Colon cancers can be identified on a variety of imaging modalities including DCBE, CT, CTC, and MRI. Both DCBE and CTC are used as screening methods for detecting colonic polyps, whereas colon cancer can be detected on CT or MRI as an incidental finding or as part of the evaluation of abdominal symptoms that are caused by the colon carcinoma.

Double-contrast barium enema is both widely available and cost-effective as a means of colorectal cancer screening.[290,313] Optical colonoscopy detects 85% to 95% of polyps and DCBE detects 50% to 90% of polyps 5 to 10 mm in diameter. Although DCBE is less sensitive than optical colonoscopy at detecting polyps less than 1 cm, it does detect most advanced adenomas and cancers.[285] DCBE has a sensitivity of 71% for polyps larger than 7 mm[314] and a sensitivity of 81% for polyps larger than 1 cm.[315] In the 2 largest national trials comparing same-day CTC and optical colonoscopy, the sensitivity of CTC for polyps ≥10 mm using optical colonoscopy as the reference standard ranges from 90% to 94.0% and for polyps ≥6 mm ranges from 80% to 89%.[7,10,316]

Routine CT and MRI do not play a role in primary screening for colorectal cancer because they are insensitive for the detection of colonic polyps and demonstrates variable sensitivity in the detection of primary colon cancer depending on tumor size.[299,317-321] However, routine CT is commonly used for the following indications: (1) evaluation of disease complications, (2) aiding surgical planning through identification of hematogenous or distant nodal metastatic disease and visualization of regional tumor extension or invasion into adjacent organs, (3) detection of recurrent disease, and (4) monitoring lesions during and after surgery, chemotherapy, or radiation therapy.[299]

Colorectal cancer can present with a variety of imaging appearances. Studies of barium enemas have shown that more than half of colon carcinomas will appear as annular or semiannular lesions, 38% as polypoid lesions, and 9% as plaquelike or carpet lesions (see Figure 2-37).[291] If the carcinoma is nonobstructive, the entire colon should be evaluated using DCBE or CTC to search for synchronous colonic neoplasms. However, when annular lesions are associated with signs of obstruction, a limited single-contrast examination is sufficient to confirm the presence of an obstructive lesion and to determine its location without causing harm to the patient.

On barium enema and CTC, adenomas and small carcinomas can appear as polyps that are indistinguishable from other causes of polyps. Rarely, routine CT will visualize large polyps as an enhancing soft-tissue nodule that has more uniform attenuation than adjacent stool (see Figure 2-38).[263]

In other cases, adenomas will appear as flat, broad-based, plaquelike lesions with little elevation of the mucosa and, on occasion, a central depression.[322,323] En face, these adenomas appear as curvilinear or undulating lines without other abnormality, which makes them very difficult to appreciate (see Figure 2-37). In Western populations, they account for approximately 10% of adenomatous polyps but in East Asia, they have a reported prevalence up to 48%.[322-326] There is some controversy as to whether these flat adenomas demonstrate an inherent increased predilection for severe dysplasia or carcinoma or if they simply carry an increased risk based on size >1 cm, similar to other adenomas.[324-330]

Flat polyps are challenging to discern on both CTC and optical colonoscopy.[325] On CTC, flat adenomas typically appear as shallow, plaquelike, broad-based lesions with height less than one-half its width (see Figure 2-39).[322,328] When they occur between folds, they present as a flat elevation or a focal area of wall thickening that protrudes into the lumen. When they present on or at the base of folds, they may appear simply as fold thickening. This can be challenging to detect on either polyp window or endoluminal views, particularly when they present as smooth fold thickening compared to irregular fold thickening.

On barium enemas, the villi of villous adenomas and carcinomas create a multitude of small crevices where oral contrast can collect. The majority of villous adenomas demonstrate a characteristic textured or granular appearance

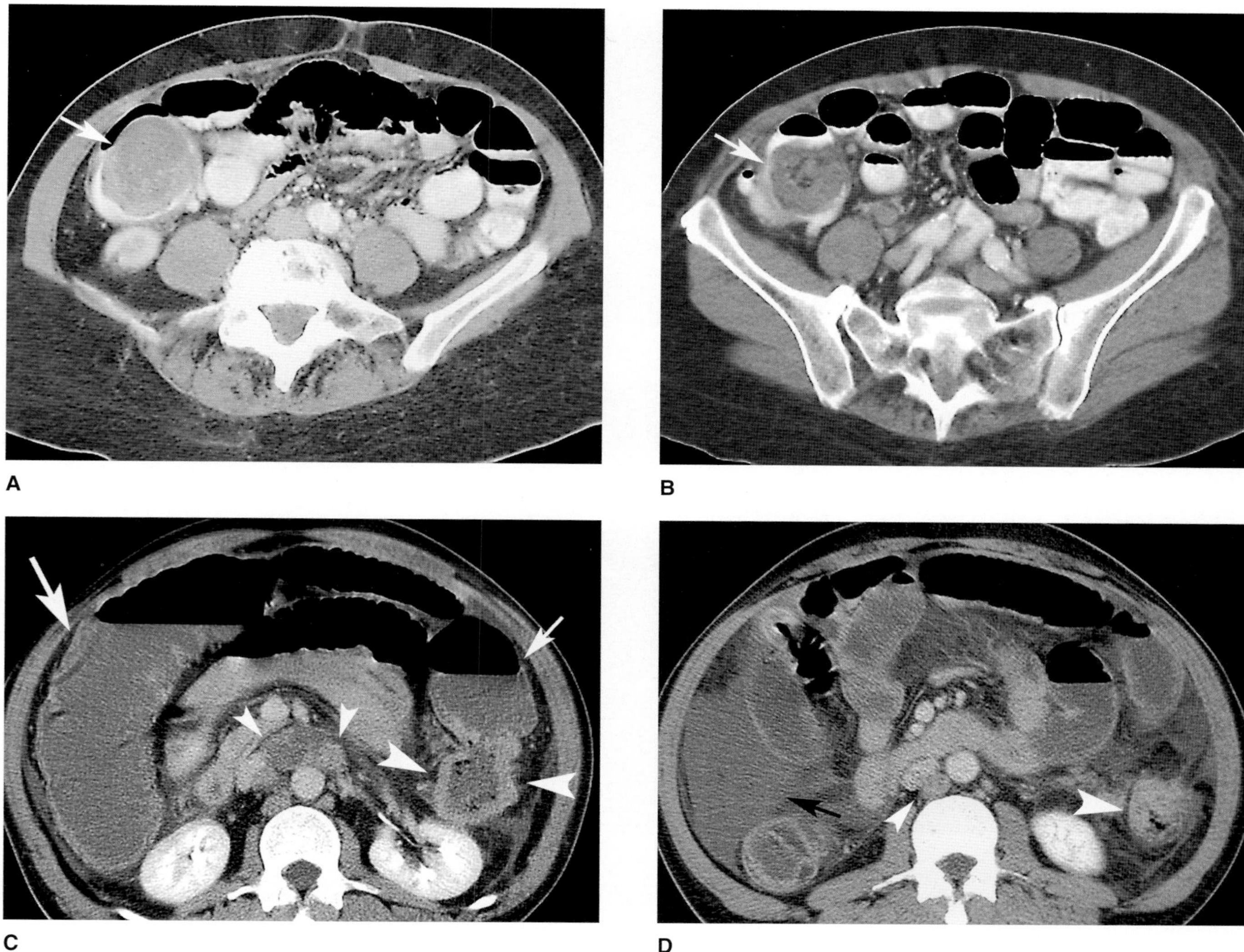

Figure 2-38 Colon Cancer Seen on CT in 2 Patients
A and **B.** This 76-year-old woman complained of abdominal pain and diarrhea. CT images demonstrate a 4-cm rounded mass (*arrows*) within the lumen of the cecum. Note the air and contrast that surrounds most of the mass. This identifies this lesion as a very large polyp or pedunculated mass. Colonoscopic biopsy was diagnostic of a poorly differentiated adenocarcinoma. **C** and **D.** This 49-year-old man complained of abdominal pain. CT images demonstrate a focal area of concentric bowel wall thickening in the mid-descending colon (*large white arrowheads*). In D, the descending colon is seen in cross section as a thick ring and in C, there is a transition from the normal thin wall of the colon (*small arrow*) to the abnormal thick wall (*arrowheads*), indicating the presence of an annular mass, probably a primary adenocarcinoma of the colon. There is infiltration of the pericolonic fat medial to the mass just above the arrowhead likely indicating local extension of the cancer. There are enlarged para-aortic lymph nodes (*small white arrowheads*), some of which appear hypoattenuating, suggesting lymphatic spread of cancer. The transverse colon (*large white arrow*) is distended, indicating bowel obstruction. Finally, there are pockets of ascites (*black arrow*) suggesting peritoneal metastasis. Surgical excision of the mass during therapy for the obstruction confirmed a diagnosis of adenocarcinoma.

on DCBE. Often, they are referred to as "carpet lesions" because of the fact that they often involve a large surface area and have a textured appearance similar to pile carpet. They are best appreciated when viewed en face and appear as coalescent nodules and plaques that produce a focal region of reticulated lines that is sharply demarcated from the normal surface mucosa.[331] In profile, these lesions have an irregular, serrated, contour in contrast with the smooth surface of the adjacent normal bowel (see Figure 2-40).[258] Villous lesions are most often located in the cecum, ascending colon, and rectum and have a propensity to undergo malignant degeneration.[332,333]

Similar to flat lesions, carpet lesions are difficult to detect with CTC.[332] On CTC, carpet lesions appear as homogenous attenuation, nodular, irregular fold thickening involving a focal region of the bowel wall.[332] Careful evaluation in the coronal, sagittal, and axial planes will improve detection of these lesions and help distinguish between

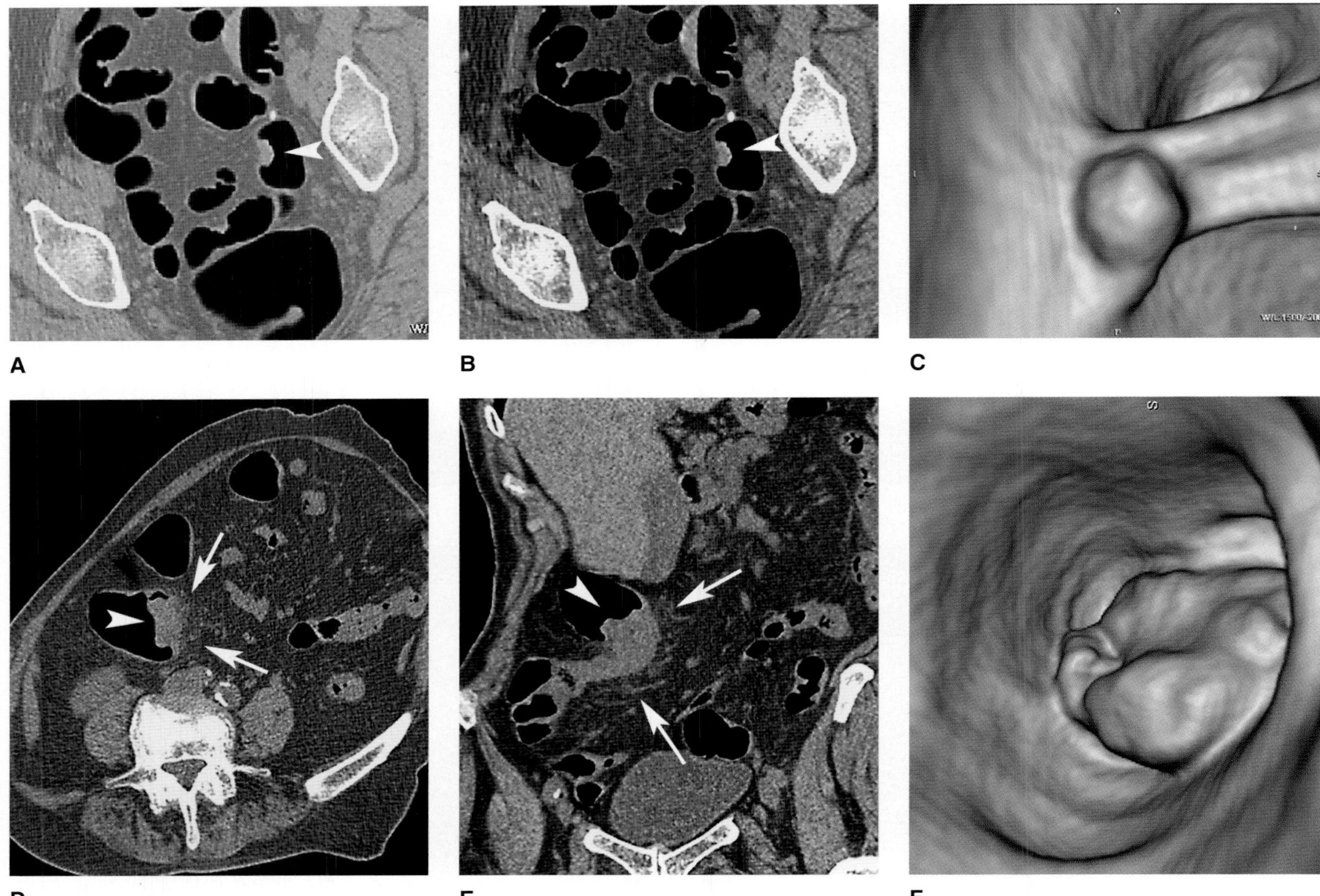

Figure 2-39 CT Colonography Appearance of Adenomas and Adenocarcinomas in 2 Patients
Sixty-nine-year-old woman with incomplete optical colonoscopy to the level of the sigmoid colon. **A.** Axial image at the level of the mid-sigmoid colon in polyp windows demonstrates a lesion projecting into the colon lumen (*white arrowhead*). **B.** Evaluation of the same level using soft-tissue window demonstrates that this lesion measures soft tissue in attenuation, reflecting a polyp (*white arrowhead*). **C.** 3D (endoluminal) appearance of the mass. On biopsy, this was found to be an adenomatous polyp. **D-F.** An 86-year-old woman on chronic anticoagulation for cardiac history presents for colon cancer screening. D. Axial CT image at the level of the ascending colon in polyp windows demonstrates a lobulated soft-tissue mass projecting into the colon lumen (*white arrowhead*) with asymmetric thickening of the colon wall (*black arrowhead*) and infiltration of the adjacent fat (*long white arrow*). E. Coronal images at the same level show that this mass is annular, involving a short segment of colon with abrupt shelflike borders (*white arrowhead*), near obliteration of the lumen, and asymmetric infiltration of the fat along the mesenteric border (*long white arrow*). F. A 3D endoluminal appearance of this mass illustrates the bulbous margins of the mass projecting into the lumen. On biopsy, this was found to represent an adenocarcinoma.

normal fold thickening and carpet lesions. Detection of these subtle lesions also requires optimal technique and a high index of suspicion (see Figure 2-40).

On barium examinations, **eccentric masses** will appear as irregularly marginated protrusions with shelflike margins into 1 side of the lumen of the bowel that resemble a saddle.[263] On CT and MRI, they will appear as a focal, irregularly marginated thickening of 1 side of the wall of the bowel in question.

Annular masses of the GI tract appear as a short segment of focal concentric thickening of the bowel wall. They are rare in the cecum and rectum because of the greater caliber of these bowel segments. On barium examination, annular adenocarcinomas demonstrate circumferential narrowing of the bowel with shelflike, overhanging borders, which resemble an "apple core" (see Figure 2-37). On CT, they are visualized as soft-tissue masses that involve the entire circumference of the bowel as confirmed on multiplanar imaging (see Figure 2-38).[263] In some cases, the mass will be centrally necrotic, with central low attenuation or gas that can mimic the appearance of an abscess.[263,299]

Colon cancers can mimic diverticulitis. On barium enemas, a long segment of luminal narrowing with smooth, tapered borders will favor a diagnosis of diverticulitis.

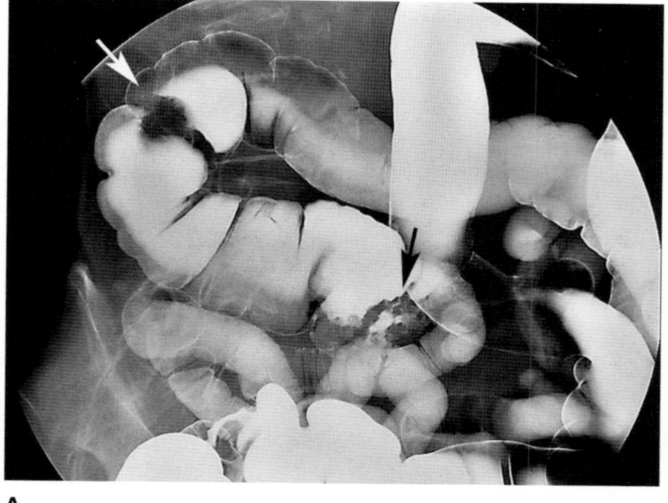

A

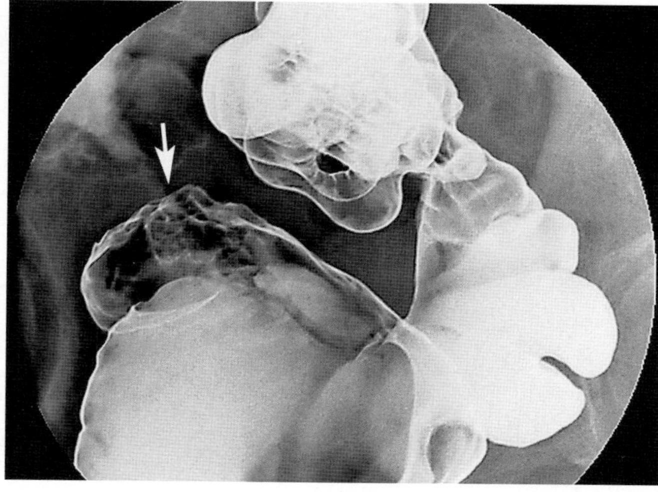

B

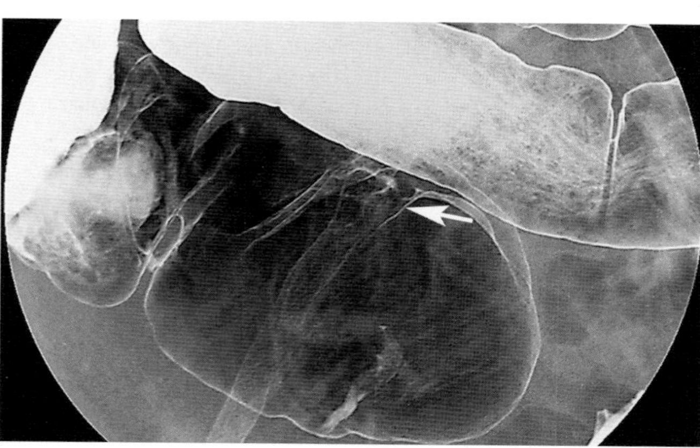

C

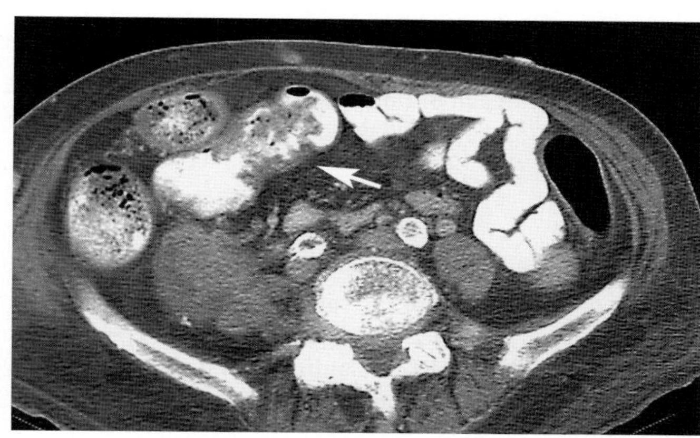

D

Figure 2-40 Carpet Lesions in 3 Patients
A. This 80-year-old woman had an annular sigmoid carcinoma diagnosed by colonoscopy. Single-contrast barium enema to evaluate the remainder of the colon shows a grapelike cluster of filling defects (*black arrow*) in the cecum, typical of a "carpet lesion" and a polypoid filling defect in the splenic flexure. Surgical biopsy demonstrated a villous adenoma and tubular adenoma, respectively. **B.** Double-contrast barium enema shows a textured surface to the wall of the rectum in this 32-year-old man. Biopsy was diagnostic of a villous adenoma. **C.** Double-contrast barium enema in this 77-year-old woman demonstrates a very subtle surface irregularity to the medial wall of the cecum. **D.** CT in the same patient as C shows a serrated plaquelike thickening of the cecal wall. Colonoscopic biopsy was diagnostic of a villous adenocarcinoma.

Conversely, a short segment of abrupt luminal narrowing with an irregular mucosal surface will favor a diagnosis of colon cancer. On CT, the presence of pericolonic fat stranding, fluid in the mesenteric root, and engorgement of the mesenteric vessels supplying the mass will favor a diagnosis of diverticulitis.[299] On the other hand, demonstration of pericolic lymph nodes will favor a diagnosis of colon cancer.[334] Despite these clues, it may not be possible to differentiate diverticulitis from colon cancer with barium enema (BE) or CT alone (see Figure 2-41). When findings are equivocal, endoscopy should be performed following treatment for diverticulitis to carry out direct tissue sampling and rule out an underlying carcinoma as the cause of these findings.[258,299]

Complications of primary colonic malignancies are well demonstrated on CT, including obstruction, perforation, and fistula formation (see Figure 2-38).[299] Intestinal obstruction is discussed later in this chapter under the heading **Bowel Dilation**. Colonic perforation can rarely result in pneumoperitoneum but typically appears as small air bubbles in the pericolic fat with adjacent fluid and mesenteric stranding.[335] On occasion, extravasation of oral contrast material can demonstrate the exact site of perforation.

A major advantage of performing preoperative CT is demonstration of local tumor involvement of adjacent organs, such as the bladder, vagina, and abdominal or pelvic musculature (see Figure 2-42).[299] Pericolic extension of tumor (T3 disease) can be suggested on CT or MRI by

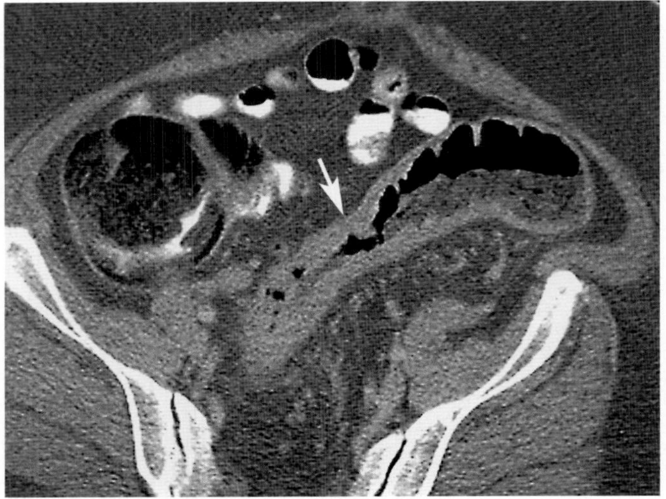

A

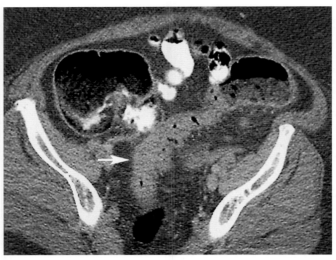

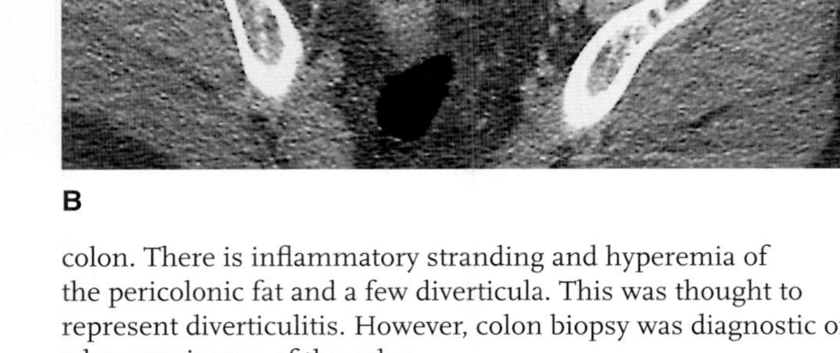

B

Figure 2-41 Adenocarcinoma Mimicking Diverticulitis This 58-year-old man complained of abdominal pain and pencil-like stools. **A** and **B.** Unenhanced axial CT images show a long segment of colonic wall thickening in the sigmoid colon. There is inflammatory stranding and hyperemia of the pericolonic fat and a few diverticula. This was thought to represent diverticulitis. However, colon biopsy was diagnostic of adenocarcinoma of the colon.

visualization of an extracolic mass, thickening and infiltration of pericolic fat, or loss of fat planes between the colon and adjacent organs (see Figures 2-38 and 2-42).[299] CT is more accurate than MRI in staging local tumor extension, particularly for rectal cancers and detection of penetration of the lamina propria.[336] However, the sensitivity of CT for local tumor extension is low (60%- 61%), with corresponding low specificity (60%-81%).[319,337] Low sensitivity for local tumor extension on CT likely reflects the inability to detect microscopic extramural tumor extension, whereas low specificity may reflect blurred fat planes due to inflammation or deep ulceration.[263]

CT and MRI are excellent at demonstrating enlarged lymph nodes in the abdomen and pelvis.[337] Knowledge of the lymphatic drainage of the colon and the site of the primary tumor can be used to predict the site of nodal metastases.[299,338,339] Lymphatic drainage parallels the venous drainage of the colon. Colon cancers first drain to the small lymph nodes on the antimesenteric border of the diseased region of colon (epicolic nodes) and then to lymph nodes in mesenteric fat just medial to the disease colon (paracolic lymph nodes) (see Figure 3-18). They then spread to the mesenteric lymph nodes adjacent to the draining arteries (mesenteric lymph nodes), then to the principal nodes at the SMA or IMA root and then finally ascend along the para-aortic and aortocaval nodes (see Figure 2-38).[338] Lymph node size greater than 1 cm has a high specificity (96%), but low sensitivity (25.9%), for detection of lymph node metastasis.[319] Unfortunately, FDG-PET has also been shown to have poor sensitivity in both T and N staging of colon cancer.[263,340,341]

All cross-sectional imaging examinations should be carefully evaluated for the presence of hematogenous metastasis. The viewer should pay careful attention to the liver, lungs, adrenals, and skeleton because these are the most common sites of metastasis.

Peritoneal tumor involvement occurs in up to 10% to 15% of patients at the time of diagnosis and approximately 40% to 70% among patients with recurrent disease.[263,342] Either ascites or nodular thickening of the peritoneum can be a sign of peritoneal spread (see Figure 2-38). Although, as discussed above, CT is the gold standard in the detection of recurrent disease, it is insensitive in the detection of early intraperitoneal metastases.[299]

The role of barium studies in evaluating for recurrent colorectal cancer is limited given that the most recurrent occurs extraluminally, next to or distant from the regions of resection of the primary tumor, rather than at the anastomosis itself.[343] Therefore, evaluation with CT or FDG-PET is of greater value in monitoring for recurrent disease than barium evaluation, or optical colonoscopy.[263,299,344]

On CT and MRI examinations, recurrent disease will appear as a soft-tissue mass in or near the surgical site. Differentiation between postsurgical change and recurrent disease is often difficult. In general, local recurrence is more masslike in appearance, whereas postsurgical fibrosis is more linear in appearance. In many cases, however, it is impossible to distinguish between postsurgical fibrosis and local recurrence on the basis of imaging appearance. When in doubt, it is reasonable to assume that abnormalities in the surgical bed that are found in the early postoperative period represent blood, granulation tissue, and scarring related to

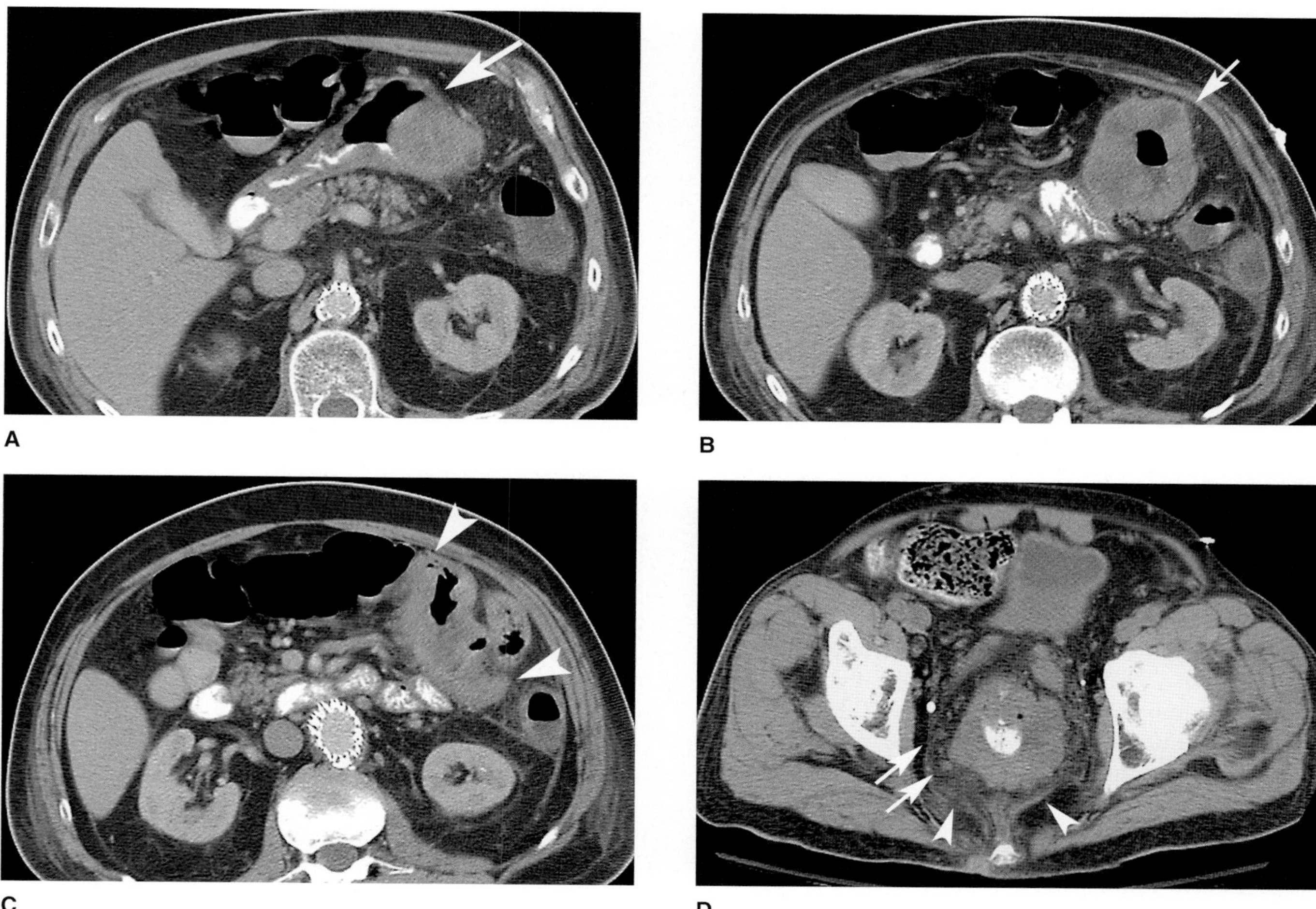

Figure 2-42 Pericolonic Extension of Colon Cancer in 2 Patients **A-C.** This 79-year-old man presented with abdominal pain. Contrast-enhanced axial CT images show a large cavitary mass (*small arrow*) that appears to involve both the stomach (*large arrow*) and the transverse colon (*arrowheads*). Differential diagnosis would include both an exophytic cavitary stomach mass such as gastric carcinoma, lymphoma, or GIST or a primary colon mass such as colon cancer, colonic lymphoma, or colonic GIST. The relatively long segment of colon wall thickening seen in **C** favors a colon primary. Surgical excision was diagnostic of an adenocarcinoma of the colon. **D.** This 69-year-old man presented with anemia. This CT image shows the rectal wall to be concentrically thickened. Other images showed this to be over a short segment of bowel. There is also fat stranding (*arrowheads*) and a cluster of small perirectal lymph nodes that are usually not present. These findings will usually indicate a rectal carcinoma with small perirectal lymph node metastasis. These findings were confirmed at surgical resection of the mass.

the recent surgery and/or radiation. This abnormality should remain stable or progressively diminish in size and conspicuity on subsequent studies. However, if on serial examinations this abnormality progresses, this should be assumed to represent local recurrence until proven otherwise.

Some studies have suggested that FDG-PET is useful in distinguishing postsurgical fibrotic/inflammatory changes from recurrent cancer and may be an alternative to serial CT or MRI examinations.[345] FDG-PET has a sensitivity of 96% and specificity of 76% for detecting recurrent colorectal cancer. Furthermore, in a meta-analysis including 8 studies with a pooled population of 698 patients, FDG-PET lead to a change management in nearly one-third of patients.[346] FDG-PET is particularly useful when recurrent disease is suspected in the setting of rising carcinoembryonic antigen (CEA) with negative CT where it has a sensitivity ranging between 70% and 100%.[76,347-350] The high utility of FDG-PET in this setting is due to both high levels of sensitivity in the detection of liver metastases as well as extrahepatic disease that often goes unnoticed in staging with CT or MRI.[76]

Rectal adenocarcinoma: Screening, diagnosis, and staging of rectal carcinoma overlaps significantly with that of colon cancer; however, rectal carcinomas does demonstrate some important differences that merit a separate discussion.

The first difference is that chemoradiation plays an important role in the preoperative management of patients with T3 and T4 disease in the United States because it downstages disease, decreases local recurrence, and allows sphincter-preserving surgery.[351,352]

The second difference is that the rectum is located in a confined anatomic space that is closer to other muscles and organs than the colon. As such, this can pose a challenge to accurate staging through imaging. CT demonstrates limited utility in local staging because of poor rectal soft-tissue contrast. T staging with CT, therefore, is relatively inaccurate in the absence of gross invasion of adjacent organs (T4); even then false-positive cases occur.[263] Greater than 50% of nodes containing metastases from rectal cancer are less than 5 mm in size.[353] Given the reliance of CT on size criteria, it is not surprising that CT is relatively insensitive for N staging (55%).[354] That said, the sensitivity of CT can be improved with the use of multiplanar reformats.[355]

MRI demonstrates superior soft-tissue contrast relative to CT. As a result, MRI is more sensitive than CT in predicting tumor invasion (97% vs 70%). However, MR is poor in distinguishing between T2 and early T3 lesions. Stranding of the mesorectal fat due to inflammation can be overstaged as T3 disease. Conversely, microscopic tumor extending into the mesorectal fat can go undetected and be understaged as T2.[263] Just as with CT, nodal staging is limited by size criteria.[353]

Endorectal ultrasound is the preferred modality for T-staging of rectal cancer in the United States with an accuracy 69% to 97%.[356] The major limitation of endorectal ultrasound is overstaging of T2 and T3 lesions because of confusion between peritumoral inflammatory changes and primary tumor.[357]

The third difference is that rectal cancer demonstrates higher rate of recurrence and morbidity than colon cancer.[358] Specifically, rectal cancer recurs in 4% to 30% of patients and is isolated in 25% to 50%.[263] Recurrent disease is difficult to detect on clinical examination and often involves major adjacent structures.

Detection of recurrent disease on MRI is challenging. Although MRI can usually differentiate between muscle and tumor using enhancement patterns, at times the distinction between tumor and posttreatment fibrosis and radiation change may be quite difficult. It is generally assumed that brisk enhancement of soft tissue in the surgical bed will represent residual or recurrent cancer, whereas poorly enhancing low T2 signal in the surgical bed will indicate the presence of postsurgical fibrosis. However, immature fibrosis can demonstrate brisk enhancement within 1 year of surgery[263] and, occasionally, pathologically proven regions of recurrent cancer can have low T2 signal.[359] As in colon cancer, FDG-PET has been shown to be useful in this setting to distinguish between treatment change and recurrent disease.

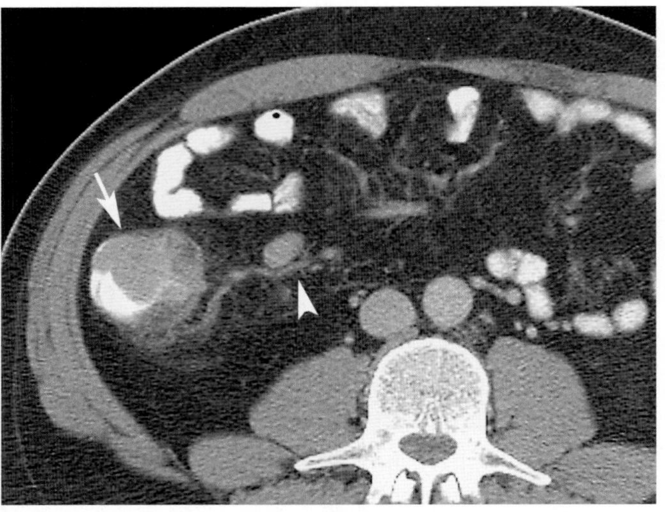

Figure 2-43 Cecal Carcinoid
CT scan in this 45-year-old woman demonstrated a semiannular mass involving the anterior wall of the cecum. There are enlarged pericecal mesenteric lymph nodes. In most cases, this would represent a primary adenocarcinoma. However, biopsy of the mass was diagnostic of a carcinoid tumor.

Carcinoid tumor

Carcinoid tumors of the colon are uncommon. The majority will arise in the rectum. Unlike the relatively more aggressive small-bowel carcinoids, carcinoid tumors of the rectum are often indolent lesions that present as incidental masses in asymptomatic patients.[85] Gastrointestinal carcinoids are discussed most completely under the previous heading **Focal Polyps and Masses of the Small Bowel** (see Figure 2-43).

Malignant melanoma

Malignant melanoma has a predilection for the small bowel, most often as a site of metastasis. Although melanoma is one of the most common malignancies to metastasize to the GI tract, it is less common in the colon (22%) than the small bowel (58%). When it does occur, only 0.8% of patients with clinically metastatic disease present with symptoms.[360] Occasionally, malignant melanoma will be discovered without evidence of a primary tumor of the skin. These are usually presumed to represent primary tumors of the bowel, but there is some evidence that they may represent metastasis with an unrecognized primary tumor.[361]

Colonic lymphoma

Primary lymphoma of the colon and rectum is very uncommon, comprising 0.4% of all colorectal malignancies and 6% to 12% of GI lymphomas.[362] When the colon is involved, lymphoma usually occurs in the cecum and the rectum. Most colonic lymphomas are B-cell in origin, T-cell lymphomas of

Imaging Notes 2-10. Imaging Features Distinguishing Colonic Lymphoma From Carcinoma

Feature	Lymphoma	Carcinoma
Distribution	Long segment	Short segment
Margins	Gradual tapering	Abrupt transition
Lymph nodes	Many, large	Fewer, smaller
Fat planes	Preserved	Infiltrated

the colon can occur rarely, although their preferential site of involvement in the GI tract is the small bowel.[93]

Lymphoma of the colon, similar to small bowel, can present with a diversity of imaging appearances on barium and CT. It may present as circumferential infiltration with or without ulceration. When the tumor is large in size, it may present as a cavitary mass with fistula formation into adjacent organs. Other appearances can range from a solitary polyp, to circumferential infiltration mimicking an annular carcinoma, to endoexoenteric tumors, which extend both endoluminally and/or project exophytically from the bowel wall. In some cases, colonic lymphoma will appear as only mucosal nodularity or fold thickening without a discrete mass.[362,363] Polypoid lymphomas typically occur near the ileocecal valve and can often result in intussusception.[364]

Distinguishing lymphoma from adenocarcinoma can be challenging. Features favoring lymphoma include (1) involvement of a long segment of bowel, particularly when the terminal ileum is included, (2) gradual transition from tumor to normal bowel, and (3) visualization of bulky mesenteric and retroperitoneal lymph nodes.[364] Additional distinguishing features include preservation of surrounding fat planes, absence of invasion into adjacent structures, and perforation without desmoplastic reaction.[365] Unlike colon carcinoma, bowel obstruction is unusual in patients with colonic lymphoma because of the absence of a desmoplastic response. Weakening of the muscularis propria can lead to aneurismal dilation of the bowel, a finding that is characteristic of bowel lymphoma. This is in contrast to the characteristic annular narrowing of the colon in adenocarcinoma.

In the colon, T-cell lymphoma is characterized by either diffuse or focal segmental wall thickening. On barium examination, T-cell lymphomas characteristically demonstrate extensive mucosal ulceration that can simulate IBD.[366] As is seen on other sites of the GI tract, T-cell lymphoma of the colon also has a predilection for perforation.[110]

Gastrointestinal stromal tumor

The anorectal region is the third most common location of GISTs.[85] The imaging appearance of anorectal GISTs is similar to that of GISTs elsewhere in the GI tract. On barium examinations, CT, and MRI, these tumors usually present as well-circumscribed mural masses that expand the rectal wall. When these tumors are small, they will present as concave masses with smooth borders and obtuse margins at the junction with the bowel wall, typical of a submucosal mass. As with GIST in other locations, larger lesions will frequently have central ulceration.[106] Larger tumors will often extend into the ischiorectal fossa, prostate, or vagina.[367] On CT, small masses will have a uniform attenuation both before and after contrast administration whereas larger masses demonstrate central low attenuation, reflecting central necrosis (see Figure 2-44). On MRI, these masses demonstrate uniform, intermediate T1 signal intensity, heterogeneous high T2 signal intensity, and heterogeneous enhancement following gadolinium administration.[368]

GI stromal tumors are discussed most completely under the headings **Polyps and Masses of the Stomach**.

Lipoma

Lipomas are uncommon, slow-growing submucosal tumors found throughout the GI tract that can be solitary or multiple in number.[123,124] Within the GI tract, the most common location for lipomas is the colon. Up to three-fourths of lipomas are found in the colon, mainly in the cecum and ascending colon.[123,125] True lipomas of the ileocecal valve are less common than lipomatous hypertrophy of the valve, but can be discerned as a discrete mass arising from the valve rather than generalized fatty enlargement of the entire valve.[124] After the colon, these tumors are most commonly found in the small bowel, particularly the ileum, and then the stomach.[123,125] Most lipomas are discovered incidentally in asymptomatic patients. However, lesions greater than 2 cm can ulcerate, causing chronic anemia, or serve as a lead point for intussusception.[123,124]

Greater than 90% of lipomas are submucosal in location and will appear as smooth, sharply marginated ovoid masses on barium studies, CT, and MRI. However, because of their location superficial to the muscularis propria, regular peristaltic contractions of the bowel can propel lipomas into the bowel lumen, resulting in a polypoid lesion on a pseudopedicle.[124] As with lipomas found in the subcutaneous soft tissues, these lesions can change shape or demonstrate compressibility during fluoroscopic examination. Lobulated surface ulcerations are a characteristic finding of lipomas on fluoroscopy; however, these usually are seen only in lesions larger than 2 cm. Overall, lipomas can be difficult to visualize on fluoroscopy because of the high voltage that obscures the low density of the lesion.[123,124] On cross-sectional imaging, lipomas demonstrate the characteristic imaging features of mature fat on every modality, including homogenous attenuation between -80 and -120 Hounsfield units (HU) on CT;[123,124] increased echogenicity of fat outlined by the bowel lumen providing a doughnut,

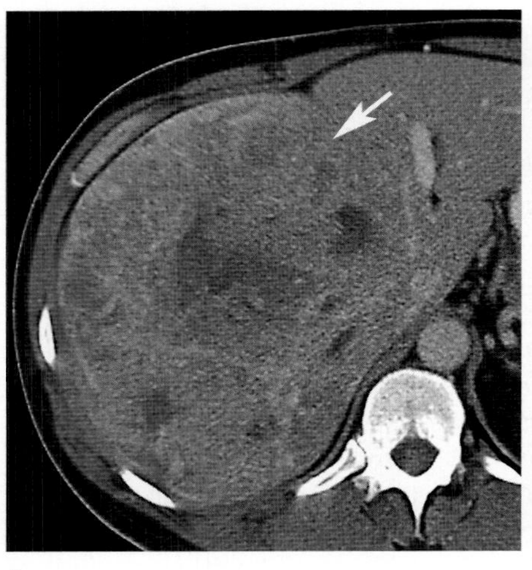
A

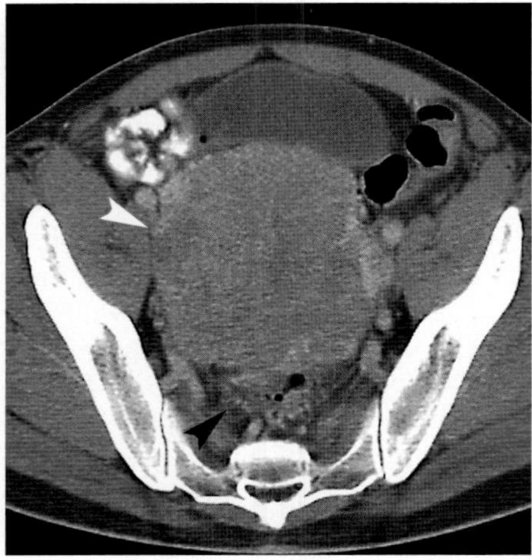
B

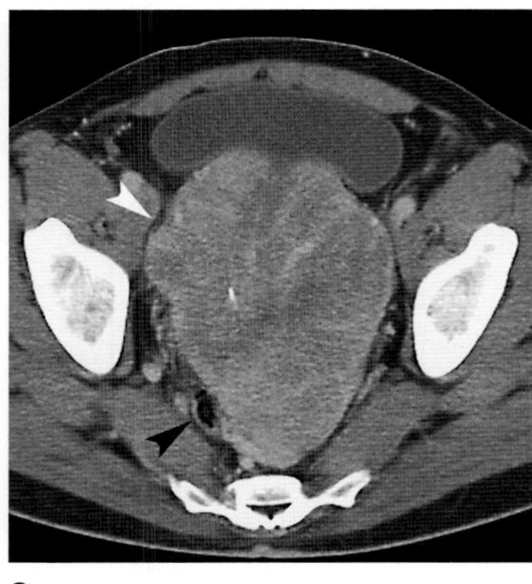
C

Figure 2-44 Malignant GIST of the Colon
This 45-year-old man complained of fatigue, nausea, and diarrhea. **A-C.** Contrast-enhanced axial CT images show a large heterogeneous mass (*white arrowheads*) in the pelvis that is directly adjacent to the sigmoid colon (*black arrowheads*). In a woman, this appearance would most often represent an exophytic uterine leiomyoma or leiomyosarcoma. However, in a man this is most likely to represent either a GIST of the colon or a soft tissue sarcoma of the retroperitoneal soft tissues. There is also a large heterogeneous mass in the liver, likely to represent a metastasis from the pelvic tumor. Biopsy of the mass was diagnostic of a GIST.

"pseudokidney," or target sign on US;[369] and signal isointense to submucosal fat on all sequences, with characteristic signal dropout on fat-suppressed images on MRI examinations (see Figure 2-45).

Other mesenchymal tumors of the colon

The vast majority of mesenchymal tumors of the colon will represent GISTs or lipomas. However, rarely, true leiomyomas, leiomyosarcomas, schwannomas, and neurofibromas occur within in the colon. These tumors will typically have an appearance that is indistinguishable from GISTs.

Focal infections of the bowel

Focal infections of the bowel are among the most common disorders of the abdomen, and imaging studies, especially CT, are currently the method of choice for their diagnosis. The 2 most common focal infectious entities are diverticulitis and appendicitis.

Diverticulitis: Pulsion diverticula, outpouchings of the colon wall occurring at the site of perforating vessels, are a common acquired abnormality of the colon. These outpouchings can become superinfected, leading to a focal infection of the bowel wall, known as diverticulitis. Diverticulosis, the presence of diverticula, is discussed in greater detail later in this chapter under the heading **Diverticula and Ulcers of the Colon.**

Diverticulitis most often occurs in the sigmoid colon, because this is the most frequent site of colonic diverticula but can be seen less frequently in every part of the colon, except the rectum. Diverticulitis typically presents as the acute onset of left lower quadrant abdominal pain and fever.[370] Of note, if the diverticulitis involves the right side of the colon, pain will be right sided and may be confused with appendicitis. Less common symptoms include alterations in bowel habits, anorexia, nausea, and vomiting. Immunocompromised individuals will often have fewer signs and symptoms of diverticulitis, presumably because of the reduced inflammatory response. As a consequence, these individuals are more likely to present later in the disease course and with complications of diverticulitis, especially perforation and pneumoperitoneum.[371]

Management of diverticulitis is dependent on the presence or absence of complications. Uncomplicated diverticulitis will resolve with dietary modification and oral or IV antibiotics in 70% to 100% of patients.[372,373] Complications of diverticulitis include the development of abscesses, fistulae, bowel obstruction, and free intra-abdominal perforation. Abscesses will develop in approximately 15% of patients.[374,375] Abscesses that are less than 2 cm in diameter will typically resolve with antibiotics alone. However, larger abscesses will usually require percutaneous or surgical drainage. Approximately one-third of patients who are successfully treated for diverticulitis will subsequently develop a second bout of diverticulitis. Unfortunately, elective surgery does not appear to reduce the incidence of subsequent episodes of diverticulitis.[373,376]

Diverticulitis initially results in inflammatory thickening of a focal segment of the bowel wall resulting in narrowing of the bowel lumen. These findings overlap with those of colon carcinoma. Therefore, differentiation of diverticulitis from colon carcinoma is a challenging but

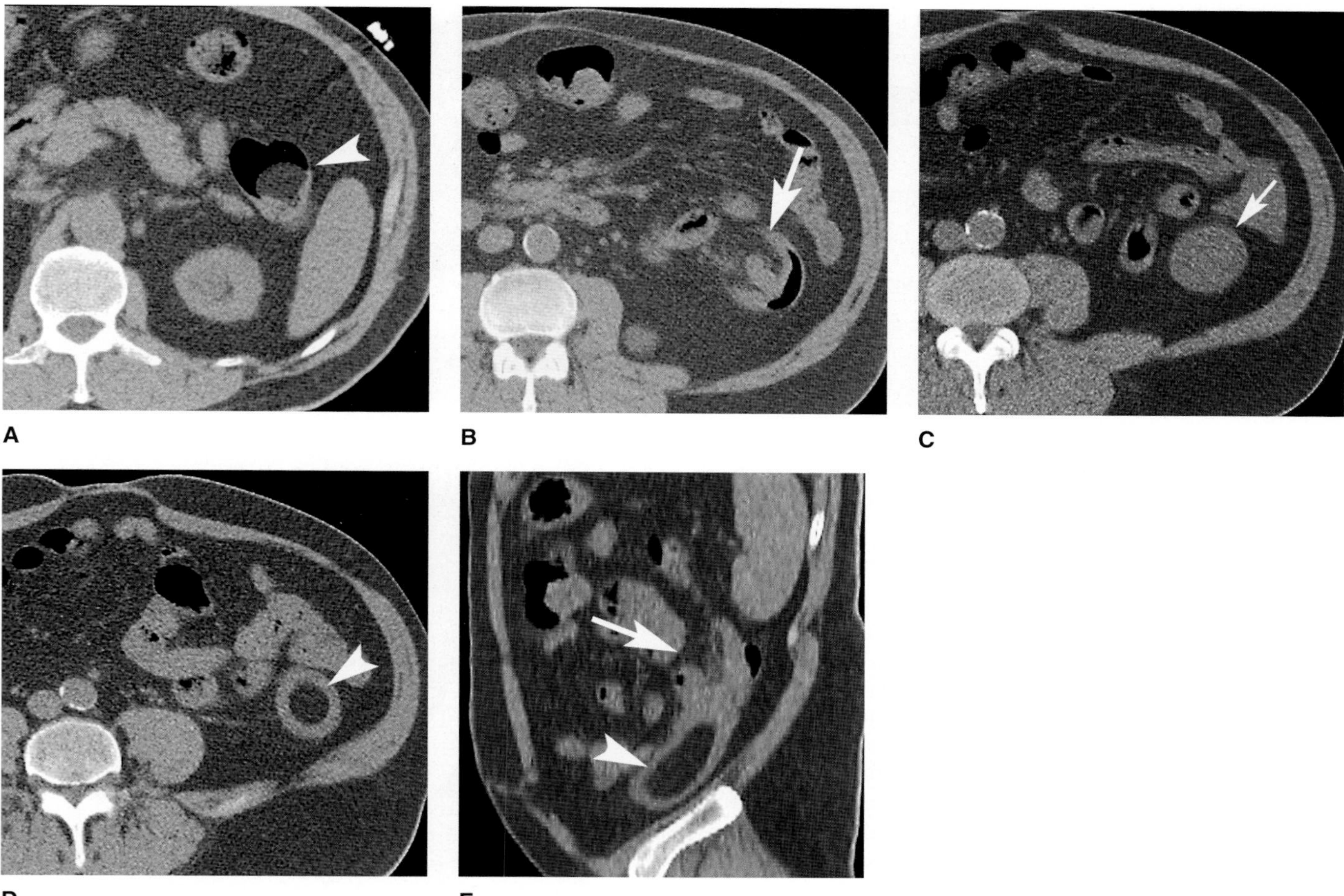

Figure 2-45 Colonic Lipoma with Transient Intussusception This 58-year-old man was asymptomatic and received 2 abdominal CT examinations 1 day apart as part of a research protocol. **A.** Noncontrast CT on day 1 shows a smoothly marginated spherical fatty mass (*arrowhead*) projecting into the lumen from the wall of the descending colon, findings typical of a small lipoma. **B-D.** Axial images on day 2 show involution of the colonic mesentery (*large arrow*) into the lumen of the colon, a portion of the nonfatty wall of the colon within the colonic lumen (*small arrow*) and the lipoma (*arrowhead*) at the leading edge of an intussusception. **E.** These findings are more readily seen on this sagittal reconstruction with lipoma (*arrowhead*) and intussuscepting mesentery (*arrow*). This patient had transient, clinically silent intussusception.

important task in the evaluation of suspected diverticulitis. On barium enema examinations, diverticulitis will characteristically appear as a long segment of inflamed bowel with smooth tapered margins and luminal narrowing of the bowel wall with preserved colonic folds (see Figure 2-46). Conversely, colon cancer will typically appear as a short segment of wall thickening with abrupt margins and loss of normal colonic folds.

CT features of diverticulitis include wall thickening, wall hyperemia, pericolonic fat stranding, mesenteric vascular engorgement, and accumulations of fluid in the bowel mesentery. In diverticulitis, wall thickening is relatively smooth and concentric as opposed to the severe, irregular, and eccentric wall thickening of colon carcinoma. As with other inflammatory processes, hyperemia of the colon wall can be visualized. An important distinguishing feature between diverticulitis and colon cancer is the extent of pericolonic fat stranding, manifest as irregular linear areas of increased attenuation in the pericolonic fat. Fat stranding is disproportionately greater than the degree of wall thickening in diverticulitis and is disproportionately less than the degree of wall thickening in colon cancer (see Figure 2-46).[377] Accumulation of small amounts of fluid in the colonic mesentery is a characteristic feature of diverticulitis and rarely found in colon cancer. This fluid typically assumes a comma shape and is known as the "comma sign."[377] Finally, engorgement of the mesenteric vessels is a common feature of inflammatory bowel disorders and can be seen with diverticulitis as well as Crohn disease and ulcerative colitis. Of note, mesenteric fluid and vascular engorgement are not features of colon cancer, and their presence in the setting of focal colonic wall thickening favors a diagnosis of diverticulitis.

Imaging Notes 2-11. Differentiation of Colon Cancer From Diverticulitis

Colon Cancer	Diverticulitis
Diverticula ±	Diverticula always present
Short segment	Longer segment
Abrupt margins	Tapered margins
Little/no fat stranding	Fat stranding very common
Mesenteric adenopathy common	Mesenteric adenopathy less common
Adjacent abscess rare	Adjacent abscess moderately common
Presentation: melena/hematochezia	Presentation: fever/abdominal pain

On any imaging evaluation, the absence of diverticula should dissuade the reader from a diagnosis of diverticulitis and should suggest alternative diagnoses.

If the infection is left untreated, complications can occur, including diverticular abscess, colovesical fistula, and perforation. CT is best for depicting these complications as compared to barium enema. Abscesses will appear as organized collections containing air fluid levels or low attenuation that corresponds to necrotic debris surrounded by thick enhancing walls. Fistulas may form between the diseased bowel segment and the bladder or adjacent small bowel. In most cases, the fistula will not be directly visualized. Occasionally, small tracts of air contrast can be seen in the soft tissues of the abdomen. Gas in the bladder can be a clue to a diagnosis of a colovesical fistula. In most cases, colonic perforation associated with diverticulitis will result in small extraluminal pockets of air or extravasation of oral contrast material. Pneumoperitoneum is a rare manifestation of diverticulitis-related perforation.[278] This is believed to be because the extensive pericolonic inflammation induced by diverticulitis seals the colon off from the peritoneum. Immunocompromised patients are more prone to the development of pneumoperitoneum related to diverticulitis, possibly because of the reduced inflammatory response.[371]

Appendicitis: Appendicitis is among the most common causes of surgically important acute abdominal pain. It is most often discovered in teenagers and young adults and is a result of obstruction of the appendiceal lumen with secondary ischemia and infection. Patients typically present with acute right lower quadrant abdominal pain, with or without fevers. Physical examination will usually show evidence of rebound tenderness, indicating secondary focal peritonitis.

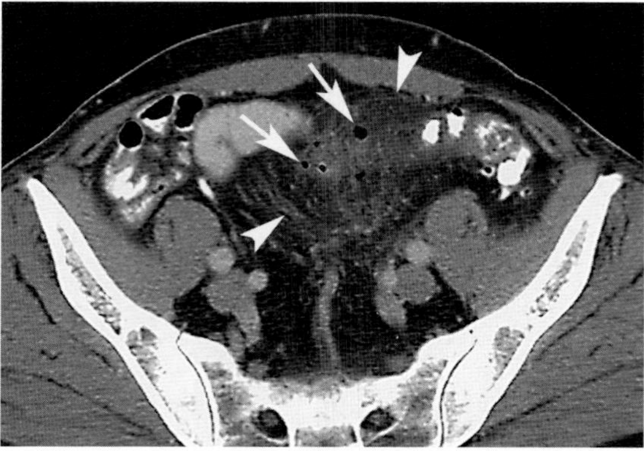

A

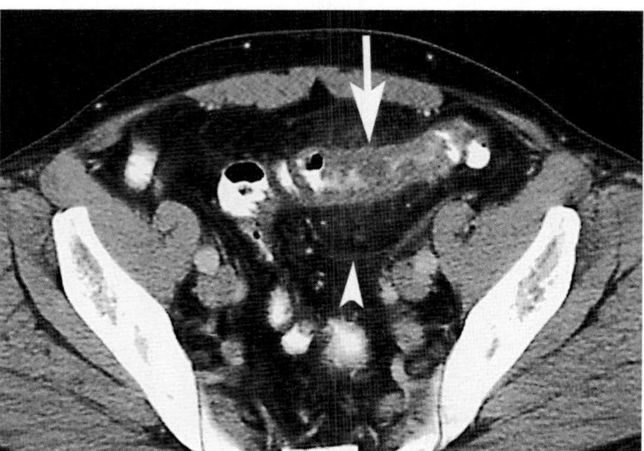

B

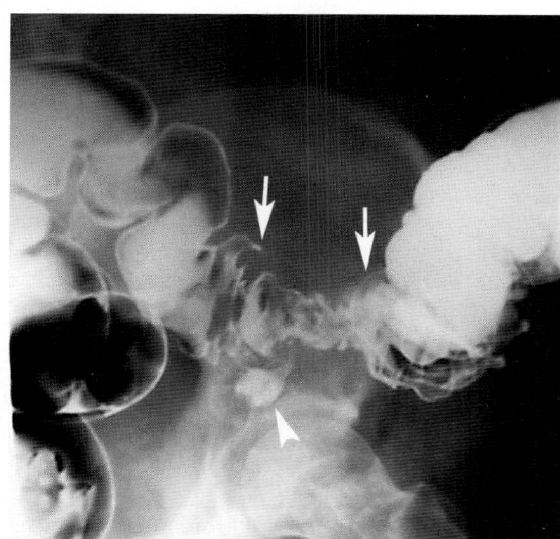

C

Figure 2-46 Diverticulitis
This 49-year-old man presented with abdominal pain, nausea, and vomiting. **A** and **B.** CT images through the pelvis show a focal region of wall thickening of the sigmoid colon (*large arrow*) with extensive pericolonic fat stranding (*arrowheads*) and several diverticula (*small arrows*). This is the characteristic appearance of sigmoid diverticulitis. **C.** Double-contrast BE from another patient shows a tapered stricture (*arrows*) of the sigmoid colon with a small extraluminal barium collection (*arrowhead*). This is the typical appearance of diverticulitis with a small abscess on barium enema.

Abdominal x-rays and barium studies have little utility in the diagnosis of acute appendicitis. All cross-sectional imaging examinations, US, CT, and MRI, are accurate in the diagnosis of acute appendicitis; however, the choice of which modality to use is dictated predominantly by the clinical scenario.[378,379] A meta-analysis of 57 studies and more than 15 000 adults and children showed CT to have a 94% sensitivity and a 95% specificity for the diagnosis of appendicitis and US to have an 88% sensitivity and a 94% specificity for acute appendicitis.[118] Another meta-analysis including 5 studies evaluating the role of MRI in suspected antenatal appendicitis demonstrate a sensitivity of 95% and a specificity of 99%.[380]

CT is the gold standard in the evaluation of appendicitis; however, US and MRI are preferred for specific populations. US is the preferred imaging modality in the evaluation of children and pregnant women given the absence of ionizing radiation. US is additionally advantageous in that it can be performed immediately and at the bedside. Because of lower availability, long examination time, and higher cost, MRI is reserved mainly for pregnant women with negative US examinations.[381]

There is considerable controversy whether the use of oral contrast, IV contrast, or both alters the sensitivity and specificity of CT for the diagnosis of acute appendicitis. CT without IV or oral contrast is similar to or slightly less sensitive than enhanced CT in this setting, and unchanged in specificity.[382-387] This is an important issue because there is a significant time delay related to the time required for oral contrast to pass from the stomach to the terminal ilium. Some studies suggest that IV contrast is the more important factor in the diagnosis of acute appendicitis, as IV contrast can be administered without delay in scanning.[386,387]

The CT and MRI diagnosis of acute appendicitis is based on demonstration of a distended appendix, with the lumen of the appendix measuring ≥6 mm.[378,388-390] Hyperenhancement of the thickened appendiceal wall and mild to moderate pericecal fat stranding are other indirect signs of appendicitis. The presence of fluid and gas in the appendix does not indicate patency of the appendiceal orifice and does not exclude a diagnosis of appendicitis. In many cases, the cecal wall immediately adjacent to the appendix will also become inflamed secondarily with resultant focal thickening relative to the remainder of the cecum, a finding known as the "arrowhead' sign (see Figures 2-47 and 2-48).[391] Occasionally, mild pericecal adenopathy will also be seen.

The ultrasonic diagnosis of acute appendicitis is made when the appendix demonstrates the following features: (1) noncompressibility, (2) immobility, and (3) external diameter ≥6 mm including the outermost layer of serosa.[392-394] The presence of an appendicolith, regardless of appendix diameter, is usually considered indicative of acute appendicitis.[393] Ancillary findings include exacerbation of pain when the appendix is compressed, increased blood flow on Doppler imaging, and hyperechoic periappendiceal fat.[392-394] An irregular or asymmetric appendiceal contour, loss of the normal layered pattern of the appendiceal wall, and absence of blood flow on Doppler imaging indicate decreased viability of the appendiceal wall.[392]

On CT, the most common cause of a false-negative examination is a paucity of abdominal fat with resultant nonvisualization of the appendix.[391] Similarly, diminished study quality can reduce the accuracy of CT diagnosis of appendicitis.

Another known cause of false-negative examinations is perforation of the appendix whereby there is a relatively normal luminal diameter on imaging because of decompression into the peritoneum.[392,393] However, in this setting the presence of a periappendiceal abscess should

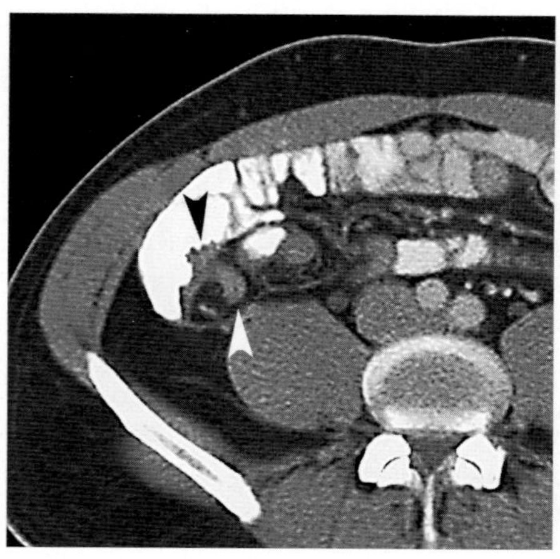
A

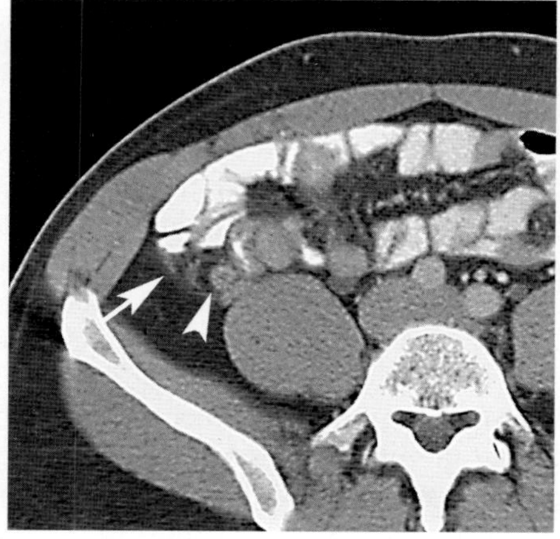
B

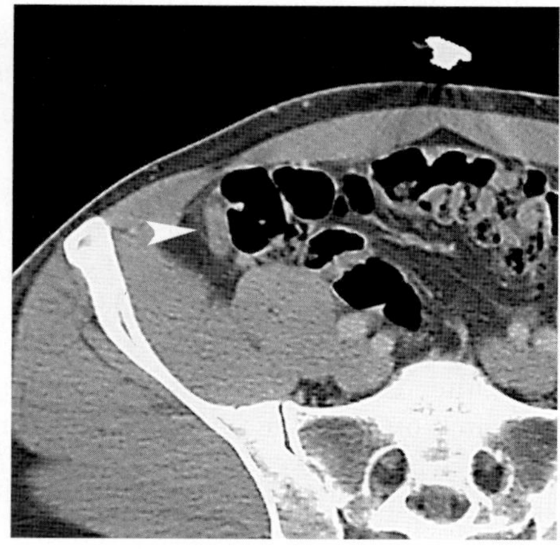
C

Figure 2-47 Appendicitis
This 36-year-old man complained of acute abdominal pain. **A-C.** CT images through the right lower quadrant demonstrate a distended, thick-walled, enhancing appendix (*white arrowheads*). The wall of the base of the cecum adjacent to the appendix is also thickened (*black arrowhead*). There is soft-tissue stranding in the periappendiceal fat (*white arrow*). This constellation of findings is diagnostic of acute appendicitis.

Imaging Notes 2-12. Imaging Findings of Acute Appendicitis

Sonography
Diagnostic findings • External diameter ≥6 mm, fixed, noncompressible appendix
Ancillary findings • Increased pain with compression • Hyperechoic peripancreatic fat • Increased color Doppler signal • Appendicolith
Signs of gangrene • Loss of the normal layered appearance of the appendix wall • Absence color Doppler signal
CT and MRI
Diagnostic findings • External diameter ≥6 mm
Ancillary findings • Wall hyperenhancement • Cecal wall thickening (arrowhead sign) • Pericecal adenopathy • Pericecal fat stranding • Appendicolith
Signs of gangrene • Nonenhancing or heterogeneously enhancing wall • Discontinuity of wall

alert the observer to the diagnosis. This will appear as an organized focal collection with enhancing walls that may contain fluid, gas, or necrotic debris. Less commonly, appendicial perforation can also result in hepatic abscess formation and SBO. An appendiceal abscess will appear on US examinations as either an inflammatory mass or localized complex fluid collection.[392]

The presence of any peritoneal fluid in a man and greater than normal peritoneal fluid in a woman should raise a suspicion for a perforated appendix. Signs of peritonitis including a generalized adynamic ileus can also be a clue to perforation.

Other common causes of false-negative CT and US examinations include tip appendicitis and stump appendicitis.[395] The reviewer should carefully evaluate the entire appendix to its bulbous tip, in order to avoid missing appendicitis that only involves the distal tip of the appendix. Stump appendicis occurs when the appendiceal stump is not invaginated into the cecum at the time of appendectomy. As such, even in the setting of prior appendicitis, the observer should evaluate the pericecal region to exclude the possibility of stump appendicitis.[395]

Regardless of the imaging modality, it is generally assumed that there is no appendicitis if no appendix is demonstrated and the study is otherwise normal. On US examinations, the lack of visualization of an appendix has an approximately 90% negative predictive value for appendicitis.[394]

Diverticula and Ulcers of the Colon

Diverticula are among the most common abnormalities detected on the imaging of the colon. Solitary ulcers can be found in the stomach and duodenum as a result of peptic ulcer disease. Colonic ulceration is seen as a manifestation of more diffuse inflammatory conditions such as Crohn disease and ulcerative colitis, which is discussed later in the chapter under the heading **Long-Segment Wall Thickening of the Small Bowel and Colon.**

Colonic diverticulosis

Most colonic diverticula are a result of pulsion by high levels of intraluminal pressure created during peristalsis of feces. There is an unusual idiopathic colonic diverticulum known as "giant colonic diverticulum."

Pulsion diverticulosis and diverticular disease: Colonic diverticulosis is characterized by outpouchings of the bowel wall and is among the most common disorders seen in Western nations. It is an age-related condition, and autopsy studies suggest that there is a prevalence of approximately 13% in individuals up to age 54, which rises up to 50% in individuals older than age 75 years.[396-398] Autopsy studies also indicate that diverticulosis is more common in women and is less common in Asian populations than in individuals from Europe and North America.[399]

Diverticula predominantly occur near sites of penetration of the vasa recta, the blood vessels to the colon. In Western nations, diverticula are found predominantly in the sigmoid colon and, in general, the left side of the colon. On the other hand, in Asian populations, they are most commonly found in the cecum and ascending colon.[399] Acquired colonic diverticula are covered only by the mucosal and serosal layer of the bowel wall and, therefore, represent pseudo-diverticula. In patients with diverticulosis, there are often concomitant changes in the muscular layers of the bowel wall, including thickening of the circular muscular layer and shortening of the longitudinal layer. The combination of diverticulosis and muscular layer changes is called "diverticular disease" and results in circumferential wall thickening. Although this thickening was initially thought to represent hypertrophy of these muscular layers, it is now known that the thickening is a result of the aberrant deposition of connective tissues, including elastin and collagen, into the smooth muscle of the colon wall.[396] Studies have also shown that colonic diverticulosis is associated with lower dietary fiber intake and obesity.[400-403]

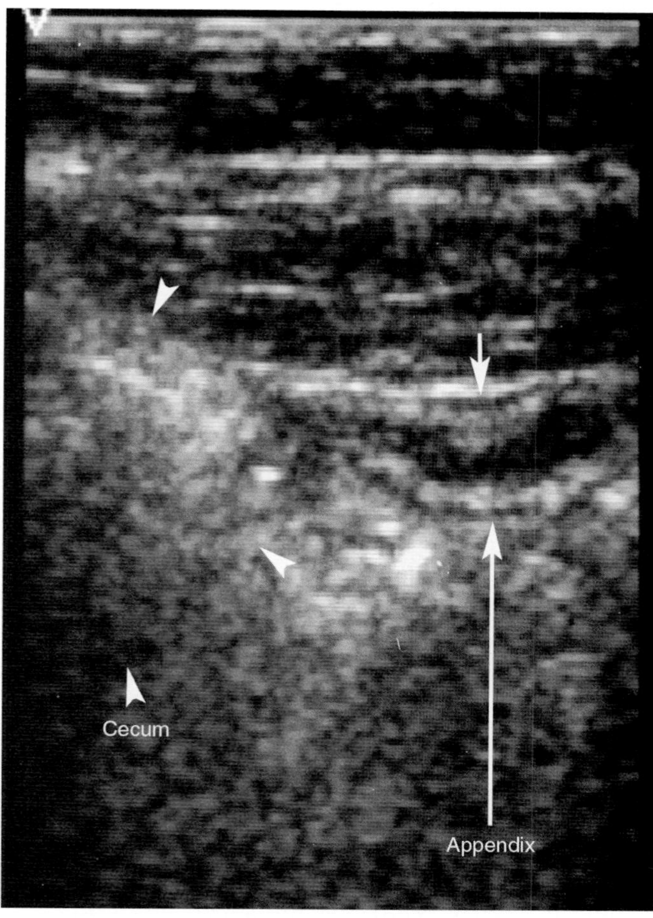

A

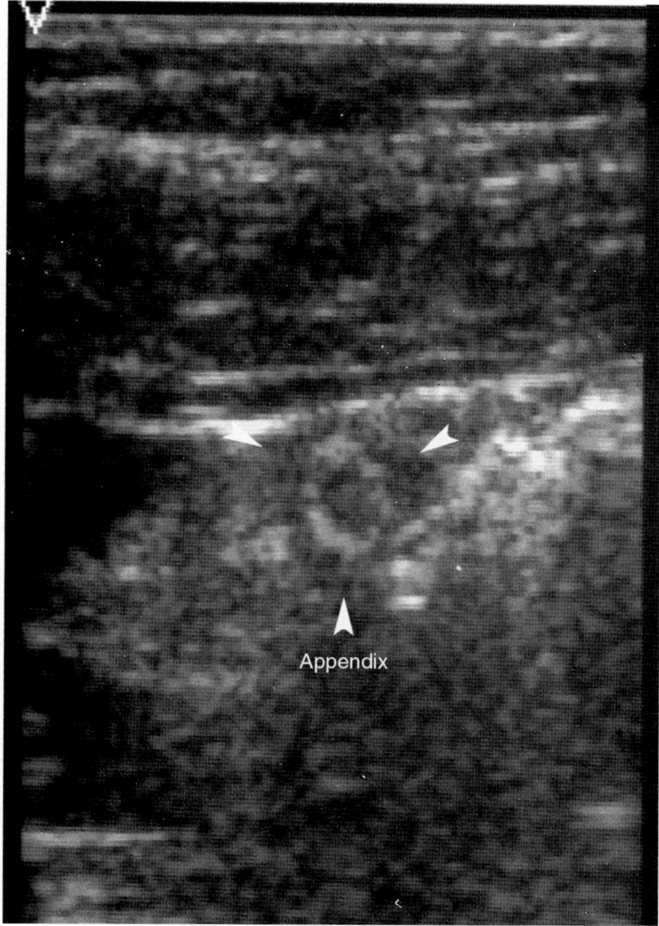

B

Figure 2-48 Appendicitis
This 22-year-old man complained of severe intermittent right lower quadrant pain and fevers. Ultrasonographic examinations for appendicitis are performed with a high-frequency transducer that shows fine detail. The ascending colon is found and then the transducer is moved to the proximal cecum, in search of the appendix. **A.** Longitudinal view of the cecum (*arrowheads*) shows a 10-mm tubular structure projecting from the cecal tip (*arrows*) this is the typical appearance of a distended appendix. The anechoic center represents fluid in the lumen of the appendix. Then there is a thickened hyperechoic mucosa and submucosa, a hypoechoic mucosal layer and a hyperechoic serosa. **B.** Longitudinal view of the appendix also shows it to be distended. These findings are diagnostic of acute appendicitis.

The traditionally accepted mechanism for diverticulosis is that peristaltic propulsion of the bowel contents causes pressure on the wall of the colon and results in forced outpouchings of the wall. It is thought that diverticula occur at the site of the perforating vessels because this location is relatively weaker than the remainder of the wall.[404,405] Furthermore, it has been suggested that low dietary fiber results in increased colonic pressures predisposing to the development of diverticulosis. However, some recent researchers are now questioning the validity of the pulsion theory of diverticulosis and suggest that other factors might be important in the development of diverticulosis, including aging, motility disorders, genetics, inflammation, and changes in the colonic microflora.[396]

The majority of patients with colonic diverticulosis are clinically asymptomatic. However, diverticulosis is associated with irritable bowel syndrome with an odds ratio of 1.8, suggesting that diverticulosis may be a cause for symptoms of irritable bowel syndrome, including bloating, abdominal pain relieved by the passage of stool, and tenemus.[406] Diverticulosis is also known to be a cause of GI bleeding, and diverticula can become superinfected, causing diverticulitis.[407] Diverticulitis has been discussed previously under the heading: **Focal Infections of the Bowel.**

On barium studies and CT and MRI examinations, diverticula will appear as smoothly marginated air-, fluid-, or barium-filled protrusions from the bowel wall (see Figure 2-49). When seen en face on barium enema, diverticula on the nondependent surface will appear as ring shadows that can mimic the appearance of nondependent colonic polyps. However, this confusion can usually be resolved by rotation of the patient. When seen obliquely on

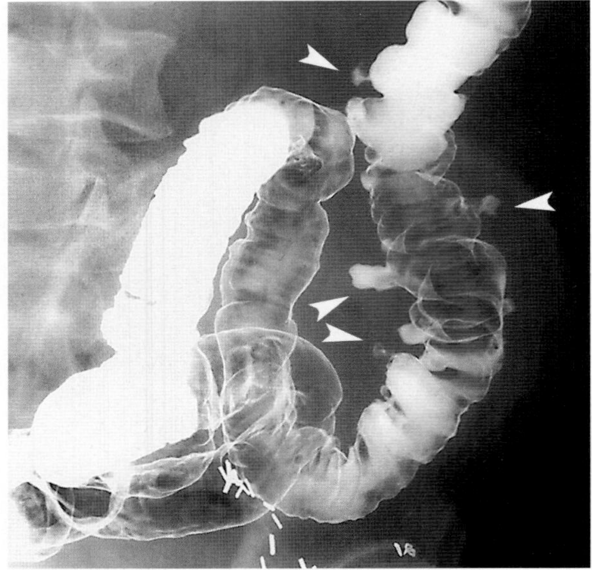

A

B

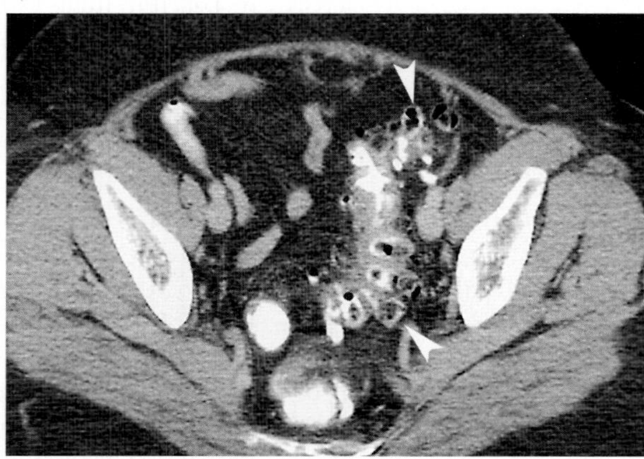

C

Figure 2-49 Diverticulosis
A. Spot film from a double-contrast barium enema shows multiple outpouchings (*arrowheads*) that are either gas or barium filled, typical of colonic diverticulosis. **B** and **C.** CT images through the lower abdomen and pelvis demonstrate multiple air-filled, contrast-filled, or stool-filled colonic outpouchings (*arrowheads*), typical of colonic diverticula.

barium enema, diverticula can have an appearance resembling a bowler hat.[266,267] A bowler hat caused by a diverticulum can be distinguished from a bowler hat caused by a polyp based on the direction in which the bowler hat points.[268] Bowler hat diverticula point away from the center of colonic lumen, whereas bowler hat polyps point toward the center of the colonic lumen. On the endoluminal or 3D images of CTC, diverticula produce a characteristic black etching artifact that encircles the entire mouth of the diverticula. This appearance is diagnostic but can be confirmed easily with 2D images.[8]

Giant colonic diverticulum: Giant colonic diverticulum is a rare disease of the colon, with fewer than 100 reported cases.[408,409] The overwhelming majority (93%) arise from the sigmoid colon. The etiology of these giant diverticula is unknown and patients present with subclinical symptoms such as vague abdominal pain. Complications are rare but include volvulus,[410] perforation,[411] diverticulitis,[412] SBO due to adhesions,[413] adhesion with the bowel or bladder,[414] and lower GI bleeding.[408] On barium enema, these diverticula demonstrate communication with the colonic lumen in approximately 50% of patients. In the remaining patients the lack of identifiable communication between the colonic lumen and the diverticulum most likely reflects inflammation of the neck. On CT, these giant diverticula are characterized by a large gas-filled cavity near the sigmoid colon.[412,415] In the absence of inflammation, they demonstrate thin, regular walls without contrast enhancement. In the setting of acute inflammation, similar to colonic diverticulitis, they will demonstrate thick enhancing walls.[412]

DIFFUSE DISORDERS OF THE SMALL BOWEL AND COLON

Diffuse disorders of the small bowel and colon primarily manifest as either long-segment thickening of the bowel wall or diffuse dilation.

Long-Segment Wall Thickening of the Small Bowel and Colon

Long-segment thickening of the small bowel and colon is a moderately common abnormality discovered on abdominal imaging. It can be seen on a variety of imaging modalities but is most often detected on abdominal plain films or CT of the abdomen. On plain films, wall thickening will manifest as an increase in the thickness of the small bowel and colonic folds. In the colon, this fold thickening has been traditionally called "thumbprinting" because the thickened folds appear as finger- or thumbwide indentations in the colonic air column (see Figure 2-50).

It is generally believed that the wall of both the small bowel and colon should measure less than 2 to 3 mm on cross-sectional imaging examinations.[278] However, on CT scans, when the lumen of the bowel is well distended, the

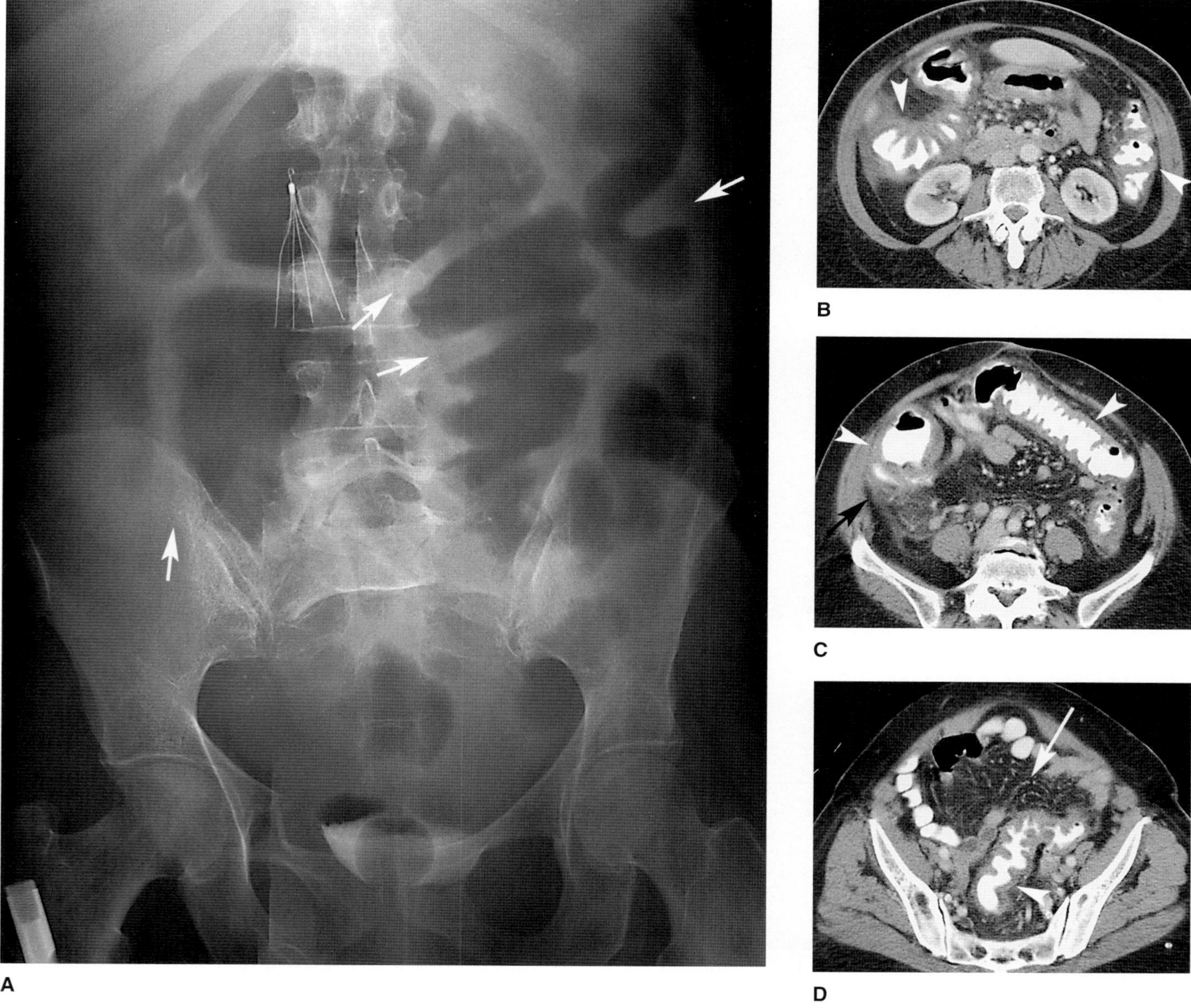

Figure 2-50 Pseudomembranous Enterocolitis
This 57-year-old man fractured his femur in a 20-foot fall. Postoperatively, he developed fevers, leucocytosis, and abdominal pain. **A.** Abdominal radiograph shows thickened folds in the cecum, transverse colon, and descending colon (*arrows*) indicating extensive colonic edema. **B-D.** CT images confirm the presence of colonic wall thickening of the entire colon (*arrowheads*). There is also some pericolonic edema (*black arrow*) and engorged mesenteric vessels (*white arrow*). *Clostridium difficile* enterocolitis is the most common cause of pancolitis in an inpatient and was the cause for this man's disorder.

wall typically appears as a nearly imperceptible thin line of tissue. In this setting, a wall greater than 1 or 2 mm will often indicate wall thickening.

Bowel wall thickening is most often a result of submucosal edema but can also be due to a variety of etiologies including intramural hemorrhage, bowel wall lymphoma, and rarely due to other infiltrative diseases of the bowel wall. Causes of small bowel and colonic edema are listed in Table 2-7. The most common causes of bowel edema are enteric and colonic infections, ischemia, IBD, and hypoproteinemia.

Infectious enteritis and colitis

Colonic infections are seen more frequently than small-bowel infections and are the most common cause of long-segment bowel wall thickening.

Pseudomembranous colitis: Pseudomembranous colitis is a severe colonic inflammation that results from toxins produced by an overgrowth of the organism *Clostridium difficile* (see Figure 2-50). In the vast majority of cases,

Table 2-7. Causes of Small-Bowel and Colonic Edema

1. Infection a. Colon i. *Clostridium difficile*[a] ii. Neutropenic colitis (Typhlitis)[b] iii. Salmonella iv. Shigella v. Yersinia vi. Amoeba vii. Cytomegalovirus[b] b. Small bowel i. Neutropenic enteritis[b] ii. Giardia iii. Cryptosporidium iv. Whiples Disease v. Tuberculosis vi. *Mycobacterium avium* complex
2. Ischemia
3. Inflammatory bowel disease a. Crohn disease b. Ulcerative colitis
4. Hypoproteinemia a. Cirrhosis b. other
5. Other causes a. Radiation enteritis

[a]Pseudomembranous enterocolitis.
[b]Immunocompromised hosts.

pseudomembranous colitis is a complication of antibiotic therapy. However, it has been associated with other conditions, including hypotensive episodes, chemotherapeutic agents, and abdominal surgery.[278] This disorder can result in significant morbidity and mortality if it is not treated aggressively.[278] Patients typically present with profuse watery diarrhea, abdominal pain, and fever.[416] Diagnosis is made through stool assays or visualization of characteristic adherent yellow plaques on endoscopy. However, in some cases, the disorder is clinically unsuspected and the diagnosis is first suggested based on imaging findings of abdominal radiographs or CT scans obtained for the evaluation of acute abdominal pain. As a consequence, radiologists should be familiar with the imaging findings of this disease. Treatment with metronidazole and vancomycin is usually effective, and less than 1% of patients require surgery.[417] However, some patients with a fulminant form of pseudomembranous colitis may not respond to medical therapy and will require colectomy or other surgical intervention.[416,418]

In most cases, both abdominal radiographs and abdominal CT will show evidence of a pancolitis manifest as diffuse colonic fold thickening on abdominal radiographs and diffuse wall thickening on CT examinations (see Figure 2-50). On CT scans, the degree of thickening can range from 3 to 32 mm.[419] Similar severe fold thickening can be seen on abdominal radiographs. The degree of thickening in pseudomembranous colitis is greater than any other inflammatory or infectious disease of the colon, with the exception of Crohn disease. In certain cases of severe wall thickening, CT examinations will demonstrate the "accordion sign." In this sign, the regular alteration of thickened folds and contrast between the folds can resemble the zigzag pattern of an accordion (see Figure 2-50).[231] In the majority of cases, pseudomembranous colitis will cause diffuse wall thickening extending from the cecum to the rectum; however, in some cases it can present as a segmental colitis.[420] This includes cases that predominantly involve the rectum and left colon and cases that predominantly involve the right colon.[278,421] The literature suggests that in up to 30% to 40% of cases, there can be isolated involvement of the right colon with sparing of the left colon.[421]

Wall thickening is the primary manifestation of pseudomembranous colitis; however, occasionally other findings can be present. The attenuation of the bowel wall can be variable. In some cases, it will appear hypoattenuating as a result of edema and in other cases can appear hyperattenuating as a result of increased contrast enhancement because of hyperemia. Colonic dilation is a variable finding in pseudomembranous colitis but, when present, can be a result of transmural inflammation or colonic ileus. Mild pericolic fat-stranding can also be present in some cases but is typically relatively mild, because this condition predominantly affects the mucosa and submucosa.[422] This absence of fat stranding can be a differentiating feature between pseudomembranous colitis and Crohn disease, which will often have greater degrees of pericolonic inflammation.

Although CT is helpful in assessing the extent and severity of the disease and evaluating for potential complications such as perforation, CT findings alone do not allow reliable prediction of which patients with pseudomembranous colitis will require surgical intervention.[420]

Neutropenic colitis (typhlitis): Neutropenic colitis, also called "typhlitis," is a relatively uncommon complication of patients with prolonged neutropenia. In most cases, the neutropenia is a result of chemotherapy for a malignancy, typically acute leukemia.[278,423] However, typhlitis can also be seen in the setting of aplastic anemia, lymphoma, AIDS, and following solid organ transplantation.[424] Patients typically present with fever, watery or bloody diarrhea, and abdominal pain.[278] Typhlitis is characterized by edema and inflammation of the bowel that characteristically involves the cecum and the ascending colon, and sometimes can also involve the terminal ileum and appendix. The combination of primary cecal and ascending colon involvement and neutropenia should suggest a diagnosis of typhlitis.

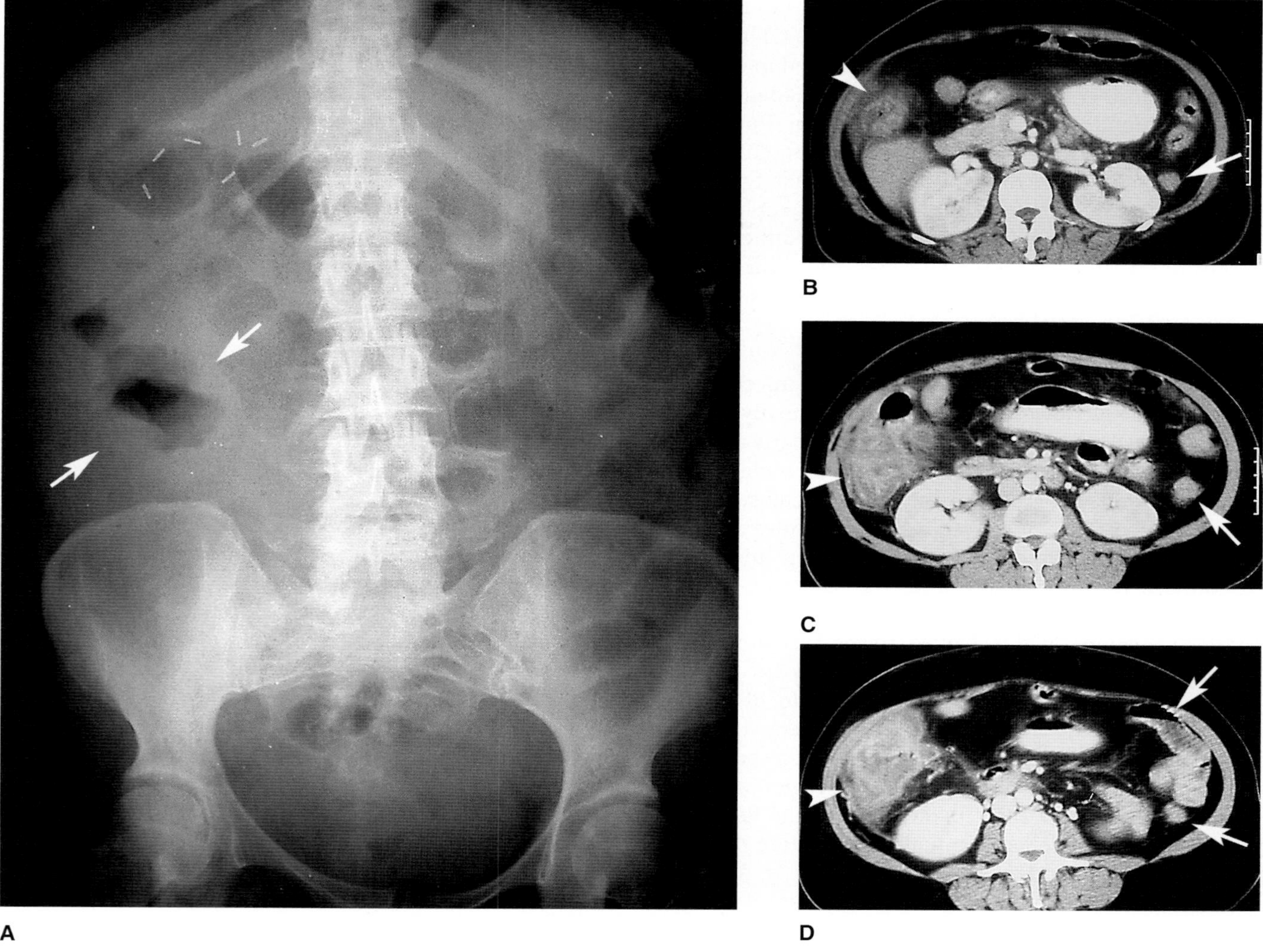

Figure 2-51 Typhlitis
This 49-year-old woman was neutropenic as a result of chemotherapy for acute myeloid leukemia when she developed fevers. **A.** Supine abdominal radiograph shows an irregular gas collection in the right lower quadrant that appears to represent a severely thick-walled gas-filled cecum. **B-D.** CT images confirm extensive wall thickening of the ascending colon with associated pericolonic fat stranding (*arrowheads*). Note the normal proximal small bowel and distal colon. In this clinical setting, this appearance is virtually diagnostic of typhlitis.

The pathophysiology of typhlitis is not completely understood but is thought to be a result of mucosal injury initiated by a combination of cytotoxic drugs, ischemia, and bowel wall hemorrhage followed by mucosal invasion by a variety of microorganisms.[424] In some cases, neoplastic infiltration can contribute to the development of disease. Mucosal invasion is a result of impaired host immune defenses related to neutropenia.[425] Once mucosal injury is initiated, the bowel becomes infected by various opportunistic pathogens, including Pseudomonas, clostridial species, and various fungal species, including Candida and Aspergillus.[426]

Resolution of typhlitis ultimately corresponds with adequate return of functioning neutrophils. Supportive treatment includes bowel rest, total parenteral nutrition, antibiotics, and aggressive fluid and electrolyte replacement. Close clinical observation of these patients is required, as some cases can develop transmural necrosis with resultant perforation that can lead to death. Surgery is indicated in patients with uncontrollable GI bleeding, obstruction, abscess, transmural necrosis, free intramural perforation, or uncontrolled sepsis.[278,427,428]

Abdominal radiographs will appear normal in some cases, but in many cases will demonstrate thickened colonic folds exclusively or predominantly involving the cecum and ascending colon (see Figure 2-51). Colonoscopy and contrast enema examinations are contraindicated in suspected typhlitis because of the risk of bowel perforation. Further, CT findings include cecal distention and circumferential wall thickening of the cecum and ascending colon. Wall thickening can be isodense compared to the normal bowel wall or can be low attenuation secondary to the edema.[429] Pericolic fat stranding is a common ancillary finding (see Figure 2-51).[278] In addition, CT can be helpful in assessing response to treatment, and in detecting complications that warrant surgical management such as pneumatosis intestinalis, pneumoperitoneum, and pericolic fluid collections.[424,428,429] Differentiation of typhlitis from other disease processes that typically involve the cecum, such as Crohn disease, tuberculosis, and several other colonic infections, can be difficult on the basis of CT findings alone. However, the clinical presentation of typhlitis is usually distinct from these other diagnoses.[278]

Tuberculosis: Tuberculosis is an uncommon infection in the United States. However, it is endemic in many countries with increasing global prevalence, particularly among immunocompromised patients, at a rate of increase of approximately 1.1% per year.[430] Although tuberculosis most often affects the respiratory system, it can involve a large number of organ systems, particularly among immunocompromised individuals, including the GI tract, which accounts for 0.7% of cases.[431,432] In 1 study from Taiwan, a quarter of patients with GI tuberculosis lacked clinical evidence of pulmonary tuberculosis.[432]

The abdomen is the most common site of extrapulmonary tuberculosis with the solid viscera affected more commonly than the GI tract.[433] When the bowel is involved, tuberculosis involves the ileocecal region in 90% of cases.[434] This preferential involvement of the ileocecal region is believed to reflect the higher proportion of lymphoid tissue in this location.[435]

Spasm and hypermobility of an incompetent ileocecal valve is the earliest finding of tuberculosis on barium examinations. Over time, the ileocecal valve becomes thickened, fixed, and irregularly shaped with an incompetent, gaping orifice.[434-438] Shallow ulceration of the bowel mucosa can be seen at this stage on DCBE examinations. Late findings of GI tuberculosis include symmetric annular stenosis and obstruction associated with shortening and retraction of the cecum and ascending colon. Typically, the lumen of the cecum will shrink and assume a conical shape whereas the normally capacious cecum will become relatively smaller than the ascending colon. This distortion of the cecum is a result of progressive granulomatous fibrosis of the affected tissues.

On CT, GI tuberculosis will present as circumferential mural thickening of the cecum and terminal ileum.[435] Occasionally, tuberculosis will cause asymmetric thickening of the medial wall of the cecum and ileocecal valve with extension of the soft-tissue mass into the adjacent tissues that engulfs the terminal ileum.[439] This form of tuberculosis can potentially be confused with infiltrating cecal neoplasms such as lymphoma. Some cases of intestinal tuberculosis will reveal multiple foci of colonic and small-bowel thickening, with associated luminal narrowing that may or may not be associated with proximal dilation. In the presence of ileocecal involvement, this multifocal pattern of wall thickening and stenosis with normal intervening bowel is suggestive of tuberculosis but can also be confused with Crohn disease.[431]

Most cases of intestinal tuberculosis will also demonstrate mesenteric lymphadenopathy, especially in the fat medial to the ileocecal valve. In fact, abdominal lymphadenopathy is the most common manifestation of abdominal tuberculosis, present in 55% to 66% of patients.[434] This adenopathy is often of greater degree than that seen with Crohn disease and other enteric infections and can be an important clue to the diagnosis of ileocecal tuberculosis on cross-sectional imaging. In many cases, tuberculous lymphadenopathy demonstrates hypoattenuating centers and hyperattenuating enhancing rims on CT, a characteristic of caseous necrosis.[434,436,440] Despite their bulky appearance, these nodes seldom cause obstruction of the adjacent bowel or ureter (see Figure 2-52).

Whipple disease: Whipple disease is a rare chronic infection due to the gram-positive intracellular bacterium *Tropheryma whipplei*, with wide-ranging multisystemic symptoms but most commonly a protein-losing enteropathy.[441] Although the disease was first reported in 1907, the first successful culture was not performed until 2000.[441] The organism is believed to be found in the general environment but the source, the mechanism of transmission, and the pathogenesis remains uncertain. It appears as though many individuals are exposed to the organism but only a few develop the disease.[441] *Tropheryma whipplei* replicates within human macrophages, resulting in apoptosis of the cell, which may be crucial for bacterial dissemination. Histologic evaluation of infected tissues, most commonly the small bowel, is characterized by massive infiltration of foamy macrophages containing periodic acid-Schiff-positive glycoprotein granules that represent the intracellular organisms.[442]

Eighty-seven percent of patients are male. Those with disease typically present with weight loss and diarrhea.[441,443] Fevers are seen in approximately 38% of patients and central lymphadenopathy is seen in approximately 52%. Joint symptoms, usually migratory arthralgias, arthritis, or both, are found in 65% to 90% of patients. Neurologic symptoms including cognitive deficits, depression, changes in libido, and abnormalities of ocular movement are variable and have been reported in 6% to 63% of patients. Cardiac, pulmonary, pleural, and cutaneous involvement can also be seen. Approximately 15% of patients will present without GI symptoms, and some studies have suggested that there may be asymptomatic carriers of the organism.[441]

Imaging demonstrates diffuse nodular thickening of small-bowel folds that can be detected on barium examinations and CT scans and barium examinations (see Figure 2-53).[442,444,445] The jejunum is typically more severely involved than the ilium. This rare disorder is also associated with enlarged low-attenuation retroperitoneal lymph nodes, which can be diagnostic of the disorder.

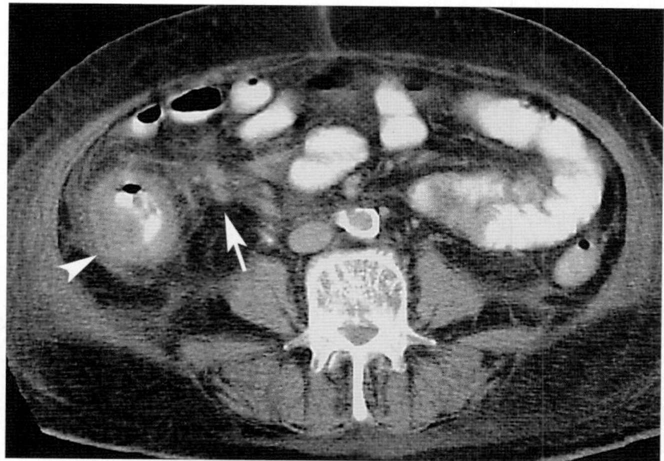

A

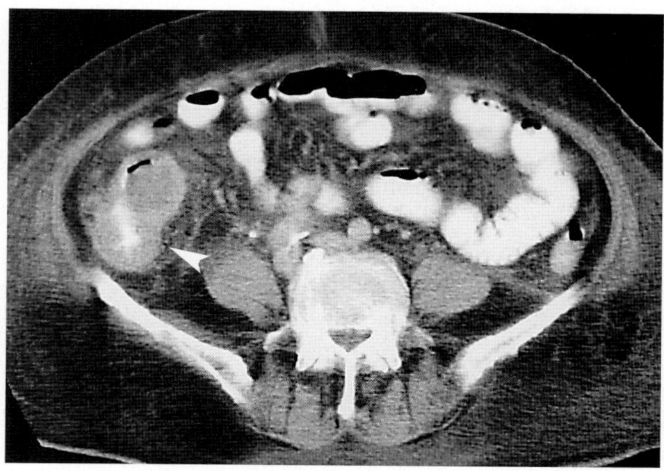

B

Figure 2-52 Abdominal Tuberculosis
This 62-year-old man with pancytopenia and fevers had emigrated from India. **A** and **B.** CT images demonstrate circumferential thickening of the cecum and ascending colon (*arrowheads*). There is also adenopathy in the small-bowel mesentery medial to the colon (*arrow*). This would usually indicate typhlitis but in this case evaluation of the abnormality was diagnostic of tuberculosis.

These nodes can have attenuation less than -40 HU, typical of lipid materials.

Other causes of infectious enteritis and colitis: There are a variety of causes of infectious enteritis and colitis, including infection from bacteria, fungi, viruses, and protozoa. A list of some of the causes of enteric infections is listed in Table 2-7. Patients will typically present with cramping abdominal pain, fever, and acute diarrhea. Stool culture is the primary method for diagnosing these infections and it is rare for patients to receive imaging. However, when clinical symptoms are not straightforward, imaging may be ordered and the diagnosis of an enteric infection can be suggested according to CT findings.[278,364]

In most cases, abdominal x-rays will appear normal or nonspecifically abnormal. However, some cases will demonstrate multiple air-fluid levels within nondistended small bowel or colon. This bowel gas pattern is suggestive of a diagnosis of enteritis or colitis. Thickening of the small-bowel or colonic folds can also be seen in some cases (see Figures 2-54 and 2-55). Further, CT scans will typically demonstrate circumferential wall thickening in a segmental or diffuse distribution of either the small bowel in enteritis or the colon in colitis. Most cases will also show homogeneous increased enhancement of the bowel wall; however, some cases will show uniform low attenuation representing edema (see Figure 2-54). Ascites or inflammation of the pericolic fat can be present in some cases.[446] As with the abdominal radiograph, multiple air-fluid levels can also be seen. There is considerable overlap of the imaging appearance of the multiple infectious causes of enteritis/colitis, and laboratory studies are necessary for a confirmation of the offending organism.[278,364]

Certain organisms tend to have characteristic distribution of the affected bowel. Infections that typically cause thickening of the terminal ileum and/or ascending colon include *Yersinia*, *Campylobacter*, *Salmonella*, and *Shigella* species in addition to tuberculosis and neutropenic colitis previously described. Diffuse infectious colitis will most often be due to *Clostridium difficile*-related pseudomembranous colitis but can also be due to cytomegalovirus and *Escherichia coli* infections.[424] Rectosigmoid wall thickening is typical of gonorrhea, herpesvirus, and *Chlamydia trachomatis*. These are organisms that are sexually transmitted, and colonic involvement is often associated with anal sex.[447] In schistosomiasis, involvement is usually confined to the descending and sigmoid colon because the adult worms have a tendency to enter the IMV.[278,364]

Ischemic bowel

Ischemic bowel is a rare but potentially life-threatening condition that is 1 of the causes of diffuse bowel wall edema. Mechanisms of intestinal ischemia include arterial occlusion (60%-70% of cases), venous occlusion (5%-10% of cases), and intestinal hypoperfusion (20%-30% of cases).[448,449] Causes of bowel ischemia include thromboembolism, hypoperfusion, bowel obstruction, neoplasms, vasculitis, abdominal inflammatory conditions, trauma, medications (chemotherapy), radiation, and corrosive injury (see Table 2-8).[450]

Patients typically present with nonspecific acute abdominal pain. However, ischemia only accounts for approximately 1% of patients presenting with acute abdominal pain.[451,452] Leucocytosis and elevated levels of lactate and/or amylase are nonspecific and often late signs of ischemia.[452]

Imaging Notes 2-13. Patterns of Bowel Wall Thickening

Distribution of Disease	Causes[a]
Pancolitis	(1) *Clostridium difficile* (pseudomembranous colitis)
	(2) Ulcerative colitis
	(3) Crohn disease
	(4) Other infections: Cytomegalovirus, *Escheirchia coli*
Terminal ileum and cecum	(1) Crohn disease
	(2) Infections: *Yersinia*, *Campylobacter*, *Salmonella*, *Shigella* sp.
	(3) Tuberculosis (also has adenopathy)
Cecum, ascending colon	(1) Crohn disease
	(2) Neutropenic enterocolitis (Typhlitis)
Rectosigmoid colon	(1) Ulcerative colitis
	(2) Crohn disease
	(3) Infectious colitis: *Gonococcus*, *Chlamydia trachomatis*, Herpes simplex
Proximal small bowel	(1) Crohn disease
	(2) Giardia infection
	(3) Celiac disease
Fold reversal	(1) Celiac disease

[a]Order of causes is in approximate frequency in the general population of the United States.

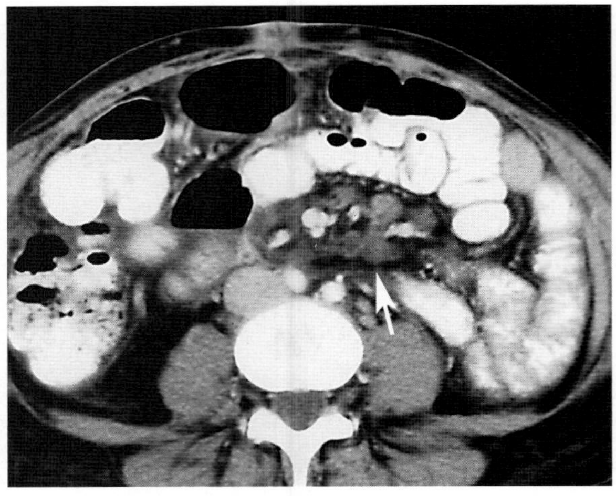

A

B

C

Figure 2-53 Whipple Disease
This 44-year-old woman complained of chronic diarrhea and lower extremity edema. **A-C.** Axial CT images demonstrate prominent small-bowel folds throughout the abdomen associated with mesenteric adenopathy (*arrow* in A) and ascites (*arrowhead* in C). Note the faint low attenuation of the lymph nodes. Small-bowel biopsy was diagnostic of Whipple disease.

Abdominal plain films and barium evaluation are not indicated in the evaluation of intestinal ischemia because they cannot differentiate between the underlying causes. However, abdominal radiographs obtained for the indication of abdominal pain in some cases will demonstrate thickened small-bowel or colonic folds (see Figure 2-56). Although nonspecific, these findings can be suggestive of bowel ischemia in the appropriate clinical situation. Similarly, barium studies of the small bowel and/or colon can also confirm the presence of nonspecific thickening of small-bowel and/or colonic folds.

The most common CT finding of acute mesenteric ischemia is bowel wall thickening that is greater than 3 mm (usually 8-9 mm) but less than 2 cm (see Figure 2-57). Thickening is caused by a combination of mural edema, congestion, hemorrhage, and/or superinfection of the ischemic bowel wall.[453-455] Bowel wall thickening is more

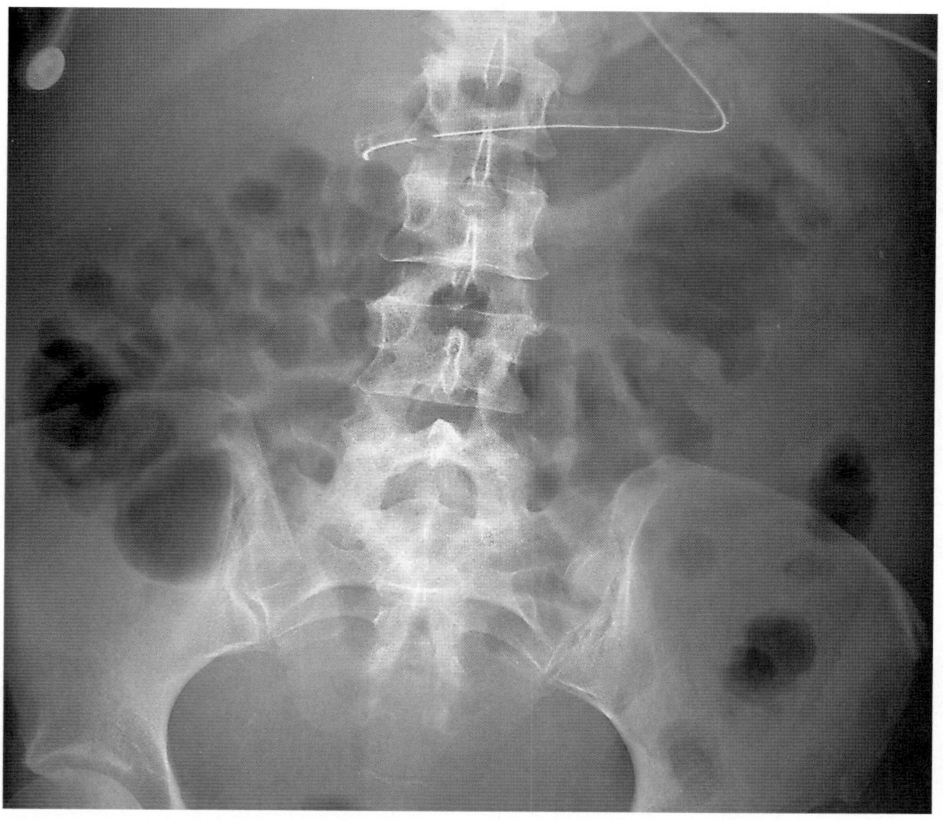

A

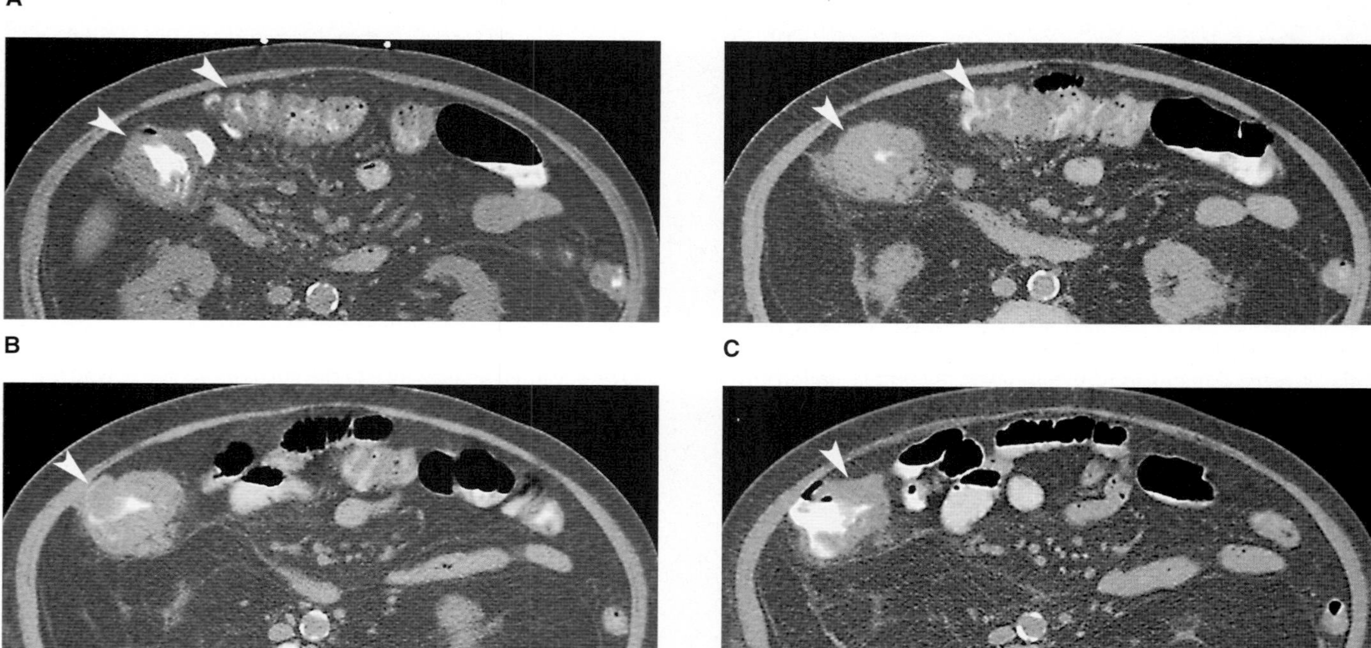

B C D E

Figure 2-54 Infectious Colitis in 2 Patients
A. This 43-year-old man complained of abdominal pain, nausea, and vomiting. Anteroposterior view of the abdomen shows mild nodular fold thickening of the transverse colon, suggesting the presence of colitis. Stool cultures were positive for *Salmonella* species. **B-E.** This 62-year-old man with a history of a heart transplant and non-Hodgkin lymphoma complained of malaise and weakness. Unenhanced axial CT images show a long segment of bowel wall thickening involving ascending and proximal transverse colons. Differential diagnosis included bowel lymphoma, adenocarcinoma, and infectious and ischemic colitis. Colonoscopic biopsies and cultures revealed an unexpected diagnosis of *Mycobacterium avium intracellulare* infection.

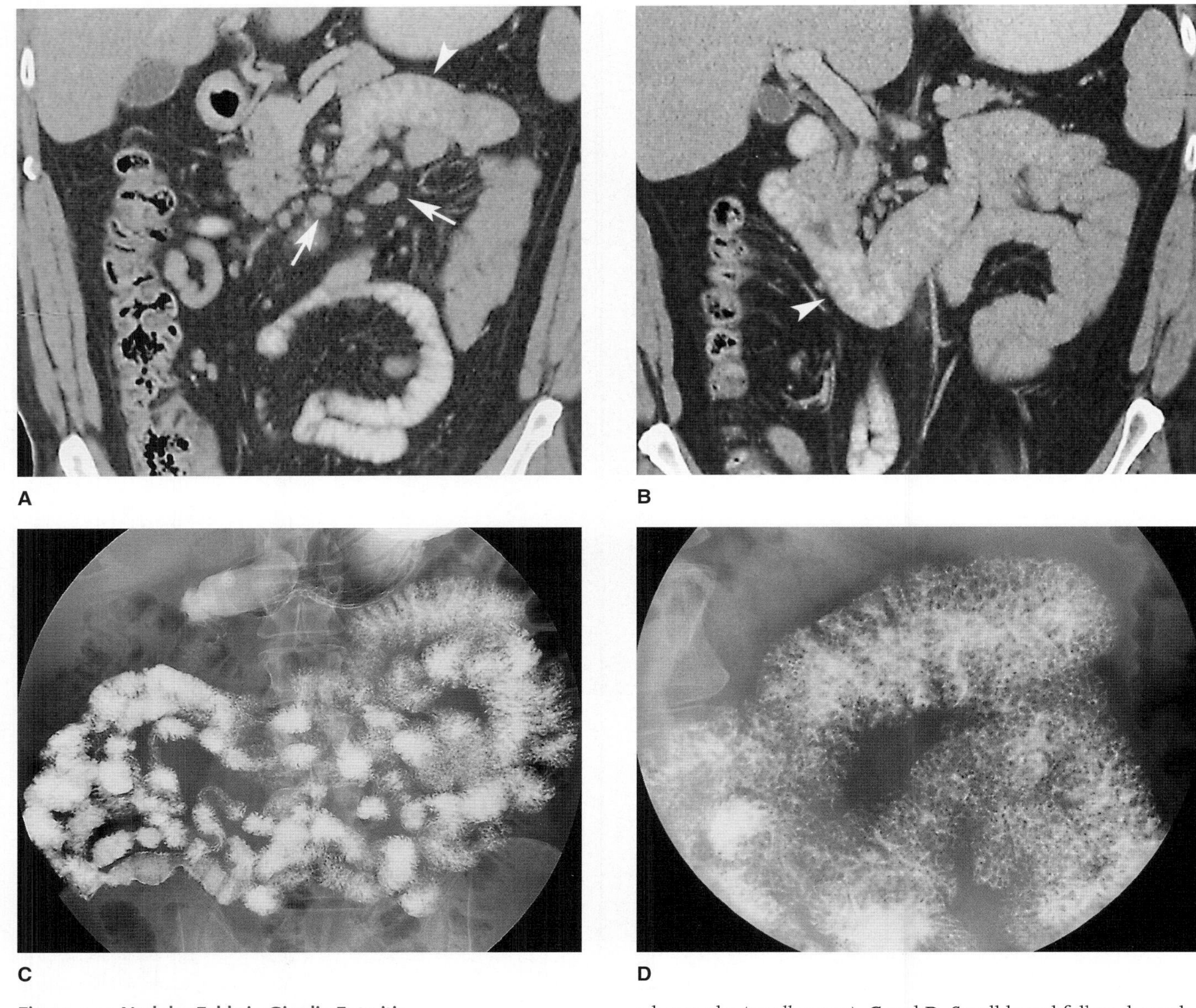

Figure 2-55 Nodular Folds in Giardia Enteritis
This 45-year-old man had recurrent DVTs due to a coagulopathy of unknown cause. **A** and **B.** Coronal reconstructions from an abdominal CT show subtly thickened folds (*arrowheads*) in the proximal small bowel associated with mild mesenteric adenopathy (*small arrows*). **C** and **D.** Small-bowel follow-through shows a feathery appearance to the small-bowel folds, which on magnified view are shown to represent innumerable small regions of nodular thickening. Small-bowel biopsy and cultures were diagnostic of giardia infection.

pronounced in ischemia caused by venous occlusion than by arterial occlusion and therefore, bowel wall thickening greater than 1.5 cm in the setting of suspected ischemia should prompt a search for venous thrombosis.[454,456] Unfortunately, bowel wall thickening is not a consistent CT finding of ischemia, and the degree of thickening does not correlate with severity.[454] Patients with transmural intestinal infarction due to arterial occlusion can present with normal bowel wall thickness.

On unenhanced examinations, ischemic bowel wall attenuation will demonstrate alternating rings of higher and lower attenuation, termed the "target sign." A low attenuation wall occurs as a result of edema, whereas a high attenuation wall will occur as a result of intramural hemorrhage. A double halo or target sign appears as an outer ring of high attenuation representing the muscularis propria, a middle ring of intermediate or low attenuation representing edema of the submucosa, and an inner ring of high attenuation representing the inflamed mucosa (see Figure 2-57).[457]

Some ancillary, but nonspecific, imaging findings that can be present in patients with bowel ischemia include bowel dilation, pericolonic fat stranding, mesenteric fluid, pneumatosis intestinalis, and portal venous gas. Bowel dilation,

Table 2-8. Causes of Intestinal Ischemia

A. Arterial Occlusion
  1. Thromboemboli
    a. Atrial fibrillation
    b. Endocarditis
    c. Other
  2. Arterial stenosis
    a. Atherosclerosis
    b. Vasculitis
    c. Fibromuscular dysplasia
    d. Other
  3. Hypercoagulable states
    a. Antiphospholipid antibody syndrome
    b. Protein C deficiency
    c. Protein S deficiency
  4. Invading malignancy

B. Venous occlusion
  1. Hypercoagulable states (see above for details)
  2. Invading malignancy
  3. Causes of extrinsic venous compression
    a. Bowel obstruction
    b. Invading malignancy

C. Hypoperfusion
  1. Heart failure
  2. Hemorrhagic or septic shock
  3. Medications affecting blood pressure
  4. Arterial stenosis coupled with other causes of diminished blood pressure

in patients with mesenteric ischemia, is due to disruption of normal peristalsis. When the degree of bowel dilation is severe, this typically reflects irreversible transmural ischemia or infarction.[453,454] Pneumatosis intestinalis and portal venous gas are uncommon findings, often indicating bowel wall necrosis, which can occasionally be seen in association with intestinal ischemia. Both abdominal radiographs and abdominal CT are capable of detecting pneumatosis and portal venous gas, but CT is more sensitive. Absence of bowel wall enhancement is a highly specific finding of mesenteric ischemia.[454] However, this finding is rarely seen because of redundancy of the mesenteric vasculature.

Computed tomographic findings in most cases can only suggest the diagnosis of intestinal ischemia. The definitive diagnosis is based on colonoscopic or surgical findings coupled with pathologic evaluation of resected specimens.

The preferred modality for the evaluation of bowel ischemia is a dual-phase CT angiographic evaluation with neutral oral contrast during arterial and portal venous phase of enhancement. This allows for evaluation of the distribution of the affected small bowel as well as the underlying cause.[454,456] Conventional angiography can

Imaging Notes 2-14. CT Evaluation of Intestinal Ischemia

Nonspecific findings
1. Bowel dilation
2. Bowel wall thickening
3. Pericolonic fat stranding
4. Mesenteric fluid

Suggestive findings
1. Pneumotosis intestinalis with or without portal venous gas
2. Bowel wall thickening in a vascular territory

Specific findings
1. Absence of contrast enhancement of the bowel wall
2. Secondary signs of intestinal ischemia plus arterial or venous occlusion of the mesenteric vessels

definitively diagnose and in some cases treat occlusive arterial and venous causes of bowel ischemia (see Figure 2-57). However, angiographic examinations are insensitive for the detection of nonocclusive mesenteric ischemia.[456]

The distribution of ischemic changes can be dependent on the underlying cause of the ischemia and will be discussed under the specific causes of intestinal ischemia.

Thromboembolism: Vascular occlusion is typically a result of thromboemboli but can also be due to in situ thrombosis or vascular invasion by adjacent malignancy.[278] This is most often seen in the elderly with atrial fibrillation but should also be suspected in younger patients with underlying diseases that can affect mesenteric blood flow, such as vasculitis and hereditary or familial coagulation disorders such as antiphospholipid syndrome, protein C deficiency, and protein S deficiency.[456] Bowel abnormalities will be found in the territory served by the occluded vessel.[278] The SMA supplies and the SMV drains the small bowel and the ascending and transverse colons. The IMA supplies and the IMV drains the descending colon and proximal sigmoid colon. Arterial or venous occlusion of these vessels will lead to edema of the bowel wall in the affected territory.

When evaluating for potential intestinal ischemia, it is important to differentiate between arterial occlusive and venous occlusive causes of bowel ischemia because these disorders are treated differently. Acute arterial mesenteric ischemia is treated surgically or by using percutaneous thrombolytic treatment.[458] On the other hand, transmural ischemia is rare in patients with venous obstruction and so these patients can often be treated conservatively with anticoagulative therapy.[459]

Hypoperfusion: Hypoperfusion or nonocclusive ischemic bowel can be caused by low perfusion pressure, by

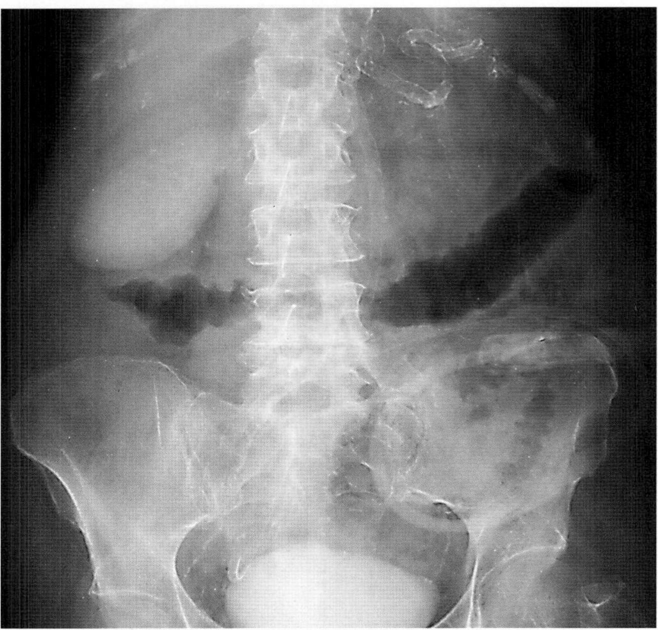

Figure 2-56 Ischemic Colitis
This 70-year-old woman on peritoneal dialysis for chronic renal failure complained of supraumbilical pain. Supine view of the abdomen shows thumbprinting in the transverse colon and thickened folds in multiple small-bowel loops most likely due to extensive small-bowel and colonic edema. Given her peritoneal dialysis, this could be a manifestation of peritonitis and given her renal failure these findings, could be a result of hypoproteinemia. However, there are also multiple vascular calcifications, indicating extensive atherosclerosis and a risk for ischemic bowel. Surgical exploration confirmed extensive ischemia of the colon and small bowel.

mesenteric arterial vasoconstriction, or a combination of both.[140] Vasoconstriction can be a reflexive response to hypotension or can be a response to a variety of vasoactive drugs including digitalis, ergot preparations, vasopressin or other pressor agents, amphetamine, and cocaine.[450] As a consequence of these factors, hypoperfusion ischemia is most often seen in the setting of heart failure with low cardiac output, hemorrhagic or septic shock, and with drugs affecting blood pressure.[460]

The splenic flexure and the rectosigmoid colon represent watershed regions at the border of 2 major vascular territories. These regions are particularly susceptible to hypoperfusion ischemia as a result of poor perfusion. It is interesting to note that hypoperfusion ischemia can affect different portions of the bowel depending on the age of the patient.[454] In elderly patients, where hypoperfusion is typically compounded by atherosclerotic vascular narrowing, ischemia is typically more severe in the distribution of the descending and sigmoid colons. In younger patients where hypoperfusion is typically a manifestation of hemorrhagic shock due to penetrating or blunt trauma, ischemia is more pronounced in the right hemicolon and small bowel.[460] The explanation for this right-sided predominance is uncertain but could reflect inconsistent development of the marginal artery of the right colon or poor collateral blood supply to the right colon.[461,462]

Restoration of normal perfusion pressure is the treatment of choice for hypoperfusion ischemia, unless the bowel has not become infarcted, in which case surgery is required.

Bowel obstruction: Ischemia can also be seen as a complication of bowel obstruction, particularly closed loop obstruction. In the setting of closed-loop obstruction, the vascular supply is directly occluded by twisting of the feeding and draining vessels with resultant increased pressure. However, in other causes of obstruction, massive distention of the bowel can apply pressure to the small vessels of the wall, reducing blood flow and resulting in hypoperfusion ischemia. Bowel obstruction and imaging features related to ischemia are discussed most completely under the heading **Bowel Dilation**.

Neoplasms: Ischemic colitis is a coexistent condition with colon carcinoma in 1% to 7% of patients. In most cases, this is a consequence of colonic obstruction with the mechanisms explained previously.[450] However, rarely, proliferation of bacteria proximal to the site of obstruction as a result of the bowel contents are believed to be a cause for ischemia.[463] In 25% of cases, CT will not be able to distinguish between wall thickening attributable to tumor infiltration and wall thickening attributable to ischemia.[464] The thicker and more irregular the thickening, the more likely it is to represent cancer. Smooth concentric thickening measuring less than 10 mm will usually indicate edema due to ischemia.

Rarely, retroperitoneal tumors, such as pancreatic carcinoma, can invade the superior or inferior mesenteric artery or vein and cause intestinal ischemia due to vascular compression or invasion or by inducing thrombosis.[450]

Vasculitis: Systemic vasculitis is a rare cause of bowel ischemia, most often as a result of polyarteritis nodosa, which accounts for 50% to 70% of bowel ischemia cases.[446] Other causes include systemic lupus erythematosus, rheumatoid arthritis, progressive systemic sclerosis, Henoch-Schönlein purpura, Wegener granulomatosis, giant cell arteritis, and fibromuscular dysplasia.[465-468] Although larger vessels can be involved, vasculitis typically involves the small peripheral mesenteric vessels. As a result, there is a critical reduction in blood flow to the bowel with resulting wall ischemia. Because vasculitis can affect discontinuous arteries of the bowel, there is often corresponding discontinuous involvement of diseased and health bowel segments as well as involvement of both the small bowel and colon simultaneously.[450] When visualized, this discontinuous pattern of disease can be a strong indicator of vasculitis as the underlying etiology. Among other causes of bowel wall edema, only Crohn disease will more commonly demonstrate this pattern of bowel wall involvement.

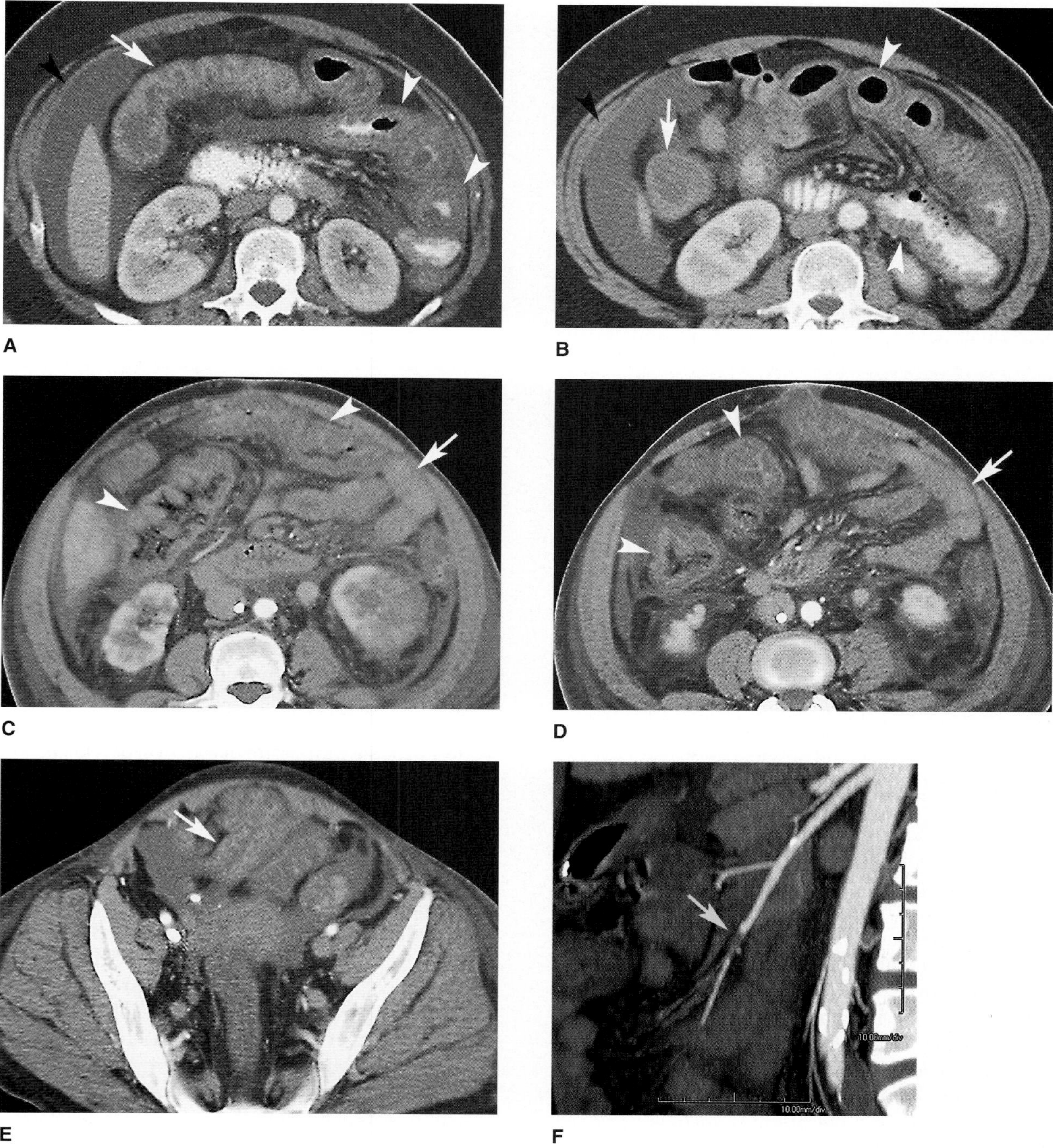

Figure 2-57 Ischemic Colitis in 2 Patients
A and **B.** This 53-year-old woman with systemic lupus erythematosus (SLE) and antiphospholipid antibody syndrome presented with abdominal pain. CT images demonstrate extensive wall thickening of the small bowel (*white arrowheads*) and colon (*arrows*) in association with ascites (*black arrowheads*) and mesenteric fluid collections. Note how the bowel wall thickening has central low attenuation a finding called the "halo" sign. CT angiographic images showed no evidence of large-vessel occlusion. This was presumed to represent a small-vessel vasculitis related to her SLE. **C-F.** This 53-year-old woman had a prosthetic mitral valve and presented with abdominal pain and an elevated lactic dehydrogenase (LDH). A-C. Contrast-enhanced axial CT images demonstrate diffuse colonic wall (*arrowheads*) and small bowel (*arrows*) wall thickening. Note the subtle target sign in the ascending and transverse colon in figure (D). There is also extensive mesenteric edema, vascular engorgement, and mild ascites present. Note the focally diminished perfusion of the left kidney in C indicating a renal infarction. These findings in conjunction with the clinical history were suspicious for mesenteric ischemia. D. CT angiogram demonstrates a filling defect within the superior mesenteric artery diagnostic of an embolus.

Radiation enteritis and colitis

Radiation-related injury to the bowel is a moderately common complication of radiation therapy for a variety of abdominal malignancies. Radiation injury at doses of less than 40 Gy is uncommon but is relatively common with doses greater than 50 Gy. Unfortunately, the doses that cause injury are very close to the doses needed to adequately treat most cancer. Rest periods between radiation sessions are important for the recovery of tissues because rapidly dividing cells are the most radiosensitive.

Bowel injury is commonly divided into early and late disease. In early radiation damage, the growing cells of the epithelial crypts are damaged by radiation, resulting in disruption of the repopulation of surface epithelium.[469] This, in turn, leads to atrophy of villi and impaired resorption, resulting in malabsorption and diarrhea. Epithelial damage also leads to inflammation and edema of the submucosal tissues and potential bacterial superinfection with further bowel wall injury. With more severe injury, mucosal ulcerations can develop. Radiation can also damage capillary endothelium, leading to further ischemic related injury. Over time, the inflammatory changes to the bowel wall from this constellation of injuries leads to collagen deposition, resulting in fibrosis and stricturing. Complete histologic recovery can take as long as 6 months. As opposed to the acute radiation change, chronic radiation damage is primarily a result of chronic bowel ischemia and necrosis from obliterative arteritis with the subsequent development of chronic ulceration and strictures.[470]

It is estimated that 2% to 5% of patients receiving abdominal or pelvic irradiation will develop radiation-related bowel injury.[471,472] Early symptoms occur 2 to 3 weeks into treatment and typically resolve within 2 to 6 months. These include anorexia, nausea, vomiting, abdominal cramps, diarrhea, and rectal bleeding.[469,473] Chronic radiation bowel injury will present 6 months to years after therapy. It is characterized mainly by dysmotility and malabsorption but occasionally can present with intestinal bleeding due to chronic ischemic complications of therapy.[469] Higher doses and larger radiation fields result in a greater incidence of radiation-induced bowel injury.[473]

Other factors that predispose patients to the development of radiation-induced bowel injury include prior surgery, coincident chemotherapy, arterial disease, diabetes, and systemic hypertension.

The most important imaging characteristic of radiation-related injuries to the bowel is their confinement to the radiation portal. Barium studies can show areas of ulceration with thickened folds in acute disease[472,474] and diminished peristalsis of the affected bowel in chronic disease.

On CT and MRI, acute radiation enteritis/colitis will typically result in bowel wall thickening due to submucosal edema that appears similar to other causes of segmental bowel wall edema (see Figure 2-58).[475] In acute disease, mucosal enhancement and the target sign can also be seen. In chronic disease, complications may be present, including bowel strictures and fistulae.[473]

Inflammatory bowel disease

Inflammatory bowel disease is a group of systemic autoimmune diseases that primarily affect the GI tract but can also affect other organ systems.[476,477] These are subdivided into Crohn disease, ulcerative colitis, and IBD-unclassified. Crohn disease and ulcerative colitis account for 85% to 90% of IBD, with the remainder being unclassified. Although some of the clinical, histologic, and radiographic characteristics of Crohn disease and ulcerative colitis overlap, it is important to distinguish between these 2 diseases when possible because of differences in their prognosis, management, and complications.[478]

Disease distribution and histopathology in IBD: Crohn disease is a transmural inflammatory disease of the mucosa characterized by discontinuous involvement of the GI tract, also known as skip lesions. It is a chronic disease with frequent relapses that can involve the entire GI tract from the mouth to the anus, and it has a predilection for the small bowel.[279] Isolated small-bowel involvement is found in 30% to 40% of patients, 90% of whom have disease affecting the terminal ileum. Both the small-bowel and colonic involvement occurs in 40% to 55% of patients, and isolated colonic involvement is demonstrated in 15% to 25% of patients.[16,281,282,479] Involvement of the proximal GI tract, including the esophagus, stomach, duodenum, and jejunum, has been reported in 20% to 40% of patients with Crohn disease but is almost never seen without concurrent ileocolic disease.[163,281] Up to 90% of patients with Crohn disease will develop perianal disease at some time during the course of their illness.[480]

In contrast to Crohn disease, ulcerative colitis is a superficial inflammatory process that only involves the mucosa of the bowel and is confined to the colon. However, approximately 15% to 20% of patients with severe ulcerative colitis have associated inflammation of the terminal ileum called "backwash ileitis." Unlike Crohn colitis, which will typically demonstrate discontinuous regions of disease, ulcerative colitis characteristically spreads contiguously from the rectum toward the proximal colon in a retrograde fashion. In fact, rectal involvement is demonstrated in the overwhelming majority of cases, with only 5% of patients demonstrating rectal sparing.[479] Approximately 15% to 20% of individuals with ulcerative colitis develop a fulminant form of the disease[161] characterized by severe symptoms and inflammation that extends beneath the colonic mucosa.[282,481,482] In these cases, colonic dilation and loss of haustra develop because of damage to the muscularis propria, a finding that is most severe in nondependent bowel segments, such as the transverse colon.[280,481,482]

Histopathologically, the earliest changes of Crohn disease are lymphoid hyperplasia and lymphedema in the mucosa and submucosa, with resultant development of small aphthoid or superficial ulcerations. Similar to Crohn disease, the earliest histopathologic changes in ulcerative colitis are small superficial erosions of the colonic mucosa, which manifest as granular mucosa, due to hyperemia and altered mucin production.[280,481,483]

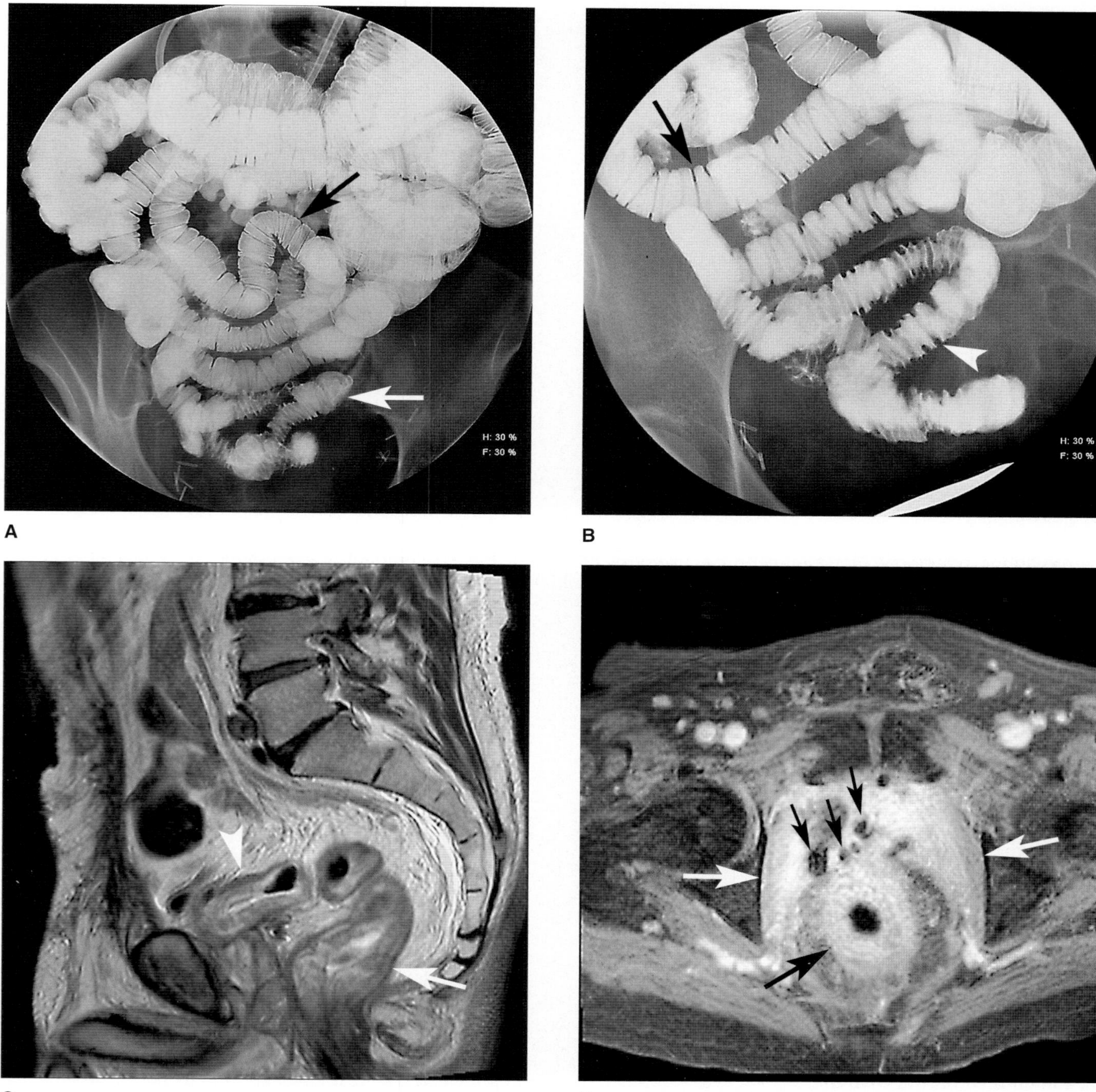

Figure 2-58 Radiation Enteritis and Colitis in 2 Patients
A and **B**. This 53-year-old woman underwent radiation therapy for endometrial carcinoma and now complains of mild abdominal pain. A. View of the abdomen from a small-bowel enema shows normal-caliber proximal small bowel (*white arrow*) with diminished-caliber pelvic small bowel in the area of the radiation portal. B. Magnified view of the pelvis shows the diminished-caliber small bowel to have thickened folds. Notice how the folds of the diseased loops (*white arrowhead*) are much thicker than the normal proximal loops (*black arrow*), indicating edema of wall of the diseased loops. This combination of findings is indicative of radiation enteritis in the region of the radiation portal. **C** and **D**. This 83-year-old man received a radical prostatectomy, cystectomy, and external beam radiation therapy for prostate cancer. C. Sagittal T2-weighted fat-saturated images of the pelvis demonstrate severe rectal (*arrows*) and distal sigmoid (*arrowhead*) wall thickening. D. Fat-saturated, postgadolinium T1-weighted sequences show severe rectal wall thickening with associated diffuse wall enhancement—findings constant with severe radiation colitis. There is also intense enhancement in the fat anterior to the rectum (*white arrows*) with absence of the prostate and multiple internal foci of susceptibility (*small black arrows*) reflecting postsurgical clips and associated inflammatory changes.

Crohn disease is distinguished from ulcerative colitis by progression of inflammation into the submucosal and adventitial tissues of the bowel wall. This transmural spread of disease results in deep ulceration of the bowel wall and, as the disease spreads into the surrounding soft tissues, can potentially lead to the development of fistulas, abscesses, intra-abdominal adhesions, inflammation of the peri-intestinal fat, and enlargement of lymph nodes.[484] In contradistinction, because ulcerative colitis is a superficial mucosal disorder, fistulas, sinus tracts, and abscesses virtually never occur.[16,481,485]

Clinical presentation of IBD: Crohn disease, ulcerative colitis, and the unclassified IBDs have similar clinical presentations. In most cases, patients first come to clinical attention between the second and fifth decades of life, with a peak distribution between 15 and 30 years of age.[16] Rarely, Crohn disease will present in the elderly. In most cases, patients with IBD will characteristically present with abdominal pain, diarrhea, and intestinal bleeding.

Often, the initial diagnosis of IBD will be suggested by findings on imaging examinations obtained to evaluate the presenting symptoms. However, definitive diagnosis of IBDs is made by histologic evaluation of tissue obtained during endoscopy from areas of diseased bowel. When disease involves the colon, esophagus, stomach, or duodenum, it is simple to obtain tissue. However, when disease exclusively involves the small bowel, it is difficult to obtain tissue. In this setting, integration of patient history, physical examination findings, and evidence of inflammation on endoscopic or imaging evaluations are used to make a presumptive diagnosis of IBD. Following initial diagnosis, findings on serial imaging examinations are frequently used to direct management by determining the presence, severity, and extent of disease, and visualization of complications such as obstruction, fistula formation, or infection.[484,486] For this reason, imaging is disease progression, regression, and recurrence.

Complications of IBD: Intra-abdominal complications of IBD include small-bowel and colonic obstruction, fistula formation, intra-abdominal abscesses, toxic megacolon, GI lymphomas, and colon carcinomas. Characteristics of bowel obstruction will be discussed in the subsequent section entitled: **Bowel Dilation**.

Intra-abdominal accesses and fistulas are common complications of Crohn disease due to the transmural spread of disease, as discussed above, but are very rare in ulcerative colitis. Development of fistulas and sinus tracts occur in 20% to 40% of patients with Crohn disease.[16,485,487] Imaging is commonly used both in the detection and the monitoring of these complications. Barium enema is best for detecting enterocolic and enteroenteric fistulas, whereas CT is more accurate for detecting perianal, enterovesical, and enterocutaneous fistulas and sinus tracts.[278,480,485,487-489]

Toxic megacolon, a potentially fatal complication, develops in less than 5% of patients with ulcerative colitis.[280,481,482] However, when it occurs, it is the most common cause of death in these patients.[16,279,280] Approximately one-third of toxic megacolon cases develop within the first 3 months of diagnosis, but this complication can occur at any point during the course of the disease.[280,481,482] Histopathologically, it is characterized by transmural inflammation and ulceration with destruction of ganglion cells in the bowel wall resulting in colonic dilation measuring at least 6 cm.[16,280] Patients will present with signs and symptoms of systemic toxicity such as fever, tachycardia, increasing diarrhea, anemia, and electrolyte abnormality.[481]

Five percent of patients with ulcerative colitis are found to have sclerosing cholangitis.[281,485] Imaging and clinical characteristics of sclerosing cholangitis are discussed in Chapter 3. A small number of patients with ulcerative colitis can also develop cirrhosis as a complication of chronic or active hepatitis or of primary sclerosing cholangitis.[485,490]

Neoplasms, including carcinoma and lymphoma, are uncommonly seen in IBD.[16,484,485,491] Both patients with ulcerative colitis and Crohn ileocolitis have an increased risk of developing colon cancer, whereas patients with Crohn disease and enteritis also have an increased risk of developing small-bowel cancer.[281,485,488,492] Risk factors for the development of carcinoma include younger age at diagnosis, greater extent and duration of disease, increased severity of inflammation, family history of colon cancer, and coexisting sclerosing cholangitis.[493,494]

Neoplasm is thought to develop when chronic inflammation results first in dysplasia and then in metaplasia, finally leading to the development of carcinoma.[494] In addition to the risk factors cited above, the risk of developing carcinoma appears to be higher in patients with ulcerative colitis than those with Crohn disease. Estimates of risk have widely varied but recent studies suggests a cumulative probability of colon carcinoma in ulcerative colitis of 2.5% at 20 years, 7.6% at 30 years, and 10.8% after 40 years of disease.[495] Although the risk of colon cancer for patients with Crohn disease is less than for patients with ulcerative colitis, it is equivalent when the extent of colonic disease in the 2 diseases is similar.[494] Distinguishing between cancerous and inflammatory lesions is difficult in this population, both on endoscopy and imaging. Despite this difficulty, most carcinoma is suspected on the basis of imaging or endoscopic surveillance and only 3% of cancers are discovered incidentally in surgical specimens performed for reasons other than cancer resection.[493] It is further heartening that modern medical and surgical therapy is likely reducing the incidence of cancer in these diseases.[494]

In addition to carcinoma, patients with IBD may also be at increased risk for developing lymphoma. In a large meta-analysis of patients with IBD who were treated with immunosuppressive therapy, there was an approximately 4-fold risk of developing lymphoma over the general population.[496] However, these results are indeterminate as population-based studies suggest that IBD does not appear to be associated with an increased risk of lymphoma.[497,498]

Imaging features of IBD: Imaging findings in IBD fit into 1 of several characteristics. The inflammation of the bowel results in submucosal edema of the bowel wall, which can be identified on abdominal plain films, barium studies, and cross-sectional imaging examinations. Double-contrast barium enema is advantageous over cross-sectional imaging in that it visualizes the surface of the colonic mucosa with fine detail. As such, it can identify a variety of abnormalities, including subtle ulcerations, larger ulcers, and extensive denudement of the mucosa. Cross-sectional imaging examinations are advantageous over barium evaluation in that they can evaluate the pericolonic tissues for evidence of inflammation, hyperemia, and adenopathy. Both barium and cross-sectional imaging examinations are able to demonstrate extramucosal complications such as sinus tracts, fistula, and abscesses.

Abdominal x-rays: Abdominal radiographs are insensitive and nonspecific in the evaluation of IBD. They are not recommended in routine evaluation of patients with IBD. However, on occasion, findings on abdominal radiographs will be the first imaging indication of the presence of either Crohn disease or ulcerative colitis. For example, abdominal radiographs may demonstrate small-bowel fold thickening in patients with Crohn disease or may demonstrate colonic thumbprinting in patients with Crohn colitis or ulcerative colitis (see Figure 2-59). These diseases can also present with the typical radiographic findings of bowel obstruction.

Imaging Notes 2-15. Imaging Features That Differentiate Crohn Disease and Ulcerative Colitis

Ulcerative Colitis	Crohn Disease
1. Continuous progresses from rectum toward proximal colon	1. Discontinuous involvement, rectum often spared
2. Symmetric circumferential of mucosa involvement,	2. Asymmetric often less than 360 degrees of involvement "pseudosacculation"
3. Disease confined to mucosa- no fistulas/ sinus tracts/abscesses	3. Transmural disease—fistulas/sinus tracts/ abscesses common
4. Collar button ulcers on background of mucosal granularity	4. Aphthoid ulcer on background of normal mucosa
5. Disease outside the colon is rare terminal ileum occasionally involved—"backwash ileitis"	5. Disease outside the colon is common terminal ileum often involved

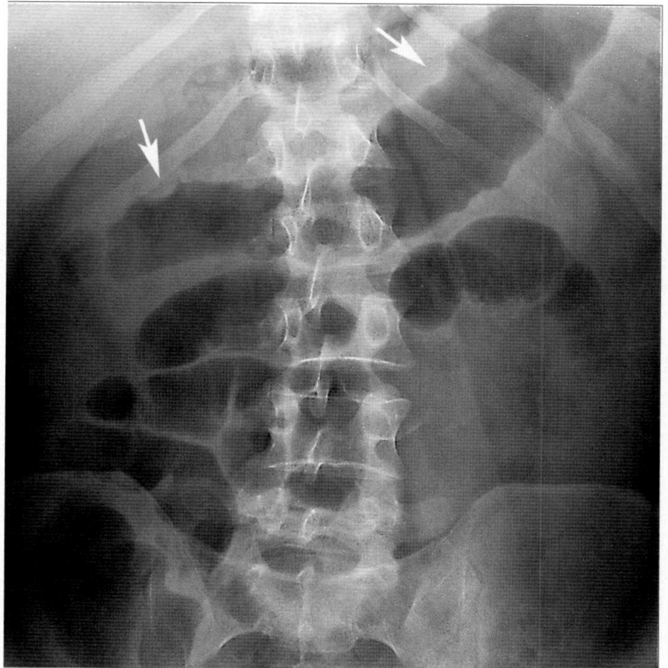

A

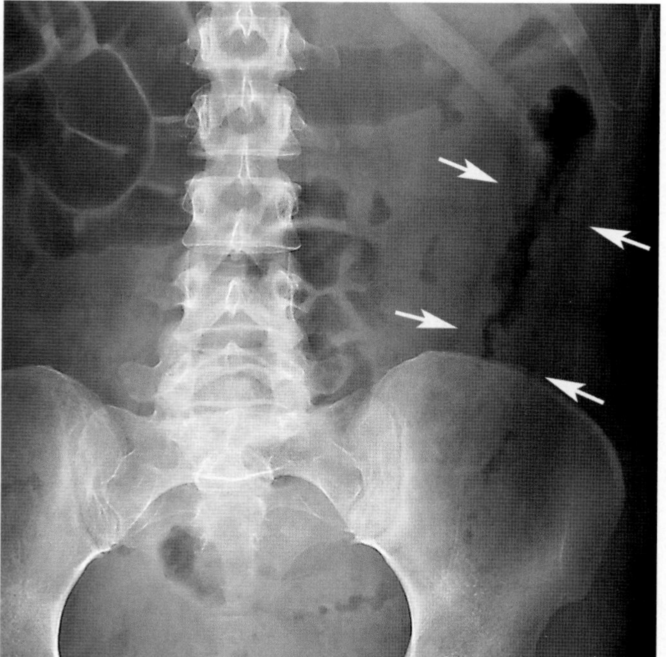

B

Figure 2-59 Crohn Disease and Ulcerative Colitis Seen on Abdominal Plain Films
A. This 25-year-old man had abdominal pain and diarrhea. Supine radiograph shows multiple foci of "thumbprinting in the transverse colon, which is most often due to colonic edema. Further evaluation was diagnostic of Crohn disease. **B.** This 27-year-old woman had blood in her stools and abdominal pain. Supine radiograph shows a thin irregular gas-filled lumen of the descending colon. The properitoneal and abdominal fat faintly outline the walls (*arrows*) of the descending colon indicating excessive wall thickening. Further evaluation resulted in a diagnosis of ulcerative colitis.

On plain films, toxic megacolon usually appears as colonic distention measuring at least 6 cm, often with associated thumbprinting.[280,485,488] In more severe cases, the mucosal surface outlined by air appears shaggy or irregular in shape. This mucosal irregularity corresponds to pseudopolyps from severe mucosal ulceration. When visualized, this portends a bad prognosis with an increased incidence of colonic perforation (see Figure 2-60).

Contrast examinations: Small-bowel follow-through and DCBEs comprise an excellent means of evaluating the bowel for the manifestations of Crohn disease and ulcerative colitis. The most important distinguishing features between Crohn disease and ulcerative colitis are the characteristic differences in distribution of the 2 diseases, such as (1) predominant small-bowel disease in Crohn disease and predominant colonic disease in ulcerative colitis, and (2) skip lesions in Crohn disease and continuous disease in ulcerative colitis. However, these diseases also have subtle differences in mucosal ulceration that are best demonstrated on endoscopy and on barium examinations using SBFT or DCBE.[281,481]

The aphthoid ulcers of early Crohn disease are seen on barium examinations as rounded 1- to 2-mm collections of barium surrounded by thin radiolucent halos of edema with normal intervening mucosa.[16,280,485] Histologically, these ulcers correspond to shallow erosions on the surface of hyperplastic lymphoid follicles in the lamina propria (see Figure 2-61).[279] In the appropriate clinical condition, these ulcers are highly suggestive of Crohn disease, but can also be seen in the acute presentation of other conditions, including tuberculosis, yersinia, amebiasis, cytomegalovirus, ischemia, and, rarely, Behçet disease.[16,280,281]

As Crohn disease advances, these small aphthous ulcers progress to form deeper ulcers that appear as stellate, serpiginous, or linear collections of barium on DCBEs. Over time, these deeper ulcers become confluent and a network of deep transverse and longitudinal ulcers develop that are separated by residual areas of edematous mucosa and surviving tissue. On DCBE, this will appear as a cobblestone or ulceronodular pattern of barium trapped within the disrupted mucosa outlining islands of mucosal edema.[16,278-280,499,500] With healing, the regions of spared mucosa form multiple linear tendrils of tissue projecting into the lumen of the colon, lesions that have been termed inflammatory pseudopolyps (see Figures 2-36 and 2-60).[16,278-281]

The severe edema and inflammation associated with Crohn disease can lead to circumferential narrowing of the small bowel that reverts to normal caliber on follow-up barium studies after treatment.[16,281] However, transmural inflammation can also lead to asymmetric scarring along the mesenteric border of the small bowel resulting in the formation of sacculations along the antimesenteric border.[16,278-280] Alternatively, circumferential scarring may be present that results in irreversible strictures in the small bowel or colon.[280,485]

In contrast to Crohn disease, the superficial erosions of ulcerative colitis typically cause a stippled, granular appearance to the surface of the colon on DCBE (see Figure 2-62).[280,481,483] As the disease advances, large ulcerations can erode into the submucosa and extend laterally beneath the diseased, but intact, mucosa. These ulcerations have a narrow neck and larger submucosal cavity that, when filled with contrast and viewed in profile, resembles a "collar button." When seen, these ulcers are characteristic of Crohn disease.[279-281] As with Crohn disease, disease progression leads to confluence of these ulcers followed by sloughing of the overlying mucosa that leaves islands of residual tissue, or pseudopolyps, that extend into the colonic lumen.[169] These mucosal remnants can rarely be identified on plain radiographs and CT images if they are outlined by air.[16,279-282,485]

Differentiation of Crohn disease and ulcerative colitis can be difficult when there is a pancolitis associated with backwash ileitis. In this setting, features that favor a diagnosis of ulcerative colitis include the following: a fixed patulous ileocecal valve; the absence of small-bowel ulceration; and a dilated, granular terminal ileum on DCBE or

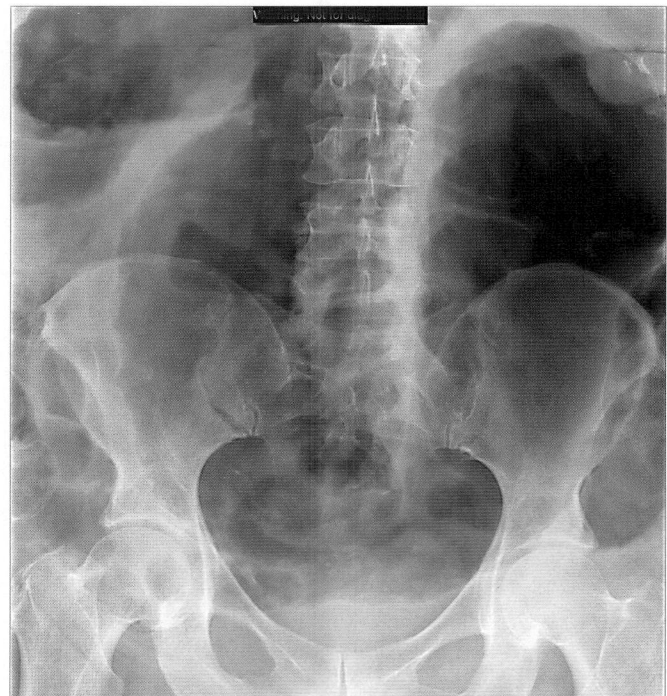

A

Figure 2-60 Toxic Megacolon
This 54-year-old woman presented with fever, abdominal pain, nausea, vomiting, and an elevated white count. **A.** Supine view of the abdomen demonstrates massive distension of the transverse colon to 13 cm at greatest diameter. The mucosa of the bowel has a nodular appearance, indicating edema or polypoid projections into the lumen.

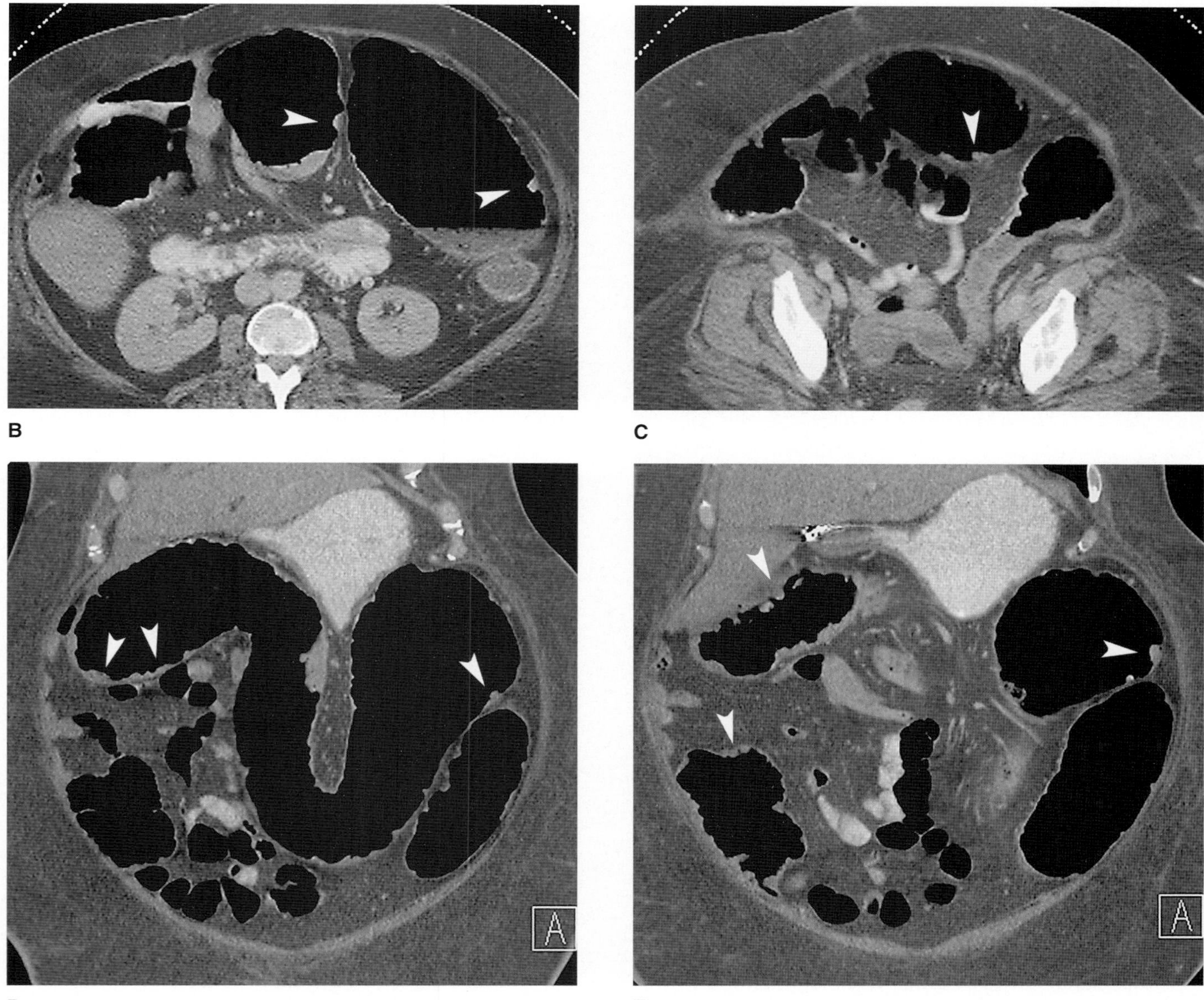

Figure 2-60 Toxic Megacolon (*Continued*)
Axial (**B** and **C**) and coronal (**D** and **E**) CT images confirm the distension of the colon and show multiple small polypoid projections into the lumen of the colon, representing pseudopolyps. This combination of findings suggests toxic megacolon. The wall of the colon is paradoxically thinned because of mucosal destruction and overdistension. In most cases, this will require surgical removal of the colon. Histologic evaluation of the bowel showed evidence of nonspecific inflammatory bowel disease.

SBFT.[16,279-281,481,501] In contrast, involvement of the terminal ileum in patients with Crohn disease is characterized by a stenotic ileocecal valve, luminal narrowing, ulceration, and fistula formation.[170]

Over time, the appearance of the colon in ulcerative colitis will alter because of chronic inflammation. Following severe episodes of colitis, healing of the colon can lead to hypertrophy of the muscularis mucosae, which when contracted, produces an ahaustral appearance to the colon.[280,282,485] Other findings of chronic disease include submucosal and extramural fat deposition due to chronic inflammation. If severe enough, extramural fat deposition may produce luminal narrowing, particularly of the rectum.[16,280,281,481,485,499] Alternatively, luminal narrowing may result from postinflammatory strictures reflecting fibrosis.[169] In constellation, these processes produce a foreshortened, narrowed, and ahaustral colon (see Figure 2-62). This appearance, termed the "lead-pipe colon," is typical of ulcerative colitis and reflects the uniform distribution of disease. In contrast, the heterogeneous inflammation and scarring of the colon in Crohn disease is unlikely to produce a uniformly narrowed colon.

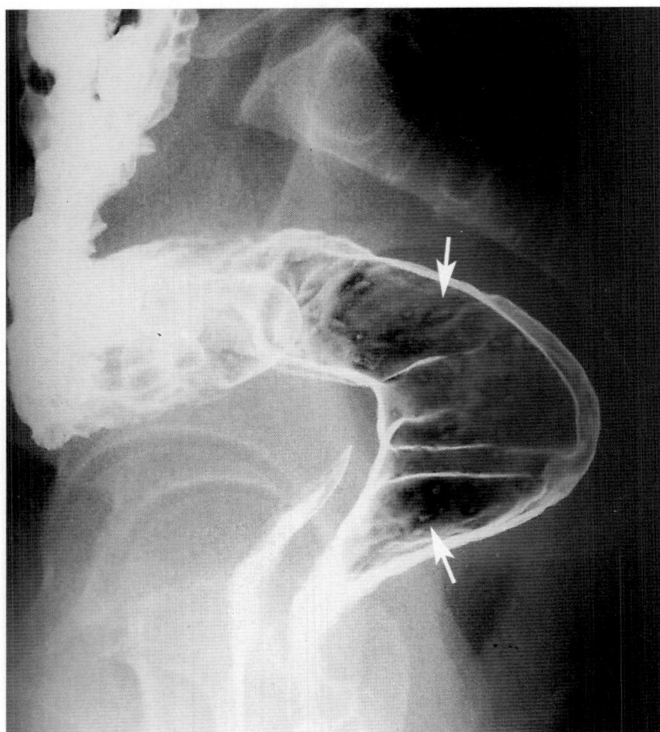

Figure 2-61 Aphthous Ulcers in Crohn Colitis
This 24-year-old woman complained of abdominal pain. Double-contrast barium enema shows multiple small aphthous ulcers in the rectum. These are seen as small barium collections surrounded by a lucent halo, representing the ulcer and surrounding edema. There is also contrast within the vagina indicating the presence of an anovaginal fistula.

Barium examination can also be useful in the detection of complications of IBD. Sinus tracts and fistulas can be seen as tracts of barium extending beyond the lumen of the bowel (see Figures 2-61 and 2-63). Abscesses can be seen as large extraintestinal collections of barium; however, in most cases cross-sectional imaging will be more sensitive in their detection.

As above, patients with ulcerative colitis are at higher risk for developing carcinoma relative to patients with Crohn disease. In fact, both early and advanced colon cancers can be difficult to detect on DCBE examinations among patients with ulcerative colitis. Early cancers often appear as flat, plaquelike lesions superimposed on inflamed mucosa.[281,502] Advanced cancers tend to be infiltrating or scirrhous lesions that can be mistaken for benign strictures on barium evaluation (see Figure 2-62).[170] Similarly, Crohn-related small-bowel carcinomas typically appear as smooth, tapered areas of narrowing that can be impossible to differentiate radiographically from benign strictures.[159] Crohn-related GI lymphomas can also be indistinguishable from areas of underlying Crohn disease on barium, CT, and MRI examination.[480,485] However, visualization of mesenteric lymph nodes on cross-sectional imaging measuring >1 cm should raise the possibility of a concomitant cancer or lymphoma in patients with IBD (see Figure 2-64).[280]

Cross-sectional imaging: CT, and to a lesser extent MRI, are the most commonly used imaging studies for the evaluation of Crohn disease and ulcerative colitis because they can identify both the distribution of intestinal wall inflammation and the presence of extramucosal findings, including pericolonic soft-tissue inflammation, lymph node enlargement, fistulas, abscesses, and adhesions.[282,481,484,503] In addition, CT is used more commonly than MRI because of its greater availability and shorter examination time. However, MR enterography has also proven highly effective in evaluation of this disease and is emerging as the preferred modality for evaluating younger patients where radiation exposure is of concern. Further, CT and MRI are particularly important in the evaluation of patients with Crohn disease, where they are commonly used in guiding management and monitoring of response to therapy.[280,488,504-506]

Detection of abnormal bowel wall enhancement is not possible when positive intraluminal contrast is used because mucosal enhancement is obscured by the high attenuation or signal within the lumen of the bowel. Instead negative intraluminal contrast, in other words, contrast that is low attenuation on CT or low signal on MRI, is necessary to accurately evaluate bowel wall enhancement.[221,484,485,489,507] The use of these agents permits visualization of the high attenuation or signal of the enhancing bowel wall distinct from the low attenuation or low signal intraluminal bowel contents. Hyperenhancement of the bowel is judged relative to the enhancement of normal nondiseased bowel wall segments.

Bowel wall thickening is the most consistent feature of both Crohn disease and ulcerative colitis on cross-sectional images.[16,36,280,485,487,488,503,508-514] Typical wall thickening in IBD is in the range of 1 to 2 cm, although, as above when the small-bowel lumen is distended a wall thickness >3 to 4 mm is considered abnormal.[231,282] In general, Crohn disease, which causes transmural inflammation, produces greater wall thickening, on average 11 mm to 13 mm, compared to ulcerative colitis, which causes only mucosal inflammation, on average 8 mm.[16,278,280,281,446,488] In addition to the degree of wall thickening, the distribution of the wall thickening is also important in differentiating between these diseases. Transmural thickening in Crohn disease is most common in the terminal ileum and in many cases will demonstrate multiple noncontiguous areas of disease (see Figure 2-65). In contrast, patients with ulcerative colitis will characteristically have uniform, continuous colonic wall thickening with absence of small-bowel wall thickening (see Figure 2-64).[16]

Bowel wall enhancement is an important adjunct finding of disease chronicity and disease activity in patients

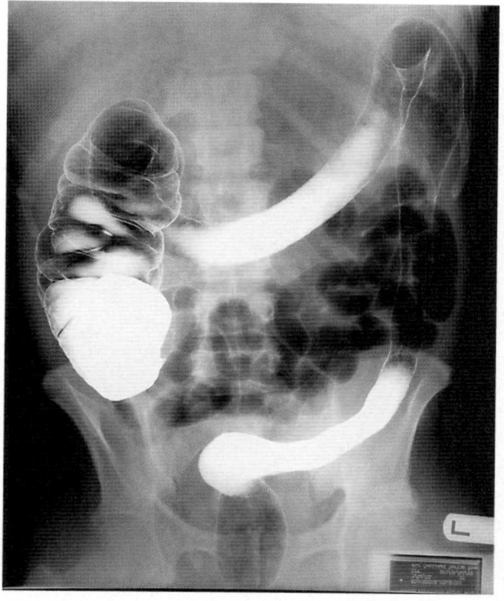

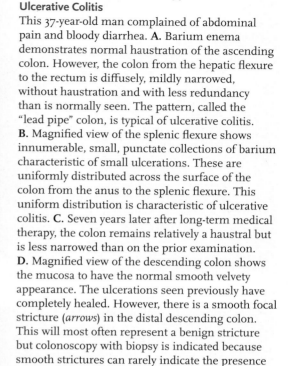

A

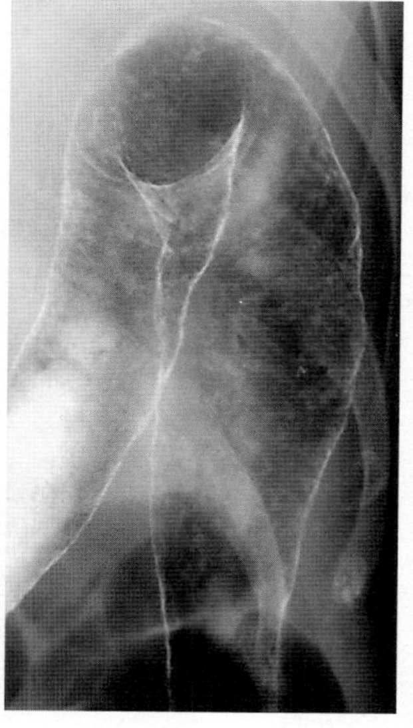

B

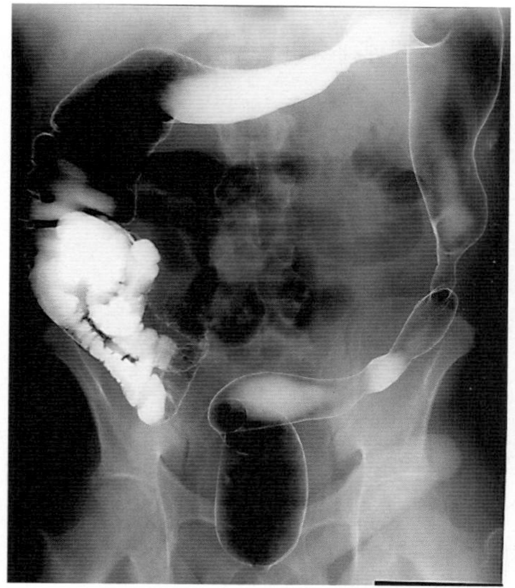

C

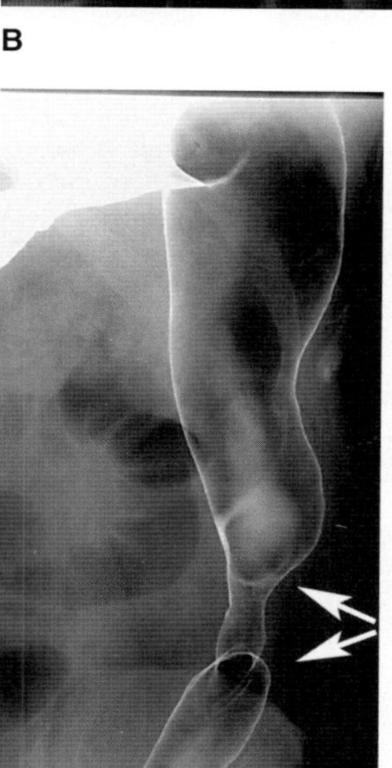

D

Figure 2-62 Lead Pipe Colon Appearance of Ulcerative Colitis
This 37-year-old man complained of abdominal pain and bloody diarrhea. **A.** Barium enema demonstrates normal haustration of the ascending colon. However, the colon from the hepatic flexure to the rectum is diffusely, mildly narrowed, without haustration and with less redundancy than is normally seen. The pattern, called the "lead pipe" colon, is typical of ulcerative colitis. **B.** Magnified view of the splenic flexure shows innumerable, small, punctate collections of barium characteristic of small ulcerations. These are uniformly distributed across the surface of the colon from the anus to the splenic flexure. This uniform distribution is characteristic of ulcerative colitis. **C.** Seven years later after long-term medical therapy, the colon remains relatively a haustral but is less narrowed than on the prior examination. **D.** Magnified view of the descending colon shows the mucosa to have the normal smooth velvety appearance. The ulcerations seen previously have completely healed. However, there is a smooth focal stricture (*arrows*) in the distal descending colon. This will most often represent a benign stricture but colonoscopy with biopsy is indicated because smooth strictures can rarely indicate the presence of a colon cancer.

with IBD that can be seen on both CT and MRI examinations. In early Crohn disease, wall thickening usually reflects edema and spasm, whereas in chronic disease wall thickening usually reflects fibrotic strictures with varying degrees of obstruction.[279,280] The differentiation between active and chronic disease is also based on the pattern and degree of bowel wall enhancement. Mural enhancement is the most sensitive finding of active Crohn disease and, when combined with wall thickening, correlates with disease activity (see Figures 2-64 and 2-65).[485,515,516] As a consequence, both of these factors are currently used to guide management of patients with Crohn disease.[505]

As on CT, the degree of mural enhancement after administration of gadolinium on MRI correlates with the degree of disease activity and the degree of inflammation.[280,510-512,517] Specifically, high T2 signal within a thickened bowel wall with corresponding enhancement indicates inflammation associated with active Crohn disease. In contrast, wall thickening without high-signal intensity on T2-weighted images or without enhancement after gadolinium indicates decreased disease activity associated with clinical remission.[280,510,514]

In some cases of IBD, the bowel wall will appear as concentric rings of higher then lower and then higher attenuation. These concentric rings have different meanings depending on the etiology of the lower attenuation central or submucosal ring. In acute disease, the concentric rings are due to differences in the enhancement pattern of the layers of the bowel wall. The outer ring of high attenuation represents hyperemia of the muscularis propria and serosa,

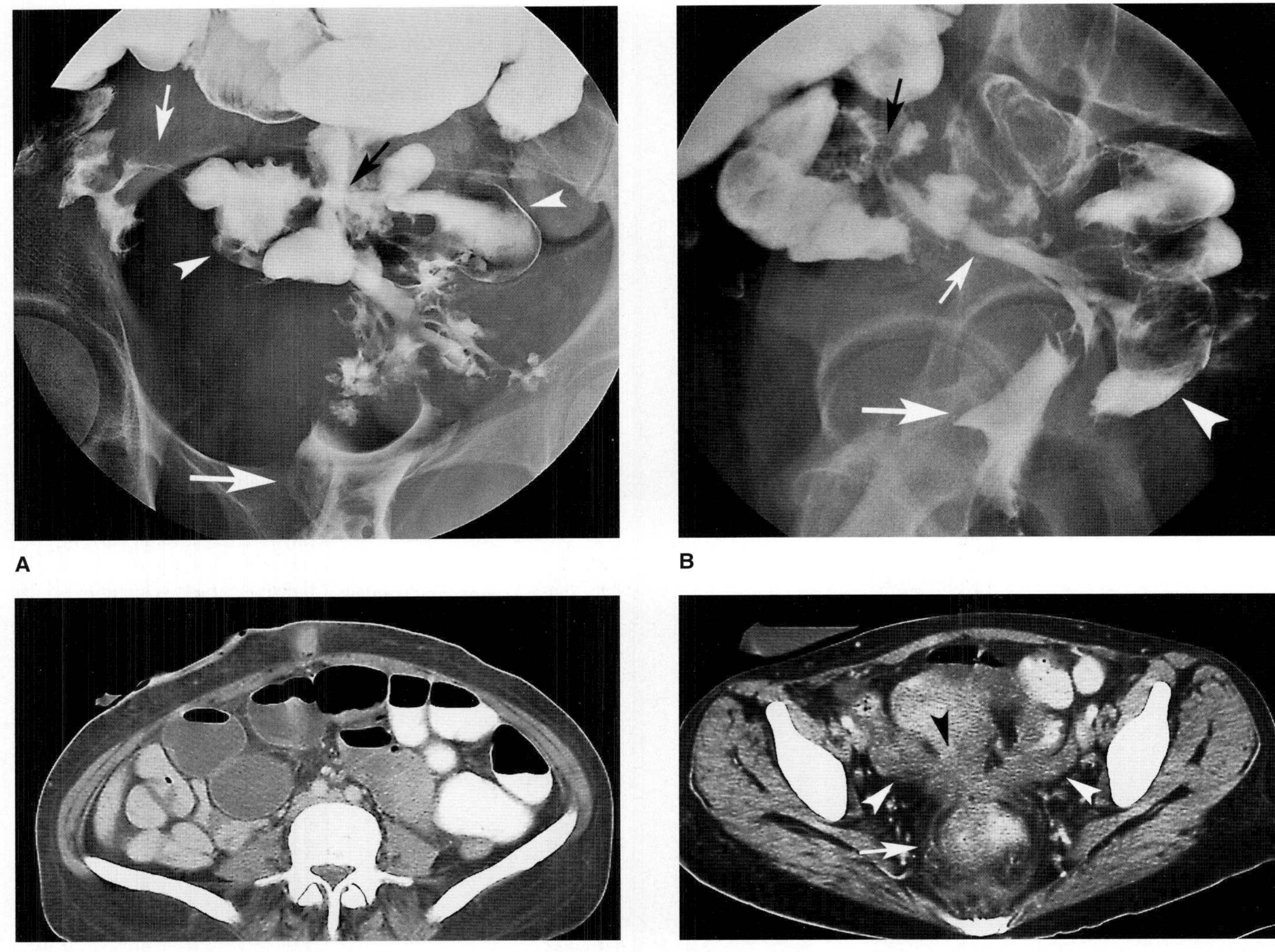

Figure 2-63 Crohn Disease with Multiple Fistula
This 35-year-old woman had active Crohn disease that required a partial colectomy. Several months after the surgery, she complained of persistent abdominal pain and a vaginal discharge. **A** and **B**. Images from a small-bowel follow-through shows tethering of multiple small-bowel loops (*small arrowheads*) around a central point (*black arrow*). A small fistulus tract can be seen extending to the cecum (*small arrow* in A) and a larger fistulous tract (*small arrow* in B) is seen extending to the vagina (*large white arrow*) and the rectum (*large arrowhead* in B). Two months later, she complained of increased abdominal pain. **C** and **D**. CT scan demonstrates extensive thickening of the rectal wall (*arrow*) with inflammatory stranding of the perirectal fat. Multiple small-bowel loops are seen tethered around a central pelvic scar (*black arrowhead*) reminiscent of the bowel loops in A. The fistulas cannot be identified. However, the proximal small-bowel loops in C are dilated, indicating obstruction due to the pelvic scarring and inflammation.

the central ring of low attenuation represents submucosal edema, and an inner ring of high attenuation represents hyperemia of the mucosa, lamina propria, and muscularis mucosa. This phenomenon is called "mural stratification," the "target" sign, or the "double halo" sign. It is a manifestation of active, acute or subacute, inflammation (see Figure 2-64).[279,446,457,488,506,518-520] These concentric rings are also visible on MRI, best demonstrated on T2-weighted images, where the mural stratification is visualized as high-signal submucosa sandwiched between the low-signal mucosa and muscularis propria layers.[171] Whereas central low density in acute disease reflects edema, central low density in chronic disease reflects submucosal fat deposition, which can be seen on enhanced or unenhanced examinations. In this situation, the outer ring represents the normal soft tissue attenuating muscularis propria and serosa, the central ring represents submucosal fat, and an inner ring represents the normal soft-tissue attenuation mucosa, lamina propria, and muscularis mucosa. This phenomenon has been called the "fat halo" sign and is a common manifestation of ulcerative colitis, seen in 60% of patients, but a relatively uncommon manifestation of Crohn disease,

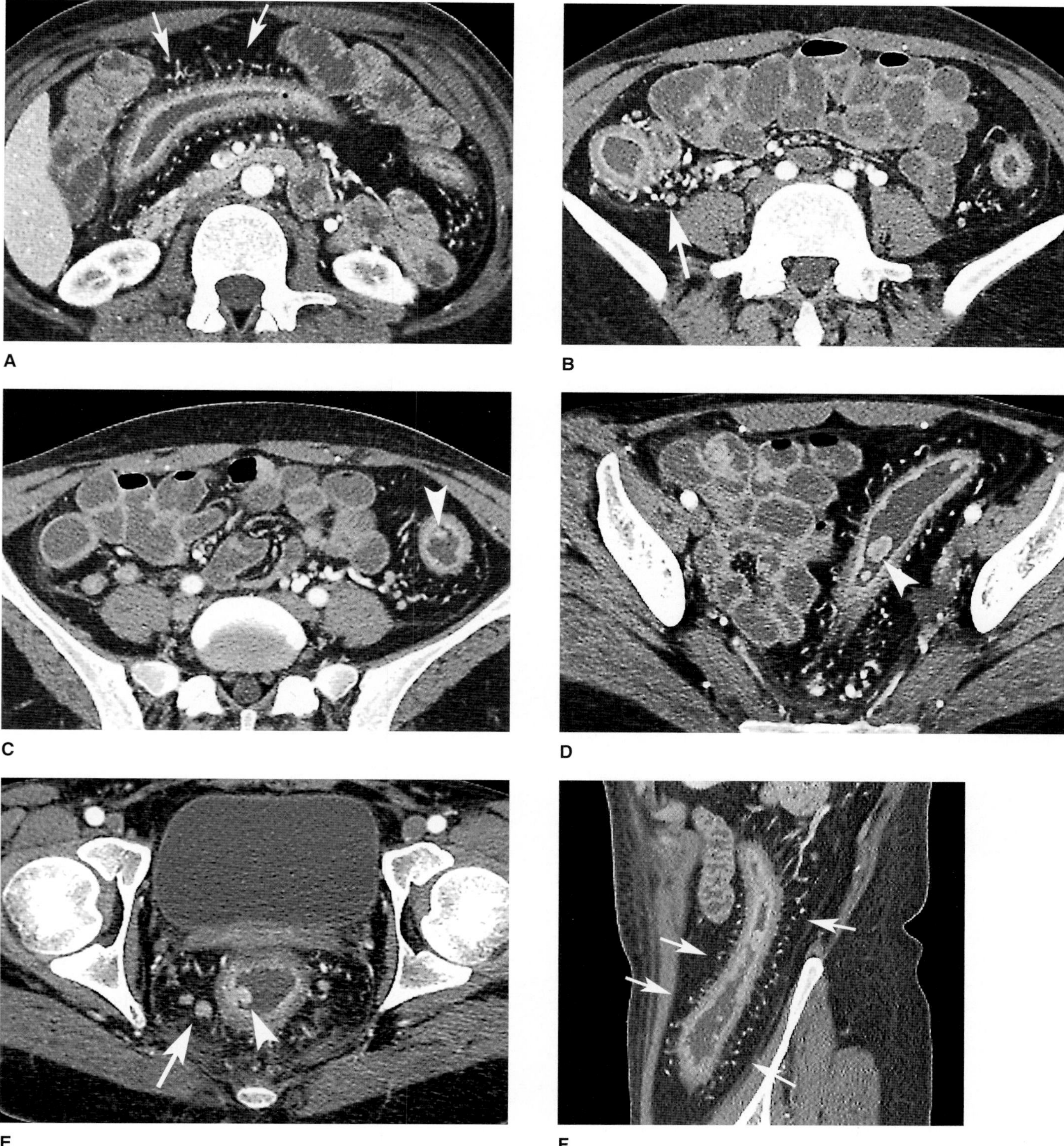

Figure 2-64 Ulcerative Colitis
This 26-year-old woman presented with severe abdominal pain and bloody diarrhea. Axial images from CT enterography (**A-E**) and sagittal reconstruction (**F**) of the descending colon demonstrate diffuse colonic wall thickening, from the anus to the cecum. The wall has alternating layers of attenuation with a hyperattenuating inner ring, a hypoattenuating middle ring, and a hyperattenuating outer ring. This phenomenon is called the target sign or mural stratification. There are small polypoid projections (*arrowheads*) into the lumen of the colon representing pseudopolyps. There are enlarged perirectal and pericecal lymph nodes (*large arrows*). Note the parallel arrays of engorged vessels extending from the wall of the transverse and descending colons (*small arrows*), a finding called the comb sign.

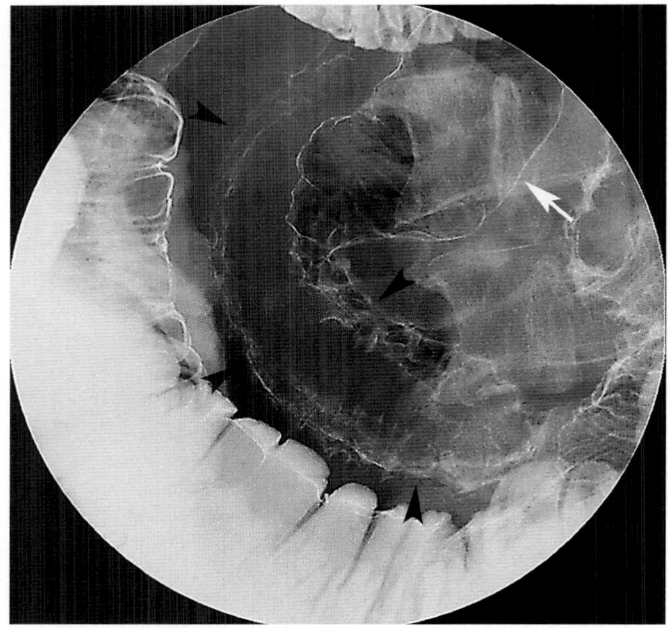

A

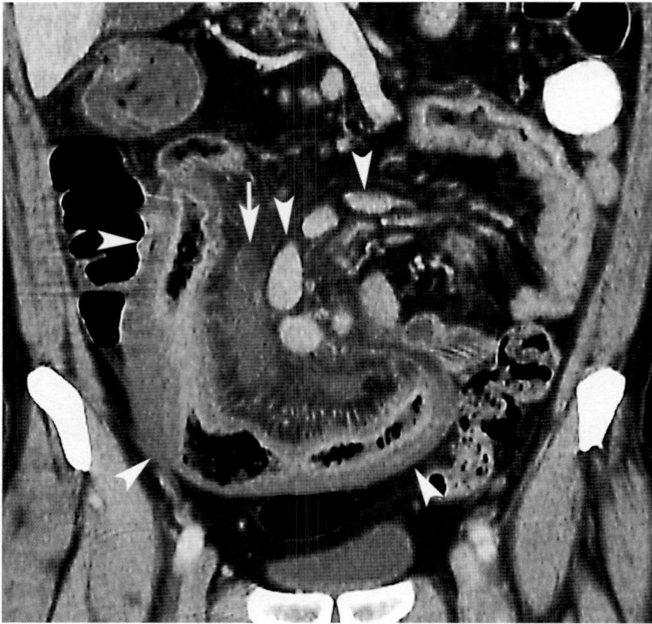

B

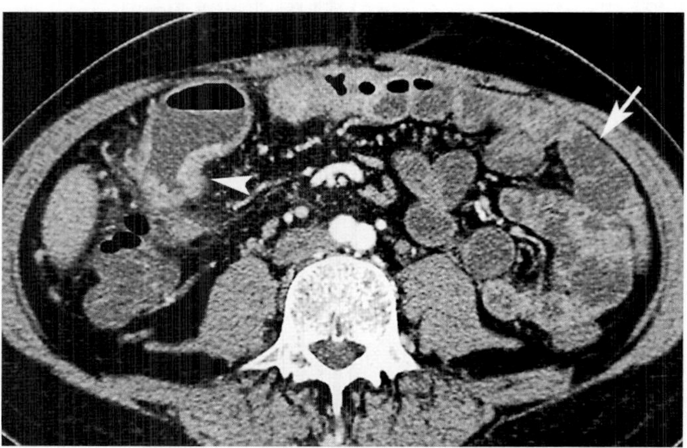

C

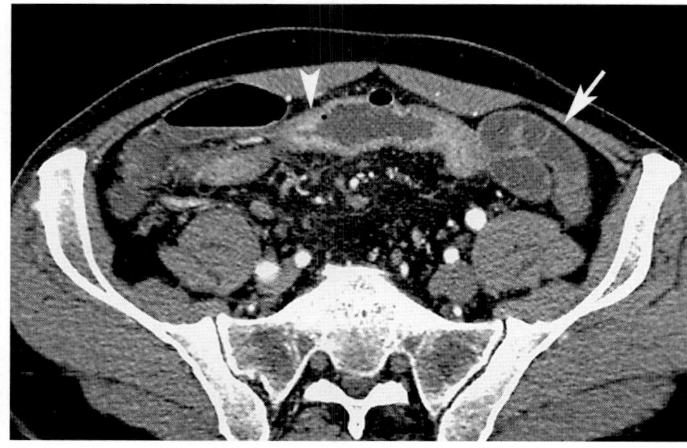

D

Figure 2-65 Crohn Disease in 2 Patients
A and **B.** This 51-year-old man presented with bloody diarrhea. A. Coronal image from an enhanced CT scan shows a terminal ilium (*large arrowheads*) with extensive mucosal thickening. Note the enhancement of the mucosa with low attenuation edema of the submucosa. There are enlarged mesenteric lymph nodes (*small arrowheads*) and edema in the root of the mesentery (*arrow*). Note the increased size of small vessels radiating from the mesenteric border of the abnormal small-bowel loop. This finding is called the "comb sign" and indicates increased blood flow due to inflammation. B. Peroral pneumocolon of the distal small bowel also shows the diseased terminal ilium (*black arrowheads*). Note the stippled appearance of the mucosal surface and compare with the normal mucosa of the more proximal ilium (*white arrow*). These small stipples represent small ulcers. **C** and **D.** This 42-year-old man complained of abdominal pain and bloody diarrhea. These CT images are part of a CT enterogram. In this examination, low attenuation oral contrast is administered in conjunction with intravenous contrast. The bowel lumen is dark and, therefore, the enhancement of the mucosa can be seen. The images show a focal region of wall thickening in the distal small bowel (*arrowheads*). Compare this with the normal thin enhancing wall of the proximal small bowel (*arrows*).

seen in only 8% of patients (see Figure 2-66).[446,521] The presence of submucosal fat was thought to be a specific indicator of previous IBD. However, this finding is now known to be nonspecific and can be seen in normal individuals. In normal patients, submucosal fat has been shown to correlate with body weight. In a study of 100 consecutive abdominopelvic CT examinations, 21% had the CT halo sign and none of these patients had a history of IBD.[522]

MRI examinations can also demonstrate the fat-halo sign as a high-signal layer in the central portion of the bowel wall on T2-weighted sequences. On non-fat-saturated T2-weighted imaging, this high signal can be due to either

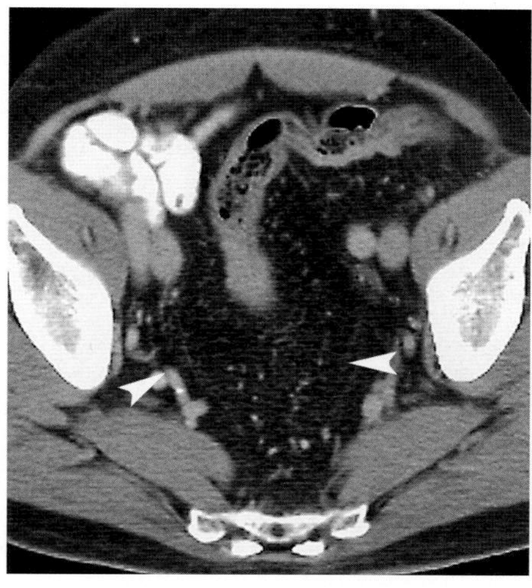

A

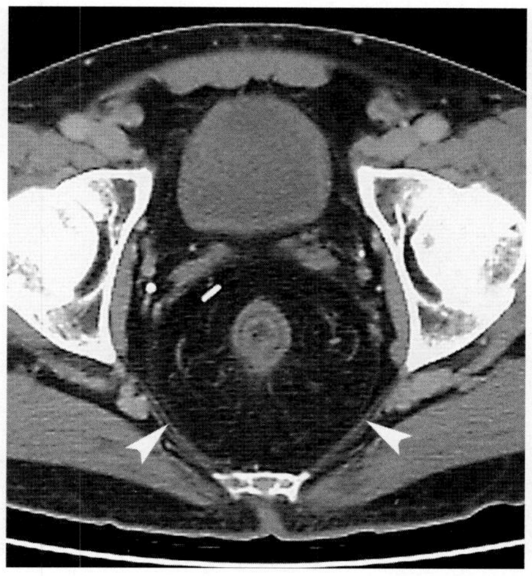

B

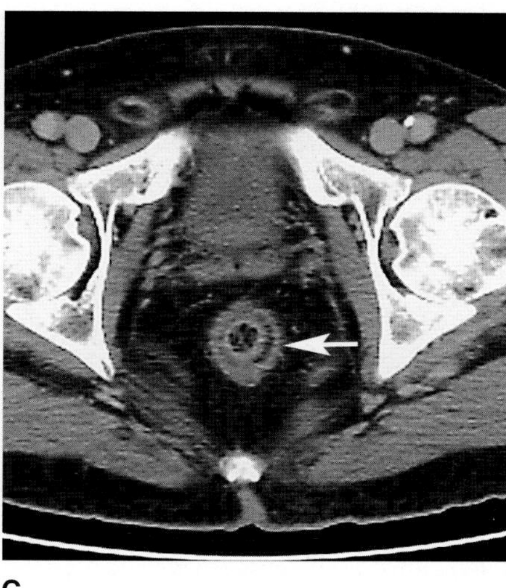

C

Figure 2-66 Fibrofatty Proliferation and the Fat Halo Sign This 57-year-old man had a history of ulcerative colitis and complained of abdominal pain. **A-C.** Unenhanced axial CT images though the pelvis demonstrate an excessive amount of fat (*arrowheads*) that surround the rectum and displace other pelvic structures. This is known as fibrofatty proliferation and is a manifestation of previous chronic bowel inflammation, most often seen in inflammatory bowel disease. Note also the layered appearance of the bowel wall. In C, this has the same attenuation as the perirectal fat. This is called the fat halo sign and is another manifestation of previous chronic bowel inflammation.

edema or fat. Using fat-suppressed T2-weighted images, however, these 2 etiologies can be distinguished. Edema will remain high-signal intensity, whereas fat infiltration will show a loss of signal intensity.[280,479,509]

Eventually over the course of this disease, bowel wall thickening will reflect fibrosis and these 3 mural layers disappear.[280,485] In this setting, the wall will enhance only mildly, if at all, indicating poor response to therapy.[280,483,505,515] Similar findings are demonstrated on MRI.[530]

There are a variety of extraintestinal manifestations of IBD that also can be a clue in diagnosing IBDs. Inflammation of the bowel results in increased mesenteric blood flow. This is seen as enlarged mesenteric blood vessels traversing the mesenteric fat to penetrate the muscularis propria of the diseased bowel. They characteristically form parallel arrays of engorged vessels that resemble a comb and are called the "comb sign" (see Figures 2-64 and 2-65).[280,487,520,523,524]

Similar to other intestinal inflammatory conditions, the pericolonic and perienteric fat can demonstrate vague increases in attenuation or streaky lines of increased attenuation traversing along the fibrous tissue planes through this fat representing edema. This finding is known as "fat stranding." This combination of the fat stranding and the comb sign is highly specific for Crohn disease on CT (see Figure 2-67).[525]

Fibrofatty proliferation of the fat surrounding an inflamed segment of bowel, also known as "creeping fat," is an extraintestinal manifestation of chronic colonic inflammation. This reflects an influx of fluid and inflammatory cells into the extraintestinal fat that leads to edema, hemorrhage, and eventually fibrosis.[16,280,446,485,506] This finding is characterized on CT as both an increased amount of fat as well as increased attenuation of the fat surrounding diseased segments of bowel (see Figure 2-66). On MRI, high T2 signal within the fibrofatty proliferation, best seen on fat-saturated sequences,[511] is a clue to the activity of the bowel disease. High T2 signal is indicative of active intestinal inflammation. However, when patients are in clinical remission, this high T2 signal resolves, leaving low-signal-intensity mesenteric fat or signal voids on fat-saturated T2-weighted sequences.[511] Since reversal of these inflammatory changes is not visualized on CT, MRI may prove to be superior to CT for monitoring the response of Crohn disease to medical therapy.

Fibrofatty proliferation of the small-bowel mesentery occurs in up to 50% of cases of Crohn disease and is virtually specific for this diagnosis. Fibrofatty proliferation of perirectal fat can also be seen with inflammatory diseases of the colon but is nonspecific and can be due to ulcerative colitis, Crohn disease, pseudomembranous colitis, and radiation colitis.[278,280,446]

Pericolonic, mesenteric, and to a lesser extent retroperitoneal lymph node abnormalities are a common finding in patients with active IBD. Typically, there will be an increase in number and size of lymph nodes draining regions of active inflammation. These lymph nodes will virtually never exceed 20 mm in diameter and in most cases remain smaller than 10 mm in short axis (see Figures 2-64 and 2-65). In the setting of active IBD, most lymph nodes between 10 and 20 mm will be a response to the inflammatory disease. However, when

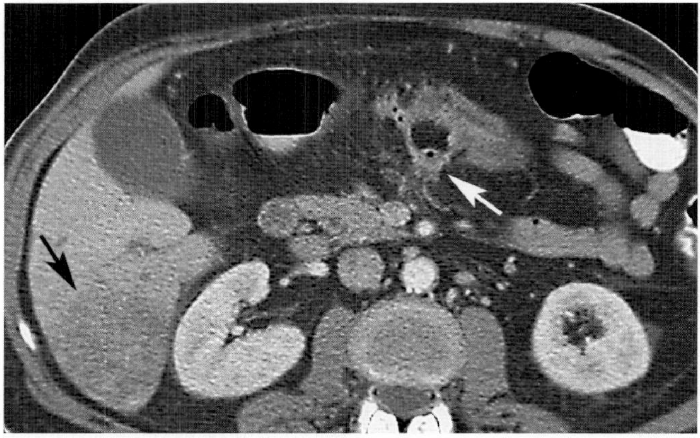
A

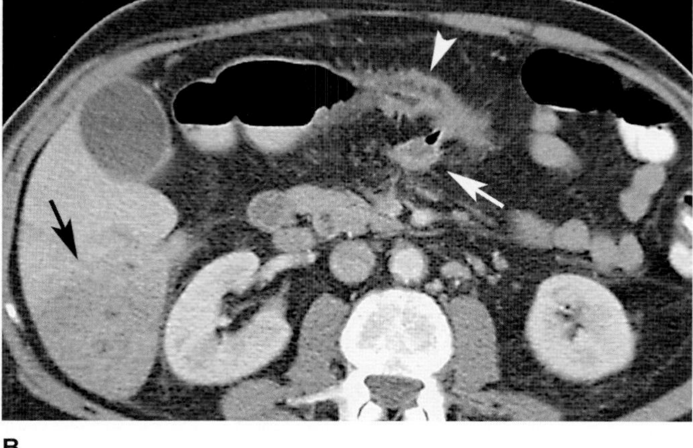
B

Figure 2-67 Crohn Disease With Sinus Tract and Abscesses This 58-year-old man with Crohn disease had persistent fevers and abdominal pain. **A** and **B.** Contrast-enhanced axial images demonstrate a small mesenteric abscess (*white arrows*) with small fistulous tracts to the transverse colon. There is a low attenuation hepatic lesion (*black arrows*) representing a developing liver abscess. Note the wall thickening and fatty attenuation submucosa in the transverse colon, indicating chronic colonic inflammation. There is also streaking of the fat surrounding the transverse colon indicating mesenteric edema.

lymph nodes greater than 10 mm are identified in the setting of chronic Crohn disease careful evaluation of the bowel should be performed to look for the development of a secondary lymphoma or carcinoma.[16,484,485,488,491]

Cross-sectional imaging is commonly used to detect and monitor the complications of IBD including sinus tracts, fistulas, abscesses and malignancies. Fistulas and sinus tracts can be seen on both CT and MRI. On CT, these fistulas and sinus tracts are demonstrated by the presence of contrast material or air within the soft tissues beyond the bowel lumen (see Figure 2-63).[278,488,506] If an enterovesical or colovesical fistula is suspected, it is helpful to obtain CT scans following the administration of oral or rectal contrast but without IV contrast. This eliminates the potential that positive contrast in the bladder may originate from the collecting system rather than the bowel.[278,488] Inclusion and evaluation of the soft tissues below the level of the pubic symphysis is also imperative in order to detect perianal disease in Crohn disease (Imaging Notes 2-15).[280,480,488,526]

Abscess and phlegmons as a result of Crohn disease can occur in many locations including the small-bowel mesentery, abdominal wall, psoas muscle, around the anus in ischiorectal fossa, and adjacent solid organs in the abdomen (see Figure 2-67).[278,446,485] Abscesses are found in one-third of patients with Crohn disease on CT where they usually occur as a complication of disease involving the small bowel rather than the colon.[485,527] CT is helpful not only in establishing the presence of these abscesses but also in guiding drainage of these collections.[278,280,488]

Hypoproteinemia

Hypoproteinemia is among the most common causes of bowel wall edema after intestinal infections, ischemia, and IBD. This is most often seen in individuals with liver disease on the basis of cirrhosis and classically involves multiple bowel segments, usually the jejunum and ascending colon.[528] Diminished plasma oncotic pressure results in transudation of fluids into the interstitial spaces of the body, including the bowel wall, which results in diffuse small-bowel and colonic wall thickening. Ascites, anasarca, and diffuse infiltration of the subcutaneous, retroperitoneal, and abdominal fat are usually concomitant findings and clues to the diagnosis of hypoproteinemia as the cause of diffuse bowel wall thickening (see Figure 2-68).

Celiac disease

Celiac disease (celiac sprue, gluten-sensitive enteropathy) is a disorder of the small intestine where genetically susceptible individuals develop intestinal inflammation and subsequent malabsorption following the ingestion of gluten. Gluten, a protein found in wheat, rye, and barley, induces an immune-mediated inflammatory response in the small-bowel mucosa leading to destruction of intestinal villi, the lengthening of intestinal crypts, and reduction in the absorption of nutrients.[529] This inflammatory response results in characteristic morphologic alterations in the distribution and frequency of small-bowel folds, which can be detected on imaging examinations. Normal individuals demonstrate a progressive decrease in the frequency of small-bowel folds from proximal jejunum to distal ilium. In patients with celiac disease, immune-mediated damage to the villi results in decreased frequency of jejunal folds to ≤3 per inch.[530,531] In an attempt to counteract the loss of resorptive area, the ileum will often hypertrophy, increasing the frequency of ileal folds to ≥3 per inch, a phenomenon called "jejunization of the ileum."[531,532] Increased wall thickness is another manifestation of celiac disease and is

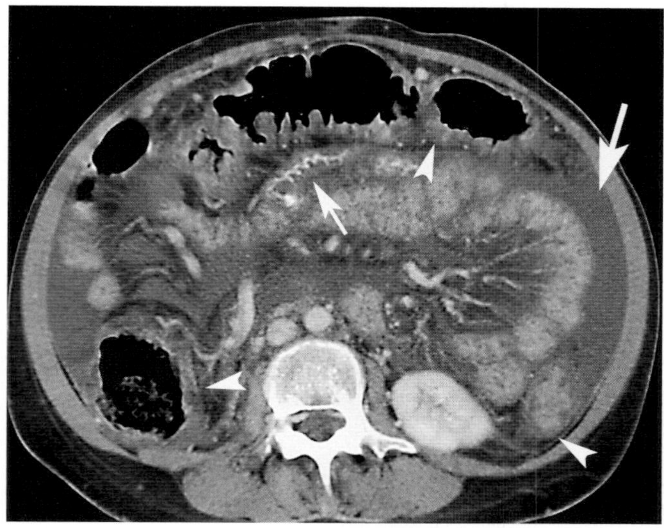

A

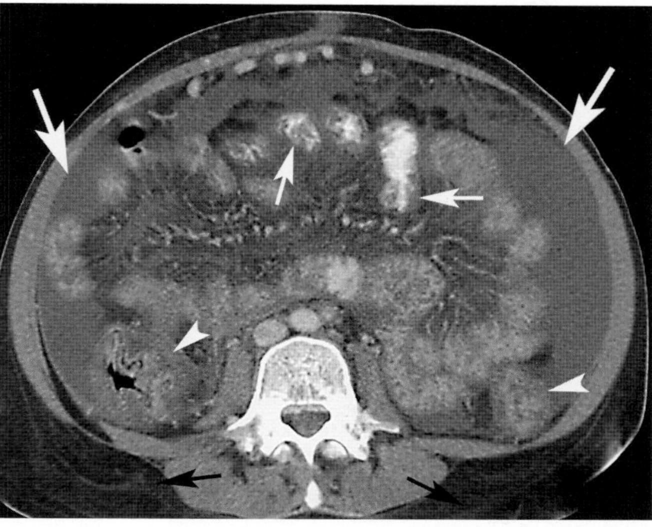

B

Figure 2-68 Bowel Edema due to Hypoproteinemia
This 23-year-old man was receiving chemotherapy for metastatic islet cell tumor. **A** and **B.** CT images demonstrate diffuse colonic wall edema (*arrowheads*) and small-bowel wall edema. The small-bowel thickening is seen best on the loops that are distended with contrast (*small arrows*) but is present in all small-bowel loops. There is also ascites (*large white arrows*) and edematous infiltration of the abdominal wall fat (*black arrows*). This constellation of findings is usually due to hypoproteinemia.

believed to be a result of edema from a low-protein state in the setting of malabsorption.[530,531,533]

There is a significant hereditary component to celiac disease with a prevalence of approximately 5% among first-degree relatives and a strong association of celiac disease with 2 human leukocyte antigen (HLA) haplotypes (DQ2 and DQ8).[534,535] The development of serologic tests for celiac disease has enabled large-scale screening studies in Europe and the United States, which reveal that the prevalence of this disease is slightly less than 1% of the general population.[535,536]

It is now recognized that there is a wide spectrum of clinical presentation in celiac disease ranging from complete lack of symptoms, to nonspecific chronic abdominal pain, to typical symptoms of malabsorption including diarrhea, steatorrhea, flatulence, weight loss, and fatigue and finally to symptoms related to malabsorption of vitamins and minerals, including anemia, osteoporosis, and arthritis. In many cases, patients' symptoms have been ascribed to irritable bowel syndrome and only later are recognized to have celiac disease.

A definitive diagnosis of celiac disease is established through small-bowel biopsy and resolution of malabsorption symptoms following the removal of gluten from the patient's diet. Early diagnosis is important because patients with untreated disease have an increased risk for developing intestinal T-cell lymphoma and adenocarcinoma.[530,537-539]

It is generally believed that the jejunoileal fold reversal is diagnostic of celiac disease and is the single most reliable finding on both routine CT examinations with oral contrast as well as CT enteroclysis for the diagnosis of celiac disease.[530,532] In 1 study of CT enteroclysis with 44 celiac disease patients and 44 healthy control subjects, jejunoileal fold reversal had a 100% specificity and a 64% sensitivity for the diagnosis of celiac disease.[532] The advantage of enteroclysis, as discussed previously, is that it produces optimal distension of the bowel compared with routine SBFT and standard enhanced CT examinations. As such enteroclysis allows for more reliable evaluation of the small-bowel fold patterns, however, small-bowel fold patterns can also be seen on standard CT examinations (see Figure 2-69). One study of 46 patients with celiac disease standard enhanced CT was able to evaluate small-bowel folds in approximately 52% of cases.[175] In fact, when small-bowel folds can be reliably evaluated, between 38% and 68% of cases demonstrated ileojejunal fold reversal.[540,541]

An advantage of CT compared to SBFT and conventional barium enteroclysis examinations is the ability to evaluate wall thickness and extraintestinal manifestations. Patients with celiac disease can demonstrate increased wall thickness of up to 11 mm in diameter with mean thicknesses of 7.7 mm in 1 study (see Figure 2-70).[540] The frequency of wall thickness greater than 4 mm ranged from 21% (7/28) in one study of standard CT to approximately 65% (29/44) in a study of CT enteroclysis.[532,541]

Another manifestation of celiac disease is luminal dilation, defined as a bowel lumen diameter of >4 cm in the jejunum and >3 cm in the ileum.[531,533] This dilation is typically most pronounced in the mid- and distal jejunum and can be seen with superimposed atonic and featureless

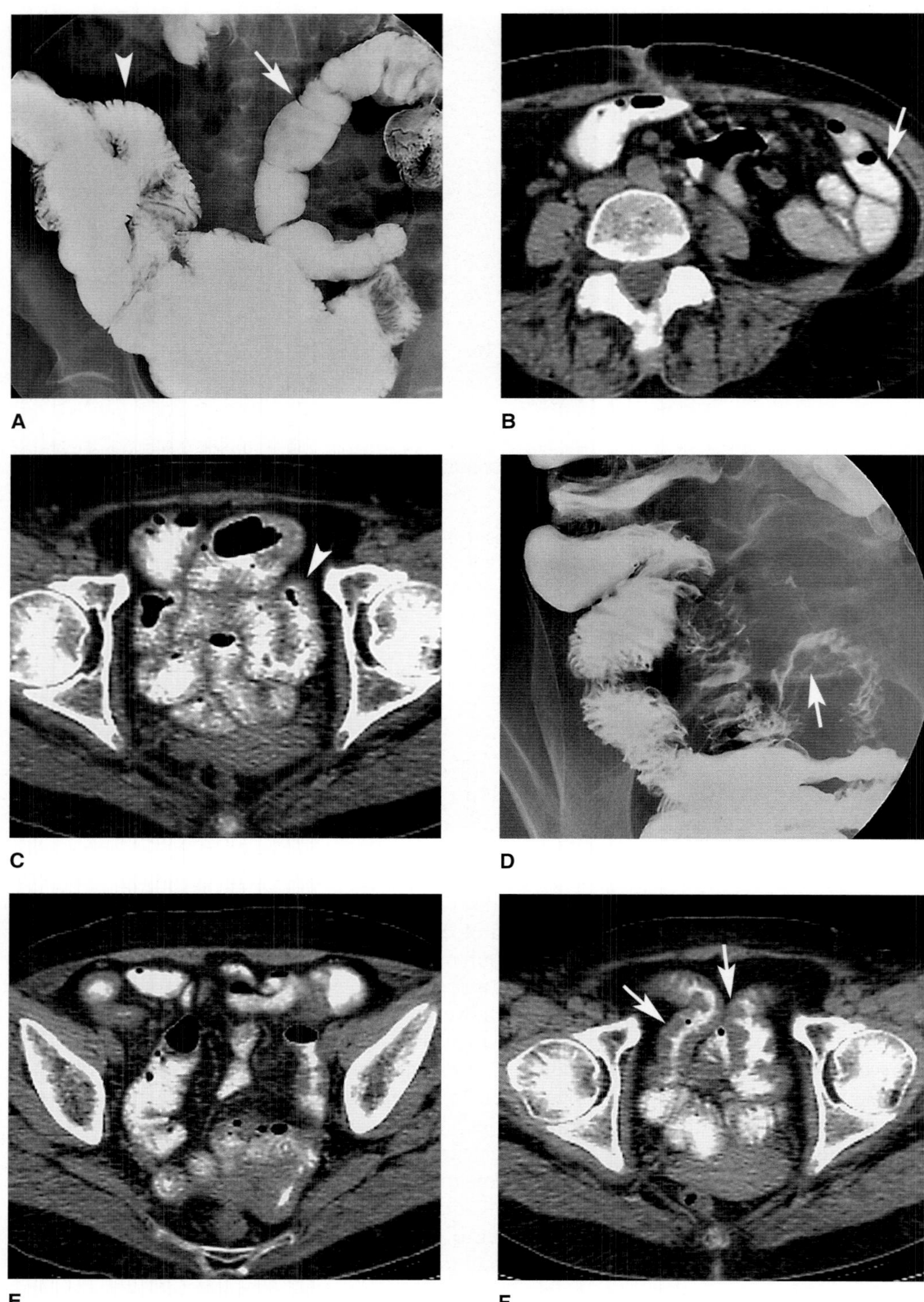

Figure 2-69 Lymphoma Complicating Celiac Disease
This 57-year-old woman had chronic diarrhea. Small-bowel follow-through (**A**) and concurrent abdominal CT (**B** and **C**) demonstrates a decreased number of small-bowel folds in the proximal small bowel (*arrow*) and an increased number of small-bowel folds in the distal small bowel (*arrowhead*), features virtually diagnostic of celiac disease. Two years later, the patient developed weight loss. Spot film from a small-bowel follow-through (**D**) and concurrent abdominal CT (**E** and **F**) now show thickening of the wall and folds of the distal small bowel (*arrows*). This is a worrisome feature and can indicate development of a lymphoma. Biopsy was diagnostic of a T-cell lymphoma.

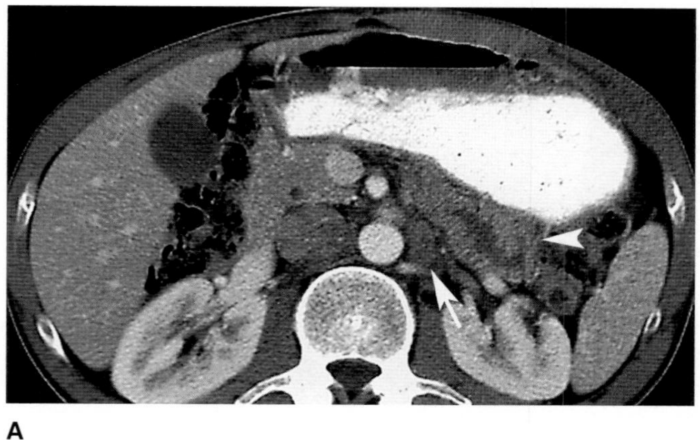

A

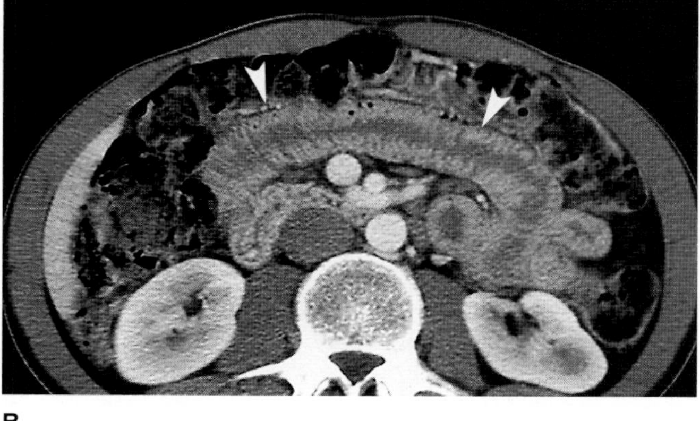

B

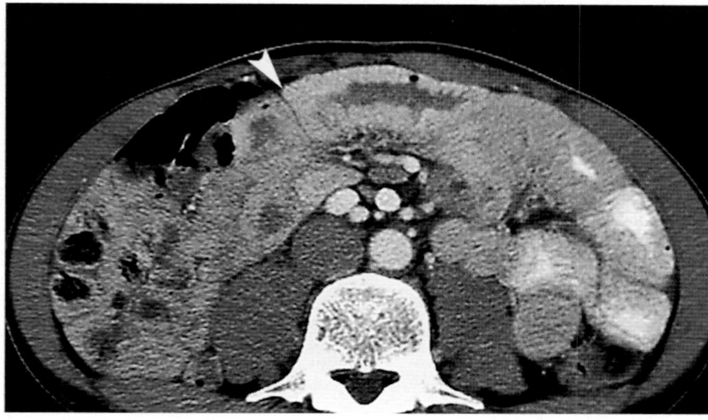

C

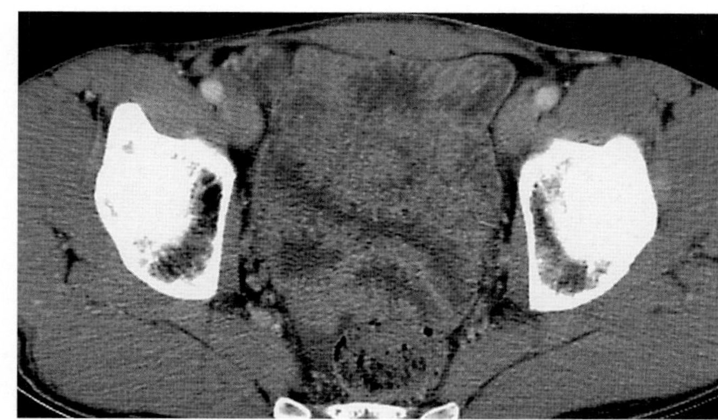

D

Figure 2-70 Celiac Sprue
This 45-year-old woman had chronic abdominal pain and bloating. Enhanced CT shows thickened proximal small-bowel wall (*arrowheads*) with an increased number of folds in the distal small bowel in image **D.** These are features that strongly suggest the diagnosis of celiac disease. There is also mild para-aortic lymphadenopathy (*arrow*) in **A.**

appearance of the small-bowel segments.[24,533,539] In addition, CT examinations of patients with celiac disease have demonstrated small-bowel luminal dilation in 24% to 66% of cases.[532,540,541]

Excess of fluid and/or air in the bowel are subjective findings that have been reported as a manifestation of celiac disease.[532,540,541] Excess fluid, characterized by dilution and/or flocculation of the intraluminal barium, has been observed in 56% to 64% of cases on CT examinations.[540,541]

Mesenteric adenopathy, defined as nodes measuring greater than 10 mm in short axis, has been variably demonstrated in 11% to 43% of patients with celiac disease on abdominal CT examinations (see Figure 2-70).[531,532,539-541] Rarely, celiac disease can be associated with an uncommon lymph node pathology called "the cavitating mesenteric lymph node syndrome." The cause of this rare complication of celiac disease is not known but has been associated with refractory celiac disease. It is characterized by moderately enlarged, centrally cystic mesenteric lymph nodes. (This unusual phenomenon is discussed in greater detail in Chapter 13, Imaging of the Lymph Nodes and Lymphatic Ducts.)

Other reported extraintestinal manifestations of celiac disease include the following: (1) increased mesenteric vessel diameter seen in up to 25% to 83% of patients on CT;[532,540,541] (2) splenic atrophy present in 30% to 50% of adults with celiac disease;[531,532] and (3) mesenteric panniculitis characterized by increased attenuation of the small-bowel mesentery fat seen in up to 6% of the general population and 11% (5/44) of patients with celiac disease in 1 study.[174] Patients with untreated celiac disease have an increased incidence of small-bowel lymphoma (see Figure 2-69).

Other causes of bowel inflammation

There are a variety of unusual causes of bowel wall inflammation that can lead to bowel wall edema. These include some chemotherapeutic medications and graft versus host disease. These 2 disorders result in toxic- or immunologic-mediated inflammation of the bowel mucosa, leading to mucosal hyperemia and submucosal edema. Imaging examinations will demonstrate similar findings of bowel wall inflammation, including bowel wall thickening, mucosal hyperenhancement, submucosal

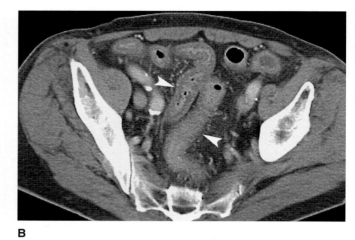

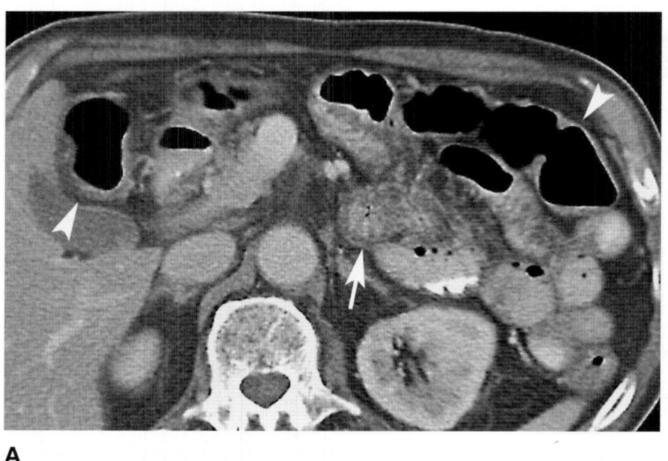

A

B

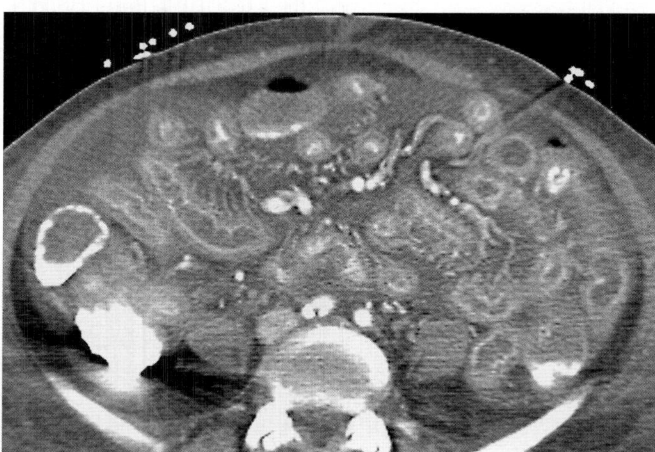

C

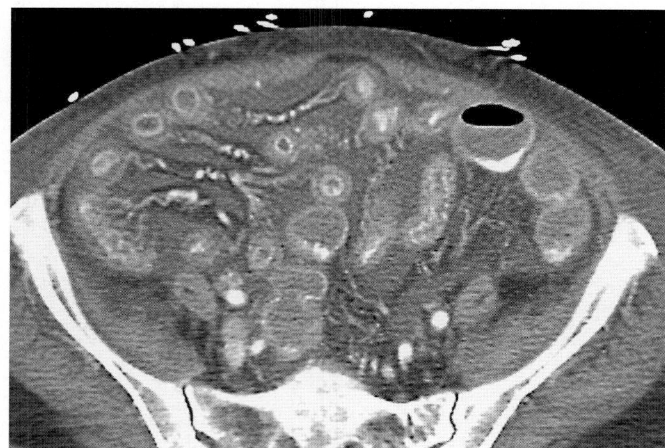

D

Figure 2-71 Other Causes of Diffuse Bowel Wall Inflammation **A** and **B**. This 80-year-old man had 3 days of abdominal pain and diarrhea after 5-fluorouracil therapy for a pancreatic carcinoma. Axial CT images show mild colonic (*arrowheads*) and small-bowel (*arrow*) wall thickening. No cause could be identified, and this was assumed to be due to 5FU bowel toxicity. **C** and **D**. This 59-year-old woman complained of nausea, vomiting, and abdominal pain after bone marrow transplant for acute myelogenous leukemia. CT enterography demonstrates intense small-bowel and colonic mucosal enhancement with submucosal edema indicating a diffuse enterocolitis. There is also moderate ascites and engorged mesenteric vessels. This patient responded to therapy for graft versus host disease.

edema, and mural stratification. They can also result in secondary pericolonic signs of inflammation including fat stranding (see Figure 2-71 and Imaging Notes 2-13).

Bowel wall hemorrhage

Intramural hemorrhage is an uncommon cause of segmental wall thickening, which can be seen in patients who are undergoing anticoagulation therapy or have an underlying bleeding diathesis. Other conditions, including alcoholism, leukemia, lymphoma, carcinoma, collagen vascular disorders, and pancreatitis can also be associated with intramural hemorrhage but are seen less frequently.[542]

Almost half of patients are asymptomatic at presentation. Those who are symptomatic typically present with vague symptoms such as nausea, vomiting, and crampy abdominal pain. GI bleeding is identified in only 30% of patients. Variability in symptoms is thought to reflect the speed with which the hemorrhage occurs as well as the volume of blood in the bowel wall.[542]

The most common sites of spontaneous intramural small-bowel hemorrhage are the duodenum and the proximal jejunum. This distribution is likely due to both the rich vascularity of the duodenum and the absence of a complete circumferential serosal layer. As a result, the duodenal wall demonstrates variable elasticity, which may facilitate expansion of intramural hematomas. In addition, the duodenal mesentery is short and relatively rigid because of fixation of the pylorus and the ligament of Treitz at the origin and termination of this bowel segment. Therefore, sudden pressure changes can result in a shearing of the bowel wall layers, resulting in a tear of the vascular plexus. This likely explains why patients with bleeding diathesis can develop intramural bowel hemorrhage through benign activities as a cough or a valsalva maneuver.[542]

Abdominal x-rays can demonstrate thickened folds in the small bowel or colon that are indistinguishable from bowel wall edema. CT will also demonstrate circumferential and symmetric bowel wall thickening involving a long segment of bowel.[231,543] In some cases, the bowel wall thickening will be nonspecific; however, in some cases the bowel wall thickening will be high in attenuation, ranging from 50 to 80 HU. This high attenuation is virtually specific for acute hemorrhage into the bowel wall. As this hemorrhage evolves, the attenuation will become isodense to the surrounding tissues at 10 days and hypodense after a few weeks. This hyperattenuation is more easily detected on unenhanced examinations. Therefore, when hemorrhage is suspected, unenhanced CT should be performed initially (see Figure 2-72).[542,543] Subsequently, IV contrast can be administered and the hematoma will appear homogenous in attenuation with no appreciable enhancement compared to the unenhanced examination.[542,543]

Infiltrating neoplasms

Infiltrating neoplasms are the least common cause of long-segment bowel wall thickening.[530] These are most often due to intestinal lymphoma but can occasionally be due to carcinomas of the bowel wall, especially in individuals with chronic inflammatory conditions such as ulcerative colitis and Crohn disease. These tumors most often present as a focal concentric or eccentric mass of the bowel wall. However, rarely, they can infiltrate along the submucosa of the GI tract and appear as long segment of symmetric bowel wall thickening (see Figures 2-69 and 2-73).[231,232,544]

Bowel Dilation

The 2 most common causes of diffuse bowel dilation are bowel obstruction and a dynamic ileus. Taken together, they are both frequent causes of hospitalization and surgical consultations, representing 20% of all surgical admissions for acute abdominal pain.[545,546] Imaging plays an important role in the diagnosis and management of these 2 conditions.

Terminology associated with bowel dilation

Mechanical blockage of forward flow of intestinal contents is variably called "bowel obstruction," "mechanical obstruction," and "mechanical ileus." Functional blockage of the bowel as a result of absent or diminished peristalsis is variably called "ileus," "adynamic ileus," "functional ileus," and "paralytic ileus." The term *ileus* is most often used to indicate bowel obstruction due to impaired peristalsis of the bowel but can occasionally be synonymous with a mechanical bowel obstruction. For example, the terms *gallstone ileus* and *meconium ileus* refer to mechanical obstruction by a gallstone and meconium, respectively. In this text, the terms *small-bowel obstruction* and *colonic obstruction* are used to indicate mechanical obstruction of the small bowel and colon, respectively, and the term *adynamic ileus* is used to indicate bowel blockage as a result of absent or diminished peristalsis.

Obstruction can be classified further into simple obstruction, meaning the lumen is variably occluded but that normal blood flow is preserved, and strangulation whereby the blood flow is compromised, leading to edema, ischemia, and eventually necrosis and perforation. Simple obstruction

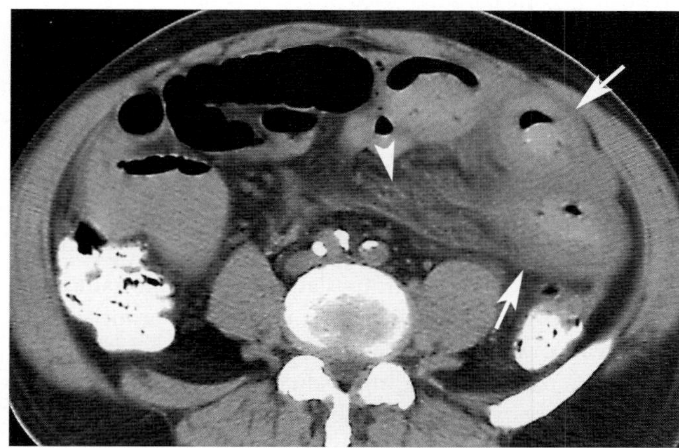

A

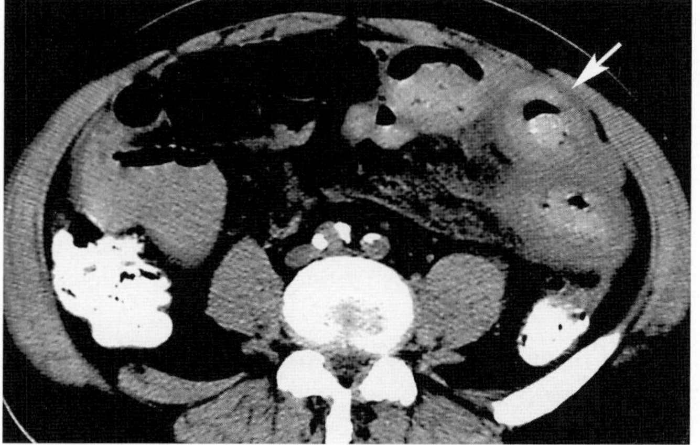

B

Figure 2-72 Bowel Wall Hematoma
This 66-year-old man was anticoagulated for a pontine stroke when he developed abdominal pain. **A.** Unenhanced CT images demonstrate circumferential wall thickening of a segment of small bowel (*arrows*) associated with mesenteric fat stranding (*arrowheads*). Note how the abnormal loop appears faintly higher attenuation than the adjacent abdominal wall. It measured 60 HU, suggesting intramural blood from a spontaneous bleed. **B.** The same image seen with a narrower window shows the high attenuation (*arrow*).

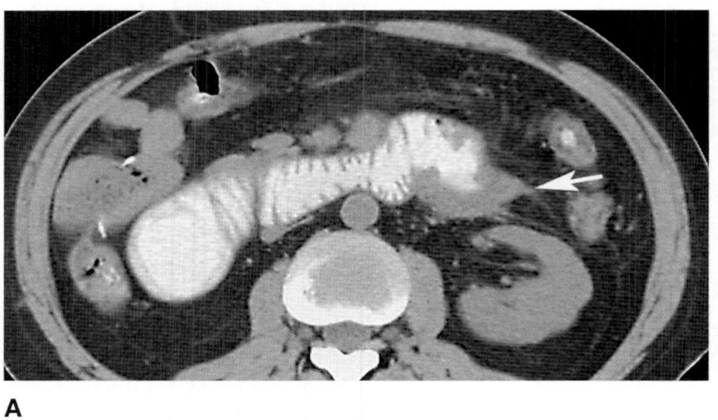

A

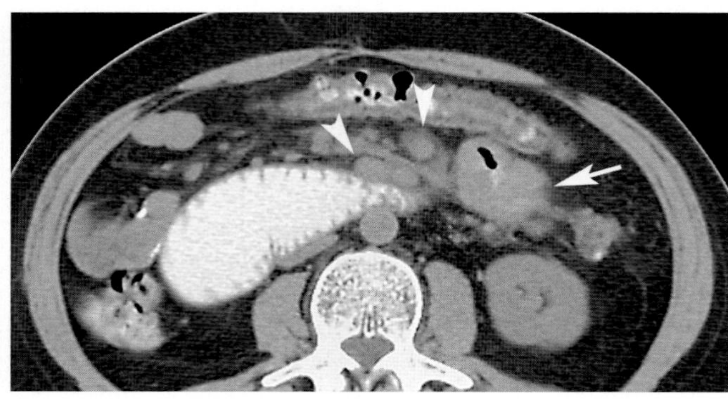

B

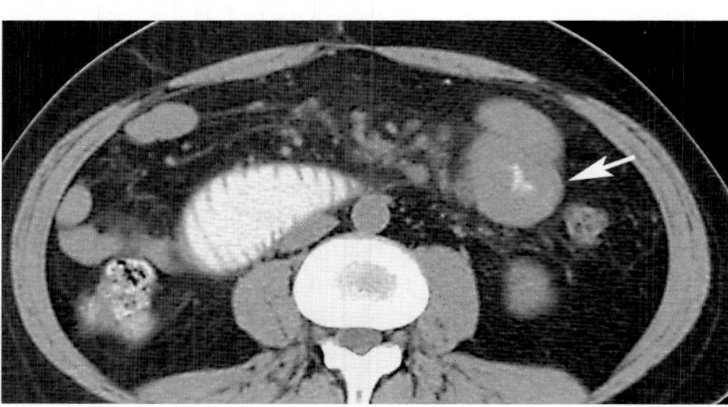

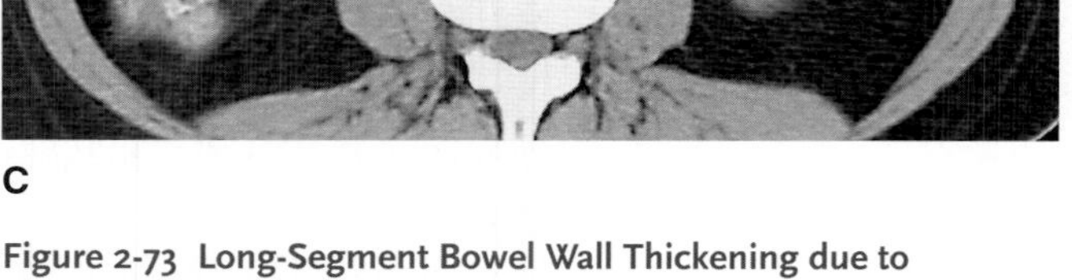

C

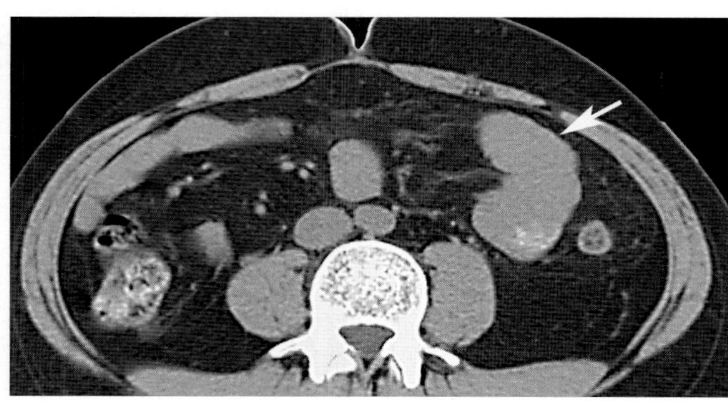

D

Figure 2-73 Long-Segment Bowel Wall Thickening due to Lymphoma
This 36-year-old man had received a heart transplant in the previous year and now presented with abdominal pain, nausea, and vomiting. **A-D.** Axial CT images demonstrate a long segment of wall thickening involving the proximal jejunum. Note the abrupt transition in **A** from normal to diseased bowel, a feature favoring a neoplastic rather than inflammatory cause for the wall thickening. Endoscopic biopsy was diagnostic of a B-cell lymphoma and is indicative of PTLD as a complication of the immunosuppression related to the heart transplant.

can further be classified into complete or partial depending on whether there is no passage or some passage of fluid or gas beyond the site of obstruction, respectively. An open-loop obstruction denotes distal blockage with open loops proximally that are amenable to decompression by vomiting or drainage by placement of a tube in the stomach or proximal small bowel. A closed-loop obstruction denotes that flow into and out of the site of obstruction is blocked leading to progressive accumulation of fluid and gas within this loop. These concepts will be discussed in detail in the following section focusing on how radiology is critical to guiding management of both bowel obstruction and adynamic ileus.

Role of imaging in guiding management of bowel obstruction

Over the past 2 decades, imaging has assumed a primary role in both the diagnosis and treatment of patients with bowel obstruction.[547] This approach has evolved due mainly to 2 factors. First, the diagnosis of SBO has improved overall as well as in the early diagnosis of strangulation in particular, using cross-sectional imaging. Second, nonsurgical treatment of bowel obstruction has also increased, typically through the use of nasointestinal decompression for patients with low-grade or uncomplicated obstruction.[548] Historically, all patients with suspected bowel obstruction were taken to the operating room because of the limited ability to diagnose complications of SBO, specifically strangulation, on clinical examination and imaging, prompting the adage "Never let the sun rise or set on a small-bowel obstruction."[549] The present role of imaging, however, has moved beyond simply determining the presence of obstruction to addressing the severity, location, and etiology of the obstruction as well as the presence of complications of obstruction such as strangulation.[547,550] This radiologic information is critical to triaging patients appropriately to conservative versus surgical management.

In the past, the imaging evaluation of suspected bowel obstruction began with a combination of a supine and erect plain film of the abdomen, an examination known as an "obstruction series." This approach is limited in sensitivity as plain films are diagnostic in only 50% to 60% of cases; equivocal in about 20% to 30%; and normal, nonspecific, or misleading in 10% to 20%. However, because these examinations are readily available, quickly obtained and low in cost they can be useful as an initial examination

Imaging Notes 2-16. Terminology of Bowel Obstruction

Adynamic ileus:	Blockage of the bowel due to diminished peristalsis
Small-bowel obstruction:	Mechanical blockage of the small bowel
Colonic obstruction:	Mechanical blockage of the colon
Strangulation:	Bowel obstruction associated with compromise of the vascular supply leading to ischemia and infarction
Close-loop obstruction:	Bowel obstruction of both inflow and outflow of a single bowel loop leading to progressive accumulation of fluid and air within the loop
Intussusception:	Telescoping of the bowel
Volvulus:	Twisting of the bowel around a point

from which to triage patients for further imaging and management.[551-553]

Currently, many centers use CT directly in the evaluation of suspected bowel obstruction because it provides detailed information about both the site and cause of bowel obstruction and can also provide alternative diagnoses when bowel obstruction is excluded. Moreover, CT has a sensitivity of 82% to 100% for high-grade and complete SBO and the early demonstration of strangulation.[554-559] As such, CT is useful in determining which patients would benefit from conservative management and close follow-up and which patients would benefit from immediate surgical intervention.

In patients with equivocal CT scans or in whom there is persistent clinical concern for obstruction despite normal CT examinations, further evaluation with small-bowel enteroclysis or CT enteroclysis may be indicated.[560] These examinations distend the bowel using high volumes of fluid that exaggerate the effects of mild or subclinical obstructions. Enteroclysis is further advantageous in that it utilizes frequent intermittent "real-time" fluoroscopic monitoring during the examination that facilitates the recognition of fixed and nondistensible segments and can point to the location of the obstruction.[561-563] In addition, CT enteroclysis is more advantageous in that it is readily available and reproducible across practice settings. However, the largest drawbacks to both routine barium and CT enteroclysis is the placement of a nasoenteric tube, with resultant patient discomfort and slow transit in dilated hypotonic bowel segments.[564]

Imaging of bowel obstruction

Abdominal plain films and abdominal CT are the primary imaging means of evaluating suspected bowel obstruction. On occasion, barium studies, including enterocleisis, SBFT, and barium enemas are used to evaluate suspected obstruction. Although CT is highly sensitive and specific in the diagnosis of high-grade bowel obstruction, CT enteroclysis is recommended as the primary method of investigation in patients with suspected low-grade or subclinical SBO in certain patients, CT enteroclysis can be therapeutic as well as diagnostic.[184]

Plain film evaluation of bowel obstruction: With respect to the bowel, the obstruction series is designed to detect 3 major abnormalities as follows: (1) air-fluid levels within the bowel, (2) dilation of air-filled bowel, and (3) pneumoperitoneum. Detection and evaluation of these findings allow for the diagnosis of SBO, colonic obstruction, adynamic ileus, enteritis, and bowel perforation. Differentiation of these clinical conditions is based on 2 principles. First, the characteristic feature of obstruction of any peristaltic tube is proximal dilation and distal collapse. Second, air-fluid levels within the bowel are never normal on abdominal plain films except in the stomach.

A horizontal beam film is necessary to detect air-fluid levels. The horizontal orientation of the x-ray beam, perpendicular to gravity, will show the border between dependent fluid and nondependent air, known as an "air-fluid level." Horizontal beam films are typically taken with the patient standing erect but can also done with the patient in a decubitus position or as a crosstable lateral radiographs, where the patient lies on his or her back with the x-ray beam oriented horizontally. The primary differential diagnoses of air-fluid levels include SBO, colonic obstruction, adynamic ileus, and enteritis/colitis (Table 2-9).

The first rule of obstruction of any peristaltic tube is proximal dilation and distal collapse. Tubular structures of the body, including the GI tract and the ureters, all undergo peristalsis regularly and spontaneously. This peristalsis propels the contents of the tube from proximal to distal locations. If there is obstruction of forward flow, the luminal contents will progressively increase proximal to the site of obstruction causing dilation. Continuation of peristalsis beyond the site of obstruction results in evacuation of the distal portion of the tube. Because no new contents are propelled into the portion of the tubular structure distal to the obstruction, that portion of the tube collapses. It is, therefore, possible to determine the site of obstruction

Table 2-9. Causes of Air-Fluid Levels in the Bowel

1. Obstruction a. Small bowel obstruction b. Colonic obstruction
2. Adynamic ileus
3. Enteritis/colitis (diarrhea)

Imaging Notes 2-17. Evaluation of Bowel Obstruction

Based on the Tenant: Proximal Dilatation and Distal Collapse
Use imaging to determine which loops of bowel are dilated • Abdominal x-rays indirectly determine which loops are dilated based on location and characteristics of bowel folds • CT, MRI, and barium studies directly evaluate the dilation of the bowel

by determining the location where the caliber of the tube changes. In SBO, there will be dilated air- and fluid-filled loops in the small-bowel proximal to the site of obstruction with collapse and a paucity of gas and fluid in the small-bowel and colon distal to the obstruction (see Figure 2-74). In colonic obstruction, there is dilation of the entire small bowel and the portion of the colon proximal to the obstruction with collapse of the distal portion of the colon (see Figure 2-75). Patients with a generalized adynamic ileus will present with dilation of the entire bowel from the duodenum to the rectum (see Figure 2-76).

To determine the site of obstruction, the observer must be able to distinguish between air-filled small bowel and air-filled colon. This is occasionally a difficult task even for an experienced observer, but there are a variety of clues that help in distinguishing small from large bowel. The most important separating feature in differentiating small bowel and the colon is the location of the bowel segments. The ascending and descending colons are retroperitoneal structures and are therefore fixed in the lateral aspects of the abdomen. Consequently, they are the most lateral colon segments and travel in a craniocaudal direction. The rectum is also retroperitoneal and fixed in location in the midpelvis. The transverse colon is suspected on a mesentery and will typically form a U-shaped tubular structure between the splenic and hepatic flexures. These colonic structures are usually readily distinguished from small-bowel loops based on their characteristic locations. Both the small bowel and sigmoid colon can occupy the midabdomen and because of their mesenteries, their position can be variable. Consequently, the sigmoid colon may be confused with small bowel (see Figure 3-4).

The different appearance of the folds of the small bowel and colon also help to differentiate these structures. Plica circularis, the folds of the small bowel, are thin, regularly spaced, uniform in size, and extend across the entire circumference of the lumen (see Figures 2-76 and 2-2). Haustra, the folds of the colon, are thick, irregularly spaced, and usually do not extend across the entire luminal diameter (see Figures 2-76 and 2-2).

The site of obstruction in the bowel can be approximated by determining which portion of the small bowel is dilated. The jejunum is largely present in the left upper and midabdomen. If air-fluid levels are confined to this location then the obstruction is usually in the jejunum. The ileum is predominantly located in the mid- and lower abdomen and pelvis. When the small bowel is dilated to this level, then the obstruction is usually in the distal ileum. When the site of obstruction is located in the distal small bowel, there is a "stepladder" appearance to the stacked segments of small bowel. Similar to the small bowel, the site of colonic obstruction can be suggested by determining the point at which the colon transitions from dilated to collapsed segments.

Although both obstruction and adynamic ileus will produce dilation of the bowel, in patients with enteritis or colitis, or other causes of diarrhea, the bowel is usually not distended but air-fluid levels will often be present on horizontal beam films (see Figure 2-77). The normal small bowel is typically less than 2.5 cm in diameter.[555] Maximal diameter of the colon varies based on location. The cecum is the most distensible portion of the colon but is usually less than 9 cm in diameter. The transverse colon is usually less than 6 cm and the descending and sigmoid colons are usually slightly smaller in caliber.[278] Bowel loops larger than these thresholds are dilated.

Duodenal obstruction causes a unique appearance termed the **double bubble sign**. In this case, only the stomach and duodenal bulb are dilated. Thus, 2 rounded air collections are seen in the upper abdomen, the larger stomach in the left upper quadrant (see Figure 2-25). This is most commonly seen in the newborn and may be due to duodenal atresia, duodenal stenosis, and rotational anomalies with or without congenital peritoneal bands, also known as Ladd bands.[565]

The "**String of Pearls**" sign refers to a row of small bubbles that resembles a string of pearls (see Figure 2-78). This sign is seen when the dilated small-bowel segments proximal to the site of obstruction are filled primarily with fluid and only a small amount of gas. In this setting, small amounts of air become trapped beneath individual plica circularis along the superior or nondependent wall of the fluid-filled dilated small bowel. On horizontal-beam radiographs, the meniscal effect of the gas outlined by the fluid gives the rounded appearance of a pearl. Although this sign can rarely be seen in adynamic ileus and gastroenteritis, it is considered virtually diagnostic of an SBO in the appropriate setting.[566-568]

CT evaluation of bowel obstruction: Multidetector CT plays a primary role in the evaluation of patients with acute obstruction of the small bowel and colon.[547] Further, CT is superior to plain film in the detection of simple and closed loop obstruction and can provide pertinent additional information including the following: (1) the anatomic site(s) of obstruction in the small bowel or colon; (2) the etiology of the obstruction; (3) the severity of obstruction; and (4) the presence or absence of findings of vascular compromise (strangulation). The reader should systematically address each of these questions in their report as these data are essential in guiding treatment to surgical and nonsurgical approaches.[556,557,569]

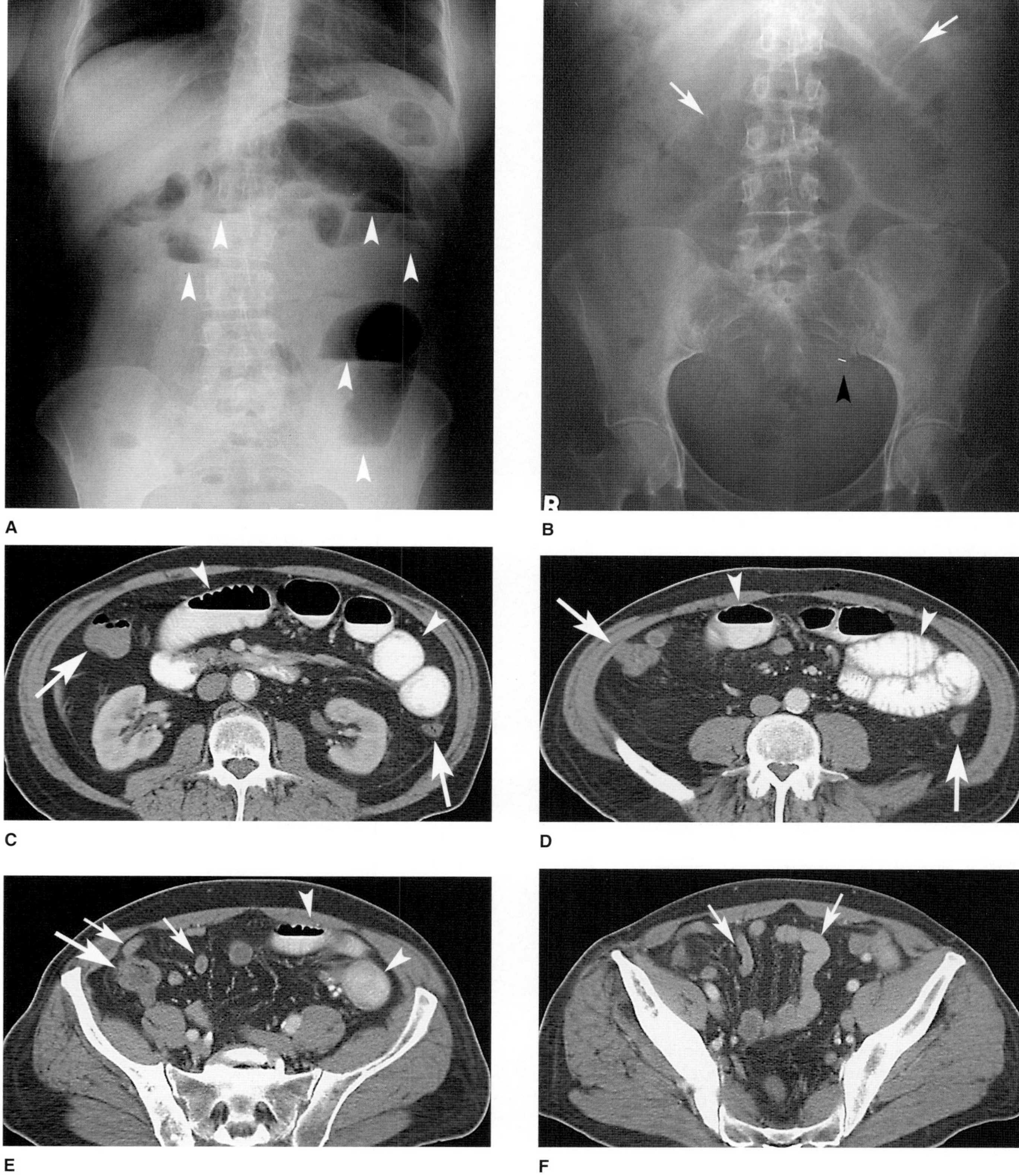

Figure 2-74 Small-bowel Obstruction
This 55-year-old woman complained of crampy abdominal pain, nausea, and vomiting. **A.** Erect abdominal radiograph demonstrates multiple air-fluid levels (*white arrowheads*). **B.** Although the loops in the upper abdomen (*white arrows*) in this supine radiograph appear large enough to represent colon, the folds are thin, regular, and pass all the way across the loop, findings characteristic of the plica circularis of small bowel. Therefore, these findings are indicative of a small-bowel obstruction. Note the single surgical clip in the left of the pelvis (*black arrowhead*) indicting prior pelvic surgery. This small-bowel obstruction is most likely due to adhesions from the prior surgery. **C-F.** CT images through the abdomen and pelvis show dilated proximal small-bowel loops (*white arrowheads*) with collapsed distal small bowel (*white arrows*) and colon (*large white arrows*) diagnostic of a small-bowel obstruction, in this case as a result of abdominal adhesions from prior surgery.

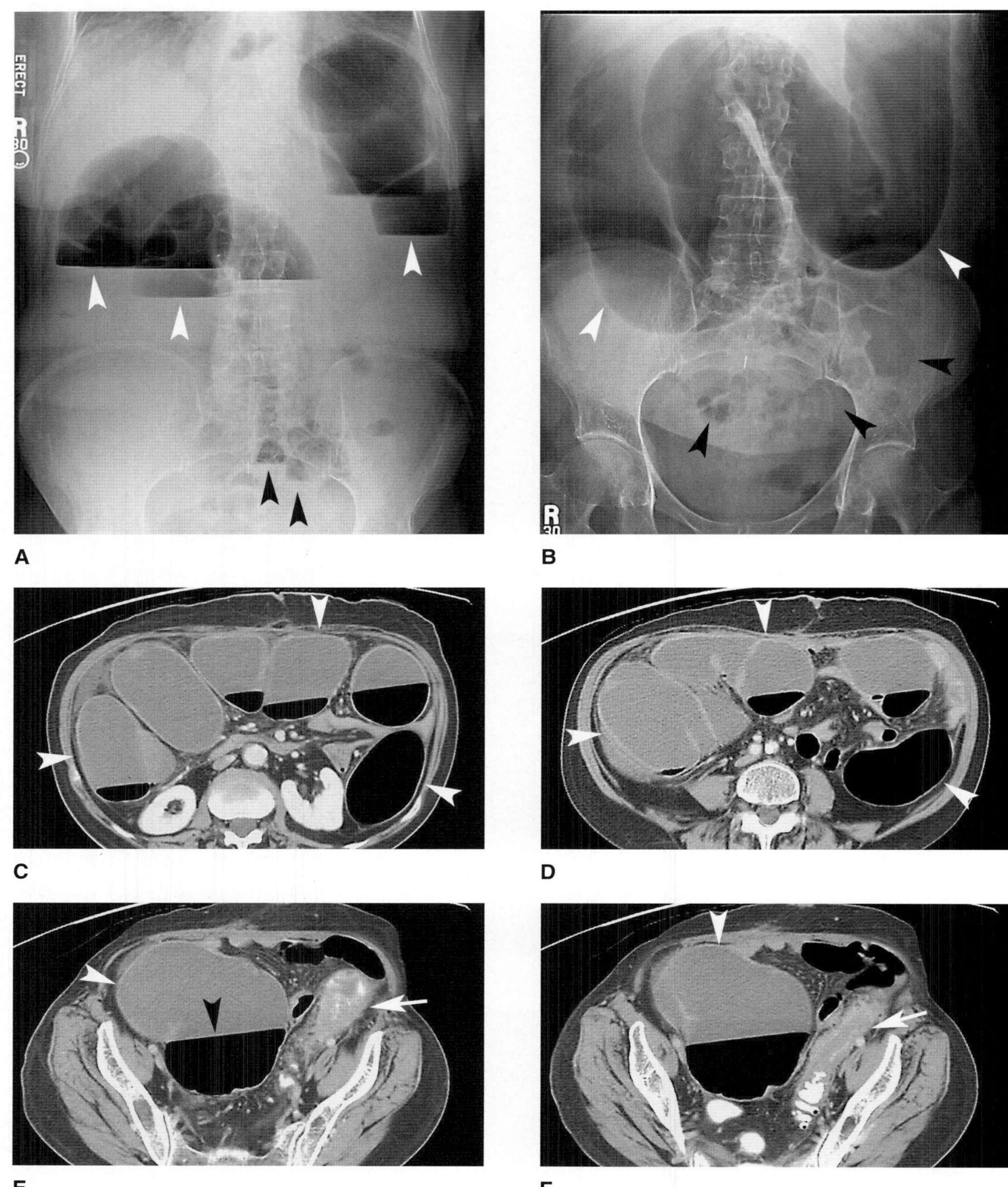

Figure 2-75 Colonic Obstruction from Diverticulitis
This 76-year-old woman with a history of ovarian cancer complained of abdominal pain and fevers. **A.** Erect view demonstrates multiple air-fluid levels in the colon (*white arrowheads*) and small bowel (*black arrowheads*). **B.** Supine view confirms the presence of a dilated, redundant transverse colon (*white arrowheads*) and multiple dilated loops of small bowel (*black arrowheads*). No gas is seen in the distal colon or rectum. These findings are typical of a colonic obstruction and in the setting of ovarian cancer could indicate obstruction due to peritoneal spread of the cancer. **C-F.** CT images were obtained in the prone position. Note that the air in the colon (*black arrowhead* in E) is below the fluid. We have inverted the images to appear in the supine position by convention. The CT examination confirms the presence of dilated loops of colon (*white arrowheads*). There is a long segment of wall thickening in the sigmoid colon (*white arrows*). There serosa appears brighter than the muscularis layer, indicating serosal enhancement and edema of the mucosa. Compare the fat adjacent to the sigmoid colon in E with the perinephric fat. The fat adjacent to the sigmoid colon has high attenuation streaks within it, called "fat stranding." This finding can be associated with malignancies but it more commonly indicates edema due to an inflammatory process. The combination of segmental thickening and fat stranding in the colon will usually indicate diverticulitis. Surgical exploration confirmed a diagnosis of diverticulitis.

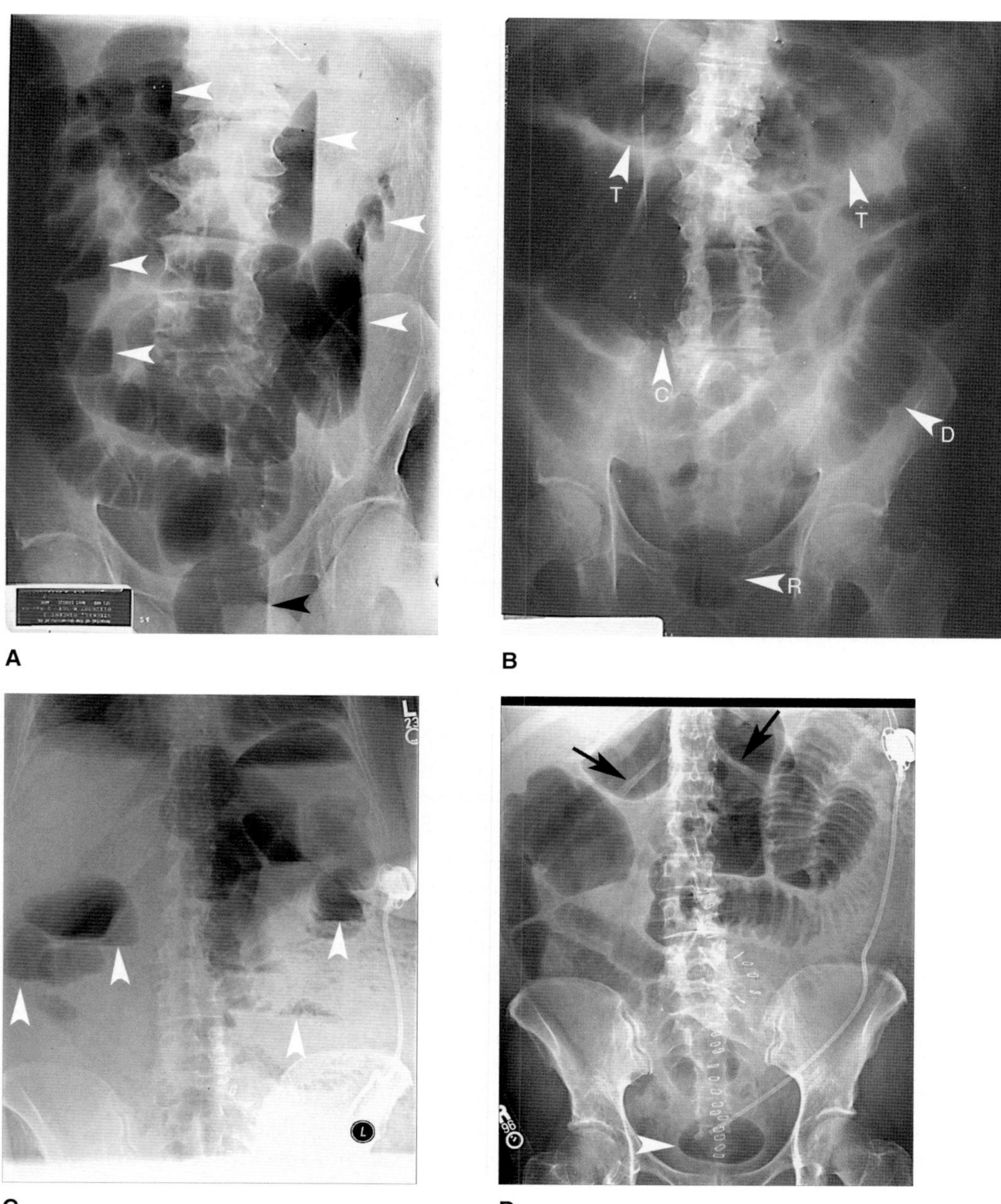

Figure 2-76 Adynamic Ileus
This 64-year-old man complained of abdominal distension following a recent laminectomy. The patient was unable to stand and so a left lateral decubitus view of the abdomen (**A**) was obtained demonstrating multiple air-fluid levels (*white arrowheads*). Notice the distended rectum with air-fluid level (*black arrowhead*). **B.** Supine radiograph demonstrates the characteristic appearance of distended cecum ("C"), transverse colon ("T"), and descending colon ("D"). The other bowel loops represent dilated small bowel. Note that the rectum ("R") contains air but is not dilated. This is because the rectum is a posterior structure and air rises out of the rectum and into the remainder of the colon. This examination shows how a decubitus radiograph can be useful in confirming free passage of air into the rectum, a finding that indicated bowel dilatation due to an adynamic ileus. This ileus is not due to the spine surgery but is a manifestation of narcotics used to treat the surgical pain. **C** and **D.** This 61-year-old woman underwent hysterectomy 2 days prior. She now complains of nausea and vomiting. C. Erect radiograph shows multiple air-fluid levels. D. Supine radiograph shows dilated loops of bowel. The loops in the left upper quadrant have thin continuous folds, closely stacked with each other, typical of small bowel. The loops in the right upper quadrant have fewer folds that appear thicker (*black arrows*), typical of the colon. Air is seen in the rectum (*white arrowhead*). This clinical history and radiographic appearance is typical of a postoperative adynamic ileus.

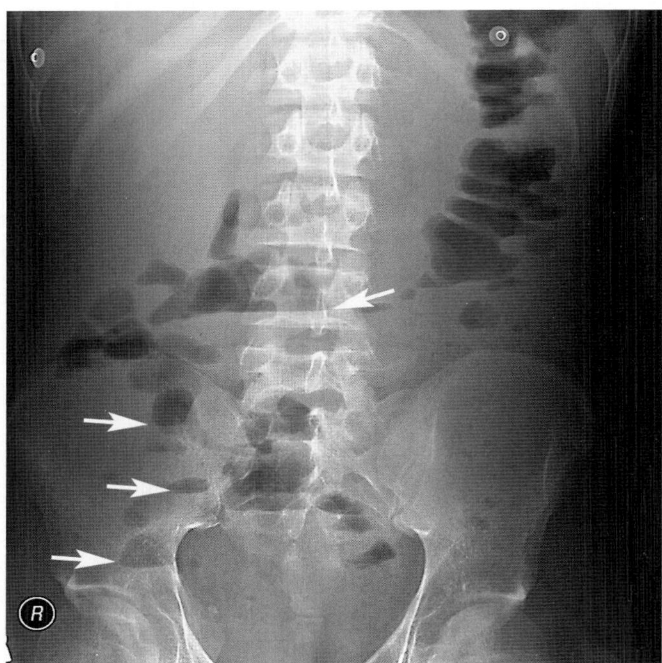

Figure 2-77 Giardia Enteritis
This 22-year-old HIV-positive man complained of abdominal pain and diarrhea. Erect radiograph demonstrates multiple air-fluid levels in nondilated small bowel and colon. This combination of findings is usually a manifestation of an enteritis. Stool cultures confirmed the presence of Giardia species.

The CT evaluation of bowel obstruction follows the same general tenants as abdominal plain films: proximal dilation and distal collapse. Computed tomographic criteria for SBO are the presence of dilated small-bowel segments, defined as segments with diameter >2.5 cm from outer wall to outer wall, proximal to the site of obstruction with normal-caliber or collapsed segments distal to the site of obstruction.[547,570] At the transition point between dilated and collapsed bowel segments, CT can evaluate for the various causes of obstruction, including an intrinsic or extrinsic mass, bowel herniation, or abnormal thickening of the bowel wall. When no abnormality is visualized at the transition point the presumed etiology of obstruction is adhesions. This is presumed both because adhesions are the most common cause of obstruction and because they are not visualized on CT.

Severity of bowel obstruction can be evaluated using the degree of distal collapse, proximal bowel dilation, the passage of oral contrast, and occasionally through the presence of the "small-bowel feces" sign. If positive oral contrast material is given, the passage of a sufficient amount of contrast material through the transition point indicates an incomplete low-grade or partial SBO.[547,571] A high-grade partial SBO is diagnosed when there is some stasis and delay in the passage of the contrast medium, so that diluted oral contrast material appears in the distended proximal bowel and minimal contrast material appears in the collapsed distal loops. Finally, a high-grade complete obstruction is defined by the absence of contrast beyond the point of obstruction.[547] High-grade obstruction, either partial and complete, can also be diagnosed on the basis of an approximately 50% difference in caliber between the proximal dilated bowel and the distal collapsed bowel.[547] This discrepancy in bowel caliber is due to accumulation of unabsorbed fluid proximal to the obstruction and complete evacuation of the bowel contents distal to the obstruction point after several days,[572] which exaggerates the discrepancy in caliber between the proximal and distal small-bowel loops.

The "**small-bowel feces**" sign can be an additional clue to the diagnosis of SBO, but as explained below, it should be interpreted with caution. The normal contents of the small bowel are liquid and air. When there is delayed small-bowel transit stasis of bowel contents, it leads to the development of particulate, feculent-appearing material with gas bubbles that resembles the appearance of stool in the colon on CT scans. This is called the small-bowel feces sign and is thought to reflect incompletely digested food, bacterial overgrowth, or increased water absorption of the distal small-bowel contents due to stasis.

Although the small-bowel feces sign can be seen in SBO, it is neither sensitive nor specific for this diagnosis.[573] The incidence of this sign in the setting of SBO is variable ranging from 7% to 55%. When present in the setting

Imaging Notes 2-18. Reporting of Bowel Obstruction

The CT interpretation of bowel obstruction should include determination of the:

1. Anatomic site(s)
2. Etiology of obstruction
3. Severity of obstruction
4. Presence or absence of vascular compromise (strangulation)

Imaging Notes 2-19. Grading of Bowel Obstruction

Grade	Contrast Beyond Transit ion Point	≥50% Difference in Caliber of Bowel Proximal and Distal to Obstruction
Incomplete, low-grade	Moderate	No
Incomplete, high-grade	Minimal	Yes
Complete, high-grade	None	Yes

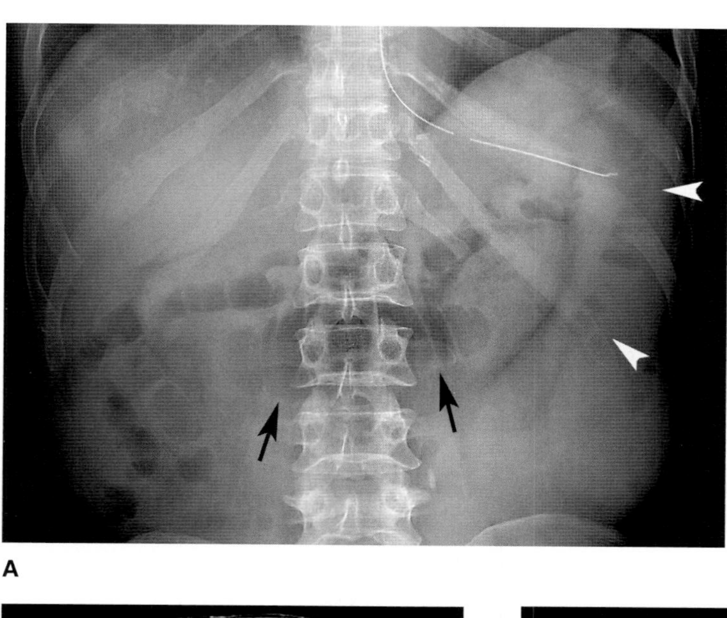

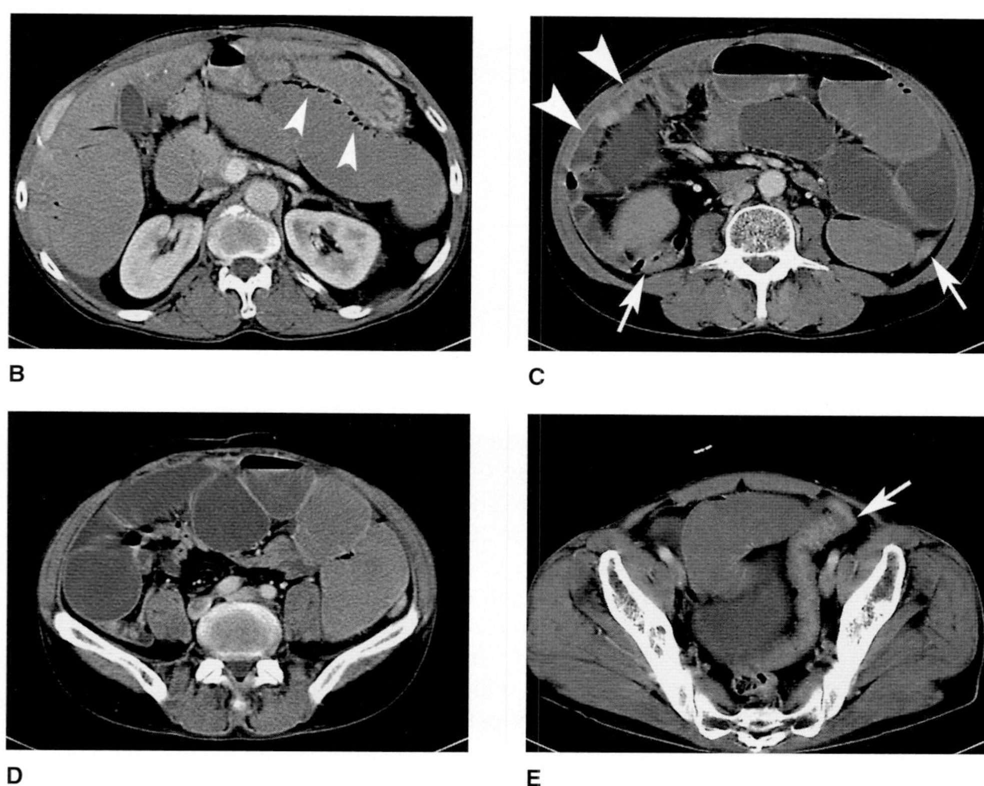

Figure 2-78 String of Pearls Sign
This 43-year-old man presented with intermittent abdominal pain. **A.** Supine radiograph shows a general paucity of bowel gas. However, there is a dilated loop with multiple thin folds characteristic of small bowel (*black arrows*) and a paucity of gas in the colon. This is strongly suggestive of a small-bowel obstruction, where the loops are predominantly fluid filled. There is a cluster of oval gas bubbles (*white arrowheads*) in a row in the left upper quadrant. This finding is known as the "string of pearls" sign and is associated with a diagnosis of small-bowel obstruction. **B-E.** CT images through the abdomen confirm the presence of multiple dilated loops of small bowel that are primarily filled with fluid. There are some collapsed loops of small bowel (*large arrowheads*) and colon (*white arrows*). This constellation of findings meets the imaging criteria for a small-bowel obstruction. Note the row of bubbles (*small arrowheads*) in B. This row is caused by air trapped under individual plica circularis. This phenomenon is what causes the "string of pearls" appearance on the abdominal x-ray. There was no identifiable cause for this obstruction and so a diagnosis of adhesions was suggested.

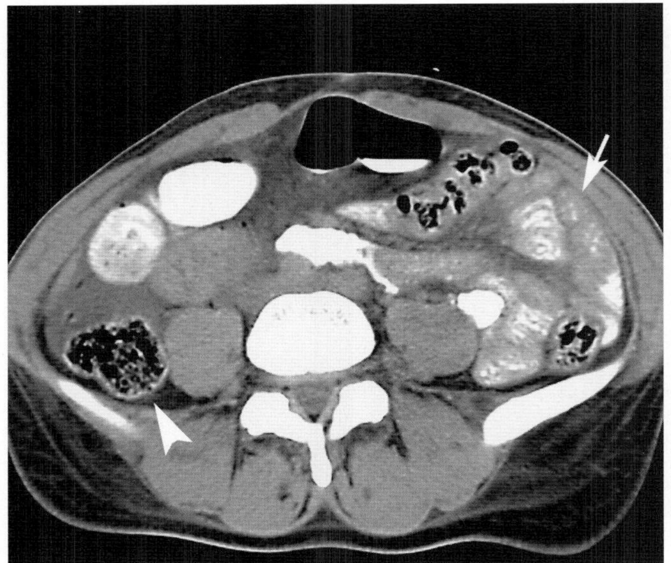

A

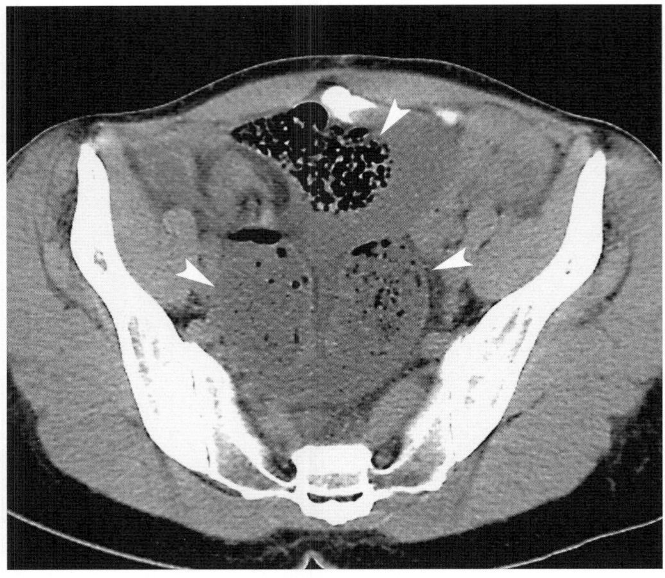

B

Figure 2-79 Small-Bowel Feces Sign
This 42-year-old woman with a history of a prior hysterectomy complained of intermittent crampy abdominal pain for several months. In image **A**, there is normal-appearing proximal small bowel (*arrow*) and colon (*large arrowhead*). Note the appearance of feces in the ascending colon. In image **B**, there is a dilated loop of small bowel containing a mixture of air and solid material (*small arrowheads*). This is an abnormal finding called the small-bowel feces sign that is most often associated with a low-grade chronic small-bowel obstruction. Surgical exploration confirmed a diagnosis of SBO due to pelvic adhesions.

of SBO, it has been observed more often in patients with moderate or severe obstruction. However, it is not able to discern between low-grade, subacute obstruction and moderate or high-grade obstruction.[547,573-575] A helpful guide to determining the significance of this sign is that when it is present in the setting of obstruction, it is typically located just at or proximal to the transition point and is therefore a clue to the location of obstruction.[573,574] On the other hand, when this sign is present in the setting of normal or mildly dilated small bowel, it is usually indicative of a diversity of etiologies of delayed intestinal transit from causes other than obstruction including the following: cystic fibrosis, infectious enteritis, rapid jejunostomy tube feedings, bezoars, and reflux of fecal matter from the cecum (see Figure 2-79 and Table 2-10).[574,576,577]

The site of obstruction or transition point is determined by identifying a caliber change between the dilated proximal and collapsed distal bowel loops. This should be accomplished in a systematic fashion starting from the terminal ileum and moving proximally through the small bowel in the setting of suspected SBO and starting from the rectum and moving proximally in the setting of suspected colon obstruction. Once the site of obstruction is identified, this should be confirmed by starting at the distal duodenum and moving distally or at the cecum and moving distally in the setting of small and large bowel obstruction, respectively. Multiplanar reformats also can be helpful in confirming the suspected site of obstruction.[558]

Barium studies in the evaluation of bowel obstruction: Routine CT demonstrates accuracy of greater than 90% in the diagnosis of high-grade SBO. However, the sensitivity and specificity of routine CT in the diagnosis of low-grade SBO is 50% and 94%, respectively. As above, when low-grade small obstruction is suspected, CT enteroclysis is superior to routine CT with sensitivity and specificity of 89% and 100%, respectively.

For the indication of suspected SBO, CT enteroclysis is usually performed with positive oral contrast. This permits performance of fluoroscopy during oral contrast

Table 2-10. Causes of the Small-Bowel Feces Sign

1. Small-bowel obstruction
2. Cystic fibrosis
3. Infectious enteritis
4. Rapid jejunostomy feeds
5. Bezoar
6. Reflux of feces from the colon

infusion, which can detect subtle delays in the passage of contrast material. This technique is particularly sensitive in the detection of adhesions, both obstructive and nonobstructive. In addition, CT enteroclysis is advantageous in patients with symptoms of proximal jejunal obstruction, particularly when the stomach may have been decompressed either through the use of a nasogastric tube or patient emesis prior to the scan.

Causes of SBO

Once the site of obstruction is discovered, the cause of the obstruction should be determined. Over the past 50 years, the etiology of SBO in Western society has shifted from predominantly hernias to adhesions, Crohn disease, and malignancy as the top 3 causes in decreasing order.[547] Hernias continue to represent the predominant cause of SBO in developing countries.[578]

Etiologies of SBO can be categorized into extrinsic, intrinsic, and intraluminal. Intrinsic bowel lesions are usually seen at the transition point and include causes of focal wall thickening that may lead to intussusception, such as Crohn disease, celiac disease, primary small-bowel neoplasms, hematomas, and ischemia. Extrinsic causes include adhesions, internal and external hernias, secondary neoplasms, endometriosis, and hematomas. Finally, intraluminal lesions are identified by their location and imaging characteristics that differ from other enteric contents and include gallstones, bezoars, and foreign bodies (see Table 2-11).[547]

Adhesions: Adhesions are the most common cause of SBO, accounting for approximately 50% to 80% of all cases. Adhesions are mostly due to prior intra-abdominal intervention, with only a minority due to peritonitis.[570,579-582] Adhesive bands are not seen directly on imaging examinations but are implied when there is an abrupt change in the caliber of the bowel without associated extrinsic mass lesion, intraluminal foreign body, or inflammatory changes at the transition point (see Figures 2-74, 2-78, and 2-79).[547] Kinking and tethering of the adjacent nonobstructed small-bowel segments also suggest the presence of adhesion (see Figure 2-80).

Table 2-11. Causes of Small-Bowel Obstruction

1. Extrinsic Causes
   a. Adhesions (50%-80%)[a]
      i. Prior surgery
      ii. Prior peritoneal inflammation
         i. Peritonitis
         ii. Pelvic inflammatory disease
         iii. Other
   b. Hernia (all subtypes) (10%)
   c. Endometrioma
   d. Hematoma
2. Intrinsic causes
   a. Neoplasm (10%)
      i. Primary tumors
      ii. Peritoneal metastasis
      iii. Direct invasion from adjacent neoplasms
      iv. Hematogenous metastasis[b]
   b. Inflammation
      i. Crohn disease (7%)
      ii. Tuberculosis
      iii. Parasites (Ascaris)
   c. Intussusception
      i. Post viral infection
      ii. Meckel diverticulum
      iii. Polyp
      iv. Lipoma
      v. Celiac disease
      vi. Other lead point.
   d. Vascular lesions
      i. Postradiation
      ii. Ischemia
3. Intraluminal causes
   a. Gallstone ileus
   b. Bezoar
   c. Foreign body
4. Congenital causes
   a. Midgut volvulus
   b. Duodenal atresia and other small-bowel atresia

[a]Numbers in parenthesis indicate the approximate percentage of SBO attributed to this cause.
[b]Metastasis acts as a lead point causing intussusception and SBO.

Hernia: Hernias of the peritoneum are responsible for approximately 10% of SBOs in developed countries. In developing countries, they are the leading cause of SBO.[578] External hernias result from a defect in the abdominal or pelvic wall at sites of congenital weakness or prior surgery. Examples of external hernias include direct and indirect inguinal, incisional, umbilical, femoral, obturator, diaphragmatic, and Spigelian hernias. Diagnosis of these hernias is usually, but not always, obvious on physical examination. When the herniated bowel is filled with air, the hernia can also be visualized on abdominal plain films as an abnormally positioned small-bowel loop, in a location exterior to the peritoneum in the setting of an SBO. On barium, these hernias are best depicted in the lateral projection but can also be detected on frontal projections where there is compression and deformity of the bowel segments entering and exiting the hernia sac. When detected, reduction can be attempted during fluoroscopic evaluation.[583] On CT examinations, hernias can be easily identified as protrusion of bowel loops through a defect in the abdominal wall (see Figure 2-81). Internal hernias are less common than external hernias and occur when there is protrusion of the viscera through the peritoneum or mesentery and into a compartment within the abdominal cavity. These hernias include,

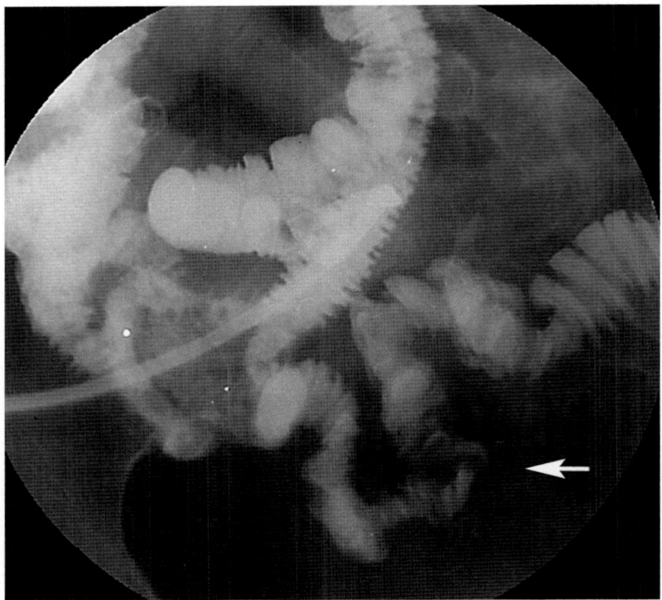

A

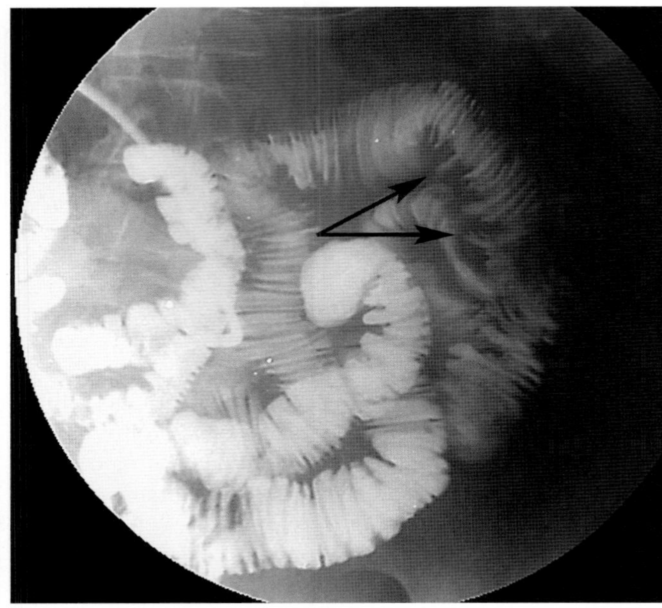

B

Figure 2-80 Adhesions
This 75-year-old man had undergone total collectomy years before as therapy for ulcerative colitis and complained of nausea and vomiting. **A** and **B.** Two spot films from a small-bowel follow-through show angulation (*white arrow*) of some loops of bowel and regions of tethering (*black arrows*). These are typical features of adhesions.

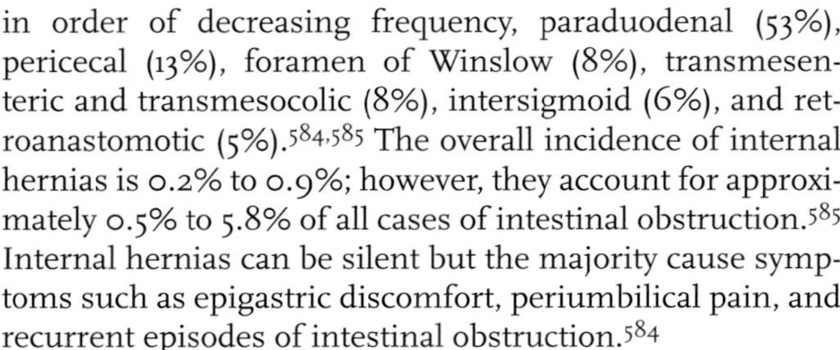

in order of decreasing frequency, paraduodenal (53%), pericecal (13%), foramen of Winslow (8%), transmesenteric and transmesocolic (8%), intersigmoid (6%), and retroanastomotic (5%).[584,585] The overall incidence of internal hernias is 0.2% to 0.9%; however, they account for approximately 0.5% to 5.8% of all cases of intestinal obstruction.[585] Internal hernias can be silent but the majority cause symptoms such as epigastric discomfort, periumbilical pain, and recurrent episodes of intestinal obstruction.[584]

Internal hernias are almost always diagnosed by imaging and are associated with a high mortality rate, exceeding 50% in some series.[585] On CT and MRI, internal hernias typically produce a saclike mass or cluster of dilated small-bowel loops in an abnormal anatomic location within the abdomen, in the presence of SBO. The vascular pedicle of these loops is often engorged, stretched, and displaced from its normal position, converging at the hernial orifice.[584]

Paraduodenal hernias are more common in men, and are located on the left in 75% of cases.[585] Left paraduodenal hernias occur when bowel prolapses through the Landzert fossa, which is present in approximately 2% of the population and is located behind the ascending (fourth portion) duodenum. On CT, they are characterized by an abnormal cluster or saclike mass of dilated small-bowel loops lying between the pancreas and stomach to the left of the ligament of Treitz. These dilated segments typically exert a mass effect on adjacent structures, including displacement of the posterior stomach wall anteriorly, of the duodenojejunal junction inferomedially, and of the transverse colon inferiorly. Abnormalities of the mesenteric vessels include engorgement, crowding, and stretching of the vessels at the entrance of the hernia sac as well as displacement of the IMV and ascending left colic artery along the anterior and medial border of the sac.[584,585]

Right paraduodenal hernias occur when bowel prolapses through the fossa of Waldeyer located immediately behind the SMA and inferior to the transverse (third portion) duodenum. On CT and MRI, these hernias will present as a cluster of dilated small-bowel loops in the right midabdomen near the root of the small-bowel mesentery. Usually, right paraduodenal hernias occur in the setting of a small-bowel malrotation with a normally or incompletely rotated colon. Accordingly, right paraduodenal hernias are

Imaging Notes 2-20. Neoplastic Mechanisms of Bowel Obstruction

Primary neoplasm
• Annular narrowing by the primary mass • Intussusception of primary neoplasm
Secondary neoplasm
• Peritoneal implants with invasion • Direct extension with invasion • Intussusception of hematogenous metastasis

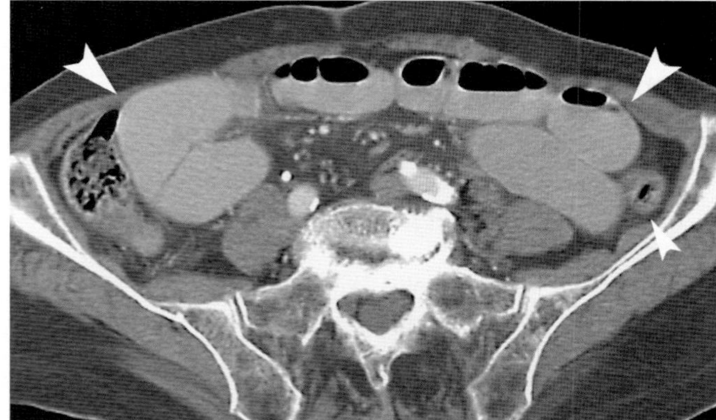

A

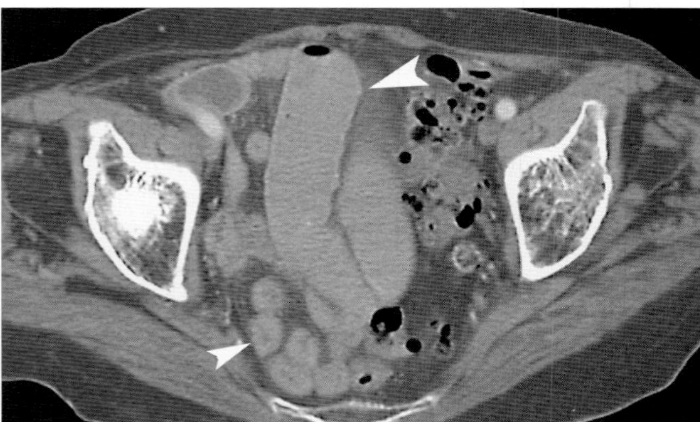

B

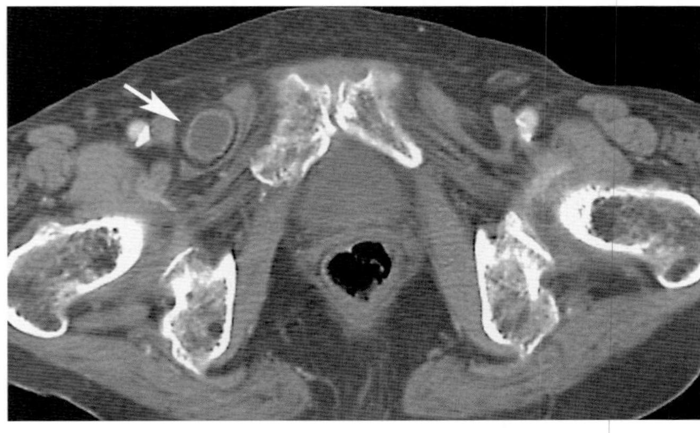

C

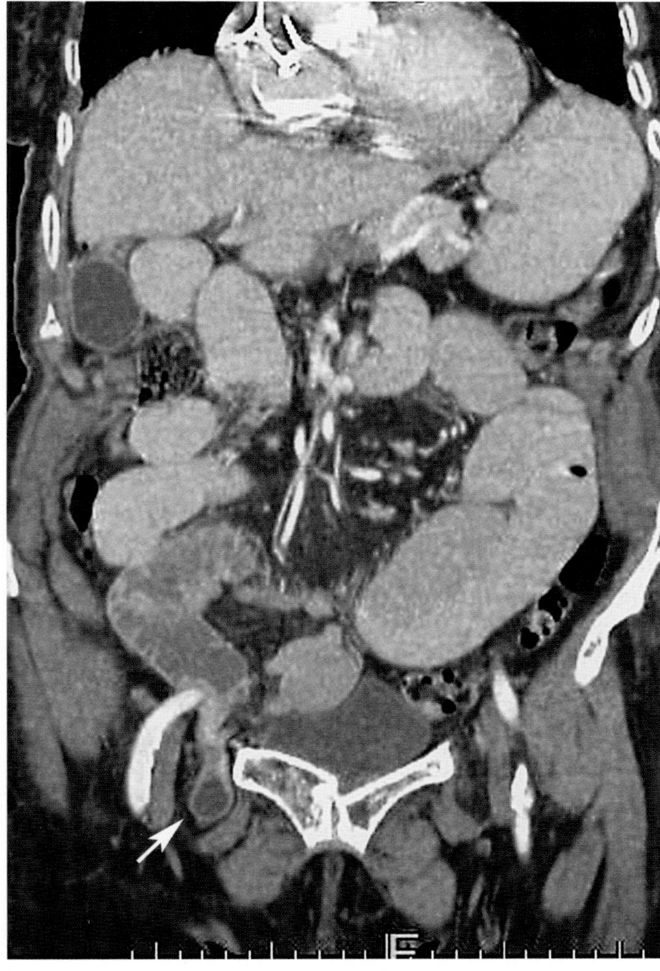

D

Figure 2-81 Small-Bowel Obstruction due to Inguinal Hernia
This 98-year-old man complained of abdominal pain, nausea, and vomiting for 2 days. **A-C.** Axial CT images demonstrate dilation of the proximal small bowel (*large arrowheads*) with collapse of the distal small bowel and colon (*small arrowheads*), diagnostic of a small-bowel obstruction. Careful observation shows protrusion of a distal small-bowel loop (*arrow*) through a right inguinal hernia. **D.** Coronal image shows the inguinal hernia (*arrow*) to better advantage.

associated with abnormal location of the SMV to the left of, and ventral to, the SMA and with absence of the normal horizontal duodenum. A hallmark of right paraduodenal hernia is visualization of the SMA and right colic vein along the anterior-medial border of the encapsulated small-bowel loops.[584,585]

Neoplasm: Neoplasms are among the most common cause of SBO and can cause obstruction through a variety of mechanisms. Serosal implants from peritoneal carcinomatosis are the most common neoplastic mechanism of SBO. This is most often due to ovarian cancer but can also be a result of appendiceal, colon, and endometrial carcinomas but is rarely due to other neoplasms such as primary peritoneal mesothelioma. These implants invade and then obstruct the small bowel. Their presence is suggested by visualization of extrinsic serosal soft-tissue nodules or masses located near the transition point.

Direct growth into the small bowel from a non-small bowel primary abdominal malignancy is a rare cause of SBO. This will appear as a large mass arising from an adjacent organ, which invades the small bowel, causing obstruction. This phenomenon is most commonly seen from tumors of the pelvic organs such as cervical or ovarian cancers. If cecal or colonic malignancy involves the ileocecal valve, it can also result in SBO.

Primary small-bowel carcinomas can grow into an annular mass similar to colon carcinoma leading to obstruction (see Figure 2-25). Primary small-bowel neoplasms are a rare cause of SBO because intrinsic small-bowel neoplasms constitute less than 2% of GI malignancies. When they occur, small-bowel neoplasms are usually advanced and are characterized by pronounced, asymmetric, and irregular mural thickening of the small-bowel wall at the transition point.[556,586]

Finally, hematogenous metastasis and small primary neoplasms can act as a lead point for small-bowel intussusception—a very rare mechanism of small-bowel and colonic obstruction whereby the bowel telescopes upon itself. This is most frequently a result of melanoma or Kaposi sarcoma metastasis. When intussusception is visualized on CT, a leading mass can be identified but should be differentiated from the soft-tissue pseudotumor of the intussusception itself.[570,579,581,582,587]

Crohn disease: Crohn disease accounts for approximately 7% of SBOs.[578] SBO in Crohn disease can be a manifestation of 3 clinical situations: (1) luminal narrowing secondary to the transmural acute inflammatory process, (2) chronic fibrotic stenosis of affected segments, and (3) adhesions, incisional hernias, or postoperative strictures in patients who have undergone previous intestinal surgery.[547,556,571,586,588,589] Distinguishing between these conditions is essential for proper patient treatment. Crohn disease is discussed more completely in the previous section **Long-Segment Wall Thickening of the Small Bowel and Colon**.

Intussusception: Intussusception is a rare cause of SBO in adults and accounts for less than 5% of cases; however, this is a relatively common cause of small-bowel and colonic obstruction in infants and young children.[571,590] In intussusception, a soft-tissue projection such as a polyp, inverted Meckel diverticulum or bowel neoplasm is pulled forward with other endoluminal contents by normal peristalsis. As this lesion is pulled forward, it brings along the bowel wall to which it is attached, causing that portion of bowel to invert and telescope within the lumen of the more distal small bowel.

Pediatric intussusception is idiopathic in up to 90% of cases. In these cases, lymphoid hyperplasia (hypertrophied Peyer patches) is believed to act as the lead point. The etiology of adult intussusception, on the other hand, remains controversial. Reviews of hospital discharge summaries and surgical reports have suggested that up to 80% of adult intussusception cases are associated with an underlying pathologic lead point such as a neoplasm, adhesion, inverted Meckel diverticulum, and foreign body.[16,571,587,591] However, studies based on CT and MRI have shown that almost 50% of adult intussusceptions visualized on CT and MRI are idiopathic. These imaging-detected intussusceptions are typically transient, resolve spontaneously, are without clinical significance, and are thought to be a result of transient dysmotility (see Figure 2-45). These transient intussusceptions are predominantly located in the small bowel and have a higher incidence in patients with celiac disease and scleroderma in whom there is a higher incidence of small-bowel dysmotility.[571,592]

Because of limited soft-tissue resolution, abdominal radiographs can only demonstrate small-bowel or colonic obstruction, which is rarely associated with intussusception. However, cross-sectional imaging including CT, US, and MRI will depict the collapsed, intussuscepted proximal bowel (intussusceptum) with the mesenteric fat and vessels lying within the wall of the distal bowel (intussuscipiens). In profile, the intussusceptum appears as a sausage-shaped structure within the lumen of the bowel and, in cross section, it produces a targetlike appearance because of the alternating layers of mucosa and mesenteric fat. In some cases, careful observation will demonstrate the underlying lesion at the lead point of the intussusceptum; however, cross-sectional imaging has a limited ability to distinguish a lead point from thickened or edematous bowel wall (see Figure 2-82).[571,592-595] In the absence of clinical symptoms, the majority of short-segment intussusceptions will represent a transient, idiopathic finding without significance and require no further evaluation (see Figure 2-45).

Midgut volvulus: Midgut volvulus is a rare cause of SBO in adults but is an important cause of SBO in infants and young children. Midgut volvulus is a direct complication of malrotation of the small bowel. In normal fetal development, the developing bowel undergoes 2 rotations that result in the duodenal sweep placing the ligament of Treitz and proximal jejunum in the left upper quadrant and the cecum and ileocecal valve in the right lower quadrant. In this alignment, the small-bowel mesentery is a long band extending from the ligament of Treitz to the ileocecal valve. This broad band of mesentery is resistant to twisting of the small bowel. In small-bowel malrotation, the small-bowel mesentery comes to a single point in the right upper quadrant at the site of the SMA rather than a long band, and the entire small bowel is located in the right side of the abdomen. At the same time the entire colon is located in the left side of the abdomen. Because the entire mesentery comes to a single point, it is possible for the entire small bowel to rotate around this point, a phenomenon known as "midgut volvulus." Midgut volvulus will typically result in obstruction of the small bowel and compromise of the blood supply of the small bowel leading to ischemia and infarction of nearly the entire small bowel.

Most cases of midgut volvulus will present in children during the first month of life. Approximately 60% to 80% of patients will present with bilious vomiting.[596,597] Emergency surgery must be performed to repair the malrotation because a delay in diagnosis can result in infarction of the

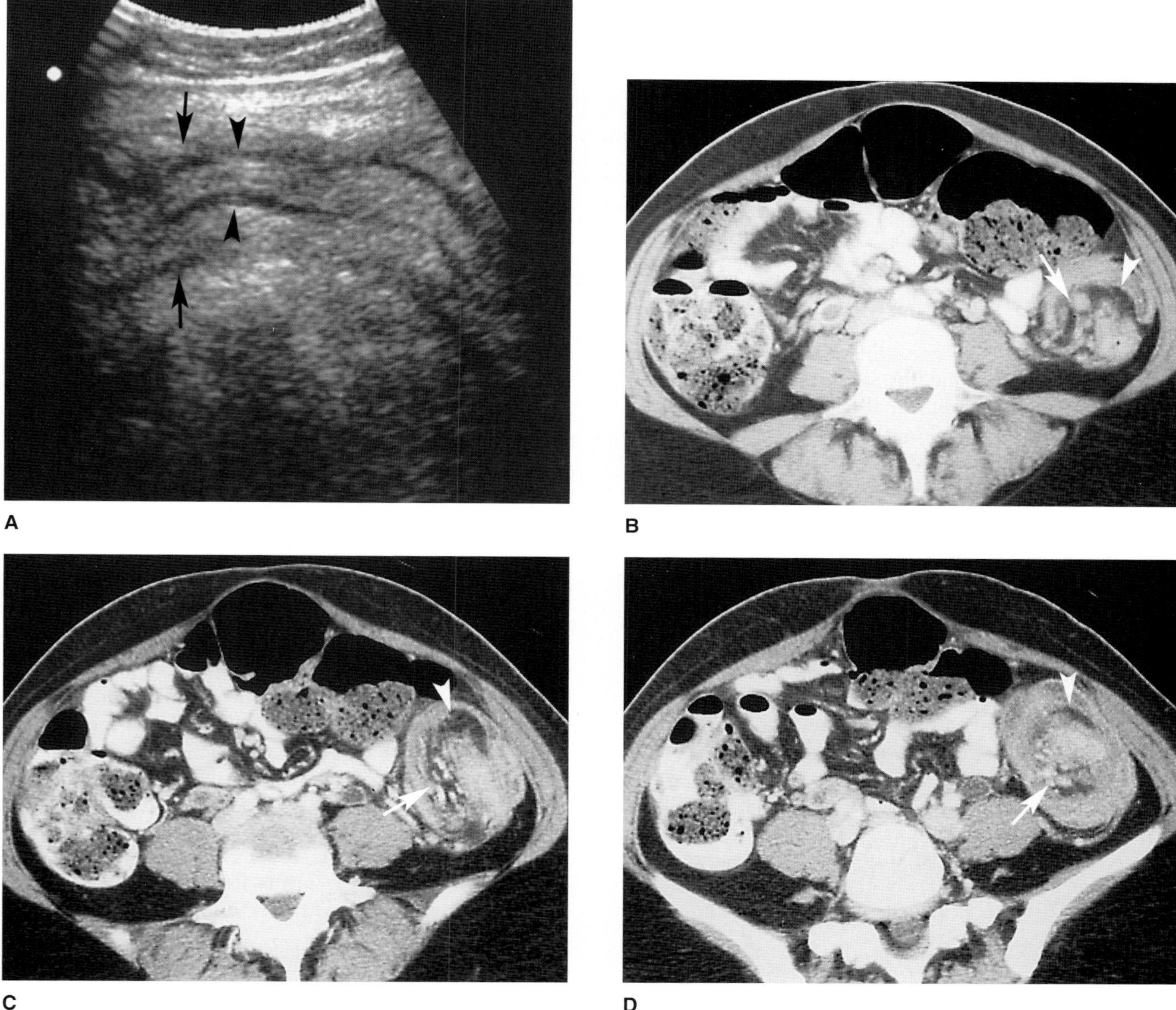

Figure 2-82 Intussusception in 2 Patients
This 26-year-old woman presented with cramp abdominal pain 2 months following cesarean section. **A.** Ultrasound of the left lower quadrant shows 2 inner lines (*arrowheads*) surrounded by 2 outer lines (*arrows*). This is the ultrasound appearance of intussusception of the bowel. **B-D.** CT images show a masslike area in the left lower quadrant. Within the mass are a curvilinear area of fat (*arrowheads*) and multiple enhancing vessels (*arrows*) that represent the mesentery of the bowel as the intussusceptum passes into the intussuscipiens. These findings are diagnostic of intussusception. Surgical exploration showed a colon cancer as the lead point of this colo-colic intussusception.

small bowel and death of the child. As the use of CT in emergency departments has increased, however, midgut volvulus has increasingly been recognized in adults. Adults can present with abdominal pain, nausea, and vomiting similar to the presentation in infants. In some adults, midgut volvulus can manifest as chronic intermittent abdominal pain that resolves when the volvulus spontaneously reduces.[596,598]

Conventional radiography is rarely helpful in the diagnosis of midgut volvulus. Fluoroscopic upper GI and small-bowel examinations are the gold standard for revealing the characteristic abnormal position of most of the small bowel in the right abdomen and the resultant abnormal location of the ligament of Treitz. Normally, on upper GI images the duodenal sweep terminates at the ligament of Treitz in the left upper quadrant of the abdomen at, or to the left of, the left L1 pedicle. In patients with malrotation, the duodenum fails to curve upward and to the left and instead remains in the right side of the abdomen. The twisted proximal small bowel has a characteristic corkscrew-like appearance on fluoroscopic images.[597]

In addition to the abnormal position of the small bowel and colon, malrotation will often result in an abnormal relationship between the SMV and the SMA. In the normal individual, the SMV is located to the right of the SMA; however, in patients with malrotation, the SMV may occupy a position directly anterior or to the left of the SMA.[597,599] US can sometimes illustrate the abnormal position of the SMV and SMA. However, a normal SMA-SMV relationship does not exclude malrotation, and the upper GI examination remains the preferred imaging modality to demonstrate malrotation of the bowel.

Computed tomographic examinations can demonstrate all of the typical manifestations of malrotation and midgut volvulus, including the abnormal relationship of the SMV to the SMA, the abnormal location of the small bowel in the right side of the abdomen, and the entire colon in the left side of the abdomen and distention of the volvulized loops (see Figure 2-83). CT can also demonstrate swirling of vessels in the mesenteric root, which can be a sign of mesenteric vovulus[597,598,600] but can also occur in normal patients. Therefore, application of the mesenteric swirl sign should be used very carefully. In most cases, swirling of the mesenteric vessels should be assumed to represent a normal variant, unless there are other findings of malrotation and midgut volvulus present. Familiarity with the CT findings of midgut volvulus is important because adult patients will typically present with nonspecific symptoms.

Gallstone ileus: In most cases, the abdominal plain film is not capable of identifying the cause of SBO. One exception to this rule is gallstone ileus. Although current usage of the term *ileus* is confined to bowel obstruction due to diminished peristalsis, historically, the ileus was subdivided into 2 groups: adynamic (paralytic) ileus and mechanical ileus. The older term *mechanical ileus* is now called either SBO or colonic obstruction. Thus, the term *gallstone ileus* should in current terminology be called "gallstone obstruction" but the older term *gallstone ileus* remains the terminology that is generally used.

Gallstone ileus is a rare complication of recurrent acute cholecystitis whereby a large gallstone erodes through the gallbladder directly into the small bowel via a biliary-intestinal fistula. As a result of its large size, the stone becomes impacted at a narrow segment of the bowel, typically the ileocecal valve, resulting in SBO. This pathophysiology results in a classic triad of findings on both plain film and CT: (1) obstructed bowel gas pattern, (2) pneumobilia secondary to the biliary-intestinal fistula, and (3) an ectopic gallstone, usually located in the right lower quadrant at the site of the ileocecal valve (see Figure 4-41).[601] Gallstone ileus has become an increasingly rare event in developed countries. This is probably due to improved diagnosis of acute cholecystitis with cross-sectional and hepatobiliary imaging.

Parasitic infection: Globally 1.5 billion people, approximately 25% of the world population, are infested with ascariasis.[602] Ascaris infection is among the most common causes of SBO in the developing world. Although ascariasis infection occurs at all ages, it is most common to affect children 2 to 10 years old with a decreasing trend over the age of 15 years.[603] Children are at higher risk for developing Ascaris-related intestinal obstruction because of the smaller diameter of the lumen of the bowel and often a greater worm load than that seen in adults.[602] In a 2-year study of a tertiary care hospital in India, 63% (131/207) SBOs in children were a result of ascaris infection.[604]

Transmission occurs primarily via ingestion of water or food contaminated with *Ascaris lumbricoides* eggs.[602]

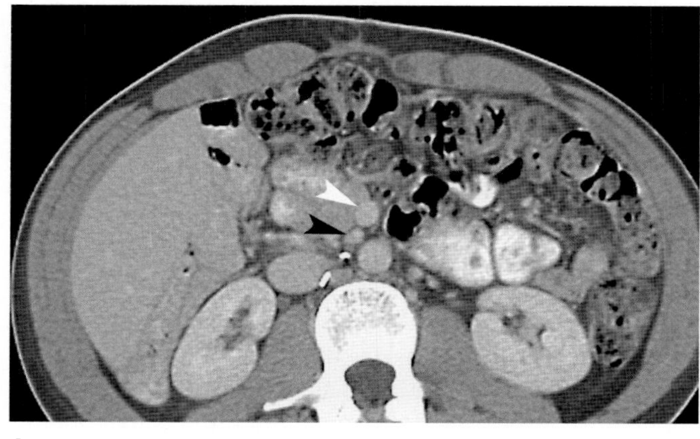

A

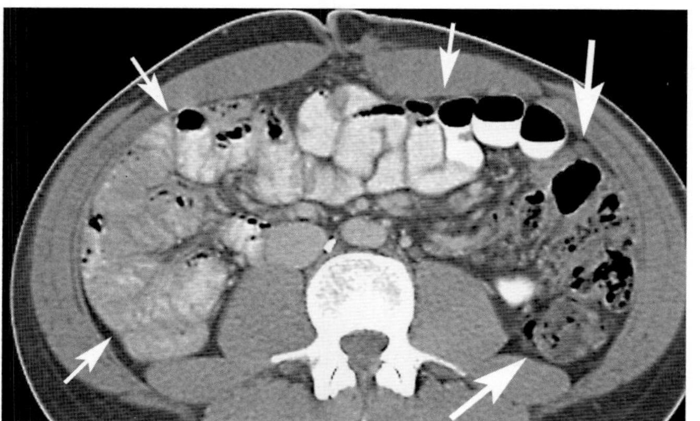

B

Figure 2-83 Malrotation Without Volvulus
This 19-year-old man was being evaluated for testicular cancer. **A.** Contrast-enhanced axial CT images shows an abnormal position of the larger SMV (*white arrowhead*), anterior rather than to the right of the smaller SMA (*black arrowhead*).

B. At the level of the umbilicus, the contrast-filled small bowel (*small arrows*) occupies the right of the abdomen and the feces-filled colon (*large arrows*) is seen only in the left of the abdomen. These findings are typical of malrotation of the bowel.

Children playing in contaminated soil can acquire the parasite from their hands. The number of adult worms per infested person relates to the degree of continued exposure to infectious eggs over time because adult worms do not multiply in the human host.

Most patients infected with *A lumbricoides* are clinically asymptomatic. Symptomatic patients present with the typical symptoms of obstruction such as abdominal pain, nausea, and vomiting. However, occasionally passage of worms in the stool or vomiting of worms can also be seen.[602] Obstruction usually requires a relatively large worm burden, estimated to be greater than 60 worms in most cases.[445] The greater the worm burden, the higher the likelihood of death due to obstruction.

Obstruction due to ascariasis typically occurs at the terminal ileum, although worms can be found throughout the bowel. Delay in the management of the intestinal obstruction can lead to bowel perforation and contamination of the peritoneum with worms and eggs.[605]

Abdominal x-rays will demonstrate the typical features of SBO. However, occasionally multiple linear or serpentine structures, representing the worms, can be seen as filling defects within the air-filled lumen of the small bowel, also called the "cigar bundle" appearance.[602] Abdominal ultrasound can demonstrate the intraluminal worms. In longitudinal section, the Ascaris worm can be seen as a linear intraluminal mass with 3 or 4 internal linear echogenic interfaces. In cross section, the worm will appear as a round or oval structure, with multiple layers resembling a target.[606-608] On real-time US, the worms demonstrate a curling movement within the lumen of the bowel.[602,608] CT and MRI can also demonstrate the presence of worms within the lumen of the bowel. They appear as approximately 0.5-cm by 10-cm linear or curvilinear filling defects within the lumen of the bowel.[609,610] In some cases, the worms will ingest the oral contrast and their gut will appear radiodense.

Duodenal and other small-bowel atresia: Small-bowel atresia is an uncommon cause of intestinal obstruction, which most commonly occurs in the duodenum. A 25-year review of intestinal atresia from a single pediatric center demonstrated 277 cases of intestinal atresia, of which 138 (50%) were in the duodenum and 128 (46%) were at sites in the jejunum and ilium.[611] Patients typically present with bilious emesis, abdominal distension, and/or feeding intolerance. Duodenal atresia is associated with Down syndrome; approximately one-quarter of patients with duodenal atresia will have associated Down syndrome.[611] The double bubble sign of duodenal obstruction will be present in the majority of patients with duodenal atresia and was evident in 78% (108/138) of cases in one series.[611] Jejunoileal atresia can be associated with gastroschisis in a minority of patients.

Other causes of SBO: There are a variety of other causes of SBOs, some of which are listed in Table 2-11. Often clinical history or physical examination will indicate the cause of an SBO. History of prior surgery, peritonitis, or pelvic inflammatory disease will suggest adhesions as a cause of obstruction. Hernias are often clinically palpable and their presence will denote this as a cause of obstruction. Some individuals will have a history of an abdominal or pelvic malignancy, which may directly invade the small bowel or metastasize via the peritoneum and produce obstruction.

Indications for emergency surgery in patients with SBO

In most cases, SBO can initially be treated with nasointestinal decompression. Evacuation of the gastric contents will progressively remove excess fluid proximal to the obstruction and result in decreased caliber of the obstructed loops. Many cases of obstruction due to adhesions can be successfully managed with nasointestinal decompression, without surgical intervention. Some other causes of SBO may require surgical intervention but in most cases can initially be treated conservatively with delayed surgical intervention when necessary. However, patients with closed-loop obstruction have a high morbidity and mortality because of the increased risk for mesenteric ischemia.[547,550,569,571] These patients require emergency laparotomy to prevent bowel perforation, sepsis, and other complications of mesenteric ischemia. Therefore, it is of critical importance that patients with imaging evidence of SBO be evaluated for the presence of closed-loop obstruction and for evidence of mesenteric ischemia of the obstructed loops.

Closed-loop obstruction: Closed-loop obstructions are diagnosed when a bowel loop of variable length is occluded at 2 adjacent points along its course. This is most commonly due to adhesive bands that cross the adjacent loops, but can also be secondary to hernias. In this process, the obstructed loops and their mesentery are fixed at a point that allows the closed loop to twist along its long axis, producing a small-bowel volvulus. Flow into and out of the closed loop is blocked, causing progressive accumulation of fluid and gas. If it is not relieved, the progressive distention of the closed loop leads to compression of the entrapped mesentery and the development of ischemia of the closed loop.[550]

On CT, closed-loop obstruction is diagnosed by characteristic fixed radial distribution of several dilated, usually fluid-filled bowel loops. These radial loops have either a C-shaped or U-shaped configuration, with the open end of the loop pointing at the site of obstruction. In addition, there will be stretched and prominent mesenteric vessels converging toward the point of torsion. This produces a "beak sign" on CT at the site of the torsion due to fusiform tapering or a "whirl sign," reflecting rotation of the bowel loops and mesenteric vessels around the fixed point of obstruction (see Figure 2-84).[550]

Strangulation: Strangulation is defined as a mechanical obstruction associated with intestinal ischemia,

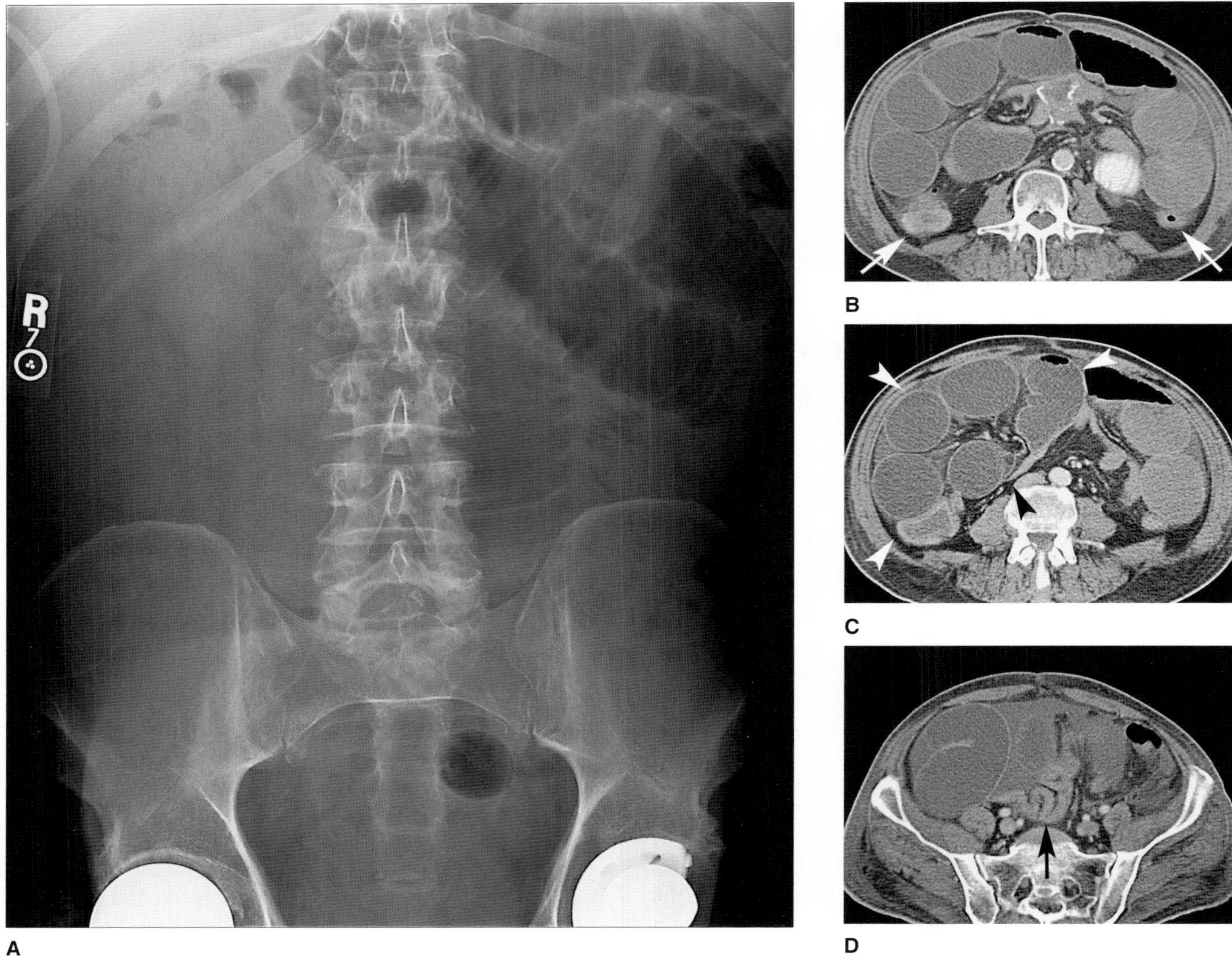

Figure 2-84 Closed Loop Obstruction
This 49-year-old man underwent a bowel resection for Burkett lymphoma 6 months previously. He now complains of intermittent severe abdominal pain. **A.** Supine view of the abdomen shows multiple dilated loops of bowel in the left upper quadrant. Note the multiple thin folds (plica circularis) in the loops characteristic of small bowel. A few tiny bubbles of gas are seen in the right upper quadrant, probably within collapsed colon. These findings are typical of a high-grade small-bowel obstruction. **B-D.** CT images through the abdomen show multiple dilated small-bowel loops with collapsed colon (*white arrows*) and collapsed distal small bowel (*black arrow*). Note how there is a cluster of loops in (C) (*arrowheads*) which appear contained in the right lower quadrant. Centrally, they form a beak (*black arrowhead*). These are CT features indicating a closed loop obstruction. Surgical exploration confirmed a closed loop obstruction due to adhesions.

which if left untreated will progress to bowel necrosis. This is seen in approximately 10% of patients with SBO and almost always occurs in the setting of a closed-loop obstruction. The distinction between closed-loop obstruction (incarceration) and strangulation (ischemia) should be emphasized as these are related phenomena but separate pathologic entities. Strangulation always develops because of a closed loop; however, a closed loop can be only partially obstructed, may not be associated with strangulation, and can resolve spontaneously.[550] This differentiation is critical to the interpretation of obstruction. When strangulation occurs in the setting of obstruction, mortality rates rise to 20% to 37%, compared with 5% to 8% for a simple obstruction.[571,612-614] This high mortality rate in strangulating obstruction is mainly attributed to a delay in establishing the correct diagnosis and initiating appropriate treatment. Because CT examinations are the primary means of diagnosing closed-loop obstruction and strangulation, imaging plays a critical role in the management of these patients.

Imaging Notes 2-21. Features of Obstruction with Strangulation (Mesenteric Ischemia)

Presence of the typical features of obstruction and any of the following features:
1. Lack of enhancement of the bowel wall following intravenous contrast
2. Thickened bowel wall
3. Target sign in the bowel wall
4. Pneumotosis intestinalis
5. Portal venous gas

CT findings suggesting the presence of mesenteric ischemia include (1) thickening of the bowel wall, (2) alterations in the attenuation of the affected bowel wall, producing a halo or "target sign," (3) pneumatosis intestinalis, and (4) portal venous gas. However, these findings are not specific for mesenteric ischemia and can be seen with infections of the small bowel. A specific finding is lack of wall enhancement; asymmetric enhancement or even delayed enhancement may also be found. Localized fluid and hemorrhage in the mesentery can also be seen in patients with mesenteric ischemia.[550,569,571] Strangulation is usually associated with adhesions or internal or external hernias.

Causes of colonic obstruction

The causes of colonic obstruction are very similar to the causes of SBO with the exception that the 2 most common causes of SBO, adhesions and hernias, virtually never cause colonic obstruction. Table 2-12 lists some of the causes of colonic obstruction. As with SBOs the combination of radiographic findings and clinical history often allows for a presumptive diagnosis.

Colonic obstruction can be diagnosed through a variety of radiologic examinations. Plain films have 84% sensitivity and 72% specificity,[615] contrast enema has 96% sensitivity and 98% specificity,[616] and multidetector CT has a sensitivity and specificity of about 90%[617,618] in the diagnosis of colonic obstruction. Colonic obstruction is an abdominal emergency with high morbidity and significant mortality. In colonic obstruction, the mural tension is highest in the cecum where the colonic radius is greatest, according to Laplace's law. Therefore, in the setting of a competent ileocecal valve, the cecum is most often the site of colonic ischemia or perforation when it is involved in a mechanical obstruction.[615] A cecal diameter greater than 9 cm is abnormal, and in the setting of colonic obstruction the cecal wall should be evaluated for early findings of ischemia.

Neoplasms: Neoplasms are responsible for 60% of colonic obstruction.[16,615,619] Unlike SBOs where neoplastic causes of obstruction are most often due to peritoneal implants or direct extension from an extraintestinal primary malignancy, colonic obstruction is most often due to primary colon carcinoma (see Figure 2-38). The mechanism of colonic obstruction by neoplasms is the same as previously described for SBO.

Table 2-12. Causes of Colonic Obstruction

1. Neoplasm
   a. Primary malignancy
   b. Direct invasion of extra-GI tumor
   c. Peritoneal metastasis
2. Volvulus
   a. Cecal
   b. Sigmoid
   c. Other
3. Diverticulitis
4. Inflammatory bowel disease
   a. Crohn disease
   b. Ulcerative colitis
5. Ischemic stricture
6. Post irradiation stricture
7. Parasites (ascaris)
8. Intussusception
9. Hirschsprung disease
10. Meconium ileus
11. Anal atresia and other colonic atresia

Colonic volvulus: Volvulus is the second leading cause of colonic obstruction, accounting for approximately 10% to 15% of cases.[16,615,619] Volvulus occurs when the bowel rotates around a single point and can, therefore, only occur in colon segments that are suspended from a mesentery. In the colon, volvulus is seen most frequently in the sigmoid colon, which accounts for 76% of cases, followed by the cecum, which accounts for 22% of cases.[596,619] Rarely, portions of the transverse colon, especially the splenic flexure, can develop volvulus. The various types of colonic volvulus often have characteristic imaging appearances at conventional radiography, which is sufficient for diagnosis in a large percentage of patients.[596]

Sigmoid volvulus: Sigmoid volvulus is an acquired condition with an increased prevalence among those with sigmoid colonic redundancy. Colonic redundancy can be due to laxative abuse usually for chronic constipation, high-fiber diet, pregnancy, chronic institutionalization, Chagas disease, Parkinson disease, and Hirschsprung disease.[596,615,621,622] Patients with colonic volvulus typically present with nonspecific abdominal pain and symptoms of obstruction and are typically older than patients with cecal volvulus.

Sigmoid volvulus will usually appear on abdominal radiograph as a markedly enlarged loop of bowel extending from the pelvis or right lower quadrant of the abdomen to the left upper quadrant of the abdomen. The dilated loop often extends beyond the level of the transverse colon, a finding termed the "northern exposure" sign.[620,623] The dilated sigmoid loop typically sharply folds in the left upper quadrant and comes to a point at the site of the twist in the right lower quadrant. Thus, the loop of the sigmoid appears as an oval air collection with a thin central line (the wall between the ascending and descending loop of the sigmoid colon) that has an appearance similar to a coffee bean and has been termed the "coffee bean" sign (see Figure 2-85).[620,624] On barium enema, contrast will abruptly terminate at the transition point of the volvulus, forming a beak-shaped cone of contrast without opacification of the dilated air-filled sigmoid colon beyond the site of obstruction (see Figure 2-85). Barium enema is additionally advantageous in that it can potentially reduce the volvulus, thereby offering both diagnosis and therapy. CT examinations will demonstrate both the abnormal position of the sigmoid colon and swirling of the mesentery at the level of the volvulus. Often coronal and sagittal reformats are useful for locating the mesenteric swirl and evaluating the orientation of the rotated bowel segment (see Figure 2-85).[596]

Cecal volvulus: In contrast to sigmoid volvulus, which is acquired, cecal volvulus is usually the consequence of a congenital abnormality. Specifically, this condition occurs when there is persistence of a cecal mesentery with resultant abnormal mobility that creates the potential for volvulus. This term is a misnomer, however, because most patients with cecal volvulus will in fact have torsion of the ascending colon located above the level of the ileocecal valve.

Patients with cecal volvulus are younger than those presenting with sigmoid volvulus (30-60 years old). Clinically they present with symptoms of obstruction, including nausea, vomiting, constipation, and acute cramping pain. Patient history typically reveals prior abdominal surgery, presence of a pelvic mass, violent coughing, atonia of the colon, extreme exertion, unpressurized air travel, recent colonoscopy, or third-trimester pregnancy.[596,625]

Abdominal radiographs of cecal volvulus will reveal a massive air collection with ovoid morphology in the left upper quadrant or midabdomen that represents the dilated cecum (see Figure 2-86). Occasionally, however, the distended cecum can be displaced to other locations within the abdomen. Depending on the acuity of the obstruction, proximal obstruction may or may not be present.[596,621] Of note, the reader should be careful not to overdiagnose the presence of cecal volvulus. When the cecum is loosely attached to its mesentery, air will rise into the nondependent portion and the cecum may fold on itself without torsion. As a consequence, patients with diminished bowel motility will often have a mildly distended air-filled cecum visualized as a dilated bowel segment in the midabdomen, a phenomenon termed a "cecal bascule." This finding does not indicate bowel obstruction and does not require surgical intervention. A diagnosis of cecal volvulus should be suggested only when the cecum is massively distended. In questionable cases, evaluation with barium enema or CT should be performed.

Contrast enema evaluation will show the distal colon to be decompressed with a beaklike tapering of the ascending colon at the site of the volvulus. In most cases, contrast will fail to pass beyond the site of volvulus. Although the contrast enema findings are characteristic of cecal volvulus, most patients are initially evaluated with CT. CT examinations will demonstrate an abnormally positioned cecum, often in the upper mid- and left abdomen, that can be traced back to the level of the volvulus. The volvulus appears as an area of swirling of the bowel and its mesentery, a finding known as the "whirl" sign.[596,626]

Diverticulitis: Diverticulitis is the third leading cause of colonic obstruction, accounting for 10% of cases (see Figure 2-75).[16,615,619] Although the third most common cause of colonic obstruction, colonic obstruction is a rare presentation of diverticulitis. Instead, patients with diverticulitis usually present with fever and abdominal pain but without evidence of obstruction. In 1 study of diverticulitis over a 20-year period, 7% of cases (29/422) presented with symptoms of obstruction requiring surgical intervention.[211] Diverticulitis is discussed earlier in this chapter under the heading **Focal Polyps or Masses of the Colon**.

Other pericolonic infection: Rarely, other causes of pericolonic abscess will also cause colonic obstruction.[627,628]

Inflammatory bowel disease: Although SBO is a common complication of IBD, colonic obstruction is relatively rare. In 1 surgical series of 306 patients, 16% required surgical relief of SBO whereas none required surgery for colonic obstruction.[629] In a second surgical series of patients with ulcerative colitis, only 3% (2/72) patients required surgery for colonic obstruction.[630] The outcome of obstruction is dependent on the underlying cause. Acute obstructions are usually caused by inflammatory narrowing and will respond to medical therapy. However, chronic obstructions are usually due to strictures and will often require surgical intervention.[631]

Fecal impaction: Fecal impaction is a common problem in the elderly and can also be found in individuals with spinal cord injury, cystic fibrosis, and Hirschsprung disease. However, only rarely is fecal impaction sufficiently severe to cause colonic obstruction. When it occurs, it is most characteristically seen in the very elderly with a mean age of 79 years.[632] Patients typically complain of abdominal pain and distention and are frequently bedridden or have chronic mental status changes. Abdominal x-rays will demonstrate dilation of the small bowel and colon. Air-fluid levels are uncommon; however, abundant feces are demonstrated within the rectum and colon.[632]

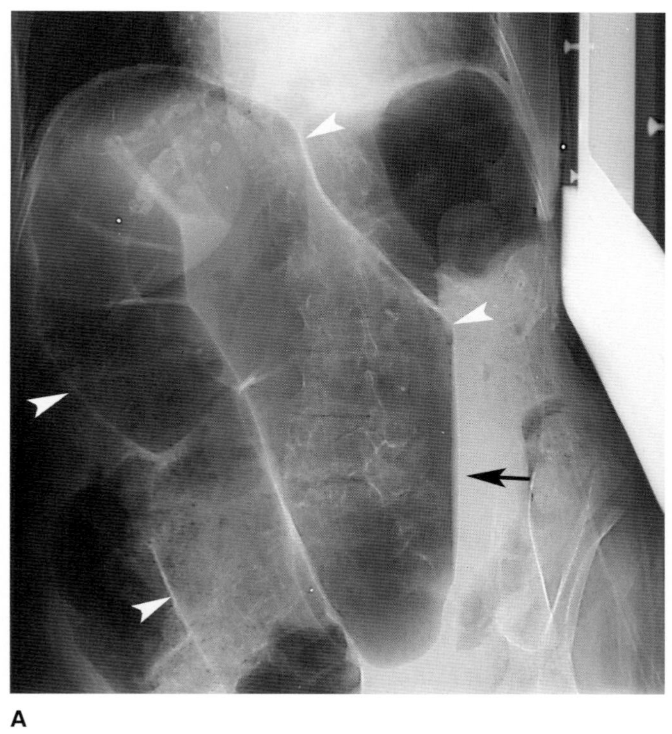

A

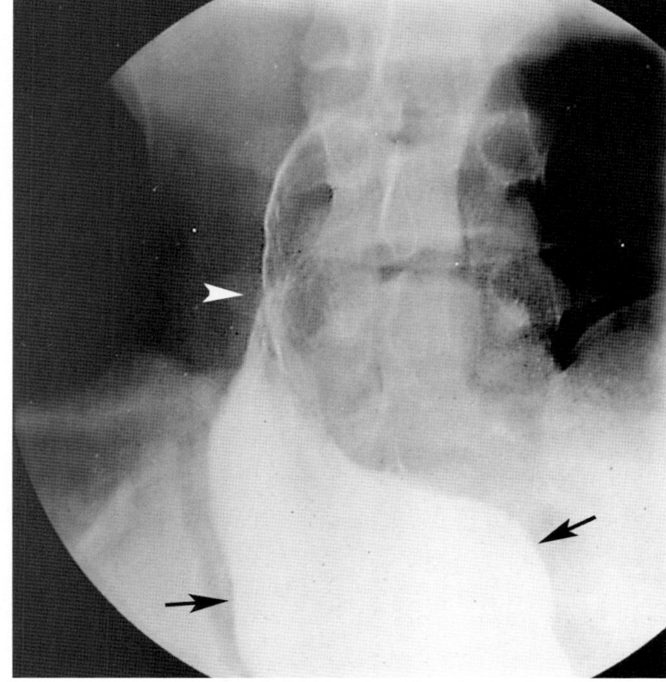

B

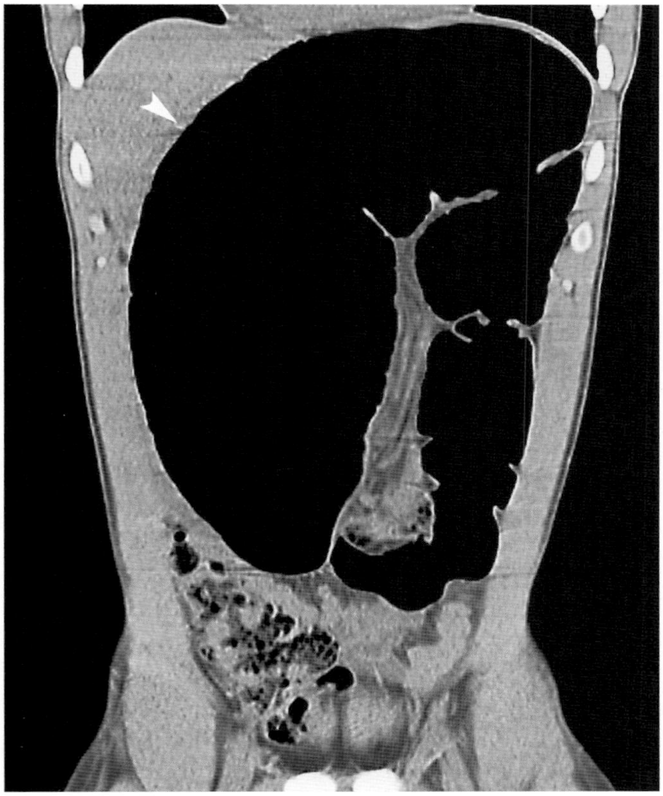

C

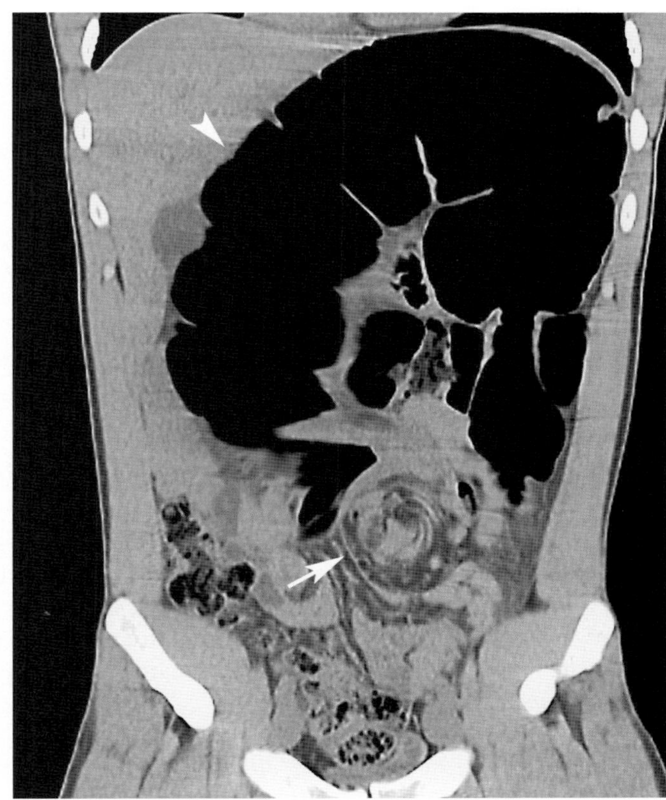

D

Figure 2-85 Sigmoid Volvulus in 3 Patients
A-D. This 91-year-old woman was transferred from a nursing home because of crampy abdominal pain. A. Left lateral decubitus film shows an air-fluid level (*black arrow*) within a markedly distended loop of colon. This loop resembles a coffee bean (*white arrows*). This appearance is diagnostic of a cecal volvulus. B. Barium enema from a different patient shows barium within the rectum (*black arrows*) and an occlusive twist at the rectosigmoid junction. **C** and **D.** This 20-year-old man was chronically presented with abdominal pain, nausea, and vomiting for 2 days. Coronal reconstructions from a noncontrast abdominal CT demonstrate a massively distended sigmoid colon (*arrowheads*) and a swirl of mesenteric vessels (*arrow*) in the left lower quadrant, diagnostic of a sigmoid volvulus.

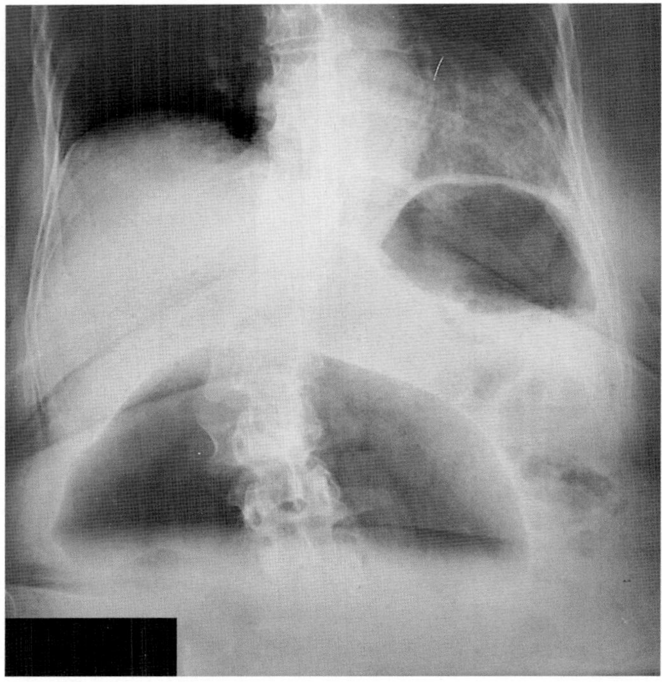

A

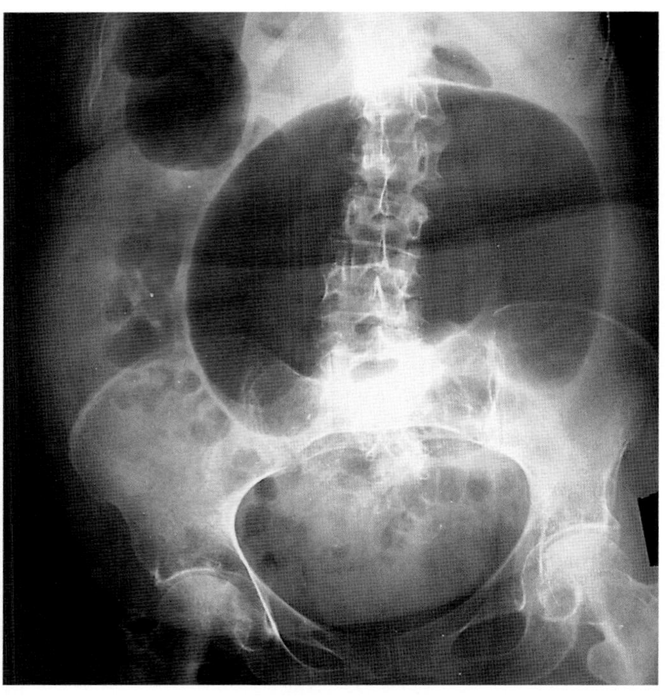

B

Figure 2-86 Cecal Volvulus
This 66-year-old man was bedridden as a result of several strokes when he complained of abdominal pain. **A.** Erect radiograph shows an air-fluid level in a large air collection in the right lower quadrant. **B.** Supine radiograph showed a 30-cm air collection in the midabdomen. There are also minimally dilated loops of small bowel in the pelvis below the air collection. This appearance is diagnostic of a cecal volvulus.

Meconium ileus and distal ileal obstruction: Meconium ileus represents obstruction at the terminal ilium or colon due to impaction of abnormally thick, tenacious, sticky meconium. It is one of the more common causes of neonatal intestinal obstruction, and the majority of cases are seen in patients with cystic fibrosis. Patients typically present with failure to pass meconium in the first 24 hours of life associated with bilious emesis and abdominal distention. Abdominal x-rays will show abnormal distention of multiple bowel loops. Barium enema will demonstrate a microcolon with obstruction of the terminal ilium.

Distal ileal obstruction, previously known as meconium ileus equivalent, represents the increased incidence of fecal impaction and obstruction in children and adults with cystic fibrosis. This disease has a mechanism similar to that of meconium ileus.

Intussusception: In most cases, intussusception occurs within the small bowel and causes SBO. However, rarely, intussusception can involve the colon and be a cause of colonic obstruction.[633] Intussusception is described most completely earlier in this chapter under the heading **Causes of SBO**.

Hirschsprung disease: Hirschsprung disease, also called congenital megacolon, is caused by failure of migration of colonic ganglion cells during gestation.[634] As a consequence, varying lengths of the distal colon remain constricted, causing functional colonic obstruction. The disease usually involves the rectosigmoid colon but can affect the entire colon and, rarely, the small intestine. Approximately 80% of patients will present in infancy with difficult bowel movements, poor feeding, poor weight gain, and progressive abdominal distention. Rarely, patients can present with persistent, severe constipation later in life. Imaging studies will show the typical features of colonic obstruction, although contrast enemas can be normal in the first few months of life.[634]

Colonic atresia: Colonic atresia is an uncommon cause of colonic obstruction in neonates and the least common site of bowel atresia. A 25-year review of intestinal atresia from a single pediatric center demonstrated only 277 cases of intestinal atresia and only 21 cases of colonic atresia.[611] Patients presented with bilious emesis, abdominal distension, and failure to pass meconium through the anus. Nearly one-quarter of patients (4/21) will have concomitant gastroschisis.[611]

Other uncommon causes of colonic obstruction: Other uncommon causes of colonic obstruction include ischemic strictures,[635] gallstone ileus,[636] bezoars,[637] endometriosis,[638] pancreatitis,[639] radiation-related strictures,[640] and diaphragmatic hernias.[641]

Table 2-13. Causes of Adynamic Ileus

1. Recent abdominal or thoracic surgery
2. Peritonitis
3. Drugs a. Narcotic b. Anticholinergics c. Other
4. Metabolic derangement a. Hypokalemia b. Hyponatremia c. Hypomagnesemia d. Hypothyroidism e. Acidosis f. Hypothermia
5. Abdominal and thoracic inflammatory processes a. Appendicitis b. Cholecystitis c. Pancreatitis d. Diverticulitis e. Pelvic inflammatory disease f. Pneumonia g. Other
6. Thoracic and abdominal trauma
7. Head trauma and neurosurgical procedures
8. Intestinal ischemia

Adynamic ileus

Adynamic ileus is a common problem among hospitalized patients. The exact physiologic mechanisms of adynamic ileus remain obscure but a variety of factors appear to increase the incidence of adynamic ileus (Table 2-13). Most common of these is abdominal and thoracic surgery.[642,643] Inflammation of the peritoneum irritates the entire bowel and causes the cessation or diminution of peristalsis. Other causes of peritonitis including peritoneal infection and inflammation will also cause a generalized adynamic ileus. Medications, usually narcotics but occasionally anticholinergic medications along with other medications, are also a common cause of adynamic ileus.[644-646] Finally, metabolic derangements such as hypokalemia and hyponatremia alter the normal metabolic activity of the bowel will also affect bowel peristalsis and cause adynamic ileus.[642]

All of the causes of ileus that have been previously mentioned will affect the entire bowel relatively uniformly and result in a "generalized" adynamic ileus. In generalized adynamic ileus, the bowel becomes dilated and fluid filled as a result of diminished peristalsis. Thus, generalized adynamic ileus is distinguished from bowel obstruction by demonstrating the presence of gas throughout the bowel, including the rectum (see Figure 2-76). It is not uncommon for the rectum to be collapsed in the supine and erect radiographs of the abdomen because in both positions it is dependent and therefore gas will rise out of it. Cross-table prone view of the rectum and left lateral decubitus views of the pelvis image the rectum in a nondependent position and often will demonstrate air in the rectum in patients with generalized adynamic ileus. Either of these views are simple methods of distinguishing a distal colonic obstruction from an adynamic ileus without the use of cross-sectional imaging.

Occasionally, adynamic ileus will involve only a focal region of the bowel. This is most often seen in adynamic ileus related to inflammatory disease of the abdomen or pelvis. Inflammatory process tends to preferentially affect peristalsis of nearby loops of bowel. Thus, in appendicitis the ileal loops can be dilated without dilation of other bowel segments and in pancreatitis, the transverse colon can be dilated without dilation of other bowel segments (see Figure 2-87). Therefore, focal adynamic ileus can mimic both SBO and colonic obstruction. The only potential clue to distinguishing between a focal adynamic ileus and small-bowel or colonic obstruction is appropriate clinical history.

Acute colonic pseudo-obstruction: Acute colonic pseudo-obstruction (ACPO) is an uncommon form of ileus characterized by massive colonic dilation. The mechanism

Imaging Notes 2-22. Bowel Gas Patterns

Finding	Pattern
Dilation and air-fluid levels	
Dilation stops in small bowel	Small-bowel obstruction Focal adynamic ileus (uncommon)
Dilation stops in colon	Colonic obstruction Focal adynamic ileus (uncommon)
Dilation throughout bowel	Generalized adynamic ileus
Normal caliber and air-fluid levels	Enteritis/colitis
Normal caliber and no air-fluid levels	Normal/Airophagia

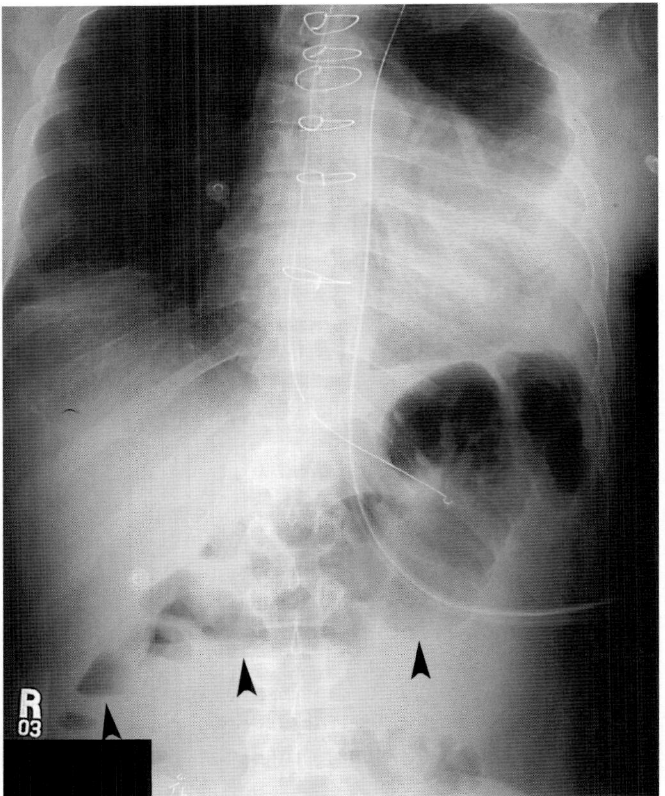

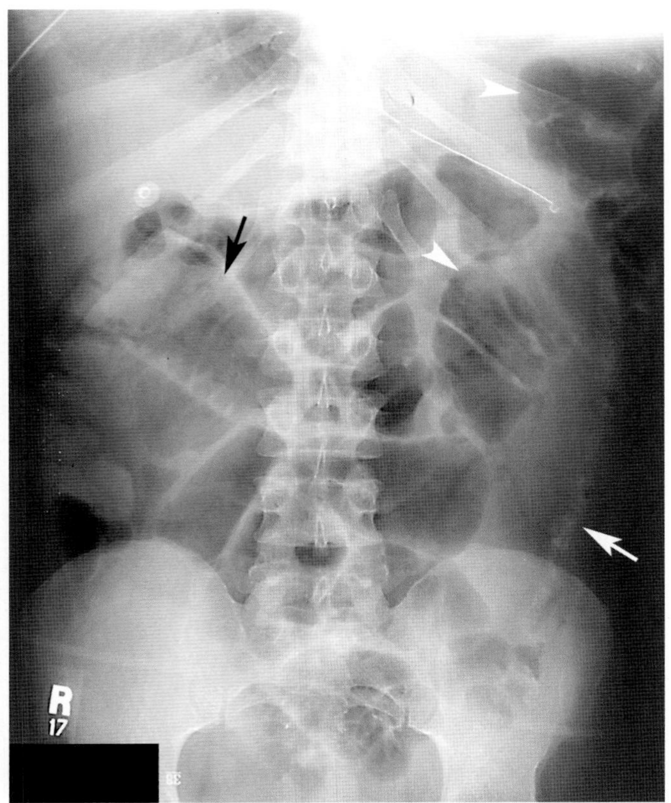

Figure 2-87 Colon Cut-off Sign
This 40-year-old man recently experienced a seizure. He now complains of boring abdominal pain. **A.** Erect radiograph demonstrates multiple air fluid levels. **B.** Supine radiograph shows dilated small bowel with multiple thin folds (*black arrow*) and dilated transverse colon and splenic flexure (*white arrowheads*). The descending colon is collapsed and contains a small amount of barium and appears as a thin string (*white arrow*). This pattern will usually indicate a colonic obstruction. However, further evaluation confirmed a diagnosis of acute pancreatitis. This is representative of a focal adynamic ileus due to local inflammation of the transverse mesocolon and jejunal small-bowel mesentery caused by the pancreatitis. This is known as the "colon cut-off" sign.

of pseudo-obstruction is most likely multifactorial because of uncoordinated, nonperistaltic, or attenuated colonic muscle contractions originating from either increased thoracic sympathetic stimulation or decreased sacral parasympathetic activity. Patients usually present with mild, diffuse, abdominal discomfort and distension as well as minimal systemic toxicity that develops slowly over several days.[647] Passage of stool or gas is absent in 50% of patients, but patients occasionally have diarrhea.[621] Most often, pseudo-obstruction presents in hospitalized patients with underlying disorders, including postoperative status, recent child birth, cardiopulmonary disease, nonoperative trauma, drugs, and electrolyte disorders.[642,648]

ACPO can only be diagnosed after exclusion of a mechanical large-bowel obstruction using barium enema or CT. Abdominal radiographs typically demonstrate massive colonic dilation, which is greater in the right colon than the left colon. This pattern of colonic dilation favors the diagnosis of ACPO rather than colonic obstruction.[227] When visualized, a colonic cut-off point favors the diagnosis of colonic obstruction; however, 40% of patients with ACPO appear to have a cut-off point most often at the splenic flexure, descending, or sigmoid colon.[616] Up to 80% of patients with ACPO have simultaneous dilation of small bowel.[649] Therefore, contrast enemas, CT, or colonoscopy is usually necessary to make this diagnosis.

Contrast enemas, using either barium or water-soluble contrast, or abdominal CT scans are often performed to exclude colonic obstruction. Abdominal CT has a sensitivity of 96% and specificity of 98% for ACPO.[616,650] CT has the additional advantages of allowing more accurate measurement of bowel diameter and a better appraisal of the condition of the mucosa to detect coexisting inflammation and ischemia.

Most patients with ACPO improve within 72 hours with supportive care. However, approximately 3% to 15% of patients with ACPO will develop a major complication, including ischemia, sepsis, and perforation. Perforation, when it occurs, is typically located in the cecum, which has the greatest level of wall tension. Surgery is reserved for patients with clinical deterioration or with evidence of colonic ischemia or perforation.[642]

UNIQUE FINDINGS RELATED TO THE BOWEL

GI bleeding, bowel perforation, pneumoperitoneum, dissection of gas in the wall of the bowel, and portal venous gas are uncommon but important complications of bowel pathology. There are also 2 unusual disorders of the bowel that can cause abdominal pain, called epiploic appendagitis and segmental omental infarction. These disorders will be reviewed.

Gastrointestinal Bleeding

Bleeding from the GI tract is a moderately common clinical problem that can be caused by a relatively wide range of disorders, including inflammation, neoplasms, dilated submucosal veins, vascular malformations, traumatic tears, and coagulopathies (see Table 2-14).[651] Approximately 75% of GI bleeding will cease spontaneously; however, bleeding can recur in up to 25% of cases.[652] Mortality rates related to GI bleeding are approximately 3% to 5%, but can be as high as 23% with massive bleeding or bleeding that recurs after hospitalization.[653]

GI bleeding is commonly divided into upper GI causes and lower GI causes. Upper GI bleeding indicates a source proximal and lower GI bleeding indicates a source distal to the ligament Treitz. Upper GI bleeding is more common than lower GI bleeding occurring in approximately 100 per 100 000 individuals and 20 per 100 000 individuals, respectively.[651]

The most common causes of upper GI bleeding are peptic ulcers accounting for approximately 35% to 60% of cases, followed by varices (4%-31%) and Mallroy-Weiss tears (4%-13%). However, the precise cause of upper GI bleeding can be unknown in up to 25% of cases.[651]

The most common cause of lower GI bleeding is diverticulosis, accounting for 33% to 50% of cases, followed by vascular ectasia (8%-20%), neoplasms (19%), and colitis (18%).[231] Meckel diverticulum is the most common cause of lower GI bleeding in children.[651]

Bleeding can present in 1 of 5 ways: (1) hematemesis, (2) melena, (3) hematochezia, (4) positive fecal occult blood tests, or (5) symptoms of blood loss or anemia such as lightheadedness and dyspnea.[651] In most cases, hematemesis will indicate an upper GI cause and hematochezia will indicate a lower GI cause. Melena will more often indicate an upper GI cause and positive occult blood tests and symptoms of blood loss or anemia can be seen with both upper and lower causes.

Endoscopy and colonoscopy are the primary methods of diagnosis of GI bleeding.[654] However, imaging can be an important adjunct test in patients where endoscopy and colonoscopy fail to identify the source of bleeding. This is most common in situations where the bleeding is intermittent and recurrent. In the past, Technetium 99m-labeled red cells [Tc-99m red blood cell (RBC)] and Technetium 99m (Tc-99m) sulfur colloid scintigraphy were the principal imaging studies used in determining the site of occult bleeding. More recently, CT examinations using angiographic technique is used to identify the presence and the site of bleeding.

Tc-99m RBC or Tc-99m sulfur colloid scintigraphy can be used to detect and localize GI bleeding. These agents circulate in the bloodstream. Extravasation of blood into the lumen of the bowel will result in increased activity in the distribution of the bowel. Location of the first site of activity indicates the site of bleeding (see Figure 2-88). Tc-99m RBC scintigraphy is approximately 93% sensitive and 95% specific for the detection of active arterial or venous bleeding and can detect bleeding rates as low as 0.2 mL/min.[655] Tc-99m RBC scintigraphy is additionally advantageous in that delayed scans can be performed up to 24 hours after administration of the radioisotope. This allows for the detection of intermittent bleeding through repeat evaluation at discrete intervals after initial scans. However, blood can travel in either a retrograde or antegrade direction between the time of bleeding and the time of imaging, which most likely accounts for false localization rates of 22%.[656] Furthermore, scintigraphic examinations cannot identify structural lesions causing the bleeding.

Computed tomographic angiography is the current accepted method for the detection of GI bleeding.[657-661] Examinations are performed following the administration of IV contrast, without the use of oral contrast. Extravasation of contrast medium results in hyperattenuating contrast in the lumen of the bowel and indicates the site of bleeding (see Figure 2-89). A meta-analysis of 9 studies with 198 patients

Table 2-14. Causes of Gastrointestinal Bleeding

1. Upper
   - a. Inflammation
     - i. Esophagitis
     - ii. Gastritis/duodenitis/peptic ulcers
   - b. Neoplasms
   - c. Esophageal and gastric varices
   - d. Vascular malformations and vascular ectasia
   - e. Superior mesenteric artery syndrome
   - f. Bleeding from pancreatic duct
   - g. Bleeding from the bile duct
2. Lower
   - a. Colitis/enteritis
     - i. Inflammatory bowel disease
     - ii. Ischemic
     - iii. Infectious
     - iv. Postradiation
   - b. Neoplasms
   - c. Hemorrhoids
   - d. Diverticular disease
     - i. Diverticulosis
     - ii. Diverticulitis
   - e. Angiodysplasia
   - f. Anal fissure
   - g. Coagulopathy
   - h. Vasculitis

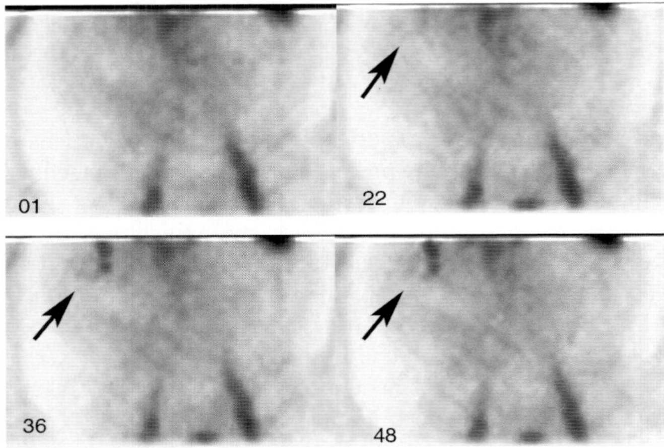

Figure 2-88 Gastrointestinal Bleeding due to a Radiation Ulcer This 66-year-old man had received radiation therapy for a cholangiocarcinoma and presented with melena, anemia, and hypotension. Images from a 99mTc red blood cell study show a faint blush of activity (*arrow*) in the right upper quadrant at 22 minutes after injection that progressively increased at 36 and 48 minutes indicating the presence of active bleeding. Colonoscopy revealed a radiation-induced ulcer in the hepatic flexure.

of CT angiography demonstrated a pooled sensitivity of 89% and specificity of 85% for the diagnosis of GI bleeding.[654] In addition to identifying the site of bleeding, CT offers the ability to identify a structural cause of the bleeding in some cases.

Mesenteric angiography can also be used to detect GI bleeding when the bleeding rates are greater than 0.5 mL/min (see Figure 2-89). Unfortunately, angiography only has a sensitivity of 40% to 86%.[652,662] In general, angiography is primarily used as a therapeutic intervention through transcatheter embolization and not a diagnostic study.

Pneumoperitoneum and Bowel Perforation

Pneumoperitoneum, often referred to as "free air," is defined by the presence of air within the peritoneal space that is outside the bowel lumen.

Causes of pneumoperitoneum

The most common causes of pneumoperitoneum are iatrogenic, including laparotomy and laparoscopy, percutaneous gastrostomy, vigorous respiratory resuscitation, peritoneal dialysis, colonoscopy, and other abdominal interventions (Table 2-15). The majority of iatrogenic causes of pneumoperitoneum leave the peritoneum sterile and without a source of further gas. In these cases, pneumoperitoneum will resolve spontaneously, without intervention and without complication.

Free air is recognized on left lateral decubitus abdominal radiographs 3 days after surgery in 44% to 60% of patients who undergo open surgery and 25% of patients who undergo laparoscopic surgery.[663,664] By day 6, 8% of patients have persistent evidence of pneumoperitoneum on optimal-quality radiographs. Although erect plain films will usually show resolution of pneumoperitoneum within 1 week, imaging identification of pneumoperitoneum can persist for several weeks following surgical intervention depending on the volume of air and absorption rate of the peritoneum.[665,666] This is especially true of CT scans, which can show pneumoperitoneum for up to 3 weeks following abdominal procedures.[239] In general, a smaller amount of pneumoperitoneum is expected in patients who undergo laparoscopic procedures, compared to open resection.[665] Regardless of the initial volume, the quantity of air should become progressively less with serial examinations.[664] If the amount of air is seen to increase over time, this should raise suspicion for the development of a complication of the recent procedure.

In the absence of a sterile iatrogenic cause for pneumoperitoneum, the recognition of free air is a cause for concern because the majority of noniatrogenic cases are associated with perforated hollow viscus and will require surgical treatment. In 5% to 15% of spontaneous cases, pneumoperitoneum will be due to causes other than perforation and does not require emergent surgery.[663,667,668]

Perforation of a hollow viscus can be due to a variety of causes and differs depending on the location of the affected bowel and the clinical setting. Gastric or duodenal ulcers are among the most common causes of bowel perforation. Colonic perforation can be due to obstruction (benign or malignant), ischemia, adynamic ileus, toxic megacolon, and inflammatory conditions, including appendicitis, diverticulitis, tuberculosis, and necrotizing enterocolitis. Although acute diverticulitis and appendicitis are both associated with intestinal perforation, free air is seldom observed with either process. This is thought to be due to containment of the free air associated with diverticulitis by the associated inflammatory reaction as well as the very small amount of gas contained within the appendix.[666]

Pneumoperitoneum in the setting of trauma should raise the possibility of bowel perforation, which can be seen in both blunt and penetrating trauma. In premature infants, the most common cause of bowel perforation is necrotizing enterocolitis.

Imaging Notes 2-23. Evaluation of Pneumoperitoneum

- Most cases of pneumoperitoneum will be iatrogenic
- Search first for causes of abdominal intervention
  - Recent surgery
  - Percutaneous gastrostomy
  - Peritoneal dialysis
  - Other
- In the absence of an iatrogenic cause, bowel perforation should be excluded
- Most common causes of bowel perforation
  - Peptic ulcer
  - Neutropenic colitis

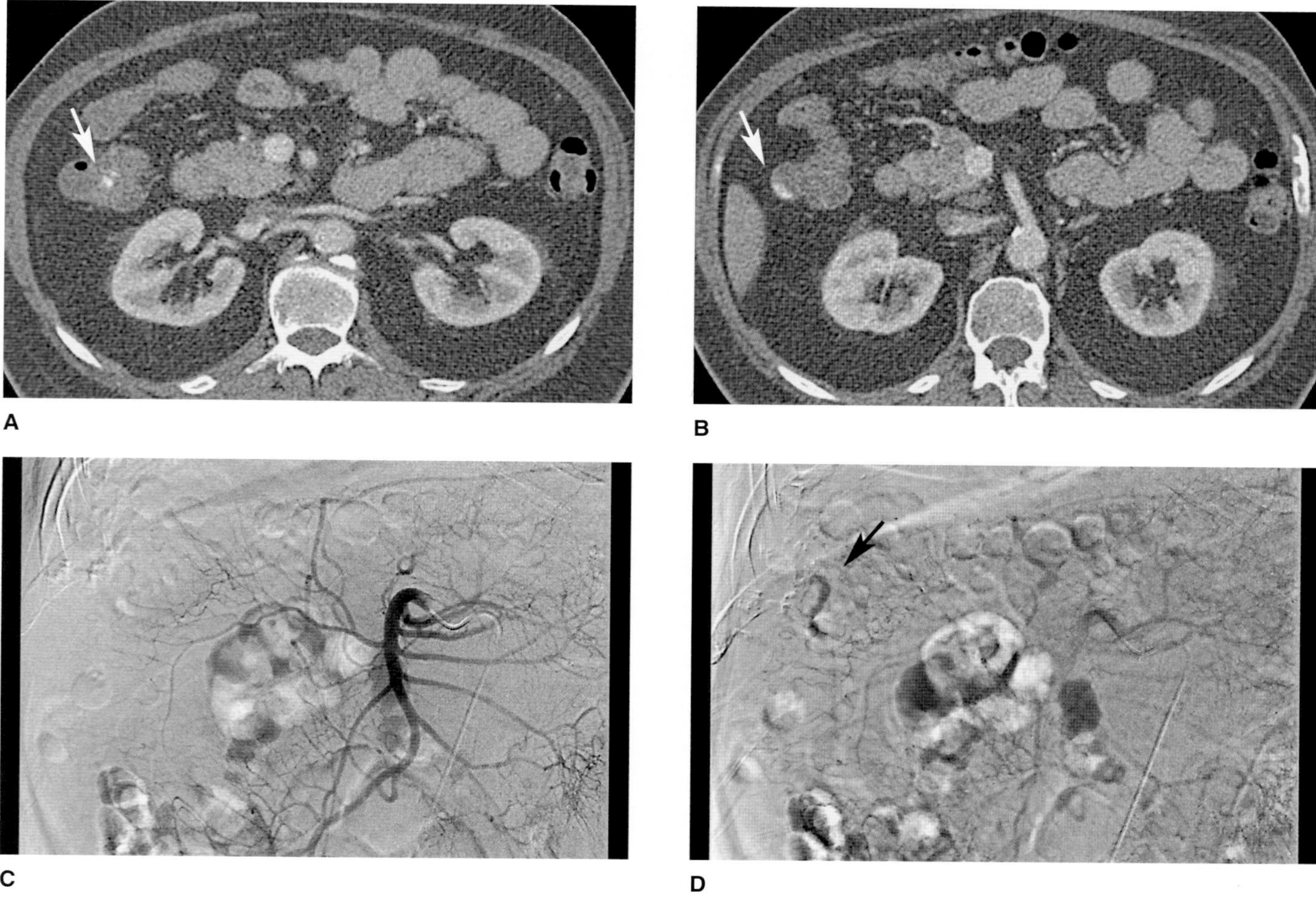

Figure 2-89 Gastrointestinal Bleeding Following Polypectomy This 63-year-old man had a polypectomy performed 1 week prior. He presented with hematochezia. **A** and **B**. CT angiogram performed without oral contrast shows a small foci of contrast (*white arrows*) in the ascending colon that had not been present on the precontrast images, indicating the presence of active bleeding. **C** and **D**. SMA angiogram performed later that day confirms the site of bleeding (*black arrow*) in the hepatic flexure. The feeding arteries were subsequently embolized.

Pulmonary barotrauma is a rare cause of pneumoperitoneum. This is caused by high pressures in the bronchial tree that results in pulmonary interstitial emphysema, which dissects into the mediastinal tissues causing pneumomediastinum and subcutaneous emphysema in the neck. Rarely, air travels in an inferior rather than superior direction and dissects into the retroperitoneum, which directly communicate with the mediastinum. Air can then perforate the parietal peritoneum and the peritoneal space.[665] In many cases, it can be impossible to distinguish barotrauma as a cause of pneumoperitoneum from bowel perforation. In general, when peritoneal signs are absent and clinical suspicion for a ruptured viscus is low, conservative management with clinical and imaging follow-up is recommended. However, if there is an increased clinical suspicion for bowel perforation, fluoroscopic evaluation with water-soluble contrast material administered via oral, rectal, or enterostomy tube may be necessary.[663]

Other miscellaneous causes of pneumoperitoneum include medications, pneumatosis coli, or pneumatosis intestinalis (discussed below) and female genital tract-related causes.[118,120] Medications leading to gastric ulcers such as corticosteroids and nonsteroidal anti-inflammatory drugs can be a cause of pneumoperitoneum. The fallopian tubes communicate with the peritoneum at one end and with the uterus at the other. Forceful transmission of air and fluid through the vagina related to douching, sexual intercourse, insufflation, water skiing, and other mechanisms can result in the transmission of air from the vagina into the peritoneum.

Imaging manifestations of pneumoperitoneum

Pneumoperitoneum can be detected by chest and abdominal radiographs, CT, and MRI.

Radiographic detection of pneumoperitoneum: Air within any space will rise to the nondependent surface of the space. Pneumoperitoneum can be visualized in profile via a horizontal beam film, either an erect chest or abdomen radiograph that includes the diaphragms or a left

Table 2-15. Causes of Pneumoperitoneum

1. Iatrogenic[a]
a. Laparotomy and laparoscopy
b. Percutaneous gastrostomy
c. Peritoneal dialysis
d. Paracentesis
e. Breakdown of surgical anastomosis
f. Other abdominal interventions
2. Bowel perforation
a. Peptic ulcer[a]
b. Penetrating and blunt trauma[a]
c. Small bowel and colonic infections
i. Neutropenic colitis (typhlitis)[a]
ii. Diverticulitis
iii. Necrotizing enterocolitis (infants)
iv. Appendicitis
v. Other bowel infections
d. Ruptured diverticulum
i. Colonic pulsion diverticula
ii. Meckel diverticulum
iii. Congenital diverticula
e. Ischemic bowel
f. Inflammatory bowel disease
i. Toxic megacolon
g. Bowel obstruction
h. Sigmoidoscopy/colonoscopy
i. Adynamic ileus
3. Pulmonary barotraumas
4. Pneumatosis intestinalis
5. Passage of air through the female genital tract
a. Intercourse
b. Douching
c. Other

[a]Most common causes.

lateral decubitus radiograph of the abdomen that includes the nondependent surface of the abdomen and the liver surface. It is generally believed that a left lateral decubitus radiograph is the most sensitive radiographic projection for the detection of pneumoperitoneum.[664]

On erect films, the pneumoperitoneum will be seen as a thin or thick black band outlining the undersurface of the diaphragm (see Figures 2-90 and 2-91). On decubitus films, air will be seen as a thin or thick black band outlining the undersurface of the abdominal wall that is easiest appreciated when outlining the liver surface on a left lateral decubitus examination. Supine and semierect films are much less sensitive for the detection of pneumoperitoneum. On semierect radiographs, air will typically rise to the central and anterior surface of the diaphragm, just beneath the heart. This is seen as a bandlike lucency across the central superior abdomen, inferior to the cardiac silhouette (see Figure 2-90).

Pneumoperitoneum can be seen on either an upright or left lateral decubitus view following the injection of as little as 1 to 2 mL of free air into the peritoneal cavity. Detection of small volumes of free air is facilitated by prolonged positioning of least 10 minutes prior to exposure.[669] Failure to maintain the patient in the erect or decubitus position for at least 10 minutes increases the likelihood that air will remain trapped in the dependent peritoneal recesses and will not be visualized.

There are several subtle signs of pneumoperitoneum that can be detected on supine radiographs. In most cases, these signs require large volumes of peritoneal gas to be detected. However, 1 study of the ability of supine films to detect pneumoperitoneum suggested that there was evidence of pneumoperitoneum on 59% (26/44) of supine examinations.[670]

The right upper quadrant sign is thought to be the most sensitive sign of free air on supine radiographs, seen in 41% to 49% of cases.[666,670,671] This sign is characterized by the presence of triangular or linear lucencies located along the diagonal surface of the liver edge. The linear collections are thought to represent gas in the right subhepatic space, whereas the triangular collections are thought to represent gas in Morrison pouch.[670]

The second most commonly seen sign on the supine radiograph is the Rigler sign found in 17% to 32% of supine radiographs of patients with pneumoperitoneum.[666,670] When a bowel loop is filled with air, the air outlines the internal border of the bowel wall. Thus, the lumen of the bowel is seen as lucent and the tissues external to the bowel appear opaque. If there is air in both the lumen of the bowel and within the peritoneum, external to the bowel, then the bowel wall will appear as a thin white line bordered by the lucent bowel lumen and the lucent peritoneum; this appearance is called Rigler's sign. Studies suggest that at least 750 mL to 1L of free air is necessary to identify this finding (see Figure 2-91).[666]

The falciform ligament is a band of peritoneum that is attached to the surface of the left lobe of the liver that contains the umbilical vein. In the normal individual, the falciform ligament is indistinguishable from the other soft tissues of the abdomen. However, in the supine position, free abdominal air will rise to the anterior surface of the abdomen and can outline the 2 sides of the falciform ligament. In this situation, the falciform ligament appears as a white band overlying the left lobe of the liver known as the falciform ligament sign (see Figure 2-91). In some situations, the peritoneal cavity may appear as an oval gas shadow known as the "Football sign," whereby the falciform ligament appears as the laces of the football. The reader should be aware that both of these findings require extensive peritoneal gas before they are visualized (see Figure 2-91).[666]

Although abdominal radiographs are advised as the initial method of evaluating for pneumoperitoneum, they are of limited sensitivity and specificity. Studies suggests that a combination of a supine and left lateral radiographs have a sensitivity of 47% to 59%[670,672] and erect films have

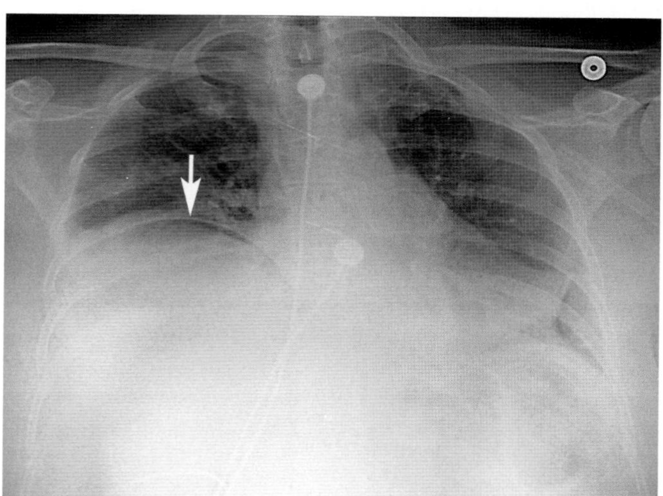

A

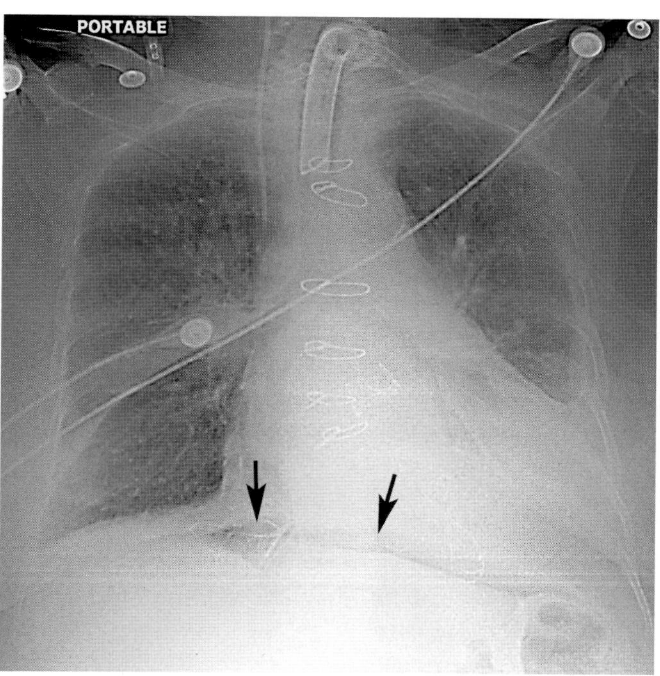

B

Figure 2-90 Pneumoperitoneum on Erect and Semierect Radiographs
A. This 65-year-old woman underwent right hemicolectomy for a colon cancer 3 days previously. Posteroanterior chest radiograph demonstrates a thin sliver of air beneath the right hemidiaphragm. This is the typical appearance of pneumoperitoneum on an erect radiograph. This air is related to the recent abdominal procedure and is an expected postoperative finding, without clinical significance. **B.** This 74-year-old woman was hospitalized with chronic heart failure following aortic valve repair. This radiograph demonstrates a bandlike lucency in the superior midabdomen. This is a common appearance of pneumoperitoneum on a semierect chest radiograph because in the semierect position the anterior portion of the diaphragm is the most nondependent portion of the abdomen.

a sensitivity of 38% for the detection of pneumoperitoneum when CT is used as the reference standard.[673] Radiographs are particularly poor at detecting small amounts of free air and are limited in obese patients.[670,673] Even when pneumoperitoneum is detected on radiographs, the etiology of this free air is usually uncertain.

CT detection of pneumoperitoneum: Computed tomographic scans have been shown to detect as little as 2.5 mL of pneumoperitoneum. As a consequence, CT scans are the gold standard in the evaluation of pneumoperitoneum.[672] Gas will predominantly collect in the nondependent portions of the peritoneum anterior to the liver just beneath the anterior abdominal wall, but can also be seen within the mesentery, lesser sac, Morrison pouch, and immediately underlying the rectus abdominis muscles.[673] This air is best visualized using lung windows.

CT will in some cases identify the cause of pneumoperitoneum, especially in the setting of bowel perforation where often the site of perforation can be discerned (see Figure 3-62). Helpful clues to determining the source of a suspected bowel perforation include (1) the location of the gas and (2) the presence or absence of an associated adynamic ileus. The largest volume of air is often located adjacent to the site of suspected perforation. Gastric and duodenal ulcers are not typically associated with an adynamic ileus, whereas colonic perforation causes a bacterial peritonitis that causes almost immediate ileus involving both the small and large bowel.

Pneumatosis intestinalis and portal venous gas: The term *pneumatosis intestinalis* means air within the bowel wall. It is important to understand that pneumatosis can be attributable to both benign causes and life-threatening causes, even in the presence of some abdominal symptoms (see Table 2-16).[674-679] Pneumatosis intestinalis is an imaging finding, not a diagnosis and requires clinical correlation in order to differentiate the etiology and prognosis.[680]

There are 2 dominant theories as to how gas enters the wall of the bowel. The mechanical theory postulates that gas enters the bowel wall either from the enteric lumen or from the lungs via the mediastinum because of increased pressure. This would explain the etiology of pneumatosis in the setting of bowel obstruction and emphysema. The bacterial theory postulates that gas produced by bacteria enters the submucosa through mucosal rents or increased mucosal permeability that produces gas in the bowel wall.[681] Bacterial overgrowth in the GI tract from a variety

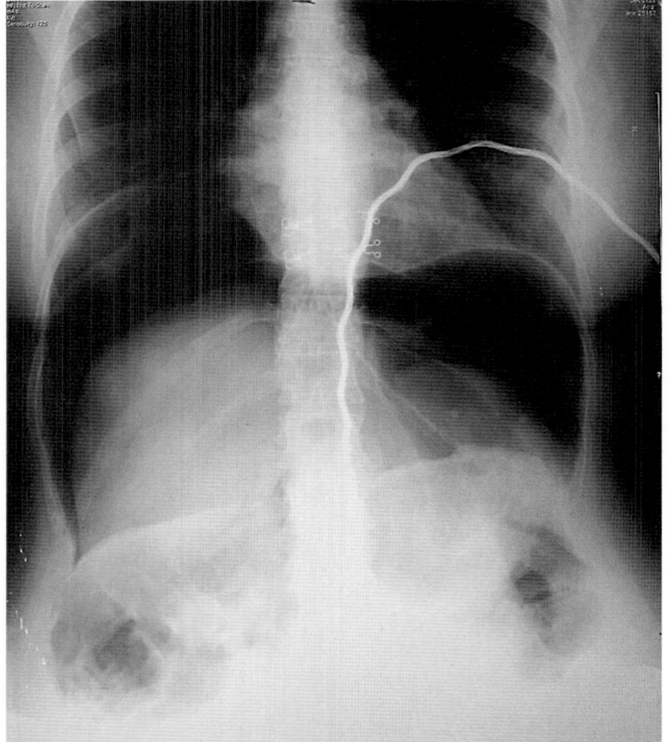

A

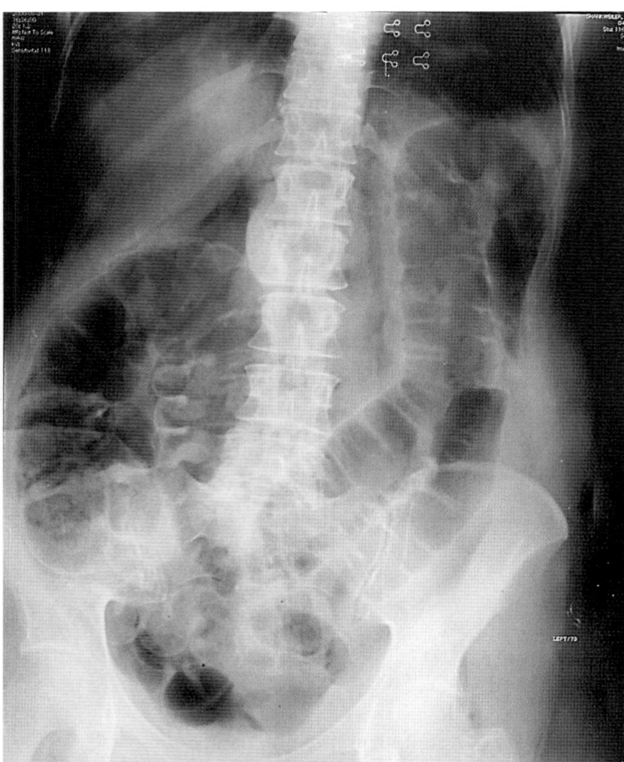

B

C

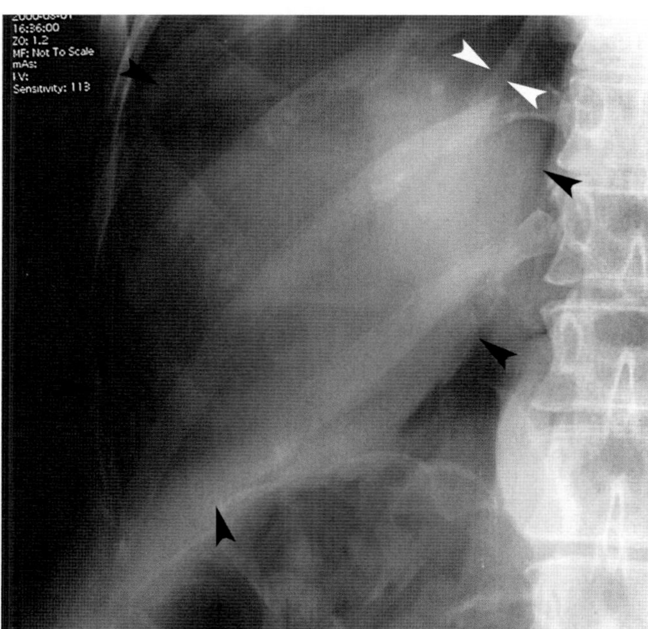

D

Figure 2-91 Pneumoperitoneum on the Supine Film
This 50-year-old man underwent sigmoidoscopy when he complained of severe abdominal pain. **A.** Erect film of the abdomen shows a massive amount of air beneath both hemidiaphragms. **B.** Supine radiograph shows an air-filled colon and 2 subtle signs of pneumoperitoneum on a supine radiograph. **C.** Magnified view of the right midabdomen shows the hepatic flexure. Note how the colon wall is seen as a thin white line (*arrowheads*). This finding is known as "Rigler" sign and is seen because there is air within the colon and also outside of the colon (pneumoperitoneum) that outline both sides of the bowel wall. **D.** Magnified view of the right upper quadrant shows air in the peritoneum outlining the borders of the liver (*black arrowheads*) and the falciform ligament (*white arrowheads*), creating the "football" sign.

Table 2-16. Causes of Pneumatosis Intestinalis

1. Life-Threatening Causes:
    a. Intestinal Ischemia
    b. Mesenteric vascular disease
    c. Intestinal obstruction (especially strangulation)
    d. Infectious enteritis/colitis[a]
    e. Toxic megacolon
    f. Trauma
    g. Organ transplantation (especially bone marrow transplant)[a]
    h. Collagen vascular disease[a]
2. Benign Causes:
    a. Pulmonary disease
        i. Asthma
        ii. Chronic obstructive pulmonary disease
        iii. Cystic fibrosis
        iv. Positive end expiratory pressure (ventilator-associated barotraumas)
    b. Systemic
        i. Scleroderma[a]
        ii. Systemic lupus[a]
        iii. AIDS
    c. Intestinal causes
        i. Infectious enteritis/colitis[a]
        ii. Intestinal obstruction[a]
        iii. Inflammatory bowel disease
            1. Crohn disease
            2. Ulcerative colitis
    d. Medication related
        i. Corticosteroids
        ii. Chemotherapy
    e. Organ Transplant
        i. Graft vs host disease
        ii. Bone marrow[a]
        iii. Solid organ transplant (kidney, liver)
    f. Primary
        i. Idiopathic (usually involves colon)
        ii. Pneumatosis cystoides intestinalis

[a]Some causes are listed under both benign and life threatening.

of causes can lead to excessive hydrogen gas production, bowel distention, and subsequently, dissection of intraluminal hydrogen gas into the bowel wall.[124-127,682] Prior literature has demonstrated that the gas collections in the bowel wall have a hydrogen content up to 50%,[681] which supports the bacterial theory because hydrogen is a byproduct of bacterial metabolism. However, the bacterial theory is not supported by the finding that long-standing pneumoperitoneum associated with pneumatosis rarely results in peritonitis.[683] It is likely that the cause of pneumatosis varies depending on the clinical condition and reflects a combination of both theories.

Patient presentation is rarely helpful in the diagnosis of pneumoperitoneum and often reflects the consequence of the underlying cause or condition.[684] However, because of benign causes, such as pulmonary disease, patients are usually asymptomatic or may have mild abdominal discomfort.[122,128-130] Conversely, the presence of peritoneal signs can imply intestinal perforation from life-threatening causes.[675]

Abdominal radiography and CT are both used for the diagnosis of pneumatosis intestinalis. However, CT is more sensitive than radiography and should be used when there are questionable findings on plain radiographs.[675,685-689] On CT examinations, pneumatosis intestinalis is best identified using lung windows. Pneumatosis typically adopts 1 of 3 appearances on radiographs and CT images: linear, bubbly, or circular patterns of gas collection. In general, the circular form of pneumotosis intestinalis (PI) is usually benign and is classically associated with pneumatosis cystoides intestinalis—a subset of pneumatosis intestinalis that almost always occurs in the colon and its mesentery (see Figure 2-92).[675,686,690] Conversely, linear or bubble-like pneumatosis intestinalis can be due to either benign or life-threatening causes (see Figure 2-93).[675] However, these are general guides rather than absolute rules, and correlation with patient symptoms is imperative in distinguishing between benign and life-threatening causes.

The presence or absence of other findings on CT scans can be helpful in distinguishing between the likelihood of benign versus life-threatening causes. The presence of a normal bowel wall will usually indicate a benign cause. Conversely, the presence of bowel wall thickening, either absent or intense mucosal enhancement, dilated bowel, arterial or venous occlusion, ascites, and hepatic portal or portomesenteric venous gas raise suspicion for pneumatosis due to a life-threatening cause.[675,691,692] Pneumatosis intestinalis confined to a specific vascular territory should raise suspicion of underlying ischemia.[252]

The extent of pneumatosis is often inversely related to the severity of the disease.[674,693] This is probably because life-threatening processes such as ischemia may develop so rapidly that there is less time to form pneumatosis than in less serious conditions. The location of pneumatosis in the colon versus the small bowel or stomach cannot be used

Imaging Notes 2-24. Features Suggesting Life-Threatening Pneumatosis Intestinalis

1. Bowel wall thickening
2. Absent or increased mucosal enhancement
3. Bowel dilation
4. Arterial or venous occlusion
5. Ascites
6. Portal venous gas

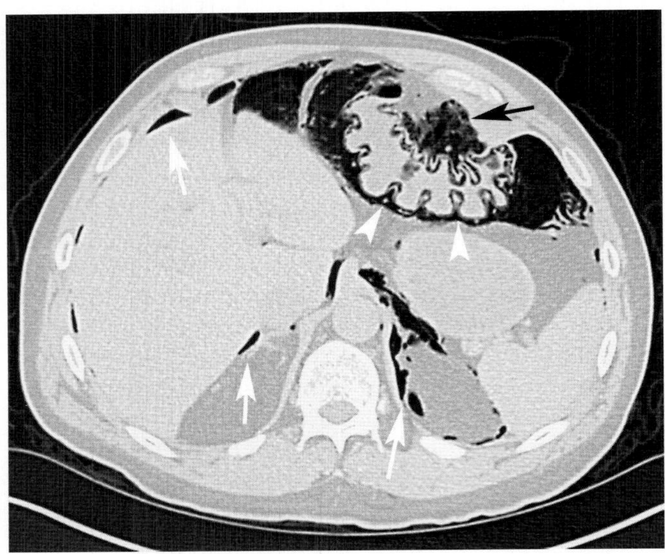

A

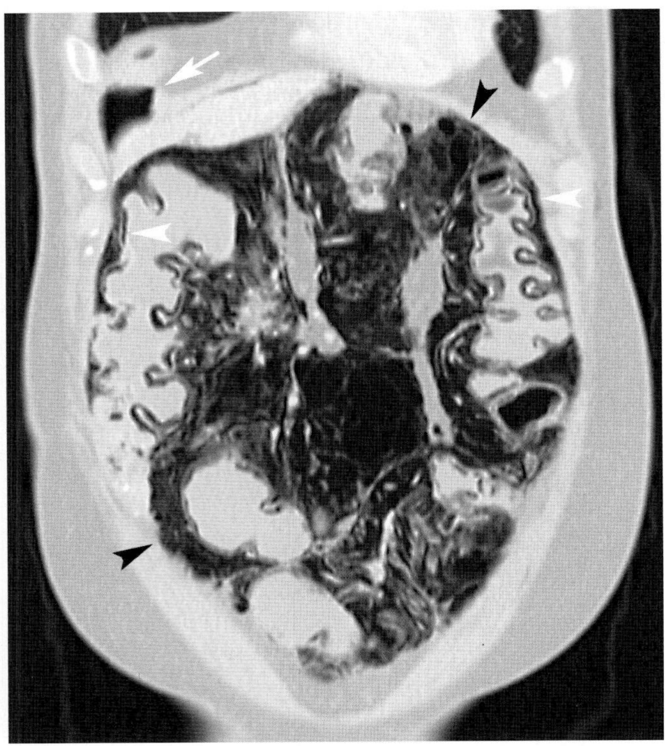

B

Figure 2-92 Pneumatosis Cystoides Intestinalis
This 63-year-old man with Crohn disease was status post ileocolica anastamosis and receiving corticosteroids when he complained of increased flatus. CT images in the axial (**A**) and coronal (**B**) planes using lung windows demonstrate both linear (*white arrowhead*) and bubbly (*black arrowhead*) pneumatosis involving essentially the entire colon. There are also scattered foci of pneumoperitoneum (*long white arrow*). Despite the extensive nature of the pneumatosis, the patient was asymptomatic, with stable vital signs and benign physical examination at the time of the scan. Following the scan, he was admitted for observation and discharged 2 days later without intervention in stable condition.

to distinguish the cause of the pneumatosis and does not indicate its clinical significance.[681,690,693]

Portal venous gas is classically visualized as branching linear or nodular gas collections in the peripheral aspect of the liver (see Figure 2-93). Further, CT is more sensitive than radiography in the detection of hepatic portal and portomesenteric venous gas (see Figure 2-94).[675,687,691,694] When visualized in the setting of pneumatosis, this finding is most often due to bowel ischemia in adults and necrotizing enterocolitis in infants. In this setting, portal venous gas reflects the passage of gas from the bowel wall into the mesenteric veins and then into the portal venous system.[692,695-697] Examples of nonischemic causes of hepatic portal or portomesenteric venous gas include mesenteric abscess formation, portomesenteric thrombophlebitis, sepsis, abdominal trauma, severe enteritis, cholangitis, chronic cholecystitis, pancreatitis, IBD, diverticulitis, and following GI surgery or liver transplantation.[675,679,688,691,696,698-702] There have also been several reports of gas in the portal vein in conditions with benign pneumatosis,[674,687,693] again emphasizing the importance of clinical correlation.

Ultrasound with color Doppler is very sensitive and specific, both in early detection and follow-up of portal venous gas. Gray-scale US typically demonstrates highly echogenic intravascular particles that move in the direction of blood flow. Alternatively, this gas can present as poorly defined patchy hepatic gas accumulation in the nondependent hepatic parenchyma (see Figure 2-94). Color Doppler tracings will often demonstrate bidirectional spikes superimposed on the background of a normal spectral portal vein tracing. These bidirectional spikes are thought to represent artifact caused by acoustic reflections from the mobile intravascular gas bubbles (see Figure 2-94).[133-135] The main drawback of US is that when portal venous gas is visualized, further exploration with CT is warranted to evaluate for pneumatosis intestinalis.

Recent literature has suggested that patients with isolated pneumatosis intestinalis are more likely to have partial or nontransmural ischemia, whereas patients with both pneumatosis and portomesenteric venous gas are more likely to have transmural infarction.[40,136] Overall survival is higher among patients with nontransmural intestinal

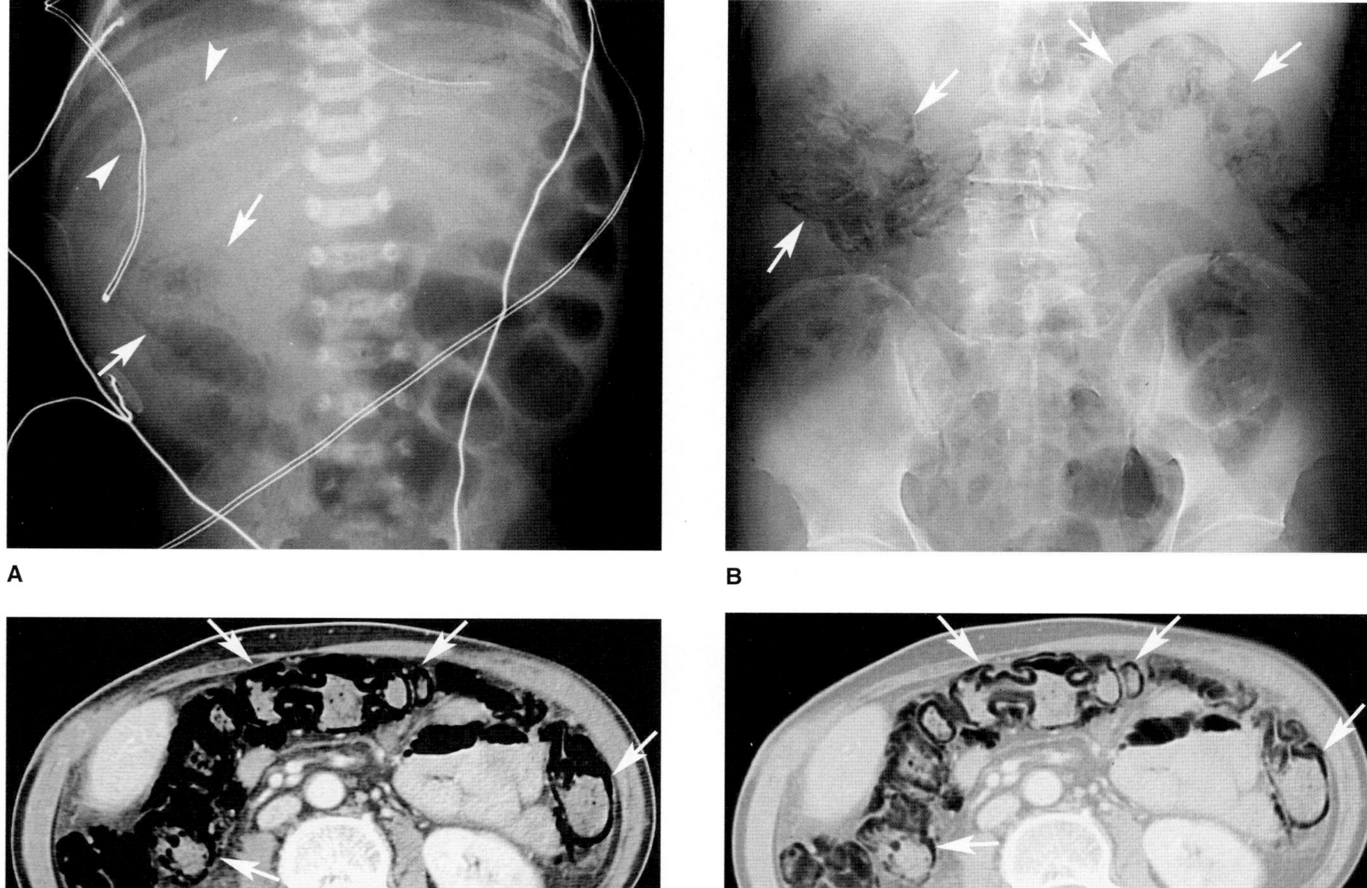

Figure 2-93 Pneumatosis Intestinalis in 2 Patients
A. This 2-week-old premature infant had fevers, abdominal distension, and increased gastric residuals. AP view of the abdomen demonstrates linear pneumatosis intestinalis (*arrows*) in the right lower quadrant. There are also small bubbles of gas in the right upper quadrant characteristic of portal venous gas. These findings are indicative of severe necrotizing enterocolitis. **B-D.** This 56-year-old man had received a liver transplant several months prior to presenting with abdominal pain. B. Supine view of the abdomen demonstrates fine curvilinear collections of gas outlining the wall of the transverse colon (*arrows*), typical of pneumatosis intestinalis. CT images in standard soft tissue windows (C) and lung windows (D) confirm the presence of extensive pneumatosis intestinalis (*arrows*). Surgical exploration confirmed the presence of intramural air within an otherwise normal colon and so the bowel was left intact without subsequent complication.

ischemia compared with those patients with transmural intestinal infarction.

UNIQUE FOCAL LESIONS OF THE BOWEL

Epiploic appendagitis and idiopathic segmental omental infarction are 2 rare complications of the mesenteric fat that present with acute abdominal pain due to infarction.[377] The clinical presentation of these diagnoses can mimic more common inflammatory conditions such as appendicitis, cholecystitis, and diverticulitis. However, both of these diagnoses demonstrate a unique appearance on CT, which allows confident diagnosis of the disorder.

Epiploic Appendagitis

The epiploic appendages are small pedunculated fatty projections that protrude from the antimesenteric border of the colon into the peritoneal cavity and extend from the cecum to the rectosigmoid junction. These appendages are approximately 1 to 2 cm thick and 2 to

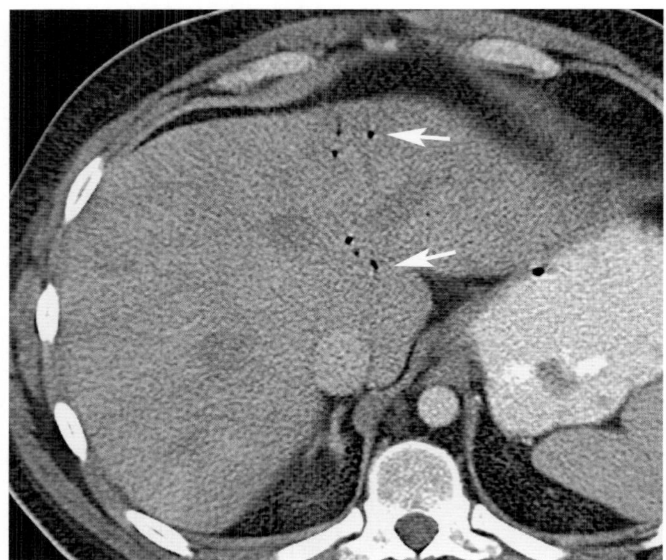

A

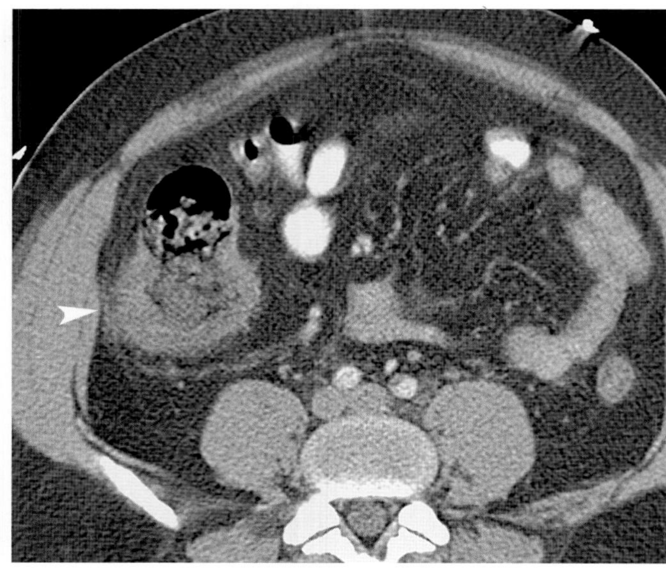

B

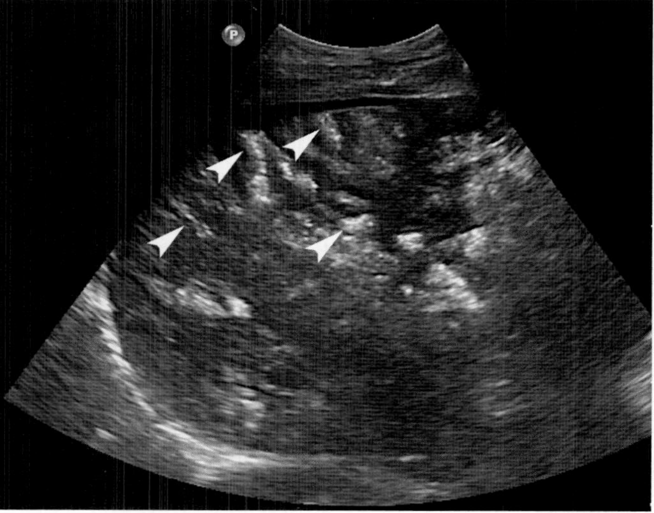

C

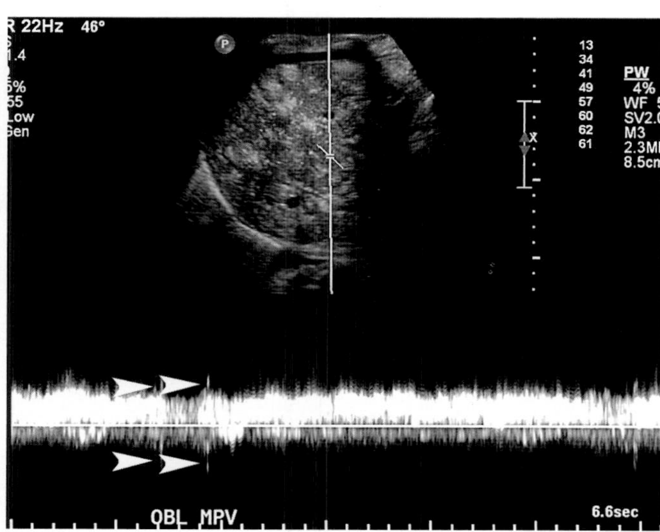

D

Figure 2-94 Portal Venous Gas in 2 Patients
A and **B.** This 32-year-old man had a congenital cardiomyopathy with chronic heart failure when he presented with right lower quadrant pain, fevers, and leucocytosis. A. Axial CT image through the liver demonstrates 6 small black dots (*arrows*) that represent air in the portal venous system. This finding usually indicates necrosis of some portion of the bowel wall with passage of bowel gas into the portal system. B. CT of the right lower quadrant shows focal thickening of the cecum consistent with bowel edema. Surgical exploration confirmed a diagnosis of necrotic ischemic cecum and ascending colon. **C** and **D.** This 47-year-old male with congestive heart failure, diabetes, and hypertension presented with distended abdomen. C. Transverse image of the right hepatic lobe demonstrates multiple linear-branching echogenic structures extending peripherally to the liver capsule (*white arrowhead*). D. Spectral Doppler interrogation of the main portal vein demonstrates portal venous waveform with superimposed bidirectional spikes (*white arrowhead*), typical of portal venous gas.

5 cm long. Usually, they are imperceptible as they blend with the surrounding mesenteric and retroperitoneal fat. Each appendage is supplied by 1 or 2 small end arteries branching from the vasa recta longa of the colon and is drained by a vein that passes through its narrow pedicle.[312,377]

Rarely the appendices epiploicae will undergo spontaneous torsion or spontaneous venous thrombosis because of their limited blood supply, pedunculated shape, and excessive mobility.[377,703,704] When they torse, they result in a focal inflammatory process called epiploic appendagitis. Patients typically present with severe, acute abdominal

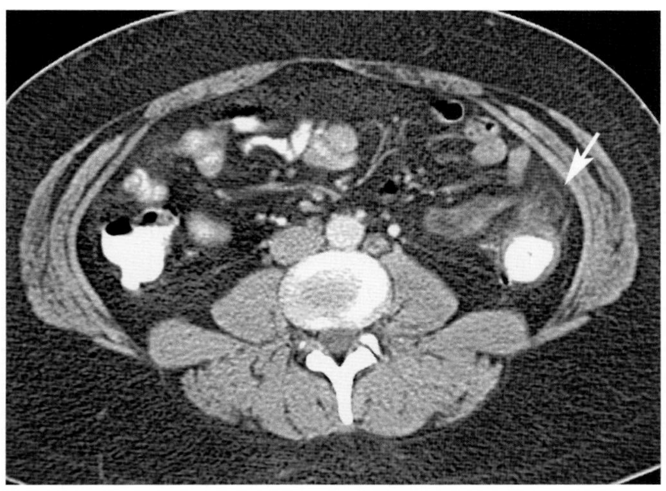

Figure 2-95 Epiploic Appendagitis
This 32-year-old woman complained of acute left lower quadrant pain. The CT image shows a ring of soft-tissue attenuation surrounding a fatty center (*arrow*) adjacent to the descending colon. There is fat stranding surrounding the ring and there is mild thickening of the adjacent colon wall. This appearance is diagnostic of epiploic appendagitis.

pain that is localized to 1 of the lower quadrants and mimics acute appendicitis or diverticulitis.

Computed tomographic findings of epiploic appendagitis are highly diagnostic and include visualization of the following: (1) a 1- to 4-cm paracolonic oval fatty mass representing the infarcted or inflamed appendix epiploica, (2) a well-circumscribed hyperattenuated rim that surrounds the mass and represents the inflamed visceral peritoneal lining, and (3) rarely a high-attenuation central dot representing engorged or thrombosed central vessels (see Figure 2-95).[377,705,706]

A hallmark of this disease process is that the paracolonic inflammatory changes are disproportionately severe relative to the mild local reactive thickening of the adjacent colonic wall.[377] This pattern of inflammation denotes that the pathologic process is centered in the mesentery adjacent to the bowel wall rather than in the bowel wall. When visualized in a paracolonic distribution, this helps to narrow the differential diagnosis to include epiploic appendagitis and diverticulitis.[377] Recognition of this unique appearance on noninvasive imaging and absence of diverticula within the region of inflammation are important because epiploic appendagitis is a self-limited process that does not require surgical intervention.[707,708]

Segmental Omental Infarction

The greater omentum is the largest peritoneal fold consisting of a double layer of peritoneum that extends inferiorly from the greater curvature of the stomach as low as the pelvis and drapes over the anterior surfaces of both the transverse colon and the pancreas. The right and left gastroepiploic arteries provide its main blood supply. On CT, the greater omentum typically appears as a layer of fat located just anterior to the transverse colon invested with small blood vessels.[377] The size of the omentum is larger in obese patients and smaller in lower-weight patients.

Segmental omental infarction preferentially occurs on the right side of the abdomen. It is believed that an embryologic variant of the blood supply to the right portion of the omentum predisposes it to venous thrombosis.[709] About 85% of cases occur in adults. Patients typically present with abdominal pain located just to the right of the umbilicus,[710] a clinical presentation that can mimic appendicitis, gallbladder disease, or pyelitis.[377] The exact etiology and pathogenesis of omental infarction is unknown; however, anomalous arterial supply to the omentum, kinking of veins secondary to increases in intraabdominal pressure, and vascular congestion after large meals have been proposed as possible mechanisms.[710] Risk factors for the development of omental infarction include obesity, recent surgery, and coughing.[709,710]

On US examinations, segmental omental infarction will appear as a solid, well-circumscribed, hyperechoic, and noncompressible mass immediately underlying the site of focal tenderness. This mass can adhere to the adjacent peritoneum. This phenomenon is best appreciated in the sagittal plane, which shows the mass to move in synchrony

Imaging Notes 2-25. CT-Identifiable Causes of GI-Related Acute Abdominal Pain

Diverticulitis
Primary finding: Focal wall thickening of the colon
Secondary findings: Fat stranding, abscess

Appendicitis
Primary finding: Distended (>7 cm) enhancing appendix
Secondary findings: Fat stranding, cecal wall thickening, abscess

Cholecystitis
Primary finding: Distended gallbladder with thickened wall (>1 mm)
Secondary findings: gallstones, fat stranding

Epiploic Appendagitis
Primary finding: Small ring of edema around fatty epiploic appendage
Secondary findings: none

Segmental Omental Infarction
Primary finding: Focal inflammatory mass in the right side of the greater omentum
Secondary findings: fat stranding in the greater omentum

with the abdominal wall during respiration rather than separately from the abdominal wall like other intraperitoneal contents.[28,710,711]

In most cases, the diagnosis of segmental omental infarction is made on CT examinations. CT will demonstrate a large ovoid or cakelike mass with heterogenous regions of mixed fat and soft-tissue attenuation within the anterior abdomen. The mass is usually located in a paraumbilical location between the rectus abdominis muscles and the transverse colon in the expected region of the greater omentum.[377,710] Ancillary findings occasionally include thickening of either or both the adjacent peritoneum and the bowel wall. Because the inflammatory process is centered in the omentum, the degree of fat stranding is disproportionately more severe than the colonic wall thickening, an important finding distinguishing segmental omental infarction from diverticulitis and other primary bowel pathologies.[377]

At times, distinguishing between omental infarction and epiploic appendagitis can be challenging because of the overlap in imaging appearance on CT. The clinical relevance of this distinction is limited, however, because management for both conditions is conservative.[377,710]

REFERENCES

1. Paulsen SR, Huprich JE, Fletcher JG, et al. CT enterography as a diagnostic tool in evaluating small bowel disorders: review of clinical experience with over 700 cases. *Radiographics.* 2006;26(3):641-657; discussion 657-662.
2. Maglinte DD, Sandrasegaran K, Lappas JC. CT enteroclysis: techniques and applications. *Radiol Clin North Am.* 2007;45(2):289-301.
3. Mazzeo S, Caramella D, Battolla L, et al. Crohn disease of the small bowel: spiral CT evaluation after oral hyperhydration with isotonic solution. *J Comput Assist Tomogr.* 2001;25(4):612-616.
4. Doerfler OC, Ruppert-Kohlmayr AJ, Reittner P, et al. Helical CT of the small bowel with an alternative oral contrast material in patients with Crohn disease. *Abdom Imaging.* 2003;28(3):313-318.
5. Wold PB, Fletcher JG, Johnson CD, et al. Assessment of small bowel Crohn disease: noninvasive peroral CT enterography compared with other imaging methods and endoscopy—feasibility study. *Radiology.* 2003;229(1):275-281.
6. Pickhardt PJ. Three-dimensional endoluminal CT colonography (virtual colonoscopy): comparison of three commercially available systems. *AJR Am J Roentgenol.* 2003;181(6):1599-1606.
7. Johnson CD, Chen MH, Toledano AY, et al. Accuracy of CT colonography for detection of large adenomas and cancers. *N Engl J Med.* 2008;359(12):1207-1217.
8. Macari M, Bini EJ, Jacobs SL, et al. Filling defects at CT colonography: pseudo- and diminutive lesions (the good), polyps (the bad), flat lesions, masses, and carcinomas (the ugly). *Radiographics.* 2003;23(5):1073-1091.
9. Lefere PA, Gryspeerdt SS, Dewyspelaere J, Baekelandt, et al. Dietary fecal tagging as a cleansing method before CT colonography: initial results polyp detection and patient acceptance. *Radiology.* 2002;224(2):393-403.
10. Pickhardt PJ, Choi JR, Hwang I, et al. Computed tomographic virtual colonoscopy to screen for colorectal neoplasia in asymptomatic adults. *N Engl J Med.* 2003;349(23):2191-2200.
11. Pickhardt PJ. Screening CT colonography: how I do it. *AJR Am J Roentgenol.* 2007;189(2):290-298.
12. Macari M, Bini EJ, Jacobs SL, et al. Significance of missed polyps at CT colonography. *AJR Am J Roentgenol.* 2004;183(1):127-134.
13. Johnson CD, Dachman AH. CT colonography: the next colon screening examination? *Radiology.* 2000;216(2):331-341.
14. Dachman AH, Kuniyoshi JK, Boyle CM, et al. CT colonography with three-dimensional problem solving for detection of colonic polyps. *AJR Am J Roentgenol.* 1998;171(4):989-995.
15. Macari M, Milano A, Lavelle M, et al. Comparison of time-efficient CT colonography with two- and three-dimensional colonic evaluation for detecting colorectal polyps. *AJR Am J Roentgenol.* 2000;174(6):1543-1549.
16. Gore RM, Levine MS, Laufer I. *Textbook of Gastrointestinal Radiology. Vol. 2.* Philadelphia: W.B. Saunders Co.; 1994:2716.
17. Pickhardt PJ. Primary 2D versus primary 3D polyp detection at screening CT colonography. *AJR Am J Roentgenol.* 2007;189(6):1451-1456.
18. Macari M, Megibow AJ. Pitfalls of using three-dimensional CT colonography with two-dimensional imaging correlation. *AJR Am J Roentgenol.* 2001;176(1):137-143.
19. Taylor SA, Halligan S, Slater A, et al. Polyp detection with CT colonography: primary 3D endoluminal analysis versus primary 2D transverse analysis with computer-assisted reader software. *Radiology.* 2006;239(3):759-767.
20. Beaulieu CF, Jeffrey RB Jr, Karadi C, et al. Display modes for CT colonography. Part II. Blinded comparison of axial CT and virtual endoscopic and panoramic endoscopic volume-rendered studies. *Radiology.* 1999;212(1):203-212.
21. Mang T, Maier A, Plank C, et al. Pitfalls in multi-detector row CT colonography: a systematic approach. *Radiographics.* 2007;27(2):431-454.
22. Yee J, Kumar NN, Hung RK, et al. Comparison of supine and prone scanning separately and in combination at CT colonography. *Radiology.* 2003;226(3):653-661.
23. Laks S, Macari M, Bini EJ. Positional change in colon polyps at CT colonography. *Radiology.* 2004;231(3):761-766.
24. Macari M, Berman P, Dicker M, et al. Usefulness of CT colonography in patients with incomplete colonoscopy. *AJR Am J Roentgenol.* 1999;173(3):561-564.
25. Morrin MM, Kruskal JB, Farrell RJ, et al. Endoluminal CT colonography after an incomplete endoscopic colonoscopy. *AJR Am J Roentgenol.* 1999;172(4):913-918.
26. Fenlon HM, McAneny DB, Nunes DP, et al. Occlusive colon carcinoma: virtual colonoscopy in the preoperative evaluation of the proximal colon. *Radiology.* 1999;210(2):423-428.
27. O'Malley ME, Wilson SR. US of gastrointestinal tract abnormalities with CT correlation. *Radiographics.* 2003;23(1):59-72.
28. Puylaert JB. Ultrasound of acute GI tract conditions. *Eur Radiol.* 2001;11(10):1867-1877.
29. Fleischer AC, Muhletaler CA, James AE Jr. Sonographic assessment of the bowel wall. *AJR Am J Roentgenol.* 1981;136(5):887-891.
30. Ledermann HP, Borner N, Strunk H, et al. Bowel wall thickening on transabdominal sonography. *AJR Am J Roentgenol.* 2000;174(1):107-117.

31. Leyendecker JR, Bloomfeld RS, DiSantis DJ, et al. MR enterography in the management of patients with Crohn disease. *Radiographics.* 2009;29(6):1827-1846.
32. Masselli G, Casciani E, Polettini E, et al. Comparison of MR enteroclysis with MR enterography and conventional enteroclysis in patients with Crohn's disease. *Eur Radiol.* 2008;18(3):438-447.
33. Rieber A, Wruk D, Potthast S, et al. Diagnostic imaging in Crohn's disease: comparison of magnetic resonance imaging and conventional imaging methods. *Int J Colorectal Dis.* 2000;15(3):176-181.
34. Siddiki HA, Fidler JL, Fletcher JG, et al. Prospective comparison of state-of-the-art MR enterography and CT enterography in small-bowel Crohn's disease. *AJR Am J Roentgenol.* 2009;193(1):113-121.
35. Lee SS, Kim AY, Yang SK, et al. Crohn disease of the small bowel: comparison of CT enterography, MR enterography, and small-bowel follow-through as diagnostic techniques. *Radiology.* 2009;251(3):751-761.
36. Low RN, Francis IR, Politoske D, et al. Crohn's disease evaluation: comparison of contrast-enhanced MR imaging and single-phase helical CT scanning. *J Magn Reson Imaging.* 2000;11(2):127-135.
37. Schmidt S, Lepori D, Meuwly JY, et al. Prospective comparison of MR enteroclysis with multidetector spiral-CT enteroclysis: interobserver agreement and sensitivity by means of "sign-by-sign" correlation. *Eur Radiol.* 2003;13(6):1303-1311.
38. Negaard A, Paulsen V, Sandvik L, et al. A prospective randomized comparison between two MRI studies of the small bowel in Crohn's disease, the oral contrast method and MR enteroclysis. *Eur Radiol.* 2007;17(9):2294-2301.
39. Schreyer AG, Geissler A, Albrich H, et al. Abdominal MRI after enteroclysis or with oral contrast in patients with suspected or proven Crohn's disease. *Clin Gastroenterol Hepatol.* 2004;2(6): 491-497.
40. Horton KM, Fishman EK. Current role of CT in imaging of the stomach. *Radiographics.* 2003;23(1):75-87.
41. Rossi M, Broglia L, Maccioni F, et al. Hydro-CT in patients with gastric cancer: preoperative radiologic staging. *Eur Radiol.* 1997;7(5):659-664.
42. Hori S, Tsuda K, Murayama S, et al. CT of gastric carcinoma: preliminary results with a new scanning technique. *Radiographics.* 1992;12(2):257-268.
43. Baert AL, Roex L, Wilms G, et al. Computed tomography of the stomach with water as an oral contrast agent: technique and preliminary results. *J Comput Assist Tomogr.* 1989;13(4): 633-636.
44. Hundt W, Braunschweig R, Reiser M. Assessment of gastric cancer: value of breathhold technique and two-phase spiral CT. *Eur Radiol.* 1999;9(1):68-72.
45. Ming SC. The classification and significance of gastric polyps. *Monogr Pathol.* 1977(18):149-175.
46. Abraham SC, Singh VK, Yardley JH, et al. Hyperplastic polyps of the stomach: associations with histologic patterns of gastritis and gastric atrophy. *Am J Surg Pathol.* 2001;25(4):500-507.
47. Abraham SC, Singh VK, Yardley JH, et al. Hyperplastic polyps of the stomach associations with histologic patterns of gastritis and gastric atrophy. *Am J Clin Pathol.* 2001;115(2):224-234.
48. Tomosulo J. Gastric polyps: Histologic types and their relationship to gastric carcinoma. *Cancer.* 1971;27:1346-1355.
49. Ming SC, Goldman H. Gastric polyps; a histogenetic classification and its relation to carcinoma. *Cancer.* 1965; 18:721-726.
50. Ming SC. The adenoma-carcinoma sequence in the stomach and colon: II. Malignant potential of gastric polyps. *Gastrointest Radiol.* 1976;1:121-125.
51. Joffe N, Antonioli D. Atypical appearances of benign hyperplastic polyps. *AJR.* 1978;131:147-152.
52. Smith HJ, Lee EL. Large hyperplastic polyps of the stomach. *Gastrointest Radiol.* 1983;8:19-23.
53. Burt RW. Gastric fundic gland polyps. *Gastroenterology.* 2003;125:1462-1469.
54. Tsuchigame T, Saito R, Ogata Y, et al. Clinical evaluation of gastric fundic gland polyps without familial polyposis coli. *Abdom Imaging.* 1995;20:101-105.
55. Iida M, Yao T, Itoh H, et al. Natural history of fundic gland polyposis in patients with familial adenomatosis coli/Gardner's syndrome. *Gastroenterology.* 1985;89:1021-1025.
56. Iida M, Yao T, Watanabe J, et al. Fundi gland polyposis in patients without familial adenomatosis coli: Its incidence and clinical features. *Gastroenterology.* 1984;86:1437-1442.
57. Watanabe H, Enjoji M, Yao T, et al. Gastric lesions in familial adenomatosis coli. *Hum Pathol.* 1978;9:269-283.
58. Nishiura M, Hirota T, Itabashi M, et al. A clinical and histopathological study of gastric polyps in familial polyposis coli. *Am J Gastroenterol.* 1984;79(2):98-103.
59. Buck J, Harned RK, Lichtenstein JE, et al. Peutz-Jeghers syndrome. *Radiographics.* 1992;12:365-378.
60. Manfredi M. Hereditary hamartomatous polyposis syndromes understanding the disease risks as children reach adulthood. *Gastroenterol Hepatol (NY).* 2010;6(3):185-196.
61. Moore JR. Gastric carcinoma: 30-year review. *Can J Surg.* 1986;29(1):25-28.
62. Parkin DM, Bray F, Ferlay J, et al. Global cancer statistics, 2002. *CA Cancer J Clin.* 2005;55(2):74-108.
63. Ba-Ssalamah A, Prokop M, Uffmann M, Pokieser P, Teleky B, Lechner G. Dedicated multidetector CT of the stomach: spectrum of diseases. *Radiographics.* 2003;23(3):625-644.
64. Watanabe H, Bass J, Sobin L. Histological Typing of Esophageal and Gastric Tumors. 2nd Ed. 1990, Berlin: Springer-Verlag.
65. Balthazar EJ, Rosenberg H, Davidian MM. Scirrhous carcinoma of the pyloric channel and distal antrum. *AJR Am J Roentgenol.* 1980;134(4):669-673.
66. Levine MS, Kong V, Rubesin SE, et al. Scirrhous carcinoma of the stomach: radiologic and endoscopic diagnosis. *Radiology.* 1990;175(1):151-154.
67. Hisamichi S. Screening for gastric cancer. *World J Surg.* 1989;13:31-37.
68. Dicken BJ, Bigam DL, Cass C, et al. Gastric adenocarcinoma: review and considerations for future directions. *Ann Surg.* 2005;241(1):27-39.
69. Oiso T. Incidence of stomach cancer and its relation to dietary habits and nutrition in Japan between 1900 and 1975. *Cancer Res.* 1975;35(11 Pt. 2):3254-3258.
70. Fukuya T, Honda H, Hayashi T, et al. Lymph-node metastases: efficacy for detection with helical CT in patients with gastric cancer. *Radiology.* 1995;197(3):705-711.

71. Montesi A, Graziani L, Pesaresi A, et al. Radiologic diagnosis of early gastric cancer by routine double-contrast examination. *Gastrointest Radiol.* 1982;7(3):205-215.
72. Gold RP, Green PH, O'Toole KM, et al. Early gastric cancer: radiographic experience. *Radiology.* 1984;152(2):283-290.
73. Laufer I, Lavine MS. *Double Contrast Gastrointestinal Radiology.* 2nd ed. Philadelphia, PA: Saunders; 1992:xii, 701.
74. Levine MS, Igor L. Stomach. In: *Double Contrast Gastrointestinal Radiology.* Philadelphia: W.B. Saunders; 2000:213-225.
75. Maruyama M, Baba Y. Diagnosis of the invasive depth of gastric cancer. *Abdom Imaging.* 1994;19(6):532-536.
76. Hustinx R. PET imaging in assessing gastrointestinal tumors. *Radiol Clin North Am.* 2004;42(6):1123-1139, ix.
77. Stahl A, Ott K, Weber WA, et al. FDG PET imaging of locally advanced gastric carcinomas: correlation with endoscopic and histopathological findings. *Eur J Nucl Med Mol Imaging.* 2003;30(2):288-295.
78. Ott K, Fink U, Becker K, et al. Prediction of response to preoperative chemotherapy in gastric carcinoma by metabolic imaging: results of a prospective trial. *J Clin Oncol.* 2003;21(24):4604-4610.
79. Mochiki E, Kuwano H, Katoh H, et al. Evaluation of 18F-2-deoxy-2-fluoro-D-glucose positron emission tomography for gastric cancer. *World J Surg.* 2004;28(3):247-253.
80. Yoshioka T, Yamaguchi K, Kubota K, et al. Evaluation of 18F-FDG PET in patients with advanced, metastatic, or recurrent gastric cancer. *J Nucl Med.* 2003;44(5):690-699.
81. Turlakow A, Yeung HW, Salmon AS, et al. Peritoneal carcinomatosis: role of (18)F-FDG PET. *J Nucl Med.* 2003;44(9):1407-1412.
82. Aaltonen LA, Hamilton Stanley R, World Health Organization, et al. Pathology and genetics of tumours of the digestive system. World Health Organization classification of tumours., Lyon, Oxford: IARC Press; Oxford University Press; 2000 (distributor. 314 p.)
83. Capella C, Solcia E, Sobin LH, et al. Endocrine tumours of the stomach. In: Hamilton SR, Aaltonen LA, eds. *World Health Organization Classification of Tumours: Pathology and Genetics of Tumours of the Digestive System.* IARC: Lyon, France; 2000:53-57.
84. Modlin I, Sandor A, Tang LH, et al. A 40-year analysis of 265 gastric carcinoids. *Am J Gastroenterol.* 1997;92:633-638.
85. Levy AD, Sobin LH. From the archives of the AFIP: Gastrointestinal carcinoids: imaging features with clinicopathologic comparison. *Radiographics.* 2007; 27(1):237-257.
86. Binstock AJ, Johnson CD, Stephens DH, et al. Carcinoid tumors of the stomach: a clinical and radiographic study. *AJR.* 2001;176:947-951.
87. Rindi G, Luinetti O, Cornaggia M, et al. Three subtypes of gastric argyrophil carcinoid and the gastric neuroendocrine carcinoma: a clinicopathologic study. *Gastroenterology.* 1993; 104:994-1006.
88. Rindi G, Bordi C, Rappel S, et al. Gastric carcinoids and neuroendocrinecarcinomas: pathogenesis, pathology, and behavior. *World J Surg.* 1996;20:168-172.
89. Balthazar EJ, Megibow A, Bryk D. Gastric carcinoid tumors: radiographic features in eight cases. *AJR.* 1997;139:1123-1127.
90. Berger MW, Stephens DH. Gastric carcinoid tumors associated with chronic hypergastrinemia in a patient with Zollinger-Ellison syndrome. *Radiology.* 1996;201:371-373.
91. Gossios K, Katsimbri P, Tsianos E. CT features of gastric lymphoma. *Eur Radiol.* 2000;10(3):425-430.
92. Yoo CC, Levine MS, Furth EE, et al. Gastric mucosa-associated lymphoid tissue lymphoma: radiographic findings in six patients. *Radiology.* 1998;208(1):239-243.
93. Ghai S, Pattison J, O'Malley ME, et al. Primary gastrointestinal lymphoma: spectrum of imaging findings with pathologic correlation. *Radiographics.* 2007;27(5):1371-1388.
94. Smith C, Kubicka RA, Thomas CR Jr. Non-Hodgkin lymphoma of the gastrointestinal tract. *Radiographics.* 1992;12(5):887-899.
95. Levine AM, Meyer PR, Begandy MK, et al. Development of B-cell lymphoma in homosexual men. Clinical and immunologic findings. *Ann Intern Med.* 1984;100(1):7-13.
96. Mengoli M, Marchi M, Rota E, et al. Primary non-Hodgkin's lymphoma of the esophagus. *Am J Gastroenterol.* 1990;85(6): 737-741.
97. Araki K, Ogata T, Kobayashi M, et al. A morphological study on the histogenesis of human colorectal hyperplastic polyps. *Gastroenterology.* 1995;109:1468-1474.
98. Craig O, Gregson R. Primary lymphoma of the gastrointestinal tract. *Clin Radiol.* 1981;32(1):63-72.
99. Menuck LS. Gastric lymphoma, a radiologic diagnosis. *Gastrointest Radiol.* 1976;1(2):157-161.
100. ReMine SG, Braasch JW. Gastric and small bowel lymphoma. *Surg Clin North Am.* 1986;66(4):713-722.
101. Levine MS, Pantongrag-Brown L, Aguilera NS, et al. Non-Hodgkin lymphoma of the stomach: a cause of linitis plastica. *Radiology.* 1996;201(2):375-378.
102. Buy JN, Moss AA. Computed tomography of gastric lymphoma. *AJR Am J Roentgenol.* 1982;138(5):859-865.
103. Miller FH,Kochman ML, Talamonti MS, et al. Gastric cancer. Radiologic staging. *Radiol Clin North Am.* 1997;35(2):331-349.
104. Ciftci AO, Tanyel FC, Kotiloğlu E, Hiçsönmez A. Gastric lymphoma causing gastric outlet obstruction. *J Pediatr Surg.* 1996;31(10):1424-1426.
105. Miettinen M, Lasota J. Gastrointestinal stromal tumors—definition, clinical, histological, immunohistochemical, and molecular genetic features and differential diagnosis. *Virchows Arch.* 2001;438(1):1-12.
106. Miettinen M, Sarlomo-Rikala M, Sobin LH, et al. Gastrointestinal stromal tumors and leiomyosarcomas in the colon: a clinicopathologic, immunohistochemical, and molecular genetic study of 44 cases. *Am J Surg Pathol.* 2000;24(10):1339-1352.
107. Suster S. Gastrointestinal stromal tumors. *Semin Diagn Pathol.* 1996;13(4):297-313.
108. Nauert TC, Zornoza J, Ordonez N. Gastric leiomyosarcoma. *AJR Am J Roentgenol.* 1982;139(2):291-297.
109. Pannu HK, Hruban RH, Fishman EK. CT of gastric leiomyosarcoma: patterns of involvement. *AJR Am J Roentgenol.* 1999;173(2):369-373.
110. Libshitz HI, Lindell MM, Dodd GD. Metastases to the hollow viscera. *Radiol Clin North Am.* 1982;20(3):487-499.
111. Dunnick NR, Harell GS, Parker BR. Multiple "bull's-eye" lesions in gastric lymphoma. *AJR Am J Roentgenol.* 1976;126(5):965-969.
112. Goldstein HM, Beydoun MT, Dodd GD. Radiologic spectrum of melanoma metastatic to the gastrointestinal tract. *AJR Am J Roentgenol.* 1977;129(4):605-612.

113. Rose HS, Balthazar EJ, Megibow AJ, et al. Alimentary tract involvement in Kaposi sarcoma: radiographic and endoscopic findings in 25 homosexual men. *AJR Am J Roentgenol.* 1982;139(4):661-666.
114. McLeod AJ, Zornoza J, Shirkhoda A. Leiomyosarcoma: computed tomographic findings. *Radiology.* 1984;152(1):133-136.
115. Sharp RM, Ansel HJ, Keel SB. Best cases from the AFIP: gastrointestinal stromal tumor. Armed Forces Institute of Pathology. *Radiographics.* 2001;21(6):1557-1560.
116. Scatarige JC, Fishman EK, Jones B, et al. Gastric leiomyosarcoma: CT observations. *J Comput Assist Tomogr.* 1985;9(2):320-327.
117. Hasegawa S, Semelka RC, Noone TC, et al. Gastric stromal sarcomas: correlation of MR imaging and histopathologic findings in nine patients. *Radiology.* 1998;208(3):591-595.
118. Rose H, Balthazar EJ, Megibow AJ, et al. Alimentary tract involvement in Kaposi sarcoma: Radiographic and endoscopic findings in 25 homosexual men. *AJR.* 1982;139:661-666.
119. Friedman SL. Gastrointestinal and hepatobiliary neoplasms in AIDS. *Gastroenterol Clin North Am.* 1988;17:465-486.
120. Saltz R, Kurtz RC, Lightdale CJ, et al. Kaposi's sarcoma: Gastrointestinal involvement correlation with skin findings and immunologic function. *Dig Dis Sci.* 1984;29:817-823.
121. Wall SD, Friendman SL, Margulis AR. Gastrointestinal Kaposi's sarcoma in AIDS: Radiographic manifestations. *J Clin Gastroenterol.* 1984;6:165-171.
122. Hadjiyane C, Lee YH, Stein L, et al. Kaposi's sarcoma presenting as linitis plastica. *Am J Gastroenterol.* 1991;86:1823-1825.
123. Thompson WM. Imaging and findings of lipomas of the gastrointestinal tract. *AJR Am J Roentgenol.* 2005;184(4):1163-1171.
124. Taylor AJ, Stewart ET, Dodds WJ. Gastrointestinal lipomas: a radiologic and pathologic review. *AJR Am J Roentgenol.* 1990;155(6):1205-1210.
125. Agha FP, Dent TL, Fiddian-Green RG, et al. Bleeding lipomas of the upper gastrointestinal tract. A diagnostic challenge. *Am Surg.* 1985;51(5):279-285.
126. Menuck L, Amberg J. Metastatic disease involving the stomach. *Am J Dig Dis.* 1975;20:903-913.
127. Klein M, Sherlock P. Gastric and colonic metastases from breast carcinoma. *Am J Dig Dis.* 1972;17:881-886.
128. Das Gupta TK, Brasfield RD. Metastatic melanoma of the gastrointestinal tract. *Arch Surg.* 1964;88:969-973.
129. Meyers M, McSweeney J. Secondary neoplasms of the bowel. *Radiology.* 1972;105:1-11.
130. Goldstein HM, Beydonn MT, Dodd GD. Radiologic spectrum of metastatic melanoma to the gastrointestinal tract. *AJR.* 1977;129:605-612.
131. Lipshutz H, Lindell M, Dodd G. Metastases to the hollow viscera. *Radiol Clin North Am.* 1982;20:487-499.
132. Caskey CI, Scatarige JC, Fishman EK. Distribution of metastases in breast carcinoma: CT evaluation of the abdomen. *Clin Imaging.* 1991;15:166-171.
133. Taal BG, Peterse H, Boot H. Clinical presentation, endoscopic features, and treatment of gastric metastases from breast carcinoma. *Cancer.* 2000;89:2214-2221.
134. Furth EE, Rubesin SE, Levine MS. Pathologic primer on gastritis: an illustrated sum and substance. *Radiology.* 1995;197(3):693-698.
135. Lanza F, Royer G, Nelson R. An endoscopic evaluation of the effects of non-steroidal anti-inflammatory drugs on the gastric mucosa. *Gastrointest Endosc.* 1975;21(3):103-105.
136. Laufer I, Trueman T. Multiple superficial gastric erosions due to Crohn's disease of the stomach. Radiologic and endoscopic diagnosis. *Br J Radiol.* 1976;49(584):726-728.
137. Ariyama J, Wehlin L, Lindstrom CG, et al. Gastroduodenal erosions in Crohn's disease. *Gastrointest Radiol.* 1980;5(2):121-125.
138. Cronan J, Burrell M, Trepeta R. Aphthoid ulcerations in gastric candidiasis. *Radiology.* 1980;134(3):607-611.
139. McLean AM, Paul RE Jr, Philipps E, et al. Chronic erosive gastritis—clinical and radiological features. *J Can Assoc Radiol.* 1982;33(3):158-162.
140. Dooley CP, Cohen H, Fitzgibbons PL, et al. Prevalence of Helicobacter pylori infection and histologic gastritis in asymptomatic persons. *N Engl J Med.* 1989;321(23):1562-1566.
141. Levine MS, Rubesin SE. The Helicobacter pylori revolution: radiologic perspective. *Radiology.* 1995;195(3):593-596.
142. Graham DY, Lew GM, Klein PD, et al. Effect of treatment of Helicobacter pylori infection on the long-term recurrence of gastric or duodenal ulcer. A randomized, controlled study. *Ann Intern Med.* 1992;116(9):705-708.
143. NIH Consensus Conference. Helicobacter pylori in peptic ulcer disease. NIH Consensus Development Panel on Helicobacter pylori in Peptic Ulcer Disease. *JAMA.* 1994;272(1):65-69.
144. Poplack, Paul RE, Goldsmith M, Matsue H, Moore JP, Norton R. Demonstration of erosive gastritis by the double-contrast technique. *Radiology.* 1975;117(3 Pt 1):519-521.
145. Laufer I. Assessment of the accuracy of double contrast gastroduodenal radiology. *Gastroenterology.* 1976;71(5):874-878.
146. Den Orth JO, Dekker W. Gastric erosions: radiological and endoscopic aspects. *Radiol Clin (Basel).* 1976;45(2-4):88-99.
147. Tragardh B, Wehlin L, Ohashi K. Radiologic appearance of complete gastric erosions. *Acta Radiol Diagn (Stockh).* 1978;19(4):634-642.
148. Catalano D, Pagliari U. Gastroduodenal erosions: radiological findings. *Gastrointest Radiol.* 1982;7(3):235-240.
149. Laufer I, Hamilton J, Mullens JE. Demonstration of superficial gastric erosions by double contrast radiography. *Gastroenterology.* 1975;68(2):387-391.
150. Levine MS, Verstandig A, Laufer I. Serpiginous gastric erosions caused by aspirin and other nonsteroidal antiinflammatory drugs. *AJR Am J Roentgenol.* 1986;146(1):31-34.
151. Laveran-Stieber RL, Laufer I, Levine MS. Greater curvature antral flattening: a radiologic sign of NSAID-related gastropathy. *Abdom Imaging.* 1994;19(4):295-297.
152. Levine MS, Creteur V, Kressel HY, Laufer I, Herlinger H. Benign gastric ulcers: diagnosis and follow-up with double-contrast radiography. *Radiology.* 1987;164(1):9-13.
153. Sun DC, Stempien SJ. The Veterans Administration Cooperative Study on Gastric Ulcer. 3. Site and size of the ulcer as determinants of outcome. *Gastroenterology.* 1971;61(4):(suppl 2):576-584.
154. Thompson G, Somers S, Stevenson GW. Benign gastric ulcer: a reliable radiologic diagnosis? *AJR Am J Roentgenol.* 1983;141(2):331-333.

155. Gelfand DW, Dale WJ, Ott DJ. The location and size of gastric ulcers: radiologic and endoscopic evaluation. *AJR Am J Roentgenol.* 1984;143(4):755-758.
156. Amberg JR, Zboralske FF. Gastric ulcers after 70. *Am J Roentgenol Radium Ther Nucl Med.* 1966;96(2):393-399.
157. Sheppard MC, Holmes GK, Cockel R. Clinical picture of peptic ulceration diagnosed endoscopically. *Gut.* 1977;18(7): 524-530.
158. Kikuchi Y, Levine MS, Laufer I, et al. Value of flow technique for double-contrast examination of the stomach. *AJR Am J Roentgenol.* 1986;147(6):1183-1184.
159. Urban BA, Fishman EK, Hruban RH. Helicobacter pylori gastritis mimicking gastric carcinoma at CT evaluation. *Radiology.* 1991;179(3):689-691.
160. Jacobs JM, Hill MC, Steinberg WM. Peptic ulcer disease: CT evaluation. *Radiology.* 1991;178(3):745-748.
161. Wagtmans M, Verspaget HW, Lamers CB, et al. Clinical aspects of Crohn's disease of the upper gastrointestinal tract: A comparison with distal Crohn's disease. *Am J Gastroenterol.* 1997;92:1467-1470.
162. Marshak RH, Maklansky D, Kurzban JD, et al. Crohn's disease of the stomach and duodenum. *Am J Gastroenterol.* 1982;77:340-343.
163. Levine MS. Crohn's disease of the upper gastrointestinal tract. *Radiol Clin North Am.* 1987;25(1):79-91.
164. Nelson SW. The discovery of gastric ulcers and the differential diagnosis between benignancy and malignancy. *Radiol Clin North Am.* 1969;7(1):5-25.
165. Levine MS. Erosive gastritis and gastric ulcers. *Radiol Clin North Am.* 1994;32(6):1203-1214.
166. Meeroff M, Gollan JRM, Meeroff JC. Gastric diverticulum. *Am J Gastroenterol.* 1967;47:89-203.
167. Martin L. Diverticula of the stomach. *Ann Intern Med.* 1936;10:447-465.
168. Schwartz AN, Goiney RC, Graney DO. Gastric diverticulum simulating an adrenal mass: CT appearance and embryogenesis. *AJR Am J Roentgenol.* 1986;146:553-554.
169. Harford W, Jeyarajah R. Diverticula of the pharynx, esophagus, stomach, and small intestine. In: Feldman M, Friedman L, Brandt LJ, eds. *Sleisenger & Fordtran's gastrointestinal and liver disease.* Philadelphia, PA: Saunders. 2006;465-477.
170. Akerlund A. Diverticula of the stomach from a roentgenological point of view. *Acta Radiol (Stockh).* 1923;2:476-485.
171. Chen C, Jaw YS, Wu DC, et al. MDCT of giant gastric folds: differential diagnosis. *AJR Am J Roentgenol.* 2010;195(5): 1124-1130.
172. Lauren P. The two histological main types of gastric carcinoma: Diffuse and so-called intestinal-typecarcinoma. *Acta Pathol Microbiol Scand.* 1965;64:31-49.
173. Raskin M. Some specific radiological findings and consideration of linitis plastica of the gastrointestinal tract. *CRC Crit Rev Clin Radiol Nucl Med.* 1976;8(1):87-106.
174. Sohn J, Levine MS, Furth EE, et al. Helicobacter pylori gastritis: radiographic findings. *Radiology.* 1995;195(3):763-767.
175. Fishman EK, Urban BA, Hruban RH. CT of the stomach: spectrum of disease. *Radiographics.* 1996;16(5):1035-1054.
176. Jensen RT. Gastrinomas: Advances in Diagnosis and Management. *Neuroendocrinology.* 2004;80(suppl 1):23-27.
177. DeVita VT, Hellman S, Rosenberg SA. *Cancer, principles & practice of oncology.* Philadelphia, PA: Lippincott Williams & Wilkins; 2005:1788-1813.
178. Wolfe MM, Jensen RT. Zollinger-Ellison syndrome: Current concepts in diagnosis and management. *N Engl J Med.* 1987;317:1200-1209.
179. Amberg J, Ellison EH, Wilson SD, et al. Roentgenographic observations in the Zollinger-Ellison syndrome. *JAMA.* 1964;190:185-187.
180. Missakian MM, Carlson HC, Huzenga KA. Roentgenographic findings in Zollinger-Ellison syndrome. *AJR.* 1965;94:429-437.
181. Nelson S, Christoforidis A. Roentgenologic features of the Zollinger-Ellison syndrome: Ulcerogenic tumor of the pancreas. *Semin Roentgenol.* 1968;3:254-266.
182. Akerstrom G, Hellman P. Surgery on neuroendocrine tumours. *Best Pract Res Clin Endocrinol Metab.* 2007;21(1): 87-109.
183. Rockall AG, Reznek RH. Imaging of neuroendocrine tumours (CT/MR/US). *Best Pract Res Clin Endocrinol Metab.* 2007;21(1):43-68.
184. Wank SA, Doppman JL, Miller D, et al. Prospective study of the ability of computed axial tomography to localize gastrinomas in patients with Zollinger-Ellison syndrome. *Gastroenterology.* 1987;92(4):905-912.
185. Balci NC, Semelka RC. Radiologic features of cystic, endocrine and other pancreatic neoplasms. *Eur J Radiol.* 2001;38(2): 113-119.
186. Doppman JL. The localization and treatment of parathyroid adenomas by angiographic techniques. *Ann Radiol (Paris).* 1980;23(4):253-258.
187. Ichikawa T, Peterson MS, Federle MP, et al. Islet cell tumor of the pancreas: biphasic CT versus MR imaging in tumor detection. *Radiology.* 2000;216(1):163-171.
188. Owen NJ, Sohaib SA, Peppercorn PD, et al. MRI of pancreatic neuroendocrine tumours. *Br J Radiol.* 2001;74(886):968-973.
189. Semelka RC, Custodio CM, Cem Balci N, Woosley JT. Neuroendocrine tumors of the pancreas: spectrum of appearances on MRI. *J Magn Reson Imaging.* 2000;11(2): 141-148.
190. Coffey RJ, Washington MK, Corless CL, Heinrich MC. Ménétrier disease and gastrointestinal stromal tumors: hyperproliferative disorders of the stomach. *J Clin Invest.* 2007;117(1):70-80.
191. Wolfsen H, Carpenter H, Talley N. Ménétrier's disease: A form of hypertrophic gastropathy or gastritis? *Gastroenterology.* 19093;104:1310-1319.
192. Occena R, Taylor SF, Robinson CC, et al. *J Pediatr Gastroenterol Nutr.* 1993;17(2):217-224.
193. Reese D, Hodgson J, Dockerty M. Giant hypertrophy of the gastric mucosa (Ménétrier's disease): A correlation of the roentgenographic, pathologic, and clinical findings. *AJR.* 1962;88:619-626.
194. Olmsted W, Cooper P, Madewell J. Involvement of the gastric antrum in Ménétrier's disease. *AJR.* 1976;126:524-529.
195. Duprey K, Ahmed S, Mishriki Y. Ménétrier disease in an acquired immunodeficiency syndrome patient. *South Med J.* 2010;103(1):93-95.
196. Wilkerson M, Meschter S, Brown R. Menetrier's disease presenting with iron deficiency anemia. *Ann Clin Lab Sci.* 1998;28(1):14-18.

197. Klein N, Hargrove R, Sleisenger M, et al. "Eosinophilic gastroenteritis". *Medicine (Baltimore)*. 1970;49(4):299-319.
198. Naylor A. *"Eosinophilic gastroenteritis"*. Eosinophilic gastroenteritis. *Scott Med J*. 1990;35(6):163-165.
199. Baig M, Qadir A, Rasheed J. A review of eosinophilic gastroenteritis. *J Natl Med Assoc*. 2006;98(10):1616-1619.
200. Goldberg H, O'Kieffe D, Jenis EH, et al. Diffuse eosinophilic gastroenteritis. *AJR*. 1973;119:342-351.
201. Wehunt WD, Lewis BS, Frankel A, et al. Eosinophilic gastritis. *Radiology*. 1976;120:85-89.
202. Sheikh RA, Baba AA, Ahmad SM, et al. Unusual presentations of eosinophilic gastroenteritis: Case series and review of literature. *World J Gastroenterol*. 2009;15(17):2156-2161.
203. Tursi A, Rella G, Inchingolo CD, et al. Gastric outlet obstruction due to gastroduodenal eosinophilic gastroenteritis. *Endoscopy*. 2007;39(suppl 1):E184.
204. Rosai J. *Ackerman's Surgical Pathology*. Vol. 2. 8th ed. St. Louis: Mosby; 1996: (xiv, 2732. 50 p.).
205. DiSario JA, Burt RW, Vargas H, et al. Small bowel cancer: epidemiological and clinical characteristics from a population-based registry. *Am J Gastroenterol*. 1994;89(5):699-701.
206. Rosai J. *Gastrointestinal tract. In:* Rosai J. ed. *Ackerman's Surgical Pathology*. St. Louis, MO: Mosby-Year Book: 1995.
207. Herbsman H, Wetstein L, Rosen Y, et al. Tumors of the small intestine. *Curr Probl Surg*. 1980;17(3):121-182.
208. Gore RM. Small bowel cancer. Clinical and pathologic features. *Radiol Clin North Am*. 1997;35(2):351-360.
209. Maglinte DD, O'Connor K, Bessette J, et al. The role of the physician in the late diagnosis of primary malignant tumors of the small intestine. *Am J Gastroenterol*. 1991;86(3):304-308.
210. Dudiak KM, Johnson CD, Stephens DH. Primary tumors of the small intestine: CT evaluation. *AJR Am J Roentgenol*. 1989;152(5):995-998.
211. Lai EC, Doty JE, Irving C, Tompkins RK. Primary adenocarcinoma of the duodenum: analysis of survival. *World J Surg*. 1988;12(5):695-699.
212. Laurent F, Raynaud M, Biset JM, et al. Diagnosis and categorization of small bowel neoplasms: role of computed tomography. *Gastrointest Radiol*. 1991;16(2):115-119.
213. Buckley JA, Fishman EK. CT evaluation of small bowel neoplasms: spectrum of disease. *Radiographics*. 1998;18(2): 379-392.
214. Maglinte DD, Gage SN, Harmon BH, et al. Obstruction of the small intestine: accuracy and role of CT in diagnosis. *Radiology*. 1993;188(1):61-64.
215. Kazerooni EA, Quint LE, Francis IR. Duodenal neoplasms: predictive value of CT for determining malignancy and tumor resectability. *AJR Am J Roentgenol*. 1992;159(2):303-309.
216. Merine D, Fishman EK, Jones B. CT of the small bowel and mesentery. *Radiol Clin North Am*. 1989;27(4):707-715.
217. Modlin IM, Lye KD, Kidd M. A 5-decade analysis of 13,715 carcinoid tumors. *Cancer*. 2003;97(4):934-959.
218. Sweeney JF, Rosemurgy AS. Carcinoid Tumors of the Gut. *Cancer Control*. 1997;4(1):18-24.
219. Capella C, Solcia E, Sobin LH, et al. Endocrine tumours of the small intestine, in World Health Organization classification of tumours: pathology and genetics of tumours of the digestive system, Hamilton SR, Aaltonen LA, Editors. IARC: Lyon, France. 2000;77-82.
220. Pantongrag-Brown L, Buetow PC, Carr NJ, et al. Calcification and fibrosis in mesenteric carcinoid tumor: CT findings and pathologic correlation. *AJR Am J Roentgenol*. 1995;164(2): 387-391.
221. Herlinger H, Maglinte DDT, Birnbaum BA. *Clinical Imaging of the Small Intestine*. 2nd ed. New York: Springer; 1999:xvi, 576.
222. Horton KM, Kamel I, Hofmann L, et al. Carcinoid tumors of the small bowel: a multitechnique imaging approach. *AJR Am J Roentgenol*. 2004;182(3):559-567.
223. Bader TR, Semelka RC, Chiu VC, et al. MRI of carcinoid tumors: spectrum of appearances in the gastrointestinal tract and liver. *J Magn Reson Imaging*. 2001;14(3):261-269.
224. Scarsbrook AF, Ganeshan A, Statham J, et al. Anatomic and functional imaging of metastatic carcinoid tumors. *Radiographics*. 2007;27(2):455-477.
225. Quan GM, Pitman A, Slavin J, et al. Soft tissue metastasis of carcinoid tumour: a rare manifestation. *ANZ J Surg*. 2004;74(3):164-166.
226. Isidori AM, Kaltsas G, Frajese V, et al. Ocular metastases secondary to carcinoid tumors: the utility of imaging with [(123)I]meta-iodobenzylguanidine and [(111)In]DTPA pentetreotide. *J Clin Endocrinol Metab*. 2002;87(4):1627-1633.
227. Robboy SJ, Scully RE, Norris HJ. Carcinoid metastatic to the ovary. A clinocopathologic analysis of 35 cases. *Cancer*. 1974;33(3):798-811.
228. Pelage JP, Soyer P, Boudiaf M, et al. Carcinoid tumors of the abdomen: CT features. *Abdom Imaging*. 1999;24(3):240-245.
229. Levine MS, Rubesin SE, Pantongrag-Brown L, et al. Non-Hodgkin's lymphoma of the gastrointestinal tract: radiographic findings. *AJR Am J Roentgenol*. 1997;168(1):165-172.
230. Koh PK, Horsman JM, Radstone CR, et al. Localised extranodal non-Hodgkin's lymphoma of the gastrointestinal tract: Sheffield Lymphoma Group experience (1989-1998). *Int J Oncol*. 2001;18(4):743-748.
231. Macari M, Balthazar EJ. CT of bowel wall thickening: significance and pitfalls of interpretation. *AJR Am J Roentgenol*. 2001;176(5):1105-1116.
232. Balthazar EJ, Noordhoorn M, Megibow AJ, et al. CT of small-bowel lymphoma in immunocompetent patients and patients with AIDS: comparison of findings. *AJR Am J Roentgenol*. 1997;168(3):675-680.
233. Byun JH, Ha HK, Kim AY, et al. CT findings in peripheral T-cell lymphoma involving the gastrointestinal tract. *Radiology*. 2003;227(1):59-67.
234. Shojaku H, Futatsuya R, Seto H, et al. Malignant gastrointestinal stromal tumor of the small intestine: radiologic-pathologic correlation. *Radiat Med*. 1997;15(3): 189-192.
235. Zua MS. Familial Adenomatous Polyposis Syndrome. *Hospital Physician*. 1999;35(5):61-68.
236. Burt RW. Inherited colorectal cancer syndrome. *American Society for Gastrointestinal Endoscopy Clinical Update*. 1998; 5:1-4.
237. Giardiello F, Welsh SB, Hamilton SR, et al. Increased risk of cancer in the Peutz. Jeghers syndrome. *N Engl J Med*. 1987;316:1151-1154.
238. Sener R, Kumcuoglu Z, Elmas N, et al. Peutz-Jeghers syndrome: CT and US demonstration ofsmall bowel polyps. *Gastrointest Radiol*. 1991;16:21-23.

239. Margulis AR, Burhenne HJ. *Practical Alimentary Tract Radiology.* St. Louis: Mosby-Year Book; 1993:xii, 512.

240. Koehler RE. Neoplasms. In: Freeny PC, Stevenson GW, eds. *Margulis and Burhenne's Alimentary Tract Radiology.* St Louis, MO: Mosby-Year Book; 1994;627-648.

241. Levine MS, Rubesin SE, Laufer I. Pattern approach for diseases of mesenteric small bowel on barium studies. *Radiology.* 2008;249(2):445-460.

242. Moss S, Calam J. Helicobacter pylori and peptic ulcers: the present position. *Gut.* 1992;33(3):289-292.

243. Rodriguez HP, Aston JK, Richardson CT. Ulcers in the descending duodenum. Postbulbar ulcers. *Am J Roentgenol Radium Ther Nucl Med.* 1973;119(2):316-322.

244. Jayaraman MV, Mayo-Smith WW, Movson JS, Dupuy DE, Wallach MT. CT of the duodenum: an overlooked segment gets its due. *Radiographics.* 2001;21 Spec No:S147-S160.

245. Cooke WT, Cox EV, Fone DJ, et al. The clinical and metabolic significance of jejunal diverticula. *Gut.* 1963;4:115-131.

246. Rossi P, Gourtsoyiannis N, Bezzi M, et al. Meckel's diverticulum: imaging diagnosis. *AJR Am J Roentgenol.* 1996;166(3):567-573.

247. Park JJ, Wolff BG, Tollefson MK, et al. Meckel diverticulum: the Mayo Clinic experience with 1476 patients (1950-2002). *Ann Surg.* 2005;241(3):529-533.

248. Matsagas MI, Fatouros M, Koulouras B, et al. Incidence, complications, and management of Meckel's diverticulum. *Arch Surg.* 1995;130(2):143-146.

249. Levy AD, Hobbs CM. From the archives of the AFIP. Meckel diverticulum: radiologic features with pathologic Correlation. *Radiographics.* 2004;24(2):565-587.

250. Bani-Hani KE, Shatnawi NJ. Meckel's diverticulum: comparison of incidental and symptomatic cases. *World J Surg.* 2004;28(9):917-920.

251. Jain TP, Sharma R, Chava SP, et al. Pre-operative diagnosis of Meckel's diverticulum: report of a case and review of literature. *Trop Gastroenterol.* 2005;26(2):99-101.

252. Craig O, Murfitt J. Radiological demonstration of Meckel's diverticulum. *Br J Surg.* 1980;67(12):881-883.

253. Hughes JA, Hatrick A, Rankin S. Computed tomography findings in an inflamed meckel diverticulum. *Br J Radiol.* 1998;71(848):882-883.

254. Mortele KJ, Govaere F, Vogelaerts D, et al. Giant Meckel's diverticulum containing enteroliths: typical CT imaging findings. *Eur Radiol.* 2002;12(1):82-84.

255. Hoff G, Foerster A, Vatn MH, et al. Epidemiology of polyps in the rectum and colon. Recovery and evaluation of unresected polyps 2 years after detection. *Scand J Gastroenterol.* 1986;21(7):853-862.

256. Arthur JF. The significance of small mucosal polyps of the rectum. *Proc R Soc Med.* 1962;55:703-705.

257. Vatn MH, Stalsberg H. The prevalence of polyps of the large intestine in Oslo: an autopsy study. *Cancer.* 1982;49: 819-825.

258. Levine MS, Rubesin SE, Laufer I, et al. Diagnosis of colorectal neoplasms at double-contrast barium enema examination. *Radiology.* 2000;216(1):11-18.

259. Williams AR, Balasooriya BA, Day DW. Polyps and cancer of the large bowel: a necropsy study in Liverpool. *Gut.* 1982;23:835-842.

260. Estrada RG, Spjut HJ. Hyperplastic polyps of the large bowel. *Am J Surg Pathol.* 1980;4:127-133.

261. Goldman H, Ming S, Hickok DF. Nature and significance of hyperplastic polyps of the human colon. *Arch Pathol.* 1970;89:349-354.

262. Ott DJ, Gelfand DW, Wu WC, Ablin DS. Colon polyp morphology on double-contrast barium enema: its pathologic predictive value. *AJR Am J Roentgenol.* 1983;141(5):965-970.

263. Gollub MJ, Schwartz LH, Akhurst T. Update on colorectal cancer imaging. *Radiol Clin North Am.* 2007;45(1):85-118.

264. Laufer IaK H. Principles of double contrast diagnosis. In: *Double Contrast Gastrointestinal Radiology.* W.B. Saunders; 2000;8-46.

265. Youker JE, Welin S. Differentiation of true polypoid tumors of the colon from extraneous material: a new Roentgen sign. *Radiology.* 1965;84:610-615.

266. Simms SM. Differential diagnosis of the bowler hat sign. *AJR Am J Roentgenol.* 1985;144(3):585-587.

267. Tobin KD, Young JW. The bowler hat: a valid sign of colonic polyps? *Gastrointest Radiol.* 1987;12(3):250-252.

268. Miller WT Jr, Levine MS, Rubesin SE, et al. Bowler-hat sign: a simple principle for differentiating polyps from diverticula. *Radiology.* 1989;173(3):615-617.

269. Bussey JHR, Veale AMO, Morson BC. Genetics of gastrointestinal polyposis. *Gastroenterology.* 1978;74:1325-1330.

270. Nandakumar G, Morgan JA, Silverberg D, Steinhagen RM. Familial polyposis coli: Clinical manifestations, evaluation, management and treatment. *Mt Sinai J Med.* 2004;71:384-391.

271. Welling DR, Beart RW. Surgical alternatives in the treatment of polyposis coli. *Semin Surg Oncol.* 1987;3:99-104.

272. Taylor SA, Halligan S, Moore L, et al. Multidetector-row CT duodenography in familial adenomatous polyposis: a pilot study. *Clin Radiol.* 2004;59(10):939-945.

273. Healy JC, Reznek RH, Clark SK, et al. MR appearances of desmoid tumors in familial adenomatous polyposis. *AJR.* 1997;169:465-472.

274. Brooks AP, Reznek RH, Nugent K, et al. CT appearances of desmoid tumours in familial adenomatous polyposis: further observations. *Clin Radiol.* 1994 49(9):601-617.

275. Howe J, Mitros F, Summers R. The risk of gastrointestinal carcinoma in familial juvenile polyposis. 1988;5(8):751-756.

276. Schreibman IR, Baker M, Amos C, et al. The hamartomatous polyposis syndromes. *A clinical and molecular review.* 2005;100: 476-490.

277. Kao KT, Patel JK, Pampati V. Cronkhite-Canada Syndrome: A Case Report and Review of Literature. *Gastroenterology Research and Practice.* 2009:1-4.

278. Horton KM, Corl FM, Fishman EK. CT evaluation of the colon: inflammatory disease. *Radiographics.* 2000;20(2):399-418.

279. Caroline DF, Friedman AC. The radiology of inflammatory bowel disease. *Med Clin North Am.* 1994;78(6):1353-1385.

280. Carucci LR, Levine MS. Radiographic imaging of inflammatory bowel disease. *Gastroenterol Clin North Am.* 2002;31(1):93-117, ix.

281. Scotiniotis I, Rubesin SE, Ginsberg GG. Imaging modalities in inflammatory bowel disease. *Gastroenterol Clin North Am.* 1999;28(2):391-421, ix.

282. Lichtenstein JE. Radiologic-pathologic correlation of inflammatory bowel disease. *Radiol Clin North Am.* 1987;25(1):3-24.

283. Use of colorectal cancer tests—United States, 2002, 2004, and 2006. *MMWR Morb Mortal Wkly Rep.* 2008;57(10):253-258.

284. Winawer SJ, Fletcher RH, Miller L, et al. Colorectal cancer screening: clinical guidelines and rationale. *Gastroenterology.* 1997;112(2):594-642.

285. Muto T, Bussey HJ, Morson BC. The evolution of cancer of the colon and rectum. *Cancer.* 1975;36(6):2251-2270.

286. Morson BC. Evolution of cancer of the colon and rectum. *Cancer.* 1974;34(3):suppl:845-849.

287. Levin B, Lieberman DA, McFarland B, et al. Screening and surveillance for the early detection of colorectal cancer and adenomatous polyps, 2008: a joint guideline from the American Cancer Society, the US Multi-Society Task Force on Colorectal Cancer, and the American College of Radiology. *CA Cancer J Clin.* 2008;58(3):130-160.

288. Kelvin FM, Maglinte DD. Colorectal carcinoma: a radiologic and clinical review. *Radiology.* 1987;164(1):1-8.

289. Fischel RE, Dermer R. Multifocal carcinoma of the large intestine. *Clin Radiol.* 1975;26(4):495-498.

290. Levine MS, Glick SN, Rubesin SE, et al. Double-contrast barium enema examination and colorectal cancer: a plea for radiologic screening. *Radiology.* 2002;222(2):313-315.

291. McCarthy PA, Rubesin SE, Levine MS, et al. Colon cancer: morphology detected with barium enema examination versus histopathologic stage. *Radiology.* 1995;197(3):683-687.

292. National Cancer Institute, DCCPS, Surveillance Research Program, Cancer Statistics Branch, released April 2008, based on the November 2007 submission.

293. Lieberman DA. Clinical practice. Screening for colorectal cancer. *N Engl J Med.* 2009;361(12):1179-1187.

294. Johns LE, Houlston RS. A systematic review and meta-analysis of familial colorectal cancer risk. *Am J Gastroenterol.* 2001;96(10):2992-3003.

295. Butterworth AS, Higgins JP, Pharoah P. Relative and absolute risk of colorectal cancer for individuals with a family history: a meta-analysis. *Eur J Cancer.* 2006;42(2):216-227.

296. Bernstein CN, Blanchard JF, Kliewer E, et al. Cancer risk in patients with inflammatory bowel disease: a population-based study. *Cancer.* 2001;91(4):854-862.

297. Pickhardt PJ, Choi JR, Hwang I, et al. Nonadenomatous polyps at CT colonography: prevalence, size distribution, and detection rates. *Radiology.* 2004;232(3):784-790.

298. Winawer SJ. Natural history of colorectal cancer. *Am J Med.* 1999;106(1A):3S-6S; discussion 50S-51S.

299. Horton KM, Abrams RA, Fishman EK. Spiral CT of colon cancer: imaging features and role in management. *Radiographics.* 2000;20(2):419-430.

300. Scott NA, Wieand HS, Moertel CG, et al. Colorectal cancer. Dukes' stage, tumor site, preoperative plasma CEA level, and patient prognosis related to tumor DNA ploidy pattern. *Arch Surg.* 1987;122(12):1375-1379.

301. Cohen AM, Minsky BD, Schilsky RL. Cancer of the colon. In: Devita VT, Hellman S, eds. *Principles and Practice of Oncology.* Philadelphia, PA: Lippincott-Raven; 1997:1177-1205.

302. August DA, Ottow RT, Sugarbaker PH. Clinical perspective of human colorectal cancer metastasis. *Cancer Metastasis Rev.* 1984;3(4):303-324.

303. Tong D, Russell AH, Dawson LE, et al. Second laparotomy for proximal colon cancer. Sites of recurrence and implications for adjuvant therapy. *Am J Surg.* 1983;145(3):382-386.

304. Willett CG, Tepper JE, Cohen AM, et al. Failure patterns following curative resection of colonic carcinoma. *Ann Surg.* 1984;200(6):685-690.

305. Easson AM, Barron PT, Cripps C, et al. Calcification in colorectal hepatic metastases correlates with longer survival. *J Surg Oncol.* 1996;63(4):221-225.

306. Kinkel K, Lu Y, Both M, et al. Detection of hepatic metastases from cancers of the gastrointestinal tract by using noninvasive imaging methods (US, CT, MR imaging, PET): a meta-analysis. *Radiology.* 2002;224(3):748-756.

307. Selzner M, Hany TF, Wildbrett P, et al. Does the novel PET/CT imaging modality impact on the treatment of patients with metastatic colorectal cancer of the liver? *Ann Surg.* 2004;240(6):1027-1034; discussion 1035-1036.

308. Rydzewski B, Dehdashti F, Gordon BA, et al. Usefulness of intraoperative sonography for revealing hepatic metastases from colorectal cancer in patients selected for surgery after undergoing FDG PET. *AJR Am J Roentgenol.* 2002;178(2):353-358.

309. de Geus-Oei LF, Vriens D, van Laarhoven HW, et al. Monitoring and predicting response to therapy with 18F-FDG PET in colorectal cancer: a systematic review. *J Nucl Med.* 2009;50(suppl 1):43S-54S.

310. Gollub MJ, Akhurst T, Markowitz AJ, et al. Combined CT colonography and 18F-FDG PET of colon polyps: potential technique for selective detection of cancer and precancerous lesions. *AJR Am J Roentgenol.* 2007;188(1):130-138.

311. Meyerhardt JA, Mayer RJ. Follow-up strategies after curative resection of colorectal cancer. *Semin Oncol.* 2003;30(3):349-360.

312. Ohlsson B, Palsson B. Follow-up after colorectal cancer surgery. *Acta Oncol.* 2003;42(8):816-826.

313. Eddy DM. Screening for colorectal cancer. *Ann Intern Med.* 1990;113(5):373-384.

314. Williams CB, Macrae FA, Bartram CI. A prospective study of diagnostic methods in adenoma follow-up. *Endoscopy.* 1982;14(3):74-78.

315. Steine S, Stordahl A, Lunde OC, Løken K, Laerum E. Double-contrast barium enema versus colonoscopy in the diagnosis of neoplastic disorders: aspects of decision-making in general practice. *Fam Pract.* 1993;10(3):288-291.

316. Pickhardt PJ. By-patient performance characteristics of CT colonography: importance of polyp size threshold data. *Radiology.* 2003;229(1):291-393; author reply 293; discussion 293.

317. Balthazar EJ, Megibow AJ, Hulnick D, Naidich DP. Carcinoma of the colon: detection and preoperative staging by CT. *AJR Am J Roentgenol.* 1988;150(2):301-306.

318. Earls JP, Colon-Negron E, Dachman AH. Colorectal carcinoma in young patients: CT detection of an atypical pattern of recurrence. *Abdom Imaging.* 1994;19(5):441-445.

319. Freeny PC, Marks WM, Ryan JA, et al. Colorectal carcinoma evaluation with CT: preoperative staging and detection of postoperative recurrence. *Radiology.* 1986;158(2):347-353.

320. Gazelle GS, Gaa J, Saini S, et al. Staging of colon carcinoma using water enema CT. *J Comput Assist Tomogr.* 1995;19(1):87-91.

321. Thompson WM, Halvorsen RA, Foster WL Jr, et al. Preoperative and postoperative CT staging of rectosigmoid carcinoma. *AJR Am J Roentgenol.* 1986;146(4):703-710.

322. Pickhardt PJ, Choi JR, Hwang I, et al. Flat colorectal lesions in asymptomatic adults: implications for screening with CT virtual colonoscopy. *AJR Am J Roentgenol.* 2004;183(5):1343-1347.

323. Sato T, Konishi F, Togashi K, et al. Prospective observation of small "flat" tumors in the colon through colonoscopy. *Dis Colon Rectum.* 1999;42(11):1457-1463.

324. Muto T, Kamiya J, Sawada T, et al. Small "flat adenoma" of the large bowel with special reference to its clinicopathologic features. *Dis Colon Rectum.* 1985;28(11):847-851.

325. Fidler J, Johnson C. Flat polyps of the colon: accuracy of detection by CT colonography and histologic significance. *Abdom Imaging.* 2009;34(2):157-171.

326. Soetikno RM, Kaltenbach T, Rouse RV, et al. Prevalence of nonpolypoid (flat and depressed) colorectal neoplasms in asymptomatic and symptomatic adults. *JAMA.* 2008;299(9):1027-1035.

327. Adachi M, Muto T, Morioka Y, Ikenaga T, Hara M. Flat adenoma and flat mucosal carcinoma (IIb type)—a new precursor of colorectal carcinoma? Report of two cases. *Dis Colon Rectum.* 1988;31(3):236-243.

328. Fidler JL, Johnson CD, MacCarty RL, et al. Detection of flat lesions in the colon with CT colonography. *Abdom Imaging.* 2002;27(3):292-300.

329. Rembacken BJ, Fujii T, Cairns A, et al. Flat and depressed colonic neoplasms: a prospective study of 1000 colonoscopies in the UK. *Lancet.* 2000;355(9211):1211-1214.

330. Adachi M, Muto T, Okinaga K, et al. Clinicopathologic features of the flat adenoma. *Dis Colon Rectum.* 1991;34(11):981-986.

331. Rubesin SE, Saul S, Lauffer I, Levine M. Carpet Lesions of the Colon. *Radiographics.* 1985;5(4):537-552.

332. Galdino GM, Yee J. Carpet lesion on CT colonography: a potential pitfall. *AJR Am J Roentgenol.* 2003;180(5):1332-1334.

333. Glick SN, Teplick SK, Balfe DM, et al. Large colonic neoplasms missed by endoscopy. *AJR Am J Roentgenol.* 1989;152(3):513-517.

334. Chintapalli KN, Esola CC, Chopra S, et al. Pericolic mesenteric lymph nodes: an aid in distinguishing diverticulitis from cancer of the colon. *AJR Am J Roentgenol.* 1997;169(5):1253-1255.

335. Phatak MG, Frank SJ, Ellis JJ. Computed tomography of bowel perforation. *Gastrointest Radiol.* 1984;9(2):133-135.

336. Zerhouni EA, Rutter C, Hamilton SR, et al. CT and MR imaging in the staging of colorectal carcinoma: report of the Radiology Diagnostic Oncology Group II. *Radiology.* 1996;200(2):443-451.

337. Acunas B, Rozanes I, Acunas G, et al. Preoperative CT staging of colon carcinoma (excluding the recto-sigmoid region). *Eur J Radiol.* 1990;11(2):150-153.

338. McDaniel KP, Charnsangavej C, DuBrow RA, et al. Pathways of nodal metastasis in carcinomas of the cecum, ascending colon, and transverse colon: CT demonstration. *AJR Am J Roentgenol.* 1993;161(1):61-64.

339. Granfield CA, Charnsangavej C, Dubrow RA, et al. Regional lymph node metastases in carcinoma of the left side of the colon and rectum: CT demonstration. *AJR Am J Roentgenol.* 1992;159(4):757-761.

340. Kantorova I, Lipska L, Belohlavek O, et al. Routine (18)F-FDG PET preoperative staging of colorectal cancer: comparison with conventional staging and its impact on treatment decision making. *J Nucl Med.* 2003;44(11):1784-1788.

341. Abdel-Nabi H, Doerr RJ, Lamonica DM, et al. Staging of primary colorectal carcinomas with fluorine-18 fluorodeoxyglucose whole-body PET: correlation with histopathologic and CT findings. *Radiology.* 1998;206(3):755-760.

342. de Bree E, Koops W, Kroger R, et al. Peritoneal carcinomatosis from colorectal or appendiceal origin: correlation of preoperative CT with intraoperative findings and evaluation of interobserver agreement. *J Surg Oncol.* 2004;86(2):64-73.

343. You YT, Chang Chien CR, Wang JY, et al. Evaluation of contrast-enhanced computed tomographic colonography in detection of local recurrent colorectal cancer. *World J Gastroenterol.* 2006;12(1):123-126.

344. Thoeni RF, Rogalla P. CT for the evaluation of carcinomas in the colon and rectum. *Semin Ultrasound CT MR.* 1995;16(2):112-126.

345. Wald C, Scheirey CD, Tran TM, et al. An update on imaging of colorectal cancer. *Surg Clin North Am.* 2006;86(4):819-847.

346. Huebner RH, Park KC, Shepherd JE, et al. A meta-analysis of the literature for whole-body FDG PET detection of recurrent colorectal cancer. *J Nucl Med.* 2000;41(7):1177-1189.

347. Hine KR, Dykes PW. Serum CEA testing in the post-operative surveillance of colorectal carcinoma. *Br J Cancer.* 1984;49(6):689-693.

348. Flanagan FL, Dehdashti F, Ogunbiyi OA, et al. Utility of FDG-PET for investigating unexplained plasma CEA elevation in patients with colorectal cancer. *Ann Surg.* 1998;227(3):319-323.

349. Libutti SK, Alexander HR Jr, Choyke P, et al. A prospective study of 2-[18F] fluoro-2-deoxy-D-glucose/positron emission tomography scan, 99mTc-labeled arcitumomab (CEA-scan), and blind second-look laparotomy for detecting colon cancer recurrence in patients with increasing carcinoembryonic antigen levels. *Ann Surg Oncol.* 2001;8(10):779-786.

350. Flamen P, Hoekstra OS, Homans F, et al. Unexplained rising carcinoembryonic antigen (CEA) in the postoperative surveillance of colorectal cancer: the utility of positron emission tomography (PET). *Eur J Cancer.* 2001;37(7):862-869.

351. Crane CH, Skibber JM, Feig BW, et al. Response to preoperative chemoradiation increases the use of sphincter-preserving surgery in patients with locally advanced low rectal carcinoma. *Cancer.* 2003;97(2):517-524.

352. Minsky BD. Sphincter preservation in rectal cancer. Preoperative radiation therapy followed by low anterior resection with coloanal anastomosis. *Semin Radiat Oncol.* 1998;8(1):30-35.

353. Kotanagi H, Fukuoka T, Shibata Y, et al. The size of regional lymph nodes does not correlate with the presence or absence of metastasis in lymph nodes in rectal cancer. *J Surg Oncol.* 1993;54(4):252-254.

354. Bipat S, Glas AS, Slors FJ, et al. Rectal cancer: local staging and assessment of lymph node involvement with endoluminal US, CT, and MR imaging—a meta-analysis. *Radiology.* 2004;232(3):773-783.

355. Kulinna C, Eibel R, Matzek W, et al. Staging of rectal cancer: diagnostic potential of multiplanar reconstructions with MDCT. *AJR Am J Roentgenol.* 2004;183(2):421-427.

356. Beets-Tan RG, Beets GL. Rectal cancer: review with emphasis on MR imaging. *Radiology.* 2004;232(2):335-346.

357. Heriot AG, Grundy A, Kumar D. Preoperative staging of rectal carcinoma. *Br J Surg.* 1999;86(1):17-28.

358. Pihl E, Hughes ES, McDermott FT, et al. Disease-free survival and recurrence after resection of colorectal carcinoma. *J Surg Oncol.* 1981;16(4):333-341.

359. Beets-Tan RG, Beets GL, Borstlap AC, et al. Preoperative assessment of local tumor extent in advanced rectal cancer: CT or high-resolution MRI? *Abdom Imaging.* 2000;25(5): 533-541.

360. Tessier DJ, McConnell EJ, Young-Fadok T, et al. Melanoma metastatic to the colon: case series and review of the literature with outcome analysis. *Dis Colon Rectum.* 2003;46(4):441-447.

361. Elsayed AM, Albahra M, Nzeako UC, et al. Malignant melanomas in the small intestine: a study of 103 patients. *Am J Gastroenterol.* 1996;91(5):1001-1006.

362. Lee HJ, Han JK, Kim TK, et al. Primary colorectal lymphoma: spectrum of imaging findings with pathologic correlation. *Eur Radiol.* 2002;12(9):2242-2249.

363. Yatabe Y, Nakamura S, Nakamura T, et al. Multiple polypoid lesions of primary mucosa-associated lymphoid-tissue lymphoma of colon. *Histopathology.* 1998;32(2):116-125.

364. Hoeffel C, Crema MD, Belkacem A, et al. Multi-detector row CT: spectrum of diseases involving the ileocecal area. *Radiographics.* 2006;26(5):1373-1390.

365. Wyatt SH, Fishman EK, Hruban RH, Siegelman SS. CT of primary colonic lymphoma. *Clin Imaging.* 1994;18(2):131-141.

366. Lee HJ, Han JK, Kim TK, et al. Peripheral T-cell lymphoma of the colon: double-contrast barium enema examination findings in six patients. *Radiology.* 2001;218(3):751-756.

367. Hama Y, Okizuka H, Odajima K, et al. Gastrointestinal stromal tumor of the rectum. *Eur Radiol.* 2001;11(2):216-219.

368. van den Berg JC, van Heesewijk JP, van Es HW. Malignant stromal tumour of the rectum: findings at endorectal ultrasound and MRI. *Br J Radiol.* 2000;73(873):1010-1012.

369. Swischuk LE, Hayden CK, Boulden T. Intussusception: indications for ultrasonography and an explanation of the doughnut and pseudokidney signs. *Pediatr Radiol.* 1985;15(6):388-391.

370. Wong WD, Wexner SD, Lowry A, et al. Practice parameters for the treatment of sigmoid diverticulitis—supporting documentation. The Standards Task Force.The American Society of Colon and Rectal Surgeons. *Dis Colon Rectum.* 2000;43:290-297.

371. Perkins JD, Shield CF 3rd, Chang FC, et al. Acute diverticulitis. Comparison of treatment in immunocompromised and nonimmunocompromised patients. *Am J Surg.* 1984;148: 745-748.

372. Detry R, James J, Kartheuser A, et al. Acute localized diverticulitis: Optimum management requires accurate staging. *Int J Colorectal Dis.* 1992;7:38-42.

373. Janes S, Meagher A, Frizelle A. Elective surgery after diverticulitis. *Br J Surg.* 2005;92:133-142.

374. Bahadursingh AM, Virgo KS, Kaminski DL, Longo WE, et al. Spectrum of disease and outcome of complicated diverticular disease. *Am J Surg.* 2003;2003:696-701.

375. Ambrosetti P, Chautems P, Soravia C, et al. Long-term outcome of mesocolic and pelvic diverticular abscesses of the left colon: a prospective study of 73 cases. *Dis Colon Rectum.* 2005;48:787-791.

376. Salem L, Veenstra DL, Sullivan SD, et al. The timing of elective colectomy in diverticulitis: A decision analysis. *J Am Coll Surg.* 2004;199:904-912.

377. Pereira JM, Sirlin CB, Pinto PS, et al. Disproportionate fat stranding: a helpful CT sign in patients with acute abdominal pain. *Radiographics.* 2004;24(3):703-715.

378. Doria AS, Moineddin R, Kellenberger CJ, et al. US or CT for Diagnosis of Appendicitis in Children and Adults? A Meta-Analysis. *Radiology.* 2006;241(1):83-94.

379. Barger RLJ, Nandalur KR. Diagnostic performance of magnetic resonance imaging in the detection of appendicitis in adults: a meta-analysis. *Acad Radiol.* 2010;17(10):1211-1216.

380. Blumenfeld YJ, Wong AE, Jafari A, Barth RA, El-Sayed YY. MR imaging in cases of antenatal suspected appendicitis—a meta-analysis. *J Matern Fetal Neonatal Med.* 2011;24(3):485-488.

381. Singh A, Danrad R, Hahn PF, Blake MA, Mueller PR, Novelline RA. MR imaging of the acute abdomen and pelvis: acute appendicitis and beyond. *Radiographics.* 2007;27(5): 1419-1431.

382. Heaston D, McClellan J, Heaston D. Community hospital experience in 600+ consecutive patients who underwent unenhanced helical CT for suspected appendicitis. *AJR.* 2000;174 [American Roentgen Ray Society 98th Annual Meeting Abstract Book suppl]:53.

383. Hill BC, Johnson SC, Owens EK, et al. CT scan for suspected acute abdominal process: impact of combinations of IV, oral, and rectal contrast. *World J Surg.* 2020;34(4):699-703.

384. Hlibczuk V, Dattaro JA, Jin Z, et al. Diagnostic accuracy of noncontrast computed tomography for appendicitis in adults: a systematic review. *Ann Emerg Med.* 2010;55(1):51-59.

385. Wise SW, Labuski MR, Kasales CJ, et al. Comparative assessment of CT and sonographic techniques for appendiceal imaging. *AJR Am J Roentgenol.* 2001;176(4):933-941.

386. Anderson SW, Soto JA, Lucey BC, et al. Abdominal 64-MDCT for suspected appendicitis: the use of oral and IV contrast material versus IV contrast material only. *AJR Am J Roentgenol.* 2009;193(5):1282-1288.

387. Jacobs JE, Birnbaum BA, Macari M, et al. Acute appendicitis: comparison of helical CT diagnosis focused technique with oral contrast material versus nonfocused technique with oral and intravenous contrast material. *Radiology.* 2001;220(3): 683-690.

388. Curtin KR, Fitzgerald SW, Nemcek AA Jr, et al. CT diagnosis of acute appendicitis: imaging finding. *Am. J. Roentgenol.* 1995;164:905-990.

389. Callahan MJ, Rodriguez DP, Taylor GA. CT of Appendicitis in Children. *Radiology.* 2002;224(2):325-332.

390. Cobben L, Groot I, Kingma L, et al. A simple MRI protocol in patients with clinically suspected appendicitis: results in 138 patients and effect on outcome of appendectomy. *Eur Radiol.* 2009;19(5):1175-1183.

391. Rao PM, Wittenberg J, McDowell RK, et al. Appendicitis: use of arrowhead sign for diagnosis at CT. 1997. 1997;202:363-366.

392. Jeffrey RBJ, Laing FC, Townsend RR. Acute appendicitis: sonographic criteria based on 250 cases. *Radiology.* 1988;167:327-329.

393. Jeffrey RB, Jain KA, Nghiem HV. Sonographic diagnosis of acute appendicitis: interpretive pitfalls. *AJR.* 1994;162:55-59.

394. Kessler N, Cyteval C, Gallix B, et al. Appendicitis: Evaluation of Sensitivity, Specificity, and Predictive Values of US, Doppler US, and Laboratory Findings. *Radiology.* 2004;230:472-478.

395. Levine CD, Aizenstein O, Wachsberg RH. Pitfalls in the CT diagnosis of appendicitis. *Br J Radiol.* 2004;77(921):721-729.

396. Commane DM, Arasaradnam RP, Mills S, et al. Diet, ageing and genetic factors in the pathogenesis of diverticular disease. *World J Gastroenterol.* 2009;15(20):2479-2488.

397. Eide TJ, Stalsberg H. Diverticular disease of the large intestine in Northern Norway. *Gut.* 1979;20:609-615.

398. Parks TG. The clinical significance of diverticular disease of the colon. *Practitioner.* 1982;226:643-648, 650-654.

399. West BA. The pathology of diverticulosis: classical concepts and mucosal changes in diverticula. *J Clin Gastroenterol.* 2006;40:S126–S131.

400. Manousos O, Day NE, Tzonou A, et al. Diet and other factors in the aetiology of diverticulosis: an epidemiological study in Greece. *Gut.* 1985;26:544-549.

401. Brodribb AJ, Humphreys DM. Diverticular disease: three studies. Part I—Relation to other disorders and fibre intake. *Br Med J.* 1976;1:424-425.

402. Rosemar A, Angerås U, Rosengren A. Body mass index and diverticular disease: a 28-year follow-up study in men. *Dis Colon Rectum.* 2008;51:450-455.

403. Dobbins C, Defontgalland D, Duthie G, et al. The relationship of obesity to the complications of diverticular disease. *Colorectal Dis.* 2006;8:37-40.

404. Painter NS, Truelove SC. The Intraluminal pressure patterns in diverticulosis of the Colon. I. Resting patterns of pressure. II. the effect of morphine. *Gut.* 1964;5:201-213.

405. Painter NS, Burkitt DP. Diverticular disease of the colon: a deficiency disease of Western civilization. *Br Med J.* 1971;2: 450-454.

406. Jung HK, Choung RS, Locke GR 3rd, et al. Diarrhea-predominant irritable bowel syndrome is associated with diverticular disease: a population-based study. *Am J Gastroenterol.* 2010;105(3):652-661.

407. Fearnhead NS, Mortensen NJ. Clinical features and differential diagnosis of diverticular disease. *Best Pract Res Clin Gastroenterol.* 2002;16:577-593.

408. Sugihara S, Fujii S, Kinoshita T, et al. Giant sigmoid colonic diverticulitis: case report. *Abdom Imaging.* 2003;28(5):640-642.

409. Naing T, Ray S, Loughran CF. Giant sigmoid diverticulum: a report of three cases. *Clin Radiol.* 1999;54(3):179-181.

410. Versaci A, Macri A, Terranova M, et al. Volvulus due to a giant sigmoid diverticulum: a rare cause of intestinal occlusion. *Chir Ital.* 2008;60(3):487-491.

411. Sutorius DJ, Bossert JE. Giant sigmoid diverticulum with perforation. *Am J Surg.* 1974;127(6):745-748.

412. Roger T, Rommens J, Bailly J, et al. Giant colonic diverticulum: presentation of one case and review of the literature. *Abdom Imaging.* 1996;21(6):530-533.

413. Ona FV, Salamone RP, Mehnert PJ. Giant sigmoid diverticulitis. A cause of partial small bowel obstruction. *Am J Gastroenterol.* 1980;73(4):350-352.

414. Mehta DC, Baum JA, Dave PB, et al. Giant sigmoid diverticulum: report of two cases and endoscopic recognition. *Am J Gastroenterol.* 1996;91(6):1269-1271.

415. Grover H, Nair S, Hertan H. Giant true diverticulum of sigmoid colon. *Am J Gastroenterol.* 1998;93(11):2267-2268.

416. Kelly CP, Pothoulakis C, LaMont JT. Clostridium difficile colitis. *N Engl J Med.* 1994;330(4):257-262.

417. Lipsett PA, Samantaray DK, Tam ML, et al. Pseudomembranous colitis: a surgical disease? *Surgery.* 1994;116(3):491-496.

418. Bradley SJ, Weaver DW, Maxwell NP, et al. Surgical management of pseudomembranous colitis. *Am Surg.* 1988;54(6):329-332.

419. Fishman EK, Kavuru M, Jones B, et al. Pseudomembranous colitis: CT evaluation of 26 cases. *Radiology.* 1991;180(1):57-60.

420. Kawamoto S, Horton KM, Fishman EK. Pseudomembranous colitis: spectrum of imaging findings with clinical and pathologic correlation. *Radiographics.* 1999;19(4):887-897.

421. Ros PR, Buetow PC, Pantograg-Brown L, et al. Pseudomembranous colitis. *Radiology.* 1996;198(1):1-9.

422. Merine D, Fishman EK, Jones B. Pseudomembranous colitis: CT evaluation. *J Comput Assist Tomogr.* 1987;11(6): 1017-1020.

423. Wagner ML, Rosenberg HS, Fernbach DJ, et al. Typhlitis: a complication of leukemia in childhood. *Am J Roentgenol Radium Ther Nucl Med.* 1970;109(2):341-350.

424. Wall SD, Jones B. Gastrointestinal tract in the immunocompromised host: opportunistic infections and other complications. *Radiology.* 1992;185(2):327-335.

425. Urbach DR, Rotstein OD. Typhlitis. *Can J Surg.* 1999;42: 415-419.

426. Gorschlüter M, Mey U, Strehl J, et al. Invasive fungal infections in neutropenic enterocolitis: a systematic analysis of pathogens, incidence, treatment and mortality in adult patients. *BMC Infect Dis.* 2006;6:35-45.

427. Moir CR, Scudamore CH, Benny WB. Typhlitis: selective surgical management. *Am J Surg.* 1986;151(5):563-566.

428. Shamberger RC, Weinstein HJ, Delorey MJ, et al. The medical and surgical management of typhlitis in children with acute nonlymphocytic (myelogenous) leukemia. *Cancer.* 1986;57(3):603-609.

429. Frick MP, Maile CW, Crass JR, et al. Computed tomography of neutropenic colitis. *AJR Am J Roentgenol.* 1984;143(4):763-765.

430. Maher D, Raviglione M. Global epidemiology of tuberculosis. *Clin Chest Med.* 2005;26(2):167-182, v.

431. Burrill J, Williams CJ, Bain G, et al. Tuberculosis: a radiologic review. *Radiographics.* 2007;27(5):1255-1273.

432. Lin PY, Wang JY, Hsueh PR, et al. Lower gastrointestinal tract tuberculosis: an important but neglected disease. *Int J Colorectal Dis.* 2009;24(10):1175-1180.

433. Lam KY, Lo CY. A critical examination of adrenal tuberculosis and a 28-year autopsy experience of active tuberculosis. *Clin Endocrinol (Oxf).* 2001;54(5):633-639.

434. Leder RA, Low VH. Tuberculosis of the abdomen. *Radiol Clin North Am.* 1995;33(4):691-705.

435. Harisinghani MG, McLoud TC, Shepard JA, et al. Tuberculosis from head to toe. *Radiographics.* 2000;20(2):449-470; quiz 528-529. 532.

436. Denton T, Hossain J. A radiological study of abdominal tuberculosis in a Saudi population, with special reference to ultrasound and computed tomography. *Clin Radiol.* 1993;47(6):409-414.

437. Healy E, Rogers S. Tuberculosis verrucosa cutis in association with bovine tuberculosis. *J R Soc Med.* 1992;85(11):704-705.

438. Bargallo N, Nicolau C, Luburich P, et al. Intestinal tuberculosis in AIDS. *Gastrointest Radiol.* 1992;17(2):115-118.

439. Zissin R, Gayer G, Chowers M, et al. Computerized tomography findings of abdominal tuberculosis: report of 19 cases. *Isr Med Assoc J.* 2001;3(6):414-418.

440. Suri S, Gupta S, Suri R. Computed tomography in abdominal tuberculosis. *Br J Radiol.* 1999;72(853):92-98.
441. Fenollar F, Puéchal X, Raoult D. Whipple's Disease. *N Engl J Med.* 2007;356:55-66.
442. Horton KM, Corl FM, Fishman EK. CT of Nonneoplastic Diseases of the Small Bowel: Spectrum of Disease. *J Comput Assist Tomogr.* 1999;23(3):417-428.
443. Fleming JL, Wiesner RH, Shorter RG. Whipple's disease: clinical, biochemical, and histopathologic features and assessment of treatment in 29 patients. *Mayo Clin Proc.* 1988:1988;63:539-551.
444. Rijke AM, Falke TH, de Vries RR. Computed tomography in Whipple disease. *J Comput Assist Tomogr.* 1983;7(6):1101-1102.
445. Herlinger H. Radiology in malabsorption. *Clin Radiol.* 1992; 45(2):73-78.
446. Philpotts LE, Heiken JP, Westcott MA, et al. Colitis: use of CT findings in differential diagnosis. *Radiology.* 1994;190(2):445-449.
447. Davis TW, Goldstone SE. Sexually transmitted infections as a cause of proctitis in men who have sex with men. *Dis Colon Rectum.* 2009;52(3):507-512.
448. Wiesner W, Hauser A, Steinbrich W. Accuracy of multidetector row computed tomography for the diagnosis of acute bowel ischemia in a non-selected study population. *Eur Radiol.* 2004;14(12):2347-2356.
449. Herbert GS, Steele SR. Acute and chronic mesenteric ischemia. *Surg Clin North Am.* 2007;87(5):1115-1134, ix.
450. Rha SE, Ha HK, Lee SH, et al. CT and MR imaging findings of bowel ischemia from various primary causes. *Radiographics.* 2000;20(1):29-42.
451. Chen SC, Wang HP, Chen WJ, et al. Selective use of ultrasonography for the detection of pneumoperitoneum. *Acad Emerg Med.* 2002;9(6):643-645.
452. Levine JS, Jacobson ED. Intestinal ischemic disorders. *Dig Dis.* 1995;13(1):3-24.
453. Wiesner W, Khurana B, Ji H, et al. CT of acute bowel ischemia. *Radiology.* 2003;226(3):635-650.
454. Horton KM, Fishman EK. Multidetector CT angiography in the diagnosis of mesenteric ischemia. *Radiol Clin North Am.* 2007;45(2):275-288.
455. Lee R, Tung HK, Tung PH, et al. CT in acute mesenteric ischaemia. *Clin Radiol.* 2003;58(4):279-287.
456. Stoker J, van Randen A, Lameris W, et al. Imaging patients with acute abdominal pain. *Radiology.* 2009;253(1):31-46.
457. Thoeni RF, Cello JP. CT imaging of colitis. *Radiology.* 2006;240(3):623-638.
458. Schoots IG, Levi MM, Reekers JA, et al. Thrombolytic therapy for acute superior mesenteric artery occlusion. *J Vasc Interv Radiol.* 2005;16(3):317-329.
459. Kumar S, Sarr MG, Kamath PS. Mesenteric venous thrombosis. *N Engl J Med.* 2001;345(23):1683-1688.
460. Ludwig KA, Quebbeman EJ, Bergstein JM, et al. Shock-associated right colon ischemia and necrosis. *J Trauma.* 1995;39(6):1171-1174.
461. Landreneau RJ, Fry WJ. The right colon as a target organ of nonocclusive mesenteric ischemia. Case report and review of the literature. *Arch Surg.* 1990;125(5):591-594.
462. Ventemiglia R, Khalil KG, Frazier OH, et al. The role of preoperative mesenteric arteriography in colon interposition. *J Thorac Cardiovasc Surg.* 1977;74(1):98-104.
463. Toner M, Condell D, O'Briain D. Obstructive colitis: ulceroinflammatory lesions occurring proximal to colonic obstruction. *Am J Surg Pathol.* 1990;14:719-728.
464. Ko GY, Ha HK, Lee HJ, et al. Usefulness of CT in patients with ischemic colitis proximal to colonic cancer. *AJR Am J Roentgenol.* 1997;168(4):951-956.
465. Storesund B, Gran JT, Koldingsnes W. Severe intestinal involvement in Wegener's granulomatosis: report of two cases and review of the literature. *Br J Rheumatol.* 1998;37(4):387-390.
466. Trimble MA, Weisz MA. Infarction of the sigmoid colon secondary to giant cell arteritis. *Rheumatology (Oxford).* 2002;41(1):108-110.
467. Senadhi V. A rare cause of chronic mesenteric ischemia from fibromuscular dysplasia: a case report. *Med Case Reports.* 2010;4:373.
468. Collin DA, Duke O. Systemic vasculitis presenting with massive bowel infarction. *J R Soc Med.* 1995;88:692-693.
469. Hauer-Jensen M, Wang J, Denham JW. Bowel Injury: Current and Evolving Management Strategies. *Seminars in Radiation Oncology.* 2003;13(3):357-371.
470. Gervaz P, Morel P, Vozenin-Brotons MC. Molecular aspects of intestinal radiation-induced fibrosis. *Curr Mol Med.* 2009;9(3): 273-280.
471. Green N, Iba G, Smith WR. Measures to minimize small intestine injury in the irradiated pelvis. *Cancer.* 1975;35(6): 1633-1640.
472. Meagher T, Nolan DJ, Galland RB, et al. The radiology of irradiated gut. *London: Edward Arnold.* 1990;88-102.
473. Haboubi NY, El-Zammar O, O'Dwyer ST, et al. Radiation bowel disease: pathogenesis and management. *Colorectal Disease.* 2000;2(6):322-329.
474. Mendelson RM, Nolan DJ. The radiological features of radiation enteritis. *Clin Radiol.* 1985;36:141-148.
475. Fishman EK, Zinreich ES, Jones B, et al. Computed tomographic diagnosis of radiation ileitis. *Gastrointest Radiol.* 1984;9:149-152.
476. Baumgart DC, Carding SR. Inflammatory bowel disease: cause and immunobiology. *Lancet.* 2007;369(9573):1627-1640.
477. Xavier RJ, Podolsky DK. Unravelling the pathogenesis of inflammatory bowel disease. *Nature.* 2007;448(7152): 427-434.
478. Guindi M, Riddell RH. Indeterminate colitis. *J Clin Pathol.* 2004;57(12):1233-1244.
479. Horsthuis K, Stokkers PC, Stoker J. Detection of inflammatory bowel disease: diagnostic performance of cross-sectional imaging modalities. *Abdom Imaging.* 2008;33(4):407-416.
480. Wills JS, Lobis IF, Denstman FJ. Crohn disease: state of the art. *Radiology.* 1997;202(3):597-610.
481. Roggeveen MJ, Tismenetsky M, Shapiro R. Best cases from the AFIP: Ulcerative colitis. *Radiographics.* 2006;26(3):947-951.
482. Sheth SG, LaMont JT. Toxic megacolon. *Lancet.* 1998;351(9101):509-513.
483. Gore RM. CT of inflammatory bowel disease. *Radiol Clin North Am.* 1989;27(4):717-729.
484. Furukawa A, Saotome T, Yamasaki M, et al. Cross-sectional imaging in Crohn disease. *Radiographics.* 2004;24(3):689-702.
485. Gore RM, Balthazar EJ, Ghahremani GG, et al. CT features of ulcerative colitis and Crohn's disease. *AJR Am J Roentgenol.* 1996;167(1):3-15.

486. Zisman TL, Rubin DT. Novel diagnostic and prognostic modalities in inflammatory bowel disease. *Gastroenterol Clin North Am.* 2009;38(4):729-752.

487. Nanakawa S, Takahashi M, Takagi K, et al. The role of computed tomography in management of patients with Crohn disease. *Clin Imaging.* 1993;17(3):193-198.

488. Jacobs JE, Birnbaum BA. CT of inflammatory disease of the colon. *Semin Ultrasound CT MR.* 1995;16(2):91-101.

489. Raptopoulos V, Schwartz RK, McNicholas MM, et al. Multiplanar helical CT enterography in patients with Crohn's disease. *AJR Am J Roentgenol.* 1997;169(6):1545-1550.

490. Broome U, Bergquist A. Primary sclerosing cholangitis, inflammatory bowel disease, and colon cancer. *Semin Liver Dis.* 2006;26(1):31-41.

491. Bansal P, Sonnenberg A. Risk factors of colorectal cancer in inflammatory bowel disease. *Am J Gastroenterol.* 1996;91(1): 44-48.

492. Matsumoto T, Iida M, Kuroki F, et al. Dysplasia in ulcerative colitis: is radiography adequate for diagnosis? *Radiology.* 1996;199(1):85-90.

493. Kiran R, Khoury W, Church JM, et al. Colorectal Cancer Complicating Inflammatory Bowel Disease: Similarities and Differences Between Crohn's and Ulcerative Colitis Based on Three Decades of Experience. *Ann Surg.* 2010;252:330-335.

494. Zisman TL, Rubin DT. Colorectal cancer and dysplasia in inflammatory bowel disease. *World J Gastroenterol.* 2008;14(17):2662-2669.

495. Rutter MD, Saunders BP, Wilkinson KH, et al. Thirty-year analysis of a colonoscopic surveillance program for neoplasia in ulcerative colitis. *Gastroenterology.* 2006;130:1030-1038.

496. Kandiel A, Fraser AG, Korelitz BI, et al. Increased risk of lymphoma among inflammatory bowel disease patients treated with azathioprine and 6-mercaptopurine. *Gut.* 2005;5(8):1121-1125.

497. Lewis J, Bilker WB, Brensinger C, et al. Inflammatory bowel disease is not associated with an increased risk of lymphoma. *Gastroenterology.* 2001;121:1080-1087.

498. Loftus E, Tremaine W, Habermann T, et al. Risk of lymphoma in inflammatory bowel disease. *Am J Gastroenterol.* 1998;95: 2308-2312.

499. Dijkstra J, Reeders JW, Tytgat GN. Idiopathic inflammatory bowel disease: endoscopic-radiologic correlation. *Radiology.* 1995;197(2):369-375.

500. Hizawa K, Iida M, Kohrogi N, et al. Crohn disease: early recognition and progress of aphthous lesions. *Radiology.* 1994;190(2):451-454.

501. Lee SD, Cohen RD. Endoscopy in inflammatory bowel disease. *Gastroenterol Clin North Am.* 2002;31(1):119-132.

502. Blackstone MO, Riddell RH, Rogers BH, et al. Dysplasia-associated lesion or mass (DALM) detected by colonoscopy in long-standing ulcerative colitis: an indication for colectomy. *Gastroenterology.* 1981;80(2):366-374.

503. Loftus EV Jr. Clinical epidemiology of inflammatory bowel disease: Incidence, prevalence, and environmental influences. *Gastroenterology.* 2004;126(6):1504-1517.

504. Gossios KJ, Tsianos EV. Crohn disease: CT findings after treatment. *Abdom Imaging.* 1997;22(2):160-163.

505. Bodily KD, Fletcher JG, Solem CA, et al. Crohn Disease: mural attenuation and thickness at contrast-enhanced CT Enterography—correlation with endoscopic and histologic findings of inflammation. *Radiology.* 2006;238(2):505-516.

506. Fishman EK, Wolf EJ, Jones B, et al. CT evaluation of Crohn's disease: effect on patient management. *AJR Am J Roentgenol.* 1987;148(3):537-540.

507. Mako EK, Mester AR, Tarjan Z, et al. Enteroclysis and spiral CT examination in diagnosis and evaluation of small bowel Crohn's disease. *Eur J Radiol.* 2000;35(3):168-175.

508. Koh DM, Miao Y, Chinn RJ, et al. MR imaging evaluation of the activity of Crohn's disease. *AJR Am J Roentgenol.* 2001;177(6):1325-1332.

509. Maccioni F, Colaiacomo MC, Parlanti S. Ulcerative colitis: value of MR imaging. *Abdom Imaging.* 2005;30(5):584-592.

510. Madsen SM, Thomsen HS, Schlichting P, et al. Evaluation of treatment response in active Crohn's disease by low-field magnetic resonance imaging. *Abdom Imaging.* 1999;24(3): 232-239.

511. Maccioni F, Viscido A, Broglia L, et al. Evaluation of Crohn disease activity with magnetic resonance imaging. *Abdom Imaging.* 2000;25(3):219-228.

512. Madsen SM, Thomsen HS, Munkholm P, Schlichting P, Davidsen B. Magnetic resonance imaging of Crohn disease: early recognition of treatment response and relapse. *Abdom Imaging.* 1997;22(2):164-166.

513. Shoenut JP, Semelka RC, Magro CM, Silverman R, Yaffe CS, Micflikier AB. Comparison of magnetic resonance imaging and endoscopy in distinguishing the type and severity of inflammatory bowel disease. *J Clin Gastroenterol.* 1994; 19(1):31-35.

514. Maccioni F, Bruni A, Viscido A, et al. MR imaging in patients with Crohn disease: value of T2- versus T1-weighted gadolinium-enhanced MR sequences with use of an oral superparamagnetic contrast agent. *Radiology.* 2006;238(2): 517-530.

515. Rollandi GA, Curone PF, Biscaldi E, et al. Spiral CT of the abdomen after distention of small bowel loops with transparent enema in patients with Crohn's disease. *Abdom Imaging.* 1999;24(6):544-549.

516. Booya F, Fletcher JG, Huprich JE, et al. Active Crohn disease: CT findings and interobserver agreement for enteric phase CT enterography. *Radiology.* 2006;241(3):787-795.

517. Sempere GA, Martinez Sanjuan V, Medina Chulia E, et al. MRI evaluation of inflammatory activity in Crohn's disease. *AJR Am J Roentgenol.* 2005;184(6):1829-1835.

518. Jones B, Fishman EK, Hamilton SR, et al. Submucosal accumulation of fat in inflammatory bowel disease: CT/pathologic correlation. *J Comput Assist Tomogr.* 1986;10(5): 759-763.

519. Gore RM. Characteristic morphologic changes in chronic ulcerative colitis. *Abdom Imaging.* 1995;20(3):275-277.

520. Scott EM, Freeman AH. Prominent omental and mesenteric vasculature in inflammatory bowel disease shown by computed tomography. *Eur J Radiol.* 1996;22(2):104-106.

521. Ahualli J. The Fat Halo Sign. *Radiology 2007.* 2007;242:945-946.

522. Harisinghani MG, Wittenberg J, Lee W, et al. Bowel Wall Fat Halo Sign in Patients Without Intestinal Disease. *AJR.* 2003;181:781-784.

523. Herlinger H, Furth EE, Rubesin SE. Fibrofatty proliferation of the mesentery in Crohn disease. *Abdom Imaging.* 1998;23(4):446-448.

524. Meyers MA, McGuire PV. Spiral CT demonstration of hypervascularity in Crohn disease: "vascular jejunization of the ileum" or the "comb sign". *Abdom Imaging.* 1995; 20(4):327-332.
525. Colombel JF, Solem CA, Sandborn WJ, et al. Quantitative measurement and visual assessment of ileal Crohn's disease activity by computed tomography enterography: correlation with endoscopic severity and C reactive protein. *Gut.* 2006;55(11):1561-1567.
526. Yousem DM, Fishman EK, Jones B. Crohn disease: perirectal and perianal findings at CT. *Radiology.* 1988;167(2):331-334.
527. Ribeiro MB, Greenstein AJ, Yamazaki Y, et al. Intra-abdominal abscess in regional enteritis. *Ann Surg.* 1991;213(1):32-36.
528. Karahan OI, Dodd GD 3rd, Chintapalli KN, et al. Gastrointestinal wall thickening in patients with cirrhosis: frequency and patterns at contrast-enhanced CT. *Radiology.* 2000;215(1):103-107.
529. Kagnoff M. Celiac disease: pathogenesis of a model immunogenetic disease. *J Clin Invest.* 2007;117(1):41-49.
530. Lomoschitz F, Schima W, Schober E, et al. Enteroclysis in adult celiac disease: diagnostic value of specific radiographic features. *Eur Radiol.* 2003;13(4):890-896.
531. Rubesin SE, Herlinger H, Saul SH, et al. Adult celiac disease and its complications. *Radiographics.* 1989;9(6):1045-1066.
532. Soyer P, Boudiaf M, Dray X, et al. CT enteroclysis features of uncomplicated celiac disease: retrospective analysis of 44 patients. *Radiology.* 2009;253(2):416-424.
533. Farthing MJ, McLean AM, Bartram CI, et al. Radiologic features of the jejunum in hypoalbuminemia. *AJR Am J Roentgenol.* 1981;136(5):883-886.
534. Lars-Egil F, Bergseng E, Hotta K, et al. Differences in the risk of celiac disease associated with HLA-DQ2.5 or HLA-DQ2.2 are related to sustained gluten antigen presentation. *Nature Immunol.* 2009;10:1096-1101.
535. Fasano A, Berti I, Gerarduzzi T, et al. Prevalence of Celiac Disease in At-Risk and Not-At-Risk Groups in the United States: A Large Multicenter Study. *Arch Intern Med.* 2003;163:286-292.
536. Rubio-Tapia A, Murray JA. Celiac disease. *Curr Opin Gastroenterol.* 2010;26(2):116-122.
537. Herlinger H, Maglinte DD. Jejunal fold separation in adult celiac disease: relevance of enteroclysis. *Radiology.* 1986;158(3):605-611.
538. Holmes GK, Prior P, Lane MR, et al. Malignancy in coeliac disease—effect of a gluten free diet. *Gut.* 1989;30(3):333-338.
539. Horton KM, Fishman EK. Uncommon inflammatory diseases of the small bowel: CT findings. *AJR Am J Roentgenol.* 1998;170(2):385-388.
540. Mallant M, Hadithi M, Al-Toma A, et al. Abdominal computed tomography in refractory coeliac disease and enteropathy associated T-cell lymphoma. *World J Gastroenterol.* 2007;13(11):1696-1700.
541. Tomei E, Diacinti D, Marini M, et al. Abdominal CT findings may suggest coeliac disease. *Dig Liver Dis.* 2005;37(6):402-406.
542. Lane MJ, Katz DS, Mindelzun RE, et al. Spontaneous intramural small bowel haemorrhage: importance of non-contrast CT. *Clin Radiol.* 1997;52(5):378-380.
543. Balthazar EJ, Hulnick D, Megibow AJ, et al. Computed tomography of intramural intestinal hemorrhage and bowel ischemia. *J Comput Assist Tomogr.* 1987;11(1):67-72.
544. Balthazar EJ. CT of the gastrointestinal tract: principles and interpretation. *AJR Am J Roentgenol.* 1991;156(1):23-32.
545. Foster NM, McGory ML, Zingmond DS, et al. Small bowel obstruction: a population-based appraisal. *J Am Coll Surg.* 2006;203(2):170-176.
546. Welch JP. Bowel Obstruction: Differential Diagnosis and Clinical Management. Philadelphia: Saunders; 1990:xvi, 711.
547. Silva AC, Pimenta M, Guimaraes LS. Small bowel obstruction: what to look for. *Radiographics.* 2009;29(2):423-439.
548. Peetz DJ Jr, Gamelli RL, Pilcher DB. Intestinal intubation in acute, mechanical small-bowel obstruction. *Arch Surg.* 1982;117(3):334-336.
549. Silen W, Hein MF, Goldman L. Strangulation obstruction of the small intestine. *Arch Surg.* 1962;85:121-129.
550. Balthazar EJ. For suspected small-bowel obstruction and an equivocal plain film, should we perform CT or a small-bowel series? *AJR Am J Roentgenol.* 1994;163(5):1260-1261.
551. Lappas JC, Reyes BL, Maglinte DD. Abdominal radiography findings in small-bowel obstruction: relevance to triage for additional diagnostic imaging. *AJR Am J Roentgenol.* 2001;176(1):167-174.
552. Nicolaou S, Kai B, Ho S, et al. Imaging of acute small-bowel obstruction. *AJR Am J Roentgenol.* 2005;185(4):1036-1044.
553. Thompson WM, Kilani RK, Smith BB, et al. Accuracy of abdominal radiography in acute small-bowel obstruction: does reviewer experience matter? *AJR Am J Roentgenol.* 2007;188(3):W233-W238.
554. Maglinte DD, Heitkamp DE, Howard TJ, et al. Current concepts in imaging of small bowel obstruction. *Radiol Clin North Am.* 2003;41(2):vi, 263-283.
555. Fukuya T, Hawes DR, Lu CC, et al. CT diagnosis of small-bowel obstruction: efficacy in 60 patients. *AJR Am J Roentgenol.* 1992;158(4):765-769; discussion 771-772.
556. Qalbani A, Paushter D, Dachman AH. Multidetector row CT of small bowel obstruction. *Radiol Clin North Am.* 2007;45(3):viii, 499-512.
557. Ros PR, Huprich JE. ACR Appropriateness Criteria on suspected small-bowel obstruction. *J Am Coll Radiol.* 2006;3(11):838-841.
558. Jaffe TA, Martin LC, Thomas J, et al. Small-bowel obstruction: coronal reformations from isotropic voxels at 16-section multi-detector row CT. *Radiology.* 2006;238(1):135-142.
559. Frager D, Medwid SW, Baer JW, et al. CT of small-bowel obstruction: value in establishing the diagnosis and determining the degree and cause. *AJR Am J Roentgenol.* 1994;162(1):37-41.
560. Maglinte DD, Kelvin FM, Rowe MG, et al. Small-bowel obstruction: optimizing radiologic investigation and nonsurgical management. *Radiology.* 2001;218(1):39-46.
561. Maglinte DD, Stevens LH, Hall RC, et al. Dual-purpose tube for enteroclysis and nasogastric-nasoenteric decompression. *Radiology.* 1992;185(1):281-282.
562. Shrake PD, Rex DK, Lappas JC, et al. Radiographic evaluation of suspected small bowel obstruction. *Am J Gastroenterol.* 1991;86(2):175-178.
563. Makanjuola D. Computed tomography compared with small bowel enema in clinically equivocal intestinal obstruction. *Clin Radiol.* 1998;53(3):203-208.
564. Maglinte DD, Sandrasegaran K, Lappas JC, et al. CT Enteroclysis. *Radiology.* 2007;245(3):661-671.

565. Schmidt H, Abolmaali N, Vogl TJ. Double bubble sign. *Eur Radiol.* 2002;12(7):1849-1853.
566. Maglinte DD, Reyes BL, Harmon BH, et al. Reliability and role of plain film radiography and CT in the diagnosis of small-bowel obstruction. *AJR Am J Roentgenol.* 1996;167(6):1451-1455.
567. Levin B. Mechanical small bowel obstruction. *Semin Roentgenol.* 1973;8(3):281-297.
568. Nevitt PC. The string of pearls sign. *Radiology.* 2000;214(1): 157-158.
569. Herlinger H, Maglinte DDT. *Clinical Radiology of the Small Intestine.* Philadelphia, PA: Saunders; 1989;497-507.
570. Furukawa A, Yamasaki M, Takahashi M, et al. CT diagnosis of small bowel obstruction: scanning technique, interpretation and role in the diagnosis. *Semin Ultrasound CT MR.* 2003;24(5):336-352.
571. Furukawa A, Yamasaki M, Furuichi K, et al. Helical CT in the diagnosis of small bowel obstruction. *Radiographics.* 2001;21(2):341-355.
572. Lee JKT. *Computed Body Tomography with MRI Correlation.* 4th ed. Philadelphia, PA: Lippincott Williams & Wilkins; 2006.
573. Lazarus DE, Slywotsky C, Bennett GL, et al. Frequency and relevance of the "small-bowel feces" sign on CT in patients with small-bowel obstruction. *AJR Am J Roentgenol.* 2004;183(5):1361-1366.
574. Jacobs SL, Rozenblit A, Ricci Z, et al. Small bowel faeces sign in patients without small bowel obstruction. *Clin Radiol.* 2007;62(4):353-357.
575. Fuchsjager MH. The small-bowel feces sign. *Radiology.* 2002;225(2):378-379.
576. Mayo-Smith WW, Wittenberg J, Bennett GL, et al. The CT small bowel faeces sign: description and clinical significance. *Clin Radiol.* 1995;50(11):765-767.
577. Quiroga S, Alvarez-Castells A, Sebastia MC, et al. Small bowel obstruction secondary to bezoar: CT diagnosis. *Abdom Imaging.* 1997;22(3):315-317.
578. Miller G, Boman J, Shrier I, et al. Etiology of small bowel obstruction. *Am J Surg.* 2000;180(1):33-36.
579. Delabrousse E, Destrumelle N, Brunelle S, et al. CT of small bowel obstruction in adults. *Abdom Imaging.* 2003;28(2): 257-266.
580. Attard JA, MacLean AR. Adhesive small bowel obstruction: epidemiology, biology and prevention. *Can J Surg.* 2007; 50(4):291-300.
581. Boudiaf M, Soyer P, Terem C, et al. Ct evaluation of small bowel obstruction. *Radiographics.* 2001;21(3):613-624.
582. Sinha R, Verma R. Multidetector row computed tomography in bowel obstruction. Part 2. Large bowel obstruction. *Clin Radiol.* 2005;60(10):1068-1075.
583. Zafar HM, Levine MS, Rubesin SE, et al. Anterior abdominal wall hernias: findings in barium studies. *Radiographics.* 2006;26(3):691-699.
584. Takeyama N, Gokan T, Ohgiya Y, et al. CT of internal hernias. *Radiographics.* 2005;25(4):997-1015.
585. Martin LC, Merkle EM, Thompson WM. Review of internal hernias: radiographic and clinical findings. *AJR Am J Roentgenol.* 2006;186(3):703-717.
586. Mak SY, Roach SC, Sukumar SA. Small bowel obstruction: computed tomography features and pitfalls. *Curr Probl Diagn Radiol.* 2006;35(2):65-74.
587. Agha FP. Intussusception in adults. *AJR Am J Roentgenol.* 1986;146(3):527-531.
588. Chiorean MV, Sandrasegaran K, Saxena R, et al. Correlation of CT enteroclysis with surgical pathology in Crohn's disease. *Am J Gastroenterol.* 2007;102(11):2541-2550.
589. Zissin R, Hertz M, Paran H, et al. Small bowel obstruction secondary to Crohn disease: CT findings. *Abdom Imaging.* 2004;29(3):320-325.
590. Reijnen HA, Joosten HJ, de Boer HH. Diagnosis and treatment of adult intussusception. *Am J Surg.* 1989;158(1):25-28.
591. Herlinger H, Maglinte DDT. Clinical Radiology of the Small Intestine. Philadelphia, PA: Saunders; 1989:xviii, 605.
592. Warshauer DM, Lee JK. Adult intussusception detected at CT or MR imaging: clinical-imaging correlation. *Radiology.* 1999;212(3):853-860.
593. Lorigan JG, DuBrow RA. The computed tomographic appearances and clinical significance of intussusception in adults with malignant neoplasms. *Br J Radiol.* 1990;63(748):257-262.
594. Iko BO, Teal JS, Siram SM, et al. Computed tomography of adult colonic intussusception: clinical and experimental studies. *AJR Am J Roentgenol.* 1984;143(4):769-772.
595. Yoshimitsu K, Fukuya T, Onitsuka H, et al. Computed tomography of ileoileocolic intussusception caused by a lipoma. *J Comput Assist Tomogr.* 1989;13(4):704-706.
596. Peterson CM, Anderson JS, Hara AK, et al. Volvulus of the gastrointestinal tract: appearances at multimodality imaging. *Radiographics.* 2009;29(5):1281-1293.
597. McAlister WH, Kronemer KA. Emergency gastrointestinal radiology of the newborn. *Radiol Clin North Am.* 1996;34(4): 819-844.
598. Bernstein SM, Russ PD. Midgut volvulus: a rare cause of acute abdomen in an adult patient. *AJR Am J Roentgenol.* 1998;171(3):639-641.
599. Shimanuki Y, Aihara T, Takano H, et al. Clockwise whirlpool sign at color Doppler US: an objective and definite sign of midgut volvulus. *Radiology.* 1996;199(1):261-264.
600. Fisher JK. Computed tomographic diagnosis of volvulus in intestinal malrotation. *Radiology.* 1981;140(1):145-146.
601. Loren I, Lasson A, Nilsson A, et al. Gallstone ileus demonstrated by CT. *J Comput Assist Tomogr.* 1994;18(2):262-265.
602. Mishra PK, Agrawal A, Joshi M, et al. Intestinal obstruction in children due to Ascariasis: A tertiary health centre experience. *Afr J Paediatr Surg.* 2008;5:65-70.
603. Haswell-Elkins M, Elkins D, Anderson RM. The influence of individual, social group and household factors on the distribution of Ascaris lumbricoides within a community and implications for control strategies. *Parasitology.* 1989;98:125-134.
604. Shiekh KA, Baba AA, Ahmad SM, et al. Mechanical small bowel obstruction in children at a tertiary care centre in Kashmir. *Afr J Paediatr Surg.* 2010;7(2):81-85.
605. Dayalan, N, Ramakrishnan MS. The pattern of intestinal obstruction with special preference toascariasis. *Indian Pediatr.* 1976;13:47-49.
606. Hoffmann H, Kawooya M, Esterre P, et al. In vivo and in vitro studies of the sonographic detection of Ascaris lumbricoides. *Pediatr Radiol.* 1997;27:226-229.
607. Peck RJ. Ultrasonography of intestinal Ascaris. *J Clin Ultrasound.* 1990;18:741-743.

608. Mahmood T, Mansoor N, Quraishy S, et al. Ultrasonographic appearance of Ascaris lumbricoides in the small bowel. *J Ultrasound Med.* 2001;20:269-274.

609. Hommeyer SC, Hamill GS, Johnson JA. CT diagnosis of intestinal ascariasis. *Abdom Imaging.* 1995;20(4):315-316.

610. Beita AO, Haller JO, Kantor A. CT Findings in pediatric gastrointestinal ascariasis. *Comput Med Imaging Graph.* 1997;21:47-49.

611. Dalla VLK, Grosfeld JL, West KW, et al. Intestinal atresia and stenosis: a 25-year experience with 277 cases. *Arch Surg.* 1998;133(5):490-496.

612. Megibow AJ. Bowel obstruction. Evaluation with CT. *Radiol Clin North Am.* 1994;32(5):861-870.

613. Chakrabarty PB, Tripathy BC, Panda K. Acute intestinal obstruction (a review of 1020 operated cases). *J Indian Med Assoc.* 1976;67(3):64-69.

614. Laws HL, Aldrete JS. Small-bowel obstruction: a review of 465 cases. *South Med J.* 1976;69(6):733-734.

615. Cappell MS, Batke M. Mechanical obstruction of the small bowel and colon. *Med Clin North Am.* 2008;92(3):viii, 575-597.

616. Chapman AH, McNamara M, Porter G. The acute contrast enema in suspected large bowel obstruction: value and technique. *Clin Radiol.* 1992;46(4):273-278.

617. Frager D, Rovno HD, Baer JW, et al. Prospective evaluation of colonic obstruction with computed tomography. *Abdom Imaging.* 1998;23(2):141-146.

618. Beattie GC, Peters RT, Guy S, et al. Computed tomography in the assessment of suspected large bowel obstruction. *ANZ J Surg.* 2007;77(3):160-165.

619. Taourel P, Kessler N, Lesnik A, et al. Helical CT of large bowel obstruction. *Abdom Imaging.* 2003;28(2):267-275.

620. Ott DJ, Chen MY. Specific acute colonic disorders. *Radiol Clin North Am.* 1994;32(5):871-884.

621. Feldman M, Friedman LS, Sleisenger MH. *Sleisenger & Fordtran's Gastrointestinal and Liver Disease: Pathophysiology, Diagnosis, Management.* 7th ed. Philadelphia, PA: Saunders; 2002. 2 v. (xli, 2385. 98 p.).

622. Jones IT, Fazio VW. Colonic volvulus. Etiology and management. *Dig Dis.* 1989;7(4):203-209.

623. Javors BR, Baker SR, Miller JA. The northern exposure sign: a newly described finding in sigmoid volvulus. *AJR Am J Roentgenol.* 1999;173(3):571-574.

624. Burrell HC, Baker DM, Wardrop P, et al. Significant plain film findings in sigmoid volvulus. *Clin Radiol.* 1994;49(5):317-319.

625. Moore CJ, Corl FM, Fishman EK. CT of cecal volvulus: unraveling the image. *AJR Am J Roentgenol.* 2001;177(1): 95-98.

626. Frank AJ, Goffner LB, Fruauff AA, et al. Cecal volvulus: the CT whirl sign. *Abdom Imaging.* 1993;18(3):288-289.

627. Ng DC, Kwok SY, Cheng Y, et al. Colonic amoebic abscess mimicking carcinoma of the colon. *Hong Kong Med J.* 2006; 12(1):71-73.

628. Filippou D, Psimitis I, Zizi D, et al. A rare case of ascending colon actinomycosis mimicking cancer. *BMC Gastroenterol.* 2005;5:1.

629. Platell C, Mackay J, Collopy B, et al. Crohn's disease: a colon and rectal department experience. *Aust N Z J Surg.* 1995;65(8):570-575.

630. Pal S, Sahni P, Pande GK, et al. Outcome following emergency surgery for refractory severe ulcerative colitis in a tertiary care centre in India. *BMC Gastroenterol.* 2005;5:39.

631. Eun SK, Won HK. Inflammatory bowel disease in Korea: epidemiological, genomic, clinical, and therapeutic characteristics. *Gut Liver.* 2010;4(1):1-14.

632. Byun YH, Park YS, Myung SJ, et al. Transient intestinal obstruction due to stool impaction in the elderly. *Korean J Gastroenterol.* 2005;46(3):211-217.

633. Khan MN, Agrawal A, Strauss P. Ileocolic Intussusception - A rare cause of acute intestinal obstruction in adults; Case report and literature review. *World J Emerg Surg.* 2008;3:26.

634. Kessman J. Hirschsprung's disease: diagnosis and management. *Am Fam Physician.* 2006;74(8):1319-1322.

635. Simi M, Pietroletti R, Navarra L, et al. Bowel stricture due to ischemic colitis: report of three cases requiring surgery. *Hepatogastroenterology.* 1995;42(3):279-281.

636. Osman N, Subar D, Loh MY, et al. Gallstone ileus of the sigmoid colon: an unusual cause of large-bowel obstruction. *HPB Surg.* 2010;2010:153740.

637. Chen JH, Chen KY, Chang WK. Intestinal obstruction induced by phytobezoars. *CMAJ.* 2010;182(17):E797.

638. Indraccolo U, Trevisan P, Gasparin P, et al. Cecal endometriosis as a cause of ileocolic intussusception. *JSLS.* 2010;14(1):140-142.

639. Pyun DK, Kim KJ, Ye BD, et al. Two cases of colonic obstruction after acute pancreatitis. *Korean J Gastroenterol.* 2009;54(3):180-185.

640. Dietz DW, Remzi FH, Fazio VW. Strictureplasty for obstructing small-bowel lesions in diffuse radiation enteritis—successful outcome in five patients. *Dis Colon Rectum.* 2001;44(12): 1772-1777.

641. Aronchick JM, Epstein DM, Gefter WB, et al. Chronic traumatic diaphragmatic hernia: the significance of pleural effusion. *Radiology.* 1988;168(3):675-678.

642. Batke M, Cappell MS. Adynamic ileus and acute colonic pseudo-obstruction. *Med Clin North Am.* 2008;92(3): 649-670, ix.

643. Holte K, Kehlet H. Postoperative ileus: a preventable event. *Br J Surg.* 2000;87(11):1480-1493.

644. Townsend CM, Sabiston DC. Sabiston Textbook of Surgery : the Biological Basis of Modern Surgical Practice. Philadelphia, PA: Saunders; 2004:2388, xxv.

645. Kurz A, Sessler DI. Opioid-induced bowel dysfunction: pathophysiology and potential new therapies. *Drugs.* 2003;63(7):649-671.

646. Fallon MT, Hanks GW. Morphine, constipation and performance status in advanced cancer patients. *Palliat Med.* 1999;13(2):159-160.

647. Kahi CJ, Rex DK. Bowel obstruction and pseudo-obstruction. *Gastroenterol Clin North Am.* 2003;32(4):1229-1247.

648. Saunders MD, Kimmey MB. Systematic review: acute colonic pseudo-obstruction. *Aliment Pharmacol Ther.* 2005;22(10): 917-925.

649. Vanek VW, Al-Salti M. Acute pseudo-obstruction of the colon (Ogilvie's syndrome). An analysis of 400 cases. *Dis Colon Rectum.* 1986;29(3):203-210.

650. De Giorgio R, Knowles CH. Acute colonic pseudo-obstruction. *Br J Surg.* 2009;96(3):229-239.

651. Lavine L. Gastrointestinal Bleeding. In: Fauci AS, et al. eds. Harrison's Principles of Internal Medicine, 17th ed. New York, NY: McGraw Hill; 2008: Chap 42.

652. Imdahl A. Genesis and pathophysiology of lower gastrointestinal bleeding. *Langenbecks Arch Surg.* 2001;386(1):1-7.

653. Longstreth GF. Epidemiology and outcome of patients hospitalized with acute lower gastrointestinal hemorrhage: a population-based study. *Am J Gastroenterol.* 1997;92(3):419-424.

654. Barnert J, Messmann H. Diagnosis and management of lower gastrointestinal bleeding. *Nat Rev Gastroenterol Hepatol.* 2009;6(11):637-646.

655. Zuckier LS. Acute gastrointestinal bleeding. *Semin Nucl Med.* 2003;33(4):297-311.

656. Fallah MA, Prakash C, Edmundowicz S. Acute gastrointestinal bleeding. *Med Clin North Am.* 2000;84(5):1183-1208.

657. Ettorre GC, Francioso G, Garribba AP, et al. Helical CT angiography in gastrointestinal bleeding of obscure origin. *AJR Am J Roentgenol.* 1997;163(3):727-731.

658. Tew K, Davies RP, Jadun CK, et al. MDCT of acute lower gastrointestinal bleeding. *AJR Am J Roentgenol.* 2004;182(2):427-430.

659. Ernst O, Bulois P, Saint-Drenant S, Leroy C, Paris JC, Sergent G. Helical CT in acute lower gastrointestinal bleeding. *Eur Radiol.* 2003;13(1):114-117.

660. Zink SI, Ohki SK, Stein B, et al. Noninvasive evaluation of active lower gastrointestinal bleeding: comparison between contrast-enhanced MDCT and 99mTc-labeled RBC scintigraphy. *AJR Am J Roentgenol.* 2008;191(4):1107-1114.

661. Jaeckle T, Stuber G, Hoffmann MH, et al. Detection and localization of acute upper and lower gastrointestinal (GI) bleeding with arterial phase multi-detector row helical CT. *Eur Radiol.* 2008:2008;18(7):1406-1413.

662. Cohn SM, Moller BA, Zieg PM, et al. Angiography for preoperative evaluation in patients with lower gastrointestinal bleeding: are the benefits worth the risks. *Arch Surg.* 1998;133(1):50-55.

663. Mularski RA, Sippel JM, Osborne ML. Pneumoperitoneum: a review of nonsurgical causes. *Crit Care Med.* 2000;28(7):2638-2644.

664. Gayer G, Hertz M, Zissin R, et al. Postoperative pneumoperitoneum as detected by CT: prevalence, duration, and relevant factors affecting its possible significance. *Abdom Imaging.* 2000;25(3):301-305.

665. Gayer G, Hertz M, Zissin R. Postoperative pneumoperitoneum: prevalence, duration, and possible significance. *Semin Ultrasound CT MR.* 2004;25(3):286-289.

666. Cho KC, Baker SR. Extraluminal air. Diagnosis and significance. *Radiol Clin North Am.* 1994;32(5):829-844.

667. Roh JJ, Thompson JS, Harned RK, et al. Value of pneumoperitoneum in the diagnosis of visceral perforation. *Am J Surg.* 1983;146(6):830-833.

668. Winek TG, Mosely HS, Grout G, et al. Pneumoperitoneum and its association with ruptured abdominal viscus. *Arch Surg.* 1988;123(6):709-712.

669. Miller RE, Nelson SW. The roentgenologic demonstration of tiny amounts of free intraperitoneal gas: experimental and clinical studies. *Am J Roentgenol Radium Ther Nucl Med.* 1971;112(3):574-585.

670. Levine MS, Scheiner JD, Rubesin SE, et al. Diagnosis of pneumoperitoneum on supine abdominal radiographs. *AJR Am J Roentgenol.* 1991;156(4):731-735.

671. Menuck L, Siemers PT. Pneumoperitoneum: importance of right upper quadrant features. *AJR Am J Roentgenol.* 1976;127(5):753-756.

672. Earls JP, Dachman AH, Colon E, et al. Prevalence and duration of postoperative pneumoperitoneum: sensitivity of CT vs left lateral decubitus radiography. *AJR Am J Roentgenol.* 1993;161(4):781-785.

673. Stapakis JC, Thickman D. Diagnosis of pneumoperitoneum: abdominal CT vs. upright chest film. *J Comput Assist Tomogr.* 1992;16(5):713-716.

674. Feczko PJ, Mezwa DG, Farah MC, et al. Clinical significance of pneumatosis of the bowel wall. *Radiographics.* 1992;12(6): 1069-1078.

675. Ho LM, Paulson EK, Thompson WM. Pneumatosis intestinalis in the adult: benign to life-threatening causes. *AJR Am J Roentgenol.* 2007;188(6):1604-1613.

676. Lund EC, Han SY, Holley HC, et al. Intestinal ischemia: comparison of plain radiographic and computed tomographic findings. *Radiographics.* 1988;8(6):1083-1108.

677. Ho LM, Mosca PJ, Thompson WM. Pneumatosis intestinalis after lung transplant. *Abdom Imaging.* 2005;30(5):598-600.

678. Hwang J, Reddy VS, Sharp KW. Pneumatosis cystoides intestinalis with free intraperitoneal air: a case report. *Am Surg.* 2003;69(4):346-349.

679. Wood BJ, Kumar PN, Cooper C, et al. Pneumatosis intestinalis in adults with AIDS: clinical significance and imaging findings. *AJR Am J Roentgenol.* 1995;165(6):1387-1390.

680. Pear BL. Pneumatosis intestinalis: a review. *Radiology.* 1998;207(1):13-19.

681. Galandiuk S, Fazio VW. Pneumatosis cystoides intestinalis. A review of the literature. *Dis Colon Rectum.* 1986;29(5): 358-363.

682. Berk JE, Bockus HL. *Bockus gastroenterology.* 4th ed. Philadelphia, PA: Saunders; 1985:1-7, v.

683. Koss LG. Abdominal gas cysts (pneumatosis cystoides intestinorum hominis); an analysis with a report of a case and a critical review of the literature. *AMA Arch Pathol.* 1952;53(6):523-549.

684. St Peter SD, Abbas MA, Kelly KA. The spectrum of pneumatosis intestinalis. *Arch Surg.* 2003;138(1):68-75.

685. Caudill JL, Rose BS. The role of computed tomography in the evaluation of pneumatosis intestinalis. *J Clin Gastroenterol.* 1987;9(2):223-226.

686. Connor R, Jones B, Fishman EK, et al. Pneumatosis intestinalis: role of computed tomography in diagnosis and management. *J Comput Assist Tomogr.* 1984;8(2):269-275.

687. Federle MP, Chun G, Jeffrey RB, et al. Computed tomographic findings in bowel infarction. *AJR Am J Roentgenol.* 1984;142(1): 91-95.

688. Hutchins WW, Gore RM, Foley MJ. CT demonstration of pneumatosis intestinalis from bowel infarction. *Comput Radiol.* 1983;7(5):283-285.

689. Kelvin FM, Korobkin M, Rauch RF, et al. Computed tomography of pneumatosis intestinalis. *J Comput Assist Tomogr.* 1984;8(2):276-280.

690. Meyers MA, Ghahremani GG, Clements JL Jr, et al. Pneumatosis intestinalis. *Gastrointest Radiol.* 1977;2(2):91-105.

691. Schindera ST, Triller J, Vock P, et al. Detection of hepatic portal venous gas: its clinical impact and outcome. *Emerg Radiol.* 2006;12(4):164-170.

692. Smerud MJ, Johnson CD, Stephens DH. Diagnosis of bowel infarction: a comparison of plain films and CT scans in 23 cases. *AJR Am J Roentgenol.* 1990;154(1):99-103.

693. Knechtle SJ, Davidoff AM, Rice RP. Pneumatosis intestinalis. Surgical management and clinical outcome. *Ann Surg.* 1990;212(2):160-165.

694. Fisher JK. Computed tomography of colonic pneumatosis intestinalis with mesenteric and portal venous air. *J Comput Assist Tomogr.* 1984;8(3):573-574.

695. Epelman M, Daneman A, Navarro OM, et al. Necrotizing enterocolitis: review of state-of-the-art imaging findings with pathologic correlation. *Radiographics.* 2007;27(2):285-305.

696. Wiesner W, Mortele KJ, Glickman JN, et al. Pneumatosis intestinalis and portomesenteric venous gas in intestinal ischemia: correlation of CT findings with severity of ischemia and clinical outcome. *AJR Am J Roentgenol.* 2001;177(6): 1319-1323.

697. Kernagis LY, Levine MS, Jacobs JE. Pneumatosis intestinalis in patients with ischemia: correlation of CT findings with viability of the bowel. *AJR Am J Roentgenol.* 2003;180(3): 733-736.

698. Liebman PR, Patten MT, Manny J, et al. Hepatic—portal venous gas in adults: etiology, pathophysiology and clinical significance. *Ann Surg.* 1978;187(3):281-287.

699. Wiesner W, Mortele KJ, Glickman JN, et al. Portal-venous gas unrelated to mesenteric ischemia. *Eur Radiol.* 2002;12(6): 1432-1437.

700. Hou SK, Chern CH, How CK, et al. Hepatic portal venous gas: clinical significance of computed tomography findings. *Am J Emerg Med.* 2004;22(3):214-218.

701. Huurman VA, Visser LG, Steens SC, et al. Persistent portal venous gas. *J Gastrointest Surg.* 2006;10(5):783-785.

702. Griffith J, Apostolakos M, and Salloum RM. Pneumatosis intestinalis and gas in the portal venous system. *J Gastrointest Surg.* 2006;10(5):781-782.

703. Ghahremani GG, White EM, Hoff FL, et al. Appendices epiploicae of the colon: radiologic and pathologic features. *Radiographics.* 1992;12(1):59-77.

704. Legome EL, Sims C, Rao PM. Epiploic appendagitis: adding to the differential of acute abdominal pain. *J Emerg Med.* 1999;17(5):823-826.

705. Rao PM, Wittenberg J, Lawrason JN. Primary epiploic appendagitis: evolutionary changes in CT appearance. *Radiology.* 1997;204(3):713-717.

706. Torres GM, Abbitt PL, Weeks M. CT manifestations of infarcted epiploic appendages of the colon. *Abdom Imaging.* 1994;19(5):449-450.

707. Legome EL, Belton AL, Murray RE, et al. Epiploic appendagitis: the emergency department presentation. *J Emerg Med.* 2002;22(1):9-13.

708. van Breda Vriesman AC, de Mol van Otterloo AJ, Puylaert JB. Epiploic appendagitis and omental infarction. *Eur J Surg.* 2001;167(10):723-727.

709. Epstein LI, Lempke RE. Primary idiopathic segmental infarction of the greater omentum: case report and collective review of the literature. *Ann Surg.* 1968;167(3): 437-443.

710. Puylaert JB. Right-sided segmental infarction of the omentum: clinical, US, and CT findings. *Radiology.* 1992;185(1):169-172.

711. Puylaert JB. Ultrasonography of the acute abdomen: gastrointestinal conditions. *Radiol Clin North Am.* 2003;41(6):1227-1242, vii.

CHAPTER

Imaging of the Liver

Mark Alan Rosen, MD, PhD
Stanley Chan, MD
Wallace T. Miller Jr., MD

NORMAL HEPATIC ANATOMY

The liver primarily lies in the right upper quadrant, underneath the right hemidiaphragm, although in most individuals the left portion of the liver will cross the midline of the upper abdomen into the left upper quadrant. With the exception of a small portion of the posterior liver bordering the diaphragm, the liver is invested by the peritoneum, and is thus a peritoneal organ. The surface anatomy of the liver is categorized by various peritoneal reflections, including the falciform ligament (residual ligaments from the embryonic coelomic cavity reflection), the ligamentum teres (peritoneal investment about the residual umbilical vein), and the ligamentum venosum (peritoneal investment about the residual ductus venosum between the left portal vein and the inferior vena cava [IVC]). Posteriorly and inferiorly, the liver is bordered by the gallbladder (within the gallbladder fossa), the duodenum, the hepatic flexure of the colon, and the IVC.

The falciform ligament connects the liver to the diaphragm, and divides the anatomic right and left lobes. The ligamentum teres extends inferiorly from the falciform ligament toward the anterior abdominal wall. The liver also has attachments through the gastrohepatic ligament (which connect the liver to the stomach, and through which the left gastric artery and vein run), and the hepaticoduodenal ligament (connecting the liver to the duodenum, and through which run the gastroduodenal artery and vein).

The liver is functionally served by 2 distinct vascular supplies, the hepatic artery and the portal vein, with blood exiting via the 3 hepatic veins (right, middle, and left) and into the IVC. Functionally, the liver is divided into right and left lobes (distinct from the anatomic lobes). The functional left lobe is supplied by the left hepatic and left portal vein branches, whereas the right lobe is supplied by the right hepatic and right portal vein branches. The boundary between the right and left lobes on cross-sectional imaging is defined by the middle hepatic vein superiorly, and the gallbladder fossa inferiorly. The left lobe is divided by the falciform ligament into the left lateral segment and the left medial segment (also termed the quadrate lobe). The right lobe is divided by the right hepatic vein into the anterior and posterior segments. The caudate lobe is a small, more isolated area of the liver between the portal vein and the ligamentum venosum and has a more variable arterial and portal vein supply, as well as variant venous drainage.

Surgically, the liver is often divided into smaller segments, defined by the Couinaud system. The Couinaud system uses the existing functional lobar anatomy and further divides these segments superiorly/inferiorly by the plane of the portal vein. Couinaud segment I represents the caudate lobe; segments II and III represent the superior and inferior portions of the left lateral segment, respectively; segments IVa and IVb represent the superior and inferior portions of the left lobe medial segment (quadrate lobe), respectively. In the right lobe, the Couinaud segments begin in the inferior aspect of the anterior right lobe and run clockwise (when the liver is viewed from the anterior aspect). Thus, segment V is the inferior right anterior segment, segment VI the inferior right posterior segment, segment VII the superior posterior right segment, and segment VIII the superior right anterior segment (see Figure 3-1).

The porta hepatis region is the root of the liver, where the proper hepatic artery, the main portal vein, and the common hepatic duct lie. The primary lymphatic drainage of the liver also lies in this region, although secondary lymphatic drainage may exist about the hepatic capsule areas, particularly across the diaphragm to the cardiophrenic lymph nodes.

IMAGING OF THE LIVER

In current radiology practice, 3 imaging techniques: ultrasonography (US), computed tomography (CT), and magnetic resonance imaging (MRI), have become the mainstay of liver imaging. The general principles of these imaging techniques are discussed in Chapter 1. However, for liver evaluation, specific technical details for optimization of these techniques are discussed below. Also, for certain disorders, these cross-sectional imaging methods may be supplemented by other imaging modalities, including angiography, cholangiography, and nuclear medicine techniques. In the field of cancer imaging (within the liver and elsewhere in the body), fluorodeoxyglucose positron emission tomography (FDG-PET) has become ubiquitous and will often be used as the primary means of cancer staging, including depiction of hepatic metastatic disease. Imaging of the biliary system is often an important component of liver assessment, either directly (through endoscopic retrograde cholangiopancreatography [ERCP] or transhepatic cholangiography [THC]), or indirectly (via magnetic resonance cholangiopancreatography [MRCP]). The appearance of biliary abnormalities with these techniques is discussed in detail in Chapter 4.

US Evaluation of the Liver

US imaging of the liver is often performed in conjunction with dedicated imaging of the gallbladder and biliary system (discussed in Chapter 4), with the patient in the fasting state to ensure adequate gallbladder distention with bile. Parenchymal evaluation with US is a routine part of any hepatobiliary US examination, and can include Doppler interrogation of the hepatic vasculature when required to exclude vascular abnormalities. Though not used routinely in clinical examinations, microbubble intravenous (IV) contrast agents can greatly enhance the US examination of the liver,[1] and has been used to more efficaciously identify and characterize focal liver lesions.[2-4]

Normal hepatic parenchyma is uniformly hypoechoic in US imaging bounded by the more hyperechoic ligaments, capsule, and diaphragmatic surface (see Figure 3-2). The vascular structures in the liver are generally anechoic on non-Doppler imaging. Intrahepatic biliary ducts are

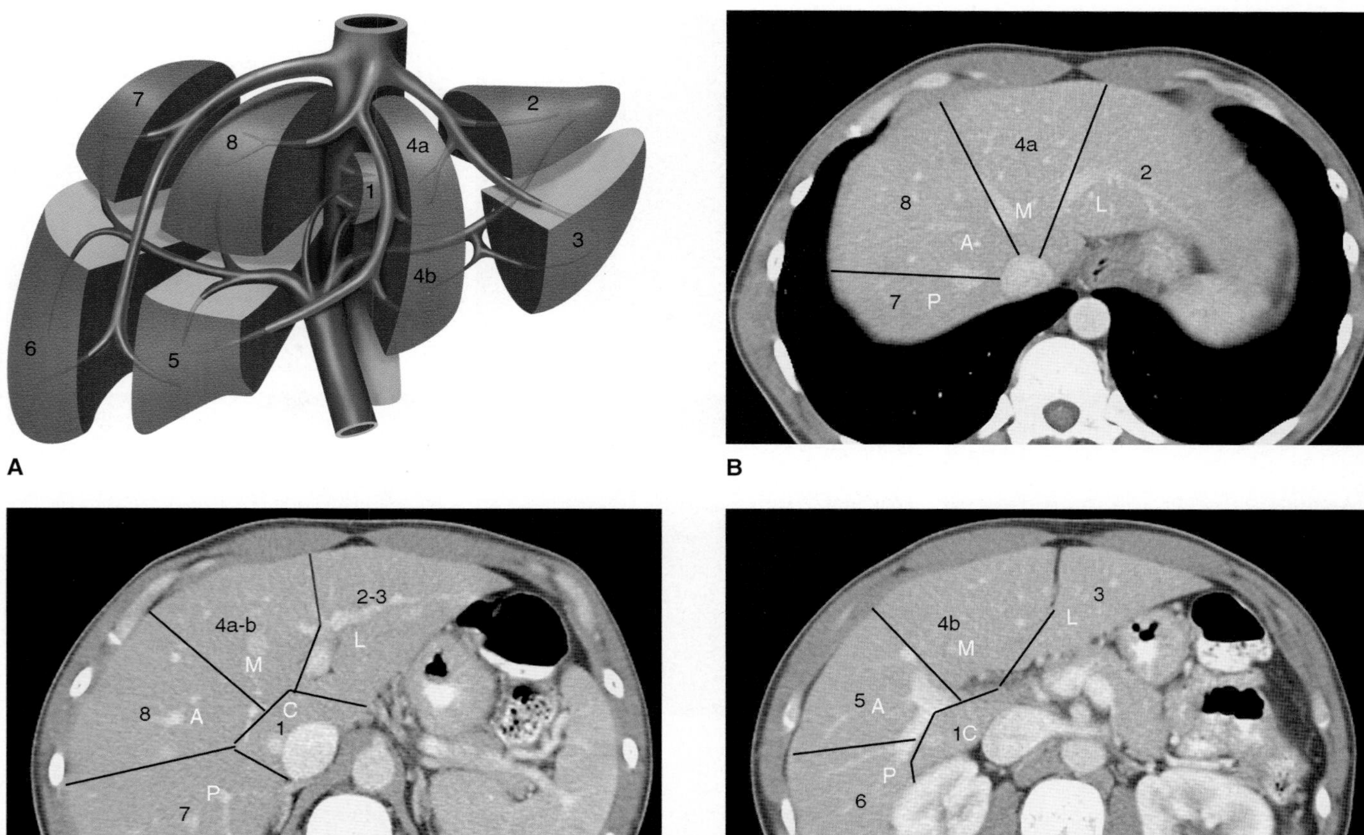

Figure 3-1 Liver Segments and the Couinaud Division of the Liver In the Couinaud system, the liver is divided vertically by radiating planes created by the hepatic veins and horizontally by the right and left portal veins, with the caudate lobe acting as a separate unit. These divisions are illustrated in the 3-dimensional figure in (**A**) and in the axial images (**B-D**) and are numbered in black lettering. The conventional division of the liver is performed only by the vertical division along the hepatic veins and are annotated with white lettering (A, anterior; P, posterior; M, medial; L, lateral). Thus, the liver is divided into right and left lobes by the middle hepatic vein. The right lobe is divided into anterior and posterior segments by the right hepatic vein, and the left hepatic lobe is divided into medial and lateral segments by the plane from the left hepatic vein to the falciform ligament. Thus, Couinaud regions 2 and 3 make up the lateral segment, Counaud regions 4a and 4b make up the medial segment, Counaud regions 5 and 8 make up the anterior segment, and Couinaud regions 6 and 7 make up the posterior segment. The small portion of the liver immediately adjacent to the inferior vena cava (C) is called the caudate lobe or segment 1 and is separated from the remainder of the liver because it drains directly into the inferior vena cava rather than through the hepatic veins like most of the remainder of the liver. (Part A: Reproduced, with permission, from Smithuis R. Liver: Segmental Anatomy. 7-5-2006 http://www.radiologyassistant.nl/en/4375bb8dc241d.)

usually not well-seen on US imaging, except when dilated, when they are noted as anechoic tubular structures. The bile ducts have relatively hyperechoic walls, whereas the portal veins have imperceptible walls on US examinations, a feature that can help identify biliary ductal dilation.

CT Evaluation of the Liver

CT imaging of the liver is almost always performed with iodinated contrast agents administered IV, except when contraindicated because of patient allergy or impaired renal function. In certain instances, for example, suspected hepatocellular carcinoma (HCC) or hypervascular liver metastases, the examination can include a dedicated "arterial-phase" image, generally acquired 20 to 30 seconds after rapid IV bolus contrast administration, in order to improve conspicuity of hypervascular liver lesions.[5,6] Precontrast imaging may also be required, for example, to exclude fatty infiltration of the liver[7,8] or to aid in determining if focally treated liver lesions (such as following

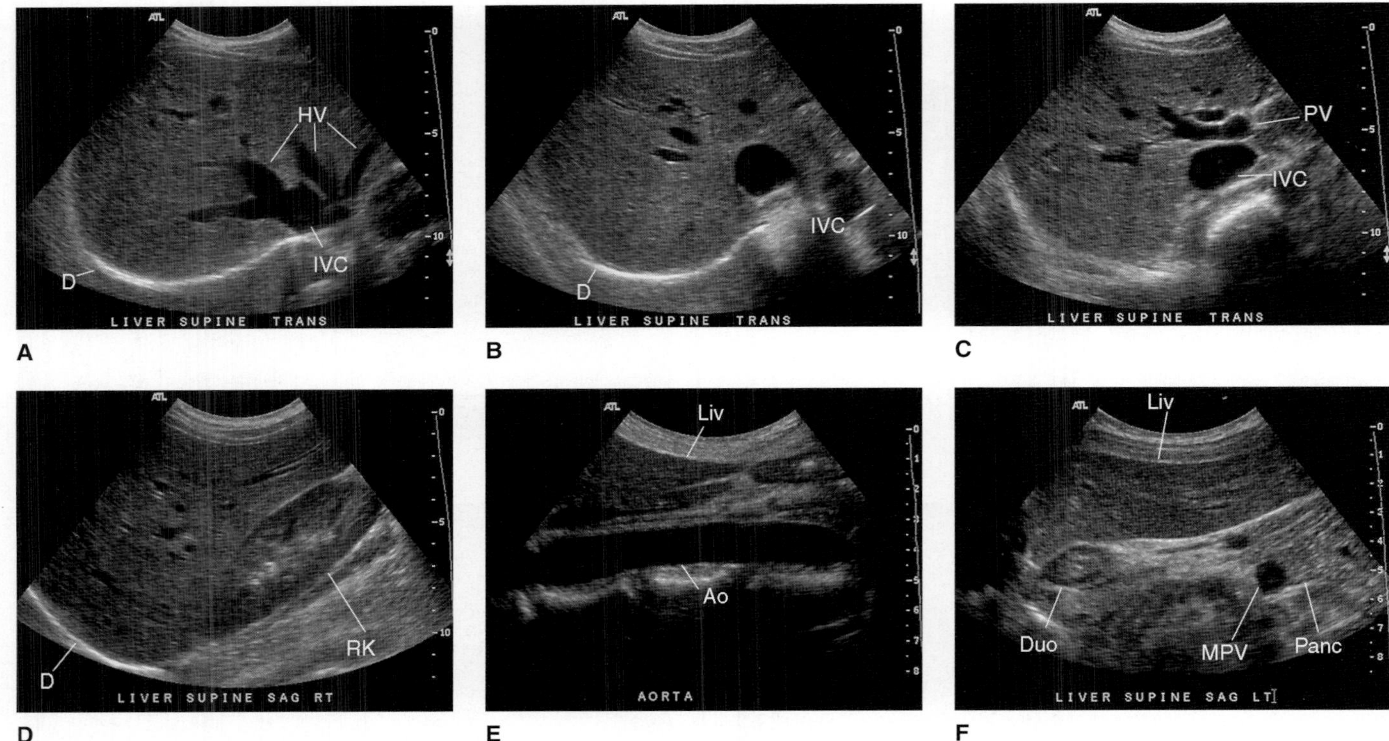

Figure 3-2 Normal US of Liver
A-C. Transaxial US images of the liver from superior to inferior locations and (**D-F**) sagittal US images of the liver from right to left. D, diaphragm; HV, hepatic veins; IVC, inferior vena cava; PV, portal veins; RK, right kidney; Ao, aorta; Liv, liver; Duo, duodenum; MPV, main portal vein; Panc, pancreas.

chemoembolization with radiopaque embolic agents) contain areas of enhancing viable tissue.[9,10] When cholangiocarcinoma is suspected or known to be present, imaging in the delayed phase of contrast (roughly 15 minutes after administration) may also be useful to improve conspicuity of these tumors.[11,12]

On CT imaging, the normal liver is relatively hyperintense, even in the absence of contrast, with more hypointense vascular structures. On contrast-enhanced imaging, the parenchyma enhances uniformly, with more hyperintense vessels, depending on the phase of dynamic contrast administration (see Figure 3-3).

MRI of the Liver

MRI of the liver will always include imaging with both T1- and T2-weighted contrast, in order to provide means of characterizing focal and diffuse liver abnormalities. T1-weighted imaging is in particular useful because of the relatively high T1 signal intensity of normal liver, and comparable high T1 signal intensity of focal lesions derived from hepatocellular lineage (ie, focal nodular hyperplasia [FNH], hepatic adenoma, and HCC). T1-weighted imaging will also in general utilize chemical shift–sensitive techniques (eg, "Dixon," or "in-phase/opposed-phase" imaging) in order to demonstrate features of fatty infiltration in focal lesions and/or background hepatic tissue.[13-15] Specialized, heavily T2-weighted (fluid-weighted) imaging to depict ductal structures, also known as MRCP is also a part of the liver MRI study, and is discussed in more detail in Chapter 4.

Gadolinium-enhanced T1-weighted imaging is routinely used in liver evaluation, except when contraindicated in the rare patient with gadolinium allergy, or in patients who are susceptible to nephrogenic sclerosing fibrosis (NSF) because of impaired renal function.[16] As MRI does not produce ionizing radiation, repeated imaging does not pose additional risk to the patient, and multiphase T1 imaging before and during IV bolus administration of gadolinium is the norm, including arterial-, portal-, and delayed-phase imaging. When imaging is performed with newer gadolinium contrast agents that undergo hepatobiliary excretion, the contrast-enhanced examination can be supplemented with delayed biliary-phase imaging. This phase of imaging has been shown to be useful for improving conspicuity and characterization of focal liver lesions.[17,18]

Iron oxide–based contrast agents are also available for liver MRI. Although these agents will also produce T1 shortening (brightening on imaging), they are often not approved for high-rate bolus injection, thus limiting their ability to act effectively as gadolinium T1 shortening agents for liver MRI. However, the iron oxide particles are selectively taken

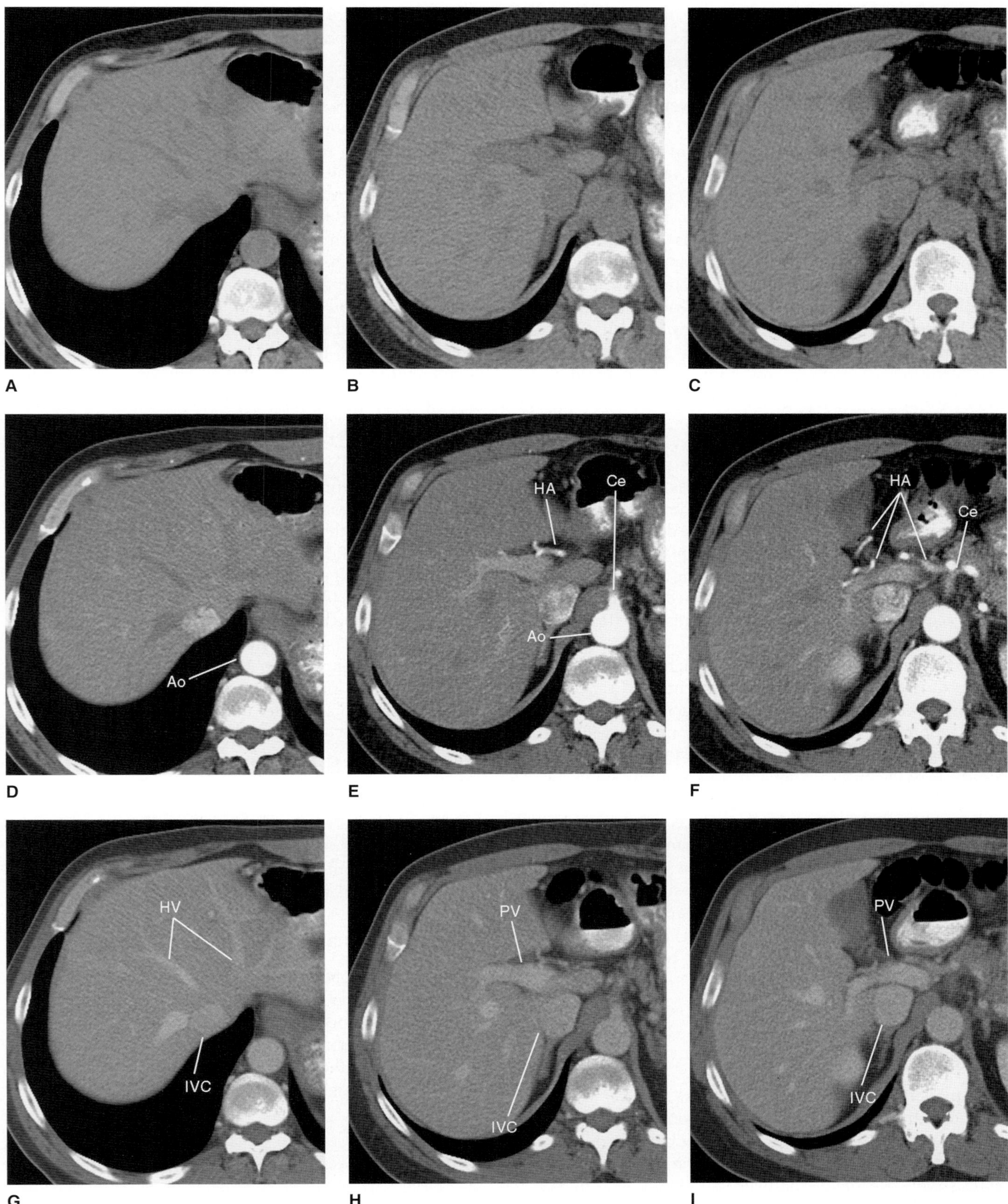

Figure 3-3 Normal CT of the Liver
A-C. Unenhanced, (**D-F**) arterial phase, and (**G-I**) portal venous phase CT images of the liver. Note how the arteries are much brighter and the veins remain unopacified in the arterial phase. During the venous phase, both the arteries and the veins are brighter than the normal liver but less so than the arteries on the arterial phase. HA, hepatic artery; Ao, aorta; Ce, celiac axis; IVC, inferior vena cava; HV, hepatic veins; PV, (main) portal vein.

up by the reticuloendothelial system, including the Kupffer cells in the liver. This leads to modest T2 and marked T2* shortening of the liver parenchyma, whereas liver lesions are spared this shortening. As such, most focal liver lesions will appear as brighter objects on T2*-weighted sequences performed after administration of these iron oxide contrast agents.[19,20] However, distribution times of these agents into the liver reticuloendothelial system may vary, and timing of optimal T2* liver imaging with these agents may vary.[21-23]

On MRI, the liver is uniformly hyperintense on T1-weighted imaging, and is hypointense on T2-weighted imaging. Intrahepatic vessels generally appear hypointense on T1 imaging, and hyperintense on T2 imaging, although rapidly flowing blood, such as in the IVC or portal vein, may appear hypointense on spin-echo imaging because of the phenomenon of "flow voids" (see Figure 3-4). Like all fluid structures, biliary ducts are low signal on T1 imaging, and very high signal on T2 imaging (the latter being the basis of MRCP, discussed in detail in Chapter 4). Post gadolinium, the T1-weighted appearance of the liver is similar to that of CT, with a uniformly enhancing liver parenchyma, and more avidly enhanced vascular structures (see Figure 3-4).

More recently, diffusion-weighted imaging (DWI) by MRI has been studied as a method for the detection and classification of liver lesions. In DWI, echo-planar T2-weighted images are acquired with and without the addition of oppositely paired diffusion gradients, applied briefly prior to signal acquisition. The diffusion gradients serve to diphase MR signal intensity from water in various tissues. In cases where the mobility of tissue water is highly restricted, the effects of the opposed diffusion gradients will cancel out each other, leaving signal intensity intact. In cases where water mobility is higher, random water motion will occur between the paired gradients, leading to incomplete compensation of the phase dispersion, and resulting signal loss.

Application of DWI in the liver has demonstrated that malignant tumors display a higher degree of restricted diffusion than background liver parenchyma.[24] This results in tumors displaying relatively brighter signal on images with stronger diffusion gradients. Resulting DWI and apparent diffusion coefficient (ADC) maps can be used to document areas of restricted diffusion, leading in some cases to improved detection and staging of malignant liver lesions.[25,26]

Multiphase Vascular Imaging of the Liver with CT and MRI

With modern CT and MRI techniques, the liver is often imaged with a dynamic or multiphase contrast protocol. In this regimen, the dynamic appearance of the liver enhancement can be shown, reflecting the unique nature of hepatic blood supply. Normally, the liver will obtain 20% to 25% of its blood supply from the hepatic artery, whereas the remaining 75% to 80% of the supply derives from the portal vein. Although this ratio can be altered in certain pathologic conditions, such as cirrhosis and portal hypertension, the basic premise of dual vascular supply, with the majority supply from the portal circulation, remains true in almost all individuals.

During bolus IV contrast enhancement, the hepatic artery receives the initial pass of high-concentration contrast from the aorta sooner than does the portal vein, because the latter receives contrast only after it has passed through the splenic and mesenteric circulation. Relative to the rather rapid transit of contrast from the aorta to the hepatic artery and then the liver, the circulation time from aorta to portal vein in the normal patient is generally 30 to 40 seconds longer. As such, the use of multiphase serial breathhold imaging during enhanced CT or MRI allows for evaluation of hepatic vascular physiology. In multiphase imaging, the liver parenchyma will enhance modestly in the early (arterial) phase of imaging but will demonstrate peak enhancement during the portal phase, when filling of the portal sinusoids with contrast yields maximal signal enhancement (see Figure 3-4).

More-delayed postcontrast imaging can also be employed, usually to define pathologies with delayed hyperenhancement. After peak portal phase enhancement, the liver and associated vascular structures will gradually lose contrast, with the blood vessels maintaining higher contrast levels and hence brighter appearance on CT or MRI. After several minutes, the degree of signal difference between liver and blood vessels will be minimal, a phenomenon that will also be seen on MRI, though the liver–blood vessel contrast generally persists for a longer time in MRI. Very delayed biliary-phase MRI may be performed with specialized gadolinium contrast agents with partial biliary excretion, as discussed later in this chapter.

UNIFOCAL, SPHERICAL LIVER LESIONS

Unifocal liver lesions can be subdivided into those that are roughly spherical in shape, typically called masses when large and nodules when small. Spherical lesions can be further subdivided into those that are cystic or cystic appearing and those that are solid appearing.

Solitary Cysts and Cystic-Appearing Lesions

Cystic or cystic-appearing nodules or masses of the liver are derived from 3 classes of lesions: idiopathic cysts, cystic or cystic-appearing neoplasms, and abscesses. The most common of these lesions are simple cysts and hemangiomas, but a variety of other neoplastic and infections lesions are represented by this category (Table 3-1).

Idiopathic cysts

Simple hepatic cysts are among the most commonly discovered abnormalities of the abdomen on cross-sectional imaging examinations. These are idiopathic abnormalities of the liver with no clinical significance, other than that they can be confused with metastasis and other hepatic neoplasms. They are more commonly multiple rather than

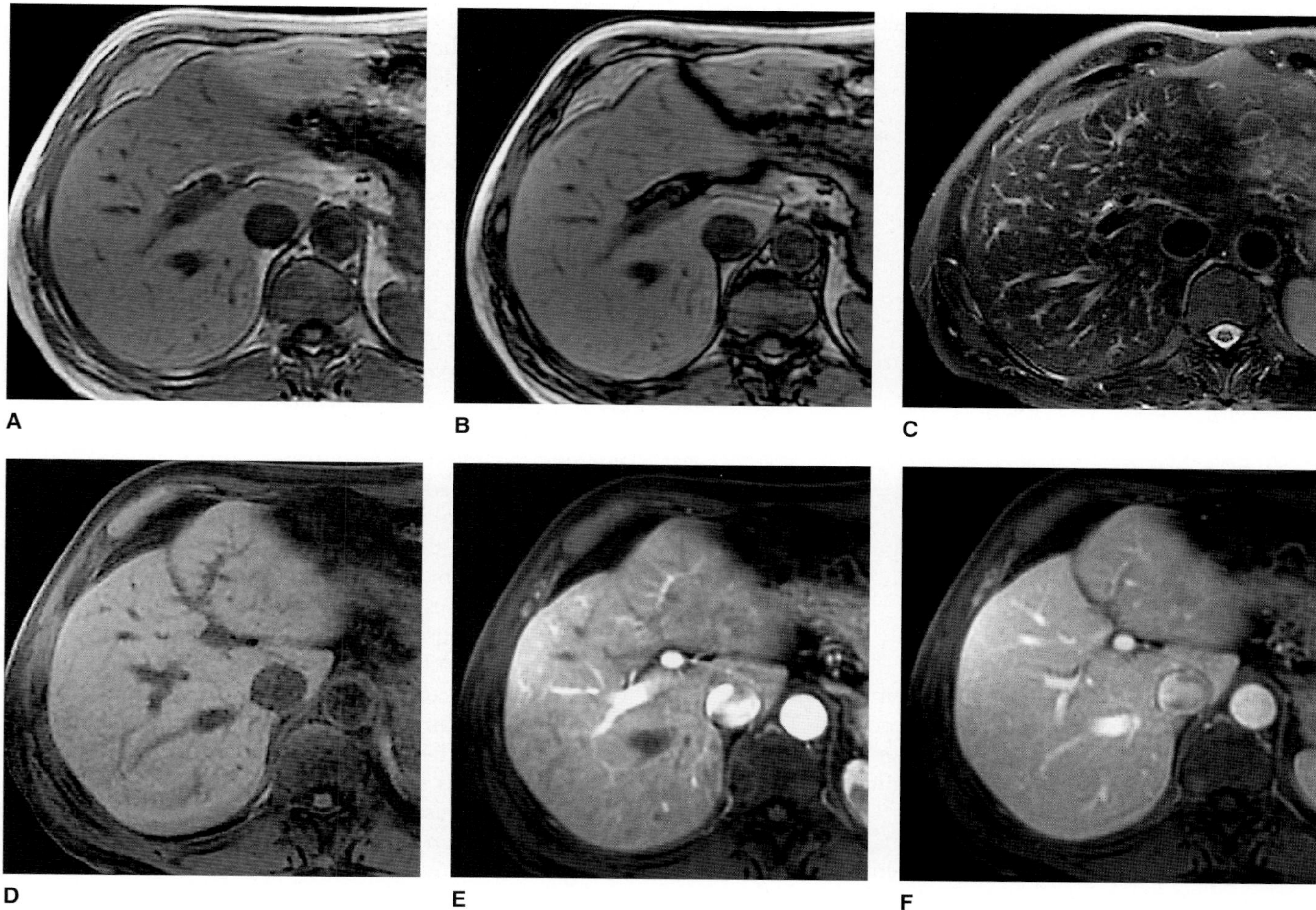

Figure 3-4 MRI of the Normal Liver
MRI of the liver seen in (**A**) T1-weighted in-phase, (**B**) T1-weighted opposed-phase, and (**C**) fat-saturated T2-weighted images. Hepatic parenchyma is bright on T1-weighted image and dark on T2-weighted images. Hepatic ducts are bright on T2-weighted images (C). Hepatic vessels are dark on T1-weighted images, whereas appearance on T2-weighted imaging is variable based on velocity and direction of blood flow. Dynamic enhanced imaging of the liver includes a (**D**) pregadolinium T1-weighted fat-saturated image, demonstrating intermediately bright hepatic parenchyma and dark vessels. Only bowel contents and pancreas (not shown) are brighter than liver on fat-saturated T1-weighted imaging. (**E**) During the late arterial phase of gadolinium-enhanced imaging, there is mild enhancement of the hepatic parenchyma, with enhancement of both hepatic arteries and variably early filling of the portal vein. (**F**) On portal-phase imaging, the portal sinusoids have filled, leading to peak liver parenchymal enhancement.

solitary[27] and are therefore discussed in detail in the subsequent heading: **Multifocal Lesions of the Liver**.

Solitary cystic or cystic appearing neoplasms

There are a variety of benign of malignant liver masses that can appear cystic on imaging examinations. The most common of these is the hepatic hemangioma, but also included are biliary hamartomas, mucinous cystadenoma/cystadenocarcinoma, epithelioid hemangioendotheliomas (EHEs), and liver metastasis.

Hemangiomas: Hemangiomas are the most common benign tumor of the liver[28] and are usually incidentally discovered on cross-sectional imaging performed for unrelated reasons. Although hemangiomas are solid vascular tumors, because they are largely composed of blood-filled channels, they can have imaging features of a cystic lesion on CT and MRI examinations. They are typically asymptomatic, and although rarely, when very large they can be painful, necessitating surgical resection.[29] In infants, large hemangiomas can result in significant shunting of blood and cause high-output congestive heart failure.[30] Their major clinical significance is the confusion with malignant hepatic masses on imaging.

On US, hepatic hemangiomas appear densely echogenic, because of the multitude of vascular channels, which act as acoustic interfaces reflecting the sound beam (see Figure 3-5).[31,32] Although the vast majority of echogenic

Table 3-1. Solitary Cystic-Appearing Nodules or Masses of the Liver

1. Idiopathic cyst a. **Simple**[a] b. **Complex**
2. Neoplasms a. **Hemangioma** b. Biliary hamartoma c. Biliary cystadenoma/cystadenocarcinoma d. Cystic and mucinous metastasis e. Epithelioid hemangioendothelioma
3. Abscesses a. **Pyogenic** b. Amoebic c. Echinococcal
4. Hematoma

[a]Lesions in bold are most common.

masses in the liver will represent hemangiomas, some malignancies can also appear hyperechoic.[33] Therefore, depending on the clinical scenario, hyperechoic masses on hepatic US may require additional imaging evaluation with CT or MRI to ensure benignity.

With the advent of dynamic helical CT scanning, multiphase contrast-enhanced CT has been shown to demonstrate with high accuracy the characteristic imaging pattern of hemangiomas. On unenhanced CT, hemangiomas will typically appear as uniform, low-attenuation nodules or masses that resemble hepatic cysts. On early (arterial-phase) imaging, hemangiomas will demonstrate incomplete globular peripheral enhancement, termed *discontinuous peripheral enhancement*. On more delayed-phase contrast CT imaging, increasing portions of the hemangioma will enhance from the periphery of the lesion to the center of the lesion, a phenomenon termed *centripetal enhancement* (see Figure 3-5).[34-38] On later phase images, the hemangioma will, typically, enhance uniformly and intensely.

More recently, MRI has become the modality of choice in many institutions for characterizing hepatic lesions as a hemangioma, avoiding the radiation exposure of multiphase CT studies. Like cysts, hemangiomas are classically markedly hyperintense to liver on T2-weighted imaging.[39,40] Furthermore, when imaged with greater degrees of T2 weighting (ie, longer echo times), hemangiomas and cysts will become more hyperintense relative to background liver, whereas metastases or other solid hepatic lesions will become less intense (see Figure 3-5). MRI can also demonstrate dense centripetal enhancement following gadolinium administration similar to that seen with CT scans.[41,42]

On occasion, the imaging appearance of hemangiomas on enhanced CT or MRI will differ from the typical features seen in most cases.[43] Very small hemangiomas will often demonstrate diffuse, uniform, early enhancement termed *flash-filling*, resembling a hypervascular solid mass.[44,45] Unlike hypervascular masses, flash-filling hemangiomas will usually remain hyperintense on more delayed imaging, paralleling the degree of aortic enhancement. When a hepatic lesion is shown to be uniformly hyperintense on early-phase contrast–enhanced imaging, portal- or delayed-phase imaging can be used to distinguish between a flash-filling hemangioma and other hypervascular solid masses. Hemangiomas will remain hyperintense on more delayed postcontrast imaging, whereas other hypervascular neoplasms will typically become more isointense with background parenchyma on portal- and delayed-phase imaging (see Figure 3-6).

Larger hemangiomas can also demonstrate an atypical imaging appearance, especially those that have undergone partial internal sclerosis. These lesions may enhance slowly, and portions may never enhance. Usually, careful inspection of the lesion on dynamic enhanced imaging will demonstrate the characteristic early nodular discontinuous peripheral enhancement.[46] When the character of a large hepatic lesion is uncertain by US or CT, MRI will often be definitive in diagnosing a hemangioma, because of both the high sensitivity of MRI to gadolinium enhancement and the added value of the T2-weighted imaging appearance. In rare circumstances, giant or sclerosed hemangiomas may require additional imaging with technetium-labeled red blood cells (RBCs), or even biopsy, to confirm the nature of these lesions.[47,48]

Traditionally, hepatic hemangiomas could be diagnosed through a nuclear medicine scan with technetium-99m–labeled RBCs (tagged RBC) study.[49] In this study, hemangiomas appeared as focally high activity nodules or masses within the liver parenchyma. However, tagged RBCs are insensitive for smaller hemangiomata.[50,51] With the improvements in liver US, the advent of dynamic

Imaging Notes 3-1. Imaging Features of Hepatic Hemangiomas

US	Hyperechoic nodule
Noncontrast CT	Hypoattenuating nodule
Noncontrast MRI	Uniformly hyperintense nodule on T2-weighted sequences
Contrast CT/MRI	Discontinuous globular peripheral enhancement
	Centripetal enhancement over time
	Uniform dense enhancement (parallels aortic enhancement)

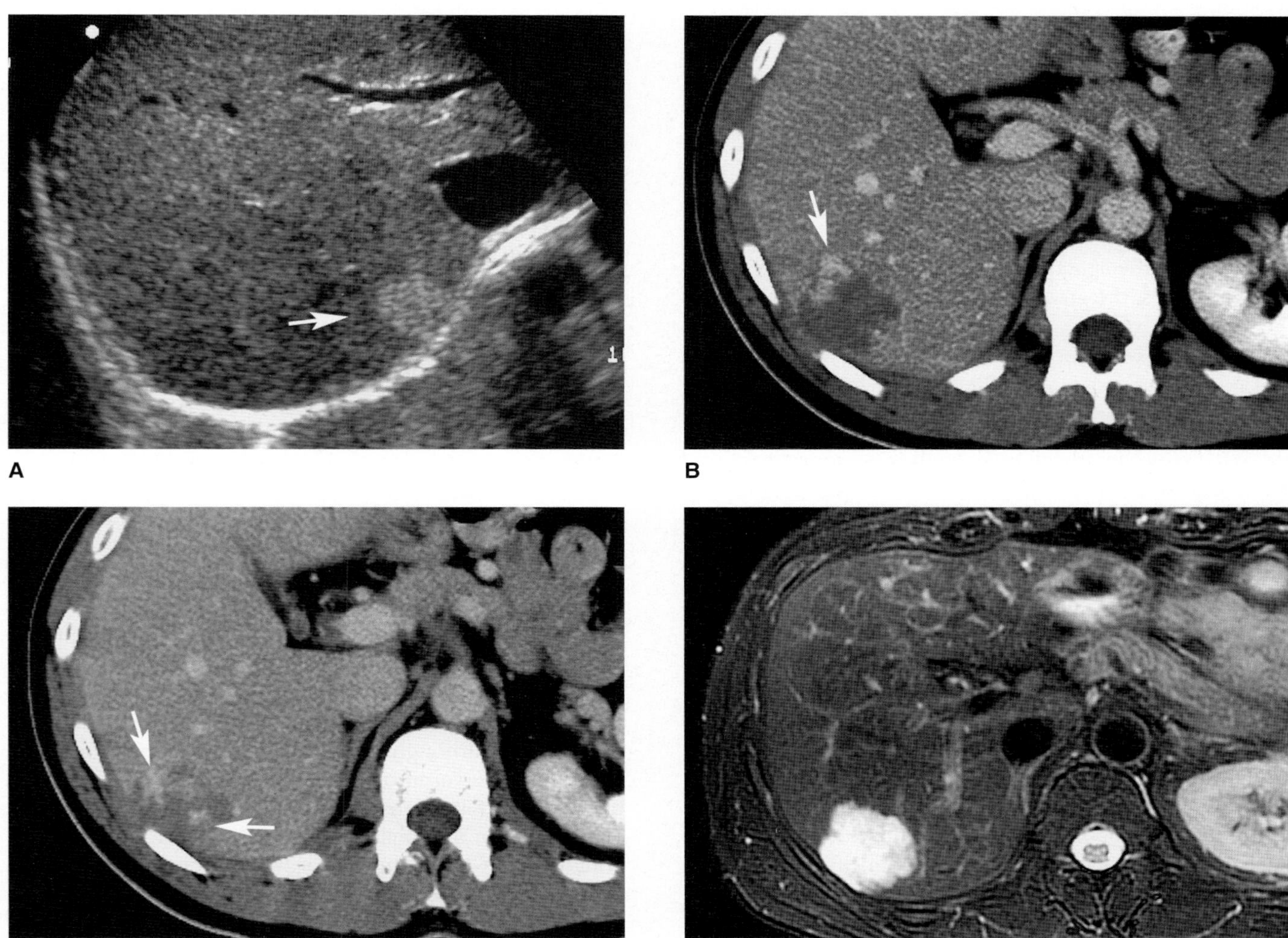

Figure 3-5 Typical Hepatic Hemangioma in 2 Patients
A. This 36-year-old woman had right upper quadrant pain. Axial US image through the liver demonstrates an echogenic mass in the right lobe of the liver. This finding will usually represent a hepatic hemangioma, which was confirmed by T2-weighted MRI (not shown). **B-D.** This 58-year-old man had rectal carcinoma. Contrast-enhanced CT scan (B and C) through the liver shows a low-attenuation mass with small puddles of contrast in the peripheral aspects of the mass (*arrows*). Although this man is at risk for hepatic metastasis, the appearance of this mass is diagnostic of a hepatic hemangioma. T2-weighted MRI examination of the liver (D) shows a lobulated, very intense (*bright white*) mass also diagnostic of a hepatic hemangioma.

helical CT, and the evolution of liver MRI, the use of labeled red cell scans to confirm the identity of suspected hemangiomas is now uncommon.

Biliary hamartoma: Biliary hamartomas are small benign tumors of the bile ducts with interspersed fibrous or hyaline stroma. These are relatively common hepatic lesions, occurring in slightly less than 1% of autopsies and characteristically appear as small simple cysts.[52-57] Occasionally, they can occur as a solitary lesion. Biliary hamartomas are discussed most completely under the heading **Multiple Cystic or Cystic-Appearing Liver Masses**.

Biliary cystadenoma and cystadenocarcinoma: Biliary cystadenoma and cystadenocarcinoma are rare mucin-producing cystic neoplasms of the biliary system that resemble mucinous cystic neoplasms of the pancreas and ovary. Biliary cystadenomas are typically seen in women, particularly in the fifth to sixth decade of life,[58] whereas malignant biliary cystadenocarcinomas can be seen in both men and women.[59] Typically, cystadenomas and cystadenocarcinomas will histologically contain both hepatobiliary epithelium and ovarian stromal tissues.[60]

Cross-sectional imaging typically demonstrates a multilocular cystic mass.[61] The fluid contents of the cyst will have the usual imaging features of fluid on US, CT,

Imaging Notes 3-2. Imaging Features of Biliary Cystadenoma/Cystadenocarcinoma

- Cystic mass with internal septations
- Cyst contents can be simple or complex fluid
- Connection to intrahepatic bile ducts can be seen in some cases
- The thicker the septations and the larger the solid components, the greater the likelihood of malignancy

and MRI. However, those cases with mucinous secretions can demonstrate more hyperintense T1 signal intensity on MRI examinations.[62] Connection to the intrahepatic ducts can be demonstrated in some cases,[63] particularly on T2-weighted MRI and MRCP sequences.[64] The walls of the biliary cystadenomas will usually be very thin, although the tumor will often demonstrate fine internal septations that can be detected on cross-sectional imaging, particularly on T2-weighted MRI and US. Contrast-enhanced imaging by CT and MRI can also demonstrate fine internal septations in some cases (see Figure 3-7). In many cases, the distinction between benign biliary cystadenomas and malignant cystadenocarcinomas is impossible. In general, the greater the proportion of solid elements and the thicker the walls, the greater the likelihood that the neoplasm is malignant. The presence of enhancing papillary nodules also increases the likelihood of malignancy.[61,63,65]

Epithelioid hemangioendothelioma: Most commonly found in women in their mid 40's, EHEs are rare malignant tumors that are typically found in the periphery of the liver.[66] They are more common than the more highly aggressive angiosarcomas, and EHEs represent 1% of all vascular hepatic neoplasms.[67] Epithelioid hemangioendotheliomas have an abundance of myxoid and fibrous stroma resulting in retraction of Glisson capsule (see Figure 3-8).[68] Epithelioid hemangioendotheliomas also have a propensity to grow into tributaries of the hepatic and portal veins, which causes occlusion of the blood supply of the neoplasm and results in self-induced ischemia.

Imaging characteristics include solitary or multifocal variants.[69] Large lesions can present as dominant masses with small satellite regions of increased vascularity. Although the vascular characteristics of EHE evoke the appearance of hemangiomas on contrast-enhanced CT and MRI, several distinct features of EHE are notable. On enhanced CT or MRI, EHEs usually demonstrate coalescing nodules of heterogenous vascularity, contrasting with the more uniform appearance of the enhancing portions of hemangiomas. T2 signal characteristics on MRI are often also distinctive, with heterogeneous areas of milder hyperintensity in EHEs rather than the more common uniformly hyperintense appearance of hemangiomas (see Figure 3-8). In addition, although focal hemangioendotheliomas can be seen, more commonly the masses show more infiltrative indistinct margins than hemangiomas.[70] The "halo" or target sign, demonstrating areas of more intermediate enhancement surrounding less-enhancing regions (an appearance not seen in hemangiomas), is often described.[71] A target appearance has also been described because of

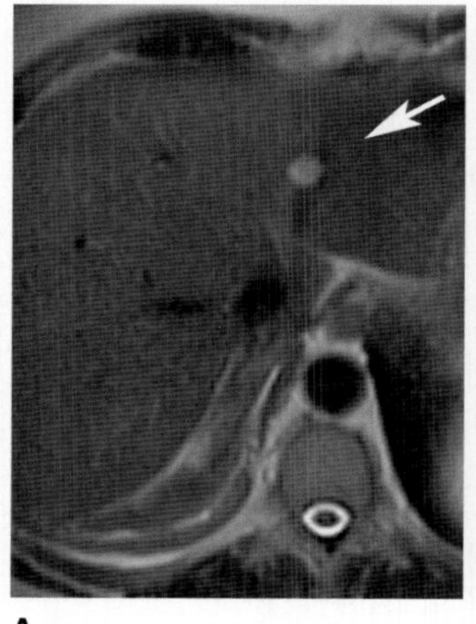
A

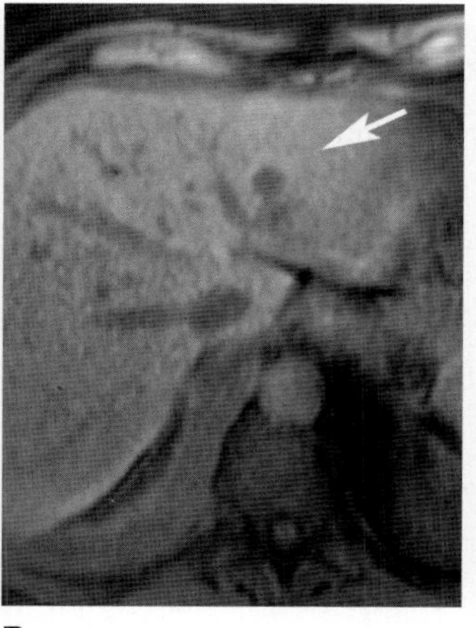
B

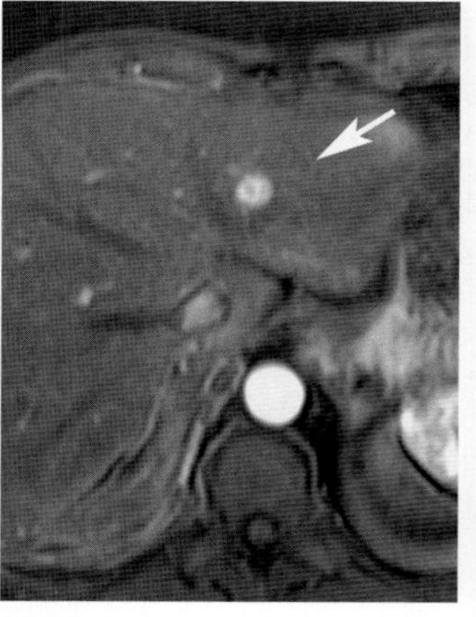
C

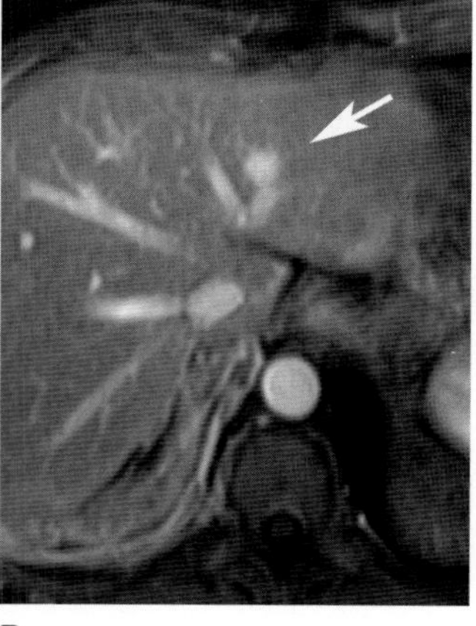
D

Figure 3-6 Flash-filling Hemangioma
This 55-year-old man had malignant mesothelioma. **A.** T2-weighted MRI sequence shows a small bright nodule typical of either a small hemangioma or simple cyst. (**B**) Pre-contrast, (**C**) hepatic arterial phase, and (**D**) portal venous phase T1-weighted postgadolinium enhanced images show immediate bright enhancement of the nodule following gadolinium enhancement. This pattern of enhancement can be seen with focal nodular hyperplasia, hepatic adenomas, hypervascular metastases, and flash-filling hemangiomas. However, the T2-weighted characteristics and persistent hyperenhancement on portal-phase imaging is typical for hemangiomas.

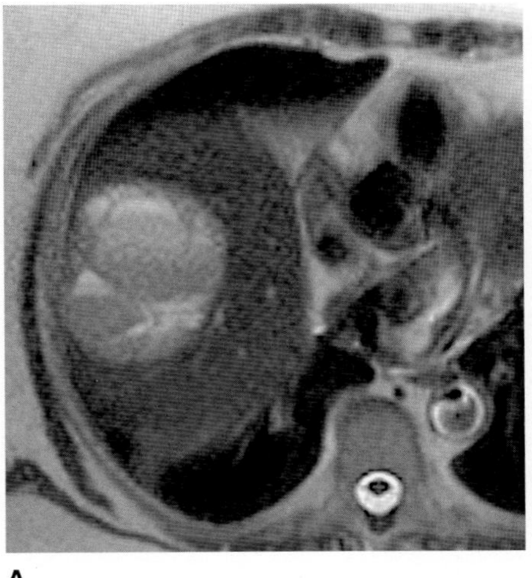
A

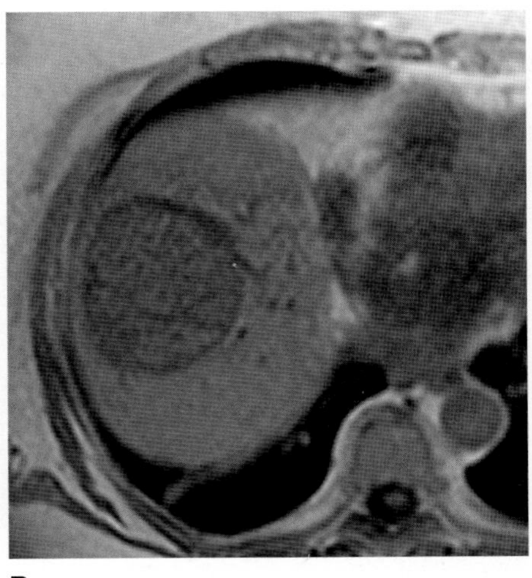
B

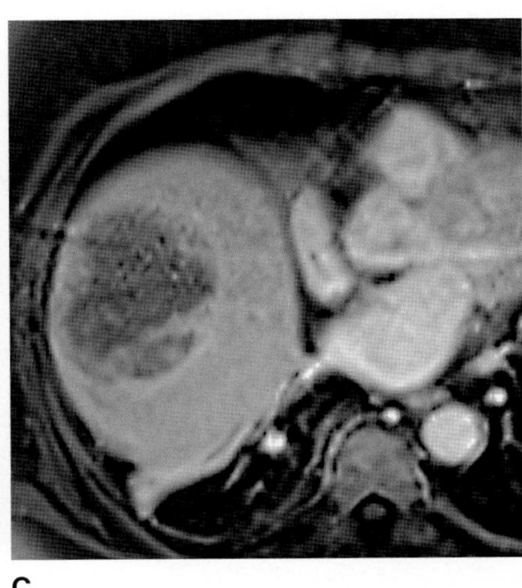
C

Figure 3-7 Biliary Cystadenoma
A. T2-weighted, (**B**) T1-weighted, and (**C**) T1-weighted post-gadolinium MR evaluation in this 84-year-old woman shows a complex multicystic mass with enhancing mural nodules and thickened septa in (C) The T2-weighted sequence also shows shading of the fluid in multiple locules, indicating the presence of a gradient of dependent debris. This is believed to represent a biliary cystadenoma, but the lesion was never biopsied.

in-growth and thrombosis of vascular channels.[72] When diagnosis is uncertain, biopsy may be required, noting that core biopsy may provide a more reliable diagnosis than fine-needle aspiration.[73,74]

Cystic and mucinous metastases: Metastatic disease to the liver commonly presents as solitary or multiple solid masses, and is described later in this chapter. However, cystic or mucinous metastases deserve special mention, as they can be casually misidentified as a benign lesion because of their partially cystic appearance.

Mucinous tumors are complex multiseptated masses filled with mucinous, gelatinous material. Solid tissue, when visible, will usually present as small papillary nodules arising from the periphery of the mass or along thickened septations. These tumors can arise from a variety of organs including the ovary, gastrointestinal (GI) tract, and pancreas and can be confused with benign cystic lesions.[75]

Malignant mucinous tumors most commonly arise from the ovary. However, these tumors generally spread by peritoneal implantation and when involving the liver will appear as a surface mass along the capsule of the liver. Hematogenous metastasis to any organ, including the liver, is unusual with mucinous adenocarcinoma of the ovary but occasionally occur. Appendiceal carcinomas are also often mucinous in nature. However, these tumors also demonstrate a propensity for peritoneal, rather than hematogenous, metastatic spread.[76] Malignant mucinous GI primary tumors, particularly stomach and colon, though less common than ovarian and appendiceal mucinous malignancies, are more likely to demonstrate hematogenous spread to the liver. When this occurs, these lesions can appear as multiple cystic lesions that can be misinterpreted as benign idiopathic cysts. Malignant cystic pancreatic neoplasms, particularly mucinous tumors, will often demonstrate hematogenous cystic metastasis to the liver.

On imaging, mucinous metastases will appear as solitary or multiple cystic lesions that casually resemble idiopathic cyst or hemangioma imaging. However, US will typically demonstrate a complex imaging appearance with septations and nodular solid areas, the latter easily confirmed by Doppler imaging. Careful evaluation of the enhancement pattern of these lesions on CT or MRI examinations will reveal peripheral enhancement without the globular discontinuous character that is typical of hemangiomas. Diffusion-weighted MRI can also be useful for distinguishing cystic metastases from other cystic lesion mimickers, revealing areas of restricted diffusion not seen in cysts and hemangiomas.[77]

Abscesses

Abscesses to the liver include pyogenic, amebic, echinococcal, and fungal causes. Fungal abscesses characteristically cause multiple tiny abscesses and will be discussed in the subsequent section titled **Multifocal Lesions of the Liver**. However, pyogenic, amebic, and echinococcal abscesses can all present as a solitary cystic mass, and will be discussed here.

Pyogenic abscesses: Bacterial (pyogenic) hepatic abscesses represent the most common infectious complication of the liver in the developed world. Although the source of many hepatic abscesses are unknown,[64] bacteria can spread hematogenously via the hepatic artery to the liver from a site of

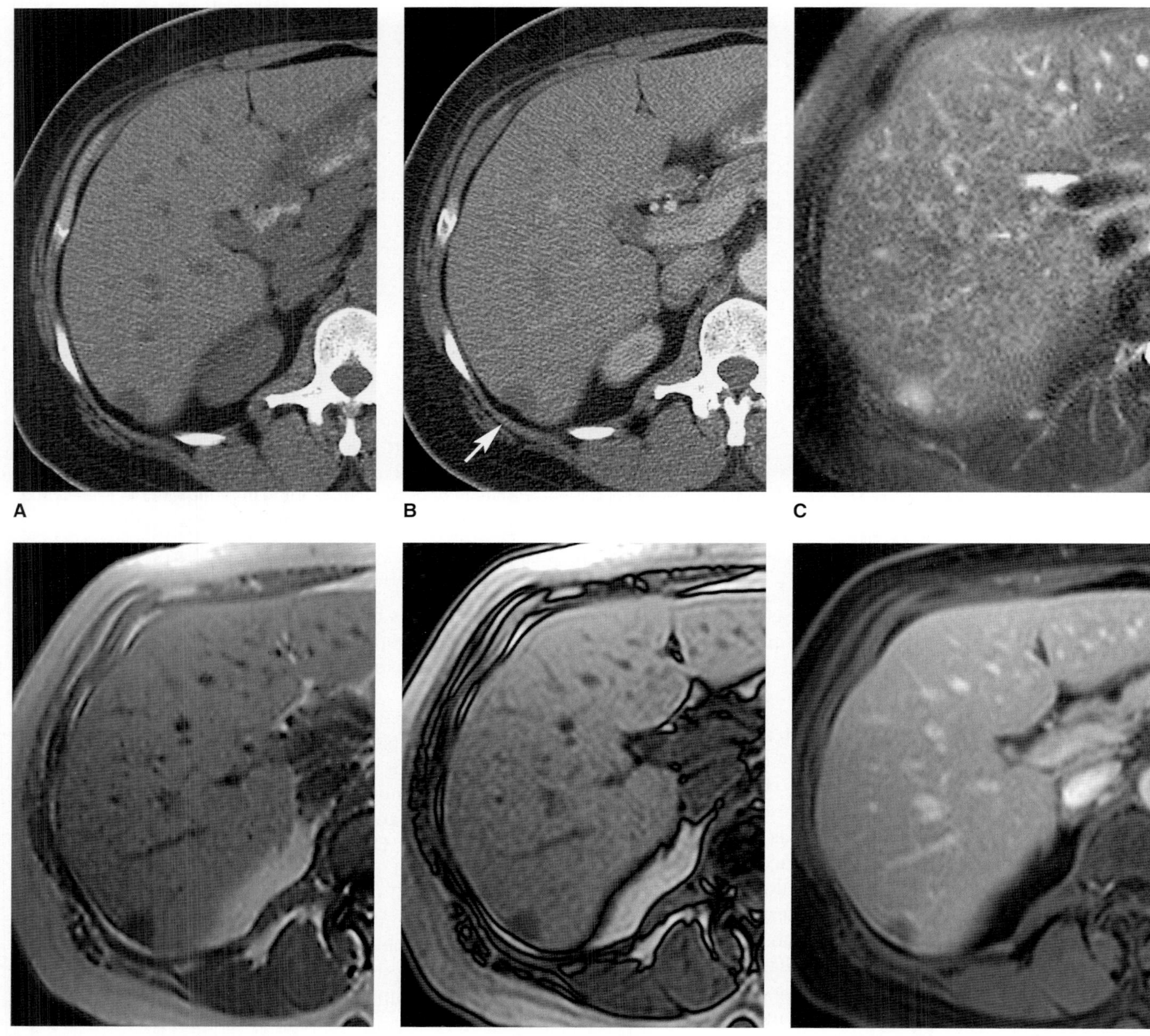

Figure 3-8 Epithelioid Hemangioendothelioma
A. Precontrast and (**B**) postcontrast axial CT images in this 53-year-old woman demonstrate a small hypoenhancing mass in the posterior segment of the liver. **C.** T2-weighted MRI sequence shows slight high attenuation of the mass. **D.** Precontrast, in-phase; (**E**) precontrast, out-of-phase; and (**F**) postcontrast T1-weighted MRI sequences show a small low signal, nonenhancing nodule. Note the subtle retraction of the hepatic capsule, seen best in B. Biopsy of the mass revealed an epithelioid hemangioendothelioma, an aggressive malignant vascular tumor. Multiple lung metastases were found on chest CT (not shown).

infection elsewhere in the body.[78,79] Hematogenous spread can also occur via the portal vein from sites of enteric infections such as appendicitis, diverticulitis, or bowel perforation.[80-84] Spread from an infected biliary tree is a third source of liver infection.[82,85] Inoculation of the liver via direct penetrating trauma or during accidental contamination during surgery is a less common source of hepatic infection.

Approximately half of pyogenic hepatic abscesses are polymicrobial.[86] *Escherichia coli* is the most common organism, though many other bacteria, both aerobic and anaerobic, can cause hepatic abscesses.[87] Abscesses that arise from seeding via the arterial or portal system will generally form in the periphery of the liver in a subcapsular location. Rarely, diffuse military involvement can also be seen.[88] Abscesses

Imaging Notes 3-3. Sources of Hepatic Abscesses

1. Hematogenous dissemination via the hepatic artery from a systemic source
   a. Endocarditis
   b. Infected catheter or in vascular hardware
   c. Other deep-tissue infection
2. Hematogenous dissemination via the portal vein from a gut infection
   a. Diverticulitis
   b. Appendicitis
   c. Abdominal abscess
3. Spread from biliary infection
4. Direct inoculation
   a. Hepatic surgery
   b. Penetrating trauma
5. Idiopathic

that arise from biliary seeding, for example, as a complication of ascending cholangitis, are typically more centrally located, and when multifocal, will be clustered to a single segment of the liver.[89,90] The segmental distribution of liver abscesses on imaging can suggest a ductal source of infection.

Patients with hepatic abscesses typically present with fever, elevated white blood cell (WBC) count, and right upper quadrant pain. Pleuritic and/or right shoulder pain can also be noted in cases of subdiaphragmatic spread. Symptoms are often insidious in onset, and can develop over several weeks. Laboratory evaluation will reveal elevation in liver enzymes, particularly alkaline phosphatase and bilirubin, with more variable transaminitis.[91]

On US examinations, pyogenic hepatic abscesses typically appear as one or several heterogeneously hypoechoic masses with ill-defined margins.[92] In one study, US examinations had an 85% sensitivity for the detection of hepatic abscesses, with most false-negative examinations due to abscesses located in the liver dome.[93]

On CT scans, pyogenic abscesses will appear as one or several hypoattenuating masses within the liver parenchyma. However, careful observation will show the center to have an attenuation greater than that of simple fluid, with measurements greater than 20 Hounsfield units (HU) (see Figure 3-9).[94] On contrast-enhanced CT, faint ill-defined enhancing rims are often present.[64] Gas bubbles or air-fluid levels are an uncommon finding on CT examinations but when present can be an important imaging clue to the diagnosis of a hepatic abscess.[95] Calcifications are rare.[96] Larger abscesses can cause portal vein thrombosis in some patients.[97]

On MRI, hepatic abscesses are low-intermediate signal intensity on T1-weighted and bright on T2-weighted images.[98] Often, mild perilesional T2 bright edema is noted around the lesion. The T2 signal intensity of the central fluid is often more moderate and heterogeneously bright than that seen with simple cysts or hemangiomas. Following the administration of IV contrast, the wall of the abscess will usually enhance. In general, MRI is more sensitive than CT for the detection of enhancement.[99-101] Diffusion-weighted imaging can be useful in discriminating abscesses from cysts. Abscesses will typically demonstrate increased signal intensity on DWIs but will generally demonstrate restricted diffusion throughout, whereas cysts and cystic/necrotic regions of tumors will more frequently demonstrate elevated ADC values.[77]

It is important to recognize that on follow-up imaging, US imaging can demonstrate residual lesions even after successful completion antibiotic therapy.[102] On CT and MRI, treated abscesses tend to decrease in size and lose their hyperenhancing rims but may persist as hypoattenuating areas on CT or hypointense areas on MRI, representing areas of granulation tissue. Partially treated, organizing abscesses can appear solid and mimic enhancing tumors on CT or MRI.[103]

Amebic abscess: Amebic abscesses are a result of mesenteric and portal venous dissemination from colonic infection with *Entamoeba histolytica*. Approximately 10% of the world's population is asymptomatically colonized with this organism that is acquired by drinking contaminated water.[104,105] In one study, nearly three-quarters of patients with liver abscess were found to have asymptomatic intestinal colonization.[106] The liver is, by far, the most common nonintestinal site of disease, and extrahepatic spread elsewhere in the abdomen or chest is often the result of rupture of a hepatic abscess.[107]

Patients with hepatic amebic abscess typically present with right upper quadrant pain, fevers, and rigors. Symptoms are often acute, although more indolent presentations can be seen manifesting as weakness and weight loss.[108] Because intestinal colonization, which precedes the development of hepatic abscesses, can be asymptomatic, gastrointestinal symptoms are more variable. Laboratory evaluation is nonspecific, and eosinophilia is rare. Stool cultures and serologic testing are now used routinely to diagnose amebic infection. Aspiration may be for diagnostic confirmation or for therapeutic drainage when risk of rupture is high.[109]

On US examinations, amebic abscess are usually seen as well-defined cystic lesions, although solid appearances early on in infection can be seen.[110] As with pyogenic abscesses, sonographic resolution can lag behind clinical response to therapy.[111,112] On CT examinations, amebic abscesses are often round or oval, and are mostly seen in the right lobe. On contrast-enhanced imaging, a thick enhancing wall is often seen.[113] On MR, lesions are uniformly dark on T1-WI with bright T2 cystic appearance.[114] There is often peri-lesion edema of the adjacent liver.[115] Contrast-enhanced appearance is similar to that of CT, with a rind of enhancement about the abscess wall.

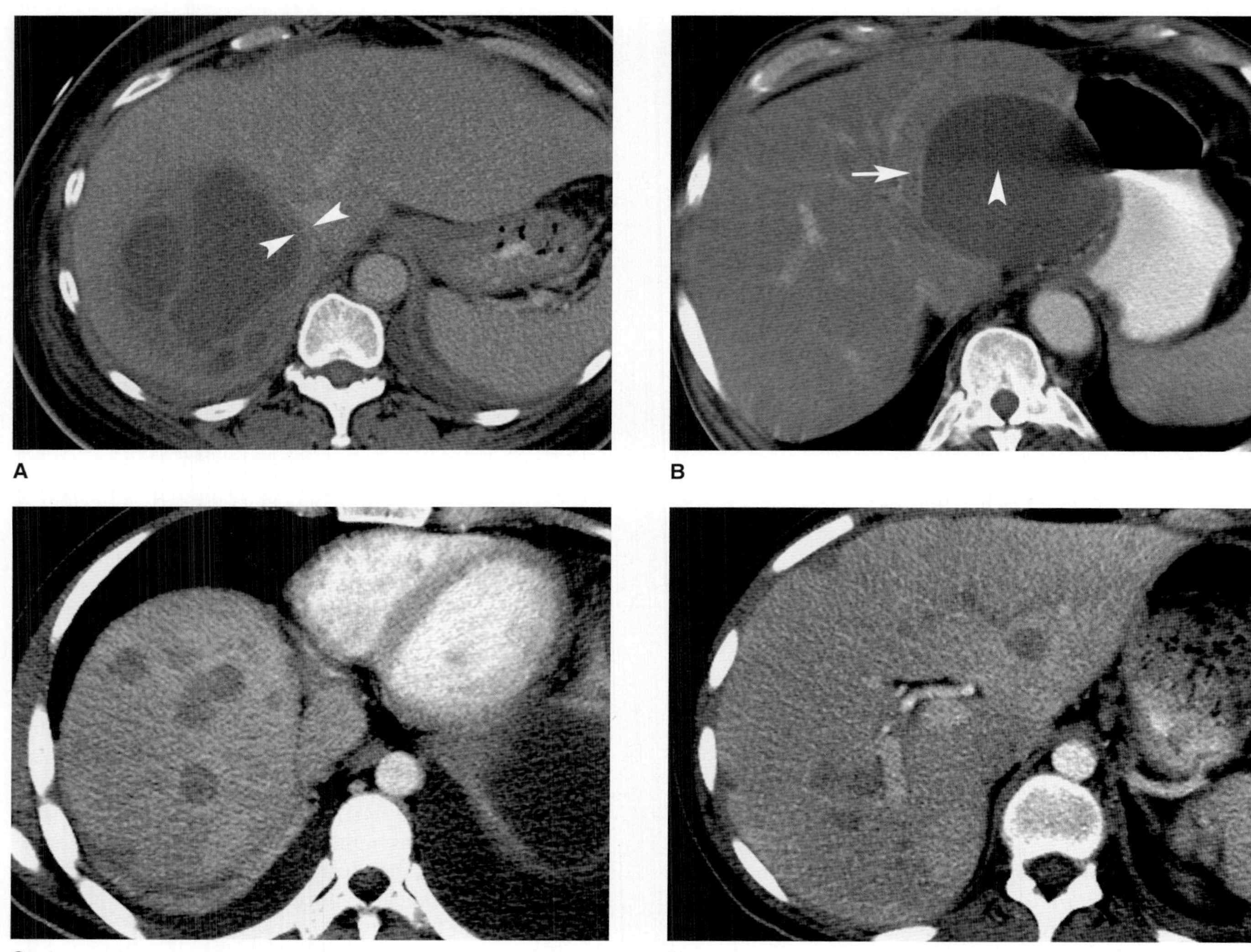

Figure 3-9 Pyogenic Liver Abscess in 3 Patients
A. This 56-year-old man complained of fever, abdominal pain, nausea, and lethargy. Contrast-enhanced CT shows a multiloculated cyst with a thick enhancing wall (*arrowheads*), features typical for a liver abscess. **B.** This 76-year-old man had persistent fevers following cecal resection for a perforated toothpick. Contrast-enhanced CT images through the liver demonstrate a large unilocular low attenuation mass (*arrows*) in the left lobe of the liver. Note the fluid debris level (*arrowhead*) within the mass, indicating a complicated cyst. Cultures of aspirated fluid from the mass demonstrated enterococcal species. **C** and **D.** This 19-year-old man with Hodgkin disease had been septic several days earlier and then complained of fever and chest pain. Contrast-enhanced CT shows multiple indistinctly marginated low attenuation nodules in the liver that were proven to represent multiple hematogenous liver abscesses.

Echinococcal cyst: Echinococcal infection is a result of the accidental ingestion of raw food contaminated with organisms contained within canine feces. *Echinococcus granulosus* and *multilocularis* are the most common species responsible for infection in humans, resulting in the cystic and alveolar forms of the disease, respectively. The organism invades the human via the gut, passing through the mesenteric and portal venous systems to infect most commonly the liver, and rarely other organs of the body such as lungs, heart, and brain.

Echinococcal abscesses of the liver will most often appear as a round or oval mass on all cross-sectional imaging examinations. Some echinococcal abscesses will appear as a unilocular cyst that can be virtually indistinguishable from idiopathic cysts. However, most echinococcal cyst will demonstrate early rim enhancement indicating the inflammatory nature of the cystic lesion.[116] In some cases, the cyst will contain small calcifications, which layer dependently within the cyst and are termed *hydatid sand*. When present, hydatid sand is an important clue to the diagnosis of echinococcal cysts and differentiates echinococcal cysts from other causes of cystic masses.[117] Many echinococcal cysts will appear as a multilocular cystic mass called the "alveolar form"

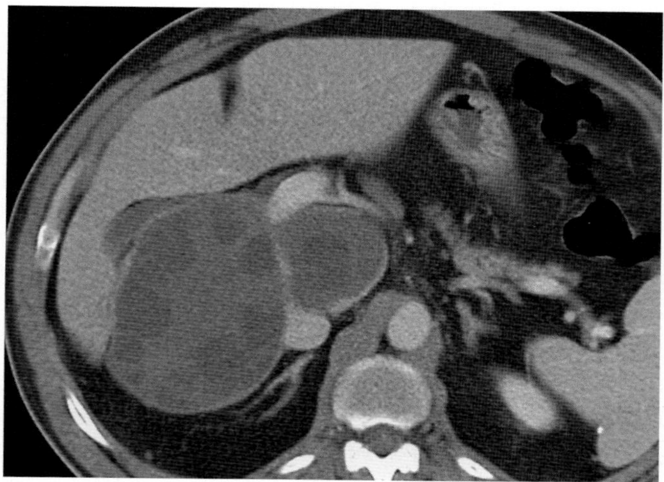

A

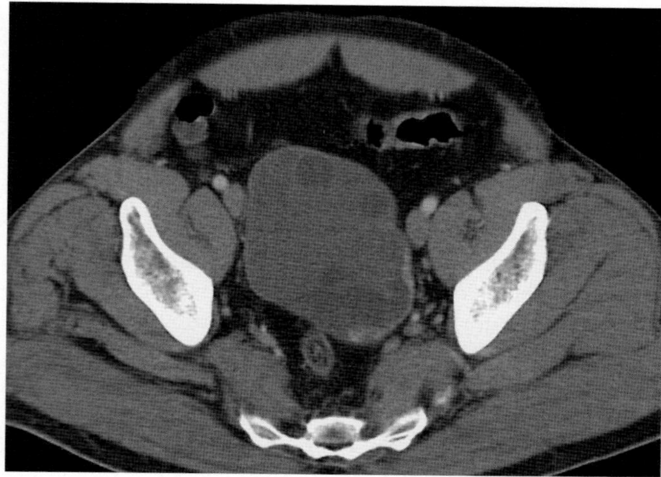

B

Figure 3-10 Echinococcal Cyst
This 51-year-old immigrant from India complained of shooting abdominal pain. **A.** Contrast-enhanced axial CT image shows a large cystic mass involving the posterior segment and caudate lobe of the liver. Note the rim of smaller cysts within the dominant cyst that represent "daughter" cysts and is diagnostic of an echinococcal cyst. **B.** There is a similar echinococcal cyst in the pelvis, indicating peritoneal spread of the infection.

of the disease.[118] The alveolar form of echinococcus has a characteristic appearance as a large cyst with many small cysts lining the internal rim of the dominant cyst. These smaller cysts are called "daughter" cysts and this appearance is pathogmnemonic of echinococcal cysts in the liver, spleen, and other organs where they arise (see Figure 3-10). MRI can demonstrate several additional imaging features of echinococcal cysts.[119] These include peripheral liver edema[100] and a low signal intensity rim.[120,121]

Solitary Solid Hepatic Masses or Nodules

The majority of solitary solid hepatic masses will represent primary or secondary neoplasms of the liver but can rarely represent other unusual conditions such as peliosis hepatis, inflammatory pseudotumor and hepatic pseudo-lesions such as focal fatty infiltration or focal fatty sparing.

Solitary solid appearing hepatic neoplasms

Solitary, solid hepatic neoplasms include hemangioma, FNH, hepatic adenoma, HCC, cholangiocarcinoma, angiosarcoma and solitary hepatic metastasis (Table 3-2).

Hemangioma: Hemangiomas have been extensively discussed in the previous section entitled: Solitary cystic or cystic-appearing neoplasms. On CT and MRI examinations these tumors will typically have imaging features indicating the presence of fluid within the lesion and will appear cystic. However, some small hemangiomas will fill with contrast so rapidly that they can appear as a uniformly enhancing solid appearing nodule on contrast-enhanced CT. Furthermore, on US examinations, the majority of hemangiomas will appear as a uniformly hyperechoic solid appearing mass.

Focal nodular hyperplasia: Focal nodular hyperplasia, as indicated by its name, represents hyperplastic proliferation of hepatic parenchyma, hepatocytes, bile canaliculi and reticuloendothelial cells, in a focal nodule. The lesion is thought to be a hyperplastic response to a central arteriovenous malformation. Focal nodular hyperplasia is the second most common benign tumor of the liver, following hemangiomas, and is a common incidental finding on imaging. It is associated with oral contraceptive use,[122]

Table 3-2. Solitary Solid-Appearing Nodules or Masses of the Noncirrhotic Liver

1. Benign primary neoplasms a. **Hemangioma**[a] b. **Focal nodular hyperplasia** c. Hepatic adenoma
2. Malignant primary neoplasms a. Cholangiocarcinoma b. Lymphoma c. Fibrolamellar HCC
3. **Metastasis**
4. Peliosis hepatis
5. Inflammatory pseudotumor
6. Pseudolymphoma
7. Pseudolesions a. **Focal fatty infiltration** b. **Focal fatty sparing**

[a]Lesions in bold are most common.

although not as strongly as with hepatic adenomas. Its lesions need no additional imaging follow-up or treatment because they represent benign proliferations of hepatocytes with no potential for malignant transformation or spontaneous hemorrhage. When FNH lesions are followed, the majority demonstrate stability over time, although regression or rarely growth has been shown.[123-126]

Definitive diagnosis of a FNH lesion is important so as to exclude other more clinically significant liver lesions. On US, FNH lesions typically appear as isoechoic nodules that faintly distort the hepatic echotexture.[127,128] Because their echotexture is nearly identical to normal parenchyma, small FNH nodules are often difficult to detect on US. Definitive diagnosis of FNH is typically made using CT and/or MRI examinations. On both unenhanced CT imaging and pregadolinium T1 MRI, FNH lesions will typically appear isointense to the background liver parenchyma (see Figure 3-11).[129] The isointense character of FNH on noncontrast T1-weighted imaging is particularly important, because metastatic lesions will typically appear hypointense relative to normal liver parenchyma. On T2-weighted imaging, FNH lesions are also generally isoechoic to liver, although faintly hyperintense pattern are seen. When visible, the central scar of an FNH lesion will be hyperintense on T2-weighted imaging, a distinguishing feature from the MR appearance of hepatic adenomas.[130]

The appearance of FNH on dynamic contrast-enhanced CT and MRI are relatively invariant.[130-132] FNH will characteristically appear as a uniformly hyperenhancing nodule on arterial-phase imaging because of the enhanced arterial supply of the nodule relative to that of normal hepatic parenchyma (see Figure 3-11). On CT arteriography, anomalous feeding artery and draining veins can be shown in some cases.[133] On portal venous-phase CT images, the nodule is usually isointense or faintly hyperintense to normal enhanced hepatic parenchyma. In many cases, even moderately large FNH nodules will be undetectable on venous phase imaging (see Figure 3-11). A consequence of this phenomenon is that previously present FNH nodules go undetected by prior venous-phase-only imaging and can be discovered as "new" hypervascular nodules on arterial-phase imaging and can be mistaken for hypervascular metastasis.

Large FNH lesions will characteristically contain a central fibrous scar, although central scars are uncommon in small FNH lesions.[131,134] Central scars often go undetected on unenhanced CT images because they are isoattenuating to liver parenchyma. However, the central scar is usually seen as a stellate central defect within the mass that is hypointense on T1-weighted imaging, and hyperintense on T2-weighted MRI. With IV contrast enhancement, the scar will typically not enhance and appear as hypoattenuating/hypointense stellate lesion within the brightly enhancing mass. With images performed after the portal venous phase of enhancement (delayed phase imaging), the mass will typically appear as a brightly enhancing stellate lesion within the less enhancing FNH nodule (see Figure 3-11).

Imaging Notes 3-4. Imaging Features of Focal Nodular Hyperplasia

Ultrasonography	Isoechoic nodule or mass
Noncontrast CT	Isoattenuating to liver parenchyma
Noncontrast MRI	Isointense T1-weighted images, T2-weighted images
Contrast CT/MRI	Hyperenhancing on arterial-phase images
	Isointense on venous-phase images

In most cases, FNH lesions can be definitively diagnosed according to their imaging characteristics on CT and MRI examinations; however, there are 2 notable exceptions. If only contrast-enhanced CT images are obtained, both small FNH lesions and small "flash filling" hemangiomas can appear as a uniformly hyperenhancing nodule within the liver parenchyma. Fortunately, as both of these lesions are benign and without clinical significance, differentiation between the lesions is unnecessary.

FNH lesions can also be confused with the rare fibrolamellar variant of HCC. This variant of HCC can also contain a central scar. Although the central scar is hypointense on T1-weighted images and resembles that seen in FNH, unlike FNH, the central scar of fibrolamellar HCC is not typically hyperintense on T2-weighted imaging. Also, fibrolamellar HCCs will typically demonstrate heterogenous enhancement, rather than demonstrate a more uniform early-enhanced appearance typical of FNH lesions.[135]

Before the widespread use of cross-sectional imaging, sulfur colloid nuclear medicine examinations were commonly used to definitively diagnose a liver mass as an FNH. Focal nodular hyperplasia has the unique characteristic among hepatic masses of containing reticuloendothelial cell, in common with the normal liver. As sulfur colloid is phagocytized by the reticuloendothelial cells of the liver, spleen, and lymph nodes, these organs demonstrate high levels of activity on sulfur colloid scans. All mass lesions other than FNH will appear as a photopenic region with the liver on sulfur colloid, whereas FNH lesions will typically take up sulfur colloid as well, therefore presenting as an area of equal or more intense tracer uptake on planar or single-photon emission computed tomographic (SPECT) imaging.[136]

Recently, the use of a newer-generation gadolinium-based MRI agents with partial hepatobiliary excretion has been shown to be useful for characterizing FNH lesions. Two such agents are currently approved for use in the United States. The first agent, gadobenate dimeglumine (MultiHance, Bracco), demonstrates approximately 2% biliary excretion in humans with normal renal and hepatic function.[137] A more recently approved agent, gadoxetate

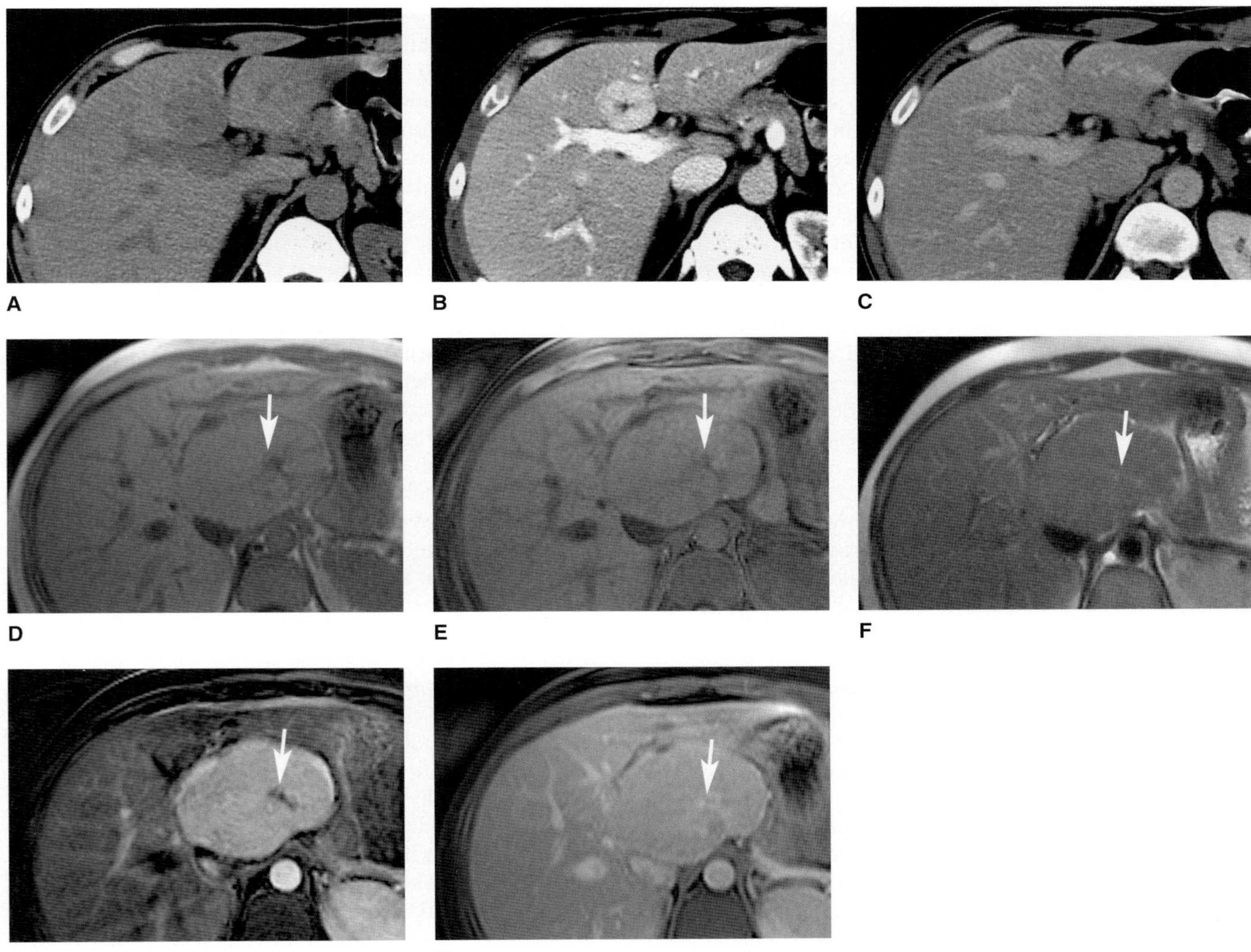

Figure 3-11 Focal Nodular Hyperplasia in 2 Patients
A-C. This 34-year-old man had a history of malignant melanoma. Noncontrast (A), arterial-phase (B), and venous-phase (C) CT images through the same location in the liver demonstrate a 2.5-cm mass in the medial segment of the liver. This is hypoattenuating on noncontrast images, hyperenhancing on arterial-phase images, and isoenhancing on venous-phase images. This appearance is common among the hepatocellular-derived tumors of the liver but is most typical of focal nodular hyperplasia. Note also the small hypoattenuating, nonenhancing central region within the mass. This is typical of a central scar and is characteristic of focal nodular hyperplasia. **D-H.** This 37-year-old woman had abdominal pain. T1-weighted (D); T1-weighted, fat saturation (E); and T2-weighted (F) MRI images through the same location in the liver demonstrate a large mass that is isointense with normal liver parenchyma. Note that there is no loss of signal in the mass following the fat saturation pulse, making a hepatic adenoma less likely. Note also the hypointense central scar (*arrow*) in (D) and (E) is hyperintense on the T2-weighted images. With intravenous contrast, the mass became hyperintense to liver on the arterial-phase (G) and isointense on venous-phase (H) images. The central scar demonstrates delayed enhancement on the venous-phase images (*arrow*). These findings are typical of focal nodular hyperplasia.

disodium (Eovist, Bayer) demonstrates approximately 50% biliary excretion.[138,139] In both cases, the delayed excretion into the biliary canaliculi provides prolonged and increased T1-weighted image enhancement after the first pass and blood pool phases of contrast accumulation have subsided. This effect has been shown to increase conspicuity of liver lesions without functioning bile canaliculi. Because FNH lesions contain biliary canaliculi, biliary-phase imaging with either agent demonstrates delayed hyperenhancement of the mass. Most other rapidly enhancing lesions in the liver will demonstrate contrast washout on the biliary-phase images.[140,141] This effect is seen earlier and is more pronounced with gadoxetate, given that this agent undergoes a greater relative degree of biliary uptake and excretion than does gadobenate. However, the use of these agents can alter the delayed-phase appearance of the central scar in FNH, rendering them hypointense to the remainder of the lesion on biliary-phase imaging.[142]

Hepatic adenoma: Hepatic adenoma is a benign tumor of hepatocytes that is most often seen in young and middle-aged women and is typically associated with the use of oral contraceptives.[143] The incidence of hepatic adenoma is directly related to the dose of estrogens within the medication and the duration of use.[144] Withdrawal of oral contraceptives will frequently lead to tumor regression.[145] Use of anabolic androgenic steroids is also associated with an increased incidence of hepatic adenoma.[146] Adenomas are also associated with glycogen storage disease types I and III.[147] Although often solitary, multiple hepatic adenomas are not uncommonly reported in patients' oral contraceptive use.[148] Multiplicity is also associated with hepatic steatosis.[149]

Hepatic adenomatosis is a distinct entity resulting in the appearance of multiple adenomas unrelated to steroid use or glycogen storage disease. The appearance of the individual lesions in hepatic adenomatosis is similar to that of "acquired" isolated tumors. However, management is more challenging as there are no options to remove the precipitating agent. Discovery of multiple hepatic adenomatous lesions unassociated with glycogen storage disease and oral contraceptive or anabolic steroid use can suggest the presence of hepatic adenomatosis.[150-152] Differentiation from other presentations such as multiple FNH lesion is critical for clinical management.

Hepatic adenomas are composed of benign hepatocytes without bile ducts and usually without Kupffer cells. Adenoma cells can contain increased intracellular lipid, a feature that can be used to identify the tumor on chemical shift–sensitive MRI (see Figure 3-12).[153] Hepatic adenomas are often detected incidentally. However, spontaneous rupture and hemorrhage of these lesions is not uncommon, especially for larger lesions (see Figure 3-13).[154-156] When spontaneous rupture occurs, patients will typically present with acute right upper quadrant pain. In these cases, hemorrhage in some cases will completely or partially obscure the lesion on cross-sectional imaging. One consequence of this is that when a young woman presents with spontaneous intrahepatic hemorrhage, an underlying adenoma should be considered as the potential etiology, even if the lesion itself is not initially apparent.

Like other tumors of hepatocellular origin, hepatic adenomas demonstrate an imaging appearance that is similar to normal hepatic parenchyma. Nonhemorrhagic hepatic adenomas will often appear as a isoechoic or faintly hypoechoic spherical lesion in the liver on US (see Figure 3-12).[157] On noncontrast CT, the lesion will be isoattenuating or slightly hypoattenuating relative to background liver.[158] The MRI appearance of hepatic adenomas can be variable but is most often nearly isointense to liver on both T1- and T2-weighted sequences (see Figure 3-12).[54,159-161]

Intravenous contrast on both CT and MRI will show moderate to strong enhancement of the nodule relative to liver on arterial-phase images, and often slightly decreased enhancement relative to liver on venous-phase images, although the degree of enhancement can be variable (see Figure 3-12). As noted previously, tumors of hepatic origin, including hepatic adenomas, will often demonstrate the presence of microscopic lipid on chemical shift–sensitive MRI. Thus, the lesion will lose signal intensity on opposed-phase images when compared with in-phase images (see Figure 3-12). The presence of spontaneous hemorrhage on either CT or MRI can also be an important clue to the diagnosis of hepatic adenoma (see Figure 3-13). Larger hepatic adenomas will often develop a central stellate scar. Scar tissue will typically demonstrate delayed enhancement on contrast-enhanced CT and MRI images.

Focal nodular hyperplasia is the most common hepatic lesion to resemble hepatic adenomas. As noted in the discussion of FNH, both sulfur colloid scanning and the hepatobiliary excreted gadolinium agents (gadobenate and gadoxetate) can be useful to distinguish between hepatic adenoma and FNH.[140,158,162-164] Both sulfur colloid and the hepatobiliary excreted gadolinium agents are taken up by FNH but not hepatic adenomas. Therefore, hepatic adenomas will appear as photopenic regions on sulfur colloid scans and will appear hypointense to enhanced liver on these delayed postgadolinium images, whereas FNH will have the same or increased activity as normal liver on sulfur colloid scans and will have increased signal on delayed-phase MRI images (see Figure 3-14).

Imaging Notes 3-5. Hepatic Masses with Intracellular Lipid

Intracellular lipid as measured by chemical shift imaging (in-phase and opposed-phase T1-weighted images) within a hepatic mass is highly associated with primary neoplasms of the hepatocyte:

1. Hepatic adenoma
2. Hepatocellular carcinoma
3. Focal nodular hyperplasia

Hepatocellular carcinoma: HCC in almost all cases is a complication of cirrhosis. As a consequence, the imaging appearance of HCC is intrinsically connected with the imaging features of cirrhosis and will be discussed with cirrhosis under the heading: **Hepatic Disorders with a Specific Appearance** later in this chapter.

Fibrolamellar HCC: Fibrolamellar HCC is a rare tumor that has several clinical and radiologic features that distinguish it from the much more common variant of HCC associated with cirrhosis. Fibrolamellar HCC tends to occur in younger patients and is not associated with underlying liver disease.[165] As such, fibrolamellar HCC can often be treated

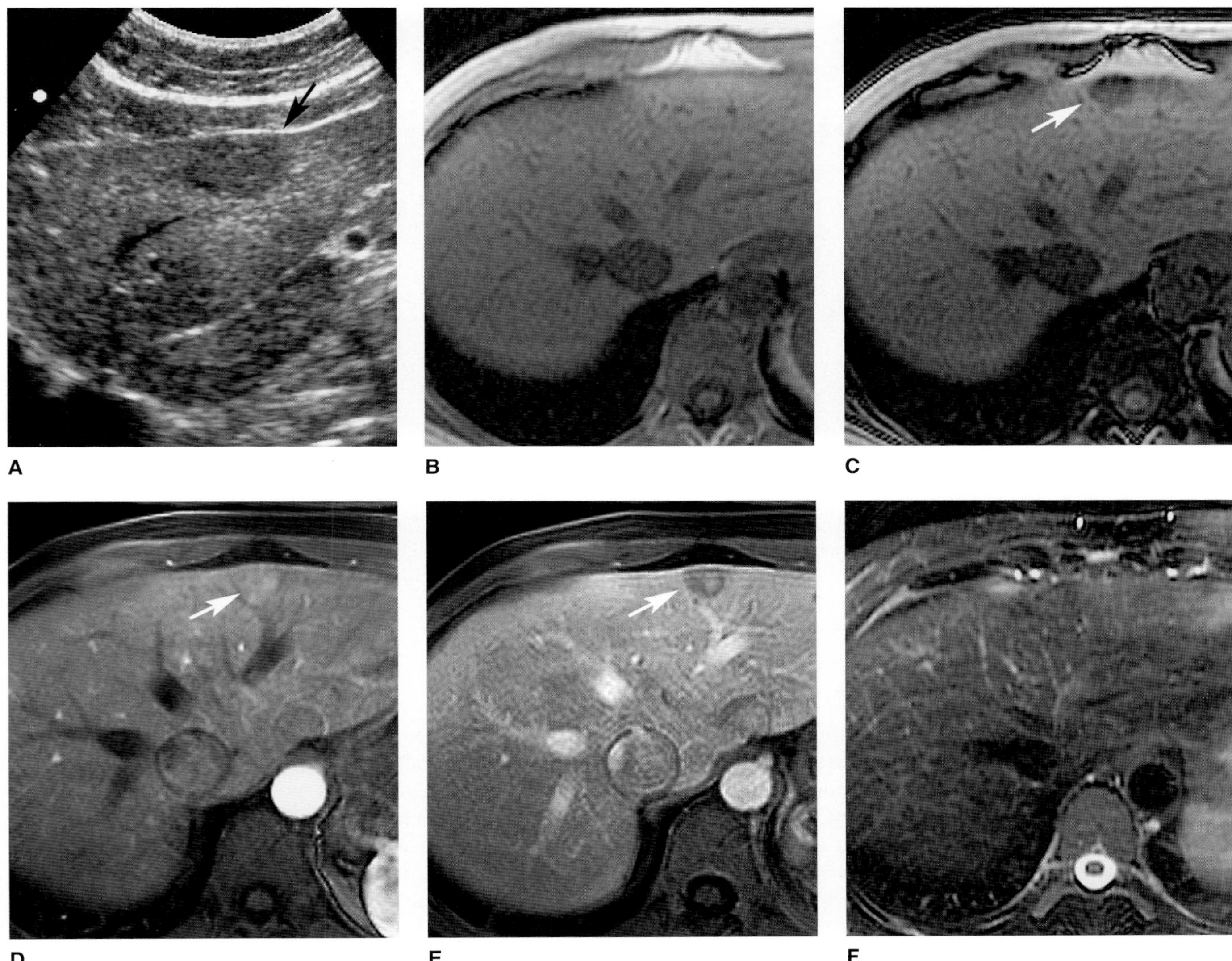

Figure 3-12 Hepatic Adenoma in 2 Patients
A. This 40-year-old woman had been using oral contraceptives when she complained of right upper quadrant pain. US of the left lobe of the liver demonstrates a slightly hypoechoic mass (*arrow*) subsequently shown to represent a hepatic adenoma. **B-F.** This 47-year-old woman used oral contraceptives and complained of abdominal pain. T1-weighted in-phase (B), T1-weighted out-of-phase (C), T1-weighted postcontrast arterial-phase (D), T1-weighted postcontrast venous-phase (E), and T2-weighted (F) sequences through the same region of the liver. A low signal mass (*arrow*) is seen in the medial segment of the liver in the out-of-phase image (C) but is isointense to liver on T1- and T2-weighted sequences and is virtually invisible on these sequences. Careful evaluation of the arterial-phase images (D) shows a slight increased enhancement of the mass (*arrow*) and venous-phase images (E) show slightly decreased enhancement of the mass (*arrow*) relative to normal liver parenchyma. This was subsequently demonstrated to represent a hepatic adenoma.

more aggressively, and patients with HCC, even when large, often have a better prognosis when compared to that of patients with advanced-stage HCC associated with liver disease.[166]

Fibrolamellar HCCs tend to be large at presentation, as small lesions are asymptomatic. Calcification is present in many cases, and is easily demonstrated by CT. Lesions are unifocal and lobular, with low signal intensity on unenhanced CT and variable low-isointense appearance on pregadolinium T1-weighted MR images. Lesions are usually marked heterogeneous on T2-weighted imaging, with relatively high signal intensity.

Fibrolamellar HCCs are notable for containing a central scar, a characteristic associated with the more common benign FNH lesion, and occasionally with giant sclerosed hemangiomas. As such, the presence of a lesion with a central scar on cross-sectional imaging can pose a diagnostic dilemma initially. However, the central scar of fibrolamellar HCC will not enhance or will enhance only mildly, in contrast with the central scar of FNH, which is generally

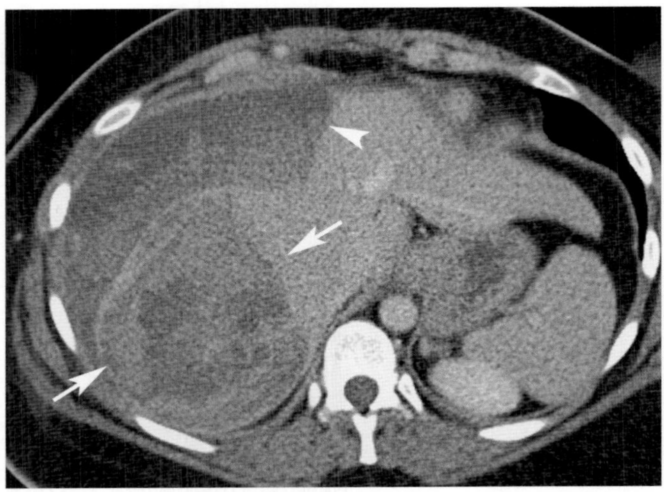

A

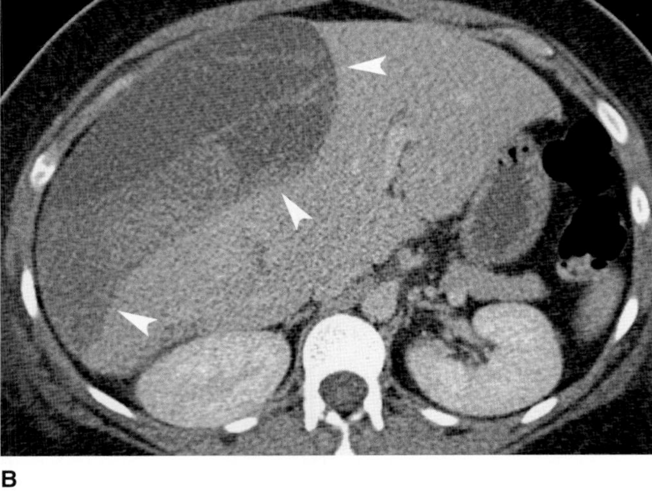

B

Figure 3-13 Ruptured Hepatic Adenoma
This 27-year-old woman developed fever and abdominal pain while on oral contraceptives. **A** and **B.** Contrast-enhanced CT shows a heterogeneous mass (*arrows*) in the right lobe of the liver. This is associated with a mixed-attenuation subcapsular fluid collection (*arrowheads*) compressing the surface of the liver. The mixed attenuation is typical of a subcapsular hematoma with differing phases of blood. Although the mass is nonspecific, the combination of the clinical history of oral contraceptive use and the presence of a subcapsular hematoma is highly suggestive of spontaneous rupture of a hepatic adenoma.

hyperenhancing on delayed-phase imaging. Furthermore, fibrolamellar HCCs typically demonstrate markedly heterogenous enhancement, a feature common to many malignant lesions. As such, fibrolamellar HCCs can often be distinguished from benign entities that also present with a central scar.[135]

Cholangiocarcinoma: Cholangiocarcinoma (CCA) is the second most common hepatic primary malignancy and is typically found in patients in their fifth and sixth decade of life.[167] This tumor can arise sporadically or be associated with a variety of chronic inflammatory disorders of the bile ducts, including sclerosing cholangitis[168] and parasitic infections of the biliary tree.[169,170] As biliary parasites are more commonly found in East Asia, cholangiocarcinoma is more frequently seen in Japan, Korea, and China than in Western countries.[171] Patients with Caroli disease (congenital dilation of the intrahepatic bile ducts; see Chapter 4) and patients with biliary stones are also at an increased risk for developing cholangiocarcinoma.[172,173]

Cholangiocarcinomas can arise from any portion of the bile ducts, both intrahepatic and extrahepatic, but most typically occur at the junction of the left and right bile ducts in the porta hepatis. Tumors at this location are termed *Klatskin tumors*. Cholangiocarcinomas are divided into types based on their growth pattern: (1) mass forming, (2) periductal infiltrating, and (3) intraductal-growing types.[174,175] The periductal and intraductal types of intrahepatic cholangiocarcinoma, as well as extrahepatic tumors, will be discussed in Chapter 4: **Imaging of the Gallbladder and Biliary System**.

In some cases, cholangiocarcinomas grow as a focal well-defined, intrahepatic mass that can be confused with other causes of hepatic masses.[176-178] However, mass-forming intrahepatic cholangiocarcinomas will often obstruct the biliary system, a feature that is more commonly seen in cholangiocarcinomas than other primary or secondary liver masses (see Figure 3-15).

If CT or MRI examinations are obtained several minutes after the injection of IV contrast, there can be delayed enhancement of cholangiocarcinomas.[179] Combination of dynamic and delayed-phase imaging can therefore improve depiction of cholangiocarcinoma.[180] This delayed enhancement is characteristic of the scirrhous nature of these lesions, with abundant fibrous tissue interspaced with malignant tumor cells.[11]

Cholangiocarcinoma is discussed most completely in Chapter 4: **Imaging of the Gallbladder and Biliary System.**

Angiosarcoma: Angiosarcoma is among the rarest primary hepatic neoplasms. It is estimated that only 25 cases will occur annually in the United States.[181] Angiosarcoma is a highly malignant tumor with a very poor prognosis. Most patients will die within a year of diagnosis.[182] They are of historical interest because they were discovered to be induced by the intravascular contrast agent: thorium dioxide (Thorotrast). Thorium dioxide colloidal solution, or Thorotrast, was introduced as a radiographic contrast agent in 1928 and used until the early 1950s. Thorotrast accumulates in the cells of the reticuloendothelial system, where it is retained throughout life. Thorium, an alpha-particle emitter with a biologic half-life of 200 to 400 years, resulted in a cumulative radiation

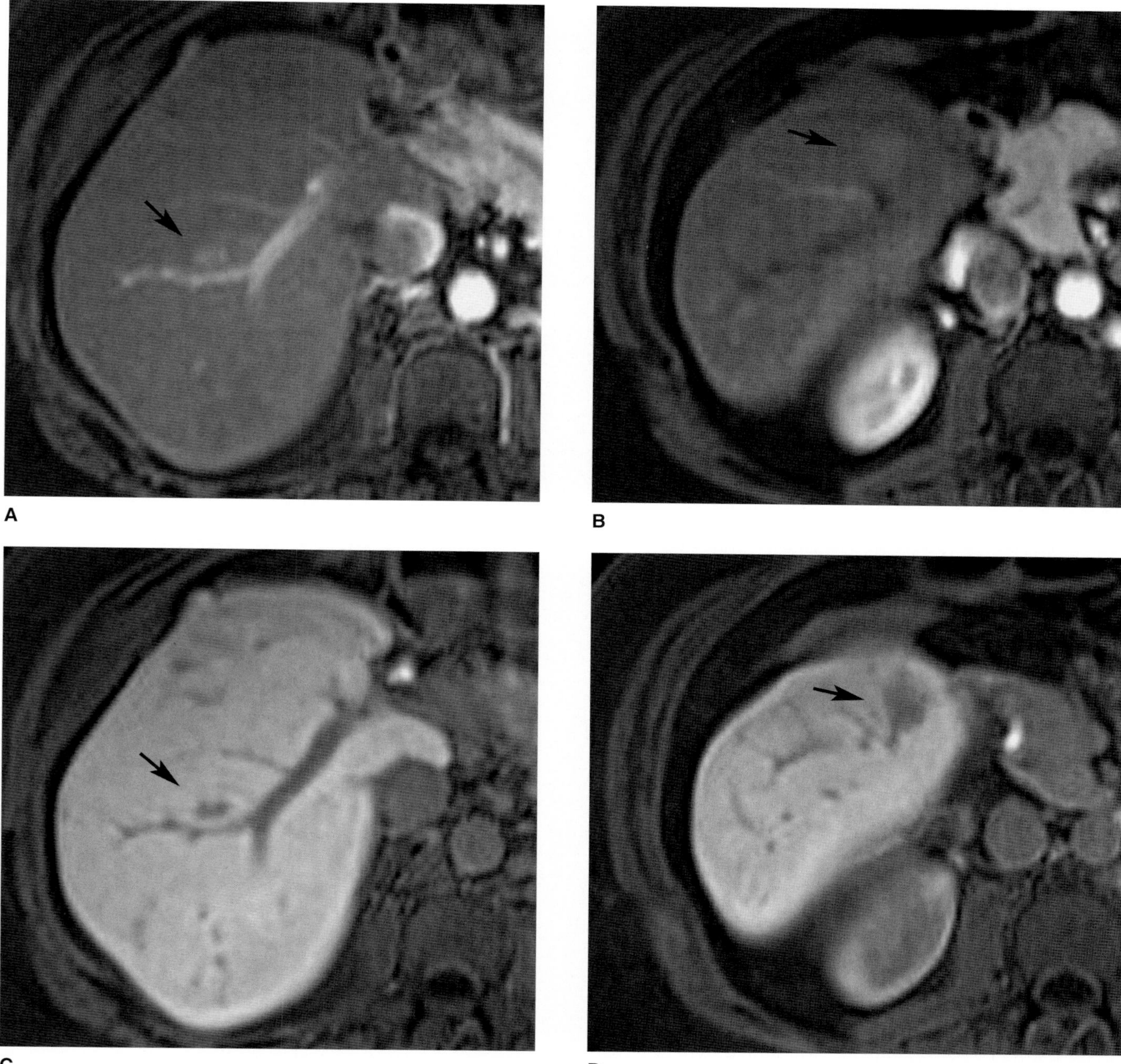

Figure 3-14 Hepatic Adenomas Demonstrated by Absence of Hepatobiliary Contrast
A 54-year-old woman with multiple known hepatic adenomas. **A** and **B**. Arterial-phase MRI demonstrates 2 small hypervascular lesions (*arrows*). **C** and **D**. Hepatobiliary phase image at 20 minutes demonstrates diffuse uptake (brightening in the liver) with washout of vessels. The adenomas are hypointense relative to background liver, reflecting the lack of biliary uptake in the tumors.

exposure leading to an increased incidence of cholangiocarcinoma, HCC, and angiosarcoma of the liver.[183] Other risk factors for angiosarcoma include arsenic and polyvinyl chloride exposure, use of anabolic steroids, and a history of hemochromatosis or cirrhosis.[184] However, most angiosarcomas develop sporadically without a known risk factor.[185]

Angiosarcoma will typically present in the seventh decade of life and is seen more commonly in men, with a male-female ratio of 4:1.[186] Patients will most often present with right upper-quadrant abdominal pain, abdominal discomfort, anorexia, or weight loss.[182] Patients will often have associated thrombocytopenia, disseminated intravascular

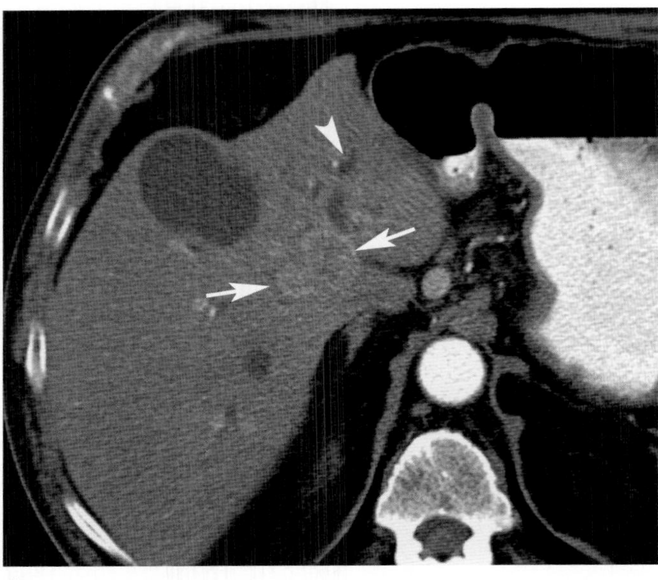
A

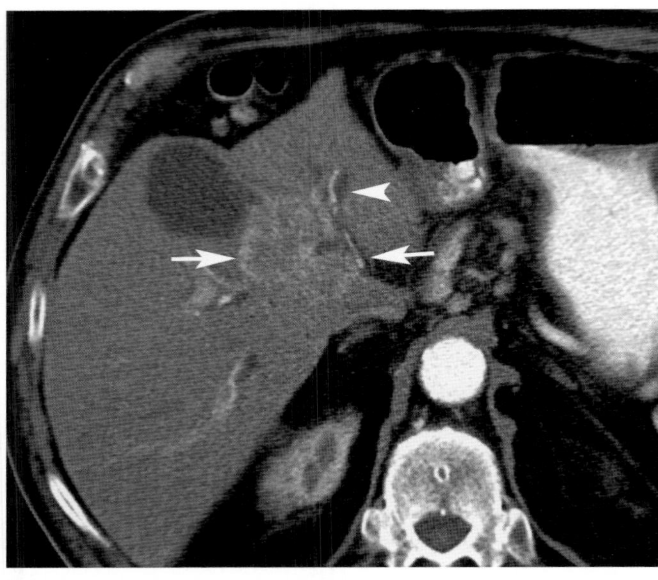
B

Figure 3-15 Cholangiocarcinoma
This 82-year-old man presented with jaundice. **A** and **B.** Contrast-enhanced CT shows mild intrahepatic ductal dilation (*arrowheads*) and a faintly enhancing mass (*arrows*) in the porta hepatis. Biopsy was diagnostic of a cholangiocarcinoma.

coagulation (DIC), and/or hemolytic anemia. Most patients will have metastasis discovered at presentation. Common sites of metastasis include the spleen and lung.[187]

Angiosarcoma is typically a multifocal neoplasm of the liver.[188] In approximately one-half of patients, angiosarcoma will appear as a large dominant mass within the liver with or without scattered smaller satellite nodules.[189] In most of the remainder, it will appear as multifocal nodular lesions scattered throughout the liver (see Figure 3-16). Rarely, angiosarcoma will appear as diffuse nodular infiltration of the liver. On CT, the masses will usually appear hypoattenuating on precontrast[190] images, occasionally with focal regions of higher attenuation.[191] On MRI examinations, angiosarcomas will typically appear hypointense on T1-weighted images and hyperintense on T2-weighted images. Small focal regions of T1-weighted hyperintensity and areas with fluid-fluid levels on T2-weighted images are commonly found and suggest the presence of intratumoral hemorrhage.[192] Following contrast administration, typically heterogeneous regions of the mass will enhance, and the extent of enhancement will increase with delayed images, although rarely tumors appeared hyperenhancing to liver parenchyma.[193]

Lymphoma: Secondary involvement of the liver by lymphomas is not uncommon, with an 8% incidence of Hodgkin disease and 25% incidence of non-Hodgkin lymphoma.[194,195] However, primary hepatic lymphoma is extremely rare. Hepatic lymphoma most often appears as diffuse hepatomegaly but can also appear as one or several focal masses.[196] When presenting as a focal mass in the liver, lymphoma will demonstrate a uniform hypoechoic appearance on US.[197] On CT, lymphoma is hypodense to liver[181] and demonstrates little enhancement following contrast administration (see Figure 4-59). On MRI, lymphoma appears hypointense on T1, with variable signal intensity

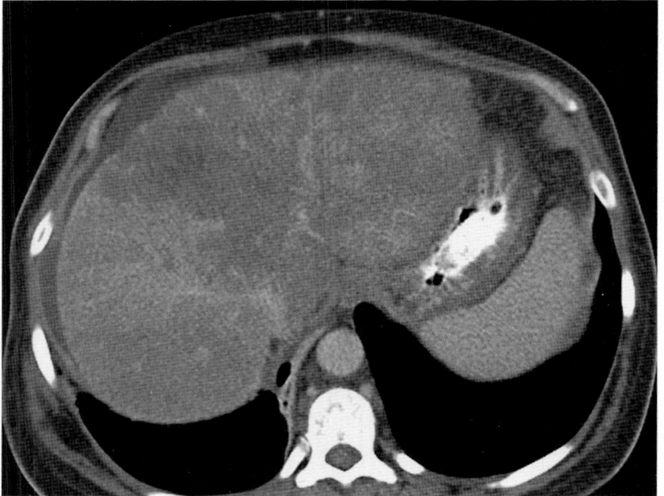

Figure 3-16 Angiosarcoma
This 55-year-old woman presented with dyspnea. Contrast-enhanced CT shows a large heterogenous mass filling and expanding the left hepatic lobe. There is also a small amount of perihepatic ascites. An infiltrative mass of this appearance will usually indicate a primary hepatic neoplasm, most often HCC. Liver biopsy was diagnostic of an epithelioid angiosarcoma.

on T2 imaging, and modest enhancement post gadolinium administration.[198,199]

Peliosis hepatis

Peliosis hepatis is a rare benign vascular lesion characterized by solitary or multifocal randomly distributed regions of sinusoidal dilation and blood-filled hepatic spaces. A variety of agents have been linked with peliosis hepatis, including chemicals such as arsenic and polyvinyl chloride, drugs such as oral contraceptives, anabolic steroids, and corticosteroids;[200] and infectious agents such as Bartonella in AIDS.[201] Peliosis hepatitis is also seen in patients with renal or cardiac transplants,[202] and malignancies such as HCC.[203]

The pathophysiology of peliosis hepatis is not known. Hypotheses regarding the etiology include the following: (1) it is a result of sinusoidal epithelial damage; (2) it is a result of pressure from obstruction of hepatic venous outflow; or (3) it is a result of hepatic necrosis.[204,205] In most cases, patients are asymptomatic and the disorder is discovered as a result of elevated liver function tests or imaging examinations performed for other reasons.[206] However, occasionally, when severe, peliosis hepatis can be symptomatic, presenting with hepatomegaly, jaundice, liver failure, and/or hemoperitoneum. It is important to consider the diagnosis of peliosis hepatis because a correct diagnosis can lead to withdrawal of the offending drug or toxin, leading to resolution of the disease and prevention of serious complications such as hepatic failure or intra-abdominal hemorrhage.[206]

Cross-sectional imaging examinations will typically demonstrate 1 or multiple focal masses or nodules within the liver parenchyma that can be confused with hepatic neoplasms, especially hemangiomas, focal nodular hyperplasia, and other hypervascular liver masses.[206-208] Hemorrhagic findings with multiple cystic dilated spaces can be a clue to the diagnosis.[209]

On US examinations, peliosis hepatis will typically appear as a uniform hyperechoic mass.[206] If the mass is complicated by hemorrhage, it can appear heterogeneously hyperechoic and, in patients with hepatic steatosis, it can appear hypoechoic because of increased echogenicity of the background liver parenchyma.

On unenhanced CT examinations, peliosis hepatis will typically appear as uniform hypoattenuating liver nodules or masses.[206] Contrast-enhanced CT will characteristically demonstrate one or multiple hepatic masses with early globular enhancement with centripetal increase in enhancement during later phases of imaging. Occasionally brisk, uniform, diffuse early enhancement can be seen.[210] Also, areas of central enhancement, termed the target sign, can be identified. On delayed-phase images, peliosis hepatis can appear homogeneously hyperintense to surrounding liver parenchyma.[211]

On MR examinations, the appearance of peliosis hepatis will depend on the age and status of the hemorrhagic component.[206] On T2-weighted sequences, peliotic lesions are typically hyperintense to liver parenchyma. Multiple small foci of even higher signal intensity are seen within the lesion, which are thought to be due to hemorrhagic necrosis. On T1-weighted sequences, the lesions are usually hypointense because of the presence of subacute blood. Enhancement patterns are similar to CT, with globular centripetal or centrifugal enhancement.

Imaging Notes 3-6. Hypervascular Lesions of the Otherwise Normal Liver

Uniformly hyperenhancing lesions in the arterial phase of enhancement in an otherwise normal-appearing liver are most often due to either flash-filling hemangiomas or regions of focal nodular hyperplasia. Less commonly, they can represent small hepatic adenomas. Rarely, they can be due to hypervascular metastasis (especially neuroendocrine neoplasms) or vascular disorders such as hemangioendotheliomas, peliosis hepatis, and arteriovenous malformations. In the cirrhotic liver, hypervascular nodules typically represent either regenerative nodules or small hepatocellular carcinomas.

Inflammatory pseudotumor

Inflammatory pseudotumor is a pathologically defined disease and specifically refers to a benign proliferation of inflammatory and myofibroblastic spindle cells. Inflammatory hepatic pseudotumors are masses consisting of proliferation of inflammatory cells and fibrous stroma that occur in children and young adults.[212] The cause of these lesions is unknown, although they have been hypothesized to represent sequelae of previous hepatic infection.

Although approximately one-third of patients with hepatic inflammatory pseudotumor are asymptomatic, the remainder will have symptoms and serum chemistries suggesting inflammation of the liver. In one study, symptoms included fever, fatigue, weight loss, abdominal pain, nausea, and vomiting of 2 weeks to 6 months in duration.[213] Laboratory studies showed elevations in C-reactive protein, sedimentation rate, and elevated WBC count in half of patients, and abnormalities in liver function were elevated in a minority. Knowledge of these signs and symptoms of inflammation can be an important clue to the diagnosis of inflammatory pseudotumor, because most solitary hepatic masses will present asymptomatically, without laboratory abnormalities.

At US, inflammatory pseudotumors have been described as both hypoechoic and hyperechoic masses with increased through transmission and visualization of multiple septa.[214,215] Nonspecific imaging characteristics are seen at CT. Commonly, the tumors are hypoattenuating to liver parenchyma on unenhanced images, and variable patterns of enhancement are seen after contrast material administration, including peripheral enhancement or enhancement of multiple internal septa.[213,215] Calcification may be seen by

Imaging Notes 3-7. Hepatic Inflammatory Pseudotumor

> Inflammatory pseudotumor typically appears as a nonspecific liver mass on cross-sectional imaging exams. However, with the exception of liver abscesses, this is the only liver mass that characteristically presents with signs and symptoms of systemic inflammation such as fever and elevations in serum white blood cell count, sedimentation rate, and C-reactive protein.

CT in some cases.[215] Variable appearances of inflammatory pseudotumors of the liver have been described at MRI as well. The lesions are typically hypointense on T1-weighted images and hyperintense on T2-weighted images, with variable enhancement patterns.[216,217] A delayed hyperenhancing fibrous pseudocapsule may be seen.[215] However, as is suggested by its name, pseudotumors can mimic focal malignant lesions, and biopsy may be the only method of definitively excluding malignancy.[218]

Pseudolymphoma

Pseudolymphoma is a term representing neoplastic-like proliferation of inflammatory cells, without evidence of clonal expansion. Most commonly seen in the skin, pseudolymphomas have been reported in multiple visceral compartments. Hepatic pseudolymphomas are relatively rare and are thought to be associated with inflammatory or autoimmune insults to the liver.[219] Pseudolymphomas usually present as a focal mass, with nonspecific imaging characteristics similar to that of lymphoma,[220] although hypervascularity has been reported.[221] The diagnosis requires pathologic evaluation with immunohistochemical and/or flow cytometry evaluation to distinguish this from true hepatic lymphoma.

Hepatic pseudolesions

Unlike inflammatory pseudotumor and pseudolymphoma that have defined pathologic characteristics, the term *pseudotumor* is ubiquitous in the radiology literature, and is nonspecifically used to refer to any masslike lesion without a neoplastic cause. In the liver, diffuse infiltrative processes sparring certain regions or cirrhosis with nodular regeneration can result in a "pseudotumor" on imaging.[222,223]

Focal and nodular steatosis: Hepatic steatosis is usually diffuse or regional in distribution. However, nodular variants are sometimes encountered.[224] Focal hepatic steatosis is a common phenomenon and is usually seen in characteristic locations, most commonly in the medial segment left lobe abutting the ligamentum teres.[225] Less typically, steatosis can present as a multinodular variant that may be confused with metastatic disease (see Figure 3-17).[226,227] The demonstration of microscopic fat on chemical shift–sensitive MRI can help avoid this diagnostic dilemma. On contrast-enhanced CT and MR, enhancing vessels can sometimes be seen coursing through steatosis regions, a finding that distinguishes these lesions from primary or secondary hepatic masses (see Figure 3-17).[228]

Focal fatty sparing: The obverse of focal hepatic steatosis, focal fatty sparing, can also occur. In this situation, there is fatty infiltration of the majority of the liver with small focal regions of sparing that on imaging can resemble a focal liver mass. Focal fatty sparing occurs most commonly around the gall bladder fossa, in the left lobe of the liver, or abutting the falciform ligament (see Figure 3-18).[229,230]

MULTIPLE MASSES OR NODULES OF THE LIVER

Like solitary masses and nodules, multifocal hepatic masses or nodules can be solid or cystic in character, features that can help distinguish the underlying cause of the lesion.

Multiple Cystic or Cystic-Appearing Liver Masses

Simple idiopathic cysts are the most common multifocal cystic-appearing lesion of the liver. Other causes include multiple hemangiomas, cystic metastasis, autosomal dominant polycystic liver disease, and multifocal liver abscesses (Table 3-3).

Idiopathic cysts

The incidence of idiopathic hepatic cysts in the general population is not known; however, 1 study of 1541 consecutive US examinations of the liver showed an 11.3% incidence of hepatic cysts.[231] There were no cysts found in 413 individuals younger than 40 years, suggesting that the incidence of idiopathic hepatic cysts increases with increasing age. The cause for this common hepatic abnormality is not known; however, they have no clinical significance, other than that they can be confused with metastasis and other hepatic neoplasms. Rarely, hepatic cysts can be symptomatic, particularly in patients with polycystic liver or kidney disease, and they can be treated by surgical unroofing procedures or catheter drainage with or without sclerosis.[232] They are composed of cuboidal epithelium surrounded by fibrous stroma and contain serous fluid.[233] Their incidence increases with age and they are more commonly multiple rather than solitary.[27] Except when very small, they unequivocally can be diagnosed by any of the cross-sectional imaging techniques through demonstration of the characteristic imaging features of a cyst. Idiopathic cysts can be subdivided into those that are simple and those that are complex.

Simple cysts: Hepatic cysts are round or oval in cross section with imperceptible walls and contain simple fluid.

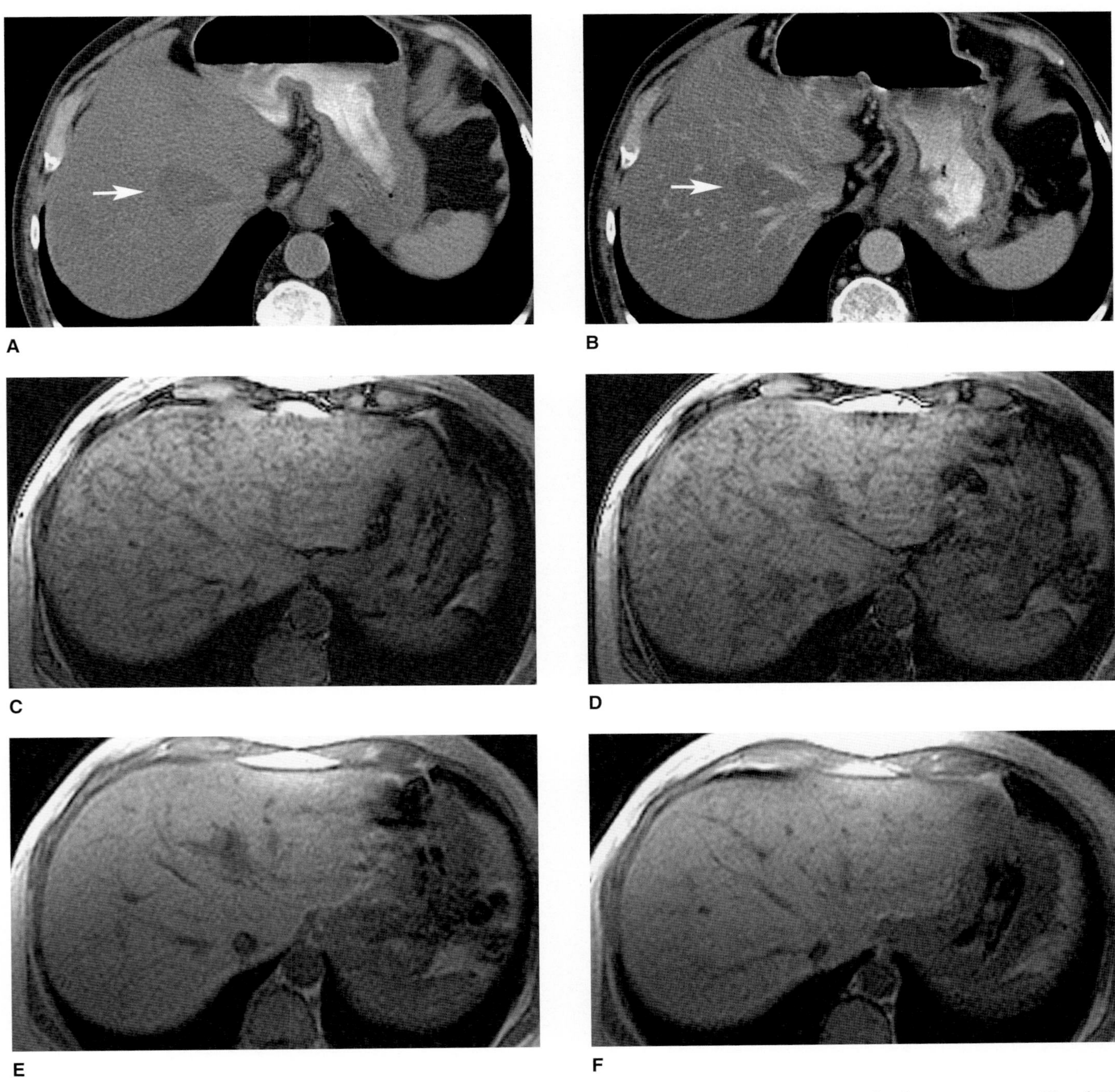

Figure 3-17 Nodular Steatosis in 2 Patients
A and **B**. This 66-year-old man was being evaluated for a renal mass. Unenhanced (A) and enhanced (B) CT images show a focal zone of decreased attenuation within the liver. Note the geographic borders and the presence of undisturbed vessels passing through the lesion. These are typical features of focal fatty infiltration. **C-F**. This 46-year-old woman had an islet cell transplant. Opposed-phase T1-weighted MRI sequence (C and D) shows innumerable small, low-signal lesions throughout the liver. In-phase T1-weighted sequence (E and F) shows no evidence of the small lesions. This combination of findings indicates the presence of fat within the lesions and represents multinodular hepatic steatosis.

On US examinations, they will appear anechoic (uniformly black) and have increased through transmission;[234] on CT examinations, they will have an attenuation between 0 and 20 HU and will not enhance with IV contrast.[235] On MRI examinations, they will be uniformly low-intermediate intensity (medium gray) on T1-weighted sequences and uniformly high intensity (bright white) on T2-weighted sequences (see Figure 3-19).[236,237]

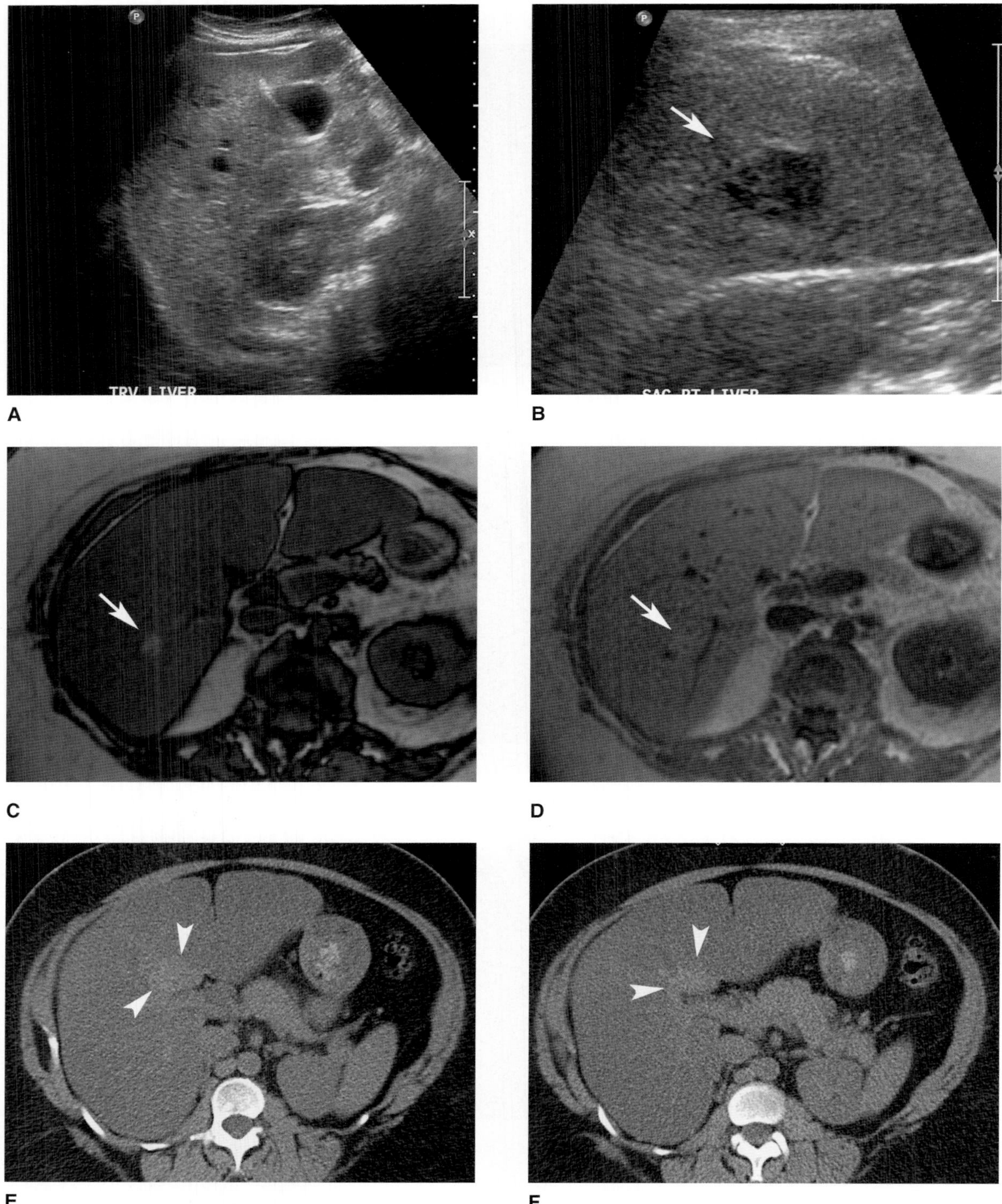

Figure 3-18 Focal Fatty Sparing Appearing as a Liver Mass in 3 Patients

A and **B.** This 38-year-old woman had right upper quadrant pain. US of the liver (A) shows diffuse hyperechogenicity, a finding associated with steatosis. Within the right hepatic lobe (B), this hypoechogenic mass (*arrow*) was discovered. Subsequent MRI (not shown) was pathognomonic for focal fatty sparing. **C** and **D**. This 62-year-old women had colon cancer with local spread to the pelvic nodes and peritoneum. Opposed-phase (C) and in-phase (D) imaging demonstrates diffuse hepatic steatosis. There is a focal nodule (*arrows*) that is both bright on opposed-phase imaging and iso-intense on in-phase imaging. No abnormality was seen on diffusion imaging, and the lesion did not hyperenhance following gadolinium. FDG-PET imaging was also negative for hepatic metastatic disease. On serial imaging, the lesion varied in size based on degree of steatosis. These findings are compatible with nodular sparing of steatosis. **E** and **F.** This 62-year-old woman had lung cancer. Unenhanced CT of the abdomen viewed with narrow windows shows a focal masslike region (*arrowheads*) adjacent to the porta hepatis that could be confused with a liver metastasis. However, the liver is diffusely low attenuation relative to the spleen, indicating hepatic steatosis. This pseudolesion represents focal fatty sparing.

Table 3-3. Multiple Cystic or Cystic-Appearing Liver Masses

1. Idiopathic cysts a. **Simple cysts**[a] b. Complex cysts
2. Polycystic liver disease
3. Multiple cystic or cystic-appearing neoplasms a. **Multiple hemangiomas** b. Biliary hamartoma c. **Cystic and mucinous metastases**
4. Multifocal abscesses a. Fungal microabscesses b. Acute disseminated tuberculosis c. Bacterial abscesses d. Amebic abscesses

[a]Most common appear in bold.

Complex cysts: Complex cysts are cysts that have septations, a thickened wall, and/or have contents other than simple fluid within them as a result of prior infections or hemorrhage (see Figure 3-19). On US, internal septations and complex mildly echogenic fluid and or debris can be shown.[238] Higher CT attenuation values can be seen internally because of increased protein content, such as from old hemorrhage.[235] On MRI, proteinaceous or hemorrhagic cysts will have T1 shortening and therefore higher T1 signal.[239,240]

Polycystic liver disease

Polycystic liver disease encompasses a spectrum of imaging presentations. A polycystic liver is often an accompanying feature of autosomal dominant polycystic kidney disease (ADPCK), presenting in upwards of 70% to 80% of such patients.[241] However, polycystic liver disease can be present as a distinct entity without renal involvement.[242] Patients with polycystic liver disease demonstrate DNA alterations that map to a different genetic locus than that of ADPCK.[243-245] Although usually asymptomatic, polycystic liver disease can cause symptoms, including abdominal pain,[246] portal hypertension,[247,248] and lower extremity swelling (because of IVC obstruction).[247,248] Even in the setting of extensive hepatic involvement, liver dysfunction is rare.[249]

Imaging of polycystic liver disease by either US, CT, or MRI will reveal the extent of liver involvement. Appearance is variable depending on the degree of hepatic involvement. The liver is generally enlarged—sometimes massively. Cysts of varying size and number are scattered throughout the liver, typically with areas of interspersed normal liver (see Figure 3-20). Most cysts are simple in appearance, although septations, hemorrhage, or thickened cyst walls can be seen. Imaging is generally done to confirm the presence of cysts as the cause of hepatomegaly, and to document the size and location of cysts when interventional or surgical therapies are planned in the setting of intractable symptoms. Often, vascular compression of the portal vein or IVC can be seen, and imaging can be used to plan directed therapy toward the lesion(s), resulting in vascular compromise.

Imaging Notes 3-8. Multiple Nodular Lesions of the Liver

- Idiopathic cysts and hemangiomas are the most common cause of multiple cystic-appearing nodules of the liver.
- Metastases are the most common cause of multiple solid-appearing nodules of the liver.

Multiple cystic or cystic-appearing neoplasms

There are 2 neoplasms that commonly appear as multiple cystic-appearing lesions in the liver: hemangiomas and biliary hamartomas. There are also some cystic or mucinous malignancies that when they metastasize to the liver cause multiple cystic liver metastasis.

Multiple hemangiomas: Multiple hemangiomas are the most common cause, after idiopathic cysts, of multiple cystic-appearing masses of the liver. Hemangiomas are solid vascular tumors, but because they are largely composed of blood-filled channels, they can have imaging features of a cystic lesion on unenhanced CT and MRI examinations. On contrast-enhanced CT and MRI, hemangiomas have a characteristic enhancement pattern, discontinuous peripheral globular enhancement, a finding pathognomonic for hemangioma. On US examinations, hepatic hemangiomas appear as a densely echogenic solid masses of the liver. Hemangiomas are discussed most completely under the prior heading: **Solitary Cysts and Cystic-Appearing Lesions**.

Biliary hamartoma: Biliary hamartomas are small benign tumors composed of dilated bile ducts with interspersed fibrous or hyaline stroma. These are relatively common hepatic lesions and can be incidentally found in slightly less than 1%of autopsies, and are not clinically significant.[52,53] Biliary hamartomas can be seen by US, contrast-enhanced CT, and MRI[52,54-57] and characteristically appear as small, usually <15-mm, simple cysts. Smaller lesions can appear to be partly or completely solid as enhancement of the lesion rim and/or septae can obscure the central fluid attenuation.[250] In general, MRI is the most accurate means of characterizing these lesions because of the sensitivity of T2-weighted MRI for small cysts regardless of size (see Figure 3-21).

Cystic and mucinous metastases: Metastatic disease to the liver commonly presents as solitary or multiple solid masses, and is described later in this chapter. However, cystic or mucinous metastases deserve special mention,

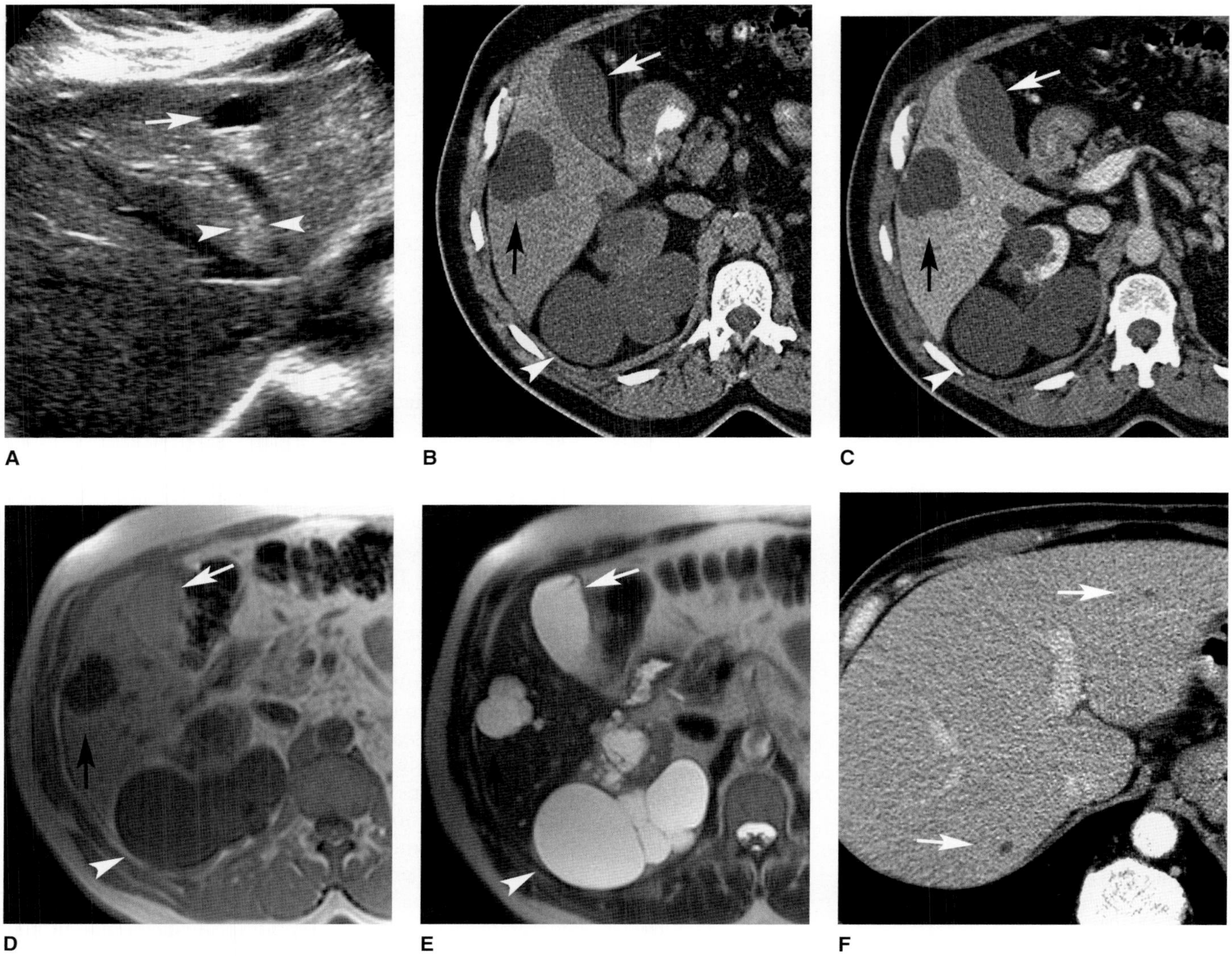

A B C

D E F

Figure 3-19 Idiopathic Hepatic Cysts in 3 Patients
A. US of the liver, in the first patient, shows a 1-cm, anechoic lesion (*arrow*) in the left lobe of the liver. This has increased through transmission (*arrowheads*) seen as a bright band extending inferiorly from the back of the cyst. All of these findings are characteristic of a simple hepatic cyst. **B.** Noncontrast CT, (**C**) postcontrast CT, (**D**) T1-weighted MRI, and (**E**) T2-weighted MRI images in a second patient demonstrate a 2.5-cm lobulated lesion (*black arrows*) in the right lobe of the liver. On CT, this is low attenuation and does not enhance with intravenous contrast. On MRI, it has a low signal on T1-weighted sequences and a very high signal on T2-weighted sequences. These are the typical features of an idiopathic cyst. Note the fine septations in the cyst in image (E), indicating a minimally complex cyst. In the retroperitoneum is a multiseptated renal cyst (*arrowheads*) that has similar CT and MRI features to the hepatic cyst. The gallbladder (*white arrow*) medial to the liver also has similar CT and MRI features, except for the T1-weighted sequence. The bile salts are not the same as simple fluid and alter the T1 relaxation of the fluid in the gallbladder, changing the signal characteristics. (**F**) Contrast-enhanced CT in a third patient demonstrates 2 tiny hypodensities (*arrows*) in the liver. Tiny liver hypodensities similar to these lesions are accidentally found in a large number of CT scans of the abdomen. In the majority of cases, they will represent small incidental liver cysts.

as they can be casually misidentified as a benign lesion because of their partially cystic appearance.

Mucinous tumors are complex multiseptated masses filled with mucinous, gelatinous material. Solid tissue, though present, can represent only small papillary nodules arising from the periphery of the mass or along thickened septations. These tumors can be confused with cystic lesions[75] and can arise from a variety of organs, including the ovary, gastrointestinal tract, and pancreas. Ovarian cancer is the most common site of mucinous neoplasms; however, they generally spread by peritoneal metastasis, and hematogenous metastasis to any organ—including the

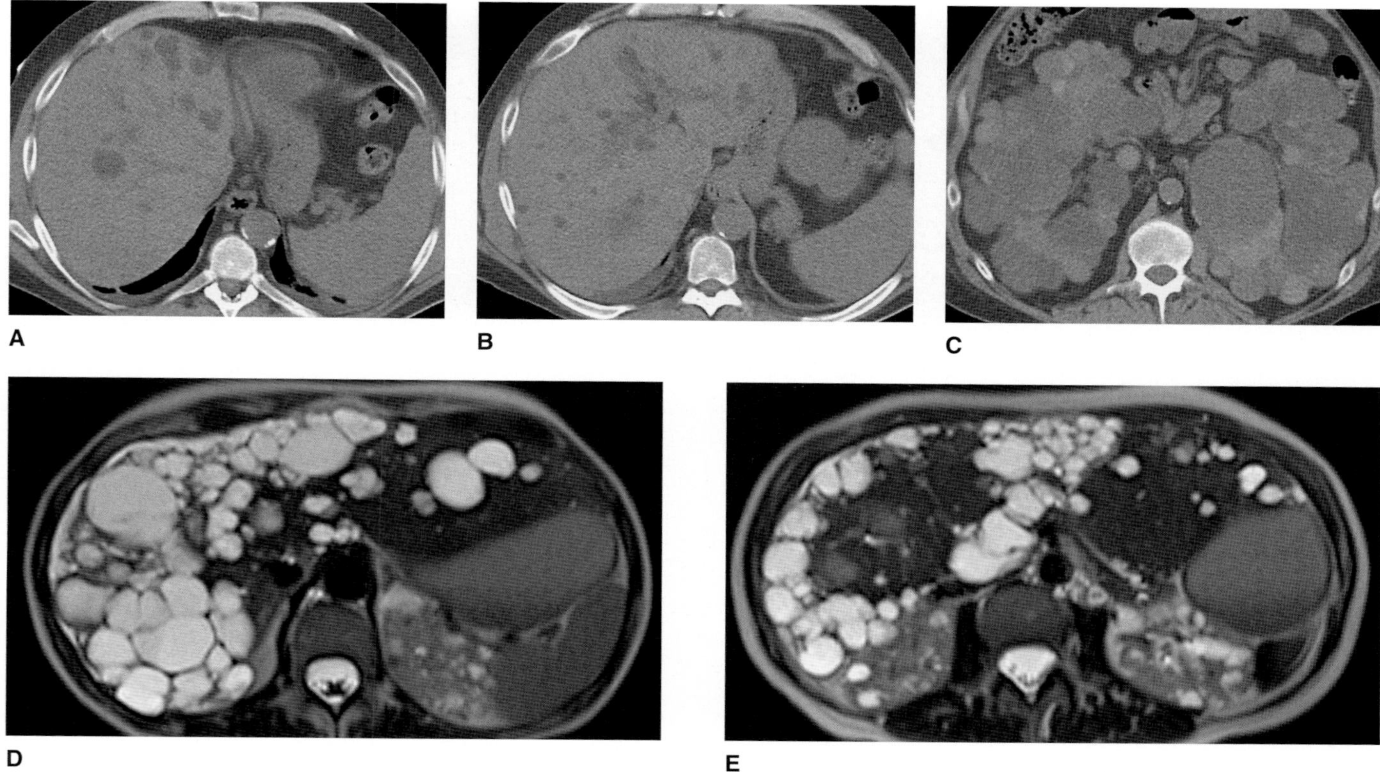

Figure 3-20 Polycystic Liver Disease in 2 Patients
A-C. This 58-year-old woman has innumerable large kidney cysts seen in (C) and many hepatic cysts seen in (A and B). This is typical of autosomal dominant polycystic kidney and liver disease. Liver cysts are typically less predominant than kidney cysts but can occasionally be severe. **D** and **E.** This 58-year-old man also has innumerable liver and kidney cysts seen on these T2-weighted MRI images. This person had normal renal function and has much less severe kidney cysts relative to liver cysts.

liver—is unusual. Appendiceal carcinomas are often mucinous in nature; however, these tumors also demonstrate a propensity for peritoneal metastasis, rather than hematogenous metastasis.[76] Gastrointestinal primary tumors, particularly stomach and colon, typically metastasize to the liver. Cystic pancreatic neoplasms, particular mucinous tumors, when malignant, will often demonstrate hematogenous metastasis to the liver.

On imaging, mucinous metastases will often appear as solitary or multiple cystic lesions that resemble idiopathic cysts or hemangiomas on US, CT, and MRI (see Figure 3-22). However, careful evaluation of the lesion on enhanced CT or MRI examinations will reveal peripheral enhancement without the globular discontinuous character that is typical of hemangiomas. Diffusion-weighted MRI can also be useful for distinguishing cystic metastases from other cystic lesion mimickers and has been discussed in detail under the heading: **Solitary Cysts and Cystic-Appearing Lesions**.[77]

Multifocal abscesses

As noted earlier in this chapter, abscesses to the liver include pyogenic, amebic, echinococcal, and fungal causes. Fungal abscesses characteristically cause multiple tiny abscesses and will be discussed here. Pyogenic, amebic, and echinococcal abscesses will often cause solitary or a few cystic masses and have been discussed previously under the heading: **Solitary Cysts and Cystic-Appearing Lesions** (see Figure 3-9).

Fungal microabscesses: Fungal liver abscesses will nearly always be a complication of disseminated candidiasis. They will usually appear as innumerable small lesions in the liver and spleen. Hepatic candidal infection is most commonly seen in immunocompromised patients, particularly febrile neutropenic patients who have undergone recent bone marrow transplantation. The appearance of these lesions on US and CT is nonspecific but is usually easily identified when multiple small lesions are seen in both the liver and spleen in the correct clinical setting (see Figure 3-23).[251-253] Rim enhancement of these lesions on CT is less pronounced than on MRI. On MRI, the moderately T2 hyperintense appearance can be useful for detection when contrast-enhanced examination is not feasible because of renal insufficiency.[100] When contrast CT or MRI is performed, early rim hyperenhancement is a common imaging feature. MRI is often preferred for diagnosis, because of the slightly higher sensitivity of T2-weighted images for the detection of small amounts of fluid.[254]

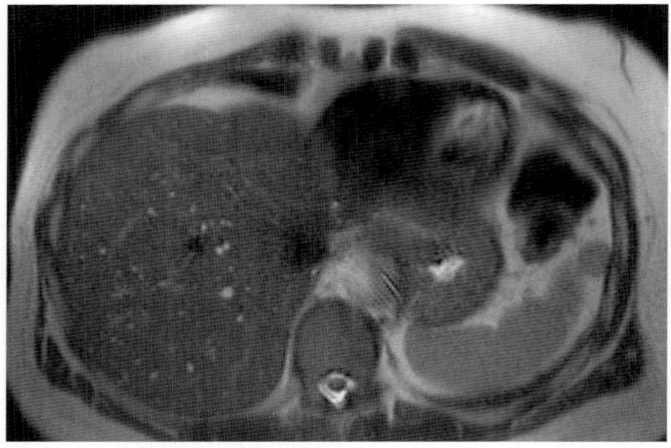

A

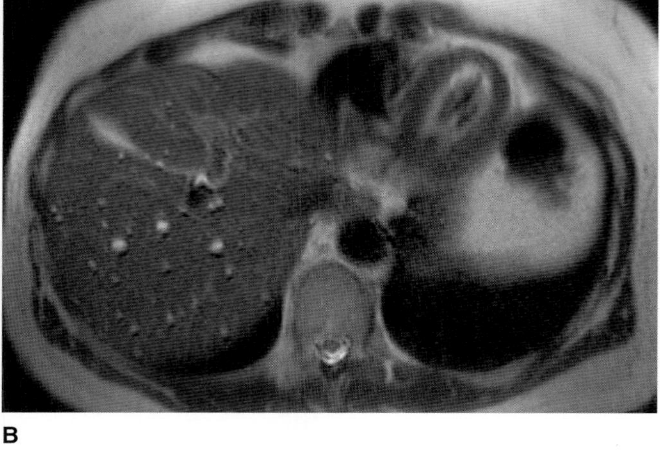

B

Figure 3-21 Probable Biliary Hamartomas
This 65-year-old man was being evaluated for a kidney mass. **A** and **B.** T2-weighted MRI images show innumerable tiny high signal cysts in the liver. Although these may represent small idiopathic cysts, this pattern of many tiny cysts will often indicate the presence of multiple small biliary hamartomas.

Following successful antifungal therapy, hepatic fungal microabscesses will typically demonstrate decreasing size and relative loss of conspicuity on follow-up CT scans.[255] However, lesions can persist following successful medical therapy in some cases.[256] On MRI, both the T2 hyperintensity and the gadolinium hyperenhancement will typically fade once effective therapy is initiated. However, small hyperintense foci of granulation tissue can remain at the sites of previous abscesses.

Multiple Solid Hepatic Masses or Nodules

Multiple solid hepatic masses or nodules will most often be due to primary or secondary neoplasms of the liver but can rarely be a result of granulomatous infection of the liver (Table 3-4).

Neoplasms appearing as multiple solid masses or nodules

Metastasis is the most common neoplasm to appear as multiple solid hepatic masses or nodules. Other neoplastic causes of this pattern include multiple FNH, multiple adenomas, and lymphoma.

Metastatic disease: Metastases are the most common malignancy of the liver. They most often originate from gastrointestinal malignancies, especially colon, stomach, and pancreatic carcinomas.[257] Lung and breast cancer are common extra-abdominal malignancies to metastasize to the liver. However, almost any malignant tumor can metastasize to the liver.

Hepatic metastasis will typically appear as multiple round or oval nodules. These lesions will usually appear smoothly marginated but can occasionally have irregular borders (see Figure 3-24). When multiple larger metastases are present, they can become confluent, forming a nonspherical lesion that can resemble a more infiltrative process (see Figure 3-24).

Hepatic metastases are typically hypoechoic to liver on US, although occasionally they can have a heterogenous echotexture or uniform hyperechoic echotexture (see Figure 3-24).[258]

On noncontrast CT, most metastasis are faintly hypodense to liver parenchyma, unless calcified. The attenuation difference between the liver and metastasis can be very small, making it very difficult to identify metastatic lesions on unenhanced CT. Use of narrow display windows can improve the detection of these more subtle lesions. Calcification (psammomatous bodies) is relatively common in mucinous colon carcinoma metastases,[259,260] with rarer reports in other tumor types.[261]

On MRI, metastases typically appear hypointense on T1-weighted imaging. On T2-weighted imaging, metastases will typically appear moderate hyperintense, a feature that in some situations can be confused with benign cysts or hemangiomas. However, the T2 hyperintensity typically decreases on more heavily T2-weighted longer echo time (TE) sequences, an important feature distinguishing metastasis from benign cysts or hemangiomas on noncontrast imaging (see Figure 3-25).[262] DWI has been shown to be helpful in identifying metastases as areas of restricted diffusion, particularly when the use of gadolinium is contraindicated or otherwise not possible (see Figure 3-26).[263-266]

The appearance of metastases on contrast-enhanced CT and MRI is variable. Most lesions are hypoattenuating or hypointense to enhanced liver on portal-phase CT

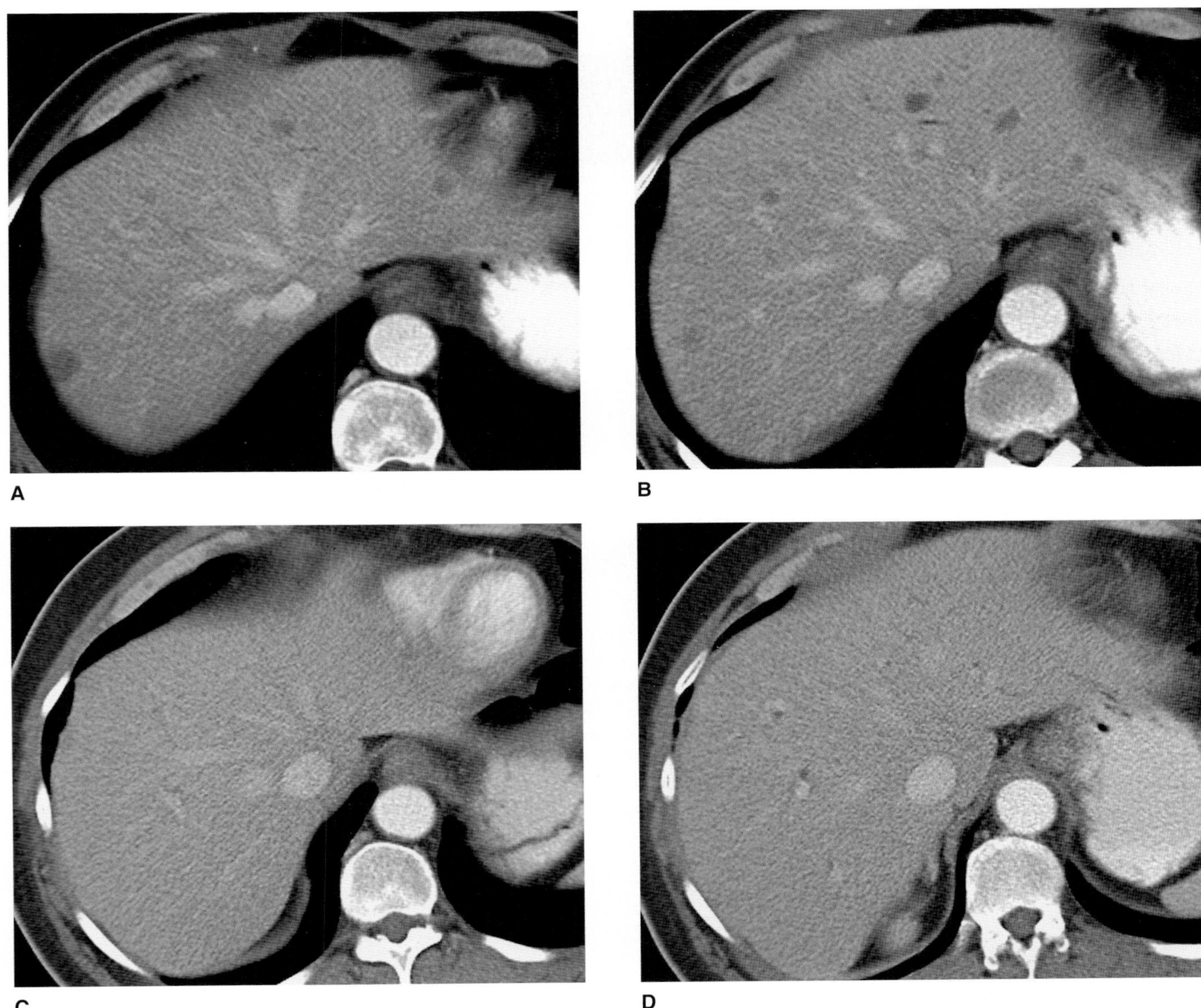

Figure 3-22 Multiple Cystic Metastasis
This 66-year-old woman had pancreatic carcinoma. **A** and **B.** Contrast-enhanced axial CT images show multiple uniformly low attenuation lesions within the liver. In most cases, these will represent small idiopathic hepatic cysts. **C** and **D.** A CT examination performed 5 months earlier shows no evidence of the small cystic lesions, identifying them as small cystic metastasis.

and MRI.[41,267] When large, the lesions are often heterogeneous, with enhancing rims, and relatively less attenuating (necrotic) cores (see Figure 3-24). Certain tumors with hypervascular characteristics, such as renal cell carcinoma, thyroid cancer, neuroendocrine tumors, and malignant melanoma can have similar portal venous enhancement to the normal liver parenchyma. This characteristic can make it difficult or impossible to appreciate hypervascular metastasis from normal liver on portal phase contrast-enhanced CT, images that are the standard phase of liver imaging on CT. In such cases, the addition of hepatic arterial-phase images by CT (or MRI) can improve lesion detection.[41,268,269] Scanning through the liver prior to contrast administration and during the arterial and portal venous phases of enhancement is called a "triple phase" study and is recommended in the evaluation of liver metastasis from hypervascular neoplasms. Care must be taken to differentiate between benign etiologies of hypervascular liver lesions (FNH, adenoma, or hemangioma) and hypervascular liver metastases. MRI may be most useful in this regard, as these lesions typically have different imaging appearance on noncontrast T1- and T2-weighted sequences.

Imaging Notes 3-9. Hypervascular Liver Masses or Nodules

					Enhancement Pattern			
					Early-Phase[e]		Late-Phase[f]	
Lesion Type	US[a]	NC-CT[b]	T1W[c]	T2W[d]	Contrast	Morphology	Contrast	Morphology
Hemangioma	↑↑	↓	↓↓	↑↑	↑↑	Peripheral nodular	↑	Uniform
Hemangioendothelioma	↓	↓↓	↓	↑	↑↑	Heterogeneous	Variable	Heterogenous
Focal nodular hyperplasia	→	→	→	↓ to →	↑↑	Uniform	→	Delayed enhancing scar
Hepatic adenoma	→	→	→	→ to ↑	↑↑	Slightly heterogeneous	↓	Homogeneous
Hepatocellular carcinoma	↓↓	↓	↓ to →	→ to ↑	Variable, often ↑↑	Homogeneous (unless large)	↓	Homogeneous (unless large)
Metastases	↓	↓	↓	↑	↑↑	Usually rim	→	Homogenous (unless large)
Arteriovenous malformations	↓↓	↓↓	↓↓	Variable	↑↑	Uniform	↑↑	Uniform
Abscess	↓	↓	↓	↑↑	↑↑	Rim	↑↑	Rim

Imaging features may be variable, especially for larger lesions. The most common imaging features are shown.
[a]Ultrasonography. Features represent echogenicity relative to surrounding liver.
[b]Noncontrast computed tomography. Features represent attenuation relative to surrounding liver on unenhanced images.
[c]T1-Weighted MRI. Features represent signal intensity relative to surrounding liver.
[d]T2-Weighted MRI. Features represent signal intensity relative to surrounding liver.
[e]Late arterial phase of liver enhancement on CT or MRI. Features represent enhancement relative to background liver.
[f]Portal-delayed phase of liver enhancement on CT or MRI. Features represent enhancement relative to background liver.
↓↓ = markedly hypo-; ↓ = moderately hypo-; → = iso-; ↑ = moderately hyper-; ↑↑ = markedly hyper-

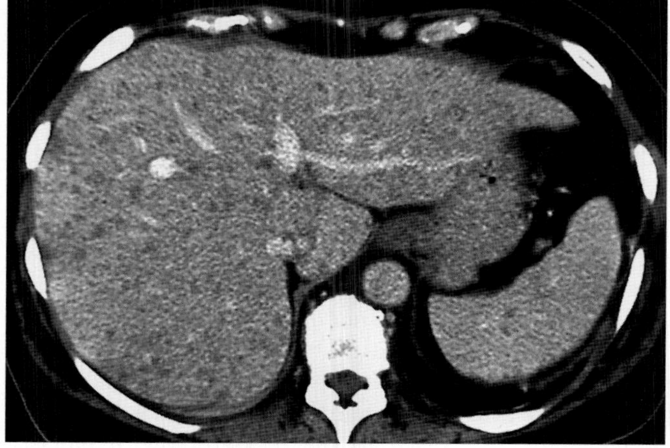
A

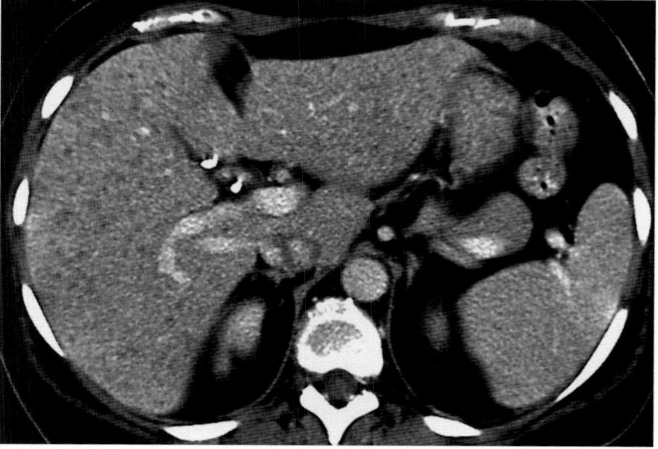
B

Figure 3-23 Candida Microabscesses of the Liver and Spleen This 52-year-old man with acute myeloid lymphoma was neutropenic as a result of chemotherapy. **A** and **B.** Contrast-enhanced CT images viewed with narrow windows reveal innumerable small low attenuation lesions in the liver and a few small low attenuation lesions in the spleen. This is the characteristic appearance of hematogenously disseminated candidiasis of the liver and spleen.

Table 3-4. Multiple Solid Hepatic Masses or Nodules

1. Neoplasms appearing as multiple solid masses or nodules a. **Metastatic disease**[a] b. **Multiple focal nodular hyperplasia** c. Multiple hepatic adenomas and hepatic adenomatosis d. Lymphoma
2. Granulomatous diseases of the liver a. Sarcoidosis b. Tuberculosis c. Histoplasmosis
3. Peliosis hepatis

[a]Most common appear in bold.

In many cases, liver metastases will demonstrate patterns of radial variation in signal intensity. Common to all of these imaging patterns is the presence of "layers," which can variably include a necrotic or hypoperfused central tumor core, a well-perfused tumor periphery, and a band of compressed hepatic parenchyma peripherally, with variable degrees of angiogenesis and/or fibrosis, and occasionally perilesional edema. Terms such as *target sign, reverse target sign, halo sign,* and *peripheral washout sign* have been used to describe these phenomena. The nature of these "lamellar" appearances varies by the type of imaging and, when applicable, the relative, timing of contrast administration (see Figure 3-24).[270]

The use of FDG-PET imaging for staging malignancy is increasing. Malignant cells have been shown to take up glucose preferentially (Warburg effect) and thus metastases can be shown as FDG-avid lesions on PET imaging.[271] When PET is used for staging of tumors, the presence of hepatic metastases is usually easily determined (see Figure 3-27). Fluorodeoxyglucose-PET has been shown to be superior to CT in identifying both hepatic and extrahepatic abdominal metastases in a variety of tumor types.[272-276] Smaller metastasis can be difficult to identify on FDG-PET because of mild background hepatic FDG uptake.[277] Furthermore, differentiation between hepatic metastases and extrahepatic nodal, peritoneal, or lung base/pleural lesions can be difficult in some cases. However, the increased use of FDG-PET in combination with low-dose CT for attenuation correction and anatomic correlation (PET-CT) has led to more confident anatomic correlation of FDG-avid lesions.[278]

Multiple focal nodular hyperplasia: Focal nodular hyperplasia is a common hyperplastic proliferation of hepatic parenchyma, hepatocytes, bile canaliculi, and reticuloendothelial cells that is thought to be a hyperplastic response to a central arteriovenous malformation. Focal nodular hyperplasia is the second most common benign tumor of the liver and is most often a solitary lesion. However, occasionally it can present as a few solid nodular lesions of the liver. Focal nodular hyperplasia has been discussed in detail under the heading: **Solitary Solid Hepatic Masses or Nodules.**

Multiple hepatic adenomas and hepatic adenomatosis: Hepatic adenomas will most often appear as a single solid mass of the liver. However, patients with the glycogen storage diseases, oral contraceptives, and patients on anabolic steroids are at risk for the development of multiple hepatic adenomas. In addition to these situations, multiple hepatic adenomas can develop in the absence of an underlying cause, a phenomenon called hepatic adenomatosis.[150-152]

The imaging characteristics of multiple adenomas is the same as for individual adenomas that is discussed in detail under the heading: **Solitary Solid Hepatic Masses or Nodules.**

Lymphoma: Secondary involvement of the liver by lymphomas most often appears as diffuse hepatomegaly but can also appear as 1 or several focal masses.[196] When presenting as a focal mass in the liver, lymphoma will demonstrate a uniform hypoechoic appearance on US.[197] On CT, lymphoma is hypodense to liver,[181] and demonstrates little enhancement following contrast administration (see Figures 3-28 and 14-28). On MRI, lymphoma appears hypointense on T1, with variable signal intensity on T2 imaging, and modest enhancement postgadolinium administration.[198,199]

Granulomatous diseases of the liver

The granulomatous diseases sarcoidosis and tuberculosis can rarely cause multiple, small solid-appearing nodules within the liver.

Sarcoidosis: Sarcoidosis is a systemic granulomatous condition that most commonly involves the lungs and thoracic lymph nodes. However, sarcoidosis can involve multiple extrathoracic organs, including the brain, eye, heart, joints, liver, and spleen. Although pathology studies indicate a high incidence of microscopic liver involvement with sarcoidosis, radiologically evident disease is only seen in about 15% of patients.[182]

On imaging examinations, hepatic sarcoidosis most often appears as hepatomegaly, but in some cases, imaging will demonstrate innumerable small nodules, which represent noncaseating granulomas (see Figure 14-34).[279] Most patients with hepatic nodules, will also have splenic nodules, which are more commonly present than hepatic nodules.[183]

US examinations can show hepatomegaly. In some cases, the hepatic parenchyma will appear more echogenic than normal and occasionally multiple small hypoechoic nodules will be seen throughout the liver.[184] On CT, the hepatic nodules of sarcoidosis will typically appear hypoattenuating to the normal liver (see Figure 14-34).[185] On MRI examinations, the nodules typically appear iso- or hypointense on T1-weighted and hypointense on T2-weighted MR

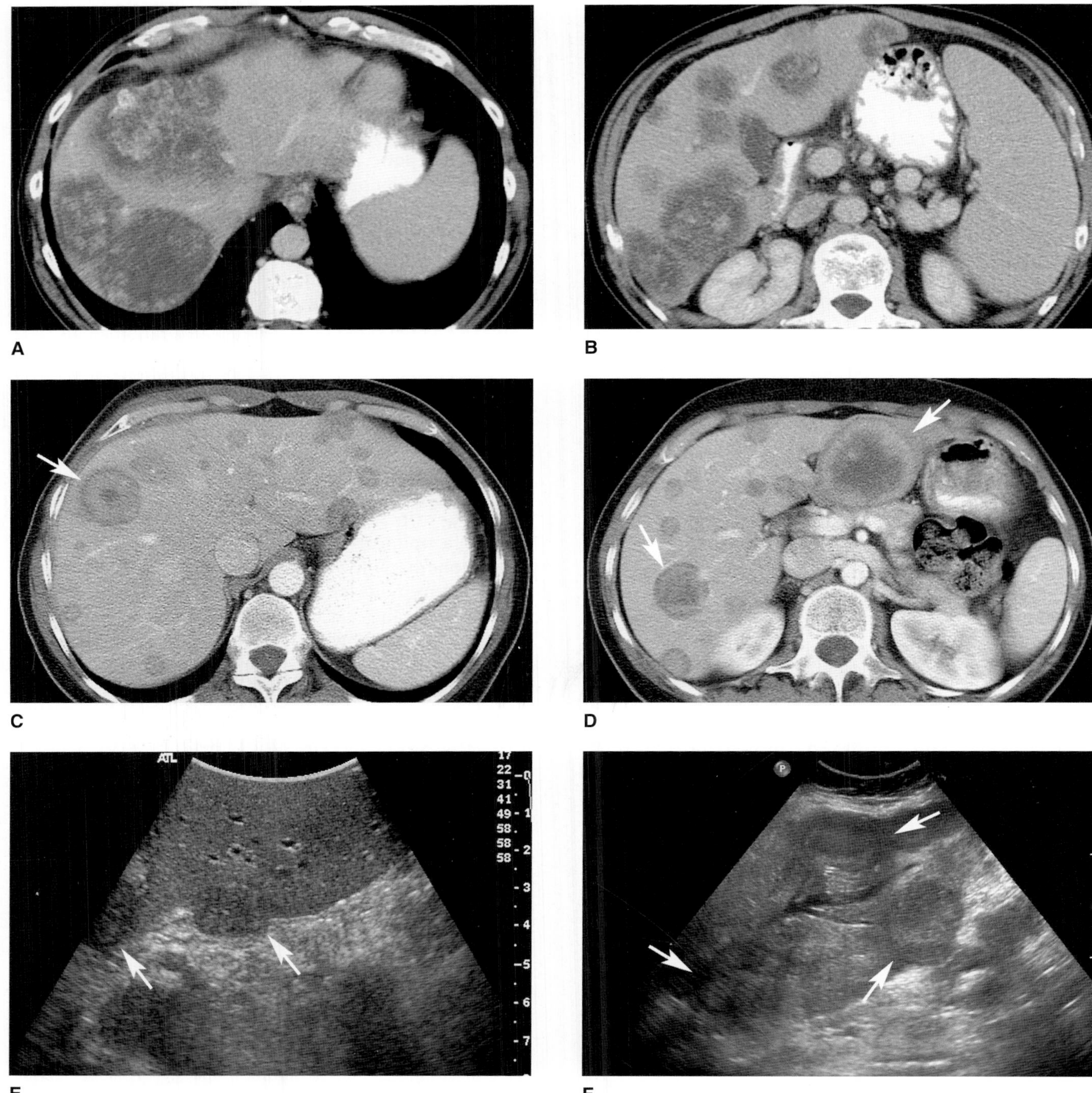

Figure 3-24 Hepatic Metastasis in 4 Patients
A and **B.** This 50-year-old man had colon cancer. Contrast-enhanced CT images through the liver demonstrate multiple hepatic hypodensities with heterogenous areas of enhancement, representing metastasis. Notice how in image (A) several metastasis have grown together to form 2 large irregularly shaped masses. **C** and **D.** This 47-year-old woman had breast cancer. CT images through the liver demonstrate multiple low attenuation lesions seen throughout the liver. Note how many of the lesions demonstrate concentric rings of attenuation, known as the "target" sign (*arrows*). This is an appearance strongly associated with liver metastasis. The central hypoattenuation represents ischemic or necrotic tumor, the higher attenuation middle ring represents viable enhancing tumor and the darker outer ring represents compressed liver parenchyma. **E.** This 49-year-old man had rectal cancer. Longitudinal US of the liver shows 2 hypoechoic masses (*arrow*) in the left lobe of the liver, the typical appearance of hepatic metastasis. **F.** This 61-year-old man had metastatic cancer of unknown primary. Axial US of the liver shows multiple heterogeneously echogenic masses (*arrows*) in the liver indicating the presence of liver metastasis.

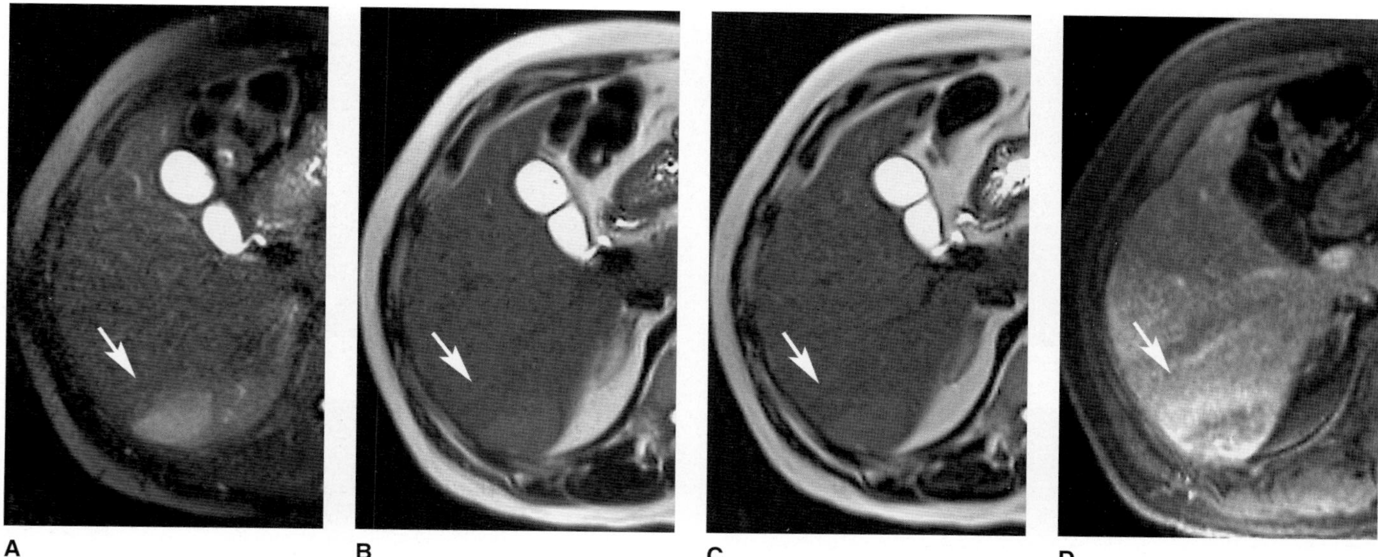

Figure 3-25 Effect of TE on Visualization of Liver Metastases This 51-year-old man had transitional cell carcinoma of the bladder, metastatic to the liver. **A.** The fat-saturated T2 image with moderate T2 weighting (TE = 89 ms) demonstrates a liver lesion with amorphous intermediate-high T2 signal intensity relative to the darker signal of normal liver. **B.** On non–fat suppressed T2 imaging with similar echo time (TE = 104 ms), the lesion conspicuity is similar, though slightly decreased because of the high signal intensity of fat. **C.** On heavily-weighted T2 imaging (TE = 179 ms), the lesion is nearly isointense to liver. **D.** Metastasis is confirmed on the postgadolinium portal-phase image.

images.[186] Sarcoid nodules typically show slow progressive enhancement on dynamic enhanced CT or MR images. In most cases, patients with imaging evidence of hepatic sarcoidosis will also have abdominal lymphadenopathy in the para-aortic, porta hepatis, and celiac chains.[182]

Tuberculosis: Hepatic involvement in tuberculosis is relatively rare. Coinfection with HIV is not uncommon. Presenting symptoms include fever, weight loss, and abdominal pain, with hepatomegaly common in physical examination.[187] Imaging findings vary, including hepatomegaly without discrete focal lesions in the military form, multifocal involvement (similar to that seen in fungal infections), and dominant single lesion.[188] In the latter case, the dominant lesion can be smooth or lobular, often with a complex cystic appearance. In other cases, hepatic tuberculomas can present with low signal on T2-weighted imaging.[189] Calcification on CT is reported in approximately 50% of cases.[96]

Histoplasmosis: Histoplasmosis is endemic in portions of the central United States. However, infection is often subclinical, and imaging reports of acute infection of the liver are few. However, healed infections often present as multiple punctuate calcifications in the liver and/or spleen, a nonspecific imaging finding.[96]

Peliosis hepatis

Peliosis hepatis is a rare benign vascular lesion characterized by solitary or multifocal randomly distributed regions of sinusoidal dilation and blood-filled hepatic spaces. The nodules are typically hyperechoic on US imaging, hypoattenuating on CT examinations, hypoattenuating on T1-weighted MRI, and heterogeneously hyperechoic on T2-weighted MRI examinations. They can have an intense but variable enhancement pattern following the administration of IV contrast. Peliosis hepatis is discussed most completely under the heading: **Solitary Solid Hepatic Masses or Nodules.**

NONSPHERICAL, FOCAL LESIONS OF THE LIVER

Most focal lesions of the liver will have an approximately spherical shape and appear as round or oval lesions on cross-sectional imaging. However, occasionally, focal abnormalities of the liver will be irregularly shaped or involve regions of the liver. This is most often due to traumatic or vascular-based abnormalities. These lesions often have a distinctive imaging appearance and clinical milieu that helps to specifically diagnose the lesion (Table 3-5).

Liver Trauma

Because of its large size, laceration to the liver is a common consequence of penetrating trauma such as stabbing or gunshot wounds. The liver is also susceptible to injury from blunt abdominal trauma such as automobile accidents or fall from a height, representing up to 10% of abdominal injuries in such settings.[190] Contrast-enhanced CT scans of the abdomen have become an essential element

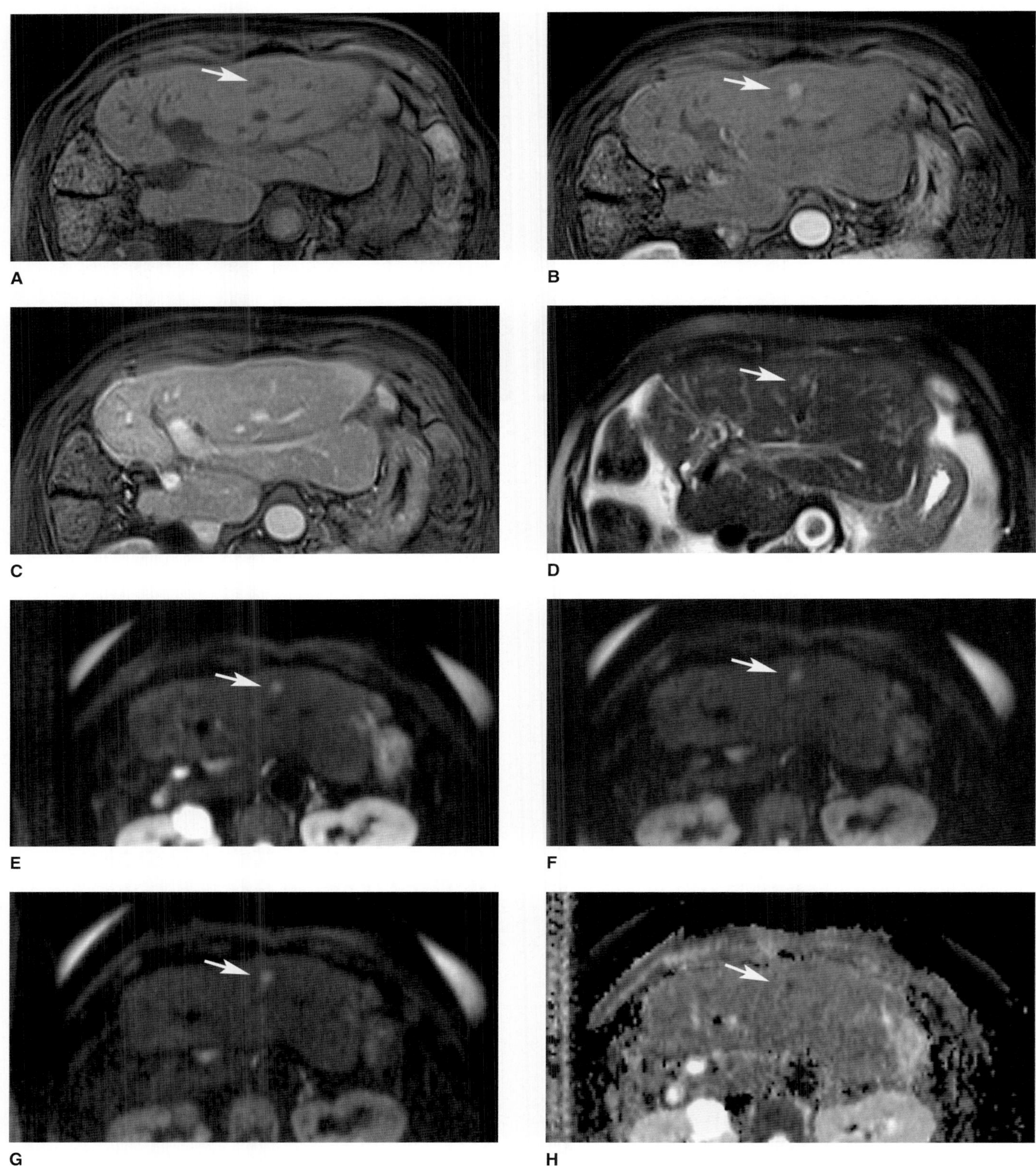

Figure 3-26 Diffusion Imaging of Liver Metastasis
This 64-year-old woman had a neuroendocrine tumor. **A.** Pre-gadolinium T1-weighted image demonstrates a faintly hypointense liver lesion that (**B**) demonstrates arterial-phase enhancement but is not seen on (**C**) portal-phase imaging. **D.** The lesion was also only faintly visible on T2-weighted imaging. **E-G.** Diffusion weighted imaging with *B* values of 50, 400, and 800 demonstrates a hyperintense lesion that does not fade on higher diffusion-weighted sequences. **H.** ADC map confirms restricted diffusion. These features are indicative of a liver metastasis.

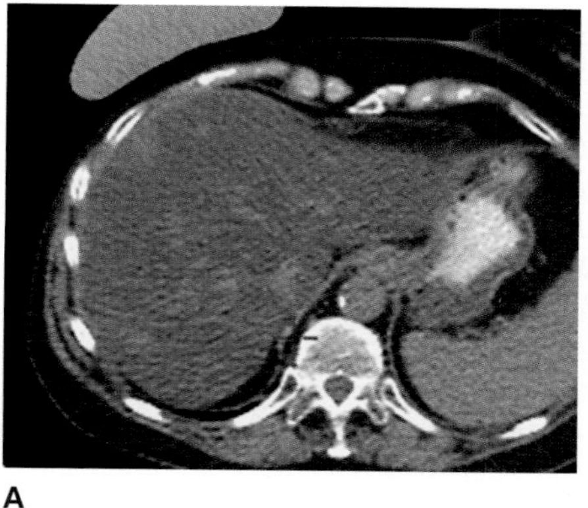
A

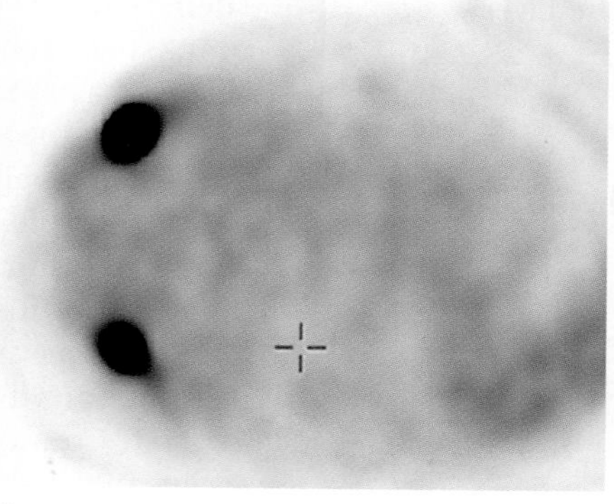
B

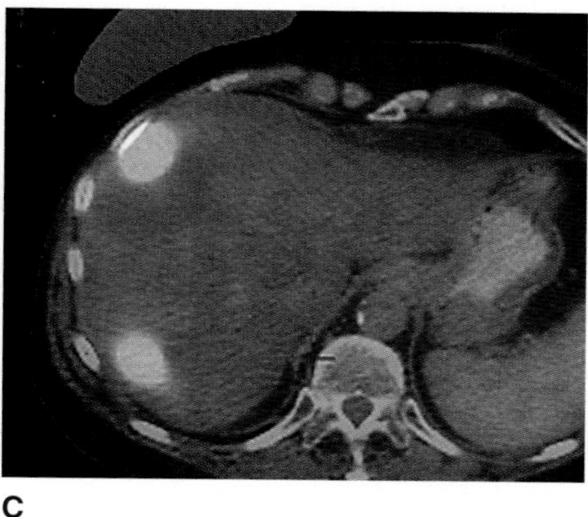
C

Figure 3-27 PET-CT of Liver Metastasis
This 58-year-old woman had breast cancer. **A.** CT images from a PET-CT show faint hypervascular lesions in the liver that are much more conspicuous on the (**B**) PET and (**C**) PET-CT fusion images that represent liver metastasis.

in the evaluation of abdominal trauma and are routinely employed to evaluate the abdominal organs for evidence of trauma,[191] although in some settings US is used as the primary imaging screen for abdominal trauma.[192] Most hepatic trauma can be treated conservatively with supportive care. However, hepatic injury with evidence of active bleeding will often require emergency embolic therapy[193] or laparotomy[280] to stop the ongoing hemorrhage.

Computed tomographic grading for liver trauma[281] ranges from minor (grade 1) injuries to major (grade 5) fragmentation and devascularization (Table 3-6). Grade 1 injuries include periportal blood tracking without visible laceration, and small subcapsular hematomas and lacerations. Deeper lacerations, larger subcapsular hematomas, and central hematomas are grade 2 or 3, depending on the size. Much larger lacerations, and segmental or bilobar fragmentation or devascularization, indicate grade 4 or 5 injury, depending on size and extent. This classification scheme has proven useful for predicting need for operative management,[282] although active arterial extravasation and degree of intraperitoneal blood also predict likelihood of significant injury and/or hemodynamic instability.[283,284]

Subcapsular hematomas are a common finding associated with trauma to the liver and can also be seen following hemorrhage of a hepatic mass such as a hepatic adenoma or HCC. Subcapsular hematomas will usually have a lenticular shape because the blood dissects between the liver capsule and liver parenchyma. Perihepatic hemorrhagic

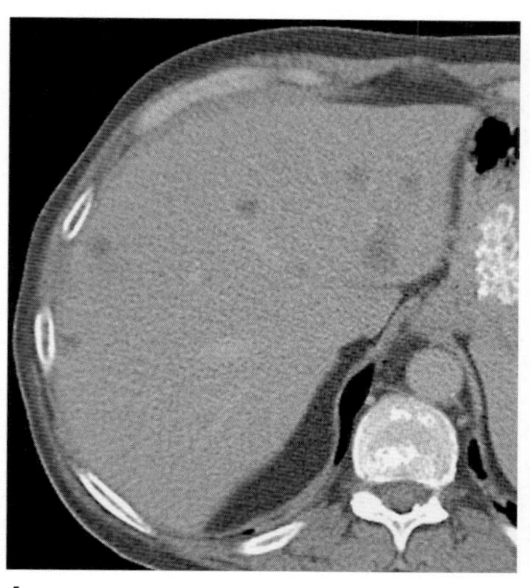
A

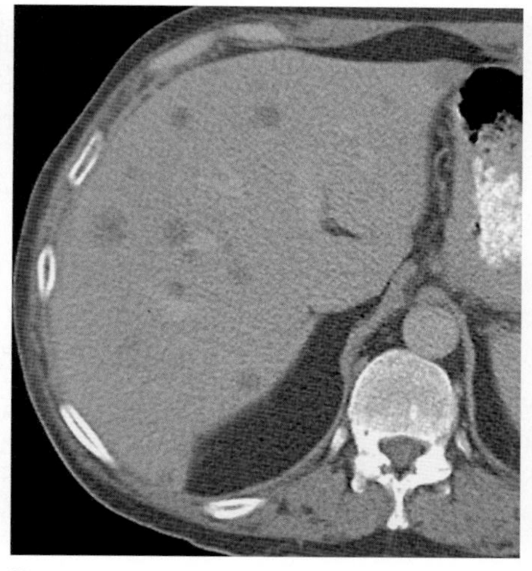
B

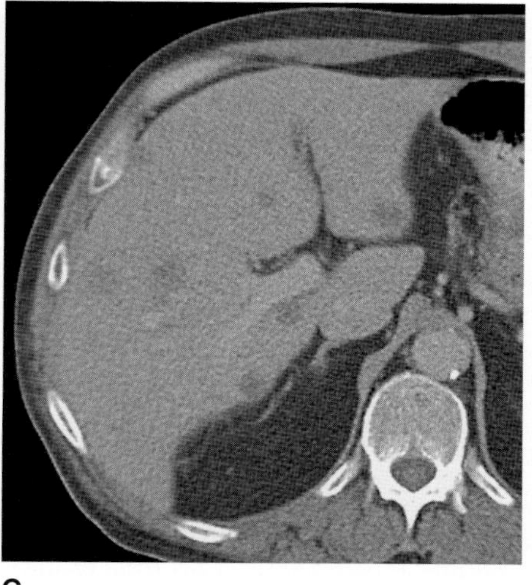
C

Figure 3-28 Multifocal Lymphoma
This 65-year-old man presented with fever, cough, and a rash. **A-C.** Contrast-enhanced CT demonstrates multiple indistinctly marginated nodules in the liver. Given this clinical history, the nodules might have represented multiple liver abscesses but further evaluation was diagnostic of an intermediate grade B-cell lymphoma.

Table 3-5. Nonspherical Focal Lesions of the Liver

1. Laceration/fracture
2. Infarction
3. Transient hepatic attenuation (intensity) difference (THAD, THID)
4. Focal fatty infiltration
5. Focal fatty sparing

ascites will usually have a more crescentic shape because the blood is not under pressure and therefore does not indent the liver parenchyma (see Figures 3-13 and 3-29).

Liver lacerations and contusions will usually appear as irregularly shaped and irregularly marginated lesions of decreased attenuation within the liver on contrast-enhanced CT. On noncontrast CT, small lacerations may be harder to identify, though larger ones are often recognized as a regional or segmental irregularly marginated hypodense lesion (see Figure 3-29). Lacerations from penetrating trauma will, by definition, extend to the liver capsule. Contusions from blunt trauma are more variable in their appearance, but in most cases will also extend to the liver capsule. Liver lacerations can also be identified on US examination as irregularly marginated hypoechoic regions, often with associated pericapsular fluid or hematoma. On contrast-enhanced CT, extravasation of contrast can be observed as small puddles of markedly increased attenuation within the area of trauma (see Figure 3-29).

When liver trauma results in severe injury to the hepatic capsule, hematoma and hemorrhagic ascites is the common result. Hematomas will often occur adjacent to the organ of injury (the so-called sentinel le clot sign).[285] Hemorrhagic ascites will appear as free fluid within the peritoneum with an attenuation measurement greater than 20 HU. Common sites of accumulation of hemorrhagic ascites in the abdomen following liver trauma includes the porta hepatic region, Morrison pouch, the right paracolic gutter, and the pelvic recesses (pouch of Douglas in women and the rectovesical pouch in men). The higher attenuation of hemorrhagic ascites can be recognized subjectively by comparing the attenuation of the ascites with the bile in the gallbladder, unopacified urine, or fluid within simple hepatic or renal cysts. The elevated attenuation greater than 20 HU can also be directly measured to confirm the hemorrhagic nature of the fluid.

Bilomas are common posttraumatic abnormalities of the liver from either blunt or penetrating trauma.[286,287] Bilomas will appear as fluid-filled structures that are usually round or oval in shape. However, occasionally they can have tubular or stellate shapes depending on the mechanism of trauma.

Table 3-6. Grading System for Hepatic Trauma

Grade 1 Capsular avulsion, superficial laceration(s) less than 1 cm deep, subcapsular hematoma less than 1 cm in maximum thickness, periportal blood tracking only
Grade 2 Laceration(s) 1-3 cm deep, central subcapsular hematoma(s) 1-3 cm in diameter
Grade 3 Laceration greater than 3 cm deep, central-subcapsular hematoma(s) greater than 3 cm in diameter
Grade 4 Massive central-subcapsular hematoma greater than 10 cm, lobar tissue destruction (maceration) or devascularization
Grade 5 Bilobar tissue destruction (maceration) or devascularization

Reproduced, with permission, from Mirvis SE, Whitley NO, Vainwright JR, Gens DR. Blunt hepatic trauma in adults: CT-based classification and correlation with prognosis and treatment. *Radiology*. 1989;171:27-32.

Spontaneous (Nontraumatic) Hemorrhage

Most spontaneous (nontraumatic) hemorrhage in the abdomen is due to underlying tumors or vascular pathology (ie, ruptured abdominal aortic aneurysm). Even in the event of excessive anticoagulation, spontaneous hemorrhage in the abdomen is typically seen in compartments other than the liver, most commonly the muscle or bowel.[288,289] Spontaneous liver hemorrhage is rare, and in most cases is due to underlying mass, especially hepatic adenoma or HCC (see Figure 3-13).[156,290] However, patients with preeclampsia are prone to the development of subcapsular liver hematomas in the setting of thrombocytopenia form HELLP syndrome.[291,292] When a nontraumatic liver hematoma is discovered on imaging, follow-up is required to exclude underlying mass.

Hepatic Infarction

The liver is supplied by 2 sources of blood, the hepatic artery and the portal vein. If 1 of these supplies is compromised, the other can compensate for the diminished blood flow. As a result, hepatic infarction is a rare event because both vascular supplies must be compromised in order to induce liver ischemia. Most patients will have a preexisting damage to 1 of the 2 blood sources before an infarction can result. For example, patients with portal vein flow disruption, such as in cirrhosis, are more susceptible to ischemic changes.

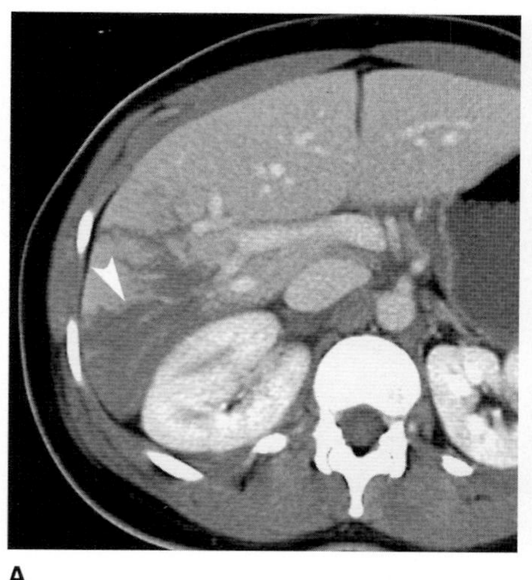
A

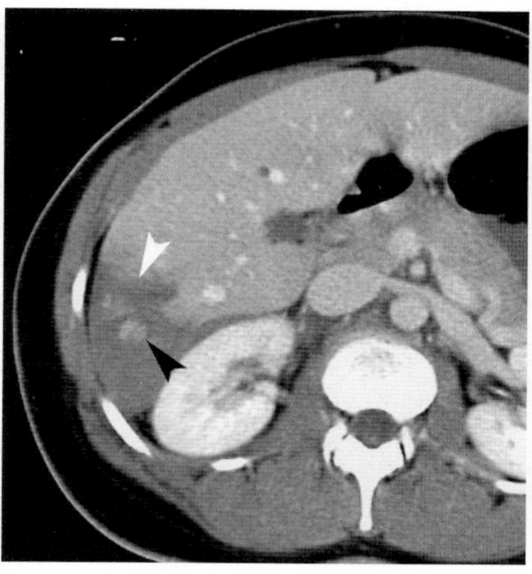
B

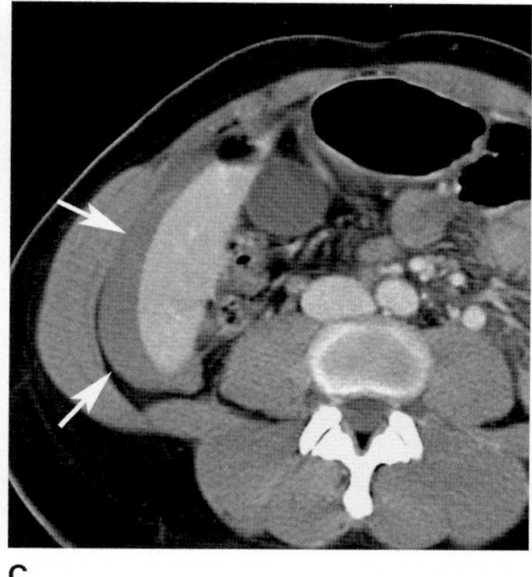
C

Figure 3-29 Liver Laceration
This 31-year-old man was involved in a motor vehicle accident. **A-C**. Contrast-enhanced CT shows an irregularly marginated hypoattenuating lesion (*white arrowheads*) in the posterior segment of the liver typical of a hepatic laceration. Note the perihepatic hemorrhagic ascites (*white arrows*) and the acute extravasation of contrast (*black arrowhead*).

Segmental hepatic ischemia is a known complication of arterial chemoembolism, especially when performed to treat HCC in cirrhotic patients (see Figure 3-30).[293] Major liver or pancreaticobiliary surgery can also lead to segmental hepatic ischemia or infarction.[294,295] Spontaneous hepatic infarction has also been demonstrated in preeclampsia patients with HELLP syndrome.[296]

Further, CT and MRI are the modalities best able to demonstrate segmental hepatic infarction. CT will typically show a wedge-shaped or cone-shaped region of decreased attenuation, with the base of the wedge or cone along the surface of the liver (see Figure 3-31).[297] On MRI, the ischemic region will have the same wedge or cone shape with base along the surface of the liver and will have a low signal on T1-weighted sequences and high signal on T2-weighted sequences.[298] The hallmark of segmental liver infarction is the lack of enhancement following administration of contract agent, indicating

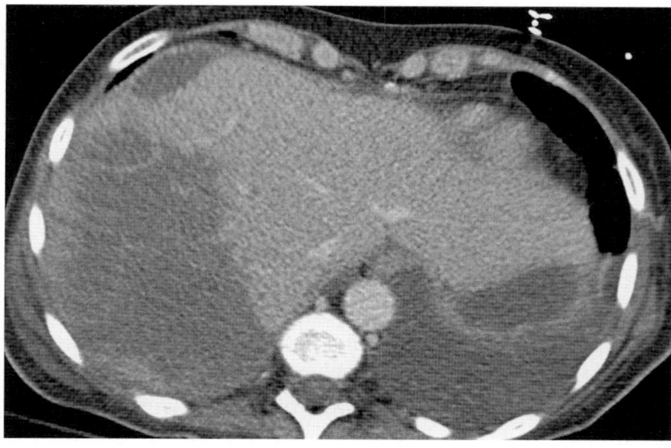
A

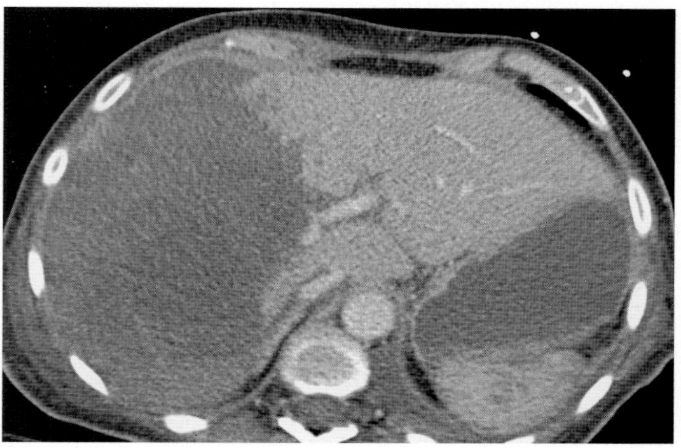
B

Figure 3-30 Hepatic Infarction
This 50-year-old man had suffered from multiple arterial thromboses due to antiphospholipid antibody syndrome and had recently undergone surgical interventions to both his superior mesenteric artery and celiac trunks when he presented with right upper quadrant pain. **A** and **B**. Contrast-enhanced axial CT images during the portal phase of enhancement show nearly the entire right lobe of the liver to be nonenhancing and decreased attenuation consistent with occlusion of the right hepatic artery and infarction of the right lobe.

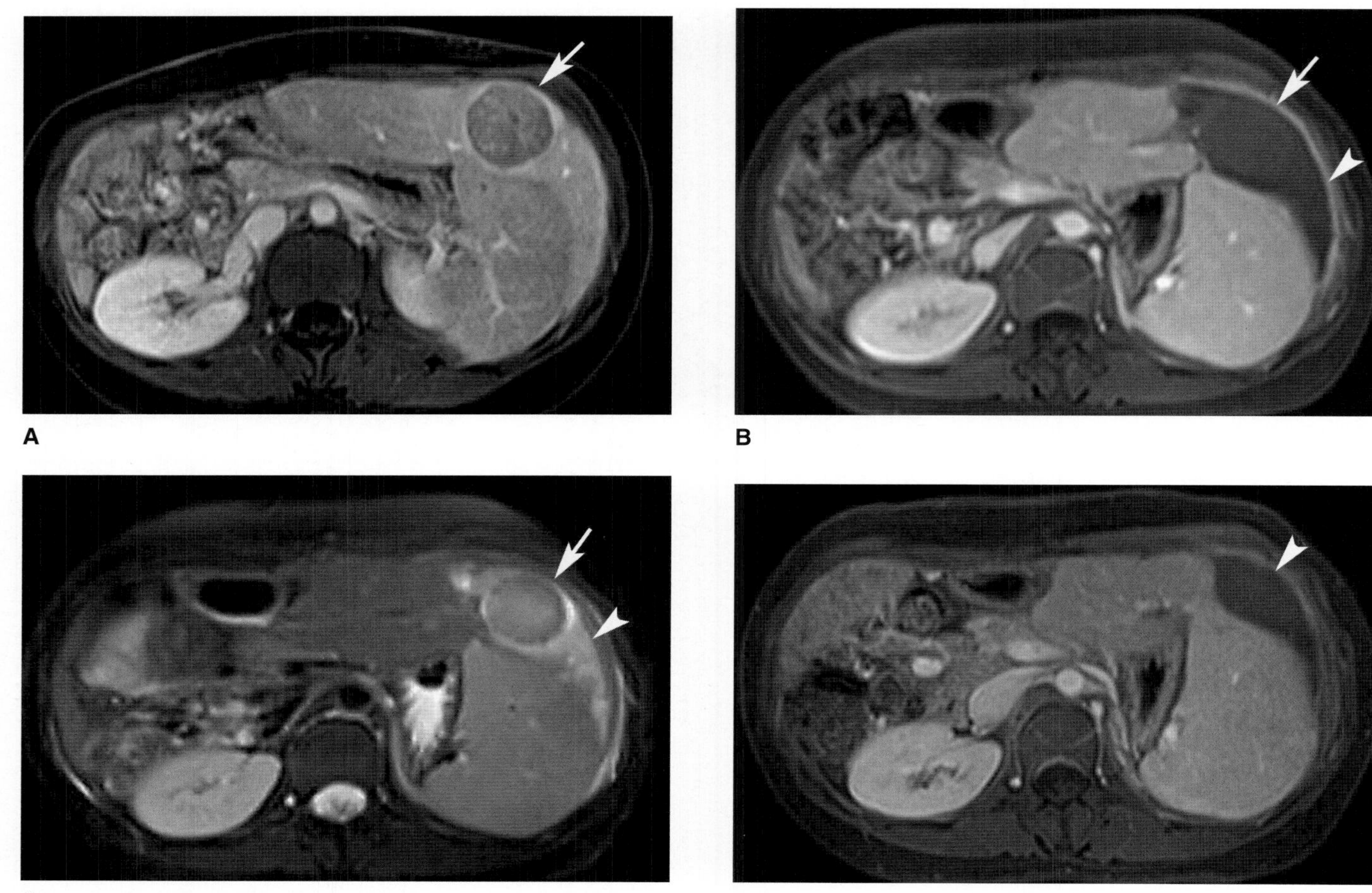

Figure 3-31 Hepatic Infarct After Chemoembolization
This 24-year-old hepatitis B patient had a right hepatectomy for HCC. **A.** Postgadolinium T1-weighted MR image shows a large left lobe tumor (*arrow*) and normal adjacent liver and spleen. **B.** Repeat post gadolinium T1-weighted MRI image 1 month after chemoembolization demonstrates extensive necrosis involving both tumor (*arrow*) and adjacent liver parenchyma (*arrowhead*). **C.** T2 image confirms coagulative tumor necrosis in tumor (*arrow*) and adjacent edematous infarction of adjacent liver (*arrowhead*). **D.** Follow-up MRI 3 months later demonstrates decreasing size of infarct (*arrowhead*).

devascularization of the liver segment. This pattern helps to distinguish segmental infarction from confluent or segmental fibrosis.

Arterial-Portal Shunting (Transient Hepatic Attenuation [or Intensity] Difference)

Arterial-portal (AP) shunting, also known as transient hepatic attenuation (or intensity) difference (THAD, THID) is a phenomenon whereby a portion of the hepatic parenchyma is supplied largely or entirely by the arterial flow. The etiology is varied, and shunting can be seen in acute inflammatory conditions such as cholecystitis or pancreatitis,[299,300] in scarring with cirrhosis,[301] adjacent to tumors or hemangiomas,[302] following focal liver therapy,[303] or in association with portal vein thrombus (see Table 3-7 and Figure 3-32).[304]

Arterial-portal shunting generally occurs when portal flows itself is disrupted, allowing for “arterialization” of the hepatic parenchyma, likely through development of collateral supply of the portal sinusoids by hepatic arterial branches.[305] This type of shunting is revealed by an area of relative hyperenhancement of the liver during the arterial phase-contrast CT or MRI, reflecting this increase in relative percentage arterial supply. Given the vascular nature of this phenomenon, the affected area will often demonstrate sharp linear margination from unaffected liver, and will in general extend in a wedge-shaped pattern, bordering the hepatic capsule (see Figure 3-32).[300]

As liver parenchyma affected by arterial-portal shunting is normal in all other ways, on the more routine portal-phase, the affected segment of the liver will look identical to that of the surrounding unaffected liver on CT scans and T1-weighted MRI sequences (see Figure 3-32). However, in

Table 3-7. Causes of Arterial-Portal Shunting

1. Portal or hepatic vein thrombosis or obstruction a. Neoplasms i. Hepatocellular carcinoma ii. Other b. Hypercoagulable states c. Other
2. Siphoning effect a. Hepatocellular carcinoma b. Hemangioma c. Focal nodular hyperplasia d. Hypervascular metastasis
3. Arterioportal shunting a. Congenital b. Neoplasms i. Hepatocellular carcinoma ii. Hemangioma iii. Other c. Trauma i. Accidental ii. Iatrogenic (interventional procedures) d. Cirrhosis
4. Local inflammation a. Hepatic abscess b. Acute cholecystitis
5. Aberrant blood supply

some cases T2-weighted images will show hyperintensity in the affected region.[306] In the case of small tumors, AP shunting can be the only or most readily visible imaging feature. Therefore, it is important to look at the apex of the region of arterial-portal shunting to exclude a mass as the underlying cause. In some cases, follow-up imaging to exclude enlarging mass at an area of AP shunting may be needed.

Certain tumors, most commonly HCC, demonstrate a propensity to invade the adjacent portal veins (see section **The Cirrhotic Liver and Hepatocellular Carcinoma** later in this chapter). In advanced cases, the presence of macroscopic portal vein invasion is clearly demonstrated. Smaller and earlier-stage tumors may demonstrate only microvascular invasion. Arterial shunting around a small HCC lesion on early-phase contrast-enhanced CT or MRI may predict this histologic finding.[307] This phenomenon can lead to erroneous overstaging if the peripheral vascular blush is included in the overall measurement of the tumor diameter.

Focal Steatosis and Focal Fatty Sparing

Although fatty infiltration of the liver is typically considered a diffuse process, it is also common to affect 1 region of the liver while sparing other portions. These focal regions of steatosis can appear spherical or have geometric distributions. Similarly, when the liver is diffusely infiltrated with fat, there can be focal regions of sparing that can have a spherical or geometric shape. Focal steatosis and focal fatty sparing are discussed most completely under the heading **Solitary Solid Hepatic Masses or Nodules**.

DIFFUSE LIVER DISEASES

Diffuse and infiltrative disorders of the liver comprise a wide variety of phenomena, including metabolic, inflammatory/toxic, and neoplastic etiologies. In many cases, the evaluation of diffuse abnormalities of the liver by cross-sectional imaging is nonspecific. Diffuse and infiltrative hepatic abnormalities can reveal irregular or diffuse changes in hepatic parenchymal appearance. At times, these are accompanied by global or lobar/segmental changes in liver size. In general, confirmation of the etiology of diffuse liver abnormalities is often dependent on the results of blood tests, or occasionally liver biopsy. However, certain common diffuse or infiltrative liver disorders reveal a characteristic imaging appearance on 1 or more cross-sectional modalities. In such cases, imaging may obviate the needs for further diagnostic evaluation.

Diffuse abnormalities of the liver include increased liver volume (hepatomegaly), decreased liver volume (cirrhosis), diffuse fatty infiltration of the liver, and iron deposition in the liver.

Hepatomegaly

In many, but not all, cases of infiltrative liver disease, liver enlargement is seen. However, there are no reliable objective criteria for the diagnosis of hepatomegaly. The subjective diagnosis of hepatomegaly can be challenging because of normal variations in the liver orientation. In some cases, the liver is relatively short in the craniocaudal direction but relatively long in the transverse dimension, such that a small tip of the left lobe wraps around the spleen. In other cases, the liver is more vertically oriented and extends into the pelvis with a relatively limited transverse diameter. One study has suggested that US is more reliable than other cross-sectional imaging techniques, because use of real-time imaging allows for a more precise linear estimate of the liver length with a sagittal midhepatic length of more than 15.5 cm correlating highly with hepatomegaly based on volumetric measures at subsequent autopsy.[308] An imaging characteristic that is very useful in the diagnosis of hepatomegaly is a change in the shape of the liver. In all situations, the liver has an overall triangular shape. When it becomes more bulbous appearing is when a diagnosis of hepatomegaly should be suggested (see Figure 3-33).

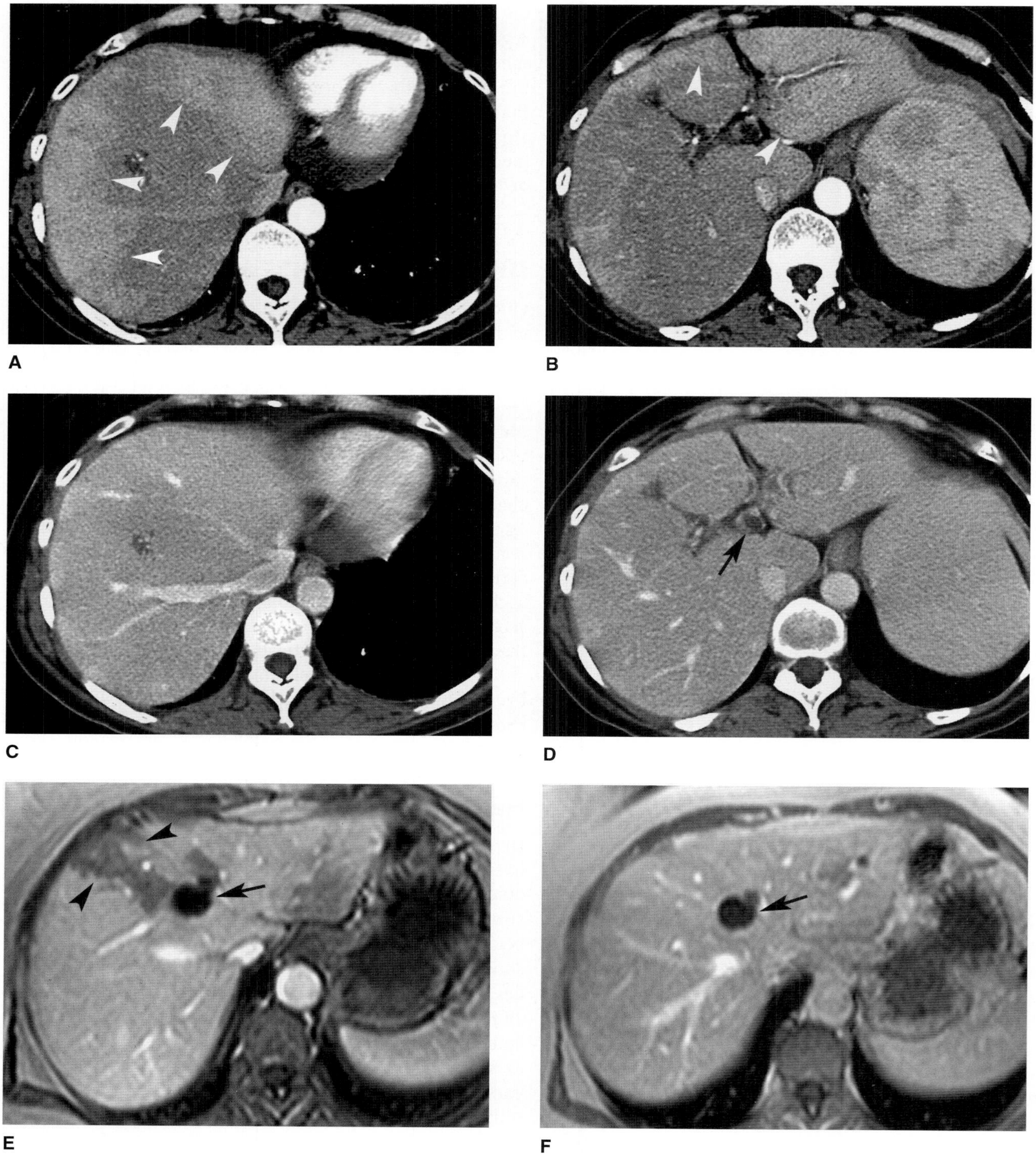

A

B

C

D

E

F

Figure 3-32 THAD Due to Portal Vein Thrombosis and THID Due to Hepatic Cyst in 2 Patients
A-D. This 47-year-old woman had pancreatitis with an infected pseudocyst. Arterial-phase images (A and B) of the liver show geographic regions of higher and lower attenuation (*arrowheads*). On the venous-phase images (C and D), these regions are no longer present. This is typical of transient hepatic attenuation difference. Careful observation of image (D) reveals a thrombus in the portal vein (*black arrow*) as the cause of the THAD. **E** and **F.** This 66-year-old woman had breast cancer. Hepatic arterial-phase (E) and portal venous-phase (F) images from a postgadolinium T1-weighted MRI examination shows a nonenhancing slightly lobulated lesion in the liver that was shown to be a lobulated cyst on T2-weighted sequences. The arterial phase shows an approximately wedge-shaped low signal lesion (*arrowheads*) distal to the cyst that disappears on the portal venous phase. This is characteristic of a transient hepatic intensity difference that, in this case, is probably caused by compression of the arterial supply to the segment of liver distal to the cyst.

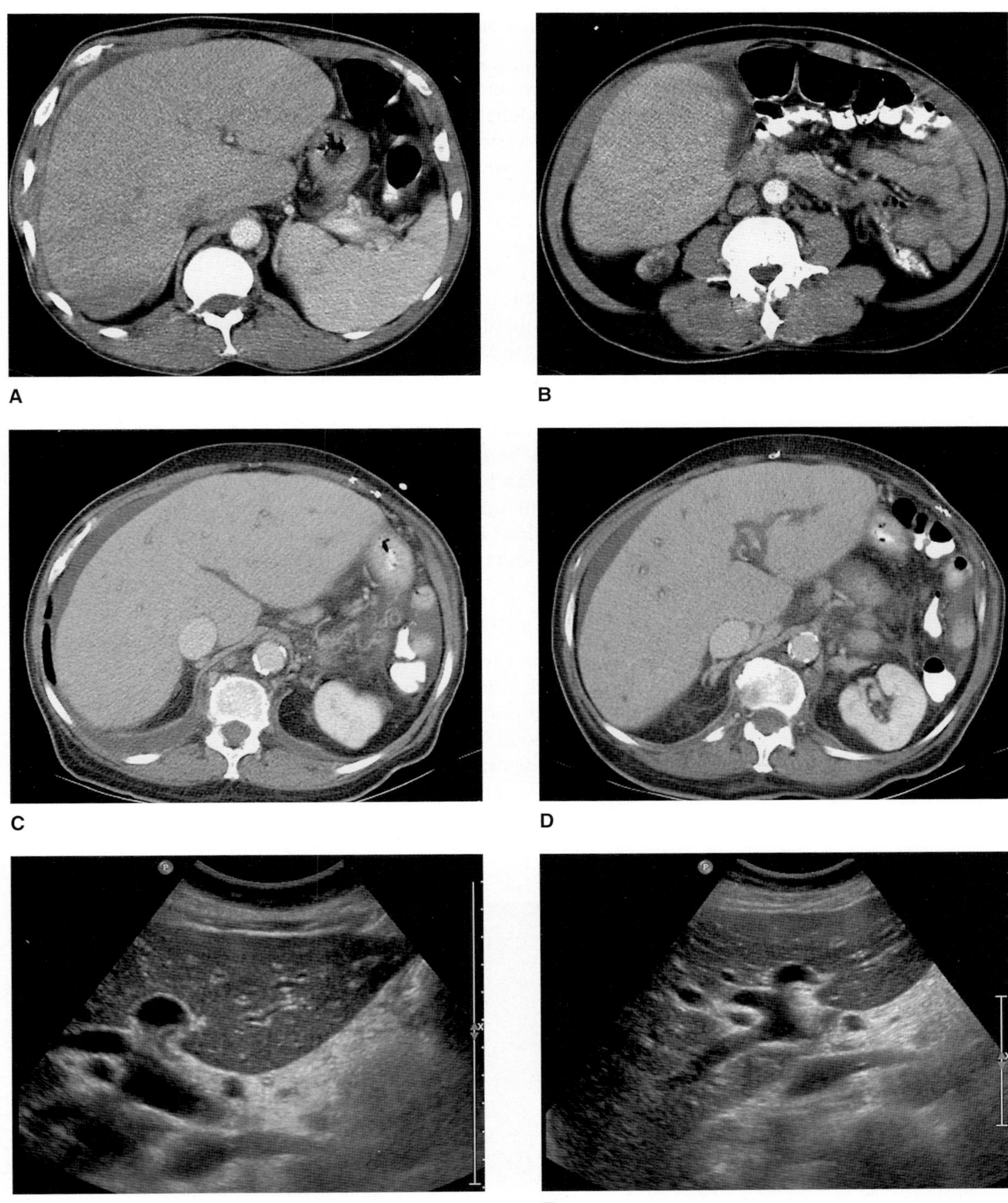

Figure 3-33 Hepatitis in 3 Patients
A and **B**. This 48-year-old man with HIV and hepatitis C infections complained of abdominal pain. Note how the liver has a bulbous appearance on these contrast-enhanced CT images (A and B). This suggests hepatomegaly with distention of the liver. The liver also has a slightly lower attenuation than the spleen, a finding suggesting diffuse hepatic edema. These findings are consistent with active hepatitis. **C** and **D**. This 72-year-old woman was being treated for chronic lymphocytic leukemia when she developed a transaminitis. Contrast-enhanced CT shows a similar bulbous appearance to the liver (C and D). There are also low attenuation rings around each of the portal veins, a finding consistent with periportal edema. These features are a manifestation of acute hepatitis, in this case, drug related. **E** and **F**. This 55-year-old woman with breast cancer and acute myeloid leukemia had elevated liver function tests. Longitudinal US shows the liver parenchyma to be considerably less echogenic than the portal triads and the surrounding abdominal fat (E and F). This is a feature suggesting diffuse hepatic edema due to hepatitis, in this case a drug toxicity.

Table 3-8. Causes of Hepatomegaly

1. Diffuse edema
   - a. Hepatitis
     - i. Infection
       1. Viruses (hepatitis A, B, C)
     - ii. Autoimmune
       1. Autoimmune hepatitis
       2. Sclerosing cholangitis
     - iii. Toxic
       1. Alcohol
   - b. Vascular obstruction
     - i. **Passive congestion (right heart failure)**[a]
     - ii. Budd-Chiari syndrome
     - iii. Hepatic veno-occlusive disease
2. Infiltrative disease
   - a. Neoplasms
     - i. **Leukemia**
     - ii. **Lymphoma**
   - b. Other infiltrative processes
     - i. Sarcoidosis
     - ii. Gaucher disease
     - iii. Glycogen storage disease
     - iv. Amyloidosis

[a]Causes in bold are most common.

Causes of hepatomegaly include acute hepatitis, lymphoma and leukemia, and nonmalignant infiltrative disorders (Table 3-8).

Acute hepatitis

Acute hepatitis can result from a variety of infectious, toxic, and autoimmune insults to the liver. In general, cross-sectional imaging does not aid in distinguishing between the various toxic or infectious causes of hepatitis but can be used to document the degree of hepatomegaly. Acute hepatocellular injury results in edema of the liver, causing increase in size of the liver. The presence of edema may be apparent on US as a diffuse decrease in echogenicity of the liver (see Figure 3-33).[309] On CT, the acutely inflamed liver can demonstrate diffuse decrease in attenuation. More frequently, edema on CT manifests as a periportal halo,[310] because of the accumulation of fluid in the periportal tracts. Periportal and diffuse edema in acute hepatitis can also be demonstrated by T2-weighted MRI.[311] On all imaging modalities, lymphadenopathy in the portohepatic region can be demonstrated.[312,313] Less commonly, acute hepatitis can be caused by severe biliary or vascular obstruction, sometimes leading to fulminant hepatic failure.[314] Imaging in this case will document the vascular or biliary abnormality, and can aid in surgical palliation (see Figure 3-33).

Hematologic malignancies

Liver involvement in hematologic malignancies, including leukemia and lymphoma, is common, with hepatic involvement more rarely seen in patients with multiple myeloma. Secondary involvement of the liver by Hodgkin and non-Hodgkin lymphomas has been found in 8% and 25% of cases at staging laparotomy, respectively.[194,195] Diffuse hepatomegaly is the most common imaging manifestation

A

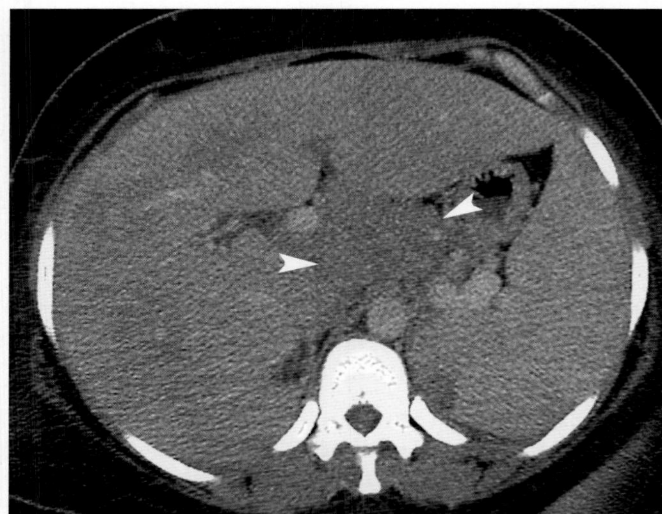

B

Figure 3-34 Lymphomatous Infiltration of the Liver
This 32-year-old woman had non-Hodgkin lymphoma. **A** and **B.** Images of the upper abdomen appear to be completely filled with the liver and spleen, indicating hepatosplenomegaly. The liver also has a bulbous appearance and the attenuation of the liver is not uniform with vague regions of lower attenuation. These finding are nonspecific but in this clinical setting indicate diffuse hepatic and splenic infiltration by lymphoma. There is also a large nodal mass (*arrowheads*) anterior to the aorta, indicating lymphadenopathy due to lymphoma.

of hepatic involvement in lymphoma but lymphoma can also appear as 1 or several focal masses (see Figure 3-34).[196] Occasionally, lymphoma can mimic periportal edema on CT or MRI.[315,316] Hepatomegaly is also the most common imaging feature of liver involvement with leukemias.[317] In general, the imaging findings are nonspecific and biopsy is often necessary for definitive diagnosis. Other causes of liver enlargement, including opportunistic infection, myeloma-associated amyloidosis, or extramedullary hematopoiesis should be considered in the evaluation of hepatomegaly in the setting of hematologic malignancy.

Sarcoidosis

Sarcoidosis is a common systemic granulomatous disease that can have imaging evidence of liver disease in 15% of patients.[182] On imaging examinations, hepatic sarcoidosis most often appears as hepatomegaly, but in some cases can demonstrate innumerable small hepatic nodules. Hepatic sarcoidosis is most completely discussed under the heading: **Multiple Solid Hepatic Masses or Nodules**.

Gaucher disease

Gaucher disease is the most common lysosomal storage disease. It is a metabolic disease secondary to glucocerebrosidase deficiency that results in accumulation of glucocerebroside in the lysosomes of monocyte-derived macrophages in tissues of the reticuloendothelial system, particularly liver, spleen, and bone. Joints and skin are also often involved.

On imaging, patients with Gaucher disease present with extreme hepatosplenomegaly (see Figure 14-35).[318] In some cases, patients can be treated by enzyme replacement therapy, and monitoring of splenic and hepatic volumes by imaging can be useful for tracking response to therapy. MRI in particular is useful for documenting the degree of bone marrow involvement and the presence of marrow infarcts.[319,320] As such, combined abdominal and musculoskeletal surveillance of patients with Gaucher disease may be employed.[321]

In addition to hepatosplenomegaly, Gaucher patients can demonstrate focal hepatic abnormalities, relating to either more focal cellular degeneration or fibrosis.[322-324] Stellate areas of hepatic T2 hyperintensity on MRI that are thought to be secondary to ischemia or fibrosis have also been reported.[325]

Glycogen storage disease

Glycogen storage disease represents a spectrum of inborn errors of metabolism that affect the processing of glycogen in the liver, muscles, and other tissues. Multiple types are defined, based on the specific enzymatic defect. Presentation is in early childhood, with growth retardation and muscle abnormalities a common presenting finding. With improved medical and dietary management, many patients live into adulthood.

Hepatic involvement is common in most, but not all, types of glycogen storage disease, depending on the exact enzymatic defect. Liver enlargement is commonly seen, with variable development of fibrosis depending on the glycogen storage disease subtype and the longevity of the affected individual. Development of hepatic adenoma is common in glycogen storage disease type Ia (von Gierke disease) and type III (Cori disease).[147,326] Other reported liver abnormalities include fatty infiltration[147] and HCC[327,328] developing in a smaller fraction of affected individuals. Surveillance with US is recommended beyond the first decade of life to monitor and manage the development of liver adenomas.[329]

Amyloidosis

Amyloidosis refers to the deposition of abnormal conglomerated insoluble protein fragments (amyloid) into tissues, leading to organ dysfunction and failure. A variety of amyloid types are defined by the nature of the protein fragment, whether the defect is primary/inherited or secondary to other disease processes. Certain amyloid conditions affect just 1 organ (eg, brain, heart) whereas others, such as primary familial amyloidosis or myeloma associated amyloidosis (AL) demonstrate multiple target organs.

Hepatic involvement in systemic amyloidoses varies,[330,331] and is generally seen less often than that of kidney and spleen.[183] When hepatic involvement occurs, pain, hepatomegaly, and cholestasis with jaundice and pruritus are seen.

The imaging features of hepatic amyloidosis are not specific.[332] Echogenicity of the liver may be heterogeneously increased.[333] Contrast enhancement on CT and MRI is often decreased, with or without focal lesions.[334,335] A striking decrease in splenic enhancement can be seen, and may suggest the diagnosis.[336] In some cases CT will demonstrate splenic and hepatic calcification.[335] In most presentations of systemic amyloidosis, renal disease is also demonstrated, and renal biopsy will allow for definitive diagnosis.

Liver Atrophy

Diminished liver size is 1 of multiple features of cirrhosis. Cirrhosis has many unique imaging characteristics and

Table 3-9. Causes of Hepatic Steatosis

1. Alcohol abuse
2. Metabolic syndrome
3. Obesity
4. Diabetes
5. Hypertriglyceridemia
6. Corticosteroids (exogenous and endogenous)
7. Hyperalimentation
8. Systemic chemotherapy
9. Glycogen storage diseases

is discussed under the heading: **Hepatic Disorders with a Specific Appearance**.

Hepatic Steatosis

Hepatic steatosis or fatty infiltration of the liver is a result of excessive deposition of triglyceride and is a nonspecific response to cell injury that can be seen in a variety of conditions[337] (Table 3-9). Steatosis is most commonly a result of excess alcohol consumption or obesity, especially when associated with metabolic syndrome. When associated with alcohol consumption, hepatic steatosis typically precedes the development of alcoholic cirrhosis.[338,339] Metabolic syndrome is a combination of medical disorders that increase the risk of developing cardiovascular disease and diabetes and affects more than 20% of the US population.[340] It is characterized by central obesity, hypertension, elevated serum triglycerides, depressed serum high-density lipoproteins (HDL), elevated fasting plasma glucose, and microalbuminuria. Hepatic steatosis is most often detected incidentally by imaging. However, occasionally, patients can present with right upper quadrant pain and fatigue or with abnormal liver function tests.

Fatty infiltration is most often a diffuse process that involves the entire liver parenchyma uniformly; however, occasionally steatosis will involve geographic regions of the liver while sparing other regions. The liver may be normal in size, although in more severe cases patients may present with hepatomegaly.[341] When steatosis is uniform, rather than regional or focal, the appearance can be difficult to appreciate. On US, the liver appears diffusely echogenic relative to that of the kidney (see Figure 3-35).[342,343] On nonenhanced CT, the liver will demonstrate hypoattenuation relative to spleen and abdominal muscles.[344] An attenuation difference (liver minus spleen) of greater than 10 HU is considered diagnostic of hepatic steatosis on noncontrast CT (see Figure 3-35).[345,346] On contrast-enhanced CT, the use of HU liver-spleen differences is less reliable, because of variation in liver and spleen attenuation related to variations in phase of contrast enhancement, and a more conservative estimate of a Hounsfield difference with spleen of more than 25 HU is generally accepted to avoid false-positive diagnoses.[347,348] On MRI, the diagnosis of steatosis is generally made reliably with chemical shift–sensitive gradient echo imaging.[349,350] Steatotic liver will demonstrate signal loss on the opposed-phase T1-weighted imaging relative to the liver signal intensity on the in-phase T1-weighted image (see Figure 3-35).

The clinical significance of the imaging finding of steatosis is variable. In general, it is not possible to differentiate simple (noninflamed) hepatic steatosis with the more clinically relevant nonalcoholic steatohepatitis (NASH).[351,352] Nonalcoholic steatohepatitis is of greater clinical concern because these patients can go on to cirrhosis, liver fibrosis, and the development of HCC. Currently, biopsy is required to differentiate nonalcoholic fatty liver disease (NAFLD) from NASH.[353]

Iron Deposition

Iron deposition within the liver can occur in the setting of increased iron circulation, or as a result of genetic disorders of iron handling. Primary hemochromatosis is a genetic disorder of the *HFE* gene, leading to abnormally high GI absorption of iron that then causes excess deposition of iron into a variety of tissues, including the liver.[354] Excess liver parenchymal iron can lead to oxidative damage to the liver and can cause cirrhosis and HCC.[355] Nongenetic forms of systemic iron overload are referred to as hemosiderosis, or secondary hemochromatosis, and can result from hemolytic conditions, or multiple transfusions.[356]

Transfusional or iron overload result in the accumulation of iron in the reticuloendothelial system, including the liver, spleen, and bone marrow.[357] Genetic (primary) hemochromatosis also results in abnormal hepatic iron accumulation, but spares the remainder of the reticuloendothelial system. However, in primary hemochromatosis, iron deposition can also occur in the pancreas and heart muscle.[358]

US has not been shown to be useful for identification of hepatic iron deposition, although long-term changes from iron damage, including fibrosis and cirrhosis can be seen. Iron deposition in the liver can be demonstrated on CT as an increase in density diffusely through the hepatic parenchyma (see Figure 3-36).[359,360] However, MRI has proven to be more sensitive and specific in detecting and quantifying liver iron deposition than CT.[361,362] Iron is a ferromagnetic substance and as a consequence, can induce local magnetic fields. This results in inhomogeneity of the local magnetic fields of the liver and spleen and results in a loss of signal in the regions around the iron deposition on both T1- and T2-weighted and gradient echo sequences. As a consequence, the liver will appear as diffusely dark in signal on MRI images, especially on T2*-weighted gradient images that are more affected by local magnetic field inhomogeneity (see Figure 3-36).

Amiodarone Deposition

Amiodarone is a medication used in the therapy of cardiac arrhythmias. The chemical composition of amiodarone includes several iodine moieties and therefore deposits of amiodarone will attenuate x-rays to a greater degree than most soft tissues. It is known that amiodarone is deposited within the liver parenchyma and can result in increased attenuation of the liver on unenhanced CT scans.[363] This deposition does not alter the MRI signal or acoustic impedance and is therefore not visible by MRI or US (see Figure 3-37).

HEPATIC DISORDERS WITH A SPECIFIC APPEARANCE

There are a variety of liver disorders that have a unique appearance signaling the presence of the disorder. These include cirrhosis, pseudocirrhosis, radiation hepatitis, hepatic congestion, and some vascular anomalies.

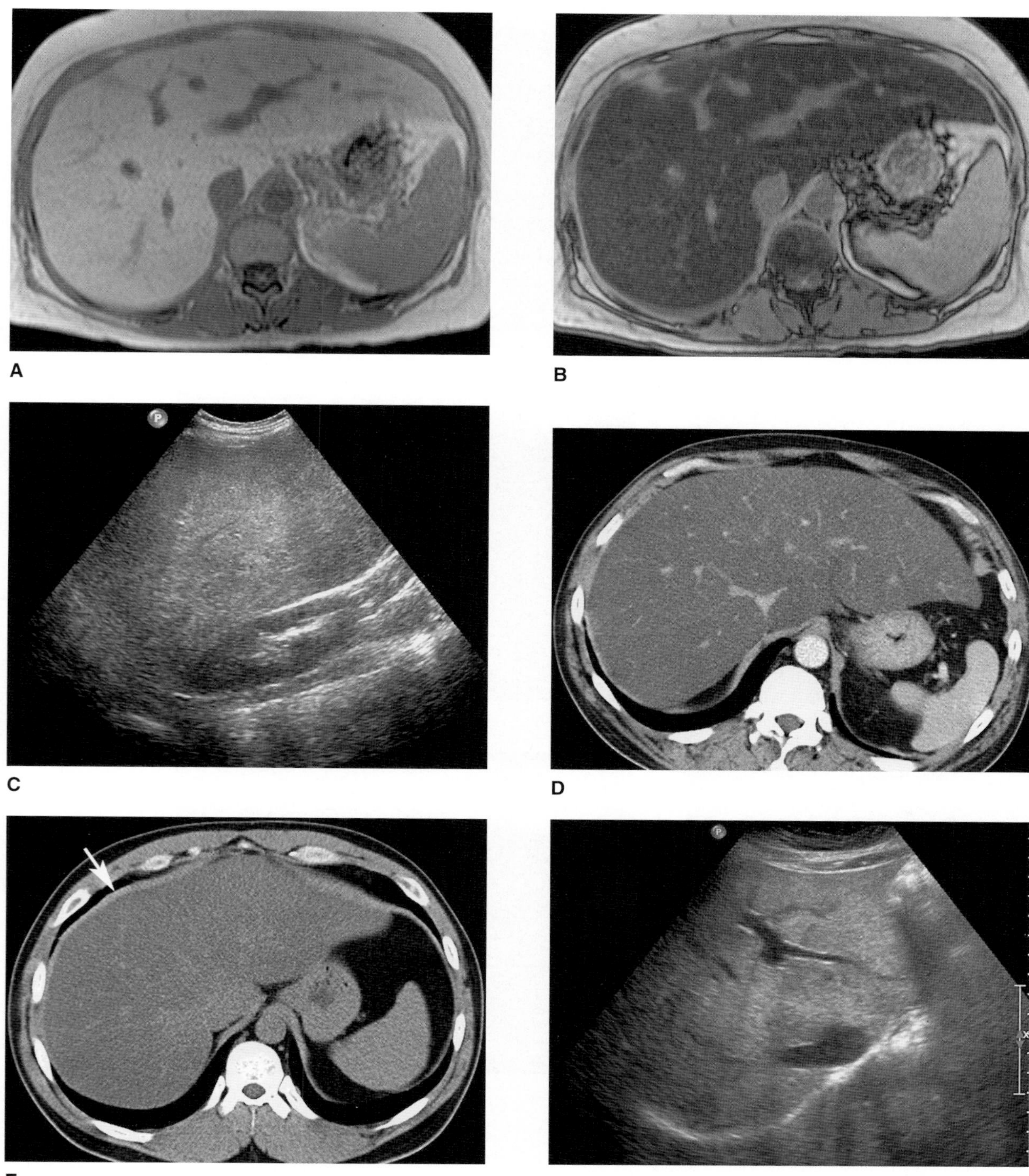

Figure 3-35 Hepatic Steatosis in 3 Patients
In-phase (**A**) and opposed-phase (**B**) T1-weighted MRI sequences in a 46-year-old man with chronic pancreatitis show dramatic signal loss of the liver on the opposed-phase images, indicating the presence of diffuse fatty infiltration. **C** and **D.** This 44-year-old man was a known alcoholic. Sagittal US (C) of the liver shows diffuse increase in echogenicity typical of diffuse fatty infiltration. Contrast-enhanced CT (D) shows a dramatic difference in attenuation between the liver and the spleen of 60 HU. Although not as accurate as unenhanced CT, this is likely to indicate the presence of hepatic steatosis. **E** and **F.** This 34-year-old man had flank pain and was being evaluated for a suspected renal calculus. The liver (E), which is normally similar in attenuation to the adjacent diaphragm muscle (*arrow*), chest wall muscles, and spleen, appears lower attenuation than these structures in this unenhanced CT examination. This is typical of hepatic steatosis. Longitudinal US (F) shows diffuse increased echogenicity of the liver typical of steatosis. Increased echogenicity due to steatosis is typically very fine and less coarse than is typically seen in cirrhosis (see Figure 3-39 Cirrhosis in 3 Patients).

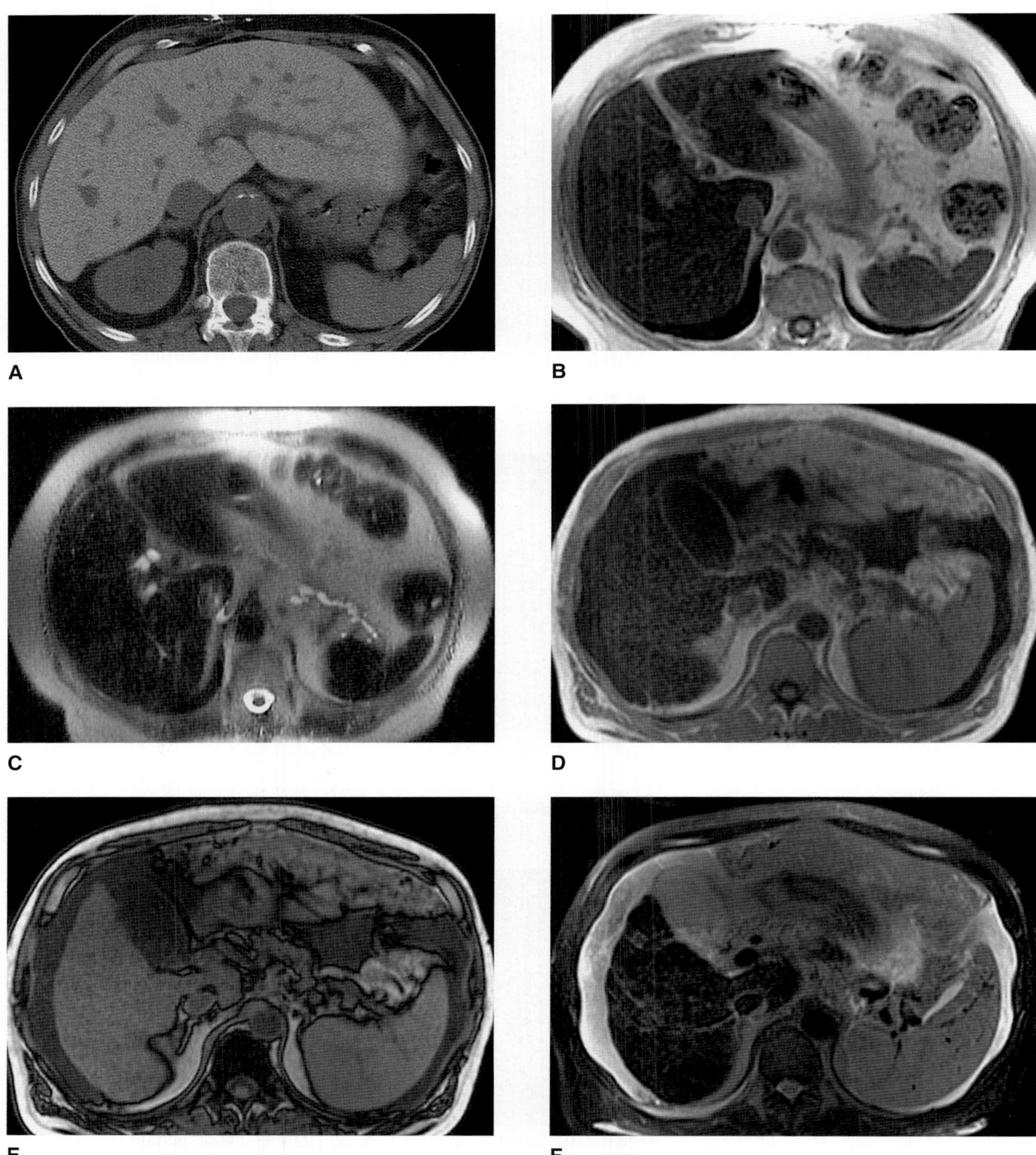

Figure 3-36 Hemosiderosis and Hemochromatosis in 3 Patients

A. This 62-year-old woman had congenital heart disease and chronic anemia requiring multiple transfusions. CT image shows the liver to be considerably more hyperattenuating than the spleen and paraspinal muscles. This is a nonspecific finding and can be due to amiodarone deposition; however, in this patient with multiple transfusions it is most likely due to iron deposition as a result of hemosiderosis. **B** and **C.** This 80-year-old woman had a history of chronic pancreatitis and multiple blood transfusions. Compare the T1-weighted MRI (B) and the T2-weighted MRI (C) of this patient with previous MRIs of the liver shown in this chapter. Note how low signal intensity of both the liver and the spleen appear in this patient in comparison with previous patients. This is the characteristic appearance of iron deposition in the liver and spleen, hemosiderosis—in this case, due to multiple prior transfusions. **D-F.** This 52-year-old man presented with elevated liver function tests. T1-weighted in-phase (D) and T1-weighted opposed-phase images (E) demonstrates substantial signal loss on in-phase imaging because of longer echo time. Similar changes are also noted in the pancreas. These features indicate a diagnosis of primary hemochromatosis. The liver has a nodular contour and there is ascites surrounding the liver and spleen, indicating cirrhosis as a complication of hemochromatosis. Fat-saturated T2-weighted imaging (F) demonstrates darkened liver relative to muscle, another finding seen with extensive hepatic iron deposition.

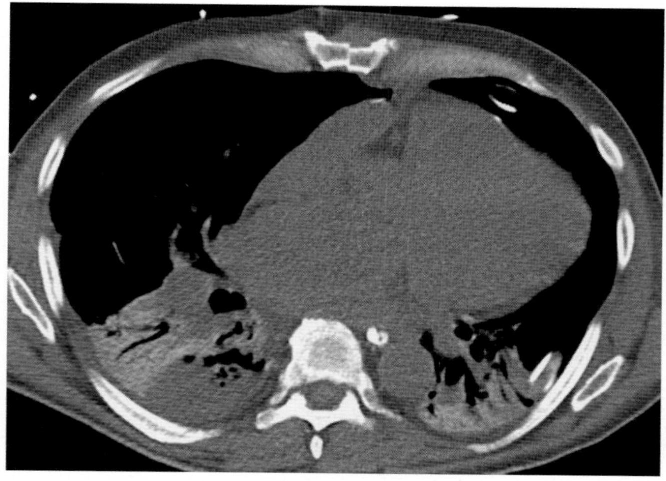

A

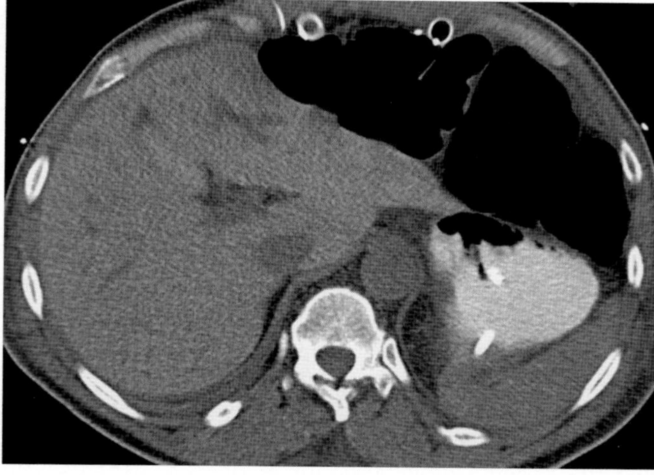

B

Figure 3-37 Amiodarone Deposition in the Liver and Lung This 50-year-old man had undergone a heart transplant and had postoperative fever. **A** and **B**. Unenhanced CT demonstrates high attenuation of the atelectatic lung parenchyma and liver relative to muscle and the spleen. The liver hyperattenuation could be due to either hemosiderosis or amiodarone deposition. However, the lung hyperintensity is only seen in amiodarone deposition. This patient had received amiodarone prior to transplant because of arrhythmias.

The Cirrhotic Liver and Hepatocellular Carcinoma

The cirrhotic liver presents a unique challenge to the diagnostic radiologist. Cirrhosis is the end stage of a variety of infectious, metabolic, or toxic insults to the liver. Although cirrhosis is a diffuse disease of the liver, it often manifests with unifocal, multifocal, regional, or vascular abnormalities on imaging, often in various combinations. As such, cirrhosis may encompass the entire morphologic spectrum of imaging abnormalities of the liver. This complexity and heterogeneity of potential imaging abnormalities produces a confusing pattern of radiologic findings, leading to challenges in accurate diagnosis of secondary pathologies within the cirrhotic liver.

Etiology and evolution of cirrhosis

The etiologies of cirrhosis are numerous (Table 3-10). Worldwide, viral hepatitis, particularly infections with the hepatitis B virus, accounts for the greatest single factor in the development of cirrhosis.[364] In Western populations, cirrhosis is more commonly caused by hepatitis C infection and alcohol abuse.[338] Other less common etiologies of cirrhosis include NASH, biliary cirrhosis, hemochromatosis, Wilson disease, autoimmune hepatitis, and idiopathic cirrhosis. In many cases, the etiology of cirrhosis can be multifactorial.

The development of cirrhosis is a gradual process, in most cases initiated by damage to the hepatocyte by viral or environmental factors. These infectious and toxic insults can lead to an acute inflammatory response leading to hepatitis or a chronic or relapsing inflammatory response resulting in chronic scarring and fibrosis, known as cirrhosis. In severe cases, the combination of hepatic cellular damage and architectural distortion can impede normal hepatic function, resulting in clinical symptoms of cirrhosis. The combination of liver scarring and hepatocyte regeneration leads to characteristic pathologic and imaging features of micronodular and macronodular changes in the structure of the liver. In some cases, whole regions of the liver can become enveloped by scarring, whereas others will regenerate freely, leading to patterns of lobar

Table 3-10. Causes of Cirrhosis

1. Alcohol abuse
2. Infectious hepatitis (see Table 3-8)
3. Autoimmune hepatitis (see Table 3-8)
4. Heritable a. Hemochromatosis b. Wilson disease
5. Vascular a. Budd-Chiari syndrome b. Chronic passive congestion c. Hepatic veno-occlusive disease
6. Other a. Nonalcoholic steatohepatitis (NASH) b. Cryptogenic cirrhosis

asymmetry that can be characteristic in certain etiologies of cirrhosis.

Not all individuals who develop liver inflammation from viral or other causes will develop cirrhosis. Antiviral therapies such as interferon treatment have been effective in delaying or preventing the development of cirrhosis.[365,366] Removal of the toxic cause of liver inflammation, such as reduction in alcoholic intake or dietary and lifestyle modification, can also be effective in preventing development of cirrhosis. Directed therapies, such as repetitive phlebotomy or iron chelation strategies in hemochromatosis,[367] can also be helpful to prevent the development of cirrhosis.

Acute viral hepatitis results in variable degrees of liver inflammation, manifested mostly by systemic illness and hepatic enzyme elevations. In many cases, acute viral hepatitis is self-limited, although a subset of patients with hepatitis B or C develop chronic infection. Ongoing insults to the liver, whether because of chronic viral infection or repetitive toxic injury, lead to an inflammatory cascade that, if unabated, initiates a pattern of progressive liver damage. However, many individuals with viral or other inflammatory causes of liver disease can be clinically asymptomatic in the early and middle stages of disease. In some cases, abnormal imaging examinations can be the first indication of liver disease.

Regardless of the etiology of hepatic insult, the end result of continued liver inflammation is scarring and fibrosis with secondary liver regeneration. Once liver fibrosis has commenced, the damage is irreversible, although medical antiviral therapies or reversal of liver exposure to the toxic agent (eg, alcohol) may prevent further damage and liver deterioration. End-stage liver disease is characterized by loss of liver function, portal hypertension, hepatorenal syndrome, and generalized clinical deterioration. Absent liver transplantation, life expectancy for patients who suffer from end-stage liver disease is less than 15% at 5 years.[368]

Secondary findings in chronic liver inflammation and early cirrhosis

During the initial stages of liver insult, whether because of viral or toxic etiologies, the liver can appear normal on cross-sectional imaging. However, occasionally viral hepatitis will lead to characteristic diffuse decreased echogenicity on US,[369] diffuse or periportal decreased attenuation on CT, or periportal or diffuse increased in liver signal on T2-weighted MRI.[370] Acute hepatitis is discussed more completely under the heading **Diffuse Liver Diseases**, subheading Acute hepatitis.

When there is ongoing inflammation, increase in periportal lymph node size and number can be seen by CT or MRI.[311,371-373] Periportal lymphadenopathy can be the most prominent radiologic abnormality in patients with ongoing hepatic inflammation and the incidental discovery of periportal lymphadenopathy on imaging examinations performed for other reasons can be the first sign of ongoing liver inflammation in an otherwise healthy patient[313] (Table 3-11).

Table 3-11. Secondary Findings of Chronic Liver Inflammation

1. Periportal lymphadenopathy
2. Fatty infiltration
3. Iron deposition (typically nodular in distribution: siderotic nodules)

Toxic or infectious insults to the liver can result in the development of diffuse fatty infiltration of the liver. Fatty infiltration is a common finding in alcoholic hepatitis[338,374] but can also develop in the setting of chronic viral infection.[375] However, in certain metabolic conditions, such as nonalcoholic liver disease (NALFD), fatty infiltration of the liver precedes the development of inflammation.[376] The relationship between lipid deposition and liver inflammation is further complicated by the fact that steatosis can itself become the inciting etiology of liver inflammation, as seen in NASH.[377] Hepatic steatosis appears as increased liver echogenicity on US examinations, decreased attenuation on CT examinations, and loss of signal on opposed-phase chemical shift–sensitive MRI images. Details of the imaging features of hepatic steatosis are discussed under the heading: **Diffuse Liver Diseases**, subheading Hepatic Steatosis.

The relationship between hepatic iron deposition and inflammation/fibrosis is also variable. Diffuse iron infiltration of the liver is characteristic of primary hemochromatosis, a condition that will often lead to end-stage liver disease in the absence of effective iron chelation therapy. However, iron accumulation of the liver can also be a secondary phenomenon due to chronic transfusions (hemosiderosis). Increased hepatic iron uptake can also occur following the development of cirrhosis when regenerative nodules sequester excess iron, leading to a pattern of multiple siderotic nodules, or hepatic siderosis. In end-stage liver disease, hepatic iron accumulation, whether primary or secondary, can decline as fibrosis gradually replaces the hepatic parenchyma. Iron deposition in the liver can rarely appear as increased liver attenuation on CT examinations but is frequently recognized as decreased liver signal on both T1 and more extensively on T2-weighted sequences on MRI (see Figure 3-38). Iron deposition is discussed more completely under the heading: **Diffuse Liver Diseases**, subheading Iron Deposition.

The end-stage cirrhotic liver

When inflammation of the liver continues unabated, fibrosis and scarring ensue. The microscopic and macroscopic changes to the liver as cirrhosis progresses are highly variable and depend in part on the etiology of liver inflammation and the degree of damage. As scarring reduces liver function, the regenerative capacity of less affected areas of

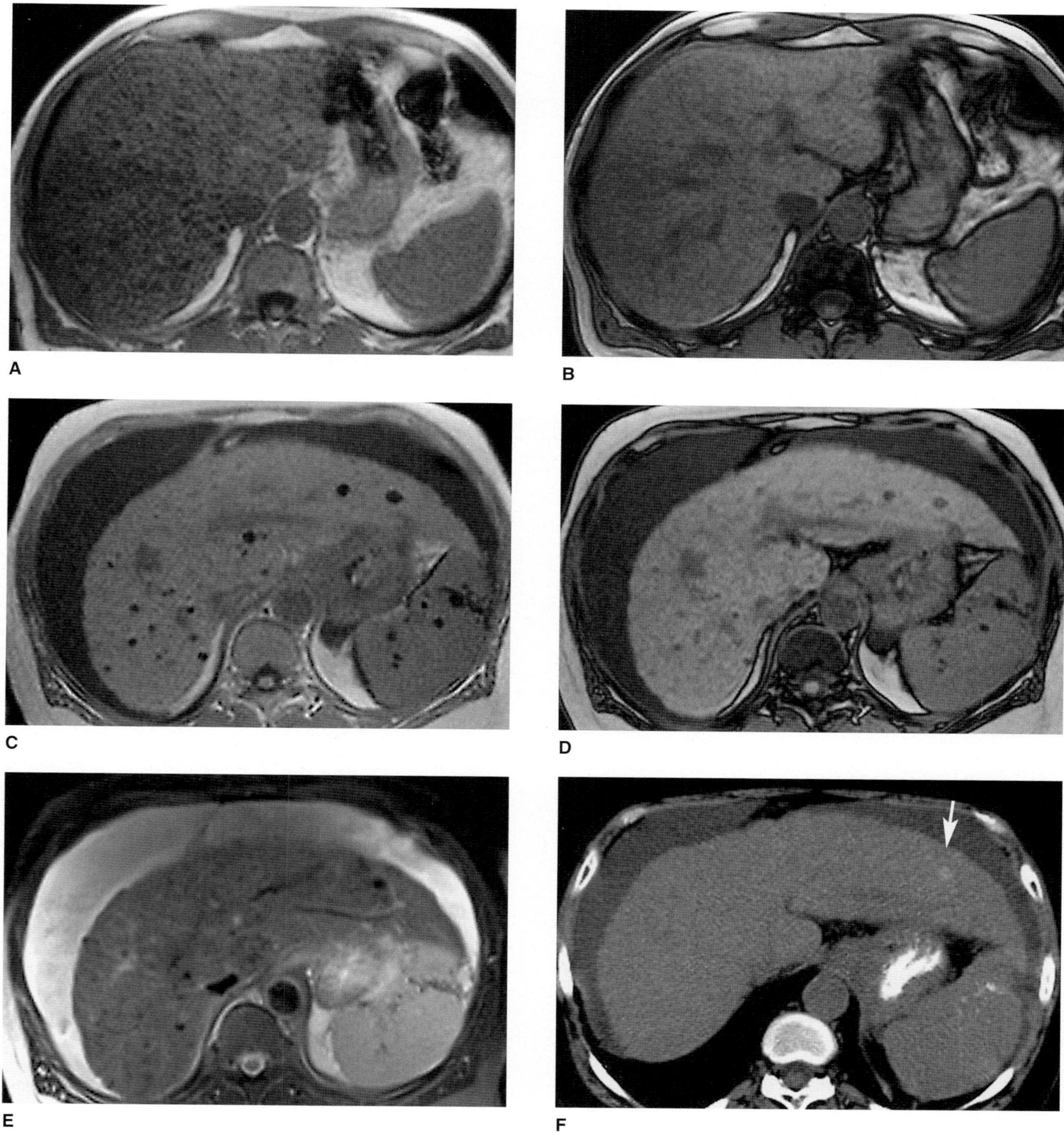

Figure 3-38 Siderotic Nodules in 2 Patients with Cirrhosis
A and **B**. This 65-year-old man developed cirrhosis as a result of hepatitis C. In-phase (A) and opposed-phase (B) T1-weighted imaging demonstrates the decrease in signal of the liver on the longer TE in-phase imaging, with a heterogeneous nodular pattern due to innumerable small siderotic nodules. There is also a high signal mass in the dome of the liver representing a HCC. **C-F.** This 61-year-old woman also developed cirrhosis due to hepatitis C infection. T1-weighted in-phase image (C), T1-weighted opposed-phase image (D), and T2-weighted image (E) demonstrate multiple hypointense nodules in the liver, characteristic of siderotic nodules. The "blooming" effect of the iron is demonstrated on the longer TE in-phase image relative to the shorter TE opposed-phase image. Unenhanced CT study (F) demonstrates hyperintensity of the larger left lobe lesion, demonstrating the effect of iron deposition in CT intensity. However smaller lesions are harder to identify on the CT study.

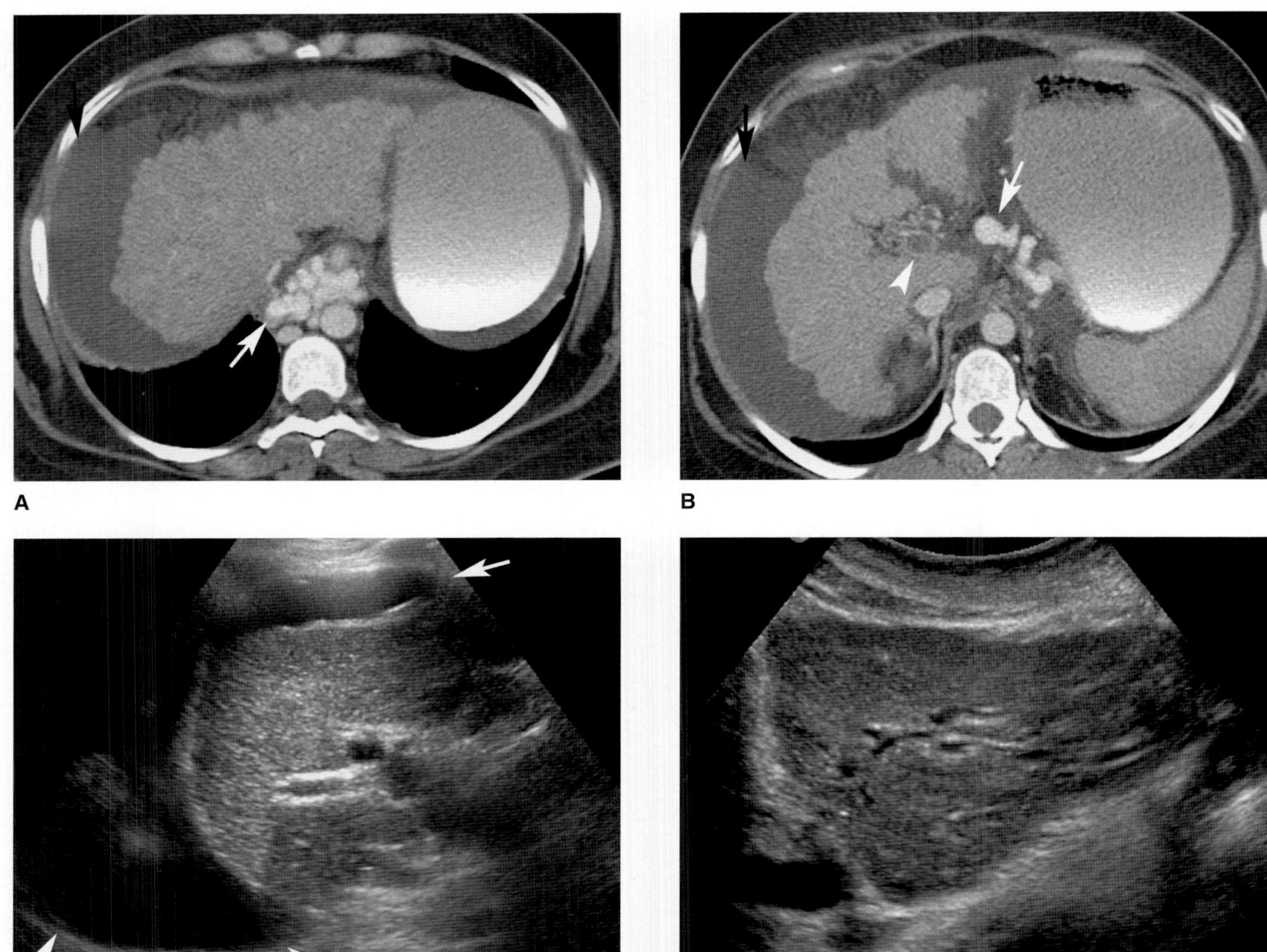

Figure 3-39 Cirrhosis in 3 Patients
A and **B.** This 28-year-old woman with autoimmune hepatitis was noted to be encephalopathic and have hematemesis. The liver is very small in size and has a multinodular appearance characteristic of advanced cirrhosis (A and B). The multiple small nodules represent regenerative nodules. A large amount of acites (*black arrows*) splenic and esophageal varices (*white arrows*) and portal vein thrombosis (*arrowhead*) are complications of the cirrhosis and ensuing portal hypertension. **C.** This 73-year-old woman was an alcohol abuser. Longitudinal US shows a small liver with a nodular surface and coarse increased echogenicity typical of advanced cirrhosis. There is also ascites (*arrow*) and a large pleural effusion (*arrowheads*) present. **D.** Longitudinal US in a 48-year-old man with hepatitis C shows a nodular contour to the surface and coarse increased echogenicity of the liver typical of cirrhosis.

the liver proceeds in an attempt to boost overall liver function. On the microscopic level, small regenerative nodules can develop between linear areas of fibrosis. As this process continues, a micronodular appearance of the liver can develop. In some cirrhotic patients, areas of less affected liver regenerate more rapidly, leading to areas of lobar hypertrophy, typically in the caudate lobe and lateral segment of the left lobe.[378,379] Macronodular regeneration can also ensue when larger regions of regenerating liver are intersected by broad bands of fibrosis. Eventually, as more severe cirrhosis develops, overall liver size will decrease, leaving a shrunken, usually nodular liver typical of end-stage liver disease.

Imaging patterns in the cirrhotic liver reflect the microscopic and macroscopic pathologic changes. Fibrosis can lead to increased echogenicity of the liver on US examinations (see Figure 3-39).[380] However, hyperechogenicity of the liver is also a hallmark of fatty infiltration and may be more highly correlated with liver fat than liver fibrosis.[381] The micronodular pattern of liver cirrhosis can be revealed on US, especially when high-resolution probes are used to interrogate the more superficial anterior surface of the liver (see Figure 3-39).[382,383]

CT is relatively insensitive to micronodular regeneration of the liver, because the nodular lesions are typically isointense on noncontrast and portal-phase contrast imaging.[384] On CT examinations, micronodular regeneration is seen best as a subtle nodular undulation of the surface of the liver (see Figure 3-39).[385] Macronodular regeneration is more clearly depicted by CT scanning. In addition, US, CT, and MRI can all depict the lobar asymmetry that may develop in patients with cirrhosis.[386-388] Metrics for defining abnormal caudate-right lobe diameters have been developed as a means of assessing for cirrhotic changes in the absence of the classic nodular appearance.[378]

Because of the exquisite soft-tissue contrast of MRI, regenerative nodules not seen by CT will often be recognized by MRI examinations, although some regenerative nodules can be difficult to identify because of poor contrast from background liver, whereas other smaller regenerative nodules can be below the resolution of MRI.[389] Further, MRI is also more sensitive than CT in detecting the presence of hepatic fibrosis. Fibrotic areas will have altered appearance relative to less affected liver with lower SI on T1-weighted images[390-391] and hyperenhancement on delayed postgadolinium imaging.[392] T2 imaging may depict high signal intensity within fibrotic areas undergoing active inflammation due to the resulting edema.[393]

More recently, noninvasive elastographic methods by US[394] and MRI[395] have been proposed to assess the compliance of the liver as an indirect measure of fibrosis. Early studies have demonstrated good correlation between elastographic measures of liver firmness and degrees of fibrotic change on biopsy,[396,397] but these methods have not yet been advanced into routine clinical use.

Imaging Notes 3-10. Imaging Features of Cirrhosis

Morphologic/ Physiologic Feature	Imaging Manifestation
Micronodular regeneration	Nodular liver surface (CT, MRI)
	Nodular inhomogeneity of parenchyma (MRI)
Diffuse fibrosis	Hyperechogenic (US)
Asymmetric hypertrophy of lobes	Hypertrophied caudate and lateral segment (US, CT, MRI)
Portal hypertension	Splenomegaly (US, CT, MRI)
	Abdominal varices (CT, MRI)
	Portal thrombosis (US, CT, MRI)
Acites	Peritoneal fluid (US, CT, MRI)

Portal hypertension, thrombosis, and ascites

As liver fibrosis develops, the portal sinusoids become obliterated, increasing resistance to portal blood flow. Progressive disease will eventually lead to portal hypertension, with resulting passive congestion of the spleen, and often the development of collateral blood flow via portal venous varices (see Figure 3-39). When portal flow bypasses the liver, hepatic encephalopathy can ensue. Hypertrophied collateral venous channels in the esophagus can lead to upper GI bleeding. Stasis in the portal venous system can promote the development of segmental or main portal vein thrombosis. Increased mesenteric pressures can alter the normal balance of fluid homeostasis in the GI tract, with the resulting development of ascites in the peritoneal cavity (see Figure 3-39). The development of ascites can also be hastened by oncotic factors related to the decrease in serum albumin concentrations as the synthetic function of the liver is compromised.

The findings of portal hypertension are readily identified by imaging. US with color Doppler can identify the patency and direction of flow within the portal veins.[398,399] CT with contrast can depict portal vein thrombosis,[400] and can be used to determine the deep extent of thrombus into the extrahepatic portal vein and splenic or superior mesenteric vein.[401] MRI both with and without contrast can also visualize portal vein thrombosis, and specialized phase-sensitive MRI techniques can also be used to determine flow direction in vessels.[402]

The development of portal hypertension signals an increase in the severity of cirrhosis, and portends poorer prognosis.[403] As such, cross-sectional imaging by US, CT, or MRI is frequently employed to confirm the presence of portal hypertension, avoiding more invasive catheter-based methods of assessing portal venous pressures. Collateral portal venous vessels are readily identified by US, CT, and MRI, as is splenomegaly.[404] Further, US can readily depict even small quantities of ascitic fluid in the various peritoneal recesses, and CT or MRI are also sensitive for ascites when larger amounts of fluid are present.

Regenerative nodules and HCC

Because of the regenerative capacity of the liver, in the setting of scarring and fibrosis, foci of liver regeneration will be seen. When focal regeneration occurs in a cirrhotic liver, a regenerative nodule (RN) is formed. Regenerative nodules are generally small[405] but can be as large as 2 cm or greater.[406] Although other forms of liver regeneration, such as FNH, occur in the absence of intrinsic liver disease, the development of regenerative nodules is specific to livers undergoing the changes of cirrhosis.

When visible on cross-sectional imaging, regenerative nodules typically have imaging characteristics that are similar to normal liver. On US, regenerative nodules can be isoechoic to normal liver (see Figure 3-40). However, because cirrhotic liver has usually increased echogenicity as a result of the presence of fibrosis, the regenerative nodules

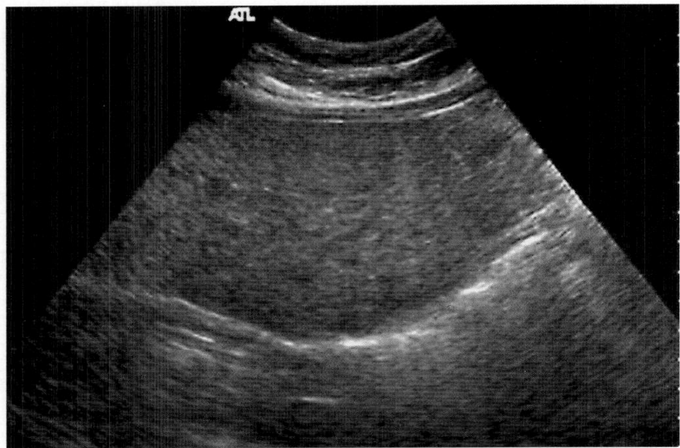

A

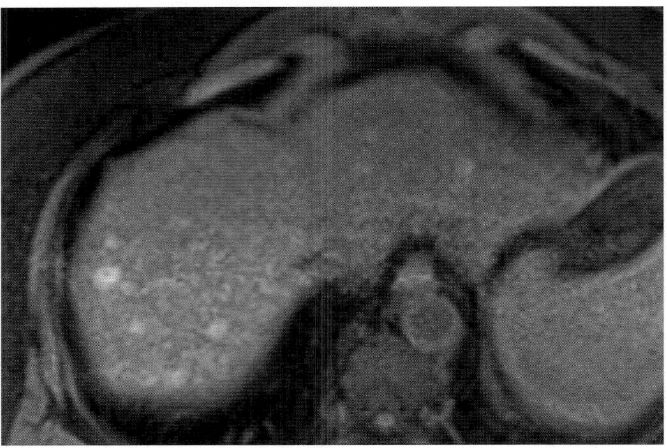

B

Figure 3-40 Regenerative Nodules on US and MRI
This 63-year-old man had elevated Liver function test (LFTS). **A.** Longitudinal US of the liver shows several hypoechoic nodules typical of regenerative nodules. There is background increased echogenicity of the liver parenchyma reflecting underlying cirrhosis with steatosis, a feature that makes the regenerative nodules more distinct. **B.** On MR, small T1 hyperintense lesions of similar size are seen. None of the lesion demonstrated arterial enhancement.

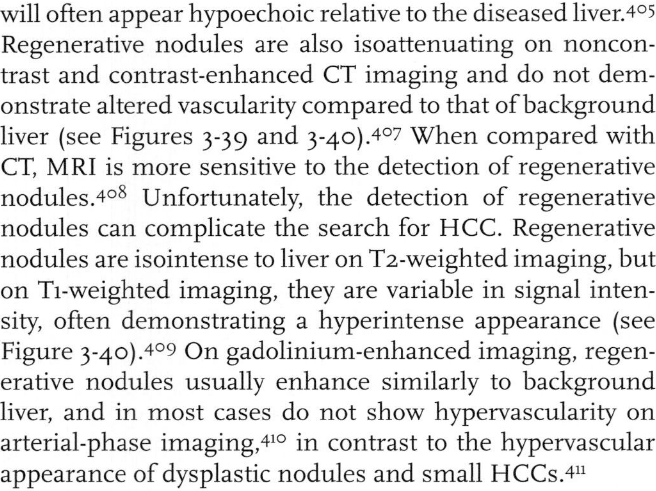

will often appear hypoechoic relative to the diseased liver.[405] Regenerative nodules are also isoattenuating on noncontrast and contrast-enhanced CT imaging and do not demonstrate altered vascularity compared to that of background liver (see Figures 3-39 and 3-40).[407] When compared with CT, MRI is more sensitive to the detection of regenerative nodules.[408] Unfortunately, the detection of regenerative nodules can complicate the search for HCC. Regenerative nodules are isointense to liver on T2-weighted imaging, but on T1-weighted imaging, they are variable in signal intensity, often demonstrating a hyperintense appearance (see Figure 3-40).[409] On gadolinium-enhanced imaging, regenerative nodules usually enhance similarly to background liver, and in most cases do not show hypervascularity on arterial-phase imaging,[410] in contrast to the hypervascular appearance of dysplastic nodules and small HCCs.[411]

Siderotic nodules are a special class of regenerative nodules with increased iron uptake. Siderotic nodules demonstrate low signal on T1- and T2-weighted images[412] and can show the susceptibility effect of iron on gradient echo T2*-weighted images. As with other regenerative nodules, siderotic nodules will not demonstrate hypervascularity on arterial-phase contrast imaging, nor delayed washout or pseudocapsule (see Figure 3-38).

Dysplastic nodules are regenerative nodules that demonstrate dysplastic changes on histologic evaluation. These lesions can demonstrate mild hypervascularity on arterial-phase MRI and be confused with small HCCs. In addition to showing mild hypervascularity, dysplastic nodules can be hyperintense on T1-weighted images, but should remain hypointense on T2-weighted images, an appearance that can overlap that of low-grade HCCs.[411] Unlike HCC, neither dysplastic nor regenerative nodules will demonstrate delayed postcontrast hypointensity to liver, nor will they demonstrate a pseudocapsule—features that are associated strictly with HCC.[413,414]

Hepatocellular carcinoma

HCC is the most common primary malignancy of the liver. Although HCC can present in patients without liver disease, these tumors most commonly arise in the setting of cirrhosis.[415] In the United States, this is usually alcohol related, though incidence due to hepatitis C virus is rising.[416,417] In other regions of the world, HCC is more often related to chronic infection with hepatitis B or parasitic hepatitis.[418,419]

Patients with early HCC are often asymptomatic. Symptoms ascribed to advanced HCC, including right upper quadrant pain, weight loss, fever, jaundice, increased abdominal girth (because of ascites), or encephalopathy, overlap with those of cirrhosis. As such, screening of high risk cirrhotic individuals for HCC is often undertaken. Screening guidelines for HCC in patients with cirrhosis, as recommended by the American Society of Liver Disease, include serum evaluation of α-fetoprotein (AFP) and liver US every 6 months. However, AFP levels can be elevated because of background liver disease, and many patients with HCC do not demonstrate elevated AFP levels. Ultrasonographic screening for HCC in the cirrhotic liver can be challenging, especially in the setting of hepatic steatosis or fibrosis. In addition, US efficacy can depend on the body habitus of the patient, and can be operator dependent. Furthermore, US can have difficulty in distinguishing between large regenerative nodules and HCC. Other imaging methods for HCC screening, specifically multiphase contrast-enhanced CT or MRI, have been proposed as alternatives to US screening.[420,421] However, cost-effectiveness of CT or MRI screening has not been demonstrated.

Most researchers agree that the sensitivity of all modalities for small (<2-cm) HCC is in the range of 50%,[422,423] although newer imaging techniques such as MRI with iron oxide or hepatobiliary contrast agents may lead to increased sensitivities.[424,425] Specificity for HCC on cross-sectional imaging is also variable. Use of strict diagnostic imaging criteria requiring the combination of arterial hyperenhancement, delayed-phase washout, and the presence of an enhancing pseudocapsule has been proposed to improve the specificities of HCC diagnosis on CT and MRI.[426]

The mechanism leading to the formation of HCC is still uncertain. A stepwise pathway has been proposed, beginning with the RN, and progressing to the RN with a focus of dysplasia, the dysplastic nodule, and then early HCC.[427,428] Others propose a de novo pathway for the etiology of HCC.[429] Regardless of the pathophysiology, HCC is almost always associated with longstanding liver cirrhosis. In individuals with hepatitis C infection, a latency of 10 to 20 years is usually required before HCC develops.[430] HCC may develop more rapidly in patients with hepatitis B infection, secondary to genomic disruption from the insertion of the viral hepatitis B DNA genome,[431] and in other etiologies of liver disease, such as hemochromatosis.[432]

A characteristic of HCC that has aided in its detection by imaging is the hypervascular nature of these lesions. As early or small HCC nodules progress, they elicit angiogenic factors that recruit neo-vessels from the hepatic arterial system. This arterialization of tumor blood flow results in hyperenhancement of small HCCs during the hepatic arterial phase of contrast enhancement on CT and MRI examinations and is one of the hallmarks of the imaging appearance of HCC. Unfortunately, a subset of HCC lesions can be hypovascular on arterial-phase images.[433,434] Furthermore, some HCC lesions grow in an infiltrative pattern, spreading via the formation of multiple small nodules extending segmentally from the liver periphery toward the center. This is termed the *cirrhotomimetic* pattern of spread and has imaging features that resemble the multinodular character of the underlying cirrhotic liver, rendering confident identification of tumor more challenging in these cases.[435]

Given the variable imaging appearance of HCC, and the heterogenous and frequently multinodular characteristics of the underlying cirrhotic liver, the imaging diagnosis of HCC can be exceedingly challenging, and there is high incidence of false-positive and false-negative imaging examinations. When larger, HCC lesions often present as hypoechoic masses (see Figure 3-41).[436] However, many smaller HCC lesions can be isoechoic to background liver. Detection of HCC may be further confused by the presence of multiple regenerative nodules, or by the increased echogenicity of the background liver due to either fibrosis or fatty infiltration. The use of US microbubble contrast agents, though not approved for the indication of detecting liver lesions, has been shown to demonstrate HCC tumors to better advantage.[437]

On noncontrast CT scans, HCC lesions, unless very large, can be virtually undetectable or indistinguishable from regenerative nodules. On routine (portal-phase) contrast-enhanced imaging, large HCCs will typically demonstrate irregular hypointensity, and variably demonstrate a hyperenhancing pseudocapsule, that represents a region of compressed hepatic parenchyma surrounding the tumor (see Figure 3-42). Small HCCs are often isointense to liver on portal-phase images and can only be detected by the presence of a hyperenhancing lesion on the hepatic arterial phase (see Figure 3-43). Delayed images, performed 1 to 5 minutes after the portal phase, in some cases will show a hypointense tumor with surrounding hyperenhancing pseudocapsule.

Imaging Notes 3-11. Imaging Characteristics of Macroscopic Nodules in Cirrhosis

Lesion	US[a]	NC-CT[b]	T1W[c]	T2W[d]	HAP[e] Enhancement	Delayed Washout	Pseudocapsule
Regenerative Nodule	↓ to →	→	→ to ↑	→	No	No	No
Siderotic Nodule	↓ to →	→	↓ to →	↓↓	No	No	No
Dysplastic Nodule	↓ to →	→	→ to↑	↓ to →	Sometimes	No	No
Small HCC	↓ to →	→	→ to ↑	Variable	Usually	Often	Usually
Large HCC	↓	↓	↓ to →	↑ to ↑↑	Heterogeneous	Yes	Usually

[a]Ultrasonography. Features represent echogenicity relative to surrounding liver.
[b]Noncontrast computer tomography. Features represent attenuation relative to surrounding liver on unenhanced images.
[c]T1-weighted MRI. Features represent signal intensity relative to surrounding liver.
[d]T2-weighted MRI. Features represent signal intensity relative to surrounding liver.
[e]Hepatic arterial phase.
↓↓ = markedly hypo-; ↓ = moderately hypo-; → = iso-; ↑ = moderately hyper-; ↑↑ = markedly hyper-.

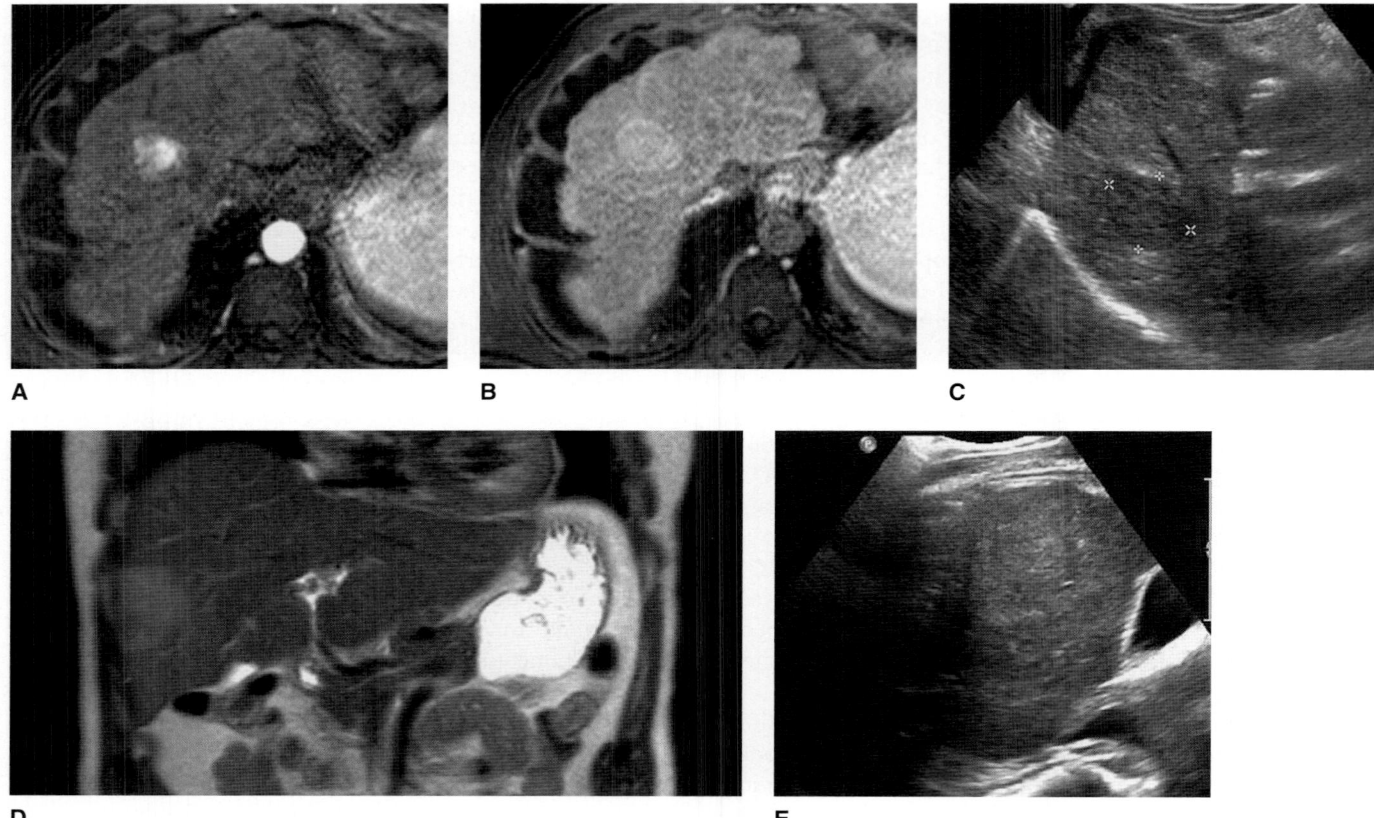

Figure 3-41 US and MRI of HCC in 2 Patients
A-C. This 54-year-old woman with hepatitis C was receiving MRI surveillance examinations. T1-weighted arterial-phase postgadolinium image (A) shows a hypervascular mass that becomes less apparent on the portal-phase image (B). Sonographic image (C) obtained during biopsy demonstrates corresponding hypoechoic nodule. **D.** This 62-year-old man with hepatitis C had this large hyperintense mass noted on this T2-weighted coronal image. US image obtained during biopsy (**E**) demonstrates an ill-defined hyperechoic lesion in the right lobe, corresponding to the known HCC.

The appearance of HCC on MRI shares many characteristics with the appearance on CT. HCCs are most often isointense to liver on unenhanced T1-weighted imaging, although hypointense and even hyperintense appearances have been described (see Figure 3-43).[409] On T2-weighted imaging, HCCs are usually isointense to liver, although the higher grade tumors tend to show some hyperintense characteristics (see Figure 3-43). As with CT, the hallmark of HCC on MRI is the presence of a hyperenhancing lesion on arterial-phase imaging that then reverts to an isointense, or more often hypointense, appearance on portal- and delayed-phase imaging (see Figure 3-43).[438] Often the hyperenhancing pseudocapsule will be seen on delayed-phase MRI, a finding highly specific for HCC when coupled with hyperenhancement on arterial-phase imaging.[439] As with CT, infiltrative HCCs are much more difficult to identify on MRI than the more common mass lesion. Infiltrative HCCs present as irregular lesions with poorly defined margins. Although infiltrative HCCs generally present with heterogeneous appearance following gadolinium administration, the heterogeneous nature of the cirrhotic liver presents a similar imaging appearance and can make even large infiltrative tumors difficult to detect. The absence of the normal regional portal venous structures can be an important clue to the presence of an infiltrative HCC (see Figure 3-43).

The presence of lipid and/or differences in iron content within a liver lesion can also be a clue to the diagnosis of HCC on MRI examinations. Hepatocyte-derived neoplasms, primarily HCC and hepatic adenomas, can contain intracellular lipid that can be recognized by chemical shift–sensitive T1-weighted images. Thus, these tumors will have a loss in signal on opposed-phase images when compared with that of in-phase images. Because hepatic adenomas are not commonly found in cirrhotic livers, the presence of lipid-containing lesions in the cirrhotic patient should raise concern for HCC. Iron accumulation or iron deficit relative to the remaining liver can also be seen in certain HCC lesions and be a clue to the presence of malignancy.[440] However, the presence of iron in a focal lesion in a cirrhotic liver is not specific for HCC. Benign siderotic nodules can also demonstrate the presence of iron in the

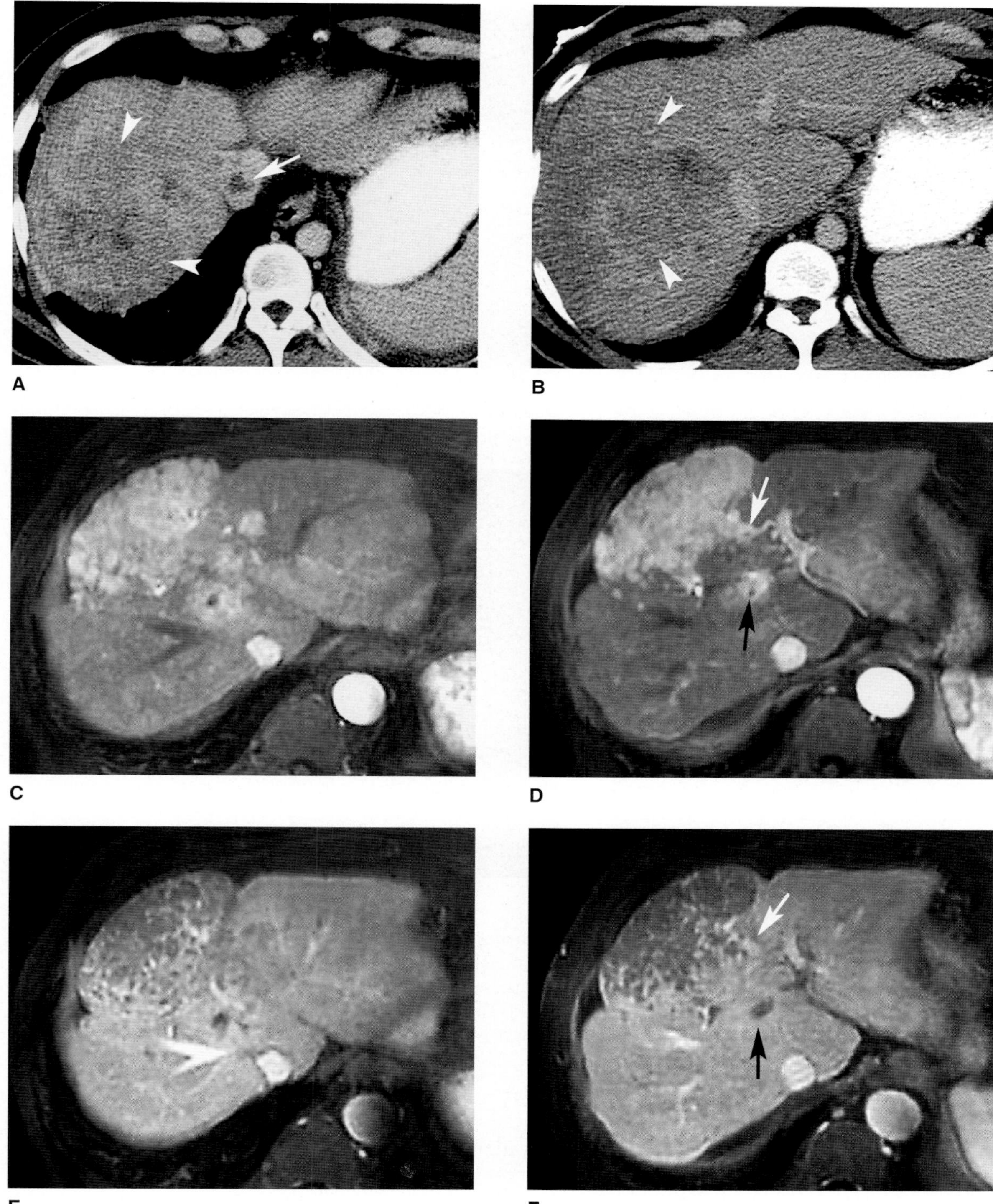

Figure 3-42 Two HCC with Venous Invasion in 2 Patients
A and **B.** This 57-year-old man with a history of hepatitis B complained of dyspnea and weight loss. CT images (A and B) reveal a faint, ill-defined, indistinctly marginated, mixed attenuation mass (*arrowheads*) in the right lobe of the liver. This is a common appearance for an advanced HCC. Note the filling defect in the inferior vena cava (*arrow*) representing tumor thrombus. **C-F.** This 81-year-old man had cryptogenic cirrhosis and HCC. Arterial-phase postgadolinium T1-weighted images (C and D) demonstrate a large hyperenhancing mass in the hepatic dome straddling the right and left lobes. In (D), enhancement is seen in branches of both the left (*white arrow*) and right (*black arrow*) portal vein. Portal-phase images (E and F) demonstrate extensive washout of the tumor. In (F), the intact left portal vein segment remains brightly enhancing (*white arrow*), whereas the tumor thrombus in the right portal vein segment demonstrates hypointensity because of washout.

A

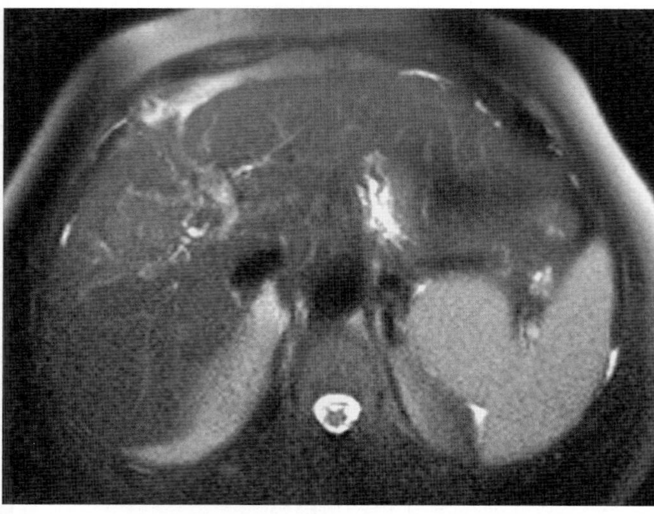

B

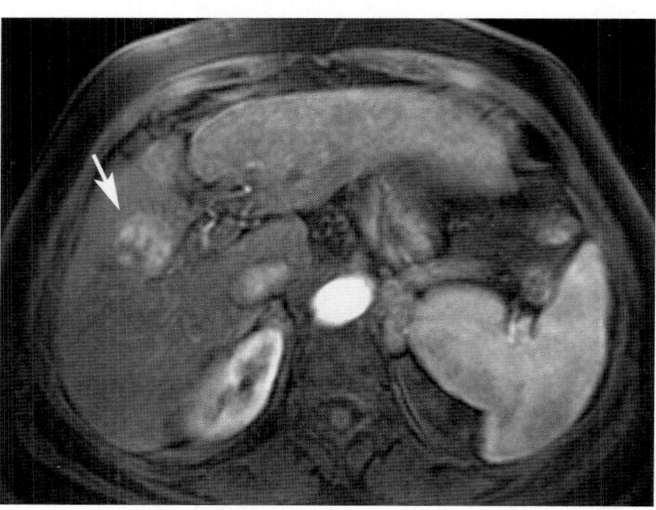

C

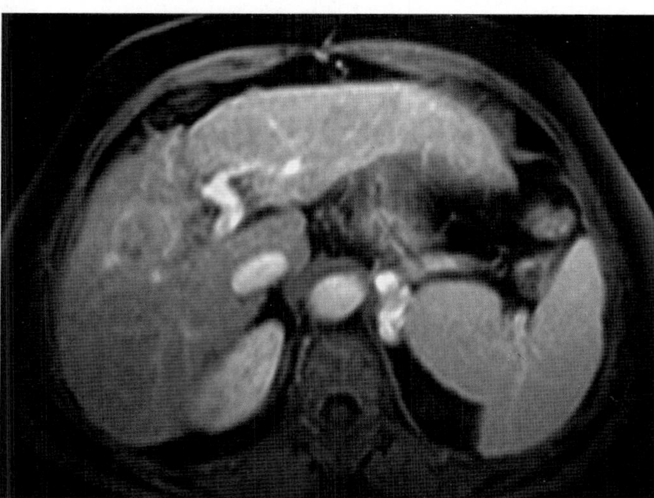

D

Figure 3-43 Two Patients with HCC
A-D. This 64-year-old man had a history of cirrhosis. T1-weighted (A), T2-weighted (B), T1-weighted postgadolinium arterial-phase (C) and T1-weighted postgadolinium venous-phase (D) images through the same location of the liver are shown. Note the multinodular appearance of the liver parenchyma in (A) typical of cirrhosis. Notice in (C), the 2-cm enhancing mass (*arrow*) in the right lobe of the liver. Try to see the mass in the other 3 images. It is faintly seen in (B and D) but is unrecognizable in (A). This represents HCC. The difficulty in recognizing this mass is typical for smaller HCCs.

nodule (see Figure 3-38). More commonly, HCC can present as a focal area of sparing in an otherwise iron-rich liver, a finding easily depicted on T2-weighted series.

Unfortunately, other focal hepatic lesions, including FNH, hepatic adenomas, hypervascular metastases, small hemangiomas, and nonneoplastic arterial-portal shunts (also common in cirrhotic livers), can exhibit 1 or several of the imaging features typical of HCC. Therefore, the diagnosis of HCC by CT or MRI requires careful evaluation of lesion appearance on all phases of contrast administration and under all imaging sequences.

Elevation in AFP levels can be an important clinical clue to the presence of HCC. Unfortunately, AFP elevation is variable in HCC, and reliance on this serum marker to confirm the diagnosis of HCC can be problematic. However, the combination of very elevated AFP levels with a liver mass that is hyperenhancing on arterial-phase imaging is highly associated with a diagnosis of HCC.[441]

HCC can invade the portal, and less commonly the hepatic, veins.[442] Vascular invasion is demonstrated as a filling defect within the lumen of a portal or hepatic vein on US examinations and contrast-enhanced CT and MRI examinations (see Figure 3-42). Multiphase CT and MRI can distinguish bland portal vein thrombus from tumor thrombus by demonstrating enhancement of the clot

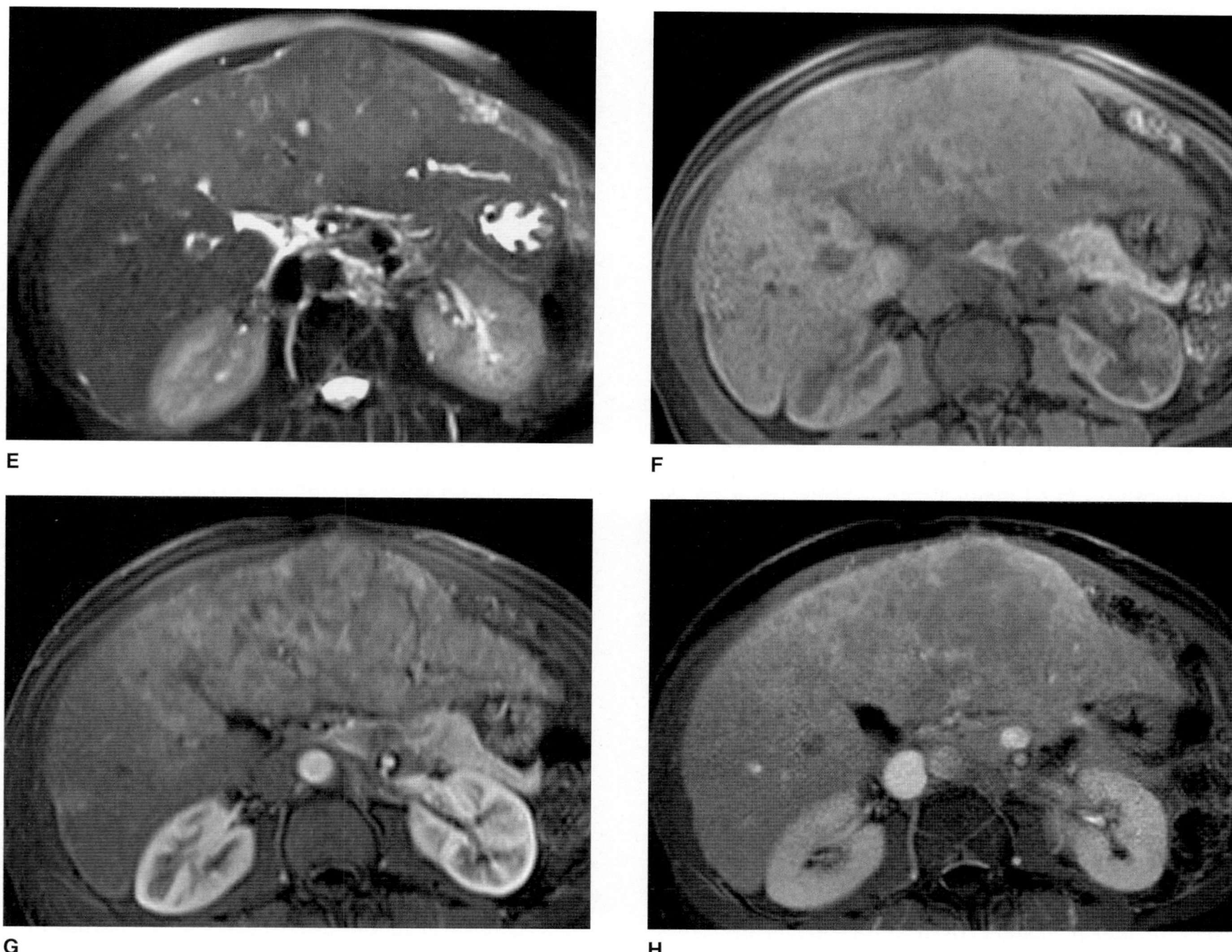

Figure 3-43 Two Patients with HCC (*Continued*)
E-H. This 62-year-old man had hepatitis C. Axial T2-weighted (E) and axial T1-weighted (F) images demonstrate lobular enlargement of the left lobe of the liver. There is faint hyperintensity on the T2-weighted sequence and faint hypointensity on the T1-weighted sequence, suggesting an infiltrative mass. Arterial-phase (G) and delayed-phase (H) postcontrast images confirm vague diffuse enhancement difference to the enlarged left lobe, hyperintense on the early phase and hypointense on the delayed phase. Biopsy was diagnostic of HCC.

in tumor thrombus (see Figure 3-43).[443] Furthermore, tumor thrombus will more often expand the vein, whereas portal veins with bland thrombus are more frequently smaller.

Lymphatic metastasis from HCC to the porta hepatis and celiac axis nodes is not uncommon.[444] Unfortunately, cirrhosis without HCC can also cause adenopathy at these sites and, therefore, lymph node enlargement in the porta hepatis and celiac axis is a nonspecific finding in patients with HCC. Hematogenous metastasis will most often involve the lungs and bone.[445]

When more than 1 hypervascular liver lesion is seen on CT or MRI of the cirrhotic liver, it becomes important to identify which lesions, if any, are likely to represent HCC, and which lesions are more likely to represent benign lesions (either dysplastic nodules or nodular arterial-portal shunts). As described earlier, the characteristic appearance of HCCs on CT or MRI includes hypervascularity on arterial-phase imaging, with delayed hypointensity ("washout") on portal- or delayed-phase imaging, and the appearance of a hyperenhancing pseudocapsule on delayed-phase imaging. Because of the higher intrinsic tissue contrast of MRI, and the exquisite sensitivity of MRI to gadolinium on T1-weighted imaging, MRI may be more sensitive to detect small HCC lesions. However, MRI is also more likely than CT to demonstrate dysplastic nodules and arterial-portal shunts. As such, there remains debate over whether MRI or CT is more accurate in identifying the number of HCC lesions. As the management of HCC depends on the size and number of HCC lesions, these issues remain an ongoing area of study.

When the diagnosis of HCC is made, imaging-based staging is a critical component in the planning of clinical management. The staging of HCC is complex, and is geared toward the determination of postsurgical, especially posttransplant outcomes. Currently, most centers that treat HCC lesions use the Milan criteria. This system based on the proposed staging by Mazzaferro, also known as the "Milan" criteria, was designed to predict the likelihood of recurrence after liver transplantation.[446] In the Milan criteria, single tumors less than 2 cm are T1 lesions. Single tumors over 2 cm but less than 5 cm are T2 lesions. Patients with 2 to 3 tumors are also considered to harbor T2 tumor burden, provided that no tumors is greater than 3 cm. Patients who harbor any tumor greater than 5 cm, or 2 to 3 tumors with at least 1 greater than 3 cm, are considered T3 patients. Patients with 4 or more tumors, or any patients with malignant portal or hepatic venous invasion on imaging, are designated as T4.

The treatment of HCC is complex. For patients with very early-stage disease (T1) and adequate liver reserve, surgical resection can be performed. Focal catheter- or needle-based ablation techniques can also be used for small tumors,[447,448] especially those patients who are not candidates for surgical therapies. For patients with slightly more advanced disease (T2), liver transplantation may be an option. Current practice of the United Network for Organ Sharing (UNOS) will allocate priority allocation of donor livers for transplantation based on the size of the largest tumor and the degree of multifocality. Under the current system, patients with T2-stage HCC may be eligible for prioritization for liver transplant, whereas T1-stage patients with a single small (<2 cm) lesion, even if biopsy proven to represent HCC, must be observed for tumor growth to be eligible for transplant. Patients with more advanced T3- and T4-stage tumors are not currently eligible for transplantation, although some exceptions are made based on more expansive criteria.[449] Treatment options for these patients include liver-directed therapies, especially catheter-based chemoembolization. For patients with extensive extrahepatic spread of tumor, newer targeted chemotherapy agents, such as sorafenib, have shown modest improvement in patient survival.[450]

Pseudocirrhosis

The term *pseudocirrhosis* is reserved for the appearance of the widely metastatic liver after a partial or complete response to systemic therapy. This appearance was first described for breast cancer,[451] but can also be seen in other treatable cancers where multifocal hepatic metastases are common.[452,453] As metastatic disease is rarely cured by chemotherapy, recurrence following the initial response may lead to a bizarre appearance of the liver with areas of contour retraction and scarring adjacent to bulging areas of viable growing tumor. As the term implies, the appearance of the pseudo-cirrhotic liver may overlap that of end-stage liver disease, and correlation with clinical history can aid the radiologist in making a diagnostic error (see Figure 3-44).

Radiation Hepatitis

Complications of radiation therapy to the liver typically occur in patients who have received at least 3500 rad and manifests itself 2 to 6 weeks after completion of radiation therapy.[454] Patients can present with right upper quadrant pain and with elevated liver function tests. Because complete liver radiation will result in unacceptable toxicity, typically only a portion of the liver is irradiated. In other cases, portions of the liver are incidentally irradiated in the setting of treatment for other conditions, such as midline abdominal radiation in lymphoma. In either setting, only those regions of the liver receiving high radiation dose will develop changes of radiation hepatitis. As a consequence, the abnormal area will be sharply demarcated based on the border of the radiation portal. This feature is characteristic of radiation-related changes in all organs and is virtually specific for the diagnosis of radiation changes. The liver affected by radiation will appear hyperechoic on US examinations.[455] On CT, there will be an area of low attenuation because of edema or fatty infiltration with decreased perfusion.[456] In patients who develop diffuse hepatic steatosis from chemotherapy, the radiated area of the liver may be spared from fatty change (see Figure 3-45).[457] On MRI, the radiated area will appear lower signal than the normal liver on T1-weighted images and high signal on T2-weighted sequences.[458] There is usually complete recovery of the affected region, but some patients' radiation damage will result in atrophy of the treated region.

Hepatic Congestion, Budd-Chiari Syndrome, and the Nutmeg Liver

Chronic venous outflow obstruction is an uncommon but important cause of chronic liver dysfunction. Obstruction of the hepatic veins can lead to microvascular ischemia as a result of liver congestion.[459,460] If sufficiently severe and long-standing, this can result in liver insufficiency and cirrhosis.

Causes of hepatic venous outflow obstruction include right-sided heart failure, Budd-Chiari syndrome, and hepatic veno-occlusive syndrome.[461] Budd-Chiari syndrome represents thrombotic or nonthrombotic hepatic venous outflow obstruction.[459] Prothrombotic conditions contributing to Budd-Chiari syndrome include protein C deficiency, protein S deficiency, paroxysmal nocturnal hematuria, Behçet disease, polycythemia vera, pregnancy/postpartum state, antiphospholipid syndrome, and oral contraceptive

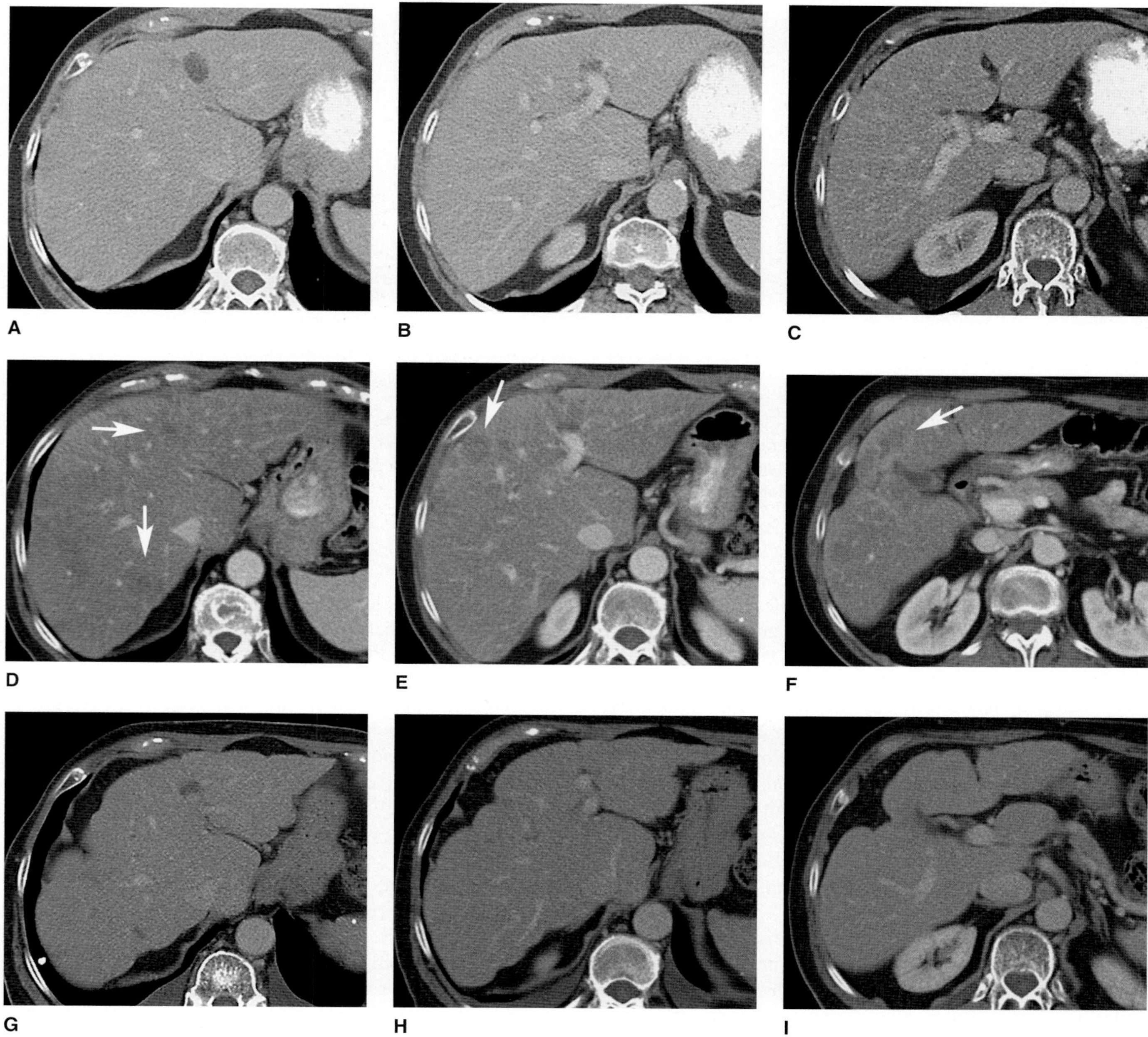

Figure 3-44 Pseudocirrhosis
This 68-year-old woman had breast cancer. **A-C.** Three axial images from a contrast-enhanced CT appear normal, except for a small simple cyst in (A). **D-F.** Two years later, there are several low-attenuation lesions within the liver, indicating the presence of liver metastasis. The patient received chemotherapy and was reevaluated a further 6 months later. **G-I.** The liver metastasis are no longer seen; however, the surface of the liver now has an irregular, nodular-appearing contour resembling the appearance of a cirrhotic liver. This is the pseudocirrhosis pattern of scarring following chemotherapy for liver metastasis.

use. Rarely, Budd-Chiari syndrome is caused by a congenital IVC web or extrinsic IVC compression from an adjacent mass (Table 3-12). Hepatic veno-occlusive syndrome is a diffuse small-vessel occlusive disease that is an uncommon complication of bone marrow transplantation.[462]

Patients with Budd-Chiari syndrome present with acute liver disease, subacute liver disease, fulminant liver disease, or chronic liver failure.[459,460,463] In the acute and subacute forms of disease, patients present with abdominal pain, hepatomegaly, jaundice, ascites, and acute renal failure. Most patients will present with the chronic form of disease characterized by progressive ascites without jaundice, and in 50% of cases with associated renal failure. A fulminant presentation is least common and is characterized by acute hepatic failure, ascites, tender hepatomegaly, jaundice, and renal failure.

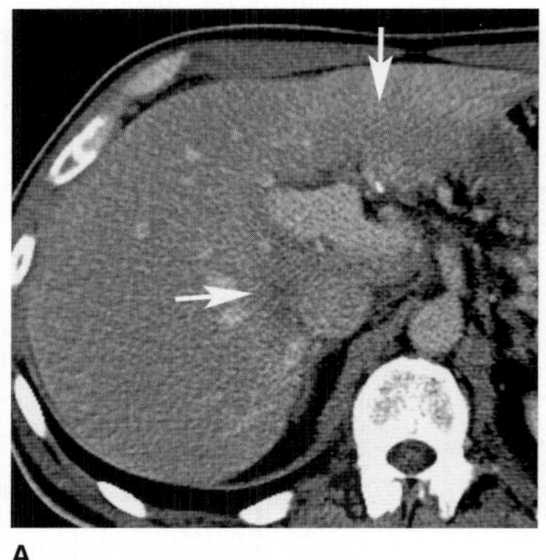
A

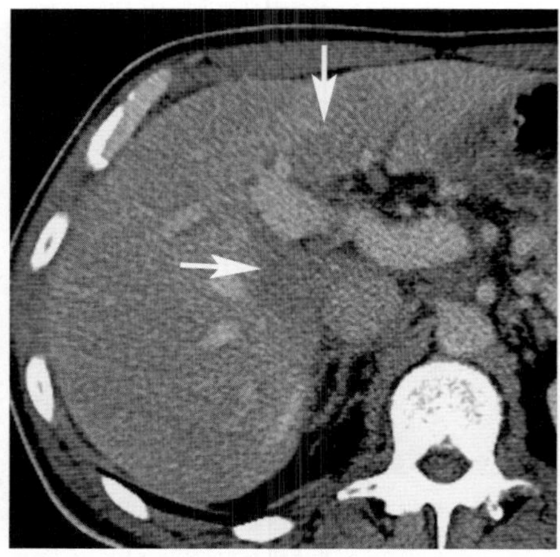
B

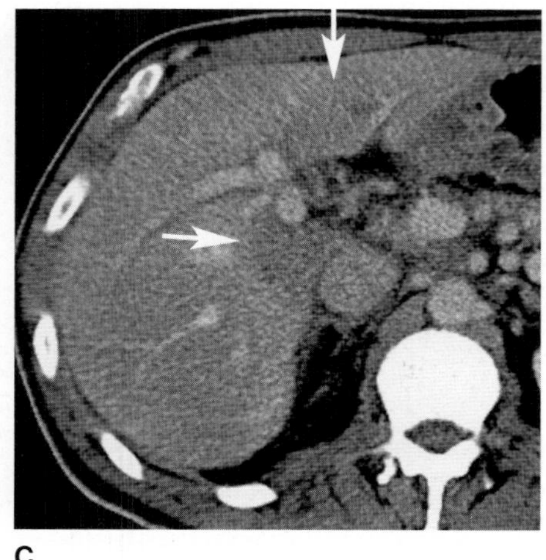
C

Figure 3-45 Radiation Changes
This 54-year-old man had received chemotherapy and radiation therapy for pancreatic carcinoma. **A-C.** Contrast-enhanced CT shows a regional zone of decreased attenuation (*arrows*) within the central liver. This vaguely forms a right angle and is the typical appearance of radiation changes as part of therapy for pancreatic carcinoma.

Patients with any cause of chronic venous outflow obstruction will have a characteristic enhancement pattern on contrast-enhanced CT and MRI, termed the *nutmeg* liver.[464-466] Instead of the normal uniform tissue enhancement, the liver has a reticular pattern of poor or delayed enhancement (see Figure 3-46). This appearance is due to impaired venous outflow, with poor progression of contrast between the hepatic portal sinusoids and the hepatic veins.[464] Segmental hepatic outflow patterns can also be shown when outflow compromise is isolated to a single hepatic vein.[467] MRI examinations will also demonstrate hyperintensity of the liver parenchyma on T2-weighted images because of hepatic edema.[468]

Budd-Chiari syndrome is distinguished from other causes of hepatic outflow obstruction by the obliteration and absence of the main portal veins or by their obstruction with thrombus or tumor. All cross-sectional imaging examinations—US, CT and MRI—can demonstrate the absence of the main portal vein flow. They can also demonstrate an extrinsic mass obstructing hepatic vein outflow or intravascular clot or tumor (see Figure 3-47). One study has suggested that contrast-enhanced MRI is slightly more accurate than CT for the detection of Budd-Chiari syndrome.[469] Ultrasonographic examinations have the added advantage of being able to detect the presence and direction of flow within the hepatic vasculature. Patients with Budd-Chiari syndrome will lack venous flow within the hepatic veins on Doppler imaging.[470] In severe cases, there may be hepatofugal flow within the main portal vein because of retrograde propagation of increased sinusoidal pressures backward into the main portal vein, leading to portal hypertension, but this finding was reported in less than 10% of patients in 1 cohort study.[471] In severe or long-standing cases of hepatic vein obstruction, ascites and splenomegaly can develop.[472]

The caudate lobe drains directly into the IVC and can bypass the obstruction in the hepatic veins present in patients with Budd-Chiari syndrome. As a consequence, the atrophy induced by chronic outflow obstruction spares the caudate lobe, which can hypertrophy in response to atrophy of the rest of the liver. Caudate lobe enlargement can be a common ancillary finding of Budd-Chiari syndrome on all cross-sectional imaging examinations, including US.[469,473]

In the setting of long-standing Budd-Chiari syndrome and other causes of chronic hepatic vein outflow obstruction, the liver can develop cirrhosis and resultant nodular regenerative hyperplasia[474] and also have an increased risk of developing HCC.[475] As with all causes of cirrhosis, regenerative nodules will be hyperattenuating on arterial-phase images and will remain isoattenuating or hyperattenuating on portal venous images, because of diminished portal venous flow and compensatory increase in hepatic arterial flow.[476] Small HCCs can be distinguished from regenerative nodules by the washout of contrast on delayed-phase images.

Vascular Malformations

Isolated vascular malformations of the liver, including both arteriovenous and venovenous lesions, are rare, and in the majority of cases are seen in conjunction with cirrhosis.[477] However, intrahepatic vascular malformations are commonly seen in hereditary hemorrhagic telangiectasia (HHT), also known as Osler-Weber-Rendu Syndrome. Affected patients demonstrate characteristic vascular skin lesions, with a large number of patients presenting with pulmonary arteriovenous malformations (AVMs), leading to early stoke or brain abscesses.[478]

Table 3-12. Causes of Budd-Chiari Syndrome

A. Hematologic disorders 1. Inherited thrombotic disorders a. Protein C deficiency b. Protein S deficiency c. Antithrombin III deficiency d. Factor V Leiden deficiency 2. Paroxysmal nocturnal hemoglobinuria 3. Polycythemia rubra vera 4. Antiphospholipid antibody syndrome 5. Essential thrombocytosis
B. Neoplasms 1. Hepatocellular carcinoma 2. Renal cell carcinoma 3. Leiomyosarcoma 4. Adrenal carcinoma 5. Wilms tumor
C. Chronic infections 1. Hydatid cysts 2. Aspergillosis 3. Amebic abscess 4. Syphilis 5. Tuberculosis
D. Chronic inflammatory diseases 1. Inflammatory bowel disease 2. Sarcoidosis 3. Connective tissue disorders a. Systemic lupus erythematosus b. Mixed connective-tissue disease c. Sjögren syndrome d. Behçet disease
E. Miscellaneous 1. Membranous webs 2. Pregnancy and postpartum 3. Oral contraceptives 4. α_1-antitrypsin deficiency 5. Trauma
F. Idiopathic

Liver involvement in HHT is often asymptomatic, with incidence reports varying between 30% and 70%.[479,480] US is usually used as the initial liver screening modality in HHT. In most cases the arteriovenous shunts are not directly detected by US examinations. Instead, the presence of the shunts can be inferred by the recognition of increased blood flow within the liver. This increased flow results in dilation and tortuosity of the main hepatic artery with increased flow velocities.[481,482] Hepatic arterial diameter greater than 7 mm has been suggested as a reliable indicator of the presence of multiple AVMs in patients with HHT.[483,484] Color Doppler examinations will also demonstrate diffuse increased vascularity in the liver parenchyma.

Dynamic enhanced CT or MRI can also be used to reveal the degree of vascular liver involvement in HHT.[485] Further, dynamic enhanced CT and MRI can demonstrate small telangiectatic liver lesions in patients with HHT,[486,487] although patients with smaller liver lesions and absence of hepatic arterial anomalies generally show no signs of liver dysfunction or symptomatic extracardiac shunting.[488,489] On contrast-enhanced CT or MRI, vascular malformations in the liver in HHT appear as blushes on contrast enhancement and/or tangled enhancing vessels. Both arterial-portal and arteriovenous malformations can be seen, with arteriovenous malformation more common.[490] The type of malformation can be determined via identification of the draining vein. Portovenous malformations can also occur but may not be as prominent based on the relatively lower flow from the feeding portal vein branch (see Figure 3-48).

Posttraumatic Fistula

Although hepatic vascular malformations are often associated with hereditary hemorrhagic telangiectasia, isolated posttraumatic arteriovenous, venovenous, and venobiliary fistulae are not uncommon. These lesions can be seen in association with penetrating trauma,[491] or as a complication of percutaneous biopsy.[492] It has been estimated that approximately 5% of percutaneous biopsies result in one of these vascular fistulae.[493] Small peripheral fistulae are typically asymptomatic, but larger central fistulae can result in portal hypertension, portal vein thrombosis, and/or symptomatic portosystemic shunting if left untreated.[494] Pseudoaneurysm formation can also occur.[495]

Doppler US is the best modality for evaluation of hepatic fistulae. Color Doppler imaging in some cases will demonstrate the fistula directly. Alternatively, asymmetry in the pulsatility and/or resistive indices of the right and left hepatic arteries on pulse-wave Doppler may signal the presence of an underlying fistula.[496] Dynamic enhanced CT or MRI can demonstrate arteriovenous fistulae as asymmetric early portal or hepatic vein filling.[497] Angiography is confirmatory and can be used to perform therapeutic embolization (see Figure 3-49).[498]

IMAGING THE POSTOPERATIVE LIVER

The liver is a frequent site of intervention, both surgical and nonsurgical. Common indications for liver interventions include treatments for malignancies, relief of biliary obstruction, debridement of infections, and treatment of vascular abnormalities. Hepatic transplantation is also increasing in frequency, including variants such as partial living liver donation. The common postprocedural and postoperative appearances to the liver are described in this section.

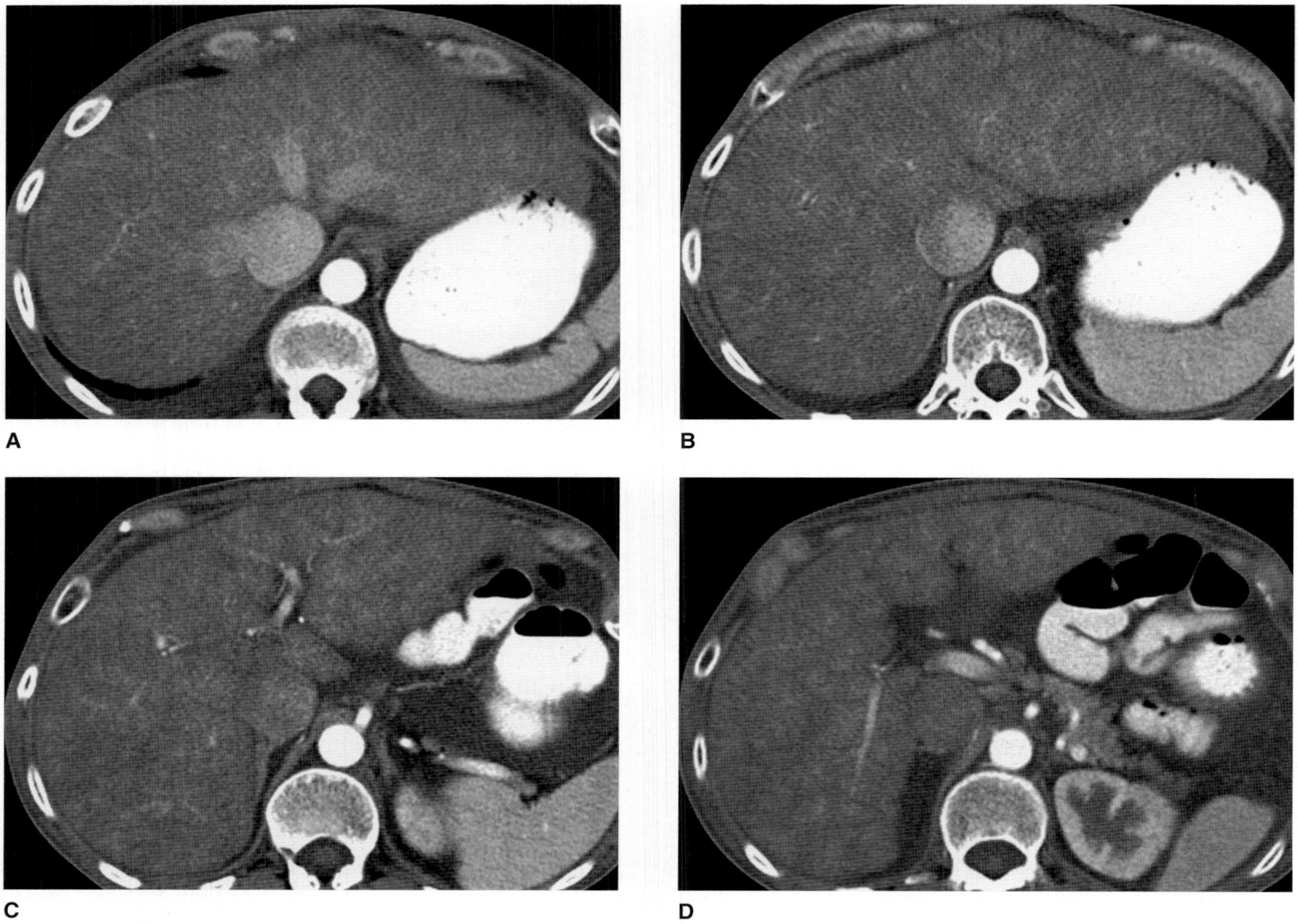

A

B

C

D

Figure 3-46 Nutmeg Liver
This 40-year-old woman had a severe cardiomyopathy with biventricular heart failure. **A-D.** Contrast-enhanced axial CT images in the portal phase show diffuse regular heterogeneity of the liver attenuation, with decreased attenuation surrounding the hepatic veins. This is a characteristic appearance of hepatic congestion due to right-sided heart failure and is called the "nutmeg liver." Note also the distended hepatic veins and reflux of contrast from the superior vena cava (SVC) into the hepatic veins, 2 other findings associated with right heart failure.

Nonsurgical Therapies

The nonsurgical interventions for liver tumor treatment can be divided into purely vascular procedures such as coil embolization for acute bleeding or other vascular pathologies, vascular-based antitumor procedures such as transarterial chemoembolization (TACE), and transarterial radioembolization, percutaneous ablation procedures for tumor treatment such as radiofrequency, chemical, and cryoablation and TIPS placement for chronic portal hypertension.

Coil embolization

Hepatic artery pseudoaneurysms can occur after liver biopsy, focal tumor ablation, or liver transplantation. They are usually asymptomatic and identified incidentally on imaging evaluation of the primary liver abnormality. When identified, pseudoaneurysms can be treated by coil embolization.[499,500] Coil embolization is also used for the treatment of variceal bleeding form portal hypertension.[501] The presence of prior coil embolization is easily depicted by abdominal x-rays and cross-sectional imaging. On CT, the coils will appear as curvilinear metallic objects within the liver parenchyma. The metallic coils vary in size and appearance, but can usually be distinguished from surgical clips by their irregular shape and their intrahepatic location of deployment. On US, coils can be seen as heavily shadowing objects within the liver parenchyma. On MRI, coils will typically generate very large areas of magnetic susceptibility out of proportion to the actual coil size, because of the irregular looped geometry of coils. This effect is easily noticeable on imaging, and often renders the

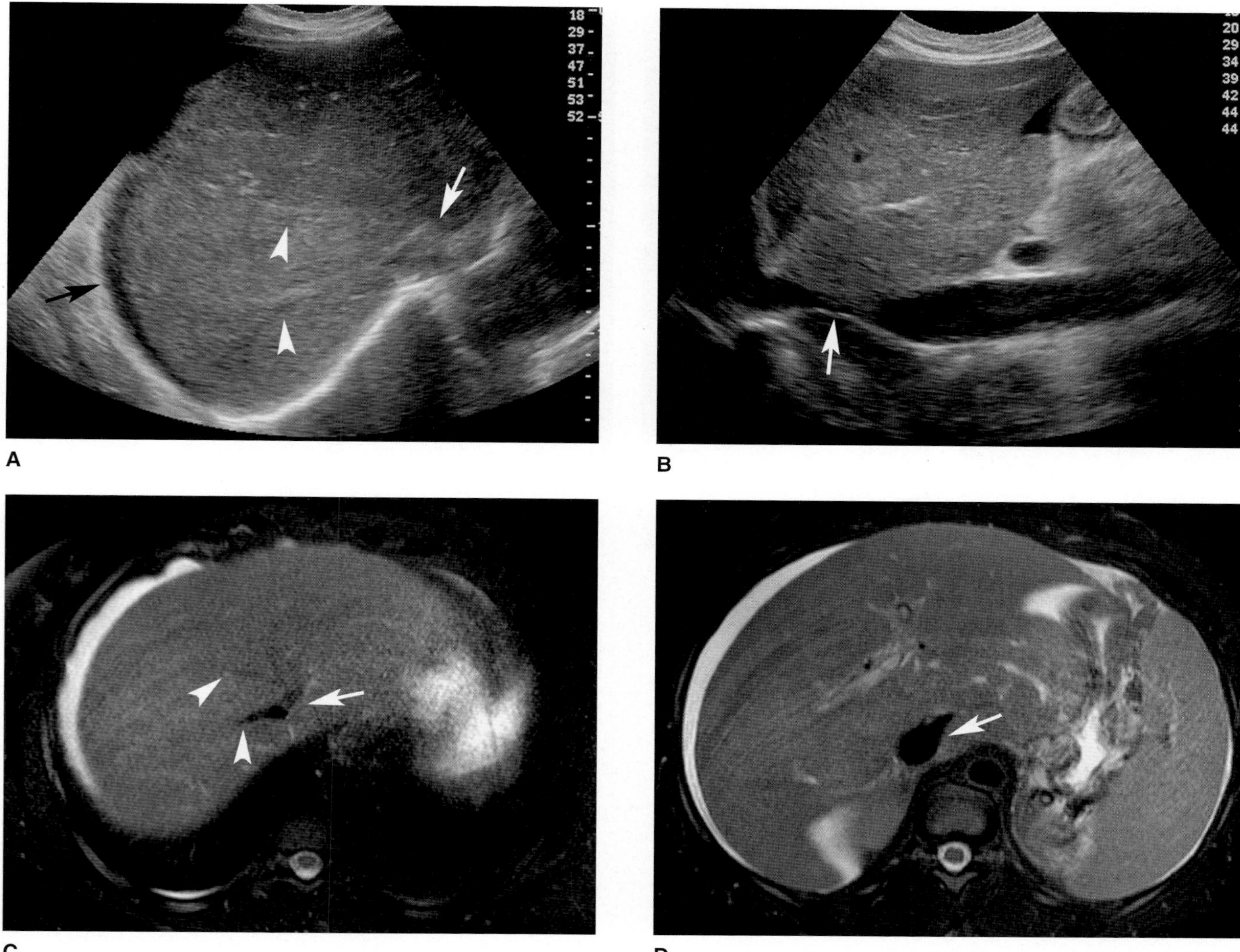

Figure 3-47 Budd-Chiari Syndrome
This 46-year-old man with polycythemia vera developed hepatic dysfunction. **A.** Transverse US through the hepatic dome shows faint echogenic cords in the expected location of the right and middle hepatic veins (*arrowheads*) and an echogenic inferior vena cava (IVC) (*arrow*). There is also a small sliver of ascites along the margin of the liver (*black arrow*). **B.** Longitudinal US of the IVC shows a short stricture (*arrow*) in the superior most aspect of the IVC. These findings are indicative of Budd-Chiari syndrome. **C.** Axial T2-weighted MRI sequence through the superior liver show virtually occluded hepatic veins (*arrowheads*) and IVC (*arrow*). **D.** At a lower level, the IVC appears normal. Note also the high signal perihepatic ascites. These findings confirm the diagnosis of Budd-Chiari syndrome.

MR examination nondiagnostic for large portions of the liver. Despite the imaging dramatic artifact, the presence of vascular coils in the liver does not itself constitute an MRI safety issue for the patient.

Transjugular intrahepatic portosystemic shunt placement

Transjugular intrahepatic portosystemic shunts (TIPS) are commonly used to control complications of portal hypertension. Routine follow-up of TIPS placement is performed by color Doppler US to document patency of the shunt and to document any evidence of stenosis.[502,503] Velocity measurements can be used to determine the functional significance of stenoses, based on maximum absolute peak flow velocity, or changes in peak flow velocity over time.[504] When significant stenoses are shown by US or are suspected clinically, repeat interventional procedures with angioplasty or placement of nested stents to maintain the proper degree of patency can be performed.[505]

On abdominal plain films, TIPS will appear as a meshwork of crossing wires in the right upper quadrant of the abdomen. On CT, they will appear as a similar complex metallic network extending from a central portal vein to 1 of

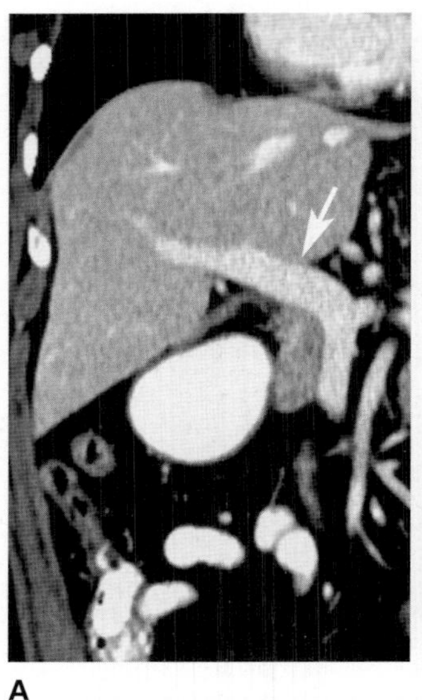

A

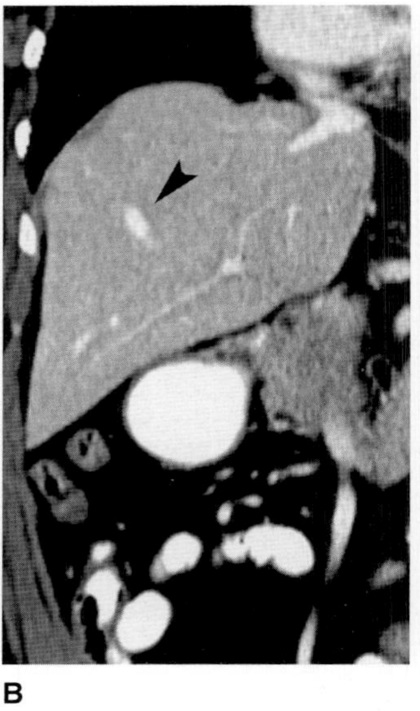

B

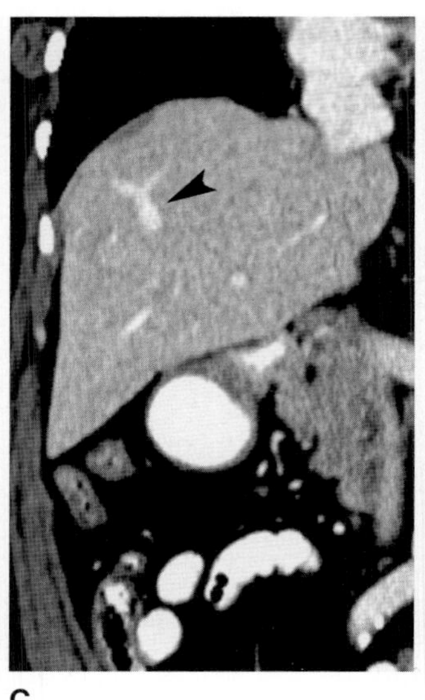

C

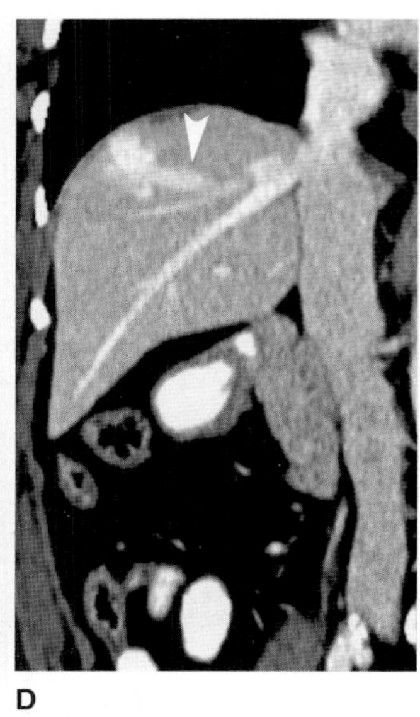

D

Figure 3-48 Portosystemic Shunt
This 76-year-old man was being evaluated for possible metastasis from lung cancer. **A-D.** Sequential coronal reconstructions of an enhanced CT from anterior to posterior show a communication between the right portal vein (*white arrow*) and the right hepatic vein (*white arrowhead*) via progressively smaller branches (*black arrowheads*) of the right portal vein.

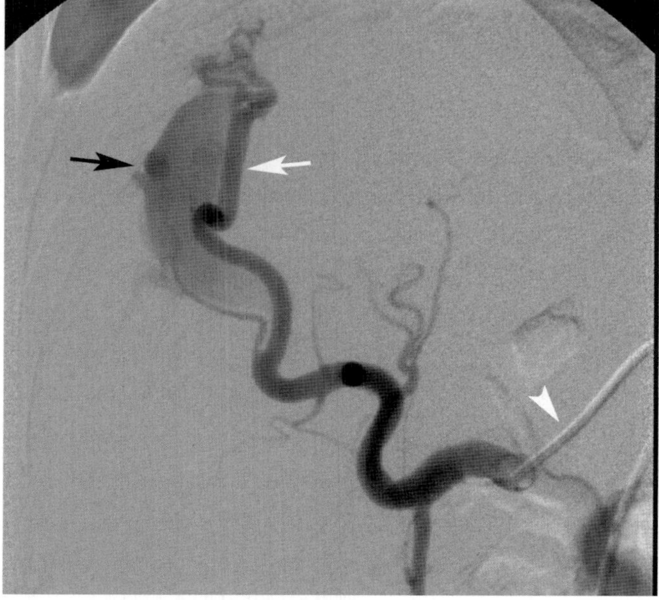

A

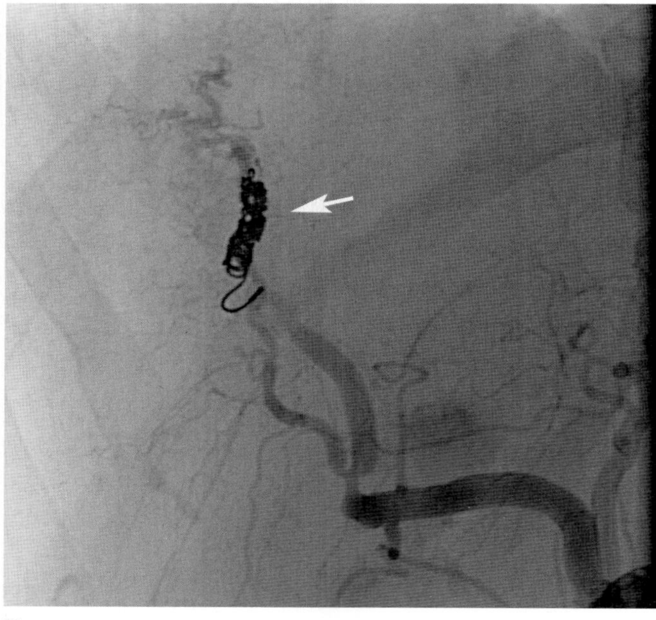

B

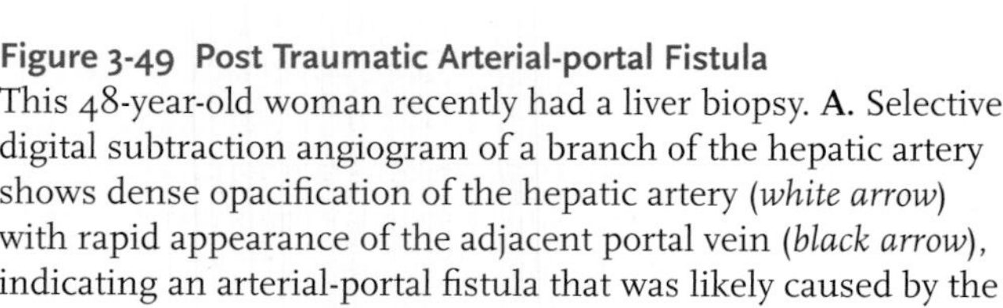

Figure 3-49 Post Traumatic Arterial-portal Fistula
This 48-year-old woman recently had a liver biopsy. **A.** Selective digital subtraction angiogram of a branch of the hepatic artery shows dense opacification of the hepatic artery (*white arrow*) with rapid appearance of the adjacent portal vein (*black arrow*), indicating an arterial-portal fistula that was likely caused by the recent needle biopsy of the liver. The angiographic catheter is also seen (*white arrowhead*) **B.** Hepatic arteriogram after coil embolization shows occlusion of the branch of the hepatic artery and absence of the portal fistula. The embolectomy coils appear as metallic coils (*arrow*).

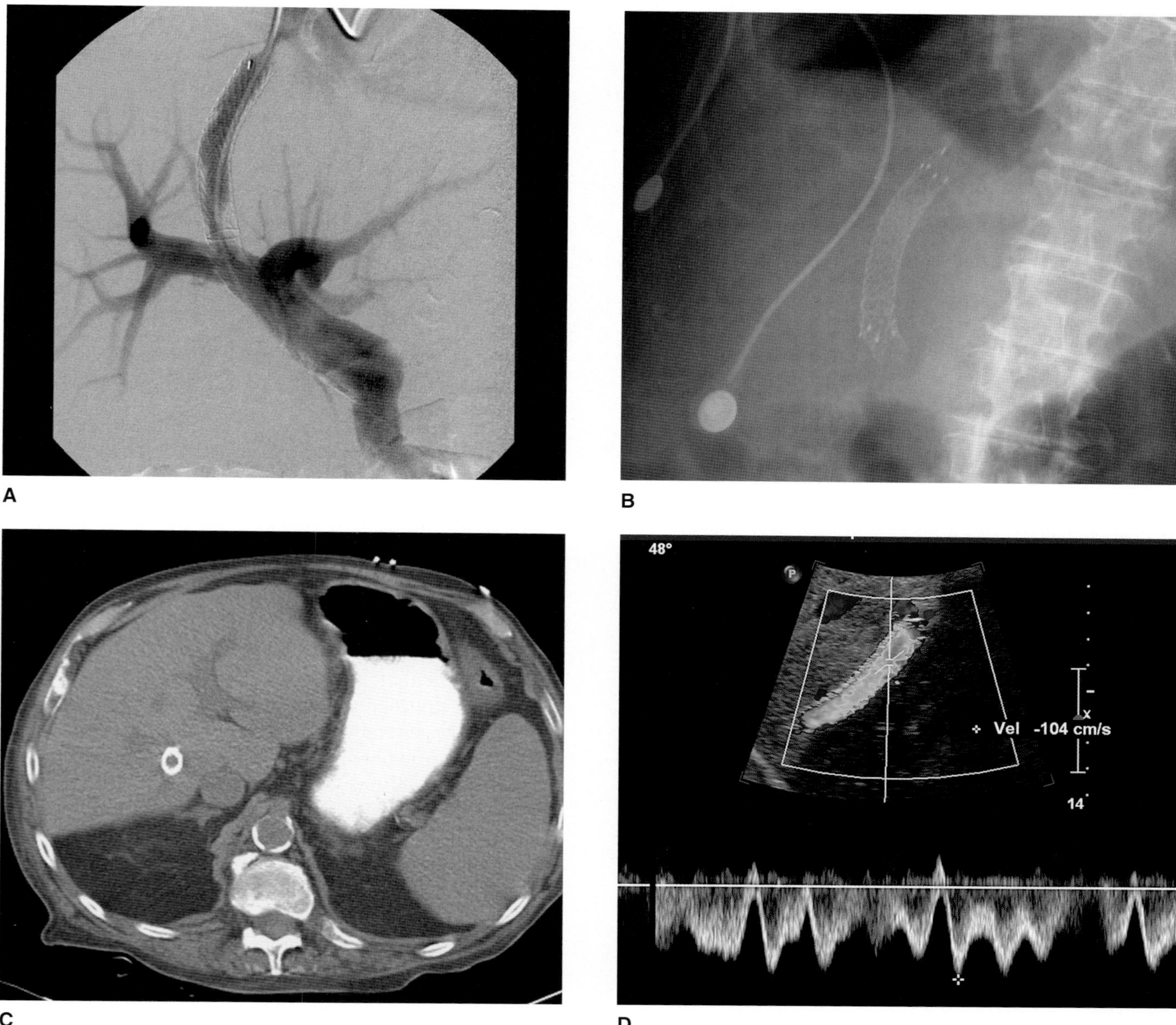

Figure 3-50 TIPS on Multiple Modalities
This 68-year-old man had end-stage cirrhosis. **A.** Angiogram performed during placement of the TIPS shows the fine mesh of the TIPS and the communication between the right portal vein and the inferior vena cava (IVC). **B.** Magnified view from an abdominal plain film shows a tubular structure composed of interlocking fine wires overlying the liver shadow, findings typical of a TIPS. **C.** Unenhanced CT shows the nodular appearance of a cirrhotic liver and a metallic ring of the TIPS in cross section. **D.** Doppler US of the TIPS shows the typical undulating flow of blood in the TIPS, caused by respirations.

the 3 hepatic veins. Like other metallic objects, TIPS will appear as a large black area of magnetic susceptibility in the superior central liver. Because of streak artifact from the metal struts, documentation of shunt patency can be difficult to obtain by contrast-enhanced CT (see Figure 3-50).[506] Similarly, artifact will often render the interior of the stent dark on MRI, even with gadolinium enhancement, an appearance that should not be confused with that of occlusion. The more recent generation of covered stents has reduced MR artifact, allowing for a partial evaluation of stent patency by MRI.[507]

Transarterial chemoembolization

TACE is commonly used in the therapy of primary and secondary liver malignancies.[508] In this procedure, an embolic mixture is instilled into a major segmental branch of the liver. The mixture commonly includes a chemotherapy mixture that can be delivered to the tumor(s) at much higher

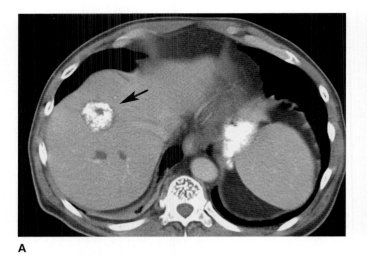

A

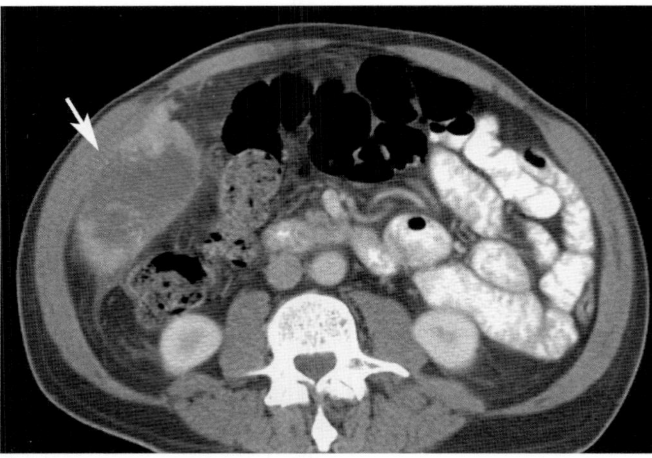

B

Figure 3-51 Post TACE Complicated by a Hepatic Infarct This 56-year-old man had HCC which was recently treated with TACE. **A.** Contrast-enhanced CT shows a very high attenuation nodule (*black arrow*) in the anterior segment of the liver. This is the typical appearance of retained Ethiodol within the HCC after successful treatment of the malignancy with TACE. **B.** Within the inferior tip of the liver is an irregularly marginated region of hypoattenuation (*white arrow*), with fat stranding in the adjacent perihepatic fat. Although nonspecific in appearance, this is likely to represent hemorrhagic infarction of the liver secondary to the TACE.

concentration than can safely be achieved systemically, although bland embolization for benign vascular tumors, such as adenomas, can also be performed.[509]

Interventional techniques vary, and the postprocedural appearance of treated liver tumors is often determined by the presence or absence of iodized oil within the embolic mixture. When used, the iodized oil, such as Ethiodol, is readily apparent on noncontrast CT scans and is often retained in treated tumors (see Figure 3-51).[510] Early postprocedural scans can be used to verify the segmental distribution of the embolic mixture, and to determine degree of uptake in known or suspected tumors.[511] The incidental nontumorous oil deposition is usually cleared over the ensuing months, although some residual nontumor accumulation is common. Tumor accumulation of the oil is generally longstanding. Successful treatment of hepatic tumors will result immediately in loss of tumor enhancement on contrast-enhanced scans, and gradual shrinkage in tumor size over time. However, the persistence of iodized oil accumulation in treated lesions can complicate the CT evaluation of residual tumor viability on postprocedural enhanced studies as the high attenuation of the embolic material can obscure the depiction of contrast enhancement.[512]

MRI is commonly used for the evaluation of tumor response to TACE, as this modality is not affected by the high attenuation of iodized oil in the tumor.[513] Occasionally, the oil accumulation can be depicted as signal dropout on opposed-phase chemical shift–sensitive imaging. The successfully treated tumor will demonstrate increased T1 signal pre-gadolinium, a finding because of the high relaxation rate of tissue that has undergone coagulative necrosis. On T2, the findings are more variable, although coagulative necrosis generally displays low T2 signal, and areas of more intermediate-high signal may represent areas of viability.[514] Gadolinium-enhanced imaging is used to depict areas of tumor viability, easily shown as internal enhancing regions on T1-weighted imaging (see Figure 3-52).[515] Rim enhancement is common after treatment and generally represents reactive hyperemia and granulation tissue rather than residual viable tumor. However, lack on visible enhancement after therapy does not always predict complete response, as explant evaluation of treated HCC lesions can show viable tumor even in lesions without enhancement on imaging.[516] More recently, DWI has been proposed as a method for evaluating treatment response to chemoembolization.[517-519]

Complications from TACE can include liver necrosis,[520] biliary stricture/biloma formation,[521] and infection (see Figure 3-51).[522] Liver infarctions after TACE appear as wedge-shaped regions of nonenhancement on CT or MRI. When segmental infarctions are seen following TACE, close clinical and imaging follow-up is needed to exclude the possibility that the infarcted area does not in actuality represent treated infiltrative tumor that was occult to cross-sectional imaging prior to therapy.

Percutaneous ablation

Percutaneous ablation is another nonsurgical option for treatment of liver tumors. Several options for ablation of tumors exist, including heating via radiofrequency ablation, freezing via cryoablation, or chemical treatment via

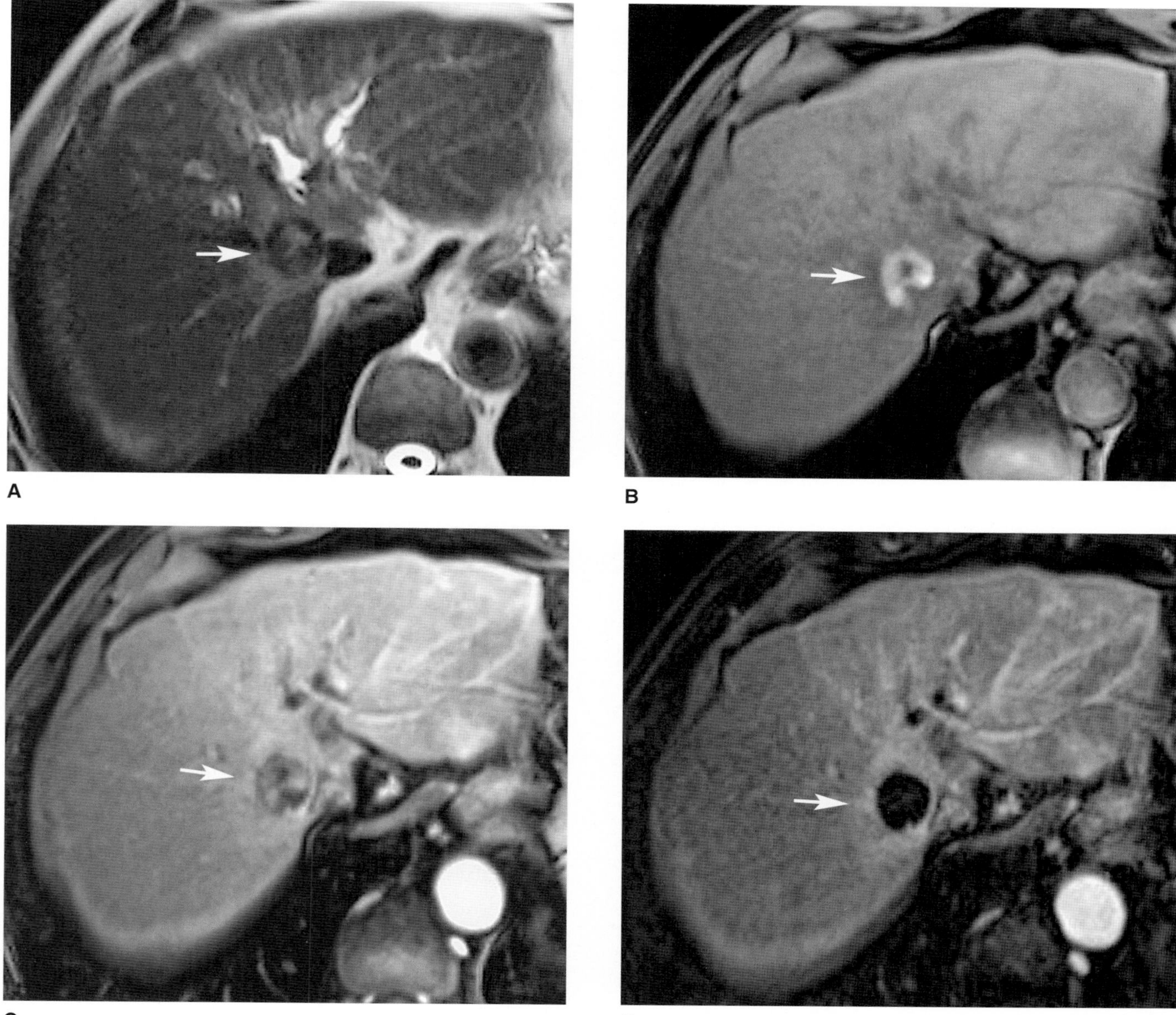

Figure 3-52 MRI Evaluation of HCC Following Chemoembolization
This 79-year-old male with HCC received chemoembolization 1 month earlier. T2-weighted image (**A**) demonstrates low signal intensity of the treated mass (*arrow*) and T1-weighted images (**B**) demonstrate high signal intensity of the treated mass (*arrow*), features characteristic of coagulative necrosis. Postgadolinium T1 image (**C**) demonstrates high signal areas only in the same distribution as in (B), suggesting absence of tumor enhancement. Subtraction image (**D**) of the precontrast from postcontrast image confirms absence of enhancement.

acetic acid or ethanol ablation.[523-525] Despite differences in the techniques, the postablation appearance of the treated liver and surrounding tissue is similar. The ablated area will appear hypoattenuating on CT scans and will show absence of enhancement following IV contrast administration. MRI examinations will show the characteristic signal intensity of coagulative necrosis on precontrast MRI, bright T1 signal, and heterogeneous dark T2 signal and will show nonenhancement following IV contrast administration. As with embolic therapies, a posttreatment rim of reactive tissue enhancement is not uncommon. Areas with persistent tumor viability after treatment will typically show a nodular pattern of contrast enhancement. In general, the area of ablation will be larger than the original tumor, so reporting of postablation therapies should differentiate between size of residual viable tumor, if any, and

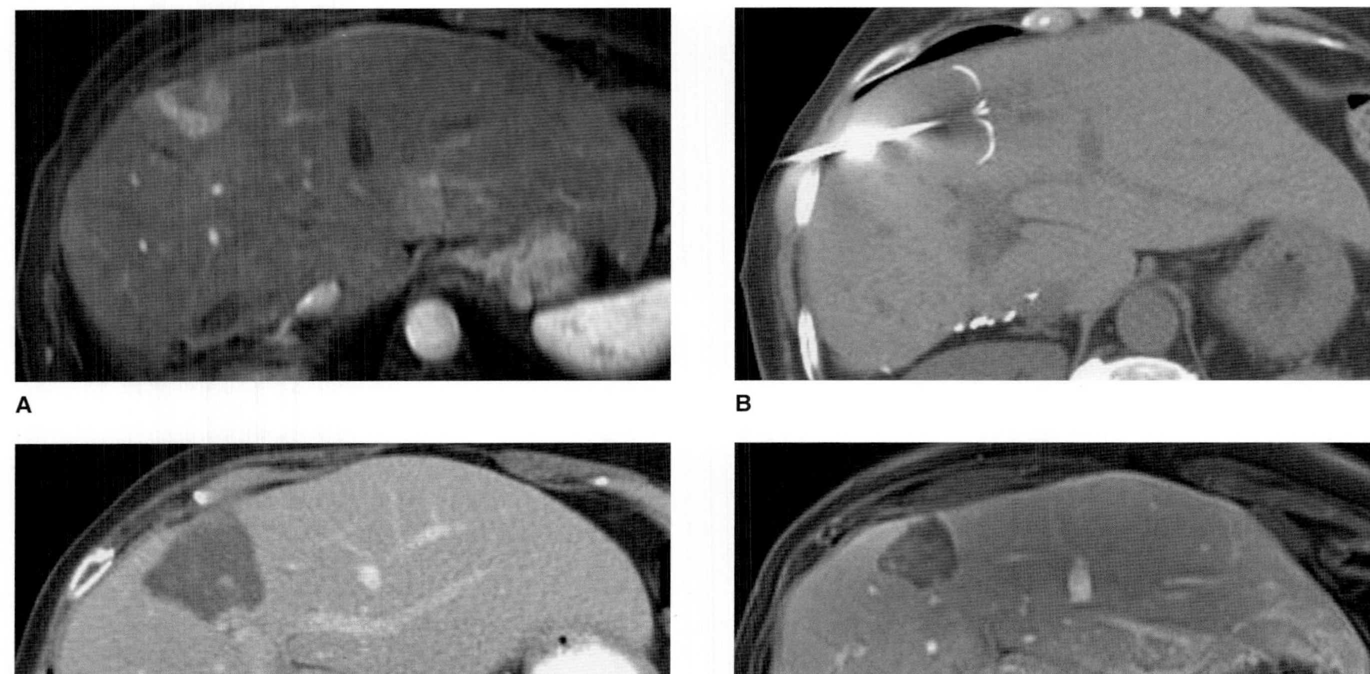

Figure 3-53 Treatment Zone Effect of RFA
This 68-year-old woman had a posterior hepatic segmentectomy for metastatic colon cancer and developed recurrent disease in the residual left lobe. **A.** MRI demonstrates new enhancing lesion. Biopsy indicated metastatic colon cancer. **B.** Image from CT-guided radiofrequency ablation (RFA) procedure. **C.** Follow-up CT demonstrates enlargement of lesion, but with increase hypodensity. **D.** Follow-up MRI 1 year later demonstrates decrease in size of lesion with absent enhancement. The apparent size of the lesion often increases following RFA. Theamount of residual enhancing tissue is a better measure of residual disease.

the area of treatment effect, especially in cases where accurate reporting of tumor size is critical for staging purposes (see Figure 3-53).[526]

Liver-specific complications of ablative therapies can include large areas of liver infarction, superinfection, biloma/biliary stricture, and venous thrombosis. Extrahepatic complications can include gall bladder or diaphragm injury and hematoma.[527,528] In cases of hematoma transgressing the liver capsule and causing hemoperitoneum, follow-up imaging should be performed to identify potential tumor seeding.

Surgical Treatment of the Liver

Surgery is often indicated for treatment of infectious[529] and neoplastic conditions of the liver.[530-532] The choice of surgical versus nonsurgical management will depend on a variety of factors, including accurate presurgical diagnosis of liver lesion(s), the presence of nonsurgical management options, comorbid conditions, and the presence and nature of extrahepatic disease. Surgical options for focal liver lesions include subsegmental (wedge) resections, lobectomies, and liver transplantation. The radiologist should be familiar with the common appearance of the postoperative liver.

Wedge resection

When a small peripheral or exophytic tumor is present, surgical excision via a wedge resection is possible.[533-535] In such cases, the nature of the surgical defect will depend on the location and size of the lesion that was excised (see Figure 3-54). Defects from wedge resection usually appear triangular on cross-sectional imaging. In the early postoperative period, fluid collections about the resection cavity are common. With time, this fluid will resorb and a variable amount of scarring will take place. Postoperative resection scars are hypointense on nonenhanced CT imaging. With contrast, the appearance is more variable. Some scars will remain hypointense to neighboring liver, whereas others will demonstrate hyperenhancement

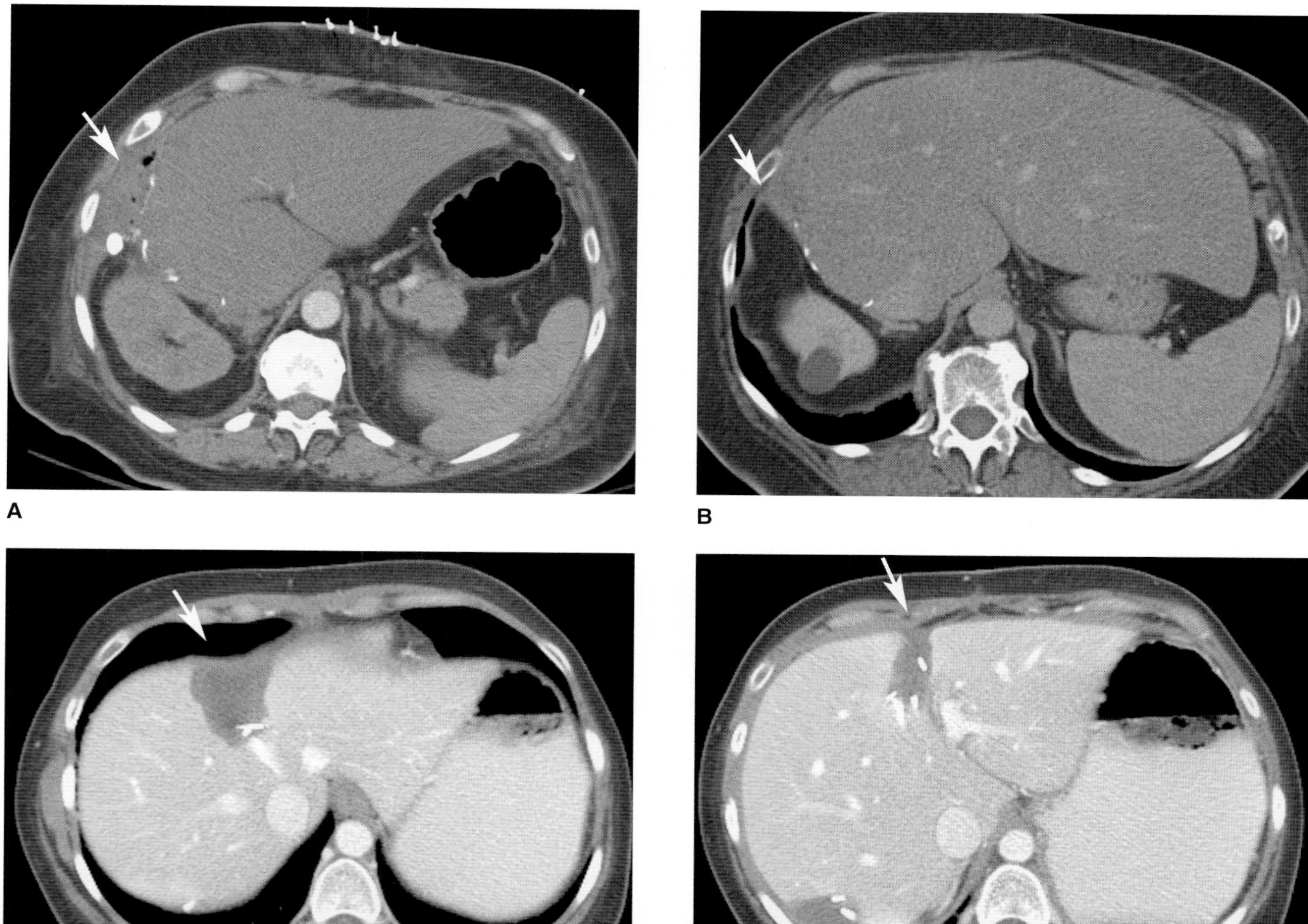

Figure 3-54 Imaging Features of Hepatic Lobectomy and Wedge Resection in 2 Patients
A and **B.** This 60-year-old woman had colon cancer with 2 metastasis to the right hepatic lobe. Contrast-enhanced CT (A) shows absence of the right hepatic lobe with a small collection of air and fluid (*arrow*) in the surgical bed. There are multiple small high attenuation surgical clips at the margin of the lobectomy and high attenuation cutaneous staples in the anterior abdominal wall. These are the typical features of a right hepatic lobectomy. Contrast-enhanced CT (B) obtained 2 years later demonstrates considerable compensatory hypertrophy of the remaining left lobe. There is a small residual scar (*arrow*) at the margin of the lobectomy. **C** and **D.** This 34-year-old woman had ovarian cancer. There are small peripheral fluid collections, associated with metallic surgical clips in the surface of the liver in the medial and posterior segments. This is a typical postsurgical appearance of hepatic wedge resections.

due to scarring. On MRI, scars and fluid are low signal intensity on T1-weighted imaging. Postoperative seromas have typical bright T2 signal of fluid unless complicated by hemorrhage. Scars are more variable on T2-weighted imaging. Immature scarring may be relatively T2 hyperintense, with mature scars darker on T2 imaging. With gadolinium administration, the scar will generally demonstrate modest enhancement, which can increase over time on multiphase imaging, a finding that is atypical for most tumors.

Hepatic segmentectomy and lobectomy

When larger or more centrally located tumors are removed surgically, a segmental or lobar resection is required. The types of segmental/lobal resection available to the liver surgeon is determined by the vascular and biliary anatomy of the liver. Resections of the left lateral segment are straightforward based on the natural cleavage plane of the falciform ligament and ligamentum teres, which separates this lobe from the remainder of the liver.[536] Resection of the posterior segment right lobe, though more complex, is also feasible, using the branch point of the posterior segment of the right portal vein to define the cleavage plane.[537]

When tumors are located more centrally, lobar resections are generally required. Both right and left lobar resections can be performed, as required by the anatomy of the tumor or tumors. Right lobar resections are not uncommon following partial responses to chemotherapeutic treatment of metastatic disease from colon cancer, because right lobe lesions often predominate when only a small number of lesions are present.[538] Left lobar resections are performed when left medial segment tumors are present.[539] On occasion, the larger trisegmental resection can be performed for more advanced primary liver tumors, such as removal of the right lobe and medial segment of the left lobe.[540] Such procedures can only be performed in patients with good hepatic reserve and large enough left lateral segments to allow for adequate hepatic function postoperatively. Surgical removal of the caudate lobe is not in general considered technically feasible, and nonsurgical therapies for tumors in this region are usually required.

When segmental or lobar resection of the liver is contemplated, the radiologist needs to provide accurate staging information to the surgeon. For metastatic disease, accurate reporting of the number and location of tumors is important, especially if bilobar disease is present. Attention to prior imaging to document location of all lesions can be important when response to chemotherapy renders previously present lesions more subtle.[541] Intraoperative US is often used during hepatic resection for metastatic disease, because intraoperative US is the most sensitive modality for the detection of small hepatic lesions, which can be treated focally at the time of segmental resection.[542]

Identification of the extent of the tumor, and the relationship of tumor margins to the critical vascular and biliary structures at the root of the liver are critical pieces of information. Tumor margin depiction in cholangiocarcinoma and infiltrative HCC can be subtle on cross-sectional imaging, and oblique reconstructed images may be required to show the anatomic relationships optimally. Attention to subtle finding of vascular encasement in the portal vein or biliary obstruction is required, as these findings may better indicate the actual extent of tumor, allowing the liver surgeon the opportunity to judge the feasibility of resection.[543] Further, MRCP images can be helpful in achieving this goal, and when there is doubt, ERCP imaging can be used as a supplement to cross-sectional imaging.

Postoperative imaging of the patient following liver resection is important for assessing local resection success and to exclude local hepatic or marginal extrahepatic tumor recurrence. The appearance of the surgical margin following segmental or lobar liver resection is similar to that of smaller wedge resection, with fluid accumulation and/or scar formation common (see Figure 3-54). Long-term follow-up may be required to exclude local tumor recurrence. In addition, FDG-PET imaging can be useful, especially in the setting of surgery for metastatic disease. However, inflammatory changes in the early postoperative period can lead to abnormal FDG-avidity despite the absence of residual tumor.[544] Cross-sectional imaging can also demonstrate false-positive findings for tumor recurrence because of focal hypodense areas and perfusional changes at the resection margin.[545]

Postoperative complications following segmental or lobar resection include bilomas, hematomas, and abscess formation. Following larger resections, it is not uncommon for the residual liver to enlarge as the regenerative capacity of the liver takes place to restore more adequate hepatic reserve. This enlargement can lead to a liver volume that approximates the normal liver, and the radiologist may not recognize that surgery has taken place (see Figure 3-54). Correlation with earlier studies and clinical history is helpful to avoid this error, and attention to the hepatic vascular anatomy can aid the radiologist in the absence of accurate clinical history to avoid this pitfall.

Evaluation of the potential partial liver donor

The imaging evaluation of the living donor for liver transplantation deserves special mention. Currently, living donor liver transplantation (LDLT) is an alternative to cadaveric (orthotopic) liver donation.[546] Because of the special consideration of the health of the living donor, guidelines exist to qualify such donors, and imaging plays a central role in this qualification process. For pediatric recipients, the left lateral segment of the adult donor is removed. As this is a less invasive surgery with fewer complications, imaging criteria for donor acceptability are less stringent. For adult recipients, the right lobe of the adult donor liver is used, sparing the left and caudate lobes.

Preoperative cross-sectional imaging is required for potential donors for volumetric assessment of the liver, to determine that such surgery does not compromise the hepatic reserve of the donor.[547] Surgical guidelines indicate that the donor must be able to retain adequate liver volume to be eligible for donation. Specialized software can be used to determine relative lobar volumes.[548] Alternatively, manual planar areas can be drawn and summed to estimate volumes.[549]

In general, ERCP, MRCP, or CT cholangiography is required to depict the biliary tree and exclude biliary variants that could preclude living donation.[550] The most common significant biliary variant is the origin of the right posterior biliary segment from the left bile duct. In this situation, a right lobe resection would render the posterior segment without a viable biliary anastomosis for drainage, and result in bile leakage.[551] Vascular variants such as aberrant right hepatic artery and accessory right hepatic veins are also common and should be noted in the radiologic report. Subjects with more severe degrees of fatty liver infiltration are also ineligible for donation, and many centers use imaging with noncontrast CT or MRI as a surrogate for liver biopsy to exclude more severe fatty liver disease.[552]

Postoperative assessment of the living donor is often used to document the status of the remaining liver, exclude biliary or vascular complications, and to document adequate regeneration of the residual liver.[553-555]

Liver Transplantation

Liver transplantation is performed for end-stage liver disease or localized HCC. Although cadaveric livers are the most common source for transplantation, the use of living donors is increasing.

Normal transplant appearance

The presence of a liver transplant can often be identified by the unique side-to-end anastomosis at the IVC, which can lead to a double IVC appearance on cross-sectional imaging (see Figure 3-55).[556] In the absence of this appearance, it can be difficult to identify the presence of a cadaveric transplanted liver on imaging, although metallic artifact in the IVC at the site of the venous anastomosis on CT or long echo time gradient echo MRI may aid the radiologist in recognizing the presence of a liver transplant. When a right lobe of the liver is used from a living donor, the appearance may mimic that of a prior left hepatectomy.

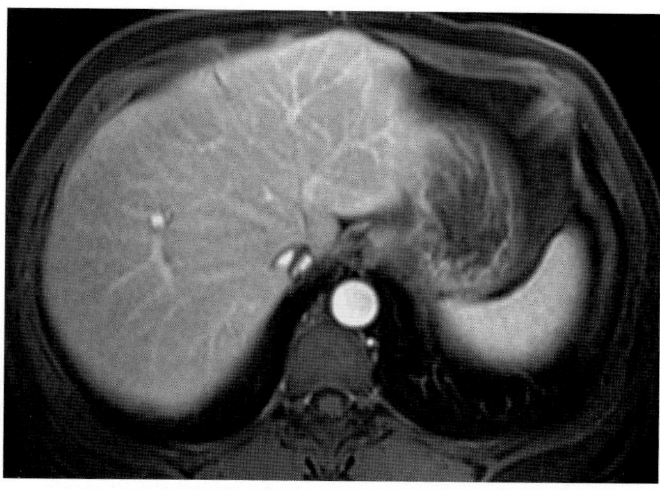

Figure 3-55 Pseudo-duplication of the IVC Following Liver Transplantation
This 44-year-old man underwent liver transplantation for HCC 18 months earlier and was getting routine surveillance imaging. Postgadolinium T1-weighted MRI demonstrates what appears to be a double IVC but represents the IVC anastomotic region with adjacent positioning of the donor intrahepatic IVC and the recipient native IVC.

Complications of liver transplantation

Within the transplanted liver, there are 4 distinct anastomoses to evaluate: the hepatic artery, the portal vein, the IVC, and the hepatic duct. Of these, the hepatic artery and the bile duct are the most common source of complications. Stenosis or occlusion at the portal vein anastomosis is rare. The findings of previous portal hypertension, including splenomegaly and venous varices, resolve slowly, if at all, after transplantation and should not be assumed to indicate the presence of portal vein anastomotic stricture.[557] The IVC anastomosis site can become stenotic and in rare cases will require intervention with angioplasty or stenting.[558,559] Severe IVC anastomotic stenosis can lead to hepatic outflow obstruction, and cause the "nutmeg liver" pattern of hepatic enhancement typical of Budd-Chiari syndrome and previously discussed under the heading: **Hepatic Disorders with a Specific Appearance** (Table 3-13).

Hepatic artery thrombosis and stenosis: Thrombosis or stenosis of the hepatic artery is the most common and most significant of the complications that arises after liver transplantation.[560] Because the biliary duct system is primarily supplied by the hepatic artery, hepatic arterial compromise can lead to bile duct ischemia or necrosis, leading to intrahepatic bilomas or abscesses.[561] The hepatic artery is most easily monitored for complications of liver transplant by US. Doppler ultrasound can document patency of the hepatic arteries and document flow velocities.[556] Sonographic findings of hepatic arterial stenosis include turbulent flow at the anastomotic site, focal accelerated velocity of greater than 2 to 3 m/s, and a tardus-parvus waveform in the distal branches of the hepatic artery (see Figure 3-56).[562] By these criteria, posttransplant Doppler US is highly accurate in identifying hepatic artery stenosis.[563] CT and MR arteriography can also be used in the assessment of hepatic arterial patency.[564]

Hepatic artery pseudoaneurysm: Pseudoaneurysms of the hepatic artery will typically occur at the anastomotic site and can lead to life-threatening hemorrhage. Ultrasonographic findings include a focal bilobed

Table 3-13. Complications of Liver Transplantation

1. Vascular complications: a. Hepatic artery and portal venous thrombosis b. Hepatic artery stenosis c. Hepatic artery pseudoaneurysm d. IVC stenosis
2. Biliary complications a. Biliary strictures b. Bile leaks
3. Posttransplant lymphoproliferative disorder (PTLD)

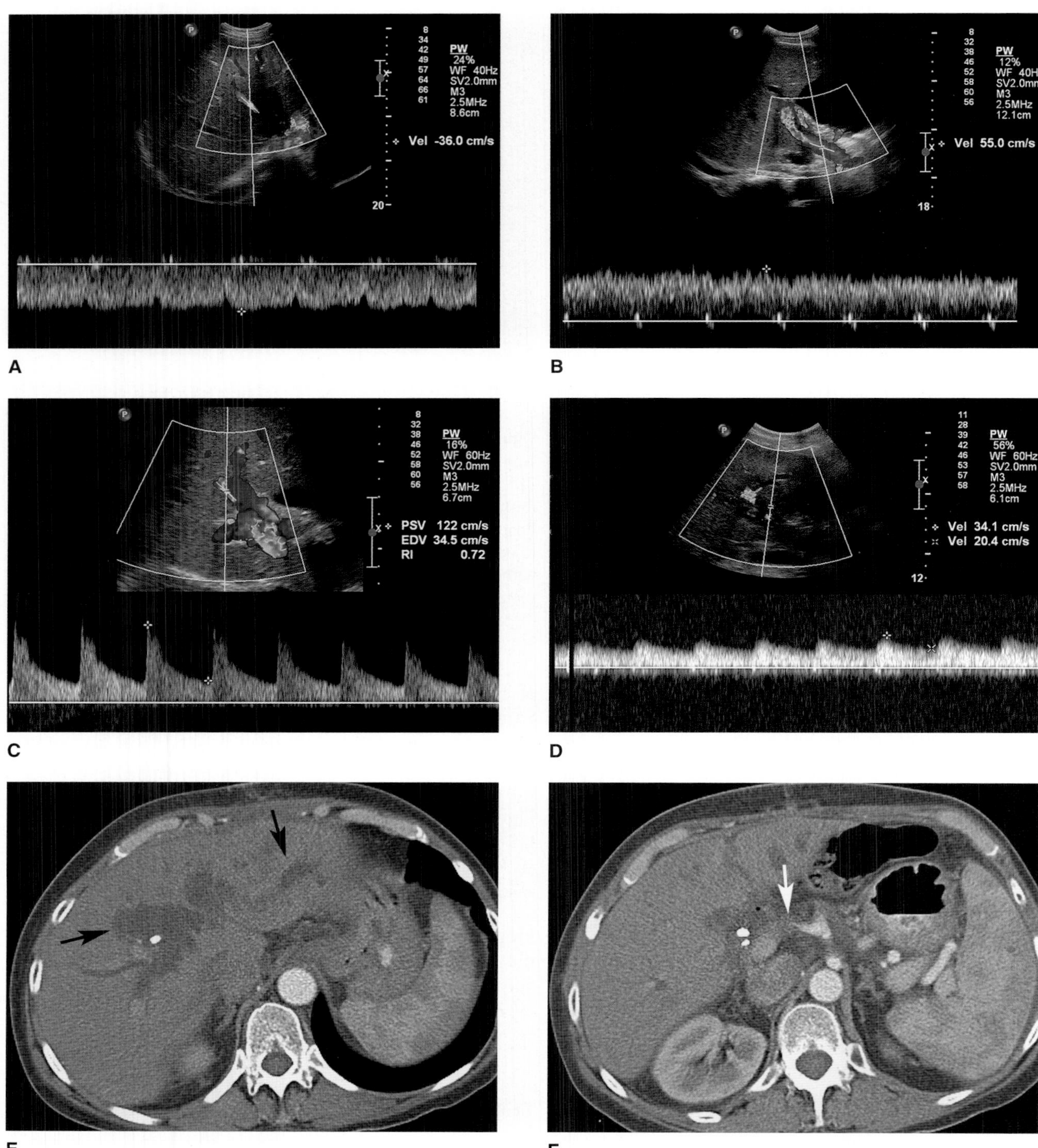

Figure 3-56 Doppler US Evaluation of Liver Transplantation
A-C. Normal Doppler US of the liver transplant. Doppler examination of the middle hepatic vein (A) shows an undulating Doppler signal typical of the respiratory variation of blood flow in the hepatic veins. Doppler examination of the main portal vein (B) shows a uniform unidirectional flow typical of portal venous blood flow. Doppler of the right hepatic artery (C) shows the characteristic sharp systolic upstroke and smooth rapid deceleration typical of normal arterial blood flow. **D-F.** This 49-year-old man had received a liver transplant a few weeks previously, when he developed increasing liver function tests. Doppler examination of the main hepatic artery (D) shows a pulsus tardus waveform with slow acceleration to the peak systolic flow and a diminished peak flow. This finding usually indicates upstream stenosis. Contrast-enhanced CT (E and F) shows multiple dilated intrahepatic bile ducts (*black arrows*) indicating the presence of a proximal biliary stricture. There is also abrupt narrowing of the proximal hepatic artery (*white arrow*) indicating hepatic arterial stenosis. Biliary stricture is a common complication of hepatic arterial stenosis/occlusion in patients following liver transplantation.

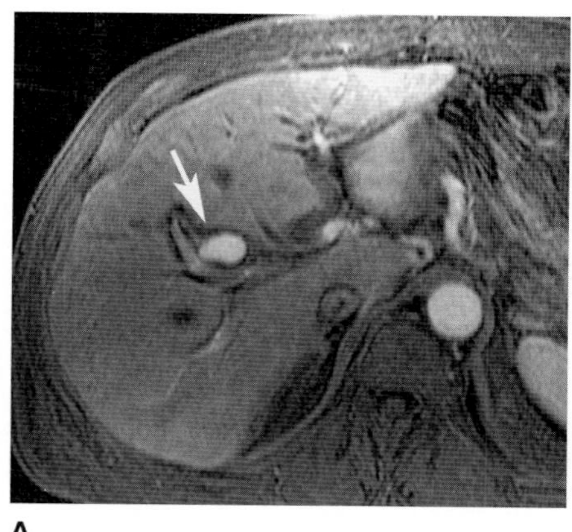
A

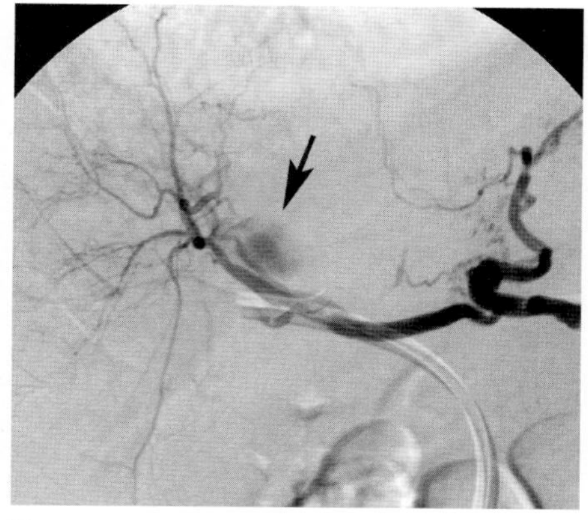
B

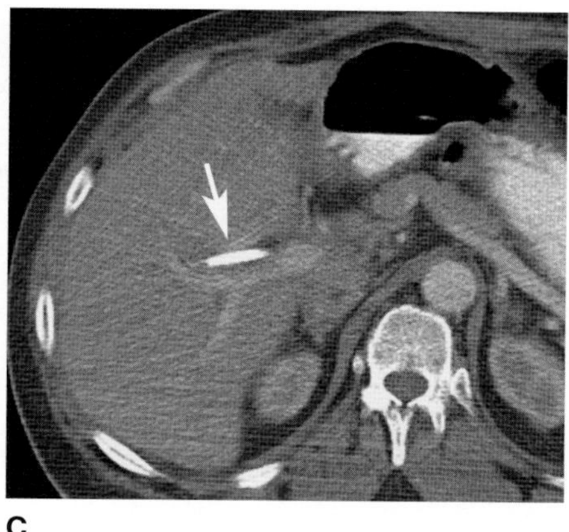
C

Figure 3-57 Hepatic Artery Pseudoaneurysm
This 61-year-old man had received a liver transplant and required prolonged placement of a biliary stent. **A.** T1-weighted post gadolinium image shows a small high attenuation nodule adjacent to the right portal vein likely representing a small pseudoaneurysm. **B.** Celiac artery angiogram confirms faint filling of a small pseudoaneurysm. **C.** Contrast-enhanced CT 2 months prior shows the presence of a biliary stent in the exact location of the pseudoaneurysm, which likely caused development of the aneurysm.

outpouching with turbulent or bidirectional flow.[565] CT and MRI will show a similar appearance of an enhancing bilobed focal outpouching.[566] Treatment with covered stents or coil embolization can be undertaken when the aneurysm is large (see Figure 3-57).[499,567]

Biliary complications: Biliary strictures are not uncommon in liver transplantation and can occur as a result of postoperative scar formation at the anastomotic site, or more centrally involving an intrahepatic bile duct as a result of biliary ischemia.[561,568] Because of anatomic differences between the donor and recipient bile ducts, caliber change in the bile duct at the anastomotic site does not in itself constitute a bile duct stricture (see Figure 3-58).[569,570] The presence or absence of intrahepatic biliary duct distension should be noted, as should change in appearance from earlier postoperative studies when available. Correlation with ERCP findings may be useful. Intrahepatic bile duct strictures or beading is a more ominous finding, suggesting ischemia due to arterial compromise, and should lead to an evaluation of the hepatic artery.

Posttransplant lymphoproliferative disorder: Posttransplant lymphoproliferative disorder (PTLD) is seen in liver transplant patients with previous exposure to Epstein-Barr virus and those who were given cyclosporine for immunosuppression.[571] The incidence of PTLD has decreased with the use of noncyclosporine immunosuppressive regimens. PTLD generally manifests in the first 2 years after transplantation and represents either a reactive or malignant lymphoproliferation resulting from a combination of T-cell immunosuppression and reactivation of dormant Epstein-Barr virus. The imaging appearance of PTLD resembles the imaging manifestations of lymphoma, and in its most severe form represents an immunosuppression-induced B-cell lymphoma. The lymphoproliferation of PTLD can occur anywhere within the body[572] and can manifest as lymphadenopathy and/or solitary or multiple masses within 1 or several organs of the body. PTLD has a predilection for the transplant organ and therefore in liver transplant recipients will commonly involve the transplanted liver, presenting as 1 or more liver masses similar to hepatic lymphoma of other causes. PTLD after liver transplant may present as lymphadenopathy or an

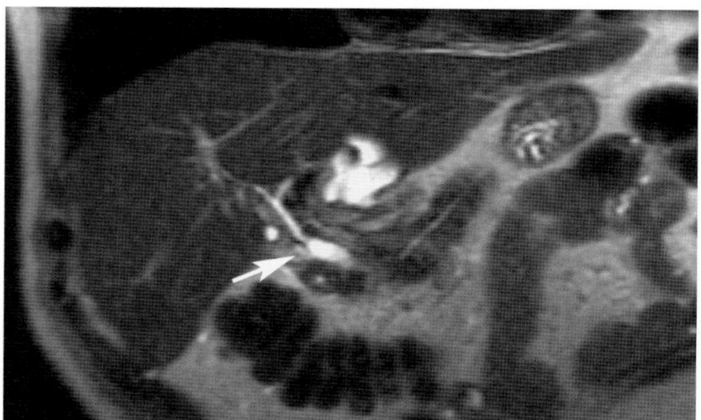

Figure 3-58 Mismatch in Bile Duct Caliber after Liver Transplantation
This 58-year-old man had undergone liver transplantation 3 years earlier. Coronal localizer T2 (HASTE) imaging demonstrates abrupt caliber change (*arrow*), with small donor common hepatic duct increasing in size abruptly at the level of the native common bile duct. Patient remained well without symptoms or laboratory findings to suggest bile duct stricture.

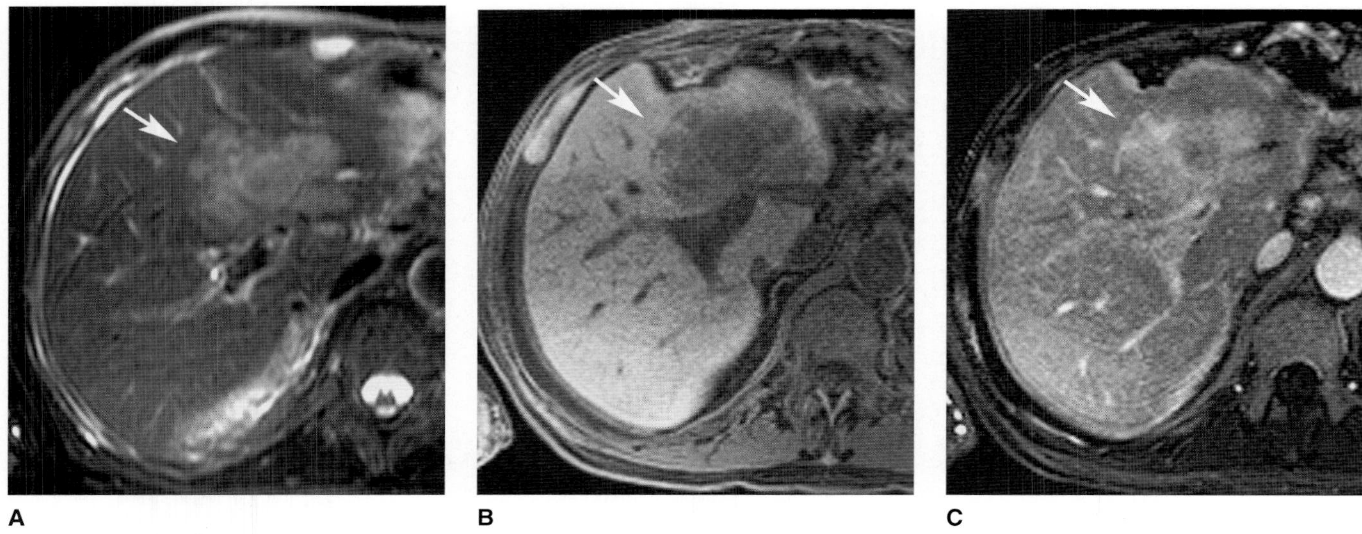

Figure 3-59 Post Transplant Lymphoproliferative Disease This 69-year-old man had received an orthotopic liver transplant a year earlier and presented with jaundice. **A.** T2-weighted, (**B**) T1-weighted, fat saturation and (**C**) T1-weighted, fat saturation, post gadolinium sequences show a focal lobulated mass near the porta hepatis. Biopsy was diagnostic of PTLD.

infiltrative mass within the porta hepatis region that does not obstruct the adjacent vascular and biliary structures (see Figure 3-59).[573,574] In cases where liver transplant was performed for HCC, differentiation from recurrent HCC may require biopsy.

REFERENCES

1. Bolondi L, Correas JM, Lencioni R, Weskott HP, Piscaglia F. New perspectives for the use of contrast-enhanced liver ultrasound in clinical practice. *Dig Liver Dis.* 2007;39(2): 187-195. Epub 2007/01/09.
2. Piscaglia F, Lencioni R, Sagrini E, Pina CD, Cioni D, Vidili G, et al. Characterization of focal liver lesions with contrast-enhanced ultrasound. *Ultrasound Med Biol.* 2010;36(4): 531-550. Epub 2010/03/31.
3. Zhou X, Liu JB, Luo Y, Yan F, Peng Y, Lin L, et al. Characterization of focal liver lesions by means of assessment of hepatic transit time with contrast-enhanced US. *Radiology.* 2010;256(2):648-655. Epub 2010/07/27.
4. Burns PN, Wilson SR. Focal liver masses: enhancement patterns on contrast-enhanced images—concordance of US scans with CT scans and MR images. Radiology. 2007;242(1):162-174. Epub 2006/11/09.
5. Oliver JH 3rd, Baron RL, Federle MP, Rockette HE Jr. Detecting hepatocellular carcinoma: value of unenhanced or arterial phase CT imaging or both used in conjunction with conventional portal venous phase contrast-enhanced CT imaging. *AJR Am J Roentgenol.* 1996;167(1):71-77. Epub 1996/07/01.
6. Oliver JH 3rd, Baron RL, Federle MP, Jones BC, Sheng R. Hypervascular liver metastases: do unenhanced and hepatic arterial phase CT images affect tumor detection? *Radiology.* 1997;205(3):709-715. Epub 1997/12/11.
7. Flournoy JG, Potter JL, Sullivan BM, Gerza CB, Ramzy I. CT appearance of multifocal hepatic steatosis. *J Comput Assist Tomogr.* 1984;8(6):1192-1194. Epub 1984/12/01.
8. Nomura F, Ohnishi K, Ochiai T, Okuda K. Obesity-related nonalcoholic fatty liver: CT features and follow-up studies after low-calorie diet. *Radiology.* 1987;162(3):845-847. Epub 1987/03/01.
9. Kim HC, Kim AY, Han JK, Chung JW, Lee JY, Park JH, et al. Hepatic arterial and portal venous phase helical CT in patients treated with transcatheter arterial chemoembolization for hepatocellular carcinoma: added value of unenhanced images. *Radiology.* 2002;225(3):773-780. Epub 2002/12/04.
10. Kim YI, Chung JW, Park JH, Kang GH, Lee M, Suh KS, et al. Multiphase contrast-enhanced CT imaging in hepatocellular carcinoma correlation with immunohistochemical angiogenic activities. *Acad Radiol.* 2007;14(9):1084-1091. Epub 2007/08/21.
11. Asayama Y, Yoshimitsu K, Irie H, Tajima T, Nishie A, Hirakawa M, et al. Delayed-phase dynamic CT enhancement as a prognostic factor for mass-forming intrahepatic cholangiocarcinoma. *Radiology.* 2006;238(1):150-155. Epub 2005/11/24.
12. Fukukura Y, Hamanoue M, Fujiyoshi F, Sasaki M, Haruta K, Inoue H, et al. Cholangiolocellular carcinoma of the liver: CT and MR findings. *J Comput Assist Tomogr.* 2000;24(5):809-812. Epub 2000/10/25.
13. Fishbein MH, Stevens WR. Rapid MRI using a modified Dixon technique: a non-invasive and effective method for detection and monitoring of fatty metamorphosis of the liver. *Pediatr Radiol.* 2001;31(11):806-809. Epub 2001/11/03.
14. Kim H, Taksali SE, Dufour S, Befroy D, Goodman TR, Petersen KF, et al. Comparative MR study of hepatic fat quantification using single-voxel proton spectroscopy, two-point dixon and three-point IDEAL. *Magn Reson Med.* 2008;59(3):521-527. Epub 2008/02/29.
15. Kovanlikaya A, Guclu C, Desai C, Becerra R, Gilsanz V. Fat quantification using three-point dixon technique: in vitro validation. *Acad Radiol.* 2005;12(5):636-639. Epub 2005/05/04.

16. Perez-Rodriguez J, Lai S, Ehst BD, Fine DM, Bluemke DA. Nephrogenic systemic fibrosis: incidence, associations, and effect of risk factor assessment—report of 33 cases. *Radiology.* 2009;250(2):371-377. Epub 2009/02/04.
17. Cruite I, Schroeder M, Merkle EM, Sirlin CB. Gadoxetate disodium-enhanced MRI of the liver: part 2, protocol optimization and lesion appearance in the cirrhotic liver. *AJR Am J Roentgenol.* 2010;195(1):29-41. Epub 2010/06/23.
18. Ringe KI, Husarik DB, Sirlin CB, Merkle EM. Gadoxetate disodium-enhanced MRI of the liver: part 1, protocol optimization and lesion appearance in the noncirrhotic liver. *AJR Am J Roentgenol.* 2010;195(1):13-28. Epub 2010/06/23.
19. Lwakatare F, Yamashita Y, Nakayama M, Takahashi M. SPIO-enhanced MR imaging of focal fatty liver lesions. *Abdom Imaging.* 2001;26(2):157-160. Epub 2001/02/15.
20. Namkung S, Zech CJ, Helmberger T, Reiser MF, Schoenberg SO. Superparamagnetic iron oxide (SPIO)-enhanced liver MRI with ferucarbotran: efficacy for characterization of focal liver lesions. *J Magn Reson Imaging.* 2007;25(4):755-765. Epub 2007/03/06.
21. Saito K, Shindo H, Ozuki T, Ishikawa A, Kotake F, Shimazaki Y, et al. Detection of hepatocellular carcinoma with ferucarbotran (resovist)-enhanced breath-hold MR imaging: feasibility of 10 minute-delayed images. *Magn Reson Med Sci.* 2008;7(3):123-130. Epub 2008/10/02.
22. Ferrucci JT, Stark DD. Iron oxide-enhanced MR imaging of the liver and spleen: review of the first 5 years. *AJR Am J Roentgenol.* 1990;155(5):943-950. Epub 1990/11/01.
23. Chen F, Ward J, Robinson PJ. MR imaging of the liver and spleen: a comparison of the effects on signal intensity of two superparamagnetic iron oxide agents. *Magn Reson Imaging.* 1999;17(4):549-556. Epub 1999/05/07.
24. Koh DM, Padhani AR. Diffusion-weighted MRI: a new functional clinical technique for tumour imaging. Br J Radiol. 2006;79(944):633-635. Epub 2006/06/24.
25. Parikh T, Drew SJ, Lee VS, Wong S, Hecht EM, Babb JS, et al. Focal liver lesion detection and characterization with diffusion-weighted MR imaging: comparison with standard breath-hold T2-weighted imaging. *Radiology.* 2008;246(3):812-822. Epub 2008/01/29.
26. Taouli B, Koh DM. Diffusion-weighted MR imaging of the liver. *Radiology.* 2010;254(1):47-66. Epub 2009/12/25.
27. Edmondson HA, Peters RL. Tumors of the liver: pathologic features. *Semin Roentgenol.* 1983;18(2):75-83. Epub 1983/04/01.
28. Takagi H. Diagnosis and management of cavernous hemangioma of the liver. *Semin Surg Oncol.* 1985;1(1):12-22. Epub 1985/01/01.
29. Belli L, De Carlis L, Beati C, Rondinara G, Sansalone V, Brambilla G. Surgical treatment of symptomatic giant hemangiomas of the liver. *Surg Gynecol Obstet.* 1992;174(6): 474-478. Epub 1992/06/01.
30. Bruce S, Downe L, Devonald K, Ellwood D. Noninvasive investigation of infantile hepatic hemangioma: a case study. *Pediatrics.* 1995;95(4):595-597. Epub 1995/04/01.
31. Bruneton JN, Drouillard J, Fenart D, Roux P, Nicolau A. Ultrasonography of hepatic cavernous haemangiomas. *Br J Radiol.* 1983;56(671):791-795. Epub 1983/11/01.
32. Klein MA, Slovis TL, Chang CH, Jacobs IG. Sonographic and Doppler features of infantile hepatic hemangiomas with pathologic correlation. *J Ultrasound Med.* 1990;9(11):619-624. Epub 1990/11/01.
33. Ignee A, Weiper D, Schuessler G, Teuber G, Faust D, Dietrich CF. Sonographic characterisation of hepatocellular carcinoma at time of diagnosis. *Z Gastroenterol.* 2005;43(3): 289-294. Epub 2005/03/15.
34. Freeny PC, Marks WM. Hepatic hemangioma: dynamic bolus CT. *AJR Am J Roentgenol.* 1986;147(4):711-719. Epub 1986/10/01.
35. Hanafusa K, Ohashi I, Himeno Y, Suzuki S, Shibuya H. Hepatic hemangioma: findings with two-phase CT. *Radiology.* 1995;196(2):465-469. Epub 1995/08/01.
36. Ito K, Honjo K, Matsumoto T, Tanaka R, Nakada T, Nakanishi T. Distinction of hemangiomas from hepatic tumors with delayed enhancement by incremental dynamic CT. *J Comput Assist Tomogr.* 1992;16(4):572-577. Epub 1992/07/01.
37. Drop A. Types and patterns of contrast enhancement of hepatic tumours (hepatoma, hemangioma and metastasis) with dynamic computed tomography. *Ann Univ Mariae Curie Sklodowska Med.* 2001;56:348-356. Epub 2002/04/30.
38. Jang HJ, Choi BI, Kim TK, Yun EJ, Kim KW, Han JK, et al. Atypical small hemangiomas of the liver: "bright dot" sign at two-phase spiral CT. *Radiology.* 1998;208(2):543-548. Epub 1998/07/29.
39. Semelka RC, Brown ED, Ascher SM, Patt RH, Bagley AS, Li W, et al. Hepatic hemangiomas: a multi-institutional study of appearance on T2-weighted and serial gadolinium-enhanced gradient-echo MR images. *Radiology.* 1994;192(2):401-406. Epub 1994/08/01.
40. Soyer P, Dufresne AC, Somveille E, Scherrer A. Hepatic cavernous hemangioma: appearance on T2-weighted fast spin-echo MR imaging with and without fat suppression. *AJR Am J Roentgenol.* 1997;168(2):461-465. Epub 1997/02/01.
41. Quillin SP, Atilla S, Brown JJ, Borrello JA, Yu CY, Pilgram TK. Characterization of focal hepatic masses by dynamic contrast-enhanced MR imaging: findings in 311 lesions. *Magn Reson Imaging.* 1997;15(3):275-285. Epub 1997/01/01.
42. Whitney WS, Herfkens RJ, Jeffrey RB, McDonnell CH, Li KC, Van Dalsem WJ, et al. Dynamic breath-hold multiplanar spoiled gradient-recalled MR imaging with gadolinium enhancement for differentiating hepatic hemangiomas from malignancies at 1.5 T. *Radiology.* 1993;189(3):863-870. Epub 1993/12/01.
43. Caseiro-Alves F, Brito J, Araujo AE, Belo-Soares P, Rodrigues H, Cipriano A, et al. Liver haemangioma: common and uncommon findings and how to improve the differential diagnosis. *Eur Radiol.* 2007;17(6):1544-1554. Epub 2007/01/30.
44. Outwater EK, Ito K, Siegelman E, Martin CE, Bhatia M, Mitchell DG. Rapidly enhancing hepatic hemangiomas at MRI: distinction from malignancies with T2-weighted images. *J Magn Reson Imaging.* 1997;7(6):1033-1039. Epub 1997/12/24.
45. Yamashita Y, Ogata I, Urata J, Takahashi M. Cavernous hemangioma of the liver: pathologic correlation with dynamic CT findings. *Radiology.* 1997;203(1):121-125. Epub 1997/04/01.
46. Vilgrain V, Boulos L, Vullierme MP, Denys A, Terris B, Menu Y. Imaging of atypical hemangiomas of the liver with pathologic correlation. *Radiographics.* 2000;20(2):379-397. Epub 2000/03/15.
47. Brown RK, Gomes A, King W, Pusey E, Lois J, Goldstein L, et al. Hepatic hemangiomas: evaluation by magnetic resonance imaging and technetium-99m red blood cell scintigraphy. *J Nucl Med.* 1987;28(11):1683-1687. Epub 1987/11/01.

48. Hosokawa A, Maeda T, Tateishi U, Satake M, Iwata R, Ojima H, et al. Hepatic hemangioma presenting atypical radiologic findings: a case report. *Radiat Med.* 2005;23(5):371-375. Epub 2005/12/14.
49. Moinuddin M, Allison JR, Montgomery JH, Rockett JF, McMurray JM. Scintigraphic diagnosis of hepatic hemangioma: its role in the management of hepatic mass lesions. *AJR Am J Roentgenol.* 1985;145(2):223-228. Epub 1985/08/01.
50. Krause T, Hauenstein K, Studier-Fischer B, Schuemichen C, Moser E. Improved evaluation of technetium-99m-red blood cell SPECT in hemangioma of the liver. *J Nucl Med.* 1993;34(3):375-380. Epub 1993/03/01.
51. Ziessman HA, Silverman PM, Patterson J, Harkness B, Fahey FH, Zeman RK, et al. Improved detection of small cavernous hemangiomas of the liver with high-resolution three-headed SPECT. *J Nucl Med.* 1991;32(11):2086-2091. Epub 1991/11/11.
52. Principe A, Lugaresi ML, Lords RC, D'Errico A, Polito E, Gallo MC, et al. Bile duct hamartomas: diagnostic problems and treatment. *Hepatogastroenterology.* 1997;44(16):994-997. Epub 1997/07/01.
53. Okeda R. Mesenchymal hamartoma of the liver—an autopsy case with serial sections and some comments on its pathogenesis. *Acta Pathol Jpn.* 1976;26(2):229-236. Epub 1976/03/01.
54. Horton KM, Bluemke DA, Hruban RH, Soyer P, Fishman EK. CT and MR imaging of benign hepatic and biliary tumors. *Radiographics.* 1999;19(2):431-351. Epub 1999/04/09.
55. Lev-Toaff AS, Bach AM, Wechsler RJ, Hilpert PL, Gatalica Z, Rubin R. The radiologic and pathologic spectrum of biliary hamartomas. *AJR Am J Roentgenol.* 1995;165(2):309-313. Epub 1995/08/01.
56. Cheung YC, Tan CF, Wan YL, Lui KW, Tsai CC. MRI of multiple biliary hamartomas. *Br J Radiol.* 1997;70(833): 527-529. Epub 1997/05/01.
57. Semelka RC, Hussain SM, Marcos HB, Woosley JT. Biliary hamartomas: solitary and multiple lesions shown on current MR techniques including gadolinium enhancement. *J Magn Reson Imaging.* 1999;10(2):196-201. Epub 1999/08/10.
58. Vogt DP, Henderson JM, Chmielewski E. Cystadenoma and cystadenocarcinoma of the liver: a single center experience. *J Am Coll Surg.* 2005;200(5):727-733. Epub 2005/04/26.
59. Lee JH, Lee KG, Park HK, Lee KS. Biliary cystadenoma and cystadenocarcinoma of the liver: 10 cases of a single center experience. *Hepatogastroenterology.* 2009;56(91-92):844-849. Epub 2009/07/23.
60. Beuran M, Venter MD, Dumitru L. Large mucinous biliary cystadenoma with "ovarian-like" stroma: a case report. *World J Gastroenterol.* 2006;12(23):3779-3781. Epub 2006/06/15.
61. Korobkin M, Stephens DH, Lee JK, Stanley RJ, Fishman EK, Francis IR, et al. Biliary cystadenoma and cystadenocarcinoma: CT and sonographic findings. *AJR Am J Roentgenol.* 1989;153(3):507-511. Epub 1989/09/01.
62. Lewin M, Mourra N, Honigman I, Flejou JF, Parc R, Arrive L, et al. Assessment of MRI and MRCP in diagnosis of biliary cystadenoma and cystadenocarcinoma. *Eur Radiol.* 2006;16(2):407-413. Epub 2005/06/29.
63. Choi BI, Lim JH, Han MC, Lee DH, Kim SH, Kim YI, et al. Biliary cystadenoma and cystadenocarcinoma: CT and sonographic findings. *Radiology.* 1989;171(1):57-61. Epub 1989/04/01.
64. Mortele KJ, Ros PR. Cystic focal liver lesions in the adult: differential CT and MR imaging features. *Radiographics.* 2001;21(4):895-910. Epub 2001/07/14.
65. Yu FC, Chen JH, Yang KC, Wu CC, Chou YY. Hepatobiliary cystadenoma: a report of two cases. *J Gastrointestin Liver Dis.* 2008;17(2):203-206. Epub 2008/06/24.
66. Lyburn ID, Torreggiani WC, Harris AC, Zwirewich CV, Buckley AR, Davis JE, et al. Hepatic epithelioid hemangioendothelioma: sonographic, CT, and MR imaging appearances. *AJR Am J Roentgenol.* 2003;180(5):1359-1364. Epub 2003/04/22.
67. Bolke E, Gripp S, Peiper M, Budach W, Schwarz A, Orth K, et al. Multifocal epithelioid hemangioendothelioma: case report of a clinical chamaeleon. *Eur J Med Res.* 2006;11(11):462-466. Epub 2006/12/22.
68. Mermuys K, Vanhoenacker PK, Roskams T, D'Haenens P, Van Hoe L. Epithelioid hemangioendothelioma of the liver: radiologic-pathologic correlation. *Abdom Imaging.* 2004;29(2):221-223. Epub 2004/08/05.
69. Miller WJ, Dodd GD 3rd, Federle MP, Baron RL. Epithelioid hemangioendothelioma of the liver: imaging findings with pathologic correlation. *AJR Am J Roentgenol.* 1992;159(1):53-57. Epub 1992/07/01.
70. Van Beers B, Roche A, Mathieu D, Menu Y, Delos M, Otte JB, et al. Epithelioid hemangioendothelioma of the liver: MR and CT findings. *J Comput Assist Tomogr.* 1992;16(3):420-424. Epub 1992/05/01.
71. Bargellini I, Vignali C, Cioni R, Petruzzi P, Cicorelli A, Campani D, et al. Hepatocellular carcinoma: CT for tumor response after transarterial chemoembolization in patients exceeding Milan criteria—selection parameter for liver transplantation. *Radiology.* 2010;255(1):289-300. Epub 2010/03/24.
72. Economopoulos N, Kelekis NL, Argentos S, Tsompanlioti C, Patapis P, Nikolaou I, et al. Bright-dark ring sign in MR imaging of hepatic epithelioid hemangioendothelioma. *J Magn Reson Imaging.* 2008;27(4):908-912. Epub 2008/02/28.
73. Gupta R, Mathur SR, Gupta SD, Durgapal P, Iyer VK, Das CJ, et al. Hepatic epithelioid hemangioendothelioma: A diagnostic pitfall in aspiration cytology. *Cytojournal.* 2010;6:25. Epub 2010/02/19.
74. Manucha V, Sun CC. Cytologic findings and differential diagnosis in hepatic Epithelioid hemangioendothelioma: a case report. *Acta Cytol.* 2008;52(6):713-717. Epub 2008/12/17.
75. Lacout A, El Hajjam M, Julie C, Lacombe P, Pelage JP. Liver metastasis of a mucinous colonic carcinoma mimicking a haemangioma in T2-weighted sequences. *J Med Imaging Radiat Oncol.* 2008;52(6):580-582. Epub 2009/01/31.
76. Low RN, Barone RM, Gurney JM, Muller WD. Mucinous appendiceal neoplasms: preoperative MR staging and classification compared with surgical and histopathologic findings. *AJR Am J Roentgenol.* 2008;190(3):656-665. Epub 2008/02/22.
77. Chan JH, Tsui EY, Luk SH, Fung AS, Yuen MK, Szeto ML, et al. Diffusion-weighted MR imaging of the liver: distinguishing hepatic abscess from cystic or necrotic tumor. *Abdom Imaging.* 2001;26(2):161-165. Epub 2001/02/15.
78. Shen MC, Lee SS, Chen YS, Yen MY, Liu YC. Liver abscess caused by an infected ventriculoperitoneal shunt. *J Formos Med Assoc.* 2003;102(2):113-116. Epub 2003/04/24.

79. Kajiya T, Uemura T, Kajiya M, Kaname H, Hirano R, Uemura N, et al. Pyogenic liver abscess related to dental disease in an immunocompetent host. *Intern Med.* 2008;47(7):675-678. Epub 2008/04/02.
80. Perez MJ, Carrillo JL, Montin IM, Castellano AD. Liver abscess due to ileocecal perforation: a case report with literature review. *Emerg Radiol.* 2007;14(4):241-243. Epub 2007/03/27.
81. Flancbaum L, Nosher JL, Brolin RE. Percutaneous catheter drainage of abdominal abscesses associated with perforated viscus. *Am Surg.* 1990;56(1):52-56. Epub 1990/01/01.
82. Andersson R, Forsberg L, Hederstrom E, Hochbergs P, Bengmark S. Percutaneous management of pyogenic hepatic abscesses. *HPB Surg.* 1990;2(3):185-188. Epub 1990/07/01.
83. Mahieu X, Boverie J, Lemaire JM, Jacquet N. Pyogenic liver abscess. Diagnostic and therapeutic approach: a case report. *Acta Chir Belg.* 1993;93(5):220-223. Epub 1993/09/01.
84. Karaca C, Pinarbasi B, Danalioglu A, Akyuz F, Kaymakoglu S, Ozdil S, et al. Liver abscess as a rare complication of Crohn's disease: a case report. *Turk J Gastroenterol.* 2004;15(1):45-48. Epub 2004/07/21.
85. Pearce NW, Knight R, Irving H, Menon K, Prasad KR, Pollard SG, et al. Non-operative management of pyogenic liver abscess. *HPB (Oxford).* 2003;5(2):91-95. Epub 2008/03/12.
86. Zibari GB, Maguire S, Aultman DF, McMillan RW, McDonald JC. Pyogenic liver abscess. *Surg Infect (Larchmt).* 2000;1(1): 15-21. Epub 2003/02/22.
87. McDonald MI, Corey GR, Gallis HA, Durack DT. Single and multiple pyogenic liver abscesses. Natural history, diagnosis and treatment, with emphasis on percutaneous drainage. *Medicine (Baltimore).* 1984;63(5):291-302. Epub 1984/09/01.
88. Mathieu D, Vasile N, Fagniez PL, Segui S, Grably D, Larde D. Dynamic CT features of hepatic abscesses. *Radiology.* 1985;154(3):749-752. Epub 1985/03/01.
89. Jeffrey RB Jr, Tolentino CS, Chang FC, Federle MP. CT of small pyogenic hepatic abscesses: the cluster sign. *AJR Am J Roentgenol.* 1988;151(3):487-489. Epub 1988/09/01.
90. Shimada H, Ohta S, Maehara M, Katayama K, Note M, Nakagawara G. Diagnostic and therapeutic strategies of pyogenic liver abscess. *Int Surg.* 1993;78(1):40-45. Epub 1993/01/01.
91. Gyorffy EJ, Frey CF, Silva J Jr, McGahan J. Pyogenic liver abscess. Diagnostic and therapeutic strategies. *Ann Surg.* 1987;206(6):699-705. Epub 1987/12/01.
92. Hui JY, Yang MK, Cho DH, Li A, Loke TK, Chan JC, et al. Pyogenic liver abscesses caused by Klebsiella pneumoniae: US appearance and aspiration findings. *Radiology.* 2007;242(3):769-776. Epub 2007/02/28.
93. Lin AC, Yeh DY, Hsu YH, Wu CC, Chang H, Jang TN, et al. Diagnosis of pyogenic liver abscess by abdominal ultrasonography in the emergency department. *Emerg Med J.* 2009;26(4):273-275. Epub 2009/03/25.
94. Wang CL, Guo XJ, Qiu SB, Lei Y, Yuan ZD, Dong HB, et al. Diagnosis of bacterial hepatic abscess by CT. *Hepatobiliary Pancreat Dis Int.* 2007;6(3):271-275. Epub 2007/06/06.
95. Kim SB, Je BK, Lee KY, Lee SH, Chung HH, Cha SH. Computed tomographic differences of pyogenic liver abscesses caused by Klebsiella pneumoniae and non-Klebsiella pneumoniae. *J Comput Assist Tomogr.* 2007;31(1):59-65. Epub 2007/01/30.
96. Mortele KJ, Segatto E, Ros PR. The infected liver: radiologic-pathologic correlation. *Radiographics.* 2004;24(4):937-955. Epub 2004/07/17.
97. Syed MA, Kim TK, Jang HJ. Portal and hepatic vein thrombosis in liver abscess: CT findings. *Eur J Radiol.* 2007;61(3):513-519. Epub 2006/12/13.
98. Nakagawara M, Hanai H, Kajimura M. Images in clinical medicine. Detection of liver abscesses by T1-weighted magnetic resonance imaging. *N Engl J Med.* 2004;351(10):1013. Epub 2004/09/03.
99. Doyle DJ, Hanbidge AE, O'Malley ME. Imaging of hepatic infections. *Clin Radiol.* 2006;61(9):737-748. Epub 2006/08/15.
100. Balci NC, Sirvanci M. MR imaging of infective liver lesions. *Magn Reson Imaging Clin N Am.* 2002;10(1):121-135, vii. Epub 2002/05/10.
101. Mendez RJ, Schiebler ML, Outwater EK, Kressel HY. Hepatic abscesses: *MR imaging findings. Radiology.* 1994;190(2):431-436. Epub 1994/02/01.
102. K CS, Sharma D. Long-term follow-up of pyogenic liver abscess by ultrasound. *Eur J Radiol.* 2010;74(1):195-198. Epub 2009/02/17.
103. Kim YK, Kim CS, Lee JM, Ko SW, Moon WS, Yu HC. Solid organizing hepatic abscesses mimic hepatic tumor: Multiphasic computed tomography and magnetic resonance imaging findings with histopathologic correlation. *J Comput Assist Tomogr.* 2006;30(2):189-196. Epub 2006/04/22.
104. Hughes MA, Petri WA Jr. Amebic liver abscess. *Infect Dis Clin North Am.* 2000;14(3):565-582, viii. Epub 2000/09/15.
105. Pritt BS, Clark CG. Amebiasis. Mayo Clin Proc. 2008;83(10):1154-1159; quiz 9-60. Epub 2008/10/03.
106. Irusen EM, Jackson TF, Simjee AE. Asymptomatic intestinal colonization by pathogenic Entamoeba histolytica in amebic liver abscess: prevalence, response to therapy, and pathogenic potential. *Clin Infect Dis.* 1992;14(4):889-893. Epub 1992/04/01.
107. Greaney GC, Reynolds TB, Donovan AJ. Ruptured amebic liver abscess. *Arch Surg.* 1985;120(5):555-561. Epub 1985/05/01.
108. Hoffner RJ, Kilaghbian T, Esekogwu VI, Henderson SO. Common presentations of amebic liver abscess. *Ann Emerg Med.* 1999;34(3):351-355. Epub 1999/08/25.
109. vanSonnenberg E, Mueller PR, Schiffman HR, Ferrucci JT Jr, Casola G, Simeone JF, et al. Intrahepatic amebic abscesses: indications for and results of percutaneous catheter drainage. *Radiology.* 1985;156(3):631-635. Epub 1985/09/01.
110. Ahmed L, el Rooby A, Kassem MI, Salama ZA, Strickland GT. Ultrasonography in the diagnosis and management of 52 patients with amebic liver abscess in Cairo. *Rev Infect Dis.* 1990;12(2):330-337. Epub 1990/03/01.
111. Berry M, Bazaz R, Bhargava S. Amebic liver abscess: sonographic diagnosis and management. *J Clin Ultrasound.* 1986;14(4):239-242. Epub 1986/05/01.
112. Ahmed L, Salama ZA, el Rooby A, Strickland GT. Ultrasonographic resolution time for amebic liver abscess. *Am J Trop Med Hyg.* 1989;41(4):406-410. Epub 1989/10/01.
113. Radin DR, Ralls PW, Colletti PM, Halls JM. CT of amebic liver abscess. *AJR Am J Roentgenol.* 1988;150(6):1297-1301. Epub 1988/06/01.
114. Ralls PW, Henley DS, Colletti PM, Benson R, Raval JK, Radin DR, et al. Amebic liver abscess: MR imaging. *Radiology.* 1987;165(3):801-804. Epub 1987/12/01.

115. Elizondo G, Weissleder R, Stark DD, Todd LE, Compton C, Wittenberg J, et al. Amebic liver abscess: diagnosis and treatment evaluation with MR imaging. *Radiology.* 1987;165(3):795-800. Epub 1987/12/01.

116. Kratzer W, Reuter S, Hirschbuehl K, Ehrhardt AR, Mason RA, Haenle MM, et al. Comparison of contrast-enhanced power Doppler ultrasound (Levovist) and computed tomography in alveolar echinococcosis. *Abdom Imaging.* 2005;30(3):286-290. Epub 2005/06/21.

117. Haddad MC, Birjawi GA, Khouzami RA, Khoury NJ, El-Zein YR, Al-Kutoubi AO. Unilocular hepatic echinococcal cysts: sonography and computed tomography findings. *Clin Radiol.* 2001;56(9):746-750. Epub 2001/10/05.

118. Czermak BV, Akhan O, Hiemetzberger R, Zelger B, Vogel W, Jaschke W, et al. Echinococcosis of the liver. *Abdom Imaging.* 2008;33(2):133-143. Epub 2007/10/04.

119. Agildere AM, Aytekin C, Coskun M, Boyvat F, Boyacioglu S. MRI of hydatid disease of the liver: a variety of sequences. *J Comput Assist Tomogr.* 1998;22(5):718-724. Epub 1998/10/01.

120. Hoff FL, Aisen AM, Walden ME, Glazer GM. MR imaging in hydatid disease of the liver. *Gastrointest Radiol.* 1987;12(1):39-42. Epub 1987/01/01.

121. Taourel P, Marty-Ane B, Charasset S, Mattei M, Devred P, Bruel JM. Hydatid cyst of the liver: comparison of CT and MRI. *J Comput Assist Tomogr.* 1993;17(1):80-85. Epub 1993/01/01.

122. Nakamuta M, Ohashi M, Fukutomi T, Tanabe Y, Hiroshige K, Nakashima O, et al. Oral contraceptive-dependent growth of focal nodular hyperplasia. *J Gastroenterol Hepatol.* 1994;9(5): 521-523. Epub 1994/09/01.

123. Nagorney DM. Benign hepatic tumors: focal nodular hyperplasia and hepatocellular adenoma. *World J Surg.* 1995;19(1):13-18. Epub 1995/01/01.

124. Di Stasi M, Caturelli E, De Sio I, Salmi A, Buscarini E, Buscarini L. Natural history of focal nodular hyperplasia of the liver: an ultrasound study. *J Clin Ultrasound.* 1996;24(7):345-350. Epub 1996/09/01.

125. Leconte I, Van Beers BE, Lacrosse M, Sempoux C, Jamart J, Materne R, et al. Focal nodular hyperplasia: natural course observed with CT and MRI. *J Comput Assist Tomogr.* 2000;24(1):61-66. Epub 2000/02/10.

126. Kuo YH, Wang JH, Lu SN, Hung CH, Wei YC, Hu TH, et al. Natural course of hepatic focal nodular hyperplasia: a long-term follow-up study with sonography. *J Clin Ultrasound.* 2009;37(3):132-137. Epub 2008/10/16.

127. Majewski A, Gratz KF, Brolsch C, Gebel M. Sonographic pattern of focal nodular hyperplasia of the liver. *Eur J Radiol.* 1984;4(1):52-57. Epub 1984/02/01.

128. Shirkhoda A, Farah MC, Bernacki E, Madrazo B, Roberts J. Hepatic focal nodular hyperplasia: CT and sonographic spectrum. *Abdom Imaging.* 1994;19(1):34-38. Epub 1994/01/01.

129. Hussain SM, Terkivatan T, Zondervan PE, Lanjouw E, de Rave S, Ijzermans JN, et al. Focal nodular hyperplasia: findings at state-of-the-art MR imaging, US, CT, and pathologic analysis. *Radiographics.* 2004;24(1):3-17; discussion 8-9. Epub 2004/01/20.

130. Mortele KJ, Praet M, Van Vlierberghe H, de Hemptinne B, Zou K, Ros PR. Focal nodular hyperplasia of the liver: detection and characterization with plain and dynamic-enhanced MRI. *Abdom Imaging.* 2002;27(6):700-707. Epub 2002/10/24.

131. Brancatelli G, Federle MP, Grazioli L, Blachar A, Peterson MS, Thaete L. Focal nodular hyperplasia: CT findings with emphasis on multiphasic helical CT in 78 patients. *Radiology.* 2001;219(1):61-68. Epub 2001/03/29.

132. Grazioli L, Morana G, Federle MP, Brancatelli G, Testoni M, Kirchin MA, et al. Focal nodular hyperplasia: morphologic and functional information from MR imaging with gadobenate dimeglumine. *Radiology.* 2001;221(3):731-739. Epub 2001/11/24.

133. Brancatelli G, Federle MP, Katyal S, Kapoor V. Hemodynamic characterization of focal nodular hyperplasia using three-dimensional volume-rendered multidetector CT angiography. *AJR Am J Roentgenol.* 2002;179(1):81-85. Epub 2002/06/22.

134. Ruppert-Kohlmayr AJ, Uggowitzer MM, Kugler C, Zebedin D, Schaffler G, Ruppert GS. Focal nodular hyperplasia and hepatocellular adenoma of the liver: differentiation with multiphasic helical CT. *AJR Am J Roentgenol.* 2001;176(6): 1493-1498. Epub 2001/05/25.

135. Blachar A, Federle MP, Ferris JV, Lacomis JM, Waltz JS, Armfield DR, et al. Radiologists' performance in the diagnosis of liver tumors with central scars by using specific CT criteria. *Radiology.* 2002;223(2):532-539. Epub 2002/05/09.

136. Welch TJ, Sheedy PF 2nd, Johnson CM, Stephens DH, Charboneau JW, Brown ML, et al. Focal nodular hyperplasia and hepatic adenoma: comparison of angiography, CT, US, and scintigraphy. *Radiology.* 1985;156(3):593-595. Epub 1985/09/01.

137. Vogl TJ, Pegios W, McMahon C, Balzer J, Waitzinger J, Pirovano G, et al. Gadobenate dimeglumine—a new contrast agent for MR imaging: preliminary evaluation in healthy volunteers. *AJR Am J Roentgenol.* 1992;158(4):887-892. Epub 1992/04/01.

138. Hamm B, Staks T, Muhler A, Bollow M, Taupitz M, Frenzel T, et al. Phase I clinical evaluation of Gd-EOB-DTPA as a hepatobiliary MR contrast agent: safety, pharmacokinetics, and MR imaging. *Radiology.* 1995;195(3):785-792. Epub 1995/06/01.

139. Giovagnoni A, Paci E. Liver. III: Gadolinium-based hepatobiliary contrast agents (Gd-EOB-DTPA and Gd-BOPTA/Dimeg). *Magn Reson Imaging Clin N Am.* 1996;4(1):61-72. Epub 1996/02/01.

140. Grazioli L, Morana G, Kirchin MA, Schneider G. Accurate differentiation of focal nodular hyperplasia from hepatic adenoma at gadobenate dimeglumine-enhanced MR imaging: prospective study. *Radiology.* 2005;236(1):166-177. Epub 2005/06/16.

141. Seale MK, Catalano OA, Saini S, Hahn PF, Sahani DV. Hepatobiliary-specific MR contrast agents: role in imaging the liver and biliary tree. *Radiographics.* 2009;29(6):1725-1748. Epub 2009/12/05.

142. Karam AR, Shankar S, Surapaneni P, Kim YH, Hussain S. Focal nodular hyperplasia: Central scar enhancement pattern using gadoxetate disodium. *J Magn Reson Imaging.* 2010;32(2):341-344. Epub 2010/08/03.

143. Rooks JB, Ory HW, Ishak KG, Strauss LT, Greenspan JR, Hill AP, et al. Epidemiology of hepatocellular adenoma. The role of oral contraceptive use. *JAMA.* 1979;242(7):644-648. Epub 1979/08/17.

144. Edmondson HA, Henderson B, Benton B. Liver-cell adenomas associated with use of oral contraceptives. *N Engl J Med.* 1976;294(9):470-472. Epub 1976/02/26.

145. Edmondson HA, Reynolds TB, Henderson B, Benton B. Regression of liver cell adenomas associated with oral contraceptives. *Ann Intern Med.* 1977;86(2):180-182. Epub 1977/02/01.

146. Socas L, Zumbado M, Perez-Luzardo O, Ramos A, Perez C, Hernandez JR, et al. Hepatocellular adenomas associated with anabolic androgenic steroid abuse in bodybuilders: a report of two cases and a review of the literature. *Br J Sports Med.* 2005;39(5):e27. Epub 2005/04/26.

147. Labrune P, Trioche P, Duvaltier I, Chevalier P, Odievre M. Hepatocellular adenomas in glycogen storage disease type I and III: a series of 43 patients and review of the literature. *J Pediatr Gastroenterol Nutr.* 1997;24(3):276-279. Epub 1997/03/01.

148. van der Windt DJ, Kok NF, Hussain SM, Zondervan PE, Alwayn IP, de Man RA, et al. Case-orientated approach to the management of hepatocellular adenoma. *Br J Surg.* 2006;93(12):1495-1502. Epub 2006/10/20.

149. Furlan A, van der Windt DJ, Nalesnik MA, Sholosh B, Ngan KK, Pealer KM, et al. Multiple hepatic adenomas associated with liver steatosis at CT and MRI: a case-control study. *AJR Am J Roentgenol.* 2008;191(5):1430-1435. Epub 2008/10/23.

150. Flejou JF, Barge J, Menu Y, Degott C, Bismuth H, Potet F, et al. Liver adenomatosis. An entity distinct from liver adenoma? *Gastroenterology.* 1985;89(5):1132-1138. Epub 1985/11/01.

151. Arsenault TM, Johnson CD, Gorman B, Burgart LJ. Hepatic adenomatosis. *Mayo Clin Proc.* 1996;71(5):478-480. Epub 1996/05/01.

152. Grazioli L, Federle MP, Ichikawa T, Balzano E, Nalesnik M, Madariaga J. Liver adenomatosis: clinical, histopathologic, and imaging findings in 15 patients. *Radiology.* 2000;216(2):395-402. Epub 2000/08/05.

153. Outwater EK, Blasbalg R, Siegelman ES, Vala M. Detection of lipid in abdominal tissues with opposed-phase gradient-echo images at 1.5 T: techniques and diagnostic importance. *Radiographics.* 1998;18(6):1465-1480. Epub 1998/11/20.

154. Gaa J, Lee MJ, Saini S. Case report: haemorrhagic hepatic adenoma—MR features. *Clin Radiol.* 1994;49(10):719-720. Epub 1994/10/01.

155. Meissner K. Hemorrhage caused by ruptured liver cell adenoma following long-term oral contraceptives: a case report. *Hepatogastroenterology.* 1998;45(19):224-225. Epub 1998/03/13.

156. Casillas VJ, Amendola MA, Gascue A, Pinnar N, Levi JU, Perez JM. Imaging of nontraumatic hemorrhagic hepatic lesions. *Radiographics.* 2000;20(2):367-378. Epub 2000/03/15.

157. Grazioli L, Federle MP, Brancatelli G, Ichikawa T, Olivetti L, Blachar A. Hepatic adenomas: imaging and pathologic findings. *Radiographics.* 2001;21(4):877-892; discussion 92-94. Epub 2001/07/14.

158. Mergo PJ, Ros PR. Benign lesions of the liver. *Radiol Clin North Am.* 1998;36(2):319-331. Epub 1998/04/01.

159. Paulson EK, McClellan JS, Washington K, Spritzer CE, Meyers WC, Baker ME. Hepatic adenoma: MR characteristics and correlation with pathologic findings. *AJR Am J Roentgenol.* 1994;163(1):113-116. Epub 1994/07/01.

160. Chung KY, Mayo-Smith WW, Saini S, Rahmouni A, Golli M, Mathieu D. Hepatocellular adenoma: MR imaging features with pathologic correlation. *AJR Am J Roentgenol.* 1995;165(2):303-308. Epub 1995/08/01.

161. Lewin M, Handra-Luca A, Arrive L, Wendum D, Paradis V, Bridel E, et al. Liver adenomatosis: classification of MR imaging features and comparison with pathologic findings. *Radiology.* 2006;241(2):433-440. Epub 2006/09/13.

162. Kume N, Suga K, Nishigauchi K, Shimizu K, Matsunaga N. Characterization of hepatic adenoma with atypical appearance on CT and MRI by radionuclide imaging. *Clin Nucl Med.* 1997;22(12):825-831. Epub 1997/12/31.

163. Zech CJ, Herrmann KA, Reiser MF, Schoenberg SO. MR imaging in patients with suspected liver metastases: value of liver-specific contrast agent Gd-EOB-DTPA. *Magn Reson Med Sci.* 2007;6(1):43-52. Epub 2007/05/19.

164. Ba-Ssalamah A, Uffmann M, Saini S, Bastati N, Herold C, Schima W. Clinical value of MRI liver-specific contrast agents: a tailored examination for a confident non-invasive diagnosis of focal liver lesions. *Eur Radiol.* 2009;19(2):342-357. Epub 2008/09/24.

165. McLarney JK, Rucker PT, Bender GN, Goodman ZD, Kashitani N, Ros PR. Fibrolamellar carcinoma of the liver: radiologic-pathologic correlation. *Radiographics.* 1999;19(2):453-471. Epub 1999/04/09.

166. Friedman AC, Lichtenstein JE, Goodman Z, Fishman EK, Siegelman SS, Dachman AH. Fibrolamellar hepatocellular carcinoma. *Radiology.* 1985;157(3):583-587. Epub 1985/12/01.

167. Khan SA, Thomas HC, Davidson BR, Taylor-Robinson SD. Cholangiocarcinoma. *Lancet.* 2005;366(9493):1303-1314. Epub 2005/10/11.

168. Schulick RD. Primary sclerosing cholangitis: detection of cancer in strictures. *J Gastrointest Surg.* 2008;12(3):420-402. Epub 2007/11/14.

169. Lim JH, Mairiang E, Ahn GH. Biliary parasitic diseases including clonorchiasis, opisthorchiasis and fascioliasis. *Abdom Imaging.* 2008;33(2):157-165. Epub 2007/10/16.

170. Rana SS, Bhasin DK, Nanda M, Singh K. Parasitic infestations of the biliary tract. *Curr Gastroenterol Rep.* 2007;9(2):156-164. Epub 2007/04/10.

171. Shin HR, Oh JK, Masuyer E, Curado MP, Bouvard V, Fang YY, et al. Epidemiology of cholangiocarcinoma: an update focusing on risk factors. *Cancer Sci.* 2010;101(3):579-585. Epub 2010/01/21.

172. Miller WJ, Sechtin AG, Campbell WL, Pieters PC. Imaging findings in Caroli's disease. *AJR Am J Roentgenol.* 1995;165(2):333-337. Epub 1995/08/01.

173. Yalcin S. Diagnosis and management of cholangiocarcinomas: a comprehensive review. Hepatogastroenterology. 2004;51(55):43-50. Epub 2004/03/12.

174. Manfredi R, Barbaro B, Masselli G, Vecchioli A, Marano P. Magnetic resonance imaging of cholangiocarcinoma. *Semin Liver Dis.* 2004;24(2):155-164. Epub 2004/06/12.

175. Chung YE, Kim MJ, Park YN, Choi JY, Pyo JY, Kim YC, et al. Varying appearances of cholangiocarcinoma: radiologic-pathologic correlation. *Radiographics.* 2009;29(3):683-700. Epub 2009/05/19.

176. Zhang Y, Uchida M, Abe T, Nishimura H, Hayabuchi N, Nakashima Y. Intrahepatic peripheral cholangiocarcinoma: comparison of dynamic CT and dynamic MRI. *J Comput Assist Tomogr.* 1999;23(5):670-677. Epub 1999/10/19.

177. Valls C, Guma A, Puig I, Sanchez A, Andia E, Serrano T, et al. Intrahepatic peripheral cholangiocarcinoma: *CT evaluation. Abdom Imaging.* 2000;25(5):490-496. Epub 2000/08/10.

178. Kim SJ, Lee JM, Han JK, Kim KH, Lee JY, Choi BI. Peripheral mass-forming cholangiocarcinoma in cirrhotic liver. *AJR Am J Roentgenol.* 2007;189(6):1428-1434. Epub 2007/11/22.

179. Rimola J, Forner A, Reig M, Vilana R, de Lope CR, Ayuso C, et al. Cholangiocarcinoma in cirrhosis: absence of contrast washout in delayed phases by magnetic resonance imaging avoids misdiagnosis of hepatocellular carcinoma. *Hepatology.* 2009;50(3):791-798. Epub 2009/07/18.

180. Leyendecker JR, Gakhal M, Elsayes KM, McDermott R, Narra VR, Brown JJ. Fat-suppressed dynamic and delayed gadolinium-enhanced volumetric interpolated breath-hold magnetic resonance imaging of cholangiocarcinoma. *J Comput Assist Tomogr.* 2008;32(2):178-184. Epub 2008/04/02.

181. Gazelle GS, Lee MJ, Hahn PF, Goldberg MA, Rafaat N, Mueller PR. US, CT, and MRI of primary and secondary liver lymphoma. *J Comput Assist Tomogr.* 1994;18(3):412-415. Epub 1994/05/01.

182. Warshauer DM, Molina PL, Hamman SM, Koehler RE, Paulson EK, Bechtold RE, et al. Nodular sarcoidosis of the liver and spleen: analysis of 32 cases. *Radiology.* 1995;195(3):757-762. Epub 1995/06/01.

183. Mortele KJ, Ros PR. Imaging of diffuse liver disease. *Semin Liver Dis.* 2001;21(2):195-212. Epub 2001/07/05.

184. Kessler A, Mitchell DG, Israel HL, Goldberg BB. Hepatic and splenic sarcoidosis: ultrasound and MR imaging. *Abdom Imaging.* 1993;18(2):159-163. Epub 1993/01/01.

185. Folz SJ, Johnson CD, Swensen SJ. Abdominal manifestations of sarcoidosis in CT studies. *J Comput Assist Tomogr.* 1995;19(4): 573-579. Epub 1995/07/01.

186. Sakai T, Maeda M, Takabatake M, Hayashi N, Ishii Y, Kitamura M, et al. MR imaging of hepatosplenic sarcoidosis. *Radiat Med.* 1995;13(1):39-41. Epub 1995/01/01.

187. Vilaichone RK, Vilaichone W, Tumwasorn S, Suwanagool P, Wilde H, Mahachai V. Clinical spectrum of hepatic tuberculosis: comparison between immunocompetent and immunocompromised hosts. *J Med Assoc Thai.* 2003;86(suppl 2):S432-S428. Epub 2003/08/22.

188. Yu RS, Zhang SZ, Wu JJ, Li RF. Imaging diagnosis of 12 patients with hepatic tuberculosis. *World J Gastroenterol.* 2004;10(11):1639-1642. Epub 2004/05/27.

189. Murata Y, Yamada I, Sumiya Y, Shichijo Y, Suzuki Y. Abdominal macronodular tuberculomas: MR findings. *J Comput Assist Tomogr.* 1996;20(4):643-646. Epub 1996/07/01.

190. Romano L, Giovine S, Guidi G, Tortora G, Cinque T, Romano S. Hepatic trauma: CT findings and considerations based on our experience in emergency diagnostic imaging. *Eur J Radiol.* 2004;50(1):59-66. Epub 2004/04/20.

191. Roberts JL, Dalen K, Bosanko CM, Jafir SZ. CT in abdominal and pelvic trauma. *Radiographics.* 1993;13(4):735-752. Epub 1993/07/01.

192. Katz S, Lazar L, Rathaus V, Erez I. Can ultrasonography replace computed tomography in the initial assessment of children with blunt abdominal trauma? *J Pediatr Surg.* 1996;31(5):649-651. Epub 1996/05/01.

193. Hagiwara A, Murata A, Matsuda T, Matsuda H, Shimazaki S. The efficacy and limitations of transarterial embolization for severe hepatic injury. *J Trauma.* 2002;52(6):1091-1096. Epub 2002/06/05.

194. Moran EM, Ultmann JE, Ferguson DJ, Hoffer PB, Ranniger K, Rappaport H. Staging laparotomy in non-Hodgkin's lymphoma. *Br J Cancer Suppl.* 1975;2:228-236. Epub 1975/03/01.

195. Ferguson DJ, Allen LW, Griem ML, Moran ME, Rappaport H, Ultmann JE. Surgical experience with staging laparotomy in 125 patients with lymphoma. *Arch Intern Med.* 1973;131(3): 356-361. Epub 1973/03/01.

196. Ginaldi S, Bernardino ME, Jing BS, Green B. Ultrasonographic patterns of hepatic lymphoma. *Radiology.* 1980;136(2):427-431. Epub 1980/08/01.

197. Wernecke K, Peters PE, Kruger KG. Ultrasonographic patterns of focal hepatic and splenic lesions in Hodgkin's and non-Hodgkin's lymphoma. *Br J Radiol.* 1987;60(715):655-660. Epub 1987/07/01.

198. Kelekis NL, Semelka RC, Siegelman ES, Ascher SM, Outwater EK, Woosley JT, et al. Focal hepatic lymphoma: magnetic resonance demonstration using current techniques including gadolinium enhancement. *Magn Reson Imaging.* 1997;15(6):625-636. Epub 1997/01/01.

199. Rizzi EB, Schinina V, Cristofaro M, David V, Bibbolino C. Non-hodgkin's lymphoma of the liver in patients with AIDS: sonographic, CT, and MRI findings. *J Clin Ultrasound.* 2001;29(3):125-129. Epub 2001/05/01.

200. Zafrani ES. An additional argument for a toxic mechanism of peliosis hepatis in man. *Hepatology.* 1990;11(2):322-323. Epub 1990/02/01.

201. Tappero JW, Mohle-Boetani J, Koehler JE, Swaminathan B, Berger TG, LeBoit PE, et al. The epidemiology of bacillary angiomatosis and bacillary peliosis. *JAMA.* 1993;269(6): 770-775. Epub 1993/02/10.

202. Cavalcanti R, Pol S, Carnot F, Campos H, Degott C, Driss F, et al. Impact and evolution of peliosis hepatis in renal transplant recipients. *Transplantation.* 1994;58(3):315-316. Epub 1994/08/15.

203. Hoshimoto S, Morise Z, Suzuki K, Tanahashi Y, Ikeda M, Kagawa T, et al. Hepatocellular carcinoma with extensive peliotic change. *J Hepatobiliary Pancreat Surg.* 2009;16(4): 566-570. Epub 2009/02/03.

204. Gushiken FC. Peliosis hepatis after treatment with 2-chloro-3'-deoxyadenosine. *South Med J.* 2000;93(6):625-626. Epub 2000/07/06.

205. Wanless I. Vascular Disorders. In: MacSween RNM BA, Portmann BC, Ishak KG, Scheuer PJ, Anthony PP, eds. *Pathology of the Liver.* 4th ed. Glasgow, UK: Churchill Living stone; 2002:553-555.

206. Iannaccone R, Federle MP, Brancatelli G, Matsui O, Fishman EK, Narra VR, et al. Peliosis hepatis: spectrum of imaging findings. *AJR Am J Roentgenol.* 2006;187(1):W43-W52. Epub 2006/06/24.

207. Tateishi T, Machi J, Morioka WK. Focal peliosis hepatis resembling metastatic liver tumor. *J Ultrasound Med.* 1998;17(9):581-584. Epub 1998/09/11.

208. Kim SH, Lee JM, Kim WH, Han JK, Lee JY, Choi BI. Focal peliosis hepatis as a mimicker of hepatic tumors: radiological-pathological correlation. *J Comput Assist Tomogr.* 2007;31(1): 79-85. Epub 2007/01/30.

209. Vignaux O, Legmann P, de Pinieux G, Chaussade S, Spaulding C, Couturier D, et al. Hemorrhagic necrosis due to peliosis hepatis: imaging findings and pathological correlation. *Eur Radiol.* 1999;9(3):454-456. Epub 1999/03/23.

210. Steinke K, Terraciano L, Wiesner W. Unusual cross-sectional imaging findings in hepatic peliosis. *Eur Radiol.* 2003;13(8):1916-1919. Epub 2003/08/28.

211. Verswijvel G, Janssens F, Colla P, Mampaey S, Verhelst H, Van Eycken P, et al. Peliosis hepatis presenting as a multifocal hepatic pseudotumor: MR findings in two cases. *Eur Radiol.* 2003;13(suppl 4):L40-L44. Epub 2004/03/17.

212. Lacaille F, Fournet JC, Sayegh N, Jaubert F, Revillon Y. Inflammatory pseudotumor of the liver: a rare benign tumor mimicking a malignancy. *Liver Transpl Surg.* 1999;5(1):83-85. Epub 1999/01/05.

213. Fukuya T, Honda H, Matsumata T, Kawanami T, Shimoda Y, Muranaka T, et al. Diagnosis of inflammatory pseudotumor of the liver: value of CT. *AJR Am J Roentgenol.* 1994;163(5): 1087-1091. Epub 1994/11/01.

214. Tai YS, Lin PW, Chen SG, Chang KC. Inflammatory pseudotumor of the liver in a patient with human immunodeficiency virus infection. *Hepatogastroenterology.* 1998;45(23):1760-1763. Epub 1998/12/05.

215. Abehsera M, Vilgrain V, Belghiti J, Flejou JF, Nahum H. Inflammatory pseudotumor of the liver: radiologic-pathologic correlation. *J Comput Assist Tomogr.* 1995;19(1):80-83. Epub 1995/01/01.

216. Ijuin H, Ono N, Koga K, Yoshida T, Ohnishi H, Miyazaki S, et al. Inflammatory pseudotumor of the liver—MR imaging findings. *Kurume Med J.* 1997;44(4):305-313. Epub 1997/01/01.

217. Mortele KJ, Wiesner W, de Hemptinne B, Elewaut A, Praet M, Ros PR. Multifocal inflammatory pseudotumor of the liver: dynamic gadolinium-enhanced, ferumoxides-enhanced, and mangafodipir trisodium-enhanced MR imaging findings. *Eur Radiol.* 2002;12(2):304-308. Epub 2002/03/01.

218. Borgonovo G, Razzetta F, Varaldo E, Cittadini G, Ceppa P, Torre GC, et al. Pseudotumor of the liver: a challenging diagnosis. *Hepatogastroenterology.* 1998;45(23):1770-1773. Epub 1998/12/05.

219. Zen Y, Fujii T, Nakanuma Y. Hepatic pseudolymphoma: a clinicopathological study of five cases and review of the literature. *Mod Pathol.* 2010;23(2):244-2450. Epub 2009/11/17.

220. Matsumoto N, Ogawa M, Kawabata M, Tohne R, Hiroi Y, Furuta T, et al. Pseudolymphoma of the liver: Sonographic findings and review of the literature. *J Clin Ultrasound.* 2007;35(5):284-288. Epub 2007/04/17.

221. Nagano K, Fukuda Y, Nakano I, Katano Y, Toyoda H, Nonami T, et al. Reactive lymphoid hyperplasia of liver coexisting with chronic thyroiditis: radiographical characteristics of the disorder. *J Gastroenterol Hepatol.* 1999;14(2):163-167. Epub 1999/02/24.

222. Nagasue N, Akamizu H, Yukaya H, Yuuki I. Hepatocellular pseudotumor in the cirrhotic liver. Report of three cases. *Cancer.* 1984;54(11):2487-2494. Epub 1984/12/01.

223. Sauerbrei EE, Lopez M. Pseudotumor of the quadrate lobe in hepatic sonography: a sign of generalized fatty infiltration. *AJR Am J Roentgenol.* 1986;147(5):923-927. Epub 1986/11/01.

224. Karcaaltincaba M, Akhan O. Imaging of hepatic steatosis and fatty sparing. *Eur J Radiol.* 2007;61(1):33-43. Epub 2006/11/23.

225. Yoshikawa J, Matsui O, Takashima T, Sugiura H, Katayama K, Nishida Y, et al. Focal fatty change of the liver adjacent to the falciform ligament: CT and sonographic findings in five surgically confirmed cases. *AJR Am J Roentgenol.* 1987;149(3):491-494. Epub 1987/09/01.

226. Halvorsen RA, Korobkin M, Ram PC, Thompson WM. CT appearance of focal fatty infiltration of the liver. *AJR Am J Roentgenol.* 1982;139(2):277-281. Epub 1982/08/01.

227. Kemper J, Jung G, Poll LW, Jonkmanns C, Luthen R, Moedder U. CT and MRI findings of multifocal hepatic steatosis mimicking malignancy. *Abdom Imaging.* 2002;27(6):708-710. Epub 2002/10/24.

228. McKenzie A, Gill G, McIntosh R, Hennessy O, Pryde D. Computed tomographic and ultrasound appearances of focal spared areas in fatty infiltration of the liver. *Australas Radiol.* 1991;35(2):166-168. Epub 1991/05/01.

229. Kissin CM, Bellamy EA, Cosgrove DO, Slack N, Husband JE. Focal sparing in fatty infiltration of the liver. *Br J Radiol.* 1986;59(697):25-28. Epub 1986/01/01.

230. Matsui O, Kadoya M, Takahashi S, Yoshikawa J, Gabata T, Takashima T, et al. Focal sparing of segment IV in fatty livers shown by sonography and CT: correlation with aberrant gastric venous drainage. *AJR Am J Roentgenol.* 1995;164(5):1137-1140. Epub 1995/05/01.

231. Larssen TB, Rorvik J, Hoff SR, Horn A, Rosendahl K. The occurrence of asymptomatic and symptomatic simple hepatic cysts. A prospective, hospital-based study. *Clin Radiol.* 2005;60(9):1026-1029. Epub 2005/08/30.

232. Tikkakoski T, Makela JT, Leinonen S, Paivansalo M, Merikanto J, Karttunen A, et al. Treatment of symptomatic congenital hepatic cysts with single-session percutaneous drainage and ethanol sclerosis: technique and outcome. *J Vasc Interv Radiol.* 1996;7(2):235-239. Epub 1996/03/01.

233. Sanfelippo PM, Beahrs OH, Weiland LH. Cystic disease of the liver. *Ann Surg.* 1974;179(6):922-925. Epub 1974/06/01.

234. Scholmerich J, Volk BA. Differential diagnosis of anechoic/hypoechoic lesions in the abdomen detected by ultrasound. *J Clin Ultrasound.* 1986;14(5):339-353. Epub 1986/06/01.

235. Murphy BJ, Casillas J, Ros PR, Morillo G, Albores-Saavedra J, Rolfes DB. The CT appearance of cystic masses of the liver. *Radiographics.* 1989;9(2):307-322. Epub 1989/03/01.

236. Semelka RC, Shoenut JP, Kroeker MA, Greenberg HM, Simm FC, Minuk GY, et al. Focal liver disease: comparison of dynamic contrast-enhanced CT and T2-weighted fat-suppressed, FLASH, and dynamic gadolinium-enhanced MR imaging at 1.5 T. *Radiology.* 1992;184(3):687-694. Epub 1992/09/01.

237. Goldberg MA, Hahn PF, Saini S, Cohen MS, Reimer P, Brady TJ, et al. Value of T1 and T2 relaxation times from echoplanar MR imaging in the characterization of focal hepatic lesions. *AJR Am J Roentgenol.* 1993;160(5):1011-1017. Epub 1993/05/01.

238. Erwin BC, Carroll BA. Ultrasonographic diagnosis of a hemorrhagic hepatic cyst clinically mimicking acute cholecystitis. *J Ultrasound Med.* 1983;2(5):237-238. Epub 1983/05/01.

239. Wilcox DM, Weinreb JC, Lesh P. MR imaging of a hemorrhagic hepatic cyst in a patient with polycystic liver disease. *J Comput Assist Tomogr.* 1985;9(1):183-185. Epub 1985/01/01.

240. Mathieu D, Paret M, Mahfouz AE, Caseiro-Alves F, Tran Van Nhieu J, Anglade MC, et al. Hyperintense benign liver lesions on spin-echo T1-weighted MR images: pathologic correlations. *Abdom Imaging.* 1997;22(4):410-417. Epub 1997/07/01.

241. Bae KT, Zhu F, Chapman AB, Torres VE, Grantham JJ, Guay-Woodford LM, et al. Magnetic resonance imaging evaluation of hepatic cysts in early autosomal-dominant polycystic kidney disease: the Consortium for Radiologic Imaging Studies of Polycystic Kidney Disease cohort. *Clin J Am Soc Nephrol.* 2006;1(1):64-69. Epub 2007/08/21.

242. Morgan DE, Lockhart ME, Canon CL, Holcombe MP, Bynon JS. Polycystic liver disease: multimodality imaging for complications and transplant evaluation. *Radiographics.* 2006;26(6):1655-1668; quiz Epub 2006/11/15.

243. Peces R, Drenth JP, Te Morsche RH, Gonzalez P, Peces C. Autosomal dominant polycystic liver disease in a family without polycystic kidney disease associated with a novel missense protein kinase C substrate 80K-H mutation. *World J Gastroenterol.* 2005;11(48):7690-7693. Epub 2006/01/27.

244. Qian Q, Li A, King BF, Kamath PS, Lager DJ, Huston J 3rd, et al. Clinical profile of autosomal dominant polycystic liver disease. *Hepatology.* 2003;37(1):164-171. Epub 2002/12/25.

245. Li A, Davila S, Furu L, Qian Q, Tian X, Kamath PS, et al. Mutations in PRKCSH cause isolated autosomal dominant polycystic liver disease. *Am J Hum Genet.* 2003;72(3):691-703. Epub 2003/01/17.

246. Erdogan D, van Delden OM, Rauws EA, Busch OR, Lameris JS, Gouma DJ, et al. Results of percutaneous sclerotherapy and surgical treatment in patients with symptomatic simple liver cysts and polycystic liver disease. *World J Gastroenterol.* 2007;13(22):3095-3100. Epub 2007/06/26.

247. Shin ES, Darcy MD. Transjugular intrahepatic portosystemic shunt placement in the setting of polycystic liver disease: questioning the contraindication. *J Vasc Interv Radiol.* 2001;12(9):1099-1102. Epub 2001/09/06.

248. Iguchi S, Kasai A, Kishimoto H, Suzuki K, Ito S, Ogawa Y, et al. Thrombosis in inferior vena cava (IVC) due to intra-cystic hemorrhage into a hepatic local cyst with autosomal dominant polycystic kidney disease (ADPKD). *Intern Med.* 2004;43(3):209-212. Epub 2004/04/22.

249. Everson GT, Helmke SM, Doctor B. Advances in management of polycystic liver disease. *Expert Rev Gastroenterol Hepatol.* 2008;2(4):563-576. Epub 2008/12/17.

250. Tohme-Noun C, Cazals D, Noun R, Menassa L, Valla D, Vilgrain V. Multiple biliary hamartomas: magnetic resonance features with histopathologic correlation. *Eur Radiol.* 2008;18(3):493-499. Epub 2007/10/16.

251. Gorg C, Weide R, Schwerk WB, Koppler H, Havemann K. Ultrasound evaluation of hepatic and splenic microabscesses in the immunocompromised patient: sonographic patterns, differential diagnosis, and follow-up. *J Clin Ultrasound.* 1994;22(9):525-529. Epub 1994/11/01.

252. Linker CA, DeGregorio MW, Ries CA. Computerized tomography in the diagnosis of systemic candidiasis in patients with acute leukemia. *Med Pediatr Oncol.* 1984;12(6):380-385. Epub 1984/01/01.

253. Pastakia B, Shawker TH, Thaler M, O'Leary T, Pizzo PA. Hepatosplenic candidiasis: wheels within wheels. *Radiology.* 1988;166(2):417-421. Epub 1988/02/01.

254. Semelka RC, Kelekis NL, Sallah S, Worawattanakul S, Ascher SM. Hepatosplenic fungal disease: diagnostic accuracy and spectrum of appearances on MR imaging. *AJR Am J Roentgenol.* 1997;169(5):1311-1316. Epub 1997/11/14.

255. Berlow ME, Spirt BA, Weil L. CT follow-up of hepatic and splenic fungal microabscesses. *J Comput Assist Tomogr.* 1984;8(1):42-425. Epub 1984/02/01.

256. Shirkhoda A, Lopez-Berestein G, Holbert JM, Luna MA. Hepatosplenic fungal infection: CT and pathologic evaluation after treatment with liposomal amphotericin *B. Radiology.* 1986;159(2):349-353. Epub 1986/05/01.

257. Gilbert HA, Kagan AR, Hintz BL, Nussbaum H. Patterns of Metastases. In: Weiss L, Gilbert HA, editors. Liver Metastases. Boston, MA: GK Hall Medical Publishers; 1982;19-39.

258. Choti MA, Kaloma F, de Oliveira ML, Nour S, Garrett-Mayer ES, Sheth S, et al. Patient variability in intraoperative ultrasonographic characteristics of colorectal liver metastases. *Arch Surg.* 2008;143(1):29-34; discussion 5. Epub 2008/01/23.

259. Hale HL, Husband JE, Gossios K, Norman AR, Cunningham D. CT of calcified liver metastases in colorectal carcinoma. *Clin Radiol.* 1998;53(10):735-741. Epub 1998/11/17.

260. Easson AM, Barron PT, Cripps C, Hill G, Guindi M, Michaud C. Calcification in colorectal hepatic metastases correlates with longer survival. *J Surg Oncol.* 1996;63(4): 221-225. Epub 1996/12/01.

261. McDonnell CH 3rd, Fishman EK, Zerhouni EA. CT demonstration of calcified liver metastases in medullary thyroid carcinoma. *J Comput Assist Tomogr.* 1986;10(6): 976-978. Epub 1986/11/01.

262. Tang Y, Yamashita Y, Namimoto T, Takahashi M. Characterization of focal liver lesions with half-fourier acquisition single-shot turbo-spin-echo (HASTE) and inversion recovery (IR)-HASTE sequences. *J Magn Reson Imaging.* 1998;8(2):438-445. Epub 1998/04/30.

263. Demir OI, Obuz F, Sagol O, Dicle O. Contribution of diffusion-weighted MRI to the differential diagnosis of hepatic masses. *Diagn Interv Radiol.* 2007;13(2):81-86. Epub 2007/06/15.

264. Goshima S, Kanematsu M, Kondo H, Yokoyama R, Kajita K, Tsuge Y, et al. Diffusion-weighted imaging of the liver: optimizing b value for the detection and characterization of benign and malignant hepatic lesions. *J Magn Reson Imaging.* 2008;28(3):691-697. Epub 2008/09/09.

265. Koh DM, Brown G, Riddell AM, Scurr E, Collins DJ, Allen SD, et al. Detection of colorectal hepatic metastases using MnDPDP MR imaging and diffusion-weighted imaging (DWI) alone and in combination. *Eur Radiol.* 2008;18(5):903-910. Epub 2008/01/15.

266. Choi JS, Kim MJ, Choi JY, Park MS, Lim JS, Kim KW. Diffusion-weighted MR imaging of liver on 3.0-Tesla system: effect of intravenous administration of gadoxetic acid disodium. *Eur Radiol.* 2010;20(5):1052-1060. Epub 2009/11/17.

267. Kanematsu M, Kondo H, Goshima S, Kato H, Tsuge U, Hirose Y, et al. Imaging liver metastases: review and update. *Eur J Radiol.* 2006;58(2):217-228. Epub 2006/01/13.

268. Bressler EL, Alpern MB, Glazer GM, Francis IR, Ensminger WD. Hypervascular hepatic metastases: CT evaluation. *Radiology.* 1987;162(1 Pt 1):49-51. Epub 1987/01/01.

269. Mahfouz AE, Hamm B, Taupitz M, Wolf KJ. Hypervascular liver lesions: differentiation of focal nodular hyperplasia from malignant tumors with dynamic gadolinium-enhanced MR imaging. *Radiology.* 1993;186(1):133-138. Epub 1993/01/01.

270. Wittenberg J, Stark DD, Forman BH, Hahn PF, Saini S, Weissleder R, et al. Differentiation of hepatic metastases from hepatic hemangiomas and cysts by using MR imaging. *AJR Am J Roentgenol.* 1988;151(1):79-84. Epub 1988/07/01.

271. Kim JW, Dang CV. Cancer's molecular sweet tooth and the Warburg effect. *Cancer Res.* 2006;66(18):8927-8930. Epub 2006/09/20.

272. Delbeke D, Vitola JV, Sandler MP, Arildsen RC, Powers TA, Wright JK Jr, et al. Staging recurrent metastatic colorectal carcinoma with PET. *J Nucl Med.* 1997;38(8):1196-1201. Epub 1997/08/01.

273. Abdel-Nabi H, Doerr RJ, Lamonica DM, Cronin VR, Galantowicz PJ, Carbone GM, et al. Staging of primary colorectal carcinomas with fluorine-18 fluorodeoxyglucose whole-body PET: correlation with histopathologic and CT findings. *Radiology.* 1998;206(3):755-760. Epub 1998/03/12.
274. Holder WD Jr, White RL Jr, Zuger JH, Easton EJ Jr, Greene FL. Effectiveness of positron emission tomography for the detection of melanoma metastases. *Ann Surg.* 1998;227(5): 764-769; discussion 9-71. Epub 1998/05/30.
275. Yeung HW, Macapinlac H, Karpeh M, Finn RD, Larson SM. Accuracy of FDG-PET in Gastric Cancer. Preliminary Experience. *Clin Positron Imaging.* 1998;1(4):213-221. Epub 2003/10/01.
276. Frohlich A, Diederichs CG, Staib L, Vogel J, Beger HG, Reske SN. Detection of liver metastases from pancreatic cancer using FDG PET. *J Nucl Med.* 1999;40(2):250-255. Epub 1999/02/20.
277. Bacigalupo L, Aufort S, Eberle MC, Assenat E, Ychou M, Gallix B. Assessment of liver metastases from colorectal adenocarcinoma following chemotherapy: SPIO-MRI versus FDG-PET/CT. *Radiol Med.* 2010. Epub 2010/06/25. Valutazione con SPIO-RM e TC-PET-FDG di metastasi epatiche di adenocarcinoma colorettale dopo chemioterapia.
278. Khandani AH, Wahl RL. Applications of PET in liver imaging. *Radiol Clin North Am.* 2005;43(5):849-860, vii. Epub 2005/08/16.
279. Koyama T, Ueda H, Togashi K, Umeoka S, Kataoka M, Nagai S. Radiologic manifestations of sarcoidosis in various organs. *Radiographics.* 2004;24(1):87-104. Epub 2004/01/20.
280. Carrillo EH, Richardson JD. The current management of hepatic trauma. *Adv Surg.* 2001;35:39-59. Epub 2001/10/03.
281. Mirvis SE, Whitley NO, Vainwright JR, Gens DR. Blunt hepatic trauma in adults: CT-based classification and correlation with prognosis and treatment. *Radiology.* 1989;171(1):27-32. Epub 1989/04/01.
282. Fang JF, Wong YC, Lin BC, Hsu YP, Chen MF. The CT risk factors for the need of operative treatment in initially hemodynamically stable patients after blunt hepatic trauma. *J Trauma.* 2006;61(3):547-553; discussion 53-54. Epub 2006/09/13.
283. Yao DC, Jeffrey RB Jr, Mirvis SE, Weekes A, Federle MP, Kim C, et al. Using contrast-enhanced helical CT to visualize arterial extravasation after blunt abdominal trauma: incidence and organ distribution. *AJR Am J Roentgenol.* 2002;178(1):17-20. Epub 2002/01/05.
284. Hahn DD, Offerman SR, Holmes JF. Clinical importance of intraperitoneal fluid in patients with blunt intra-abdominal injury. *Am J Emerg Med.* 2002;20(7):595-600. Epub 2002/11/21.
285. Lubner M, Menias C, Rucker C, Bhalla S, Peterson CM, Wang L, et al. Blood in the belly: CT findings of hemoperitoneum. *Radiographics.* 2007;27(1):109-125. Epub 2007/01/20.
286. Howard R, Bansal S, Munshi IA. Biloma: a delayed complication of blunt hepatic injury. *J Emerg Med.* 2008;34(1):33-25. Epub 2007/11/03.
287. Demetriades D, Karaiskakis M, Alo K, Velmahos G, Murray J, Asensio J. Role of postoperative computed tomography in patients with severe liver injury. *Br J Surg.* 2003;90(11): 1398-1400. Epub 2003/11/05.
288. Abbas MA, Collins JM, Olden KW. Spontaneous intramural small-bowel hematoma: imaging findings and outcome. *AJR Am J Roentgenol.* 2002;179(6):1389-1394. Epub 2002/11/20.
289. Federle MP, Pan KT, Pealer KM. CT criteria for differentiating abdominal hemorrhage: anticoagulation or aortic aneurysm rupture? *AJR Am J Roentgenol.* 2007;188(5):1324-1330. Epub 2007/04/24.
290. Merine D, Fishman EK, Zerhouni EA. Spontaneous hepatic hemorrhage: clinical and CT findings. *J Comput Assist Tomogr.* 1988;12(3):397-400. Epub 1988/05/01.
291. Barton JR, Sibai BM. Gastrointestinal complications of pre-eclampsia. *Semin Perinatol.* 2009;33(3):179-188. Epub 2009/05/26.
292. Wicke C, Pereira PL, Neeser E, Flesch I, Rodegerdts EA, Becker HD. Subcapsular liver hematoma in HELLP syndrome: Evaluation of diagnostic and therapeutic options—a unicenter study. *Am J Obstet Gynecol.* 2004;190(1):106-112. Epub 2004/01/30.
293. Meakem TJ 3rd, Unger EC, Pond GD, Modiano MR, Alberts DR. CT findings after hepatic chemoembolization. *J Comput Assist Tomogr.* 1992;16(6):916-920. Epub 1992/11/01.
294. Furukawa H, Kosuge T, Shimada K, Yamamoto J, Ushio K. Helical CT of the abdomen after pancreaticoduodenectomy: usefulness for detecting postoperative complications. *Hepatogastroenterology.* 1997;44(15):849-855. Epub 1997/05/01.
295. Smith GS, Birnbaum BA, Jacobs JE. Hepatic infarction secondary to arterial insufficiency in native livers: CT findings in 10 patients. *Radiology.* 1998;208(1):223-239. Epub 1998/07/01.
296. Zissin R, Yaffe D, Fejgin M, Olsfanger D, Shapiro-Feinberg M. Hepatic infarction in preeclampsia as part of the HELLP syndrome: CT appearance. *Abdom Imaging.* 1999;24(6): 594-596. Epub 1999/10/20.
297. Holbert BL, Baron RL, Dodd GD 3rd. Hepatic infarction caused by arterial insufficiency: spectrum and evolution of CT findings. *AJR Am J Roentgenol.* 1996;166(4):815-820. Epub 1996/04/01.
298. Itai Y, Ohtomo K, Kokubo T, Minami M, Yoshida H. CT and MR imaging of postnecrotic liver scars. *J Comput Assist Tomogr.* 1988;12(6):971-975. Epub 1988/11/01.
299. Takayasu K, Moriyama N, Muramatsu Y, Tajiri H. Transient perihilar attenuation difference in the liver on dynamic CT secondary to portal vein thrombosis: report of two cases. *Gastroenterol Jpn.* 1989;24(2):205-208. Epub 1989/04/01.
300. Yamasaki M, Furukawa A, Murata K, Morita R. Transient hepatic attenuation difference (THAD) in patients without neoplasm: frequency, shape, distribution, and causes. *Radiat Med.* 1999;17(2):91-96. Epub 1999/07/10.
301. Tamura S, Kihara Y, Yuki Y, Sugimura H, Shimizu T, Adjei ON, et al. Pseudo lesions on CTAP secondary to arterio-portal shunts. *Clin Imaging.* 1997;21(5):359-365. Epub 1997/10/08.
302. Byun JH, Kim TK, Lee CW, Lee JK, Kim AY, Kim PN, et al. Arterioportal shunt: prevalence in small hemangiomas versus that in hepatocellular carcinomas 3 cm or smaller at two-phase helical CT. *Radiology.* 2004;232(2):354-360. Epub 2004/06/25.
303. Catalano O, Esposito M, Nunziata A, Siani A. Multiphase helical CT findings after percutaneous ablation procedures for hepatocellular carcinoma. *Abdom Imaging.* 2000;25(6): 607-614. Epub 2000/10/12.
304. Colagrande S, Carmignani L, Pagliari A, Capaccioli L, Villari N. Transient hepatic attenuation differences (THAD) not connected to focal lesions. *Radiol Med.* 2002;104(1-2):25-43. Epub 2002/10/19.

305. Quiroga S, Sebastia C, Pallisa E, Castella E, Perez-Lafuente M, Alvarez-Castells A. Improved diagnosis of hepatic perfusion disorders: value of hepatic arterial phase imaging during helical CT. *Radiographics*. 2001;21(1):65-81; questionnaire 288-294. Epub 2001/02/07.

306. Kanematsu M, Kondo H, Semelka RC, Matsuo M, Goshima S, Hoshi H, et al. Early-enhancing non-neoplastic lesions on gadolinium-enhanced MRI of the liver. *Clin Radiol*. 2003;58(10):778-786. Epub 2003/10/03.

307. Kim SR, Imoto S, Nakajima T, Ando K, Mita K, Fukuda K, et al. Scirrhous hepatocellular carcinoma displaying atypical findings on imaging studies. *World J Gastroenterol*. 2009;15(18): 2296-2299. Epub 2009/05/14.

308. Gosink BB, Leymaster CE. Ultrasonic determination of hepatomegaly. *J Clin Ultrasound*. 1981;9(1):37-44. Epub 1981/01/01.

309. Kurtz AB, Rubin CS, Cooper HS, Nisenbaum HL, Cole-Beuglet C, Medoff J, et al. Ultrasound findings in hepatitis. *Radiology*. 1980;136(3):717-723. Epub 1980/09/01.

310. Lawson TL, Thorsen MK, Erickson SJ, Perret RS, Quiroz FA, Foley WD. Periportal halo: a CT sign of liver disease. *Abdom Imaging*. 1993;18(1):42-46. Epub 1993/01/01.

311. Matsui O, Kadoya M, Takashima T, Kameyama T, Yoshikawa J, Tamura S. Intrahepatic periportal abnormal intensity on MR images: an indication of various hepatobiliary diseases. *Radiology*. 1989;171(2):335-338. Epub 1989/05/01.

312. Gimondo P, Mirk P, Messina G, Pizzi C. Abdominal lymphadenopathy in benign diseases: sonographic detection and clinical significance. *J Ultrasound Med*. 1996;15(5):353-359; quiz 61-62. Epub 1996/05/01.

313. Gore RM, Vogelzang RL, Nemcek AA Jr. Lymphadenopathy in chronic active hepatitis: CT observations. *AJR Am J Roentgenol*. 1988;151(1):75-78. Epub 1988/07/01.

314. Taylor GA. Acute hepatic disease. *Radiol Clin North Am*. 1997;35(4):799-814. Epub 1997/07/01.

315. Coakley FV, O'Reilly EM, Schwartz LH, Panicek DM, Castellino RA. Non-Hodgkin lymphoma as a cause of intrahepatic periportal low attenuation on CT. *J Comput Assist Tomogr*. 1997;21(5):726-728. Epub 1997/09/19.

316. Karcaaltincaba M, Haliloglu M, Akpinar E, Akata D, Ozmen M, Ariyurek M, et al. Multidetector CT and MRI findings in periportal space pathologies. *Eur J Radiol*. 2007;61(1):3-10. Epub 2006/11/25.

317. Gore RM, Shkolnik A. Abdominal manifestations of pediatric leukemias: sonographic assessment. *Radiology*. 1982;143(1): 207-210. Epub 1982/04/01.

318. Hainaux B, Christophe C, Hanquinet S, Perlmutter N. Gaucher disease. Plain radiography, US, CT and MR diagnosis of lungs, bone and liver lesions. *Pediatr Radiol*. 1992;22(1):78-79. Epub 1992/01/01.

319. Terk MR, Esplin J, Lee K, Magre G, Colletti PM. MR imaging of patients with type 1 Gaucher disease: relationship between bone and visceral changes. *AJR Am J Roentgenol*. 1995;165(3):599-604. Epub 1995/09/01.

320. DeMayo RF, Haims AH, McRae MC, Yang R, Mistry PK. Correlation of MRI-Based bone marrow burden score with genotype and spleen status in Gaucher disease. *AJR Am J Roentgenol*. 2008;191(1):115-123. Epub 2008/06/20.

321. Terk MR, Dardashti S, Liebman HA. Bone marrow response in treated patients with Gaucher disease: evaluation by T1-weighted magnetic resonance images and correlation with reduction in liver and spleen volume. *Skeletal Radiol*. 2000;29(10):563-571. Epub 2000/12/29.

322. Hadas-Halpern I, Deeb M, Abrahamov A, Zimran A, Elstein D. Gaucher disease: spectrum of sonographic findings in the liver. *J Ultrasound Med*. 2010;29(5):727-733. Epub 2010/04/30.

323. Patlas M, Hadas-Halpern I, Reinus C, Zimran A, Elstein D. Multiple hypoechoic hepatic lesions in a patient with Gaucher disease. *J Ultrasound Med*. 2002;21(9):1053-1055. Epub 2002/09/10.

324. Poll LW, Vom Dahl S. Image of the month. Hepatic Gaucheroma mimicking focal nodular hyperplasia. *Hepatology*. 2009;50(3): 985-986. Epub 2009/08/29.

325. Hill SC, Damaska BM, Ling A, Patterson K, Di Bisceglie AM, Brady RO, et al. Gaucher disease: abdominal MR imaging findings in 46 patients. *Radiology*. 1992;184(2):561-566. Epub 1992/08/01.

326. Lee P, Mather S, Owens C, Leonard J, Dicks-Mireaux C. Hepatic ultrasound findings in the glycogen storage diseases. *Br J Radiol*. 1994;67(803):1062-1066. Epub 1994/11/01.

327. Gossmann J, Scheuermann EH, Frilling A, Geiger H, Dietrich CF. Multiple adenomas and hepatocellular carcinoma in a renal transplant patient with glycogen storage disease type 1a (von Gierke disease). *Transplantation*. 2001;72(2):343-344. Epub 2001/07/31.

328. Franco LM, Krishnamurthy V, Bali D, Weinstein DA, Arn P, Clary B, et al. Hepatocellular carcinoma in glycogen storage disease type Ia: a case series. *J Inherit Metab Dis*. 2005;28(2):153-162. Epub 2005/05/07.

329. Rake JP, Visser G, Labrune P, Leonard JV, Ullrich K, Smit GP. Guidelines for management of glycogen storage disease type I - European Study on Glycogen Storage Disease Type I (ESGSD I). *Eur J Pediatr*. 2002;161(suppl 1):S112-S119. Epub 2002/10/10.

330. Gertz MA, Kyle RA, Thibodeau SN. Familial amyloidosis: a study of 52 North American-born patients examined during a 30-year period. *Mayo Clin Proc*. 1992;67(5):428-440. Epub 1992/05/01.

331. Gertz MA, Kyle RA. Hepatic amyloidosis: clinical appraisal in 77 patients. *Hepatology*. 1997;25(1):118-121. Epub 1997/01/01.

332. Kim SH, Han JK, Lee KH, Won HJ, Kim KW, Kim JS, et al. Abdominal amyloidosis: spectrum of radiological findings. *Clin Radiol*. 2003;58(8):610-620. Epub 2003/07/31.

333. Monzawa S, Tsukamoto T, Omata K, Hosoda K, Araki T, Sugimura K. A case with primary amyloidosis of the liver and spleen: radiologic findings. *Eur J Radiol*. 2002;41(3):237-241. Epub 2002/02/28.

334. Dursun M, Ayyildiz O, Yilmaz S, Bilici A. An unusual presentation of primary amyloidosis. *Saudi Med J*. 2004;25(10):1478-1481. Epub 2004/10/21.

335. Suzuki S, Takizawa K, Nakajima Y, Katayama M, Sagawa F. CT findings in hepatic and splenic amyloidosis. *J Comput Assist Tomogr*. 1986;10(2):332-334. Epub 1986/03/01.

336. Mainenti PP, Camera L, Nicotra S, Cantalupo T, Soscia E, Di Vizio D, et al. Splenic hypoperfusion as a sign of systemic amyloidosis. *Abdom Imaging*. 2005;30(6):768-772. Epub 2005/08/13.

337. Angulo P. Nonalcoholic fatty liver disease. *N Engl J Med*. 2002;346(16):1221-1231. Epub 2002/04/19.

338. Tan HH, Virmani S, Martin P. Controversies in the management of alcoholic liver disease. *Mt Sinai J Med.* 2009;76(5):484-498. Epub 2009/09/30.

339. Schwenzer NF, Springer F, Schraml C, Stefan N, Machann J, Schick F. Non-invasive assessment and quantification of liver steatosis by ultrasound, computed tomography and magnetic resonance. *J Hepatol.* 2009;51(3):433-445. Epub 2009/07/17.

340. Ford ES, Giles WH, Dietz WH. Prevalence of the metabolic syndrome among US adults: findings from the third National Health and Nutrition Examination Survey. *JAMA.* 2002;287(3):356-359. Epub 2002/01/16.

341. Oliva MR, Mortele KJ, Segatto E, Glickman JN, Erturk SM, Ros PR, et al. Computed tomography features of nonalcoholic steatohepatitis with histopathologic correlation. *J Comput Assist Tomogr.* 2006;30(1):37-43. Epub 2005/12/21.

342. Saverymuttu SH, Joseph AE, Maxwell JD. Ultrasound scanning in the detection of hepatic fibrosis and steatosis. *Br Med J (Clin Res Ed).* 1986;292(6512):13-15. Epub 1986/01/04.

343. Webb M, Yeshua H, Zelber-Sagi S, Santo E, Brazowski E, Halpern Z, et al. Diagnostic value of a computerized hepatorenal index for sonographic quantification of liver steatosis. *AJR Am J Roentgenol.* 2009;192(4):909-914. Epub 2009/03/24.

344. Jain KA, McGahan JP. Spectrum of CT and sonographic appearance of fatty infiltration of the liver. *Clin Imaging.* 1993;17(2):162-168. Epub 1993/04/01.

345. Piekarski J, Goldberg HI, Royal SA, Axel L, Moss AA. Difference between liver and spleen CT numbers in the normal adult: its usefulness in predicting the presence of diffuse liver disease. *Radiology.* 1980;137(3):727-729. Epub 1980/12/01.

346. Jacobs JE, Birnbaum BA, Shapiro MA, Langlotz CP, Slosman F, Rubesin SE, et al. Diagnostic criteria for fatty infiltration of the liver on contrast-enhanced helical CT. *AJR Am J Roentgenol.* 1998;171(3):659-664. Epub 1998/09/02.

347. Johnston RJ, Stamm ER, Lewin JM, Hendrick RE, Archer PG. Diagnosis of fatty infiltration of the liver on contrast enhanced CT: limitations of liver-minus-spleen attenuation difference measurements. *Abdom Imaging.* 1998;23(4):409-415. Epub 1998/07/15.

348. Panicek DM, Giess CS, Schwartz LH. Qualitative assessment of liver for fatty infiltration on contrast-enhanced CT: is muscle a better standard of reference than spleen? *J Comput Assist Tomogr.* 1997;21(5):699-705. Epub 1997/09/19.

349. Lee JK, Dixon WT, Ling D, Levitt RG, Murphy WA Jr. Fatty infiltration of the liver: demonstration by proton spectroscopic imaging. Preliminary observations. *Radiology.* 1984;153(1): 195-201. Epub 1984/10/01.

350. Siegelman ES. MR imaging of diffuse liver disease. Hepatic fat and iron. *Magn Reson Imaging Clin N Am.* 1997;5(2):347-365. Epub 1997/05/01.

351. Saadeh S, Younossi ZM, Remer EM, Gramlich T, Ong JP, Hurley M, et al. The utility of radiological imaging in nonalcoholic fatty liver disease. *Gastroenterology.* 2002;123(3):745-750. Epub 2002/08/29.

352. Kalra N, Duseja A, Das A, Dhiman RK, Virmani V, Chawla Y, et al. Chemical shift magnetic resonance imaging is helpful in detecting hepatic steatosis but not fibrosis in patients with nonalcoholic fatty liver disease (NAFLD). *Ann Hepatol.* 2009;8(1):21-25. Epub 2009/02/18.

353. Neuschwander-Tetri BA. Nonalcoholic steatohepatitis: an evolving diagnosis. *Can J Gastroenterol.* 2000;14(4):321-326. Epub 2000/05/08.

354. Andrews NC. Disorders of iron metabolism. *N Engl J Med.* 1999;341(26):1986-1995. Epub 1999/12/23.

355. Olynyk JK, St Pierre TG, Britton RS, Brunt EM, Bacon BR. Duration of hepatic iron exposure increases the risk of significant fibrosis in hereditary hemochromatosis: a new role for magnetic resonance imaging. *Am J Gastroenterol.* 2005;100(4):837-841. Epub 2005/03/24.

356. Yoon DY, Choi BI, Han JK, Han MC, Park MO, Suh SJ. MR findings of secondary hemochromatosis: transfusional vs erythropoietic. *J Comput Assist Tomogr.* 1994;18(3):416-419. Epub 1994/05/01.

357. Pomerantz S, Siegelman ES. MR imaging of iron depositional disease. *Magn Reson Imaging Clin N Am.* 2002;10(1):105-120, vi. Epub 2002/05/10.

358. Ptaszek LM, Price ET, Hu MY, Yang PC. Early diagnosis of hemochromatosis-related cardiomyopathy with magnetic resonance imaging. *J Cardiovasc Magn Reson.* 2005;7(4): 689-692. Epub 2005/09/03.

359. Ueda J, Kobayashi Y, Kenko Y, Koike H, Kubo T, Takano Y, et al. Distribution of water, fat, and metals in normal liver and in liver metastases influencing attenuation on computed tomography. *Acta Radiol.* 1988;29(1):33-39. Epub 1988/01/01.

360. Jager HJ, Mehring U, Gotz GF, Neise M, Erlemann R, Kapp HJ, et al. Radiological features of the visceral and skeletal involvement of hemochromatosis. *Eur Radiol.* 1997;7(8):1199-1206. Epub 1997/01/01.

361. Guyader D, Gandon Y, Robert JY, Heautot JF, Jouanolle H, Jacquelinet C, et al. Magnetic resonance imaging and assessment of liver iron content in genetic hemochromatosis. *J Hepatol.* 1992;15(3):304-308. Epub 1992/07/01.

362. Gandon Y, Guyader D, Heautot JF, Reda MI, Yaouanq J, Buhe T, et al. Hemochromatosis: diagnosis and quantification of liver iron with gradient-echo MR imaging. *Radiology.* 1994;193(2):533-538. Epub 1994/11/01.

363. Patrick D, White FE, Adams PC. Long-term amiodarone therapy: a cause of increased hepatic attenuation on CT. *Br J Radiol.* 1984;57(679):573-576. Epub 1984/07/01.

364. Kew MC. Epidemiology of chronic hepatitis B virus infection, hepatocellular carcinoma, and hepatitis B virus-induced hepatocellular carcinoma. *Pathol Biol (Paris).* 2010;58(4): 273-277. Epub 2010/04/10.

365. Yuen MF, Lai CL. Treatment of chronic hepatitis B: Evolution over two decades. *J Gastroenterol Hepatol.* 2011;26(suppl 1): 138-143. Epub 2011/01/14.

366. Teoh NC, Farrell GC, Chan HL. Individualisation of antiviral therapy for chronic hepatitis C. *J Gastroenterol Hepatol.* 2010;25(7):1206-1216. Epub 2010/07/03.

367. Waalen J, Beutler E. Hereditary hemochromatosis: screening and management. *Curr Hematol Rep.* 2006;5(1):34-40. Epub 2006/03/16.

368. Schuppan D, Afdhal NH. Liver cirrhosis. *Lancet.* 2008; 371(9615):838-851. Epub 2008/03/11.

369. Giorgio A, Amoroso P, Fico P, Lettieri G, Finelli L, de Stefano G, et al. Ultrasound evaluation of uncomplicated and complicated acute viral hepatitis. *J Clin Ultrasound.* 1986;14(9):675-679. Epub 1986/11/01.

370. Itoh H, Sakai T, Takahashi N, Kitada M, Saito M, Kataoka M, et al. Periportal high intensity on T2-weighted MR images in acute viral hepatitis. *J Comput Assist Tomogr.* 1992;16(4): 564-567. Epub 1992/07/01.

371. Outwater E, Kaplan MM, Bankoff MS. Lymphadenopathy in sclerosing cholangitis: pitfall in the diagnosis of malignant biliary obstruction. *Gastrointest Radiol.* 1992;17(2):157-160. Epub 1992/01/01.

372. Bilaj F, Hyslop WB, Rivero H, Firat Z, Vaidean G, Shrestha R, et al. MR imaging findings in autoimmune hepatitis: correlation with clinical staging. *Radiology.* 2005;236(3): 896-902. Epub 2005/08/25.

373. Cassani F, Zoli M, Baffoni L, Cordiani MR, Brunori A, Bianchi FB, et al. Prevalence and significance of abdominal lymphadenopathy in patients with chronic liver disease: an ultrasound study. *J Clin Gastroenterol.* 1990;12(1):42-46. Epub 1990/02/01.

374. Hamer OW, Aguirre DA, Casola G, Sirlin CB. Imaging features of perivascular fatty infiltration of the liver: initial observations. *Radiology.* 2005;237(1):159-169. Epub 2005/08/16.

375. Mitchell DG, Navarro VJ, Herrine SK, Bergin D, Parker L, Frangos A, et al. Compensated hepatitis C: unenhanced MR imaging correlated with pathologic grading and staging. *Abdom Imaging.* 2008;33(1):58-64. Epub 2007/03/28.

376. Charatcharoenwitthaya P, Lindor KD. Role of radiologic modalities in the management of non-alcoholic steatohepatitis. *Clin Liver Dis.* 2007;11(1):37-54, viii. Epub 2007/06/05.

377. Gupte P, Amarapurkar D, Agal S, Baijal R, Kulshrestha P, Pramanik S, et al. Non-alcoholic steatohepatitis in type 2 diabetes mellitus. *J Gastroenterol Hepatol.* 2004;19(8):854-858. Epub 2004/07/10.

378. Awaya H, Mitchell DG, Kamishima T, Holland G, Ito K, Matsumoto T. Cirrhosis: modified caudate-right lobe ratio. *Radiology.* 2002;224(3):769-774. Epub 2002/08/31.

379. Vilgrain V, Condat B, Bureau C, Hakime A, Plessier A, Cazals-Hatem D, et al. Atrophy-hypertrophy complex in patients with cavernous transformation of the portal vein: CT evaluation. *Radiology.* 2006;241(1):149-155. Epub 2006/08/16.

380. Gurkaynak G, Yildirim B, Aksoy F, Temucin G. Sonographic findings in noncirrhotic portal fibrosis. *J Clin Ultrasound.* 1998;26(6):309-313. Epub 1998/06/26.

381. Mathiesen UL, Franzen LE, Aselius H, Resjo M, Jacobsson L, Foberg U, et al. Increased liver echogenicity at ultrasound examination reflects degree of steatosis but not of fibrosis in asymptomatic patients with mild/moderate abnormalities of liver transaminases. *Dig Liver Dis.* 2002;34(7):516-522. Epub 2002/09/19.

382. Freeman MP, Vick CW, Taylor KJ, Carithers RL, Brewer WH. Regenerating nodules in cirrhosis: sonographic appearance with anatomic correlation. *AJR Am J Roentgenol.* 1986;146(3):533-536. Epub 1986/03/01.

383. Di Lelio A, Cestari C, Lomazzi A, Beretta L. Cirrhosis: diagnosis with sonographic study of the liver surface. *Radiology.* 1989;172(2):389-392. Epub 1989/08/01.

384. Freeny PC, Grossholz M, Kaakaji K, Schmiedl UP. Significance of hyperattenuating and contrast-enhancing hepatic nodules detected in the cirrhotic liver during arterial phase helical CT in pre-liver transplant patients: radiologic-histopathologic correlation of explanted livers. *Abdom Imaging.* 2003;28(3): 333-346. Epub 2003/04/30.

385. Keedy A, Westphalen AC, Qayyum A, Aslam R, Rybkin AV, Chen MH, et al. Diagnosis of cirrhosis by spiral computed tomography: a case-control study with feature analysis and assessment of interobserver agreement. *J Comput Assist Tomogr.* 2008;32(2):198-203. Epub 2008/04/02.

386. Giorgio A, Amoroso P, Lettieri G, Fico P, de Stefano G, Finelli L, et al. Cirrhosis: value of caudate to right lobe ratio in diagnosis with US. *Radiology.* 1986;161(2):443-445. Epub 1986/11/01.

387. Okazaki H, Ito K, Fujita T, Koike S, Takano K, Matsunaga N. Discrimination of alcoholic from virus-induced cirrhosis on MR imaging. *AJR Am J Roentgenol.* 2000;175(6):1677-1681. Epub 2000/11/25.

388. Zhou XP, Lu T, Wei YG, Chen XZ. Liver volume variation in patients with virus-induced cirrhosis: findings on MDCT. *AJR Am J Roentgenol.* 2007;189(3):W153-W159. Epub 2007/08/24.

389. Krinsky GA, Lee VS. MR imaging of cirrhotic nodules. *Abdom Imaging.* 2000;25(5):471-482. Epub 2000/08/10.

390. Ohno A, Ohta Y, Ohtomo K, Hirata K, Takatsuki K, Mochida S, et al. Magnetic resonance imaging in chronic liver disease evaluated in relation to hepatic fibrosis—clinical and experimental results. *Radiat Med.* 1990;8(5):159-163. Epub 1990/09/01.

391. Aube C, Moal F, Oberti F, Roux J, Croquet V, Gallois Y, et al. Diagnosis and measurement of liver fibrosis by MRI in bile duct ligated rats. *Dig Dis Sci.* 2007;52(10):2601-2609. Epub 2007/04/13.

392. Semelka RC, Chung JJ, Hussain SM, Marcos HB, Woosley JT. Chronic hepatitis: correlation of early patchy and late linear enhancement patterns on gadolinium-enhanced MR images with histopathology initial experience. *J Magn Reson Imaging.* 2001;13(3):385-391. Epub 2001/03/10.

393. Vitellas KM, Tzalonikou MT, Bennett WF, Vaswani KK, Bova JG. Cirrhosis: spectrum of findings on unenhanced and dynamic gadolinium-enhanced MR imaging. *Abdom Imaging.* 2001;26(6):601-615. Epub 2002/03/22.

394. Sandrin L, Fourquet B, Hasquenoph JM, Yon S, Fournier C, Mal F, et al. Transient elastography: a new noninvasive method for assessment of hepatic fibrosis. *Ultrasound Med Biol.* 2003;29(12):1705-1713. Epub 2003/12/31.

395. Huwart L, Sempoux C, Salameh N, Jamart J, Annet L, Sinkus R, et al. Liver fibrosis: noninvasive assessment with MR elastography versus aspartate aminotransferase-to-platelet ratio index. *Radiology.* 2007;245(2):458-466. Epub 2007/10/18.

396. Yoneda M, Mawatari H, Fujita K, Endo H, Iida H, Nozaki Y, et al. Noninvasive assessment of liver fibrosis by measurement of stiffness in patients with nonalcoholic fatty liver disease (NAFLD). *Dig Liver Dis.* 2008;40(5):371-378. Epub 2007/12/18.

397. Asbach P, Klatt D, Schlosser B, Biermer M, Muche M, Rieger A, et al. Viscoelasticity-based Staging of Hepatic Fibrosis with Multifrequency MR Elastography. *Radiology.* 2010. Epub 2010/08/04.

398. Koslin DB, Berland LL. Duplex Doppler examination of the liver and portal venous system. *J Clin Ultrasound.* 1987;15(9):675-686. Epub 1987/11/01.

399. Koslin DB, Mulligan SA, Berland LL. Duplex assessment of the portal venous system. *Semin Ultrasound CT MR.* 1992;13(1):22-33. Epub 1992/02/01.

400. Marn CS, Francis IR. CT of portal venous occlusion. *AJR Am J Roentgenol.* 1992;159(4):717-726. Epub 1992/10/01.

401. Vogelzang RL, Gore RM, Anschuetz SL, Blei AT. Thrombosis of the splanchnic veins: CT diagnosis. *AJR Am J Roentgenol.* 1988;150(1):93-96. Epub 1988/01/01.

402. Applegate GR, Thaete FL, Meyers SP, Davis PL, Talagala SL, Recht M, et al. Blood flow in the portal vein: velocity quantitation with phase-contrast MR angiography. *Radiology.* 1993;187(1):253-256. Epub 1993/04/01.

403. Merkel C, Bolognesi M, Berzigotti A, Amodio P, Cavasin L, Casarotto IM, et al. Clinical significance of worsening portal hypertension during long-term medical treatment in patients with cirrhosis who had been classified as early good-responders on haemodynamic criteria. *J Hepatol.* 2010;52(1):45-53. Epub 2009/11/17.

404. Sharma MP, Dasarathy S, Misra SC, Saksena S, Sundaram KR. Sonographic signs in portal hypertension: a multivariate analysis. *Trop Gastroenterol.* 1996;17(2):23-29. Epub 1996/04/01.

405. Kanematsu M, Hoshi H, Yamada T, Murakami T, Kim T, Kato M, et al. Small hepatic nodules in cirrhosis: ultrasonographic, CT, and MR imaging findings. *Abdom Imaging.* 1999;24(1):47-55. Epub 1999/02/06.

406. Dodd GD 3rd, Baron RL, Oliver JH 3rd, Federle MP. Spectrum of imaging findings of the liver in end-stage cirrhosis: Part II, focal abnormalities. *AJR Am J Roentgenol.* 1999;173(5):1185-1192. Epub 1999/11/30.

407. Taylor AJ, Carmody TJ, Quiroz FA, Erickson SJ, Varma RR, Komorowski RA, et al. Focal masses in cirrhotic liver: CT and MR imaging features. *AJR Am J Roentgenol.* 1994;163(4): 857-862. Epub 1994/10/01.

408. de Ledinghen V, Laharie D, Lecesne R, Le Bail B, Winnock M, Bernard PH, et al. Detection of nodules in liver cirrhosis: spiral computed tomography or magnetic resonance imaging? A prospective study of 88 nodules in 34 patients. *Eur J Gastroenterol Hepatol.* 2002;14(2):159-165. Epub 2002/05/01.

409. Earls JP, Theise ND, Weinreb JC, DeCorato DR, Krinsky GA, Rofsky NM, et al. Dysplastic nodules and hepatocellular carcinoma: thin-section MR imaging of explanted cirrhotic livers with pathologic correlation. *Radiology.* 1996;201(1): 207-214. Epub 1996/10/01.

410. Rode A, Bancel B, Douek P, Chevallier M, Vilgrain V, Picaud G, et al. Small nodule detection in cirrhotic livers: evaluation with US, spiral CT, and MRI and correlation with pathologic examination of explanted liver. *J Comput Assist Tomogr.* 2001;25(3):327-336. Epub 2001/05/15.

411. Krinsky GA, Theise ND, Rofsky NM, Mizrachi H, Tepperman LW, Weinreb JC. Dysplastic nodules in cirrhotic liver: arterial phase enhancement at CT and MR imaging—a case report. *Radiology.* 1998;209(2):461-464. Epub 1998/11/10.

412. Murakami T, Nakamura H, Hori S, Nakanishi K, Mitani T, Tsuda K, et al. CT and MRI of siderotic regenerating nodules in hepatic cirrhosis. *J Comput Assist Tomogr.* 1992;16(4):578-582. Epub 1992/07/01.

413. Onaya H, Itai Y. MR imaging of hepatocellular carcinoma. *Magn Reson Imaging Clin N Am.* 2000;8(4):757-768. Epub 2001/01/10.

414. Ishigami K, Yoshimitsu K, Nishihara Y, Irie H, Asayama Y, Tajima T, et al. Hepatocellular carcinoma with a pseudocapsule on gadolinium-enhanced MR images: correlation with histopathologic findings. *Radiology.* 2009;250(2):435-443. Epub 2008/12/20.

415. Regan LS. Screening for hepatocellular carcinoma in high-risk individuals. A clinical review. *Arch Intern Med.* 1989;149(8):1741-1744. Epub 1989/08/01.

416. Hassan MM, Frome A, Patt YZ, El-Serag HB. Rising prevalence of hepatitis C virus infection among patients recently diagnosed with hepatocellular carcinoma in the United States. *J Clin Gastroenterol.* 2002;35(3):266-269. Epub 2002/08/23.

417. El-Serag HB. Hepatocellular carcinoma and hepatitis C in the United States. *Hepatology.* 2002;36(5 suppl 1):S74-S83. Epub 2002/10/31.

418. Shekhar KC. Tropical gastrointestinal disease: hepatosplenic schistosomiasis—pathological, clinical and treatment review. *Singapore Med J.* 1994;35(6):616-621. Epub 1994/12/01.

419. Andre F. Hepatitis B epidemiology in Asia, the Middle East and Africa. *Vaccine.* 2000;18(suppl 1):S20-S22. Epub 2000/02/23.

420. Arguedas MR, Chen VK, Eloubeidi MA, Fallon MB. Screening for hepatocellular carcinoma in patients with hepatitis C cirrhosis: a cost-utility analysis. *Am J Gastroenterol.* 2003;98(3):679-690. Epub 2003/03/26.

421. Federle MP. Use of radiologic techniques to screen for hepatocellular carcinoma. *J Clin Gastroenterol.* 2002;35 (5 suppl 2):S92-S100. Epub 2002/10/24.

422. Krinsky GA, Lee VS, Theise ND, Weinreb JC, Morgan GR, Diflo T, et al. Transplantation for hepatocellular carcinoma and cirrhosis: sensitivity of magnetic resonance imaging. *Liver Transpl.* 2002;8(12):1156-1164. Epub 2002/12/11.

423. Forner A, Vilana R, Ayuso C, Bianchi L, Sole M, Ayuso JR, et al. Diagnosis of hepatic nodules 20 mm or smaller in cirrhosis: Prospective validation of the noninvasive diagnostic criteria for hepatocellular carcinoma. *Hepatology.* 2008;47(1):97-104. Epub 2007/12/12.

424. Kitao A, Zen Y, Matsui O, Gabata T, Kobayashi S, Koda W, et al. Hepatocellular Carcinoma: Signal Intensity at Gadoxetic Acid-enhanced MR Imaging—Correlation with Molecular Transporters and Histopathologic Features. *Radiology.* 2010. Epub 2010/07/29.

425. Ahn SS, Kim MJ, Lim JS, Hong HS, Chung YE, Choi JY. Added value of gadoxetic acid-enhanced hepatobiliary phase MR imaging in the diagnosis of hepatocellular carcinoma. *Radiology.* 2010;255(2):459-466. Epub 2010/04/24.

426. Pomfret EA, Washburn K, Wald C, Nalesnik MA, Douglas D, Russo M, et al. Report of a national conference on liver allocation in patients with hepatocellular carcinoma in the United States. *Liver Transpl.* 2010;16(3):262-278. Epub 2010/03/09.

427. Sakamoto M, Hirohashi S, Shimosato Y. Early stages of multistep hepatocarcinogenesis: adenomatous hyperplasia and early hepatocellular carcinoma. *Hum Pathol.* 1991;22(2) :172-178. Epub 1991/02/01.

428. Romeo R, Colombo M. The natural history of hepatocellular carcinoma. *Toxicology.* 2002;181-182:39-42. Epub 2002/12/31.

429. Hussain SM, Zondervan PE, JN IJ, Schalm SW, de Man RA, Krestin GP. Benign versus malignant hepatic nodules: MR imaging findings with pathologic correlation. *Radiographics.* 2002;22(5):1023-1036; discussion 37-39. Epub 2002/09/18.

430. Liang TJ, Heller T. Pathogenesis of hepatitis C-associated hepatocellular carcinoma. *Gastroenterology.* 2004;127 (5 suppl 1):S62-S71. Epub 2004/10/28.

431. Tabor E. Pathogenesis of hepatitis B virus-associated hepatocellular carcinoma. *Hepatol Res.* 2007;37(suppl 2): S110-S114. Epub 2007/09/20.

432. Kowdley KV. Iron, hemochromatosis, and hepatocellular carcinoma. *Gastroenterology.* 2004;127(5 suppl 1):S79-S86. Epub 2004/10/28.

433. Honda H, Kaneko K, Maeda T, Kuroiwa T, Fukuya T, Yoshimitsu K, et al. Small hepatocellular carcinomas undetected on two-phased incremental computed tomography. Angiographic and clinicopathologic findings. *Invest Radiol.* 1995;30(8):458-465. Epub 1995/08/01.

434. Yoshimatsu S, Inoue Y, Ibukuro K, Suzuki S. Hypovascular hepatocellular carcinoma undetected at angiography and CT with iodized oil. *Radiology.* 1989;171(2):343-347. Epub 1989/05/01.

435. Han YS, Choi DL, Park JB. Cirrhotomimetic type hepatocellular carcinoma diagnosed after liver transplantation—eighteen months of follow-up: a case report. *Transplant Proc.* 2008;40(8): 2835-2836. Epub 2008/10/22.

436. Choi BI, Kim CW, Han MC, Kim CY, Lee HS, Kim ST, et al. Sonographic characteristics of small hepatocellular carcinoma. *Gastrointest Radiol.* 1989;14(3):255-261. Epub 1989/01/01.

437. Xu HX, Xie XY, Lu MD, Liu GJ, Xu ZF, Zheng YL, et al. Contrast-enhanced sonography in the diagnosis of small hepatocellular carcinoma < or =2 cm. *J Clin Ultrasound.* 2008;36(5):257-266. Epub 2007/12/20.

438. Carlos RC, Kim HM, Hussain HK, Francis IR, Nghiem HV, Fendrick AM. Developing a prediction rule to assess hepatic malignancy in patients with cirrhosis. *AJR Am J Roentgenol.* 2003;180(4):893-900. Epub 2003/03/21.

439. Grazioli L, Olivetti L, Fugazzola C, Benetti A, Stanga C, Dettori E, et al. The pseudocapsule in hepatocellular carcinoma: correlation between dynamic MR imaging and pathology. *Eur Radiol.* 1999;9(1):62-67. Epub 1999/02/05.

440. Balci NC, Befeler AS, Bieneman BK, Fattahi R, Saglam S, Havlioglu N. Fat containing HCC: findings on CT and MRI including serial contrast-enhanced imaging. *Acad Radiol.* 2009;16(8):963-968. Epub 2009/04/24.

441. Ryder SD. Guidelines for the diagnosis and treatment of hepatocellular carcinoma (HCC) in adults. *Gut.* 2003;52(suppl 3):iii1-iii8. Epub 2003/04/15.

442. Honda H, Onitsuka H, Adachi E, Ochiai K, Gibo M, Yasumori K, et al. Hepatocellular carcinoma: prospective assessments of the T-factor with CT, US, and MR imaging. *Abdom Imaging.* 1993;18(3):247-252. Epub 1993/01/01.

443. Shah ZK, McKernan MG, Hahn PF, Sahani DV. Enhancing and expansile portal vein thrombosis: value in the diagnosis of hepatocellular carcinoma in patients with multiple hepatic lesions. *AJR Am J Roentgenol.* 2007;188(5):1320-1323. Epub 2007/04/24.

444. Watanabe J, Nakashima O, Kojiro M. Clinicopathologic study on lymph node metastasis of hepatocellular carcinoma: a retrospective study of 660 consecutive autopsy cases. *Jpn J Clin Oncol.* 1994;24(1):37-41. Epub 1994/02/01.

445. Katyal S, Oliver JH 3rd, Peterson MS, Ferris JV, Carr BS, Baron RL. Extrahepatic metastases of hepatocellular carcinoma. *Radiology.* 2000;216(3):698-703. Epub 2000/08/31.

446. Mazzaferro V, Regalia E, Doci R, Andreola S, Pulvirenti A, Bozzetti F, et al. Liver transplantation for the treatment of small hepatocellular carcinomas in patients with cirrhosis. *N Engl J Med.* 1996;334(11):693-639. Epub 1996/03/14.

447. Roche A. Therapy of HCC—TACE for liver tumor. *Hepatogastroenterology.* 2001;48(37):3-7. Epub 2001/03/28.

448. Lau WY, Leung TW, Yu SC, Ho SK. Percutaneous local ablative therapy for hepatocellular carcinoma: a review and look into the future. *Ann Surg.* 2003;237(2):171-179. Epub 2003/02/01.

449. Yao FY, Ferrell L, Bass NM, Watson JJ, Bacchetti P, Venook A, et al. Liver transplantation for hepatocellular carcinoma: expansion of the tumor size limits does not adversely impact survival. *Hepatology.* 2001;33(6):1394-1403. Epub 2001/06/08.

450. Llovet JM, Ricci S, Mazzaferro V, Hilgard P, Gane E, Blanc JF, et al. Sorafenib in advanced hepatocellular carcinoma. *N Engl J Med.* 2008;359(4):378-390. Epub 2008/07/25.

451. Young ST, Paulson EK, Washington K, Gulliver DJ, Vredenburgh JJ, Baker ME. CT of the liver in patients with metastatic breast carcinoma treated by chemotherapy: findings simulating cirrhosis. *AJR Am J Roentgenol.* 1994;163(6):1385-1388. Epub 1994/12/01.

452. Kang SP, Taddei T, McLennan B, Lacy J. Pseudocirrhosis in a pancreatic cancer patient with liver metastases: a case report of complete resolution of pseudocirrhosis with an early recognition and management. *World J Gastroenterol.* 2008;14(10):1622-1624. Epub 2008/03/12.

453. Robinson PJ. The effects of cancer chemotherapy on liver imaging. *Eur Radiol.* 2009;19(7):1752-1762. Epub 2009/02/25.

454. Sempoux C, Horsmans Y, Geubel A, Fraikin J, Van Beers BE, Gigot JF, et al. Severe radiation-induced liver disease following localized radiation therapy for biliopancreatic carcinoma: activation of hepatic stellate cells as an early event. *Hepatology.* 1997;26(1):128-134. Epub 1997/07/01.

455. Garra BS, Shawker TH, Chang R, Kaplan K, White RD. The ultrasound appearance of radiation-induced hepatic injury. Correlation with computed tomography and magnetic resonance imaging. *J Ultrasound Med.* 1988;7(11):605-609. Epub 1988/11/01.

456. Itai Y, Murata S, Kurosaki Y. Straight border sign of the liver: spectrum of CT appearances and causes. *Radiographics.* 1995;15(5):1089-1102. Epub 1995/09/01.

457. Cutillo DP, Swayne LC, Fasciano MG, Schwartz JR. Absence of fatty replacement in radiation damaged liver: CT demonstration. *J Comput Assist Tomogr.* 1989;13(2):259-261. Epub 1989/03/01.

458. Unger EC, Lee JK, Weyman PJ. CT and MR imaging of radiation hepatitis. *J Comput Assist Tomogr.* 1987;11(2):264-268. Epub 1987/03/01.

459. Aydinli M, Bayraktar Y. Budd-Chiari syndrome: etiology, pathogenesis and diagnosis. *World J Gastroenterol.* 2007;13(19):2693-2696. Epub 2007/06/15.

460. Darwish Murad S, Plessier A, Hernandez-Guerra M, Fabris F, Eapen CE, Bahr MJ, et al. Etiology, management, and outcome of the Budd-Chiari syndrome. *Ann Intern Med.* 2009;151(3): 167-175. Epub 2009/08/05.

461. Moulton JS, Miller BL, Dodd GD 3rd, Vu DN. Passive hepatic congestion in heart failure: CT abnormalities. *AJR Am J Roentgenol.* 1988;151(5):939-942. Epub 1988/11/01.

462. DeLeve LD, Shulman HM, McDonald GB. Toxic injury to hepatic sinusoids: sinusoidal obstruction syndrome (veno-occlusive disease). *Semin Liver Dis.* 2002;22(1):27-42. Epub 2002/04/03.

463. Marudanayagam R, Shanmugam V, Gunson B, Mirza DF, Mayer D, Buckels J, et al. Aetiology and outcome of acute liver failure. *HPB (Oxford).* 2009;11(5):429-434. Epub 2009/09/22.

464. Camera L, Mainenti PP, Di Giacomo A, Romano M, Rispo A, Alfinito F, et al. Triphasic helical CT in Budd-Chiari syndrome: patterns of enhancement in acute, subacute and chronic disease. *Clin Radiol.* 2006;61(4):331-337. Epub 2006/03/21.

465. Erden A, Erden I, Yurdaydin C, Karayalcin S. Hepatic outflow obstruction: enhancement patterns of the liver on MR angiography. *Eur J Radiol.* 2003;48(2):203-208. Epub 2003/12/19.

466. Holley HC, Koslin DB, Berland LL, Stanley RJ. Inhomogeneous enhancement of liver parenchyma secondary to passive congestion: contrast-enhanced CT. *Radiology.* 1989;170 (3 Pt 1):795-800. Epub 1989/03/01.

467. Fitoz S, Atasoy C, Yagmurlu A, Akyar S. Segmental hyperattenuation in the liver as a result of right hepatic vein thrombosis: an unusual complication of central venous catheterization. *Australas Radiol.* 2002;46(3):299-301. Epub 2002/08/28.

468. Noone TC, Semelka RC, Siegelman ES, Balci NC, Hussain SM, Kim PN, et al. Budd-Chiari syndrome: spectrum of appearances of acute, subacute, and chronic disease with magnetic resonance imaging. *J Magn Reson Imaging.* 2000;11(1):44-50. Epub 2000/02/17.

469. Miller WJ, Federle MP, Straub WH, Davis PL. Budd-Chiari syndrome: imaging with pathologic correlation. *Abdom Imaging.* 1993;18(4):329-335. Epub 1993/01/01.

470. Singh V, Sinha SK, Nain CK, Bambery P, Kaur U, Verma S, et al. Budd-Chiari syndrome: our experience of 71 patients. *J Gastroenterol Hepatol.* 2000;15(5):550-554. Epub 2000/06/10.

471. Chawla Y, Kumar S, Dhiman RK, Suri S, Dilawari JB. Duplex Doppler sonography in patients with Budd-Chiari syndrome. *J Gastroenterol Hepatol.* 1999;14(9):904-907. Epub 1999/10/27.

472. Boozari B, Bahr MJ, Kubicka S, Klempnauer J, Manns MP, Gebel M. Ultrasonography in patients with Budd-Chiari syndrome: diagnostic signs and prognostic implications. *J Hepatol.* 2008;49(4):572-580. Epub 2008/07/16.

473. Noone TC, Semelka RC, Woosley JT, Pisano ED. Ultrasound and MR findings in acute Budd-Chiari syndrome with histopathologic correlation. *J Comput Assist Tomogr.* 1996;20(5):819-822. Epub 1996/09/01.

474. Brancatelli G, Federle MP, Grazioli L, Golfieri R, Lencioni R. Large regenerative nodules in Budd-Chiari syndrome and other vascular disorders of the liver: CT and MR imaging findings with clinicopathologic correlation. *AJR Am J Roentgenol.* 2002;178(4):877-883. Epub 2002/03/22.

475. Moucari R, Rautou PE, Cazals-Hatem D, Geara A, Bureau C, Consigny Y, et al. Hepatocellular carcinoma in Budd-Chiari syndrome: characteristics and risk factors. *Gut.* 2008;57(6):828-835. Epub 2008/01/26.

476. Rha SE, Lee MG, Lee YS, Kang GH, Ha HK, Kim PN, et al. Nodular regenerative hyperplasia of the liver in Budd-Chiari syndrome: CT and MR features. *Abdom Imaging.* 2000;25(3): 255-258. Epub 2000/05/24.

477. Bodner G, Peer S, Karner M, Perkmann R, Neuhauser B, Vogel W, et al. Nontumorous vascular malformations in the liver: color Doppler ultrasonographic findings. *J Ultrasound Med.* 2002;21(2):187-197. Epub 2002/02/09.

478. Govani FS, Shovlin CL. Hereditary haemorrhagic telangiectasia: a clinical and scientific review. *Eur J Hum Genet.* 2009;17(7): 860-871. Epub 2009/04/02.

479. Buscarini E, Plauchu H, Garcia Tsao G, White RI Jr, Sabba C, Miller F, et al. Liver involvement in hereditary hemorrhagic telangiectasia: consensus recommendations. *Liver Int.* 2006;26(9):1040-1046. Epub 2006/10/13.

480. Buonamico P, Suppressa P, Lenato GM, Pasculli G, D'Ovidio F, Memeo M, et al. Liver involvement in a large cohort of patients with hereditary hemorrhagic telangiectasia: echo-color-Doppler vs multislice computed tomography study. *J Hepatol.* 2008;48(5):811-820. Epub 2008/03/07.

481. Cloogman HM, DiCapo RD. Hereditary hemorrhagic telangiectasia: sonographic findings in the liver. *Radiology.* 1984;150(2):521-522. Epub 1984/02/01.

482. Naganuma H, Ishida H, Niizawa M, Igarashi K, Shioya T, Masamune O. Hepatic involvement in Osler-Weber-Rendu disease: findings on pulsed and color Doppler sonography. *AJR Am J Roentgenol.* 1995;165(6):1421-1425. Epub 1995/12/01.

483. Caselitz M, Bahr MJ, Bleck JS, Chavan A, Manns MP, Wagner S, et al. Sonographic criteria for the diagnosis of hepatic involvement in hereditary hemorrhagic telangiectasia (HHT). *Hepatology.* 2003;37(5):1139-1146. Epub 2003/04/30.

484. Milot L, Kamaoui I, Gautier G, Pilleul F. Hereditary-hemorrhagic telangiectasia: one-step magnetic resonance examination in evaluation of liver involvement. *Gastroenterol Clin Biol.* 2008;32(8-9):677-685. Epub 2008/09/02.

485. Memeo M, Stabile Ianora AA, Scardapane A, Suppressa P, Cirulli A, Sabba C, et al. Hereditary haemorrhagic telangiectasia: study of hepatic vascular alterations with multi-detector row helical CT and reconstruction programs. *Radiol Med.* 2005;109(1-2):125-138. Epub 2005/02/25.

486. Memeo M, Stabile Ianora AA, Scardapane A, Buonamico P, Sabba C, Angelelli G. Hepatic involvement in hereditary hemorrhagic telangiectasia: CT findings. *Abdom Imaging.* 2004;29(2):211-220. Epub 2004/08/05.

487. Siddiki H, Doherty MG, Fletcher JG, Stanson AW, Vrtiska TJ, Hough DM, et al. Abdominal findings in hereditary hemorrhagic telangiectasia: pictorial essay on 2D and 3D findings with isotropic multiphase CT. *Radiographics.* 2008;28(1):171-184. Epub 2008/01/22.

488. Ianora AA, Memeo M, Sabba C, Cirulli A, Rotondo A, Angelelli G. Hereditary hemorrhagic telangiectasia: multi-detector row helical CT assessment of hepatic involvement. *Radiology.* 2004;230(1):250-259. Epub 2003/12/03.

489. Wu JS, Saluja S, Garcia-Tsao G, Chong A, Henderson KJ, White RI Jr. Liver involvement in hereditary hemorrhagic telangiectasia: CT and clinical findings do not correlate in symptomatic patients. *AJR Am J Roentgenol.* 2006;187(4):W399-W405. Epub 2006/09/21.

490. Khalid SK, Garcia-Tsao G. Hepatic vascular malformations in hereditary hemorrhagic telangiectasia. *Semin Liver Dis.* 2008;28(3):247-258. Epub 2008/09/25.

491. Van Haeften FF, Broker FH. Post-traumatic intrahepatic arteriovenous fistula. *Injury.* 1984;15(5):311-315. Epub 1984/03/01.

492. Sato M, Ishida H, Konno K, Komatsuda T, Hamashima Y, Naganuma H, et al. Longstanding arterioportal fistula after laparoscopic liver biopsy. *Abdom Imaging.* 1999;24(4):383-385. Epub 1999/07/03.

493. Saad WE, Davies MG, Ryan CK, Rubens DJ, Patel NC, Lee DE, et al. Incidence of arterial injuries detected by arteriography following percutaneous right-lobe ultrasound-guided core liver biopsies in human subjects. *Am J Gastroenterol.* 2006;101(11):2641-2645. Epub 2006/10/14.

494. Guzman EA, McCahill LE, Rogers FB. Arterioportal fistulas: introduction of a novel classification with therapeutic implications. *J Gastrointest Surg.* 2006;10(4):543-550. Epub 2006/04/22.

495. Galeon M, Goffette P, Van Beers BE, Pringot J. Post-traumatic intrahepatic pseudoaneurysm: diagnosis with helical CT angiography and management with embolization. *J Belge Radiol.* 1997;80(6):287-288. Epub 1998/02/28.

496. Bolognesi M, Sacerdoti D, Bombonato G, Chiesura-Corona M, Merkel C, Gatta A. Arterioportal fistulas in patients with liver cirrhosis: usefulness of color Doppler US for screening. *Radiology.* 2000;216(3):738-743. Epub 2000/08/31.

497. Balci NC, Semelka RC, Sandhu JS. Intrahepatic arterioportal fistula: gadolinium-enhanced 3D magnetic resonance angiography findings and angiographic embolization with steel coils. *Magn Reson Imaging.* 1999;17(3):475-478. Epub 1999/04/09.

498. Kowdley KV, Aggarwal AM, Sachs PB. Delayed hemorrhage after percutaneous liver biopsy. Role of therapeutic angiography. *J Clin Gastroenterol.* 1994;19(1):50-53. Epub 1994/07/01.

499. Millonig G, Graziadei IW, Waldenberger P, Koenigsrainer A, Jaschke W, Vogel W. Percutaneous management of a hepatic artery aneurysm: bleeding after liver transplantation. *Cardiovasc Intervent Radiol.* 2004;27(5):525-528. Epub 2004/09/24.

500. Datta RV. Intrahepatic pseudoaneurysm after radiofrequency ablation of liver lesion. *Int Surg.* 2008;93(6):381-384. Epub 2008/11/01.

501. Ford JM, Shah H, Stecker MS, Namyslowski J. Embolization of large gastric varices using vena cava filter and coils. *Cardiovasc Intervent Radiol.* 2004;27(4):366-369. Epub 2004/09/04.

502. Longo JM, Bilbao JI, Rousseau HP, Garcia-Villareal L, Vinel JP, Zozaya JM, et al. Transjugular intrahepatic portosystemic shunt: evaluation with Doppler sonography. *Radiology.* 1993;186(2):529-534. Epub 1993/02/01.

503. Chong WK, Malisch TW, Mazer MJ. Sonography of transjugular intrahepatic portosystemic shunts. *Semin Ultrasound CT MR.* 1995;16(1):69-80. Epub 1995/02/01.

504. Middleton WD, Teefey SA, Darcy MD. Doppler evaluation of transjugular intrahepatic portosystemic shunts. *Ultrasound Q.* 2003;19(2):56-70; quiz 108-110. Epub 2003/09/16.

505. Latimer J, Bawa SM, Rees CJ, Hudson M, Rose JD. Patency and reintervention rates during routine TIPSS surveillance. *Cardiovasc Intervent Radiol.* 1998;21(3):234-239. Epub 1998/06/17.

506. Puttemans T, Agneessens E, Mathieu J. T.I.P.S.: follow-up imaging and revision procedure. *Acta Gastroenterol Belg.* 2000;63(2):174-178. Epub 2000/08/05.

507. Itkin M, Patel A, Trerotola SO, Litt HI. MRI of TIPS with covered stent-grafts: In vitro analysis using a flow phantom and initial clinical experience. *AJR Am J Roentgenol.* 2009;192(6):W317-W320. Epub 2009/05/22.

508. Palma LD. Diagnostic imaging and interventional therapy of hepatocellular carcinoma. *Br J Radiol.* 1998;71(848):808-818. Epub 1998/11/26.

509. Kobayashi S, Sakaguchi H, Takatsuka M, Suekane T, Iwai S, Morikawa H, et al. Two cases of hepatocellular adenomatosis treated with transcatheter arterial embolization. *Hepatol Int.* 2009;3(2):416-420. Epub 2009/08/12.

510. Ohishi H, Uchida H, Yoshimura H, Ohue S, Ueda J, Katsuragi M, et al. Hepatocellular carcinoma detected by iodized oil. Use of anticancer agents. *Radiology.* 1985;154(1):25-29. Epub 1985/01/01.

511. Chung J, Yu JS, Chung JJ, Kim JH, Kim KW. Haemodynamic events and localised parenchymal changes following transcatheter arterial chemoembolisation for hepatic malignancy: interpretation of imaging findings. *Br J Radiol.* 2010;83(985):71-81. Epub 2009/07/08.

512. Schima W, Ba-Ssalamah A, Kurtaran A, Schindl M, Gruenberger T. Post-treatment imaging of liver tumours. *Cancer Imaging.* 2007;7 Spec No A:S28-S36. Epub 2007/10/09.

513. Semelka RC, Worawattanakul S, Mauro MA, Bernard SA, Cance WG. Malignant hepatic tumors: changes on MRI after hepatic arterial chemoembolization—preliminary findings. *J Magn Reson Imaging.* 1998;8(1):48-56. Epub 1998/03/21.

514. Bartolozzi C, Lencioni R, Caramella D, Falaschi F, Cioni R, DiCoscio G. Hepatocellular carcinoma: CT and MR features after transcatheter arterial embolization and percutaneous ethanol injection. *Radiology.* 1994;191(1):123-128. Epub 1994/04/01.

515. Kim S, Mannelli L, Hajdu CH, Babb JS, Clark TW, Hecht EM, et al. Hepatocellular carcinoma: assessment of response to transarterial chemoembolization with image subtraction. *J Magn Reson Imaging.* 2010;31(2):348-355. Epub 2010/01/26.

516. Marin HL, Furth EE, Olthoff K, Shaked A, Soulen MC. Histopathologic outcome of neoadjuvant image-guided therapy of hepatocellular carcinoma. *J Gastrointestin Liver Dis.* 2009;18(2):169-176. Epub 2009/07/01.

517. Yu JS, Kim JH, Chung JJ, Kim KW. Added value of diffusion-weighted imaging in the MRI assessment of perilesional tumor recurrence after chemoembolization of hepatocellular carcinomas. *J Magn Reson Imaging.* 2009;30(1):153-160. Epub 2009/06/27.

518. Mannelli L, Kim S, Hajdu CH, Babb JS, Clark TW, Taouli B. Assessment of tumor necrosis of hepatocellular carcinoma after chemoembolization: diffusion-weighted and contrast-enhanced MRI with histopathologic correlation of the explanted liver. *AJR Am J Roentgenol.* 2009;193(4):1044-1052. Epub 2009/09/23.

519. Kamel IR, Liapi E, Reyes DK, Zahurak M, Bluemke DA, Geschwind JF. Unresectable hepatocellular carcinoma: serial early vascular and cellular changes after transarterial chemoembolization as detected with MR imaging. *Radiology.* 2009;250(2):466-473. Epub 2009/02/04.

520. Tarazov PG, Polysalov VN, Prozorovskij KV, Grishchenkova IV, Rozengauz EV. Ischemic complications of transcatheter arterial chemoembolization in liver malignancies. *Acta Radiol.* 2000;41(2):156-160. Epub 2000/03/31.

521. Kim HK, Chung YH, Song BC, Yang SH, Yoon HK, Yu E, et al. Ischemic bile duct injury as a serious complication after transarterial chemoembolization in patients with hepatocellular carcinoma. *J Clin Gastroenterol.* 2001;32(5):423-427. Epub 2001/04/25.

522. Hashimoto T, Mitani T, Nakamura H, Hori S, Kozuka T, Kobayashi Y, et al. Fatal septic complication of transcatheter chemoembolization for hepatocellular carcinoma. *Cardiovasc Intervent Radiol.* 1993;16(5):325-327. Epub 1993/09/01.

523. Vogl TJ, Muller PK, Mack MG, Straub R, Engelmann K, Neuhaus P. Liver metastases: interventional therapeutic techniques and results, state of the art. *Eur Radiol.* 1999;9(4):675-684. Epub 1999/06/04.

524. Livraghi T, Goldberg SN, Lazzaroni S, Meloni F, Solbiati L, Gazelle GS. Small hepatocellular carcinoma: treatment with radio-frequency ablation versus ethanol injection. *Radiology.* 1999;210(3):655-661. Epub 1999/04/20.

525. Tatli S, Acar M, Tuncali K, Morrison PR, Silverman S. Percutaneous cryoablation techniques and clinical applications. *Diagn Interv Radiol.* 2010;16(1):90-95. Epub 2009/12/10.

526. Gervais DA, Kalva S, Thabet A. Percutaneous image-guided therapy of intra-abdominal malignancy: imaging evaluation of treatment response. *Abdom Imaging.* 2009;34(5):593-609. Epub 2008/11/19.

527. Curley SA, Izzo F, Delrio P, Ellis LM, Granchi J, Vallone P, et al. Radiofrequency ablation of unresectable primary and metastatic hepatic malignancies: results in 123 patients. *Ann Surg.* 1999;230(1):1-8. Epub 1999/07/10.

528. Gelczer RK, Charboneau JW, Hussain S, Brown DL. Complications of percutaneous ethanol ablation. *J Ultrasound Med.* 1998;17(8):531-533. Epub 1998/08/11.

529. Hsieh HF, Chen TW, Yu CY, Wang NC, Chu HC, Shih ML, et al. Aggressive hepatic resection for patients with pyogenic liver abscess and APACHE II score > or =15. *Am J Surg.* 2008;196(3):346-350. Epub 2008/08/23.

530. Mazziotti A, Grazi GL, Cavallari A. Surgical treatment of hepatocellular carcinoma on cirrhosis: a Western experience. *Hepatogastroenterology.* 1998;45(suppl 3):1281-1287. Epub 1998/09/08.

531. Roayaie S, Guarrera JV, Ye MQ, Thung SN, Emre S, Fishbein TM, et al. Aggressive surgical treatment of intrahepatic cholangiocarcinoma: predictors of outcomes. *J Am Coll Surg.* 1998;187(4):365-372. Epub 1998/10/23.

532. Bramhall SR, Gur U, Coldham C, Gunson BK, Mayer AD, McMaster P, et al. Liver resection for colorectal metastases. *Ann R Coll Surg Engl.* 2003;85(5):334-339. Epub 2003/11/05.

533. Hashizume M, Shimada M, Sugimachi K. Laparoscopic hepatectomy: new approach for hepatocellular carcinoma. *J Hepatobiliary Pancreat Surg.* 2000;7(3):270-275. Epub 2000/09/12.

534. Gibbs JF, Litwin AM, Kahlenberg MS. Contemporary management of benign liver tumors. *Surg Clin North Am.* 2004;84(2):463-480. Epub 2004/04/06.

535. Belli G, Fantini C, D'Agostino A, Belli A, Langella S. Laparoscopic hepatic resection for completely exophytic hepatocellular carcinoma on cirrhosis. *J Hepatobiliary Pancreat Surg.* 2005;12(6):488-493. Epub 2005/12/21.

536. Carswell KA, Sagias FG, Murgatroyd B, Rela M, Heaton N, Patel AG. Laparoscopic versus open left lateral segmentectomy. *BMC Surg.* 2009;9:14. Epub 2009/09/09.

537. Kobayashi A, Imamura H, Miyagawa S, Shimada R, Makuuchi M, Kawasaki S. Extended right posterior segmentectomy for metastatic liver tumors. *Surgery.* 1997;121(6):698-703. Epub 1997/06/01.

538. Lindner P, Cahlin C, Friman S, Hafstrom L, Klingenstierna H, Lonn L, et al. Extended right-sided liver resection for colorectal liver metastases—impact of percutaneous portal venous embolisation. *Eur J Surg Oncol.* 2006;32(3):292-296. Epub 2006/01/26.

539. Kosuge T, Andersson R, Yamazaki S, Makuuchi M, Takayama T, Mukai K, et al. Surgical management of biliary cystadenocarcinoma. *Hepatogastroenterology.* 1992;39(5):417-419. Epub 1992/10/01.

540. Chan KL, Tam PK. Successful right trisegmentectomy for ruptured hepatoblastoma with preoperative transcatheter arterial embolization. *J Pediatr Surg.* 1998;33(5):783-786. Epub 1998/06/02.

541. Benoist S, Nordlinger B. The role of preoperative chemotherapy in patients with resectable colorectal liver metastases. *Ann Surg Oncol.* 2009;16(9):2385-2390. Epub 2009/06/26.

542. Shah AJ, Callaway M, Thomas MG, Finch-Jones MD. Contrast-enhanced intraoperative ultrasound improves detection of liver metastases during surgery for primary colorectal cancer. *HPB (Oxford).* 2010;12(3):181-187. Epub 2010/07/02.

543. Endo I, Shimada H, Sugita M, Fujii Y, Morioka D, Takeda K, et al. Role of three-dimensional imaging in operative planning for hilar cholangiocarcinoma. *Surgery.* 2007;142(5):666-675. Epub 2007/11/06.

544. McGahan JP, Khatri VP. Imaging findings after liver resection by using radiofrequency parenchymal coagulation devices: initial experiences. *Radiology.* 2008;247(3):896-902. Epub 2008/05/20.

545. Goshima S, Kanematsu M, Matsuo M, Kondo H, Yokoyama R, Hoshi H, et al. Early-enhancing nonneoplastic lesions on gadolinium-enhanced magnetic resonance imaging of the liver following partial hepatectomy. *J Magn Reson Imaging.* 2004;20(1):66-74. Epub 2004/06/29.

546. Merion RM. Current status and future of liver transplantation. *Semin Liver Dis.* 2010;30(4):411-421. Epub 2010/10/21.

547. Frericks BB, Kirchhoff TD, Shin HO, Stamm G, Merkesdal S, Abe T, et al. Preoperative volume calculation of the hepatic venous draining areas with multi-detector row CT in adult living donor liver transplantation: Impact on surgical procedure. *Eur Radiol.* 2006;16(12):2803-2810. Epub 2006/05/20.

548. Frericks BB, Caldarone FC, Nashan B, Savellano DH, Stamm G, Kirchhoff TD, et al. 3D CT modeling of hepatic vessel architecture and volume calculation in living donated liver transplantation. *Eur Radiol.* 2004;14(2):326-333. Epub 2003/12/11.

549. Hermoye L, Laamari-Azjal I, Cao Z, Annet L, Lerut J, Dawant BM, et al. Liver segmentation in living liver transplant donors: comparison of semiautomatic and manual methods. *Radiology.* 2005;234(1):171-178. Epub 2004/11/27.

550. Sirvanci M, Duran C, Ozturk E, Balci D, Dayangac M, Onat L, et al. The value of magnetic resonance cholangiography in the preoperative assessment of living liver donors. *Clin Imaging.* 2007;31(6):401-405. Epub 2007/11/13.

551. Catalano OA, Singh AH, Uppot RN, Hahn PF, Ferrone CR, Sahani DV. Vascular and biliary variants in the liver: implications for liver surgery. *Radiographics.* 2008;28(2): 359-378. Epub 2008/03/20.

552. Rinella ME, McCarthy R, Thakrar K, Finn JP, Rao SM, Koffron AJ, et al. Dual-echo, chemical shift gradient-echo magnetic resonance imaging to quantify hepatic steatosis: Implications for living liver donation. *Liver Transpl.* 2003;9(8):851-856. Epub 2003/07/29.

553. Kamel IR, Erbay N, Warmbrand G, Kruskal JB, Pomfret EA, Raptopoulos V. Liver regeneration after living adult right lobe transplantation. *Abdom Imaging.* 2003;28(1):53-57. Epub 2002/12/17.

554. Marcos A, Fisher RA, Ham JM, Shiffman ML, Sanyal AJ, Luketic VA, et al. Liver regeneration and function in donor and recipient after right lobe adult to adult living donor liver transplantation. *Transplantation*. 2000;69(7):1375-1379. Epub 2000/05/08.

555. Nadalin S, Testa G, Malago M, Beste M, Frilling A, Schroeder T, et al. Volumetric and functional recovery of the liver after right hepatectomy for living donation. *Liver Transpl.* 2004;10(8):1024-1029. Epub 2004/09/25.

556. Singh AK, Nachiappan AC, Verma HA, Uppot RN, Blake MA, Saini S, et al. Postoperative imaging in liver transplantation: what radiologists should know. *Radiographics*. 2010;30(2): 339-351. Epub 2010/03/17.

557. Ohira M, Ishifuro M, Ide K, Irei T, Tashiro H, Itamoto T, et al. Significant correlation between spleen volume and thrombocytopenia in liver transplant patients: a concept for predicting persistent thrombocytopenia. *Liver Transpl.* 2009;15(2):208-215. Epub 2009/01/30.

558. Simo G, Echenagusia A, Camunez F, Quevedo P, Calleja IJ, Ferreiroa JP, et al. Stenosis of the inferior vena cava after liver transplantation: treatment with Gianturco expandable metallic stents. *Cardiovasc Intervent Radiol*. 1995;18(4):212-216. Epub 1995/07/01.

559. Pfammatter T, Williams DM, Lane KL, Campbell DA Jr, Cho KJ. Suprahepatic caval anastomotic stenosis complicating orthotopic liver transplantation: treatment with percutaneous transluminal angioplasty, Wallstent placement, or both. *AJR Am J Roentgenol*. 1997;168(2):477-480. Epub 1997/02/01.

560. Kim BS, Kim TK, Jung DJ, Kim JH, Bae IY, Sung KB, et al. Vascular complications after living related liver transplantation: evaluation with gadolinium-enhanced three-dimensional MR angiography. *AJR Am J Roentgenol*. 2003;181(2):467-474. Epub 2003/07/24.

561. Meersschaut V, Mortele KJ, Troisi R, Van Vlierberghe H, De Vos M, Defreyne L, et al. Value of MR cholangiography in the evaluation of postoperative biliary complications following orthotopic liver transplantation. *Eur Radiol*. 2000;10(10): 1576-1581. Epub 2000/10/25.

562. Choi JY, Lee JY, Lee JM, Kim SH, Lee MW, Han JK, et al. Routine intraoperative Doppler sonography in the evaluation of complications after living-related donor liver transplantation. *J Clin Ultrasound*. 2007;35(9):483-490. Epub 2007/06/23.

563. Rinaldi P, Inchingolo R, Giuliani M, Di Stasi C, De Gaetano AM, Maresca G, et al. Hepatic artery stenosis in liver transplantation: Imaging and interventional treatment. *Eur J Radiol*. 2011. Epub 2011/03/29.

564. Boraschi P, Donati F, Cossu MC, Gigoni R, Vignali C, Filipponi F, et al. Multi-detector computed tomography angiography of the hepatic artery in liver transplant recipients. *Acta Radiol*. 2005;46(5):455-461. Epub 2005/10/18.

565. Marshall MM, Muiesan P, Srinivasan P, Kane PA, Rela M, Heaton ND, et al. Hepatic artery pseudoaneurysms following liver transplantation: incidence, presenting features and management. *Clin Radiol*. 2001;56(7):579-587. Epub 2001/07/12.

566. Kim HJ, Kim KW, Kim AY, Kim TK, Byun JH, Won HJ, et al. Hepatic artery pseudoaneurysms in adult living-donor liver transplantation: efficacy of CT and Doppler sonography. *AJR Am J Roentgenol*. 2005;184(5):1549-1555. Epub 2005/04/28.

567. Ginat DT, Saad WE, Waldman DL, Davies MG. Stent-graft placement for management of iatrogenic hepatic artery branch pseudoaneurysm after liver transplantation. *Vasc Endovascular Surg*. 2009;43(5):513-517. Epub 2009/07/31.

568. Boraschi P, Donati F, Gigoni R, Urbani L, Femia M, Cossu MC, et al. Ischemic-type biliary lesions in liver transplant recipients: evaluation with magnetic resonance cholangiography. *Transplant Proc*. 2004;36(9):2744-2747. Epub 2004/12/29.

569. Ito K, Siegelman ES, Stolpen AH, Mitchell DG. MR imaging of complications after liver transplantation. *AJR Am J Roentgenol*. 2000;175(4):1145-1149. Epub 2000/09/23.

570. Girometti R, Cereser L, Como G, Zuiani C, Bazzocchi M. Biliary complications after orthotopic liver transplantation: MRCP findings. *Abdom Imaging*. 2008;33(5):542-554. Epub 2007/09/14.

571. Duvoux C, Pageaux GP, Vanlemmens C, Roudot-Thoraval F, Vincens-Rolland AL, Hezode C, et al. Risk factors for lymphoproliferative disorders after liver transplantation in adults: an analysis of 480 patients. *Transplantation*. 2002;74(8):1103-1109. Epub 2002/11/20.

572. Xu QS, Ye S, Zhou YQ, Sheng JF, Ye K, Zheng SS. Posttransplantation lymphoproliferative disorder involving the central nervous system in liver transplant recipients. *Hepatobiliary Pancreat Dis Int*. 2008;7(5):551-554. Epub 2008/10/10.

573. Shaw AS, Ryan SM, Beese RC, Sidhu PS. Ultrasound of non-vascular complications in the post liver transplant patient. *Clin Radiol*. 2003;58(9):672-680. Epub 2003/08/29.

574. Kaushik S, Fulcher AS, Frable WJ, May DA. Posttransplantation lymphoproliferative disorder: osseous and hepatic involvement. *AJR Am J Roentgenol*. 2001;177(5):1057-1059. Epub 2001/10/20.

CHAPTER

Imaging of the Gallbladder and Biliary System

Stephanie Carruth Kurita, MD
Mark Alan Rosen, MD, PhD
Wallace T. Miller Jr., MD

ANATOMY OF THE GALLBLADDER

The gallbladder is a fluid-filled organ located inferior to the liver adjacent to the interlobar fissure in the gallbladder fossa and serves as a reservoir for bile. Bile is secreted by the liver into small ducts, which join to form the right and left common hepatic ducts that drain the right and left lobes of the liver. The right and left hepatic ducts join to form the common hepatic duct. With ingestion of food and the release of cholecystokinin by the digestive tract, the gallbladder contracts and releases bile into the cystic duct, which joins the common hepatic duct to form the common bile duct. The common bile duct drains bile into the duodenum to aid in the digestive process.

IMAGING OF THE GALLBLADDER

With all imaging modalities, elective examinations of the gallbladder should be performed with the patient fasting for 6 to 12 hours in order to have maximal physiologic distention of the gallbladder. In most situations, ultrasonography (US) will be the initial imaging modality used in the evaluation of the gallbladder and biliary tree. The normal appearance of the gallbladder on ultrasound is an anechoic structure with a thin wall located beneath the liver and adjacent to the interlobar fissure. The normal thickness of the gallbladder wall should not exceed 3 mm, and the maximum transverse diameter of the gallbladder is 4 cm (see Figure 4-1). Occasionally, there can be a fold near the gallbladder fundus called a Phrygian cap, a normal variant (see Figure 4-2).

Cholescintigraphy utilizing technetium-99m-iminodiacetic acid is another important imaging tool in the evaluation of biliary diseases, especially acute and chronic cholecystitis (see Figure 4-3). The radiopharmaceuticals have the same uptake and excretion as bilirubin, and sequential imaging over time will first demonstrate the agent in the liver parenchyma, followed by radiolabel in the biliary tree, gallbladder, common bile duct, and duodenum. In most cases, the gallbladder will begin to fill with radiotracer by approximately 10 minutes following injection, and the small bowel will fill by approximately 60 minutes post injection.

Unenhanced and enhanced computed tomography (CT) is rarely chosen as the initial evaluation for gallbladder

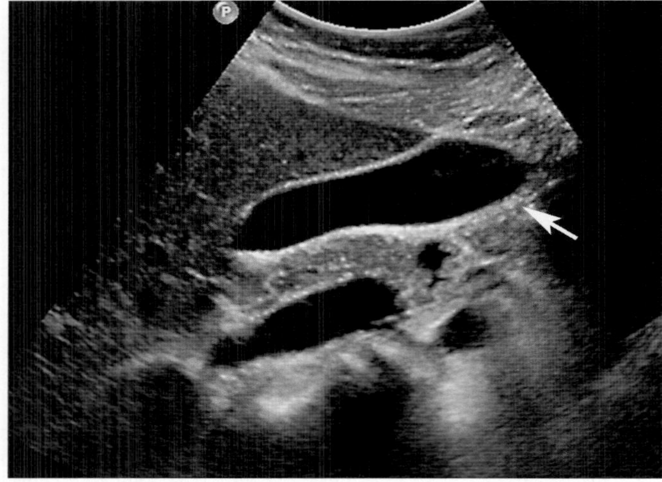

A

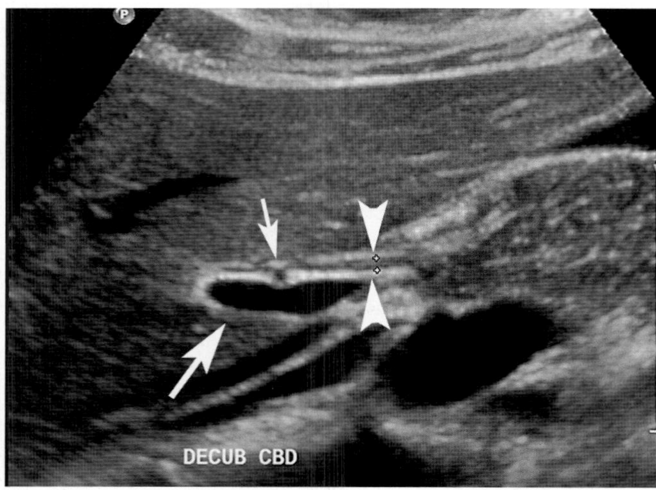

B

Figure 4-1 US of Normal Gallbladder and Biliary Tree
This 20-year-old woman had right upper quadrant pain. **A.** US of the gallbladder (*arrow*) shows an anechoic sack-like structure with a thin echogenic wall, typical of the normal gallbladder. **B.** Oblique image directed toward the right shoulder shows the characteristic appearance of the common bile duct (*arrowheads*) anterior to the portal vein (*large arrow*) and the crossing hepatic artery (*small arrow*). The common bile duct measures 2 mm. The normal intrahepatic ducts are too small to identify.

disease; however, because the normal gallbladder is routinely visualized in CT examinations performed for other purposes, many gallbladder disorders will be identified on CT examinations. The gallbladder appears as an oval, fluid-filled structure just inferior to the liver. The gallbladder wall is seen as a thin, 1- to 2-mm, slightly enhancing line surrounding the fluid-filled lumen (see Figure 4-4).

Magnetic resonance imaging (MRI) is rarely used for gallbladder imaging but may be used as a problem-solving tool when gallbladder abnormalities are identified on other examinations. Furthermore, normal and abnormal gallbladders may be seen on MRI when abdominal MR examinations are performed for other indications. On T2-weighted images, the gallbladder wall has low signal

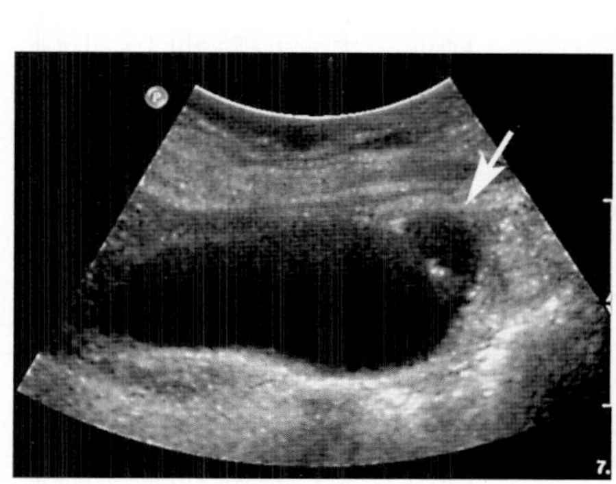

A

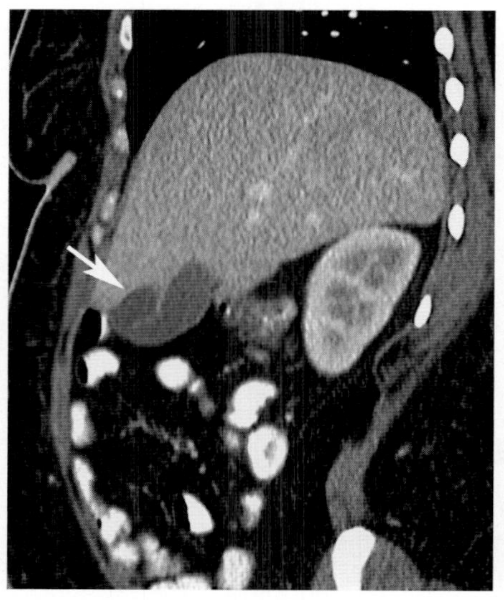

B

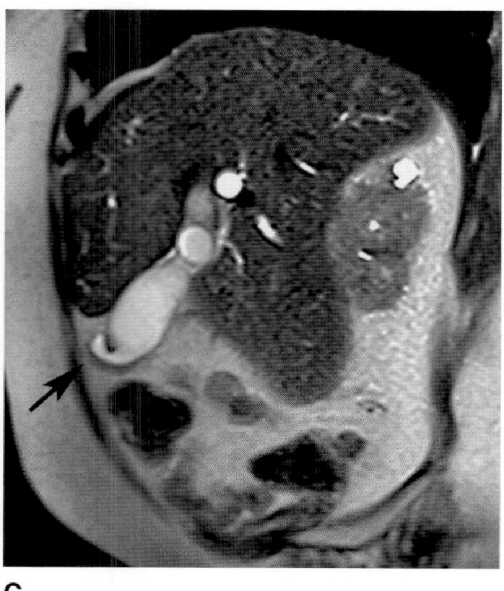

C

Figure 4-2 Phrygian Cap
A. Longitudinal US of the gallbladder. **B.** Sagittal reconstruction from an enhanced CT. **C** Sagittal T2-weighted MRI sequence from 3 separate individuals all show a small fundal fold (*arrow*). This is a normal variant called a Phrygian cap.

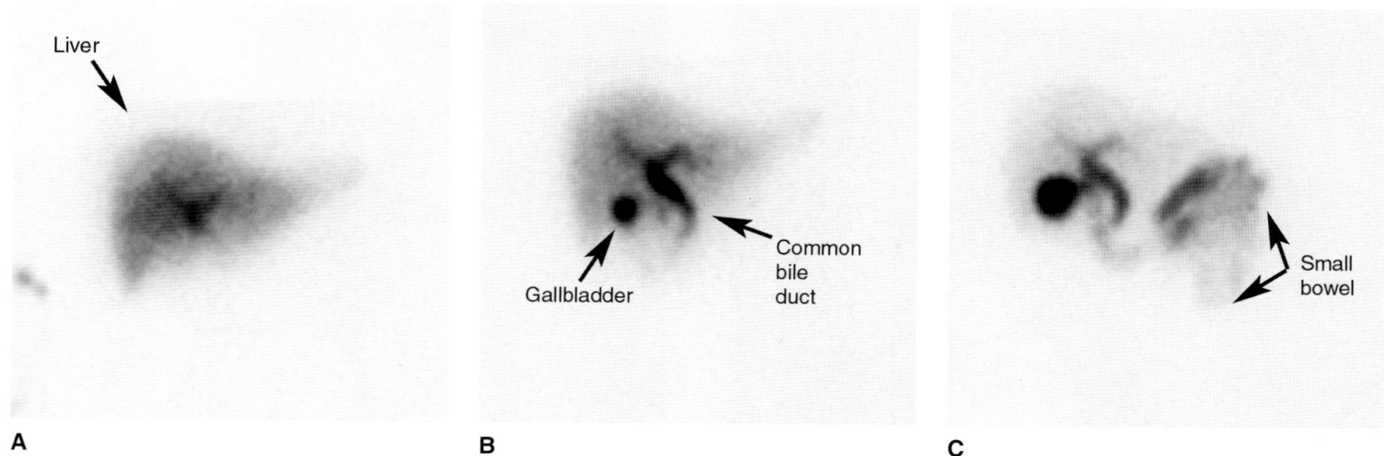

Figure 4-3 Hepatobiliary Iminodiacetic Acid (HIDA) Scan Tc99M HIDA is an agent that is excreted within the bile. Imaging will show the biodistribution of this agent, including the liver, gallbladder, common bile duct, and small bowel. **A.** Image taken at 15 minutes after injection shows distribution within the liver. **B.** Image taken 30 minutes after injection shows the agent filling the gallbladder and being excreted in the common bile duct. **C.** Image taken at 60 minutes after injection shows near complete clearance of the Tc99M HIDA from the liver and passage of the agent into the small bowel.

intensity, and on T1-weighted images, the wall has intermediate signal intensity (see Figure 4-5). The gallbladder wall should be a thin structure, which enhances uniformly after administration of contrast. The cystic duct insertion into the hepatic duct can usually be visualized with T2WI and with magnetic resonance cholangiopancreatography (MRCP; see Biliary section). Normal bile has high signal intensity on fluid-sensitive sequences and variable signal on T1-weighted images.[2]

DISEASES OF THE GALLBLADDER

As with other organs, we will divide diseases of the gallbladder into focal and diffuse disorders.

Focal Lesions of the Gallbladder

Focal lesions of the gallbladder wall can be subdivided into large masses and small polypoid lesions. Focal lesions are most often due to neoplasms of the gallbladder epithelium or as a result of inflammation or cholesterol deposits.

Gallbladder masses

Gallbladder neoplasms are rare tumors, most often seen in elderly individuals. They usually represent primary neoplasms of the gallbladder epithelium but in rare cases can be due to metastasis to the gallbladder wall or lymphoma.

Gallbladder carcinoma: Approximately 6500 new cases of gallbladder carcinoma are diagnosed annually in the United States. The peak incidence occurs in the sixth and seventh decades of life, and there is a 4:1 female-to-male ratio.[3] Although gallbladder carcinoma has an overall low prevalence, it is the most common malignant tumor of the biliary tract and the fifth most common malignancy in the alimentary tract after colorectal, pancreatic, gastric, and esophageal carcinoma.[4-7] In most cases, gallbladder neoplasia is believed to be a result of chronic inflammation of the gallbladder, usually because of the presence of gallstones, which are present in the majority of patients with gallbladder cancer.[4,8-10] Larger gallstones, those that are more likely to induce inflammation, are also seen with greater frequency in patients with gallbladder cancer. Diffuse gallbladder wall calcification, called a "porcelain" gallbladder, has been associated with an increased incidence of gallbladder carcinoma in some studies but not others. Porcelain gallbladder is illustrated later in the text under the heading: **Unique Disorders of the Gallbladder**.

Early gallbladder carcinoma is usually asymptomatic. When symptoms are present, they are usually indistinguishable from cholelithiasis and cholecystitis such as right upper quadrant pain and/or jaundice.[4] The presentation of gallbladder carcinoma makes the diagnosis of early gallbladder carcinoma very rare, and thus most malignant tumors of the gallbladder are unresectable at the time of diagnosis.[4,6,11-14]

Gallbladder carcinoma can take one of 3 imaging appearances: (1) as a large mass that replaces the entire gallbladder (40%-60% of cases), (2) as focal or diffuse thickening of the gallbladder wall (20%-30% of cases), or (3) as a gallbladder polyp.

Sonographically, a large mass replacing the gallbladder appears heterogeneous and variably echogenic (see Figure 4-6).[4] Similarly, on CT the mass will appear as a large, low-attenuation, irregularly marginated mass

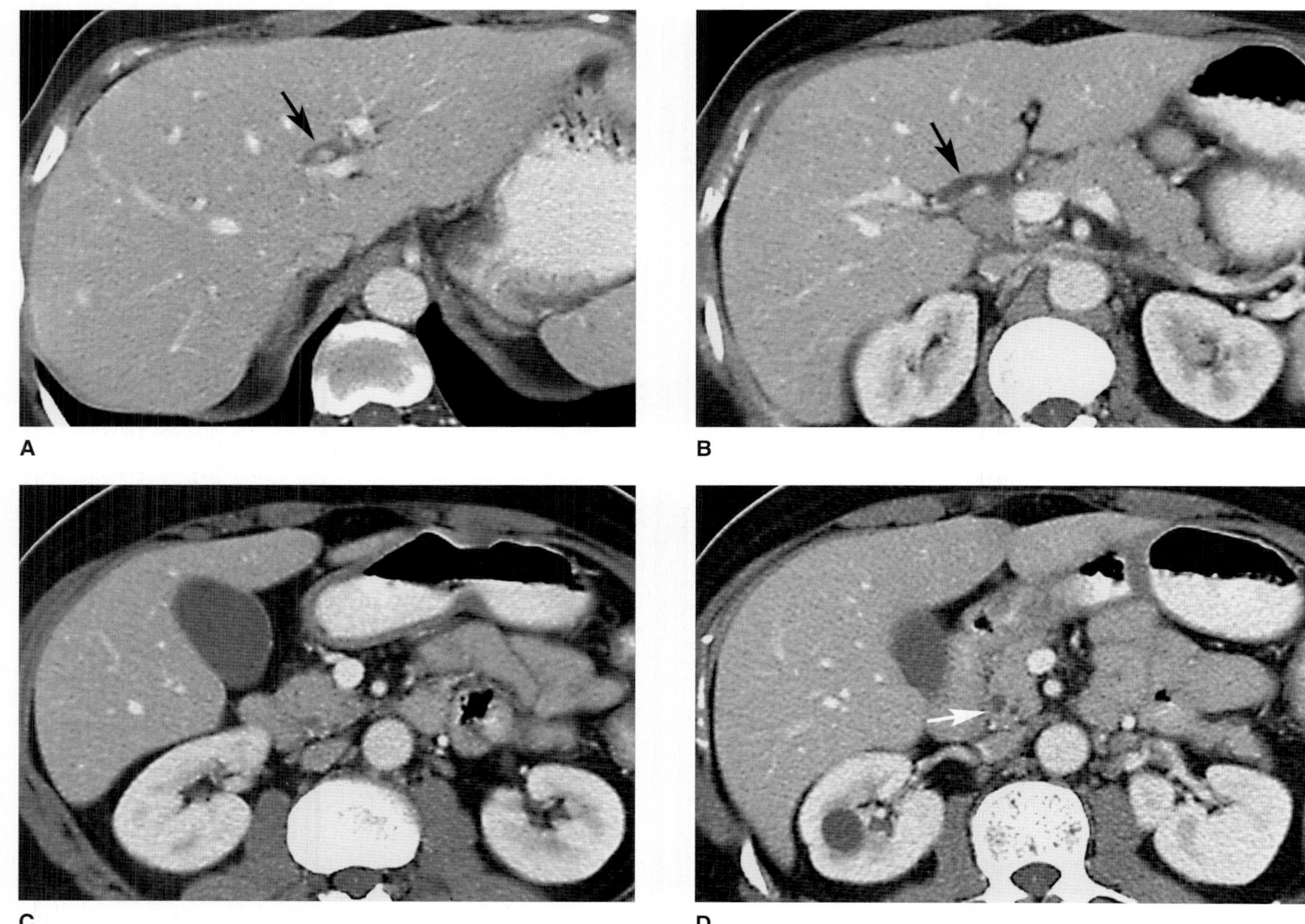

Figure 4-4 CT of Normal Gallbladder and Biliary Tree
A-D. Contrast-enhanced CT of the upper abdomen shows a few low attenuation tubes in the central liver (*black arrows*) representing normal intrahepatic bile ducts. Peripheral bile ducts are too small to see. The gallbladder is seen as a low attenuation ovoid in (C) and the common bile duct can be seen as a small low attenuation oval in the head of the pancreas (*white arrow* in D).

replacing the gallbladder. Following contrast enhancement, viable tumor will enhance; however, the tumor mass may contain low-attenuation areas of necrosis.[15] Further, MRI usually demonstrates the mass as hypointense on T1-weighted images and hyperintense on T2-weighted images with respect to liver parenchyma.[4] With gadolinium enhancement, the tumor will demonstrate ill-defined early enhancement on dynamic images.[15]

Diffuse gallbladder wall thickening can be difficult to distinguish from chronic cholecystitis;[4,16] however, several researchers suggest that malignant infiltration is thicker and more irregular than inflammatory wall thickening.[17-19] On US examinations, the thickened wall can appear either hypoechoic or hyperechoic (see Figure 4-7).[20] On CT and MRI, the wall of the gallbladder will generally appear thickened but will otherwise have similar imaging characteristics to the normal wall. The use of contrast-enhanced CT is helpful for distinguishing complicated cholecystitis from gallbladder carcinoma because demonstration of associated lymphadenopathy, hepatic invasion, and metastatic lesions highly favors gallbladder carcinoma.[15,21-23]

Lastly, gallbladder carcinoma may present as an intraluminal mass or polyp within the gallbladder lumen. On US, the nonmobile mass may be of homogeneous or heterogeneous echogenicity and will not demonstrate shadowing.[4] Prospective differentiation between carcinoma, a cholesterol polyp, and gallbladder adenoma is not always possible (see Figures 4-7 and 4-8). However, in some situations, cross-sectional imaging will show a large fungating mass within the gallbladder lumen readily identifiable as a polypoid carcinoma.

In addition to diagnosing the condition, cross-sectional imaging is also useful in staging gallbladder carcinoma. Staging will require either MRI or CT examinations. Direct spread into the adjacent liver is best evaluated

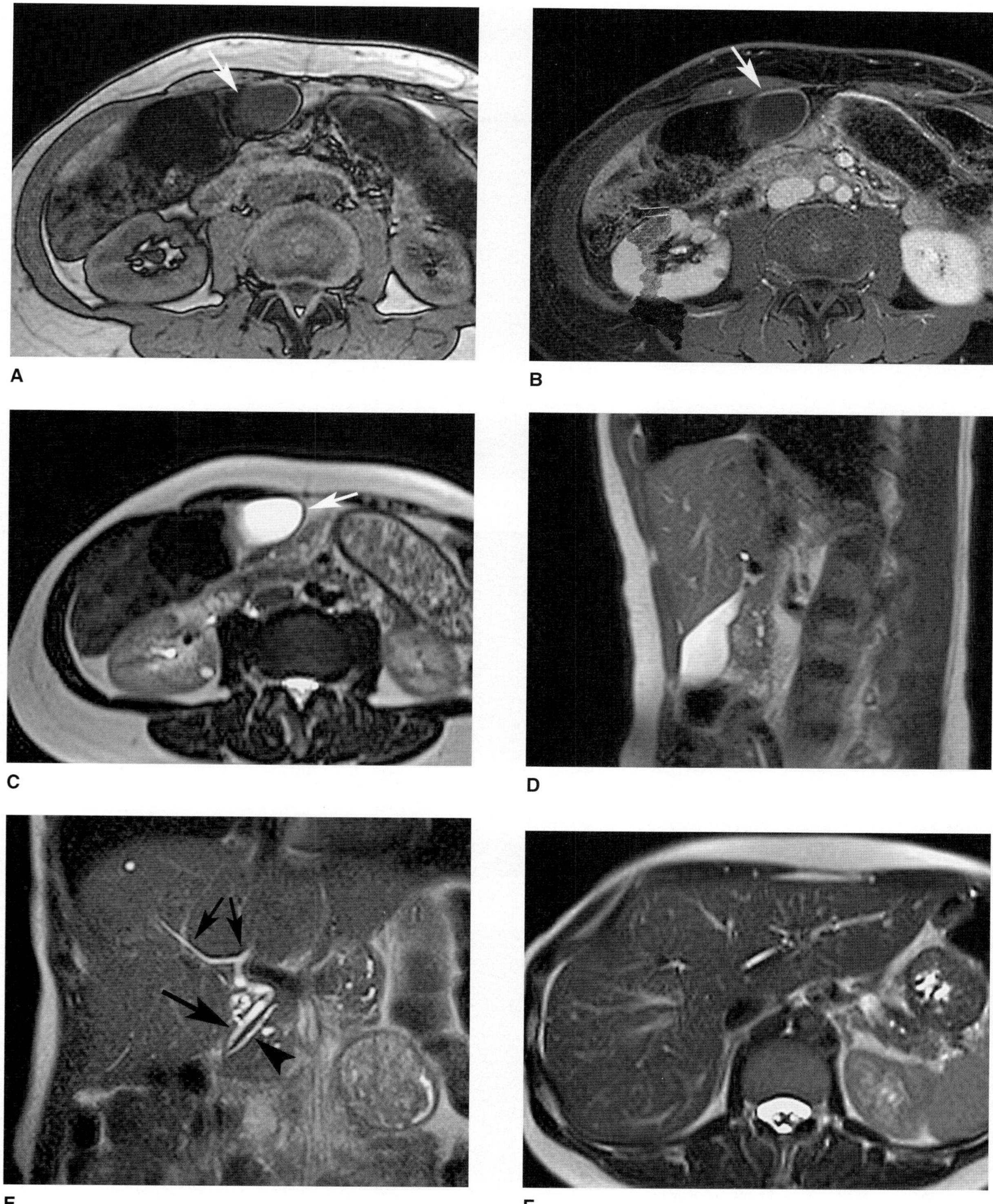

Figure 4-5 MRI of Normal Gallbladder and Biliary System
Axial T1-weighted image (**A**) before and (**B**) after gadolinium contrast shows a portion of the gallbladder (*white arrows*). Bile is normally dark on T1-weighted images, although bile that is saturated with cholesterol or contains sludge may be T1 hyperintense. The normal gallbladder wall is intermediate signal intensity on T1-weighted imaging and enhances moderately after gadolinium. **C.** Axial heavily T2-weighted images of the gallbladder demonstrate the uniform high T2 signal intensity of bile. Bile duct wall is thin, uniform, and dark on T2-weighted imaging (*small white arrow*). **D.** Sagittal T2-weighted image shows longitudinal view of gallbladder. **E.** Coronal T2-weighted image shows portions of the common bile duct (*large black arrow*) and pancreatic duct (*black arrowhead*). **F.** Axial T2-weighted image through the liver shows portion of the left intrahepatic ducts. On routine T2-weighted imaging, both biliary ducts and veins can demonstrate bright signal intensity against the dark liver.

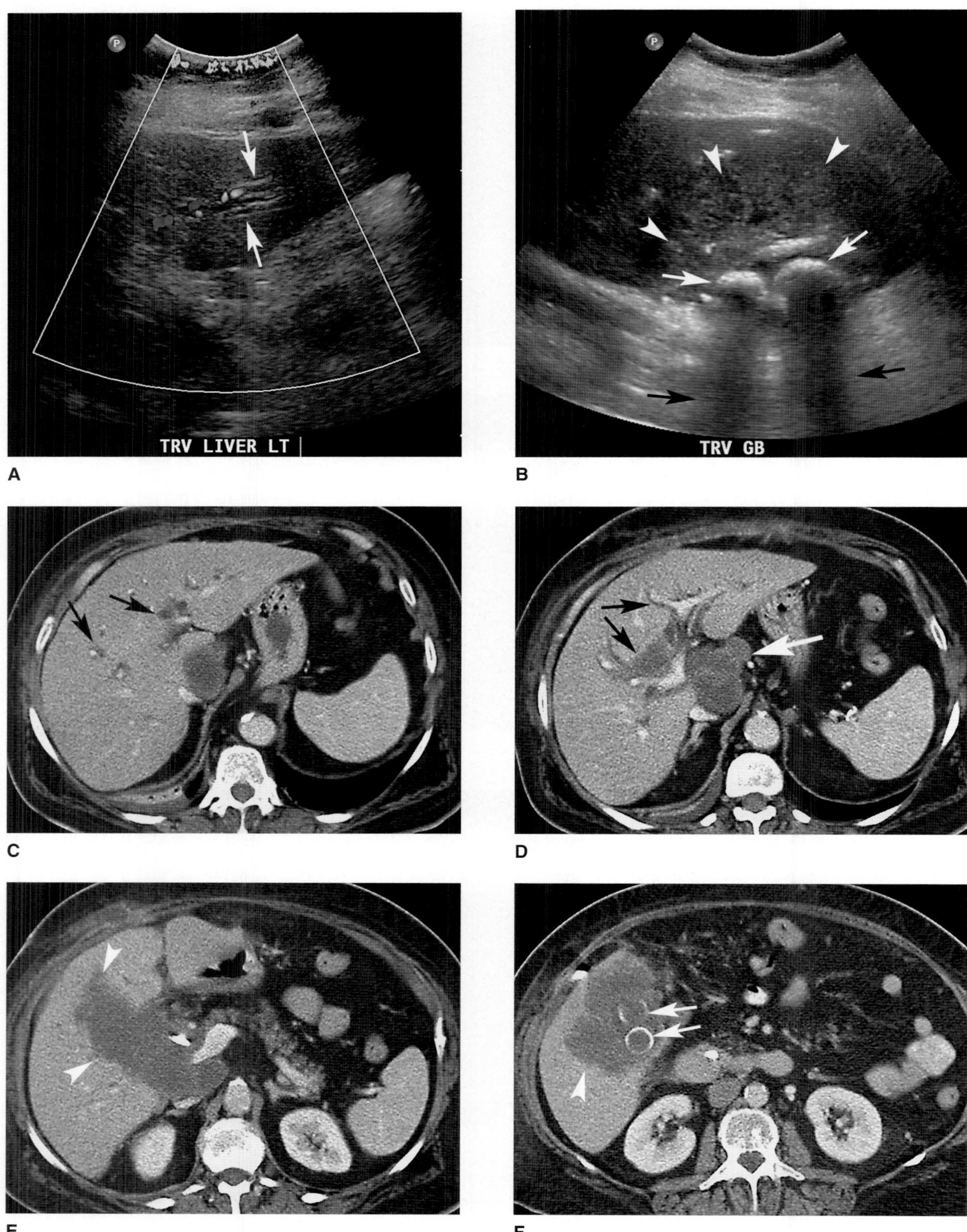

Figure 4-6 Gallbladder Carcinoma
This 68-year-old woman presented with jaundice. **A.** Color-flow US examination of the liver shows normal hepatic vasculature (*colored lines*) and multiple dilated intrahepatic ducts (*arrows*). **B.** US examination of the gallbladder demonstrates echogenic stones (*white arrows*) that cause acoustic shadowing (*black arrows*). Surrounding the stones is a hyperechoic mass (*arrowheads*), rather than anechoic bile that would normally be present in the gallbladder. **C-F.** CT images confirm the

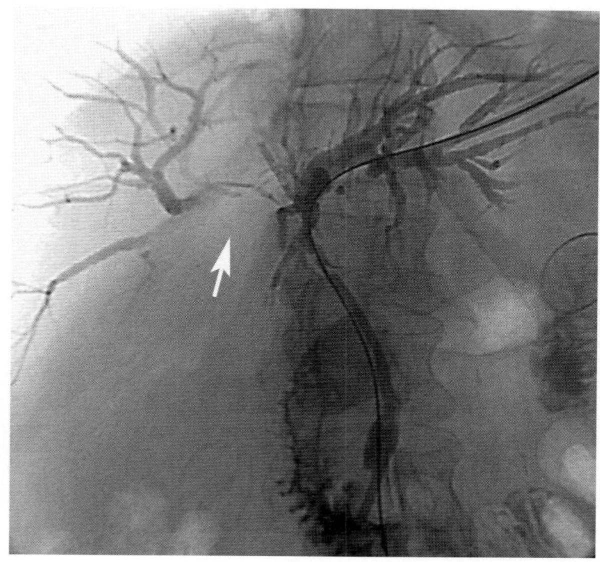

G

Figure 4-6 Gallbladder Carcinoma (*Continued*) presence of abnormally dilated intrahepatic biliary ducts (*black arrows*), a large hypoechoic mass in the gallbladder fossa (*arrowheads*) and gallstones (*white arrows*) and also demonstrates celiac axis adenopathy (*large white arrow*). **G.** Percutaneous cholangiogram also shows dilated intrahepatic biliary ducts with absence of ducts at the porta hepatis (*arrow*) at the site of malignant occlusion.

with dynamic contrast-enhanced MR evaluation. Arterial-phase enhancement extending beyond the gallbladder wall indicates serosal invasion while enhancement limited to the wall suggests subserosal invasion only.[24] In addition, CT and MRI can demonstrate extrahepatic or intrahepatic biliary obstruction and invasion of other adjacent structures such as the duodenum, pancreas, and colon. Lymphatic spread of gallbladder carcinoma will generally involve the hepatoduodenal ligament to the lymph nodes surrounding the pancreatic head with involvement of the celiac, superior mesenteric, and para-aortic lymph nodes.[15] Lymph nodes generally are enlarged and demonstrate heterogeneous contrast enhancement (see Figure 4-6).[15,25] Hematogenous metastasis is most often seen in the liver,[15,26] with pulmonary, skeletal, pancreatic, renal, adrenal, and brain metastases occurring rarely.[15]

Other gallbladder malignancies: There are other rare malignancies that can also occur in the gallbladder. Lymphoma of the gallbladder can be due to primary non-Hodgkin lymphoma or can be secondary to systemic lymphoma.[2,27,28] Primary lymphoma of the gallbladder is very rare. Findings on all cross-sectional imaging modalities are difficult to distinguish from gallbladder carcinoma and include irregular gallbladder wall thickening or a mass in the gallbladder fossa with possible hepatic extension.[2] Kaposi sarcoma of the gallbladder has also been described and can result in gallbladder wall thickening on cross-sectional imaging; however, imaging features are nonspecific.[29] Other rare malignancies include rhabdomyosarcoma,[30] carcinoid, and metastases.[15]

Gallbladder polyps

The term *polyp* means a growth projecting from the wall of a cavity lined with a mucous membrane. Approximately 5% of adults will have a small polyp demonstrable on cross-sectional imaging. In most cases, gallbladder polyps are clinically silent lesions that are discovered by imaging examinations. Polypoid lesions of the gallbladder can be described by 2 categories: pseudopolyps and true neoplasms (Table 4-1).[31-33]

Cholesterol polyps and focal adenomyomatosis: Gallbladder pseudopolyps are benign, nonneoplastic growths of the wall of the gallbladder. These are most often cholesterol polyps that represent focal deposition of cholesterol within the mucosa of the gallbladder wall. Pathologically, cholesterol polyps are projections of the mucosa containing lipid-laden macrophages covered by normal gallbladder epithelium. Cholesterol polyps are typically small, usually less than 5 mm, are often multiple in number, and are most commonly discovered in younger patients.[34] Most small polyps will represent cholesterol polyps. These lesions usually show no enhancement on CT and MRI and no color flow on US within the polyp. A specific diagnosis of a cholesterol polyp can be made on US or MRI if the polyp has characteristic features of cholesterol within the polyp. On US, the typical feature of cholesterol is the ring-down artifact, a cascade of decreasing-size echogenic lines deep into the polyp (see Figure 4-9). On MRI, some cholesterol polyps will show a central region of high T1 signal, indicating the presence of lipid (see Figure 4-10).

Adenomyomatosis is benign hyperplasia of the gallbladder mucosa associated with cholesterol deposition. It is characterized by proliferation of the gallbladder wall mucosa with invaginations called Rokitansky-Aschoff sinuses. Adenomyomatosis can involve the entire wall of the gallbladder, the generalized form; involve a distinct region of the gallbladder, the segmental form; or involve a single deposit, the focal form. When focal, it can have the appearance of a pseudopolyp.[35] Polyps related to adenomyomatosis are sometimes called hyperplastic polyps. Cholesterolosis and adenomyomatosis will be further discussed under the heading: **Diffuse and Focal Gallbladder Wall Thickening**.

Gallbladder adenoma and other small focal neoplasms: Less commonly, polypoid lesions represent neoplasms. Neoplastic polyps are usually either benign adenomas or small malignant gallbladder adenocarcinomas. Other less common histologies include papillomas, lipomas, and leiomyomas (see Figures 4-8, 4-11, and 4-12).

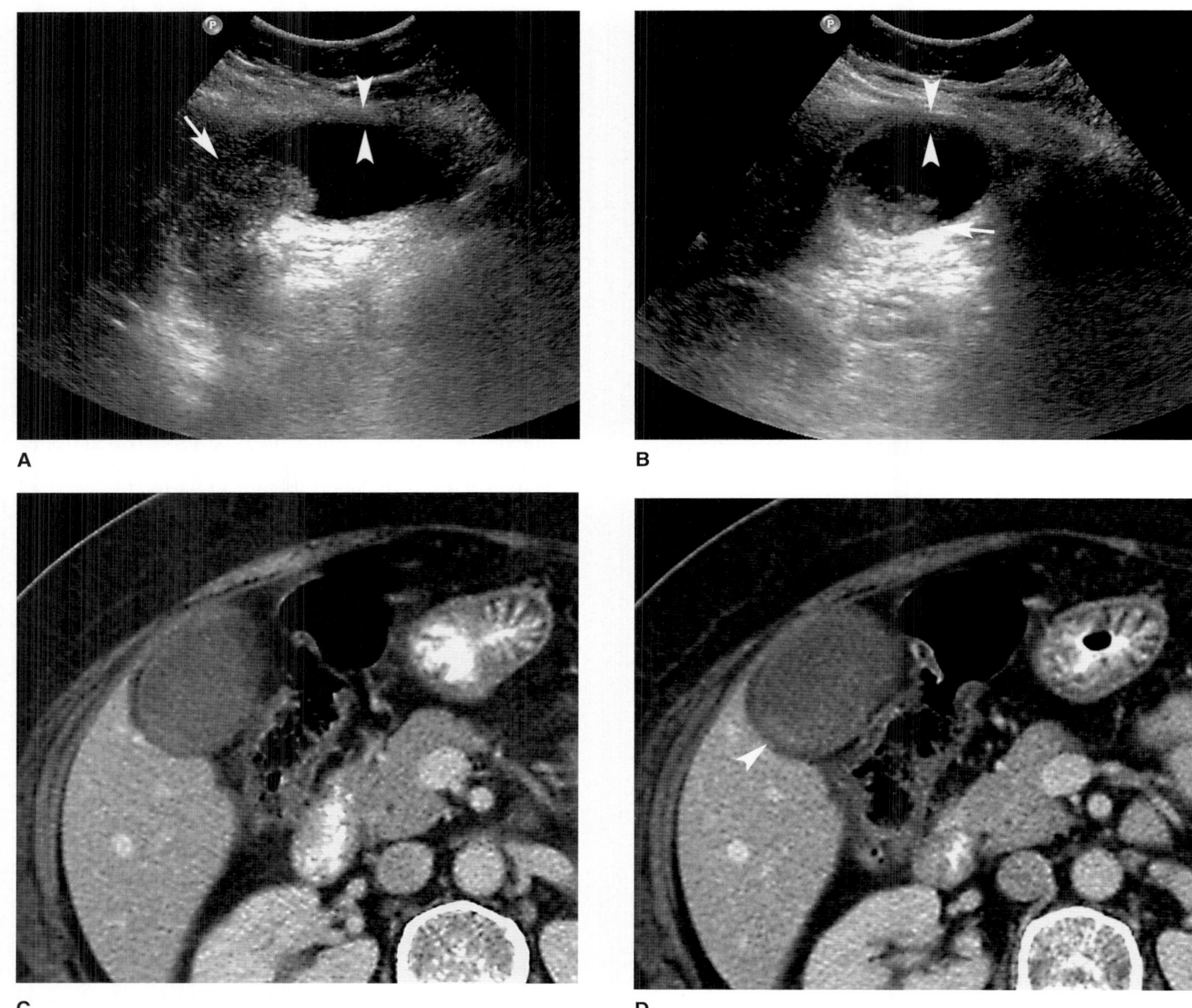

Figure 4-7 Gallbladder Carcinoma A With Endoluminal Polyp and Diffuse Wall Thickening
This 65-year-old woman presented with epigastric pain and weakness. **A**. Longitudinal and (**B**) transverse US of the gallbladder demonstrates extensive gallbladder wall thickening (*arrowheads*) associated with an irregularly marginated polypoid mass projecting into the neck of the gallbladder. Note the absence of shadowing, indicating that the intraluminal mass is soft tissue and not stones. **C** and **D**. Enhanced CT confirms the irregular thickening (*arrowhead*) of the gallbladder wall. The polypoid intraluminal growth is much more difficult to recognize. Note the faint increased attenuation of the lumen in C relative to D, indicating the intraluminal growth of the tumor. Surgical excision was diagnostic of a gallbladder carcinoma.

Metastasis: Metastases to the gallbladder are rare. Malignant melanoma and breast carcinoma are the 2 malignancies most likely to metastasize to the gallbladder, with melanoma being, by far, the most common and accounting for more than 50% of gallbladder metastases.[2,36] They will usually appear as a focal nodule or mass involving the wall of the gallbladder (see Figure 4-13).[36] In most cases, other sites of metastasis involving other abdominal organs and lymph nodes will provide clues that a gallbladder mass or polyp represents metastatic disease.

Imaging features of gallbladder polyps: Both neoplastic and inflammatory gallbladder polyps will appear as small round or oval structures projecting from the wall into the lumen of the gallbladder on all cross-sectional imaging examinations.[31] Polyps can be distinguished from stones by

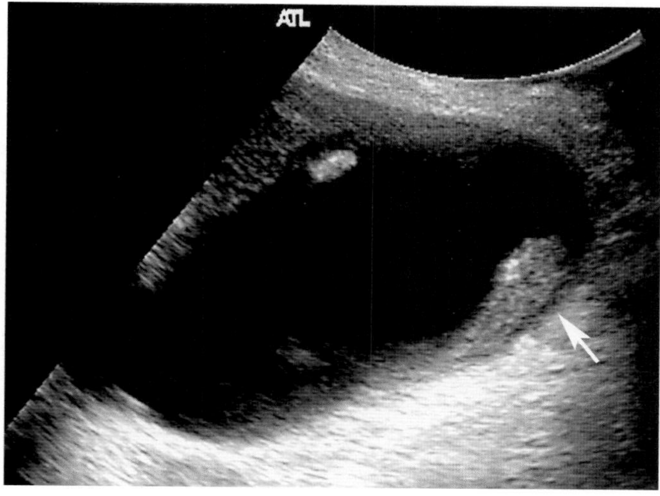

A

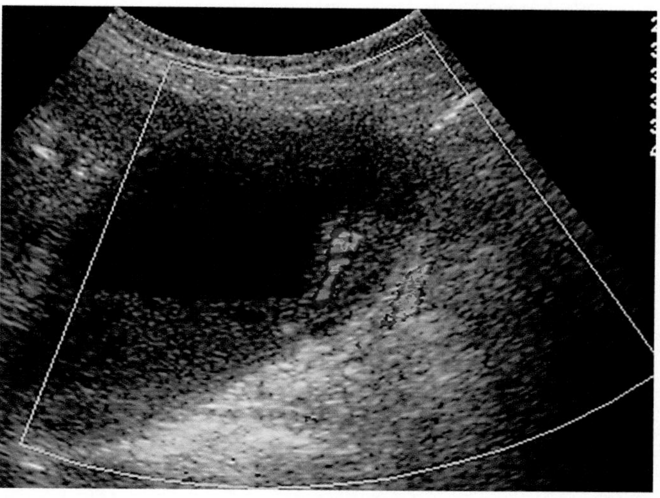

B

Figure 4-8 Polypoid Gallbladder Carcinoma
This 89-year-old woman had a history of breast carcinoma. Longitudinal US of the gallbladder during (**A**) grey-scale and (**B**) color flow imaging shows a large polyp of the posterior wall (*arrow*) that has detectable blood flow within the stalk. Evidence of blood flow will usually indicate a gallbladder neoplasm such as an adenoma, carcinoma, or metastasis. Evaluation of the surgical specimen was diagnostic of a small carcinoma.

their fixation to the gallbladder wall. Further, CT and MRI will show the polyp to enhance with intravenous contrast. On US examinations, polyps appear as a small nonmobile echogenic pedunculated nodule and, unlike gallstones, do not cause shadowing (see Figures 4-8 and 4-10 through 4-13).[37] Occasionally, especially in larger polyps, the soft-tissue nature of the polyp can be recognized by demonstration of blood flow into the polyp on Doppler imaging (see Figures 4-8 and 4-12). Size is an important predictor of malignancy, with 40% to 88% prevalence of malignancy in polyps larger than 1 cm.[24,38] Features that increase probability of malignancy also include the presence of a solitary polyp, age of patient greater than 60 years, sessile lesion, gallstones, and rapid rate of growth.[24,38-41] Because of the poor prognosis of gallbladder malignancies, it is important to distinguish between benign and malignant gallbladder polyps. It is recommended that polyps less than 5 mm require no further follow-up, and polyps measuring between 5 and 10 mm should be followed up to document stability.[31,42] Lesions greater than 1 cm should be resected in most cases (Table 4-1).

Cholesterol polyps can sometimes be distinguished from other causes by the characteristic ring-down artifact on US and high T1 signal on MRI.

Diffuse Thickening of the Gallbladder Wall

Diffuse thickening of the wall of the gallbladder is defined as a transverse diameter greater than 3 mm. This is a nonspecific finding and can be found in a variety of conditions, some unrelated to intrinsic gallbladder disease and can be seen in both symptomatic and asymptomatic patients. Diffuse gallbladder wall thickening is typically the result of (1) edema, (2) chronic inflammation, (3) hyperplasia, or

Table 4-1. Causes of Gallbladder Polyps

1. Neoplasms
   a. Adenoma
   b. Adenocarcinoma
   c. Leiomyoma
   d. Lipoma
   e. Metastasis (melanoma, breast)
2. Pseudotumors
   a. **Cholesterol polyp**[a]
   b. **Adenomyomatosis (hyperplastic polyp)**
   c. Inflammatory polyp

[a]Entities in bold are common.

Imaging Notes 4-1. Recommended Management of Gallbladder Polyps

<5 mm	Low-risk malignant	No further investigation necessary
5-10 mm	Intermediate-risk malignant	Imaging follow-up to confirm stability
>10 mm	40%-88% malignant	Surgical resection

Cholesterol polyps can also be positively identified by the presence of ring-down artifact on US and central high T1 signal on MRI.

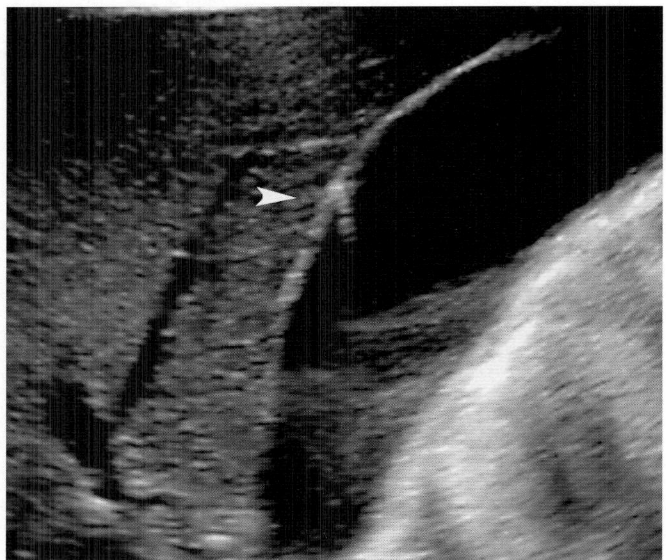

Figure 4-9 Cholesterol Polyp With Ring-Down Artifact
This 33-year-old man presented with right upper quadrant pain. Longitudinal US of the gallbladder shows a cascading line of echoes (*arrowhead*) projecting from the anterior wall. This is typical of ring-down artifact and is a characteristic feature of cholesterol deposits in the gallbladder wall. A single focus will often indicate the presence of a small cholesterol polyp.

Imaging Notes 4-2. Imaging Findings in Acute Cholecystitis

1. Distended GB
2. Thickened GB wall
3. Hyperemic GB wall
4. Pericholecystic fluid
5. Pericholecystic fat stranding
6. Sonographic "Murphy sign"
7. Lack of filling of GB by radionuclide

(4) infiltrating tumor (Table 4-2). Pseudothickening of the gallbladder wall can be seen shortly after eating when the gallbladder is collapsed.

Gallbladder wall edema

Gallbladder wall edema can be due to (1) inflammation of the gallbladder wall, (2) inflammation of the tissues surrounding the gallbladder, or (3) causes of generalized edema. On US, gallbladder wall edema typically has a layered appearance, with both hyperechoic and hypoechoic elements (see Figure 4-14).[43,44] On CT, a thickened gallbladder wall will often demonstrate a hypodense layer of subserosal edema (see Figure 4-15).[43,45] On MRI examinations, gallbladder edema appears as a thickened wall that may appear striated, including layers of alternating signal intensities.[46]

Acute cholecystitis: Acute cholecystitis is the inflammation and edema that results from obstruction of the cystic duct. In most cases, this will be due to an obstructing gallstone but will, in some cases, occur without an obvious obstructing lesion, termed *acalculous* cholecystitis. Gallstone-related cholecystitis is more commonly seen in women than men and typically occurs in middle age. Patients will usually present with colicky, right upper quadrant pain and fever.[43]

Acalculous cholecystitis, seen most frequently in children and the elderly, is associated with chronic bile stasis such as a debilitated postoperative state, use of parenteral nutrition, narcotic use, and starvation. Patients can present with abdominal pain and fever similar to calculus cholecystitis or can present with sepsis, without localizing signs.[43]

In acute cholecystitis, cross-sectional imaging with US, CT, or MRI will demonstrate a distended gallbladder with a thickened wall.[46,47] Fluid surrounding the gallbladder called "pericholecystic fluid" is often present. Inflammatory fat stranding of the adjacent right upper quadrant fat is also a frequent associated finding seen on CT or MRI (see Figure 4-15). With color-flow Doppler, there is normally little or no flow in the gallbladder wall. In patients with acute cholecystitis, many will have increased blood flow on color-flow Doppler imaging (see Figures 4-16 and 4-17).[43] This hyperemia can also be seen on CT and MRI examinations as increased enhancement of the wall of the gallbladder, which is normally only minimally enhancing. Additionally, MR demonstrates pericholecystic enhancement in more than 70% of patients with acute cholecystitis (see Figure 4-15).[24] Finally, pain elicited by pressure directly over the gallbladder during the sonographic evaluation, called a positive sonographic "Murphy sign," is usually present.[43] In most cases, a gallstone will be demonstrated in the neck of the gallbladder, but in cases of acalculous cholecystitis, no gallstone will be seen (see Figure 4-15).

Radionuclide hepatobiliary imaging is also an important tool in the evaluation of acute cholecystitis. As previously described, a radiolabeled agent that is excreted in the bile is intravenously injected into the bloodstream. Sequential imaging over time will first demonstrate the agent in the liver parenchyma, followed by radiolabel in the biliary tree, gallbladder, common bile duct, and duodenum. Failure of the gallbladder to fill indicates obstruction of the cystic duct and in most cases will indicate acute cholecystitis (see Figures 4-18 and 4-19).[48] False-positive examinations can occur with prolonged fasting or with the use of hyperalimentation. Augmentation with morphine or cholecystokinin, which induces spasm of the sphincter of Oddi,

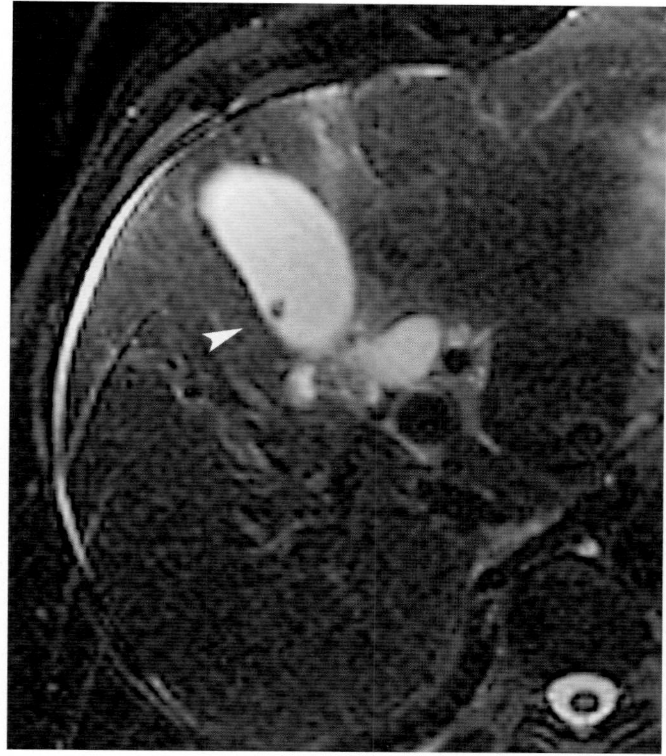

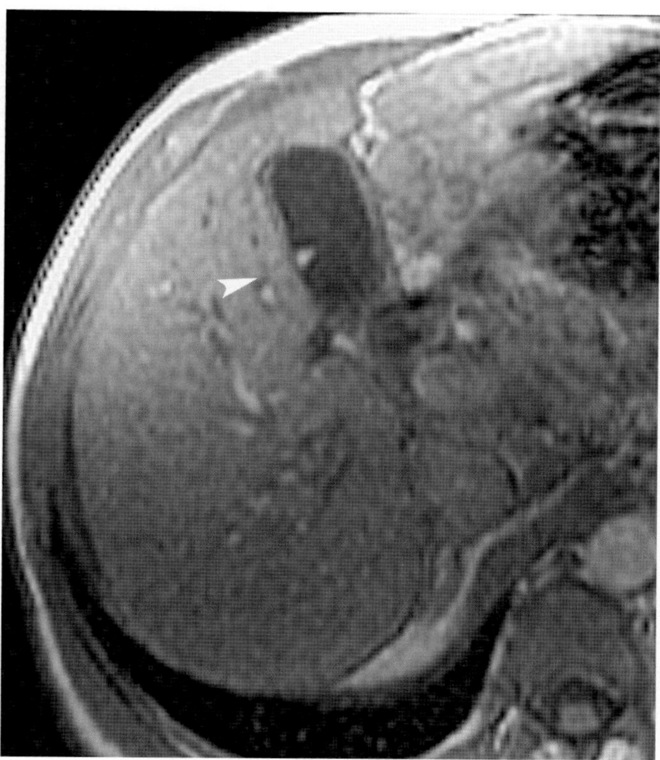

Figure 4-10 Cholesterol Polyp with High T1 Signal
This 45-year-old man had elevated liver function tests. **A.** T2-weighted MRI image through the gallbladder shows a low-signal polyp within the high-signal bile. This is a nonspecific finding and could represent any cause of gallbladder polyp. A cholesterol polyp would be the most likely cause, given the small size. **B.** T1-weighted MRI image demonstrates very high signal in the center of the polyp, similar to the signal of subcutaneous fat and indicating the presence of lipid material. This is a characteristic feature of a cholesterol polyp.

has been shown to decrease false-positive rates.[49] Another specific finding that is seen in 25% to 35% of patients with acute cholecystitis is the "rim sign," which is increased uptake adjacent to the gallbladder fossa on cholescintigraphy. This sign also identifies patients who are at increased risk for complications, including gangrene and gallbladder perforation (see Figure 4-19).[49]

Gangrenous cholecystitis is a complication of acute cholecystitis and is associated with increased morbidity and mortality. Pathologically, it includes intramural hemorrhage, necrosis, and formation of microabscesses. If perforation occurs, pericholecystic abscesses or peritonitis can also be observed. Perforation is reported to occur in 10% of patients with acute cholecystitis.[50] Older men with cardiovascular disease[24] and patients with diabetes mellitus[51] are at increased risk of developing gangrene in the setting of acute cholecystitis. Sonographically, gangrenous cholecystitis will usually appear as asymmetric gallbladder wall thickening containing course intraluminal echoes (see Figure 4-20).[50] In some cases, CT will demonstrate gas within the gallbladder wall or absence of gallbladder wall enhancement in addition to other findings of acute cholecystitis. In addition, MR demonstrates segmental absence of mucosal enhancement suggesting complicating gangrene.[24] In some cases, gallbladder perforation will only be apparent by the presence of excessive pericholecystic fluid, ascites, or abdominal abscesses. However, in many cases, focal absence of the gallbladder wall will indicate the presence of perforation (see Figure 4-21).

Extracholecystic inflammation: Inflammation occurring outside the gallbladder can secondarily cause diffuse gallbladder wall thickening, either by direct spread of inflammation or because of an immunologic reaction to the extracholecystic inflammation.[43,52] Theoretically, any cause of inflammation can extend to the gallbladder, but the most common causes include hepatitis, pancreatitis, and pyelonephritis (see Figure 4-22).[43] Diffuse wall thickening has also been reported in patients diagnosed with mononucleosis[53] and in patients with acquired immunodeficiency syndrome (AIDS) (see Figure 4-23).[45]

Causes of generalized edema: Systemic diseases can lead to generalized total body edema of which gallbladder wall thickening is one part. Common causes include congestive heart failure, cirrhosis, and renal failure. Any

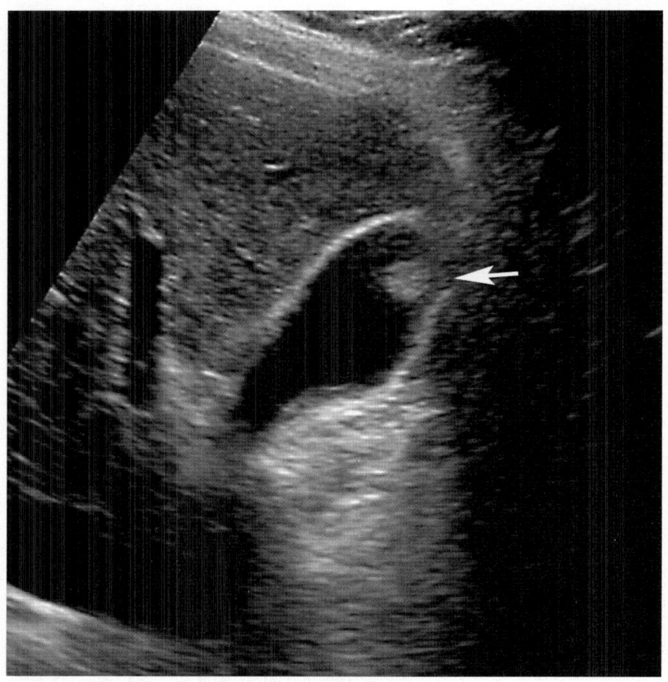

A

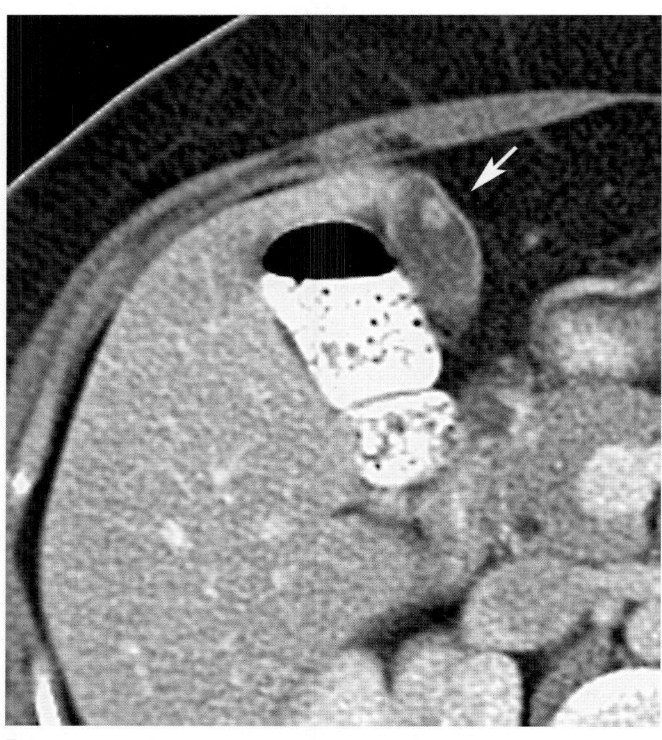

B

Figure 4-11 Gallbladder Polyp
This 27-year-old woman complained of abdominal pain and bloating. **A.** US examination of the gallbladder demonstrates an echogenic, nonshadowing nodule in the fundus of the gallbladder. **B.** Enhanced CT confirms the presence of an enhancing nodule projecting from the wall of the gallbladder fundus. These are the typical findings of a gallbladder polyp, most likely a small adenoma.

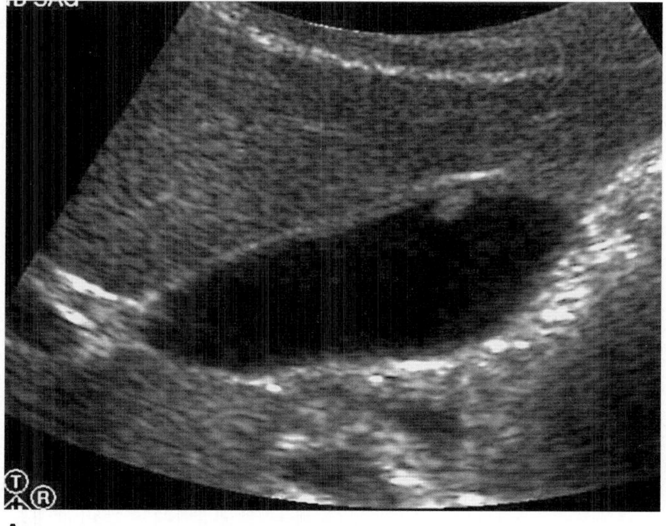

A

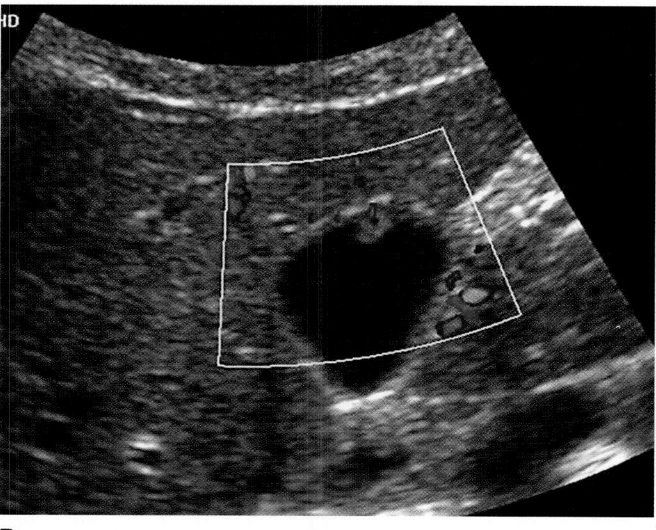

B

Figure 4-12 Adenomatous Polyp of the Gallbladder
This 24-year-old woman was being evaluated for fatty liver disease. **A.** Longitudinal US of the gallbladder shows a focal, nondependent, nonshadowing nodule attached to the anterior wall of the gallbladder typical of a small polyp. **B.** Transverse images show slight color flow in the base of the polyp. This finding suggests that this is likely a neoplasm, probably a small adenoma. This lesion has remained stable on serial imaging studies.

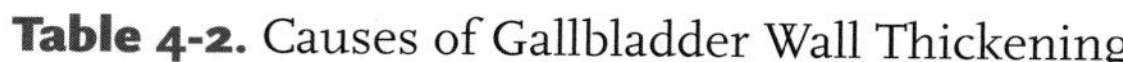

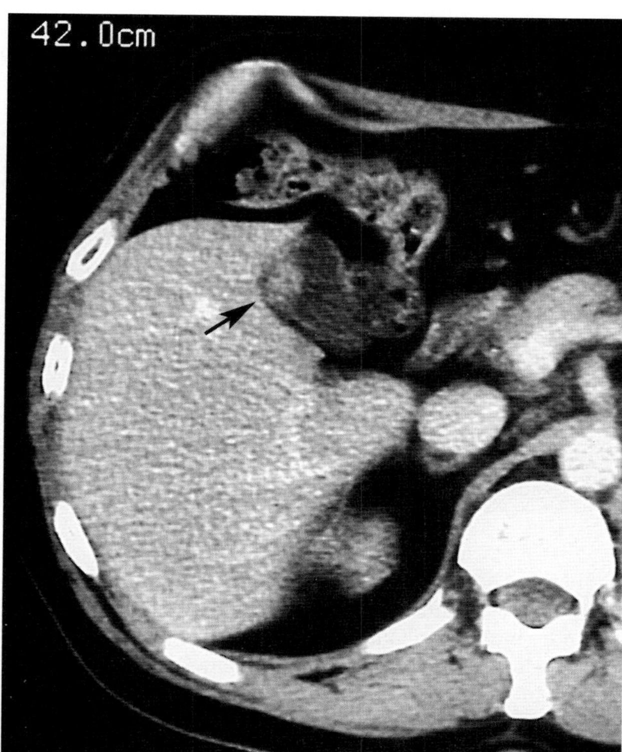

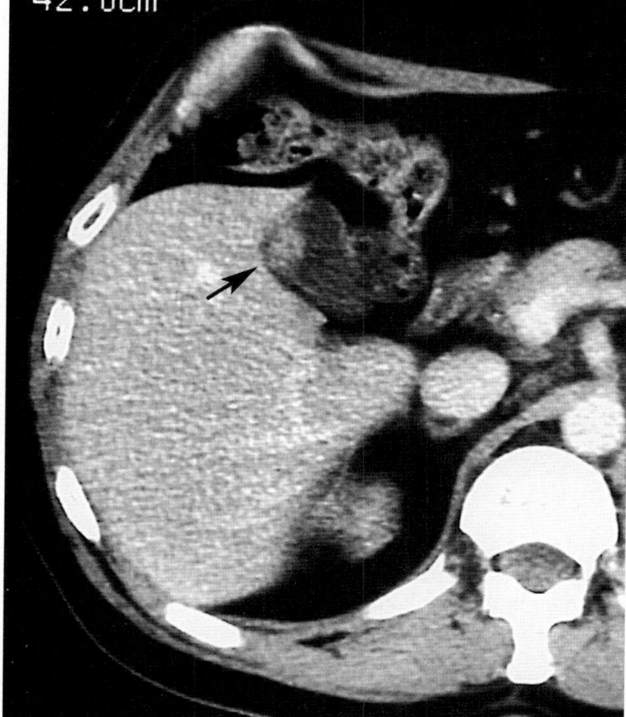

Figure 4-13 Gallbladder Metastasis from Malignant Melanoma
This 48-year-old man had a history of malignant melanoma. Image of the gallbladder from an enhanced CT demonstrates a focal enhancing polypoid lesion with slight adjacent wall thickening. This lesion was not present on a study 1 year previously and was assumed to represent a gallbladder metastasis.

Table 4-2. Causes of Gallbladder Wall Thickening

1. Edema
    a. Acute cholecystitis
    b. Extracholecystic inflammation
        i. Hepatitis
        ii. Pancreatitis
        iii. Pyelonephritis
        iv. Infectious mononucleosis
        v. AIDS
    c. Systemic conditions
        i. Congestive heart failure
        ii. Cirrhosis
        iii. Renal failure
2. Chronic inflammation
    a. Chronic Cholecystitis
    b. Xanthogranulomatous cholecystitis
3. Hyperplasia
    a. Adenomyomatosis
    b. Cholesterolosis
4. Infiltrating neoplasm
    a. Gallbladder carcinoma
    b. Lymphoma
5. Pseudothickening due to collapsed GB

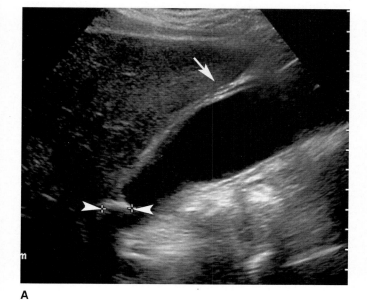

A

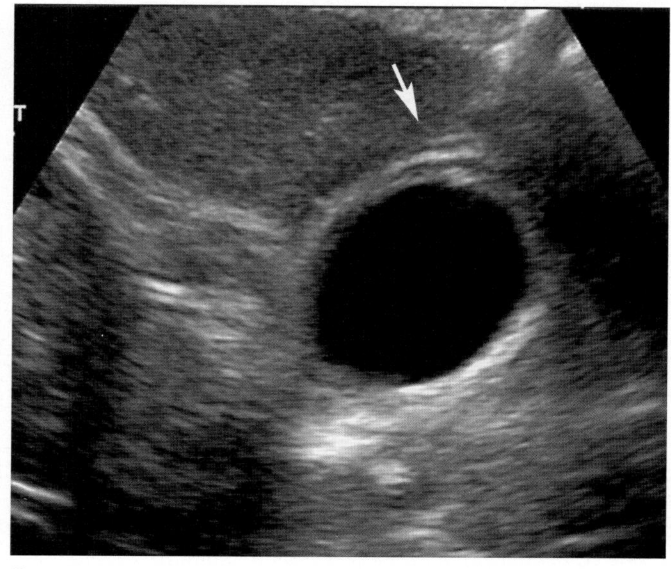

B

Figure 4-14 Striated Gallbladder
This 34-year-old woman complained of right upper quadrant pain. **A**. Longitudinal US and (**B**) transverse US of the gallbladder demonstrate an enlarged, thick-walled gallbladder with a stone logged in the neck (*arrowheads*). Note the longitudinal striations of the wall (*arrows*). These are features typical of acute cholecystitis.

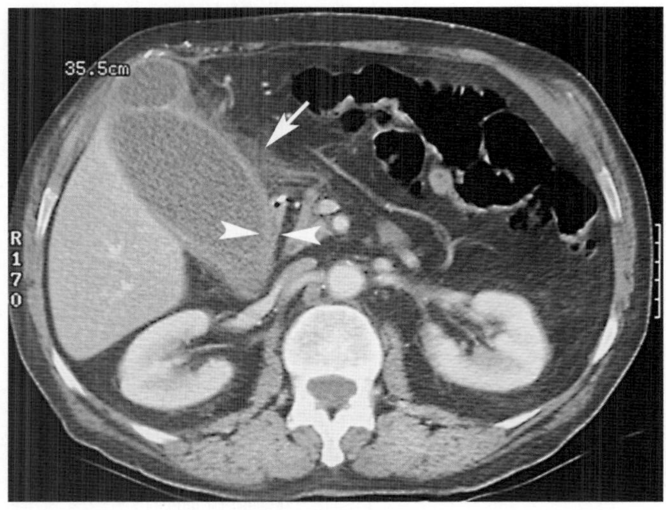

A

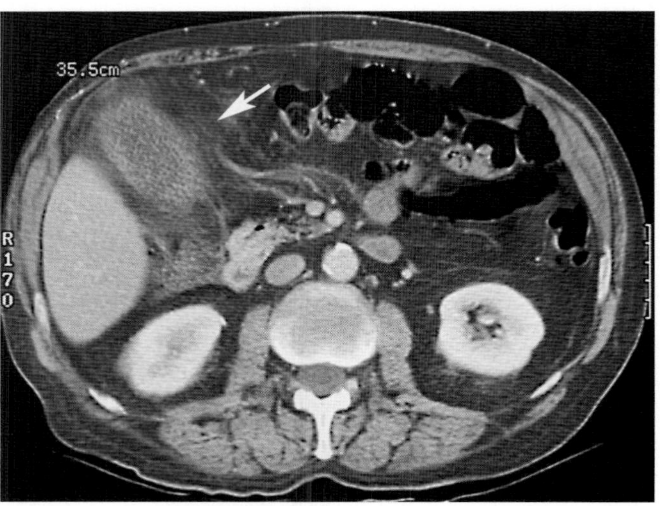

B

Figure 4-15 Acute Cholecystitis
This 70-year-old man complained of right sided chest pain. **A** and **B.** Contrast-enhanced CT images demonstrate a markedly distended gallbladder with diffuse gallbladder wall thickening (*arrowheads*). Careful observation of the wall in (A) shows a hyperattenuating mucosa with hypoattenuating (edematous) submucosa. There is also inflammatory stranding of the adjacent pericholecystic fat (*arrows*). Note also how the wall of the gallbladder brightly enhances with contrast. These are findings characteristic of acute cholecystitis. No stones were seen on CT and the pathologic specimen demonstrated cholecystitis without evidence of obstructing stone.

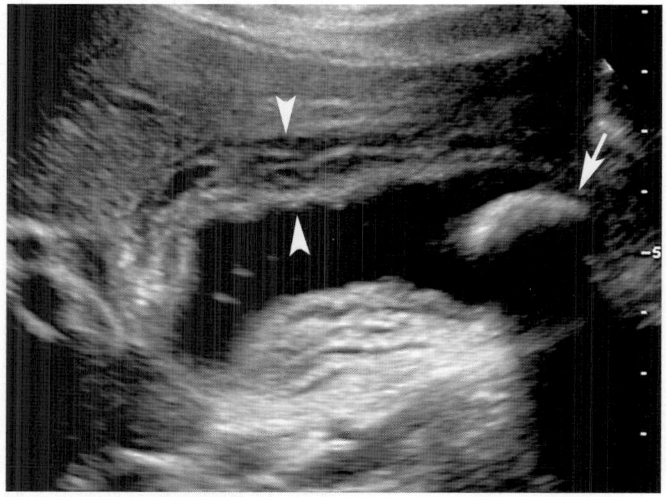

A

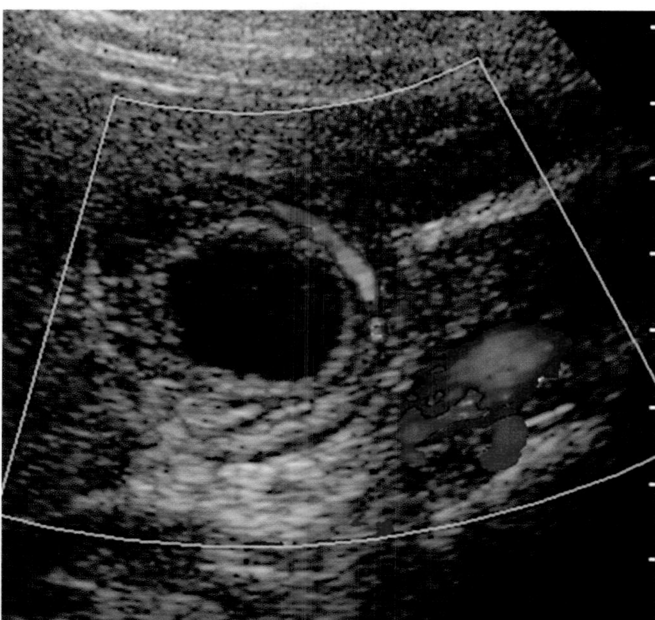

B

Figure 4-16 Striated Gallbladder with Hyperemia
This 24-year-old woman had intermittent right upper quadrant pain. **A.** Longitudinal US of the gallbladder demonstrates diffuse wall thickening (*arrowheads*) with longitudinal striations. A gallstone (*arrow*) with shadowing is seen in the fundus and a similar stone was seen in the gallbladder neck (not shown). **B.** Transverse color flow US of the gallbladder confirms the striated wall thickening and shows increased blood flow. Notice how the gallbladder is not distended, a feature that may indicate chronic rather than acute cholecystitis. The pathologic specimen demonstrated chronic cholecystitis.

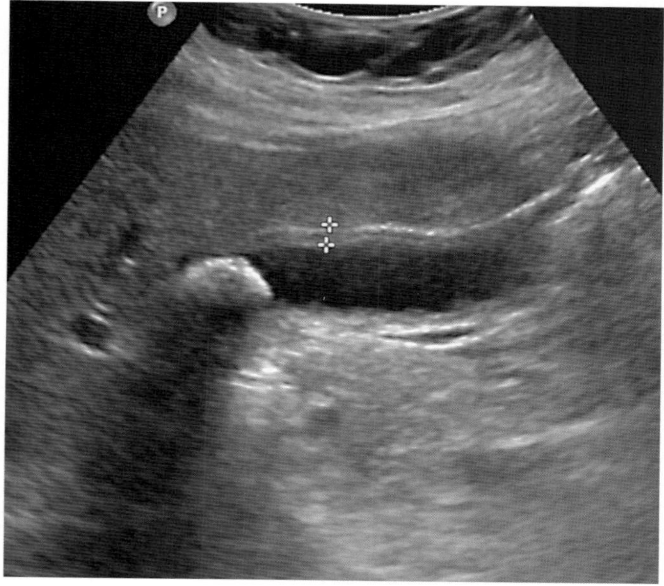

A

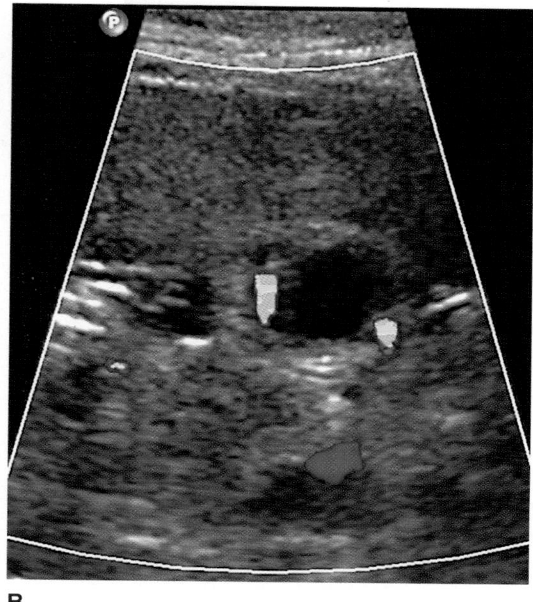

B

Figure 4-17 Acute Cholecystitis with Hyperemia
This 38-year-old woman complained of right upper quadrant pain, nausea, and vomiting. **A.** Longitudinal US of the gallbladder shows diffuse wall thickening (calipers) with a large shadowing stone in the neck of the gallbladder. **B.** Transverse color flow image of the gallbladder shows a thickened wall with increased flow. The normal gallbladder wall will normally be nearly completely without color flow. These findings are typical of acute cholecystitis.

etiology of hypoproteinemia will cause nonspecific thickening of the gallbladder wall. This finding is particularly prominent in alcoholics. In most cases, there will be evidence of edema in other locations, such as the subcutaneous fat and intra-abdominal fat, and often there will be ascites (see Figure 4-24). These findings are clues that the gallbladder wall thickening is a result of generalized edema.

Scarring and hyperplastic thickening of the gallbladder wall

Thickening of the wall of the gallbladder can be a result of chronic scarring in patients with chronic cholecystitis or as a result of mucosal hyperplasia in the hyperplastic cholecystoses: adenomyomatosis and cholesterolosis.

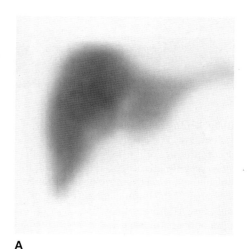

A

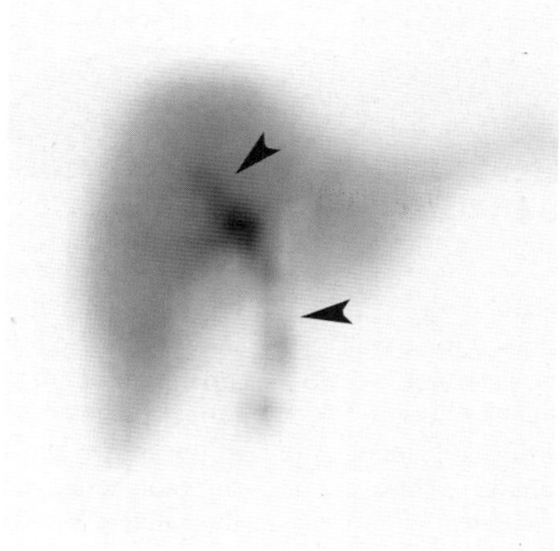

B

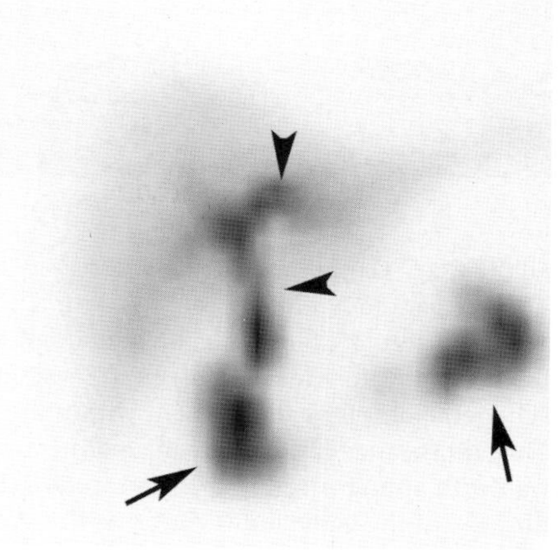

C

Figure 4-18 Acute Cholecystitis
This 49-year-old woman presented with right upper quadrant pain. **A.** In the early phase following Tc-HIDA administration, the agent is taken up by the hepatocytes and a faint outline of the liver is identified. **B.** Fifteen minutes later, the radiopharmaceutical has begun to outline the central bile ducts (*arrowheads*). **C.** After approximately 45 minutes, the radiopharmaceutical has been excreted in the bowel (*arrows*). Note that the gallbladder remains unopacified. These findings indicate obstruction of the cystic duct and are typical of acute cholecystitis.

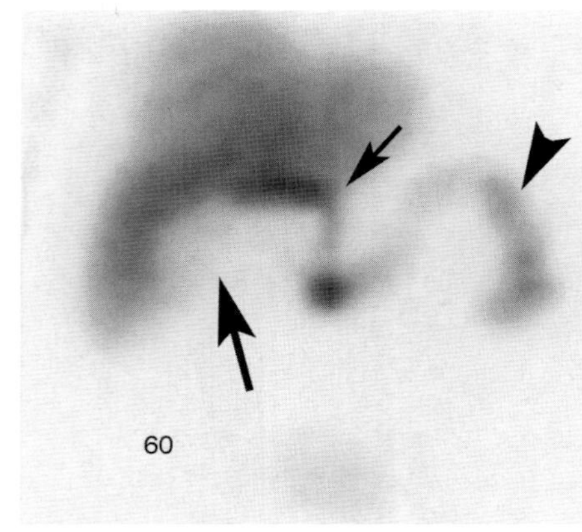

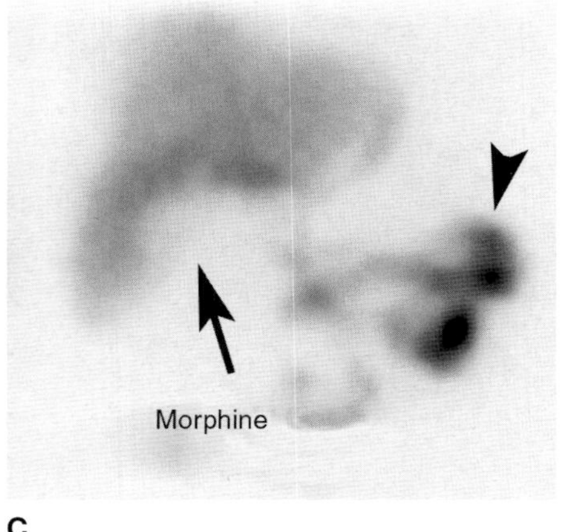

A B C

Figure 4-19 Rim Sign of Acute Cholecystitis
This patient presented with right upper quadrant pain, nausea, and vomiting. Tc-99m HIDA at (**A**) 30 and (**B**) 60 minutes postinjection and (**C**) following the injection of IV morphine shows absence of radiotracer in the gallbladder (*large arrow*) despite activity in the common bile duct (*small arrow*) and bowel (*arrowhead*). There is also increased radiotracer in the liver adjacent to the gallbladder fossa, a finding known as the "rim sign." The presence of the rim sign increases the accuracy of hepatobiliary studies for the presence of acute cholecystitis. (Courtesy of Jacob Dubroff, MD, PhD.)

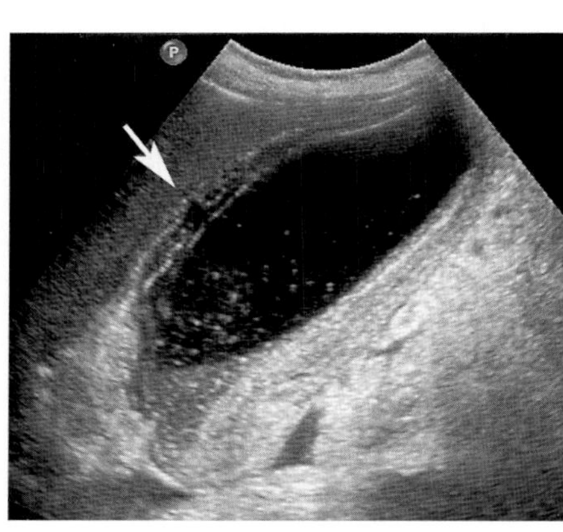

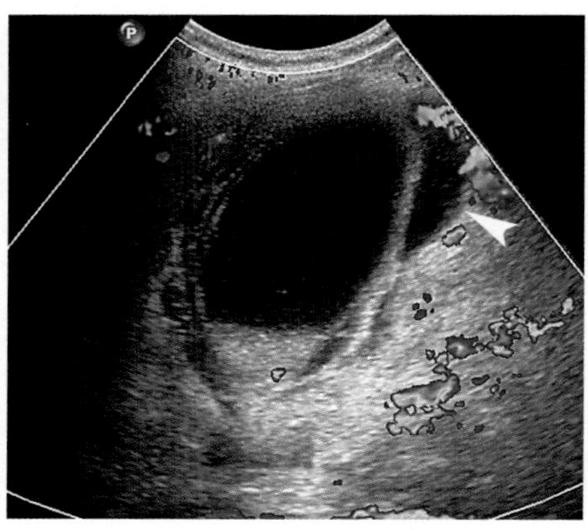

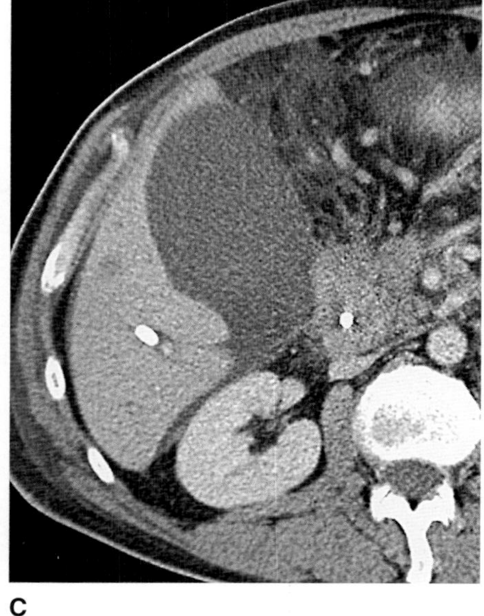

A B C

Figure 4-20 Gangrenous Cholecystitis
This 51-year-old woman presented with jaundice and fever. **A.** Longitudinal US of the gallbladder demonstrates diffuse wall thickening, with a focal defect in the wall (*arrow*). Extensive echogenic debris is also present within the gallbladder lumen. This appearance can be indicative of necrosis of the gallbladder wall with an increased risk of perforation. **B.** Transverse color flow US of the gallbladder confirms the presence of wall thickening and also demonstrates absence of blow flow in the wall. Inflammatory wall thickening of this degree will usually be associated with increased flow. The absence of increased flow could also indicate compromise of the gallbladder wall. A small amount of pericholecystic fluid is also seen (*arrowhead*). **C.** CT image of the gallbladder shows a dysmorphic appearance of the gallbladder with absence of the normal enhancement of the gallbladder wall, suggesting compromise of blood flow to the gallbladder. Evaluation of the surgical specimen confirmed a diagnosis of gangrenous cholecystitis.

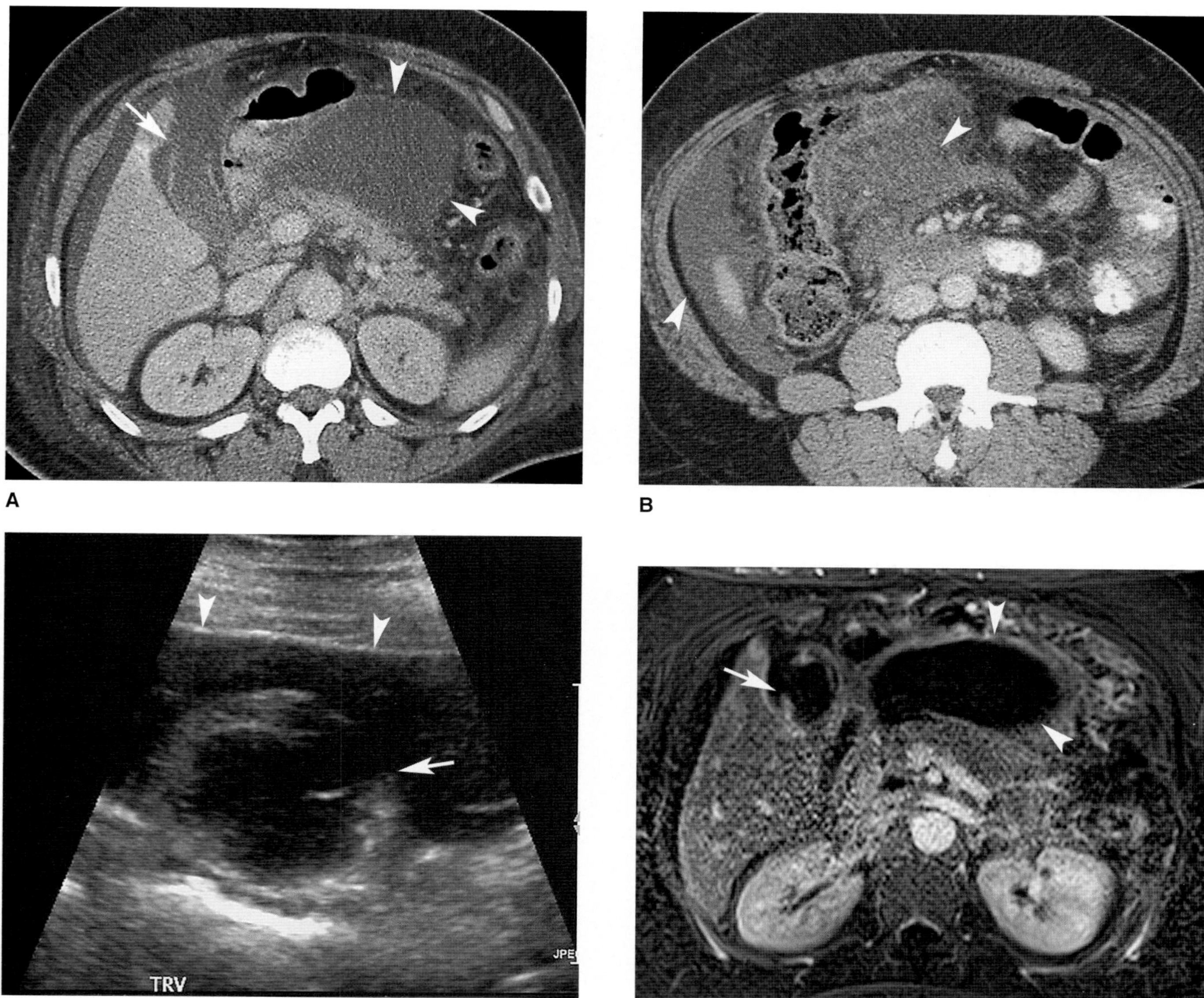

Figure 4-21 Gallbladder Perforation
This 59-year-old man developed persistent fevers after undergoing chemoembolization of hepatocellular carcinoma. CT (**A** and **B**), US (**C**), and postgadolinium T1MR (**D**) images demonstrate a focal defect in the wall of the gallbladder (*arrows*) and widespread ascites, indicative of a perforated gallbladder.

Chronic cholecystitis: Chronic cholecystitis is a result of transient, repeated obstruction of the gallbladder, usually from gallstones, causing repeated attacks of mild acute cholecystitis that leads to fibrosis and diminished function of the gallbladder. Histologically, chronic cholecystitis is seen as atrophy or hyperplastic inflammation of the mucous membrane usually with mononuclear infiltrate in the lamina propria.[54] Patients generally present with recurrent intermittent biliary colic. On all imaging modalities, the gallbladder appears diminished in size, irregularly shaped, and thick walled and typically contains gallstones (see Figures 4-16, 4-25, and 4-26). Xanthogranulomatous cholecystitis is a variant of chronic cholecystitis that is distinguished from standard chronic cholecystitis by numerous lipid-laden macrophages in the gallbladder wall. The pathology is not fully understood but may result from obstruction of the Rokitansky-Aschoff sinuses in the wall of the gallbladder with inspissations of bile, leading to rupture and inflammation of the gallbladder wall and surrounding tissues. Histiocytes phagocytize the insoluble cholesterol and bile lipids, leading to the characteristic feature of this disease.[55-58] Imaging features are usually nonspecific. On US examinations, these include a thickened echogenic gallbladder wall and gallstones. Occasionally, sludge is seen within the gallbladder lumen. Hypoechoic nodules and bands in the gallbladder wall also have been reported.[59-62]

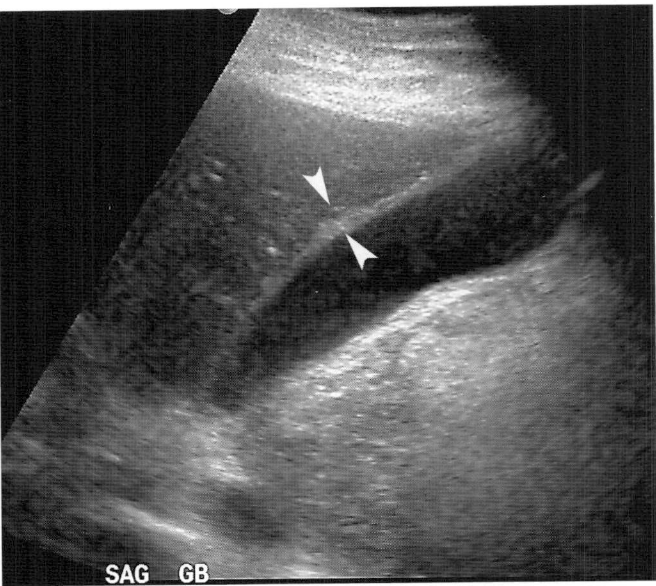

Figure 4-22 Secondary Thickening of the Gallbladder Wall From Adjacent Inflammation
This 34-year-old woman had acute pancreatitis and abdominal pain. Longitudinal US of the gallbladder shows diffuse wall thickening (*arrowheads*) due to pericholecystic inflammation as a result of the patient's pancreatitis.

The CT appearance can be indistinguishable from other causes of gallbladder wall thickening. Only when intramural hypoattenuating nodules are seen in the thickened gallbladder wall can xanthogranulomatous cholecystitis be reliably differentiated from gallbladder carcinoma.[63] Rare reports of MRI of xanthogranulomatous cholecystitis failed to differentiate this entity from gallbladder carcinoma.[59,64]

Cholesterolosis and adenomyomatosis: Adenomyomatosis and cholesterolosis are together known as the hyperplastic cholecystoses. They represent gallbladder wall thickening due to hyperplasia rather than inflammation. When focal, this will result in the formation of a gallbladder polyp and when extensive, it will result in focal or diffuse thickening of the gallbladder wall. The etiology for cholesterolosis and adenomyomatosis is unknown. They are found most often in women and are usually detected in the fourth and fifth decades. Patients can be asymptomatic or have right upper quadrant pain.

Cholesterolosis is characterized by deposition of triglycerides, cholesterol precursors, and cholesterol esters within macrophages of the lamina propria, epithelium, and stroma of the gallbladder wall.[65-70] A specific diagnosis of cholesterolosis or "strawberry gallbladder" can occasionally be made when US examination shows multiple small echogenic foci, representing small cholesterol crystals, within the wall of the gallbladder with associated comet-tail reverberation artifact also called "ring-down artifact" (see Figure 4-27). Further, CT and MRI cannot specifically diagnose cholesterolosis and demonstrate nonspecific thickening of the gallbladder wall, without pericholecystic fluid or fat stranding. This will typically appear low attenuation on CT scans but is difficult to distinguish from gallbladder wall edema (see Figure 4-28).

Adenomyomatosis of the gallbladder is characterized by hypertrophy of the gallbladder smooth muscle and overgrowth and invagination of the gallbladder mucosa. The

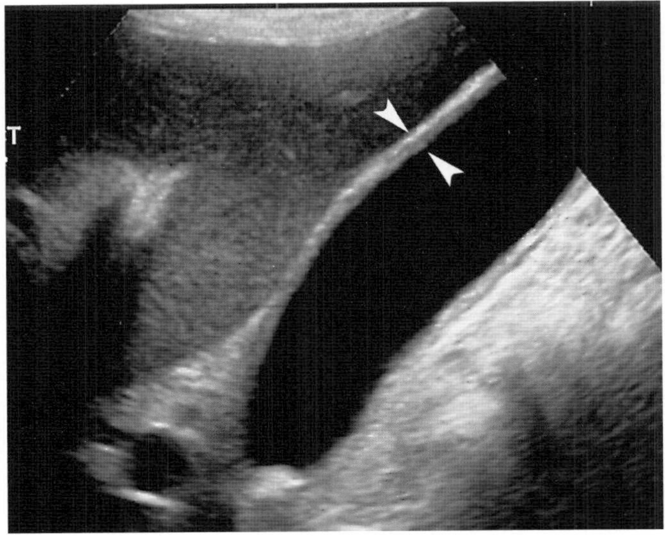

A

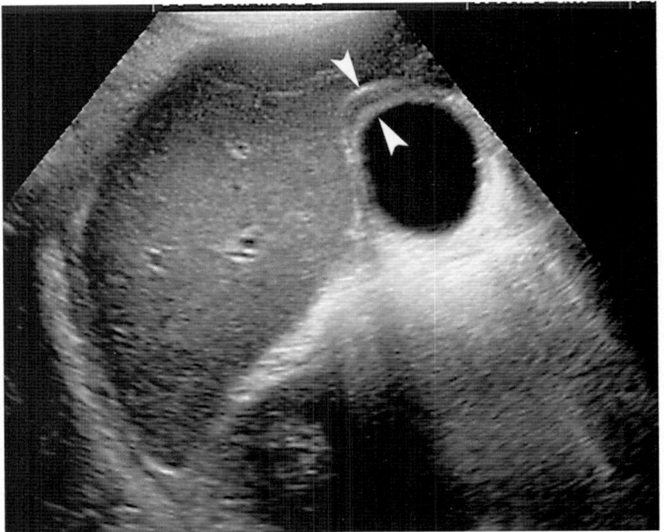

B

Figure 4-23 Gallbladder Thickening in AIDS
This 46-year-old man with AIDS had mental status changes and elevated liver function tests. Longitudinal (**A**) and transverse (**B**) images of the gallbladder show smooth diffuse thickening of the gallbladder wall (*arrowheads*). Although this could be a manifestation of many causes, in this case this is probably a direct result of the patient's AIDS.

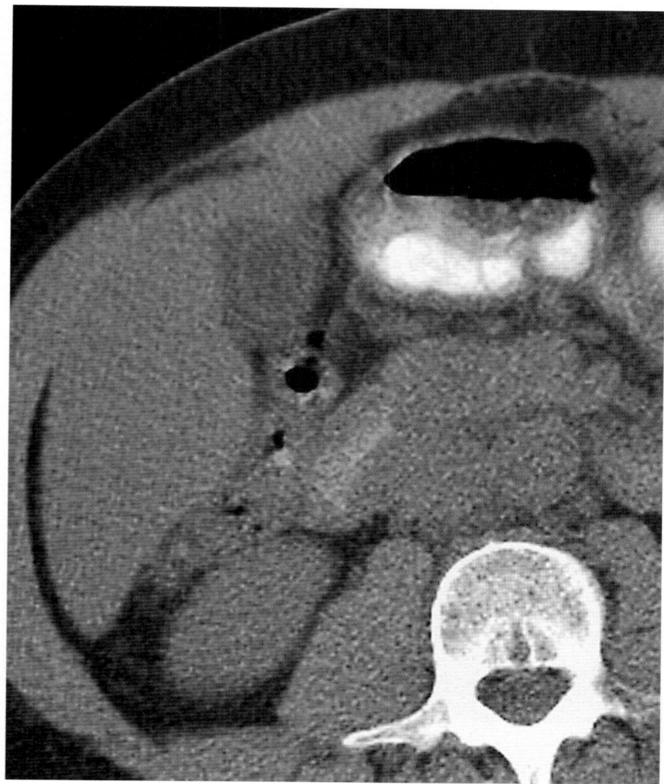

A

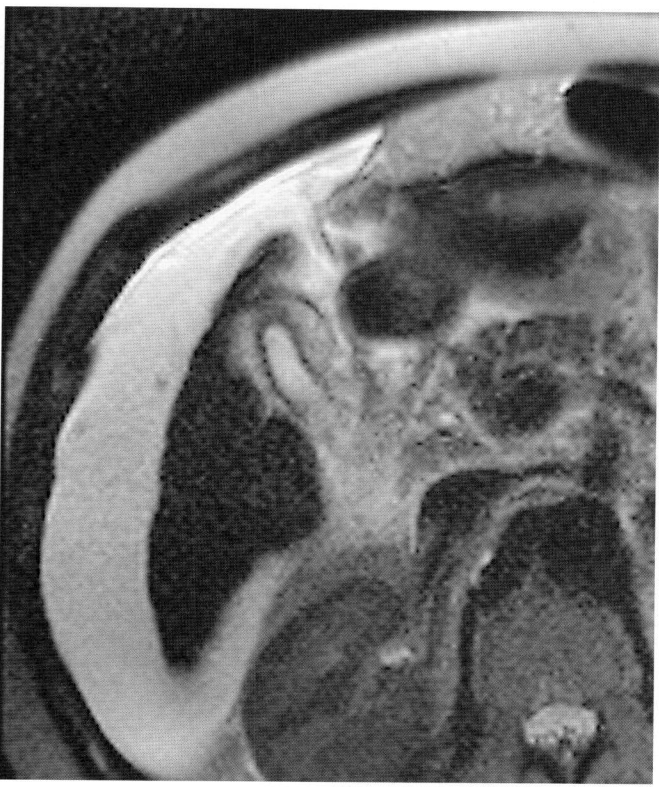

B

Figure 4-24 GB Thickening due to Hypoproteinemia
This 55-year-old man was malnourished as a result of cirrhosis. **A.** Unenhanced CT examination demonstrates the gallbladder wall to be diffusely thickened and low attenuation, indicating the presence of gallbladder wall edema. **B.** T2-weighted MRI sequence 3 years later shows increased gallbladder wall thickening and also demonstrates new presence of ascites. These findings were related to hypoproteinemia.

invagination of mucosa causes the formation of small intramural diverticula known as Rokitansky-Aschoff sinuses. Adenomyomatosis can involve the gallbladder in a segmental or diffuse distribution. It is a benign condition occurring in up to 9% of cholecystectomy specimens.[43,71] A specific diagnosis of adenomyomatosis can be made if the Rokitansky-Aschoff sinuses are visualized on imaging examinations. On US examinations, these will appear as multiple tiny, anechoic cysts within the wall of the gallbladder or as a corrugated appearance of the wall thickening due to the invagination of the Rokitansky-Aschoff sinuses (see Figure 4-29). Adenomyomatosis can also contain small cholesterol crystals and produce the comet-tail reverberation artifact similar to cholesterolosis. On MRI examinations, the diverticula will be seen as multiple tiny hyperintense cysts, linearly arranged in the gallbladder wall on T2-weighted sequences (see Figure 4-30). In most cases, the Rokitansky-Aschoff sinuses cannot be seen by CT scans (see Figure 4-28).

Malignant gallbladder wall thickening

Malignant gallbladder wall thickening can be a result of gallbladder carcinoma, lymphoma, or rarely other neoplasms, including Kaposi sarcoma.[29]

Imaging Notes 4-3. Distinguishing Features in Gallbladder Wall Thickening

Disorder	Examination	Feature
Acute cholecystitis	US, CT, MRI	Wall hyperemia
	US	Sonographic "Murphy sign"
Systemic edema	CT, MRI	Edema in tissues distant from GB[a]
Cholesterolosis	US	Comet tail artifact,
		High signal lipid on T1W MRI
Adenomyomatosis	US, MRI	Small cysts[b] in wall of GB on US
GB carcinoma	US, CT, MRI	Irregular wall
	US, CT, MRI	Severe thickening >1 cm

[a]Gallbladder
[b]Rokitansky-Aschoff sinuses

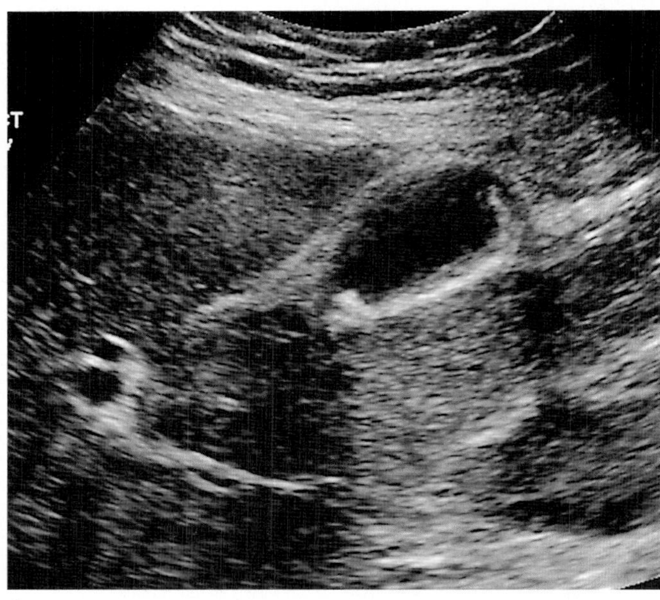

A

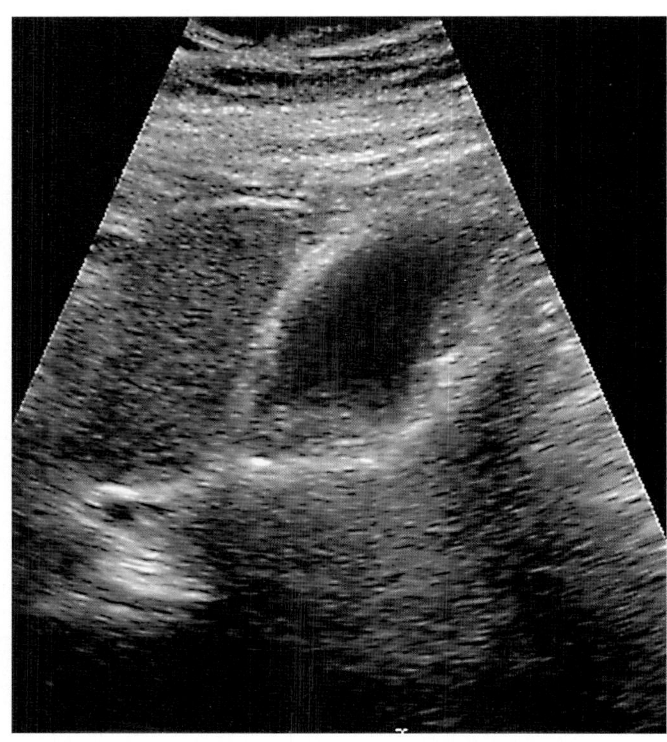

B

Figure 4-25 Chronic Cholecystitis
This 66-year-old woman presented with nausea, vomiting, and abdominal pain. **A** and **B.** Two views of the gallbladder from a US examination show a thick-walled irregularly shaped gallbladder. The pathologic specimen was characteristic of chronic cholecystitis.

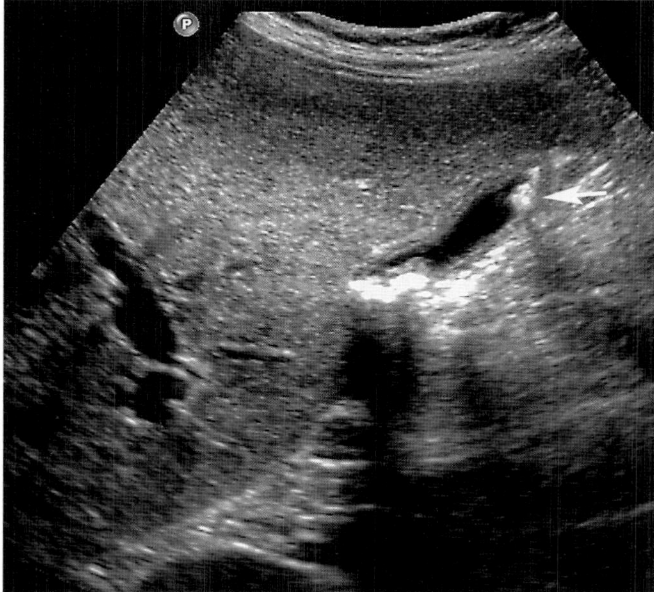

Figure 4-26 Chronic Cholecystitis With a Shrunken Gallbladder
This 61-year-old man was being evaluated for hepatitis C cirrhosis. Longitudinal US of the gallbladder shows a small thick-walled gallbladder with multiple small stones (*arrow*). Although unproven, this is likely a result of chronic cholecystitis.

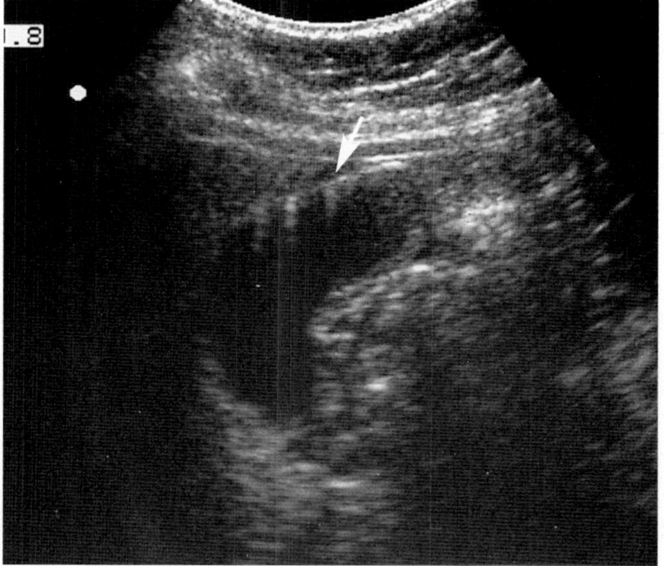

Figure 4-27 Cholesterolosis With Comet-Tail Reverberation
This 43-year-old woman complained of right upper quadrant pain. Longitudinal sonogram of the gallbladder demonstrates 3 cascading echo trains (*arrow*) that extend from the anterior wall of the gallbladder. This is the appearance of comet-tail reverberation and is a characteristic sonographic feature of cholesterolosis.

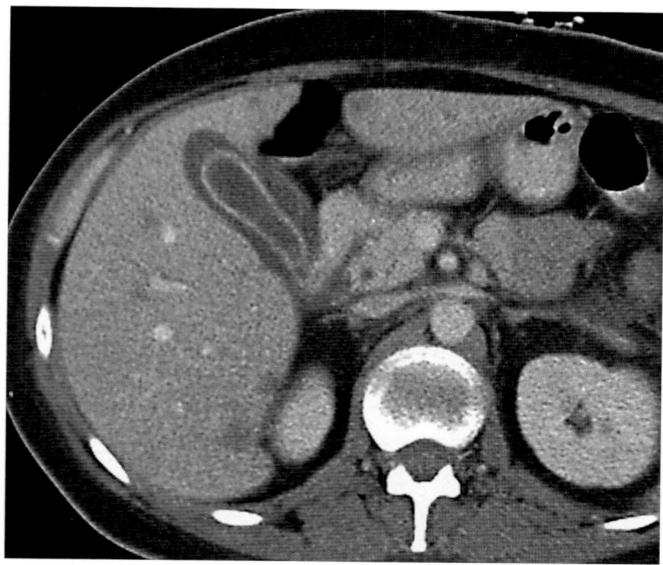

Figure 4-28 Cholesterolosis Causing Low Attenuation Wall Thickening
This 35-year-old woman had refractory T-cell lymphoma. Contrast-enhanced CT demonstrates hyperemic gallbladder mucosa with a thickened low attenuation submucosa. As a result of persistent pain, the gallbladder was removed and the thickened wall was found to be due to cholesterolosis. It is difficult to distinguish this appearance from diffuse wall thickening due to edema. However, chronicity of this finding should suggest cholesterolosis.

Gallbladder carcinoma: As noted previously, gallbladder carcinoma can occasionally present as focal or diffuse thickening of the gallbladder wall that can be indistinguishable from other causes of focal thickening (see Figures 4-31 and 4-32). This is an uncommon cause of gallbladder wall thickening and, when it occurs, the wall is usually excessively thickened with diameters of the wall greater than 10 mm. Also, unlike other causes of gallbladder wall thickening, thickening due to gallbladder carcinoma will usually have irregular margins and variable thickness.

Lymphoma: Lymphoma of the gallbladder is a rarely reported malignancy and can represent primary non-Hodgkin lymphoma from mucosa-associated lymphoid tissue or can be a result of gallbladder involvement in a patient with widespread systemic lymphoma. Approximately 20 cases of primary lymphoma have been reported.[2,72,73] Distinction between gallbladder carcinoma and gallbladder lymphoma on US, CT, or MRI is not usually possible.

Unique Disorders of the Gallbladder

Unique disorders of the biliary system are related to biliary function and malfunction. As the gallbladder is a reservoir for biliary secretions, stasis can result in the formation of gallstones and gallbladder sludge. When infection or obstruction occurs, surgical removal is indicated, which can result in postoperative complications.

Gallstones and gallbladder sludge

The gallbladder is a repository for biliary secretions that contracts in response to ingestion of food. With stasis, the bile can become increasingly concentrated, with diminished water content, known as "sludge" appears as echogenic material in the dependent portions of the gallbladder on US and increased attenuation material within the dependent portion of the gallbladder on CT (see Figures 4-33 and 4-34).[74] Layering material is seen on multiple MRI sequences with variable signal intensity. In most cases, bile stasis and sludge is a result of fasting. In certain situations, biliary secretions can form concretions known as gallstones. Gallstones are predominantly composed of cholesterol with small amounts of bile pigments and proteins and are called "cholesterol gallstones."[51] Cholesterol gallstones are seen more frequently in women than men and are also associated with obesity. Cholesterol gallstones may develop surface deposits of precipitated calcium carbonate.

Calcium bilirubinate (pigment) gallstones are less commonly encountered and are seen in patients with excessive hemolysis, especially patients with hemoglobinopathies such as sickle cell disease and hemolytic anemia. They can also be seen in patients with cirrhosis, where unconjugated bilirubin may be present in bile at higher than normal concentrations.[51] Additionally, pigment stones can result from bile colonized with bacteria, resulting in bacterial hydrolysis of conjugated bilirubin. [75]

Pigment gallstones always contain some calcification and will, in most cases, be radio-opaque on abdominal x-rays and CT scans (see Figure 4-35). Cholesterol gallstones are only radio-opaque if there is surface calcification on top of the cholesterol nidus. These stones will appear as one or several concentric rings of calcification on abdominal x-rays and CT scans (see Figures 4-36 and 4-37). US is the most sensitive imaging examination for the detection of both cholesterol and pigment gallstones and is the study of choice when a diagnosis of gallbladder calculus is suspected.[51] Both cholesterol and pigment stones are very hard substances and a have high acoustic impedance, reflecting nearly the entire ultrasound beam. They appear as an echogenic structure within the gallbladder with acoustic shadowing of structures deep to the gallbladder (see Figure 1-12).[51] As a result of its greater tissue contrast, CT will detect many gallstones that are radiolucent on abdominal x-rays. They will usually appear as increased attenuation structures with a calcific rim within the lumen of the gallbladder. Occasionally the center of the gallstone will fracture to be filled by decreased attenuation, nitrogen gas (see Figure 4-37). This is a finding that also can be seen on some abdominal x-rays. Rarely, some cholesterol gallstones will appear less attenuating than the surrounding bile because of the lipid character

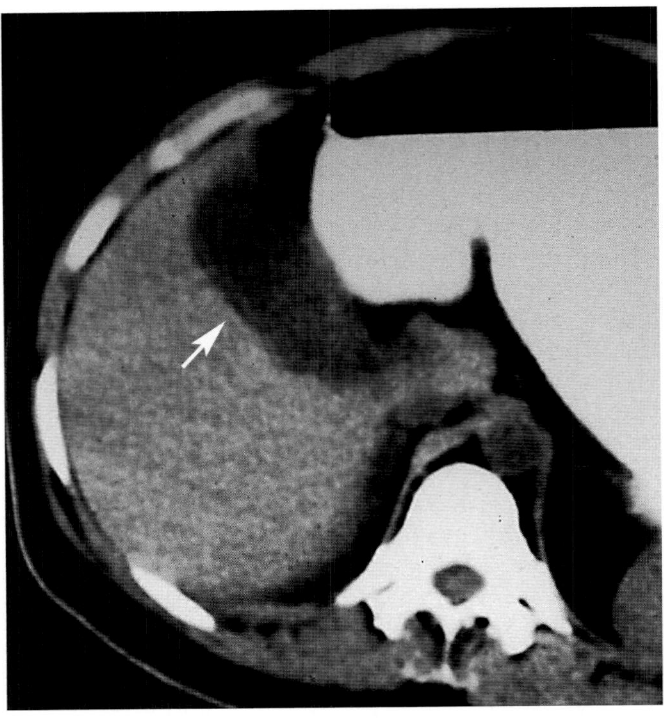

A

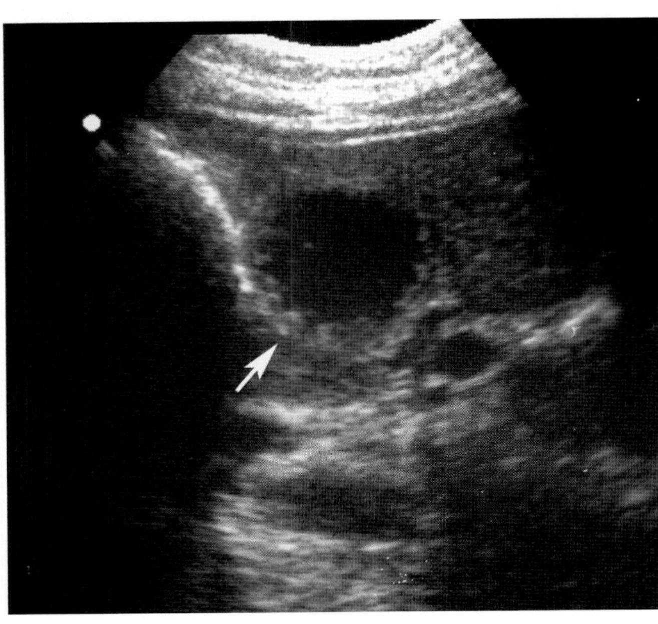

B

Figure 4-29 Adenomyomatosis
This 69-year-old woman had elevated liver function tests. Enhanced CT (**A**) and US (**B**) examinations both demonstrate a thickened gallbladder wall (*arrows*). On US, this wall has a corrugated appearance. The small clefts in the gallbladder wall represent Rokitansky-Aschoff sinuses and are diagnostic of adenomyomatosis of the gallbladder.

of cholesterol (see Figure 4-38). Further, MRI can readily identify gallstones regardless of their composition. Characteristically, calculi demonstrate low signal intensity on T1- and T2-weighted images compared to the surrounding bile. Occasionally gallstones may be difficult to identify on T1-weighted images if the bile is of low signal intensity, but stones will be more conspicuous on T2-weighted images (see Figure 4-39).[24]

Porcelain gallbladder

Diffuse gallbladder wall calcification, called a "porcelain" gallbladder, is a rare postinflammatory condition of the gallbladder that has characteristic imaging features. This phenomenon has been associated with an increased incidence of gallbladder carcinoma in some studies but not others.

A porcelain gallbladder can routinely be visualized on plain abdominal radiographs as a curvilinear calcification in the right upper quadrant corresponding to the shape of the gallbladder (see Figure 4-40). The thickness of the calcification may be thin, thick, or somewhat amorphous. The wall calcifications of a porcelain gallbladder are also readily demonstrated by CT but can be difficult to recognize on MRI examinations (see Figure 4-41). On US, it will appear as a large region of shadowing in the gallbladder fossa with absence of the normal gallbladder (see Figure 4-40).

Gallbladder fistulization

Rarely, fistula can occur between the gallbladder and surrounding structures of the gastrointestinal (GI) tract, including the duodenum and the colon. Causes of gallbladder fistulization may include neoplasms, infections, or erosion from stones. A special case of gallbladder fistulization occurs when a large gallstone erodes into the duodenum. The gallstone may pass through the GI tract without sequela but may cause obstruction at the level of the terminal ileum (see Figure 4-42). Fistulization to colon may cause recurrent cholangitis.

BILE DUCT IMAGING AND ANATOMY

Biliary disorders include an array of malignant and inflammatory disorders. In most cases they will be detected as a result of signs and symptoms of biliary obstruction.

Imaging the Biliary System

US is usually the initial imaging study of choice to evaluate the biliary system for suspected pathology. On US

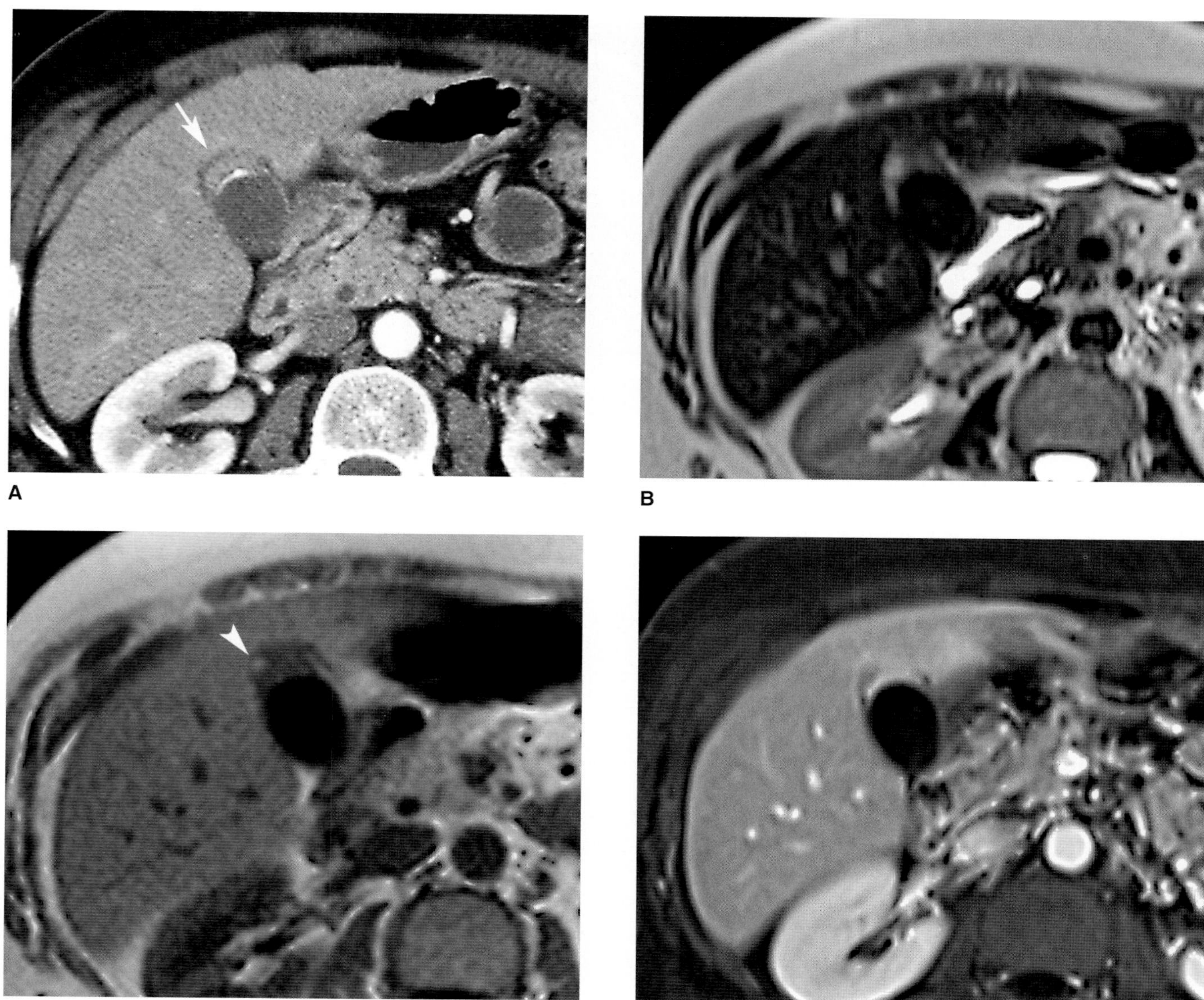

Figure 4-30 Adenomyomatosis Causing Focal Gallbladder Wall Thickening
This 54-year-old man with lung cancer had increased activity on a PET scan in the gallbladder fossa. **A.** Enhanced CT demonstrates focal enhancing thickening (*arrow*) of the gallbladder wall with a thin rim of calcification. Differential diagnosis would include gallbladder cancer, focal adenomyomatosis, chronic cholecystitis, and possibly a metastasis. **B.** T2-weighted MRI sequence confirms the focal region of thickening. **C.** T1-weighted MRI sequence shows a small hyperintense focus (*arrowhead*) within the region of thickening, indicating the presence of lipid material. This is indicative of cholesterol and positively identifies the wall thickening as due to adenomyomatosis. **D.** Postgadolinium T1-weighted sequence shows avid enhancement of the focal adenomyomatosis.

examination, the extrahepatic duct is easily visualized longitudinally, coursing over the portal vein, as an anechoic structure with thin walls (see Figure 4-1). Doppler evaluation can be used to help identify the portal vein and distinguish it from an adjacent dilated extrahepatic bile duct. US is also useful for identifying the intrahepatic bile ducts, small anechoic tubular structures located immediately adjacent to the intrahepatic portal veins.

With continuing improvement in CT technology, it is normal to visualize central intrahepatic bile ducts as tubular low-attenuation structures adjacent to the central portal veins (see Figure 4-4). The intrahepatic ducts are usually better seen in the right lobe than in the left lobe. Peripheral intrahepatic bile ducts should not be routinely visualized on normal examination. When there is specific pathology or attention toward the biliary tree during CT

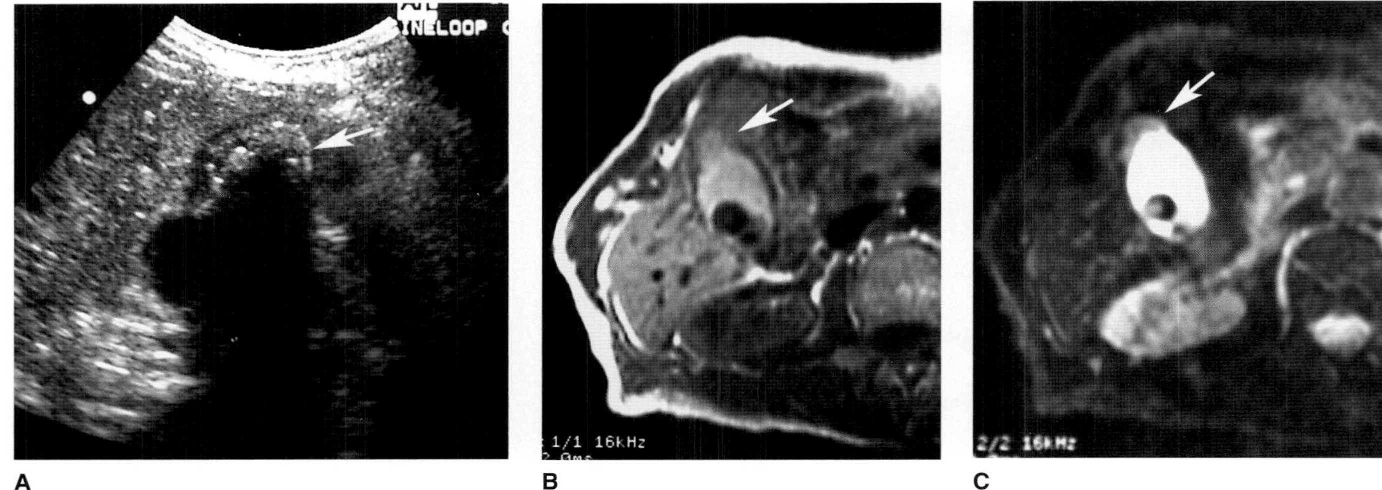

A B C

Figure 4-31 Gallbladder Carcinoma Appearing as Wall Thickening
This 70-year-old man complained of increasing right upper quadrant pain. Longitudinal view of the gallbladder (**A**) demonstrates extensive thickening of the anterior wall (*arrow*) of greater than 1 cm. There is shadowing beneath this thickened wall, indicating the presence of calcification. Axial T1-weighted (**B**) and T2-weighted (**C**) MRI examinations show focal thickening of the anterior wall of the gallbladder (*arrow*) with normal lateral and posterior walls. Focal thickening of this type can occasionally be due to adenomyomatosis but is most suggestive of a gallbladder malignancy. Biopsy was diagnostic of adenocarcinoma. Gallstones are also seen within the lumen of the gallbladder in B and C.

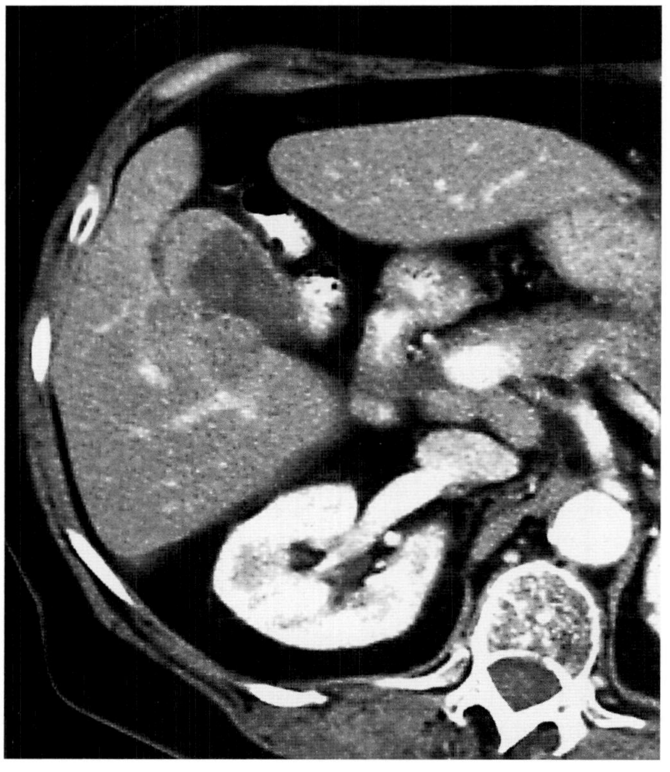

A

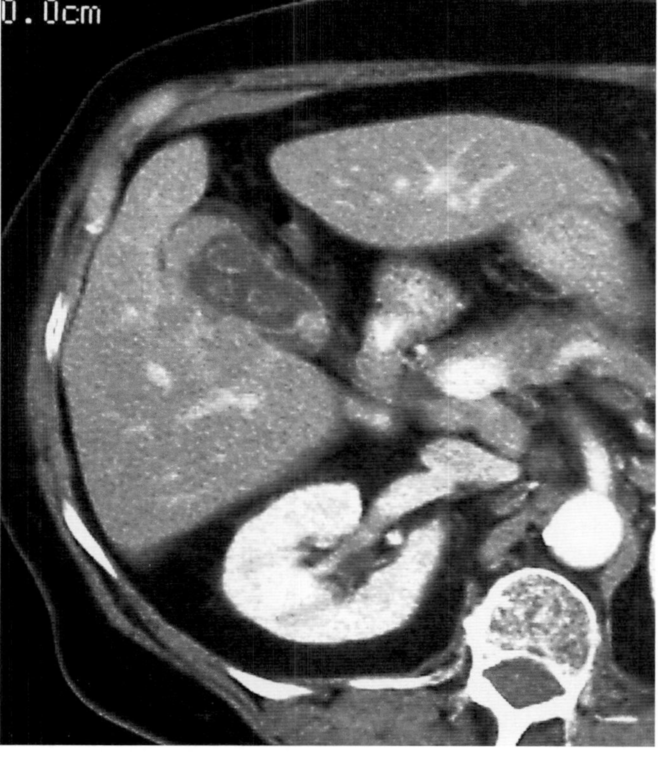

B

Figure 4-32 Gallbladder Carcinoma Appearing as Focal Wall Thickening
This 75-year-old woman had nausea and vomiting. **A** and **B.** Enhanced CT demonstrates focal thickening of the fundus of the gallbladder, with multiple intraluminal gallstones. There are also enlarged para-aortic lymph nodes suggesting local lymphatic metastasis. Needle biopsy of the lymph nodes was diagnostic of adenocarcinoma consistent with gallbladder carcinoma.

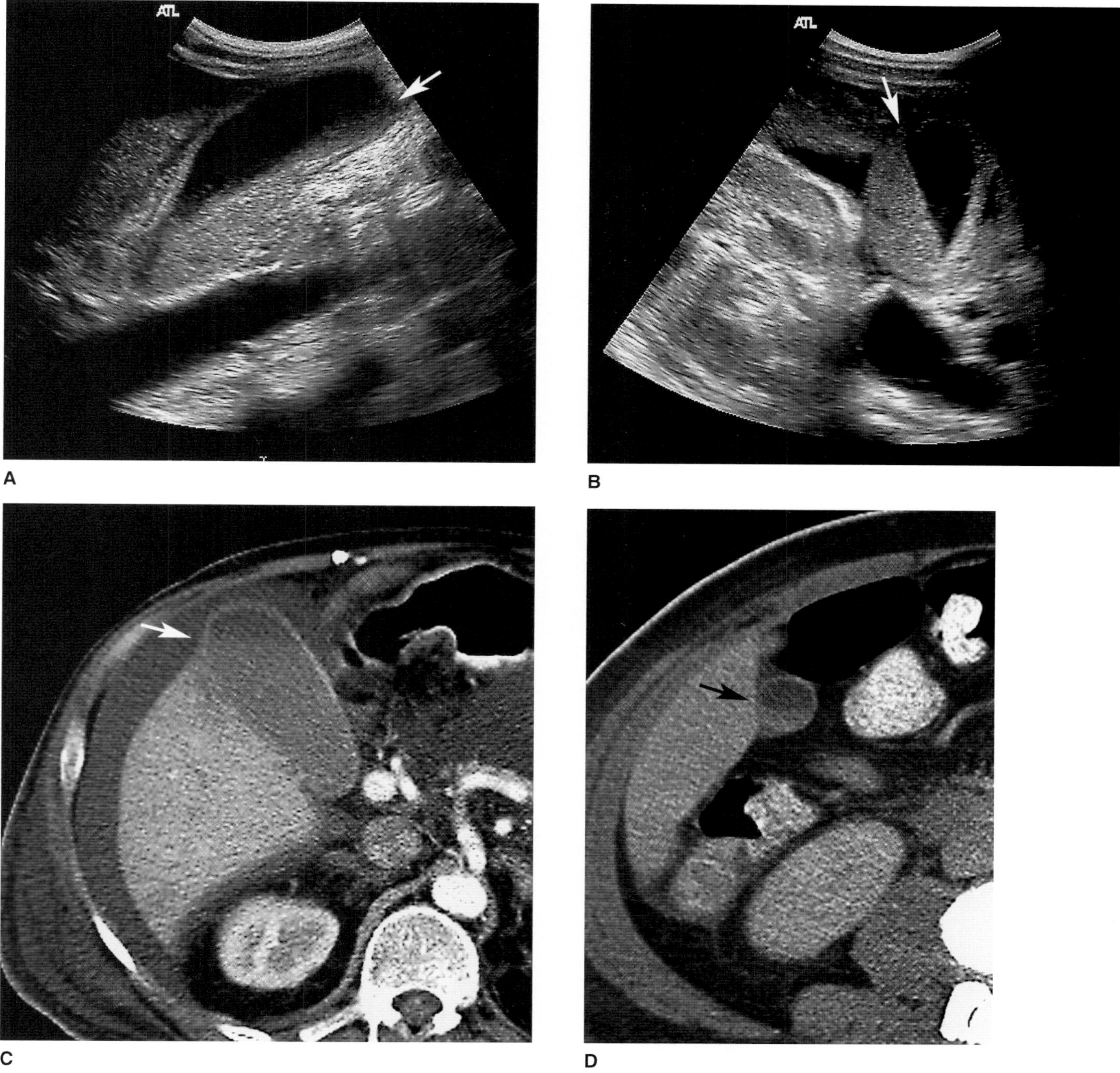

Figure 4-33 Gallbladder Sludge
Longitudinal (**A**) and transverse (**B**) US of the gallbladder from one individual and CT scans (**C** and **D**) from 2 additional patients show fluid debris levels within the gallbladder (*arrow*). This debris is known as gallbladder sludge and is typically found in patients who have been fasting.

study, the examination can be supplemented to include a CT-cholangiographic study. Further, CT cholangiography is performed by approximately 60 minutes following administration of an iodinated contrast agent with hepatobiliary uptake. At this time, the biliary system is then well opacified by the contrast, enabling clear visualization of the ducts. In routine intravenous-enhanced CT, the majority of the previously administered iodinated contrast is located in the biliary system at the time of imaging.

On MRI, both the extrahepatic and intrahepatic ducts can be identified as high signal structures on T2-weighted imaging. Because of the higher intrinsic tissue contrast of T2-weighted MRI relative to that of CT, it is common

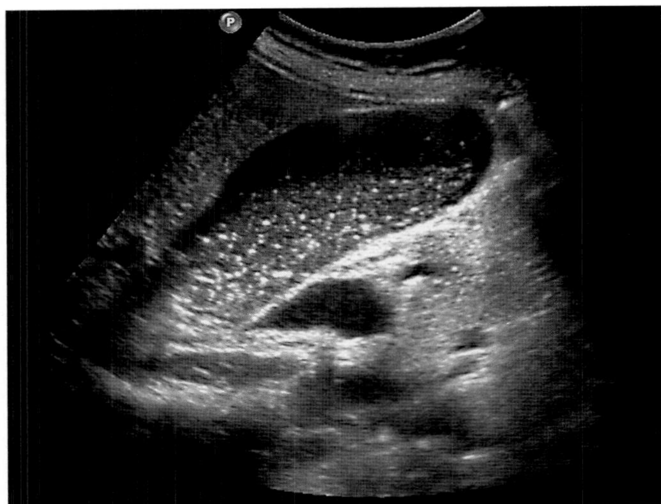

Figure 4-34 Starry Sky Appearance of Gallbladder Sludge
This 35-year-old woman with refractory T-cell lymphoma had elevated liver function tests. Longitudinal US of the gallbladder shows a speckled or "starry sky" appearance to the dependent debris, one of the US appearances of sludge and represents cholesterol microcrystals.

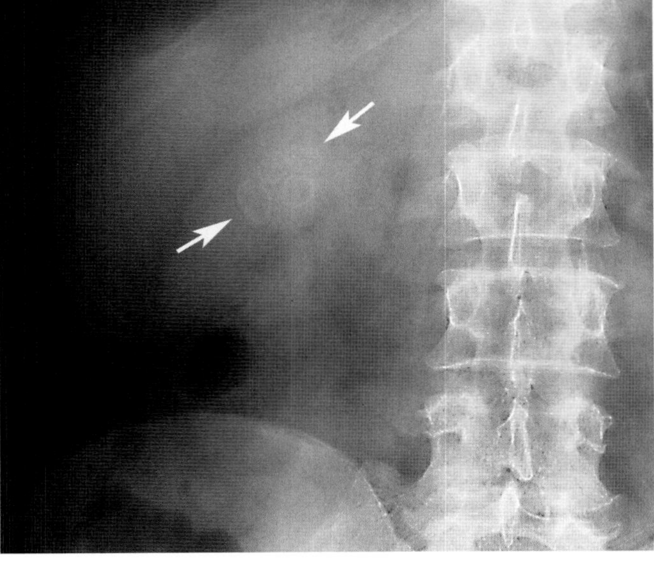

Figure 4-36 Gallstones
Magnified view of the right upper quadrant of the abdomen shows 4 faint rim calcifications (*arrows*). This is the typical appearance of multiple gallstones.

to see a greater number of small intrahepatic ducts on T2-weighted cross-sectional MR images than on axial CT images. However, small intrahepatic veins are also bright on T2-weighted MRI, so that only the main branches of the intrahepatic ducts are visible (see Figure 4-5). Magnetic resonance cholangiopancreatography (MRCP) represents a specialized type of MRI in which very heavily T2-weighted series are acquired in order to highlight the biliary system from other structures, including vessels. Although MRCP imaging is not specific for biliary ductal imaging, it will

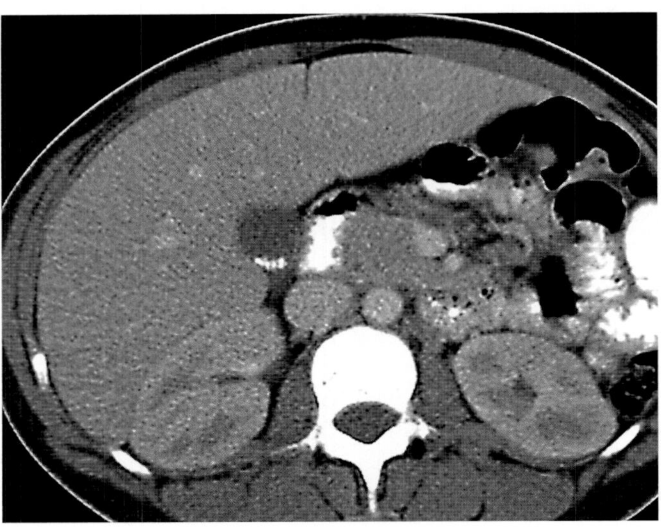

Figure 4-35 Pigment Gallstone
This 28-year-old woman with sickle cell disease had postpartum fever. Enhanced CT demonstrates a row of small calcified gallstones in the dependent portion of the gallbladder. These are typical of small pigment gallstones in this woman with sickle cell disease.

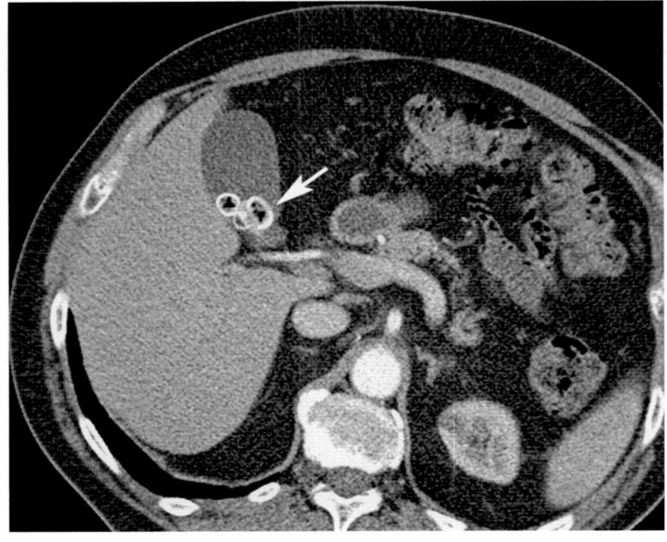

Figure 4-37 Calcified Gallstones
CT image of the upper abdomen demonstrates 3 rim calcified gallstones (*arrow*). The center of the gallstone appears black, indicating central gas within the gallstone that occasionally occurs in some cholesterol gallstones.

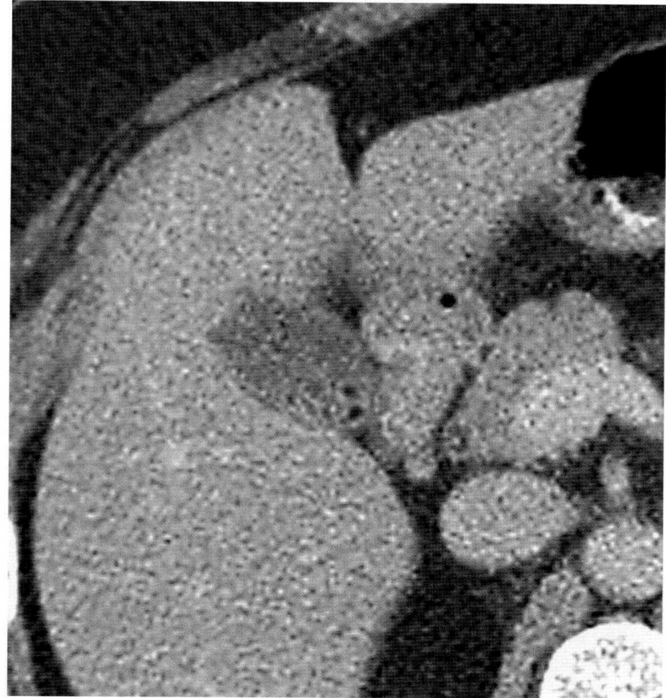

Figure 4-38 Low Attenuation Cholesterol Gallstones
CT through the gallbladder fossa demonstrates several faintly calcified gallstones. The central portions of the gallstones are low attenuation typical of cholesterol gallstones. With their low attenuation, cholesterol gallstones can be difficult to distinguish from the bile in the gallbladder.

highlight any fluid-containing structure, including cystic lesions, bowel lumen, and renal collecting systems. In addition, MRCP can be performed in either 2-dimensional (slab) mode, or 3-dimensional, high-resolution mode. In the latter case, maximal-intensity projection images (MIPs) are created to highlight the biliary anatomy in projection mode (see Figure 4-43).

Direct evaluation of the biliary system is possible with the injection of dense radio-opaque contrast during fluoroscopic and radiographic imaging. Direct access to the biliary system may be through percutaneous injection of the intrahepatic bile ducts (percutaneous transhepatic cholangiography [PTC]) or through retrograde access of the common bile duct (often in concomitant access of the pancreatic duct during endoscopic evaluation (endoscopic retrograde cholangiopancreatography [ERCP]).

Normal and Variant Biliary Anatomy

The biliary tree is divided into intrahepatic and extrahepatic ducts. On US, intrahepatic ducts are considered normal when the diameter measures less than approximately 40% of the adjacent portal vein. There is no universal definition for evaluating the size of extrahepatic bile ducts. Factors such as age and postcholecystectomy status can result in mild dilation of the extrahepatic ducts; however, an upper limit of 7 mm in transverse diameter has been used by some institutions.[1] Following cholecystectomy, the normal common bile duct can be as large as 10 mm. In most individuals, the intrahepatic biliary tree is represented by the bifurcation of the common hepatic duct into the right and left ducts, which then go on to divide into the 4 main

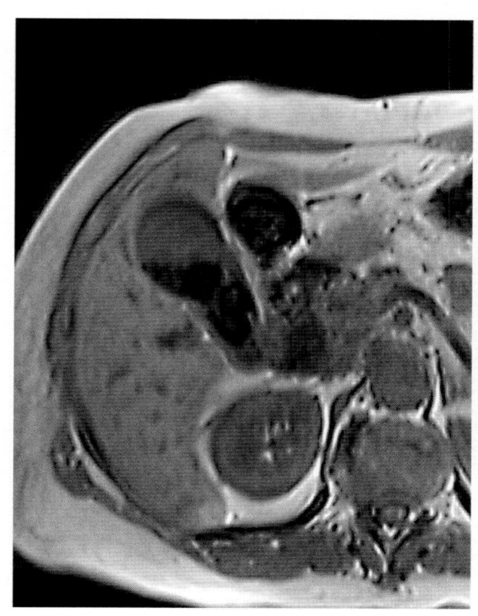

A

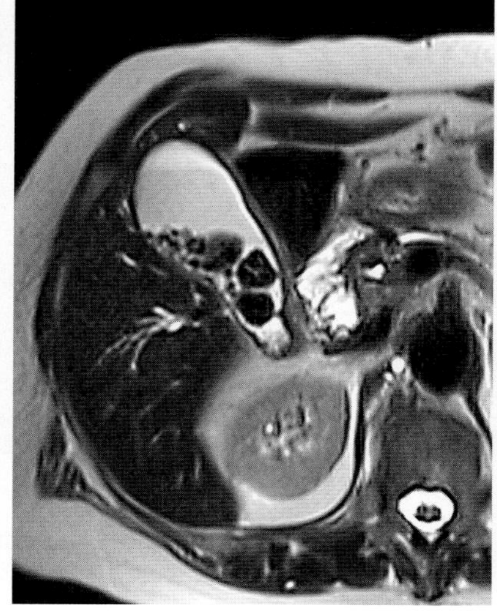

B

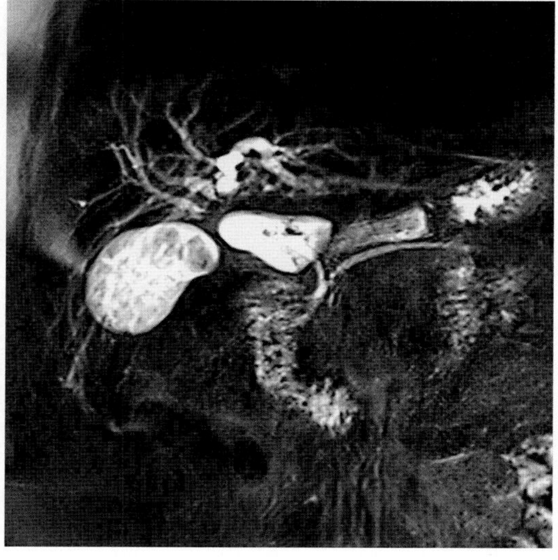

C

Figure 4-39 MRI of Gallstones
T1-weighted (A) and T2-weighted (B) MRI sequences show multiple faceted low-signal gallstones within the gallbladder lumen. MR cholangiogram (C) also shows multiple filling defects within the gallbladder typical of gallstones.

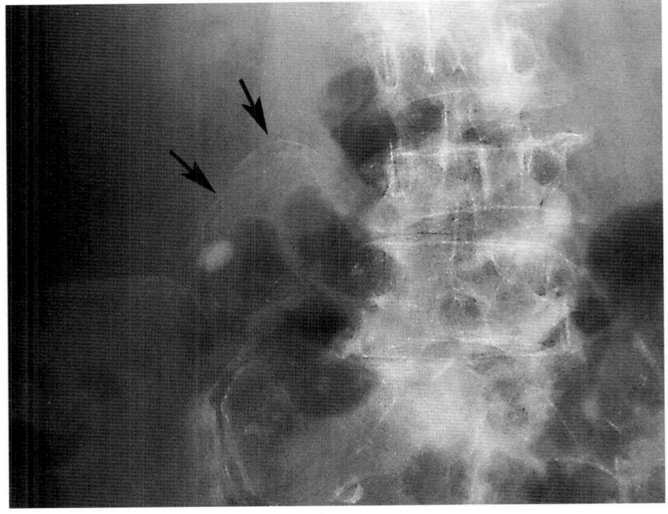

A

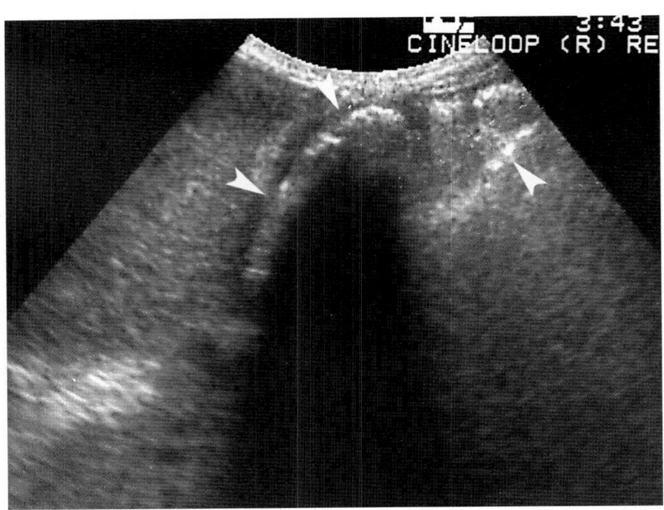

B

Figure 4-40 Porcelain Gallbladder
This 88-year-old woman complained of abdominal pain. **A.** Abdominal radiograph shows a faint curvilinear calcification (*black arrows*) in the right upper quadrant, an appearance diagnostic of a porcelain gallbladder. The oval opacity is a radiopaque pill. **B.** US examination shows a thick curvilinear area of increased echogenicity (*white arrowheads*) with complete shadowing of the deeper structures. This finding is also typical of a porcelain gallbladder.

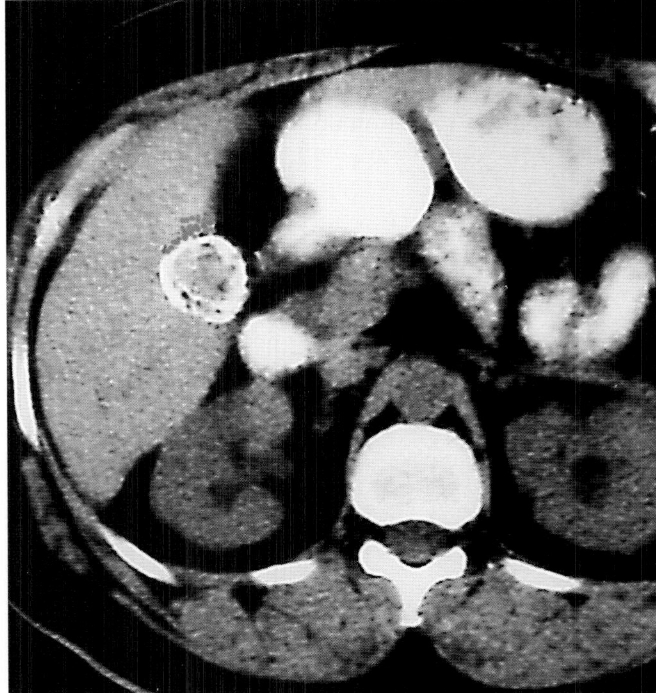

A

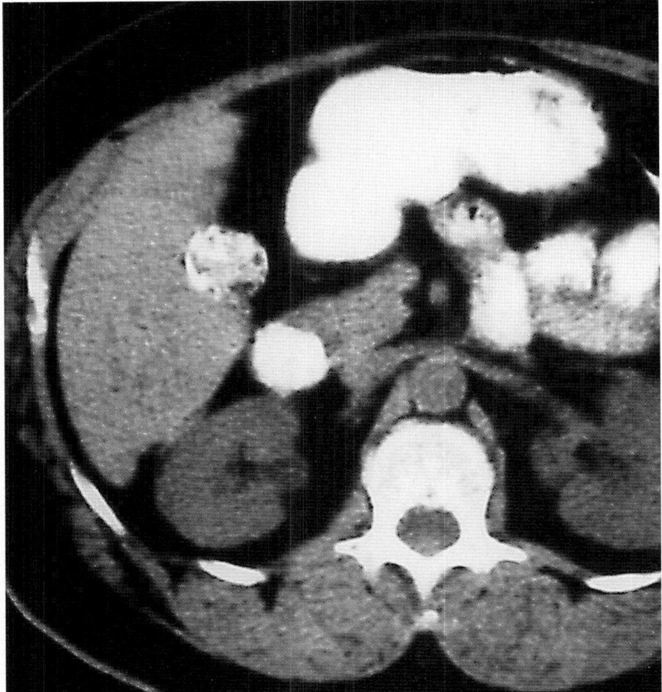

B

Figure 4-41 CT of Porcelain Gallbladder
This 69-year-old woman had vague abdominal pain. **A** and **B.** Unenhanced CT shows thick irregular calcification of the wall of the gallbladder diagnostic of a porcelain gallbladder.

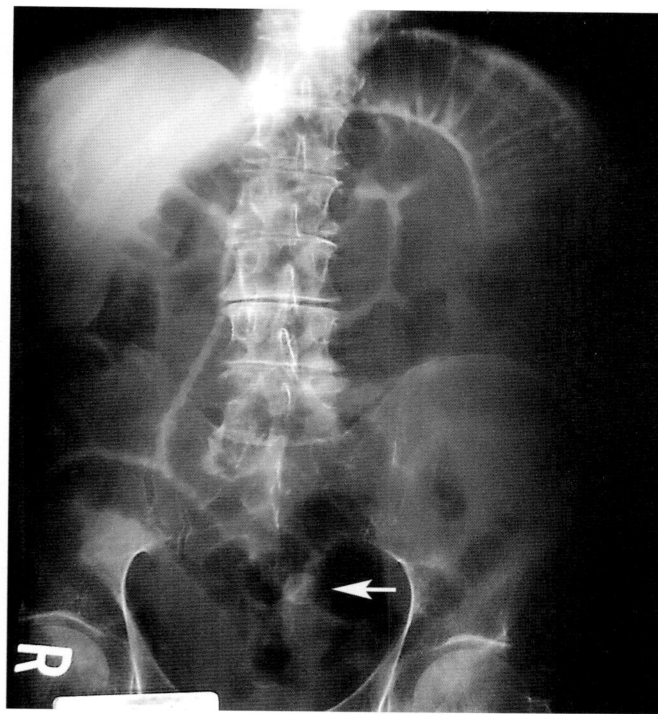

Figure 4-42 Gallstone Ileus
This elderly man presented with intermittent abdominal pain. Anteroposterior view of the abdomen demonstrates multiple dilated loops of small bowel and a calcified stone (*arrow*) in the midpelvis. Surgical exploration was diagnostic of small bowel obstruction of the distal ilium by a large gallstone.

segmental ducts (right posterior, right anterior, left medial, and left lateral). Common variants include aberrant origin of the right posterior duct from the left hepatic duct, or trifurcation of the common hepatic duct into 3 branches (right posterior, right anterior, and left). These variants in general do not predispose to pathologic conditions. However, careful mapping of the biliary anatomy is required for surgical planning, such as in partial hepatectomy for liver donation, so as to minimize inadvertent postoperative bile leaks.

PATHOLOGY OF THE BILE DUCTS

Common pathologies involving the biliary tree include congenital or acquired anatomic dilation (choledochal cysts), impacted biliary stones (choledocholithiasis), benign biliary strictures, benign extrinsic biliary compression, and malignant biliary strictures—the majority of which are secondary to cholangiocarcinomas and tumors of the ampulla of Vater. Choledocholithiasis and benign and malignant strictures usually present with symptoms of biliary ductal dilation. Pathologies that most commonly involve the smaller intrahepatic bile duct radicals, such as bilomas, biliary hamartomas, biliary cystadenomas, and biliary cystadenocarcinomas, do not usually result in biliary dilation but instead produce focal hepatic lesions and are discussed in Chapter 3.

Biliary diseases most often come to clinical attention as right upper quadrant pain, jaundice, or laboratory evidence of cholestasis such as elevations of bilirubin, serum alkaline phosphatase, or γ-glutamyl transpeptidase. Right upper quadrant pain can be a result of disorders of a variety of organs but most often is related to acute cholecystitis or choledocholithiasis with obstruction of the cystic duct or bile ducts.

Bile ductal dilation can also be identified incidentally on cross-sectional imaging preformed for other causes. When bile duct dilation is noted incidentally on imaging, careful correlation with physical and laboratory findings is required to elucidate potential occult biliary disease.

Bile Ductal Dilation

Bile duct dilation in most cases will indicate obstruction of the biliary system to the level where the dilation stops or indicates prior obstruction of the biliary system. US is the imaging method of choice for evaluating the common bile duct and can image this structure in nearly all individuals (see Figure 4-44). However, US in some cases will fail to demonstrate the most distal aspects of the common bile duct because of shadowing from gas-containing bowel. Therefore, in some cases, imaging evaluation of the extrahepatic ductal system will require additional imaging with CT or MRI.

The normal common bile duct is less than 7 mm in diameter but can increase in diameter following cholecystectomy or with aging. Occasionally, asymptomatic individuals without clinical evidence of biliary pathology will present with a common bile duct of up to 10 mm on cross-sectional imaging performed for other reasons. If the biliary dilation is limited to the extrahepatic ducts, this finding will usually represent a normal variant and has no clinical significance. However, if more severe extrahepatic ductal dilation is noted, or if the patient has mild dilation and clinical signs of obstruction such as jaundice or elevated liver function tests, thorough evaluation for additional findings of a cause of biliary ductal dilation is required.

Although, cross-sectional imaging is quite sensitive for extrahepatic bile duct dilation, it can sometimes fail to detect the cause of bile duct dilation, especially obstruction at the most distal aspect of the duct. The presence of extrahepatic ductal dilation without evidence of an obstructing mass can be due to unrecognized choledocholithiasis, subtle distal common bile duct strictures, or small tumors in the pancreatic head, duodenum, and at the ampulla of Vater. When neither routine cross-sectional imaging nor MRCP can identify the cause of suspected biliary obstruction, invasive techniques such as ERCP or PTC will be required. These studies are more sensitive for biliary strictures and intraluminal abnormalities than standard cross-sectional imaging and also useful for diagnostic tissue sampling and

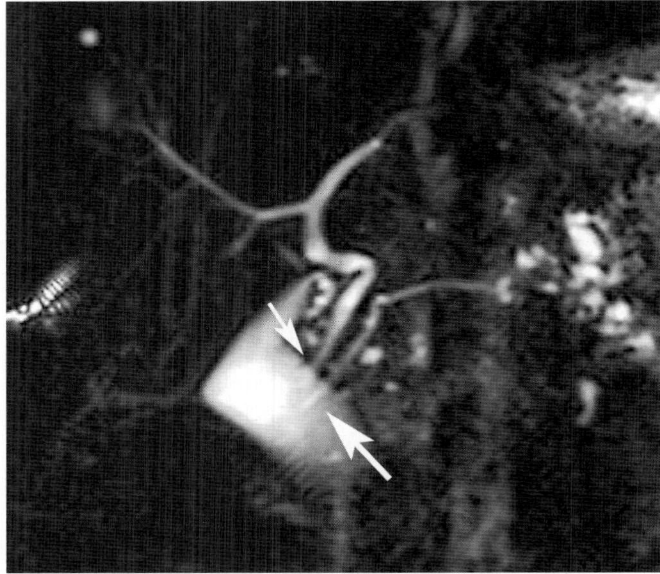
A

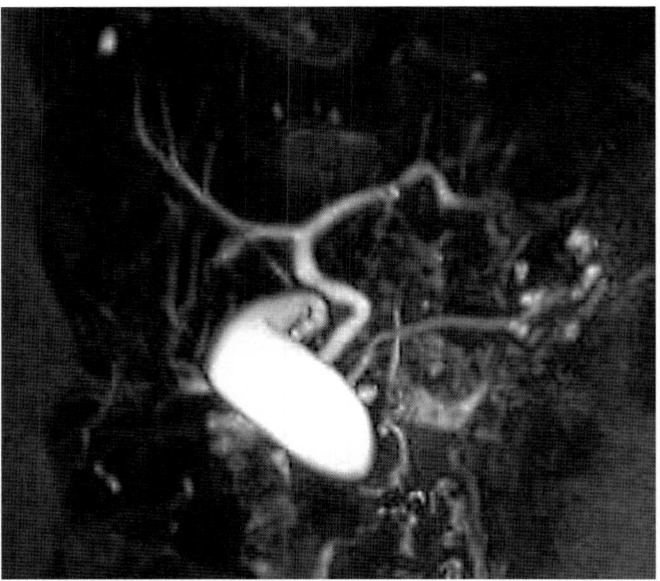
B

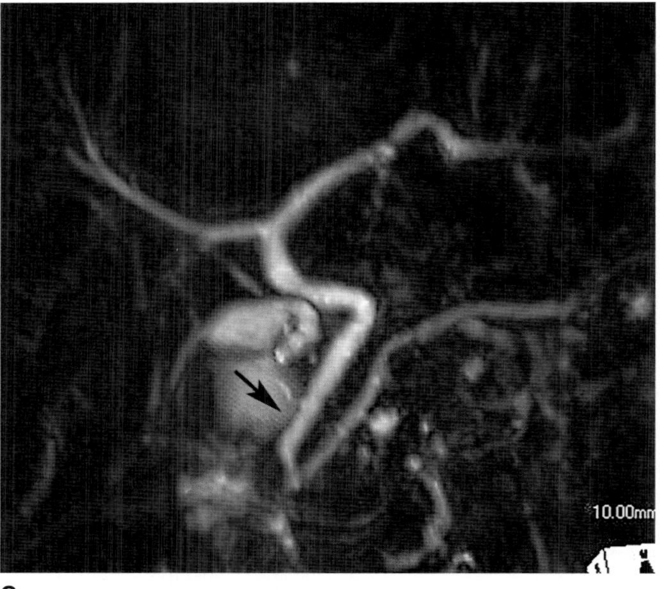

C

Figure 4-43 Normal Magnetic Resonance Cholangiopancreatography (MRCP)
A. Slab MRCP. Heavily T2-weighted image with a thick (typically 40-80 mm) single slice ("slab") demonstrates biliary ductal system and overlying structures (eg, gall bladder). The slab summation allows partial projection through overlying structures, such as distal common bile duct (*small arrow*) and pancreatic duct (*large arrow*), which can be seen in part behind the gall bladder. Oblique projections may or may not relieve this type of overlap. **B.** Maximum-intensity projection (MIP) MRCP image from a respiratory-gated 3-dimensional multi-slice sequence. The distal common bile duct and pancreatic duct are obscured by the gall bladder, with no partial transparency as in panel A. **C.** MIP image from the same image set as in panel B, with altered rotation and thinner reconstruction slab, allowing visualization of the distal common bile duct (*black arrow*) and pancreatic duct (*white arrow*), but with more limited evaluation of the central biliary tree. These images require real-time manipulation on a 3-dimensional workstation to optimize visualization of pertinent anatomy.

therapeutic intervention (stone removal, stricture stenting) at the time of the procedure to provide relief of the obstruction (see Figure 4-45).[76]

On unenhanced CT, both the intrahepatic bile ducts and the hepatic vessels will be low attenuation relative to liver parenchyma and it can be difficult to recognize mildly dilated ducts as distinguished from unopacified hepatic blood vessels, but in most cases the ducts will have a lower attenuation than the adjacent portal veins (see Figure 4-46). With contrast enhancement, the vessels become high attenuation relative to liver, and the dilated ducts are easily recognized because of their low attenuation (see Figure 4-47).

On T2-weighted images, biliary fluid will appear high intensity (bright white) relative to the hepatic parenchyma (see Figure 4-47). Detection of branching high-intensity tubules can indicate ductal dilation. Unfortunately, depending on the imaging parameters employed, the hepatic vessels can also appear high intensity and be confused with dilated bile ducts. This is especially true if flow-sensitive bright blood imaging techniques, such as balanced (T1/T2*) gradient echo techniques. On diffusion-weighted imaging, both blood vessels and bile ducts will lose signal with application of diffusion gradients. Therefore, in general, heavily T2-weighted (TE > 200 ms) are used in conjunction with high-resolution 3D or slab 2D techniques to identify smaller intrahepatic ducts via their relationship to the larger intrahepatic and extrahepatic ductal system on these projection and volumetric techniques.

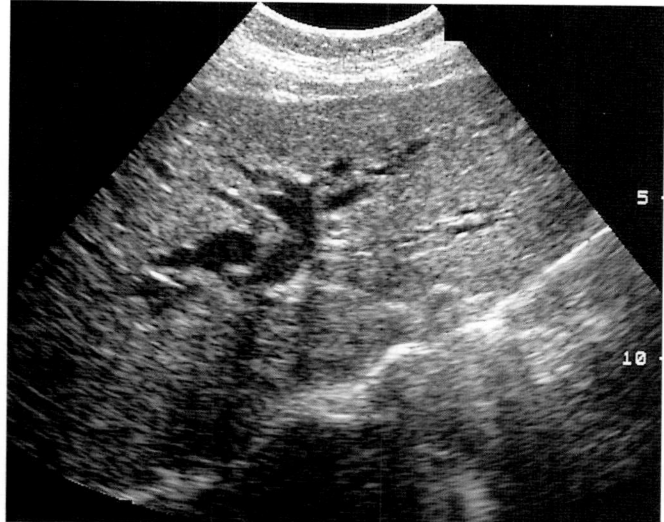

A

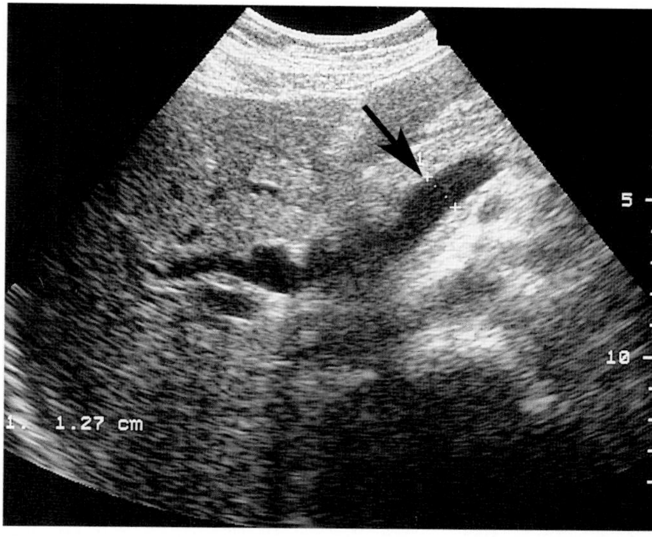

B

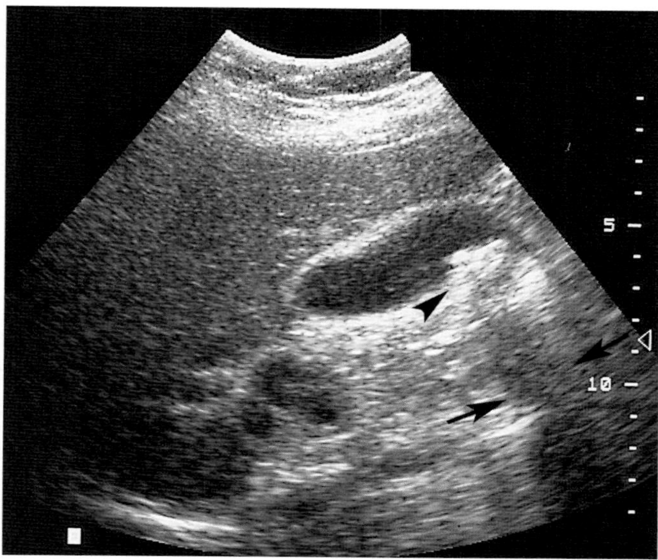

C

Figure 4-44 Choledocholithiasis with Biliary Dilation
This 18-year-old woman complained of several months of right upper quadrant abdominal pain. **A.** Transverse US demonstrated intrahepatic biliary ductal dilation. **B.** The common bile duct (*large arrow*) measures 13 mm. **C.** Multiple gallstones are seen within the gallbladder (*arrowhead*). Note the shadowing behind the gallstones (*small arrows*). Although no stone is demonstrated in the common bile duct, the presence of a stone can be inferred from the bile duct dilation. A stone was endoscopically removed from the distal common bile duct.

Bile duct obstruction

Bile duct obstruction can result from a variety of causes, including gallstones, malignancies, infections, autoimmune disorders, and congenital abnormalities (Table 4-3).

Choledocholithiasis: Choledocholithiasis is the most common cause of biliary obstruction. In most cases, gallstones will also be present within the gallbladder, and the patient will present with signs and symptoms of acute biliary ductal obstruction such as elevations in bilirubin, alkaline phosphatase, or γ-glutamyl transpeptidase associated with right upper quadrant pain. Bile duct stones are very small structures and are very difficult to detect with cross-sectional imaging. When common duct stones are suspected, the distal common bile duct should be carefully evaluated for the presence of a stone. In most cases, US fails to adequately visualize the distal common bile duct, and the presence of a stone can only be inferred from the presence of dilation of the common bile duct and stones in the gallbladder (see Figure 4-44). If the distal common bile duct can be visualized, a common duct stone will appear as a hyperechoic, shadowing structure within the distal duct, with proximal ductal dilation. On CT scans, calcified common duct stones will be seen as a few-millimeter-size hyperattenuating structures within the low attenuating common bile duct but most noncalcified stones will be missed (see Figures 4-47 and 4-48). Heavily T2-weighted MRI sequences will show the common duct stone to appear as a few-millimeter, low-signal structure within high-attenuation distal common bile duct lumen (see Figure 4-47). In general, MRCP is now the diagnostic study of choice for the evaluation of suspected choledocholithiasis. On the

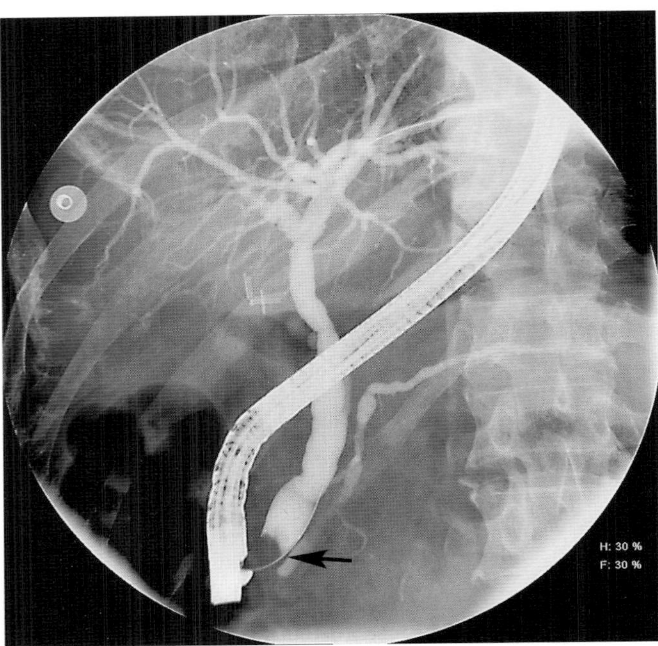

Figure 4-45 Ampullary Carcinoma
This 69-year-old man presented with jaundice. ERCP demonstrates a sharply marginated filling defect (*arrow*) in the distal common bile duct. Note the shouldered margins of the lesion relative to the duct. Differential diagnosis would include a radiolucent stone and small ampullary tumor. Biopsy was diagnostic of a small ampullary carcinoma.

other hand, ERCP and PTC are primarily used for interventions requiring the removal of biliary stones and are usually not necessary for the diagnosis of choledocholithiasis; however, occasionally all noninterventional imaging studies fail to diagnose the presence of biliary stones, which are subsequently diagnosed by ERCP or PTC (see Figure 4-49). For details about types and etiologies of gallstones, please see the heading **Unique Disorders of the Biliary System** previously discussed in this chapter.

Mirizzi syndrome is a rare cause of biliary obstruction that results from one or several gallstones lodged in the cystic duct or gallbladder neck causing common bile duct obstruction and obstructive jaundice. In order for this to occur, the cystic duct must run parallel to the extrahepatic bile duct. It is important to identify this anatomic variation preoperatively to avoid inadvertent ligation of the common bile duct during cholecystectomy (see Figure 4-50).[77-79] The obstruction may be caused directly by the gallstone or by the inflammatory reaction surrounding the affected duct. If the impaction is not resolved, erosion of the walls of the cystic duct and common bile duct can rarely result in the formation of a fistulous connection between the Hartman pouch of the gallbladder (the outpouching of the gallbladder wall at the junction of the neck and cystic duct) and adjacent common bile duct (cholecystocholedochal fistula) or stricture.

Malignant biliary obstruction: Malignancy is another common cause of bile duct obstruction, especially pancreatic carcinoma involving the head of the pancreas but also other pancreatic malignancies, intrahepatic and extrahepatic cholangiocarcinomas, hepatocellular carcinoma, other hepatic malignancies, ampullary carcinomas, duodenal carcinomas, metastasis, and lymphoma. Except for ampullary carcinoma and some cholangiocarcinomas, most of these malignancies will be easily detected by cross-sectional imaging, centered in the organ in which they arose.

Cholangiocarcinoma: Cholangiocarcinoma is an adenocarcinoma arising from bile duct epithelium. These are typically infiltrating tumors that spread along the biliary tracts and are often only minimally conspicuous. These neoplasms induce a substantial amount of fibrosis in the surrounding tissues, a feature that causes prolonged delayed enhancement of the tumor with intravenous contrast and can be an important clue to identifying these tumors.[80] Cholangiocarcinoma is associated with chronic inflammation of the biliary epithelium[81] and is, therefore, seen with increased frequency in patients with biliary stones, primary sclerosing cholangitis, infections with clonorchiasis species, choledochal cysts, and Caroli disease.[80] Cholangiocarcinoma can be classified into intrahepatic and extrahepatic cholangiocarcinoma. Intrahepatic cholangiocarcinoma can be divided further into hilar and peripheral cholangiocarcinoma and is classified as mass-forming (the most common), periductal infiltrating, and intraductal.[81]

The most common site of tumor involvement is the confluence of the right and left hepatic ducts, commonly called a Klatskin tumor.[82] In many cases, no discrete mass is identified within the porta hepatis, and so these tumors typically present as dilated intrahepatic ducts without imaging evidence of communication between the right and left hepatic ducts (see Figure 4-51).[37] Occasionally, careful observation will demonstrate focal thickening of the walls of the central bile ducts, greater than 5 mm, or faint enhancing tumor in the central ducts associated with the presence of distal duct obstruction on contrast-enhanced CT or MRI examinations (see Figures 4-52 and 4-53).[81]

Appearance as an exophytic mass can be occasionally identified, most commonly in cholangiocarcinomas of peripheral bile ducts. These tumors appear as a discrete mass within the hepatic parenchyma and will usually demonstrate obstruction of the ducts distal to the mass (see Figures 4-54 and 4-55). This is an important clue to peripheral cholangiocarcinomas. Although other hepatic neoplasms can cause bile duct obstruction, none do it with the frequency of cholangiocarcinoma. Among the least common manifestations of cholangiocarcinoma is the appearance of a small polypoid lesion projecting into the lumen of the bile duct.

Most cholangiocarcinomas will have typical imaging characteristics depending on the morphologic type (mass-forming, periductal infiltrating, or intraductal). Peripheral cholangiocarcinomas are the type of cholangiocarcinoma most likely to be mass-forming.[81] On US, the mass-forming

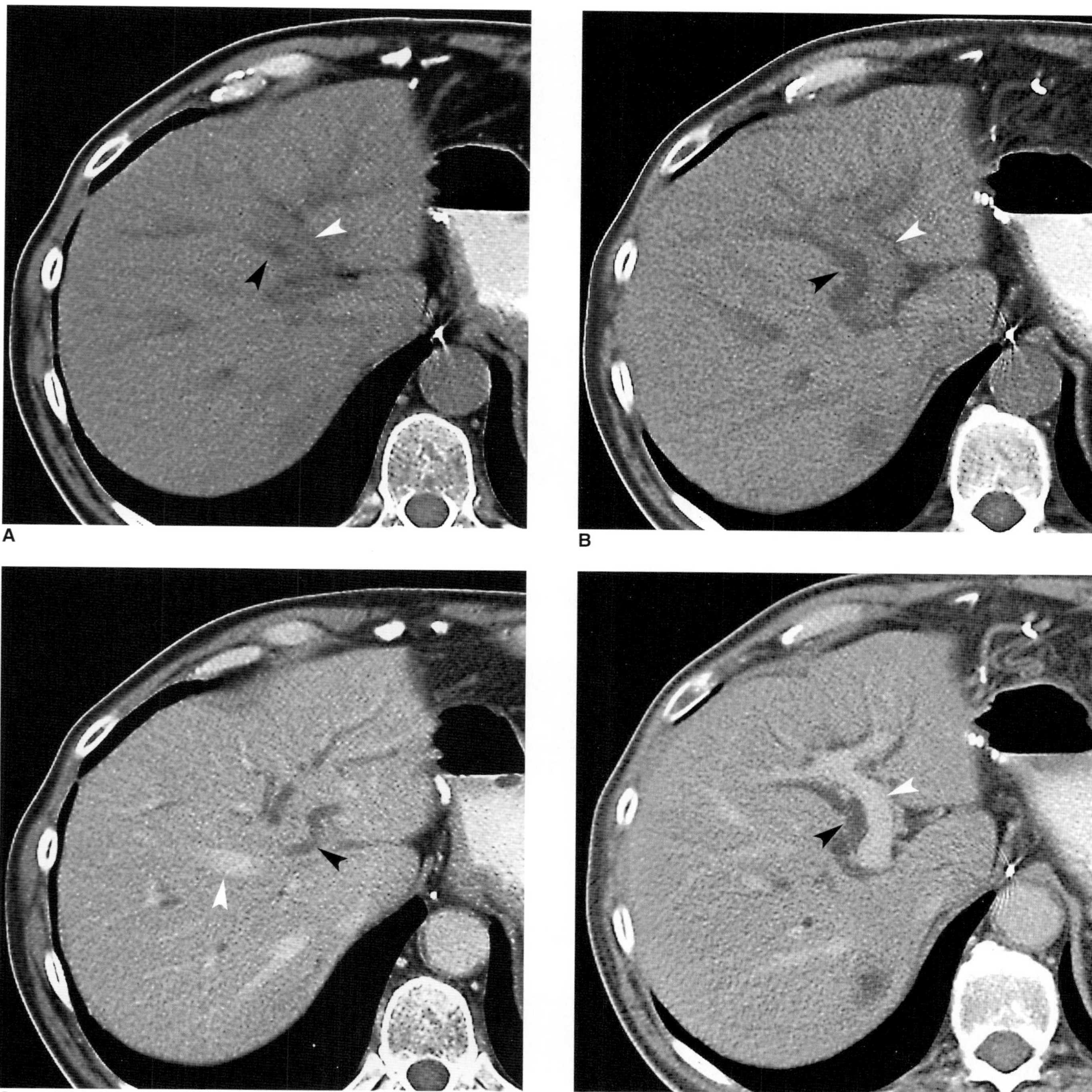

Figure 4-46 Bile Duct Dilation on Unenhanced and Enhanced CT This 68-year-old man presented with jaundice and back pain. **A** and **B.** Unenhanced CT shows 2 distinct attenuations in the portal triads, low attenuation branching structures (*black arrowheads*) that represent moderately dilated bile ducts and slightly higher attenuation branching structures (*white arrowheads*) that represent the portal veins. **C** and **D.** The dilated bile ducts (*black arrowheads*) are seen to greater advantage on post contrast-enhanced images. Images of the pancreas demonstrated a small mass in the head of the pancreas (not shown), which was later proven to represent an adenocarcinoma.

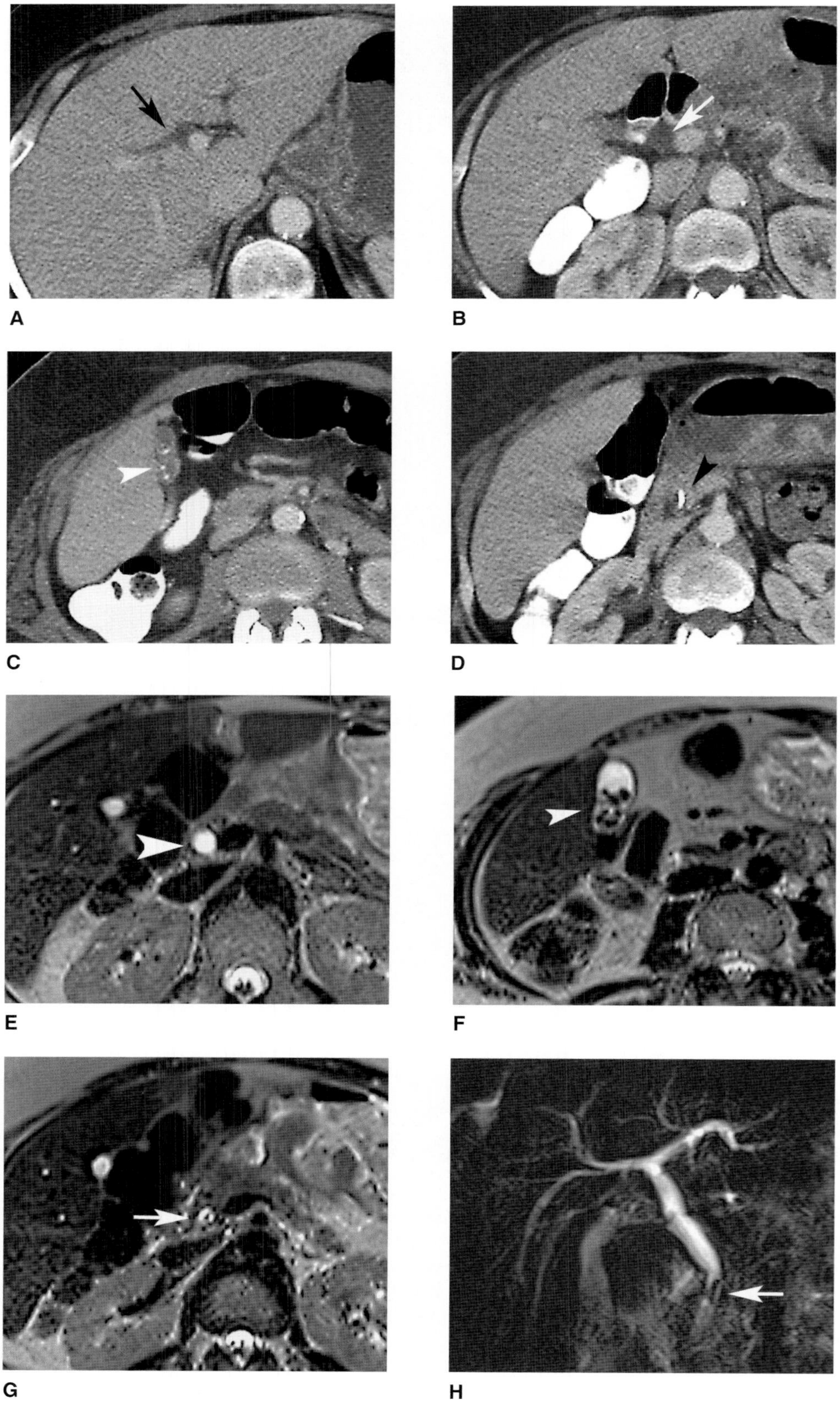

A

B

C

D

E

F

G

H

Figure 4-47 Choledocholithiasis This 58-year-old man presented with 2 weeks or right upper quadrant pain. US examination (not shown) demonstrated gallstones and dilation of the common bile duct. **A-D.** Contrast-enhanced CT examination shows gallstones within the gallbladder (*white arrowhead*), normal intrahepatic bile ducts (*black arrow*) but mild dilation of the common bile duct (*white arrow*). Within the pancreatic head is a small linear calcification (*black arrowhead*) indicating the presence of a distal common bile duct stone. **E-G.** Highly T2-weighted axial MR images confirm the presence of gallstones (*small white arrowhead*), mild dilation of the common bile duct (*large white arrowhead*), and a partially obstructing stone in the distal common bile duct (*small white arrow*). **H.** Note how much easier it is to see the stone in the distal common bile duct on this MRCP.

Table 4-3. Causes of Bile Duct Dilation

1. **Gallstones**[a]
2. **Prior surgery**
3. Malignancy a. **Pancreatic carcinoma** b. Other pancreatic malignancies c. Cholangiocarcinoma d. Ampullary carcinoma e. Duodenal carcinoma f. Hepatocellular carcinoma g. Metastasis h. Lymphoma
4. Infections a. *Clonorchis sinensis* b. *Ascaris lumbricoides*
5. Inflammatory and postinflammatory strictures a. Prior gallstone passage b. Sclerosing cholangitis c. Ascending cholangitis d. Pancreatitis
6. Congenital a. Choledochal cysts b. Biliary atresia
7. Other a. Sphincter of Oddi spasm

[a]Most common causes are listed in bold.

type will usually appear as a homogeneous mass with an irregular well-defined margin. A peripheral hypoechoic rim is seen in approximately 35% of tumors.[81,83] The echogenicity of the tumor will depend on tumor size, with greater than 3 cm appearing hyperechoic and tumors less than 3 cm being hypo- or isoechoic.[81,84] The CT appearance of the mass-forming type is a mass with homogeneous attenuation and irregular peripheral enhancement with gradual centripetal enhancement, capsular retraction, possibly satellite nodules, and vascular encasement (see Figures 4-54 and 4-55).[80,81,85-87] Delayed enhancement is seen in areas with marked fibrosis. Hepatolithiasis and ductal dilation with obliteration of the portal vein and atrophy of the involved segment can also be seen.[81,88] On MR, the mass demonstrates an irregular margin, with high signal intensity on T2-weighted images and low signal intensity on T1-weighted images with peripheral centripetal enhancement and delayed enhancement in areas with fibrous stroma.[81,89,90]

The appearance of the periductal infiltrating type has also been described. Most hilar cholangiocarcinomas are of this type.[81,93-95] On US, the infiltrating type of cholangiocarcinoma can appear as a small masslike lesion or diffuse bile duct thickening. The bile duct lumen can be occluded depending on the tumor involvement.[81,91,92]

On CT, there is diffuse periductal thickening with increased enhancement due to tumor infiltration along with dilated or irregular narrowed ducts and peripheral ductal dilation. During the arterial phase of hepatic enhancement, cholangiocarcinomas can appear faintly hyperattenuating to liver but on portal-phase imaging, the tumor will often be isoattenuating relative to normal liver parenchyma, rendering the tumor mass essentially

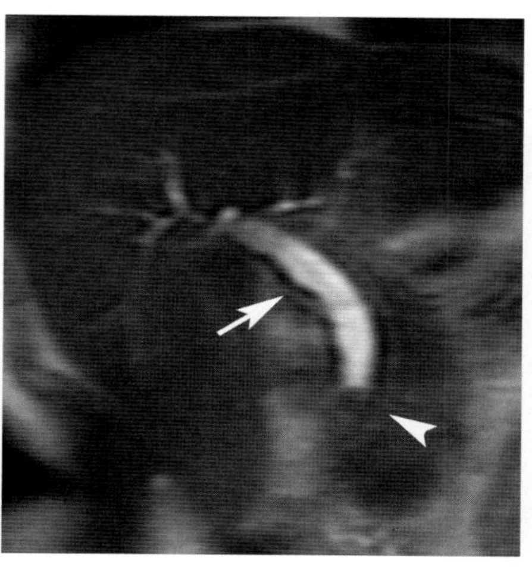

A

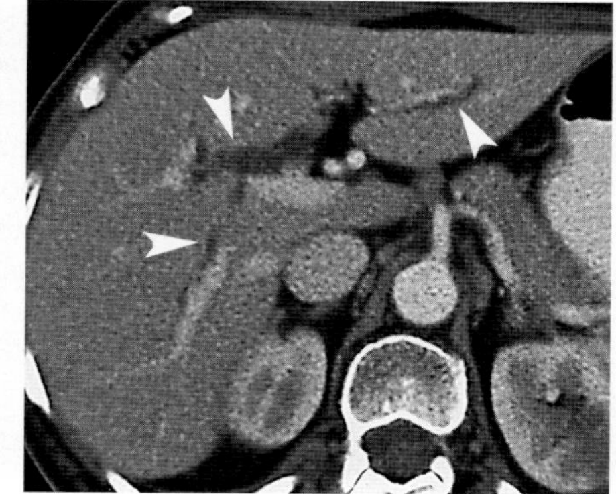

B

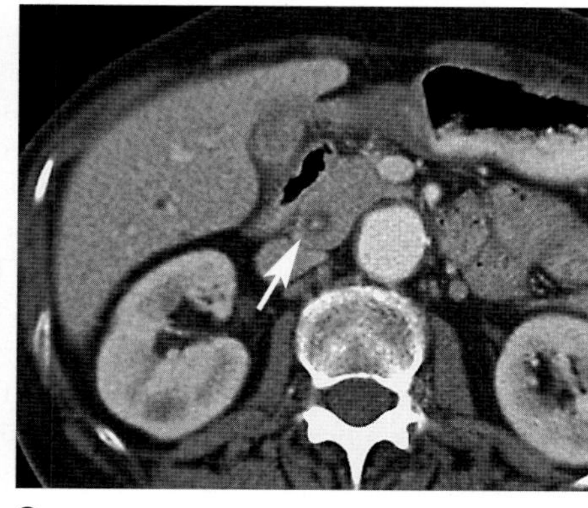

C

Figure 4-48 Choledocholithiasis
This 60-year-old woman presented with weight loss and an increased serum alkaline phosphatase and gamma-glutamyl transpeptidase (GGT). **A.** Coronal MRCP shows intrahepatic and extrahepatic (*arrow*) biliary ductal dilation to a level near the sphincter of Oddi. Notice the sharp occlusion of the distal common bile duct, suggesting an intraluminal filling defect. **B** and **C.** Enhanced CT images demonstrate low attenuation, branching, tubular structures (*arrowheads*) in the central liver, typical of intrahepatic biliary ductal dilation. There is also a small high-attenuation filling defect (*arrow*) within the distal common bile duct, within the head of the pancreas, typical of a biliary ductal stone.

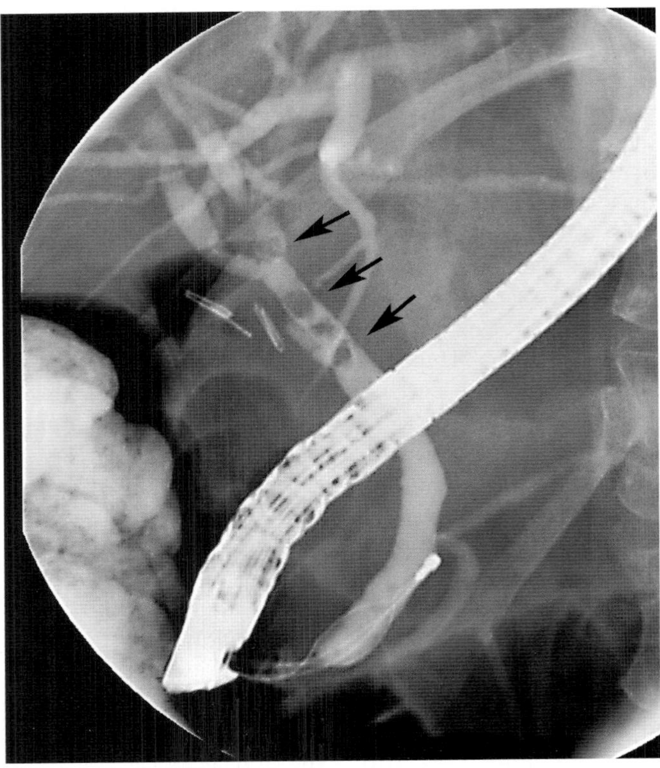
A

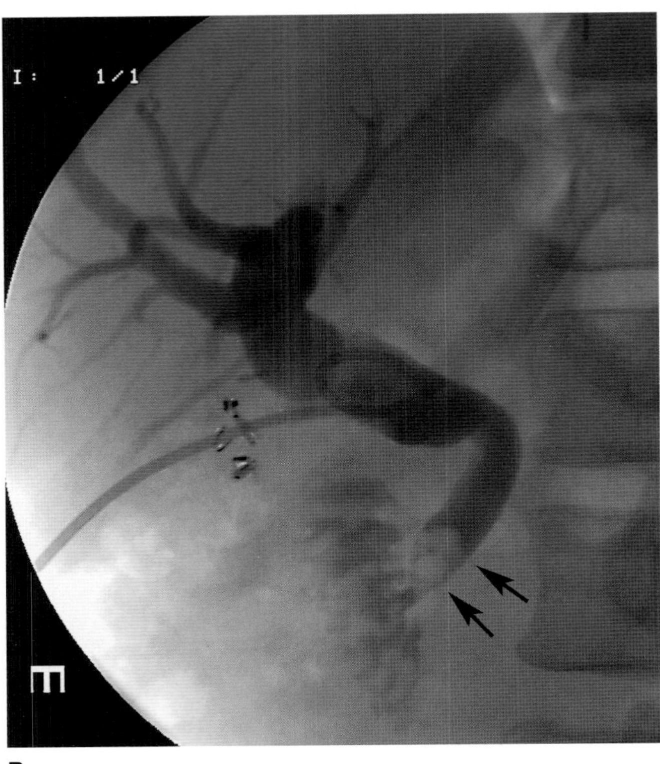

B

Figure 4-49 Choledocholithiasis by ERCP and PTC
A. Images obtained during ERCP show multiple filling defects (*arrows*) within the common hepatic duct indicating retained stones after cholecystectomy. These images were taken in preparation for stone removal. **B.** This patient had persistent pain following cholecystectomy. CT and US examinations showed persistent bile duct dilation but failed to identify a cause. PTC through a T-tube reveals retained stones in the distal common bile duct as filling defects (*arrows*) within the contrast column.

invisible (see Figures 3-15 and 4-53). Delayed-phase imaging at 3 to 5 minutes following contrast enhancement will typically show the tumor to be hyperenhancing relative to the normal liver parenchyma. This is the phase of imaging at which the periductal infiltrating forms of cholangiocarcinoma is most evident; unfortunately, this phase is not part of most typical imaging protocols and requires the observer to suspect the presence of the tumor and perform delayed-phase imaging. This delayed enhancement is characteristic of scarring of any type and is a result of the scirrhous character of cholangiocarcinomas.

Even though CT has greater spatial resolution, MRI examinations are the study of choice for evaluating suspected cholangiocarcinomas because the tumor is more conspicuous both before and after contrast enhancement.[21] In addition, MRI examinations allow for production of MR cholangiograms, an important adjunctive imaging process. Cholangiocarcinomas are typically isointense with liver parenchyma on T1-weighted sequences and will appear hypointense on T2-weighted sequences because of the surrounding scirrhous reaction. Following intravenous contrast administration, cholangiocarcinomas will have similar imaging characteristics with CT contrast enhancement: faintly hyperintense during arterial phases, isointense during portal phases, and hyperintense on delayed-phase imaging (see Figure 4-52). The intraductal type can present with localized or diffuse ductectasia occasionally with an echogenic intraductal component on ultrasound. On CT and MR, there are several appearances. There can be diffuse marked ductal dilation with an intraductal mass that can be either hypoattenuating or isoattenuating on precontrast imaging, with enhancement on postcontrast imaging, an intraductal polypoid mass within a focal dilated duct, an intraductal castlike lesion, or a focal stricture with mild proximal ductal dilation.[81]

Ampullary neoplasms: Periampullary tumors are defined as arising within 1 cm of the ampulla of Vater and include tumors of the ampulla, distal bile duct, pancreas, and duodenum. In a series of 647 consecutive periampullary tumors over a 20-year period by Michelassi et al, 85% were adenocarcinomas of the head of the pancreas, 6 % were cholangiocarcinomas of the distal common bile duct, and 4% were tumors of the ampulla itself.[96,97]

Ampullary adenomas and adenocarcinomas are neoplasms that arise from the glandular epithelium at the

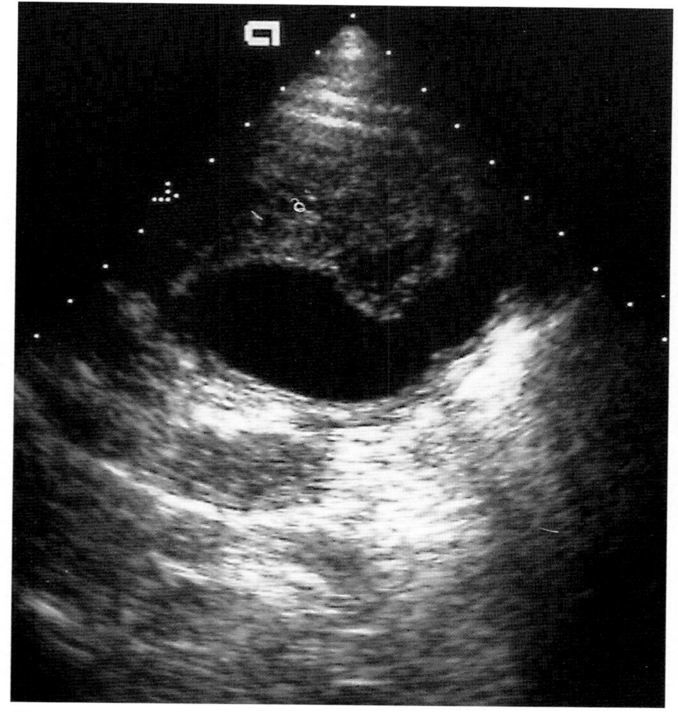

A

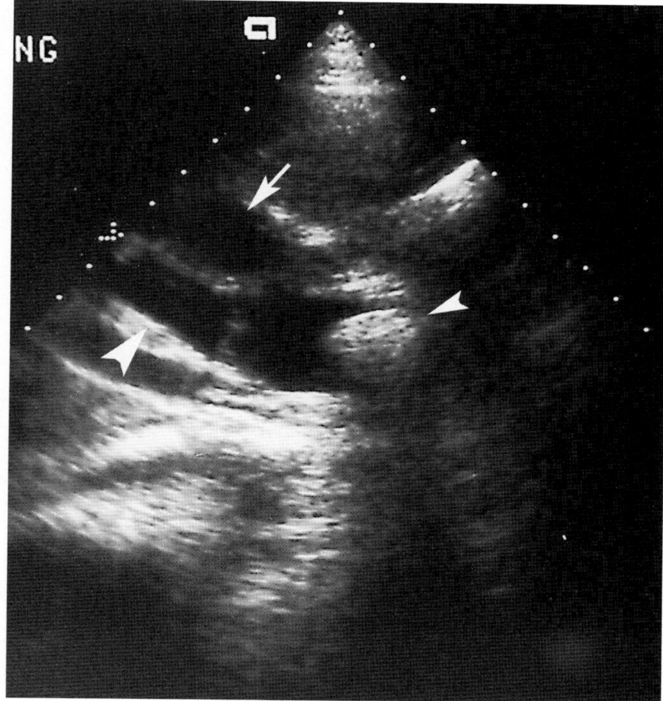

B

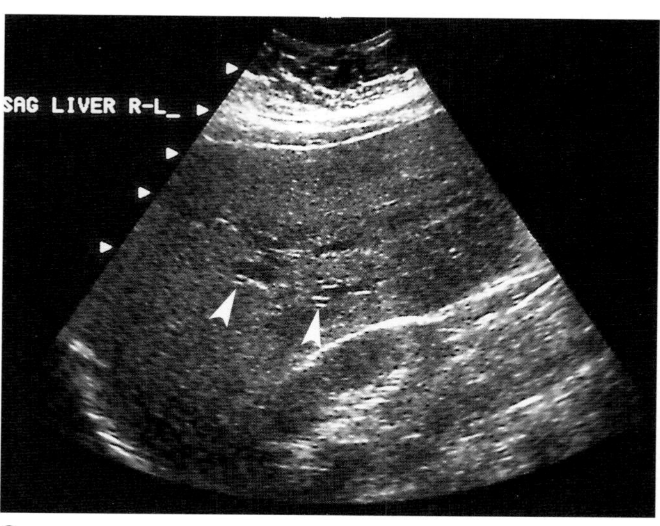

C

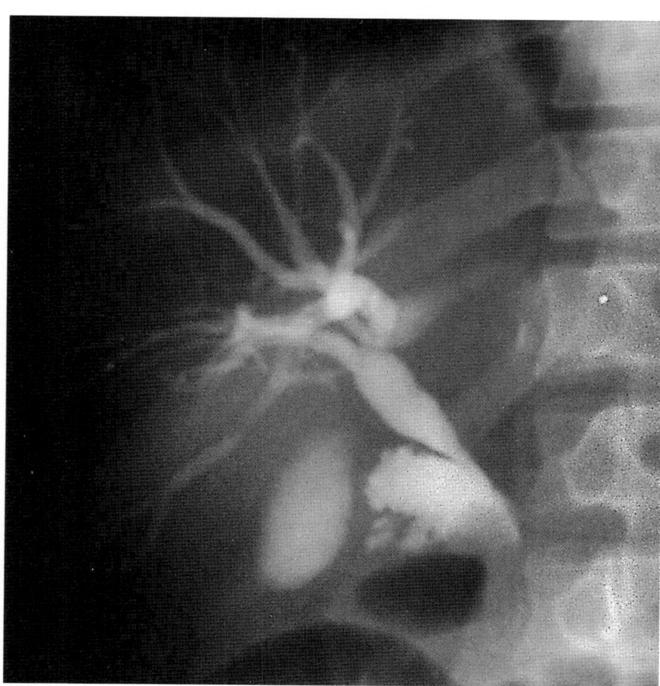

D

Figure 4-50 Mirizzi Syndrome
This middle-aged man presented with fever, jaundice, and right upper quadrant pain. **A.** US of the biliary system shows a distended gallbladder and cystic duct with diffuse thickening of the gallbladder wall. **B.** The cystic duct (*large arrowhead*) has a long course, and a large echogenic stone (*small arrowhead*) with shadowing is discovered at the distal end of the duct. There is also a dilated common bile duct (*small arrow*). **C.** Sagittal images of the liver demonstrate multiple dilated intrahepatic ducts (*arrowheads*) with their echogenic walls distinguishing them from hepatic and portal veins. This constellation of findings suggests Mirizzi syndrome. **D.** Percutaneous transhepatic cholangiogram shows dilation of the intrahepatic and extrahepatic bile ducts. The cystic duct is massively distended and there is a stone at the junction of the cystic duct and common bile duct. This appearance is diagnostic of Mirizzi syndrome.

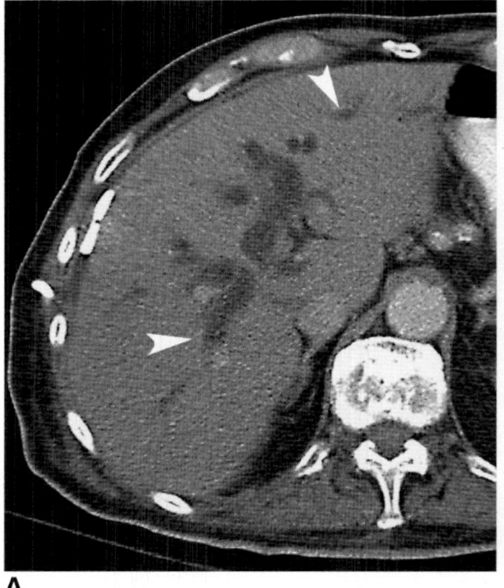
A

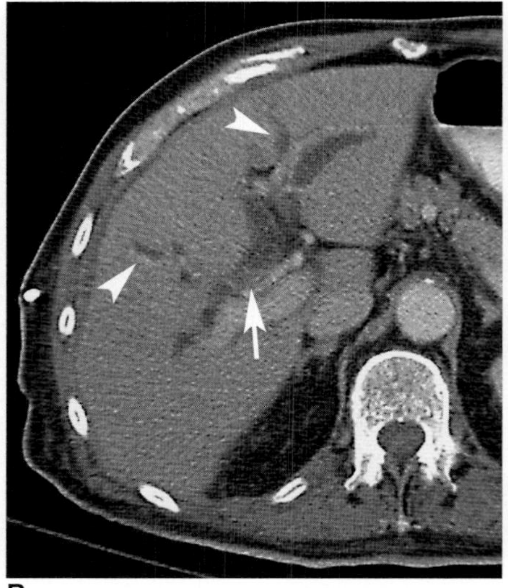
B

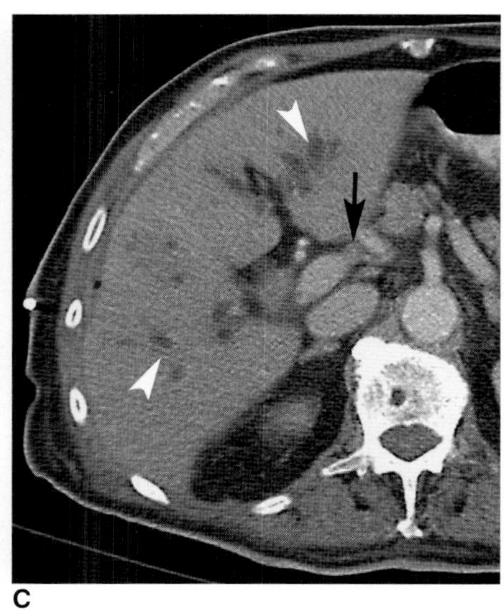
C

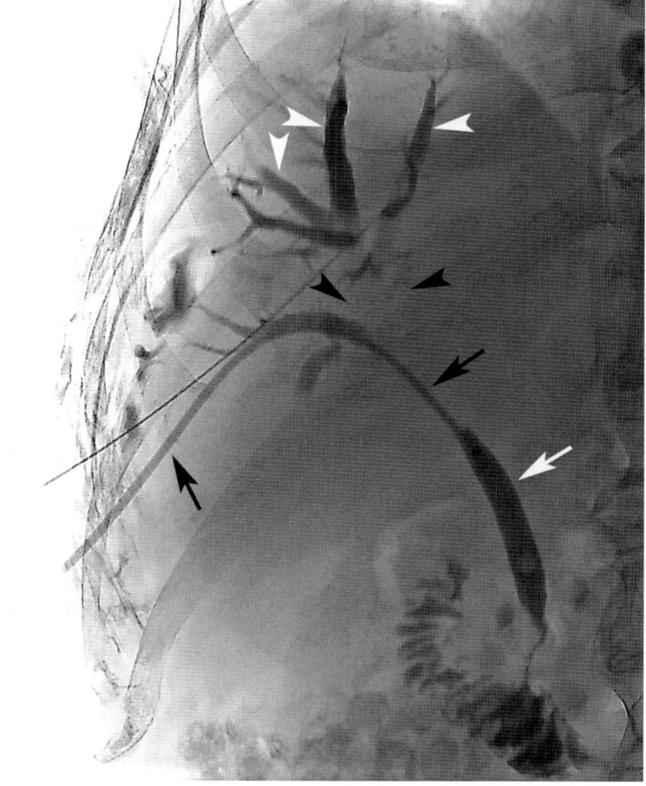
D

Figure 4-51 Cholangiocarcinoma
This 86-year-old man presented with jaundice and abdominal pain. **A-C.** CT images in the late portal phase of enhancement demonstrate multiple low-attenuation tubular structures in the liver, characteristic of dilated small and large intrahepatic biliary ducts (*arrowheads*). The common bile duct (*black arrow*) is normal in caliber, indicating obstruction at the porta hepatis. No obvious mass is identified although there is minimal soft tissue (*white arrow*) in the porta hepatis. This is the typical appearance of a central cholangiocarcinoma. The tumor infiltrates along the bile ducts and is difficult to visualize. **D.** Percutaneous transhepatic cholangiogram confirms dilated intrahepatic ducts (*white arrowheads*) with a normal diameter common bile duct (*white arrow*). The central portions of the ducts are occluded (*black arrowheads*). A percutaneous biliary drain has been placed across the obstructed bile duct (*black arrows*).

ampulla of Vater within the medial wall of the second portion of the duodenum into which the common bile duct and main pancreatic duct drain.[96] These tumors occur in both men and women with a male-to-female ratio of 2:1[96-98] and an average age of 60 years.[97-100] Symptoms are due to biliary ductal obstruction and include intermittent jaundice and acholic stools.[101] Partial obstruction can lead to ascending cholangitis with symptoms of fever, chills, and right upper quadrant pain.[102] Associated pancreatic ductal obstruction causing pancreatitis has also been described.[103] Patients with adenomas and adenocarcinomas in other sites of the GI tract, including those with familial adenomatous polyposis syndromes, are at increased risk for developing ampullary tumors.[24,96,104-109]

Ampullary neoplasms are usually small at the time of diagnosis, probably because of the relatively early onset of symptoms, with the average size 3 cm or less.[96,98,102] If the tumor is confined to the ampulla, it may be difficult to

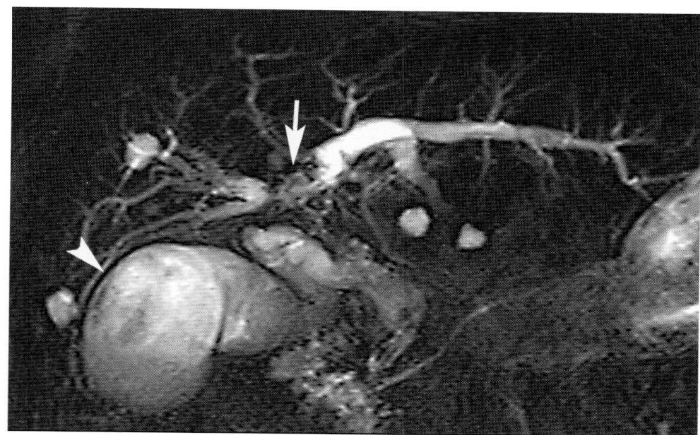

A

Figure 4-52 Cholangiocarcinoma With Bile Duct Enhancement This 85-year-old man presented with jaundice. **A.** MR cholangiogram shows dilated peripheral bile ducts as bright enhancing tubes and a dilated gallbladder (*arrowhead*). Note the narrowing of the central bile ducts in the porta hepatis (*white arrow*) a finding associated with the Klatskin-type cholangiocarcinoma. **B.** T2-weighted MRI through the porta hepatis shows mildly dilated peripheral bile ducts, with increased soft tissue surrounding the central bile ducts. T1-weighted MRI (**C**) before and (**D**) after gadolinium administration shows enhancement of the central bile ducts. These findings are highly associated with cholangiocarcinoma, which was subsequently proven by endoscopic brush biopsy.

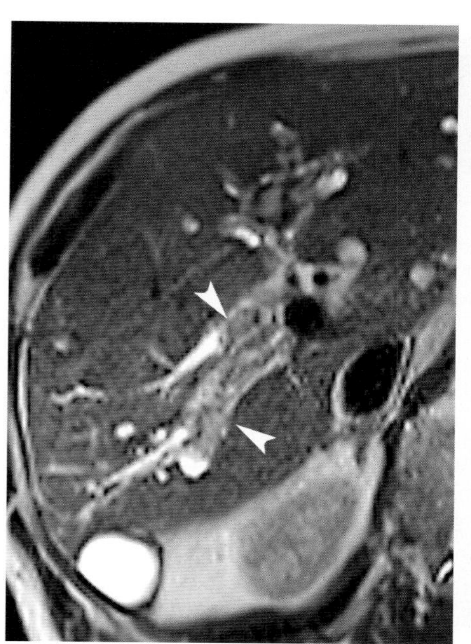

B

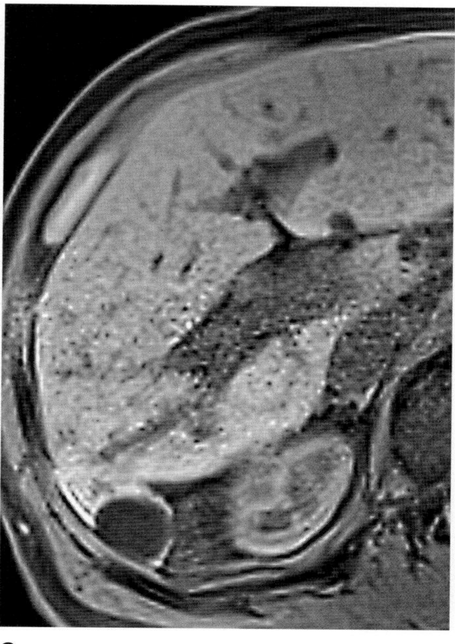

C

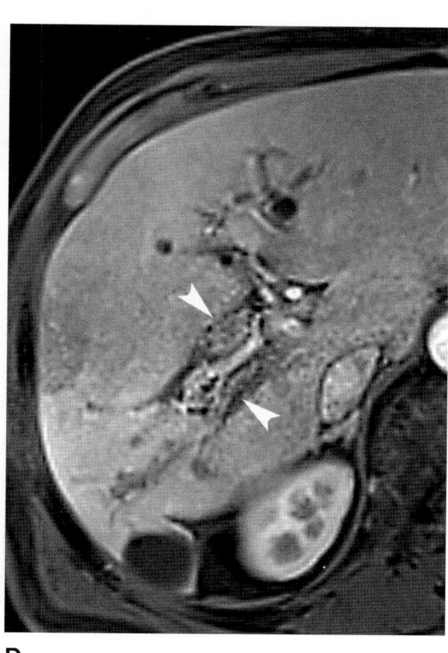

D

visualize on endoscopy.[110,111] When visible, endoscopic findings are usually a prominent papilla or submucosal mass with nonvisualization of the tumor itself. Blind biopsy with cytologic and histologic evaluation of material obtained is usually required for definitive diagnosis.[96]

The biliary or pancreatic duct dilation caused by these tumors is usually the only finding on cross-sectional imaging, including US, CT, and MR. The double-duct sign (dilation of the common bile duct and pancreatic duct) can be readily apparent but the tumor is not visualized in most cases.[96,112,113] In some cases, a small soft-tissue mass will be detected at the ampulla of Vater on CT, but this is usually due to the tumor protruding into the duodenum that is distended by contrast material (see Figure 4-56).[96] On MR, visible ampullary carcinomas are of low signal intensity relative to the pancreas on both T1- and T2-weighted images and enhance to a lesser extent than pancreas on immediate enhanced images. On delayed postcontrast sequences, these lesions demonstrate heterogeneous enhancement with variable rim enhancement.[24,114] Cholangiopancreatography by either MRCP, ERCP, or PTC will demonstrate sharp shouldering rather than gradual tapering of the distal common bile duct, suggesting the presence of a neoplasm, but this diagnosis is difficult because the short transmural segment of the pancreaticobiliary tree contains little to no fluid (see Figure 4-45).[24] Unfortunately, this shouldering can be mimicked by gallstone impacted in the distal common bile duct. Fortunately, both impacted stones and periampullary tumors will require evaluation/therapy by ERCP.

Pancreatic malignancy: As stated above, pancreatic cancer is the most common malignant cause of bile duct obstruction.[96-97] In most cases, CT and MRI will readily identify a mass in the pancreatic head as the cause of biliary obstruction (see Figure 4-57). Rarely, the pancreatic tumor can locally invade the distal common bile duct and infiltrate along the duct, making it very difficult to differentiate between a primary pancreatic neoplasm and a

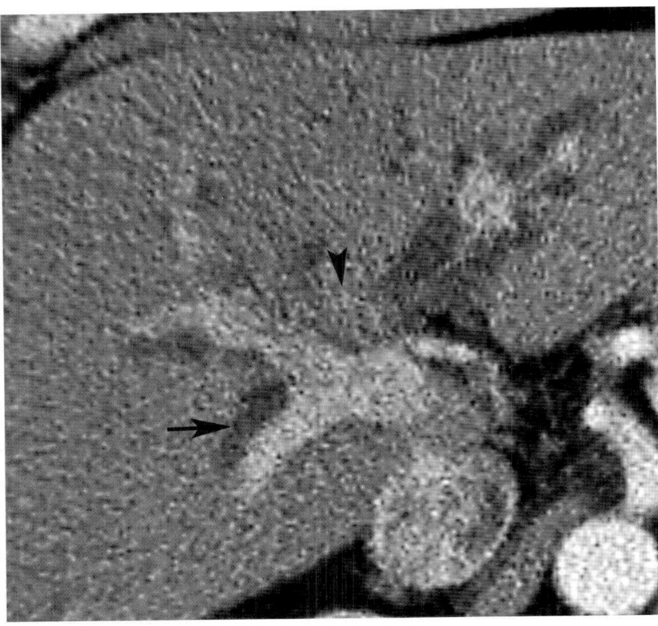

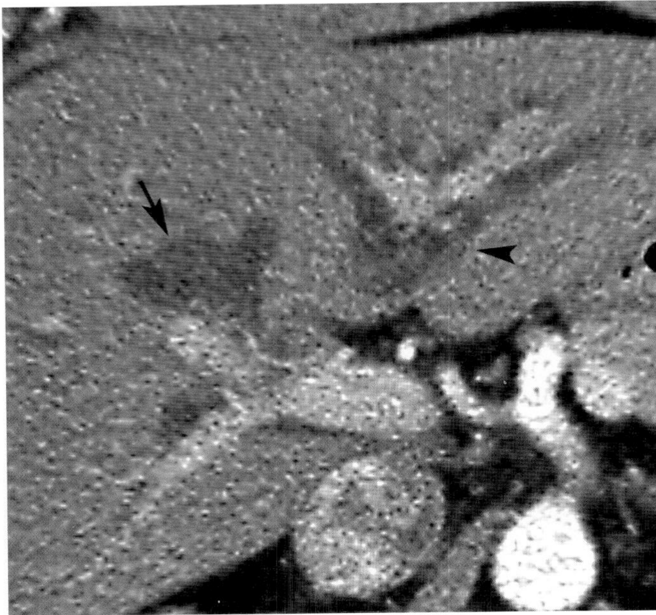

Figure 4-53 Cholangiocarcinoma With Subtle Wall Enhancement This 50-year-old man presented with jaundice. **A** and **B**. CT images in the early portal phase of enhancement demonstrate diffuse bile duct dilation. Note how the central ducts (*arrowheads*) appear slightly higher attenuation than the peripheral ducts (*arrows*). This represents enhancing intraluminal tumor. Biopsy was diagnostic of cholangiocarcinoma.

primary biliary tumor that has invaded the pancreatic head. Enlarged peripancreatic lymph nodes can also make delineating tissue planes extremely challenging.

Other extrabiliary neoplasms: Occasionally, other malignancies can result in biliary obstruction. As previously stated, primary hepatocellular carcinoma or hepatic metastases are sometimes impossible to differentiate from cholangiocarcinoma (see Figure 4-58).[81] Rarely, lymphoma has also been described as a cause for biliary obstruction (see Figure 4-59).[115] Duodenal carcinoma and other retroperitoneal cancers can also cause obstruction of the common bile duct.

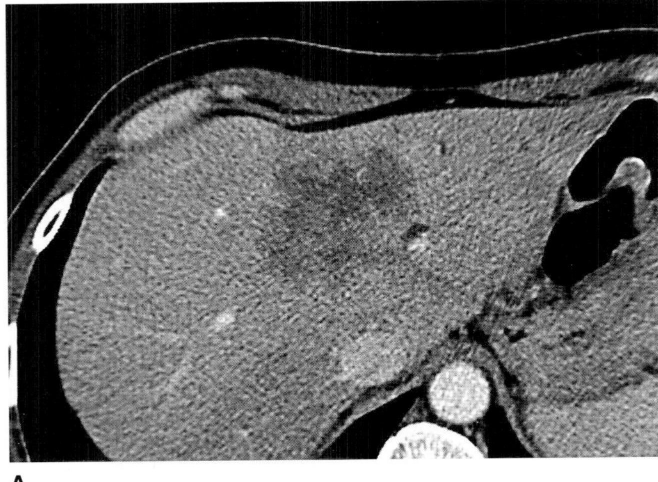

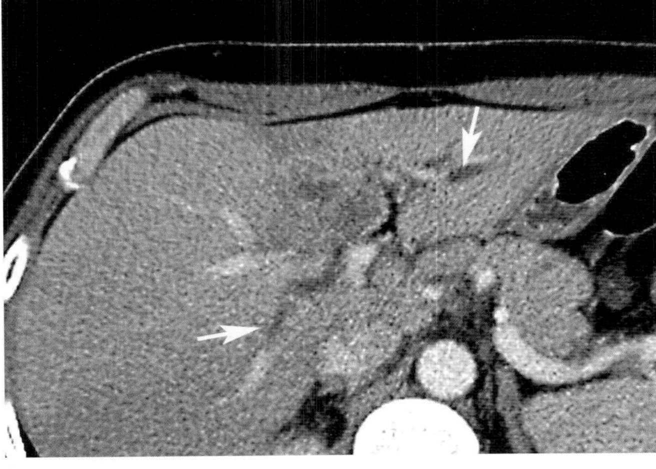

Figure 4-54 Cholangiocarcinoma Appearing as a Discrete Mass This 51-year-old woman presented with abnormal liver function tests. **A** and **B**. Images from an enhanced CT scan demonstrate an indistinctly marginated mass in the central liver causing mild bile duct dilation (*arrows*). In this early phase of contrast enhancement, the peripheral portion of the mass enhances preferentially. Biopsy was diagnostic of cholangiocarcinoma.

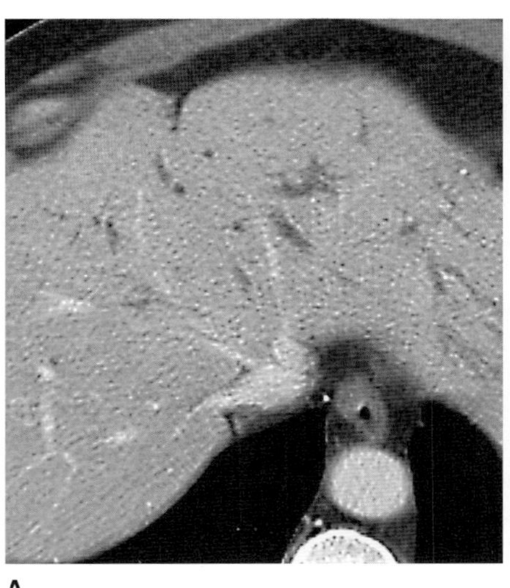
A

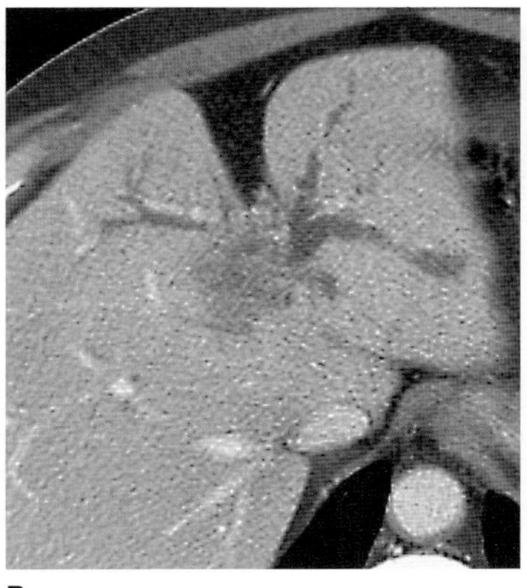
B

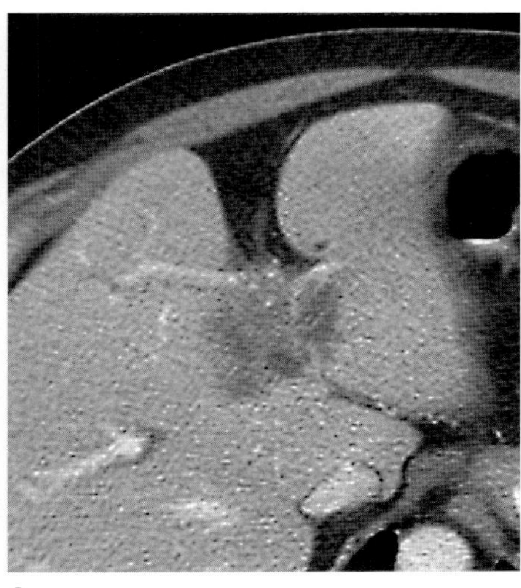
C

Figure 4-55 Cholangiocarcinoma with Bile Duct Dilation
This 72-year-old man presented with new-onset jaundice. **A-C.** CT images demonstrate multiple low attenuation branching tubes typical of dilated bile ducts. In the central liver is an irregularly marginated mass with peripheral enhancement, typical of a cholangiocarcinoma.

Disorders of the sphincter of oddi: Disorders of the sphincter of Oddi that can result in intermittent biliary obstruction include papillary dysfunction and stenosis. As with stenosis seen in other parts of the biliary system, ampullary stenosis results from bouts of inflammation at the ampulla of Vater and usually is due to the passage of gallstones. Papillary dysfunction can be related to spasm of the sphincter or abnormal sphincteric peristalsis.[24,116]

Inflammatory biliary strictures: There are a variety of inflammatory causes of biliary strictures, including prior surgery, prior choledocholithiasis, autoimmune diseases,

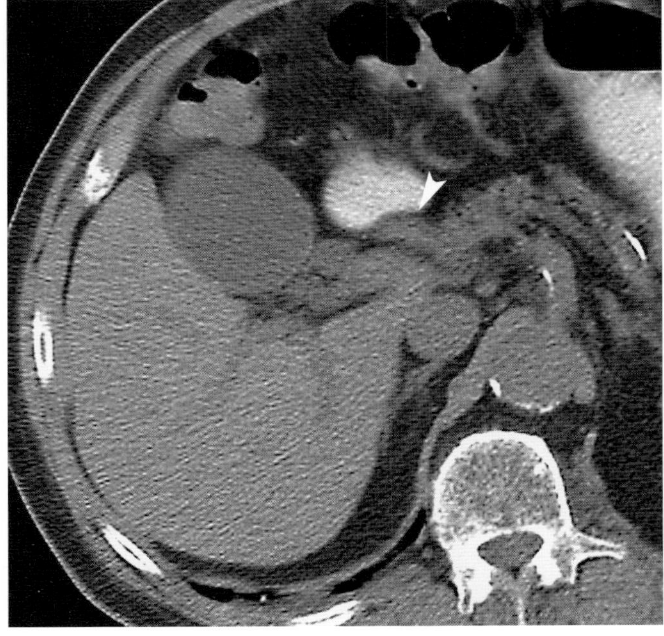
A

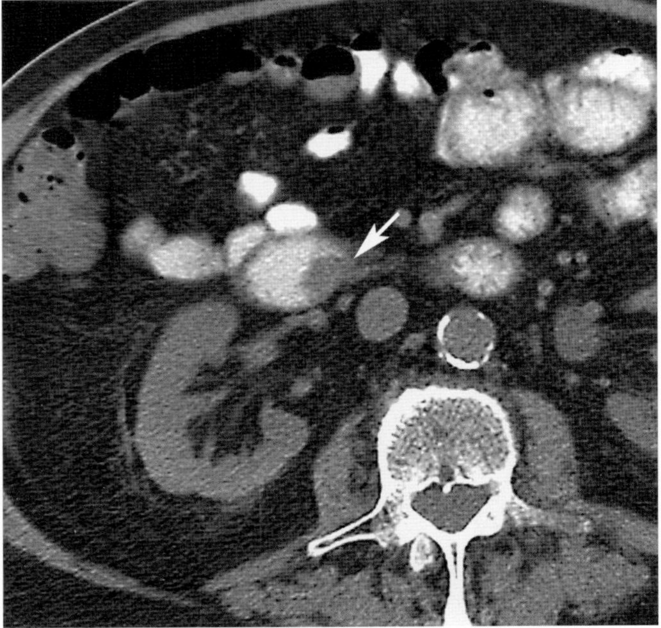
B

Figure 4-56 Ampullary Carcinoma Detected by CT
This 86-year-old man presented with intermittent abdominal pain and jaundice. **A** and **B.** Images from an unenhanced CT demonstrate mild dilation of the common bile duct (*arrowhead*) and a small polypoid tumor (*white arrow*) in the duodenum at the location of the sphincter of Oddi, characteristic of an ampullary carcinoma.

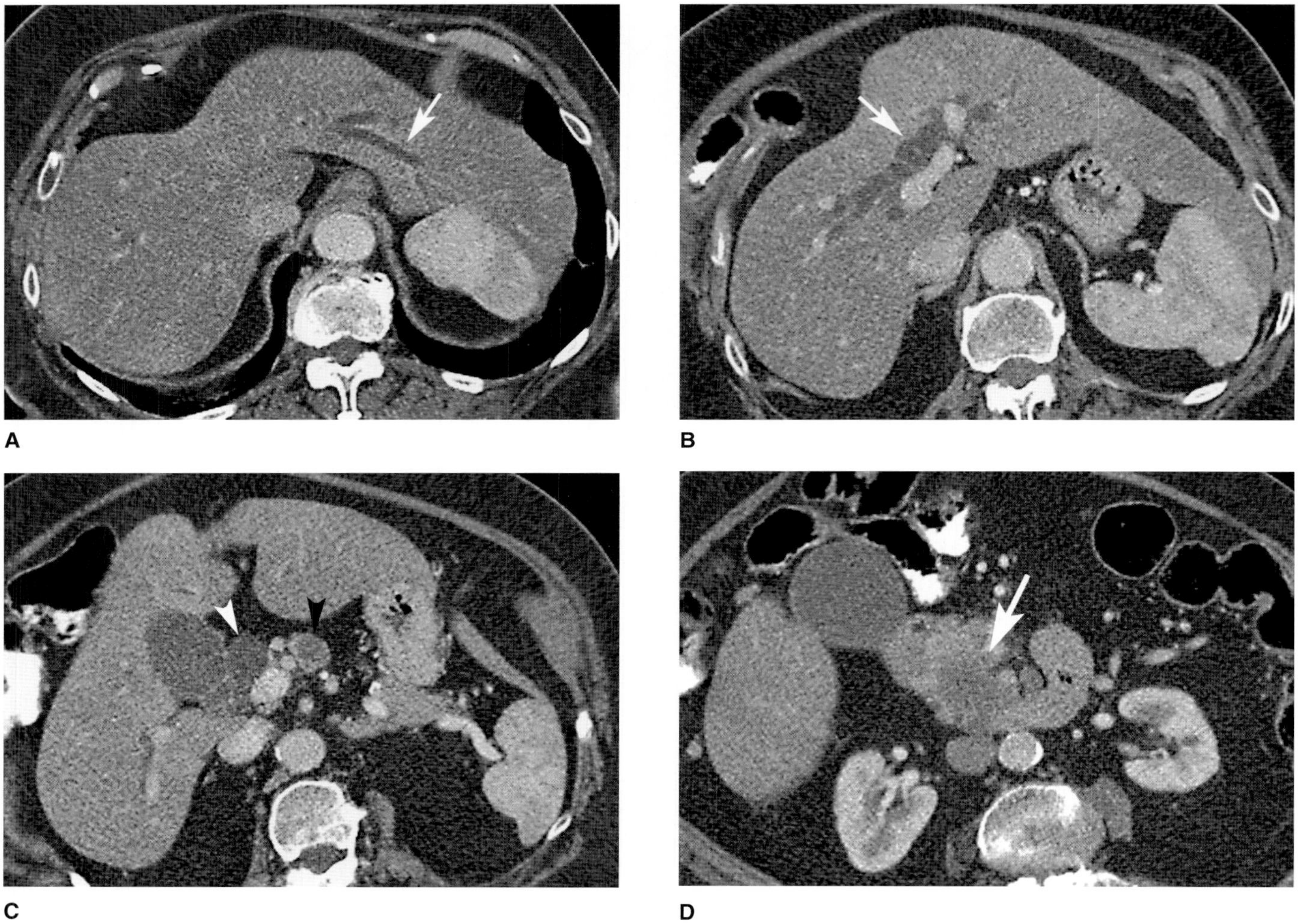

A

B

C

D

Figure 4-57 Biliary Obstruction Due to Pancreatic Carcinoma This 70-year-old woman presented with jaundice and dizziness. **A-D.** Contrast-enhanced CT images demonstrate dilation of the intrahepatic (*small arrows*) and extrahepatic (*white arrowhead*) bile ducts, indicating an extrahepatic biliary obstruction. In the head of the pancreas is an inhomogeneous mass (*large arrow*) typical of a pancreatic adenocarcinoma. There is also metastatic adenopathy near the celiac axis (*black arrowhead*).

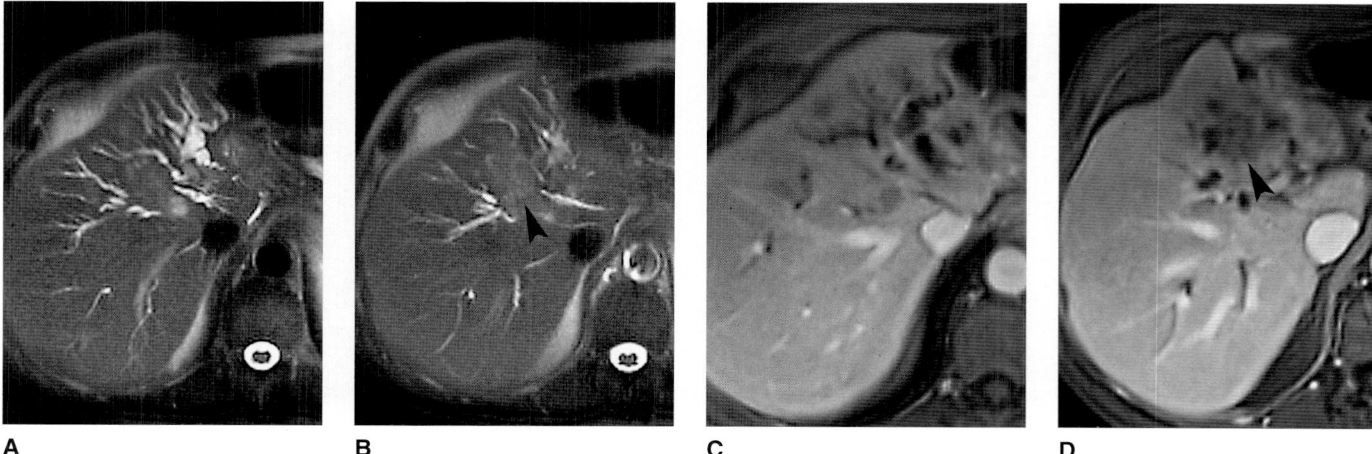

A B C D

Figure 4-58 Biliary Obstruction by Metastasis This 60-year-old man had pancreatic carcinoma. **A** and **B.** T2-weighted sequences demonstrate normal right bile ducts but dilated left ducts. There is a faint hyperintense mass (*arrowhead*) in the left side of the porta hepatis representing a metastasis. **C** and **D.** Post gadolinium T1-weighted images confirm obstruction of the left biliary radicals by a central metastasis (*arrowhead*).

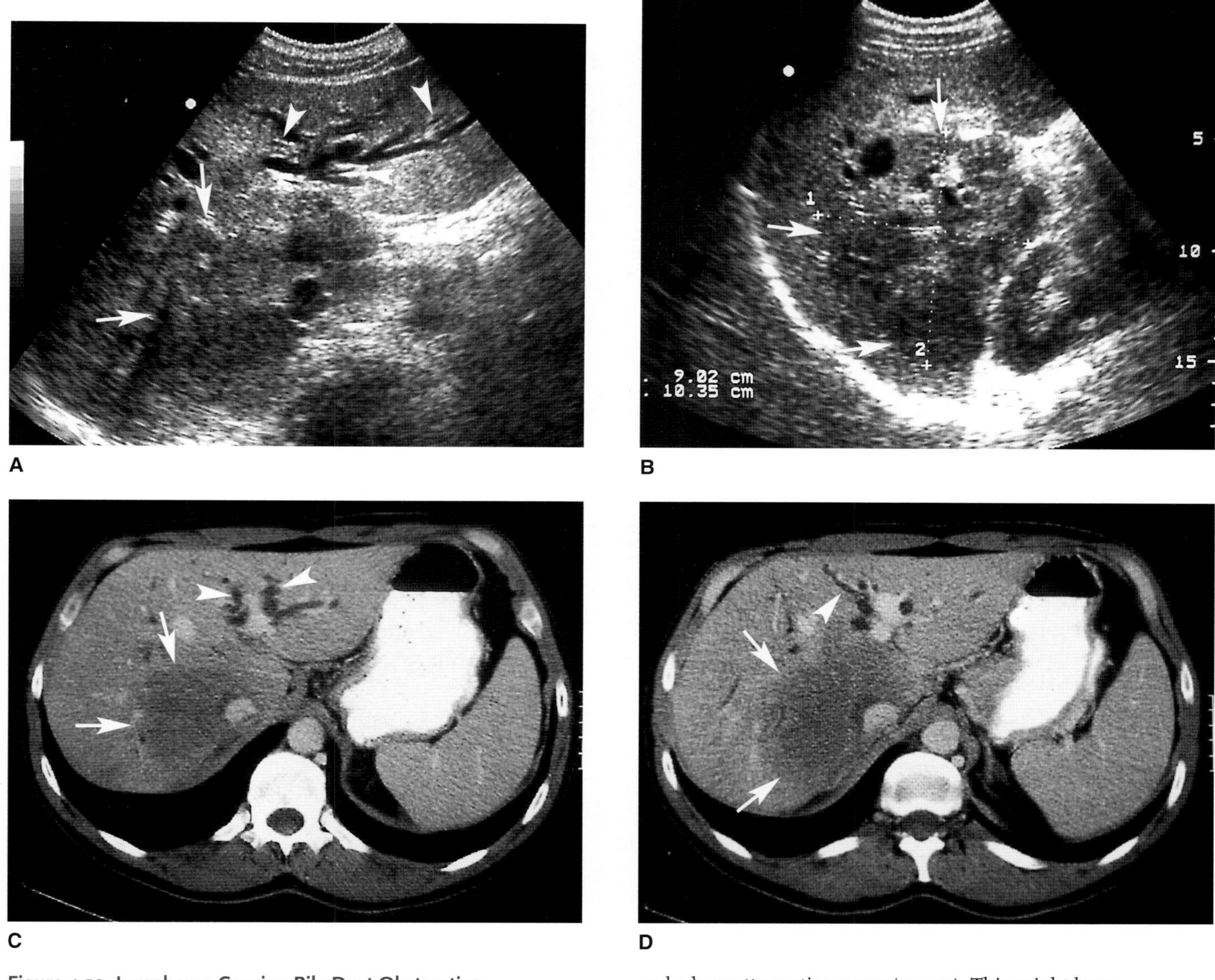

Figure 4-59 Lymphoma Causing Bile Duct Obstruction
This 38-year-old man presented with painless jaundice. **A** and **B.** US of the liver demonstrates mild intrahepatic ductal dilation (*arrowheads*) and a slightly hypoechoic mass (*arrows*). **C** and **D.** CT scan confirms the presence of ductal dilation (*arrowheads*) and a hypoattenuating mass (*arrows*). This might have represented any one of a number of primary hepatic neoplasms but surgical biopsy was diagnostic of primary hepatic lymphoma. No adenopathy or other imaging abnormality was identified.

biliary infections, radiation therapy, and blunt abdominal trauma (Table 4-4).

Biliary surgery: Stricture of the bile ducts is relatively uncommon after biliary surgery but is still among the most common causes of bile duct obstruction. These surgeries include open and laparoscopic cholecystectomy, liver transplantation, Whipple procedures, and surgical extraction of bile duct stones. Postoperative biliary strictures manifest by intrahepatic and extrahepatic biliary dilation defined as a diameter of more than 3 or 8 mm, respectively, with abrupt narrowing,[117-119] nonvisualization of part of the duct, or focal narrowing of the duct with clear identification of the duct on both sides of the narrowing.[117] The most common cause of postoperative strictures is cholecystectomy, with strictures occurring in approximately 1 of every 400 to 500 cholecystectomies.[120] Approximately 2.6% of patients develop biliary strictures after pancreaticoduodenectomy, whether it is performed for benign or malignant disease.[121] Patients generally present with intermittent cholangitis with or without jaundice.

Biliary strictures are among the most common surgical complications of liver transplantation and can develop within several months to several years after surgery. Strictures characteristically occur at 2 sites. Most common are strictures at the surgical anastomosis as a result

Table 4-4. Causes of Inflammatory Biliary Strictures

1. Prior biliary surgery
2. Prior choledocholithiasis
3. Sclerosing cholangitis
4. Biliary infections
a. Ascending pyogenic cholangitis b. *Clonorchis sinensis* c. *Ascaris lumbricoides* d. *AIDS-related cholangitis*
5. Eosinophilic cholangitis
6. Abdominal trauma
7. Radiation therapy
8. Chronic pancreatitis

of excessive scarring (see Figure 4-60).[117] Nonanastomotic strictures are caused by vascular compromise and resultant ischemia. Up to 50% of nonanastomotic strictures are caused by thrombosis of the hepatic artery. Other causes include prolonged preservation time, infectious cholangitis, and rejection. Nonanastomotic strictures usually involve a significant ductal segment and are located near the hilum.[117]

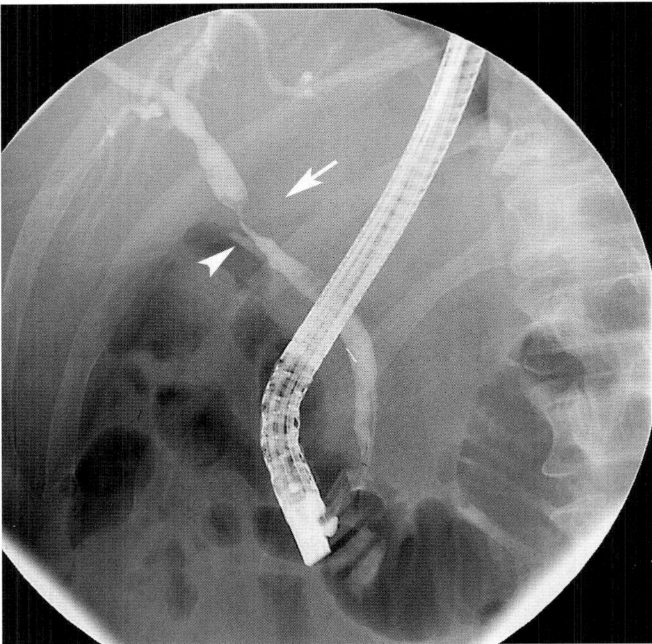

Figure 4-60 Biliary Stricture Following Liver Transplantation This 51-year-old who had undergone liver transplantation had rising biliary function tests. ERCP shows a smooth tapered stricture (*white arrow*) at the site of the biliary anastomosis. This is a known complication of liver transplantation. Note the small blind-ending cystic duct remnant (*arrowhead*) just distal to the site of the stricture.

Traditionally, percutaneous transhepatic cholangiography or ERCP has been performed in patients in whom a postoperative bile duct injury is suspected (see Figure 4-60). Because both of these modalities are invasive and have limited ability to visualize portions of the biliary tree, MRCP has become the imaging modality of choice at many institutions in evaluation for postsurgical bile duct abnormalities.

Choledocholithiasis: In addition to obstruction due to the stone itself, prior choledocholithiasis can also cause obstruction due to chronic inflammation and fibrosis, leading to biliary strictures.[123] Patients present with right upper quadrant pain. Cross-sectional imaging demonstrates dilated bile ducts without evidence of a mass. MRCP, ERCP, and PTC will show a smooth tapered stricture of the affected bile duct without other lesion (see Figure 4-61).

Sclerosing cholangitis: Sclerosing cholangitis is a rare, idiopathic, autoimmune disorder resulting in progressive inflammation of the biliary tree, causing fibrosis and multiple strictures of the bile ducts. Biliary damage leads to cirrhosis, portal hypertension, and liver failure in the majority of patients, and 10% to 15% of patients will develop cholangiocarcinoma.[124] Approximately 70% of the time, sclerosing cholangitis will be associated with inflammatory bowel disease, usually ulcerative colitis but occasionally Crohn disease.[124] In the remainder of cases, sclerosing cholangitis will be an isolated finding. Patients typically present in the fourth and fifth decades. Because of the association with inflammatory bowel disease, many patients are initially diagnosed prior to the development of symptoms. Those with symptoms can present with pruritis, jaundice, or fatigue.[124,125] Liver function enzymes are usually elevated.[124-126]

Sclerosing cholangitis appears as alternating areas of narrowing and dilation of the bile ducts that resemble a string of beads, best appreciated by MRCP, ERCP, and PTC (see Figure 4-62). The beaded appearance of the bile ducts is more difficult to appreciate on cross-sectional imaging because the ducts traverse over multiple cross sections. On cross-sectional imaging, the ducts will have a variable diameter, rather than the normal smooth tapering seen with other ductal dilation. In some cases, the ducts appear as multiple cysts along the expected course of the larger bile ducts. CT and MRI can also demonstrate inflammation of the bile ducts as linear areas of enhancement along the portal triads (see Figure 4-63).

Infectious cholangitis: Infectious cholangitis is most often due to ascending infection from the duodenum. Bacterial cholangitis is typically a complication of partial or complete biliary obstruction and is often a result of post surgical or post inflammatory strictures or choledocholithiasis.[127,128] Patients will usually present with abdominal pain, jaundice and, in some cases, sepsis.[127] Hepatic abscesses

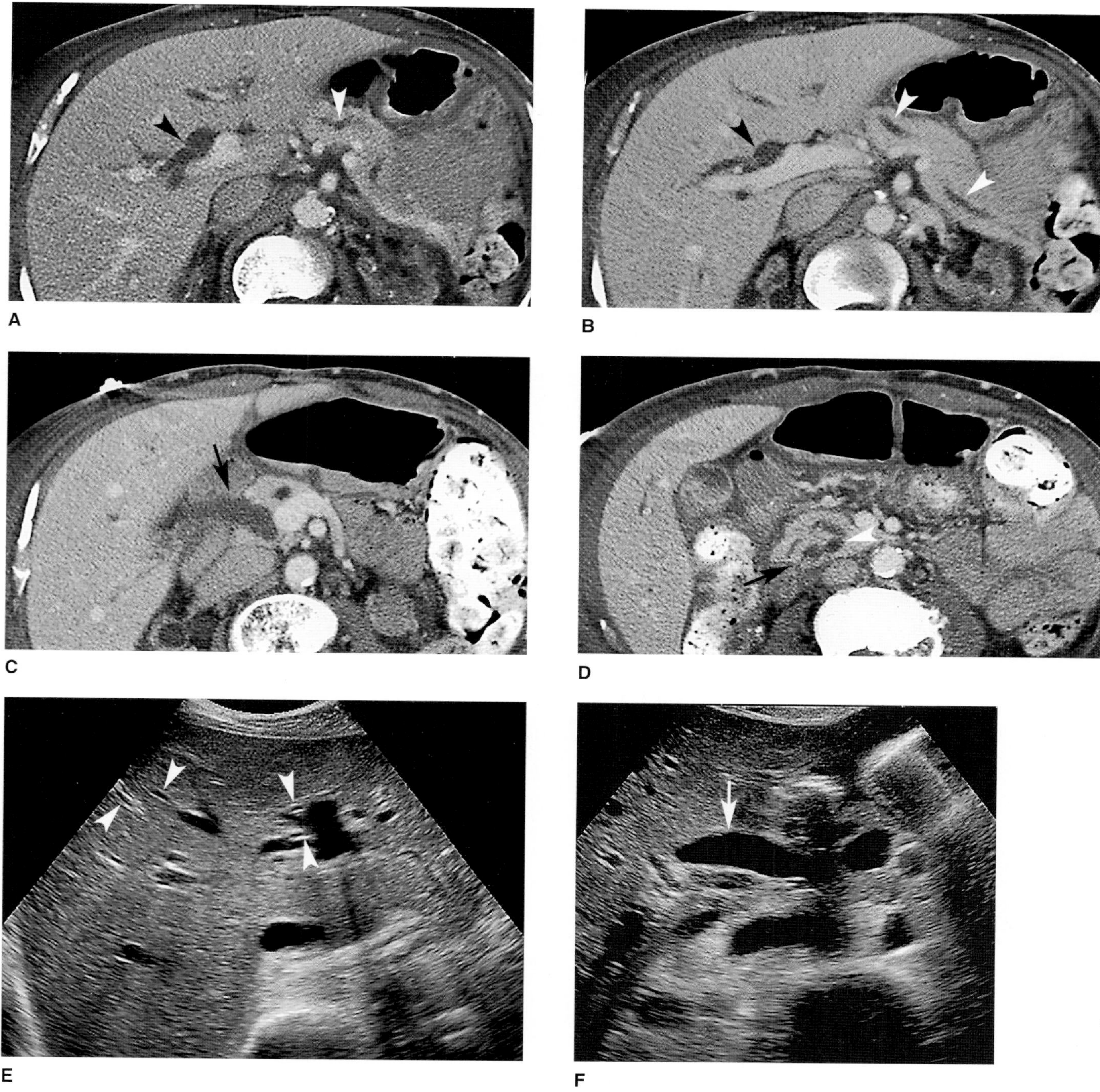

Figure 4-61 Biliary Stricture Due to Prior Choledocholithiasis This 57-year-old woman with a history of prior gallstones and chronic renal failure was being evaluated for the presence of adenopathy. **A-D.** Enhanced CT scan demonstrates dilated intrahepatic (*black arrowheads*) and extrahepatic (*black arrows*) bile ducts and a dilated pancreatic duct (*white arrowheads*), suggesting an obstruction near the sphincter of Oddi. No mass is seen in the pancreatic head on image (D). **E-H.** US examination confirms the presence of intrahepatic (*white arrowheads*) and extrahepatic (*small white arrow*) bile duct dilation and pancreatic duct dilation (*large white arrowheads*) and no mass in the pancreatic head. The examination also demonstrates multiple gallstones that were not seen on the CT scan.

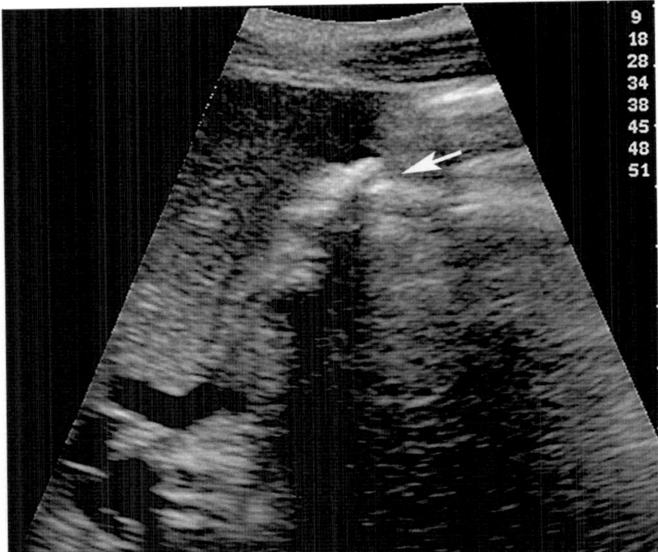

G

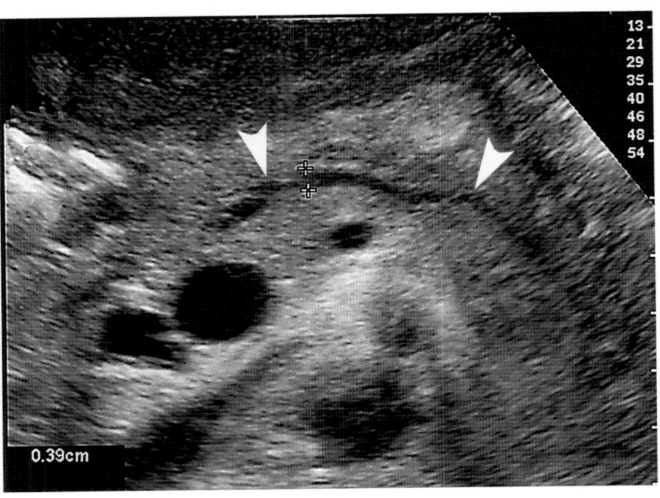

H

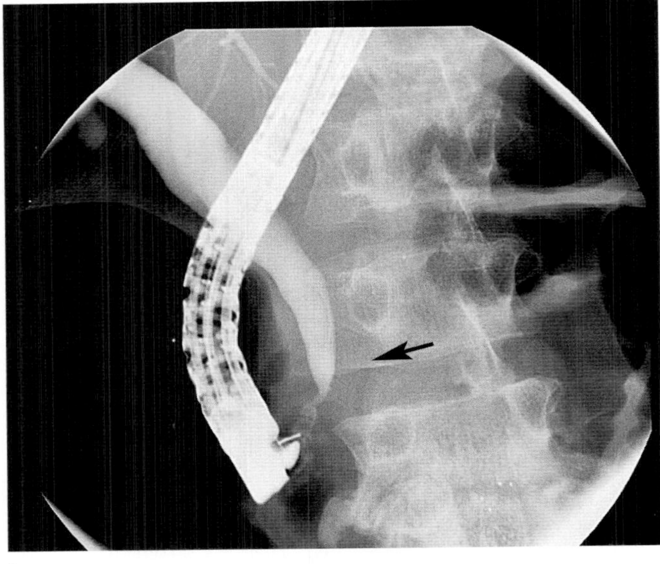

I

Figure 4-61 Biliary Stricture Due to Prior Choledocholithiasis (*Continued*)
I. ERCP shows a smooth tapered stricture (*black arrow*) at the distal common bile duct probably due to prior stone passage.

are an important complication of ascending cholangitis and are one of the reasons for cross-sectional imaging of patients with suspected cholangitis.[129] Uses of imaging include determining the level and etiology of obstruction as well as evaluating for possible complicating abscesses (see Figure 4-64).[24] Imaging findings on CT, US, and MR include extrahepatic and/or intrahepatic biliary ductal dilation with or without stones. Note that biliary ductal dilation is usually in the central liver as opposed to dilation in the peripheral liver that is seen with primary sclerosing cholangitis.[128]

In Asia and Africa, the parasitic infections: *Ascaris lumbricoides and Clonorchis sinensis* are important causes of bile duct obstruction and chronic liver disease.[130,131] *Clonorchis* infection is often known as "oriental cholangiohepatitis." These organisms ascend into the biliary tree from the small bowel where they cause inflammation and subsequent fibrosis of bile ducts.[24,132,133] They also cause multiple pigmented biliary calculi in the majority of patients. Both fibrotic strictures and biliary calculi can lead to chronic bile duct obstruction and recurrent secondary pyogenic cholangitis. Patients usually present with recurrent abdominal pain, jaundice, and fever requiring removal of stones and debris. Cross-sectional imaging will demonstrate multifocal regions of intrahepatic bile duct dilation (see Figure 4-65). MRCP, ERCP, and PTC will demonstrate multiple biliary strictures with intraluminal debris and stones.

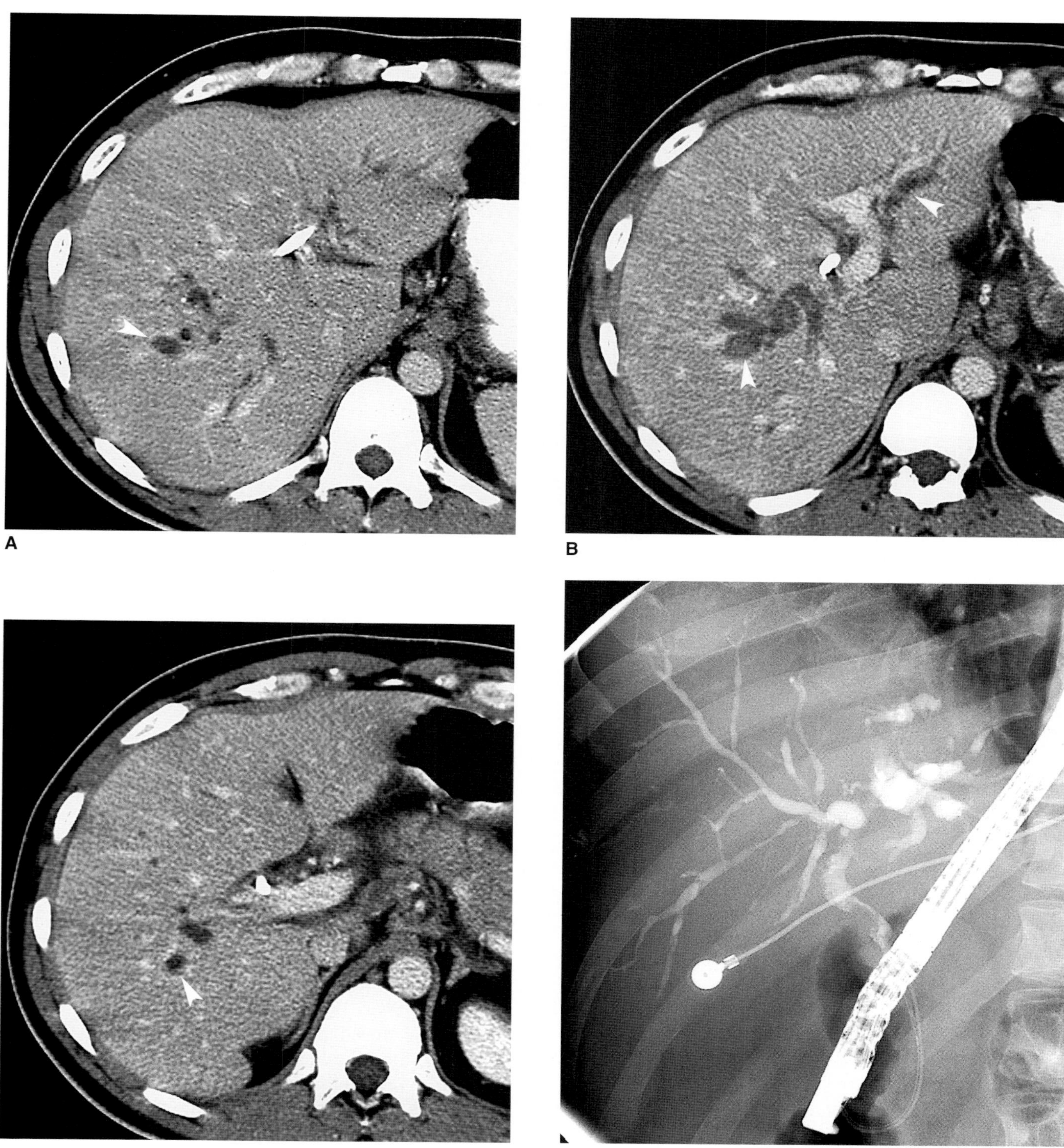

Figure 4-62 ERCP of Sclerosing Cholangitis
A-C. Contrast-enhanced CT in this patient with sclerosing cholangitis demonstrates multiple regions of bile duct dilation (*white arrowheads*). Note how the ducts are variable diameter and in some slices appear to be small cysts adjacent to the portal triads. This is the cross-sectional equivalent of beaded ducts. **D.** ERCP demonstrates the alternating dilated and stenotic appearance typical of "beading" of the bile ducts in sclerosing cholangitis.

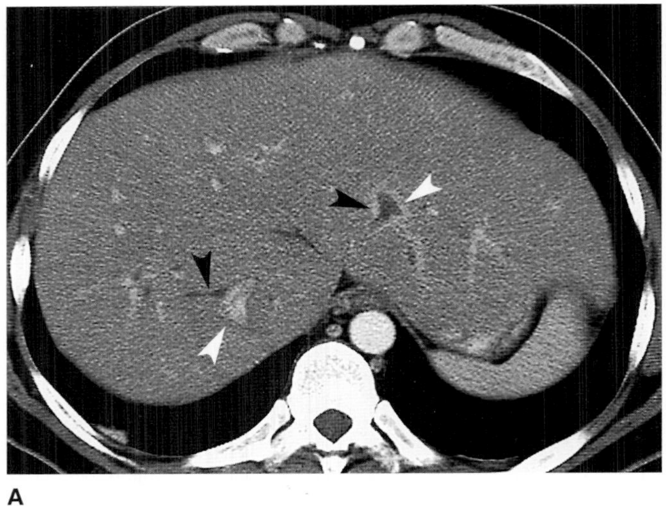

A

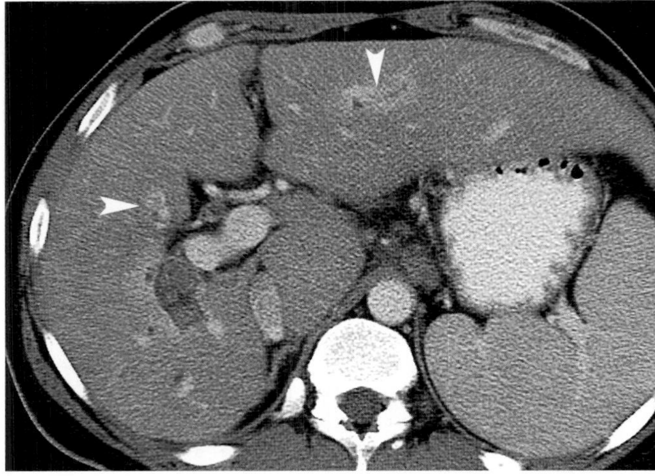

B

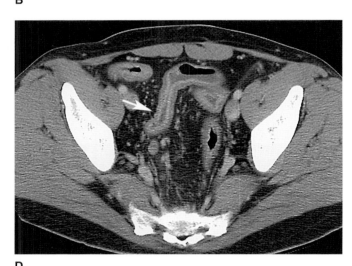

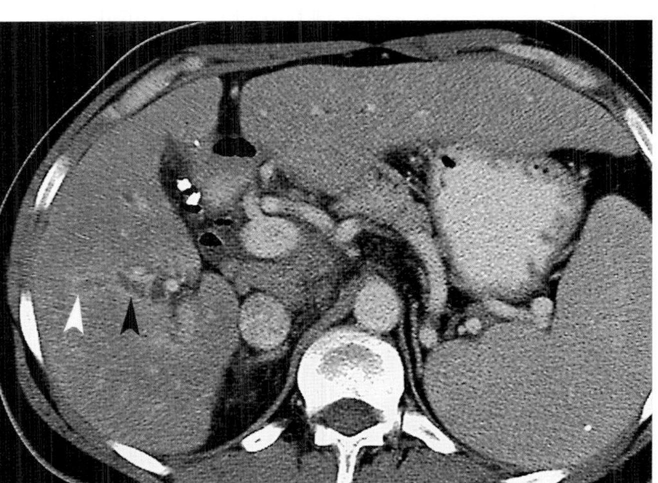

C

D

Figure 4-63 Sclerosing Cholangitis
This 40-year-old man had ulcerative colitis. **A-C.** Contrast-enhanced CT images through the liver demonstrate mild intrahepatic biliary ductal dilation (*black arrowheads*). There is also diffuse enhancement of the bile ducts seen as areas of increased attenuation surrounding the bile ducts (*white arrowheads*) that indicates diffuse inflammation of the bile ducts. In the setting of a patient with ulcerative colitis, these findings are indicative of sclerosing cholangitis. **D.** Image through the pelvis also shows enhancement of the sigmoid wall (*white arrow*) consistent with colonic inflammation in ulcerative colitis.

AIDS-Related cholangitis: Acalculous inflammation of the biliary system is a rare but well-documented complication in patients with AIDS. AIDS-related cholangitis is thought to be a complication of *Cryptosporidium* and/or cytomegalovirus infection and acalculous inflammation of the biliary tree.[134] Patients typically present with right upper quadrant pain and/or epigastric pain, jaundice, or abnormal liver enzymes.[134]

Ultrasonographic evaluation generally shows dilation of the common bile duct and, occasionally, the intrahepatic bile ducts with thickening of the duct walls.[134,135] A terminal ductal stricture is occasionally identified. Gallbladder wall thickening can be seen in some individuals. Computed tomographic findings are similar to US, and CT appears to be better at demonstrating the intrahepatic ductal dilation but less sensitive in demonstrating the bile duct wall thickening.[134] Pruning, an appearance resembling a shrub after it has lost the outermost leaves, of the distal common bile ducts can also been seen on CT. Patients can present with isolated strictures involving the extrahepatic or intrahepatic biliary ducts or ductal irregularities throughout the biliary tree. Both CT and US often demonstrate extrabiliary disease, including splenomegaly and enlarged portohepatic nodes.[134] The overall appearance can closely resemble findings of papillary stenosis and sclerosing cholangitis.

Eosinophilic cholangitis: Eosinophilic cholangiopathy is a rarely reported cause of benign biliary obstruction with an unknown cause. Histologically, there is transmural

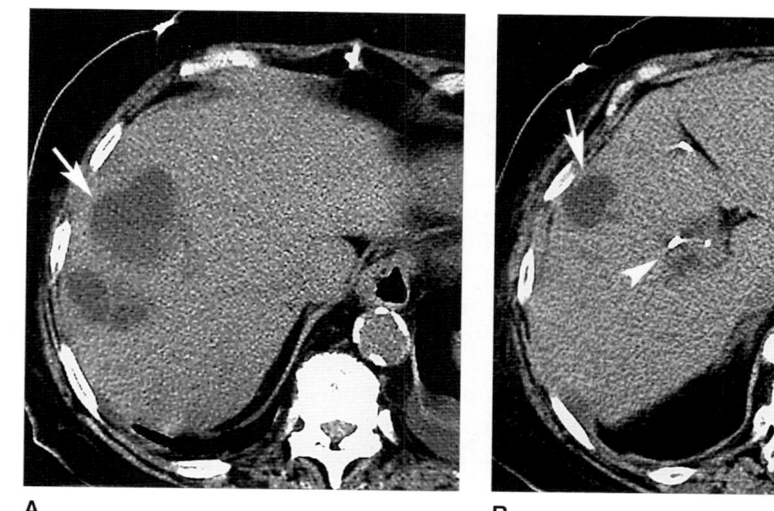

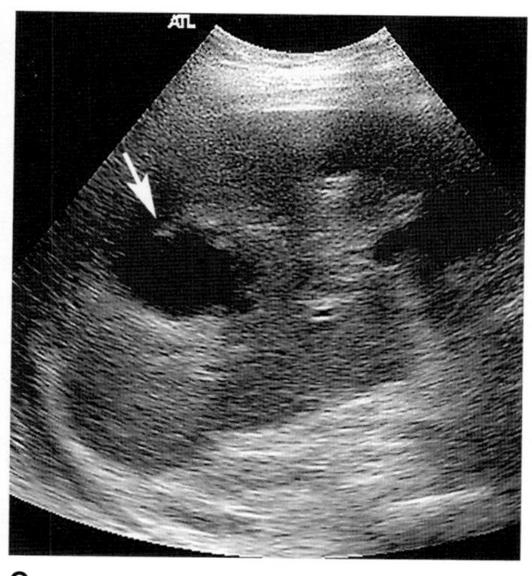

Figure 4-64 Hepatic Abscesses Due to Ascending Cholangitis This 86-year-old woman developed fever and jaundice in the first few days following cholecystectomy. **A** and **B.** Unenhanced CT images demonstrate a cluster of fluid collections (*white arrows*) in the liver that had not been on previous examinations and consistent with hepatic abscesses due to ascending cholangitis. **C.** Sagittal US also reveals an anechoic, irregularly marginated fluid collection (*white arrow*) with internal debris, typical of an abscess.

eosinophilic infiltration of the biliary tract, which can affect the gallbladder and/or the bile ducts. There can be peripheral eosinophilia.[136] There are no specific radiologic signs for eosinophilic cholangiopathy. It should be considered in patients with eosinophilia and biliary obstruction.

When eosinophilic cholangiopathy is limited to the gallbladder, treatment with steroids may help patients avoid cholecystectomy. On US, CT, and MR, this appears as acalculous cholecystitis with gallbladder distention, gallbladder wall thickening, and pericholecystic fluid.[136] When it involves the

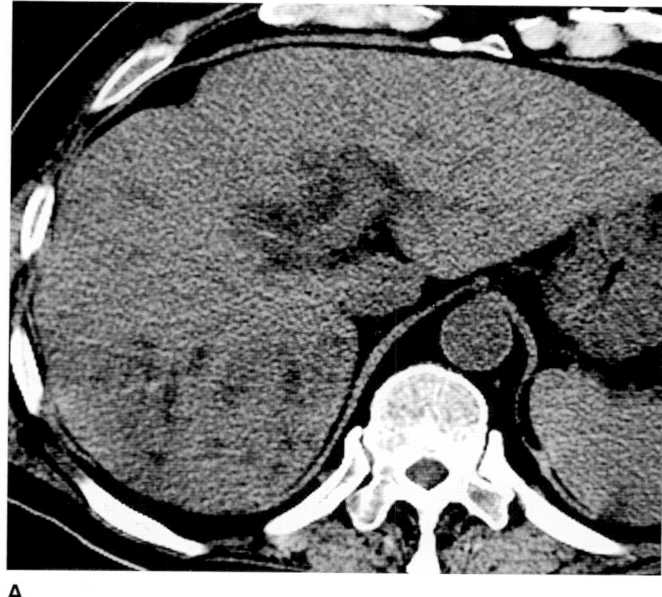

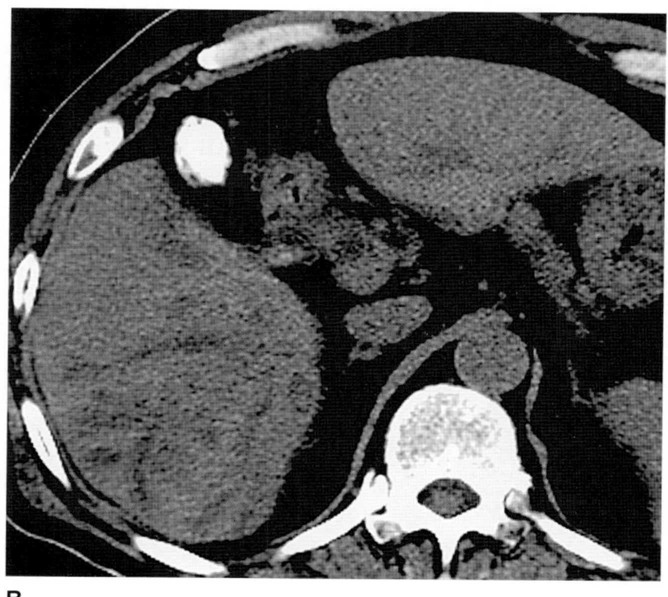

Figure 4-65 Oriental Cholangiohepatitis
This 66-year-old man, immigrant from Southeast Asia, presented with fever and right upper quadrant pain. **A** and **B.** Unenhanced CT images demonstrate intrahepatic biliary dilation involving primarily the posterior segment. The extrahepatic ducts were normal in caliber. Further evaluation was diagnostic of oriental cholangiohepatitis.

biliary tree, there is nonspecific segmental or diffuse bile wall thickening, sometimes with biliary obstruction. On ERCP, there is irregularity of the bile duct wall, which may be in a beaded pattern mimicking primary sclerosing cholangitis.[136]

Other causes of bile duct stricture: Blunt abdominal trauma and radiation therapy have rarely been reported as causes of biliary strictures. Strictures resulting from external beam radiation therapy characteristically appear in the radiation field.[137] Both blunt abdominal trauma and strictures from radiation therapy are nonspecific in appearance and present as abrupt termination of the common bile duct with proximal ductal dilation. Correlation with patient history is often necessary. These findings usually have a delayed presentation and can appear many years after the initial insult.[138] Chronic pancreatitis can occasionally cause periampullary stenosis.[139]

Choledochal cysts

Congenital cystic dilation of the bile ducts is a rare phenomenon collectively known as choledochal cysts. This dilation has been classified into 5 categories (see Figure 4-66). Type I cysts represent fusiform cystic dilation of the common bile duct (see Figures 4-67 and 4-68). Type II cysts are diverticular outpouching of the common bile duct (see Figure 4-69). Type III choledochal cysts are cystic protrusions of the common bile duct into the duodenum, also known as a choledochoceles (see Figure 4-70). Type IV cysts have been further subclassified. Type IVA cysts are dilation of both the intrahepatic and extrahepatic bile ducts. Type IVB cysts involve dilation of multiple segments of the extrahepatic bile duct with a normal intrahepatic biliary tree. Lastly, Type V choledochal cysts are multiple cystic dilations of the intrahepatic bile ducts, with normal extrahepatic bile ducts, a phenomenon called Caroli disease (see Figure 4-71). Caroli disease is an autosomal recessive disorder resulting in multifocal saccular dilation of the intrahepatic bile ducts.[140] Ductal stones, hepatic fibrosis, and portal hypertension resulting in variceal bleeding are some associated complications.[140,141] Patients also have an increased risk of developing cholangiocarcinoma. Caroli disease is also associated with autosomal dominant polycystic kidney disease.[142-145]

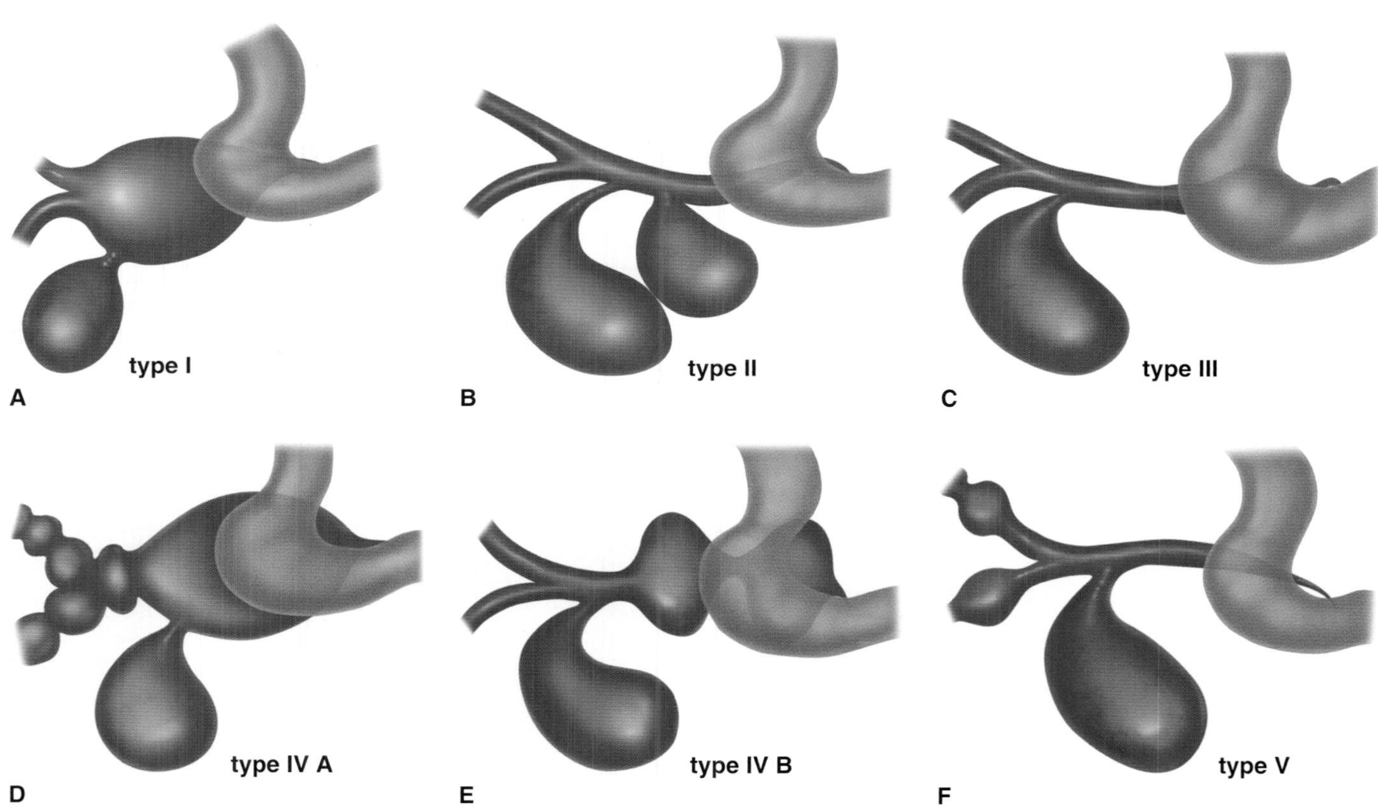

Figure 4.66 Choledochal Cysts
The biliary system is shaded green and the duodenum is shaded pink. **A.** Type I choledochal cyst: fusiform dilation of the common bile duct. **B.** Type II choledochal cyst: saccular outpouching from the common bile duct. **C.** Type III choledochal cyst: choledochocele or cystic protrusion of common bile duct into the duodenum. **D.** Type IVA choledochal cyst: dilation of both the intrahepatic and extrahepatic duct. **E.** Type IVB choledochal cyst: multiple cystic dilations of the common bile duct with normal intrahepatic duct. **F.** Type V choledochal cyst: Caroli disease or multiple cystic dilations of the intrahepatic ducts.

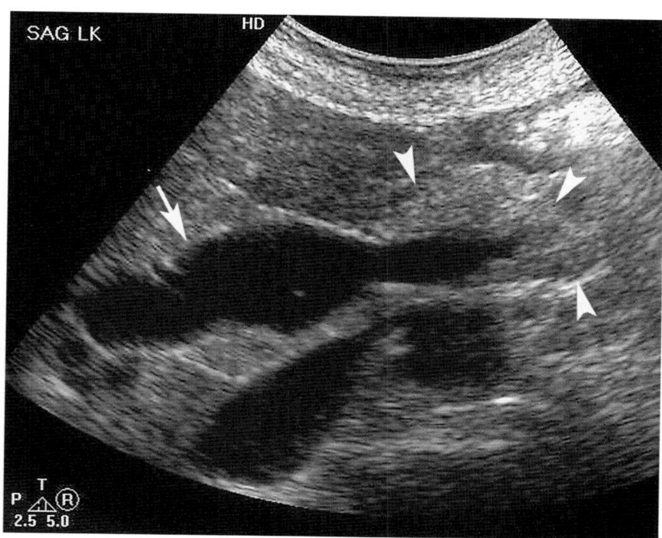

Figure 4-67 US of Choledochal Cyst
US of the common bile duct (*arrow*) in this 62-year-old man demonstrates fusiform dilation of the proximal bile duct with a tapered, narrowed distal common bile duct within the head of the pancreas (*arrowheads*). The intrahepatic ducts appeared normal. This is the typical appearance of a type I choledochal cyst.

Choledochal cysts are thought to be the result of a congenital abnormal connection between the pancreatic duct and the common bile duct that results in the chronic reflux of pancreatic secretions into the bile duct, causing irritation and subsequent dilation.[141] Although the majority will be diagnosed in infancy and childhood, occasionally they are first discovered during adulthood. The prevalence of choledochal cysts is higher in female patients. The classic triad of abdominal pain, right upper quadrant mass, and jaundice has been described but is present in less than one-third of patients.[141]

The classic US appearance of a choledochal cyst is a cystic or fusiform structure in the porta hepatis with apparent communication with the common hepatic duct and a normal-appearing gallbladder (see Figure 4-67).[141] In this case, CT and MRI evaluation is more accurate in the evaluation of the intrahepatic biliary tree and the distal common bile, duct, which is occasionally obscured by bowel gas during US evaluation (see Figures 4-68 and 4-69).[141,146] Further, MRCP, ERCP, and PTC can be more accurate in identifying the intrahepatic forms of choledochal cysts (Type IVA and Caroli disease) because the cystic intrahepatic ducts can be confused with intrahepatic cysts. Confirmation with hepatobiliary scintigraphy is occasionally performed

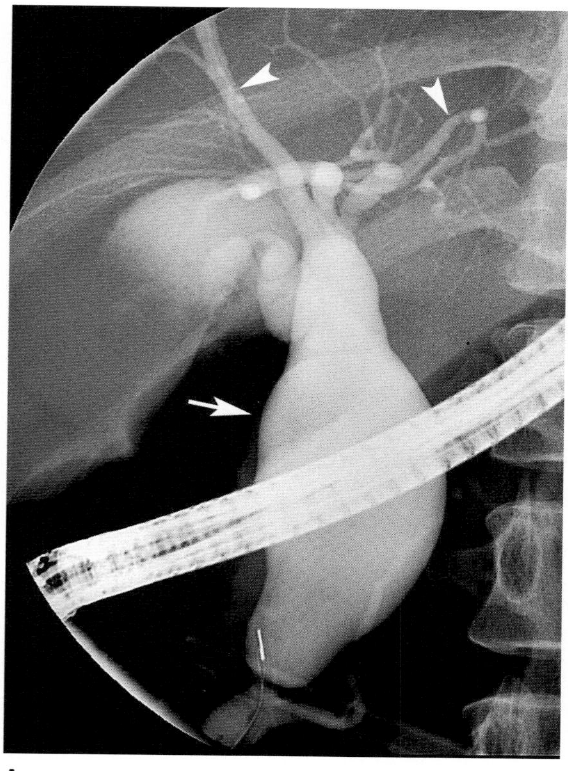
A

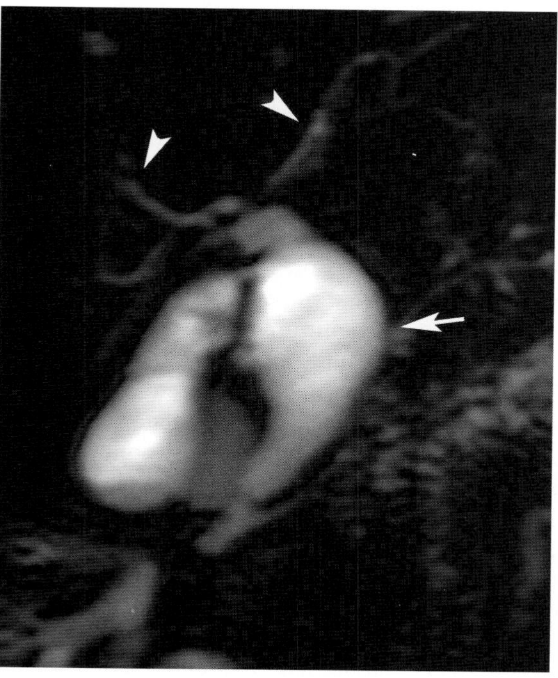
B

Figure 4-68 Choledochal Cyst Type I by ERCP and MRCP
ERCP (**A**) and MRCP (**B**) of this 59-year-old woman demonstrates fusiform dilation of the common bile duct (*arrows*) with normal-appearing intrahepatic ducts (*arrowheads*), typical of a type I choledochal cyst. The shape of the choledochal cyst is different on ERCP from that on MRCP because the cyst is distended under the pressure of injection with ERCP, whereas it is in the normal physiologic state in MRCP.

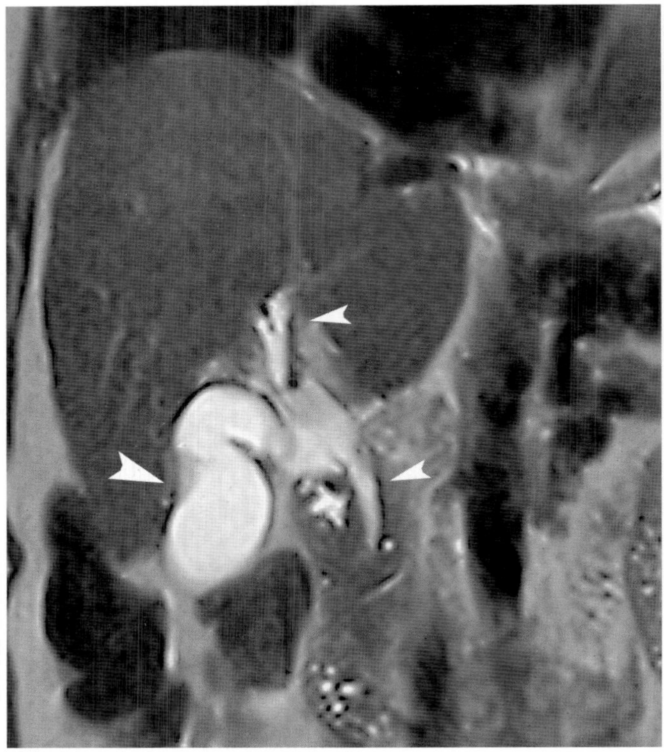

A

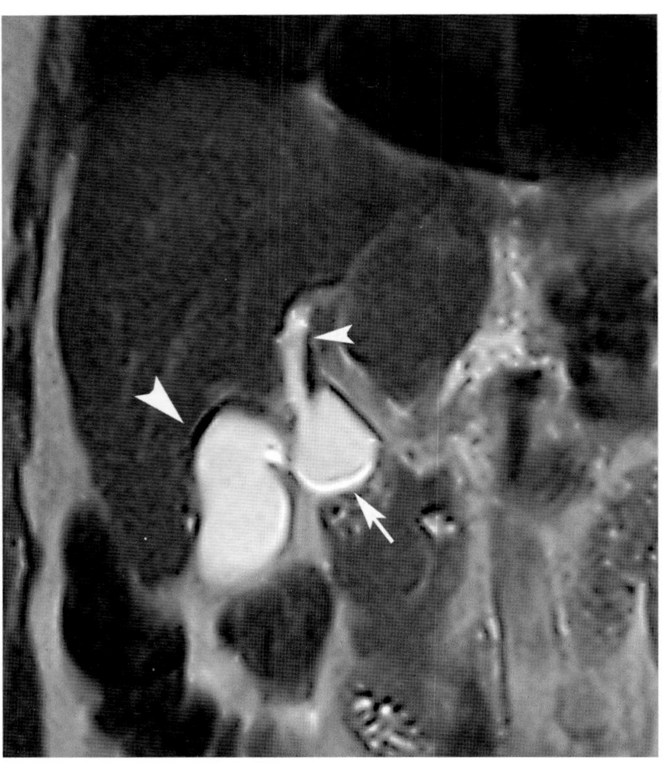

B

Figure 4-69 Type II Choledochal Cyst
A and **B**. Sequential coronal T2-weighted MRI images demonstrate normal proximal and distal common bile ducts (*small arrowheads*) and normal gallbladder (*large arrowhead*) with a saccular outpouching (*arrow*) from the mid common bile duct, features diagnostic of a type II choledochal cyst.

and demonstrates accumulation and stasis of tracer in the dilated ducts and choledochal cyst.[141,147]

The US features of Caroli disease include bile duct dilation with intraluminal protrusions. On CT, there is a classic "central dot sign" which is a high attenuation dot visualized in the dilated intrahepatic bile ducts on unenhanced CT which enhance avidly after contrast administration.[142] This enhancing focus is also seen on gadolinium-enhanced MR. The central dots correspond to intraluminal portal veins on ultrasound. Cholangiography demonstrates saccular or fusiform dilations of portions of the intrahepatic ducts that sometimes contain intraluminal filling defects corresponding to intrahepatic calculi.[140]

Periportal Edema

Edema of the portal triads can be due to a variety of conditions, many of which are not related to the biliary system. However, periportal edema can superficially resemble and be confused with biliary ductal dilation, and so we will discuss the disorder here.

Periportal edema occurs when there is increased production of hepatic extracellular fluid or decrease in the ability for lymphatics to remove excess fluid. Some common causes include congestive heart failure, hepatitis, systemic hypervolemia, abdominal trauma, or post liver transplantation (Table 4-5).[148] A distinguishing feature between periportal edema and biliary dilation is that periportal edema will appear as periportal lucency that surrounds the portal triad on all sides where dilated bile ducts lie only on one side of the portal triad (see Figures 4-72, 4-73, and 4-74).[148]

UNIQUE DISORDERS OF THE BILE DUCTS

Pneumobilia

Pneumobilia is nearly always a result of prior instrumentation of the biliary system that renders the sphincter of Oddi incompetent. This includes sphincterotomy following ERCP and surgeries that result in resection of the sphincter of Oddi, most often a Whipple procedure. Rarely, pneumobilia can be a result of ascending infection, biliary-enteric fistula, emphysematous cholecystitis, and noniatrogenic incompetence of the sphincter of Oddi.

Abdominal plain films and chest radiographs will demonstrate pneumobilia as branching tubular hypodensities within the central liver. This is distinguished from portal venous gas that will collect in the periphery of the

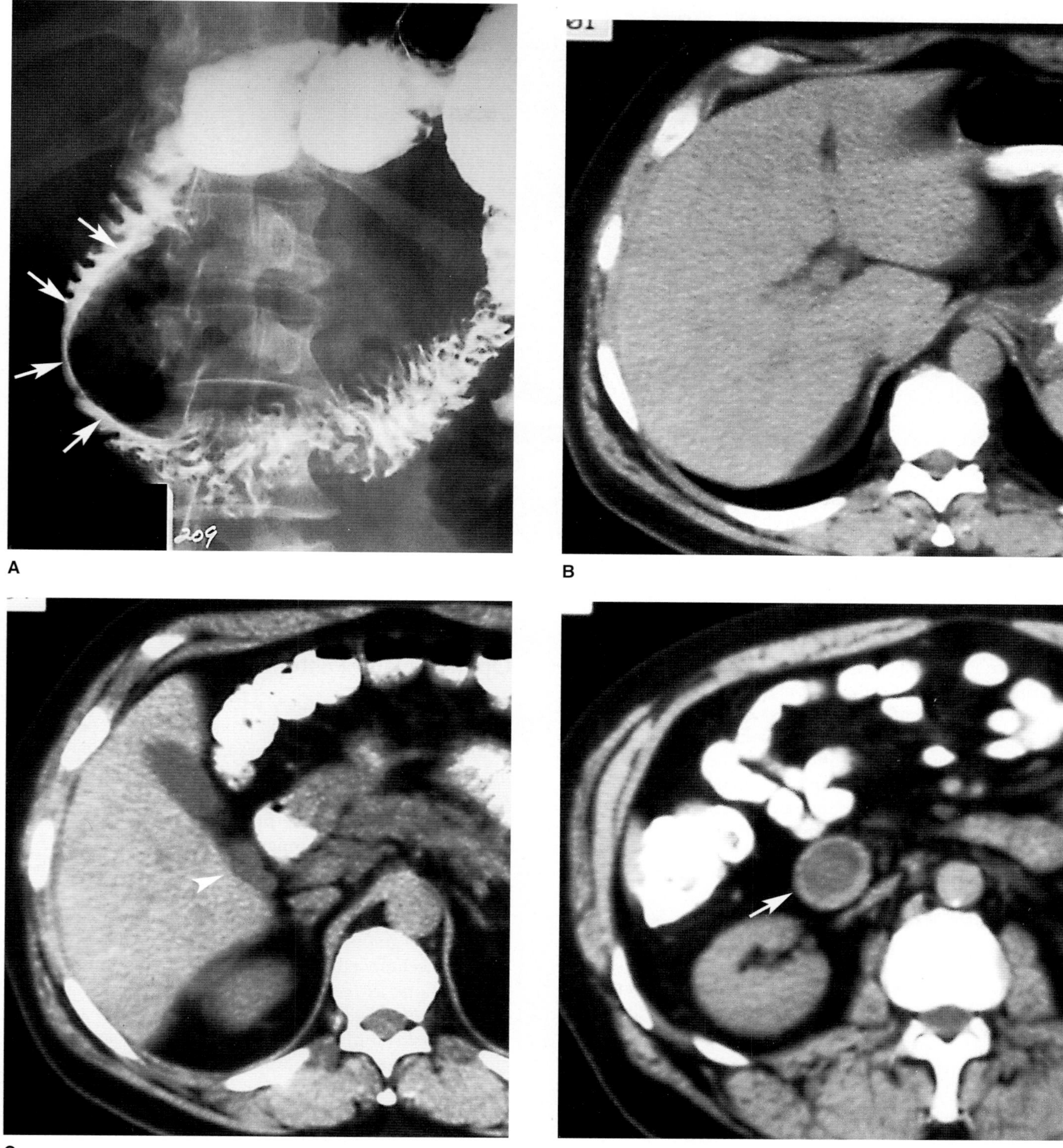

Figure 4-70 Choledochocele
This 56-year-old man had a history of alcoholic pancreatitis and complained of abdominal pain. **A.** Image of the duodenum from an upper GI examination shows smoothly marginated intraluminal mass (*arrows*) in the second portion of the duodenum. **B.** CT through the central liver shows no evidence of intrahepatic biliary dilation. **C.** Image through the gallbladder fossa shows the common bile duct (*arrowhead*) to be borderline enlarged. **D.** At the junction of the second with the third portion of the duodenum there is a cystic mass (*arrow*) projecting into the lumen of the duodenum. This is near the sight of the ampulla of Vater and represented a choledochocele.

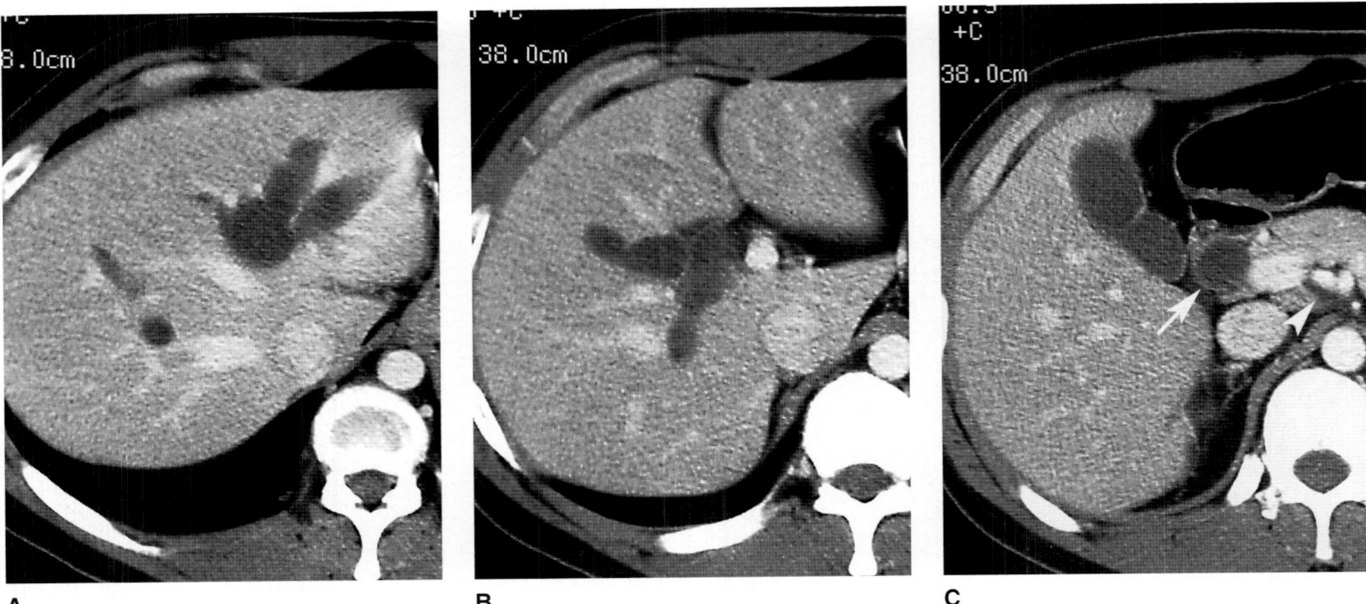

Figure 4-71 CT of Caroli Disease
This 25-year-old man presented with abdominal pain. Liver function tests were normal. **A** and **B.** Enhanced CT images demonstrate moderate multifocal dilation of the central biliary ducts with normal-appearing peripheral ducts. **C.** The mid common bile duct (*arrow*) is markedly dilated but with a normal caliber duct (*arrowhead*) as it enters the pancreas. The combination of normal liver function tests and normal peripheral and dilated central ducts is consistent with the diagnosis of Caroli disease.

liver (see Figures 4-75 and 4-76). Computed tomographic examinations will readily demonstrate hypoattenuating air within the lumen of the bile ducts, and MRI will show the air as signal voids on all pulse sequences (see Figures 4-75 and 4-77). This will most often collect in the anterior portions of the liver because air will rise into nondependent structures. US will demonstrate linear and branching echogenic structures in the distribution of bile ducts (see Figure 4-75).

POSTOPERATIVE FINDINGS RELATED TO BILIARY SURGERY

Cholecystectomy, Whipple procedure, and liver transplantation are the most common surgeries to involve the biliary system.

Table 4-5. Causes of Periportal Edema

1. Congestive heart failure
2. Hepatitis
3. Hypervolemia
4. Abdominal trauma
5. Post liver transplantation

Operative and Postoperative Hardware

The most common surgery performed on the biliary system is cholecystectomy. This procedure can be performed as an open surgery or laparoscopically, depending on the indication. The postsurgical findings are usually similar regardless of how the procedure was performed.

Normal postoperative findings after cholecystectomy include a cystic duct remnant, which is usually 1 to 2 cm long; however, remnants of up to 6 cm in length have been reported.[77,117] The diameter of the common bile duct can increase after cholecystectomy. A maximum diameter of 13 mm with gradual tapering is within normal range.[117,122] Cholecystectomy clips are apparent on plain film, and CT examinations as linear metallic densities in the gallbladder fossa (see Figure 4-78). On US, the clips appear as linear shadowing structures. On MRI, cholecystectomy clips appear as metallic artifacts in the gallbladder fossa. Usually, surgical clips and the absence of the gallbladder are the only findings in patients status post cholecystectomy. Occasionally, there can be mild ductal dilation following the surgery that persists with the common hepatic duct measuring up to 10 to 13 mm in internal diameter (see Figure 4-78).[149] The other surgery affecting the biliary system that is commonly encountered is the pancreaticoduodenectomy, also known as the Whipple procedure. The operation includes removal of the pancreatic head, duodenum, gallbladder, and gastric antrum with drainage of the biliary system through a choledochojejunostomy. The Whipple procedure is traditionally thought of as surgery

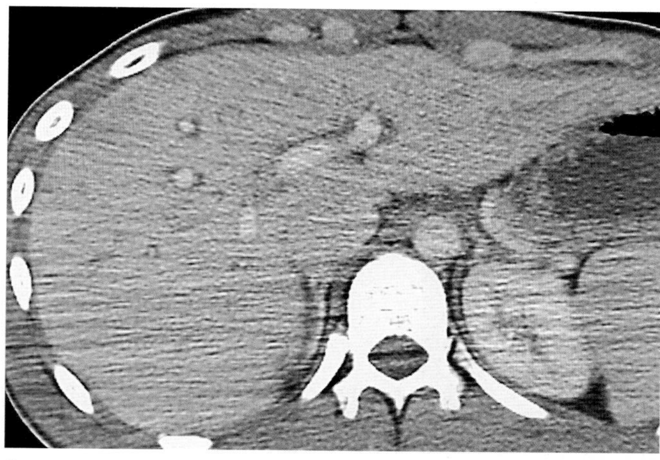

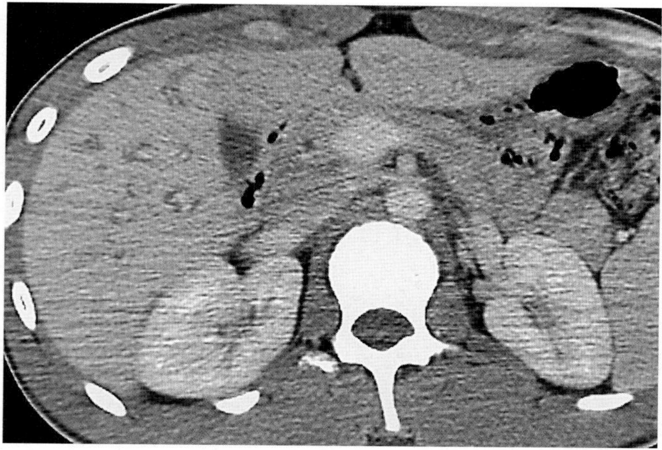

Figure 4-72 Periportal Edema in a Trauma Patient
This 18-year-old man was in a motor vehicle accident. **A** and **B.** Enhanced CT demonstrates low attenuation regions surrounding the high-attenuation enhancing portal veins. When only on one side of the portal vein, this low attenuation region will usually indicate bile duct dilation. However, when found surrounding portal veins, this finding is indicative of periportal edema. In the setting of trauma, periportal edema will usually be a manifestation of volume overload common in the acute trauma setting but can be a direct manifestation of liver trauma.

for tumors involving the pancreatic head, but it can also be performed for cholangiocarcinoma or duodenal masses requiring resection. Postsurgical changes from the choledochojejunostomy include a loop of small bowel in the gallbladder fossa usually with some degree of pneumobilia, most commonly affecting the left hepatic lobe. The loop of small bowel forming the choledochojejunostomy does not fill with oral contrast and can appear as a low attenuation masslike opacity in the porta hepatis (see Figures 4-75 and 4-79). This should not be confused with recurrent tumor or a postoperative collection. Mild bile duct dilation can imply a stricture at the choledochojejunostomy but is often

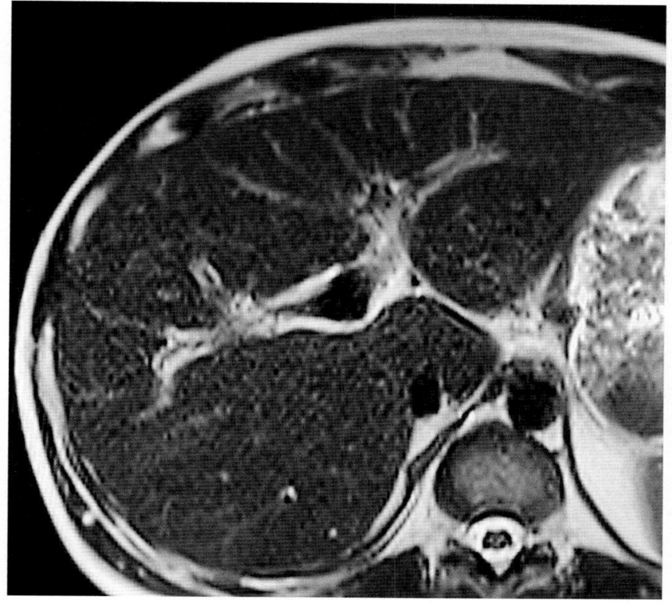

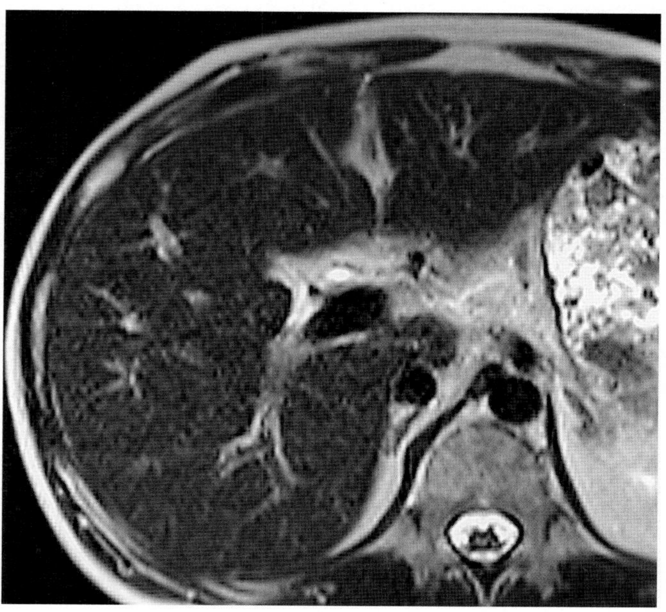

Figure 4-73 Periportal Edema Due to Chemotoxicity
This 30-year-old man with acute lymphoid leukemia (ALL) had elevated liver function tests. **A** and **B.** T2-weighted MRI sequence images show the low signal in the portal veins surrounded by high-signal edema in the portal triads, findings typical of periportal edema. This was an imaging manifestation of hepatotoxicity because of his chemotherapy for ALL.

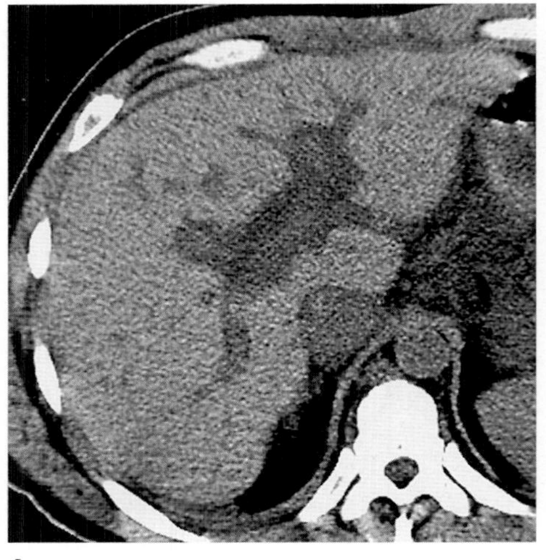

A

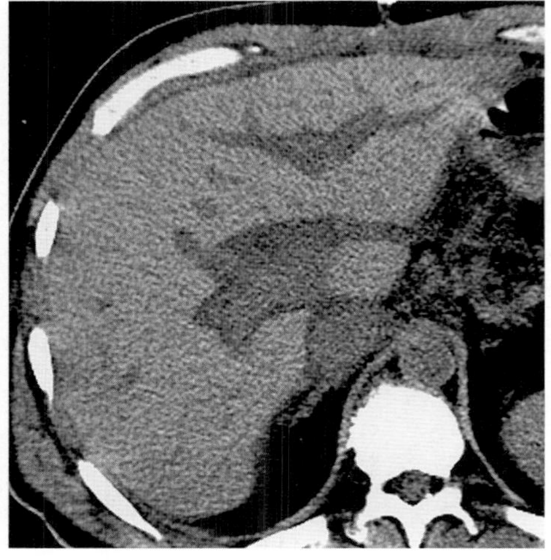

B

Figure 4-74 Periportal Edema Following Liver Transplantation
This 54-year-old man had received a liver transplant. **A** and **B.** Unenhanced CT shows the portal veins to be surrounded by lower attenuation periportal edema. This is probably due to disruption of the lymphatic drainage during liver transplantation and is usually a clinically irrelevant finding.

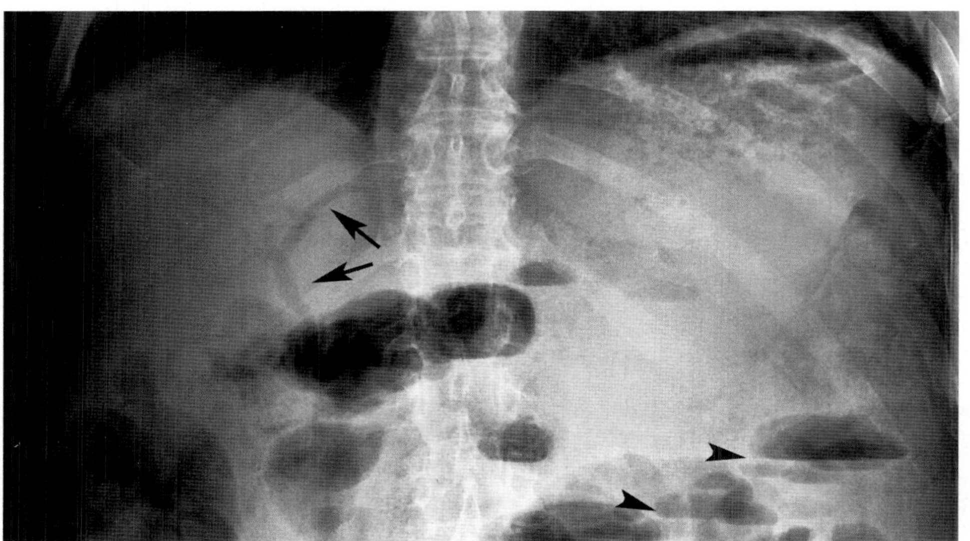

A

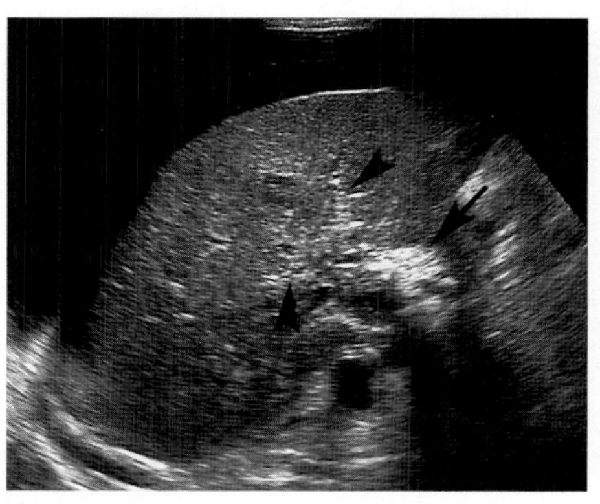

B

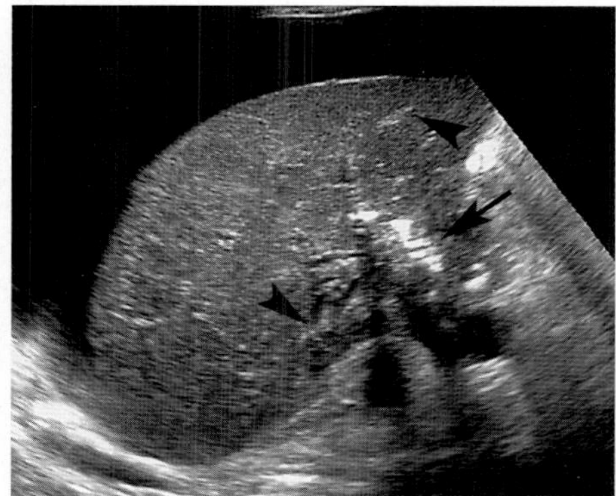

C

Figure 4-75 Pneumobilia Following Whipple Procedure
This 64-year-old man had recently undergone a Whipple procedure. **A.** Abdominal plain film also shows the pneumobilia (*arrows*) as branching hypodensity in the right upper quadrant. There are also small-bowel air-fluid levels due to an adynamic ileus (*arrowheads*). **B** and **C.** Transverse US images in the same patient demonstrate indistinct branching and linear regions of echogenicity (*black arrowheads*)—the characteristic appearance of pneumobilia on US examinations. Note the large echogenic region in the porta hepatis (*black arrow*). This is air within the choledochojejunostomy.

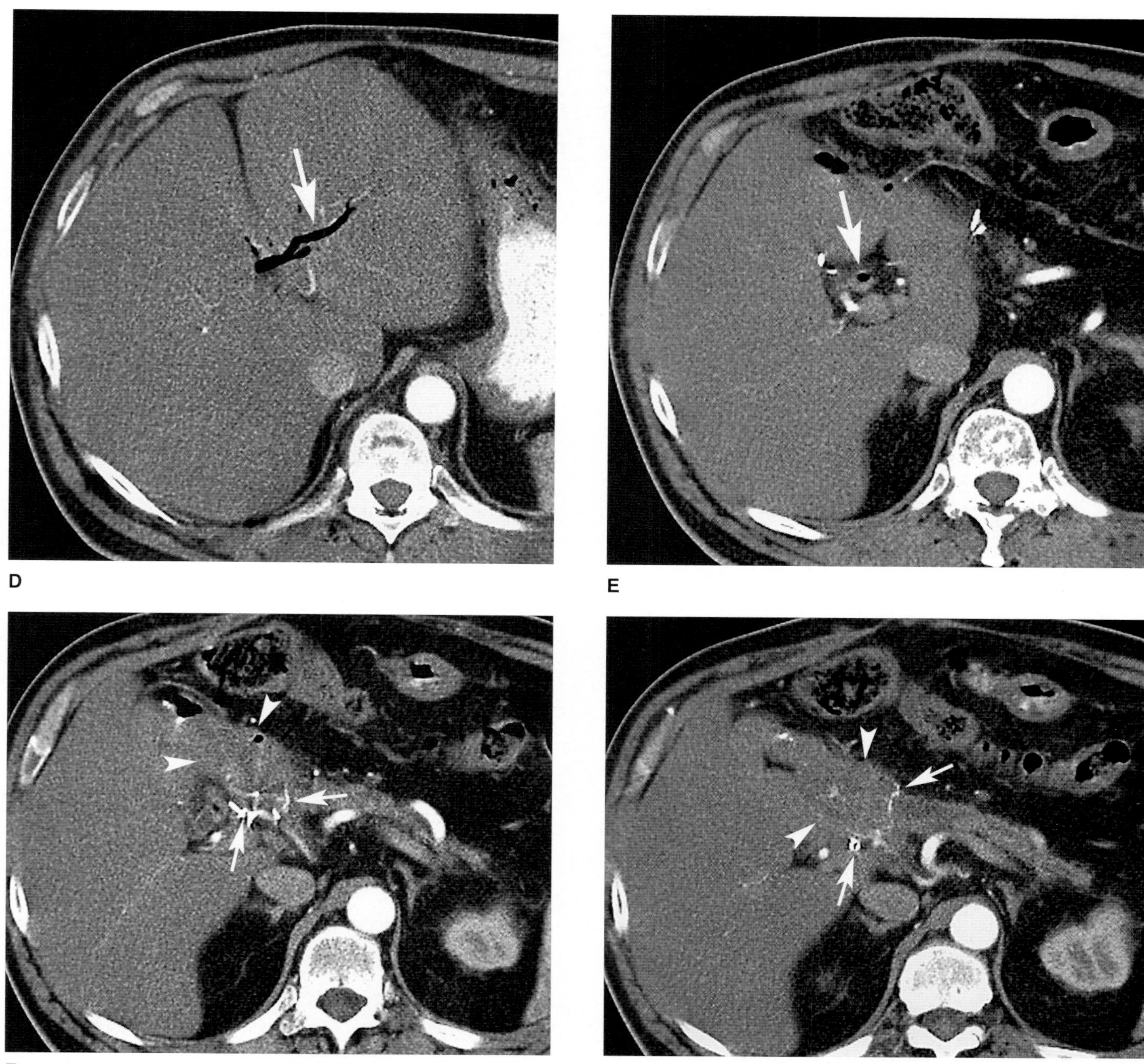

Figure 4-75 Pneumobilia Following Whipple Procedure (*Continued*) **D** and **E**. Contrast-enhanced CT images through the liver shows lines and small dots of gas in the central liver (*large arrows*) typical of pneumobilia. **F** and **G**. There is an amorphous mass within the porta hepatis (*white arrowheads*). There are small hyperattenuating foci representing surgical clips and enteric staple lines (*small arrows*). This is the typical appearance of a choledochojejunostomy. These loops of small bowel lack oral contrast and can be confused with recurrent tumor.

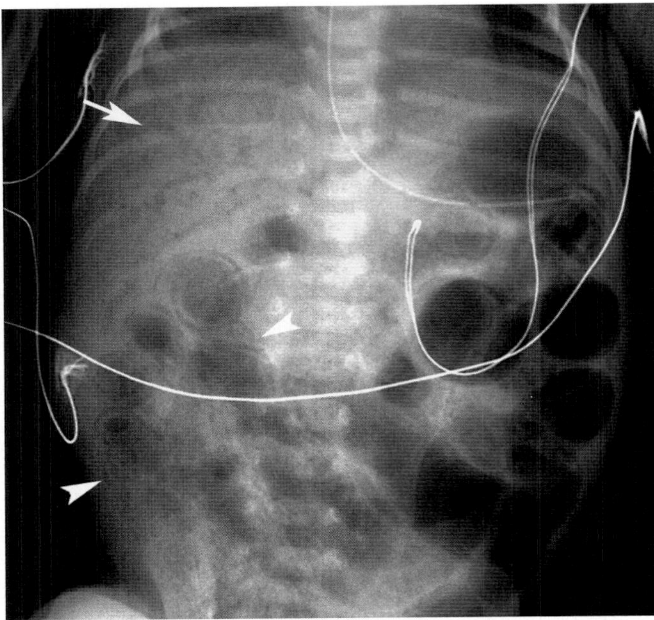

Figure 4-76 Portal Venous Gas Associated with Necrotizing Enterocolitis
This 8-day-old premature infant had increased residuals and abdominal distention. Anteroposterior view of the abdomen demonstrates multiple linear lucencies (*arrowheads*) paralleling the bowel loops, indicating pneumatosis intestinalis and typical of necrotizing enterocolitis in premature infants. There are also multiple branching lucencies overlying the liver shadow (*arrow*) typical of portal venous gas. Note how the more central portal veins are not gas filled. Biliary air typically involves the central ducts, whereas portal venous gas involves the more distal venules.

present without elevation of liver function tests, in which case it is of no significance (see Figure 4-78).

Complications of Biliary Surgery

There are many complications that can occur as a result of both laparoscopic and open cholecystectomy. Complications of laparoscopy in general include abdominal wall bleeding, abdominal vessel injury, GI perforation, solid visceral injury, and wound infection. General complications of cholecystectomy include bile duct injury, bile leakage, and infection. It is important for radiologists to be aware of the radiographic manifestations of these potential complications.[150]

The complications from laparoscopic procedures are usually readily apparent on cross-sectional imaging. Abdominal wall injury and bleeding will present as hematoma at the trochar site. GI perforation will present with increasing abdominal pain and with pneumoperitoneum that progressively increases over time. Occasionally the site of bowel injury will be visualized directly. A solid visceral injury will appear as a low attenuation region within the affected organ. Wound infections will most often appear as excessive infiltration of the subcutaneous fat, sometimes with rim-enhancing fluid collections in the anterior abdominal wall.

Complications from cholecystectomy can be more difficult to evaluate. An injury to the bile duct can be due to accidental clipping of the common hepatic duct and usually presents with jaundice, nausea, and vomiting. Usually, CT, MRI, MRCP, and ERCP examinations will demonstrate bile duct dilation and site of obstruction from an aberrant surgical clip.

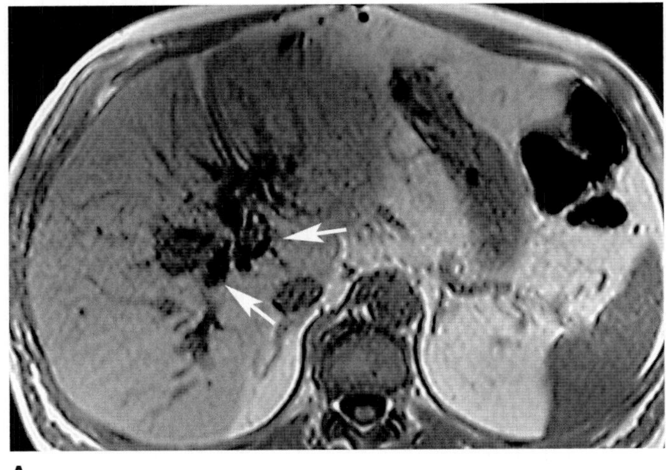

A

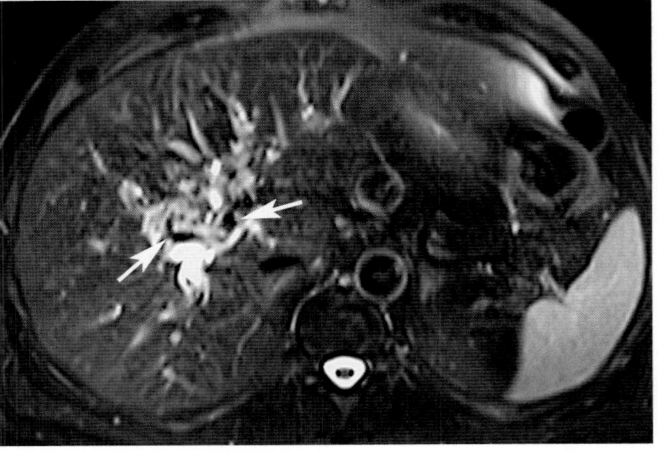

B

Figure 4-77 Pneumobilia on MRI
This 64-year-old man had recently undergone a Whipple procedure. **A**. T1-weighted and (**B**) T2-weighted MRI sequences both show areas of signal void (*arrows*) within the regions of the portal triads. These are within the central bile ducts and are typical of pneumobilia on MRI examinations.

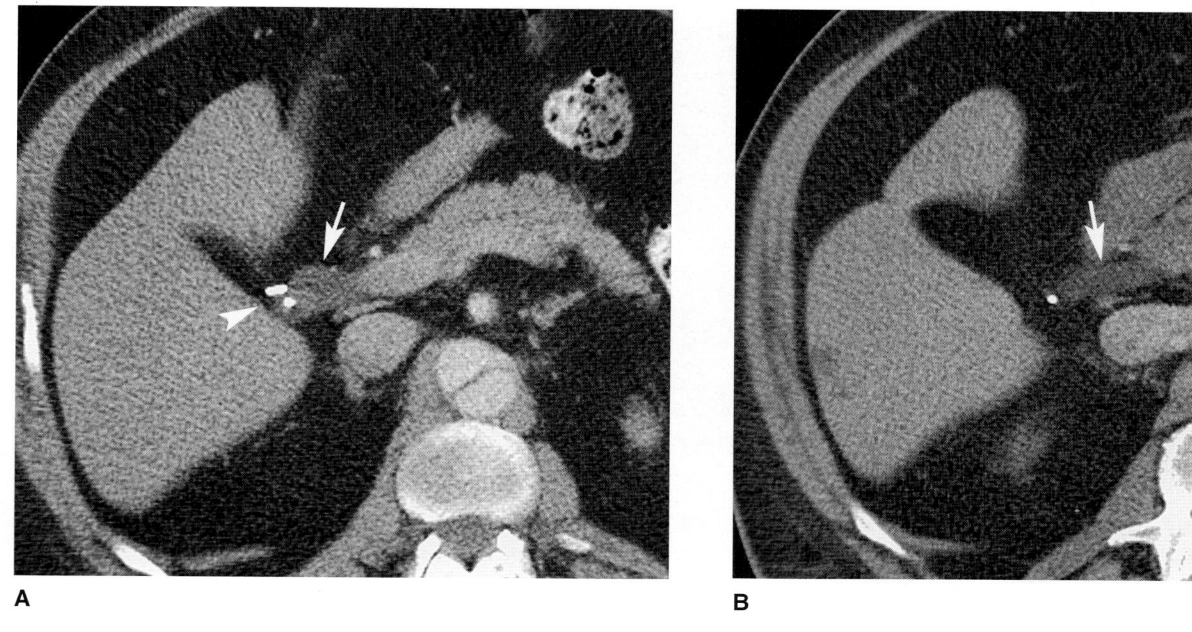

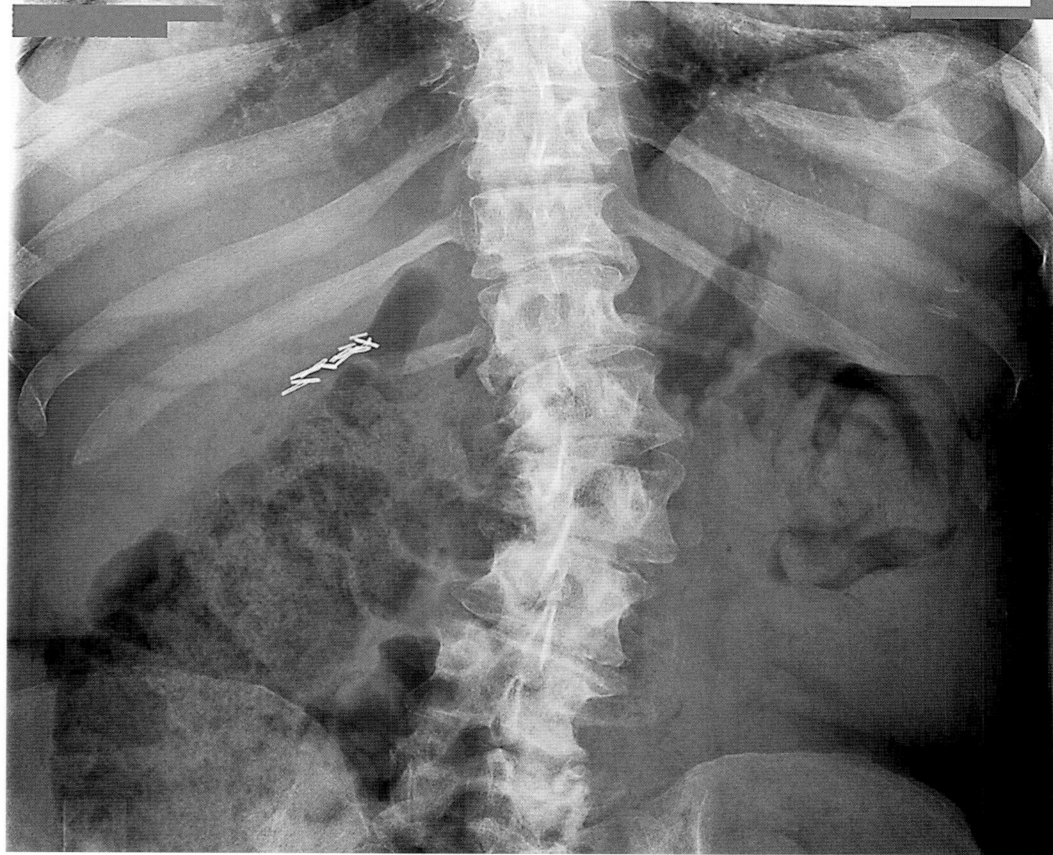

Figure 4-78 Cholecystectomy
A and **B**. Contrast-enhanced CT shows hyperattenuating surgical clips (*arrowhead*) in the gallbladder fossa and mild common bile duct dilation (*arrow*) of 10 mm. These are typical findings following cholecystectomy. There is also a dissection of the abdominal aorta. **C**. Abdominal plain film in a different patient shows the typical location of surgical clips after cholecystectomy.

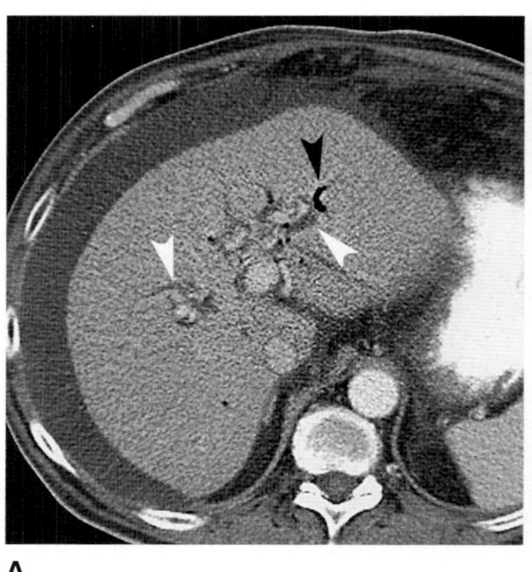

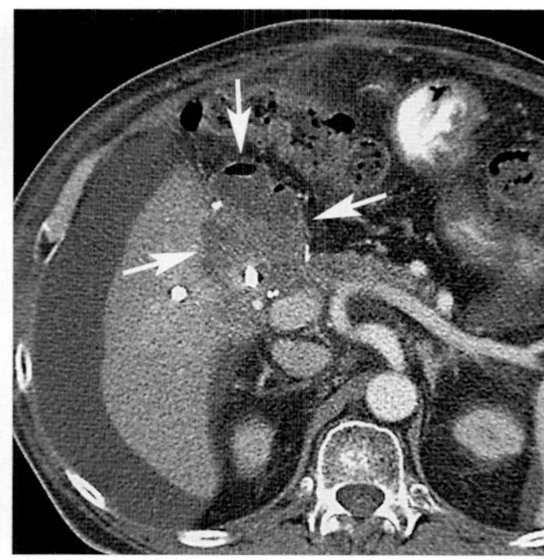

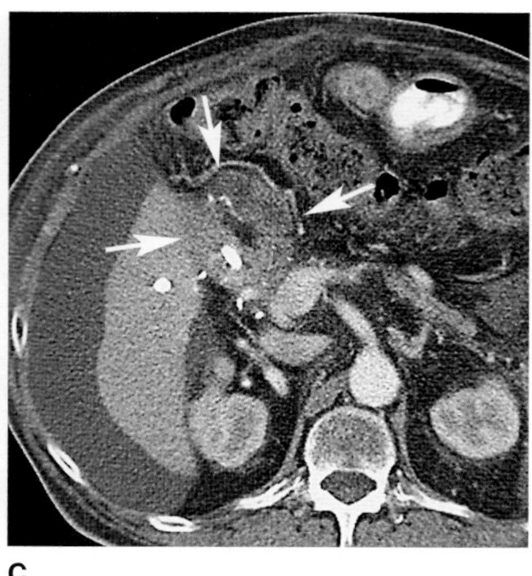

Figure 4-79 Whipple Procedure
This 64-year-old man had undergone a Whipple procedure for carcinoma of the pancreas. **A.** There is pneumobilia (*black arrowhead*) and mild intrahepatic bile duct dilation (*white arrowheads*). Liver function tests were normal. **B** and **C.** Within the porta hepatis is an amorphous mixed fluid and soft-tissue attenuation mass (*arrows*). This represents the choledochojejunostomy and should not be confused with recurrent tumor.

Bile leaks from biliary surgery are also occasionally encountered. Cross-sectional imaging will demonstrate with fluid collections near the site of the bile leak. Hepatobiliary studies will reveal leakage of radiotracer into a nonanatomic location. This will often be the gallbladder fossa and can be confused with the normal gallbladder if the reader is not aware of the previous surgery (see Figure 4-80). A loculated fluid collection from a bile leak, a biloma, can be drained percutaneously. Lastly, postoperative abscesses can be seen following cholecystectomy, Whipple procedures, and other biliary surgery. The radiologic findings are identical to abscesses seen from other etiologies and include a rim-enhancing fluid collection with surrounding inflammatory changes usually containing foci of gas. In most cases, the abscess will be present within the surgical field.

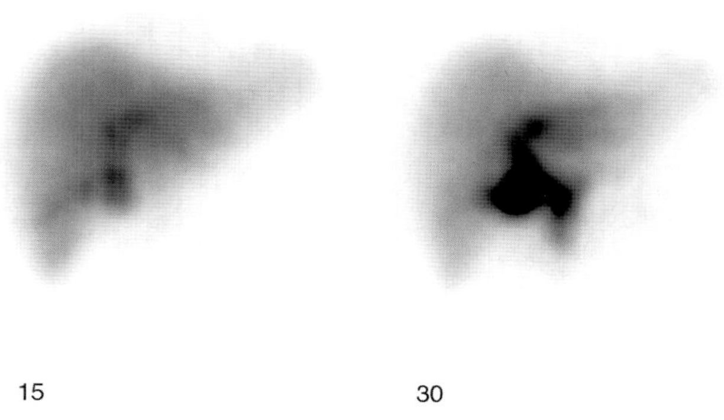

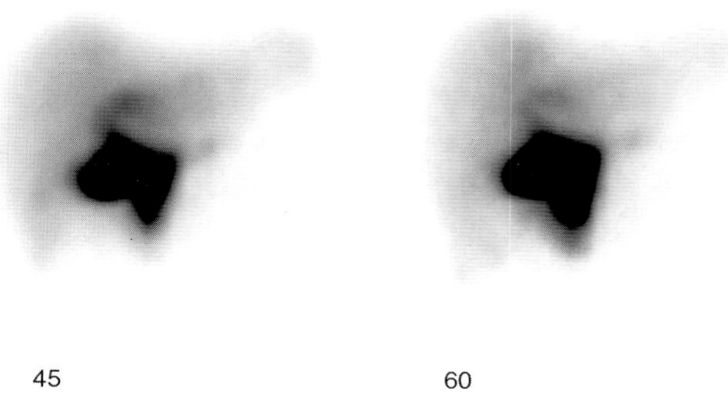

Figure 4-80 Biloma
This patient had recently undergone cholecystectomy. A fluid collection was noted in the operative bed on a postoperative CT (not shown). Tc-99m HIDA examination demonstrates an amorphous collection of tracer in the gallbladder fossa, indicating the presence of a bile leak. (Courtesy of Jacob Dubroff, MD, PhD.)

REFERENCES

1. Parulekar SG. Ultrasound evaluation of common bile duct size. *Radiology.* 1979;133:703-707.
2. Catalano OA, Sahani DV, Kalva SP, et al. MR imaging of the gallbladder: a pictorial essay. *Radiographics.* 2008;28:135-155.
3. Grand D, Horton KM, Fishman EK. CT of the gallbladder: spectrum of disease. *AJR Am J Roentgenol.* 2004;183:163-170.
4. Rooholamini SA, Tehrani NS, Razavi MK, et al. Imaging of gallbladder carcinoma. *Radiographics.* 1994;14:291-306.
5. Klein JB, Finck FM. Primary carcinoma of the gallbladder: review of 28 cases. *Arch Surg.* 1972;104:769-777.
6. Hamrick RE Jr, Liner FJ, Hastings PR, et al. Primary carcinoma of the gallbladder. *Ann Surg.* 1982;195:270-273.
7. Roberts JW, Daugherty SF. Primary carcinoma of the gallbladder. *Surg Clin North Am.* 1986;66:743-749.
8. Yum HY, Fink AL. Sonographic findings in primary carcinoma of the gallbladder. *Radiology.* 1980;134:693-696.
9. Kane RA, Jacobs R, Katz J, Costello P. Porcelain gallbladder: ultrasound and CT appearance. *Radiology.* 1984;152:137-141.
10. Robbins SL. *Pathology*. 3rd ed. Philadelphia, PA: Saunders; 1987:957-959.
11. Vaittinen E. Carcinoma of the gallbladder: a study of 390 cases diagnosed in Finland 1953-1967. *Ann Chir Gynaecol Fenn.* 1970; 59(suppl 168):1-81.
12. Adson MA. Carcinoma of the gallbladder. *Surg Clin North Am.* 1973;53:1203-1216.
13. Bergdahl L. Gallbladder carcinoma first diagnosed at microscopic examination of gallbladders removed for presumed benign disease. *Ann Surg.* 1980;191:19-22.
14. Fahim RB, McDonald JR, Richards JC, et al. Carcinoma of the gallbladder: a study of its modes of spread. *Ann Surg.* 1962; 156:114-124.
15. Levy AD, Murakata LA, Rohrmann CA Jr. Gallbladder carcinoma: radiologic-pathologic correlation. *Radiographics.* 2001;21:295-314.
16. Sako M, Ohtsuki S, Hitora S, et al. Diagnostic imaging of thickening of the gallbladder wall: angiographic approach to differentiation between cancer and chronic cholecystitis. *Rinsho Hoshasen (Japan J Clin Radiol).* 1985;30:697-704.
17. Lane J, Buck JL, Zeman RK. Primary carcinoma of the gallbladder: a pictorial essay. *Radiographics.* 1989;9:209-227.
18. Dalla Palma L, Rizzatto G, Pozzi-Mucelli RS, et al. Grayscale ultrasonography in the evaluation of carcinoma of the gallbladder. *Br J Radiol.* 1980;53:662-667.
19. Jeffrey RB, Laing FC, Wong W, et al. Gangrenous cholecystitis: diagnosis by ultrasound. *Radiology.* 1983;148:219-221.
20. Ruiz R, Teyssou H, Fernandez N, et al. Ultrasonic diagnosis of primary carcinoma of the gallbladder: a review of 16 cases. *J Clin Ultrasound.* 1980;8:489-495.
21. Franquet T, Montes M, Ruiz de Azua Y, et al. Primary gallbladder carcinoma: imaging findings in 50 patients with pathologic correlation. *Gastrointest Radiol.* 1991;16:143-148.
22. Weiner SN, Koenigsberg M, Morehouse H, et al. Sonography and computed tomography in the diagnosis of carcinoma of the gallbladder. *AJR Am J Roentgenol.* 1984;142:735-739.
23. Smathers RL, Lee JK, Heiken JP. Differentiation of complicated cholecystitis from gallbladder carcinoma by computed tomography. *AJR Am J Roentgenol.* 1984;143:255-259.
24. Siegelman ES. *Body MR.* 1st ed. Philadelphia, PA: Elsevier-Saunders ;2001:63-119.
25. Ohtani T, Shirai Y, Tsukada K, et al. Carcinoma of the gallbladder: CT evaluation of lymphatic spread. *Radiology.* 1993;189:875-880.
26. Sons HU, Borchard F, Joel BS. Carcinoma of the gallbladder: autopsy findings in 287 cases and review of the literature. *J Surg Oncol.* 1985;28:199-206.
27. Bickel A, Eitan A, Tsilman B, et al. Low-grade B cell lymphoma of mucosa-associated lymphoid tissue (MALT) arising in the gallbladder. *Hepatogastroenterology.* 1999;46:1643-1646.
28. Chim CS, Liang R, Loong F, et al. Primary mucosa-associated lymphoid tissue lymphoma of the gallbladder. *Am J Med.* 2002;112:505-507.
29. Pantongrag-Brown L, Nelson AM, Brown AE, et al. Gastrointestinal manifestations of acquired immunodeficiency syndrome: radiologic-pathologic correlation. *Radiographics.* 1995;15:1155-1178.
30. Donnelly LF, Bisset GS III, Frush DP. Embryonal rhabdomyosarcoma of the biliary tree. *Radiology.* 1998;208: 621-623.
31. Zielinski MD, Atwell TD, Davis PW, et al. Comparison of surgically resected polypoid lesions of the gallbladder to their pre-operative ultrasound characteristics. *J Gastrointest Surg.* 2009;13:19-25.
32. Okamoto M, Okamoto H, Kitahara F, et al. Ultrasonographic evidence of association of polyps and stones with gallbladder cancer. *Am J Gastroenterol.* 1999;94(2):446-450.
33. Meyers RP, Shaffer EA, Bech PL. Gallbladder polyps: epidemiology, natural history, and management. *Can J Gastroenterol.* 2002;16:187-194.
34. Choi JH, Yun JW, Yong-Sung K, et al. Pre-operative predictive factors for gallbladder cholesterol polyps using conventional diagnostic imaging. *World J Gastroenterol.* 2008;14(44):6831-6834.
35. Sermon A, Himpens J, Leman G. Symptomatic adenomyomatosis of the gallbladder—report of a case. *Acta Chir Belg.* 2003;103:225-229.
36. Martel JA, McLean CA, Rankin RN. Best cases from the AFIP: melanoma of the gallbladder. *Radiographics.* 2009;29:291-296.
37. Middleton WD, Kurtz AB, Hertzberg BS. *Ultrasound: the requisites.* 2nd ed. St Louis, MO: Mosby;2004:28-46, 87-101.
38. Terzi C, Sokmen S, Seckin S, et al. Polypoid lesions of the gallbladder: report of 100 cases with special reference to operative indications. *Surgery.* 2000;127:622-627.
39. Mainprize K, Gould S, Gilbert J. Surgical management of polypoid lesions of the gallbladder. *Br J Surg.* 2000;87: 414-417.
40. Sugiyama M, Atomi Y, Kuroda A, et al. Large cholesterol polyps of the gallbladder: diagnosis by means of US and endoscopic US. *Radiology.* 1995;169:493-497.
41. Furukawa H, Kosuge T, Shimada K, et al. Small polypoid lesions of the gallbladder: differential diagnosis and surgical indications by helical computed tomography. *Arch Surg.* 1998;133:735-739.
42. Kozuka S, Tsubone M, Yasui A, et al. Relation of adenoma to carcinoma in the gallbladder. *Cancer.* 1982;50:2226-2234.
43. Van Breda Vriesman AC, Engelbrecht MR, Smithuis RHM, et al. Diffuse gallbladder wall thickening: differential diagnosis. *AJR Am J Roentgenol.* 2007;188:495-501.

44. Rumack CM, Wilson SR, Charboneau JW. *Diagnostic ultrasound*. 2nd ed. St Louis, MO: Mosby; 1998:175-200.
45. Zissin R, Osadchy A, Shapiro M, et al. CT of a thickened-wall gallbladder. *Br J Radiol*. 2003;76:137-143.
46. Altun E, Semelka RC, Elias J Jr, et al. Acute cholecystitis: MR findings and differentiation from chronic cholecystitis. *Radiology*. 2007;244:174-183.
47. Ko CW, Lee SP. Biliary sludge and cholecystitis. *Best Pract Res Clin Gastroenterol*. 2003;17:383-396.
48. Ralls PW, Colletti PM, Halls JM, et al. Prospective evaluation of 99m-Tc-IDA cholescintigraphy and gray-scale ultrasound in the diagnosis of acute cholecystitis. *Radiology*. 1982;144: 369-371.
49. Ziessman HA, O'Malley JP, Thrall JH. *Nuclear medicine: the requisites*. 3rd ed. Philadelphia, PA: Elsevier-Mosby ; 2006: 159-214.
50. Jeffrey RB, Laing FC, Wong W, et al. Gangrenous cholecystitis: diagnosis by ultrasound. *Radiology*. 1983;148:219-221.
51. Bortoff GA, Chen MY, Ou DJ, et al. Gallbladder stones: imaging and intervention. *Radiographics*. 2000;20:751-766.
52. Kaftori JK, Pery M, Green J, et al. Thickness of the gallbladder wall in patients with hypoalbuminemia: a sonographic study of patients on peritoneal dialysis. *AJR Am J Roentgenol*. 1987;148:117-118.
53. Yamada K, Yamada H. Gallbladder wall thickening in mononucleosis syndromes. *J Clin Ultrasound*. 2001;29: 322-325.
54. Cerny E, Husek K, Jelinkova I, et al. Validity of diagnostic criteria of chronic cholecystitis. *Scripta Medica*. 2000;73: 283-288.
55. Kim PN, Lee SH, Gong GY, et al. Xanthogranulomatous cholecystitis: radiologic findings with histologic correlation that focuses on intramural nodules. *AJR Am J Roentgenol*. 1999;172:949-953.
56. Itai Y, Araki T, Yoshikawa, et al. Computed tomography of gallbladder carcinoma. *Radiology*. 1980;137:713-718.
57. Reyes CV, Jablokow VR, Reid R. Xanthogranulomatous cholecystitis: report of seven cases. *Am Surg*. 1981;47:322-325.
58. Dao AH, Wong SW, Adkins RB Jr. Xanthogranulomatous cholecystitis: a clinical and pathologic study of twelve cases. *Am Surg Pathol*. 1981;5:653-659.
59. Parra JA, Acinas O, Bueno J, et al. Xanthogranulomatous cholecystitis: clinical, sonographic, and CT findings in 26 patients. *AJR Am J Roentgenol*. 2000;174:979-983.
60. Lichtman JB, Varma VA. Ultrasound demonstration of xanthogranulomatous cholecystitis. *J Clin Ultrasound*. 1987;15:342-345.
61. Casas D, Perez-Andres R, Jimenez JA, et al. Xanthogranulomatous cholecystitis: a radiological study of 12 cases and review of the literature. *Abdom Imaging*. 1996;21:456-460.
62. Kim PN, Ha HK, Kim YH, et al. US findings of xanthogranulomatous cholecystitis. *Clin Radiol*. 1998;53: 290-292.
63. Chun KA, Ha HK, Yu ES, et al. Xanthogranulomatous cholecystitis: CT features with emphasis on differentiation from gallbladder carcinoma. *Radiology*. 1997;203:93-97.
64. Furuta A, Ishibashi T, Takahashi S, et al. MR imaging of xanthogranulomatous cholecystitis. *Radiat Med*. 1996;14:315-319.
65. Berk RN, van der Vegt JH, Lichtenstein LE. The hyperplastic cholecystoses: cholesterolosis and adenomyomatosis. *Radiology*. 1983;146:593-601.
66. McCarty WC. Pathology of the gallbladder and some associated lesions: a study of specimens from 365 cholecystectomies. *Ann Surg*. 1910;51:651-669.
67. Feldman M, Feldman M Jr. Cholesterolosis of the gallbladder: an autopsy study of 165 cases. *Gastroenterology*. 1954;27: 641-648.
68. Hoefsloot FAM. Histologic investigations of cholecystosis In: Hulst SGT, Ruijs JHJ, eds. *Symposium on functional and acalculous anomalies of the gallbladder: a multidisciplinary approach*. Amsterdam: *Excerpta Medica*; 1979:59-66.
69. Holzbach RT, Marsh M, Tang P. Cholesterolosis: physical-chemical characteristics of human and diet-induced canine lesions. *Exp Mol Pathol*. 1977;27:324-328.
70. Tilvis RS, Aro J, Strandberg TE, et al. Lipid composition of bile and gallbladder mucosa in patients with acalculous cholesterolosis. *Gastroenterology*. 1982;82:607-615.
71. Levy AD, Murakat LA, Abbott RM, et al. Benign tumors and tumorlike lesions of the gallbladder and extrahepatic bile ducts: radiologic-pathologic correlation. *Radiographics*. 2002;22: 387-413.
72. Bickel A, Eitan A, Tsilman B, et al. Low-grade B cell lymphoma of mucosa-associated lymphoid tissue (MALT) arising in the gallbladder. *Hepatogastroenterology*. 1999;46:1643-1646.
73. Chin CS, Liang R, Loong F, et al. Primary mucosa-associated lymphoid tissue lymphoma of the gallbladder. *Am J Med*. 2002;112:505-507.
74. Bolondi L, Gaiani S, Testa S, Labò G. Gall bladder sludge formation during prolonged fasting after gastrointestinal tract surgery. *Gut*. 1985;26(7):734-738.
75. Stewart L, Smith AL, Pelligirini CA, et al. Pigment gallstones form as a composite of bacterial microcolonies and pigment solids. *Ann Surg*. 1987;206(3):242-249.
76. Vitellas KM, Keogan MT, Spritzer CE, et al. MR cholangiopancreatography of bile and pancreatic duct abnormalities with emphasis on the single-shot fast spin-echo technique. *Radiographics*. 2000;20:939-957.
77. Turner MA, Fulcher AS. The cystic duct: normal anatomy and disease processes. *Radiographics*. 2001;21:3-22.
78. Htoo MM. Surgical implications of stone impaction in the gallbladder neck with compression of the common hepatic duct (Mirizzi syndrome). *Clin Radiol*. 1983;34:651-655.
79. Cruz FO, Barriga P, Tocornali J, et al. Radiology of the Mirizzi syndrome: diagnostic importance of the percutaneous transhepatic cholangiogram. *Gastrointest Radiol*. 1983; 8:249-253.
80. Han JK, Choi BI, Kim AY, et al. Cholangiocarcinoma: pictorial essay of CT and cholangiographic findings. *Radiographics*. 2002;22:173-187.
81. Chung YE, Kim MJ, Park YN, et al. Varying appearances of cholangiocarcinoma: radiologic-pathologic correlation. *Radiographics*. 2009;29:683-700.
82. Thorsen MK, Quiroz F, Lawson TL, et al. Primary biliary carcinoma: CT evaluation. *Radiology*. 1984;152:479-483.
83. Wernecke K, Henke L, Vassallo P, et al. Pathologic explanation for hypoechoic halo seen on sonograms of malignant liver tumors: an in vitro correlative study. *AJR Am J Roentgenol*. 1992;159(5):1011-1016.

84. Wibulpolprasert B, Dhiensiri T. Peripheral cholangiocarcinoma: sonographic evaluation. *J Clin Ultrasound.* 1992;20(5):303-314.
85. Lim JH. Cholangiocarcinoma: morphologic classification according to growth pattern and imaging findings. *AJR Am J Roentgenol.* 2003;181(3):819-827.
86. Ros PR, Buck JL, Goodman ZD, et al. Intrahepatic cholangiocarcinoma: radiologic-pathologic correlation. *Radiology.* 1988;167(3):689-693.
87. Choi BI, Lee JH, Han MC, et al. Hilar cholangiocarcinoma: comparative study with sonography and CT. *Radiology.* 1989;172(3):689-692.
88. Vilgrain V, Van Beers BE, Flejou JF, et al. Intrahepatic cholangiocarcinoma: MRI and pathologic correlation in 14 patients. *J Comput Assist Tomogr.* 1997;21(1):59-65.
89. Valls C, Guma A, Puig I, et al. Intrahepatic peripheral cholangiocarcinoma: CT evaluation. *Abdom Imaging.* 2000;25(5):490-496.
90. Asayama Y, Yoshimitsu K, Irie H, et al. Delayed phase dynamic CT enhancement as a prognostic factor for mass-forming intrahepatic cholangiocarcinoma. *Radiology.* 2006;238(1):150-155.
91. Mittelstaed CA. Ultrasound of the bile ducts. *Semin Roentgenol.* 1997;32(3):161-171.
92. Robledo R, Muro A, Prieto ML. Extrahepatic bile duct carcinoma: US characteristics and accuracy in demonstration of tumors. *Radiology.* 1996;198(3):869-873.
93. Park HS, Lee JM, Kim SH, et al. CT differentiation of cholangiocarcinoma from periductal fibrosis in patients with hepatolithiasis. *AJR Am J Roentgenol.* 2006;187(2):445-453.
94. Lim JH, Park CK. Pathology of cholangiocarcinoma. *Abdom Imaging.* 2004;29(5):540-547.
95. Han JK, Lee JM. Intrahepatic intraductal cholangiocarcinoma. *Abdom Imaging.* 2004;29(5):558-564.
96. Buck JL, Elsayed AM. From the archives of the AFIP: ampullary tumors: radiologic-pathologic correlation. *Radiographics.* 1993;13:193-212.
97. Michelassi F, Erroi F, Dawson PJ, et al. Experience with 647 consecutive tumors of the duodenum, ampulla, head of the pancreas, and distal common bile duct. *Ann Surg.* 1989;210:544-556.
98. Yamaguchi K, Enjoji M, Ysuneyoshi M. Pancreatoduodenal carcinoma: a clinicopathologic study of 304 patients and immunohistochemical observation for CEA and CA 19-9. *J Surg Oncol.* 1991;47:148-154.
99. Perzin KH, Bridge MF. Adenomas of the small intestine: a clinicopathologic review of 51 cases and a study of their relationship to carcinoma. *Cancer.* 1981;48:799-819.
100. Celik C, Venditti JA Jr, Satchidan S, et al. Villous tumors of the duodenum and ampulla of Vater. *J Surg Oncol.* 1986;33:268-272.
101. Fenoglio-Preiser CM, Pascal RR, Perzin KH. Tumors of the intestines. In: *Atlas of tumor pathology*, series 2, fasc 27. Washington, DC: Armed Forces Institute of Pathology;1990:173.
102. Yamaguchi K, Enjoji M, Kitamura K. Non-icteric ampullary carcinoma with a favorable prognosis. *Am J Gastroenterol.* 1990;85:994-999.
103. Wise RH Jr, Stanley RJ. Case report: carcinoma of the ampulla of Vater presenting as acute pancreatitis. *J Comput Assist Tomogr.* 1984;8:158-161.
104. Guyton DP, Schreiber H. Intestinal polyposis and periampullary carcinoma: changing concepts. *J Surg Oncol.* 1985;29:158-159.
105. Berk T, Friedman LS, Goldstein SD, et al. Relapsing acute pancreatitis as the presenting manifestation of an ampullary neoplasm in a patient with familial polyposis coli. *Am J Gastroenterol.* 1985;80:627-629.
106. Jagelman DG, DeCosse JJ, Bussey HJ. Upper gastrointestinal cancer in familial adenomatous polyposis. *Lancet.* 1988;1(8595):1149-1151.
107. Nannery WM, Barone JG, Abouchedid C. Familial polyposis coli and Gardner's syndrome. *N J Med.* 1990;87:731-733.
108. Cohen SB. Familial polyposis coli and its extracolonic manifestations. *J Med Genet.* 1982;19:193-203.
109. Ono C, Iwama T, Mishima Y. A case of familial adenomatous polyposis complicated by thyroid carcinoma, carcinoma of the ampulla of Vater, and adrenocortical adenoma. *Jpn J Surg.* 1991;21:234-240.
110. Ponchon T, Berger F, Chavaillon A, et al. Contribution of endoscopy to diagnosis and treatment of tumors of the ampulla of Vater. *Cancer.* 1989;64:161-167.
111. Nakao NL, Siegel JH, Stenger RJ, et al. Tumors of the ampulla of Vater: early diagnosis by intraampullary biopsy during endoscopic cannulation—two case presentations and a review of literature. *Gastroenterology.* 1982;83:459-464.
112. Zenman RK, Burrell MI. *Gallbladder and bile duct imaging: a clinical radiologic approach.* New York: Churchill Livingstone;1987:575.
113. Pandolfo I, Scribano E, Blandino A, et al. Tumors of the ampulla diagnosed by CT hypotonic duodenography. *J Comput Assist Tomogr.* 1990;14:199-200.
114. Smelka RC, Kelekis NL, Gesine J, et al. Ampullary carcinoma: demonstration by current MR techniques. *J Magn Reson Imaging.* 1997;7:153-156.
115. Baron RL, Stanley RJ, Lee JKT, et al. A prospective comparison of the evaluation of biliary obstruction using computed tomography and ultrasonography. *Radiology.* 1982;145:91-98.
116. Takehara Y. Fast MR imaging for evaluating the pancreaticobiliary system. *Eur J Radiol.* 1999;29:211-232.
117. Hoeffel C, Azizi L, Lewin M, et al. Normal and pathologic features of the postoperative biliary tract at 3D MR cholangiopancreatography and MR imaging. *Radiographics.* 2006;26:1603-1620.
118. Pavone P, Laghi A, Catalano C, et al. MR cholangiography in the examination of patients with biliary-enteric anastomoses. *AJR Am J Roentgenol.* 1997;169:807-811.
119. Bowie JD. What is the upper limit of normal for the common bile duct on ultrasound: how much do you want it to be? *Am J Gastroenterol.* 2000;95:897-900.
120. Williams HJ Jr, Bender CE, May GR. Benign postoperative biliary strictures: dilation with fluoroscopic guidance. *Radiology.* 1987;163:629-634.
121. House MG, Cameron JL, Schulick RD, et al. Incidence and outcome of biliary strictures after pancreaticoduodenectomy. *Ann Surg.* 2006;243:571-578.
122. Feng B, Song Q. Does the common bile duct dilate after cholecystectomy? Sonographic evaluation in 234 patients. *AJR Am J Roentgen.* 1995;165:859-861.

123. Brugge WR, Saleemuddin A, Pande H, Nikoomanesh P. Bile duct strictures. http://emedicine.medscape.com/article/186850-overview.
124. Vitellas KM, Keogan MT, Freed KS, et al. Radiologic manifestations of sclerosing cholangitis with emphasis on MR cholangiopancreatography. *Radiographics.* 2008;20:959-975.
125. Ueno Y, LaRusso NF. Primary sclerosing cholangitis. *J Gastroenterol.* 1994;29:531-543.
126. Lindor KD, Wiesner RH, MacCarty RL, et al. Advances in primary sclerosing cholangitis. *Am J Med.* 1990;89:73-80.
127. Balthazar EJ, Birnbaum BA, Naidich M. Acute cholangitis: CT evaluation. *J Comput Assist Tomogr.* 1993;17:283-289.
128. Bader TR, Braga L, Beavers KL, et al. MR imaging findings of infectious cholangitis. *Magn Reson Imaging.* 2001;19:781-788.
129. Urban BA, Fishman EK. Tailored helical CT evaluation of acute abdomen. *Radiographics.* 2000;20:725-749.
130. Seel D, Park Y. Oriental infestational cholangitis. *Am J Surg.* 1983;146:366-370.
131. Lim J. Oriental cholangiohepatitis: pathologic, clinical, and radiologic features. *AJR Am J Roentgenol.* 1991;157:1-8.
132. Kim MJ, Cha SW, Mitchell DG, et al. MR imaging findings in recurrent pyogenic cholangitis. *AJR Am J Roentgenol.* 1999;173:1545-1549.
133. Park MS, Yu JS, Kim KW, et al. Recurrent pyogenic cholangitis: comparison between MR cholangiography and direct MR cholangiography. *Radiology.* 2001;220:677-682.
134. Dolmatch BL, Laing FC, Federle MP, et al. AIDS-related cholangitis: radiographic findings in nine patients. *Radiology.* 1987;163:313-316.
135. Kavin H, Jonas RB, Chowdhury L, et al. Acalculous cholecystitis and cytomegalovirus infection in the acquired immunodeficiency syndrome. *Ann Intern Med.* 1986;104:53-54.
136. Vauthey JN, Loyer E, Chokshi P, et al. Case 57: eosinophilic cholangiopathy. *Radiology.* 2003;227:107-112.
137. Campbell W, Kirk G, Clements WB. Radiation-induced stricture of the common bile duct. *Internet J Surg.* 2008;17(2).
138. Yoon KH, Ha HK, Kim MH, et al. Biliary stricture caused by blunt abdominal trauma: clinical and radiologic features in five patients. *Radiology.* 1998;207:737-741.
139. Kim MJ, Mitchell DG, Ito K, et al. Biliary dilatation: differentiation of benign from malignant causes—value of adding conventional MR imaging to MR cholangiopancreatography. *Radiology.* 2000;214:173-181.
140. Brancatelli G, Federle MP, Vilgrain V, et al. Fibropolycystic liver disease: CT and MR imaging findings. *Radiographics.* 2005;25:659-670.
141. Kim OH, Chung HJ, Choi BG. Imaging of the choledochal cyst. *Radiographics.* 1995;15:69-88.
142. Choi BI, Yeon KM, Kim SH. Caroli disease: central dot sign in CT. *Radiology.* 1990;174:161-163.
143. Caroli J, Sonpault R, Kossakowski J, et al. La dilatation polydystique congenital des voies biliaires intra-hepatiques: essai de classification. *Semin Hop Paris.* 1958;34:128-135.
144. Mall JC, Ghahremani GG, Boyer JL. Caroli's disease associated with congenital hepatic fibrosis and renal tubular ectasia. *Gastroenterology.* 1974;66:1029-1035.
145. Mujahed Z, Glenn F, Evans JA. Communicating cavernous ectasia of the intrahepatic ducts (Caroli's disease). *AJR Am J Roentgenol.* 1971;113:21-26.
146. Katyal D, Lees GM. Choledochal cysts: a retrospective review of 28 patients and a review of the literature. *Can J Surg.* 1992; 35:584-588.
147. Sty JR, Sullivan P, Wagner R, et al. Hepatic scintigraphy in Caroli's disease. *Radiology.* 1978;124:732.
148. Ros PR, Mortele KJ. *CT and MRI of the abdomen and pelvis: a teaching file.* 2nd ed. Philadelphia, PA: Lippincott ;2006:35.
149. Graham MF, Cooperberg PL, Cohen MM, et al. The size of the normal common hepatic duct following cholecystectomy: an ultrasonographic study. *Radiology.* 1980;135:137-139.
150. Wright TB, Bertino RB, Bishop AF, et al. Complications of laparoscopic cholecystectomy and their interventional radiologic management. *Radiographics.* 1993;13:119-128.

CHAPTER

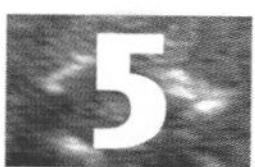

Imaging of the Pancreas

Edward R. Oliver, MD, PhD
Wallace T. Miller Jr., MD

ANATOMY OF THE PANCREAS

The pancreas is an accessory digestive gland with both exocrine and endocrine functions. Approximately 80% of the gland is exocrine in function and composed of ductal and acinar cells whereas 2% of the pancreas is composed of the endocrine islets cells of Langerhans.[1] The remainder of the gland is composed of stromal tissue.

During development, the pancreas derives from 2 separate anlage: the dorsal and ventral pancreatic buds. The dorsal anlage gives rise to the pancreatic neck, body, and tail, whereas the ventral anlage forms the pancreatic head and uncinate process.[2] Each pancreatic bud develops its own draining duct and at approximately 7 weeks of gestation, the 2 anlage rotate and fuse thereby giving the characteristic comma-shaped configuration.

The adult pancreas is a long thin organ that measures 15 to 25 cm in length.[3] The mean anteroposterior dimensions of the head, body, and tail are greatest during the third decade, when they measure approximately 2.9 cm, 1.9 cm, and 1.8 cm, respectively.[4] There is progressive atrophy of the gland throughout adulthood, with the head, body, and tail measuring approximately 2.1 cm, 1.4 cm, and 1.3 cm during the eighth decade of life.[4] The pancreas lies within the retroperitoneum at the level of L1-2 and is divided into 5 portions: the uncinate process, head, neck, body, and tail.[3] The pancreatic head is bordered laterally on the right and inferiorly by the second and third portions of the duodenum. The uncinate process extends from the head and lies posterior to the superior mesenteric vein. The neck of the pancreas lies anterior to the confluence of the splenic vein and superior mesenteric vein and the body and tail extend into the left upper quadrant anterior to the splenic vein, with the pancreatic tail located in the splenic hilum.

The main pancreatic duct, the duct of Wirsung, originates within the dorsal pancreatic anlage and is commonly referred to as the dorsal duct. This duct traverses the length of the pancreas and receives the distal common bile duct within the pancreatic head in proximity to the greater duodenal papilla. Approximately 20 to 35 secondary pancreatic duct branches drain into the main duct along its length and the majority of the pancreatic secretions empty into the duodenum through the main duct and greater duodenal papilla. The accessory pancreatic duct, the duct of Santorini, develops within the anterosuperior pancreatic head in what was originally the ventral pancreatic bud. Accessory pancreatic duct anatomy is variable. In some cases, the accessory duct empties into the minor duodenal papilla whereas in others it partially regresses or empties into the main duct. One congenital variant of ductal anatomy, pancreas divisum, is discussed in greater detail in a later section.

IMAGING OF THE PANCREAS

Computed tomography (CT), magnetic resonance imaging (MRI), and ultrasonography (US) are the 3 common imaging modalities by which the pancreas is evaluated. Imaging of the normal gland by these modalities is reviewed below.

CT is the most common modality by which the pancreas is evaluated, owing largely to its noninvasive nature and speed. The use of thin multidetector CT scanners has further improved evaluation, allowing for greater resolution and for multiplanar imaging. Most enhanced CT protocols of the abdomen and pelvis administer a positive oral contrast agent (barium or water-soluble contrast) and an iodinated intravenous contrast and view images at a nominal slice thickness of 5 mm during the portal venous phase of enhancement, approximately 70 seconds after the bolus of contrast is given. However, the protocol employed at our institution in the case of suspected pancreatic neoplasm calls for the use of a negative oral contrast agent (eg, water) and multiple scans. Positive oral contrast is not used as it commonly obscures the pancreatic head and duodenal papilla. A noncontrast scan is performed of the abdomen at a nominal slice thickness of 5 mm first to localize the level of the pancreas. Intravenous contrast is administered and the pancreas is scanned at a nominal slice thickness of 3 mm during the late arterial (pancreatic) phase of enhancement (40 seconds following contrast bolus). Finally, the entire abdomen is scanned at a slice thickness of 5 mm during the portal venous phase of enhancement (70 seconds after initiation of the contrast bolus).

On unenhanced CT, pancreatic parenchyma is homogenous and has an attenuation close to that of spleen and muscle but less than that of liver.[3] Following the administration of intravenous contrast, the pancreas demonstrates avid uniform enhancement owing to its high vascularity (see Figure 5-1). In younger individuals, the normal pancreas should demonstrate a smooth contour with the body and tail narrower than the head. With aging, fat deposition leads to an lobulated contour; however, the body and tail should remain narrower than the head as in younger patients (see Figure 5-2).[4] The main pancreatic duct may be identified as a low-attenuation linear structure running the length of the gland (see Figure 5-1). The normal duct diameter is 2 to 3 mm; however, failure to identify the main duct on CT is not uncommon and of no clinical significance.

MRI evaluation of the pancreas is best performed on a high field strength magnet (≥1.0 Tesla), which provides a high signal-to-noise ratio and allows for fast breath-hold imaging.[5] Increased fat-water frequency shift is also desired as it affords adequate chemical fat suppression.[5] Axial T1-weighted gradient echo breath-hold sequences with and without fat suppression are effective sequences with which to evaluate the pancreas and peripancreatic tissues. Fat suppression provides the greatest contrast between normal and abnormal pancreatic tissue, whereas nonsuppressed sequences allow for the evaluation of extension of disease into the extrapancreatic tissues. Enhanced imaging is performed using 2- or 3-dimensional fat-suppressed gradient echo imaging with scans performed during the capillary and interstitial phases of enhancement, which occur 15 seconds and 45 seconds after contrast arrives in the abdominal aorta.[6] Fast spin echo T2-weighted sequences are effective in the evaluation of islet cell tumors, peripancreatic fluid collections, cystic lesions, and liver metastases.[5] Although T2-weighted sequences are also useful in evaluating the ducts, heavily T2-weighted sequences (MR cholangiopancreatography [MRCP]) are particularly powerful in demonstrating the ductal anatomy and pathology.[6]

The normal pancreas is hyperintense to liver and muscle on noncontrast T1-weighted images and slightly hyperintense to muscle on T2-weighted sequences (see Figure 5-3).[8,9] In older individual, pancreatic parenchyma may demonstrate decreased T1 signal relative to liver, a finding that may be represent age-related fibrosis.[5] Fat suppression increases the difference between the signal intensity of the pancreas and surrounding fat on T1-weighted images but has little effect in T2-weighted sequences.[7] Nevertheless, fat-suppressed T2-weighted sequences are particularly helpful in demonstrating liver metastases and islet cell tumors.[5] Immediately after the administration of gadolinium contrast, the pancreas demonstrates avid homogenous enhancement, with the pancreatic signal intensity greater than that of liver and adjacent fat (see Figure 5-3).[5,8] The pancreatic signal intensity is similar to fat approximately 1 minute after contrast administration and less than fat 2 minutes after contrast administration.[5] T2-weighted images and MRCP readily demonstrate the main pancreatic duct as a linear high-signal structure traversing the pancreatic gland. The normal duct measures 2 to 3 mm and side branch ducts are not identified unless enlarged (see Figure 5-4).[6]

US is an inexpensive and fast way to evaluate the pancreas. Disadvantages include operator dependence and frequent nonvisualization of the entire pancreas either secondary to large body habitus or due to obscuration of the gland by overlying bowel gas. Sonography is best performed in thin patients, during the fasting state and with a high frequency (5-8 MHz) transducer.

At US, the pancreas usually exhibits a homogenous appearance with an echotexture that is isoechoic or hyperechoic to liver (see Figure 5-5).[1] Fatty replacement of the pancreas is commonplace with aging and obesity and results in increased echogenicity of the pancreatic parenchyma. In cases of fatty replacement, the echogenicity of the gland may approach that of the adjacent retroperitoneal fat.[1,11] The normal pancreatic duct appears as a linear hypoechoic structure extending through the pancreas (see Figure 5-6). The normal pancreatic duct diameter has

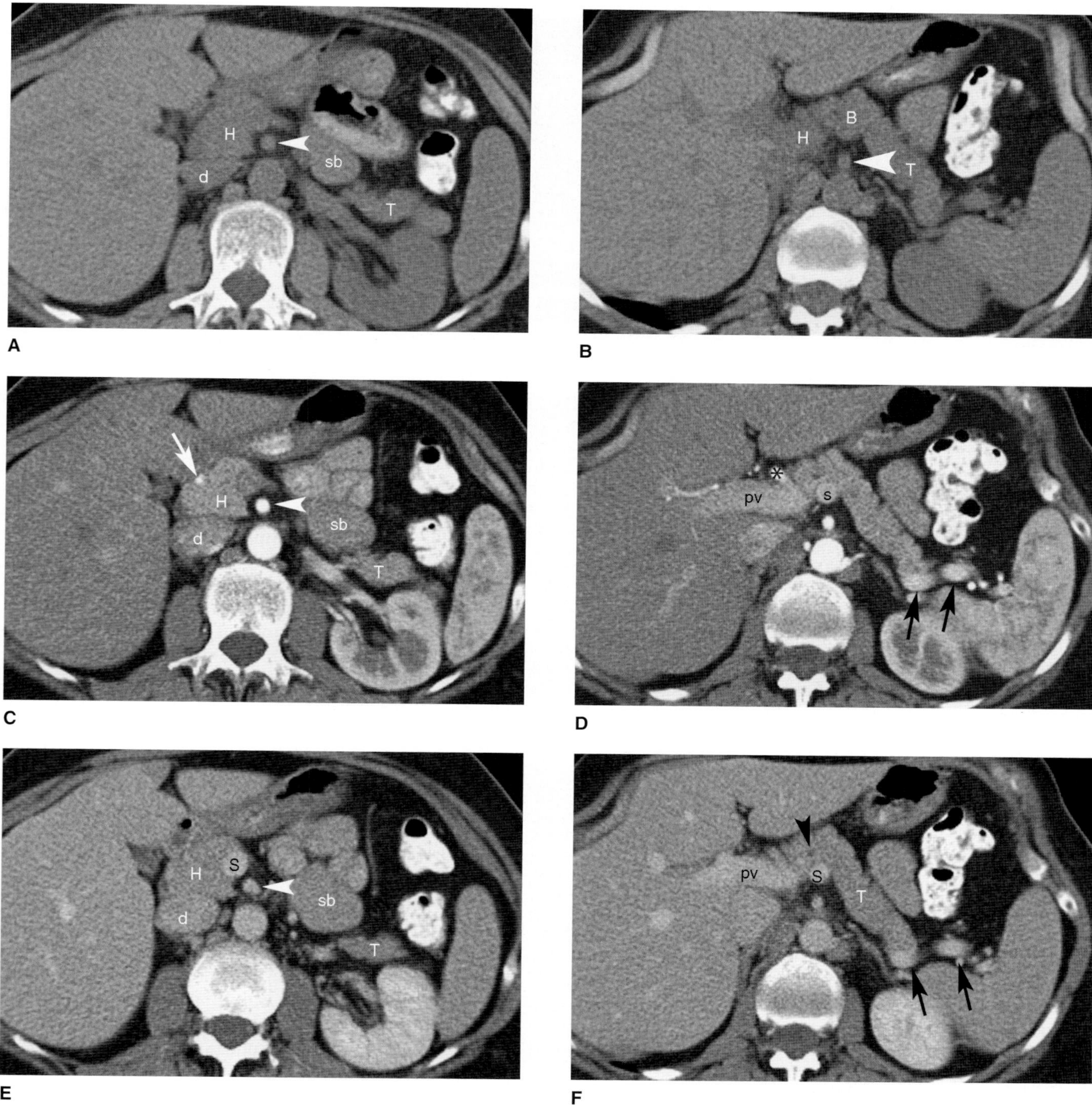

Figure 5-1 Normal Pancreas
This 41-year-old woman presented with elevated biliary enzymes. A triple phase protocol was performed. In all 3 series, the pancreas has a gently lobulated contour with the gland tapering along its length. Unenhanced images (**A** and **B**) demonstrate the pancreas (H, head; B, body; T, tail) to have an attenuation similar to spleen and muscle but an attenuation slightly less than liver parenchyma. During the arterial phase of enhancement (**C** and **D**), the pancreas demonstrates avid uniform enhancement, with an attenuation slightly greater than liver and muscle. The relationship of the pancreas to the superior mesenteric artery (*white arrowhead*) and superior mesenteric vein(s) is well appreciated. The gastroduodenal artery (*white arrow* in C) is noted passing anterior to the pancreatic head. **E** and **F**. Delayed imaging during the portal venous enhancement shows uniform enhancement with attenuation slightly less than that of liver. The main pancreatic duct is partially visualized in cross section (*black arrowhead*). The position of the pancreas anterior to the splenic vein (*black arrows*) is partially seen on the provided arterial and venous phase images. Additional annotations: sb, loop of small bowel; d, duodenum; s, superior mesenteric vein; *, common hepatic artery.

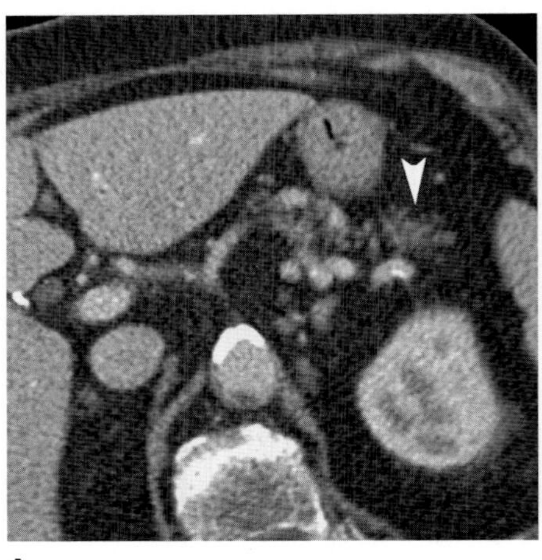

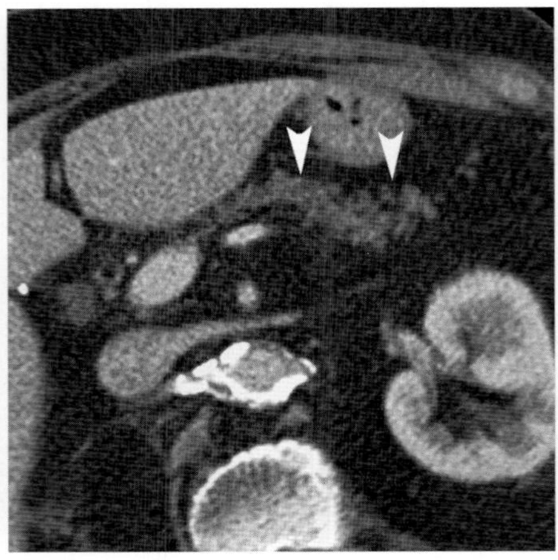

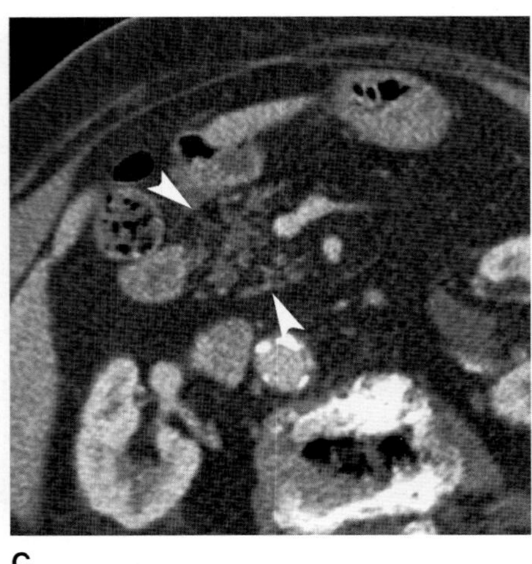

Figure 5-2 Age-Related Pancreatic Atrophy
A-C. CT angiogram of the abdomen and pelvis was performed in this 85-year-old woman for evaluation of an infrarenal aortic aneurysm. Delayed imaging demonstrates marked atrophy of the pancreas (*white arrowheads*).

been reported to be between 2 and 2.5 mm;[12,13] however, measurements slightly greater than these (~3 mm) may be considered normal if the duct walls are smooth and parallel and the duct tapers peripherally.[1] As with MRI, side branch ducts are not visible unless dilated. Sonographic evaluation of the pancreas is ideally performed during the fasting state as overlying bowel gas often obscures the pancreas. In cases where bowel gas limits evaluation of the pancreas, placing the patient in a right lateral decubitus position may improve visualization as overlying gas moves to the nondependent position.

DISEASES OF THE PANCREAS

Pancreatitis and its sequelae, chronic pancreatitis, pancreatic neoplasms, and pancreatic trauma are the primary disorders of the pancreas. Imaging findings of pancreatic disorders include solid masses, cystic masses, disruption of the gland, ductal dilation, diffuse enlargement, atrophy, calcifications, and fatty infiltration.

Solid Masses of the Pancreas

Focal masses of the pancreas will usually represent pancreatic neoplasms. However, rarely pancreatic contusions and acute pancreatitis will appear as a solid pancreatic mass.

Neoplasms of the pancreas

There are 4 groups of tumors that account for the majority of primary malignancies of the pancreas: adenocarcinoma, islet cell tumors, solid-pseudopapillary tumor, and a group of tumors called the cystic pancreatic malignancies. The cystic pancreatic malignancies will usually appear as a cystic mass and will be discussed in detail in a subsequent section. Metastases and lymphoma are other neoplasms that can rarely appear as a solid pancreatic mass (Table 5-1).

Adenocarcinoma: Pancreatic ductal adenocarcinoma is the most common malignancy of the exocrine pancreas, accounting for approximately 95% of pancreatic malignancies,[8] and is also the most common mass of the pancreas. The American Cancer Society estimates that approximately 37,680 Americans will be diagnosed with pancreatic cancer in 2008. An estimated 34,290 Americans will die from the disease during the same period. Certain risk factors are associated with pancreatic cancer and include age >45 years, cigarette use, obesity, diabetes mellitus, and chronic pancreatitis. The prognosis for pancreatic adenocarcinoma is poor. Approximately 80% of cases are inoperable at the time of diagnosis[9] and most of these patients will die within 6 months. The traditional 5-year survival rate following surgical resection has been reported as approximately 5%;[16,17] however, survival rates vary in multiple series, with one series reporting a 5-year survival rate of 0.2%[10] and one series reporting a postresection survival rate of 10%.[11] Although differences in institutional experience may account for the variable survival rate, it has been suggested that other pancreatic neoplasms (ie, nonpancreatic ductal adenocarcinoma) and even benign conditions may be incorrectly diagnosed as pancreatic adenocarcinoma and thereby artificially inflate the postsurgical pancreatic adenocarcinoma survival rates in some series.[10]

Pancreatic adenocarcinomas are rarely symptomatic at early stages and therefore are usually large in size and at an advanced stage when they present. Jaundice, usually secondary to obstruction of the common bile duct, is the most common symptom at presentation and occurs in more than 90% of patients (see Figure 4-57).[12] Other common symptoms include abdominal pain, weight loss, nausea, and anorexia.[12] Rarely, patients will present with waxing

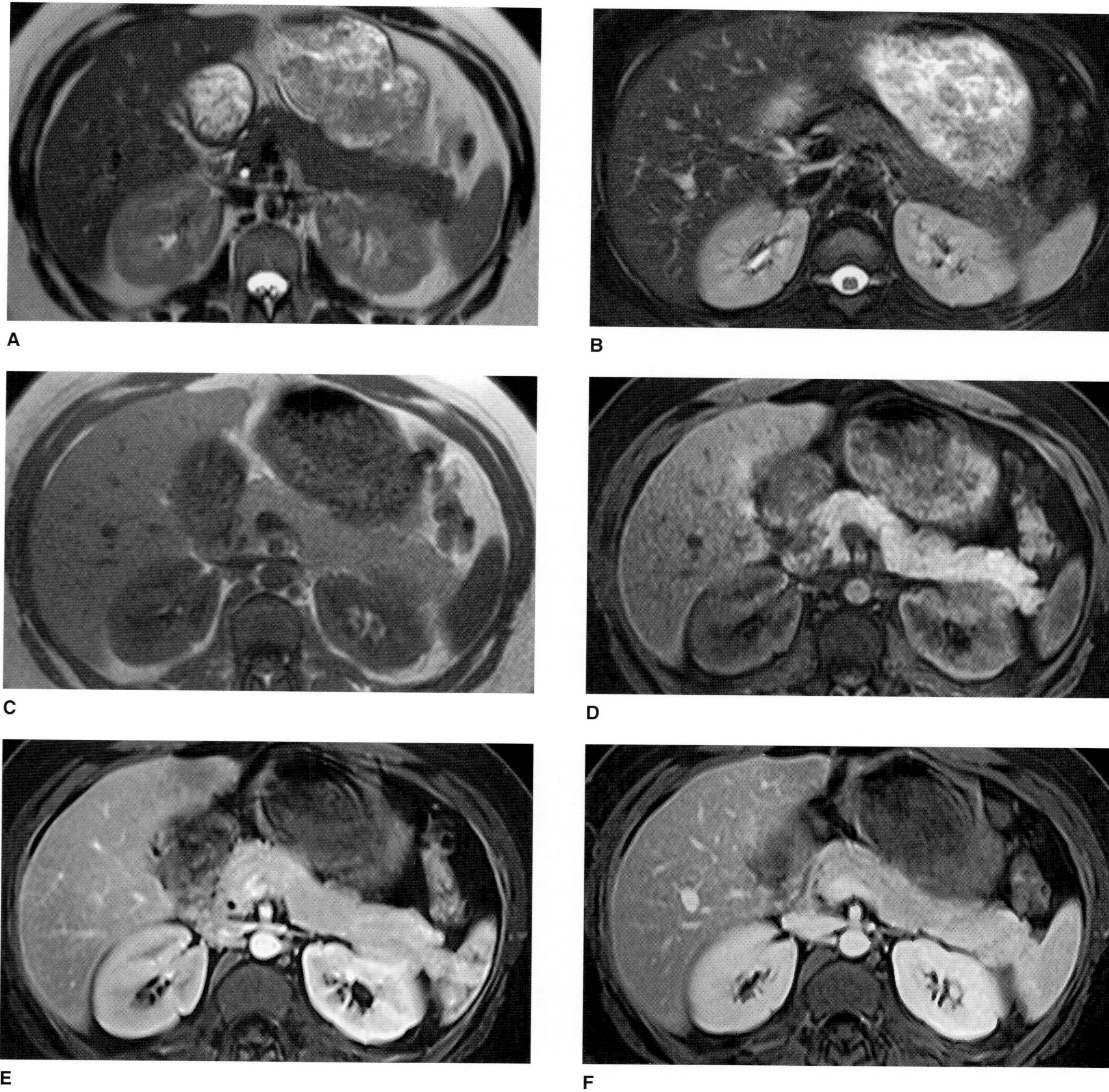

Figure 5-3 MRI of Normal pancreas
A. Abdominal pain was the presenting complaint in this 25-year-old woman. On T2-weighted images (HASTE sequence, TR 700 ms, TE 104 ms), the pancreas is slightly hyperintense to muscle. In this image, the common bile duct is identified as a hyperintense focus in the pancreatic head and a portion of the main pancreatic duct is seen as a thin hyperintense line in the pancreatic tail. **B.** On fat-suppressed T2-weighted images (FSE, TR 6680 ms, TE 98 ms), the pancreas is only slightly more hyperintense to surrounding fat-suppressed peripancreatic fat. **C.** On nonenhanced T1-weighted images (TR 142 ms, TE 4.8 ms), the pancreas is slightly hyperintense to liver and hyperintense to muscle. **D.** On nonenhanced fat-suppressed T1-weighted gradient echo images (TR 3.6 ms, TE 1.8 ms), the pancreas is hyperintense to liver and muscle and well distinguished from the peripancreatic fat. **E.** Following the administration of gadolinium contrast, the pancreas demonstrates avid enhancement in the arterial phase and is hyperintense to liver (TR 3.6 ms, TE 1.8 ms). **F.** During the venous phase of enhancement, the pancreas is slightly hyperintense to liver (TR 3.6 ms, TE 1.8 ms).

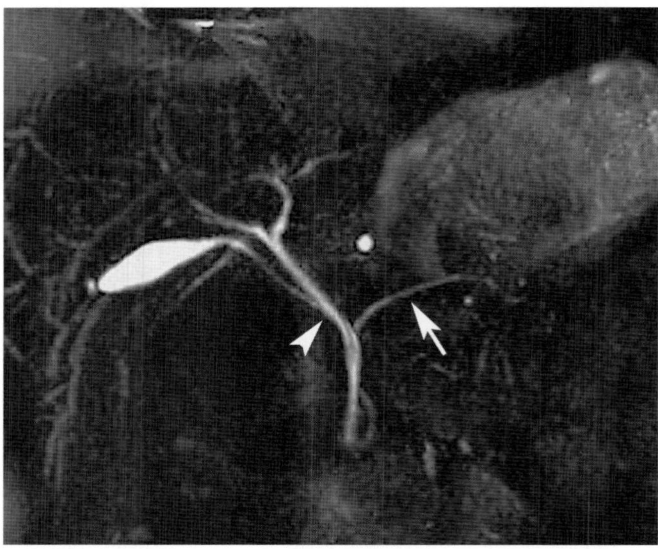

Figure 5-4 Normal MRCP
An MR/MRCP was ordered for suspected biliary obstruction. Coronal maximum-intensity projection (MIP) of high-resolution heavily T2-weighted sequence demonstrates a normal pancreatic duct (*arrow*) and the common hepatic duct (*arrowhead*). Normal pancreatic and biliary ductal anatomy is present. A small simple hepatic cyst in the caudate lobe is identified as a small focus of intense signal superiorly. The high-resolution source images should always be reviewed as small filling defects (eg, stones or neoplasms) may not be well demonstrated on MIP or thick slab sections.

and waning thromboses.[9] Tumors of the pancreatic head may come to clinical attention earlier than those within the body and tail secondary to symptomatic involvement of the bile duct and ampulla.[12] Jaundice is not usually seen in tumors of the pancreatic tail unless they have metastasized.

Cross-sectional imaging demonstrates an indistinctly marginated mass centered within a portion of the pancreatic parenchyma that can range from a few centimeters to as much as 10 cm in diameter. Approximately 60% of adenocarcinomas arise in the pancreatic head, whereas 15% and 5% develop in the body and tail, respectively.[21,22] Diffuse pancreatic involvement occurs in roughly 20% of cases.

Pancreatic adenocarcinomas are hypovascular and desmoplastic tumors. On unenhanced CT, the tumor is usually isoattenuating to normal pancreatic parenchyma and, therefore, inconspicuous unless it significantly alters the normal pancreatic contour. Contrast administration greatly improves tumor detection, with the tumor's hypovascular and desmoplastic characteristics usually resulting in a hypoattenuating appearance relative to normal pancreas (see Figures 4-56 and 5-7).[23,24] Tumor conspicuity is greater during the pancreatic phase of enhancement, with an average attenuation difference between tumor and pancreas of 67 Hounsfield units (HUs) compared to 39 HU during the portal venous phase of enhancement.[13] Multidetector CT with 3-dimensional reconstructions has improved the overall diagnostic accuracy of tumor resectability, with reported accuracies of 73% to 95%.[25-28] The

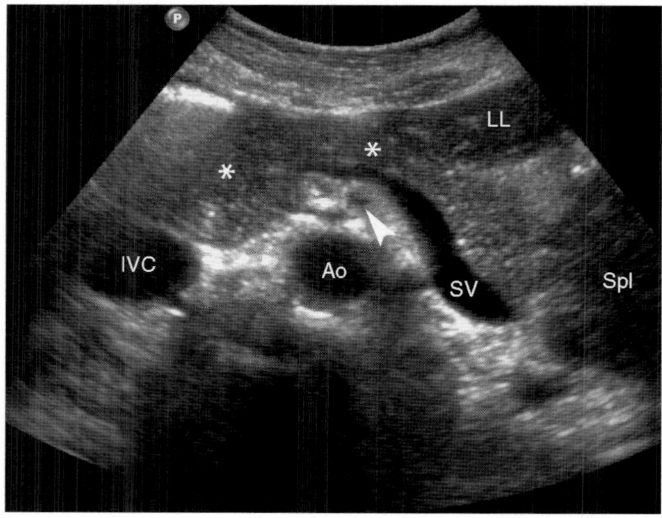

A

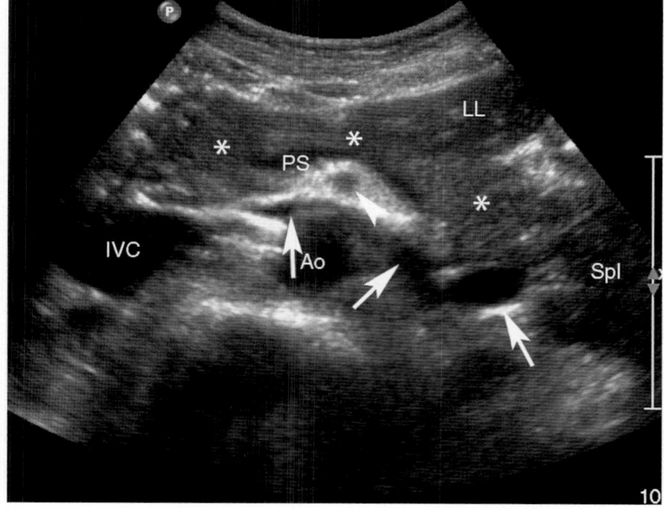

B

Figure 5-5 US of Normal Pancreas
This 33-year-old woman was being evaluated for possible gallbladder polyp. **A** and **B.** The pancreas head, body, and tail are well visualized (*asterisks*). In this patient, the pancreas is hyperechoic relative to the liver (LL, left hepatic lobe) and spleen (Spl). The pancreas lies anterior to the splenic vein (SV) and mesenteric vessels (*arrowhead*, superior mesenteric artery). IVC, inferior vena cava; Ao, Aorta; PS, portal splenic confluence. *Arrows* in (B) denote the course of the left renal vein.

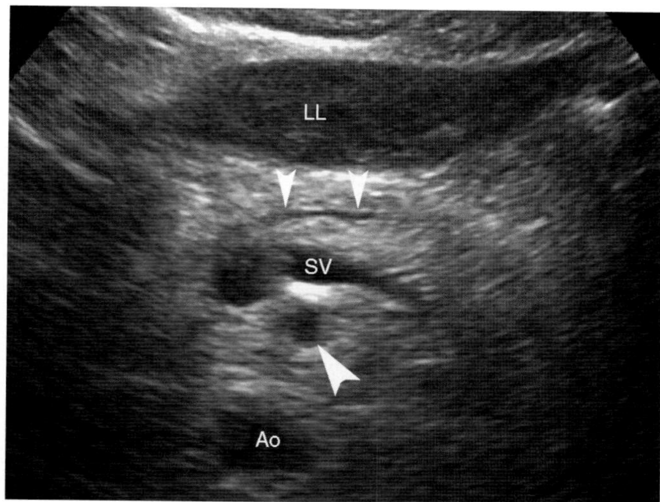

Figure 5-6 Normal Main Pancreatic Duct
This 61-year-old man was being evaluated for possible biliary obstruction. The main pancreatic duct is identified as a thin anechoic line passing through the pancreatic body in this image (*small arrowheads*). The duct diameter was normal at 2 mm. LL, left hepatic lobe; Ao, aorta; SV, splenic vein. *Large arrowhead* denotes the superior mesenteric artery.

use of these techniques also provides important information regarding the vascular anatomy and their relationship to pancreatic lesions.

Occasionally, pancreatic adenocarcinoma may be isoattenuating relative to normal pancreatic parenchyma and inconspicuous. In one small study, as many as 11% of pancreatic adenocarcinomas could not be differentiated from normal pancreas on the basis of attenuation.[14] In each of these cases, ancillary findings of underlying malignancy were detected, allowing for correct diagnosis. These include dilation of the distal main pancreatic duct with an abrupt caliber change at the tumor, the so-called interrupted duct sign; atrophy of the pancreatic parenchyma distal to the tumor; and contour abnormality of the pancreas (see Figure 5-8). Although none of these secondary signs is specific to malignancy, adenocarcinoma should be considered if any of these findings are encountered.

MR represents another modality commonly employed for the evaluation of adenocarcinoma of the pancreas. Tumors are characteristically hypointense on fat-suppressed T1-weighted, non–fat suppressed T1-weighted, and postgadolinium T1-weighted MR sequences.[30,31] The tumor may be uniform in character or variably necrotic. Regions of cystic necrosis may appear as areas of high signal on T2-weighted MR images (see Figures 5-9 and 5-10). MRCP is a powerful MR application that is at least as specific and possibly slightly more sensitive than endoscopic retrograde pancreatography in diagnosing pancreatic adenocarcinoma.[32] In addition, MRCP is particularly helpful in the evaluation of cases where tumors obstruct the pancreatic duct and/or biliary duct. Furthermore, small inconspicuous tumors can manifest as subtle contour abnormalities of the pancreatic duct on MRCP, thereby aiding in the detection of early tumors.

Transabdominal US is often the initial imaging modality utilized in cases of suspected biliary tract pathology and can detect some pancreatic adenocarcinomas. On US, pancreatic cancer is typically hypoechoic relative to normal parenchyma (see Figure 5-9). Detection of these lesions, however, is often limited to large lesions and those arising in the pancreatic head. As US is less sensitive in detecting pancreatic cancer, CT or MRI is recommended for evaluation of suspected malignancy and staging.

Surgical resection is the only cure for pancreatic adenocarcinoma and tumor resectability depends on the absence of locally advanced and metastatic disease. Therefore, it is

Table 5-1. Solid Pancreatic Masses

A. Neoplasms 1. Adenocarcinoma 2. Islet cell tumors a. Insulinoma b. Glucagonoma c. Gastrinoma d. Somatostatinoma e. VIPoma f. Carcinoid tumor 3. Metastasis 4. Lymphoma
B. Focal Pancreatitis
C. Pancreatic Contusion

Imaging Notes 5-1. Imaging Features of Pancreatic Adenocarcinoma

Direct Signs	
Indistinctly marginated mass	
CT:	Hypoattenuating 89%—Isoattenuating 11%
MRI:	Hypointense on T1 (fat suppressed and nonsuppressed)
	Hypointense on post gad T1
	Variable on T2
US:	Hypoechoic
Focal widening or enlargement of the pancreas	
Indirect Signs	
Abrupt termination of dilated pancreatic duct (interrupted duct sign)	
Atrophy of the distal pancreas	

Imaging Notes 5-2. Findings Indicating Surgical Unresectability of Pancreatic Carcinoma

1. Vascular invasion (celiac axis, hepatic artery, SMA, SMV, portal vein)
   a. Interruption of perivascular fat plane
   b. >180 degrees of contact between vessel and cancer
   c. Narrowing or distortion of vessel
   d. Dilation of peripancreatic veins (suggestive)
2. Distant metastasis
   a. Liver
   b. Peritoneal
   c. Other

important for the reader to evaluate each imaging examination for features that would contraindicate surgical intervention. Direct extension of tumor that involves the local vasculature such as the celiac axis, hepatic artery, superior mesenteric artery and vein, and portal vein renders the tumor nonresectable. Imaging findings that indicate vascular involvement include tumoral obliteration of the perivascular fat plane, contact of greater than 180 degrees between the tumor and vessel, and narrowing or distortion of the vessel (see Figures 5-10, 5-11, and 5-12).[27,33] In the absence of these findings, the presence of isolated dilated peripancreatic veins is highly suggestive of occult vascular involvement.[34-36] Metastatic disease, including peritoneal implants and liver metastases, also precludes curative resection.

Pancreatic adenocarcinoma is staged according to the TNM system, and the American Joint Committee on Cancer recently released the seventh edition of its cancer staging manual.[15] No changes were made to the TNM staging system for exocrine neoplasms of the pancreas, which already had been validated with respect to predicting survival (see Table 5-2).[16] Helical CT has been shown to be the most accurate modality in the TNM system of staging pancreatic adenocarcinoma.[39] T classification is determined by tumor size and extent. T0 refers to the absence of evidence of primary tumor. Tis represents carcinoma in situ; however, very few pancreatic adenocarcinomas are discovered at this very early stage. T1 and T2 tumors correspond to those confined to the pancreas, with size being the discriminating factor: tumors less than or equal to 2 cm in greatest dimension are considered T1 and tumors greater than 2 cm are considered T2. In T3 disease, the tumor extends beyond the pancreas into the adjacent peripancreatic tissues, including the duodenum, stomach, biliary system, adrenal glands, spleen and perirenal fat; however, there is no involvement of the celiac axis or superior mesenteric artery (see Figure 5-13). T4 disease is unresectable and corresponds to involvement of adjacent vascular structures, specifically the celiac axis and superior mesenteric artery. TX is reserved for those instances when the main tumor cannot be assessed.

N classification is determined by the extent of nodal disease. The absence of regional (peripancreatic) lymph node involvement is classified as N0, whereas involvement

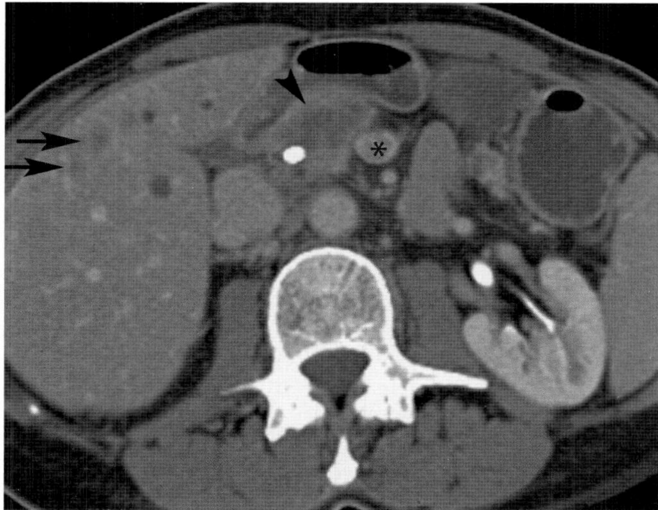

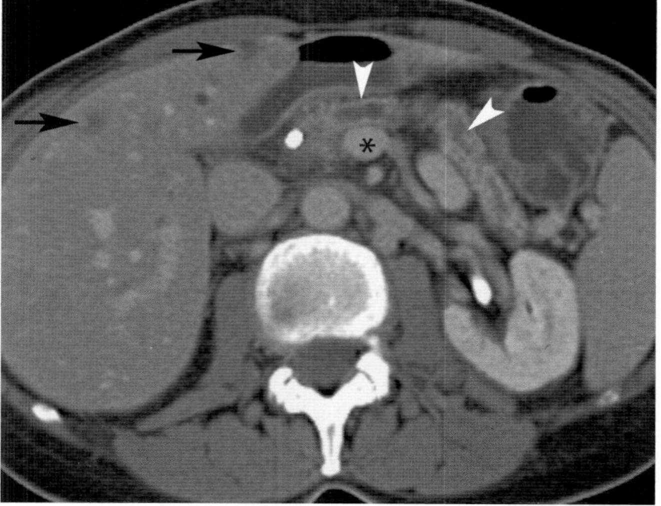

Figure 5-7 Pancreatic Head Adenocarcinoma with Obstructive Pancreatic Atrophy
A and **B.** Contrast-enhanced CT images show a heterogeneously hypoenhancing mass in the pancreatic head (*black arrowhead*). There is dilation of the peripheral main pancreatic duct and obstructive atrophy of the pancreas (*white arrowheads*). The pancreatic head adenocarcinoma contacts but does not encase the superior mesenteric vein (*asterisk*). Low attenuation lesions in the liver (*black arrows*) represent liver metastases. The high attenuation focus in the pancreatic head represents an internal biliary stent.

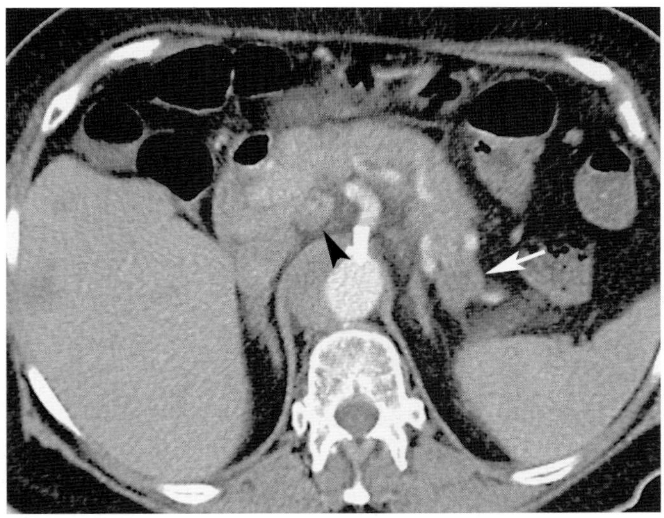

A

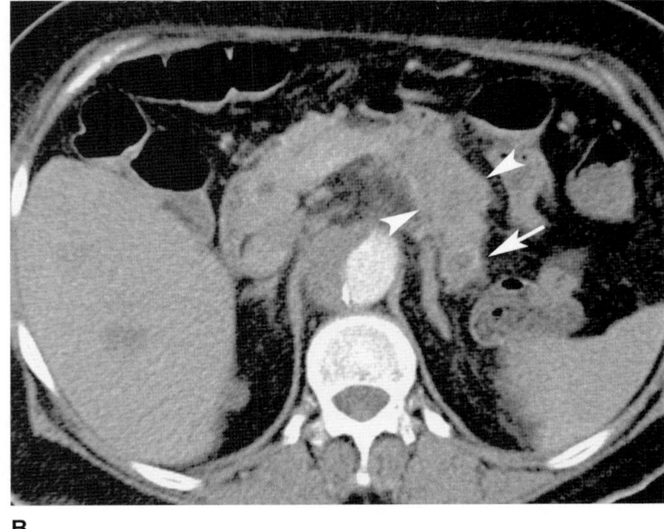

B

Figure 5-8 Pancreatic Adenocarcinoma With Hepatic Metastases A CT angiogram of the chest was performed to evaluate a suspected aortic stent graft endoleak in this 77-year-old woman. **A** and **B.** Extended cuts through the upper abdomen revealed a very subtle mass (*white arrowheads*) in the pancreatic tail, which is isoattenuating to minimally hypoattenuating to normal pancreas. Parenchymal atrophy with main pancreatic duct dilation is present distal to the mass (*arrows* in A and B). Also present are multiple hypoattenuating hepatic lesions. An enlarged celiac axis lymph node is present (*black arrowhead* in A). The imaging findings were highly suspicious for pancreatic adenocarcinoma with hepatic metastases and regional nodal metastasis. Hepatic metastasis was confirmed through percutaneous biopsy of one of the hepatic lesions. A celiac axis vascular stent is noted in A.

of regional lymph nodes is classified as N1. In cases where regional lymph node involvement cannot be assessed, the N category is classified as NX. Nodal involvement directly relates to overall prognosis; however, lymph node diameter is a poor indicator for nodal metastasis and has a low accuracy in establishing the N category. As such, pathologic sampling is always performed in cases of resectable pancreatic cancer.[40-43] Despite this limitation, any abnormalities of either size or number of regional lymph nodes should be reported because imaging identification of lymph nodes suspicious for metastasis provides surgical guidance to nodes that should be sampled and maximizes lymph node yield (see Figure 5-8).[17]

Finally, the presence or absence of distant metastases determines the M category and corresponds to the spread of disease to distant lymph nodes (ie, nonregional lymph nodes) and other organs, such as liver and lung. M0 disease corresponds to the absence of metastatic disease whereas M1 disease corresponds to the presence of distant metastatic disease. MX is reserved for cases in which distant metastatic disease cannot be assessed. Although helical CT was shown to be the most accurate imaging modality for the detection of metastatic disease,[39] peritoneal implants and small hepatic metastases are frequently too small to detect. Nevertheless, careful evaluation for hepatic metastases and peritoneal deposits should be performed because recognition of their presence results in upstaging of disease and can result in the avoidance of unnecessary surgery and its associated morbidity and mortality.

Islet cell tumors: Neuroendocrine neoplasms constitute a small subset of pancreatic neoplasms and include insulinomas, gastrinomas, glucagonomas, somatostatinomas, VIPomas, and serotonin-secreting (ie, carcinoid) tumors. Although these tumors are commonly referred to as "islet cell tumors," these neoplasms arise from neuroendocrine cells that are of a ductal and non–islet cell origin.[18] These may be sporadic in etiology but are also associated with a number of hereditary conditions, including multiple endocrine neoplasia type I (MEN1), neurofibromatosis type I, tuberous sclerosis, and von *Hippel-Lindau syndrome*.[46,47] Neuroendocrine tumors are clinically classified into 2 broad categories, syndromic and nonsyndromic, based on whether or not a clinical syndrome results from

---

Imaging Notes 5-3. Neuroendocrine tumors of the pancreas most often occur sporadically. However, occasionally their occurrence is as part of one of several hereditary syndromes including:

1. Multiple endocrine neoplasia type I (MEN1)
2. Neurofibromatosis type I
3. Tuberous sclerosis
4. von Hippel-Lindau syndrome

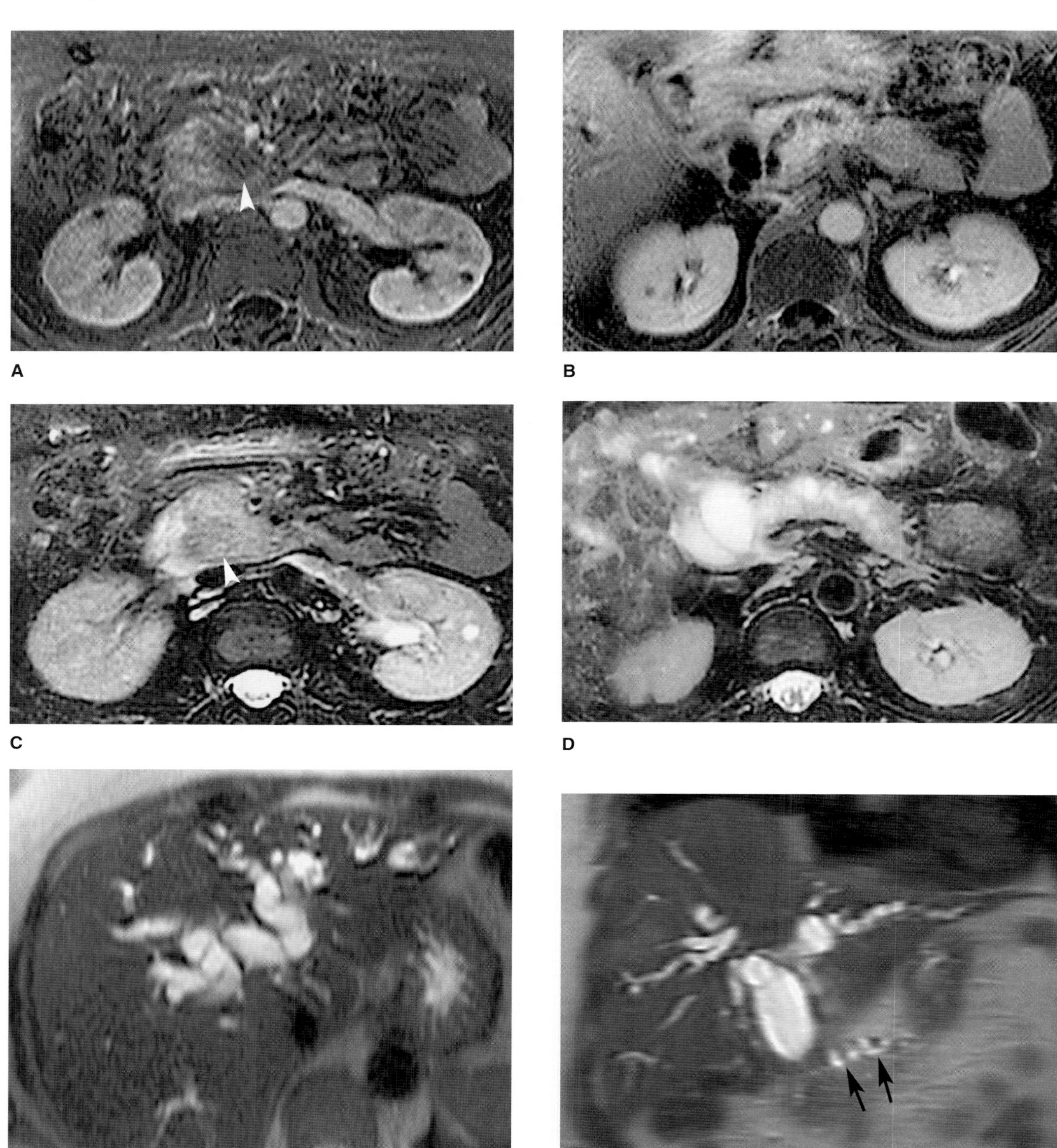

Figure 5-9 Pancreatic Adenocarcinoma causing Biliary and Pancreatic Duct Obstruction

A 54-year-old woman with adenocarcinoma of the pancreatic head. **A** and **B.** Contrast-enhanced fat-suppressed T1-weighted image reveals a mass (*white arrowhead* in A) within the medial pancreatic head that is hypointense relative to normal pancreatic parenchyma in the lateral pancreatic head (**A**). Main pancreatic duct dilation in (B) is manifested by a beaded low-signal structure running through the pancreatic body. **C.** Fat-suppressed T2-weighted image demonstrates decreased signal intensity of the mass (*arrowhead*) relative to the remainder of the pancreatic head. **D.** Fat suppressed T2-weighted image through the pancreatic body reveals an enlarged main pancreatic duct. Marked extrahepatic and intrahepatic biliary dilation is also partially visualized. **E** and **F.** Axial and coronal T2-weighted image reveals marked extrahepatic and intrahepatic biliary dilation. Pancreatic duct dilation is partially visualized (*arrows*).

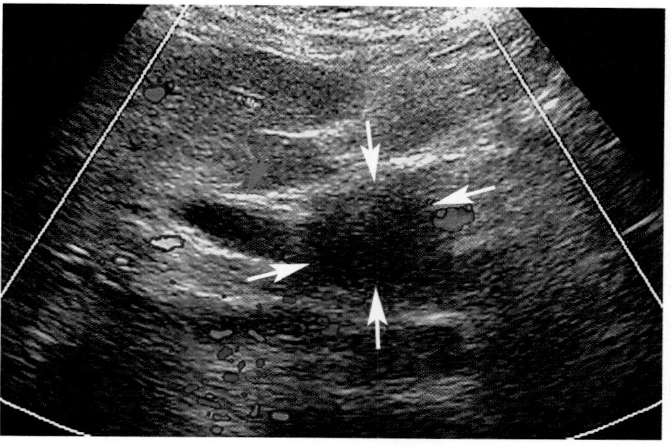

G

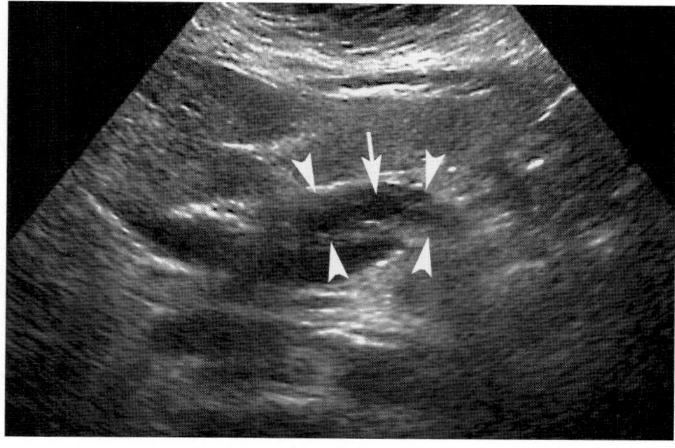

H

Figure 5-9 Pancreatic Adenocarcinoma causing Biliary and Pancreatic Duct Obstruction (*Continued*)
G. Sagittal US of the abdomen at the level of the common bile duct shows dilation of the duct to 10 mm (*green arrow*), which terminates at the obstructing hypoechoic pancreatic adenocarcinoma (*arrows*). **H.** Transverse US of the epigastrium shows the pancreatic body (*arrowheads*) with a dilated pancreatic duct (*arrow*).

the production of hormones. These terms are preferable to the more commonly used designations *hyperfunctioning* and *nonfunctioning* tumors as all neuroendocrine tumors produce some amount of hormones.[19]

Approximately 85% of neuroendocrine tumors are syndromic and named based on the dominant hormone produced.[20] These patients typically present with symptoms of endocrine disturbance such as hypoglycemia with an insulinoma, recurrent and multiple gastric ulcers with a gastrinoma (Zollinger-Ellison syndrome), or new-onset diabetes mellitus with a glucagonoma. VIPomas are named for the secretion of vasoactive intestinal polypeptide (VIP), which results in the secretion of electrolytes and fluid and a characteristic profuse watery diarrhea. Somatostatinomas are

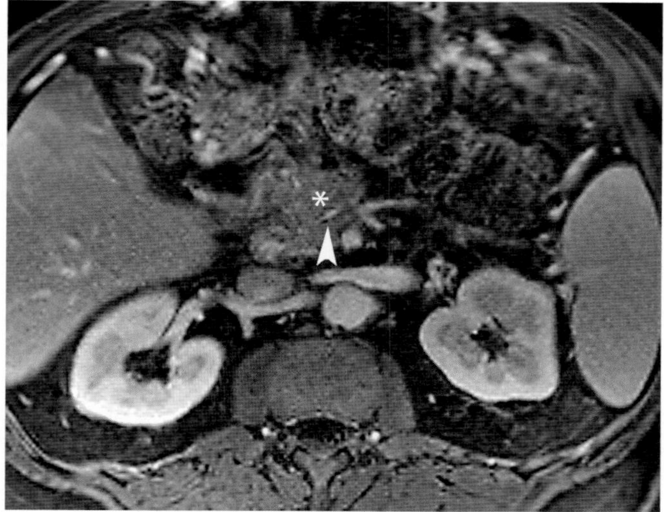

A

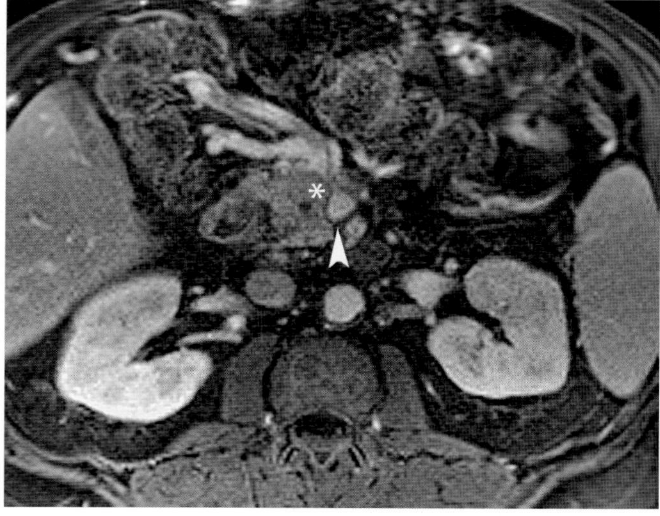

B

Figure 5-10 Pancreatic Adenocarcinoma With Vascular Encasement
This 60-year-old man was diagnosed with pancreatic adenocarcinoma of the pancreatic head/neck. **A** and **B.** Postcontrast fat-suppressed T1-weighted MR images demonstrate an ill-defined hypointense mass in the pancreatic head/neck (*asterisk*). A small amount of normal-enhancing pancreatic head parenchyma is seen in B. There is marked narrowing of the superior mesenteric vein (A) with only a slitlike appearance of the vessel (*white arrowhead*). The superior mesenteric vein (B) peripheral to the mass is slightly dilated secondary to the narrowing (*white arrowhead*). This patient was not a surgical candidate secondary to the vascular encasement.

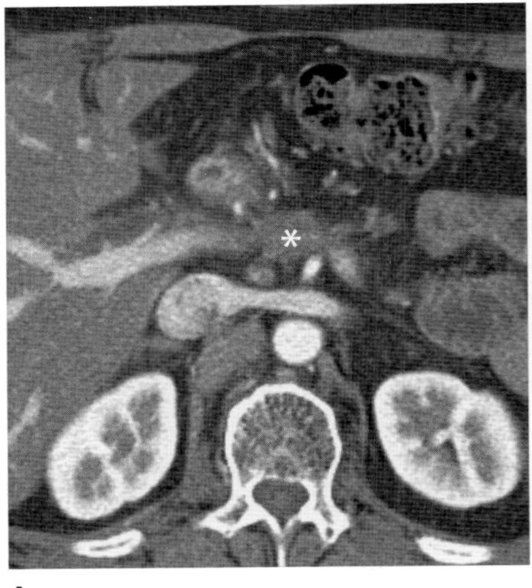

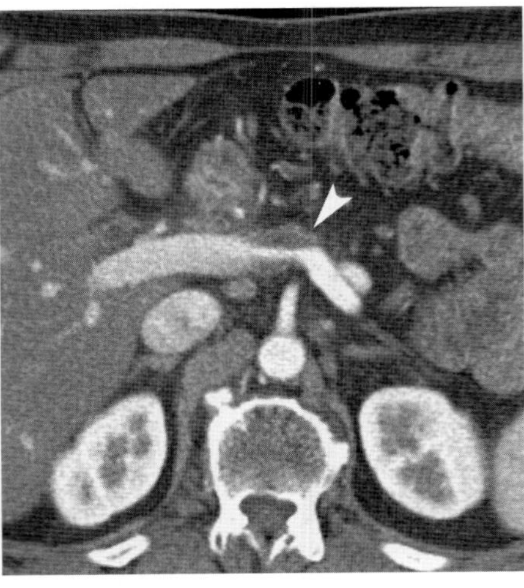

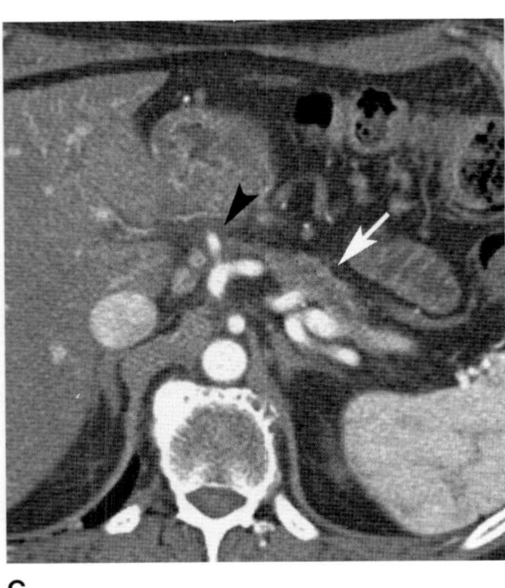

Figure 5-11 Pancreatic Adenocarcinoma With Vascular Encasement This 54-year-old man was diagnosed with pancreatic adenocarcinoma of the uncinate process. **A-C**. CT images obtained during the arterial phase of enhancement reveal a mass within the uncinate process (*asterisk*). There is circumferential encasement of the junction of the splenic and portal veins (B) with marked narrowing of the involved vessel (*white arrowhead*). There is soft-tissue density (C) surrounding the proximal common hepatic artery (*black arrowhead*), consistent with additional vascular encasement (compare the attenuation of the perivascular tissue to that of uninvolved mesenteric fat). Partially visualized is dilation of the peripheral main pancreatic duct (*white arrow*). The patient is not a surgical candidate given the degree of vascular encasement.

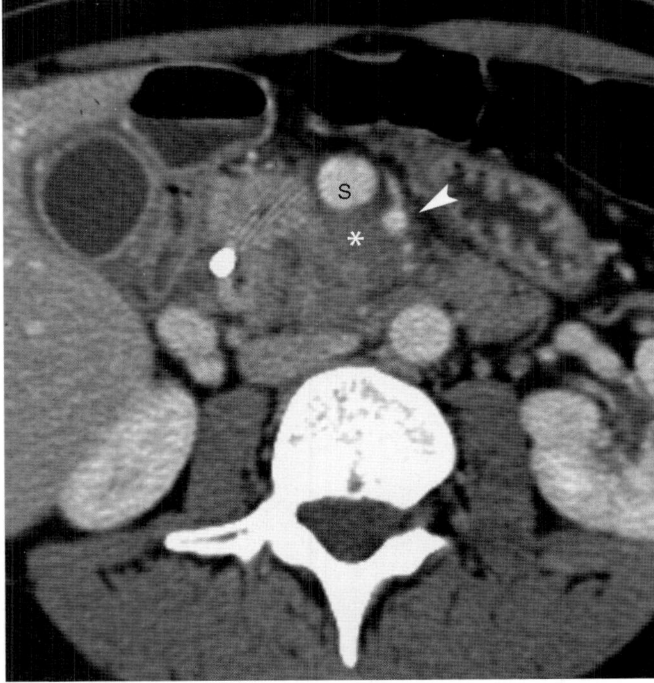

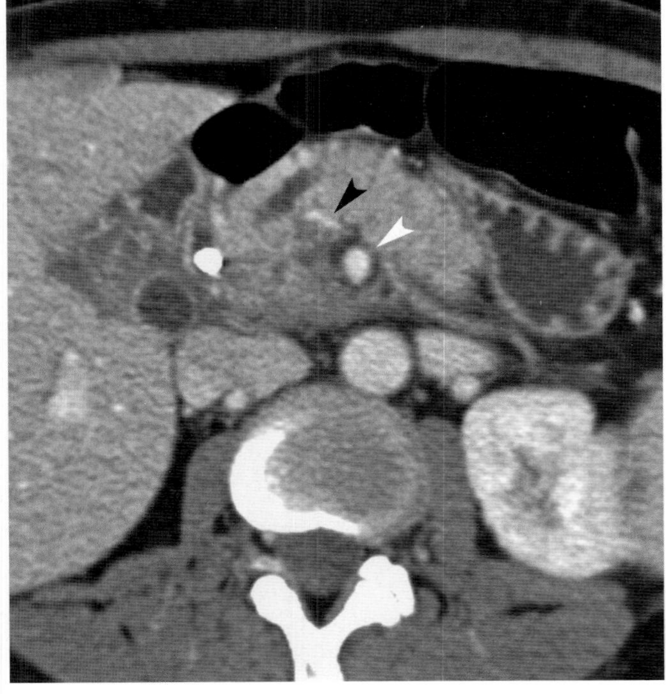

Figure 5-12 Pancreatic Adenocarcinoma with Vascular Encasement This 49-year-old woman was diagnosed with pancreatic adenocarcinoma of the uncinate process. **A**. Arterial-phase CT image demonstrates a hypoenhancing uncinate process mass involving the superior mesenteric artery (*white arrowhead*) from the 5-11 o'clock position. The superior mesenteric vein(s) is dilated and the mass abuts the vein from the 4-8 o'clock position (90 degree encasement). **B**. A more cephalad section from the same CT study reveals marked narrowing of the superior mesenteric vein (*black arrowhead*) by the hypoattenuating mass, which explains the dilation of vein more peripherally. The superior mesenteric artery is denoted by the *white arrowhead* in (B). The main pancreatic duct is partially visualized in the pancreatic neck and dilated secondary to obstruction by the mass. A biliary stent is noted in the pancreatic head. The patient is not a surgical candidate given the degree of vascular encasement.

Table 5-2. Staging Classification of Pancreatic Adenocarcinoma and Pancreatic Neuroendocrine Neoplasms

TX	Main tumor cannot be assessed
T0	No findings of primary tumor
Tis	Carcinoma in situ
T1	Confined to the pancreas, ≤2cm
T2	Confined to the pancreas, >2 cm
T3	Involvement of peripancreatic tissues[a]
T4	Direct involvement of local vessels[b]
NX	Regional lymph node involvement cannot be assessed
N0	No regional (peripancreatic) nodal involvement
N1	Regional (peripancreatic) nodal involvement
MX	Distant lymph node and organ metastasis cannot be assessed
M0	No distant lymph node spread or organ metastasis
M1	Distant lymph node spread or organ metastasis
Stage 0	Tis, N0, M0
Stage IA	T1, N0, M0
Stage IB	T2, N0, M0
Stage IIA	T3, N0, M0
Stage IIB	T1-3, N1, M0
Stage III	T4, N0-1, M0
Stage IV	T1-4, N0-1, M1

[a]Duodenum, stomach, CBD, adrenal glands, spleen, perirenal fat
[b]Hepatic artery, portal vein, SMA, SMV, splenic artery, splenic vein
Data from the *AJCC Cancer Staging Handbook*, 7th edition.

rare tumors that result in a variety of signs and symptoms including diarrhea, diabetes mellitus, cholelithiasis, and achlorhydria or hypochlorhydria. Carcinoid tumors of the pancreas are rare and are composed of enterochromaffin cells. These account for less than 1% of gastrointestinal (GI) carcinoid tumors[21] and only rarely produce symptoms relating to hypersecretion of serotonin, such as bronchospasm, diarrhea, and flushing (see Table 5-3).[8] Syndromic islet cell neoplasms are characteristically small in size (<2 cm) because the symptoms of endocrine dysfunction lead to early evaluation (see Figures 5-14 and 5-15).[49-52]

Nonsyndromic tumors account for approximately 15% of neuroendocrine tumors.[21] Although nonsyndromic neuroendocrine tumors may not present with symptoms of an endocrinopathy, they can be symptomatic when they have achieved a sufficiently large size. Symptoms tend to be nonspecific and are usually a result of mass effect, such as abdominal pain and jaundice from bile duct obstruction.[45,53] Nonsyndromic neuroendocrine tumors of the pancreas are often moderately large at presentation, measuring between 3 and 24 cm in diameter (see Figures 5-16 and 5-17).[45,49,52,53]

Since the release of the seventh edition of the American Joint Committee on Cancer's Staging Manual, neuroendocrine tumors of the pancreas are now staged using the same TNM system as exocrine tumors of the pancreas.[15] The reader is referred to the section on TNM staging of pancreatic adenocarcinoma for further discussion (Table 5-2).

Insulinomas are the most common neuroendocrine tumor of the pancreas, accounting for approximately 60% of neuroendocrine tumors (see Figure 5-17).[21] This neuroendocrine tumor may be associated with the type I multiple endocrine neoplasia (MEN1) in 7.6% to 10% of cases.[22] The "classic" clinical presentation for insulinomas is the Whipple triad: (1) fasting serum glucose <50 mg/dL, (2) symptoms related to hypoglycemia (eg, headaches, syncope, and seizures), and (3) symptom resolution following glucose administration. Almost all patients present with neurologic symptoms related to hypoglycemia, which include confusion, personality changes, tremors, palpitations, pallor, and diaphoresis.[48,55] In one study, 12% of symptomatic patients presented in a hypoglycemic coma.[23] Insulinomas can be found in all portions of the pancreas. Approximately 90% are benign;[24] however, when malignant, metastases are frequently present at the time of diagnosis.[25] Single insulinomas are managed with surgical resection or enucleation whereas advanced disease usually necessitates extensive tumor debulking to correct the patient's hypoglycemia.

Gastrinomas are the second most common neuroendocrine tumor of the pancreas and account for approximately 20% of pancreatic neuroendocrine tumors.[21] This tumor is most commonly located within the region bordered by the common bile duct, second or third portions of the duodenum, and the pancreatic head, a region known as the "gastrinoma triangle." Thus, gastrinomas of this region can be pancreatic or extrapancreatic in origin. Excessive secretion of gastrin may result in the Zollinger-Ellison syndrome, a condition characterized by peptic ulcer disease and diarrhea (see Figure 5-15). Gastrinomas may present sporadically or in association with MEN1 in up to 25% of cases (see Figure 5-16).[26] Approximately 60% to 80% of gastrinomas are malignant and about 30% to 60% are metastatic at the time of diagnosis.[47,59] Definitive treatment of gastrinomas is surgical resection; however, medical therapy with proton pump inhibitors is frequently employed to minimize acid hypersecretion prior to surgical resection or in cases where surgery is not possible.

Glucagonomas are uncommon neuroendocrine tumors, accounting for approximately 3% of islet cell tumors.[21] Malignancy is common and approximately 60% of patients present with liver metastases.[20] The "4D syndrome" (dermatosis, diarrhea, depression, and deep vein thrombosis) is the classic clinical syndrome associated with

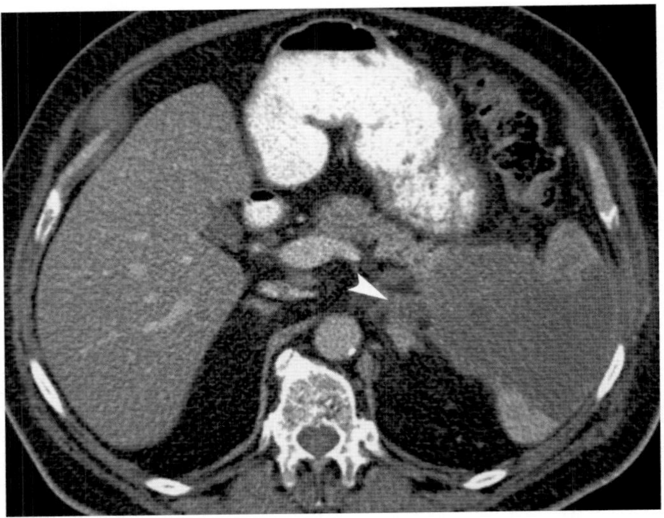

A

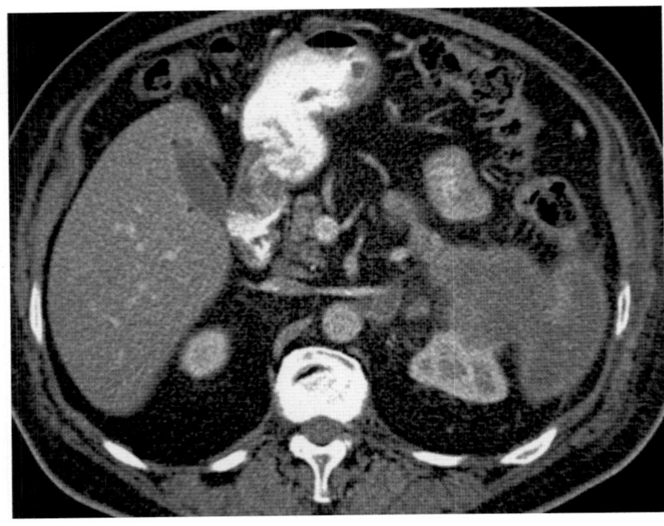

B

Figure 5-13 Invasive Pancreatic Adenocarcinoma
There is no available history for this 64-year-old man with pathologically proven invasive pancreatic adenocarcinoma. Enhanced CT demonstrates a large mass arising from the pancreatic tail with direct invasion of the spleen, (**A**) left adrenal gland (*arrowhead*), and (**B**) left kidney. Multiple hepatic metastases were also present (not shown).

glucagonomas and a characteristic rash, termed *necrolytic migratory erythema*, is present in 75% to 90% of patients.[20] Some patients will present with diabetes mellitus (see Figure 5-18).[27] These tumors are typically larger than other islet cell tumors and are more frequently present in the body and tail.[47,48]

VIPomas account for approximately 2% of islet cell tumors. These tumors secrete VIP, and elevated VIP levels can result in the Verner-Morrison syndrome, which has also been referred to as the **w**atery **d**iarrhea **h**ypokalemia **a**chlorhydria (WDHA) syndrome and pancreatic cholera syndrome.[20] VIPomas are usually greater than 3 cm in size[20] and most frequently located within the pancreatic tail.[14,61] Up to 50% of patients have liver metastases at the time of clinical presentation.[28]

Table 5-3. Syndromes Associated with Islet Cell Tumors

Syndrome	Neoplasm
Hypoglycemia	Insulinoma
Multiple peptic ulcers and diarrhea (Zollinger-Ellison syndrome)	Gastrinoma
Rash, diarrhea, depression, DVT[a]	Glucagonoma
New onset diabetes mellitus	Glucagonoma
Watery diarrhea, hypokalemia, achlorhydira	VIPoma
Flushing, hypertension	Carcinoid tumor

[a]Deep venous thrombosis

The vast majority of neuroendocrine tumors demonstrate similar imaging findings. Small neuroendocrine tumors are typically of a uniform consistency on all cross-sectional imaging modalities, whereas larger lesions may be heterogeneous. Imaging features that should raise concern for malignancy include calcifications, large size (>5 cm), and invasion of adjacent structures.[45,47,52] Metastases, when present, are diagnostic of malignancy.

On unenhanced CT scans, islet cell tumors are characteristically isoattenuating to pancreatic parenchyma.[47,62] Calcifications are uncommon and occur in only 20% of islet cell tumors and are associated with larger size as well as malignancy (see Figure 5-18).[45,49] With intravenous contrast administration, these neoplasms demonstrate marked contrast enhancement because of their rich blood supply (see Figures 5-14 to 5-18).[45,52] Smaller lesions typically demonstrate homogeneous enhancement, whereas larger lesions may demonstrate rim or heterogeneous enhancement.[46,47,49,62] In most cases, the tumor is most conspicuous on the arterial phase of CT evaluation and appears as an avidly enhancing mass.[45,46,63,64] On portal venous phase imaging, the neoplasm will often become isoenhancing relative to normal parenchyma although, less frequently, it may be either hyperenhancing or hypoenhancing relative to normal pancreas.[46,63]

On unenhanced MRI examinations, neuroendocrine tumors are typically T1 hypointense and T2 hyperintense relative to normal pancreas (see Figures 5-16 and 5-17).[45,65,66] Avid enhancement is usually identified following the administration of gadolinium,[31,45,47] with insulinomas most often demonstrating uniform enhancement, gastrinomas peripheral rim enhancement, and noninsulinoma

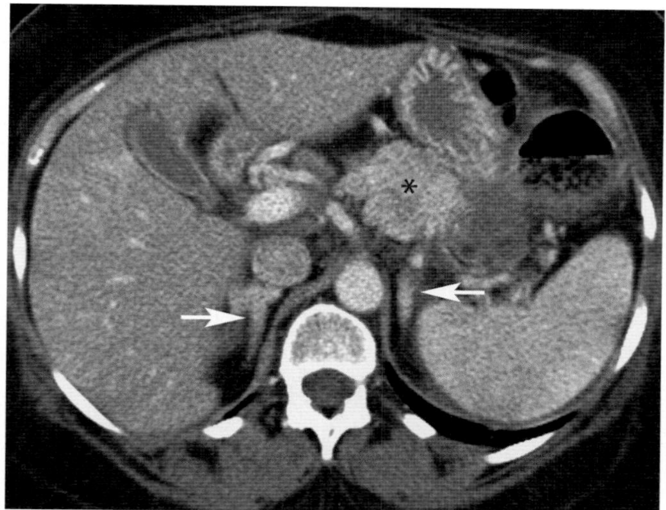

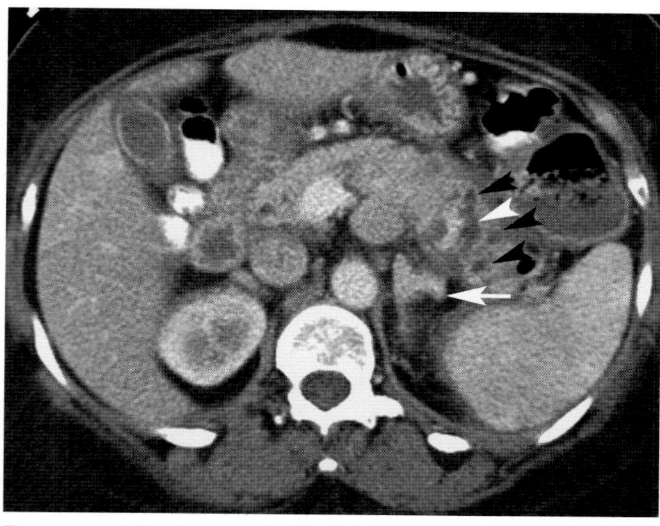

Figure 5-14 ACTH and Gastrin Secreting Pancreatic Neuroendocrine Tumor
This 47-year-old woman presented with hypokalemia, hypertension, duodenal ulcers, truncal obesity and abdominal striae. **A** and **B**. Contiguous enhanced CT images reveal a mass arising from the pancreatic body (*asterisk*) that enhances slightly more than normal pancreatic parenchyma. There is dilation of the main pancreatic duct peripheral to the mass (*white arrowhead*) and ductal tributaries (*black arrowheads*). Surgical resection of the mass yielded ACTH- and gastrin-positive neuroendocrine carcinoma. Bilateral adrenal enlargement is noted (*white arrows* in A and B), consistent with adrenal hyperplasia from excessive ACTH secretion by the neoplasm.

/nongastrinoma tumors heterogeneous enhancement.[45,65] In the case of detecting small (<2 cm) islet cell tumors, MRI may be particularly helpful as one group demonstrated an 85% sensitivity using fat suppressed T1-weighted spoiled gradient echo and fast spin echo T2-weighted sequences.[66]

If detected on US examinations, neuroendocrine tumors appear as uniform hypoechoic pancreatic masses (see Figure 5-18).[49,67] Although endoscopic US has been shown to have a similar high sensitivity for the detection of suspected neuroendocrine tumors compared to multidetector CT, there are several drawbacks to the use of endoscopic US such as its invasiveness, operator dependence, and limited ability in detecting metastatic lesions.[49,67] Intraoperative US, however, has been shown to have very high sensitivity and value in confirming the location of neuroendocrine lesions identified preoperatively by other modalities.[67,68]

In some cases, cross-sectional imaging will not detect the site of syndromic tumors because of their small size and similar imaging appearance to normal pancreatic tissue. Selective angiography may be of utility in detecting these small, functioning islet cell tumors.[18] Moreover, venous sampling at the time of angiography may be performed to detect secretory products and further localize the functional islet cell tumor to a region of the pancreas.

Metastases to the pancreas: Metastases to the pancreas are relatively uncommon, occurring in an estimated 3% to 12% of patients with advanced malignancy.[69-71] A wide

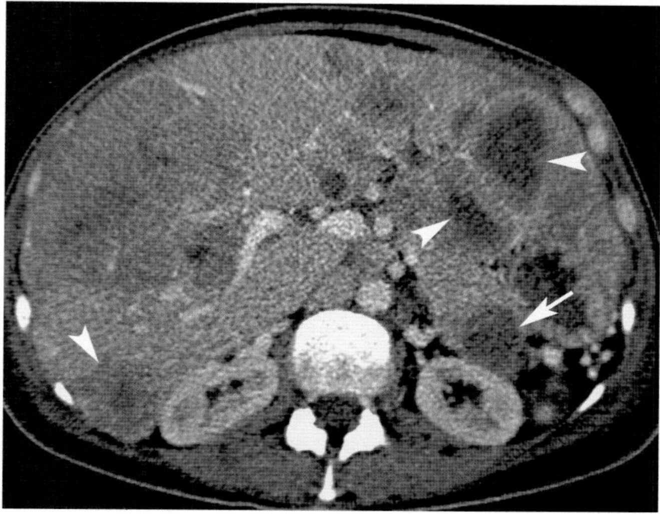

Figure 5-15 Pancreatic Tail Gastrinoma
This 38-year-old woman presented with a history of 20-pound weight loss and symptoms of Zollinger-Ellison syndrome. Contrast-enhanced CT demonstrates a hypoattenuating mass in the pancreatic tail (*arrow*). The liver was markedly enlarged by numerous hypoattenuating metastases, several of which are identified (*arrowheads*). Splenic metastases were also present (not shown). Biopsy of a hepatic lesion revealed well-differentiated neuroendocrine neoplasm, and serum gastrin levels were markedly elevated.

A

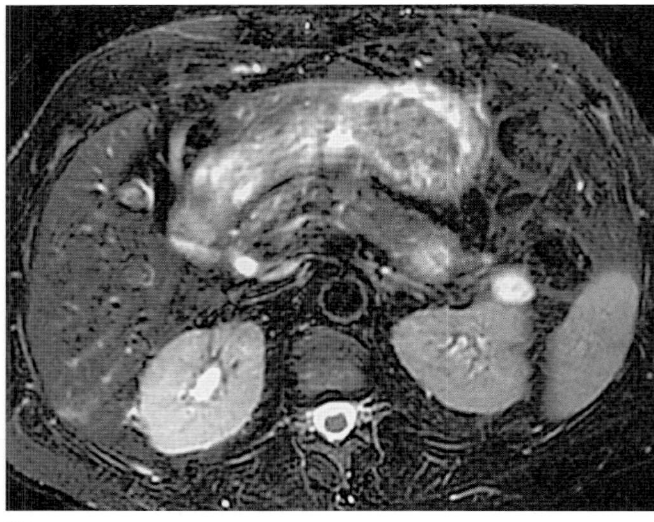

B

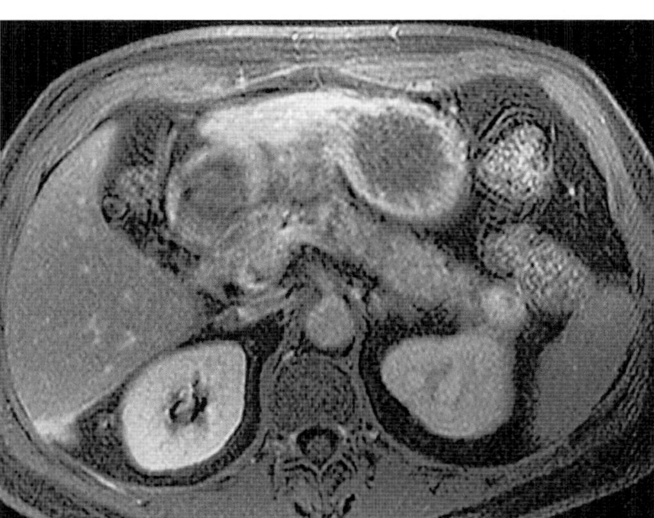

C

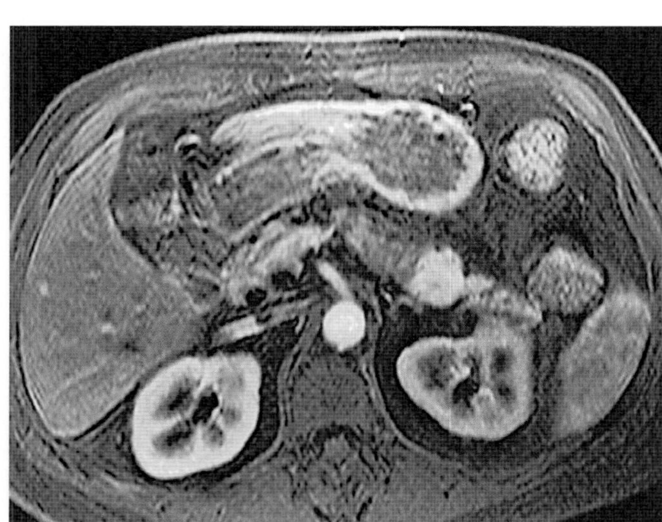

D

Figure 5-16 Multiple Pancreatic Gastrinomas in a Patient with MEN1 A 57-year-old woman with history of multiple endocrince neoplasia 1 (MEN1) and elevated serum gastrin. MRI of the abdomen demonstrates 2 masses in the pancreatic body and tail. **A.** T2-weighted sequence demonstrates 2 focal masses in the distal pancreas that are hyperintense to the remainder of the pancreas. **B.** Fat-suppressed T2-weighted sequence reveals greater conspicuity of the lesions. **C.** On fat-suppressed T1-weighted imaging, these lesions are slightly hyperintense to normal pancreas. **D.** Postgadolinium fat-suppressed T1-weighted image during the arterial phase of enhancement demonstrates marked enhancement of the more proximal lesion. The distal lesion (not shown) also demonstrated avid enhancement. The imaging findings combined with the history of MEN1 are consistent with neuroendocrine tumor of the pancreas, specifically gastrinoma in light of an elevated serum gastrin.

range of primary neoplasms have been described spreading to the pancreas, with the most common primary tumors being renal cell carcinoma, bronchogenic carcinoma, breast carcinoma, melanoma, and GI carcinoma.[29] In one series, renal cell carcinoma and bronchogenic carcinoma accounted for more than 50% of pancreatic metastases.[30] In most patients, pancreatic metastases are asymptomatic and discovered during the imaging evaluation for metastatic disease. Some patients may present with symptoms similar to that of primary pancreatic malignancy with abdominal and/or back pain, weight loss, bowel obstruction, or jaundice;[71,72] however, the history of known primary malignancy and imaging findings usually suggests the correct diagnosis.

Metastases can occur in any part of the pancreas with no particular predilection and are most likely to appear as a circumscribed solitary mass.[72,73] On unenhanced CT, the lesions are isoattenuating to slightly hypoattenuating to normal pancreas.[29] Following the administration of intravenous contrast, metastatic deposits typically demonstrate

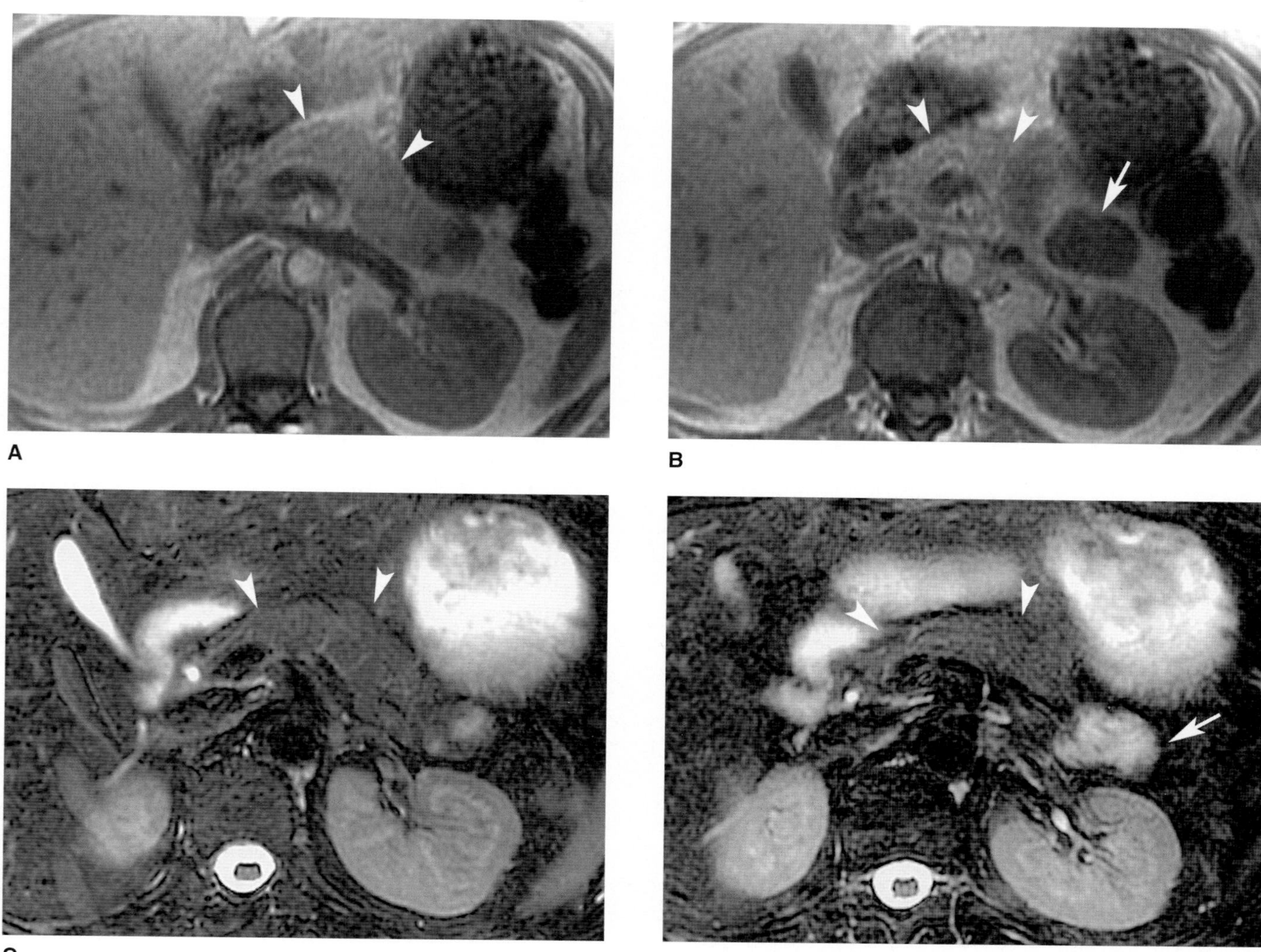

Figure 5-17 Insulinoma
This 50-year-old woman was being evaluated because of a suspected renal mass. **A** and **B.** T1-weighted MRI sequence shows the normal high signal pancreas (*arrowheads*) with a low signal mass (*arrow*) in the tail of the pancreas. **C** and **D.** T2-weighted, fat-suppressed MRI images of the same location shows the gland (*arrowheads*) to appear dark but the mass (*arrow*) to be very bright. This is a characteristic feature of islet cell tumors of the pancreas and other neuroendocrine tumors throughout the body.

increased enhancement relative to the uninvolved pancreas (see Figures 5-19 and 5-20).[73,74] Heterogeneous or peripheral enhancement is most commonly observed,[73,74] especially in tumors greater than 1.5 cm in size.[29] In one series, isoenhancement or hypoenhancement was observed in less than 25% of cases.[30] On MR, metastases are usually hypointense to normal pancreas on T1-weighted and fat-suppressed T1-weighted images and hyperintense to normal pancreas on T2-weighted sequences.[29] Postgadolinium sequences demonstrate peripheral enhancement of larger lesions and uniform enhancement of smaller metastases.[29] US is less sensitive than CT or MR in detecting intrapancreatic metastases. Nevertheless, metastases may be identified as hypoechoic or slightly hyperechoic lesions producing focal enlargement of the gland.[31] Pancreatic duct or bile duct dilation may also be detected by US depending on the site of the metastases.[31]

A solitary intrapancreatic metastasis to the pancreas may easily be misdiagnosed as pancreatic adenocarcinoma, especially in the absence of known extrapancreatic primary neoplasm. As pancreatic adenocarcinoma most commonly demonstrates decreased and delayed enhancement relative to normal pancreas, the presence of an enhancing lesion should, at the very least, raise suspicion for metastasis or islet cell tumor. Consideration of intrapancreatic metastasis is important as surgical resection may afford prolonged survival and portend a better prognosis.[32]

Pancreatic lymphoma: Primary pancreatic lymphoma is a rare form of extranodal non-Hodgkin lymphoma with less

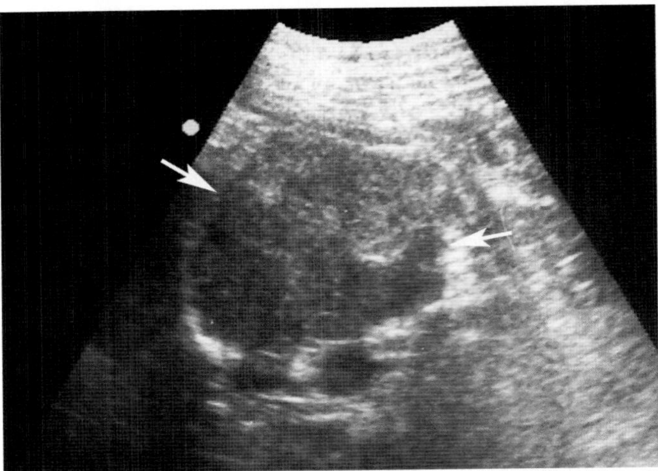

A

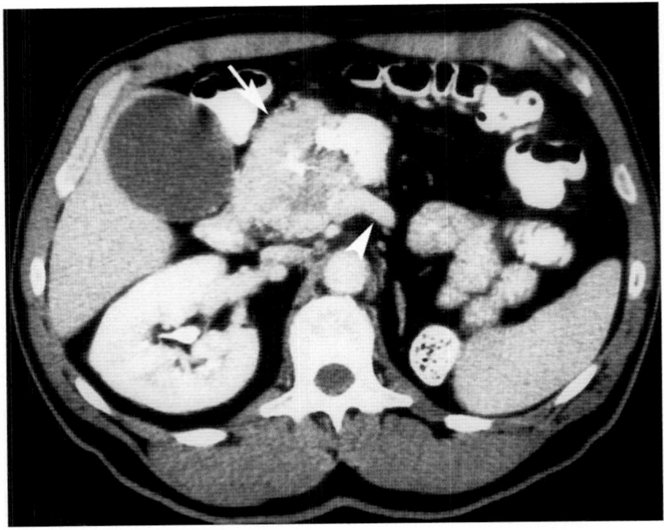

B

Figure 5-18 Glucagonoma
This 57-year-old woman presented with jaundice and worsening control of her diabetes mellitus. **A.** US of her right upper quadrant demonstrated mild biliary ductal dilation (not shown) and a sharply marginated mass in the head of the pancreas (*arrows*). **B.** CT scan shows a large uniform solid enhancing mass in the head of the pancreas (*arrow*) with central calcification. Note the region where the pancreatic body should be present anterior to the splenic vein (*arrowhead*) is uniformly fatty without glandular tissue, indicating atrophy of the distal gland. Surgical specimen was diagnostic of an islet cell tumor consistent with a glucagonoma. (Note there is also incidentally discovered atrophy of the left kidney.)

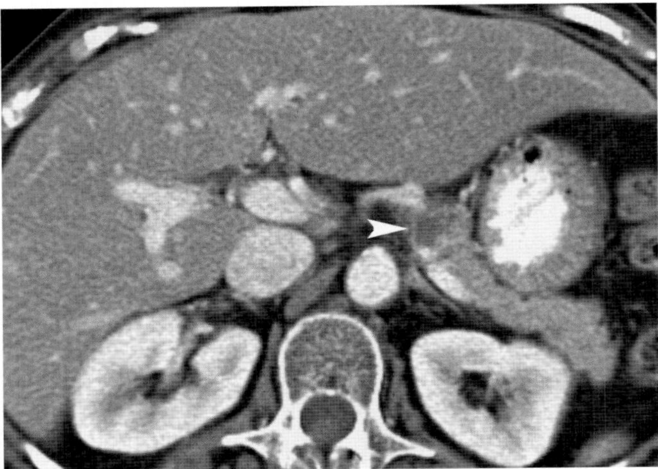

Figure 5-19 Pancreatic Metastasis
This 53-year-old woman presented with a history of non–small cell lung cancer. A predominantly hypoattenuating pancreatic mass was detected in the proximal pancreatic body (*arrowhead*). Multiple hepatic lesions were also detected and consistent with metastatic disease. It was unclear, however, whether the pancreatic lesion represented metastatic disease or a second primary malignancy. Biopsy of the pancreatic mass was performed but inconclusive. Chemotherapy directed at the lung cancer was initiated on follow-up imaging the pancreatic mass and hepatic lesions had improved, strongly suggesting the pancreatic lesion was a pancreatic metastasis.

than 1% arising from the pancreas.[76,77] Secondary involvement of the pancreas via contiguous extension of retroperitoneal lymphomatous disease or other adjacent structures is more common and may be seen in up to one-third of cases of non-Hodgkin lymphoma.[78,79] Primary pancreatic lymphoma occurs more commonly in men than women and within in the fifth to sixth decades of life.[80] Patients typically present with nonspecific complaints, most commonly abdominal pain and weight loss; other presenting symptoms include jaundice, gastric outlet obstruction, or small bowel obstruction.[33] Classic constitutional symptoms of fevers and night sweats are rare and have been reported to occur in as few as 2% of patients.[76,81]

The most common manifestation of primary pancreatic lymphoma is that of a pancreatic mass.[34] Occasionally, diffuse involvement of the pancreas may occur, resulting in a diffusely enlarged gland which may be extremely difficult to distinguish from acute pancreatitis.[64,82,83] Pancreatic duct dilation is uncommon but may been seen.[21]

CT is the most common modality by which pancreatic lymphoma is characterized and evaluated. On unenhanced CT, pancreatic lymphoma is hypoattenuating to isoattenuating to pancreas,[83-85] and following the administration of intravenous contrast, there is decreased enhancement relative to normal pancreatic parenchyma (see Figure 5-21).[64,83,85]

On MRI, the focal form of pancreatic lymphoma manifests as a homogenous hypointense lesion on T1-weighted images and a heterogeneous low- to moderately

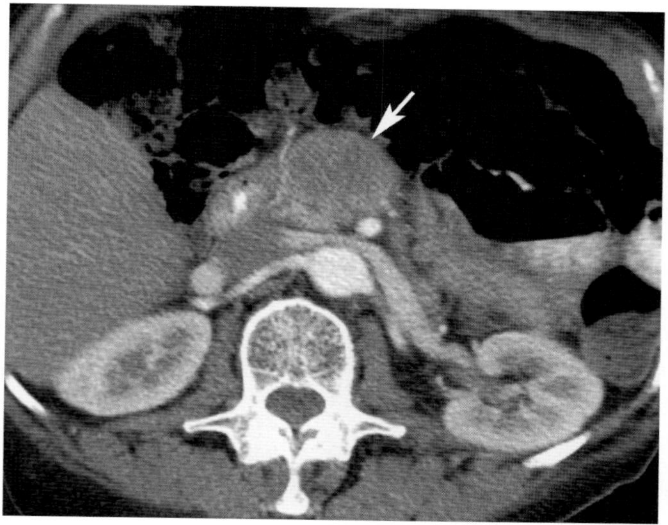

A

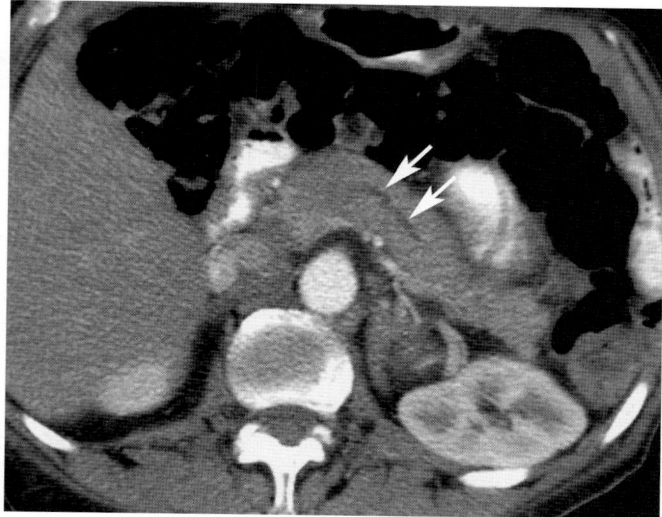

B

Figure 5-20 Pancreatic Metastasis
Contrast-enhanced abdominal CT of a 60-year-old man with history of right lung small cell carcinoma. **A.** CT image through the pancreatic neck shows a heterogeneous pancreatic neck mass (*arrow*), which is slightly hypodense to normal pancreatic parenchyma. **B.** CT section inferior to (A) and through the pancreatic body demonstrates dilation of the main pancreatic duct (*arrows*). Fine needle aspiration of the lesion revealed metastatic small cell carcinoma. Pancreatic adenocarcinoma would be a differential consideration.

intense lesion on T2-weighted images.[81,82] Postgadolinium sequences demonstrate subtle enhancement (see Figure 5-21).[34] The diffuse infiltrating form of pancreatic lymphoma demonstrates similar MR signal characteristics to the focal form and although there is primarily uniform contrast uptake, small foci of nonenhancement may be observed.[34] Mild pancreatic and biliary duct dilation, if present, is well depicted on MRCP images.[81,82]

Pancreatic lymphoma may be difficult to distinguish from pancreatic adenocarcinoma; however, a few imaging findings may help differentiate the two. One imaging clue that may suggest the diagnosis of lymphoma is no or only mild main pancreatic ductal dilation in the presence of a bulky pancreatic head tumor.[76,82,83,85] In addition, lymphadenopathy below the level of the renal veins is uncommon in pancreatic adenocarcinoma and is strongly suggestive of lymphoma.[76,82,83,85]

Cystic pancreatic tumors that appear solid on imaging: Serous cystadenoma is a benign tumor of the pancreas composed of small epithelial cysts. In some situations, the cysts are so small that the tumor appears solid on cross-sectional imaging. This is especially true of CT and US examinations whereas MRI, with its greater tissue contrast, may demonstrate the microcystic nature of the mass.[86,87] This tumor is reviewed in detail under the heading: **Cystic Masses of the Pancreas**.

Focal pancreatitis

Both acute and chronic pancreatitis can rarely cause a pancreatic mass that mimics pancreatic neoplasms. There is also a special form of focal chronic pancreatitis called "groove pancreatitis" that has characteristic imaging features.

Acute focal pancreatitis: Rarely, acute pancreatitis will involve the gland in a focal fashion that mimics a pancreatic mass. This localized form of acute pancreatitis has been shown to more commonly involve the pancreatic head and uncinate process.[88,89] In general, CT findings of this focal form of acute pancreatitis include enlargement of the involved pancreas. Adjacent peripancreatic stranding can also be present (see Figures 5-22, 5-23, and 5-24). On the other hand, MRI findings of localized acute pancreas include decreased signal relative to uninvolved pancreas on fat-suppressed T1 sequences. Associated peripancreatic fluid may also be present, which appears on T1-weighted sequences as low signal within the normally high-signal retroperitoneal fat and on fat-suppressed T2-weighted sequences as high signal within the peripancreatic fat (see Figure 5-24).[5]

At US, focal acute pancreatitis may appear as a hypoechoic lesion that mimics malignancy; however, it does not alter the normal contour of the gland or significantly impact the pancreatic or biliary ducts.[35] Although the latter distinguishing sonographic features suggest a benign etiology, pancreatic adenocarcinoma remains a diagnosis of exclusion.

Chronic focal pancreatitis: Chronic pancreatitis may also present as a focal pancreatic mass, indistinguishable from a pancreatic neoplasm. These chronic inflammatory

Imaging Notes 5-4. Distinguishing Features of Solid Pancreatic Masses

Lesion	Noncon. CT	MRI	Art. Phase	Ven Phase
Adenocarcinoma	Iso-/Hypo	Hypo T1 Iso to Hyper T2	Hypo	Hypo
Islet Cell tumor	Iso	Hypo T1 Hyper T2	Very Hyper	Iso to Hyper
Metastasis	Iso-/hypo	Hypo T1 Hyper T2	Very Hyper	Iso
Lymphoma	Iso-/hypo	Hypo T1 Iso-/hyper T2	Hypo	Hypo
Serous cystadenoma	Hypo	Hypo T1 Hyper T2 Small cysts seen	Variable	Variable
Acute pancreatitis	Hypo	Iso to Hyper	Hypo	Hypo
Chronic pancreatitis				

masses commonly arise in the pancreatic head and typically manifest as low attenuation masses on CT and hypointense masses on both T1- and T2-weighted MR sequences (see Figure 5-25). Contrast-enhanced MR fails to differentiate chronic focal pancreatitis from pancreatic adenocarcinoma because both may demonstrate decreased heterogeneous enhancement.[90,91] The similar enhancement pattern is thought to be a result of fibrosis within both chronic pancreatic inflammation and pancreatic malignancy. Other imaging features of pancreatic inflammatory masses that mimic pancreatic adenocarcinoma include obstruction of the common bile duct and main pancreatic duct ("double duct sign"), vascular encasement, and peripancreatic fat infiltration.[36]

Although it is often difficult to differentiate inflammatory pancreatic masses from pancreatic malignancies, the presence of the "penetrating duct sign" may suggest a diagnosis of an inflammatory mass. First described with US, this sign refers to the presence of a patent main pancreatic duct passing through a pancreatic mass; this finding was found to be associated more with inflammatory pancreatic masses than with pancreatic adenocarcinoma.[92-94] The "penetrating duct sign" also has been described at MRI evaluation and, although the study size was small, the MRI penetrating duct sign also was found to be associated more with inflammatory pancreatic masses than pancreatic adenocarcinoma.[37] MRCP imaging findings of this sign include a nonobstructed T2 hyperintense pancreatic duct that may or may not demonstrate smooth narrowing as it passes through a pancreatic mass. Although the presence of this finding is suggestive of an inflammatory pancreatic mass, further evaluation with tissue sampling is still required.

Groove pancreatitis: Groove pancreatitis is a localized form of chronic pancreatitis that involves the pancreaticoduodenal groove, the potential space between the duodenum, pancreatic head, and common bile duct.[96-99] Most patients are men in their fifth or sixth decades of life and typically present with abdominal pain, vomiting, weight loss, or jaundice.[38] Two forms of groove pancreatitis exist, the pure form and the segmental form.[39] In the former,

Imaging Notes 5-5. Penetrating Duct Sign

A normal or minimally narrowed pancreatic duct passing through a pancreatic mass is the penetrating duct sign. This sign is usually indicative of a benign cause of a pancreatic mass, usually focal chronic pancreatitis.

Imaging Notes 5-6. Groove Pancreatitis

Groove pancreatitis represents a special form of chronic pancreatitis that manifests as a focal mass centered on the pancreaticoduodenal groove, the potential space between the duodenum, pancreatic head, and common bile duct. This mass can mimic duodenal carcinoma, cholangiocarcinoma of the distal common bile duct and peripancreatic lymphadenopathy.

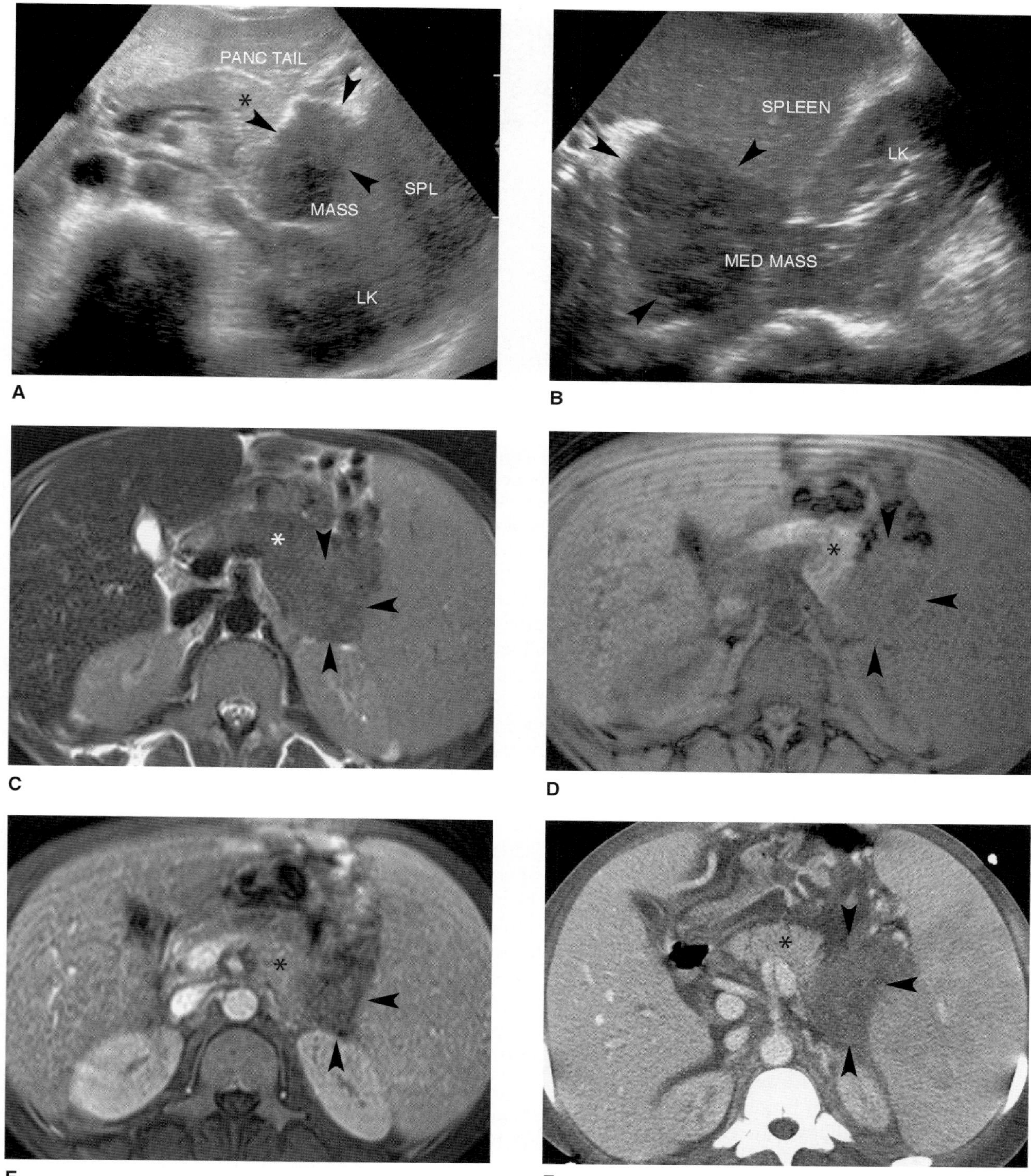

Figure 5-21 Pancreatic B-cell Lymphoma
This 34-year-old HIV-positive man presented with left upper quadrant pain and glomerulonephritis. **A** and **B**. Imaging evaluation began with retroperitoneal US, which demonstrates a large (~5 cm) hypoechoic mass (*arrowheads*) located between the pancreatic tail (*asterisk*), spleen, and left kidney (LK). The study cannot resolve whether the mass originates from the pancreas, left adrenal gland, or spleen, and further evaluation with CT or MRI was recommended. **C**. T2-weighted, (**D**) fat-suppressed unenhanced T1-weighted and (**E**) fat-suppressed enhanced T1-weighted MR sequences revealed the mass (*arrowheads*) originating from the pancreatic tail (*asterisk*). The mass is T2-isointense and T1-hypointense relative to pancreatic parenchyma. **E**. Minimal enhancement is observed following the administration of gadolinium. **F**. Enhanced CT demonstrates a hypoattenuating mass arising from the pancreatic tail (*asterisk*). Aspiration biopsy was positive for Burkitt cell lymphoma. Splenomegaly is noted on MRI and CT.

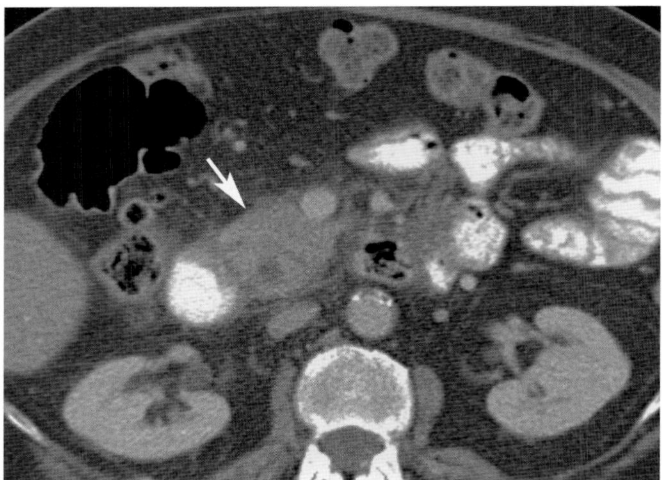
A

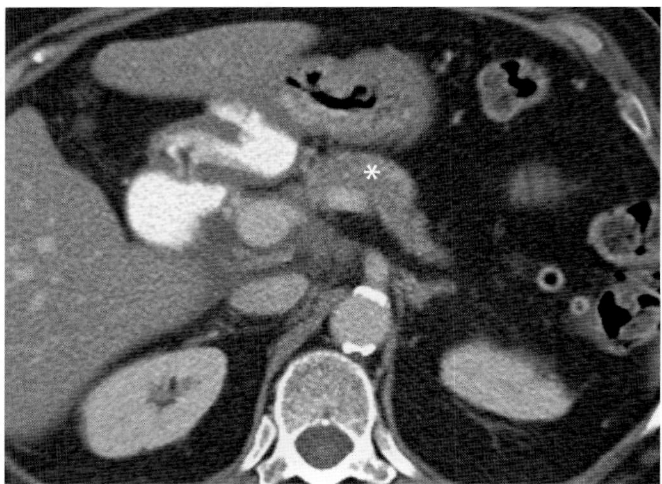
B

Figure 5-22 Focal Acute Pancreatitis
This 64-year-old woman had a history retained gallstone status post cholecystecomy. Attempts at gallstone retrieval by ERCP failed. **A** and **B.** Contrast-enhanced CT demonstrates enlargement of the pancreatic head (*white arrow*) relative to the rest of the pancreas (*asterisk*). The intrapancreatic common bile duct is also enlarged. The imaging findings are consistent with focal acute pancreatitis.

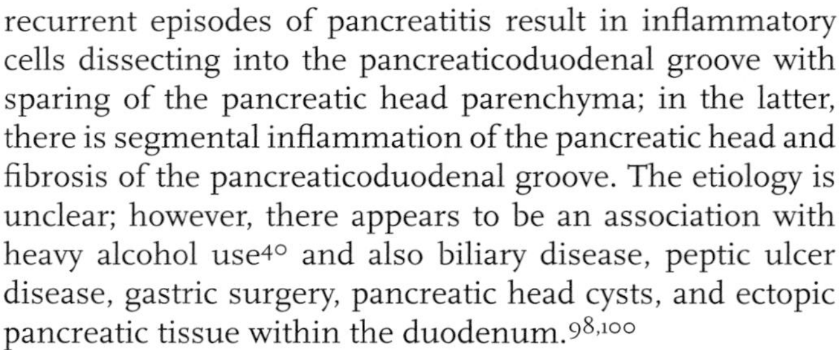

recurrent episodes of pancreatitis result in inflammatory cells dissecting into the pancreaticoduodenal groove with sparing of the pancreatic head parenchyma; in the latter, there is segmental inflammation of the pancreatic head and fibrosis of the pancreaticoduodenal groove. The etiology is unclear; however, there appears to be an association with heavy alcohol use[40] and also biliary disease, peptic ulcer disease, gastric surgery, pancreatic head cysts, and ectopic pancreatic tissue within the duodenum.[98,100]

At cross-sectional imaging, groove pancreatitis manifests as a mass centered in the pancreaticoduodenal groove. On CT, the mass is of decreased attenuation relative to the uninvolved pancreas, and following contrast administration, there is decreased enhancement relative to normal pancreas parenchyma.[97,100] Cysts within the mass and mild dilation of the common bile duct may also be present.[100,102] On MRI, a sheetlike mass is typically observed between the pancreatic head and duodenum that is T1 hypointense.[103,104] Signal intensity of the mass on T2-weighted sequences may be hyperintense, isointense, or hypointense relative to normal pancreas and this variability may reflect the acuity of the mass, with high T2 signal representing edema in the acute setting and low T2 signal representing the presence of fibrosis in the chronic setting.[102,103] Contrast-enhanced MR also reveals delayed and heterogeneous enhancement.[41] Additional MR findings include duodenal wall thickening and T2-hyperintense cysts within the duodenum or groove ranging in size from 5 mm to 3 cm.[103,104] In addition, MRCP is particularly useful as groove pancreatitis often results in duodenal stenosis, which may preclude adequate opacification at endoscopic retrograde cholangiopancreatography (ERCP). At MRCP, a long smooth segmental stenosis or medial displacement of the distal common bile duct may be seen.[103,104] Ultrasonographic findings include a hypoechoic mass with cysts between the head of the pancreas and duodenum, narrowing of the duodenum above the papilla of Vater, and irregularity of the duodenal surface.[38] Mild to moderate dilation of the common bile duct may also be present.[42]

Differential considerations for groove pancreatitis include duodenal adenocarcinoma, cholangiocarcinoma, and lymphadenopathy. An upper GI series may be particularly helpful in excluding duodenal adenocarcinoma, whereas MRCP can help exclude cholangiocarcinoma as the presence of a long smooth common bile duct stenosis would argue for groove pancreatitis.[99,104] In many cases, however, tissue sampling is required for accurate diagnosis as the imaging findings of groove pancreatitis overlap those of malignancy.

Pancreatic trauma

Trauma to the pancreas occasionally will manifest as a focal abnormality, especially when the trauma is minor. At imaging, these injuries may be subtle, with pancreatic contusions and hematomas taking the form of focal enlargement of the pancreas or irregularity of the pancreatic contour.[105,106] Although focal injuries to the pancreas may mimic a pancreatic mass, the clinical history of trauma should alert the radiologist to the traumatic etiology of the pancreatic findings. Pancreatic trauma is discussed in greater detail under the heading: **Disruption of the Gland: Pancreatic Trauma**.

Focal fatty sparing and focal fatty infiltration

With aging and some other conditions, the glandular elements of the pancreas regress and are replaced by fat.

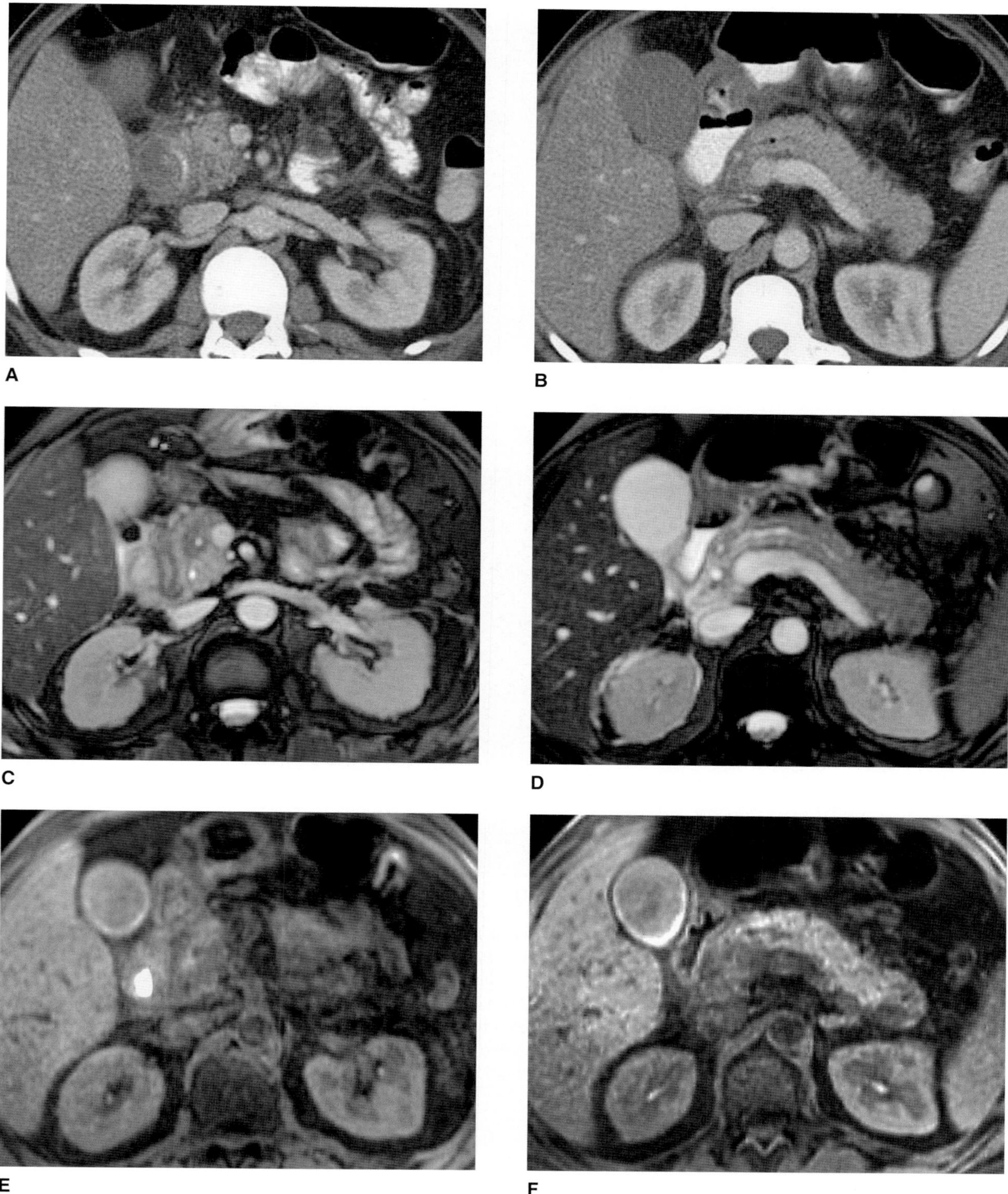

Figure 5-23 Focal Acute Pancreatitis
This 53-year-old man initially presented with abdominal pain and elevated serum lipase. Contrast-enhanced CT demonstrate enlargement of (**A**) the pancreatic head relative to (**B**) the pancreatic body and tail. Attenuation of the pancreatic head is decreased relative to the attenuation of the body and tail and is consistent with edema of the pancreatic head. A small focus of gas is noted in the main pancreatic duct and was related to instrumentation. Fat-suppressed T2-weighted MRI sequences demonstrate enlargement and increased T2 signal within (**C**) the pancreatic head relative to (**D**) the pancreatic tail and body. **E** and **F**. Fat suppressed T1-weighted sequences demonstrate pancreatic head enlargement and decreased T1-signal relative to the remainder of the gland. The T2 and T1 signal abnormalities of the pancreatic head correlate with edema. The combined imaging findings are consistent with focal acute pancreatitis of the pancreatic head.

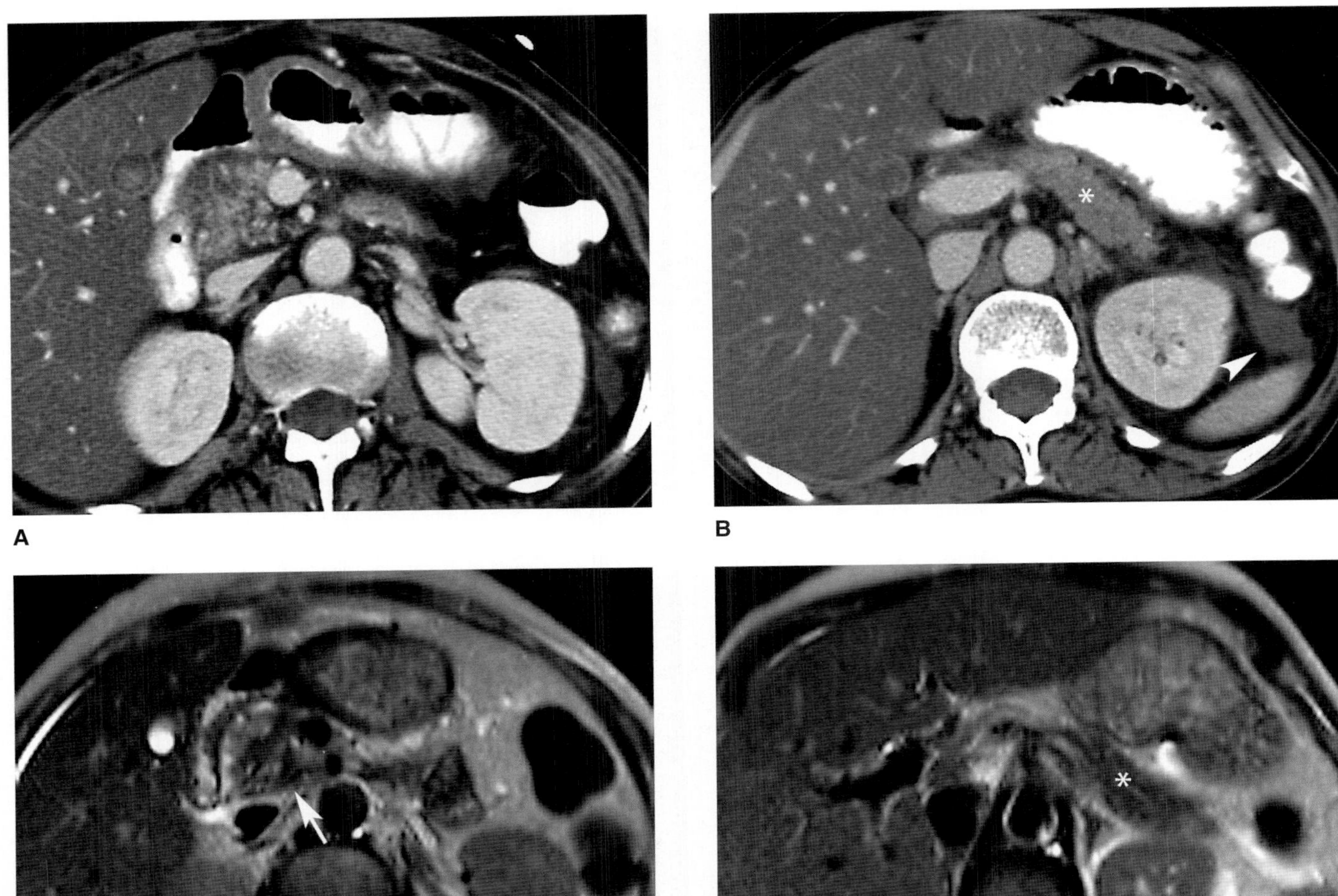

Figure 5-24 Focal Acute Pancreatitis
This 43-year-old woman presented with a history of abdominal pain, alcohol use, and a markedly elevated lipase. **A.** Contrast-enhanced CT demonstrate heterogeneous enlargement of the pancreatic head, consistent with edema. **B.** The remainder of the pancreas (*asterisk*) is spared and normal in attenuation and size. (A and B) A small amount of fluid is identified in the left pararenal space (*arrowhead*). **C** and **D**. Fast-spin echo T2-weighted MR images demonstrate increased signal within (C) the pancreatic head (*arrow*), consistent with edema. (D) The pancreatic body (*asterisk*) is normal in signal intensity. The combined CT and MRI findings represent focal acute pancreatitis of the pancreatic head. Hepatic steatosis is noted in A and B and characterized by diffusely decreased attenuation of the hepatic parenchyma.

Focal sparing of fat deposition or focal fat deposition can occasionally occur in the pancreatic head and can mimic a pancreatic mass. Imaging features that can help distinguish focal fatty sparing from a true mass lesion are (1) lack of mass effect, (2) preservation of the normal glandular architecture of the soft-tissue abnormality, and (3) lack of pancreatic or biliary ductal dilation.[43] Focal fatty sparing or focal fatty deposition can be positively identified with the use of in-phase and out-of-phase T1 MRI sequences. The out-of-phase images will demonstrate image dropout in the fatty portion of the pancreas with preservation of signal in the normal gland (see Figures 5-26 and 5-27). Fatty infiltration of the pancreas is discussed in greater detail under the heading **Fatty Infiltration of the Pancreas** later in this chapter.

Cystic Masses of the Pancreas

Small pancreatic cysts are probably the most common finding discovered at cross-sectional imaging. Studies indicate

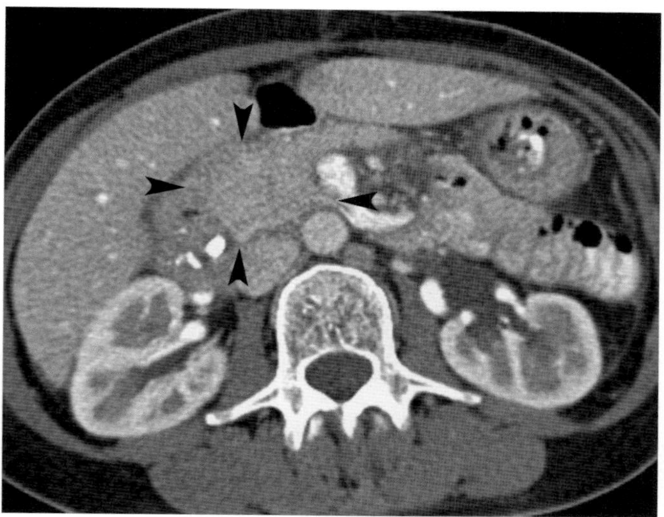

A

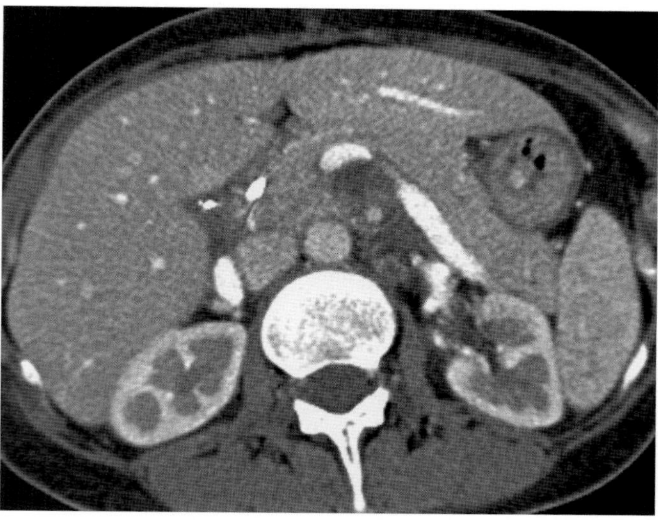

B

Figure 5-25 Focal Chronic Pancreatitis
This 51-year-old woman presented with 3 weeks of jaundice and weight loss and CT evaluation was performed to evaluate for suspected pancreatic adenocarcinoma. **A.** There is diffuse enlargement of the pancreatic head (*arrowheads*) relative to (**B**) the pancreatic body and tail. (A and B) No differential enhancement is present on the arterial phase or venous phase (not shown) of enhancement. Focal pancreatitis of the pancreatic head was favored although infiltrating neoplasm could not be excluded. The patient subsequently underwent Whipple procedure and pathology revealed findings of chronic pancreatitis and no neoplasm.

that between 1.2% and 2.5% of CT scans and up to 19.9% of MRI examinations will discover a small pancreatic cyst.[44-46] Older studies have suggested that these cysts are most often pseudocysts related to pancreatitis, but more recent studies suggest that they are predominantly benign or low-grade malignant cystic neoplasms.[47,48] Other cystic lesions include abscesses, hematomas, and simple epithelial cysts (Table 5-4).

Cystic pancreatic neoplasms

There are 3 cystic tumors of the pancreas that are either benign neoplasms or low-grade malignancies: serous cystadenomas, mucinous cystic neoplasms, and intraductal papillary mucinous neoplasms (IPMNs). In one series of cystic pancreatic lesions, 17% were serous cystadenomas, 28% were mucinous cystic neoplasms, and 27% were IPMNs, and only 3.8% were pseudocysts.[48] In most cases, these neoplasms are asymptomatic lesions that are incidentally found during an imaging examination for an unrelated problem. The cystic pancreatic neoplasms can be confused with pancreatic pseudocysts. The absence of other findings associated with pancreatitis such as a thickened, edematous pancreas or inflammation of the peripancreatic fat may be a clue to the diagnosis of a cystic pancreatic neoplasm.

Serous cystadenoma: serous cystadenomas are rare benign neoplasms that account for approximately 1% to 2% of exocrine pancreatic neoplasms and 17% of cystic pancreatic neoplasms.[8,48] These lesions are most commonly seen in women (female-male ratio >1.5:1) and in individuals greater than 60 years of age.[49] Given their increased prevalence in older women, these lesions have been referred to as "grandmother lesions."[50] Serous cystadenomas most commonly are found in the pancreatic body and tail, although they may arise within the pancreatic head.[51]

Although the majority of serous cystadenomas are asymptomatic, patients will occasionally present with nonspecific symptoms, such as vomiting and abdominal discomfort, which can be produced by mass effect on surrounding abdominal structures. When large, these lesions can present as palpable abdominal masses. Rare instances of hemoperitoneum and portal venous hypertension secondary to splenic vein compression have also been reported.[49]

Three morphologic types of serous cystadenomas occur: polycystic, oligocystic, and honeycomb. The polycystic variant occurs in 70% of patients, the honeycomb variant in 20% of cases, and the oligocystic variant in the remainder.[51] In both the polycystic and honeycomb patterns, there are typically more than 6 cysts separated by thin fibrous septations. The individual cysts are lined by cuboidal epithelium, contain glycogen-rich serous fluid, and vary in size from a few millimeters to 2 cm in diameter.[86,110-111] A fibrous central scar is usually present. There is no communication with the main pancreatic duct or its branches. In the oligocystic variant, the individual cysts can measure larger than 2 cm and differentiation from pseudocysts and mucinous cystic neoplasms may not be possible, and further evaluation with tissue sampling may be necessary.[51]

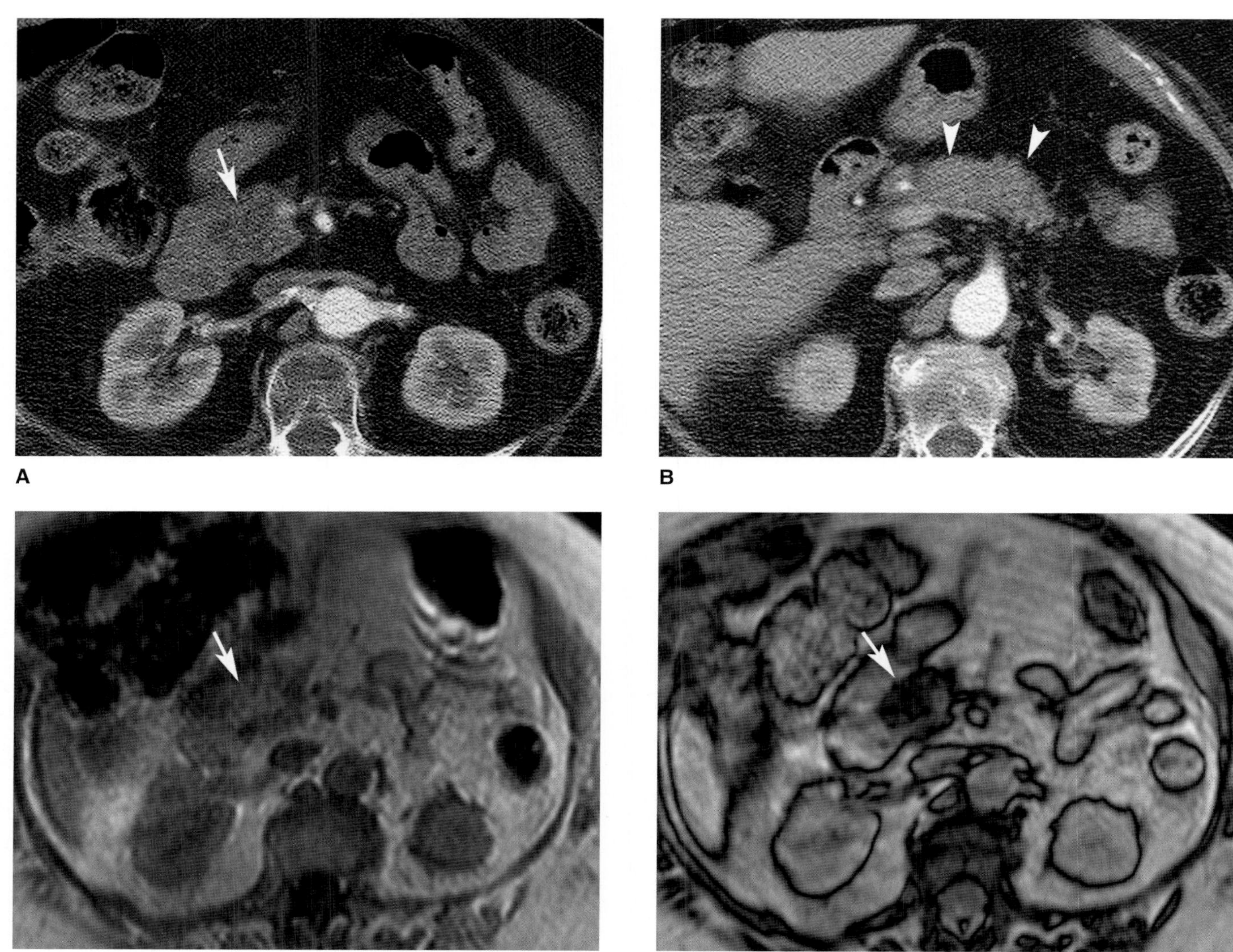

Figure 5-26 Focal Fatty Infiltration
This 77-year-old man had a history of lung cancer. **A** and **B**. Note the low attenuation region in the head of the pancreas (*arrows*) compared with the normal attenuation of the body of the pancreas (*arrowhead*) in this enhanced CT scan. It was thought that the low attenuation mass could represent either a metastasis or primary pancreatic malignancy. In-phase (**C**) and out-of-phase (**D**) T1-weighted MRI sequences demonstrate signal dropout in the mass indicative of focal fatty infiltration.

At CT, polycystic serous cystadenomas manifest as lobulated low-attenuation multiseptated cystic pancreatic masses (see Figure 5-28). The attenuation of the cysts follows fluid on unenhanced scans. Calcifications within the central scar are detected at imaging in 20% to 30% of cases, and the identification of central "starburst" calcifications within the scar is pathognomonic for serous microcystic adenoma.[110,112] Variable enhancement of the fibrous septa is observed following the administration of contrast. In the case of honeycomb serous cystadenomas, the lesions are frequently solid in appearance owing to the presence of numerous subcentimeter cysts that cannot be individually resolved.[86,87] In such cases, MR evaluation may be helpful for demonstrating the presence of fluid.[51] In the case of oligocystic serous cystadenomas, scant low-attenuation cysts larger than 2 cm are present.

On MRI, serous cystadenomas most commonly appear as a lobulated cystic mass. The cystic components appear as small foci of high T2 and low T1 signal intensity and the central scar demonstrates decreased T1 and T2 signal (see Figure 5-28).[110,113] Occasionally, increased T1 signal may be identified within the cystic portions of the mass and indicates intralesional hemorrhage.[50] As with CT, the fibrous septa demonstrate variable enhancement.[52] The presence of central scar calcifications may manifest as areas of decreased T1 and T2 signal. In addition, MRI is

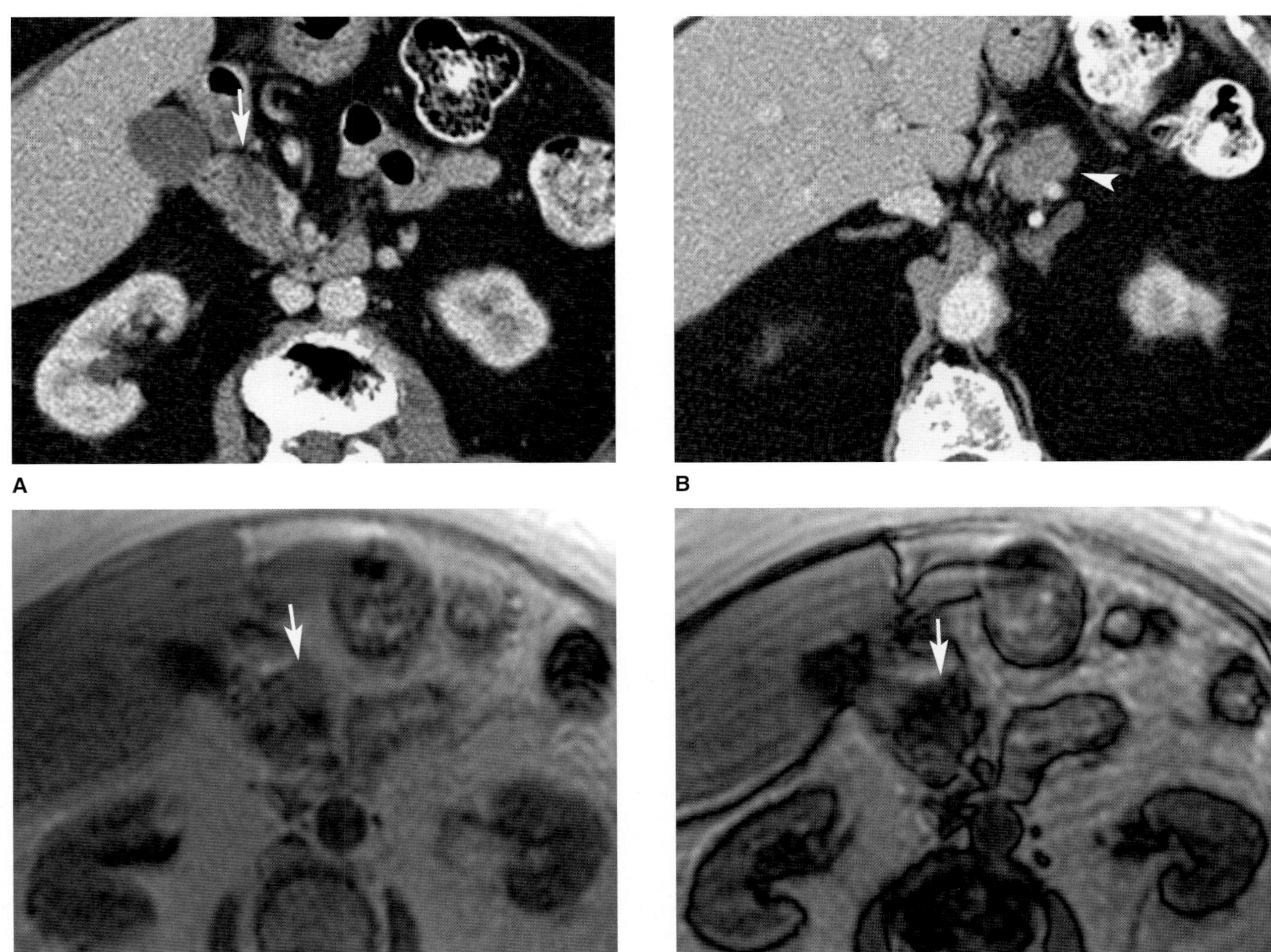

Figure 5-27 Focal Fatty Infiltration
This 75-year-old woman had a history of colon cancer. **A** and **B**. Note the low attenuation region in the head of the pancreas (*arrowhead*) compared with the normal attenuation of the body of the pancreas (*arrow*) in this enhanced CT scan. The low attenuation region was thought to represent a small multicystic mass. In-phase (**C**) and out-of-phase (**D**) T1-weighted MRI sequences demonstrate signal dropout in the mass indicative of focal fatty infiltration.

more sensitive for the presence of the septations of polycystic serous cystadenomas than CT and in some cases can demonstrate the true multilocular nature of the mass. As mentioned previously, serous microcystic adenomas may occasionally mimic a solid mass when composed of tiny microscopic cysts, and MRI often provides further insight into the identity of these lesions because the fluid-filled cysts appear as tiny foci of T2 hyperintensity.[86,87]

US reveals a well-circumscribed multilobulated mass. The cystic portions are hypoechoic and demonstrate associated increased through transmission whereas the fibrous portions are hyperechoic.[50] Calcifications may be identified as hyperechoic foci with associated posterior shadowing. In cases where the lesion is composed of very small cysts, the numerous microscopic cyst interfaces may mimic a solid mass[50] and MRI may be helpful for further evaluation.

Mucinous cystic neoplasms: Mucinous cystic tumors of the pancreas are rare lesions accounting for approximately 2.5% of exocrine pancreatic neoplasms and 28% of cystic pancreatic neoplasms.[8,48] They are slightly more common in women than men and present at a mean age of approximately 50 years. Given their tendency to occur in women of a slightly younger age than that typically seen with serous microcystic adenomas, the mucinous lesions have been termed "mother" lesions.[50] The majority of these

Table 5-4. Causes of Cystic Pancreatic Masses

1. Neoplasms
   a. Serous cystadenoma
   b. Mucinous cystic neoplasm
   c. Intrapapillary mucinous tumor (IPMT)
   d. Solid pseudopapillary tumor
2. Complications of Pancreatitis
   a. Pseudocyst
   b. Abscess
3. Trauma
   a. Hematoma
4. Epithelial cysts associated with congenital disorders
   a. Von Hippel-Lindau disease
   b. Autosomal dominant polycystic kidney disease
   c. Cystic fibrosis

lesions are asymptomatic although when symptomatic they typically present with the same constellation of nonspecific symptoms as seen with serous cystadenomas.[51] Unlike serous microcystic adenomas, mucinous neoplasms are considered surgical lesions because they all have a malignant potential.[53]

Histologically, mucinous cystic neoplasms are composed of mucin-producing columnar cells and resemble ovarian mucinous cystic neoplasms. These lesions are found predominantly in the body and tail of the pancreas[110,114] and will usually appear as a unilocular mass or a multiseptated cystic mass with at least 1 cyst greater than 2 cm in diameter.[45,110] Because the lesion does not originate from pancreatic ductal epithelium, no communication with the pancreatic duct is present.

Unenhanced CT typically reveals a smoothly lobulated cystic mass with low attenuation contents (see Figures 5-29 and 5-30). Unlike serous microcystic adenomas, these lesions are composed of fewer (<6) but larger (>2 cm) cysts.[54] Occasionally, intralesional debris and hemorrhage will be present and the cyst will have an attenuation greater than 20 HU. These lesions typically demonstrate enhancing septa and septal nodules following the administration of intravenous contrast (see Figure 5-30). Associated findings include dilation of the main pancreatic duct and pancreatic atrophy distal to the lesion. Peripheral eggshell calcifications are specific for mucinous cystic neoplasms and highly predictive of malignancy; however, these are not a common finding at CT imaging.[114,115] Features suggestive of a malignant mucinous neoplasm (ie, mucinous cystadenocarcinoma) include septations, wall, and/or septal calcifications and a wall thickness greater than 2 mm. (see Figure 5-31).[55] The presence of more than 1 of these features increases the likelihood of malignancy and when all 3 features are present, there is a 95% probability that the lesion is malignant.[55] Adjacent tissues should be assessed for signs of malignant invasion.

Imaging Notes 5-7. Imaging Features Predictive of Malignancy in Mucinous Cystic Neoplasms

Multiple septations
Wall or septal calcification
Wall thickness >2 mm

MR is superior to CT in characterizing the complex internal architecture of mucinous cystic neoplasms.[51] A lobulated cystic mass is identified with increased T2 signal intensity (see Figure 5-29).[52] Variable T1 signal intensity is present depending on the relative amounts of intralesional simple fluid and protein.[45,113] Any calcifications will manifest as decreased T1 and T2 signal intensity. Gadolinium administration reveals irregular enhancing septa and nodules.[18] Pancreatic atrophy and duct dilation may also be identified distal to the lesion.[50]

US typically reveals a cystic mass within the parenchyma.[18] The cystic contents may be simple and anechoic or may demonstrate echogenic debris and/or hemorrhage. Septa, mural nodules, and calcifications can be identified in some cases;[18] however, further evaluation by CT or MRI is usually required to optimally characterize these lesions.

Intraductal papillary mucinous neoplasms: Intraductal papillary mucinous neoplasms are rare neoplasms of the pancreas and account for 1% to 2% of exocrine pancreas tumors and approximately 28% of cystic neoplasms.[48,56] They arise from the pancreatic duct epithelium and range from benign IPMN adenomas to malignant IPMN carcinomas.[57] Histologically, IPMNs appear as papillary projections of mucin-secreting columnar epithelial cells. The papillomatous overgrowth of mucin-secreting cells is responsible for the hallmark features of this lesion: excess mucin secretion causing dilation of the involved pancreatic ducts. Two distinct forms of IPMNs exist: (1) those that involve the main pancreatic duct and (2) those that involve only side branch pancreatic ducts. The former variant is described under the heading **Pancreatic Ductal Dilation** whereas the latter is described here.

Side branch IPMNs are more commonly observed in men aged 60 to 70 years and are frequently located in the pancreatic head and uncinate process.[58] Mucinous distention of a side branch duct results in the formation of a cystic lesion with associated atrophy of the surrounding parenchyma.[59] Like other cystic pancreatic neoplasms, many cases will be accidentally discovered by cross-sectional imaging. However, because this tumor involves the pancreatic duct, it can be a cause for recurrent pancreatitis secondary to pancreatic duct obstruction from thick mucinous secretions.[56] Side branch IPMNs have a 15% 5-year risk of developing high-grade dysplasia or invasive carcinoma.[60]

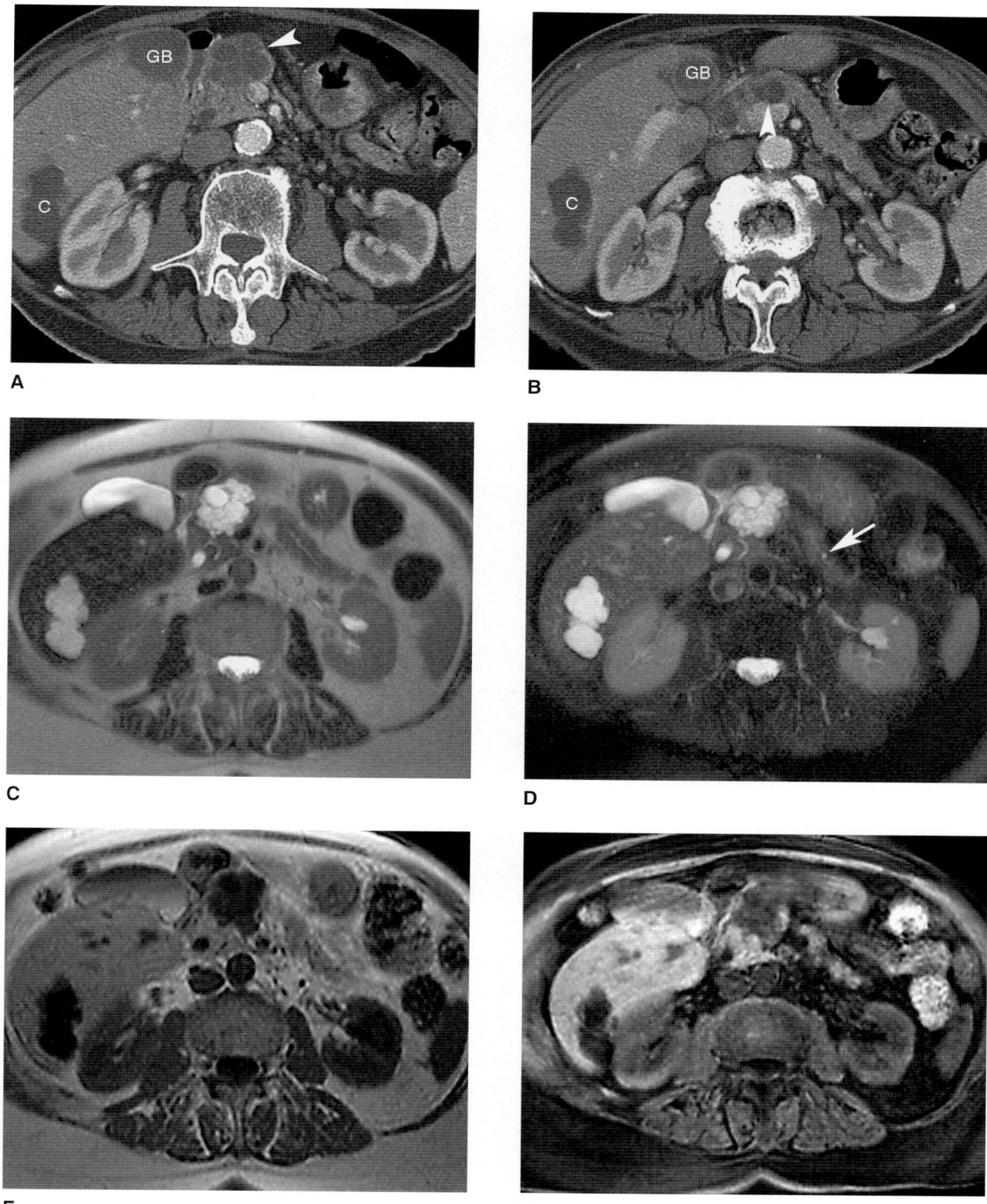

Figure 5-28 Microcystic Serous Cystadenoma
A CT study of the chest was performed in this 84-year-old woman with a history of breast carcinoma. **A** and **B**. Partially visualized was a large cystic lesion arising from the junction of the pancreatic neck and body (*arrowheads*) for which MRI was recommended for further evaluation. T2-weighted (**C**), fat-suppressed T2-weighted (**D**), T1-weighted (**E**), and contrast-enhanced fat-suppressed T1-weighted (**F**) sequences demonstrate a multiloculated lesion consisting of many small (less than 2 cm) cystic spaces. The contents of the lesion follow simple fluid on all sequences and there is no enhancement of the lesion following contrast administration (**F**). No pancreatic duct dilation is present and thin-section imaging through the lesion did not reveal any communication with the pancreatic duct (not shown). The combined imaging findings are characteristic of a microcystic serous cystadenoma. A 2-mm nonaggressive pancreatic cystic lesion is noted in the pancreatic tail (*arrow* in D). GB, gallbladder; C, hepatic cyst.

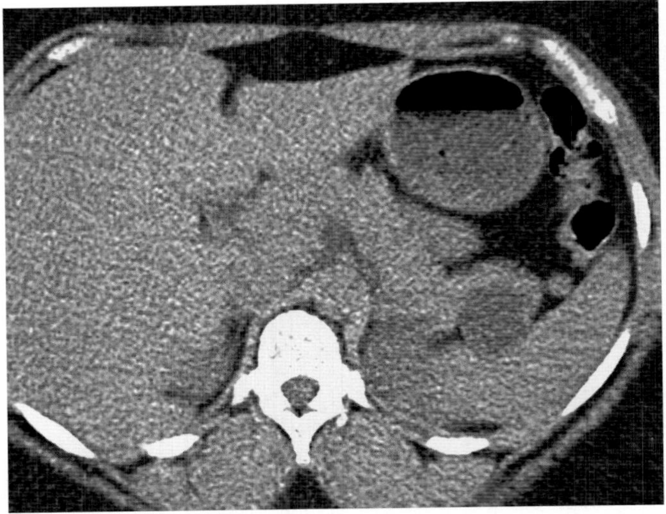

A

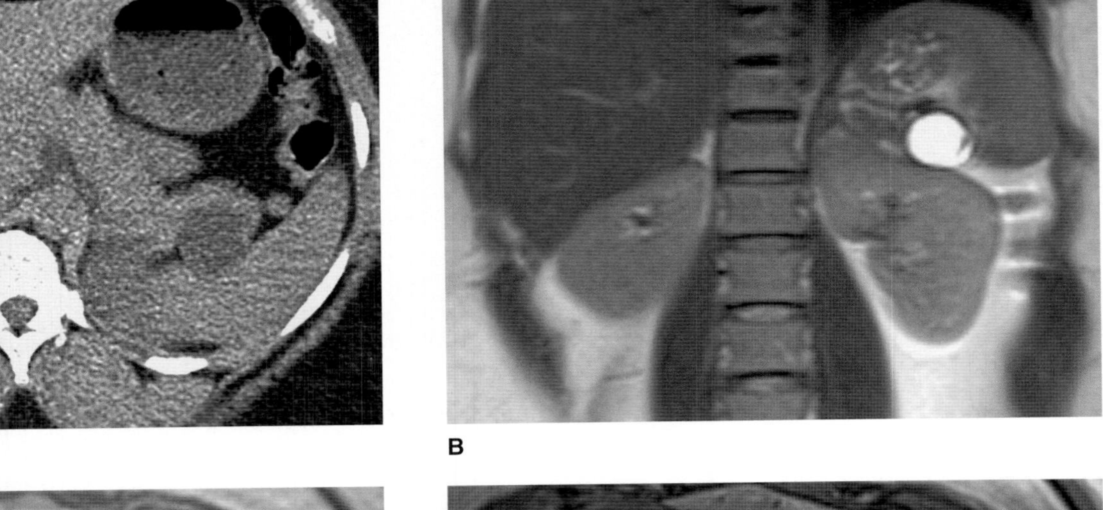

B

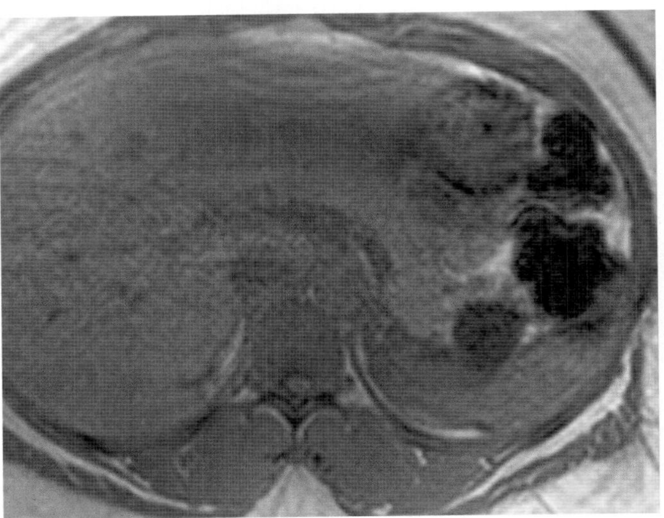

C

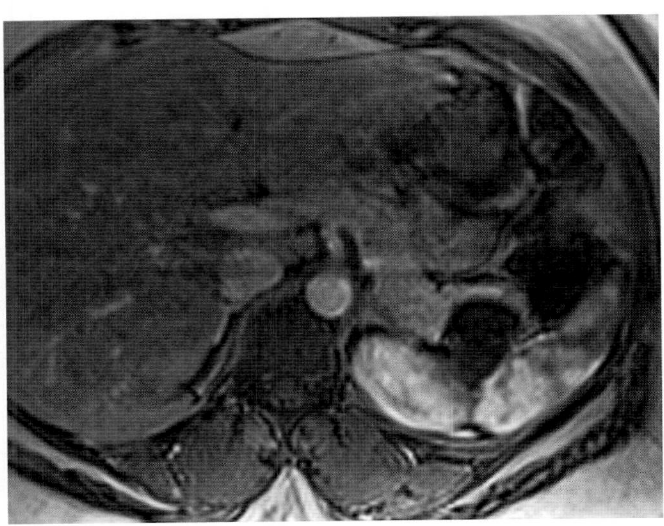

D

Figure 5-29 Mucinous Cystadenoma
This 33-year-old woman presented with low back pain. **A**. An unenhanced CT examination was performed to evaluate for suspected renal calculus. A 3-cm low-attenuation cystic lesion arising from the pancreatic tail was detected. Coronal T2-weighted (**B**), axial T1-weighted (**C**), and enhanced T1-weighted (**D**) MR sequences confirm a unilocular cystic lesion arising from the pancreatic tail. No nodular or enhancing components are identified. Pancreatic pseudocyst would be the most common cause of a cystic pancreatic lesion; however, there was no history of pancreatitis. Differential considerations would also include a mucinous cystic neoplasm, such as mucinous cystadenoma or mucinous cystadenocarcinoma. Distal pancreatectomy was performed and revealed mucinous cystadenoma with ovarian stroma.

Both microcystic and macrocystic patterns of side branch IPMNs exist.[119,121] The microcystic pattern of side branch IPMNs typically appear as clusters of small 1- to 2-mm cysts with thin septa, thus mimicking the appearance of a serous microcystic adenoma. Macrocystic side branch IPMNs appear as unilocular or multilocular lesions and are similar in appearance to mucinous cystic neoplasms (see Figure 5-32). Distinguishing these side branch lesions from serous or mucinous neoplasms is often possible with the use of MRCP, which is the modality of choice for the evaluation of suspected side branch IPMNs as it is most sensitive in defining its morphologic features, such as nodules, septa, and communication with the main pancreatic duct.[86,122] Thin-section multidetector CT (with curved reformations), though less sensitive, is another useful modality in evaluating side branch IPMNs.[86,122]

Management of side branch IPMNs is based on lesion size and the presence of additional associated findings.[121,123,124] Lesions that are 3 cm or less in size and without mural nodules or involvement of the main pancreatic duct

Imaging Notes 5-8. Intrapapillary Mucinous Tumors

Intraductal papillary mucinous tumors can usually be distinguished from other cystic pancreatic lesions by the demonstration of communication with the pancreatic duct.

may be followed with imaging. Lesions greater than 3 cm in size and/or lesions with suspicious features such as mural nodules, main duct dilation, or interval growth should be considered suspicious for malignancy and resected.

Solid pseudopapillary tumors: Solid pseudopapillary tumors (SPTs), formerly termed *solid and pseudopapillary epithelial neoplasms*, are rare low-grade malignant neoplasms of the pancreas that usually present in young women, most commonly in the second and third decades of life.[14,125] As these lesions occur primarily in young women, some have termed this entity the "daughter" lesion.[50] These lesions have often been reported to be most common in the pancreatic tail and in women of African and Asian descent;[126-128] however, the veracity of these characteristics have been challenged.[61]

Solid pseudopapillary tumors may become symptomatic when large, and patients present most commonly with an abdominal mass and/or abdominal discomfort.[62] Invasion of adjacent structures and hepatic metastases have been reported but are uncommon,[126,129,130] and the presence of metastatic lesions does not seem to preclude cure.[63] Even rarer are instances of high-grade malignant lesions.[132]

Macroscopically, SPTs are well-encapsulated masses that may be solid, mixed cystic and solid, or cystic with a thick wall.[126,128] Histologically, these lesions are composed of cells forming solid, pseudopapillary, and/or hemorrhagic pseudocystic structures.[131,133] These are not "true cysts" as no true epithelial lining is present.[63] The cellular origin of this entity remains unclear.

Imaging Notes 5-9. Age Associations of Cystic Pancreatic Neoplasms

Three cystic neoplasms are typically seen in women of different ages.

Neoplasm	Age Range	Moniker
Serous cystadenoma	>60	Grandmother tumor
Mucinous cystic neoplasm	~50	Mother tumor
Solid pseudopapillary tumor	20-30	Daughter tumor

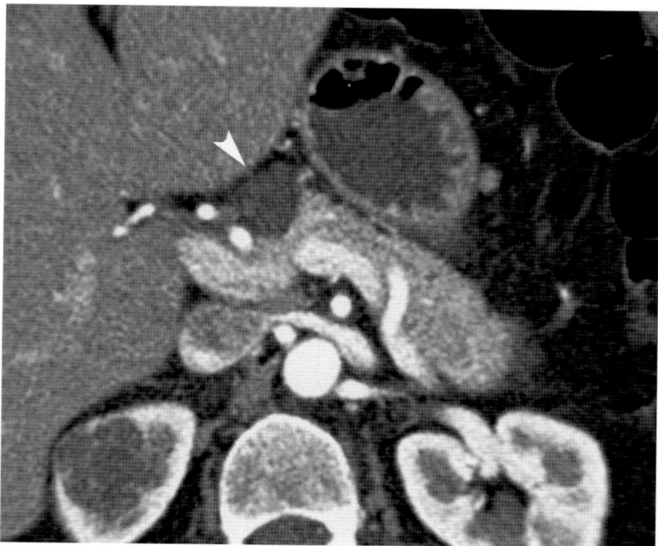

Figure 5-30 Mucinous cystadenoma
This 63-year-old woman had a cystic pancreatic lesion that was progressively enlarging on follow up studies. Enhanced CT obtained during the arterial phase of enhancement demonstrates a 2.5-cm low-attenuation cystic lesion at the junction of the pancreatic neck and body (*arrowhead*). There are subtle enhancing nodular foci within the lesion that were called prospectively. No dilation of the pancreatic duct is present. The lesion was surgically resected, and pathology revealed mucinous cystadenoma. A Bosniak category IIF cystic lesion in the right kidney is noted.

Moreover, SPTs typically appear as large mixed cystic and solid masses within the pancreatic parenchyma. Evaluation with CT typically shows a well-circumscribed complex lesion of central fluid attenuation and peripheral soft-tissue attenuation.[126,134-136] Areas of high attenuation, representing foci of hemorrhage, are also usually seen.[126,136] Calcifications may be identified peripherally or centrally.[135,136] On MRI, a heterogeneous lesion is revealed that is T1 hyperintense, corresponding to hemorrhage, and most frequently T2 hyperintense.[126,128,129] Fluid-fluid levels or fluid-debris levels may be present. In addition, MRI may demonstrate a peripheral rim of low T1 and T2 signal, corresponding to the fibrous capsule and characteristic of an SPT.[126,128,129] Following the administration of gadolinium contrast, mild peripheral enhancement is usually identified followed by enhancement of the solid elements on portal venous phase imaging.[61] US is not particularly helpful in distinguishing the lesion from other cystic lesions of the pancreas, as these lesions appear as well-circumscribed complex cystic and solid masses (see Figure 5-33).[126,134]

Simple unilocular cysts

With modern thin-section CT and MRI, small, <20-mm, unilocular cysts are commonly found within the substance of the pancreas of older individuals. The etiology

Imaging Notes 5-10. Imaging Characteristics of Cystic Pancreatic Masses

Lesion	Cyst Number	Cyst Size	Other Features
Serous cystadenoma	Multilocular Honeycomb pattern occ. unilocular	1 mm-2 cm	Central calcified scar
Mucinous cystic tumor	Unilocular or multilocular	At least one cyst > 2 cm	Enhancing nodules occ panc duct dil occ panc atrophy
Side Branch IPMT	Multilocular occ. unilocular	1 mm to >2 cm	Communication with pancreatic duct
Solid pseudopapillary tumor	Unilocular Occ multilocular	Variable	Thick enhancing wall Blood products on MRI Fluid-debris levels Low T1/low T2 fibrous capsule
Necrotic adenocarcinoma	Unilocular	>2 cm	Thick enhancing wall Irregular internal wall
Pseudocyst	Unilocular	Variable	Thin sharply def. wall
Abscess	Unilocular	Variable Usually >2 cm	Thick irregular wall Signs of pancreatitis

of these cysts is often uncertain but in one study where incidentally noted pancreatic cysts underwent resection, 25% were found to represent main duct IPMNs and 23% were found to be side branch IPMNs.[137] Of the remaining resected cystic lesions, 18% were mucinous cystic neoplasms, 13% were serous cystadenomas, 5% were SPTs, 4% were neuroendocrine neoplasms, and 2% were ductal adenocarcinomas.

The majority of these lesions are clinically irrelevant and will not require intervention. In one study, only 8% of their cases developed changes in the cyst that lead to surgical resection.[64] In another study of 90 patients with incidental cysts and a mean follow-up of 48 months, malignancy was demonstrated in only 1 patient, 7 years from diagnosis.[65,66] As a consequence of these and other studies, experts advocate a conservative approach of periodic surveillance with CT or MRCP in cases of incidentally discovered small (<30 mm), asymptomatic cysts that lack nodules or solid components.[123,137] Resection is recommended for those that increase in size, become symptomatic, or develop solid components (see Figure 5-34).[123,137]

Imaging Notes 5-11. Incidental Small Pancreatic Cysts

> Small pancreatic cysts are incidentally found in a moderate number of CT and MRI examinations. These are usually stable lesions that are clinically insignificant but require radiographic follow-up to confirm stability. In one study of surgically excised lesions, approximately 50% represented small main duct or side branch intraductal papillary mucinous tumors. The remainder represented mucinous cystic neoplasms (18%), serous cystadenomas (13%), SPTs (5%), neuroendocrine neoplasms (4%), and ductal adenocarcinomas (2%).

Epithelial cysts

Epithelial cysts of the pancreas are an uncommon finding in the pancreas and are nearly always associated with hereditary syndromes such as Von Hippel-Lindau disease, autosomal dominant polycystic kidney disease, and cystic fibrosis. When found, they tend to be multiple and demonstrate the cross-sectional imaging characteristics of cysts (see Figure 5-35).

Complications of pancreatitis

Acute pancreatitis occasionally results in complications that focally involve the pancreatic gland, with the most common of these being acute pancreatic pseudocysts. Additional complications of a focal nature include pancreatic abscess, organizing pancreatic necrosis, and central pancreatic necrosis.

Pancreatic pseudocyst: Acute pancreatic pseudocysts are well-circumscribed peripancreatic collections of pancreatic enzymes and secretions contained by a thin fibrous pseudocapsule of granulation tissue. Formation of the pseudocapsule requires approximately 4 to 6 weeks and, therefore, the term should be reserved for those fluid collections with duration of greater than 4 weeks and with a well-defined

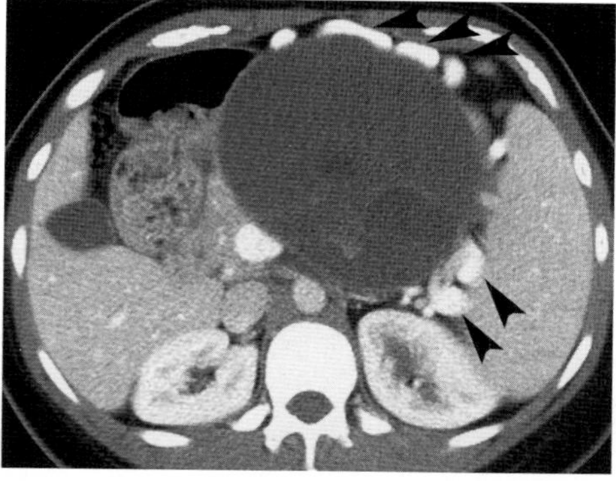
A

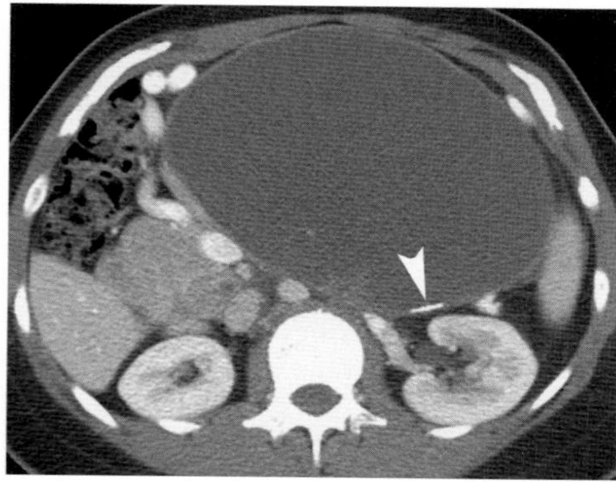
B

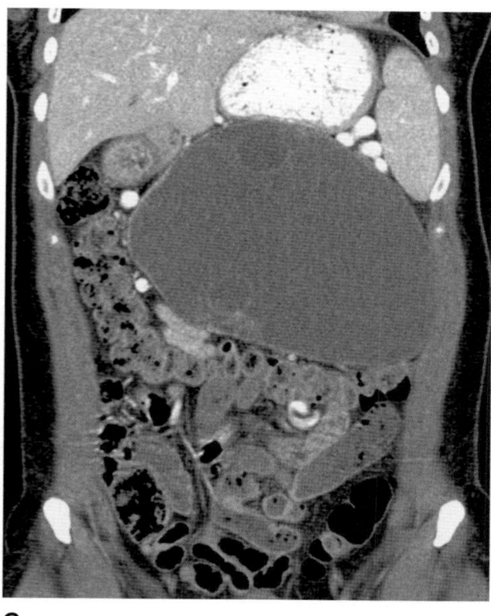
C

Figure 5-31 Mucinous cystadenocarcinoma
Abdominal distention was the presenting complaint in this 33-year-old woman. **A** and **B**. Enhanced CT revealed a very large cystic mass arising from the pancreatic body. Thin septations and a peripheral calcification (*white arrowhead*) are present. Large varices in **A** (*black arrowheads*) are present and the result of extrinsic compression of the splenic vein by the cystic mass. **C**. Coronal reformation demonstrates the extent of the mass. Mucinous cystic neoplasm was the primary consideration. This lesion was resected, with pathology revealing mucinous cystadenocarcinoma without local invasion. No imaging findings of metastatic disease were present on this or subsequent studies.

pseudocapsule. Pseudocysts less than 4 cm in diameter commonly regress spontaneously whereas those greater than 5 cm in diameter will often necessitate drainage or decompression to avoid complications[138-140] because their persistence places the patient at risk of infection, hemorrhage, and pseudoaneurysm formation.[70,141,142] Imaging features are not able to distinguish acute from chronic pseudocysts; however, detection of a pseudocyst in a patient without a history of recent acute pancreatitis will usually indicate a chronic pseudocyst. Chronic pseudocysts are usually clinically asymptomatic but can occasionally cause signs or symptoms, such as persistent abdominal pain, nausea, or vomiting due to gastric outlet obstruction, jaundice due to biliary obstruction, fevers, leukocytosis, or a palpable abdominal mass. [70,140,143,144]

Pancreatic pseudocysts appear as simple or minimally complex cysts in or near the pancreas. They are of varying sizes and are oval or round in shape.[67] Pseudocysts will manifest on CT as low-attenuation (<15 HU) cystic collections with a thin (1-2 mm), symmetric fibrous capsule (see Figure 5-36).[68] Direct communication with the main pancreatic duct can be seen.[69] The presence of high-attenuation (>45-50 HU) contents within the cyst is consistent with hemorrhage.[70] On MRI, uncomplicated pseudocysts will demonstrate decreased T1 signal and increased T2 signal.[71] Pseudocysts complicated by hemorrhage will manifest increased T1 and T2 signal.[71] If large enough, US will detect the lesion and demonstrate a hypoechoic collection with increased through transmission.[72] Small amounts of layering debris may also be identified by US.

When reporting pancreatic pseudocysts, several imaging features deserve mention as they suggest management by surgery or transcutaneous drainage.[70,140,143,144] These include progressive enlargement, size greater than 5 cm, hemorrhage, and signs of mass effect on adjacent structures (eg, biliary dilation and gastric outlet obstruction). Clinical indicators for intervention include persistent pain, infection, and abdominal mass.

Distinguishing pancreatic pseudocysts from cystic neoplasms of the pancreas can be difficult; however, a clinical history of recent acute pancreatitis should suggest the diagnosis of a pseudocyst. Furthermore, the presence of a thin symmetric capsule argues against a cystic neoplasm of the pancreas as cystic neoplasms typically demonstrate thicker and more irregular margins.[70]

Imaging Notes 5-12. Features of Pancreatic Pseudocysts Suggesting the Need for Drainage

1. Progressive enlargement
2. Size greater than 5 cm
3. Mass effect on adjacent structures
   a. Biliary dilatation
   b. Gastric outlet obstruction

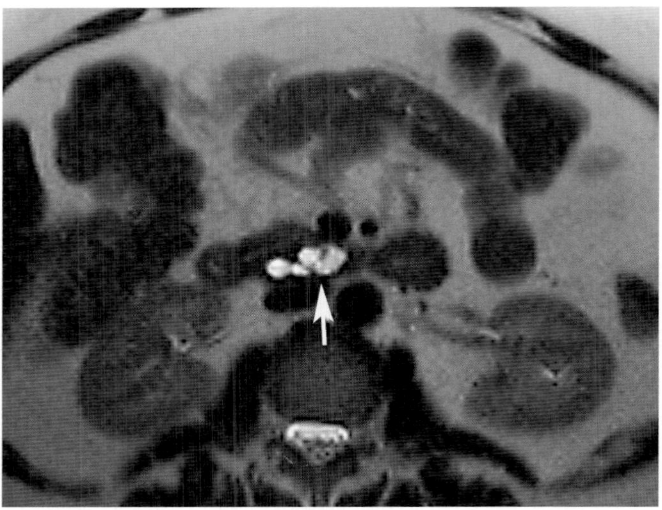

A

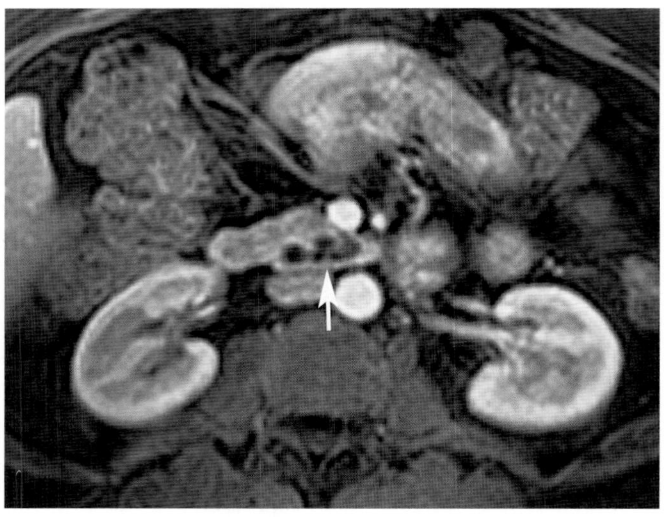

B

Figure 5-32 Intraductal Papillary Mucinous Tumor
A. T2-weighted and (**B**) post-gadolinium T1-weighted MRI images in this 59-year-old woman demonstrate a small mass (*arrow*) in the head of the pancreas. This is high signal on T2-weighted sequences, with multiple small septations indicating a multiseptated cystic lesion. The post-gadolinium images show enhancement of the normal pancreas and kidneys but no enhancement of the mass. This is consistent with a small cystic pancreatic neoplasm, most likely a small intraductal papillary tumor. This lesion had remained unchanged on multiple prior MRI examinations over several years.

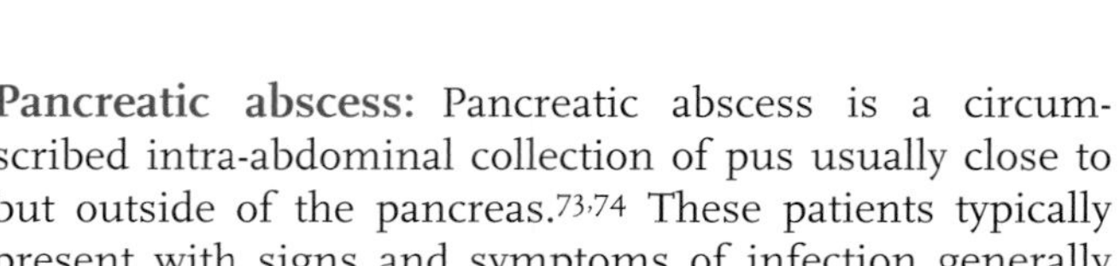

Pancreatic abscess: Pancreatic abscess is a circumscribed intra-abdominal collection of pus usually close to but outside of the pancreas.[73,74] These patients typically present with signs and symptoms of infection generally 4 to 6 weeks following the onset of acute pancreatitis.[73] The presence of a circumscribed peripancreatic collection in a patient with history of antecedent acute pancreatitis and an appropriate clinical picture distinguishes pancreatic

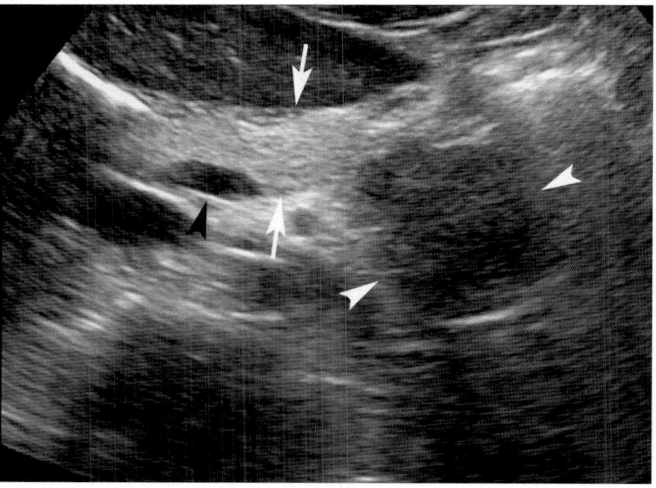

A

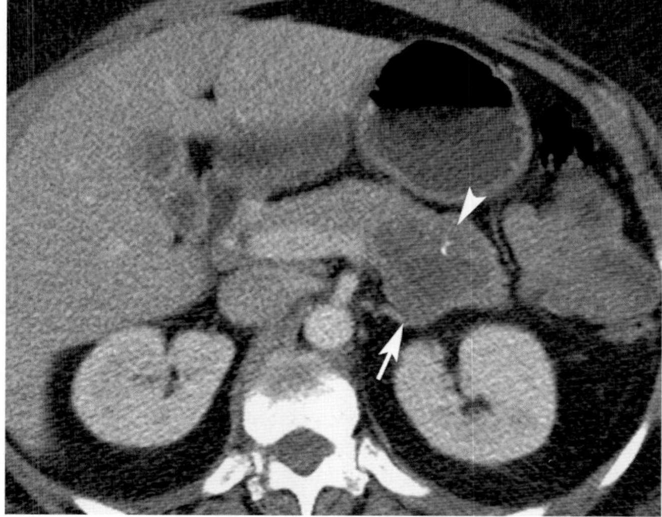

B

Figure 5-33 Solid Pseudopapillary Tumor
This 37-year-old woman had a history of hepatitis. **A.** US demonstrates the normal-appearing echogenic pancreatic body (*white arrows*) and anechoic portal vein (*black arrowhead*). But there is also a hypoechoic mass in the tail of the pancreas (*white arrowhead*). **B.** Contrast-enhanced CT shows a hypoechoic mass in the tail of the pancreas (*arrow*) with a small focus of calcification (*arrowhead*). These findings are consistent with a cystic pancreatic neoplasm. Surgical excision was diagnostic of a solid pseudopapillary tumor.

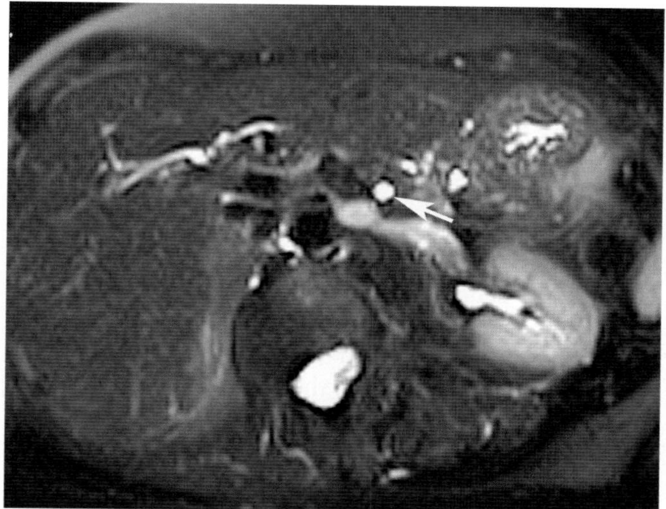

A

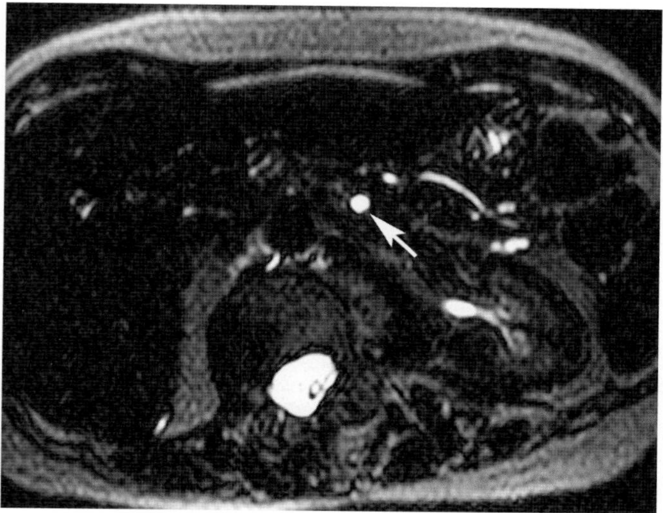

B

Figure 5-34 Stable nonaggressive unilocular pancreatic cyst **A** and **B**. Fat-suppressed T2-weighted images demonstrate no interval change in the appearance or size of a 5-mm unilocular pancreatic cyst noted in the body of the pancreas (*arrow*). Additional images revealed no communication with the pancreatic duct. The time interval between (A) and (B) was 3.5 years. Given the appearance and stability of the cyst, this is easily classified as nonaggressive pancreatic cyst. Additional nonaggressive unilocular cysts throughout the pancreas (not shown) remained unchanged over the imaging interval.

abscess from infected pancreatic necrosis. The implications of this distinction are not trivial as there is higher mortality associated with infected necrosis, and management options may differ.[74,95,145,146] It should be noted that abscess formation following elective pancreatic surgery is more properly defined as a postoperative abscess and not pancreatic abscess.[74]

On CT, pancreatic abscess appears as a poorly defined or partially circumscribed complex peripancreatic collection. The attenuation of the collection contents are greater than simple fluid, typically ranging from 20 to 50 HU.[75] The presence of gas bubbles within the collection is not entirely specific for abscess; however, their absence does not exclude the diagnosis of abscess in the appropriate clinical setting (see Figure 5-37).[70] Peripheral enhancement following contrast enhancement is typically present. In general, MRI imaging findings of pancreatic abscess include low signal intensity on T1-weighted images and intermediate to high T2 signal intensity on T2-weighted images.[76] If there is high protein content, T1 signal may be increased. Thick peripheral enhancement is seen following the administration of gadolinium. Although CT is more sensitive than MR in detecting gas, gas bubbles within the collection may manifest as foci of very low signal on T2-weighted sequences.[76]

Disruption of the Gland: Pancreatic Trauma

Traumatic injury to the pancreas is relatively uncommon, occurring in 2% to 12% of patients with blunt-force trauma to the abdomen.[77,81,147] In the setting of blunt trauma, pancreatic injury invariably results from a direct blow to the epigastrium, with motor vehicle collisions accounting for the vast majority of blunt traumatic injury to pancreas in adults.[147] Bicycle injuries and child abuse are common

Imaging Notes 5-13. Differentials for a Solitary Cystic Pancreatic Mass

Cyst Characteristics	Causes
Unilocular, thin walled	Pseudocyst Oligocystic serous cystadenoma Mucinous cystic neoplasm Side branch IPMN Epithelial cyst (Hereditary syndromes)
Unilocular, thick walled	Abscess Necrotic Adenocarcinoma
Multilocular, thin walled	Serous cystadenoma Mucinous cystic neoplasm Solid pseudopapillary tumor Side branch IPMN
Multilocular, thick walled	Malignant mucinous cystic neoplasm Solid pseudopapillary tumor
Uni-/Multilocular, mural nodule	Mucinous cystic neoplasm Side branch IPMN

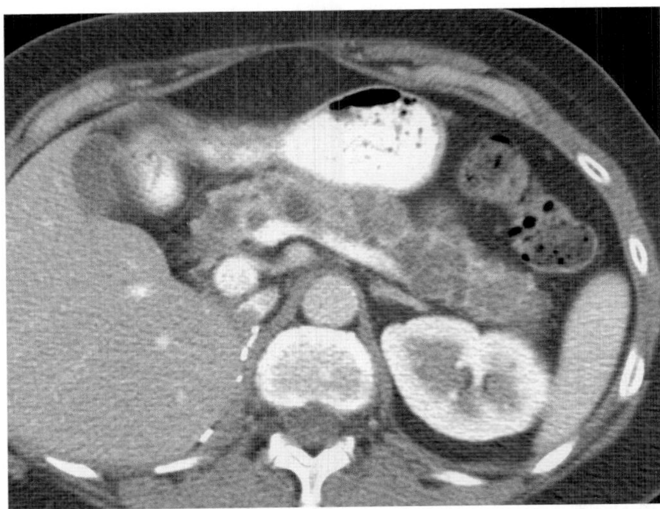

Figure 5-35 Pancreatic Cysts due to Von Hippel-Lindau Syndrome This patient with von Hippel-Lindau syndrome was being evaluated for surveillance of renal cell carcinoma. Contrast-enhanced CT through the midbody of the pancreas demonstrates multiple pancreatic cysts.

causes of pancreatic trauma in children and infants, respectively.[77] Penetrating trauma (eg, gunshot and stab wounds) accounts for other sources of pancreatic injuries.

Isolated pancreatic injury rarely occurs with blunt abdominal trauma. Injuries to the liver, duodenum, and superior mesenteric vessels are often associated with injuries to the pancreatic head and neck, whereas splenic injuries are associated with pancreatic tail injuries.[78] Early mortality is often secondary to these associated injuries, in particular vascular injuries.[79] Delayed morbidity and mortality are often related to complications arising from main pancreatic duct disruption, and include pancreatitis, necrosis, and pseudocyst and peripancreatic abscess formation.[79,147] Delayed diagnosis of main pancreatic duct injury places the patient at increased risk for pancreatic complications, and several factors have been identified predisposing to missed or delayed diagnosis of pancreatic injury, including the nonspecific nature of symptoms and clinical findings seen in pancreatic trauma.[80] The presence of few or no other abdominal injuries also appears to be a contributing factor in cases of delayed diagnosis.

Contrast-enhanced CT is the first-line imaging modality in assessing abdominal trauma but is only of moderate sensitivity in detecting pancreatic injury.[148,149] Direct signs of pancreatic trauma include laceration, complete transection, and comminution of the pancreas, which all may be manifested as low-attenuation lines through the gland (see Figure 5-38). Hematoma and active extravasation of intravenous contrast may be identified at the site of parenchymal disruption. Secondary signs of pancreatic injury include diffuse enlargement of the pancreas, heterogenous enhancement, peripancreatic fat stranding, fluid between the pancreas and splenic vein, and thickening of the left anterior renal fascia.[147] As no pancreatic abnormality may be detected initially, a repeat CT study may be helpful in cases of suspected pancreatic trauma.[78]

Disruption of the main pancreatic duct is poorly evaluated by CT although the severity of pancreatic injury may suggest its presence. In fact, one group developed a CT grading system of pancreatic laceration that parallels the surgical grading system of pancreatic injury (see Table 5-5).[81] The grade of injury is determined by the depth of the laceration, with superficial lacerations involving less

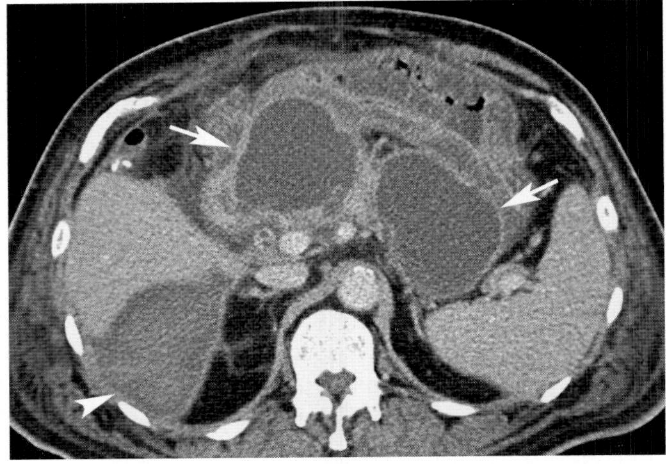

A

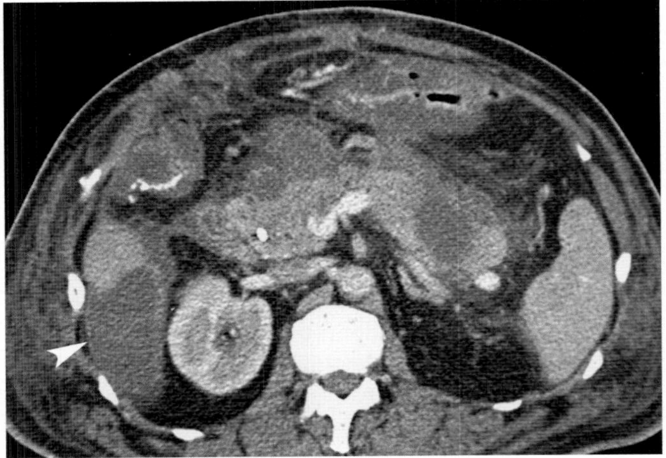

B

Figure 5-36 Pancreatic Pseudocyst
This 69-year-old man developed abdominal pain following ERCP. **A** and **B.** Enhanced CT demonstrates 2 large rim-enhancing fluid collections (*arrows*) in the body and tail of the pancreas. This is a common appearance of pancreatic pseudocysts. There is also peripancreatic fat stranding and an area of hemorrhagic acites (*arrowheads*) posterior to the liver.

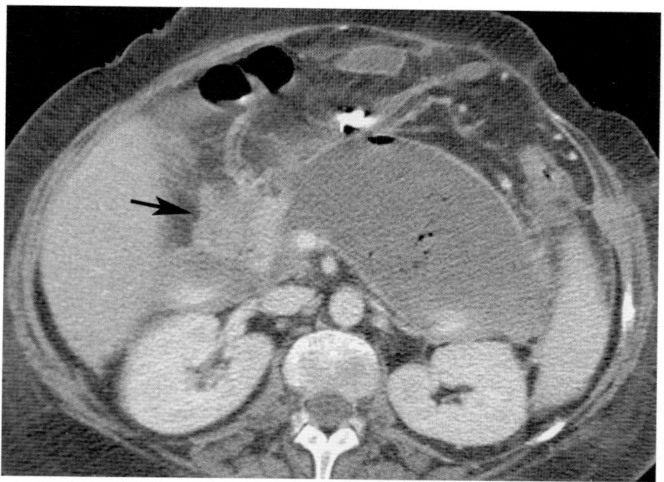

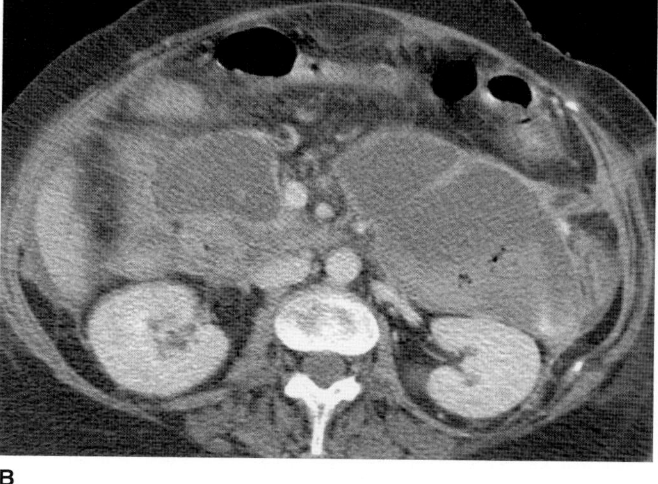

Figure 5-37 Pancreatic Abscess
This 48-year-old woman had undergone ERCP when she developed abdominal pain, fever, and increased amylase and lipase. **A** and **B.** Enhanced CT demonstrates a large rim-enhancing fluid collection in the expected location of the pancreatic body and tail. The fluid collection contains multiple small bubbles of gas, indicating the presence of infection. A small portion of the residual pancreatic head (*arrow*) is seen in A.

than 50% of the gland and deep lacerations involving 50% or more of the gland. Location of the injury is another factor in categorizing the severity of pancreatic injury, with the superior mesenteric artery serving as the boundary between proximal and distal pancreas.

According to this classification schema, CT grade A pancreatic injuries include those with findings of pancreatitis or superficial lacerations to any portion of the pancreas; grade BI injuries include deep lacerations to the distal pancreas; grade BII represent transections to the distal pancreas; grade CI injuries represent deep lacerations to the proximal pancreas; and grade CII injuries represent transections of the proximal pancreas. This CT grading system was found to correlate well with the presence of main pancreatic duct disruption at laparotomy, with CT grade B and C injuries being predictive of pancreatic duct injury.[81]

In cases where pancreatic duct laceration is suspected, ERCP or MRCP are indicated for further evaluation. ERCP is the traditional modality by which the pancreatic duct is directly evaluated.[150] In addition to providing diagnostic information regarding the integrity of the pancreatic duct, ERCP possesses the added advantage of possible therapeutic stenting in cases where the ductal injury is mild and does not necessitate surgical repair. The appropriateness of stenting in the acute setting, however, has been questioned as complications from early stenting often result and include pancreatic duct stricture formation and a subsequent inability to remove the stent.[82] Drawbacks relating to diagnostic ERCP include limited availability in the emergent setting as well as the need for the patient to be clinically stable for the examination. Laceration to the pancreatic duct will manifest as disruption of the duct with extravasation of contrast at the site of injury. In cases of complete transection, the amount of extravasated contrast tends to be large and flows inferiorly and superiorly from the site of disruption, whereas in incomplete transactions only a small amount of contrast tends to leak and does so in only one direction.[150] In cases of side branch injury, opacification of the entire main pancreatic duct may be observed well before contrast leakage is identified within pancreatic parenchyma.[150]

MRCP is the alternative modality in evaluating the pancreatic duct.[7,106,151] Advantages of MRCP include its noninvasive nature and its ability to evaluate the full extent of the main pancreatic duct.[83] The heavily weighted T2 sequences of MRCP demonstrate discontinuity of the duct, which is frequently associated with T2 hyperintense pseudocysts.[106,151] Dilation of the duct distal to the ductal injury may also be observed.[83] Another advantage of MRCP over ERCP is that evaluation of the duct may be complemented with conventional MRI of the pancreas, which can provide diagnostic information regarding the degree of parenchymal injury. Lacerations manifest as T2 hyperintense and T1 hypointense lines through the pancreas.[83]

Diffuse Processes of the Pancreas

Diffuse abnormalities of the pancreas include enlargement, atrophy, fatty infiltration, calcification and iron deposition of the gland, and diffuse dilation of the pancreatic duct.

Diffuse pancreatic enlargement

Acute and autoimmune pancreatitis are the most common causes of diffuse pancreatic enlargement although

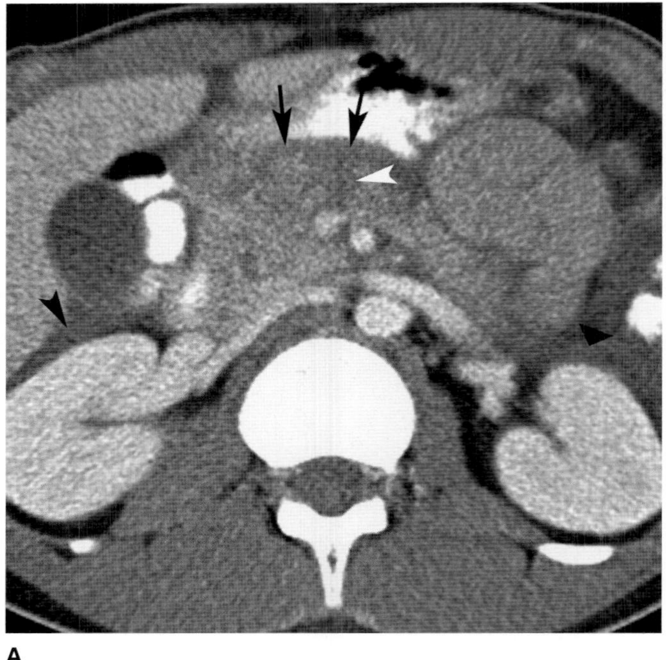

A

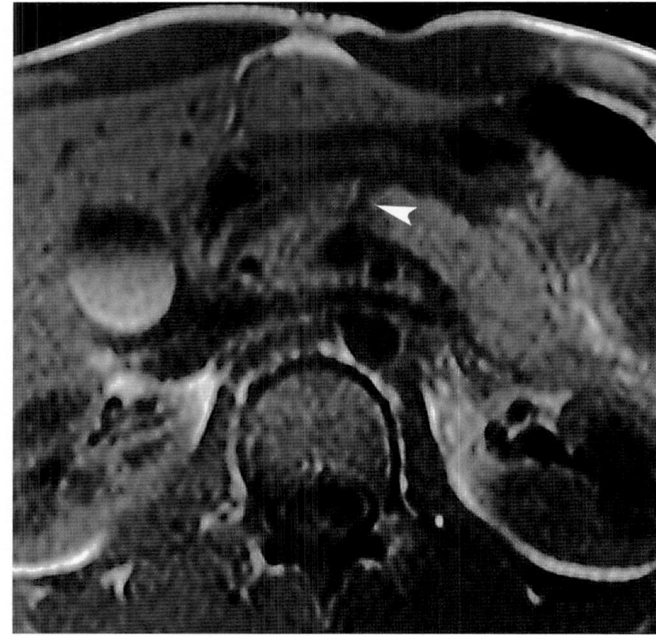

B

C

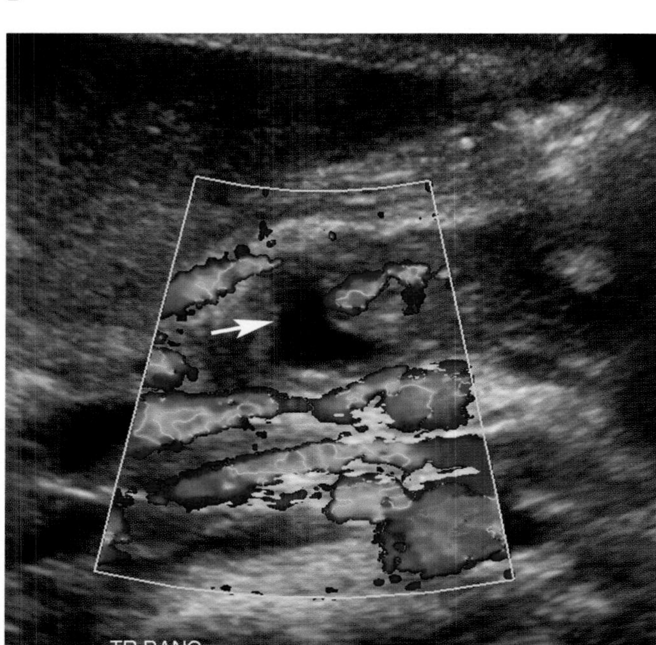

D

Figure 5-38 Pancreatic Laceration
This 16-year-old male was assaulted and suffered trauma to the abdomen. **A.** Contrast-enhanced CT demonstrates a low attenuation line through the pancreatic neck (*white arrowhead*), consistent with a pancreatic laceration. Secondary signs of pancreatic trauma are present, including peripancreatic fluid anterior to the pancreas (*black arrows*) and fluid in the anterior pararenal spaces bilaterally (*black arrowhead*). **B.** Fat-suppressed T1-weighted MR image reveals a low signal line through the pancreatic neck (*white arrowhead*), corresponding to the pancreatic laceration. **C.** Fat-suppressed T2-weighted MR image demonstrates increased signal within the pancreatic head and neck (*asterisk*), consistent with edema. High signal fluid is present anterior to the pancreas (*white arrows*) and within the retroperitoneum (*black arrowheads*). **D.** Transabdominal US at the level of the pancreatic neck reveals an anechoic avascular area (*arrow*) in the pancreatic neck, consistent with known laceration.

Table 5-5. Grading System for Pancreatic Trauma

Grade	CT Findings
A	Gland edema, peripancreatic fat stranding, superficial[a] lacerations
B1	Deep laceration distal[b] pancreas
B2	Transection of distal pancreas
C1	Deep laceration to proximal pancreas
C2	Transection of proximal pancreas

[a]Superficial lacerations involve less than 50% of the thickness of the gland while deep lacerations involve 50% or more of the thickness of the gland.
[b]The superior mesenteric artery serves as the boundary between the proximal and distal pancreas.

Table 5-7. Causes of Acute Pancreatitis

1. Alcohol abuse
2. Cholelithiasis
3. Idiopathic (possibly due to biliary sludge)
4. Trauma
5. Lipoproteinemia
6. Sepsis
7. Vasculitis
8. Congenital anomalies a. Annular pancreas b. Pancreas divisum
9. Medications

occasionally other causes, such as pancreatic lymphoma and trauma, may result in a diffusely enlarged gland (Table 5-6).

Acute pancreatitis: Acute pancreatitis is an acute inflammation of the pancreas caused by premature activation of pancreatic enzymes into the pancreatic parenchyma and surrounding tissues with resultant autodigestion of the pancreas and surrounding fat.

In the United States, alcohol abuse and cholelithiasis account for the vast majority of cases of acute pancreatitis. There is regional variability in the degree to which each of these 2 causes constitute the precipitating event, with alcohol abuse accounting for a greater number of cases in urban areas and Veterans Affairs hospitals, and cholelithiasis resulting in more cases in suburban and rural hospitals.[84] Other causes of acute pancreatitis include trauma, lipoproteinemia, sepsis, vasculitis, and some medications. No etiology can be identified for 10% to 30% of cases of acute pancreatitis and these are therefore considered "idiopathic."[152] Several studies suggest that these cases of idiopathic acute pancreatitis in fact may be secondary to biliary sludge (see Table 5-7).[152-156] In all cases, a concerted effort should be made to determine the etiology of acute pancreatitis so that recurrent episodes of acute pancreatitis and its associated complications may be prevented.

The exact pathogenesis of acute pancreatitis is incompletely understood; however, the accepted theory is that a precipitating event causes injury to the pancreatic acinar cell, leading to inappropriate activation and release of pancreatic enzymes into the pancreatic parenchyma and peripancreatic structures.[85,157] This initial injury then results in generalized inflammatory response, mediated by a cascade of chemokines and other inflammatory mediators. In approximately 75% of patients, damage is confined to the pancreatic parenchyma or the peripancreatic structures and these patients will most often experience a self-limited uneventful clinical course, a phenomenon that can be called "simple pancreatitis." A more severe and systemic inflammatory response occurs in the remaining cases, which places the patient at high risk for multiorgan dysfunction and death.[85] Deaths secondary to acute pancreatitis fall within two temporal categories, early and late.[86] In the former, the exaggerated systemic inflammatory response causes multiorgan system dysfunction and death usually within the first week. Those patients surviving this more acute clinical course typically proceed to extensive pancreatic and retroperitoneal necrosis, which is then complicated by infection, sepsis, and a continued systemic inflammatory response with resultant late multiorgan failure and death. Death rates as high as 50% can be seen in this smaller subset of cases with severe complicated pancreatitis.[85,158,159]

Common presenting symptoms include mid epigastric pain that can radiate to the back, nausea, vomiting, fever, and tachycardia. Severe cases can present with shock and hypotension. The diagnosis of simple pancreatitis is based on clinical symptoms, physical examination, and laboratory evaluation of serum amylase and lipase. The role for imaging in patients with pancreatitis lies in the evaluation for complications, specifically pseudocyst formation, pancreatic necrosis, hemorrhage, and pseudoaneurysm formation.

In general, CT is the imaging modality of choice in pancreatitis because of its speed, ready availability, and accuracy

Table 5-6. Causes of Diffuse Pancreatitic Enlargement

1. Acute pancreatitis
2. Autoimmune pancreatitis
3. Blunt trauma
4. Lymphoma

in evaluating the pancreas and surrounding abdominal and retroperitoneal structures. Nevertheless, consideration should be given to alternate methods of imaging, especially in younger individuals, as radiation dose exposure is not trivial. Thus, MRI is often a suitable alternative as the abdominal and retroperitoneal structures may be evaluated without radiation exposure. Further, MRI performed with MRCP is of additional utility as causes of pancreatitis, such as cholelithiasis, annular pancreas and pancreas divisum, can be identified.[7,113,160-162] US is somewhat limited in the evaluation of acute pancreatitis.[67] Nevertheless, US can play a secondary role in the evaluation of pancreatitis as it may identify gallstones and biliary ductal dilation secondary to choledocholithiasis, thereby helping identify those patients for which ERCP may be appropriate.

Simple pancreatitis: In some cases of enzymatically proven acute pancreatitis, imaging of the gland will appear normal on all imaging modalities. However, in most cases edema of the gland, results in diffuse enlargement (see Figure 5-39). Since there is progressive atrophy of the pancreatic gland with aging, identifying pancreatic enlargement on the basis of measurements alone can underdiagnose simple pancreatitis. Therefore it is important to look for secondary signs of pancreatitis, such as the loss of the normal lobulated pancreatic contour and evidence of pancreatic edema. On CT, pancreatic edema will appear as decreased attenuation of the pancreas.[74,88,163,164] On MR, pancreatic edema will result in increased signal intensity on T2-weighted sequences and decreased signal intensity on unenhanced T1-weighted sequences (see Figure 5-40). Primarily because of its greater sensitivity for the presence of edema, unenhanced MRI has been demonstrated to be more sensitive than CT in detecting mild acute simple pancreatitis.[87] When imaged by US, the pancreatic edema will appear as decreased echogenicity of the normally very echogenic pancreas (see Figure 5-41).[72]

In addition to the radiographic changes of the pancreatic parenchyma, CT and MRI will often demonstrate edema in the peripancreatic fat, appearing as streaky lines radiating from the pancreas or nonorganized peripancreatic and retroperitoneal fluid with imaging characteristics typical of water (see Figure 5-42).

Other imaging modalities such as abdominal and chest plain radiographs are not used in the evaluation of acute pancreatitis; however, one specific plain radiograph finding, the "colon cutoff sign," deserves special mention as this may suggest the diagnosis.[165-167] The colon cutoff sign is a classic plain film finding characterized by a colonic ileus with distention of the transverse colon, focal narrowing of the splenic flexure, and a paucity of bowel gas in the descending and distal colon. This finding owes to spasm of the splenic flexure secondary to inflammation spreading from the pancreas to the phrenicocolic ligament (see Figure 5-43).

Complications of pancreatitis: In 1992, the International Symposium of Acute Pancreatitis convened to formally define a number of terms related to the complications of acute pancreatitis.[74] These include *acute fluid collections, acute pancreatic pseudocysts, pancreatic abscesses,* and several forms of *pancreatic necrosis.* Standardization of these terms was deemed necessary as considerable variability in the use of these terms existed previously, which often led to imprecise and poor communication. Several terms should be avoided as they have resulted in confusion and/or inappropriate management.[74] These include *pancreatic phlegmon*

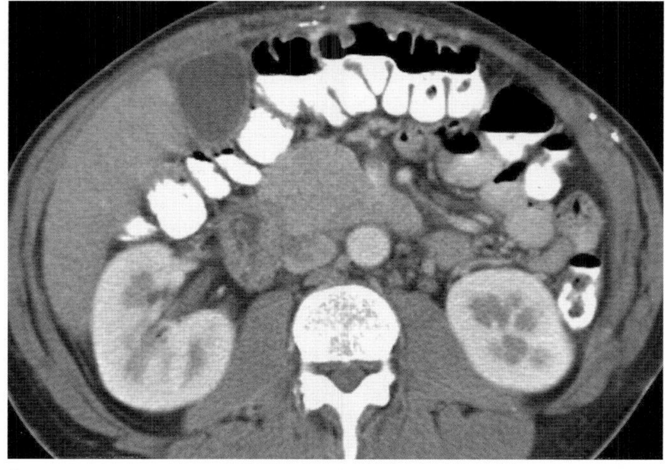

A

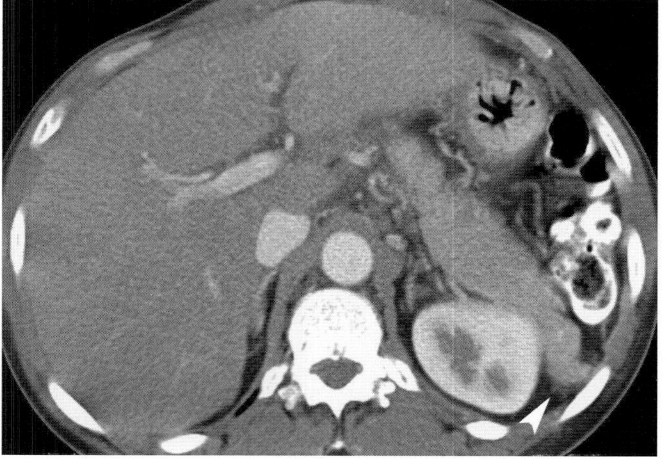

B

Figure 5-39 Simple Pancreatitis
Abdominal pain was the presenting complaint in this 55-year-old alcoholic man. Serum amylase and lipase were both elevated. **A** and **B.** Contiguous enhanced CT images through the pancreas demonstrate diffuse enlargement of the pancreas. A small amount of peripancreatic stranding is seen (B), which is best identified along the pancreatic tail (*arrowhead*). The pancreas enhances uniformly and there is no evidence of parenchymal necrosis. The combined clinical, laboratory, and imaging findings are consistent with simple acute pancreatitis.

Imaging Notes 5-14. Complications of Pancreatitis

Complication	Imaging Features
Acute fluid collections: Peripancreatic/retroperitoneal fluid collections without fibrous capsule	Irregularly shaped retroperitoneal fluid collections
Acute pancreatic pseudocysts Noninfected peripancreatic/ retroperitoneal fluid collections with a fibrous capsule	Round/oval encapsulated, thin walled fluid collection
Pancreatic abscesses Infected encapsulated peripancreatic/ retroperitoneal fluid collection	Round/oval encapsulated, usually thick wall fluid collection. Occ gas within collection
Pancreatic necrosis Nonviable, necrotic pancreatic tissue	Non-enhancing region of pancreas CT—low attenuation MRI—high T2 signal
Subtypes pancreatic necrosis	
Organizing pancreatic necrosis Encapsulated pancreatic collection Containing debris, semisolid tissue	Heterogenous cystic intrapancreatic collection can contain internal debris, solid elements
Central pancreatic necrosis Focal midpancreatic fluid collection Viable, pancreatic tissue proximal and distal to collection	Sausage-shaped fluid collection in mid gland enhancing head and tail of pancreas disrupted pancreatic duct
Extrapancreatic necrosis Necrosis peripancreatic fat	Uniformly enhancing pancreas heterogeneous pancreatic collection

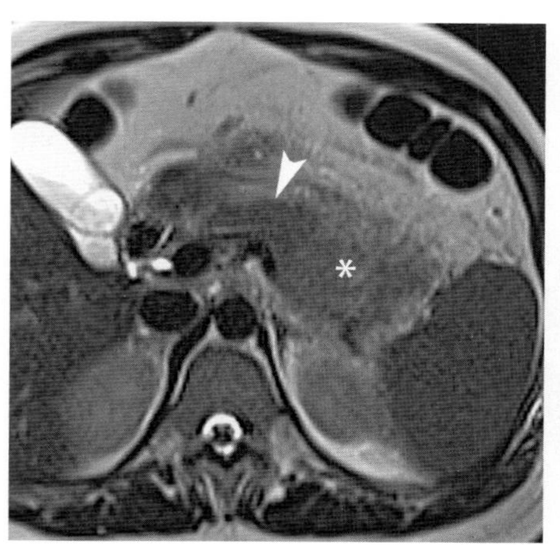
A

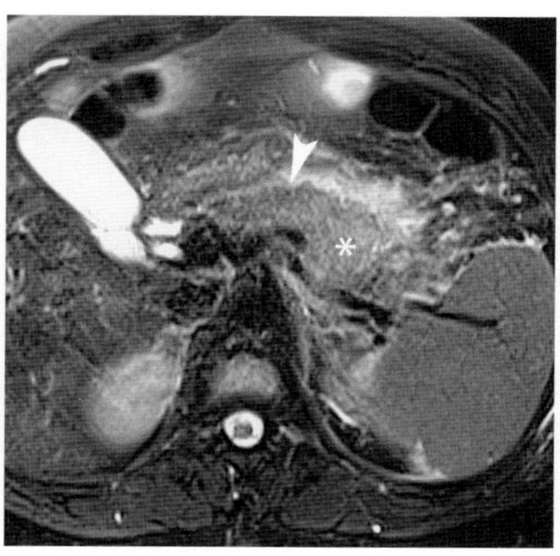
B

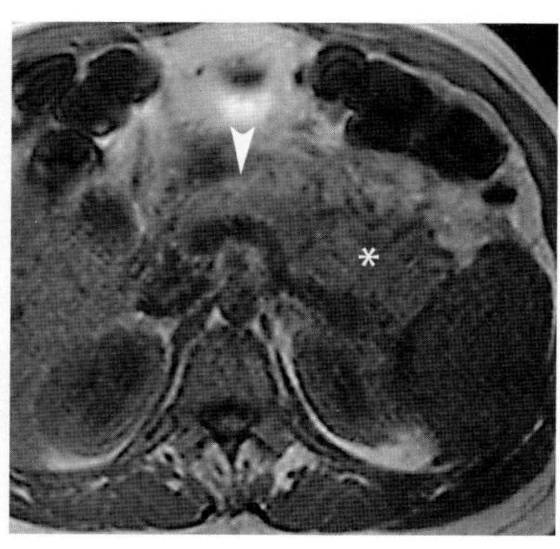
C

Figure 5-40 Acute Pancreatitis
MRI findings of acute pancreatitis are well demonstrated on this 29-year-old woman. There is enlargement of the distal pancreatic body and tail and there is signal abnormality within the involved gland characteristic of edema. Specifically, increased signal is observed in the enlarged pancreatic body and tail (*asterisk*) on T2-weighted (**A**) and fat-suppressed T2-weighted (**B**) sequences. Normal pancreatic body is denoted by the *white arrowheads.* Nonenhanced T1-weighted images (**C**) demonstrate decreased signal within the affected gland (*asterisk*), consistent with edema. Again, normal pancreatic body is indicated by the *white arrowhead.* There were no findings of pancreatic necrosis as uniform enhancement of the gland was observed on postcontrast sequences (not shown).

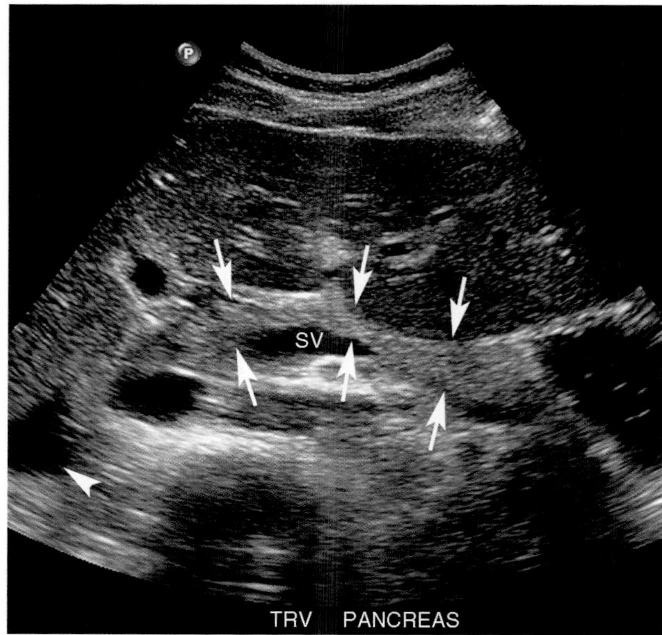

A

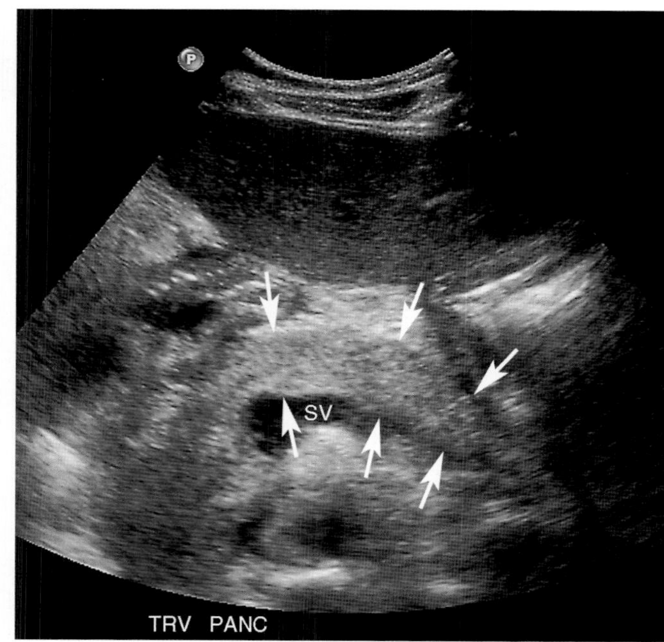

B

Figure 5-41 Ultrasound of Acute Pancreatitis
This 31-year-old female was admitted for Tylenol overdose and fulminant hepatic failure. She subsequently developed abdominal pain and elevated serum lipase and amylase levels, consistent with acute pancreatitis. **A.** US of the pancreas (*arrows*) obtained on admission demonstrates no sonographic findings of acute pancreatitis. A small amount of perihepatic ascites is noted (*arrowhead*). **B.** Abdominal US performed 9 days later demonstrates interval enlargement of the pancreas (*arrows*). Pancreatic parenchymal echogenicity is maintained. Images in (A) and (B) were obtained at equivalent levels through the pancreatic neck and body. SV, splenic vein.

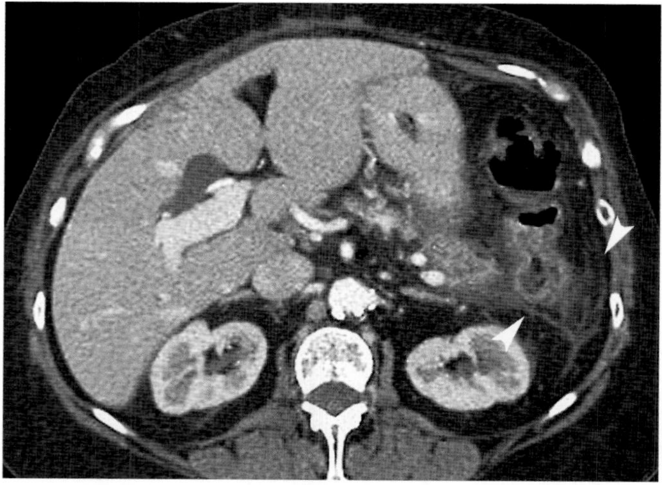

A

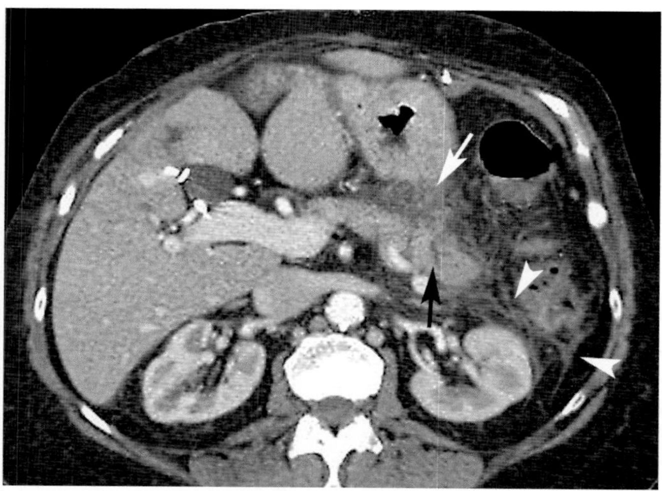

B

Figure 5-42 Simple Pancreatitis
This 47-year-old male complained of abdominal pain. **A** and **B.** CT images demonstrate edema of the tail of the pancreas seen as areas of low attenuation (*black arrow*), edema of the tissues surrounding the tail of the pancreas (*white arrow*), and stranding of the retroperitoneal fat (*arrowheads*). This is the typical appearance of uncomplicated pancreatitis.

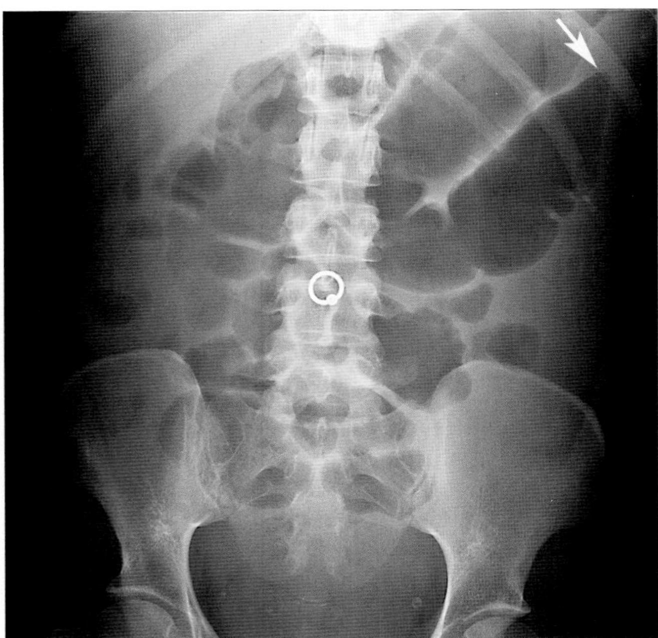

Figure 5-43 Colon Cutoff Sign
Abdominal radiograph of the same 31-year-old woman in Figure 5-40 admitted for Tylenol overdose and fulminant hepatic failure with subsequent acute pancreatitis. There is gaseous distention of the colon to the level of the splenic flexure (*arrow*) with no gas identified in the descending colon. This abrupt transition in colonic caliber has been termed the "colon cutoff sign" and may be identified in cases of acute pancreatitis.

and *infected pseudocyst*. Furthermore, the term *hemorrhagic pancreatic necrosis* should be avoided in radiologic reports as this is a gross morphologic definition made at surgery or autopsy.

Acute fluid collections: Acute fluid collections are commonly seen in acute pancreatitis and may be present in 30% to 50% of severe cases of pancreatitis.[138,168] These arise during the early phase of pancreatitis, are located in the retroperitoneal soft tissues, and lack a fibrous capsule or surrounding granulation tissue, which distinguishes them from pseudocysts and abscess. Dissection of pancreatic enzymes can lead to acute fluid collections remote from the pancreas extending along the retroperitoneal fascial planes (eg, lesser sac and anterior pararenal space) in addition to close proximity to the pancreas (see Figure 5-36). These collections may spontaneously regress or proceed to form pseudocysts or abscesses.[138,168]

Pancreatic pseudocysts and pancreatic abscess: *Acute pancreatic pseudocysts* are well-defined collections of pancreatic enzymes and secretions with a thin fibrous pseudocapsule whereas *pancreatic abscesses* represent peripancreatic collections of pus. These complications of acute pancreatitis typically present as focal lesions and are covered in greater detail under the heading: **Cystic Masses of the Pancreas**.

Pancreatic necrosis: Pancreatic necrosis connotes areas of nonviable pancreatic parenchyma secondary to autodigestion by released pancreatic enzymes. This occurs in cases of more severe pancreatitis and may be multifocal or diffuse in distribution. Sterile and infected forms of pancreatic necrosis occur and cannot be distinguished by imaging alone.[73,169,170] Transcutaneous needle aspiration is necessary to document the presence of superimposed infection.[68,73,171,172] Conservative management is appropriate in cases of sterile necrosis. Infected necrosis often requires debridement because of the high risk of death without intervention.[88,146]

On CT and MRI examinations, pancreatic necrosis is indicated by absent enhancement and can be seen in up to 21% of cases of acute pancreatitis.[88] This term is generally restricted to those cases in which there is a well-marginated area of decreased enhancement of at least 3 cm or decreased enhancement of at least 30% of the pancreas,[74,89] as considerably higher degrees of morbidity and mortality are seen above these thresholds.[89] On unenhanced CT, the pancreas normally demonstrates an attenuation value of approximately 30 to 50 HU; following the administration of contrast, the pancreas uniformly enhances with attenuation values of approximately 100 to 150 HU.[169,173] Focal or diffuse areas of devitalized pancreatic parenchyma will lack this expected uniform enhancement and appear as areas of low attenuation (see Figures 5-44 and 5-45). Areas that do not demonstrate at least 30 HU of enhancement should be considered highly suspicious for necrosis.[90] Occasionally, necrosis can be complicated by hemorrhage and the presence of high-attenuation acute blood may obscure areas of necrosis on enhanced scans. Therefore, combined unenhanced and enhanced CT scans may be helpful in cases of suspected necrosis with hemorrhage.

Although CT is considered to be the reference standard for evaluating pancreatic necrosis, several studies have demonstrated MRI to be equivalent, with MRI exhibiting similar imaging findings, namely, the absence of parenchymal enhancement on postcontrast T1-weighted sequences.[91,174,175] Necrosis may also be identified on T2-weighted sequences as a sharply defined area of increased T2 signal intensity.[91,174,176] Although one recent study demonstrated that nonenhanced MRI is comparable to contrast-enhanced CT in detecting early acute pancreatitis,[176] evaluation of the pancreas following the administration of gadolinium may still be necessary as it may be difficult to differentiate areas of necrosis from peripancreatic fluid collections on T2-weighted sequences.[91] In cases of necrosis complicated by acute hemorrhage, increased T1 and T2 signal relative to pancreas and increased signal on fat-suppressed T1 imaging may be observed.[176,177]

Three special forms of pancreatic necrosis deserve mention: organizing pancreatic necrosis, central gland necrosis, and extrapancreatic necrosis. Organizing pancreatic necrosis and central gland necrosis are discussed in this section as they tend to be focal abnormalities whereas extrapancreatic necrosis is discussed in the section on "Diffuse Processes of the Pancreas."

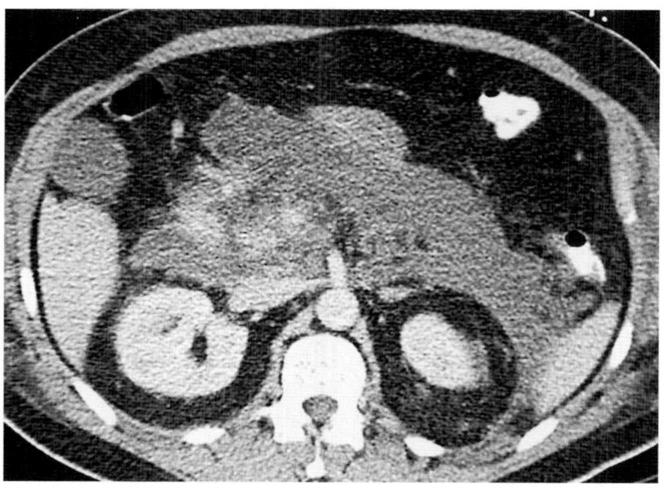
A

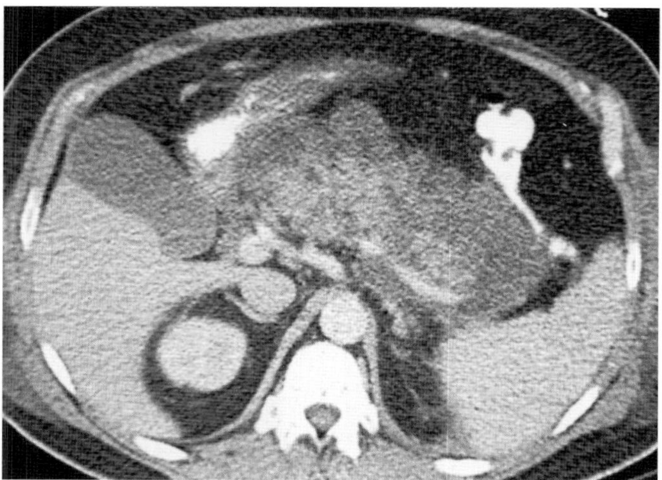
B

Figure 5-44 Necrotizing pancreatitis
This 60-year-old man presented with severe abdominal pain and hypotension. (**A**) Contrast-enhanced CT demonstrates enlargement of the pancreatic head and (**B**) body. Portions of the pancreatic head and body do not enhance, consistent with necrosis. A large amount of peripancreatic fluid is present, which is identified tracking into the left anterior pararenal space (B). No peripheral enhancement of the peripancreatic collection is present to suggest infection; however, this cannot be excluded by imaging alone. The combined findings represent necrotizing pancreatitis.

Organizing pancreatic necrosis: The term and concept of organizing pancreatic necrosis was introduced after the International Symposium of Acute Pancreatitis.[92,178,179] This refers to the development of an encapsulated peripancreatic collection in the setting of underlying pancreatic necrosis. This entity was first described in a series of patients who developed pancreatic necrosis and were treated conservatively.[92] Unlike pancreatic pseudocysts, abscesses, and necrosis, which are considered acute processes, organizing pancreatic necrosis is a subacute process, with the contents of the collection representing varying stages of liquefying pancreatic and peripancreatic tissue. Recognizing organizing pancreatic necrosis is important as the presence of necrotic debris places the patient at high risk for complicating infection. Moreover, the identification of organizing pancreatic necrosis necessitates more aggressive intervention (eg, combined large-bore endoscopic drainage catheters, irrigation, and intrapancreatic lavage catheter) as simple aspiration is often inadequate in removing the necrotic debris.[92]

Organizing pancreatic necrosis may appear very similar to pseudocysts on CT, MR, and US examinations; however, several findings can allow for discrimination between these two entities. Serial examinations typically demonstrate a developing heterogeneous cystic lesion with a partial or complete wall.[92,93,97] They replace the necrotic portions of the pancreatic bed and tend not to be peripancreatic in location.[93] As this entity evolves, the heterogeneous contents may become more homogenous as its necrotic contents undergo further liquefaction.[92,93,179] As liquefaction proceeds, the attenuation of the cystic contents approaches that of fluid on CT.[179] The detection of any debris by imaging within a cystic lesion should suggest organizing pancreatic necrosis in a patient with history of pancreatitis and pancreatic necrosis. In one study, MRI was shown to be superior to CT in detecting necrotic debris with a sensitivity and specificity of 100%.[179] Although it is not recommended that MRI be routinely used in the evaluation of severe acute pancreatitis, MRI evaluation has been suggested in those patients where necrotic debris is suspected and for which drainage is considered.[93,179]

Central pancreatic necrosis: Central pancreatic necrosis refers to necrosis of the body or body and portions of the head and/or tail.[94] Histologically, very little liquid is present and the lesion consists primarily of gelatinous necrotic pancreatic tissue. Central pancreatic necrosis usually causes disruption of the main pancreatic duct and because the functioning distal gland continues to secrete pancreatic juices, there is spillage of these secretions into the necrotic segment.[95] Complications of this ongoing leakage of pancreatic juices include organizing pancreatic necrosis, and fistulas as well as pancreatic ascites and pleural effusions.[97,180] Aggressive management, including distal pancreatectomy, may be required.[95,97,181-183]

Central pancreatic necrosis was originally described as an intrapancreatic collection having a "sausage shaped" configuration with a rim of peripheral pancreatic tissue, which contains the necrotic collection.[94] The imaging features may also mimic pancreatic pseudocysts. On CT, central gland necrosis is characterized by low-attenuation pancreatic tissue adjacent to normally enhancing pancreatic tail.[94] These findings should raise concern for pancreatic duct disruption.[96] Evaluation with ERCP typically

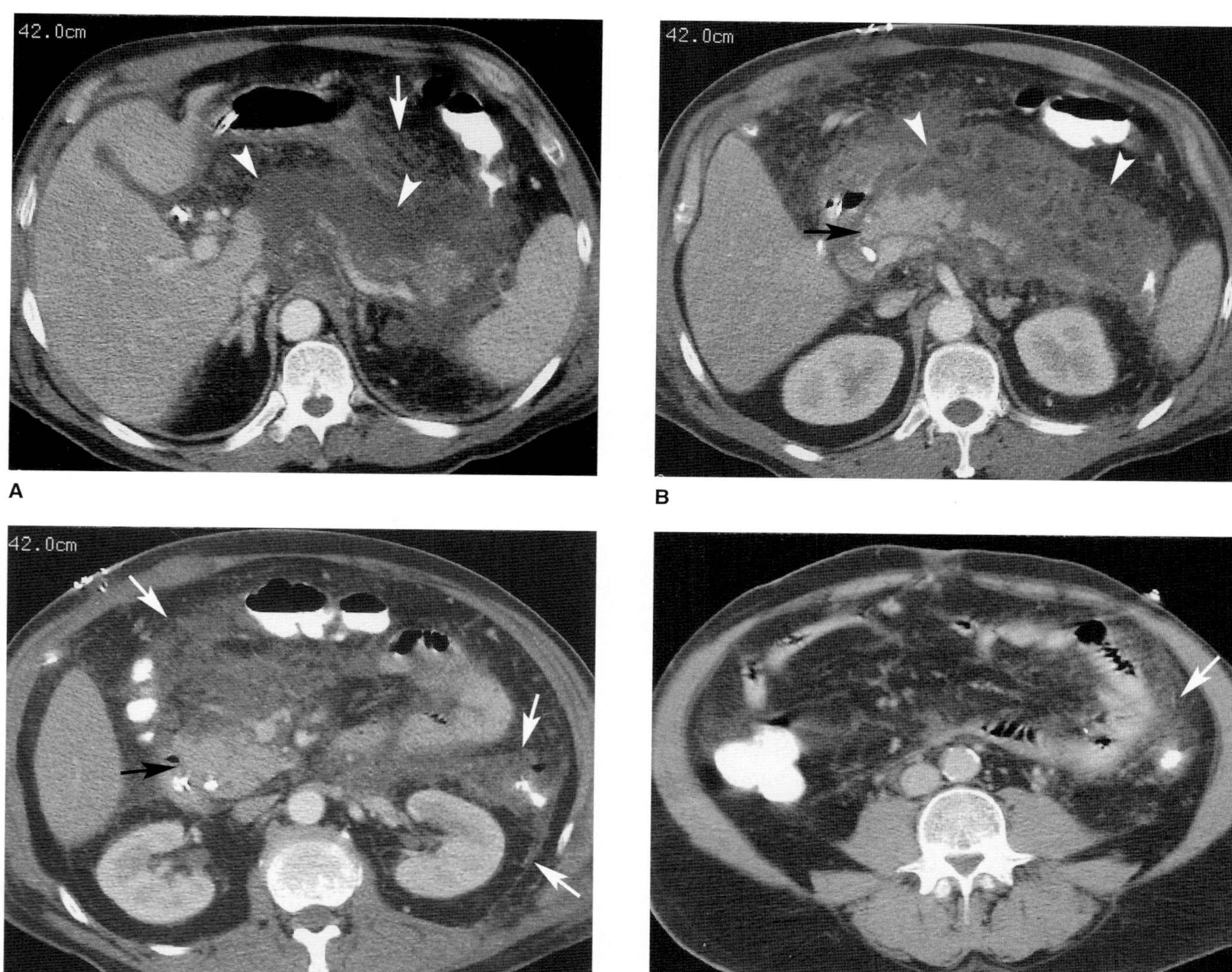

Figure 5-45 Acute Pancreatitis with Pancreatic Necrosis
This 57-year-old man presented with abdominal pain, nausea, vomiting, and hypotension. **A-D.** Enhanced CT images through the upper abdomen demonstrate an enlarged mixed attenuation pancreas (*arrowheads*). There is a small portion of the pancreas that enhances normally (*black arrows*). The remainder is low attenuation typical of pancreatic necrosis. There is also extensive infiltration of the peripancreatic fat and retroperitoneal fat planes (*white arrows*) indicating edema of the surrounding soft tissues.

demonstrates duct obstruction at the site of the intrapancreatic fluid, and extrapancreatic extravasation of contrast at the site of duct obstruction may also be seen.[96] In addition, MRCP has been suggested as an alternative method in evaluating the integrity of the pancreatic duct.[97]

Extrapancreatic necrosis: Extrapancreatic necrosis, a third subtype of pancreatic necrosis, is characterized by necrosis of the peripancreatic and retroperitoneal fat without associated pancreatic necrosis.[97,98] The extent of the extrapancreatic necrosis is not limited to the peripancreatic tissues and may extend into the paracolic gutters and pelvis. Although the etiology of extrapancreatic necrosis is unclear, the prevailing hypothesis is that pancreatic enzymes are released into adjacent tissues with resultant fat necrosis, hemorrhage, and infection.[98] Interestingly, there appears to be decreased morbidity and mortality associated with extrapancreatic necrosis compared to cases of pancreatic necrosis.[98] Not surprisingly, though, the morbidity and mortality associated with extrapancreatic necrosis seems directly related to the extent of extrapancreatic necrosis.[98]

To date, the imaging findings of extrapancreatic pancreatic necrosis have only been described for contrast-enhanced CT.[97,98] The key imaging features of extrapancreatic necrosis are a uniformly enhancing pancreas with a homogenous or heterogeneous peripancreatic collection. Diffuse pancreatic enlargement may also be noted (see Figure 5-46). Unfortunately, CT is limited in its ability to determine the extent of peripancreatic fat necrosis and is unable to discriminate between simple collections from those with necrotic debris.[67,68,98] Therefore, even simple-appearing peripancreatic collections should be viewed as potentially containing necrotic components that may be already infected or at considerable risk for infection. Should surgical management be required, alerting the surgeon to the suspicion for extrapancreatic necrosis is important as manipulation of the pancreas should be avoided at necrosectomy in order to avoid further pancreatic injury.[98] Moreover, the radiologic extent of necrosis should be reported to ensure that those areas are sufficiently explored and debrided.[98]

Autoimmune pancreatitis: Autoimmune pancreatitis is a rare form of chronic pancreatitis and was originally described in a subset of patients with chronic pancreatitis.[99] These patients were noted to have an atypical presentation that was characterized by minimal abdominal pain, hypergammaglobulinemia, and a destructive inflammatory sclerosis of the pancreas. More recently, autoimmune pancreatitis has become more widely recognized as a form of chronic pancreatitis and although the exact pathogenesis of this entity remains incompletely understood, the prevailing hypothesis is that this results from an autoimmune process.

Autoimmune pancreatitis is most commonly seen in elderly men and is currently characterized by a number of clinical, laboratory, histologic, and imaging findings.[184,185] Patients may be asymptomatic or present with only mild abdominal pain. Occasionally, patients may present with painless obstructive jaundice, which results from intrapancreatic narrowing of the common bile duct.[186] This entity can be confused with obstruction due to pancreatic adenocarcinoma.[187,188] Laboratory findings include elevated levels of serum γ-globulin, IgG, and/or IgG4. Autoantibodies and elevated pancreatic enzymes are also commonly observed. Histologically, autoimmune pancreatitis is characterized by lymphocytic infiltration and parenchymal fibrosis.[185,189,190] Response to corticosteroid therapy is a hallmark of autoimmune pancreatitis.

At imaging, there is typically diffuse enlargement of the pancreas[96,100,184,186,191] and loss of the normal lobulated pancreatic contour,[191] findings that are somewhat subjective but that can be identified by CT and MRI. This diffuse enlargement has been referred to as a sausage-like appearance.[96] Occasionally, there may be more focal or segmental enlargement of the pancreas, which may be difficult to discriminate from pancreatic malignancy.[100,186,191] Contrast-enhanced CT will typically demonstrate decreased enhancement of the involved pancreas on the pancreatic phase of enhancement but similar enhancement on the hepatic phase of enhancement.[100] Although these CT findings may mimic pancreatic adenocarcinoma, the results of one recent study suggest that distinguishing autoimmune

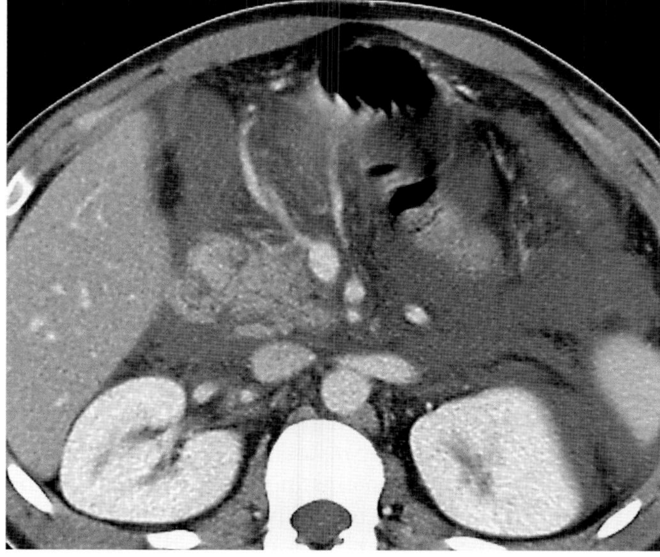
A

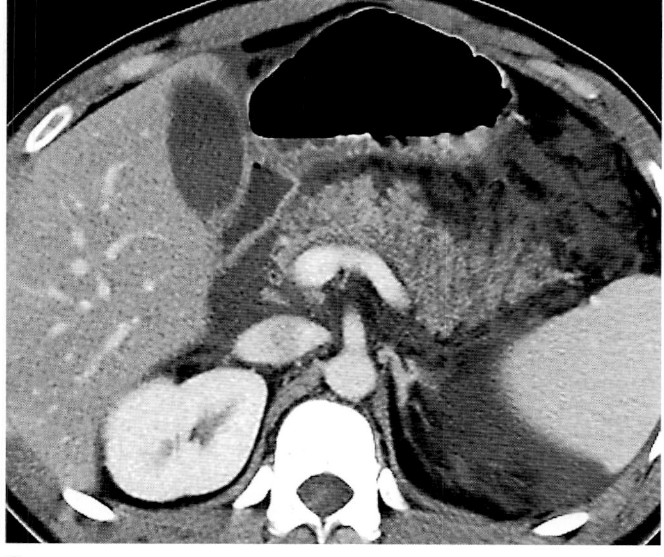
B

Figure 5-46 Extrapancreatic Necrosis in Acute Pancreatitis This 21-year-old man developed acute pancreatitis after a drinking binge on St. Patrick's Day. The pancreatic head (**A**) and body (**B**) demonstrate diffuse enlargement. There is no evidence of pancreatic necrosis as the pancreas demonstrates uniform enhancement. Extensive peripancreatic fluid collections are present and there is inflammatory stranding of the mesenteric fat—finding suggesting extrapancreatic necrosis. There is also moderate acites surrounding the spleen.

pancreatitis from pancreatic adenocarcinoma may be possible using the enhancement pattern.[100] Specifically, these authors found that although the two demonstrate similar attenuation on unenhanced scans and during the pancreatic phase of enhancement, the mean attenuation value of the parenchyma in autoimmune pancreatitis (90 HU) was significantly greater than that of pancreatic adenocarcinoma (64 HU) during the portal venous phase of enhancement. On MRI, there is decreased T1 signal and slightly increased T2 signal of the affected pancreas, and postgadolinium sequences will demonstrate decreased and heterogeneous enhancement on early and late phases of enhancement.[96,186,191] A peripheral rim of tissue can be identified by CT and MRI in some cases.[96,186,192] This peripheral rind is believed to represent an inflammatory infiltrate[96] and is low attenuation on contrast-enhanced CT and hypointense relative to the pancreas on T1- and T2-weighted sequences.[96,186] Diffuse or segmental narrowing of the main pancreatic duct is another feature of autoimmune pancreatitis and this may be detected at ERCP and MRCP.[186,191] Diffuse intrahepatic biliary strictures also may be detected at MRCP.[191] Resolution of these imaging findings following corticosteroid therapy is strongly suggestive of a diagnosis of autoimmune pancreatitis.

Pancreatic lymphoma: Occasionally, lymphoma may involve the entire pancreas and manifest as a diffusely enlarged gland. Such cases are difficult to distinguish from acute pancreatitis both clinically and radiographically. As noted previously, pancreatic lymphoma is hypoattenuating to isoattenuating to normal pancreas on unenhanced CT and hypoattenuating to normal pancreas following contrast administration;[83,85] however, the lack of normal enhancing pancreas may complicate interpretation. The signal characteristics of diffuse pancreatic lymphoma are similar to the focal form, namely homogenous low T1 signal and heterogeneous low to moderate T2 signal relative to normal pancreas.[81,82] Post contrast administration, small foci of nonenhancement may be present[34] and may be the only clue to diffuse pancreatic lymphoma.

Pancreatic trauma: Traumatic injury to the pancreas can result in diffuse pancreatic enlargement, which CT, MRI, and US will demonstrate. In the vast majority of cases, an accompanying history of trauma provides an explanation for the imaging findings. Pancreatic trauma is covered more completely under the heading: **Disruption of the Gland: Pancreatic Trauma**.

Pancreatic atrophy

As individuals age, the volume of pancreatic glandular tissue will usually diminish, resulting in a thinner gland. The gland will also decrease in attenuation as a result of fatty infiltration of the gland (see Figure 5-47). In most cases, this process has no clinical significance. Obstruction of the pancreatic duct will also lead to focal atrophy of the gland distal to the obstruction. This can be seen as a result of pancreatic neoplasms and prior acute pancreatitis (see Figure 5-7) Chronic pancreatitis will frequently result in an atrophic gland, which can be sufficiently severe to lead to pancreatic exocrine and endocrine insufficiency[101] Pancreatic atrophy can also be a complication of abdominal irradiation (see Table 5-8 and Figure 5-48).

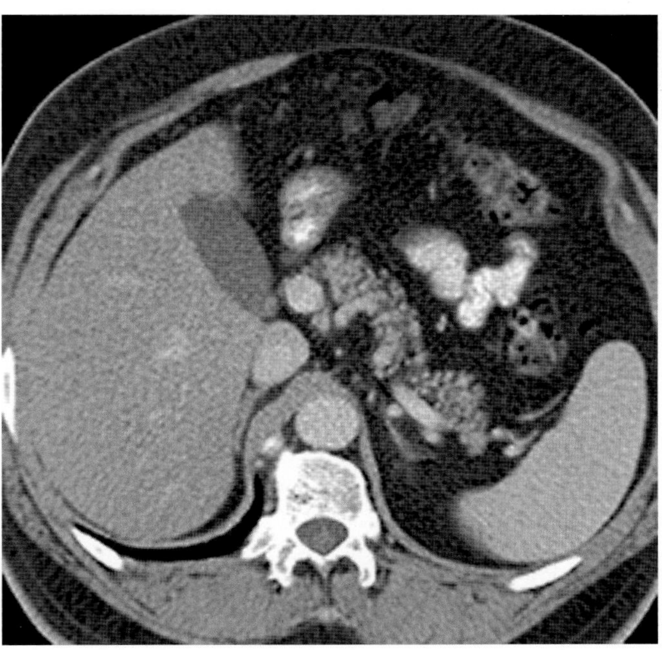

Figure 5-47 Pancreatic Atrophy
Diffuse pancreatic atrophy was noted in this 50-year-old man with a history of Hodgkin lymphoma. In addition to considerable thinning of the gland, fat is seen infiltrating into the gland.

Fatty infiltration of the pancreas

As noted earlier, fatty infiltration of the pancreas is a common phenomenon associated with aging of the pancreas. It may also be seen with a number of other conditions, including obesity, corticosteroid therapy, diabetes mellitus, and chronic pancreatitis (see Table 5-9).[102]

Premature fatty infiltration of the pancreas and pancreatic insufficiency is usually a result of one of several congenital disorders, most commonly cystic fibrosis.[102,193,194]

Table 5-8. Causes of Pancreatic Atrophy

1. Normal aging
2. Chronic duct obstruction a. Neoplasms b. Prior acute pancreatitis
3. Chronic pancreatitis

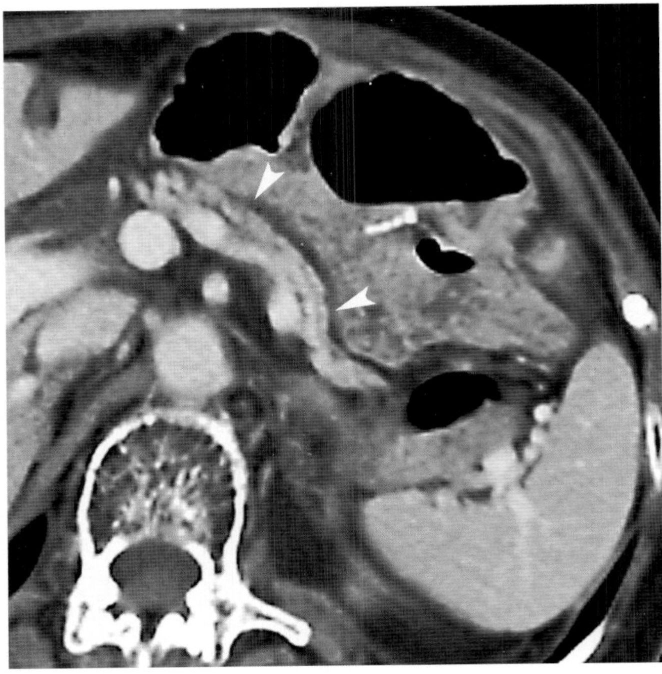

A

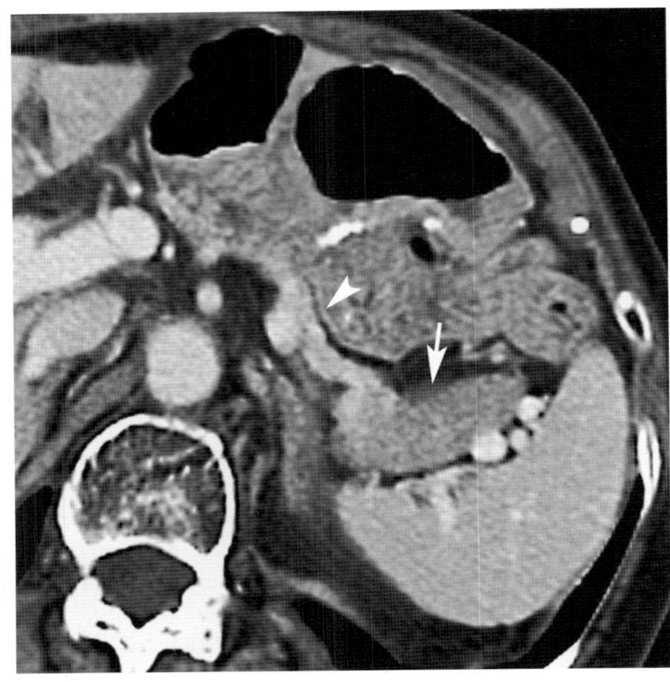

B

Figure 5-48 Pancreatic Atrophy Due to Radiation Therapy This 69-year-old man had received surgery and irradiation for gastric cancer. Note the difference between the normal-appearing tail (*arrow*) and atrophic body (*arrowheads*) of the pancreas. This was a consequence of irradiation to the gastric antrum.

Schwachman-Diamond syndrome, which is characterized by exocrine pancreatic insufficiency, metaphyseal dysostosis, and neutropenia, is a rare congenital disorder that can be a cause of premature fatty infiltration.[102,195-197] Johanson-Blizzard syndrome is another rare congenital disease characterized by fatty infiltration of the pancreas as well congenital deafness, nasal alar hypoplasia, hypothyroidism, mental retardation, growth retardation, absent permanent teeth, and malabsorption.[102,196,197]

Occasionally, fatty deposition within the pancreas will be heterogeneous. This typically appears as either focal areas of fat deposition within an otherwise normal-appearing gland or focal areas of normal glandular tissue in an otherwise fatty replaced gland. In the majority of cases, this focal fatty deposition or focal fatty sparing will occur within the pancreatic head or uncinate process. This process has been attributed to the different origin of the head of the pancreas from the dorsal pancreas when compared with the origin of the body and tail of the pancreas from the ventral pancreas.[43]

Imaging features of fatty infiltration of the pancreas include increased echogenicity of the infiltrated gland on US.[102,193,197] On CT, a pancreas with diffuse low attenuation is seen similar to fat (see Figure 5-49).[102,193,197] On MR, a normal or enlarged gland with marked T1 hyperintensity may be demonstrated.[194,196] Opposed-phase imaging will demonstrate loss of signal intensity, which may be particularly helpful in cases of focal fatty infiltration or focal fatty sparing (see Figures 5-26 and 5-27).[103]

Focal fatty sparing of the pancreatic head can occasionally mimic a pancreatic mass within a fatty replaced pancreas. Imaging features that can help distinguish focal fatty sparing from a true mass lesion are (1) lack of mass effect, (2) preservation of the normal glandular architecture of the soft tissue abnormality, and (3) lack of pancreatic or biliary ductal dilation.[43]

Iron deposition in the pancreas: hemochromatosis

Idiopathic hemochromatosis is an autosomal recessive condition characterized by increased iron absorption and deposition of the excess iron within tissues and organs. The

Table 5-9. Causes of Fatty Infiltration of the Pancreas

1. Aging
2. Metabolic disorders a. Obesity b. Diabetes mellitus c. Corticosteroid excess
3. Congenital disorders a. Cystic fibrosis b. Schwachman-Diamond syndrome c. Johanson-Blizzard syndrome

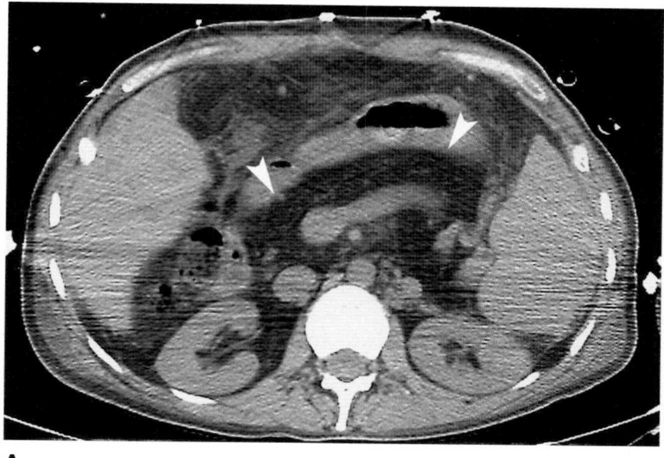

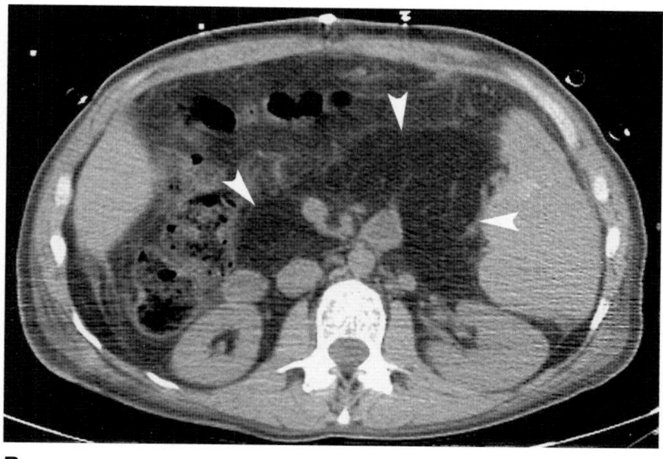

Figure 5-49 Fatty Pancreas in Cystic Fibrosis
This 31-year-old man had cystic fibrosis. **A** and **B**. Unenhanced CT images show a normal-volume pancreas that has been completely replaced by fat (*arrowheads*). This is a known complication of cystic fibrosis.

liver and pancreas are the primary targets of iron deposition. Other tissues and organs commonly involved include the skin, synovium, and heart. The progressive accumulation of iron eventually leads to organ dysfunction, which in the case of the pancreas is commonly diabetes mellitus.

Hemosiderosis represents the nonspecific deposition of iron. This can result from transfusional iron overload, ineffective hematopoiesis, and thalassemia. In hemosiderosis, iron deposition is usually limited to the reticuloendothelial system (ie, Kupffer cells of the liver, spleen, and bone marrow); however, if the reticuloendothelial system becomes saturated, iron deposition within organ parenchyma can occur.[104]

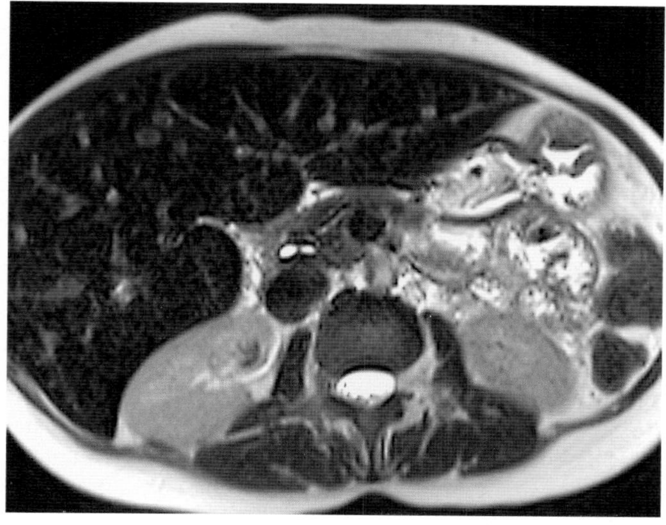

Figure 5-50 Transfusion-Related Hemosiderosis
This 34-year-old woman has a history of thalassemia intermedia with previous transfusions and no chelation therapy. Contiguous T2-weighted images demonstrate marked loss of liver signal and decreased signal within the pancreatic head and uncinate process, consistent with iron deposition. Hepatomegaly is also noted.

The imaging features of pancreatic involvement relate to the presence of iron. On CT, this manifests as increased attenuation of the pancreas as seen in the affected liver.[105] MRI demonstrates decreased signal intensity on T1-weighted images as well as T2-weighted images because of the paramagnetic effects of iron (see Figures 5-50 and 5-51).[104,105,198] Loss of parenchymal signal is particularly pronounced on T2*-weighted gradient echo sequences because of the susceptibility artifact from parenchymal iron.[104,198] The presence or absence of reticuloendothelial system involvement is usually helpful in determining whether the process is due to hemochromatosis or secondary to hemosiderosis. Specifically, sparing of the spleen and bone marrow would be consistent with hemochromatosis, whereas their involvement would be compatible with hemosiderosis.[104]

Imaging Notes 5-15. Iron Deposition in the Pancreas

Iron deposition in the pancreas can be secondary to either idiopathic hemochromatosis or secondary hemosiderosis as a result of transfusions, thalassemia, and other disorders leading to red blood cell lysis. Hemochromatosis and hemosiderosis can be distinguished by the distribution of iron in the spleen and bone marrow, which is present in these organs in patients with hemosiderosis and absent in patients with hemochromatosis.

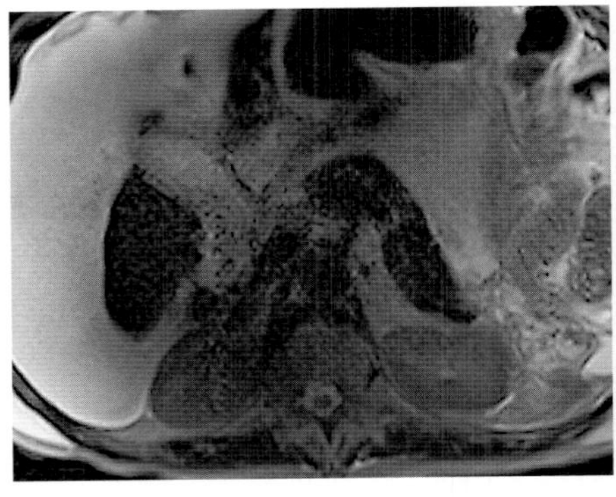
A

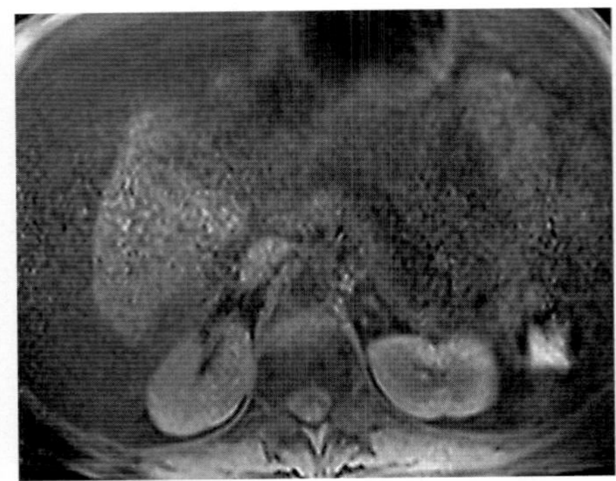
B

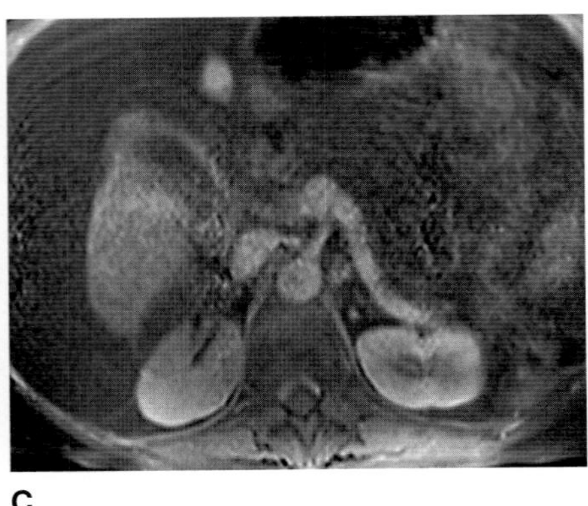
C

Figure 5-51 Transfusion-Related Hemosiderosis
This 59-year-old man had a history of transfusion-dependent anemia and end-stage liver disease secondary to chronic hepatitis C infection. T2-weighted (**A**) and fat-suppressed pregadolinium and postgadolinium enhanced T1-weighted images (**B** and **C**) demonstrate marked loss of pancreatic signal secondary to iron deposition within the pancreas. On the T2-weighted image, a thin line of signal separates the pancreas from the splenic vein flow void and represents a thin layer of retroperitoneal fascia. On the T1-weighted sequences, hypointense signal conforming to the contour of the pancreas is identified anterior to the splenic vein. Decreased T2 signal is also identified within the partially visualized liver secondary to iron deposition.

Diffuse calcifications: chronic pancreatitis

Chronic pancreatitis is a manifestation of prolonged repeated episodes of pancreatic inflammation and fibrosis that leads to irreversible damage of the exocrine and endocrine pancreas. Acute pancreatitis does not lead to chronic pancreatitis and so these diseases appear to be separate disorders. The most common etiology of chronic pancreatitis in the United States is chronic alcohol abuse, whereas in approximately one-third of cases the etiology of chronic pancreatitis is unknown.[106] It can also be associated with cholelithiasis, hyperlipidemia, hyperparathyroidism, cystic fibrosis, and pancreas divisum (Table 5-10). The similarity in risk factors between acute pancreatitis and chronic pancreatitis suggests that some individuals will be predisposed to the acute disorder and others to the chronic disorder, but few will incur both. Patients typically present with chronic or recurrent abdominal pain or steatorrhea. Nausea and weight loss are also common symptoms.

Table 5-10. Causes of Chronic Pancreatitis

1. Alcohol abuse
2. Idiopathic
3. Cholelithiasis
4. Hyperlipidemia
5. Hyperparathyroidism
6. Cystic fibrosis
7. Pancreas divisum

Diffuse pancreatic calcifications are a specific sign of chronic pancreatitis and are present in approximately one-half of cases.[107] These calcifications are located within the ducts and result from the deposition of calcium carbonate in inspissated protein.[108] Imaging findings other than pancreatic calcifications include pancreatic ductal dilation (68%), pancreatic atrophy (54%), and fluid collections (30%).[107] One recent group recently evaluated the specificity of these 4 findings and found a specificity of 77% for chronic pancreatitis when at least 2 of these 4 imaging findings are present and a specificity of 79% when at least 3 of the 4 findings are present.[109]

CT is the most sensitive modality for the detection of pancreatic calcifications and will show high-attenuation calcifications that pepper an atrophic pancreatic gland (see Figures 5-52, 5-53, and 5-54). Abdominal plain films may reveal flocculent-appearing calcifications in the epigastric and left upper quadrant regions of the abdomen, in the distribution of the pancreas (see Figure 5-54). On US, pancreatic calcifications typically manifest as shadowing echogenic foci in the expected location of the pancreas. Further, MRI is less sensitive for the detection of pancreatic calcifications; however, filling defects may be seen within the T2 intense ducts and correspond to the intraductal calculi. Although MRI is less sensitive than CT in detecting pancreatic calcifications, its utility lies in its ability to detect earlier changes of chronic pancreatitis.[108,199,200] Specifically, fat-suppressed T1-weighted images will demonstrate decreased T1 signal intensity of the normally high signal gland, and this alteration in signal results from parenchymal fibrosis.[31,199,200] Postgadolinium T1-weighted sequences will demonstrate decreased and heterogeneous pancreatic enhancement, which normally is avid and homogeneous.[9,201] T2-weighted sequences are particularly

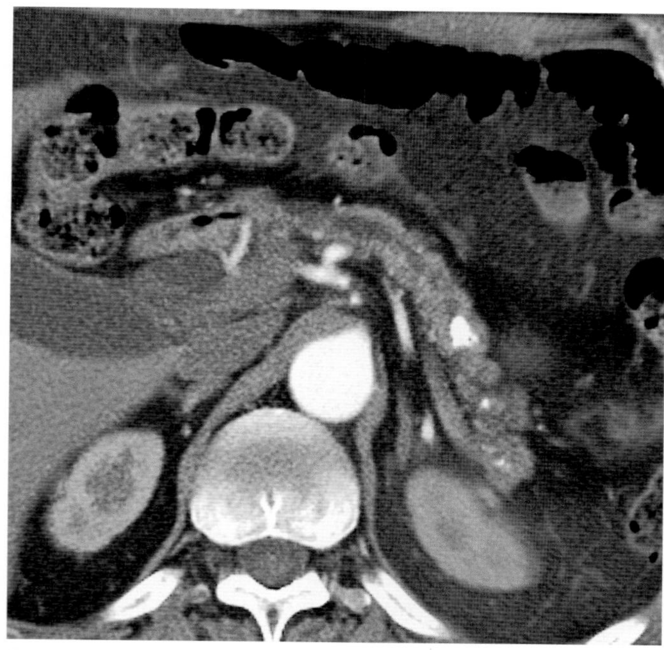

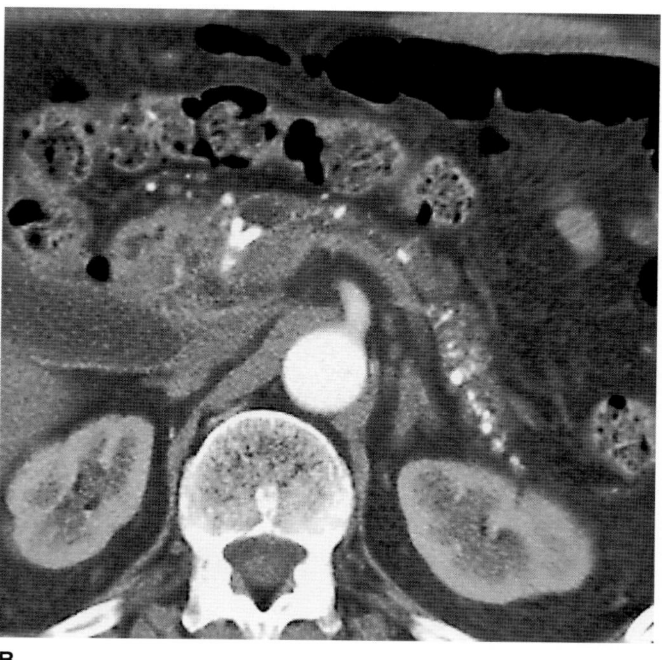

Figure 5-52 Chronic Pancreatitis
Chest pain was the presenting complaint in this 71-year-old man. **A** and **B**. Enhanced CT during the arterial phase of enhancement demonstrates pancreatic parenchymal atrophy and diffuse calcifications and dilation of the main pancreatic duct. No obstructing mass is present and the combined findings are characteristic of chronic pancreatitis.

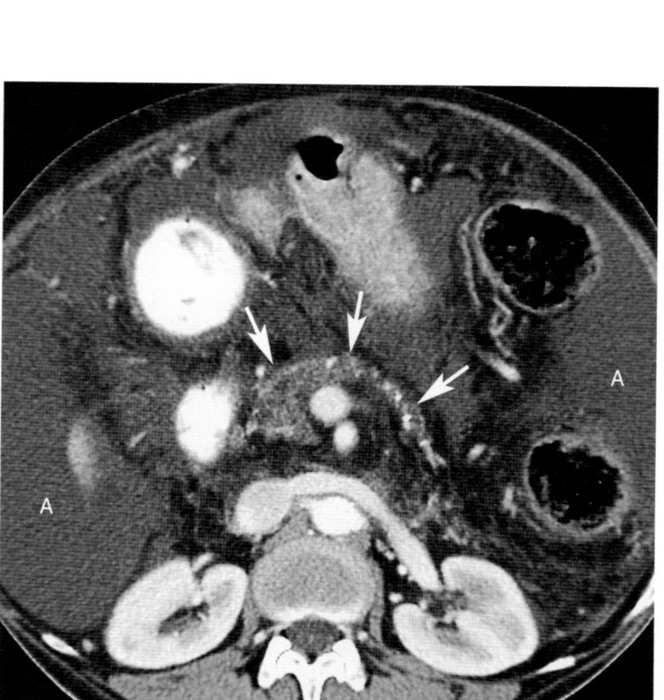

Figure 5-53 Chronic Pancreatitis
Marked pancreatic parenchymal atrophy and diffuse pancreatic calcifications (*arrows*) are classic findings of chronic pancreatitis in this cirrhotic patient. A large amount of ascites (labeled **A**) is present and a result of the patient's cirrhosis.

valuable in demonstrating other changes seen in later stages of chronic pancreatitis, including parenchymal atrophy, pancreatic duct dilation and stricture formation, intraductal calculi, and pseudocysts.[31,108]

Diffuse pancreatic ductal dilation

Adenocarcinoma of the pancreatic head and impacted gallstones within the intrapancreatic common bile duct are the most common etiologies of pancreatic ductal dilation (see Figures 5-7 and 5-9). These two entities always should be considered, especially when accompanied by biliary ductal dilation. Additional causes of pancreatic ductal dilation include IPMNs and chronic pancreatitis and strictures from prior choledocholithiasis (see Figure 4-61).

Intraductal papillary mucinous neoplasms: As described earlier, IPMNs are uncommon tumors that arise from the epithelium of the main pancreatic duct or side branch ducts, the latter of which are discussed under the heading: **Focal Lesions of the Pancreas**. Main pancreatic duct IPMNs demonstrate no sex predilection and have a peak incidence in the sixth decade.[59] The tumor can cause focal segmental dilation or diffuse dilation of the main pancreatic duct as a result of the excessive secretion of mucin.[59] Up to 40% of main pancreatic duct IMPNs demonstrate malignant invasion at the time of diagnosis[51] whereas the remainder contain elements of simple

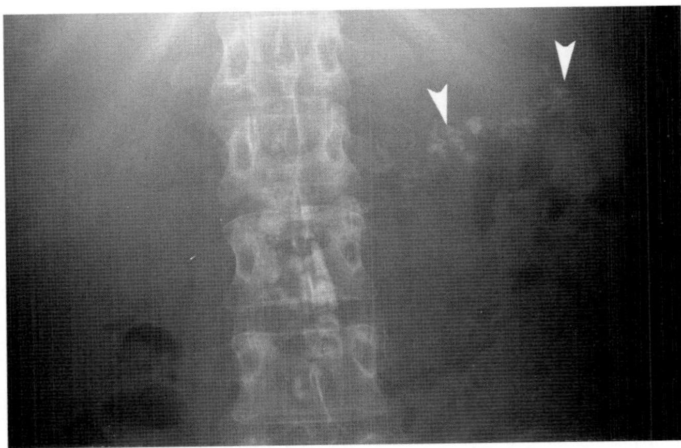

A

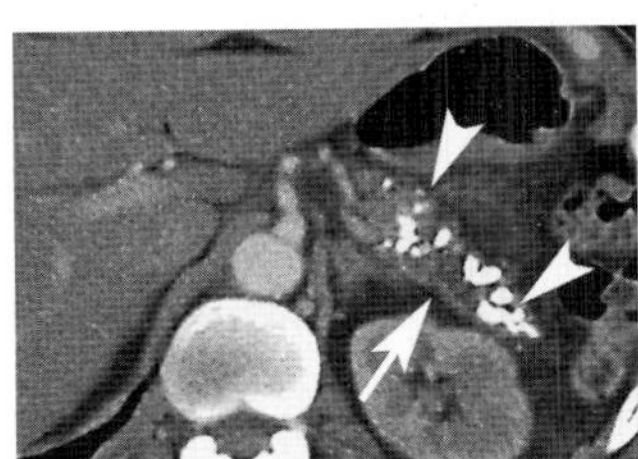

B

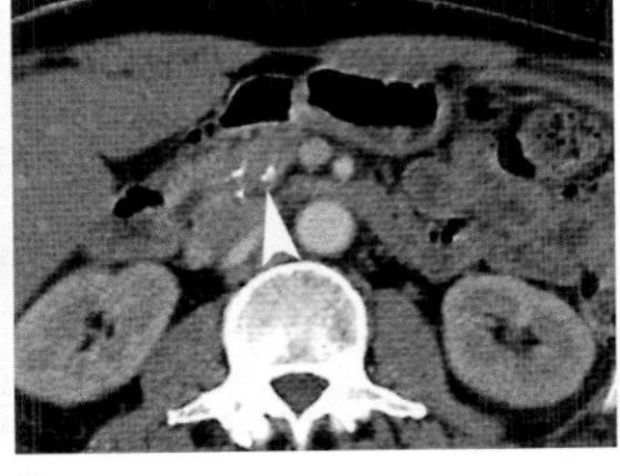

C

Figure 5-54 Chronic Pancreatitis
This 66-year-old man complained of abdominal pain. **A.** View of the upper abdomen demonstrates flocculent-appearing calcifications (*arrowheads*) in the left upper quadrant in the distribution of the pancreas. **B** and **C.** Enhanced CT images confirm the presence of chunky calcifications in the pancreas (*arrowheads*) and show fatty atrophy of a portion of the midtail of the pancreas (*arrow*). These findings are diagnostic of chronic pancreatitis.

hyperplasia, dysplasia, carcinoma in situ, and/or carcinoma.[202,203] Surgical resection of all main branch IMPNs is recommended as these lesions have a greater likelihood of malignancy.[204-206] Features suggestive of malignancy include the presence of mural nodules and main pancreatic duct dilation greater than 7 mm.[121,204]

On imaging examinations, IPMNs appear as dilation of the main or branch pancreatic ducts. On CT, the involved pancreatic duct is low in attenuation.[58] T2-weighted MR sequences demonstrate the abnormal pancreatic duct to be high in signal intensity; however, T1-weighted sequences reveal variable T1 signal intensity owing to the varying degrees of mucin hydration (see Figure 5-55).[207,208] On US, hypoechoic dilation of the pancreatic duct is identified.[58]

Both contrast-enhanced thin section CT and T2-weighted MRI sequences are particularly helpful in demonstrating small papillary growths and/or mural nodules within the dilated duct, which represent tumor or mucinous debris.[86,122] Main duct IPMNs may be difficult to distinguish from the findings of chronic pancreatitis as a dilated main pancreatic duct and associated pancreatic atrophy are present in both. Nevertheless, the identification of a major papilla bulging into the duodenum allows for the imaging diagnosis of an IPMN.[59]

Chronic pancreatitis: Dilation of the main pancreatic duct is a common finding in chronic pancreatitis and is usually accompanied by findings of pancreatic atrophy and calcifications. As described above, imaging demonstrates an increase in pancreatic duct caliber, which is low attenuation on CT, high T2 signal intensity on MRI, and anechoic on US (see Figure 5-52).

Congenital Disorders of the Pancreas

There are primarily two congenital variants of pancreatic anatomy, pancreas divisum and annular pancreas.

Pancreas divisum

Pancreas divisum is the most common pancreatic congenital variant, occurring in up to 10% of individuals.[110,209] This variant results from the failure of the dorsal and ventral ducts to fuse during embryonic development. The dorsal duct drains the majority of the pancreas through the minor papilla whereas the shorter ventral duct drains the pancreatic head through the major papilla.[110] Occasionally, a narrow communication may occur between the dorsal and ventral ducts and is termed *incomplete pancreas divisum.*

The clinical significance of pancreas divisum is controversial. The vast majority of patients with this variant are asymptomatic. However, in one study, 20 of 78 patients (25.6%) with unexplained recurrent pancreatitis were found to have pancreas divisum.[111] vThis led to the initial hypothesis that the minor papilla was inadequate to drain the pancreas, leading to obstruction with resultant symptoms and bouts of recurrent pancreatitis.[111] The fact that the vast majority of patients with this variant is asymptomatic contradicts this theory, and the prevailing hypothesis is that symptomatic patients possessing this congenital variant also have stenosis of the minor papilla.[112] According to this hypothesis, stenosis of the minor papilla superimposed on pancreas divisum results in obstruction of the primary drainage route of the pancreas.

The primary modality of diagnosing pancreas divisum has been ERCP,[110,114] although MRCP also has been shown to be highly sensitive and specific.[113] At ERCP, only the ventral duct will opacify following cannulation of the major papilla. As other causes can lead to incomplete opacification of the dorsal duct (eg, pancreatic adenocarcinoma), the diagnosis of pancreas divisum can only be made after injection of the minor papilla opacifies the dorsal duct and demonstrates no communication between the dorsal and ventral ducts.[110] MRCP will demonstrate separate dorsal and ventral ducts draining into the duodenum with the dorsal duct passing anterior to the common bile duct (see Figures 5-56 and 5-57).[7,114,162] Although maximum-intensity projections are routinely obtained with MRCP,

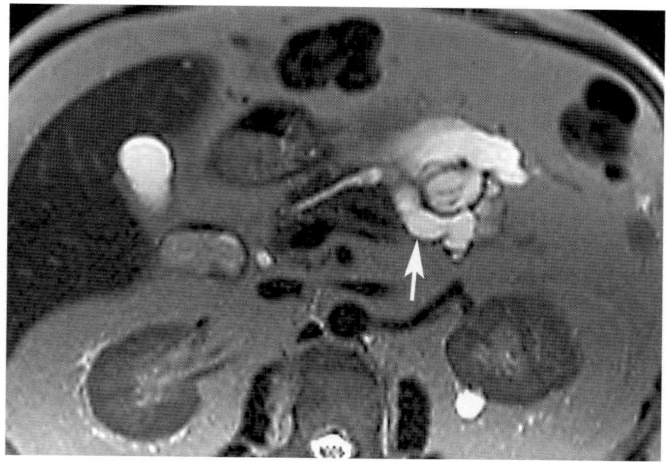
A

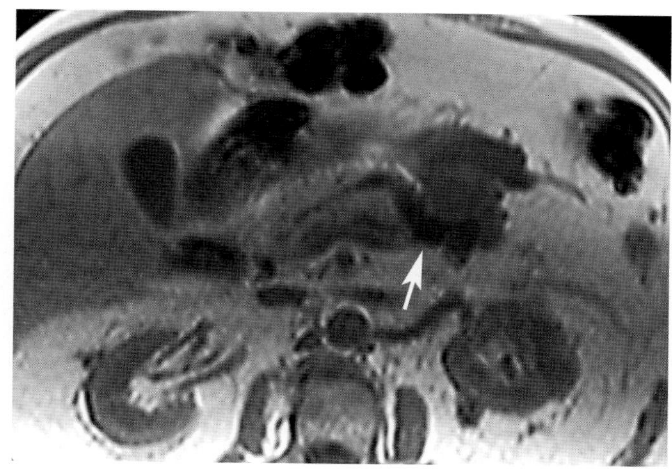
B

Figure 5-55 Main duct intraductal papillary mucinous neoplasm (IPMN)
A. T2-weighted and (**B**) T1-weighted MR images demonstrate a multilobulated cystic lesion arising from the anterior aspect of the pancreatic tail in this 81-year-old man. The cystic contents follow simple fluid on T1- and T2-weighted sequences. There is dilation of the main pancreatic duct (*arrows*). No enhancing nodular components were identified following the administration of intravenous contrast (not shown). Distal pancreatectomy and splenectomy were performed and pathology demonstrated intraductal papillary mucinous neoplasm without carcinoma but with associated pathologic findings of chronic pancreatitis.

pancreas divisum appears to be more easily detected on the axial source images.[113] In many cases, the separate ventral and dorsal ducts can be seen on standard MRI and CT planar images if the reader is careful to look for them (see Figure 5-58).

Annular pancreas

Annular pancreas is a rare congenital anomaly characterized by pancreatic tissue completely or partially surrounding the duodenum.[114] The annular pancreatic duct may drain into the ventral pancreatic duct, dorsal pancreatic

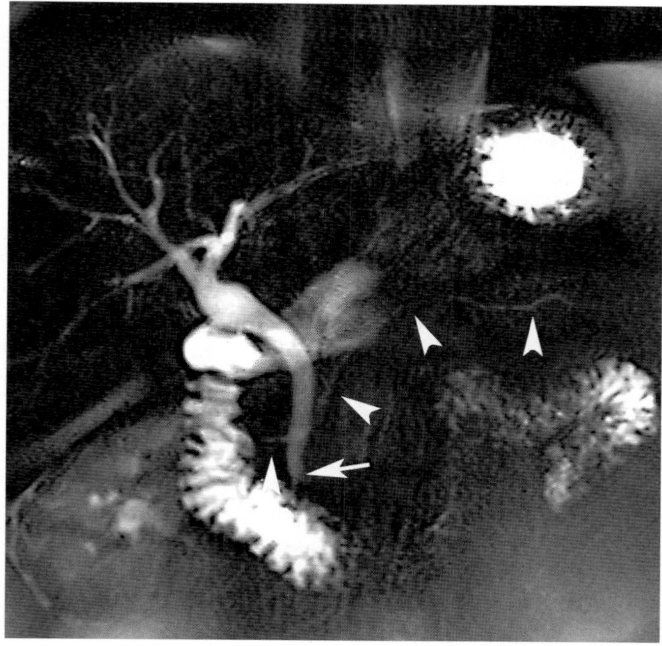
A

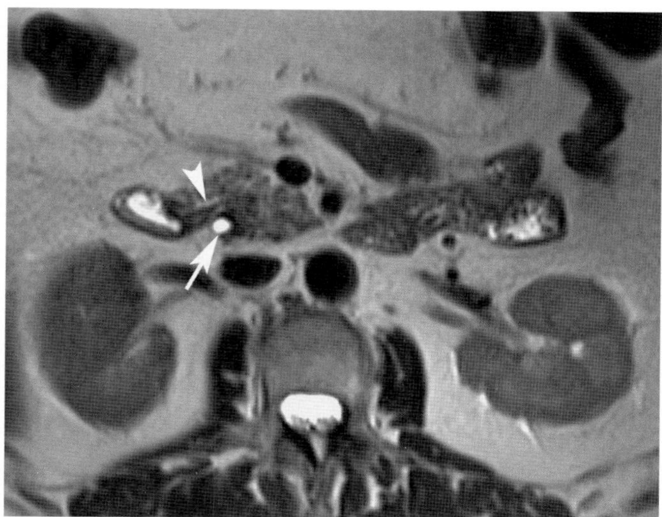
B

Figure 5-56 Pancreas Divisum on MRCP
MRI with MRCP was performed in this 59-year-old woman with incidental pancreas divisum. **A.** 3D heavily T2-weighted coronal MRCP demonstrates the no connection between the dorsal pancreatic duct (*arrowheads*) and the intrapancreatic common bile duct (*arrow*). **B.** Axial T2-weighted image confirms this finding and that the dorsal pancreatic duct (*arrowhead*) passes anterior to the intrapancreatic common bile duct (*arrow*).

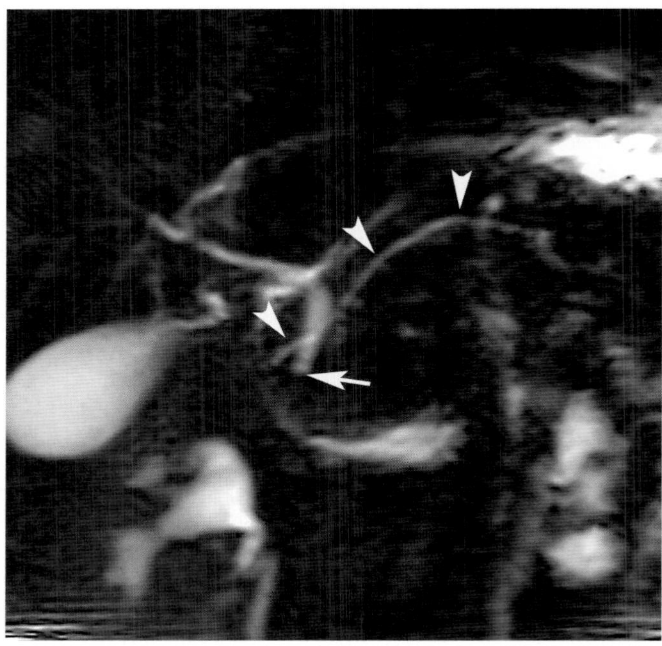

A

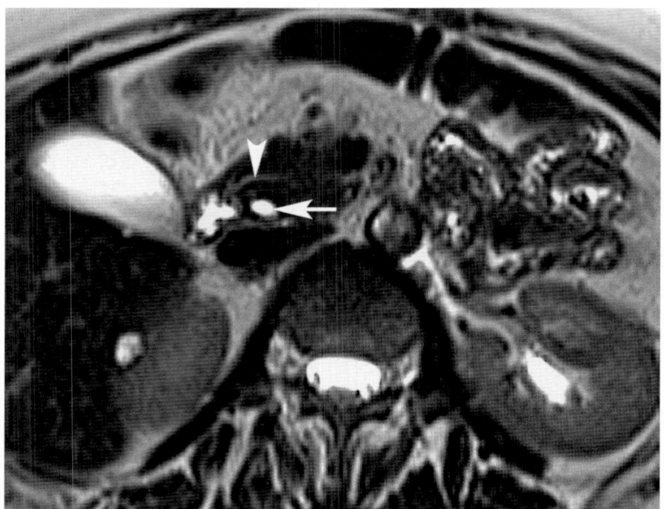

B

Figure 5-57 Pancreas Divisum on MRCP
MRI with MRCP was performed in this 75-year-old woman with malignant mixed mullerian tumor and incidental pancreas divisum. **A.** 3D heavily T2-weighted coronal MRCP demonstrates the dorsal pancreatic duct (*arrowheads*) to be separate from the intrapancreatic common bile duct (*arrow*). **B.** Axial T2-weighted image confirms this finding and that the dorsal pancreatic duct (*arrowhead*) passes anterior to the intrapancreatic common bile duct (*arrow*). A simple cyst is partially visualized in the right kidney.

duct, the common bile duct or the duodenal papilla.[115] The precise mechanism of development of annular pancreas is unclear and several theories have been proposed. One theory suggests that adherence of the right ventral pancreatic anlage to the duodenum leads to annular pancreas.[114,210] Another theory holds that persistence or hypertrophy of the left pancreatic anlage results in annular pancreas.[114,211] A third theory argues that abnormal adherence of the ventral anlage followed by rotation of the duodenum results in this congenital anomaly.[115]

Approximately one-half of cases of annular pancreas present during the neonatal period with gastric outlet obstruction.[116] Many of the patients who present in infancy will have associated congenital abnormalities, such as trisomy 21, GI malrotation, and tracheoesophageal fistula.[116,212,213] The remainder of individuals present later in childhood or adulthood with a variety of signs and symptoms, including pain, duodenal obstruction or pancreatitis.[117]

Duodenal obstruction characteristically results in gaseous distention of the stomach and proximal duodenum, creating the "double bubble" sign on abdominal radiographs.[116] The double bubble is not specific for the cause of duodenal obstruction and the differential diagnosis includes annular pancreas, duodenal atresia, and midgut volvulus. US of the neonate can demonstrate a fluid-distended proximal duodenum and a descending duodenum surrounded by echogenic pancreatic tissue.[116] Upper GI series in both children and adults may reveal varying degrees of circumferential narrowing of the descending duodenum.[116,214] Further, CT and MR evaluation of affected individuals demonstrate pancreatic tissue encircling the duodenum (see Figures 5-59 and 5-60).[116,214,215] Finally, ERCP and MRCP can demonstrate the annular pancreatic duct completely encircling the second portion of the duodenum and draining into the ventral or dorsal duct, pancreatic duct, the common bile duct, or the duodenal papilla.[216-218]

POSTOPERATIVE FINDINGS RELATED TO PANCREATIC SURGERY

Whipple Procedure

Pancreaticoduodenectomy (Whipple procedure) is a complex and aggressive surgery performed in cases of resectable cancers of the pancreatic head and other periampullary cancers (eg, distal common bile duct cholangiocarcinoma and duodenal carcinoma). The standard Whipple procedure is characterized by radical resection of the pancreatic head, neck, and uncinate process as well as resection of the gastric antrum, duodenum, proximal jejunum, gallbladder, and distal common bile duct. Lymph node dissection is also performed. Surgical reconstruction consists of retrocolic gastrojejunostomy, pancreaticoenterostomy, and choledochojejunostomy. The pancreaticoenterostomy may

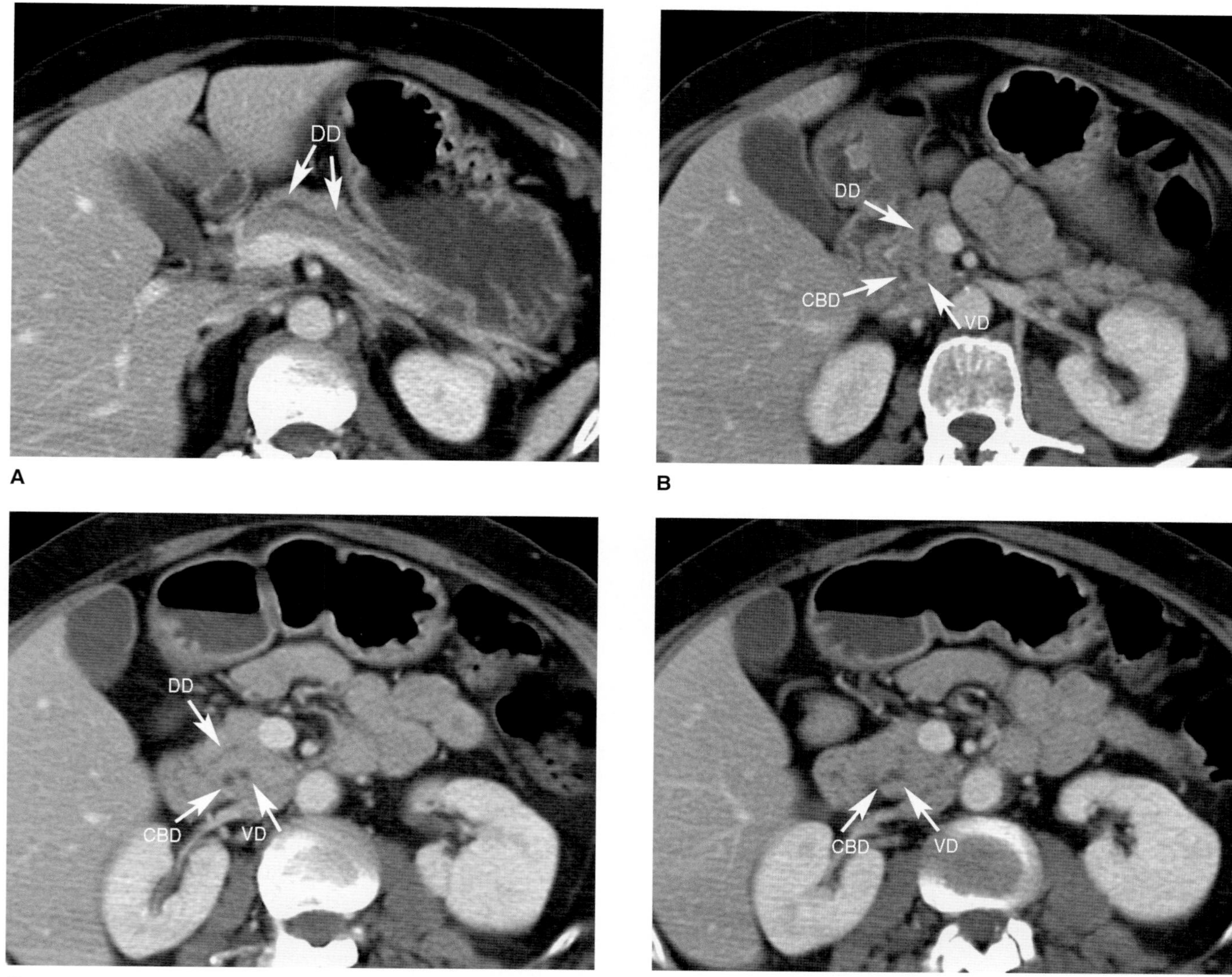

Figure 5-58 Pancreas Divisum on CT
Pancreas divisum was incidentally detected in this 46-year-old man who was involved in a motor vehicle collision. **A-D.** Enhanced CT through the pancreas demonstrate the dorsal pancreatic duct (DD) draining the neck, body and tail of the pancreas. The dorsal duct passes anteriorly to the common bile duct (CBD) in (**C**) and courses toward the duodenum where it empties via the minor papilla (not shown). The dorsal pancreatic duct does not communicate with the ventral duct (VD), which is seen draining the uncinate process and pancreatic head (B-D). The ventral duct courses toward the common bile duct where they join and empty into the major papilla (not shown).

take the form of an end-to-side anastomosis of the pancreatic remnant to either the afferent jejunal limb or the posterior wall of the stomach. Another surgical variation is the pylorus-sparing Whipple procedure in which the gastric antrum is spared, the duodenum is divided 1 to 2 cm distal to the pylorus, and a duodenojejunostomy is performed. In addition to surgical treatment of pancreatic adenocarcinoma, adjuvant radiation therapy is frequently employed.

CT is the most common modality by which the postsurgical pancreas is evaluated. Evaluation in the perioperative setting (<30 days) is almost always for the detection of complications, whereas delayed imaging (>30 days) is most typically performed for the detection or recurrent or metastatic disease.

In the immediate postoperative setting, common expected postsurgical findings include trace amounts of thin-walled or amorphous free fluid and increased attenuation of the perivascular mesenteric fat.[118,121] In one retrospective study, small fluid collections were seen in approximately 30% of patients, whereas perivascular mesenteric fat stranding was seen in 60% of patients.[118] Other common expected postsurgical findings include pneumobilia, transient reactive lymphadenopathy, and mild intrahepatic biliary dilation, the latter two of which may be present

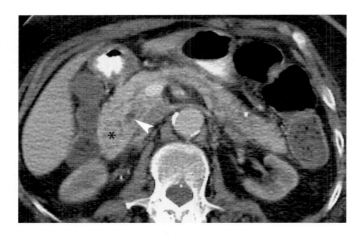

Figure 5-59 Annular Pancreas
This 54-year-old woman presented with chronic left lower quadrant pain. Enhanced CT performed during the parenchymal phase of enhancement incidentally demonstrated an annular pancreas. Pancreatic parenchyma is identified surrounding the duodenum, the wall of which is identified as an ovoid hypodense ring (*asterisk*). The common bile duct is denoted by the *arrowhead*.

in up to 25% of patients (see Figure 5-61).[118] Postsurgical pneumoperitoneum is to be expected; however, this should progressively decrease. Temporary feeding tubes within the pancreaticoenterostomy and intra-abdominal drains may be present in the immediate postoperative period but are frequently removed by the second postoperative week.

Postsurgical complications are common following Whipple procedure but tend to be limited to the perioperative period. One series demonstrated complications in 46% of postsurgical patients and a postsurgical mortality of 4%.[119] The most common complication directly related to the pancreas is leakage at the pancreaticoenterostomy anastomosis, which may be observed in an estimated 10% to 24% of patients,[120] and this usually occurs 1 to 2 weeks after surgery.[121] Although any of the surgical anastomoses may fail, anastomotic failure of the pancreaticoenterostomy is of particular import because it can result in release of pancreatic enzymes into the abdomen. Further, CT findings that should raise suspicion for pancreaticoenterostomy leak include the development of paraanastomotic fluid or ascites or increasing pneumoperitoneum. Identification of air within a paraanastomotic collection should add further suspicion that the collection represents a pancreaticojejunal anastomotic leak;[120] however, it should be noted that an anastomotic leak cannot be diagnosed with complete certainty by imaging alone unless leakage of oral or biliary contrast is observed.[121]

Other post-Whipple complications directly involving the pancreas include acute pancreatitis and rarely necrotizing pancreatitis of the pancreatic remnant.[118,119,121] The imaging features of these are similar to those seen in the nonsurgical pancreas and are reviewed in greater detail in their respective subsections of the diffuse pancreatic process section.

A number of other postsurgical complications are commonly seen in the immediate postoperative period. These include delayed gastric emptying (17%) and intra-abdominal abscess formation (10%), which are manifested by gastric distention and complex and/or rim-enhancing collections, respectively.[119,121] Less common complications include GI hemorrhage (5%) and intra-abdominal bleeding (3%), and these demonstrate the expected CT findings

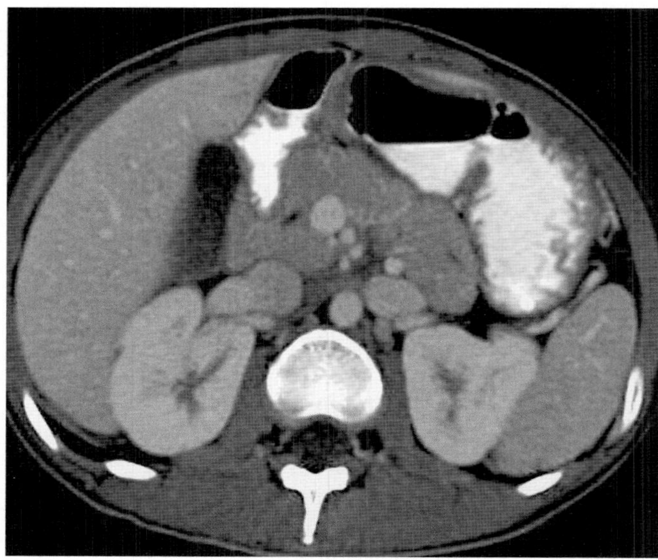
A

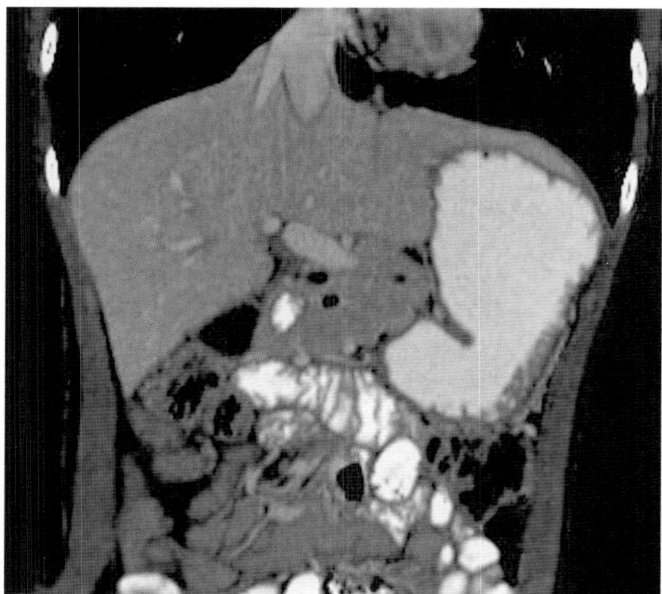
B

Figure 5-60 Annular Pancreas
This 24-year-old woman had episodes of recurrent right upper quadrant pain and pancreatitis. (**A**) Axial and (**B**) coronal reconstruction from an enhanced CT demonstrates pancreatic tissue surrounding the descending duodenum, diagnostic of annular pancreas.

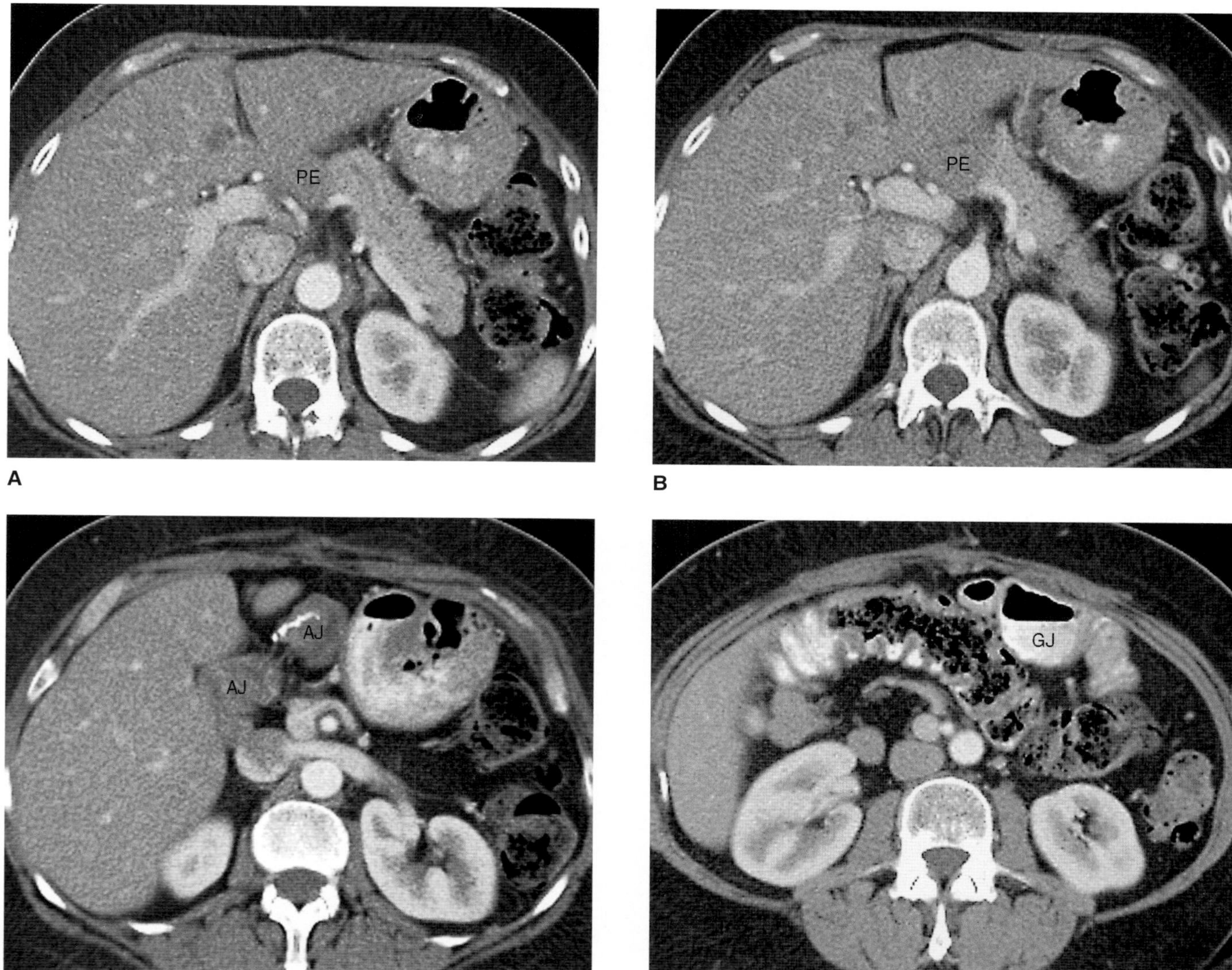

Figure 5-61 Surgical Appearance Post Whipple Procedure This 53-year-old man underwent Whipple procedure for adenocarcinoma of the pancreatic head. **A** and **B**. The characteristic reconstructive CT findings of Whipple procedure are illustrated including pancreaticoenterostomy (PE). There is minimal prominence of the pancreatic duct, likely post surgical in etiology. Findings of hepaticojejunostomy are present in (**C**), characterized by the afferent jejunal limb (AJ) in the hepatic hilum and extending anteriorly. The surgical staple line of the blind ending afferent jejunal limb is partially visualized in C. Note the masslike appearance of the afferent jejunal limb; this should not be confused for portohepatic lymphadenopathy or masses. An antecolic gastrojejunostomy is shown in (**D**), which is a variant of the more common retrocolic gastrojejunostomy performed after gastric antral resection.

of high-attenuation collections and/or vascular extravasation of contrast on enhanced scans. Uncommon complications include hepatic artery injury, organ ischemia, splenic infarction, and pseudomembranous colitis.[121]

Unfortunately, recurrent disease is common and, in one study, was observed in 47% of patients who underwent Whipple procedure.[118] Evaluation for recurrent disease is commonly performed using a combined serologic and imaging approach. Serum levels of the CA19-9 tumor antigen are evaluated, with recurrent or metastatic disease resulting in elevation of these levels. Delayed CT imaging is the modality of choice to evaluate for gross tumor recurrence although elevation of the CA19-9 marker may precede the imaging findings of recurrence.[122] The average time at which recurrent disease presents is approximately 270 days after surgery.[122] Earlier recurrence has been found to be associated with positive surgical margins but not lymph node metastases.[122]

The most common site of recurrent disease is the pancreatic bed, which appears as masses of soft-tissue density.[122] Recurrent disease may also manifest as soft tissue density surrounding the retroperitoneal vascular structures.[123] The development of ascites more than 1 month after surgery is another finding that is highly suspicious of tumor recurrence.[118] The most common sites of metastatic disease include the liver, lung, and para-aortic lymph nodes.[118,122]

A few imaging pitfalls may complicate radiologic interpretation of the post-Whipple patient, and knowledge of the postsurgical anatomy and pitfalls is important. In the post-Whipple patient, nonopacified loops of bowel and the afferent jejunal limb are frequently located at the liver hilus and have the potential for being misinterpreted as masses (see Figure 5-61).[121,122] Unfortunately, the administration of oral contrast alone is often insufficient to distinguish loops of bowel from masses, especially in the case of the afferent jejunal limb. Other clues (eg, presence of intraluminal gas or valvulae conniventes) and techniques (eg, multiplanar reformations) may be helpful in providing further clarification of hepatic hilar structures. In the specific case of the afferent jejunal limb, the use of biliary contrast media has been shown to be particularly helpful, with one group demonstrating successful opacification of the afferent limb in 95% of patients.[124] Another potential pseudomass may be found at the pancreaticojejunal anastomosis and is related to surgical technique. In this instance, it is the surgical invagination of the pancreas into the afferent jejunal limb that simulates a mass.[122]

Another mimic of recurrent disease is postsurgical fibrosis or radiation-related changes within the surgical bed, which frequently manifests as soft tissue density. Unfortunately, there are few imaging clues that allow these to be definitively characterized as posttreatment changes except for stability. Therefore, in patients with soft-tissue density within the surgical bed and around adjacent mesenteric vessels, follow-up is recommended. In one study, posttreatment changes were never found to progress but remained stable or improved over successive follow-up studies.[122]

Distal Pancreatectomy

Surgical resection of the pancreatic body and/or tail (ie, distal pancreatectomy) is performed for cases of isolated neoplastic and nonneoplastic lesions of the distal pancreas. Although the surgery may be performed for any pancreatic neoplasm, pancreatic adenocarcinoma is the most common indication for distal pancreatectomy.[125]

At surgery, the distal pancreas is resected along with the spleen. As leakage of pancreatic enzymes and juices from the surgical site is the most common complication of distal pancreatectomy, the pancreatic stump is frequently sutured to avoid this complication.[125]

Postsurgical imaging demonstrates absence of the pancreatic body and/or tail and spleen. Sutures or surgical clips within the surgical bed may also be present, which appear as radiodense and echogenic foci on CT and US, respectively, and as foci of susceptibility on MR (see Figure 5-62).

Pancreas Transplant

Pancreas transplantation is the only treatment capable of achieving true physiologic glycemic control in the diabetic patient.[219] This surgical procedure has become increasingly common, with more than 23 000 transplants having been performed since the first reported case in 1966.[126] The vast majority of pancreas transplants recipients have type

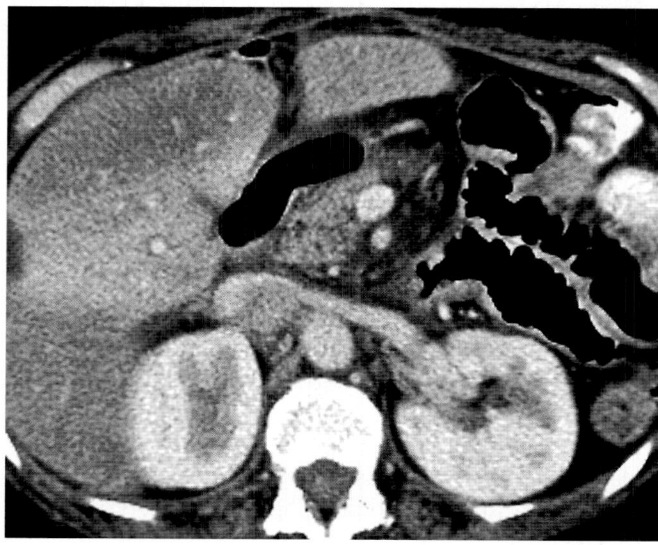

A

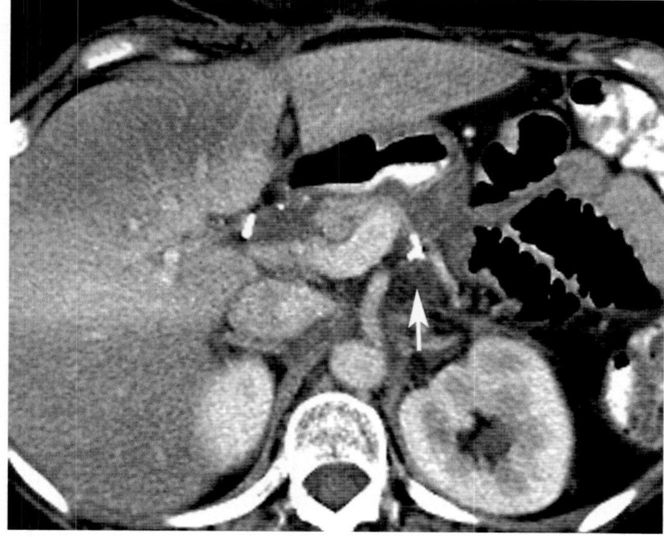

B

Figure 5-62 Distal Pancreatectomy
This 54-year-old woman is status post distal pancreatectomy and splenectomy for invasive adenocarcinoma of the pancreas. **A** and **B.** Contrast-enhanced CT shows the pancreatic tail and spleen have been surgically resected and surgical clips are identified at the pancreatic surgical margin. The pancreatic head is seen in (A) and demonstrates mild age-related atrophy.

I diabetes mellitus, whereas a smaller proportion, approximately 7%, have type II diabetes.[126,220] Depending on the individual's specific needs and organ availability, patients may receive a pancreas transplant only, a simultaneous pancreas and kidney transplant, or a pancreas after a kidney transplant.

The surgical procedure involves en bloc removal of the donor pancreas, duodenum, superior mesenteric vessels, splenic artery, and portal vein.[128,219,221] A vascular Y graft composed of the donor's common, internal, and external iliac arteries is also removed. The internal and external iliac arteries of the Y graft are anastomosed to the superior mesenteric and splenic arteries of the transplant, respectively. The pancreas transplant is placed intraperitoneally in 1 of 2 surgical variations: the enteric drainage technique and the systemic bladder drainage technique. In both variations, an arterial anastomosis is made between the recipient's common iliac artery and the Y graft's common iliac artery. In the enteric drainage technique, the transplant is positioned intraperitoneally with a venous anastomosis between the allograft's portal vein and either the recipient's right common iliac vein or the portal vein. Drainage of the pancreatic secretions occurs through a side-to-side anastomosis created between the first through third portions of the donor duodenum and the native proximal jejunum. In the systemic bladder drainage technique, the pancreas is placed within the pelvis and a venous anastomosis is created between the transplant's portal vein and the recipient's common iliac vein or inferior vena cava. The segment of donor duodenum is then anastomosed to the bladder. Although a longer vascular graft is required for portal enteric transplantation, this is the favored approach to pancreas transplantation as it results in a lower complication rate.[129,222] Complications specifically associated with the systemic bladder technique are commonly related to bladder infection.[129,222] Other complications include metabolic acidosis secondary to the loss of bicarbonate as well as fistulas, calculi, and urethral rupture.

Imaging of the pancreas allograft is commonly performed by either CT or US in the immediate postoperative period. In the setting of a simultaneous pancreas and kidney transplant, CT evaluation is often performed with oral contrast but without intravenous contrast in order to avoid renal transplant compromise.[127] Noncontrast CT evaluation of the allograft is limited but usually performed to detect early postoperative complications, such as intra-abdominal collections or abscesses. In the cases where contrast is administered, the normal allograft demonstrates uniform parenchymal enhancement[128] although the degree of enhancement may be to a lesser extent than expected in a normal native pancreas and to a lesser degree than the adjacent renal transplant (if present) (see Figure 5-63).[129] Evaluation of the bowel and enteric anastomosis is best evaluated by CT; however, it should be noted that opacification of the donor duodenum with oral contrast frequently does not occur.[128,129,223] Peri-allograft collections are commonly present in the first month post transplant; however, by themselves they are nonspecific and should be interpreted in the context of the clinical setting.[129]

US is the other modality typically utilized in evaluating the allograft in the immediate postoperative period although nonvisualization of the transplant may occur in up to 20% of transplant recipients secondary to overlying bowel gas.[129] On US, the normal transplant pancreas is usually uniform in echotexture and less echogenic than the surrounding omental and peritoneal fat.[127,128] The allograft is often less echogenic than the native pancreas for 2 reasons: (1) because the allograft is often edematous and (2) the native pancreas has often undergone fatty replacement.[129] Color and spectral Doppler evaluation of the transplant are particularly helpful in the evaluation of the allograft's vascular supply. Although intraparenchymal resistive indices are routinely obtained in the evaluation of renal transplants, they are not good predictors of pancreatic allograft rejection.[127,129] Normal paraanastomotic arterial velocities may be as high as 400 cm/s in the immediate postoperative setting but these high velocities are likely secondary to perianastomotic edema and usually fall below 300 cm/s on follow-up studies.[129] Normal portal venous velocities are between 10 and 60 cm/s.[129]

On MRI, the normal allograft demonstrates the expected T1 and T2 signal characteristics of a normal native pancreas. On contrast-enhanced MRI/MRA, uniform parenchymal enhancement and patency of the transplant's

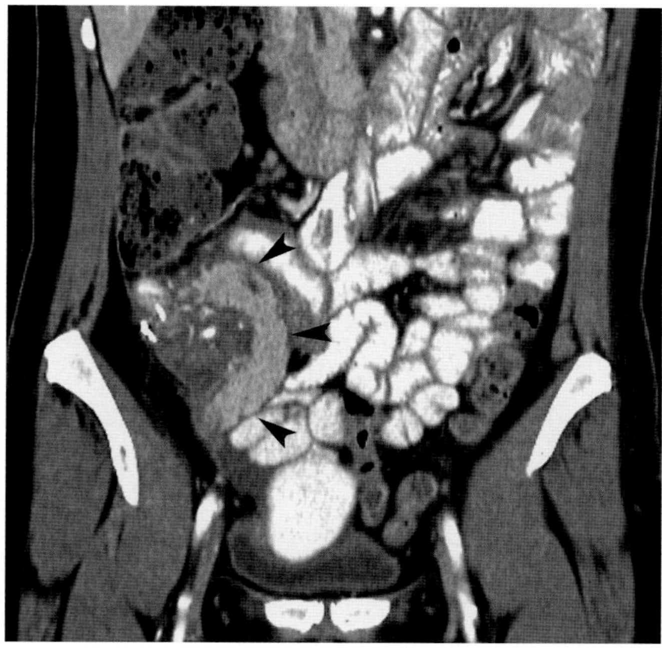

Figure 5-63 Satisfactory Appearance of Pancreas Transplant This 39-year-old woman underwent simultaneous pancreas and kidney transplantation. The donor pancreas is vertically oriented intraperitoneally in the right lower quadrant (*arrowheads*). There is uniform enhancement of the graft and the attenuation of the parenchyma is identical to that expected of a native pancreas.

vascular supply are observed.[128,131,221] Heavily T2-weighted sequences may also be performed to evaluate the pancreatic duct, which should be similar in appearance to a normal pancreas.[128]

Complications relating to pancreas transplant fall into 2 broad categories: (1) complications relating to general abdominal surgeries and (2) complications relating to pancreas transplantation. Complications in the former category include intra-abdominal collections, infection, enteric anastomotic leaks, and small bowel obstruction and are discussed elsewhere. Complications unique to pancreas allografts include rejection, allograft vascular complications, pseudocyst formation, and pancreatitis.

Allograft rejection is a profoundly disappointing but common outcome. In one series of pancreas and kidney transplants performed from 1996 to 2005, the 1-year pancreas graft survival rate was 79% to 85%.[130] A second smaller series analyzing pancreas and kidney transplants from 1998 to 2002 demonstrated a similar 1-year pancreas graft survival rate of 87% to 92%, with an acute rejection rate of 4% to 11%.[224] Graft rejection results from an alloimmune arteritis leading to small vessel occlusion. When present, clinical signs of acute rejection include abdominal pain, fever, and hyperglycemia. Evaluation of suspected acute rejection may include biopsy and/or expectant management with immunosuppressants. It is believed that unrecognized or unsuccessfully treated repeated bouts of acute rejection may lead to chronic graft rejection.[131]

The imaging findings of acute graft rejection are nonspecific. In the case of CT and US, rejection may manifest as diffuse or focal graft enlargement or edema.[127] On dynamic contrast-enhanced MRI, the typical appearance is that of decreased and inhomogeneous enhancement of the allograft.[221,225] MRI findings of chronic rejection are a small pancreas with decreased signal on T1- and T2-weighted sequences secondary to allograft fibrosis.[131] Magnetic resonance angiography (MRA) evaluation of chronic rejection reveals small vessels but normal enhancement.

Vascular complications, most notably vascular thrombosis, are a common cause of allograft dysfunction and may be evaluated by contrast-enhanced CT, contrast-enhanced MRA, and Doppler and spectral US.[128,131,221,223,226] Clinical symptoms of vascular thrombosis, if present, include abdominal pain and hyperglycemia.[131] Initial treatment is anticoagulation; however, if there are imaging signs of allograft infarction or necrosis, treatment is pancreatectomy. Short segments of thrombus occasionally may be identified within the donor superior mesenteric artery stump and portal vein stump. These are often incidental findings and considered to be of doubtful clinical consequence if the portion of the thrombosed vessel is peripheral to the pancreas.[129,131] Nevertheless, propagation of thrombus may occur and result in allograft compromise.[131] In these instances, serial short-term interval follow-up is often performed with or without anticoagulation.

Contrast-enhanced CT provides the greatest spatial resolution of the pancreatic allograft's vascular supply. On the arterial and delayed venous phases of enhancement, thrombus manifests as intraluminal filling defects in the arteries and veins, respectively (see Figure 5-64).[128,223] Contrast-enhanced MRA may also be used to evaluate the allograft's vascular supply. On precontrast T1-weighted sequences,

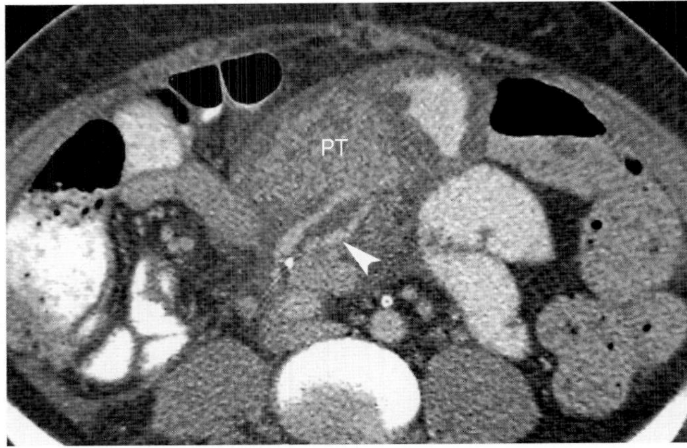

A

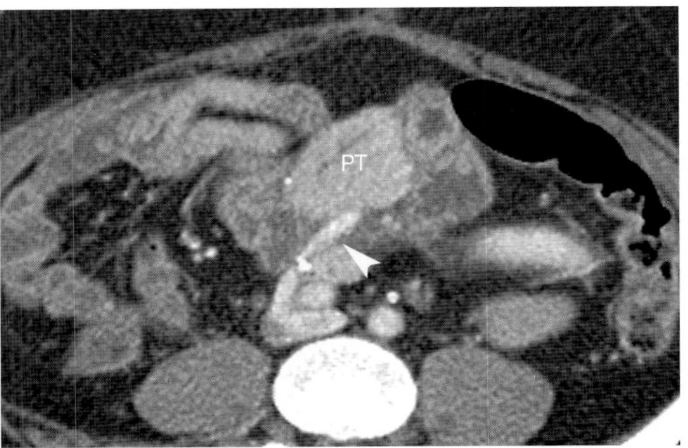

B

Figure 5-64 Transplant Pancreatitis
Acute pancreatitis of a pancreas transplant secondary to thrombosis of the venous graft. This 42-year-old man was status post simultaneous pancreas and kidney transplantation and presented with abdominal pain and fever. **A.** Contrast-enhanced CT reveals the pancreas transplant (PT) to be enlarged and decreased in attenuation. The margins are indistinct and there are surrounding inflammatory changes, consistent with acute pancreatitis. The etiology of the acute graft pancreatitis is identified within the venous graft, which is enlarged by low attenuation thrombus (*arrowhead*). **B.** Contrast-enhanced CT performed after anticoagulation therapy shows the inflammatory changes of the pancreas transplant (PT) to have resolved. The venous graft (*arrowhead*) is no longer enlarged and contrast is identified within the lumen at the site of prior thrombus.

thrombus may demonstrate increased signal if the clot contains methemoglobin.[131,221] Following the administration of gadolinium, thrombus manifests as nonopacification of the vessel.[131,221] On color and spectral Doppler US, vascular thrombosis is observed as absent flow.[127]

Other vascular complications include pseudoaneurysm and arterial venous fistula. Pseudoaneurysm may arise at the sites of surgical anastomosis, prior biopsy, or in cases of graft infection.[129,221] The imaging findings related to these complications are more completely reviewed in the vascular imaging chapter.

Posttransplant pancreatitis and pseudocyst formation may also complicate pancreas allografts.[132] The imaging manifestations of these sequela are similar to those observed in a native pancreas and the reader is referred to those sections for further discussion.

One final complication specific to the allograft is posttransplant lymphoproliferative disorder (PTLD), which ranges from a benign polyclonal B cell hyperplasia to malignant lymphoma. This is a late term complication that arises in 1% to 2.5% of transplant recipients.[227] The primary imaging feature of PTLD is diffuse allograft enlargement,[133] a finding also common to pancreatitis or graft rejection. Less commonly, PTLD may manifest as a focal allograft mass.[133] Although the imaging findings may not distinguish PTLD from pancreatitis or graft rejection, other clinical and imaging findings may prove helpful and include persistent allograft enlargement despite immunosuppressive therapy and extra-allograft involvement, such as lymphadenopathy and hepatomegaly.[129,133]

REFERENCES

1. Atri M, Finnegan P. The pancreas. In: Rumack CM, Wilson SR, Charboneau JW, eds. *Diagnostic Ultrasound*. St. Louis: Elsevier Mosby; 2005:213-267.
2. Belber JP, Bill K. Fusion anomalies of the pancreatic ductal system differentiation from pathologic states. *Radiology*. 1977; 122:637-642.
3. Hoff FL, Gabriel H, Hammond NA, Gore RM. Pancreas: normal anatomy and examination techniques. In: Gore RM, Levine MS, eds. *Textbook of Gastrointestinal Radiology*. Philadelphia, PA: Saunders Elsevier; 2008:1839-1853.
4. Heuck A, Maubach PA, Reiser M, et al. Age-related morphology of the normal pancreas on computed tomography. *Gastrointest Radiol*. 1987;12:18-22.
5. Pamuklar E, Semelka RC. MR imaging of the pancreas. *Magn Reson Imaging Clin N Am*. 2005;13:313-330.
6. Fulcher AS, Turner MA. MR pancreatography: a useful tool for evaluating pancreatic disorders. *Radiographics*. 1999;19:5-24; discussion 41-44; quiz 148-149.
7. Winston CB, Mitchell DG, Outwater EK, Ehrlich SM. Pancreatic signal intensity on T1-weighted fat saturation MR images: clinical correlation. *J Magn Reson Imaging*. 1995;5: 267-271.
8. Solcia E, Capella C, Kloppel G. Tumors of the exocrine pancreas. In: Rosai J, Sorbin L, eds. *Atlas of Tumor Pathology, 3rd series, fasc 20*. Washington, DC: Armed Forces Institute of Pathology; 1997:31-144.
9. Hruban RH, Fukushima N. Pancreatic adenocarcinoma: update on the surgical pathology of carcinomas of ductal origin and PanINs. *Mod Pathol*. 2007;20(suppl 1):S61-S70.
10. Carpelan-Holmstrom M, Nordling S, Pukkala E, et al. Does anyone survive pancreatic ductal adenocarcinoma? A nationwide study re-evaluating the data of the Finnish Cancer Registry. *Gut*. 2005;54:385-387.
11. Conlon KC, Klimstra DS, Brennan MF. Long-term survival after curative resection for pancreatic ductal adenocarcinoma. Clinicopathologic analysis of 5-year survivors. *Ann Surg*. 1996;223:273-279.
12. Kalser MH, Barkin J, MacIntyre JM. Pancreatic cancer. Assessment of prognosis by clinical presentation. *Cancer*. 1985;56:397-402.
13. Lu DS, Vedantham S, Krasny RM, Kadell B, Berger WL, Reber HA. Two-phase helical CT for pancreatic tumors: pancreatic versus hepatic phase enhancement of tumor, pancreas, and vascular structures. *Radiology*. 1996;199:697-701.
14. Prokesch RW, Chow LC, Beaulieu CF, Bammer R, Jeffrey RB Jr. Isoattenuating pancreatic adenocarcinoma at multi-detector row CT: secondary signs. *Radiology*. 2002;224:764-768.
15. Greene FL, Page DL, Fleming ID, et al. *Ajcc cancer staging handbook*. New York: Springer, 2009.
16. Bilimoria KY, Bentrem DJ, Ko CY, et al. Validation of the 6th edition AJCC Pancreatic Cancer Staging System: report from the National Cancer Database. *Cancer*. 2007;110:738-744.
17. Jones L, Russell C, Mosca F, et al. Standard Kausch-Whipple pancreatoduodenectomy. *Dig Surg*. 1999;16:297-304.
18. Balci NC, Semelka RC. Radiologic features of cystic, endocrine and other pancreatic neoplasms. *Eur J Radiol*. 2001;38:113-119.
19. Horton KM, Hruban RH, Yeo C, Fishman EK. Multi-detector row CT of pancreatic islet cell tumors. *Radiographics*. 2006;26: 453-464.
20. Hoff AO, Cote GJ, Gagel RF. Management of neuroendocrine cancers of the gastrointestinal tract: islet cell carcinoma of the pancreas and other neuroendocrine carcinomas. In: Abbruzzese JL, Evans DB, Willett CG, Fenoglio-Preiser C, eds. *Gastrointestinal Oncology*. New York: Oxford University Press; 2004:780-800.
21. Shah S, Mortele KJ. Uncommon solid pancreatic neoplasms: ultrasound, computed tomography, and magnetic resonance imaging features. *Semin Ultrasound CT MR*. 2007;28:357-370.
22. Service FJ, McMahon MM, O'Brien PC, Ballard DJ. Functioning insulinoma—incidence, recurrence, and long-term survival of patients: a 60-year study. *Mayo Clin Proc* 1991;66:711-719.
23. Dizon AM, Kowalyk S, Hoogwerf BJ. Neuroglycopenic and other symptoms in patients with insulinomas. *Am J Med*. 1999;106:307-310.
24. Cirillo F, Falconi M, Bettini R. Clinical manifestations and therapeutic management of hyperfunctioning endocrine tumors. In: Procacci C, Megibow AJ, eds. *Imaging the Pancreas: Cystic and Rare Tumors*. Berlin: Springer; 2003.
25. Kloppel G, Heitz PU. Morphology and functional activity of gastroenteropancreatic neuroendocrine tumours. *Recent Results Cancer Res*. 1990;118:27-36.
26. Spilcke-Liss E, Simon P, Lerch MM, Wallaschofski H. Pancreatic endocrine tumors in multiple endocrine neoplasia syndrome. In: Beger H, Warshaw A, Buchler M, et al., eds. *The Pancreas: An Integrated Textbook of Basic Science, Medicine, and Surgery*. Malden, MA: Blackwell; 2008:802-812.

27. Mallinson CN, Bloom SR, Warin AP, Salmon PR, Cox B. A glucagonoma syndrome. *Lancet.* 1974;2:1-5.

28. Perry RR, Vinik AI. Clinical review 72: diagnosis and management of functioning islet cell tumors. *J Clin Endocrinol Metab.* 1995;80:2273-2278.

29. Merkle EM, Boaz T, Kolokythas O, Haaga JR, Lewin JS, Brambs HJ. Metastases to the pancreas. *Br J Radiol.* 1998;71:1208-1214.

30. Klein KA, Stephens DH, Welch TJ. CT characteristics of metastatic disease of the pancreas. *Radiographics.* 1998; 18:369-378.

31. Boudghene FP, Deslandes PM, LeBlanche AF, Bigot JM. US and CT imaging features of intrapancreatic metastases. *J Comput Assist Tomogr.* 1994;18:905-910.

32. Z'Graggen K, Fernandez-del Castillo C, Rattner DW, Sigala H, Warshaw AL. Metastases to the pancreas and their surgical extirpation. *Arch Surg* 1998;133:413-417; discussion 418-419.

33. Nayer H, Weir EG, Sheth S, Ali SZ. Primary pancreatic lymphomas: a cytopathologic analysis of a rare malignancy. *Cancer.* 2004;102:315-321.

34. Merkle EM, Bender GN, Brambs HJ. Imaging findings in pancreatic lymphoma: differential aspects. *AJR Am J Roentgenol.* 2000;174:671-675.

35. Loren I, Lasson A, Fork T, et al. New sonographic imaging observations in focal pancreatitis. *Eur Radiol.* 1999;9:862-867.

36. Ito K, Koike S, Matsunaga N. MR imaging of pancreatic diseases. *Eur J Radiol.* 2001;38:78-93.

37. Ichikawa T, Sou H, Araki T, et al. Duct-penetrating sign at MRCP: usefulness for differentiating inflammatory pancreatic mass from pancreatic carcinomas. *Radiology.* 2001;221:107-116.

38. Levenick JM, Gordon SR, Sutton JE, Suriawinata A, Gardner TB. A comprehensive, case-based review of groove pancreatitis. *Pancreas.* 2009;38:e169-e175.

39. Stolte M, Weiss W, Volkholz H, Rosch W. A special form of segmental pancreatitis: "groove pancreatitis." *Hepatogastroenterology.* 1982;29:198-208.

40. Sanada Y, Yoshida K, Itoh H, Kunita S, Jinushi K, Matsuura H. Groove pancreatitis associated with true pancreatic cyst. *J Hepatobiliary Pancreat Surg.* 2007;14:401-409.

41. Blasbalg R, Baroni RH, Costa DN, Machado MC. MRI features of groove pancreatitis. *AJR Am J Roentgenol.* 2007;189:73-80.

42. Mohl W, Hero-Gross R, Feifel G, et al. Groove pancreatitis: an important differential diagnosis to malignant stenosis of the duodenum. *Dig Dis Sci.* 2001;46:1034-1038.

43. Jacobs JE, Coleman BG, Arger PH, Langer JE. Pancreatic sparing of focal fatty infiltration. *Radiology.* 1994;190:437-439.

44. Spinelli K, Fromwiller T, Daniel R, et al. Cystic pancreatic neoplasms: observe or operate. *Ann Surg.* 2004;239:651-659.

45. Laffan T, Horton K, Klein A, et al. Prevalence of unsuspected pancreatic cysts on MDCT. *AJR Am J Roentgenol.* 2008;191: 802-807.

46. Zhang X, Mitchell D, Dohke M, Holland G, Parker L. Pancreatic cysts: depiction on single-shot fast spin-echo MR images. *Radiology.* 2002;223:547-553.

47. Kim YH, Saini S, Sahani D, Hahn PF, Mueller PR, Auh YH. Imaging diagnosis of cystic pancreatic lesions: pseudocyst versus nonpseudocyst. *Radiographics.* 2005;25:671-685.

48. Fernández-del Castillo C, Targarona J, Thayer S, Rattner D, Brugge W, Warshaw A. Incidental pancreatic cysts: clinicopathologic characteristics and comparison with symptomatic patients. *Arch Surg.* 2003;138:427-434.

49. Buck JL, Hayes WS. From the archives of the AFIP. Microcystic adenoma of the pancreas. *Radiographics.* 1990;10:313-322.

50. Sidden CR, Mortele KJ. Cystic tumors of the pancreas: ultrasound, computed tomography, and magnetic resonance imaging features. *Semin Ultrasound CT MR.* 2007;28:339-356.

51. Sarr MG, Murr M, Smyrk TC, et al. Primary cystic neoplasms of the pancreas. Neoplastic disorders of emerging importance-current state-of-the-art and unanswered questions. *J Gastrointest Surg.* 2003;7:417-428.

52. Mergo PJ, Helmberger TK, Buetow PC, Helmberger RC, Ros PR. Pancreatic neoplasms: MR imaging and pathologic correlation. *Radiographics.* 1997;17:281-301.

53. Adsay N. Cystic neoplasia of the pancreas: pathology and biology. *J Gastrointest Surg.* 2008;12:401-404.

54. Sahani DV, Kadavigere R, Saokar A, Fernandez-del Castillo C, Brugge WR, Hahn PF. Cystic pancreatic lesions: a simple imaging-based classification system for guiding management. *Radiographics.* 2005;25:1471-1484.

55. Procacci C, Carbognin G, Accordini S, et al. CT features of malignant mucinous cystic tumors of the pancreas. *Eur Radiol.* 2001;11:1626-1630.

56. Taouli B, Vilgrain V, O'Toole D, Vullierme MP, Terris B, Menu Y. Intraductal papillary mucinous tumors of the pancreas: features with multimodality imaging. *J Comput Assist Tomogr.* 2002;26:223-231.

57. Longnecker DS, Adler G, Hruban RH, Kloppel G. Intraductal papillary mucinous neoplasms of the pancreas. In: Hamilton SR, Aaltonen LA, eds. *WHO Classification of Tumors of the Digestive System.* Lyon, France: IARC Press; 2000:237-240.

58. Procacci C, Graziani R, Bicego E, et al. Intraductal mucin-producing tumors of the pancreas: imaging findings. *Radiology.* 1996;198:249-257.

59. Procacci C, Megibow AJ, Carbognin G, et al. Intraductal papillary mucinous tumor of the pancreas: a pictorial essay. *Radiographics.* 1999;19:1447-1463.

60. Levy P, Jouannaud V, O'Toole D, et al. Natural history of intraductal papillary mucinous tumors of the pancreas: actuarial risk of malignancy. *Clin Gastroenterol Hepatol.* 2006; 4:460-468.

61. Cantisani V, Mortele KJ, Levy A, et al. MR imaging features of solid pseudopapillary tumor of the pancreas in adult and pediatric patients. *AJR Am J Roentgenol.* 2003;181:395-401.

62. Papavramidis T, Papavramidis S. Solid pseudopapillary tumors of the pancreas: review of 718 patients reported in English literature. *J Am Coll Surg.* 2005;200:965-972.

63. Adsay NV. Cystic lesions of the pancreas. *Mod Pathol.* 2007;20: S71-S93.

64. Allen P, D'Angelica M, Gonen M, et al. A selective approach to the resection of cystic lesions of the pancreas: results from 539 consecutive patients. *Ann Surg.* 2006;244:572-582.

65. Lahav M, Maor Y, Avidan B, Novis B, Bar-Meir S. Nonsurgical management of asymptomatic incidental pancreatic cysts. *Clin Gastroenterol Hepatol.* 2007;5:813-817.

66. Berland LL, Silverman SG, Gore RM, et al. Managing incidental findings on abdominal CT: White Paper of the ACR Incidental Findings Committee. *J Am Coll Radiol.* 2010;7:754-773.

67. Balthazar EJ, Freeny PC, vanSonnenberg E. Imaging and intervention in acute pancreatitis. *Radiology.* 1994;193:297-306.

68. Balthazar EJ. Acute pancreatitis: assessment of severity with clinical and CT evaluation. *Radiology.* 2002;223:603-613.

69. Pitchumoni CS, Agarwal N. Pancreatic pseudocysts. When and how should drainage be performed? *Gastroenterol Clin North Am.* 1999;28:615-639.

70. Balthazar EJ. Complications of acute pancreatitis: clinical and CT evaluation. *Radiol Clin North Am.* 2002;40:1211-1227.

71. Piironen A. Severe acute pancreatitis: contrast-enhanced CT and MRI features. *Abdom Imaging.* 2001;26:225-233.

72. Jeffrey RB Jr. Sonography in acute pancreatitis. *Radiol Clin North Am.* 1989;27:5-17.

73. Banks PA. Practice guidelines in acute pancreatitis. *Am J Gastroenterol.* 1997;92:377-386.

74. Bradley EL 3rd. A clinically based classification system for acute pancreatitis. Summary of the International Symposium on Acute Pancreatitis, Atlanta, GA, September 11-13, 1992. *Arch Surg.* 1993;128:586-590.

75. Balthazar EJ, Ranson JH, Naidich DP, Megibow AJ, Caccavale R, Cooper MM. Acute pancreatitis: prognostic value of CT. *Radiology.* 1985;156:767-772.

76. Noone TC, Semelka RC, Worawattanakul S, Marcos HB. Intraperitoneal abscesses: diagnostic accuracy of and appearances at MR imaging. *Radiology.* 1998;208:525-528.

77. Fischer JH, Carpenter KD, O'Keefe GE. CT diagnosis of an isolated blunt pancreatic injury. *AJR Am J Roentgenol.* 1996;167:1152.

78. Bigattini D, Boverie JH, Dondelinger RF. CT of blunt trauma of the pancreas in adults. *Eur Radiol.* 1999;9:244-249.

79. Bradley EL 3rd, Young PR Jr, Chang MC, et al. Diagnosis and initial management of blunt pancreatic trauma: guidelines from a multiinstitutional review. *Ann Surg.* 1998;227:861-869.

80. Leppaniemi AK, Haapiainen RK. Risk factors of delayed diagnosis of pancreatic trauma. *Eur J Surg.* 1999;165:1134-1137.

81. Wong YC, Wang LJ, Lin BC, Chen CJ, Lim KE, Chen RJ. CT grading of blunt pancreatic injuries: prediction of ductal disruption and surgical correlation. *J Comput Assist Tomogr.* 1997;21:246-250.

82. Lin BC, Chen RJ, Fang JF, Hsu YP, Kao YC, Kao JL. Management of blunt major pancreatic injury. *J Trauma.* 2004;56:774-778.

83. Soto JA, Alvarez O, Munera F, Yepes NL, Sepulveda ME, Perez JM. Traumatic disruption of the pancreatic duct: diagnosis with MR pancreatography. *AJR Am J Roentgenol.* 2001;176:175-178.

84. Miller FH, Keppke AL, Balthazar E. Pancreatitis. In: Gore RM, Levine MS, eds. *Textbook of Gastrointestinal Radiology.* Philadelphia, PA: Saunders Elsevier, 2008:1885.

85. Bhatia M, Wong FL, Cao Y, et al. Pathophysiology of acute pancreatitis. *Pancreatology.* 2005;5:132-144.

86. Werner J, Feuerbach S, Uhl W, Buchler MW. Management of acute pancreatitis: from surgery to interventional intensive care. *Gut.* 2005;54:426-436.

87. Amano Y, Oishi T, Takahashi M, Kumazaki T. Nonenhanced magnetic resonance imaging of mild acute pancreatitis. *Abdom Imaging.* 2001;26:59-63.

88. Beger HG, Rau B, Mayer J, Pralle U. Natural course of acute pancreatitis. *World J Surg.* 1997;21:130-135.

89. Balthazar EJ, Robinson DL, Megibow AJ, Ranson JH. Acute pancreatitis: value of CT in establishing prognosis. *Radiology.* 1990;174:331-336.

90. Larvin M, Chalmers AG, McMahon MJ. Dynamic contrast enhanced computed tomography: a precise technique for identifying and localising pancreatic necrosis. *BMJ.* 1990;300:1425-1428.

91. Saifuddin A, Ward J, Ridgway J, Chalmers AG. Comparison of MR and CT scanning in severe acute pancreatitis: initial experiences. *Clin Radiol.* 1993;48:111-116.

92. Baron TH, Thaggard WG, Morgan DE, Stanley RJ. Endoscopic therapy for organized pancreatic necrosis. *Gastroenterology.* 1996;111:755-764.

93. Petrakis I, Vrachassotakis N, Kogerakis N, Koutsoumpas V, Chalkiadakis G. Subacute pancreatic necrosis. *Panminerva Med.* 2000;42:279-286.

94. Banks PA, Gerzof SG, Sullivan JG. Central cavitary necrosis: differentiation from pancreatic pseudocyst on CT scan. *Pancreas.* 1988;3:83-88.

95. Freeny PC, Hauptmann E, Althaus SJ, Traverso LW, Sinanan M. Percutaneous CT-guided catheter drainage of infected acute necrotizing pancreatitis: techniques and results. *AJR Am J Roentgenol.* 1998;170:969-975.

96. Tann M, Maglinte D, Howard TJ, et al. Disconnected pancreatic duct syndrome: imaging findings and therapeutic implications in 26 surgically corrected patients. *J Comput Assist Tomogr.* 2003;27:577-582.

97. Bollen TL, van Santvoort HC, Besselink MG, van Es WH, Gooszen HG, van Leeuwen MS. Update on acute pancreatitis: ultrasound, computed tomography, and magnetic resonance imaging features. *Semin Ultrasound CT MR.* 2007;28:371-383.

98. Sakorafas GH, Tsiotos GG, Sarr MG. Extrapancreatic necrotizing pancreatitis with viable pancreas: a previously under-appreciated entity. *J Am Coll Surg* 1999;188:643-648.

99. Sarles H, Sarles JC, Camatte R, et al. Observations on 205 confirmed cases of acute pancreatitis, recurring pancreatitis, and chronic pancreatitis. *Gut* 1965;6:545-559.

100. Takahashi N, Fletcher JG, Hough DM, et al. Autoimmune pancreatitis: differentiation from pancreatic carcinoma and normal pancreas on the basis of enhancement characteristics at dual-phase CT. *AJR Am J Roentgenol.* 2009;193:479-484.

101. Clain JE, Pearson RK. Diagnosis of chronic pancreatitis. Is a gold standard necessary? *Surg Clin North Am.* 1999;79:829-845.

102. Nijs EL, Callahan MJ. Congenital and developmental pancreatic anomalies: ultrasound, computed tomography, and magnetic resonance imaging features. *Semin Ultrasound CT MR.* 2007;28:395-401.

103. Isserow JA, Siegelman ES, Mammone J. Focal fatty infiltration of the pancreas: MR characterization with chemical shift imaging. *AJR Am J Roentgenol.* 1999;173:1263-1265.

104. Siegelman ES, Mitchell DG, Semelka RC. Abdominal iron deposition: metabolism, MR findings, and clinical importance. *Radiology.* 1996;199:13-22.

105. Jager HJ, Mehring U, Gotz GF, et al. Radiological features of the visceral and skeletal involvement of hemochromatosis. *Eur Radiol.* 1997;7:1199-1206.

106. Steer ML, Waxman I, Freedman S. Chronic pancreatitis. *N Engl J Med.* 1995;332:1482-1490.

107. Luetmer PH, Stephens DH, Ward EM. Chronic pancreatitis: reassessment with current CT. *Radiology.* 1989;171:353-357.

108. Siddiqi AJ, Miller F. Chronic pancreatitis: ultrasound, computed tomography, and magnetic resonance imaging features. *Semin Ultrasound CT MR.* 2007;28:384-394.

109. Campisi A, Brancatelli G, Vullierme MP, Levy P, Ruzniewski P, Vilgrain V. Are pancreatic calcifications specific for the diagnosis of chronic pancreatitis? A multidetector-row CT analysis. *Clin Radiol.* 2009;64:903-911.

110. Lehman GA, Sherman S. Diagnosis and therapy of pancreas divisum. *Gastrointest Endosc Clin N Am.* 1998;8:55-77.

111. Cotton PB. Congenital anomaly of pancreas divisum as cause of obstructive pain and pancreatitis. *Gut.* 1980;21:105-114.

112. Klein SD, Affronti JP. Pancreas divisum, an evidence-based review: part I, pathophysiology. *Gastrointest Endosc.* 2004;60: 419-425.

113. Bret PM, Reinhold C, Taourel P, Guibaud L, Atri M, Barkun AN. Pancreas divisum: evaluation with MR cholangiopancreatography. *Radiology.* 1996;199:99-103.

114. Mortele KJ, Rocha TC, Streeter JL, Taylor AJ. Multimodality imaging of pancreatic and biliary congenital anomalies. *Radiographics* 2006;26:715-731.

115. Kamisawa T, Yuyang T, Egawa N, Ishiwata J, Okamoto A. A new embryologic hypothesis of annular pancreas. *Hepatogastroenterology.* 2001;48:277-278.

116. Nijs E, Callahan MJ, Taylor GA. Disorders of the pediatric pancreas: imaging features. *Pediatr Radiol.* 2005;35:358-373; quiz 457.

117. Urayama S, Kozarek R, Ball T, et al. Presentation and treatment of annular pancreas in an adult population. *Am J Gastroenterol.* 1995;90:995-999.

118. Mortele KJ, Lemmerling M, de Hemptinne B, De Vos M, De Bock G, Kunnen M. Postoperative findings following the Whipple procedure: determination of prevalence and morphologic abdominal CT features. *Eur Radiol.* 2000;10: 123-128.

119. Miedema BW, Sarr MG, van Heerden JA, Nagorney DM, McIlrath DC, Ilstrup D. Complications following pancreaticoduodenectomy. Current management. *Arch Surg.* 1992;127:945-949; discussion 949-950.

120. Hashimoto M, Koga M, Ishiyama K, et al. CT features of pancreatic fistula after pancreaticoduodenectomy. *AJR Am J Roentgenol.* 2007;188:W323-W327.

121. Smith SL, Hampson F, Duxbury M, Rae DM, Sinclair MT. Computed tomography after radical pancreaticoduodenectomy (Whipple's procedure). *Clin Radiol.* 2008;63:921-928.

122. Bluemke DA, Abrams RA, Yeo CJ, Cameron JL, Fishman EK. Recurrent pancreatic adenocarcinoma: spiral CT evaluation following the Whipple procedure. *Radiographics.* 1997;17: 303-313.

123. Lepanto L, Gianfelice D, Dery R, Dagenais M, Lapointe R, Roy A. Postoperative changes, complications, and recurrent disease after Whipple's operation: CT features. *AJR Am J Roentgenol.* 1994;163:841-846.

124. Stumpp P, Kloppel R, Kahn T. Imaging after a whipple operation: improving visibility of the afferent jejunal loop in spiral computed tomography using biliary contrast medium. *J Comput Assist Tomogr.* 2005;29:394-400.

125. Scialpi M, Scaglione M, Volterrani L, et al. Imaging evaluation of post pancreatic surgery. *Eur J Radiol.* 2005;53:417-424.

126. Gruessner AC, Sutherland DE. Pancreas transplant outcomes for United States (US) and non-US cases as reported to the United Network for Organ Sharing (UNOS) and the International Pancreas Transplant Registry (IPTR) as of June 2004. *Clin Transplant.* 2005;19:433-455.

127. Nikolaidis P, Amin RS, Hwang CM, et al. Role of sonography in pancreatic transplantation. *Radiographics.* 2003;23:939-949.

128. Freund MC, Steurer W, Gassner EM, et al. Spectrum of imaging findings after pancreas transplantation with enteric exocrine drainage: Part 1, posttransplantation anatomy. *AJR Am J Roentgenol.* 2004;182:911-917.

129. Sandrasegaran K, Lall C, Berry WA, Hameed T, Maglinte DD. Enteric drainage pancreatic transplantation. *Abdom Imaging.* 2006;31:588-595.

130. Andreoni KA, Brayman KL, Guidinger MK, Sommers CM, Sung RS. Kidney and pancreas transplantation in the United States, 1996-2005. *Am J Transplant.* 2007;7:1359-1375.

131. Dobos N, Roberts DA, Insko EK, Siegelman ES, Naji A, Markmann JF. Contrast-enhanced MR angiography for evaluation of vascular complications of the pancreatic transplant. *Radiographics.* 2005;25:687-695.

132. Freund MC, Steurer W, Gassner EM, et al. Spectrum of imaging findings after pancreas transplantation with enteric exocrine drainage: Part 2, posttransplantation complications. *AJR Am J Roentgenol.* 2004;182:919-925.

133. Meador TL, Krebs TL, Cheong JJ, Daly B, Keay S, Bartlett S. Imaging features of posttransplantation lymphoproliferative disorder in pancreas transplant recipients. *AJR Am J Roentgenol.* 2000;174:121-124.

134. Balthazar EJ, Subramanyam BR, Lefleur RS, et al. Solid and papillary epithelial neoplasm of the pancreas. Radiographic, CT, sonographic, and angiographic features. *Radiology.* 1984;150(1):39-40.

135. Casadei R, Santini D, Calculli L, et al. Pancreatic solid-cystic papillary tumor: clinical features, imaging findings and operative management. *JOP.* 2006;7(1):137-144.

136. Choi BI, Kim KW, Han MC, et al. Solid and papillary epithelial neoplasms of the pancreas: CT findings. *Radiology.* 1988;166(2):413-416.

137. Ferrone CR, Correa-Gallego C, Warshaw AL, et al. Current trends in pancreatic cystic neoplasms. *Arch Surg.* 2009;144(5):448-454.

138. Bradley EL, Gonzalez AC, Clements JL Jr. Acute pancreatic pseudocysts: incidence and implications. *Ann Surg.* 1976; 184(6):734-737.

139. Sankaran S, Walt AJ. The natural and unnatural history of pancreatic pseudocysts. *Br J Surg.* 1975;62(1):37-44.

140. Yeo CJ, Bastidas JA, Lynch-Nyhan A, et al. The natural history of pancreatic pseudocysts documented by computed tomography. *Surg Gynecol Obstet.* 1990;170(5): 411-417.

141. Burke JW, Erickson SJ, Kellum CD, et al. Pseudoaneurysms complicating pancreatitis: detection by CT. *Radiology.* 1986;161(2):447-450.

142. Gadacz TR, Trunkey D, Kieffer RF Jr. Visceral vessel erosion associated with pancreatitis. Case reports and a review of the literature. *Arch Surg.* 1978;113(12):1438-1440.

143. Frey CF. Pancreatic pseudocyst—operative strategy. *Ann Surg.* 1978;188(5):652-662.

144. vanSonnenberg E, Wittich GR, Casola G, et al. Percutaneous drainage of infected and noninfected pancreatic pseudocysts: experience in 101 cases. *Radiology.* 1989;170(3 Pt 1):757-761.
145. Bittner R, Block S, Buchler M, et al. Pancreatic abscess and infected pancreatic necrosis. Different local septic complications in acute pancreatitis. *Dig Dis Sci.* 1987;32(10):1082-1087.
146. Larvin M. Management of infected pancreatic necrosis. *Curr Gastroenterol Rep.* 2008;10(2):107-114.
147. Gupta A, Stuhlfaut JW, Fleming KW, et al. Blunt trauma of the pancreas and biliary tract: a multimodality imaging approach to diagnosis. *Radiographics.* 2004;24(5):1381-1395.
148. Ilahi O, Bochicchio GV, Scalea TM. Efficacy of computed tomography in the diagnosis of pancreatic injury in adult blunt trauma patients: a single-institutional study. *Am Surg.* 2002;68(8):704-707; discussion 707-708.
149. Nelson MG, Jones DR, Vasilakis A, et al. Computed tomographic diagnosis of acute blunt pancreatic transection. *W V Med J.* 1994;90(7):274-278.
150. Kim HS, Lee DK, Kim IW, et al. The role of endoscopic retrograde pancreatography in the treatment of traumatic pancreatic duct injury. *Gastrointest Endosc.* 2001;54(1):49-55.
151. Fulcher AS, Turner MA, Yelon JA, et al. Magnetic resonance cholangiopancreatography (MRCP) in the assessment of pancreatic duct trauma and its sequelae: preliminary findings. *J Trauma.* 2000;48(6):1001-1007.
152. Saraswat VA, Sharma BC, Agarwal DK, et al. Biliary microlithiasis in patients with idiopathic acute pancreatitis and unexplained biliary pain: response to therapy. *J Gastroenterol Hepatol.* 2004;19(10):1206-1211.
153. Lee SP, Nicholls JF, Park HZ. Biliary sludge as a cause of acute pancreatitis. *N Engl J Med.* 1992;326(9):589-593.
154. Levy MJ, Geenen JE. Idiopathic acute recurrent pancreatitis. *Am J Gastroenterol.* 2001;96(9):2540-2555.
155. Marotta PJ, Gregor JC, Taves DH. Biliary sludge: a risk factor for 'idiopathic' pancreatitis? *Can J Gastroenterol.* 1996;10(6): 385-388.
156. Ros E, Navarro S, Bru C, et al. Occult microlithiasis in 'idiopathic' acute pancreatitis: prevention of relapses by cholecystectomy or ursodeoxycholic acid therapy. *Gastroenterology.* 1991;101(6):1701-1709.
157. Karne S, Gorelick FS. Etiopathogenesis of acute pancreatitis. *Surg Clin North Am.* 1999;79(4):699-710.
158. McKay CJ, Buter A. Natural history of organ failure in acute pancreatitis. *Pancreatology.* 2003;3(2):111-114.
159. Uhl W, Warshaw A, Imrie C, et al. IAP Guidelines for the Surgical Management of Acute Pancreatitis. *Pancreatology.* 2002;2(6):565-573.
160. Laokpessi A, Bouillet P, Sautereau D, et al. Value of magnetic resonance cholangiography in the preoperative diagnosis of common bile duct stones. *Am J Gastroenterol.* 2001;96(8): 2354-2359.
161. Larena JA, Astigarraga E, Saralegui I, et al. Magnetic resonance cholangiopancreatography in the evaluation of pancreatic duct pathology. *Br J Radiol.* 1998;71(850):1100-1104.
162. Soto JA, Barish MA, Yucel EK, et al. Pancreatic duct: MR cholangiopancreatography with a three-dimensional fast spin-echo technique. *Radiology.* 1995;196(2):459-464.
163. Hill MC, Barkin J, Isikoff MB, et al. Acute pancreatitis: clinical vs. CT findings. *AJR Am J Roentgenol.* 1982;139(2):263-269.
164. Morgan DE, Baron TH. Practical imaging in acute pancreatitis. *Semin Gastrointest Dis.* 1998;9(2):41-50.
165. Brascho DJ, Reynolds TN, Zanca P. The radiographic "colon cut-off sign" in acute pancreatitis. *Radiology.* 1962;79:763-769.
166. Pickhardt PJ. The colon cutoff sign. *Radiology.* 2000;215(2): 387-389.
167. Schwartz S, Nadelhaft J. Simulation of colonic obstruction at the splenic flexure by pancreatitis: roentgen features. *Am J Roentgenol Radium Ther Nucl Med.* 1957;78(4):607-616.
168. Siegelman SS, Copeland BE, Saba GP, et al. CT of fluid collections associated with pancreatitis. *AJR Am J Roentgenol.* 1980;134(6):1121-1132.
169. Banks PA. Acute pancreatitis: medical and surgical management. *Am J Gastroenterol.* 1994;89(8 Suppl): S78-S85.
170. Bassi C. Infected pancreatic necrosis. *Int J Pancreatol.* 1994;16(1):1-10.
171. Charbonney E, Nathens AB. Severe acute pancreatitis: a review. *Surg Infect (Larchmt).* 2008;9(6):573-578.
172. Gerzof SG, Banks PA, Robbins AH, et al. Early diagnosis of pancreatic infection by computed tomography-guided aspiration. *Gastroenterology.* 1987;93(6):1315-1320.
173. Kivisaari L, Somer K, Standertskjold-Nordenstam CG, et al. Early detection of acute fulminant pancreatitis by contrast-enhanced computed tomography. *Scand J Gastroenterol.* 1983;18(1):39-41.
174. Lecesne R, Taourel P, Bret PM, et al. Acute pancreatitis: interobserver agreement and correlation of CT and MR cholangiopancreatography with outcome. *Radiology.* 1999;211(3):727-735.
175. Ward J, Chalmers AG, Guthrie AJ, et al. T2-weighted and dynamic enhanced MRI in acute pancreatitis: comparison with contrast enhanced CT. *Clin Radiol.* 1997;52(2):109-114.
176. Stimac D, Miletic D, Radic M, et al. The role of nonenhanced magnetic resonance imaging in the early assessment of acute pancreatitis. *Am J Gastroenterol.* 2007;102(5):997-1004.
177. Martin DR, Karabulut N, Yang M, et al. High signal peripancreatic fat on fat-suppressed spoiled gradient echo imaging in acute pancreatitis: preliminary evaluation of the prognostic significance. *J Magn Reson Imaging.* 2003;18(1): 49-58.
178. Baron TH. Defined nomenclature of pancreatic fluid collections. *Gastrointest Endosc.* 2003;57(2):287-288; author reply 288.
179. Morgan DE, Baron TH, Smith JK, et al. Pancreatic fluid collections prior to intervention: evaluation with MR imaging compared with CT and US. *Radiology.* 1997;203(3):773-778.
180. Bollen TL, Besselink MG, van Santvoort HC, et al. Toward an update of the atlanta classification on acute pancreatitis: review of new and abandoned terms. *Pancreas.* 2007;35(2):107-113.
181. Jacobs JE, Birnbaum BA. Computed tomography evaluation of acute pancreatitis. *Semin Roentgenol.* 2001;36(2):92-98.
182. Paulson EK, Vitellas KM, Keogan MT, et al. Acute pancreatitis complicated by gland necrosis: spectrum of findings on contrast-enhanced CT. *AJR Am J Roentgenol.* 1999;172(3): 609-613.
183. Stanten R, Frey CF. Comprehensive management of acute necrotizing pancreatitis and pancreatic abscess. *Arch Surg.* 1990. 125(10):1269-1274; discussion 1274-1275.

184. Bodily KD, Takahashi N, Fletcher JG, et al. Autoimmune pancreatitis: pancreatic and extrapancreatic imaging findings. *AJR Am J Roentgenol.* 2009;192(2):431-437.

185. Okazaki K, Kawa S, Kamisawa T, et al. Clinical diagnostic criteria of autoimmune pancreatitis: revised proposal. *J Gastroenterol.* 2006;41(7):626-631.

186. Yang DH, Kim KW, Kim TK, et al. Autoimmune pancreatitis: radiologic findings in 20 patients. *Abdom Imaging.* 2006;31(1):94-102.

187. Smith CD, Behrns KE, van Heerden JA, et al. Radical pancreatoduodenectomy for misdiagnosed pancreatic mass. *Br J Surg.* 1994;81(4):585-589.

188. van Gulik TM, Reeders JW, Bosma A, et al. Incidence and clinical findings of benign, inflammatory disease in patients resected for presumed pancreatic head cancer. *Gastrointest Endosc.* 1997;46(5):417-423.

189. Okazaki K, Chiba T. Autoimmune related pancreatitis. *Gut.* 2002;51(1):1-4.

190. Uchida K, Okazaki K, Konishi Y, et al. Clinical analysis of autoimmune-related pancreatitis. *Am J Gastroenterol.* 2000;95(10):2788-2794.

191. Sahani DV, Kalva SP, Farrell J, et al. Autoimmune pancreatitis: imaging features. *Radiology.* 2004;233(2):345-352.

192. Takahashi N, Fletcher JG, Fidler JL, et al. Dual-phase CT of autoimmune pancreatitis: a multireader study. *AJR Am J Roentgenol.* 2008;190(2):280-286.

193. Daneman A, Gaskin K, Martin DJ, et al. Pancreatic changes in cystic fibrosis: CT and sonographic appearances. *AJR Am J Roentgenol.* 1983;141(4):653-655.

194. Ferrozzi F, Bova D, Campodonico F, et al. Cystic fibrosis: MR assessment of pancreatic damage. *Radiology.* 1996;198(3): 875-879.

195. Bom EP, van der Sande FM, Tjon RT, et al. Shwachman syndrome: CT and MR diagnosis. *J Comput Assist Tomogr.* 1993;17(3):474-476.

196. Lacaille F, Mani TM, Brunelle F, et al. Magnetic resonance imaging for diagnosis of Shwachman's syndrome. *J Pediatr Gastroenterol Nutr.* 1996;23(5):599-603.

197. Robberecht E, Nachtegaele P, Van Rattinghe R, et al. Pancreatic lipomatosis in the Shwachman-Diamond syndrome. Identification by sonography and CT-scan. *Pediatr Radiol.* 1985;15(5):348-349.

198. Siegelman ES, Mitchell DG, Outwater E, et al. Idiopathic hemochromatosis: MR imaging findings in cirrhotic and precirrhotic patients. *Radiology.* 1993;188(3):637-641.

199. Miller FH, Keppke AL, Wadhwa A, et al. MRI of pancreatitis and its complications: part 2, chronic pancreatitis. *AJR Am J Roentgenol.* 2004;183(6):1645-1652.

200. Semelka RC, Shoenut JP, Kroeker MA, et al. Chronic pancreatitis: MR imaging features before and after administration of gadopentetate dimeglumine. *J Magn Reson Imaging.* 1993;3(1):79-82.

201. Johnson PT, Outwater EK, Pancreatic carcinoma versus chronic pancreatitis: dynamic MR imaging. *Radiology.* 1999;212(1):213-218.

202. Loftus EV Jr, Olivares-Pakzad BA, Batts KP, et al. Intraductal papillary-mucinous tumors of the pancreas: clinicopathologic features, outcome, and nomenclature. Members of the Pancreas Clinic, and Pancreatic Surgeons of Mayo Clinic. *Gastroenterology.* 1996;110(6):1909-1918.

203. Tenner S, Carr-Locke DL, Banks PA, et al. Intraductal mucin-hypersecreting neoplasm "mucinous ductal ectasia": endoscopic recognition and management. *Am J Gastroenterol.* 1996;91(12):2548-2554.

204. Kawamoto S, Lawler LP, Horton KM, et al. MDCT of intraductal papillary mucinous neoplasm of the pancreas: evaluation of features predictive of invasive carcinoma. *AJR Am J Roentgenol.* 2006;186(3):687-695.

205. Salvia R, Festa L, Butturini G, et al. Pancreatic cystic tumors. *Minerva Chir.* 2004;59(2):185-207.

206. Tanaka M, Sawai H, Okada Y, et al. Clinicopathologic study of intraductal papillary-mucinous tumors and mucinous cystic tumors of the pancreas. *Hepatogastroenterology.* 2006;53(71): 783-787.

207. Koito K, Namieno T, Ichimura T, et al. Mucin-producing pancreatic tumors: comparison of MR cholangiopancreatography with endoscopic retrograde cholangiopancreatography. *Radiology.* 1998;208(1):231-237.

208. Sugiyama M, Atomi Y, Hachiya J, Intraductal papillary tumors of the pancreas: evaluation with magnetic resonance cholangiopancreatography. *Am J Gastroenterol.* 1998;93(2): 156-159.

209. Agha FP, Williams KD, Pancreas divisum: incidence, detection, and clinical significance. *Am J Gastroenterol.* 1987;82(4):315-320.

210. Lecco TM. Zur morrphologie des pankreas annulare (in German). Sitzungs berichte der Akademie der Wissenschaften Mathematischnatur, Wien. 1910;119:391-406.

211. Baldwin WM, Specimen of annular pancreas. *Anat Rec.* 1910;4:299-304.

212. Vaughn DD, Jabra AA, Fishman EK. Pancreatic disease in children and young adults: evaluation with CT. *Radiographics.* 1998;18(5):1171-1187.

213. Zyromski NJ, Sandoval JA, Pitt HA, et al. Annular pancreas: dramatic differences between children and adults. *J Am Coll Surg.* 2008;206(5):1019-1025; discussion 1025-1027.

214. Jadvar H, Mindelzun RE. Annular pancreas in adults: imaging features in seven patients. Abdom Imaging. 1999;24(2):174-177.

215. Desai MB, Mitchell DG, Munoz SJ. Asymptomatic annular pancreas: detection by magnetic resonance imaging. *Magn Reson Imaging.* 1994;12(4):683-685.

216. Hidaka T, Hirohashi S, Uchida H, et al. Annular pancreas diagnosed by single-shot MR cholangiopancreatography. *Magn Reson Imaging.* 1998;16(4):441-444.

217. Kamisawa T, Tu Y, Egawa N, et al. MRCP of congenital pancreaticobiliary malformation. *Abdom Imaging.* 2007; 32(1):129-133.

218. Yogi Y, Shibue T, Hashimoto S. Annular pancreas detected in adults, diagnosed by endoscopic retrograde cholangiopancreatography: report of four cases. *Gastroenterol Jpn.* 1987. 22(1):92-99.

219. White SA, Shaw JA, Sutherland DE. Pancreas transplantation. *Lancet.* 2009;373(9677):1808-1817.

220. Nath DS, Gruessner AC, Kandaswamy R, et al. Outcomes of pancreas transplants for patients with type 2 diabetes mellitus. *Clin Transplant.* 2005;19(6):792-797.

221. Hagspiel KD, Nandalur K, Burkholder B, et al. Contrast-enhanced MR angiography after pancreas transplantation: normal appearance and vascular complications. *AJR Am J Roentgenol.* 2005;184(2):465-473.

222. Sollinger HW, Odorico JS, Knechtle SJ, et al. Experience with 500 simultaneous pancreas-kidney transplants. *Ann Surg.* 1998. 228(3):284-296.

223. Dachman AH, Newmark GM, Thistlethwaite JR Jr, et al. Imaging of pancreatic transplantation using portal venous and enteric exocrine drainage. *AJR Am J Roentgenol.* 1998; 171(1):157-163.

224. Larson TS, Bohorquez H, Rea DJ, et al. Pancreas-after-kidney transplantation: an increasingly attractive alternative to simultaneous pancreas-kidney transplantation. *Transplantation.* 2004;77(6):838-843.

225. Krebs TL, Daly B, Wong-You-Cheong JJ, et al. Acute pancreatic transplant rejection: evaluation with dynamic contrast-enhanced MR imaging compared with histopathologic analysis. *Radiology.* 1999;210(2):437-442.

226. Eubank WB, Schmiedl UP, Levy AE, et al. Venous thrombosis and occlusion after pancreas transplantation: evaluation with breath-hold gadolinium-enhanced three-dimensional MR imaging. *AJR Am J Roentgenol.* 2000;175(2):381-385.

227. Paraskevas S, Coad JE, Gruessner A, et al. Posttransplant lymphoproliferative disorder in pancreas transplantation: a single-center experience. *Transplantation.* 2005;80(5):613-622.

CHAPTER

Imaging of the Kidney

Susan Hilton, MD
Nicholas Papanicolaou, MD, FACR

ANATOMY

The adult kidney is about 11 cm long, 2.5 cm thick, and weighs between 120 and 170 g.[1] The left kidney is usually located 1 to 2 cm cephalad to the right kidney. The normal kidneys are smooth, bean-shaped structures with convex contours, except anteromedially, where the open fat-containing renal hila transmit the structures of the renal vascular pedicle. The renal hilum is the entry to the renal sinus, a fat-containing cavity surrounded by the renal parenchyma. The renal sinus contains the renal arteries, veins, lymphatics, and pelvocaliceal structures. The kidney is enveloped by perirenal fat, which in turn is invested by anterior and posterior fascial layers, known as Gerota fascia. The renal hilar fat, renal sinus fat, and perirenal fat are all continuous. The anterior and posterior layers of Gerota fascia fuse laterally to form the lateroconal fascia. The kidneys are located within the perirenal space, 1 of 3 major compartments of the retroperitoneum, deemed the anterior pararenal space (containing the retroperitoneal portion of the duodenum, ascending and descending colon, pancreas, and root of the small bowel mesentery), perirenal space, and posterior pararenal space (containing only fat).[2] The renal parenchyma is composed of cortex and medulla.

IMAGING STUDIES

Current radiographic imaging techniques for evaluating the kidneys include renal ultrasonography (US), intravenous urography (IVU), computed tomography (CT), magnetic resonance imaging (MRI), angiography, and radionuclide imaging.

Advantages of renal US include lack of use of ionizing radiation and low cost. Doppler US is useful to evaluate the renal vasculature, the blood supply and vascular pattern of renal mass lesions, and the vasculature of renal transplant kidneys. On US examination, the normal renal cortex has been described as typically less echogenic than that of liver or spleen, but the results of Platt suggest that the majority of patients whose kidneys exhibit cortical echogenicity equal to that of liver or spleen also have normal renal function.[3] The renal pyramids can often be seen in thin patients. When seen, the medullary pyramids appear hypoechoic relative to the renal cortex. The kidney is a very vascular structure and so color flow imaging will demonstrate intense color flow activity within the central portion of the kidney (see Figure 6-1).

CT is the main imaging modality for evaluation of renal masses and infiltrative renal disorders, and has largely supplanted IVU. Further, CT urography, which consists of CT scans obtained before and after administration of intravenous contrast material, including imaging of the entire urinary tract during the excretion phase, has become the modality of choice for evaluating painless gross or microscopic hematuria. (CT urography will be discussed in detail in Chapter 7: Imaging of the Urinary System.)

On CT examination performed without intravenous contrast, the normal renal parenchyma measures approximately 30 to 50 Hounsfield units (HU), with no discernible difference in density between the cortex and medulla. After intravenous contrast is given as a rapid bolus injection, the kidney can be temporally imaged during several distinct phases, each of which allows optimal visualization of specific anatomic structures and pathologic processes. Arterial-phase images, obtained at 20 to 30 seconds after the start of the intravenous contrast injection, provide detailed depiction of the renal arterial vasculature. During the cortical, or corticomedullary phase (CMP), at approximately 40 seconds after the start of contrast injection, contrast resides in the cortical capillaries, peritubular cells, proximal convoluted tubules, and columns of Bertin, and the cortex of the kidney brightly enhances. During the nephrographic phase, which begins at approximately 100 seconds after the start of contrast injection, the renal parenchyma enhances homogeneously. During the excretory phase, at approximately 3 minutes after the start of injection, the collecting structures of the kidney are densely opacified (see Figure 6-2).

MRI of the kidneys is also useful for characterizing renal masses and is valuable for determining the extent of tumor thrombus in patients with extension of renal carcinoma into the inferior vena cava (IVC). The renal cortex has a shorter T1 than the medulla because of its lower water content. Therefore, corticomedullary differentiation may

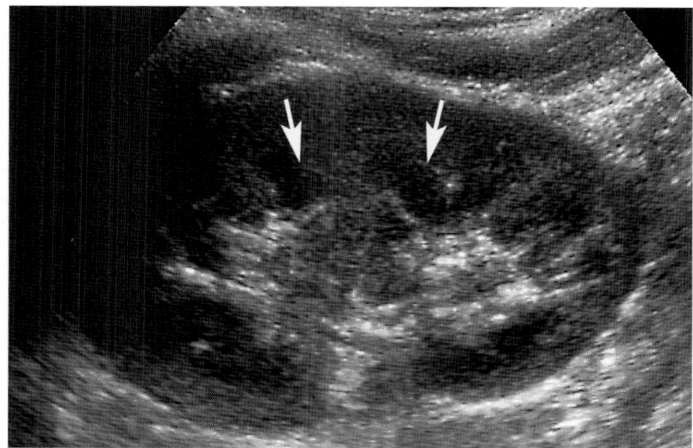

A

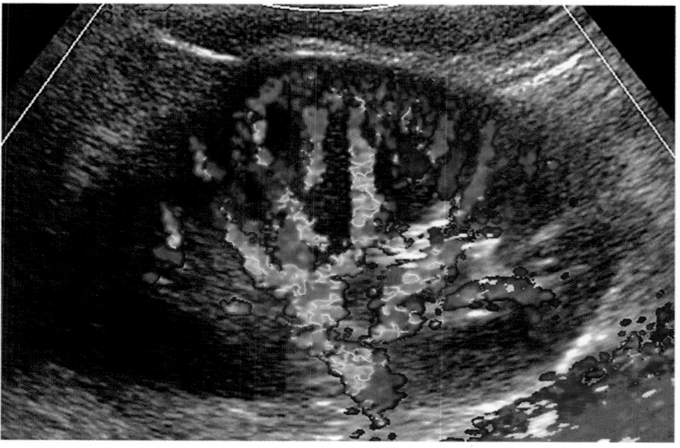

B

Figure 6-1 Normal Renal Ultrasound
Longitudinal US of the left kidney with (**A**) grayscale and (**B**) color flow US shows the normal appearance of the kidney. A. There is normal corticomedullary differentiation, with the medullary pyramids seen as hypoechoic structures (*arrows*). The combined renal sinus fat, nondilated collecting system, and major branches of the renal artery and vein are seen as an echogenic center that is invaginated by medullary pyramids. B. Color flow demonstrates brisk central flow of blood.

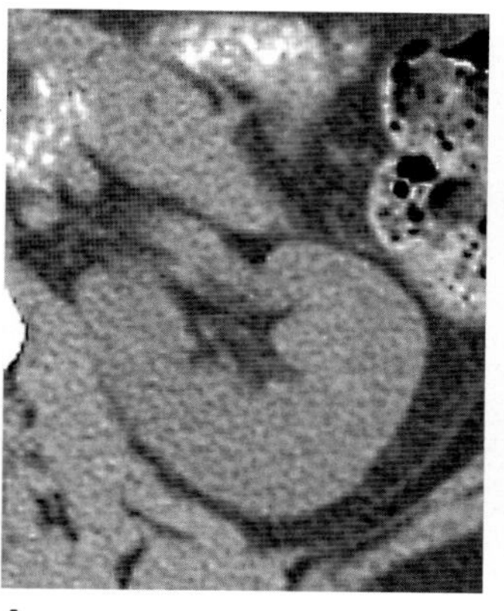
A

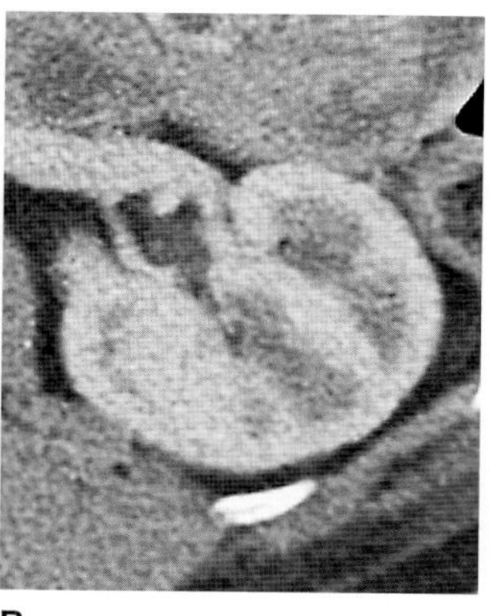
B

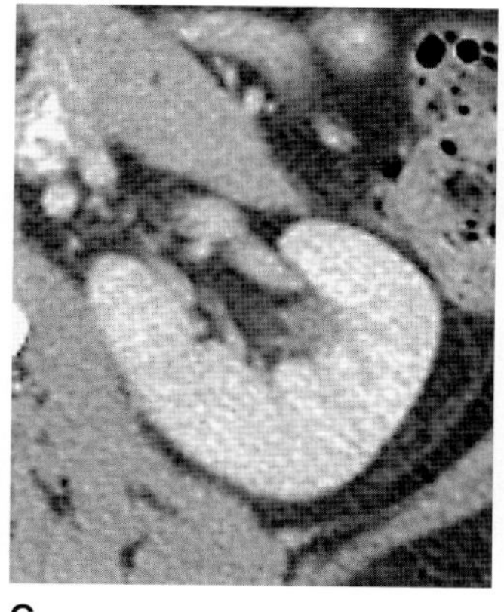
C

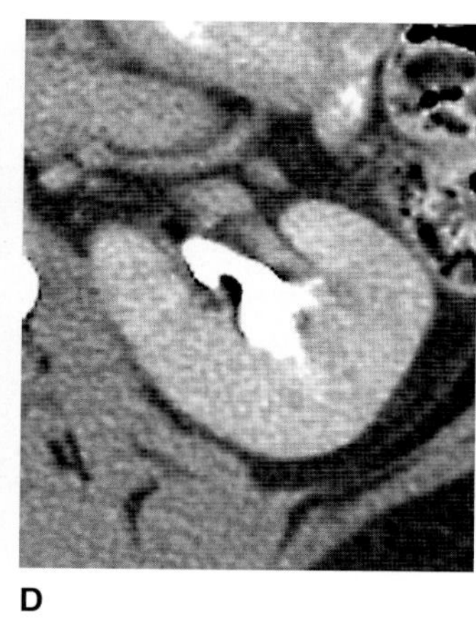
D

Figure 6-2 Phases of Contrast Enhancement
Four axial CT images of the left kidney. **A.** Unenhanced, (**B**) corticomedullary phase (different patient from A, C, and D), (**C**) nephrographic phase, and (**D**) excretory phase images of the left kidney show the changing appearance of the kidney before and after the administration of intravenous contrast. A. Prior to intravenous contrast, all of the soft tissues, except fat, have a similar attenuation. B. Approximately 40 seconds after contrast administration, the cortex of the kidney brightly enhances. The renal medulla, which receives less blood flow than the renal cortex, is less enhanced. C. Approximately 100 seconds after contrast administration, the renal parenchyma enhances homogeneously. D. After a few minutes, the kidney begins to excrete contrast into the collecting system. The calyces and the renal pelvis are filled with contrast and appear bright white. The renal cortex and medulla appear uniform in attenuation and are still slightly brighter (still enhancing) when compared with the unenhanced image.

be seen on T1-weighted images: the lower signal medullary pyramids (which appear darker on the images) are surrounded by the higher signal cortex (which appears brighter on the images). This differentiation is less visible on T2-weighted images. With intravenous administration of paramagnetic contrast agent, such as Gd-DTPA (gadolinium–diethylene-triamine-pentaacetic acid), which is completely filtered in the glomerulus and excreted by the kidneys, contrast dynamics as the agent passes through the kidney are similar to CT. On T1-weighted images, in the first 10 to 20 seconds after intravenous injection, signal intensity (SI) increases in the renal cortex, because of appearance of Gd-DTPA during marked arterial perfusion of the cortex, which receives the majority of the blood supply to the kidney. (This increased SI on T1-weighted imaging is due to T1 shortening effects of gadolinium.) Maximum SI is observed approximately 20 ± 50 seconds after the first signs of cortical perfusion. With the onset of glomerular filtration and dilution in the extravascular space, the SI slowly decreases. In the medulla, an increase in SI is typically seen approximately 10 ± 20 seconds later than in the cortex, with maximum SI reaching similar or slightly higher values than the cortex. At 30 ± 40 seconds after the first visible signs of medullary perfusion, the SI decreases steeply to a minimum value.[4]

The SI changes that may be observed in the renal medulla on contrast-enhanced MRI display one important difference from CT contrast dynamics. Reabsorption of water in the proximal tubule, loop of Henle, and collecting duct results in a hyperconcentration of Gd-DTPA; the SI drop seen in the medullary pyramids is a result of the T2-shortening effects of gadolinium that predominate at this high concentration.[5] Subsequently, when the contrast agent passes into the calyces and is diluted with non–contrast-containing glomerular filtrate, the SI in the medulla again increases to intensity similar to the cortex. With excretion into the calyces, there is an SI decrease in the region of the renal pelvis (see Figure 6-3).

Radioisotope studies of the kidneys include the radioisotope renogram, for evaluation of renal function, the diuretic renogram for evaluation of urinary tract obstruction, radionuclide renal perfusion studies for evaluation of patients with suspected renovascular hypertension (usually performed with administration of captopril, an angiotensin-converting enzyme inhibitor) or the status of a renal transplant, and radionuclide renal function studies.

Although positron emission tomography (PET) has become a powerful tool for imaging a number of malignancies, applications of PET using ^{18}F-fluorodeoxyglucose (FDG) in the urinary tract have been limited by the normal urinary excretion of FDG and the fact that renal cell carcinoma may not be FDG avid.

FOCAL KIDNEY LESIONS

Focal renal lesions can be due to neoplasm, infection, trauma, vascular cause, including infarction or hemorrhage, cyst, or uncommonly, localized forms of inflammatory conditions including xanthogranulomatous pyelonephritis and malacoplakia (Table 6-1). These focal lesions can be broadly subdivided into solid and cystic lesions.

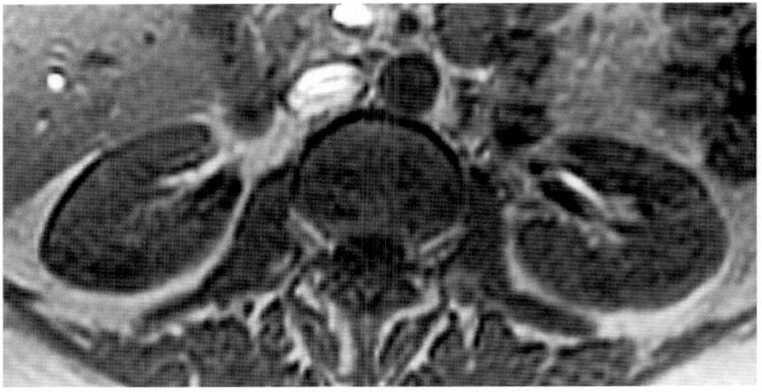

A

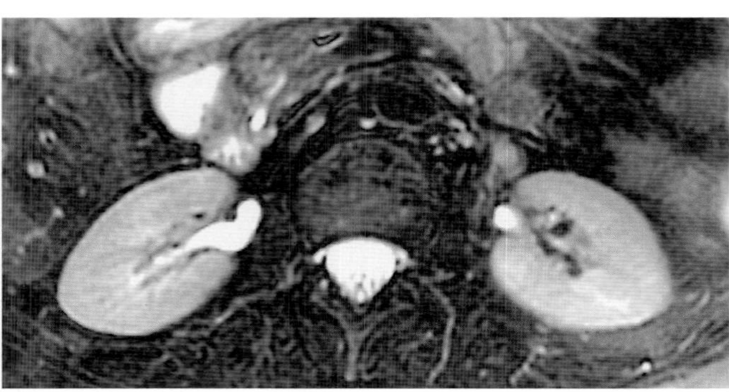

B

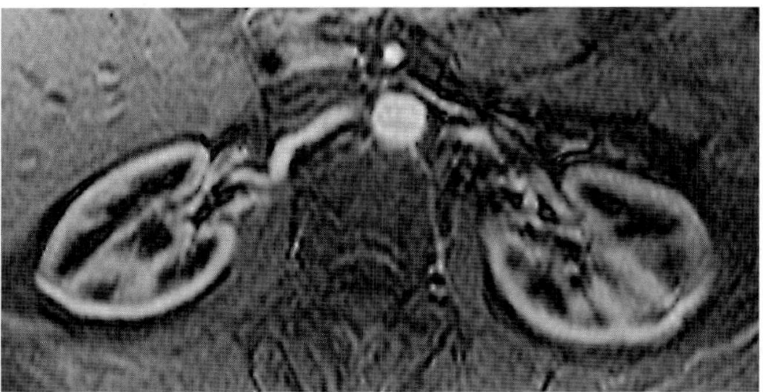

C

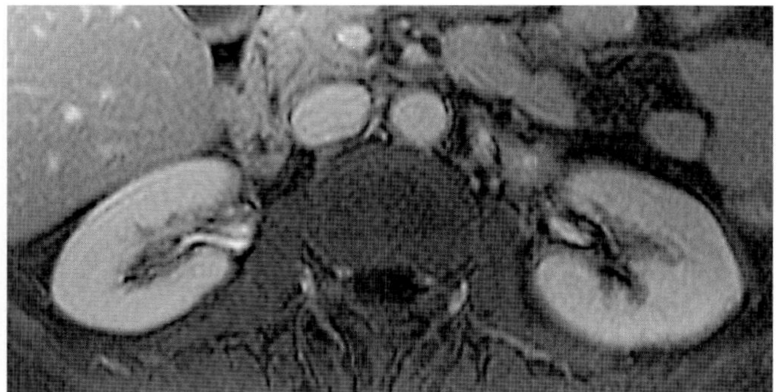

D

Figure 6-3 Normal Renal MRI
Normal kidneys on T1-weighted (**A**), fat-saturated T2-weighted (**B**), and axial fat-saturated postgadolinium T1-weighted images (**C** and **D**). Renal parenchyma is usually hypointense on T1-weighted images (A) and hyperintense on T2-weighted images (B) relative to normal liver. Note that fluid appears hyperintense on T2-weighted images, including the urine in the renal collecting system and the CSF in the spinal canal. Following administration of intravenous gadolinium, renal enhancement follows a similar pattern to that seen on CT (Figure 6-2), initially with greater enhancement of the cortex than the medulla (C, corticomedullary phase), followed by more homogeneous enhancement (D, nephrographic phase).

Solid Renal Lesions

Neoplasms are the most common cause of solid renal lesions; however, focal traumatic lesions, infarcts, and some other inflammatory lesions often also appear solid on imaging exams.

Neoplasms

At least 85% of solid renal masses are due to renal cancer. As the size of a solid renal tumor increases, there is a significantly greater likelihood that the tumor is malignant rather than benign, and among malignant tumors, that it is of clear cell subtype and higher nuclear grade.[6] Other malignant solid renal mass lesions include lymphoma and metastatic lesions to the kidney from extrarenal primary tumor sites. Benign solid renal masses include oncocytoma, benign mesenchymal neoplasms including angiomyolipomas (common) and leiomyoma (rare), papillary adenoma, metanephric adenoma (MA), and unspecified categories (Table 6-2).

Renal cell carcinoma: Renal cell carcinoma (RCC) originates from the renal tubular epithelium. Classification of histologic subtypes of renal carcinoma has evolved from a

Imaging Notes 6-1. Renal Tumor Size and histopathology

The larger the solid renal mass:
1. the greater the likelihood it is malignant.
2. the greater the likelihood of clear cell histology.

Table 6-1. Focal Kidney Lesions: Categories

Neoplasm
Infection
Trauma
Vascular
Cyst
Localized form of inflammatory conditions (uncommon)

Table 6-2. Benign Renal Neoplasms

Renal parenchymal
Solid
Oncocytoma
Metanephric adenoma
Papillary adenoma
Cystic
Cystic nephroma
Mixed epithelial and stromal tumor
Mesenchymal
Leiomyoma
Angiomyolipoma

Table 6-3. Histologic Subtypes of Renal Carcinoma

Type	Frequency	Prognosis
Conventional (clear cell) carcinoma	70%-75% of renal cancers	Second worst prognosis; 5-y survival of 55%-60%
Papillary carcinoma	10%-15% of renal cancers	High 5-y survival: 80%-90%
Chromophobe renal carcinoma	5% of renal cancers	Best prognosis: 5-y survival approximately 90%
Unclassified	4%-5% of renal cancers	Uncertain
Collecting duct carcinoma	<1% of renal cancers	Worst prognosis: 5-y survival rate <5%

morphologically based system to a scheme that attempts to incorporate the appearance of the lesions on light microscopy with the current understanding of tumor genetics. The Heidelberg classification,[7] adopted by the World Health Organization in collaboration with the Union Internationale Contre le Cancer (UICC) and the American Joint Committee on Cancer (AJCC) in 1997, includes 4 subtypes: conventional (clear cell) carcinoma (70%-75% of renal cancers), papillary carcinoma (10%-15%), chromophobe carcinoma (5%), collecting duct carcinoma (<1%), and an unclassified category (4%-5%) (see Table 6-3).[8] Patients with collecting duct carcinoma have the worst prognosis, with a 5-year survival rate of less than 5%. Clear cell carcinoma has the second worst prognosis, with 5-year survival of 55% to 60%. Papillary carcinoma is associated with a high 5-year survival rate (80%-90%), and patients with chromophobe renal carcinoma have the best prognosis, with a 5-year survival of approximately 90%.[9] Papillary renal cancers are characterized by abnormalities of chromosomes 7 and 17 and loss of chromosome Y.

Renal cell carcinoma can arise sporadically or as part of a hereditary condition, most often hereditary papillary renal carcinoma or Von Hippel-Lindau syndrome (VHL). Hereditary papillary renal carcinoma is inherited with an autosomal dominant pattern, associated with multifocal papillary renal cell carcinoma.[10] VHL disease is a familial multiple cancer syndrome in which there is a predisposition to a number of neoplasms, including clear cell renal cell carcinomas, renal cysts, retinal hemangiomas, hemangioblastomas of the cerebellum and spinal cord, pheochromocytomas, and pancreatic carcinomas and cysts (see Figure 6-4). Renal cysts are frequently multiple and

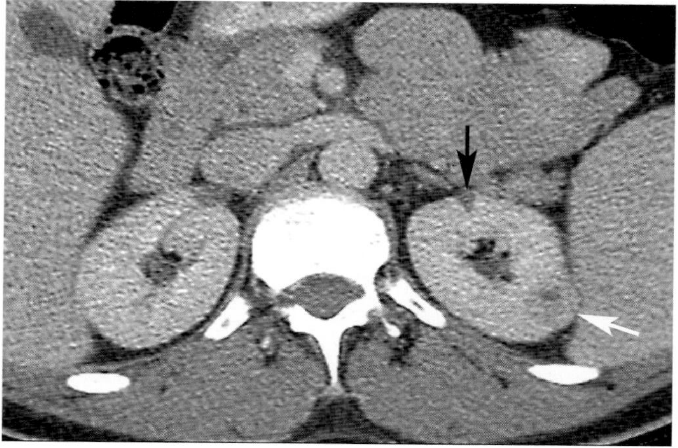

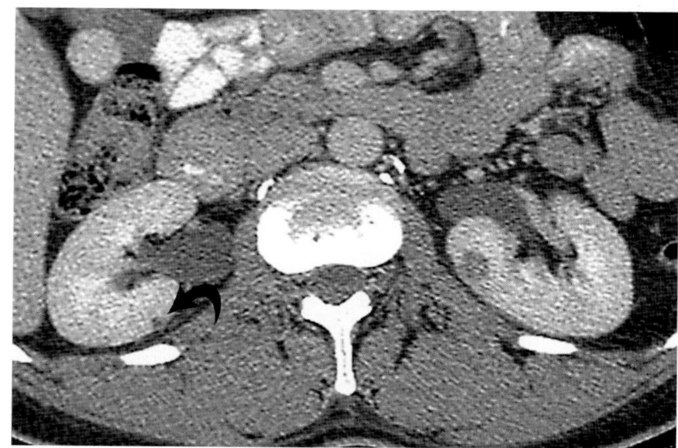

Figure 6-4 Von Hippel-Lindau syndrome (VHL)
Thirty-five-year-old man with VHL. **A** and **B**. Axial images from contrast-enhanced abdominal CT scan demonstrates multiple small lesions. Some of the lesions are cysts (*black arrow*); other lesions are cysts containing small foci of solid enhancing tissue (*curved arrow*), and some lesions are frankly solid (*white arrow*). (The patient also had a history of Hodgkin lymphoma; foci of high-density anterior to the spine in (B) represent retained contrast from a previous lymphangiogram.)

bilateral, often containing renal carcinoma. Renal cell carcinoma develops in nearly 40% of patients with VHL and is a major cause of death among these patients.[11] Defects in the VHL suppressor gene are found in 60% of the sporadic cases of clear cell carcinoma.

In addition to histologic subtyping, the use of nuclear grading of renal cancer with the Fuhrman classification system[12] is widely accepted and has been shown to confer prognostic significance. This system defines 4 nuclear grades (1-4) in order of increasing nuclear size, irregularity, and nucleolar prominence. Nuclear grading is applied mainly to clear cell and papillary cancers. Nuclear grade 4 is sometimes referred to as the sarcomatoid variant of renal carcinoma.

Patients with renal carcinoma are usually more than 40 years old at diagnosis, and the disease occurs predominantly in the seventh and eighth decades of life. Renal cell carcinoma occurs nearly twice as often in men as in women. The most common presentations are hematuria (50%-60% of patients), abdominal pain (40%), and a palpable mass in the flank or abdomen (30%-40%). However, the combination of these 3 symptoms as a "classic triad" at presentation occurs in less than 10% of patients. Patients can present with nonspecific symptoms such as fever, night sweats, malaise, and weight loss. The recent widespread use of cross-sectional imaging of the abdomen has resulted in an increase in the number of incidentally detected renal cancers. Currently, the majority of renal cancer diagnoses are made by detection of an incidental renal mass,[13] as compared with 10% or less before these imaging tools became commonly used.[11]

Renal cell carcinoma exhibits variable appearances on cross-sectional imaging, ranging from a solid mass that can contain areas of central necrosis, to a predominantly cystic mass with mural nodular components. A useful strategy for the evaluation of renal masses is to divide them on the basis of their growth pattern into ball-type or bean-type masses, a concept developed at the Armed Forces Institute of Pathology by David S. Hartman, MD, and Pablo R. Ros, MD, MPH.[13] Clear cell RCC is the prototypic ball lesion with (1) well-defined margins, (2) spherical shape, and (3) contour-deforming. Aggressive forms of transitional cell carcinoma (TCC) represent the prototypic bean lesion with (1) poorly defined margins, (2) infiltrative, nonspherical shape, and (3) non–contour deforming (see Figure 6-5). However, an exception to this rule is the approximately 5% of conventional RCCs that have an infiltrative growth pattern; these are often aggressive cancers that have already spread at the time of presentation.

Renal cancer can vary in size from several centimeters to tens of centimeters in diameter. As tumor size increases, there is an increase in the odds of having a malignant rather than a benign tumor, a clear cell rather than a papillary RCC, and a high-grade RCC rather than a low-grade RCC (see Figure 6-6).[6,14] Although small tumors, <3 cm in diameter, frequently present at a curable stage with low likelihood of metastasis, there are reports showing a definite incidence of high nuclear grade and tumor extension beyond the renal capsule in some small renal tumors.[15] These data lend support to the argument for aggressive treatment over surveillance management of small lesions.

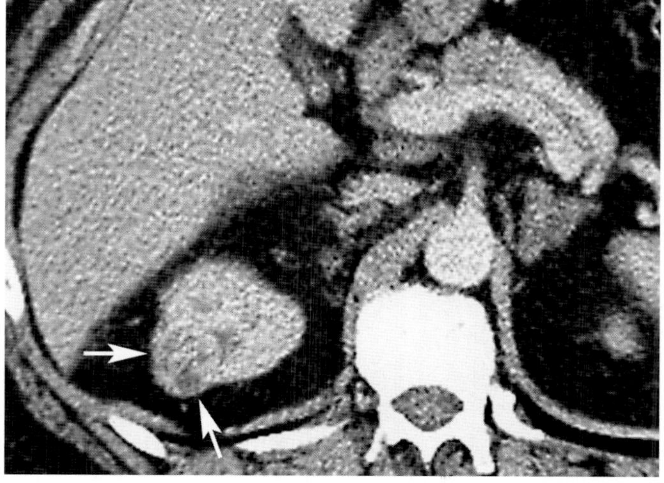

A

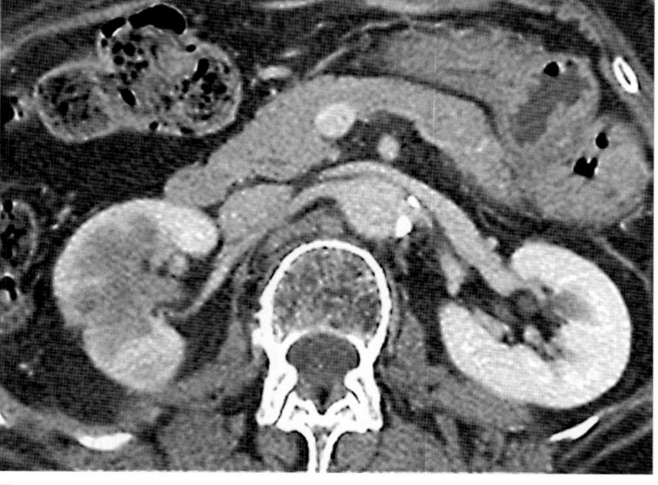

B

Figure 6-5 "Ball"-type versus "Bean"-type Renal Mass
A. Axial image from a contrast-enhanced CT scan, at the level of the right upper kidney. This spherical, sharply circumscribed, contour-deforming mass (*arrows*) is typical of a "ball"-type lesion and represented a clear cell renal carcinoma. An incidental left adrenal nodule found to represent an adenoma is also noted.

B. Axial image from a contrast-enhanced CT urogram, at the level of the renal hila. A hypoenhancing, centrally located, infiltrating mass is seen, typical of a "bean"-type lesion, and represents a poorly differentiated transitional cell carcinoma of the right renal collecting system.

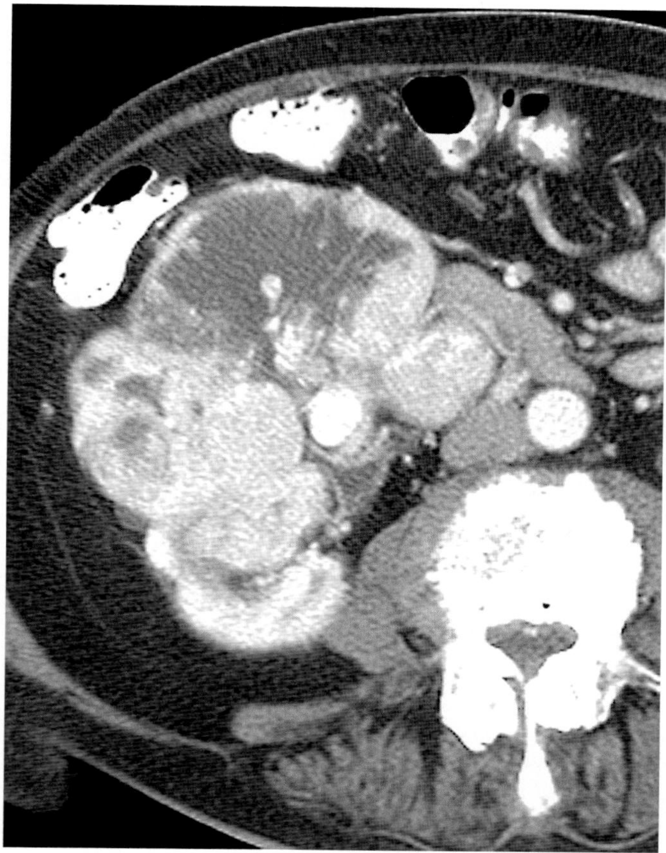

A

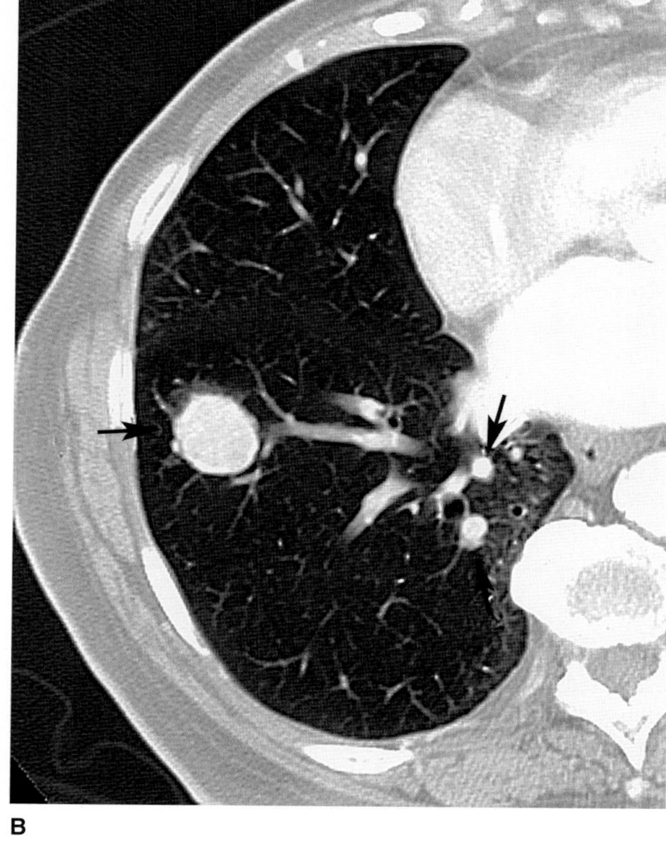

B

Figure 6-6 Large Renal Cell Carcinoma with Lung Metastases Large right renal carcinoma. **A.** Axial image from a contrast-enhanced CT scan, at the level of the right mid-kidney. A large, heterogeneously enhancing renal mass is demonstrated. **B.** An image from the same CT examination, at the level of the lung bases, demonstrates right lower lobe lung nodules (*arrows*) representing metastases.

Computed tomographic scanning is the mainstay imaging modality for assessment of renal lesions suspected to represent renal carcinoma. The CT study should be performed using thin sections (3 mm or thinner, which can be easily achieved with multidetector helical scanners), performed both before and after intravenous contrast is given, in a multiphase sequence. Scanning parameters (slice thickness, pitch, tube current, peak voltage) of the unenhanced and contrast-enhanced examinations should be held constant for the multiple phases, in order to minimize variation in HU density. The initial unenhanced images are used to detect calcification and obtain baseline HU density measurements of the mass. Arterial-phase images can be obtained using thin, 1.5-mm-or-less, axial sections, when detailed evaluation of the renal arterial vasculature is necessary. The cortical, or corticomedullary (CM), phase scan allows differentiation of normal variants of renal parenchyma from renal masses and depicts tumor hypervascularity. Peak enhancement of renal vessels during early CMP also provides information on vascular anatomy. However, small hypovascular lesions of the renal medulla can escape detection during this phase, as these lesions can be of similar density to the unenhanced renal medulla. The nephrographic phase is most optimal for detection and characterization of small renal masses.[16] During the excretory phase, at approximately 3 minutes after the start of injection, the collecting structures of the kidney are densely opacified. The excretory phase allows assessment of the relationship of the mass to the renal collecting system, especially important in planning for partial nephrectomy or ablative treatment (see Figure 6-7).

The most important criterion used in differentiating surgical from nonsurgical renal masses is the determination of enhancement, which is a significant increase in density in HU after intravenous contrast administration.[17] Enhancement indicates vascularity within the mass and is highly predictive of neoplasm. In the past, with conventional (nonhelical) CT scanners, a difference of 10 HU was suggested as evidence of enhancement. However, it is now recognized HU readings obtained on the newer helical scanners demonstrate wider variability, attributed to beam hardening created by enhancing tissue adjacent to a lesion being

Imaging Notes 6-2. Phases of Renal Contrast Enhancement on CT

Phase	Time After Start of Injection	Best for Detection of
Nonenhanced	Before injection	Renal calcifications, baseline density of mass
Arterial	20-30 s	Renal arterial abnormalities
Cortical	40 s	Differentiate normal parenchyma from renal mass
Nephrographic	100 s	Parenchymal mass lesions, enhancement of mass
Excretory	180 s	Collecting system abnormalities

evaluated, especially if the enhancing tissue partially or completely surrounds a small lesion.[18] Although there is no universally agreed upon threshold for enhancement, it has been proposed by many authors that the previous 10 HU threshold be raised to at least 15 to 20 HU. A mass that increases in density by only 10 to 20 HU should be considered indeterminate, and requires further characterization (see Figure 6-8).[17]

Several authors have attempted to differentiate subtypes of renal carcinoma based on radiologic imaging patterns. The most consistent differentiating feature is the brisk enhancement of clear cell carcinoma as compared to the other subtypes (see Figure 6-9).[9,19] Other features, including homogeneous or heterogeneous pattern of enhancement, the presence or absence of calcification, and tumor-spreading pattern overlap among the subtypes of renal cell carcinoma, although a combination of features of a given lesion may suggest a specific subtype. It is well known that papillary renal carcinomas are typically hypoenhancing (see Figure 6-8).[20] Chromophobe tumors tend to display homogeneous enhancement, with an intermediate degree of enhancement as compared to clear cell and papillary subtypes (see Figure 6-10).

MRI is useful for characterization of renal masses and can be used as a problem-solving tool for masses that prove difficult to characterize with other imaging modalities. Further, MRI is also useful as an alternative imaging modality for patients with history of sensitivity to iodinated intravenous contrast. Improved signal-to-noise ratios of higher (1.5 Tesla) field strength units and the use of fat suppression techniques improve lesion conspicuity. Signal characteristics of renal mass lesions on MRI vary with the presence of necrotic or hemorrhagic elements, and iron deposits. Enhancement with intravenous contrast (Gd-DTPA) is assessed with spin-echo or T1-weighted sequences performed before and after contrast administration. As with CT, the presence of enhancement within a renal lesion on MRI after the administration of intravenous contrast material is the most reliable criterion for distinguishing solid masses from cysts. At MRI on opposed-phase images, up to 60% of clear cell renal carcinomas show relative focal and diffuse loss of SI, because of intracytoplasmic lipid content

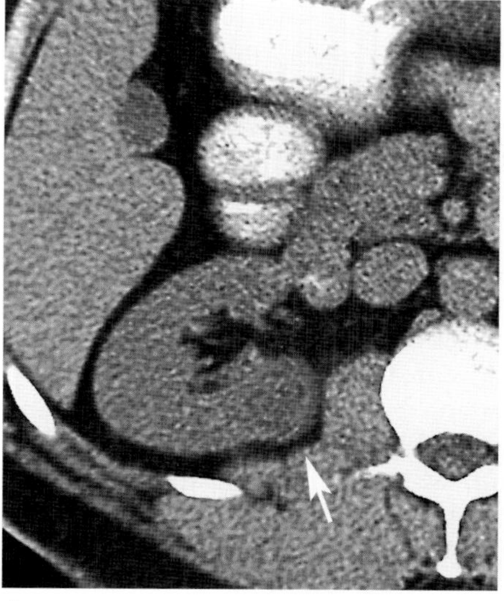
A

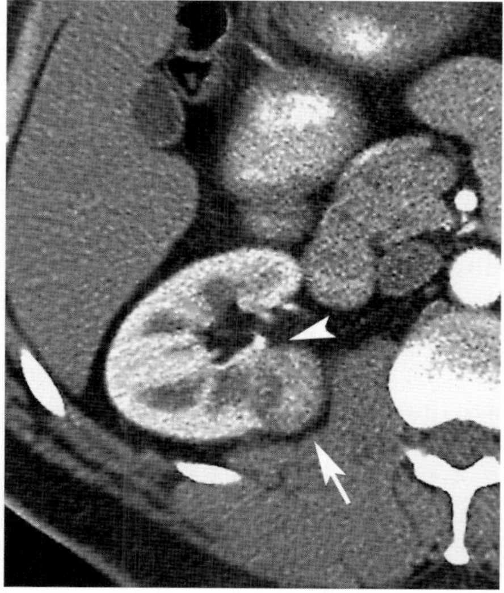
B

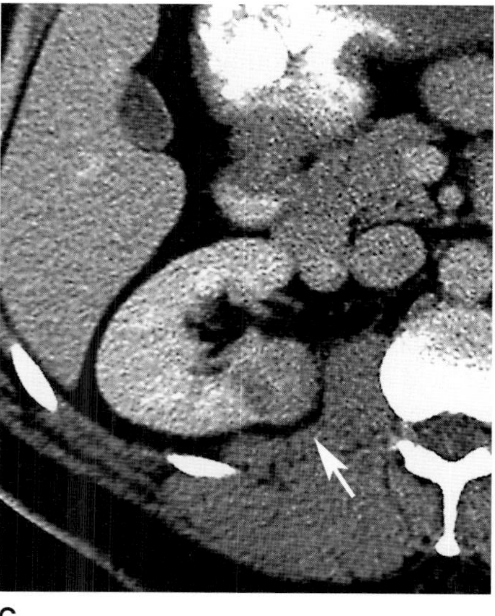
C

Figure 6-7 Small Renal Cell Carcinoma
This 52-year-old man had a palpably enlarged liver. CT images (**A**) precontrast, (**B**) arterial-phase, and (**C**) nephrographic-phase images demonstrate an incidentally detected 2.8-cm, enhancing renal mass (*arrows*). The lesion, which displays central enhancement, is most conspicuous on the contrast-enhanced images. This is most likely a small renal cell carcinoma. Metastasis is unlikely given its sharply defined and exophytic appearance.

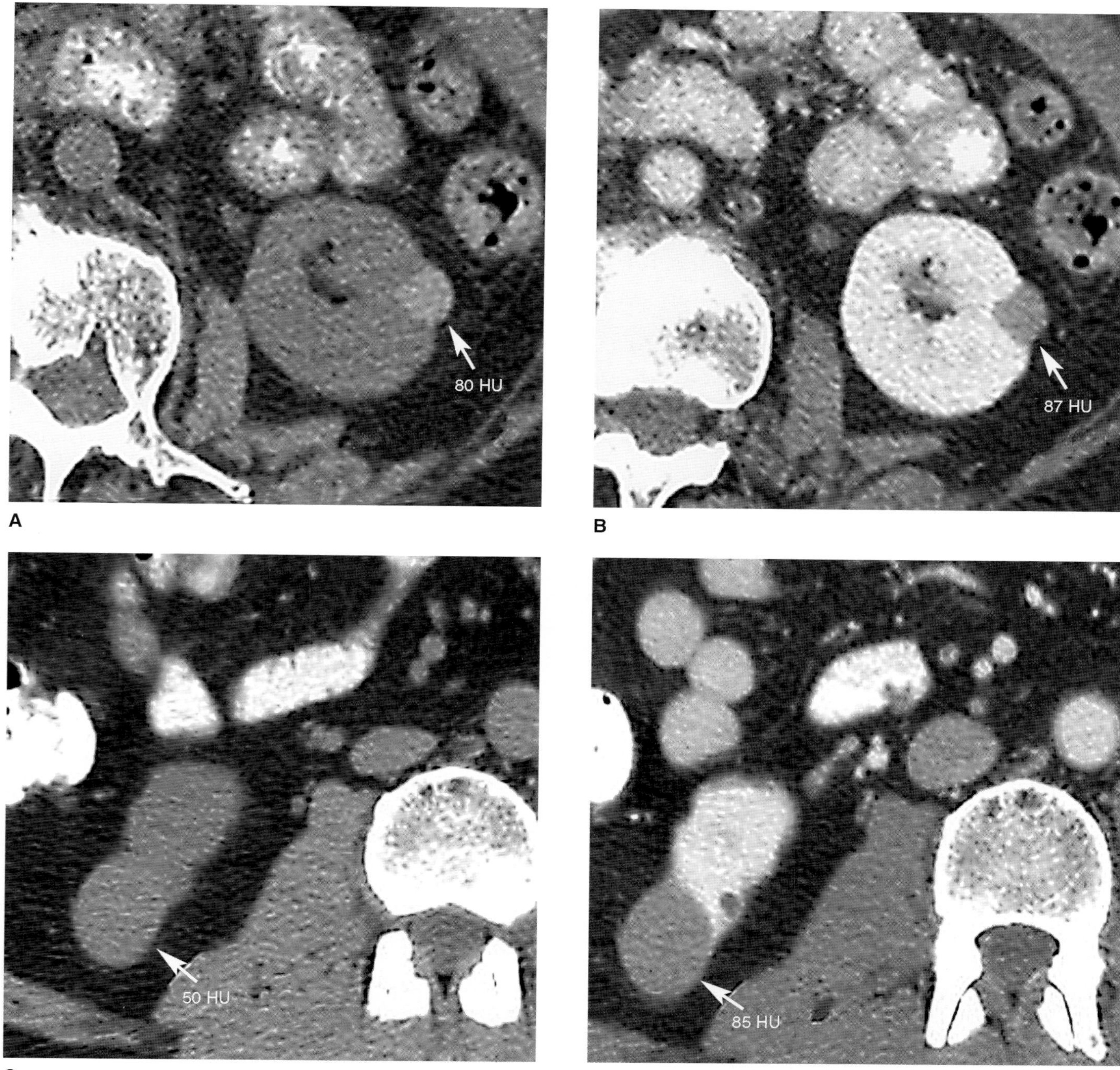

Figure 6-8 Hyperdense Cyst versus Enhancing Renal Cell Carcinoma
A. This small, left renal mass is homogenously denser than normal unenhanced renal parenchyma (*arrow*). **B.** It does not enhance after intravenous contrast administration and is therefore in keeping with a hyperdense cyst. **C.** This mass (*arrow*) is slightly denser than the normal renal parenchyma before intravenous contrast administration. **D.** Its density increases after intravenous contrast administration by more than 30 HU, in keeping with a renal neoplasm, in this case a papillary renal cell carcinoma.

of these tumors (see Figure 6-11).[21] This lipid should be distinguished from the focal fat shown in angiomyolipomas. Angiomyolipomas with a predominant fatty component are isointense relative to fat with all MRI sequences. Use of opposed-phase images will allow diagnosis of some renal carcinomas that are difficult to distinguish from transitional cell carcinoma (TCC) or oncocytoma, as neither oncocytomas nor TCC display intracellular lipid. (However, lack of lipid content in a lesion does not exclude the possibility of RCC.)[22]

Interpretation of CT or MRI studies for evaluation of renal carcinoma should include staging of the tumor based

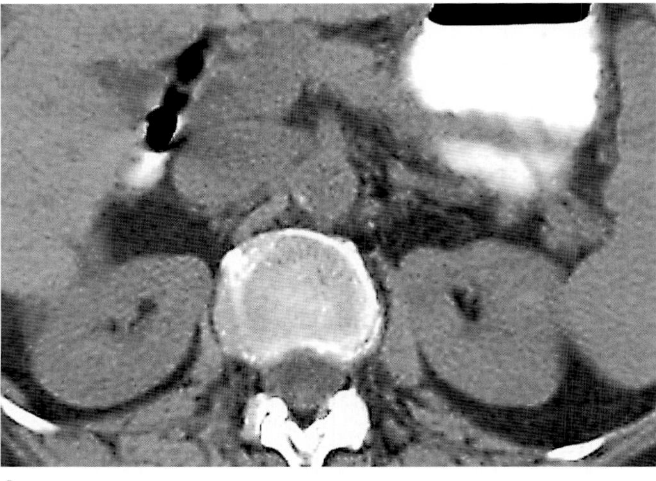

A

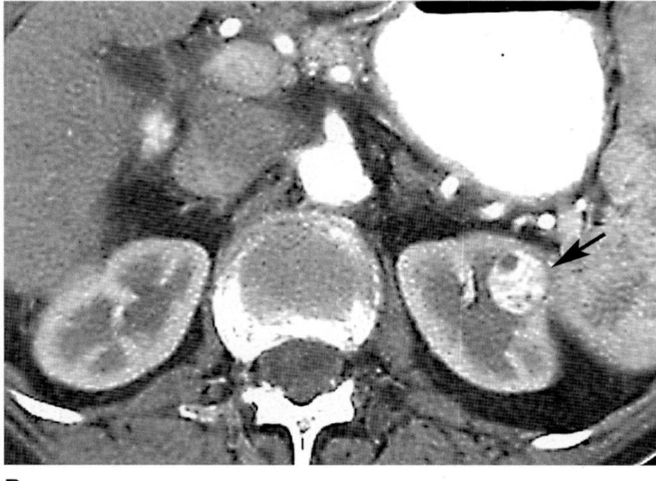

B

Figure 6-9 Briskly Enhancing Clear Cell Carcinoma
A. Axial CT image before intravenous contrast, at the level of the left upper renal pole. The mass is barely discernable from the surrounding renal tissue. **B.** Contrast-enhanced axial CT section at the same level demonstrates a spherical mass (*arrow*), with marked enhancement typical of clear cell carcinoma. This mass is completely free of the renal sinus fat and is amenable to partial nephrectomy.

on the imaging results. In the United States, the TNM staging system[23] is commonly used (Table 6-4). It has been observed that CT has a staging accuracy for renal carcinoma of up to 91%.[24] It should be kept in mind, however, that enlarged retroperitoneal regional lymph nodes can be due to benign reactive change rather than metastatic disease in up to 50% of cases;[25] care should be taken not to upstage patients to stage III solely on the basis of enlarged regional retroperitoneal lymph nodes without compelling evidence for tumor involvement (see Figure 6-12). Similarly, a mild degree of perirenal fat stranding is nonspecific and should not be assumed to represent tumor transgression beyond the renal capsule, that is, T3 and thus, stage III, disease. Evaluation for the possibility of tumor extension into the renal vein (RV) and IVC is important for treatment planning. Knowledge of the level of tumor thrombus extension into the IVC is important for preoperative planning. Four categories of IVC thrombus extension have been defined: from the RV into the infrahepatic IVC for a distance of 1 to 2 cm (level I), from the RV to not beyond the subhepatic IVC (level II), from the RV into the intrahepatic IVC or to the suprahepatic IVC but not into the right atrium (level III), from the RV into the IVC with extension into the right atrium (level IV) (see Figure 6-13). The surgical

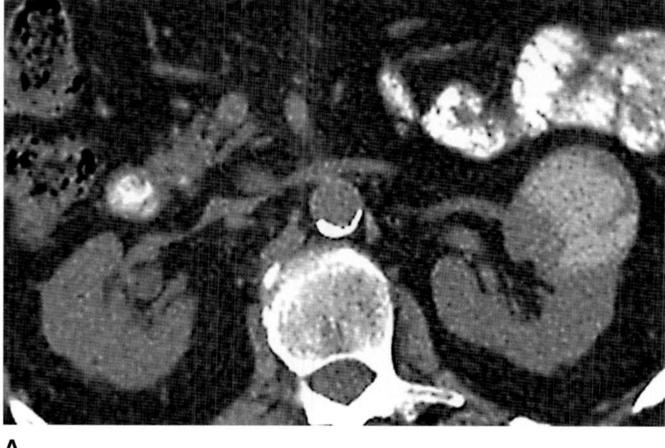

A

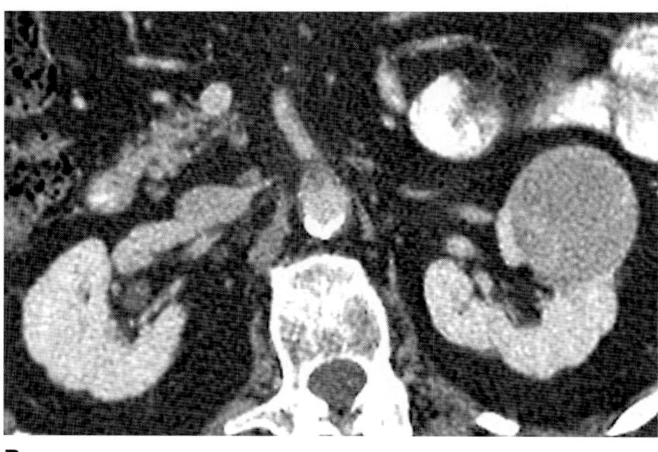

B

Figure 6-10 Chromophobe Carcinoma
A. Axial CT section, before intravenous contrast administration shows partially hyperdense mass in the left anterior mid-kidney. **B.** Contrast-enhanced section through the mass shows mild enhancement of the lesion. The noncalcified portion of the mass enhanced from 42 to 105 HU.

Imaging Notes 6-3. Categories of IVC Tumor Thrombus

Category	Description
I	From the renal vein (RV) into the infrahepatic IVC for a distance of 1-2 cm
II	From the RV to not beyond the subhepatic IVC
III	From the RV into the intrahepatic IVC or to the suprahepatic IVC but not into the right atrium
IV	From the RV into the IVC with extension into the right atrium

approach for thrombectomy, including type of incision (abdominal, thoracoabdominal, or including sternotomy) and election to use cardiopulmonary bypass, depends on the level of IVC tumor involvement delineated by preoperative imaging.[26] Traditionally, for delineation of extent of tumor thrombus within the IVC, MRI has been the imaging study of choice, largely because of its multiplanar imaging capability. However, with advances in CT technology that achieve multiphase imaging with thin sections and high-quality multiplanar and 3-D reconstruction, CT may be equally accurate.[27]

Surgical partial nephrectomy for treatment of stage I tumors is now accepted as a standard treatment.[28,29] Originally, partial nephrectomy was an option only for tumors that measured <4 cm in diameter and were without evidence of renal sinus fat extension. However, more recent reports suggest that use of a size cutoff of 7 cm results in no difference in outcome as compared to the 4 cm threshold (see Figure 6-9). A recent report describes preliminary experience with the use of laparoscopic partial nephrectomy to treat renal hilar tumors.[30]

Thermal tumor percutaneous ablative techniques, either radiofrequency (RF) or cryoablation, have attained an important role in the treatment of renal tumors for patients who are not surgical candidates. The success of these ablative procedures has led to their increased use to treat renal carcinoma in patients without significant comorbidities who prefer to undergo minimally invasive treatment rather than surgery.

Percutaneous renal RF ablation is performed by placing an electrode within the renal tumor under imaging guidance. A high-frequency alternating current passes from the active portion of the electrode into the surrounding tissues, causing frictional heating followed by cell death. Cryoablation freezes the tumor tissue; cell death results from intracellular ice formation and osmotic imbalance. Internally cooled electrodes of cryoablation allow coagulative necrosis without tissue charring, an advantage of cryoablation over RF ablation.

Radiologic imaging is performed both during and after these procedures, using CT or MRI. For both CT and MRI, it is important to perform imaging before and after the administration of intravenous contrast. A typical MRI protocol would include T1- and T2-weighted images as well as T1-weighted images obtained before and after the administration of intravenous gadolinium-based contrast material. Fat-suppressed T2-weighted images increases conspicuity of fluid collections.[31]

The postablation bed and periablational region demonstrate a predictable appearance that can be differentiated from complications or tumor recurrence. During CT-guided RF ablation, perirenal stranding develops, and the pararenal fascia may become thickened. Some hemorrhage can

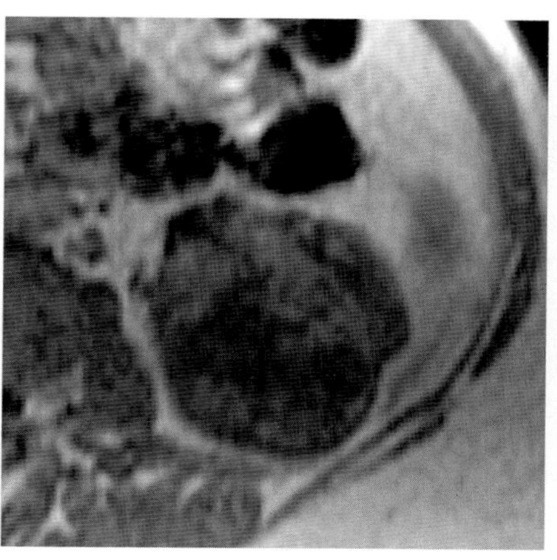
A

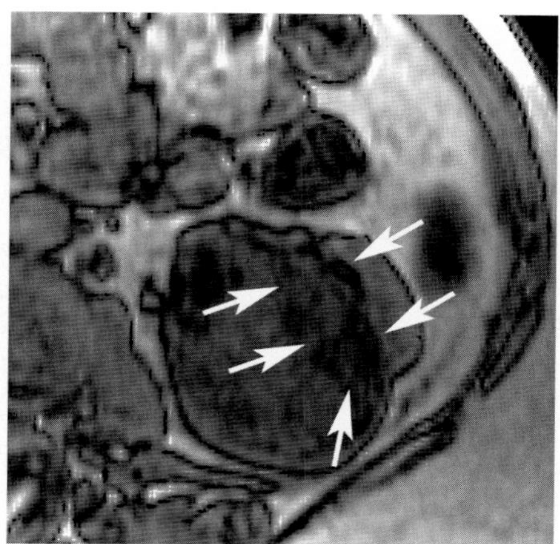
B

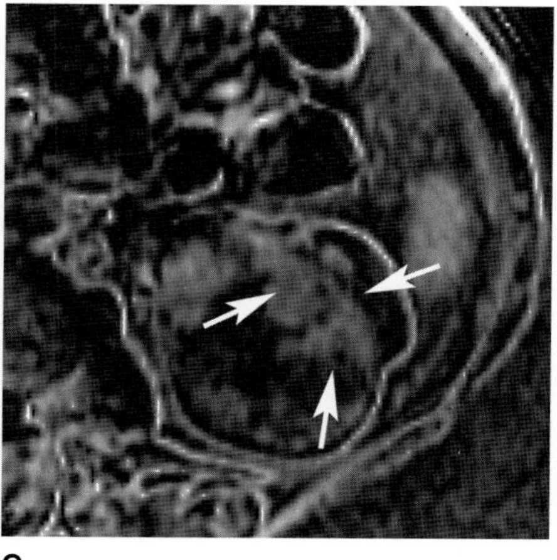
C

Figure 6-11 Clear Cell Renal Carcinoma With Lipid on MRI
A. Axial section from a T1-weighted sequence demonstrates a left renal mass with heterogeneous SI. **B.** Axial section from a T1-weighted opposed phase sequence, demonstrates a drop in SI in portions of the mass (areas appear darker, indicated by *arrows*), in keeping with intracellular lipid content. **C.** Axial subtraction image, obtained by electronically subtracting image (B) from image (A). The areas of signal loss shown in (B) now appear relatively bright (*arrows*).

Table 6-4. AJCC Staging of Renal Cancer

Definition of TNM	
Primary Tumor (T)	
TX	Primary tumor cannot be assessed
T0	No evidence of primary tumor
T1	≤7 cm, limited to kidney
T1a	≤4 cm, limited to kidney
T1b	4-7 cm, limited to kidney
T2	>7, limited to the kidney
T3	Invasion of major veins, adrenal gland, or perinephric tissues within Gerota fascia
T3a	Invasion of adrenal gland, renal sinus fat, and/or perinephric fat within Gerota fascia
T3b	Extension into renal vein or its segmental branches or IVC below the diaphragm
T3c	Extension into IVC above the diaphragm or invasion of IVC wall
T4	Tumor invades beyond Gerota fascia
Regional Lymph Nodes (N)	
NX	Regional lymph nodes cannot be assessed
N0	No regional lymph node metastases
N1	Metastases in a single regional lymph node
N2	Metastasis in more than one regional lymph node
Distant Metastasis (M)	
MX	Distant metastasis cannot be assessed
M0	No distant metastasis
M1	Distant metastasis

Stage Grouping			
Stage I	T1	N0	M0
Stage II	T2	N0	M0
Stage III	T1-2	N1	M0
	T3	N0-1	M0
Stage IV	T4	N0	M0
	T4	N1	M0
	Any T	N2	M0
	Any T	Any N	M1

Data from the *AJCC Cancer Staging Handbook*, 7th Edition.

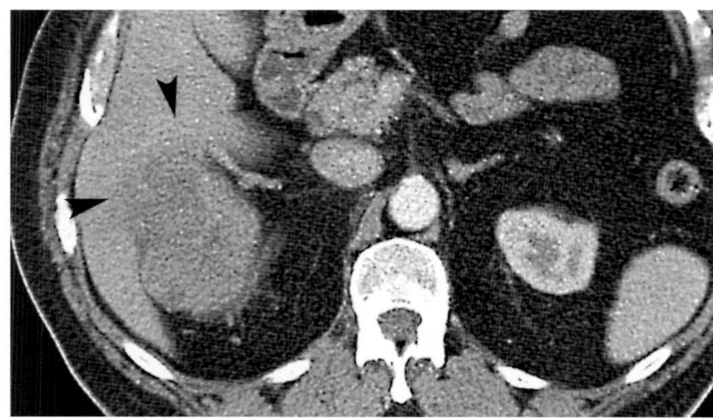

A

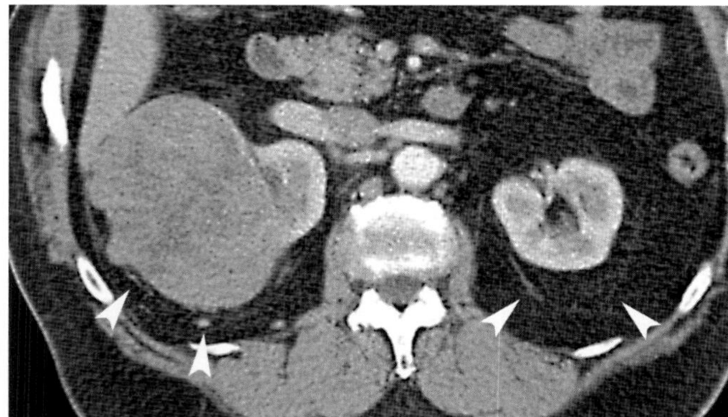

B

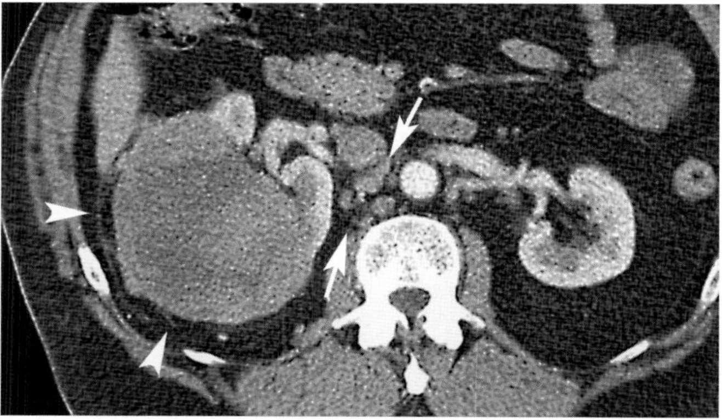

C

Figure 6-12 Large Renal Cell Carcinoma
This 72-year-old man had hematuria and weight loss. **A-C.** Enhanced CT demonstrates an inhomogeneously enhancing mass in the upper pole of the right kidney. Although there is no fat plane between the superior extent of the mass and the liver raising concern for hepatic invasion, additional imaging, preferably with MRI, should be obtained to provide confirmatory evidence of hepatic invasion to avoid upstaging the patient in error. Note the thin white line in the fat surrounding the kidneys bilaterally (*white arrows*), representing Gerota fascia. Several small bright nodular densities in the retroperitoneal fat about the mass likely represent recruited blood vessels, often seen in association with large renal cancers. The *white arrows* in (C) identify a cluster of mildly enlarged para-aortic lymph nodes; although these could represent metastasis, in up to 50% of cases these will represent reactive lymph nodes without tumor.

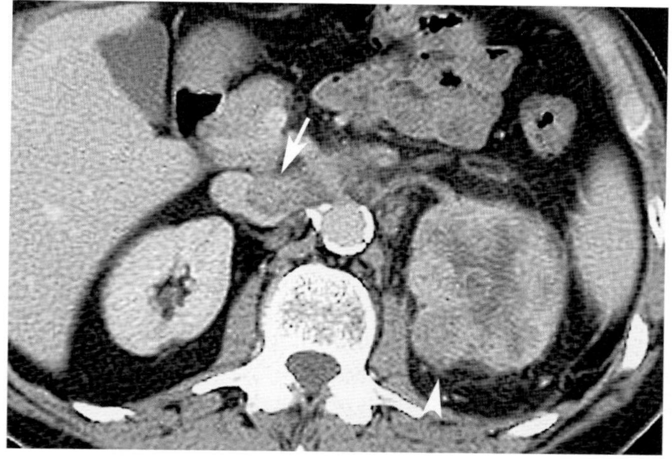

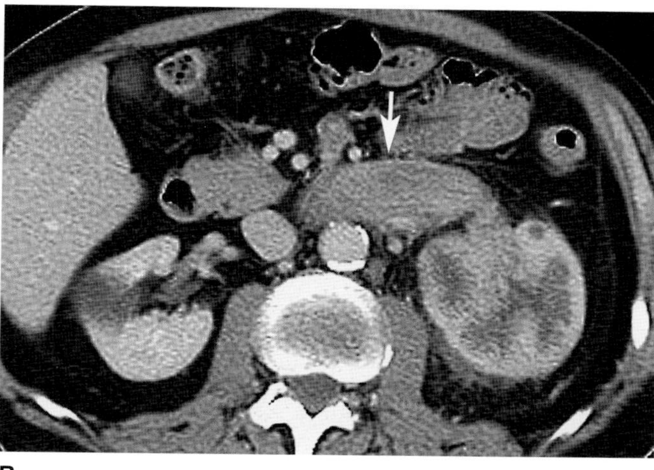

Figure 6-13 Renal Carcinoma With Renal Vein Invasion
This 60-year-old man complained of fatigue. **A** and **B.** Contrast-enhanced CT images shows a large inhomogeneous infiltrating and partially exophytic mass (*arrowhead*) projecting from the upper pole of the left kidney later proven to represent a renal carcinoma. There is extension of enhancing tumor into the left RV to the confluence with the IVC (*arrows*). Note in (B) that the left kidney is larger in size, has perinephric edema, and exhibits a delayed nephrogram. These are features of the left RV obstruction by the left upper pole mass. CT of the chest also demonstrated lung metastasis.

occur, and small locules of gas can be seen in adjacent tissue. On an immediate postprocedure contrast-enhanced CT scan, there should be no evidence of tumor enhancement. At MRI, the tumor loses SI on T2-weighted images obtained during RF ablation, becoming significantly hypointense relative to its pretreatment appearance. The SI of the treated tumor on T1-weighted images obtained at low field strength has been reported as variable immediately following ablation. During cryoablation on CT, a clearly defined region of decreased attenuation develops as the tumor is frozen. On MRI during cryoablation the ice ball appears as a well-demarcated signal void on T1-weighted MR images.[31] Postprocedure CT or MRI is useful to detect complications of thermal tumor ablation procedures, the most common being hemorrhage but also including strictures and urine leaks.

On surveillance MRI scans performed after RF ablation, the ablation site often exhibits a bull's-eye appearance, with a peritumoral rim of variable SI. On well-registered subtraction MRI images, subtracting pre– from post–intravenous contrast data sets, no central enhancement should be evident, although at least 1 study indicates that a thin peripheral rim of enhancement can present in the absence of residual tumor.[32] On surveillance CT, the RF ablation bed should also show no evidence of enhancement. Residual tumor is suggested when enhancing nodules or crescents are noted in the vicinity of the treated tumor on contrast-enhanced CT scans or MR images (see Figure 6-14).[33] The size of the ablation zone can appear to increase in the early period (1-2 m) after RF ablation, especially with small (≤3-cm³) tumors.[32] Although most treated lesions gradually regress after RF ablation, the presence of a residual mass alone does not indicate residual neoplasm. With cryoablation, as with RF ablation, no central enhancement of the tumor on contrast-enhanced CT or MRI should be present, although some authors have reported a peripheral enhancing rim to be a common MRI finding in the first few months after cryoablation. Masses after cryoablation tend to undergo much more dramatic involution than those treated with RF ablation.

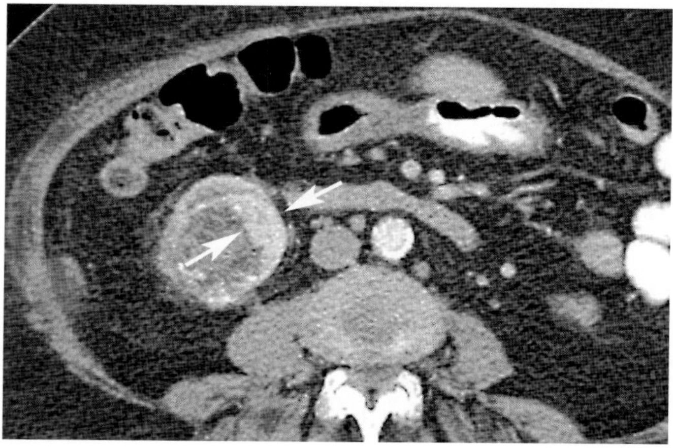

Figure 6-14 Residual Tumor After RF Ablation
Eighty-one-year-old woman with biopsy-proven right renal cell carcinoma, status post transcatheter embolization and RF ablation. A crescent-shaped area of enhancement (*arrows*) is noted at the medial aspect of the tumor mass indicating residual tumor.

Oncocytoma, renal metanephric adenoma, and papillary adenoma: Oncocytoma, renal metanephric adenoma, and papillary adenoma are 3 benign epithelial tumors of the kidney. Renal oncocytoma is a benign renal epithelial neoplasm that represents 3% to 5% of all primary epithelial neoplasms that occur in the adult kidney.[34] The age distribution for oncocytoma and renal cell carcinoma is similar with a peak incidence in the sixth and seventh decades. The tumor is often incidentally found but can also present as a renal mass or with hematuria. An oncocytoma often appears as a solid enhancing renal cortical mass that is indistinguishable from a small renal carcinoma on US, CT, and MRI exams. However, in up to one-third of cases, oncocytomas will contain a characteristic central stellate scar. The central scar can be seen on contrast-enhanced CT as a stellate central low density, but this sign often cannot be distinguished from central necrosis in RCC. On MRI, when the central scar is present, it appears as a stellate area of low SI on T1-weighted images and high SI on T2-weighted images.[21] Unfortunately, the appearance of oncocytomas on MRI is often nonspecific. Oncocytomas can be quite large, up to 25 cm, at presentation (see Figure 6-15). Bilateral and multifocal oncocytomas are seen in 2 unusual situations: renal oncocytosis and in patients with the rare syndrome: Birt-Hogg-Dubé.

Metanephric adenoma (MA) is a rare benign renal neoplasm that is histologically characterized by a monotonous population of small, embryonal (metanephric) cells. This tumor most commonly occurs as an incidental finding in patients during their fifth or sixth decades.[35] Masses due to MA are typically solid and hypoenhancing, indistinguishable from renal carcinomas. Some metanephric adenomas that reach large size can exhibit central necrosis.[36]

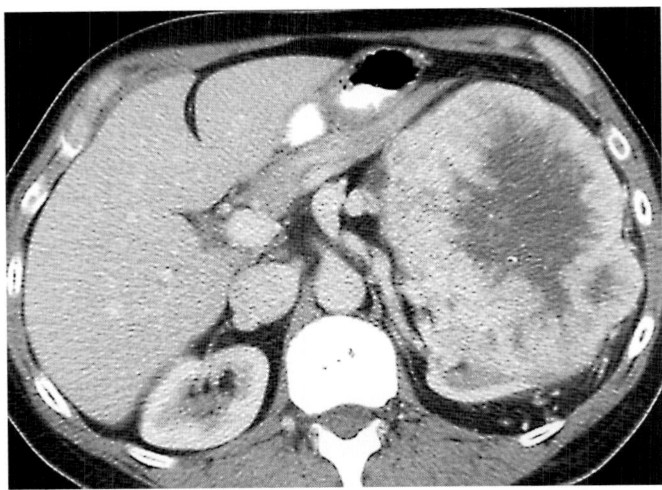

Figure 6-15 Large Renal Oncocytoma
Intravenous contrast-enhanced axial CT image shows large enhancing left renal mass containing central stellate low-density scar. The mass measured 19 cm at the largest diameter and represented an oncocytoma at surgical pathology.

The American Joint Committee on Cancer defines the term *papillary adenoma* for lesions that are <5 mm and histologically resemble low-grade papillary RCC.[37] There are few examples of these in the radiologic imaging literature, likely owing to the tiny size of these lesions and the consequent low likelihood that they will be treated surgically.

With current imaging technologies, these 3 benign renal neoplasms cannot be reliably preoperatively distinguished from renal cell carcinoma.

Leiomyoma: Renal leiomyomas are benign mesenchymal smooth muscle tumors that commonly arise from the renal capsule and derive their blood supply from capsular vessels. The tumor is usually a peripherally located, enhancing mass with an exophytic growth pattern.[34,38]

Angiomyolipoma: Angiomyolipoma (AML) is a benign mesenchymal tumor of the kidney containing varying amounts of adipose tissue, smooth muscle cells, and thick-walled blood vessels. Angiomyolipomas are grouped under a family of tumors characterized by the proliferation of perivascular epithelioid cells (PEComas).[38] The majority of AMLs occur sporadically and are typically found in women in the fourth and fifth decades. Sporadic AMLs are usually small, asymptomatic, and incidentally discovered during cross-sectional imaging. However, larger angiomyolipomas can present with flank pain due to spontaneous hemorrhage and/or gross hematuria.

Approximately 20% of AMLs are associated with the phacomatosis tuberous sclerosis (TS) or with the related lung disease lymphangioleiomyomatosis (LAM).[39] When associated with these diseases, AMLs are commonly bilateral and are often larger than those that occur sporadically and occur in younger patients, typically age 25 to 35 years, with no sex predilection. During the imaging workup of renal angiomyolipomas, the radiologist may be the first to recognize the characteristic thin-walled cysts of pulmonary LAM, a slowly progressive, ultimately severe lung disease that can occur as part of the TS complex (see Figure 6-16).

Angiomyolipoma commonly appears as a heterogeneous renal parenchymal mass with varying proportions of macroscopic fat, intralesional small aneurysms, and hypervascular soft tissue. Macroscopic fat is typically diffusely hyperechoic on US, and a renal mass that is uniformly hyperechoic on US suggests a diagnosis of AML (see Figure 6-17). However, it should be noted that some renal carcinomas also can appear echogenic on US exams; therefore CT or MRI is generally advised to confirm the presence of suspected intralesional fat (see Figures 6-17 and 6-18). Macroscopic fat within the lesion is best identified using either CT without intravenous contrast or MRI with fat suppression. Unfortunately, a small percentage of AMLs do not contain sufficient macroscopic fat to be detected on imaging studies; these lesions cannot be distinguished from other solid renal tumors, including renal carcinoma (see Figure 6-19).

Although the finding of macroscopic fat on CT is of tremendous use for diagnosis of AML, a few notes of caution

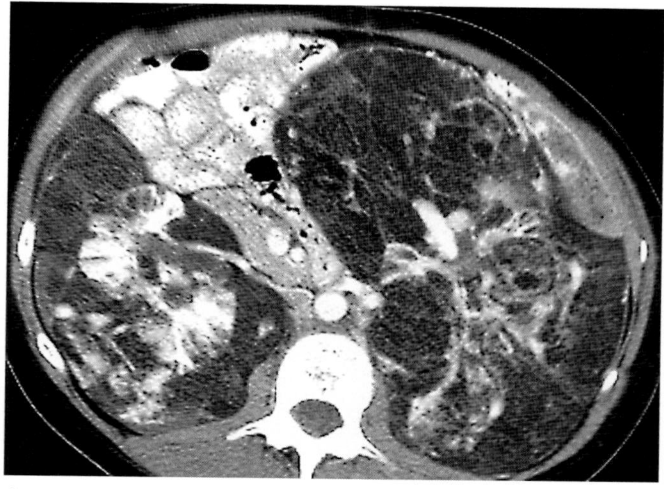

A

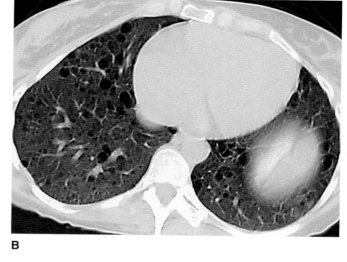

B

Figure 6-16 Tuberous Sclerosis-Associated Angiomyolipomas With Lymphangioleiomyomatosis
This 34-year-old woman had a history of TS. **A.** Contrast-enhanced axial CT image demonstrates massively enlarged kidneys with near replacement of the renal parenchyma by extensive angiomyolipomas. **B.** Image at the lung bases demonstrates typical thin-walled pulmonary cysts.

are advised. The visible fat should be clearly within the substance of the lesion, as retroperitoneal fat can be engulfed by a renal carcinoma, simulating an AML. Also, the fat within the lesion should be sharply defined. Central necrosis within a carcinoma can occasionally undergo saponification, and thus measure fat density on CT images. Any intratumoral calcification within a lesion is rare in AML and therefore suggestive of malignancy.[40]

Lymphoma: Non-Hodgkin lymphomas can involve the kidneys. In most cases, there will be associated extrarenal findings such as widespread adenopathy or large masses that will suggest the diagnosis of lymphoma. Primary renal lymphoma that is isolated to the renal parenchyma with no systemic manifestations, findings that can mimic a renal carcinoma, is uncommon, accounting for less than 1% of cases of extranodal lymphoma. Involvement of the kidneys by Hodgkin disease is exceedingly uncommon, seen in less than 1% of patients at presentation.[41] Renal lymphoma will be discussed most completely under the heading: **Multifocal Renal Lesions**, later in this chapter.

Kidney Metastasis: Renal metastases are the most common malignant neoplasms of the kidney found at autopsy.[42] However, renal metastases are uncommonly seen on cross-sectional imaging studies. When found, they will most often appear as multiple, bilateral, or less commonly, solitary unilateral, infiltrative renal masses, in the setting of a patient with a known primary malignancy. Presentation of metastasis to the kidney as a solitary renal mass is uncommon but can occur; a mass due to metastasis to the kidney is usually poorly defined and infiltrative in appearance. A sharply circumscribed solitary solid mass in a patient with a known extrarenal malignancy should be viewed as suspicious for a primary renal neoplasm.

Focal pyelonephritis

Although acute bacterial pyelonephritis most often appears normal on imaging studies or as a diffuse process involving 1 or both kidneys, in some cases pyelonephritis can present with 1 or more focal zones of involvement. A focal site of pyelonephritis can appear masslike. A focal zone of pyelonephritis is usually seen as an ill-defined, wedge-shaped area of decreased attenuation radiating from the papilla in the medulla to the cortical surface (see Figure 6-20). This wedge-shaped area probably represents a site of poorly or nonfunctioning parenchyma due to vasospasm, tubular obstruction, and/or interstitial edema. Associated findings that should suggest the correct diagnosis of focal pyelonephritis include striations within the zone of low density and perirenal fat stranding.

Renal traumatic lesions

Injury to the kidney can be produced by either blunt or penetrating trauma.[43,44] Helical CT, preferably multidetector CT, is the modality of choice for evaluation of blunt renal injury.[44] For suspected renal vascular injury, an arteriographic phase scan be included, with injection of intravenous contrast at 4 to 5 mL/s, otherwise the CT study can be performed following intravenous injection of contrast at a rate of 2 to 4 mL/s. In addition to obtaining scans in the nephrographic phase, it is important to also obtain scans in the delayed phase (5-10 min) to assess for urine leakage as a result of injury to the pelvicaliceal system. IVU is now used only to assess gross function and evaluate the

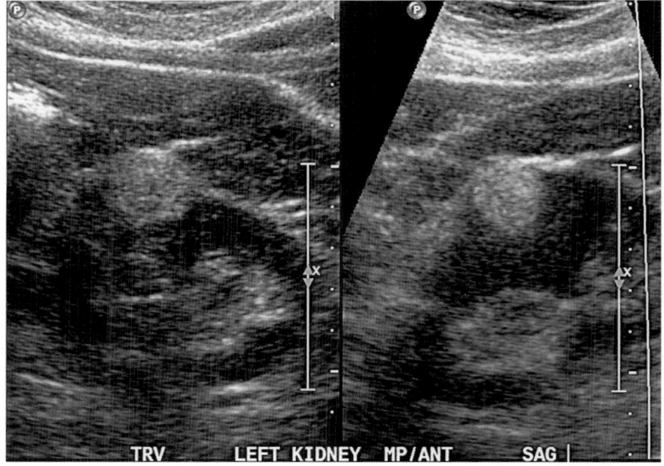

A

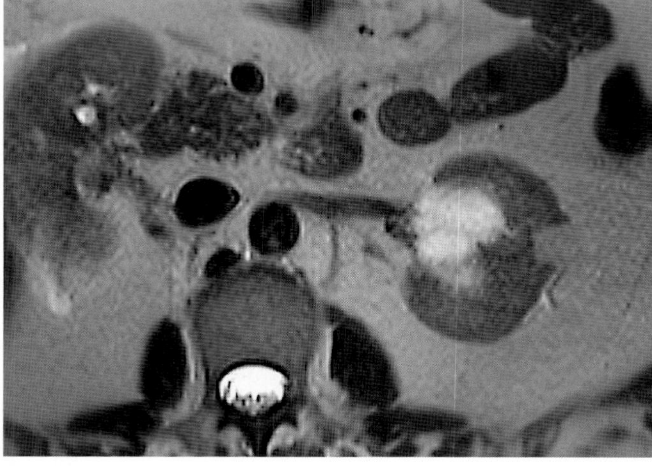

B

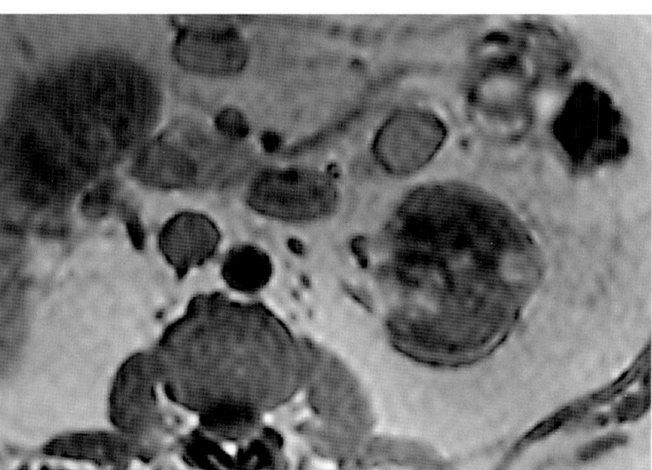

C

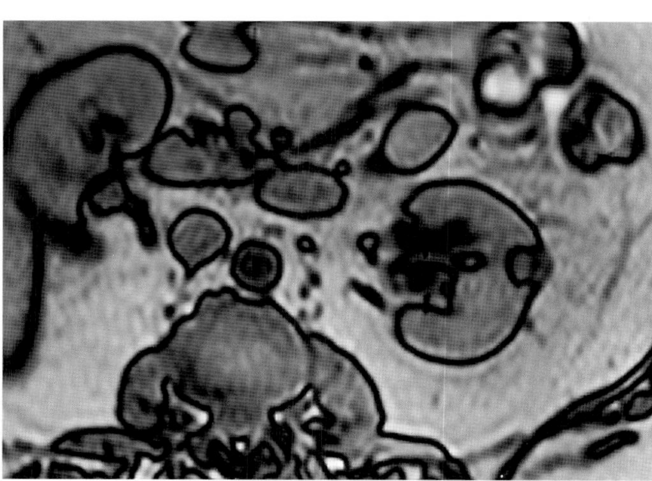

D

Figure 6-17 Angiomyolipoma on US and MRI
This 62-year-old woman had this US for reasons other than the evaluation of the kidney. **A.** Transverse and longitudinal examination of the left kidney demonstrates an echogenic solid mass. **B.** T2-weighted, (**C**) T1-weighted in-phase, and (**D**) T1-weighted out-of-phase images of the kidney show a mass with the same imaging characteristics of the retroperitoneal fat. The out-of-phase image shows the typical etching artifact around the mass when fat pixels (in the mass) are adjacent to water pixels (in the kidney). Both US and MRI imaging features are typical of a fat-rich angiomyolipoma.

uninjured kidney in hemodynamically unstable patients. Angiography can be used for diagnosis or for therapeutic embolization in hemodynamically stable patients. US and MRI has a limited role for evaluation of renal parenchymal trauma.[44]

Blunt trauma to the kidney can result in a range of injuries, including contusion, laceration, subcapsular hematoma, disruption of the renal collecting system leading to extravasation of urine, damage to the vascular supply leading to extravasation of blood, pseudoaneurysm, AV fistula, and/or renal infarction. Blunt renal injuries are classified according to the American Association of Trauma Surgeons (AAST) grading scale (see Table 6-5).[45] Conservative, nonoperative management of renal injuries is favored because of the higher nephrectomy rate for patients who undergo exploratory surgery.[46] Life-threatening bleeding is an absolute indication for surgical management. Other indications for surgery include thrombosis or avulsion of the renal artery, uncontrolled urinary extravasation, or need to débride extensively devitalized tissue (usually grade IV and grade V injuries).

Penetrating renal injuries to the flank and back can be managed according to the AAST grading scale of imaging findings. However, anterior stab wounds and anterior gunshot wounds require surgical exploration because of the risk of undetected solid organ, mesenteric, or bowel injury.

The various types of kidney injuries exhibit specific appearances on CT. A contusion is a soft-tissue injury without tear in the parenchyma. On CT, this appears as a region of poorly defined low attenuation within the kidney parenchyma. A laceration appears as a linear or branching low

Imaging Notes 6-4. Types of Renal Injuries

Injury	Definition	Appearance
Contusion	Soft-tissue injury without laceration	Intraparenchymal region of poorly defined low density
Hematoma	Collection of blood	40-80 HU
Active extravasation	Active arterial bleeding	Seen at early phase contrast-enhanced CT as focal high-density areas representing a collection of extravascular contrast, 91-274 HU
Pseudoaneurysm	Contained pulsatile collection due to arterial wall injury	Densely opacifies with contrast. Not bounded by vessel wall, can undergo sudden rupture
AV fistula	Arterial injury with venous communication	Diagnosis made with early opacification of communicating vein
Infarction	Nonperfused tissue	Wedge-shaped areas of nonenhancement; cortical rim sign characteristic

attenuation area on noncontrast and contrast-enhanced CT (see Figures 6-21 and 6-22). A hematoma is a collection of blood that is of low attenuation relative to enhancing renal parenchyma, measuring 40 to 80 HU, on contrast-enhanced CT. On unenhanced CT, acute hematomas can appear higher attenuation than normal parenchyma. Hematomas commonly collect in a subcapsular location and will appear as a lenticular or crescentic area adjacent to the renal cortex but can occasionally occur within the renal parenchyma (see Figure 6-21). Although interesting to differentiate, these simple parenchymal injuries are all managed with supportive, nonoperative care. However, vascular and collecting system injuries will often require surgical intervention, and therefore their detection is essential.

Vascular disruption with adjacent active extravasation of contrast is seen in the early phase of CT exams as globular or irregularly shaped focal high attenuation areas, measuring 91 to 274 HU (see Figure 6-23). A pseudoaneurysm results from injury to the arterial wall and appears as a well-defined, high-attenuation, spherical contrast collection communicating with a renal artery. Early opacification of the communicating vein, seen as high attenuation contrast within the vein in the early phase images is an important clue to the diagnosis of a traumatic A-V fistula. The interpreter should follow

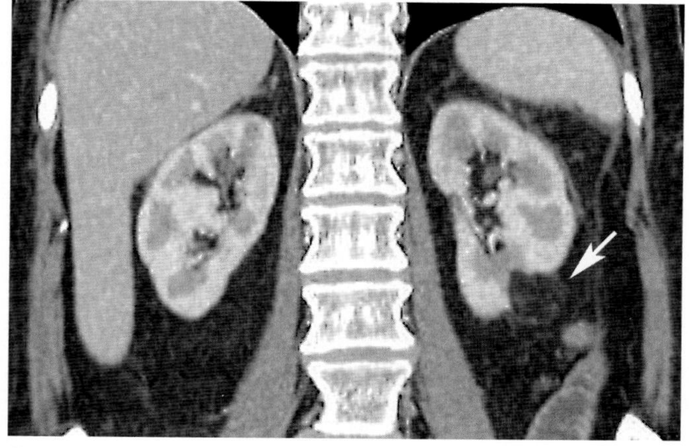

A

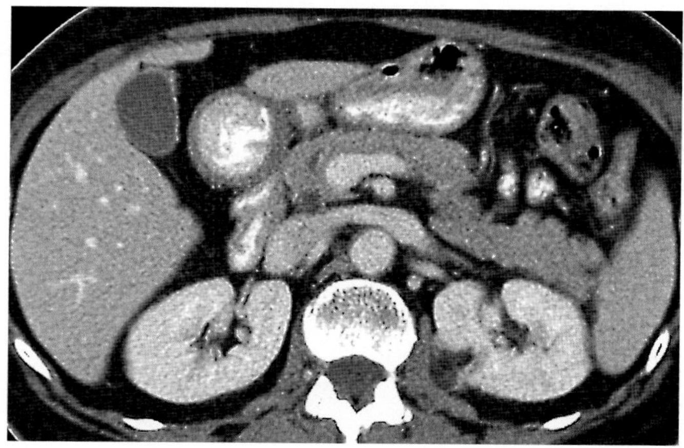

B

Figure 6-18 CT of Angiomyolipoma in 2 Patients
A. This 44-year-old man presented with abdominal pain. This coronal oblique reconstruction of the abdomen demonstrates a small low attenuation mass projecting from the lower pole of the left kidney. The pie-shaped defect in the renal parenchyma indicates that the mass is of renal parenchymal origin. Note that the attenuation of the mass is identical to the retroperitoneal fat. Fat within this renal mass is diagnostic of an angiomyolipoma. **B.** Intravenous contrast-enhanced axial CT image in a second patient demonstrates a fat-density left renal mass containing areas of enhancement, most prominent at its periphery.

A B

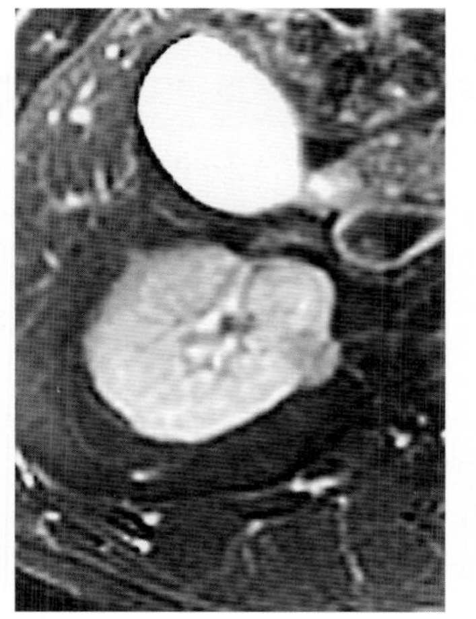

C

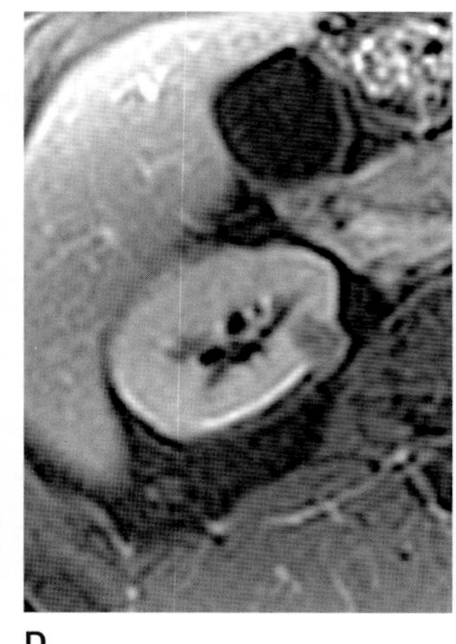

D

Figure 6-19 Lipid-Poor Angiomyolipoma
This 52-year-old man received an enhanced CT for reasons unrelated to the kidneys. **A.** Enhanced CT demonstrates a uniformly enhancing solid mass without evidence of macroscopic fat. Axial (**B**) T1-weighted; (**C**) fat-saturated, T2-weighted; and (**D**) fat-saturated, T1 postgadolinium MRI sequences also show a small solid mass without evidence of macroscopic fat. In most cases, a lesion with this imaging appearance will represent a small renal cell carcinoma. Surgical biopsy was diagnostic of an angiomyolipoma. (Thanks to Lisa Jones, MD, PhD, for the loan of this case).

the opacified vein back to the site of A-V fistula. Injury to the vascular pedicle will cause reduction or absence of perfusion of the kidney. This will be seen as lack of enhancement of the renal parenchyma (see Figures 6-23 and 6-24).[47]

Diagnosis of collecting system injury is primarily based on the detection of extravasated urine. Unenhanced and early phase images will demonstrate a fluid attenuation, 0 to 20 HU, well-defined, irregularly shaped collection in the renal sinus or perirenal soft tissues. Delayed images, after the opacification of the collecting system, will demonstrate accumulation of high attenuation contrast in at least a portion of the collection (see Figures 6-22 and 6-25).

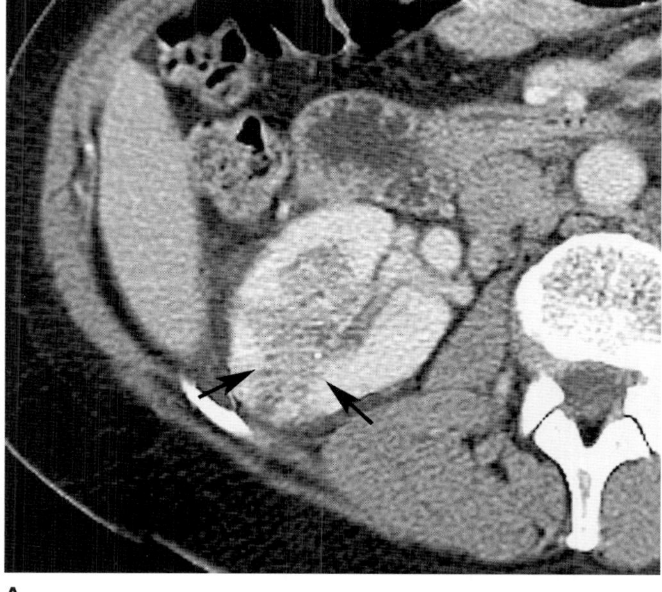

A

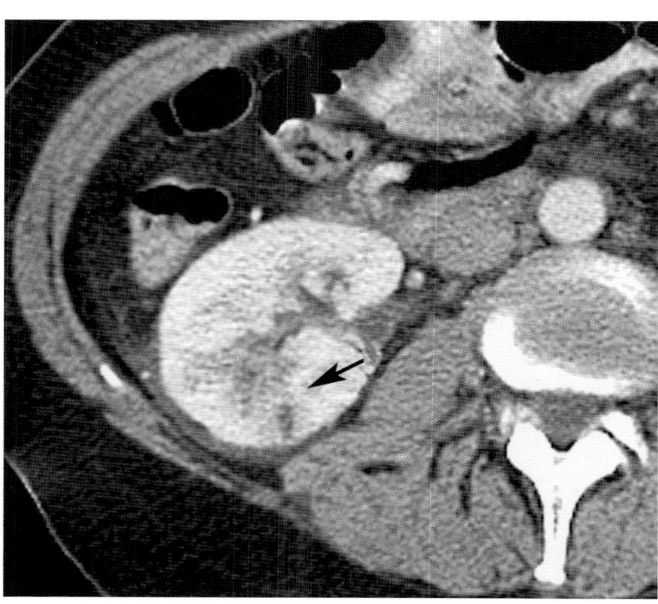

B

Figure 6-20 Focal Pyelonephritis, Right Mid-kidney
The patient was a 57-year-old woman with weakness and fevers to 104 for 5 days. **A** and **B.** Contrast-enhanced axial CT images demonstrate a slightly enlarged right kidney, perinephric fluid, and several adjacent areas of poorly defined low density (*arrows*) consistent with focal pyelonephritis.

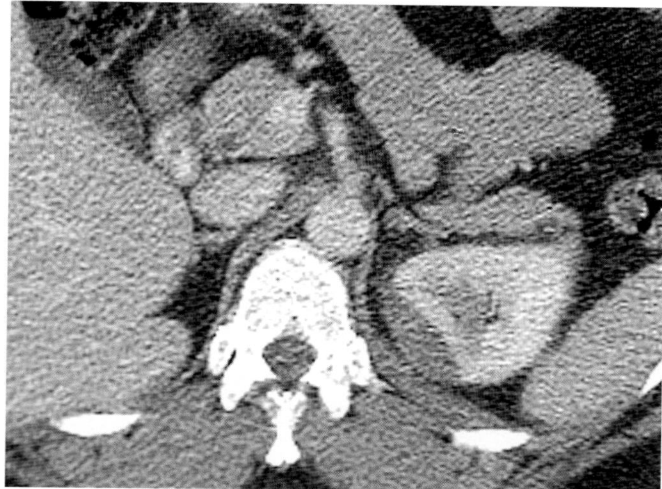

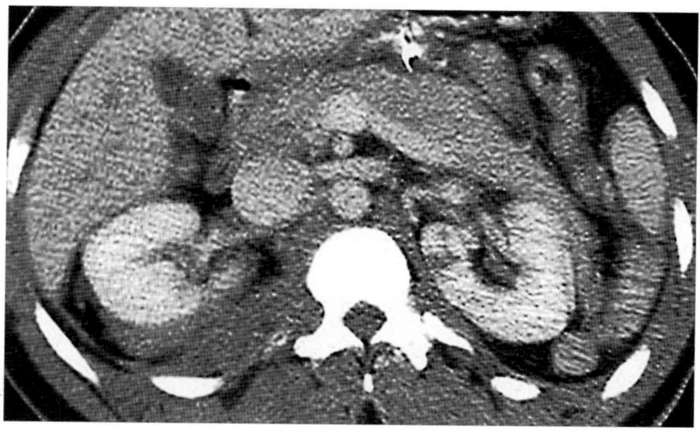

Figure 6-21 AAST Grade I and Grade II Renal Injuries in 2 Patients
A. The first patient is a 51-year-old woman who sustained blunt abdominal trauma. Contrast-enhanced axial CT image demonstrates a lenticular-shaped collection of blood compressing the adjacent renal parenchyma, typical of a small subcapsular hematoma. **B.** The second patient is a 48-year-old man who sustained blunt abdominal trauma. Contrast-enhanced axial CT image demonstrates a crescentic collection of blood surrounding the right kidney, characteristic of a perinephric hematoma. There is also a 9-mm linear defect in the medial left kidney, typical of a small laceration.

Table 6-5. Renal Injury Scale of the American Association of Surgeons in Trauma (AAST)

Grade	Injury Description
1	• Microscopic or gross hematuria with normal imaging studies or • Renal contusion and/or • Nonexpanding subcapsular hematoma without parenchymal laceration
2	• Nonexpanding perirenal hematoma confined to the retroperitoneum • Superficial cortical lacerations (<1 cm depth)
3	• Lacerations >1 cm depth in renal cortex **without** extension into the collecting system or urinary extravasation
4	• Lacerations with extension into collecting system and/or • Urinary extravasation and/or • Injuries to main renal artery or vein with contained hemorrhage and/or • Thrombosis of segmental renal artery without parenchymal laceration
5	• Lacerations that completely shatter the kidney and/or • Injuries to renal hilum with devascularization of the kidney and/or • Traumatic renal arterial disruption or occlusion

Modified from CT Findings in Blunt Renal Trauma by Harris AC, Zwirewich CV, Lyburn ID, et al. CT findings in blunt renal trauma. *Radiographics.* 2001;21 Spec No:S201–S214.

Renal infarct

Renal infarction is an uncommon cause of acute abdominal pain that when present often eludes clinical diagnosis. Renal infarcts can also be clinically silent. Some of the causes of renal infarction include emboli, renal artery dissection, renal vein thrombosis (RVT), vasculitis, and renal trauma. Although IVU can demonstrate an absence of enhancement

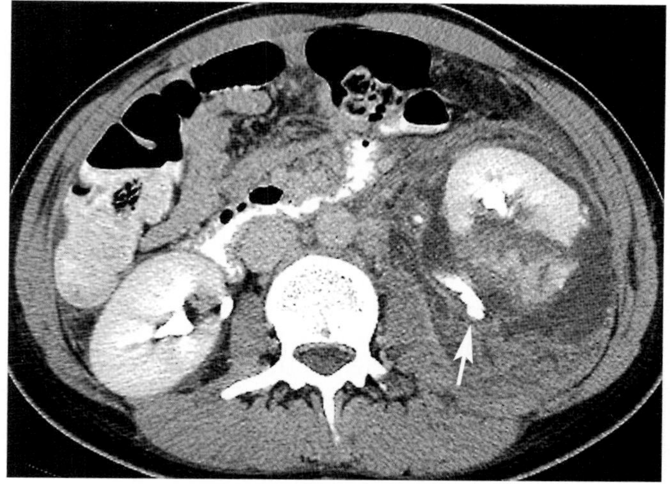

Figure 6-22 AAST Grade IV Injury
This 32-year-old woman was transferred from an outside hospital 3 days after falling from a ladder. Contrast-enhanced axial CT demonstrates through-and-through laceration of left kidney with separation of renal fragments, perirenal hematoma, and leakage of opacified urine (*arrow*) from renal collecting system injury.

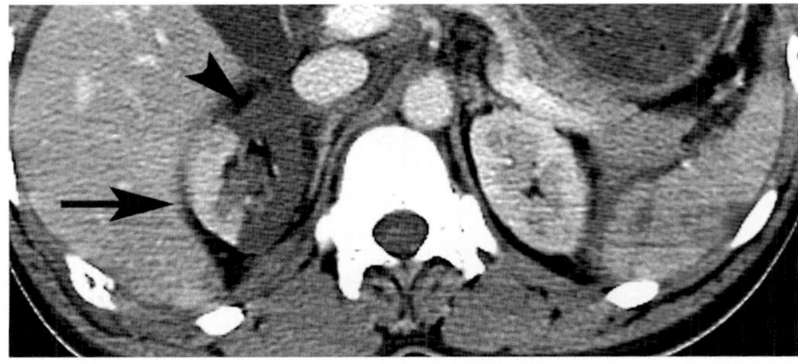

A

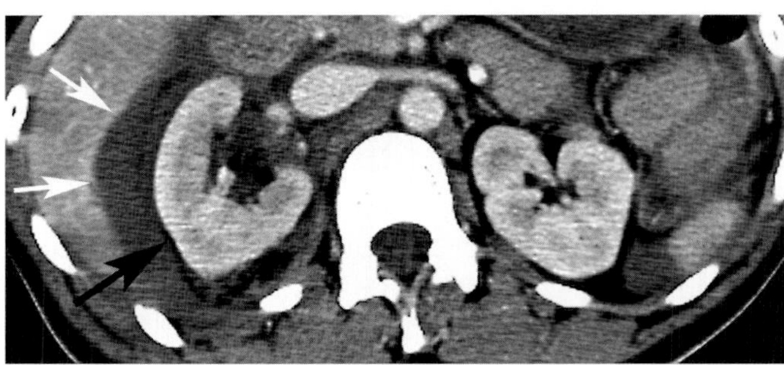

B

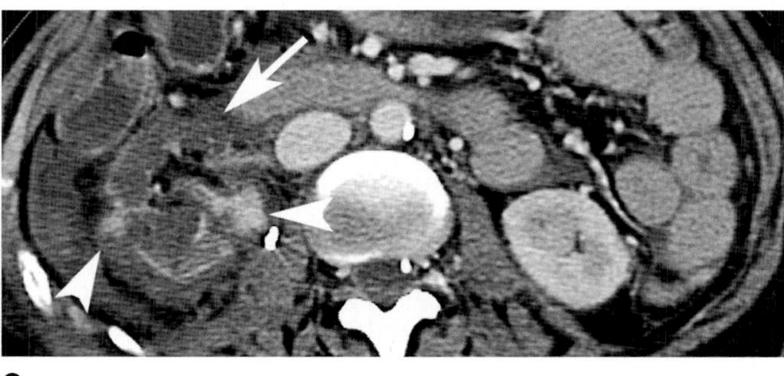

C

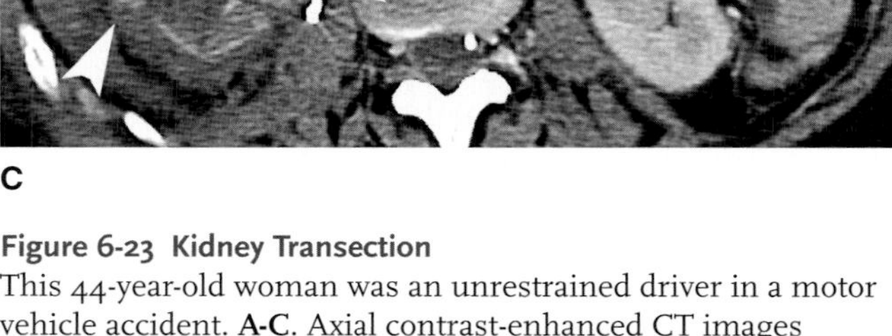

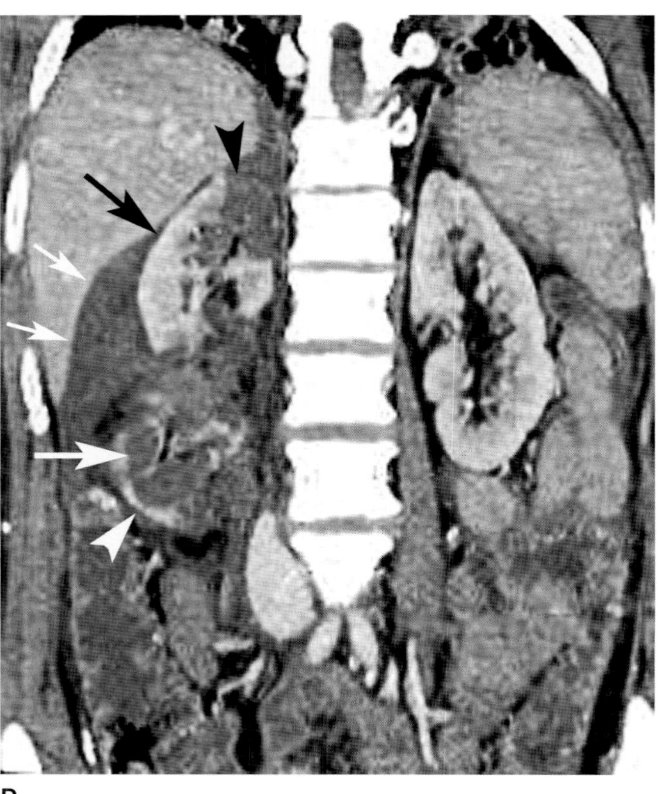

D

Figure 6-23 Kidney Transection
This 44-year-old woman was an unrestrained driver in a motor vehicle accident. **A-C.** Axial contrast-enhanced CT images and (**D**) coronal oblique reconstruction from an enhanced CT shows a normal-appearing left kidney. The upper pole of the right kidney is nonenhancing indicating a posttraumatic infarction (*black arrowheads*). The middle region of the right kidney is normally enhancing (*black arrow*) and the lower pole (*white arrow*) is nonenhancing and completely separated from the upper two-thirds of the kidney, indicating a transection of the kidney. C. There is high-attenuation intravenous contrast (*white arrowhead*) surrounding the lower pole of the right kidney. This is indicative of acute arterial extravasation. There is also hemoperitoneum (*small white arrows*).

of the affected portion of the kidney, the most sensitive imaging test for detection of nonperfused renal parenchyma is intravenous contrast-enhanced CT or MRI. Typical renal infarcts appear as wedge-shaped areas of nonenhancement with the base of the wedge extending to the renal cortex and the apex toward the renal hilum. The presence of a thin enhancing cortical rim, the "cortical rim sign," is characteristic, because of preservation of renal capsular arterial flow; however, the cortical rim sign is reported to be present in only approximately 50% of renal infarcts.[48] Infarcts of multiple solid organs, including the kidney, are a clue to a diagnosis of emboli as the cause for renal infarction (see Figure 6-26). With larger and/or global renal infarction, the involved kidney is edematous and enlarged (see Figure 6-23). With global renal infarction, IVU demonstrates no contrast opacification of the involved kidney (see Figure 6-24).

Cystic Lesions of the Kidney

Cystic lesions of the kidney are a common imaging finding, the majority of which will represent simple cortical renal cysts. However, occasionally renal cysts may be related to other processes such as a variety of inherited syndromes, chronic renal failure, and congenital ureteral obstruction. Abscesses contain fluid and therefore can mimic renal cysts. Renal neoplasms can be partly or nearly entirely cystic. Complex cystic

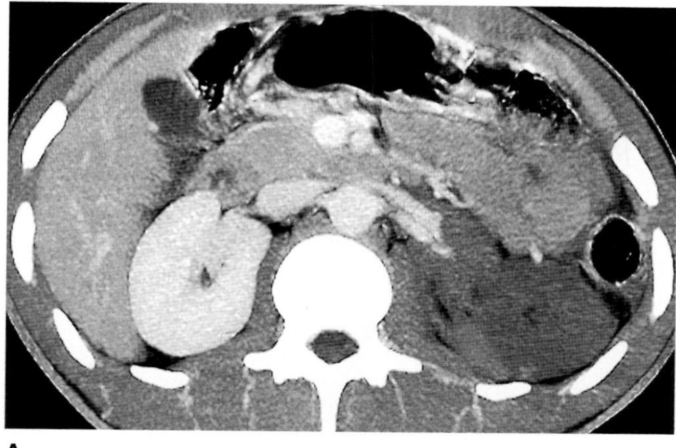

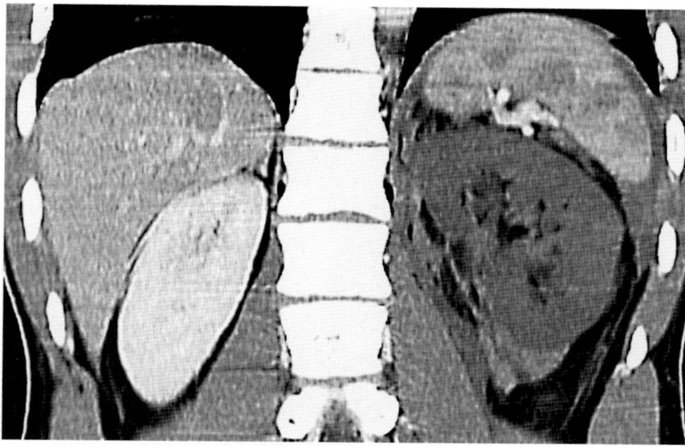

Figure 6-24 AAST Grade V Renal Injury
This 21-year-old man jumped from a roof. Contrast-enhanced axial (**A**) and coronal (**B**) CT images demonstrate nonperfusion of the left kidney with abrupt cutoff of the left renal artery, in keeping with a left renal pedicle avulsion. A small amount of high-density acute hemorrhage is seen about the left lower renal pole.

lesions should not be labeled as "cysts," as in the term "complex cyst." This designation creates confusion and can lead to unfortunate misunderstanding/mismanagement of cystic masses that can represent malignances or abscesses.

The Bosniak classification of cystic renal masses

The Bosniak classification of renal cystic lesions was first introduced in 1986 and updated in 2005, as a system to classify lesion morphology and enhancement characteristics, in order to assist in determining how these lesions should be treated.[49] Simple cysts are known to represent benign lesions; however, complicated cysts, which do not exhibit paper-thin walls or simple fluid density, have the potential to represent a cystic neoplasm. The majority of atypical cysts will represent simple cysts that have degenerated as a result of prior hemorrhage or other insult such as trauma or infection. However, some cystic renal lesions can exhibit elements that render them indistinguishable from malignant renal neoplasms. The Bosniak classification functions as an aid to decision making in the management of these lesions. Using the system, a given cystic lesion can be categorized as belonging to 1 of 4 categories, with an increasing risk of malignancy (Table 6-6).

Category I lesions are simple cysts. On US, CT, and MRI examinations, simple cysts will appear round or oval

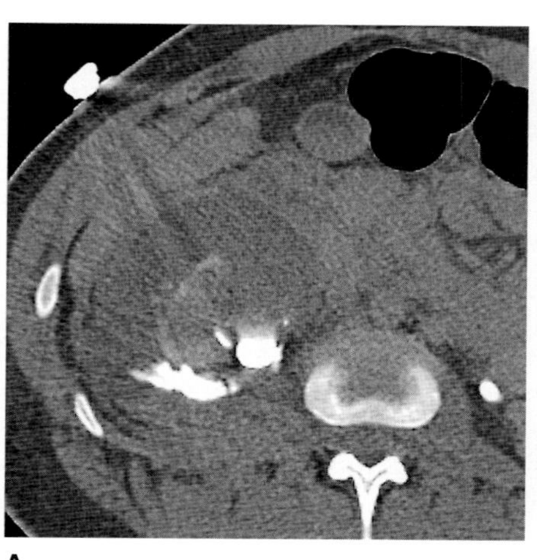

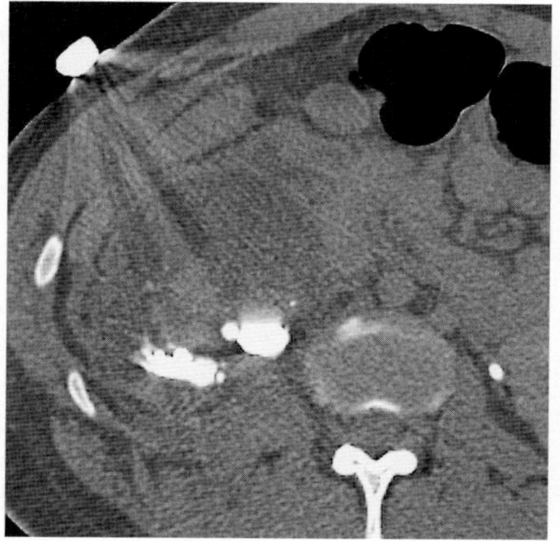

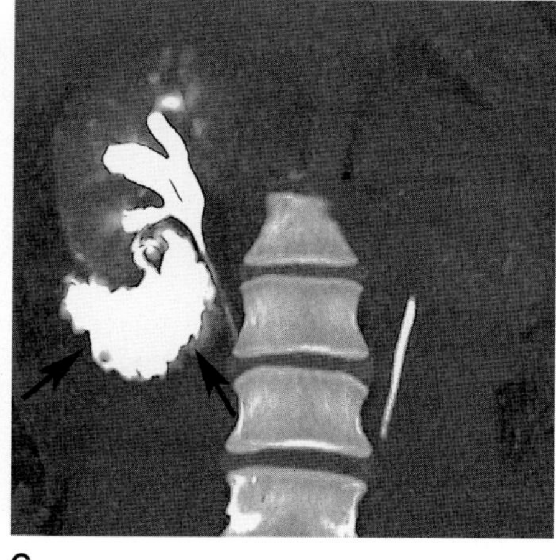

Figure 6-25 Traumatic Urinoma
The patient is a 22-year-old woman who sustained blunt trauma in a motor vehicle accident. Two axial sections (**A** and **B**) through the right lower renal pole and (**C**) a coronal reconstruction from an excretion phase series of a CT urogram. There is extravasation of dense excreted contrast about the lower pole of the right kidney, from a disrupted lower pole infundibulum. The background of the images appears "washed out" because the images are purposely viewed at low-contrast, "wide window" settings in order to discern detail within the bright areas of excreted contrast. The leak resolved after several months of ureteral stent treatment.

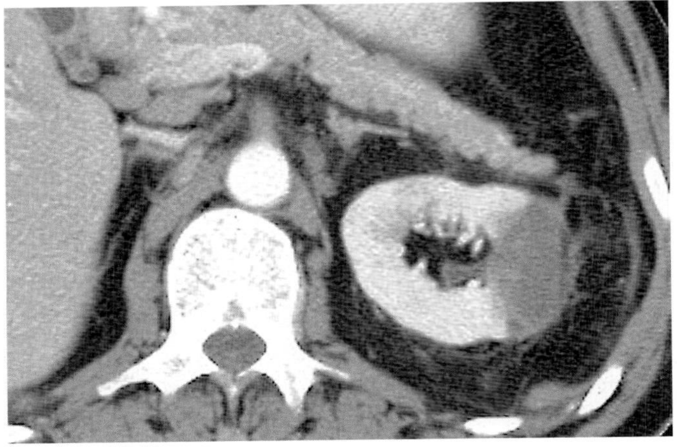

A

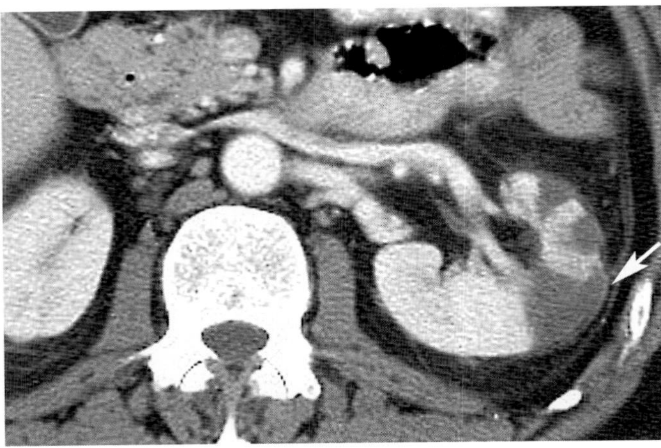

B

Figure 6-26 Renal Infarcts
The patient is a 48-year-old man with hemolytic anemia. He had undergone prior splenectomy and now showed signs of septicemia. **A** and **B**. Contrast-enhanced axial CT images demonstrate multiple wedge-shaped zones of nonperfusion in the left kidney typical of renal infarcts. A subtle thin rim of enhancement is seen (*arrows*), in keeping with capsular collateral flow.

with a thin or imperceptible wall and internal characteristics of simple fluid. On CT and MRI, simple cysts will have the additional feature of displaying no contrast enhancement following the intravenous administration of contrast (see Figure 6-27).

Category II lesions are minimally complex cysts, with **few** hairline septations (see Figure 6-28). Fine calcification or a short segment of slightly thickened calcification can be present in the wall or septa of the cyst. Uniformly high attenuation lesions <3 cm in diameter that are well marginated and do not enhance are included in this group (see Figure 6-29).

Imaging Notes 6-5. Imaging Characteristics of Simple Renal Cysts

CT
- Round
- Homogeneous fluid density: 0-20 HU
- Thin imperceptible wall
- Sharp interface with the adjacent renal parenchyma
- No enhancement with intravenous contrast administration

US
- Anechoic
- Paper-thin wall
- Increased through transmission

MRI
- Dark on T1-weighted images
- Bright on T2 -weighted images
- No enhancement with intravenous contrast
- Thin wall

These cysts are variably called hyperdense, or hemorrhagic or proteinaceous cysts, and are hyperattenuating because they contain either hemorrhagic or proteinaceous debris that raise the attenuation of the contents of the cysts. Category I and II cysts are considered benign and require no further follow-up.

Category IIF lesions contain multiple hairline septa or minimal smooth thickening of the wall or septa. The walls or septa can contain calcification that can be thick and nodular, but no measurable contrast enhancement is present. Totally intrarenal nonenhancing high-attenuation renal lesions >3 cm are also included in this category. The vast majority of these lesions will be benign. However, because there is a low risk of malignancy, it is felt that serial follow-up studies are warranted to confirm benignity.

Category III cystic lesions have thickened nodular or smooth walls or septa in which measurable enhancement is present (see Figure 6-30). These lesions require surgical resection. Some will prove to be benign at surgical pathology, for example: hemorrhagic cysts, chronic infected cysts, and multiloculated cystic nephroma; however, others will prove to be renal carcinomas.

Category IV lesions are clearly malignant. Features of malignancy include shaggy internal walls of the cystic mass, inhomogeneous enhancement of the solid elements of the mass, and/or thick mural nodules (see Figure 6-31). Although the Bosniak classification was originally applied using CT, the principles of this morphologic schema can be applied using MRI and US.

Simple renal cysts

Most renal cysts are sporadic, idiopathic, acquired lesions of the kidney. The etiology of these lesions remains obscure. The incidence of idiopathic renal cysts increases with age and as many as one-third to one half of older adults will have simple cysts identified on cross-sectional imaging.[50,51]

Table 6-6. Bosniak Classification of Cystic Renal Masses

Category	Description	Management
I	Simple cyst	No further follow-up
II	Minimally complex cysts: • few hairline septations, • fine calcification or a short segment of slightly thickened calcification of the wall or septa Hyperattenuating cysts • nonenhancing, uniformly high attenuation, <3 cm	No further follow-up
IIF	Can contain multiple hairline septa or minimal smooth thickening of the wall or septa; moreover, wall or septa can contain calcification that can be thick and nodular, but no measurable contrast enhancement present. Totally intrarenal nonenhancing high-attenuation renal lesions >3 cm also included in this category.	Follow-up imaging
III	Thickened irregular or smooth walls or septa in which measurable enhancement is present.	Surgical removal
IV	Clearly malignant features, contains areas of solid nodular soft tissue.	Surgical removal

Idiopathic cysts have no clinical significance other than the potential confusion with other focal lesions. Sporadic simple cysts are asymptomatic and do not affect renal function.

These lesions have the typical imaging features of simple cysts on US, CT, and MRI as previously described. On IVU, a simple cyst appears as a lucent renal parenchymal mass. If the cyst extends exophytically from the kidney, a "beak" or "claw" sign may be evident, indicating a lesion of renal origin with a smooth, sharp interface with the renal parenchyma. Unfortunately, IVU cannot reliably characterize the internal architecture of these masses. Therefore, suspected renal cysts should be confirmed by 1 of the cross-sectional imaging studies. US is best suited for this purpose, as it is inexpensive, lacks exposure to ionizing radiation, and is definitive in most cases (see Figure 6-32).

Some idiopathic cysts will hemorrhage, become infected, or sustain other insults that alter the cyst and transform it into a complicated cyst. These morphologic changes in cyst features are addressed by the Bosniak classification of cystic renal masses.

Localized renal cystic disease: Localized renal cystic disease is characterized by replacement of all or a localized region of the kidney by multiple cysts of various sizes, separated by islands of normal parenchyma. Although the cysts can merge as a multiseptated conglomerate, what distinguishes localized renal cystic disease from a cystic neoplasm is that they do not form an encapsulated mass or demonstrate mural nodularity (see Figure 6-33).[52] It is important to recognize this lesion as a benign conglomeration of cysts rather than a cystic neoplasm. The cause of localized renal cystic disease is not known.

Cysts associated with systemic conditions

Some cysts are associated with underlying diseases such as autosomal dominant polycystic kidney disease, VHL, TS, and cystic disease associated with chronic renal failure/dialysis. These disorders nearly always cause multiple renal cysts and are discussed under the heading: **Multifocal Renal Lesions.**

Cystic renal neoplasms

Cystic renal neoplasms should be distinguished from large renal carcinomas that have undergone central cystic necrosis. Carcinomas with central cystic necrosis remain recognizable as thick-walled solid masses. Renal neoplasms with cystic morphology include cystic nephroma and the rare multilocular cystic variant of RCC.

Imaging Notes 6-6. Cystic Renal Neoplasms

Neoplasm	Comments
Malignant	
Cystic renal carcinoma	Predominantly cystic mass with mural nodular components
Multilocular cystic renal carcinoma	Considered a relatively low-grade tumor
Benign	
Cystic nephroma, formerly termed multilocular cystic nephroma	Seen in young boys or middle-aged women, indistinguishable from carcinoma in most cases, therefore usually Bosniak category III. May extend into renal pelvis
Mixed epithelial and stromal (MEST) tumor	Seen in women. Bosniak category III

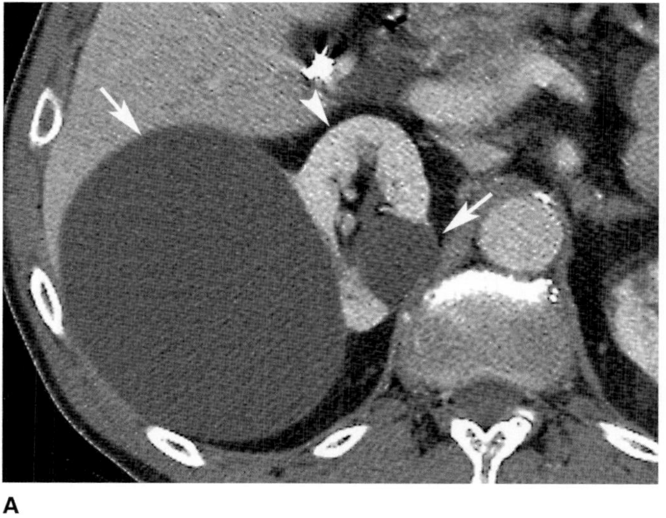

A

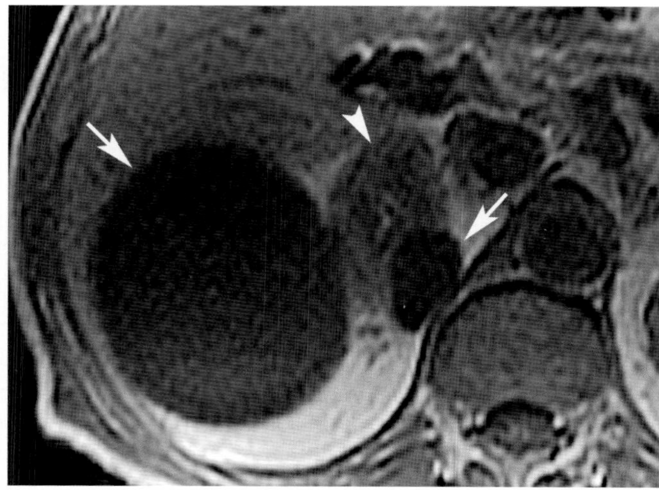

B

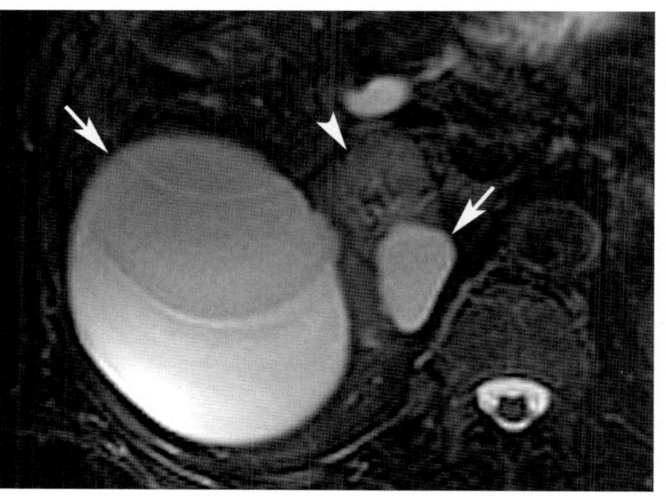

C

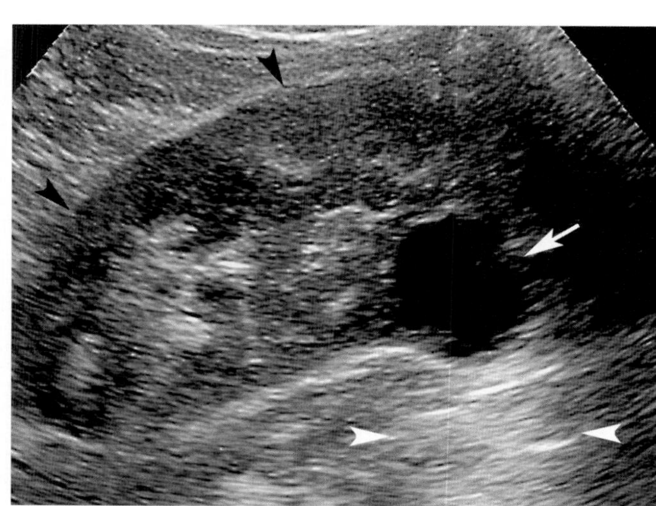

D

Figure 6-27 Simple Renal Cysts
A. Enhanced axial CT image shows 2 oval, nonenhancing low-attenuation masses (*arrows*) in the right kidney (*arrowhead*) The masses measured 12 and 14 HU, in keeping with fluid. These are the typical CT features of renal cysts. **B.** Axial T1-weighted and (**C**) T2-weighted MRI images of the same renal cysts demonstrate uniform low SI on the T1 weighted sequence and uniform high SI on T2-weighted sequences. These are the characteristic features of simple cysts by MRI. (The curved lines running through the larger renal cyst in (C) are phase-encoding artifact.) **D.** Longitudinal US examination through the left kidney (*black arrowheads*) of a different patient shows an anechoic (*uniformly black*), round mass (*white arrow*) in the lower pole of the kidney. Note the white band (*white arrowheads*) that projects in the tissues directly behind the mass, a finding indicating enhanced sound transmission. Cysts and other fluid-containing structures have the property that they attenuate sound to a lesser degree than adjacent tissues, resulting in an artifactual increase in the intensity of the echoes deep to the fluid, a feature known as "through transmission" or "posterior acoustic enhancement." These are US features diagnostic of a simple renal cyst.

Cystic nephroma: Cystic nephroma is a benign cystic neoplasm, first described in 1892, which has been referred to by other names, including multilocular cystic nephroma. The cystic components of cystic nephroma are of variable size and are lined with flat low cuboidal or hobnail epithelial cells, and septa are thin with variable cellularity. The cystic nephroma has a bimodal age distribution. Below the age of 5 years, cystic nephroma occurs most frequently in males, whereas in the adult there is a female predominance (91%), occurring most commonly between the ages of 40 and 60 years. Imaging studies demonstrate a septated cystic mass with multiple loculations, hairlike septa, peripheral and curvilinear calcifications, irregular borders, and minimal contrast enhancement (see Figure 6-34). Extension into the central sinus and into the renal pelvis can also be found. Based on imaging findings, these lesions most often fall into Bosniak category III, indistinguishable from carcinomas, requiring surgical removal for confirmation of benign nature.[53]

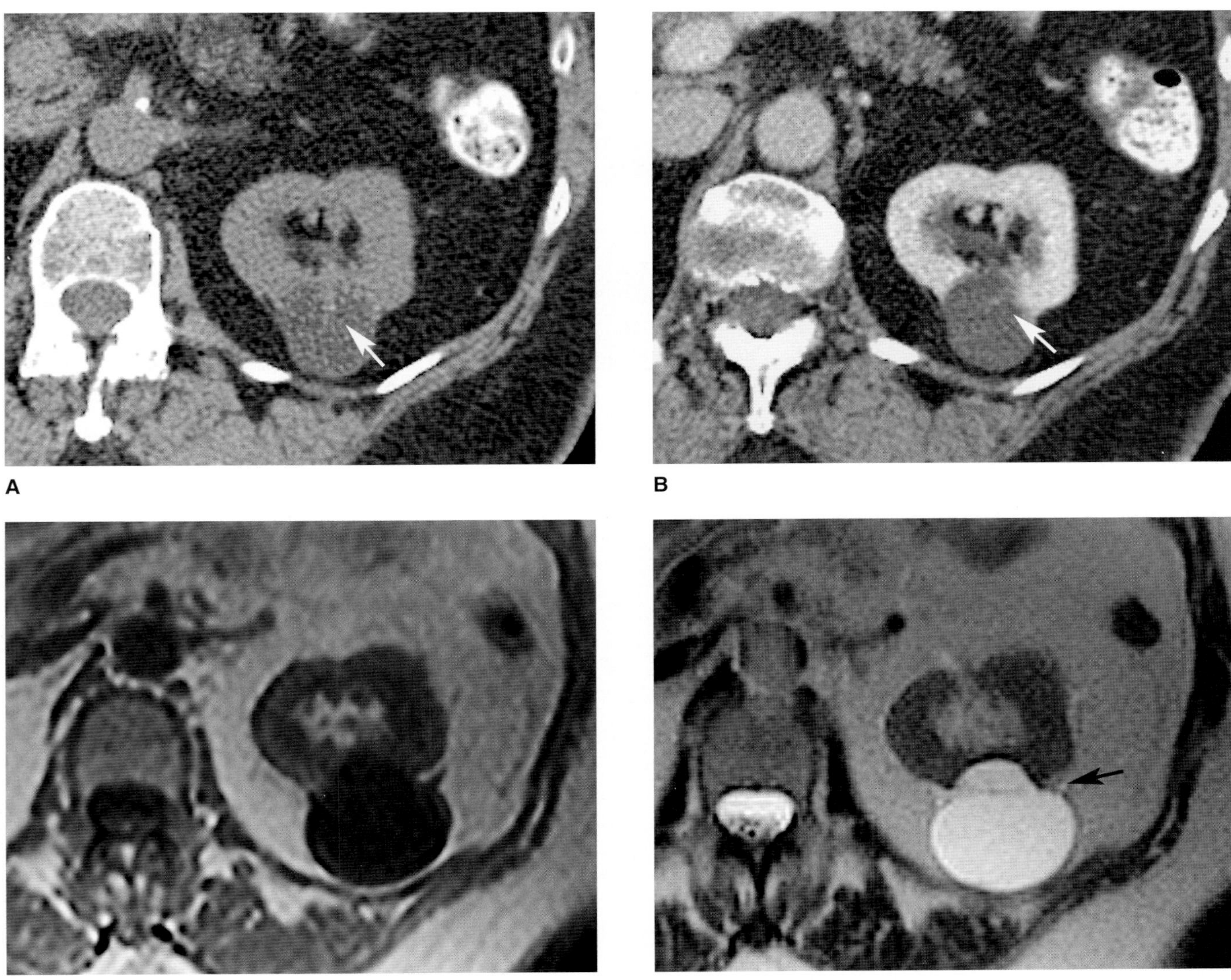

Figure 6-28 Bosniak II Renal Cyst
This 72-year-old woman had a right nephrectomy for renal cell carcinoma. **A**. Unenhanced and (**B**) contrast-enhanced axial CT images through the left kidney show a small cyst with a tiny soft-tissue attenuation focus (*white arrow*) in the superior aspect of the cyst. **C**. Axial T1-weighted fat-saturated and (**D**) single-shot axial T2-weighted MRI images show also show a minimally complicated cyst. The T2-weighted image shows a thin septation (*black arrow*) within the cysts. These findings are consistent with a benign, minimally complicated, Bosniak II cyst.

Multilocular cystic renal cell carcinoma: Multilocular cystic RCC is a rare variant of RCC, accounting for 1% to 4% of all RCCs, which was first recognized in 1982. Multilocular cystic RCC is a tumor found in adults with a mean age of presentation of 51 years. Usually, it is asymptomatic, and incidentally discovered. When compared with conventional RCC, multilocular cystic RCC has an excellent prognosis and is considered a low-grade malignancy when strict criteria are applied. Recurrence and metastasis have not been reported. Imaging findings include a multilocular cystic tumor with wall and septal contrast enhancement without any expansile tumor nodule. Asymmetric septal thickening can be seen. Twenty percent of tumors show septal or wall calcification.[53]

Mixed epithelial and stromal tumor: The mixed epithelial and stromal tumor (MEST) is a benign renal neoplasm that was first defined in 1988. Previously referred to by several names, including hamartoma and adult mesoblastic nephroma, the nomenclature of MEST was introduced by Michal and Syrucek in 1998.[34] The MEST is characterized by a proliferation of epithelium and stroma and by admixed solid and cystic regions that have variable cellularity and growth patterns. Several reports suggest that the MEST is closely related to female hormonal status. The tumor nearly always occurs in women, especially in perimenopausal women (median age, 52 y), usually presenting with flank pain and hematuria or found

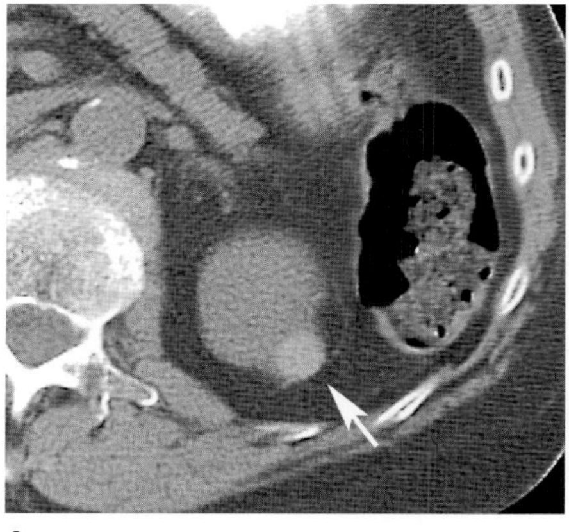
A

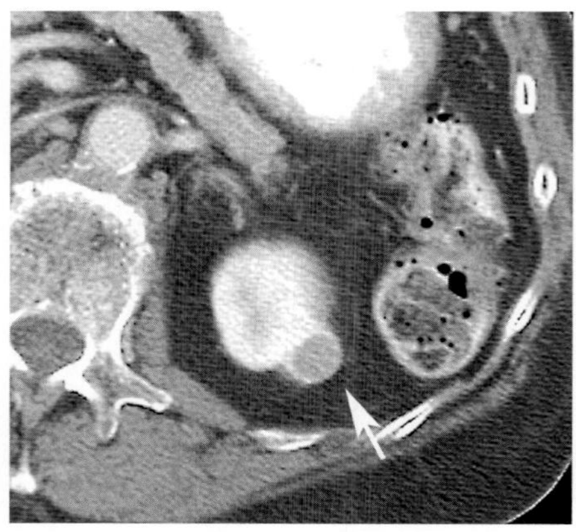
B

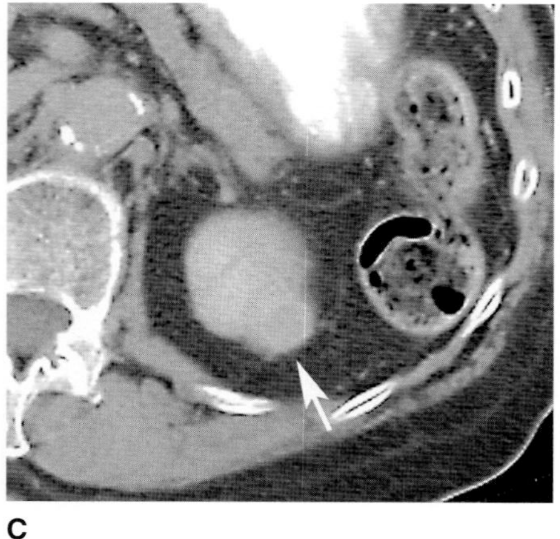
C

Figure 6-29 Hyperdense Cyst
This 82-year-old woman had a renal cell carcinoma of the right kidney resected several years prior. **A.** Unenhanced, (**B**) nephrographic-phase, and (**C**) excretory-phase axial CT images through the upper pole of the left kidney demonstrate a small renal nodule (*arrow*) that is hyperattenuating to the renal parenchyma on the unenhanced image and demonstrates thin rim of renal cortical enhancement in the nephrographic phase. However, the attenuation of the center of the nodule measured approximately 48 HU on all 3 sequences. This is a typical appearance of a "hyperdense" cyst, with the high density (relative to simple fluid) due to proteinaceous or hemorrhagic content.

incidentally. Imaging studies show a Bosniak category III or IV lesion with septa, curvilinear calcifications, and a delayed, enhancing solid components. Areas of decreased signal on T2-weighted MR images, reflecting a fibrotic component, can also be seen. In the largest series including imaging to date ($n = 10$), CT showed 70% of the lesions had solid enhancing components and included 3 Bosniak category IV lesions.[53]

Renal abscess

Renal abscess can develop as a complication of pyelonephritis or as a result of septic emboli from intravascular sources of infection such as infective endocarditis. Patients will typically present with fever and flank pain similar to patients with pyelonephritis. A renal abscess will typically appear as a unilocular, thick-walled round or oval fluid collection within the renal parenchyma. The walls of the abscess will usually be indistinctly marginated and will enhance with contrast on CT and MRI examinations. Inflammatory stranding and edema of the perirenal fat, seen on CT or MRI, is a helpful imaging sign that suggests that the lesion is inflammatory in origin (see Figure 6-35). In most cases, the diagnosis of a renal abscess will be obvious given the combination of clinical presentation and imaging appearance.

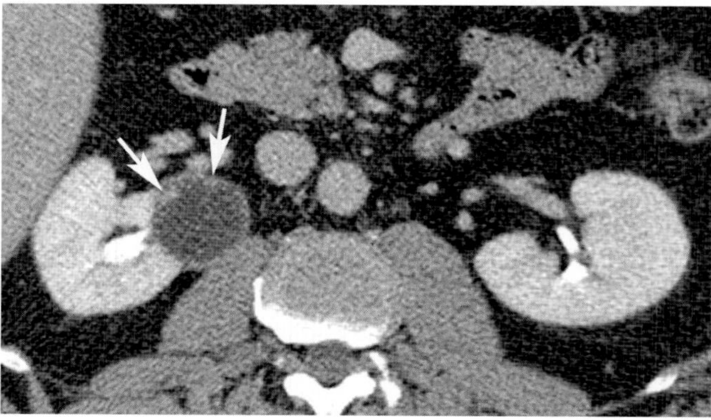

Figure 6-30 Bosniak Category III Renal Lesion
Contrast-enhanced axial CT image demonstrates a predominantly cystic mass in the medial right kidney. The mass has a thick wall and mural nodules (*arrows*). At surgery, the lesion was found to represent a clear cell renal carcinoma.

Multicystic dysplastic kidney

Multicystic dysplastic kidney (MCDK) is an uncommon congenital disorder of the kidney due to obstruction of the fetal ureter before 8 to 10 weeks of gestation. The affected kidney consists of a disorganized conglomerate of irregularly arranged cysts and fibrous tissue without functioning renal parenchyma. The cysts do not communicate, and the renal collecting system and renal vessels are atretic or absent. The hydronephrotic type of MCKD is a less common variant that results from incomplete ureteral obstruction later in gestation. In this form of MCKD, the cysts communicate with the renal pelvis. Cross-sectional imaging will demonstrate a small, multicystic mass in the renal fossa with absence of a normal kidney. Areas of dystrophic calcification are not uncommon and there is very little enhancing soft tissue or nodularity seen (see Figure 6-36).

MULTIFOCAL RENAL LESIONS

Many of the entities discussed in the previous section on focal renal lesions can present with multifocal involvement of 1 or both kidneys.

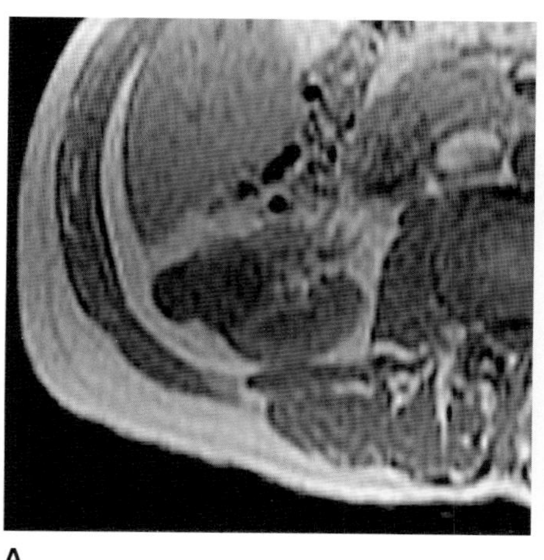

A

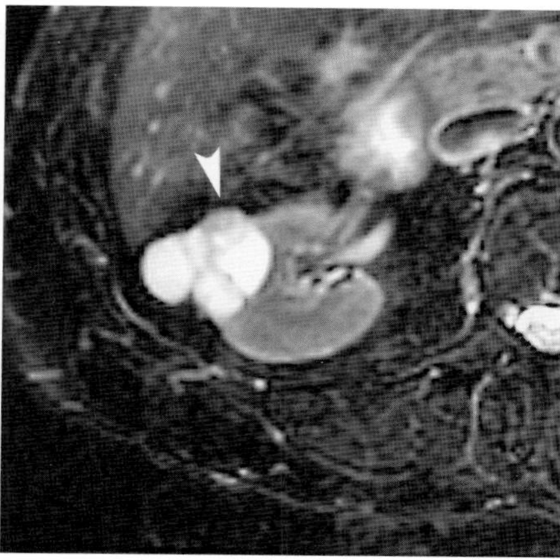

B

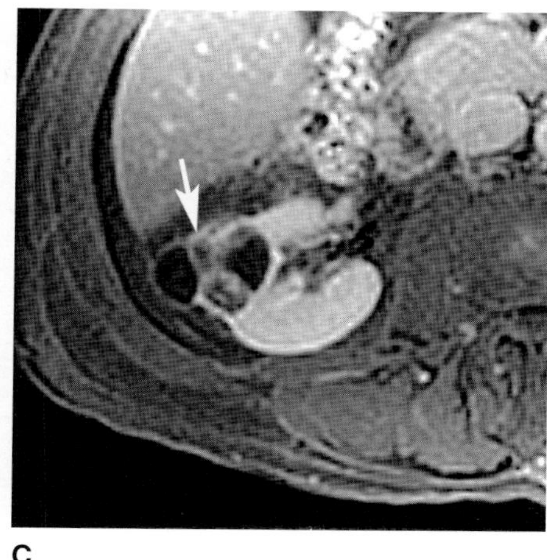

C

Figure 6-31 Bosniak IV Cystic Mass
Axial T1-weighted image (**A**) demonstrates a predominantly cystic complex mass projecting from the mid right kidney. Axial T2-weighted image (**B**) with fat suppression demonstrates thick internal septations, and marked nodularity, seen most prominently in the anterior aspect of the mass (*arrowhead*). **C.** Gradient echo axial image obtained after intravenous gadolinium administration demonstrates enhancement of the nodules and septations. This lesion likely represented a cystic renal cell carcinoma but was lost to follow-up.

Multiple Solid Renal Masses

Multiple solid enhancing nodules that do not contain macroscopic fat on imaging studies can represent lymphoma, metastatic disease, or multifocal primary renal neoplasms (Table 6-7). Multiple fat-containing masses will indicate the presence of multiple angiomyolipomas.

Renal lymphoma

Both Hodgkin and non-Hodgkin lymphomas are systemic disorders that can involve many sites throughout the body. The genitourinary system, especially the kidney, is often affected by extranodal lymphoma, being the second most commonly affected anatomic entity next to the

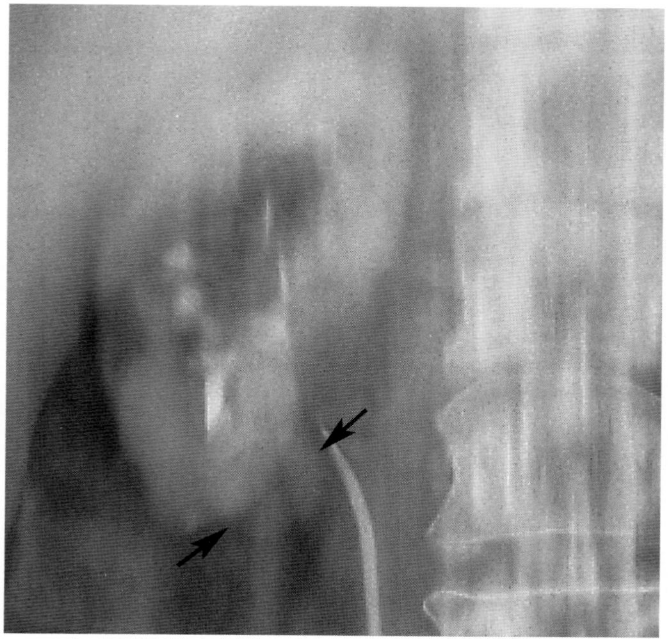

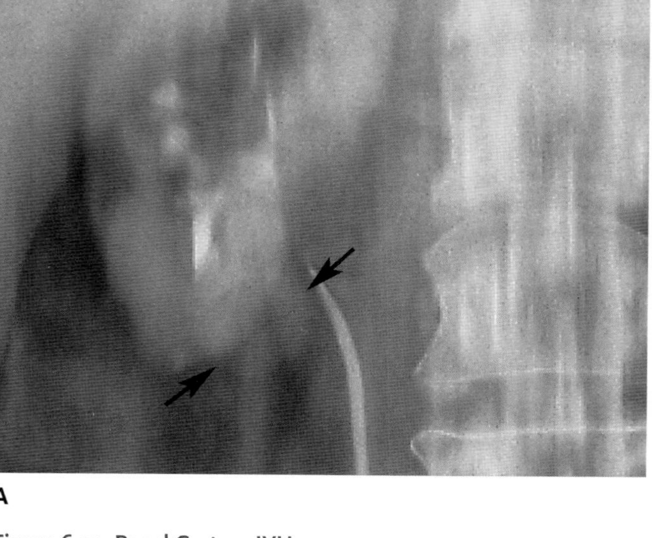

A

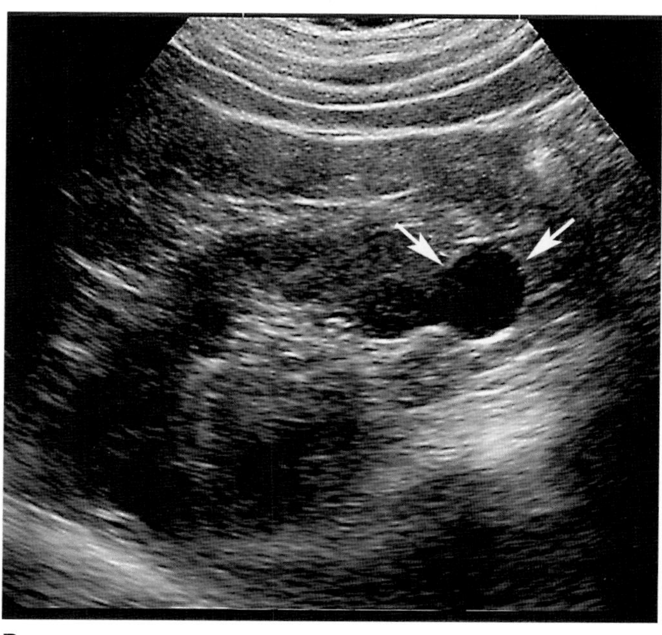

B

Figure 6-32 Renal Cyst on IVU
Sixty-five-year-old man with history of bladder cancer and flank pain. **A.** Tomographic image from and IVU demonstrates a subtle round exophytic lucent mass (*arrows*) in the right lower renal pole. **B.** Sagittal image demonstrates the lesion (*arrows*) to be thin-walled, anechoic, and with increased through-transmission, in keeping with a simple cyst.

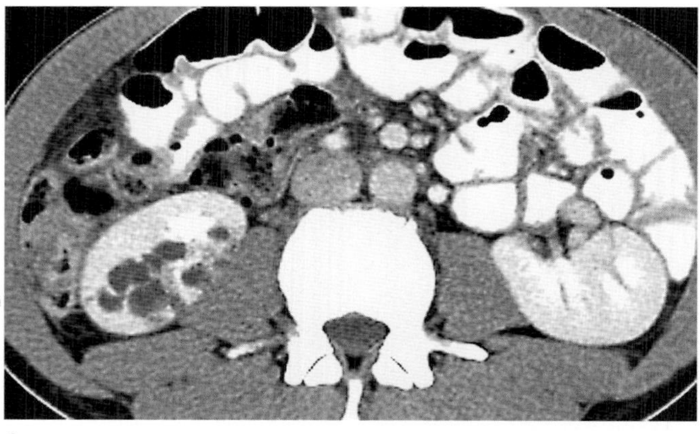
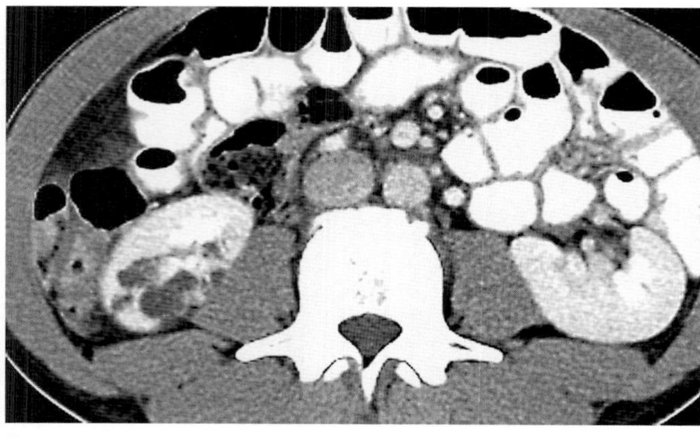

Figure 6-33 Localized Renal Cystic Disease
A and **B.** Contrast-enhanced axial CT images demonstrate a cluster of multiple small cysts in the right kidney, separated by islands of normal renal parenchyma. The lesions were stable for over 2 years, and an incidental finding in this patient with a history of gastric cancer.

hematopoietic and reticuloendothelial organs.[41] Reports based on autopsy series of patients who have succumbed to lymphoma describe foci of disease in the kidneys in approximately one-third of cases; however, imaging studies demonstrate renal abnormalities in only 3% to 8% of patients undergoing routine evaluation for staging or during the course of therapy.[41] This discrepancy may at least in part be due to the fact that the statistics on frequency of positive CT findings for lymphoma were generated before the advent of modern multidetector helical CT. Renal lymphoma usually occurs in the setting of widespread non-Hodgkin lymphoma, typically B-cell–type intermediate- and high-grade tumors such as American Burkitt lymphoma. In most of these cases, renal lymphoma is asymptomatic and detection seldom influences staging and treatment. Primary renal lymphoma that is isolated to the renal parenchyma with no systemic manifestations is uncommon, accounting for less than 1% of cases of extranodal lymphoma. Involvement of the kidneys by Hodgkin disease is exceedingly uncommon and seen in less than 1% of patients at presentation.[41]

Multi–detector row CT is the imaging modality of choice for the evaluation of patients with suspected renal lymphoma, although MRI is useful in patients with history of iodine hypersensitivity. US is less sensitive than CT or MRI for detection of renal lymphoma. On US, lymphomatous renal or perirenal masses are typically hypoechoic. On CT, lymphoma is typically hypovascular, appearing low attenuation on contrast-enhanced images. Further, PET and combined PET-CT have been shown to be very useful for detection of lymphoma; increased metabolic activity in

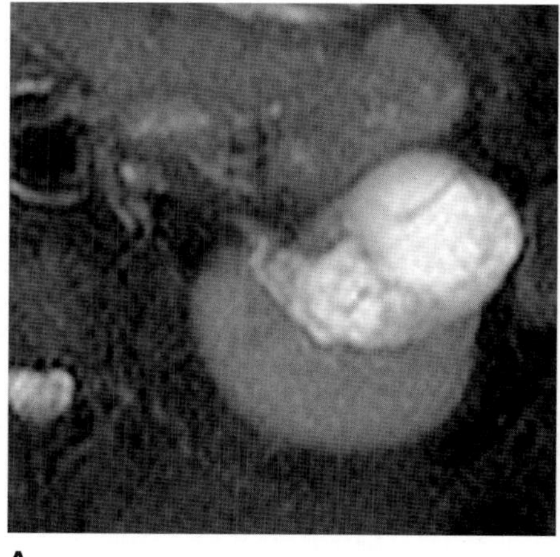
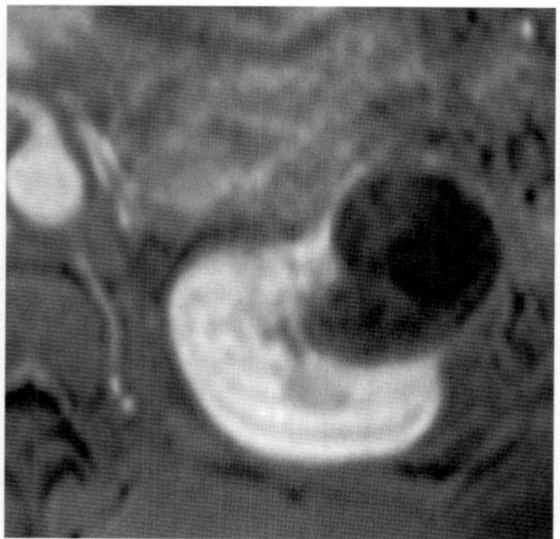
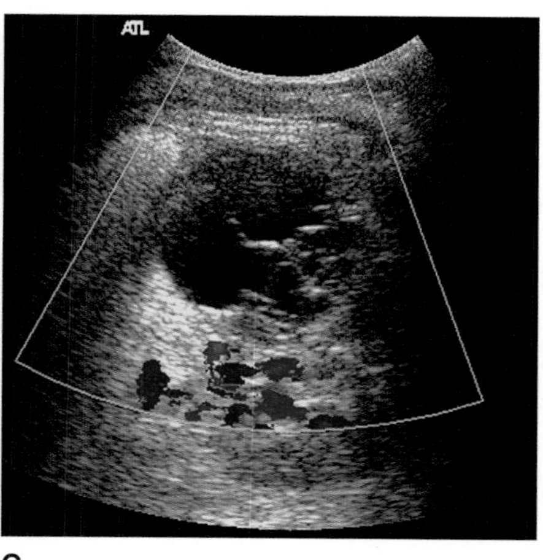

Figure 6-34 Cystic Nephroma
A. Fat-saturated axial T2-weighted MR image demonstrates cystic left renal mass, containing numerous septations. **B.** Fat-saturated axial T1-weighted MR image obtained after intravenous gadolinium administration shows faintly enhancing septae, within low SI cystic lesion. **C.** Color Doppler US image demonstrates multilocular cystic lesion corresponding to lesion on MRI, with no demonstrable vascularity. At the time of these studies, the lesion had remained stable in appearance for 6 years and most likely represents a cystic nephroma.

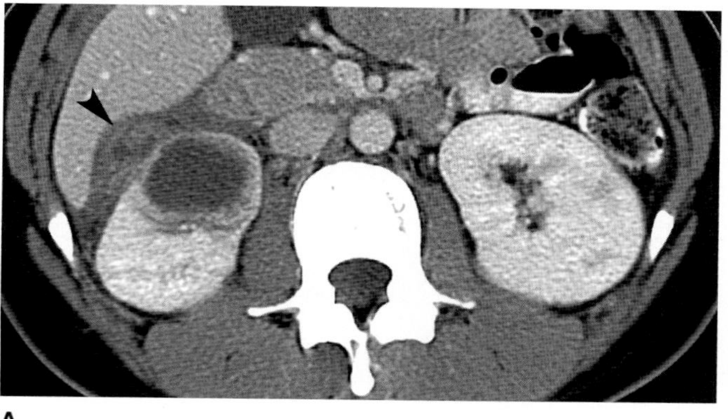
A

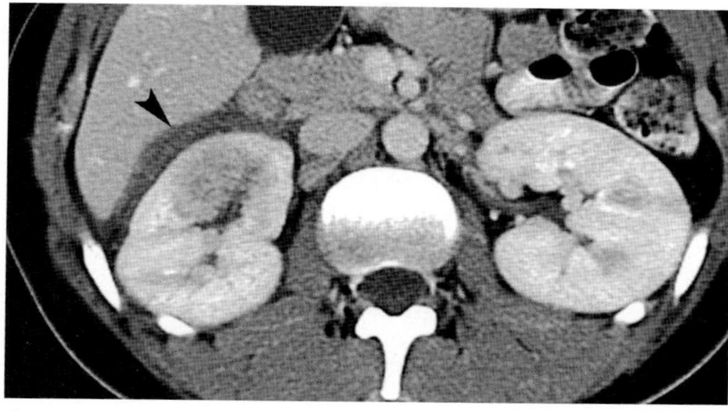
B

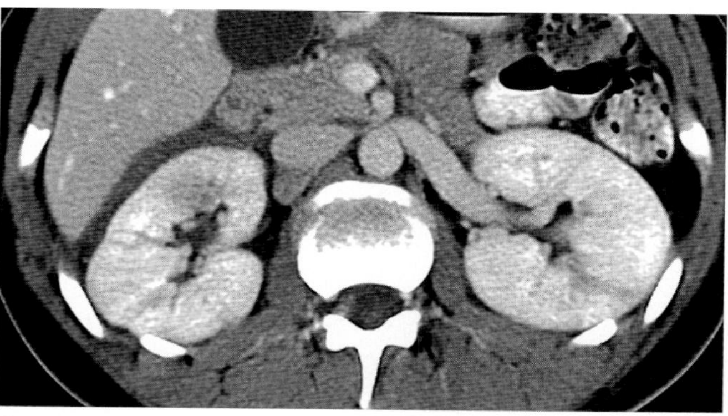
C

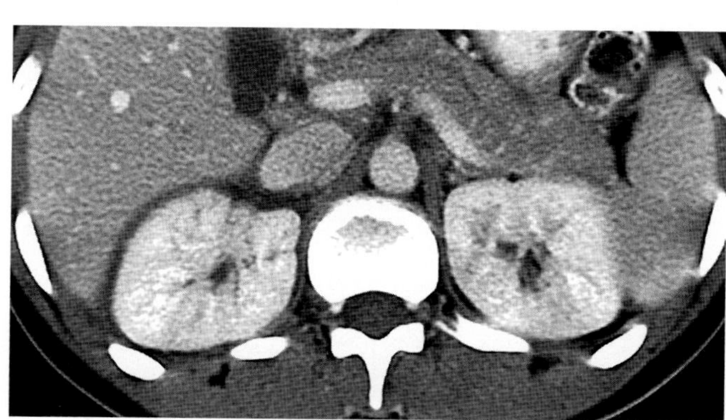
D

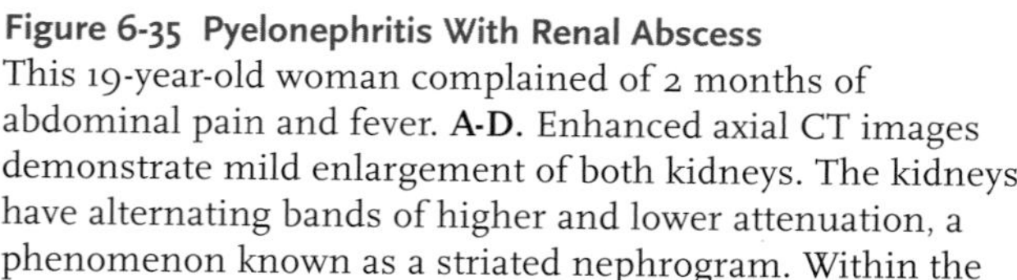

Figure 6-35 Pyelonephritis With Renal Abscess
This 19-year-old woman complained of 2 months of abdominal pain and fever. **A-D.** Enhanced axial CT images demonstrate mild enlargement of both kidneys. The kidneys have alternating bands of higher and lower attenuation, a phenomenon known as a striated nephrogram. Within the upper pole of the right kidney is a round fluid-filled mass with an indistinct margin and an enhancing rim (*white arrow*). Given the presence of pyelonephritis, this is most likely to represent a renal abscess. There is also a rim-enhancing perinephric collection (*black arrowheads*) indicating spread of infection into the perinephric tissues.

lymphomatous lesions can be evident before the lesion is evident on anatomic cross-sectional imaging.

There are a number of patterns of lymphomatous disease on imaging studies. The most common appearance of renal lymphoma is that of multiple parenchymal masses of variable size; this pattern is seen in 50% to 60% of cases (see Figure 6-37). Contiguous extension to the kidneys or perinephric space from large retroperitoneal mass is the

Imaging Notes 6-7. Patterns of Lymphomatous Involvement on Imaging Studies

Pattern	Comments
Multiple parenchymal masses	Most common pattern; seen in 50%-60% of cases
Contiguous extension to the kidneys or perinephric space from large retroperitoneal mass	Second most common pattern; seen in 25%-30% of cases
Solitary mass	Seen in 10%-25% of patients. Mass usually hypovascular—distinction from clear cell renal carcinoma
Global enlargement of the affected kidney without distortion of the normal shape of the kidney(s)	Represents lymphomatous infiltration of the renal interstitium
Infiltrative mass replacing renal sinus fat	Uncommon
Isolated perinephric lymphoma	Unusual; seen in <10% of cases

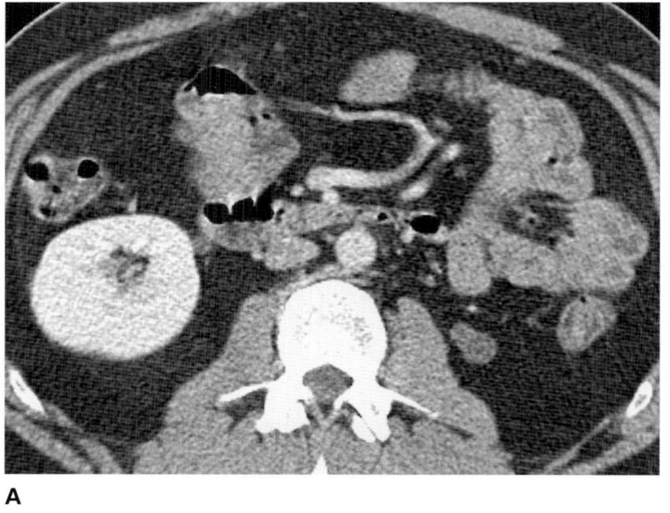

A

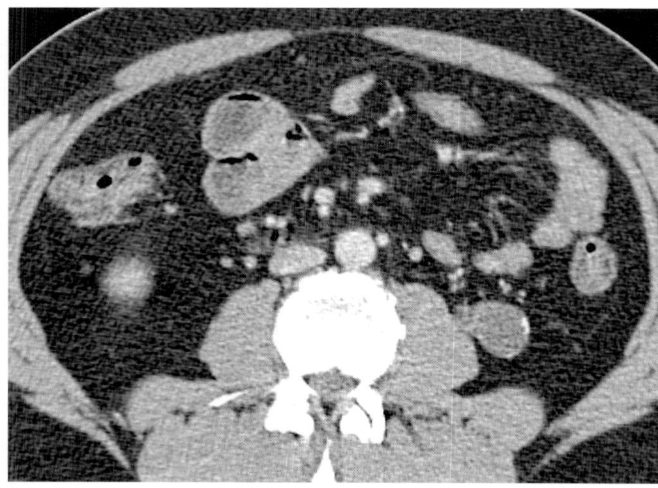

B

C

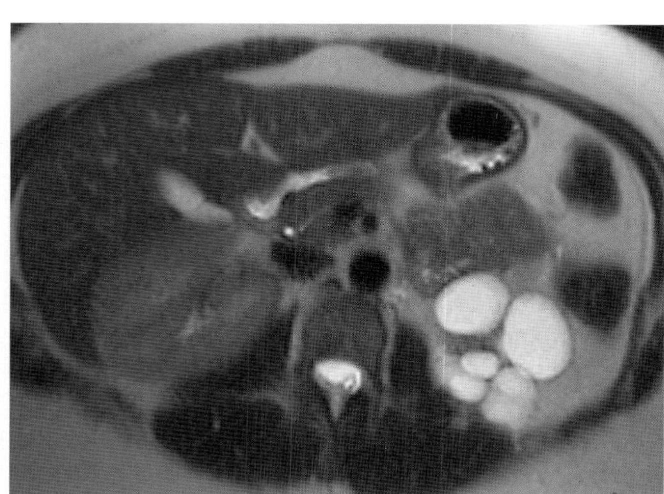

D

Figure 6-36 Multicystic Dysplastic Kidneys in 3 Patients
A and **B.** This 29-year-old man presented with nonspecific abdominal complaints. Contrast-enhanced axial CT images demonstrate a small multicystic remnant of the left kidney, with 1 cyst containing rim calcification. **C.** This newborn infant had an abnormality on prenatal US. Images of the left kidney show a small kidney nearly completely replaced by many small cysts. The remaining regions of soft tissue are inhomogeneous and dysplastic appearing. The normal renal architecture is missing. **D.** T2-weighted MRI in a third person shows a similar multicystic mass with limited residual soft tissue. These cases are all typical of incidentally detected MCDK.

second most common pattern (25%-30% of cases) (see Figures 6-38 and 6-39). This imaging appearance is highly suggestive of lymphoma; biopsy should be definitive and provide specific cell typing. Although perirenal spread from retroperitoneal or renal lymphoma is not uncommon, isolated perinephric lymphoma is unusual, accounting for less than 10% of cases. Renal lymphoma manifests as a solitary mass in 10% to 25% of patients (see Figure 6-40). The hypovascular enhancement pattern of lymphoma is a feature that allows differentiation from conventional renal carcinoma, but does not allow differentiation from other renal neoplasms such as chromophobe or papillary carcinoma. Percutaneous needle biopsy has a definite role in patients with a solitary renal mass suspected to represent lymphoma because recognition of a diagnosis of lymphoma will prevent unnecessary surgical resection. Global enlargement of the affected kidney without distortion of the normal shape of the kidneys can be seen as a result of diffuse lymphomatous infiltration of the renal interstitium. In such cases, intravenous contrast-enhanced CT demonstrates heterogeneous renal parenchymal enhancement, loss of the normal differential enhancement between the cortex and the medulla in the corticomedullary phase, and infiltration of the renal sinus fat or multiple poorly enhancing renal lesions may be visible. US will typically demonstrate a globally enlarged hypoechoic kidney. Uncommonly, lymphoma can preferentially involve the renal sinus. This is manifested on CT as an infiltrative mass replacing the

Imaging Notes 6-8. Differential Diagnosis of Solitary Hypovascular Solid Renal Mass

Renal papillary carcinoma
Chromophobe carcinoma
Lymphoma
Metastasis

Table 6-7. Multiple Kidney Nodules or Masses: Differential Diagnosis

1. Lymphoma
2. Metastases
3. Multiple renal cell carcinomas (consider hereditary papillary renal cancer, Von Hippel-Lindau syndrome)
4. Multiple angiomyolipomas (consider tuberous sclerosis)

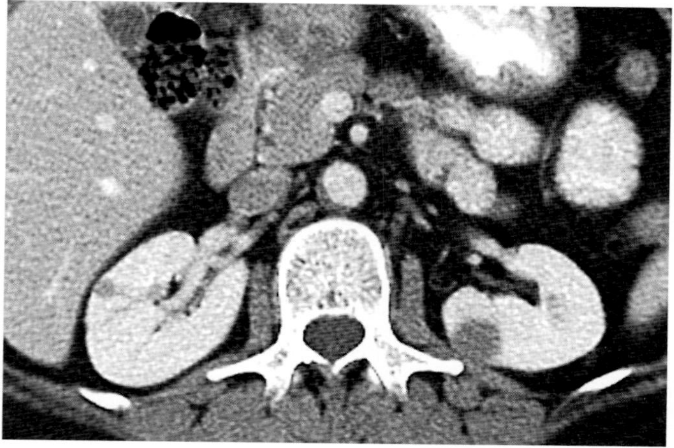
A

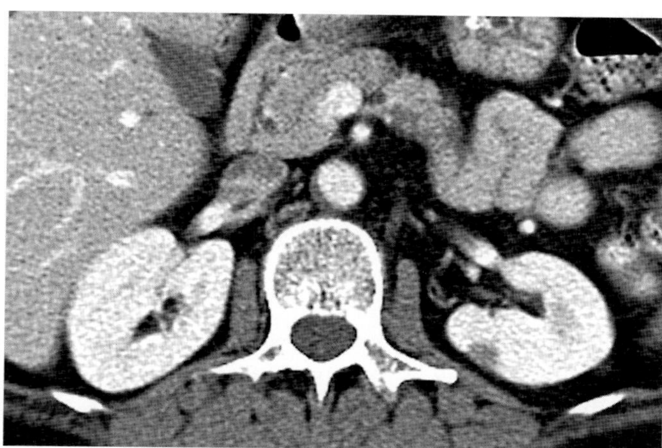
B

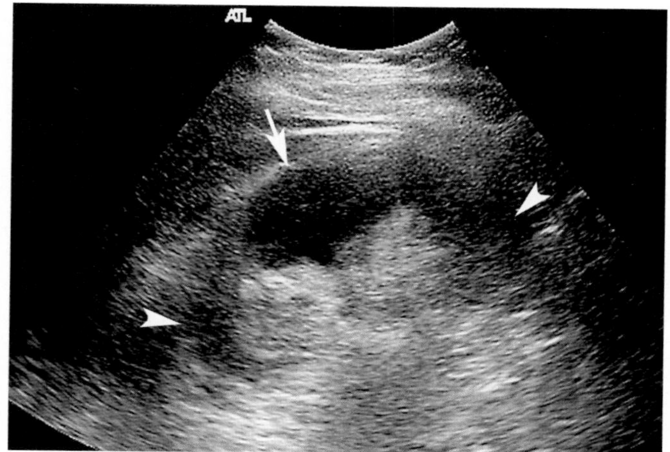

C

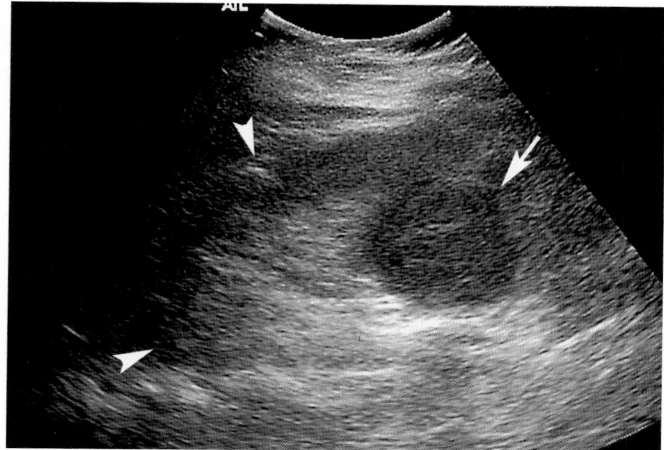
D

Figure 6-37 Multiple Renal Masses due to Non-Hodgkin Lymphoma in 2 Patients
A. Contrast-enhanced axial CT image through the level of the mid-kidneys demonstrates bilateral hypodense renal masses. **B.** CT image at the same anatomic level 5 weeks after treatment demonstrates decrease in size of the left renal mass, and the right renal mass is no longer visible. **C** and **D.** Longitudinal US images of the left kidney (*arrowheads*) in a second patient with follicular lymphoma show 2 hypoechoic masses (*arrows*), 1 in the interpolar region and the second in the lower pole. The uniform hypoechoic masses are a typical appearance of lymphoma on US examinations. Renal lymphoma can potentially be confused with renal cysts because of the hypoechoic-anechoic nature of the masses. (Thanks to Lisa Jones, MD, PhD, for the loan of the US images).

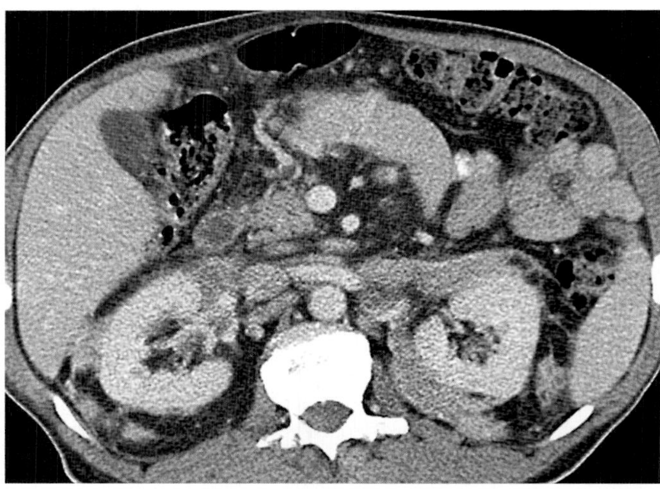

A

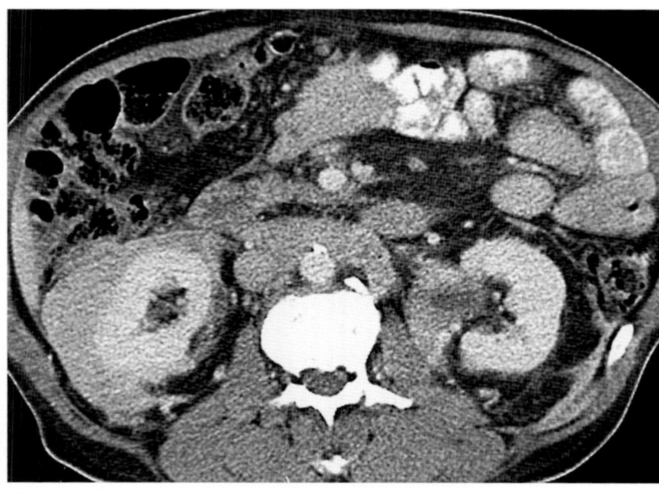

B

Figure 6-38 Contiguous Extension to Kidneys From Retroperitoneal Mass due to Non-Hodgkin Lymphoma
A and **B.** Contrast-enhanced axial CT images demonstrate extensive plaque-like tissue within both perinephric spaces, the renal sinuses, and about the central retroperitoneal vessels, representing lymphoma.

renal sinus fat (see Figure 6-41). Regardless of the renal manifestation of lymphoma, the presence of retroperitoneal adenopathy can be an important clue to the diagnosis of lymphoma.

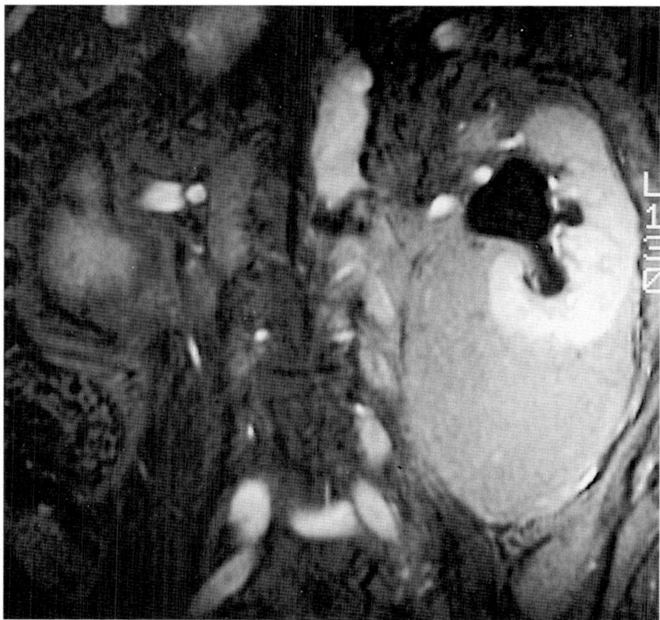

Figure 6-39 Renal Lymphoma
This 48-year-old man had an elevated serum lactic dehydrogenase. Coronal gadolinium-enhanced MRI shows a large mass surrounding the inferior pole of the left kidney. This appearance of a mass engulfing but not destroying the kidney is highly suggestive of lymphoma, usually a non-Hodgkin lymphoma.

Kidney metastasis

A renal metastasis is the most common malignant neoplasm of the kidney found at autopsy.[42] However, renal metastases are uncommonly seen on cross-sectional imaging studies. Renal metastases are most often asymptomatic; they typically do not produce hematuria or azotemia. The most common primary tumors to metastasize to the kidneys are lung, breast, gastrointestinal tract, melanoma, and hematologic malignancies. In most cases, patients with renal metastasis will have a clinically known extrarenal cancer. On

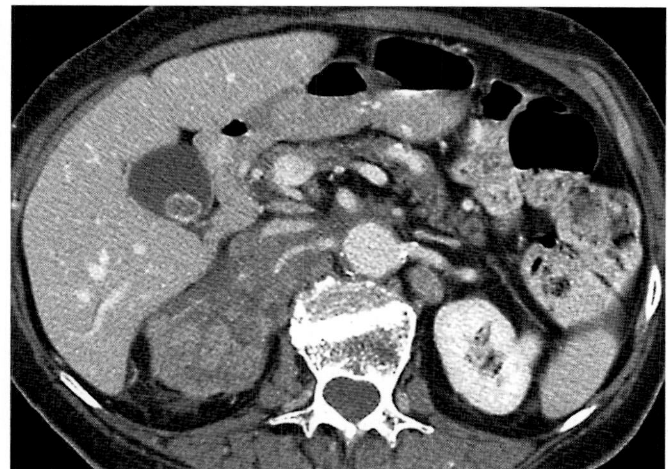

Figure 6-40 Solitary Renal Mass due to Non-Hodgkin Lymphoma
Contrast-enhanced axial CT image demonstrates a right renal mass that extends medially into the retroperitoneum and encases the renal vessels. An enlarged left para-aortic lymph node, and a gallstone, are also present.

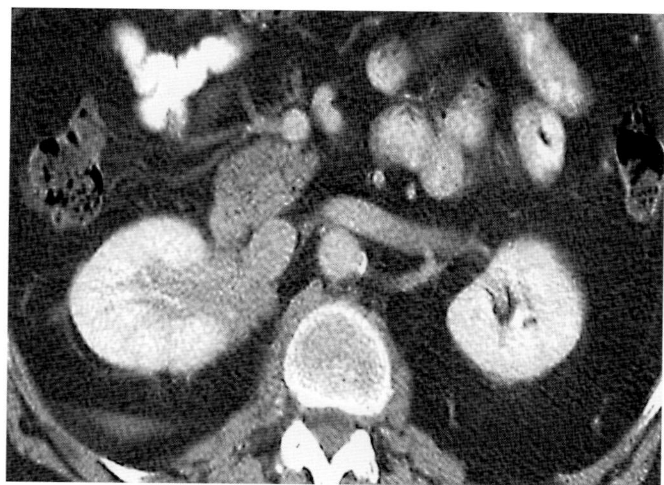

Figure 6-41 Non-Hodgkin Lymphoma of the Renal Sinus
Contrast-enhanced axial CT image demonstrates replacement of the right renal sinus fat by an infiltrating mass.

contrast-enhanced CT, the lesions are usually small, multifocal, and bilateral, exhibiting an infiltrative growth pattern. The lesions are hypoenhancing relative to the background of renal parenchyma (see Figure 6-42).[13] In a patient with a known extrarenal cancer, multiple renal nodules or masses will nearly always represent metastasis. However, a solitary renal mass in a patient with a known extrarenal cancer could represent either a metastasis or a primary renal neoplasm.

Multiple primary renal cell carcinomas

Multiple primary renal cell carcinomas are an uncommon event. When they occur, they will usually indicate an underlying genetic syndrome such as VHL or hereditary papillary renal cancer (see Figure 6-4). **Multiple** renal cell carcinomas and the associated hereditary syndromes have previously been discussed in detail under the heading: **Solitary Renal Mass.**

Angiomyolipomas associated with lymphangioleiomyomatosis and tuberous sclerosis

Multiple renal parenchymal masses containing macroscopic fat enable the diagnosis of multiple angiomyolipomas. Multiple angiomyolipomas are uncommon as a sporadic event and should raise strong suspicion of LAM or TS (see Figures 6-16 and 6-43). Angiomyolipomas, LAM, and TS have previously been discussed in detail under the heading: **Solitary Renal Mass.**

Multiple Solid Nonspherical Renal Lesions

Renal infarction and renal traumatic injuries can both cause multifocal abnormalities in the kidney. The characteristics of these lesions are similar to the unifocal lesions previously described. The alternating higher and lower

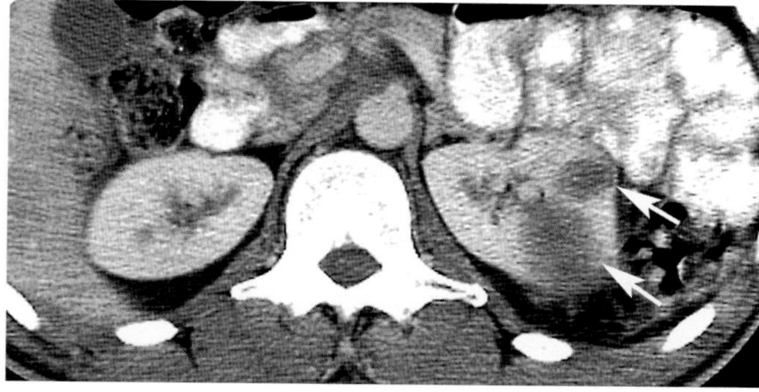

A

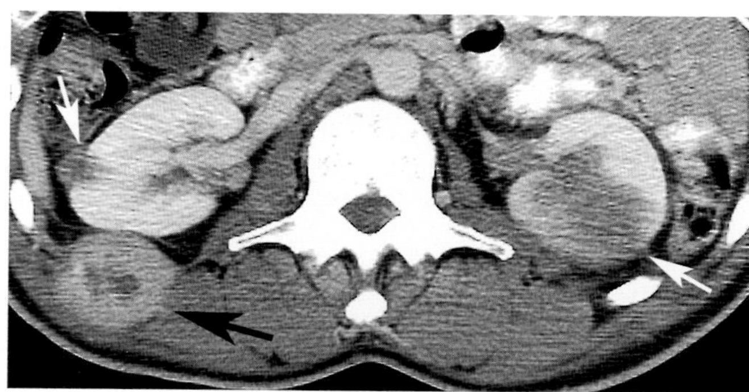

B

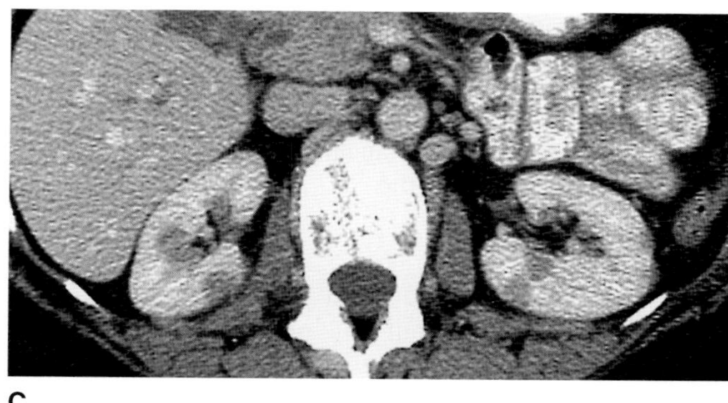

C

Figure 6-42 Renal Metastases in 2 Patients
A and **B.** This 41-year-old man was being evaluated for metastatic lung cancer. Enhanced CT demonstrates multiple poorly marginated low-attenuation lesions (*white arrows*) within both kidneys. This appearance is most often due to renal metastasis or renal lymphoma. Note the additional, enhancing soft tissue metastasis to the musculature of the back (*black arrow*). **C.** This patient had metastatic breast cancer to bone, skin, kidneys, and liver. Contrast-enhanced axial CT image demonstrates bilateral renal nodules due to metastases.

attenuation of enhanced kidneys associated with pyelonephritis is discussed later in the chapter under the heading: **Kidney Disorders with a Specific Appearance.**

Multiple Cystic Renal Masses

Multiple renal cysts can be due to idiopathic simple renal cysts or as a result of several systemic disorders. In some

Imaging Notes 6-9. Cysts associated with Renal Cystic Diseases or Systemic Diseases

Disease	Comments	Morphology/Imaging Features
Autosomal-dominant polycystic kidney disease (APCD)	Most common form of cystic kidney disease; autosomal-dominant mode of inheritance, with 100% penetrance.	Markedly enlarged kidneys, containing multiple bilateral cysts that can be complicated by hemorrhage
Multicystic dysplastic kidney (MCDK)	Cause believed to be obstruction of fetal ureter before 8-10 weeks' gestation	Disorganized conglomerate of irregularly arranged cysts and fibrous tissue without functioning renal parenchyma, usually unilateral
Tuberous sclerosis (TS) complex	Autosomal dominant inheritance; clinical features include mental retardation, seizures, or characteristic facial skin lesions. Patients develop multiple renal angiomyolipomas.	Renal cysts typically <3 cm size, indistinguishable from simple cortical cysts on imaging.
Von Hippel-Lindau (VHL) disease	Genetically transmitted disorder; CNS and retinal hemangioblastomas, renal carcinomas, pheochromocytomas, islet cell tumors of the pancreas, cysts of various organs including the kidneys	Renal cysts seen in approximately 75% of patients; renal carcinomas occur in 25%-45% of patients. Renal cysts in VHL typically small, ranging in size from 0.5 to 3 cm, morphology ranges from simple cysts to eccentric nodules within cyst walls.
Acquired renal cystic disease (ARCD)	Progressive development of multiple cysts in patients with chronic renal failure. Propensity to develop low-grade renal neoplasms.	Kidneys small; cysts small, often contain dystrophic calcification, and commonly undergo hemorrhage.

cases, the features of the cysts and other imaging findings can point to the cause for the multiple cysts.

Idiopathic renal cysts

The presence of multiple renal cysts on cross-sectional imaging in a given patient will most often signify idiopathic simple renal cysts, often of no clinical significance. They will appear as multiple variable-sized cysts, ranging in size from submillimeter to several centimeters, randomly distributed in 1 or both kidneys. A large number of cysts, more than 10 to 15 in number, should raise suspicion of an underlying genetic or metabolic cause.

Cysts associated with systemic conditions

In some cases, the presence of multiple cysts will be an indicator of an underlying disease or syndrome including autosomal dominant polycystic kidney disease, VHL, TS, acquired renal cystic disease due to dialysis.

Imaging Notes 6-10. Number of renal cysts and likelihood of underlying cause

More than 10-15 renal cysts should raise suspicion of an underlying genetic or metabolic cause for the cysts.

Autosomal-dominant polycystic kidney disease: Autosomal-dominant polycystic kidney disease, also known as adult polycystic kidney disease (APCD), is the

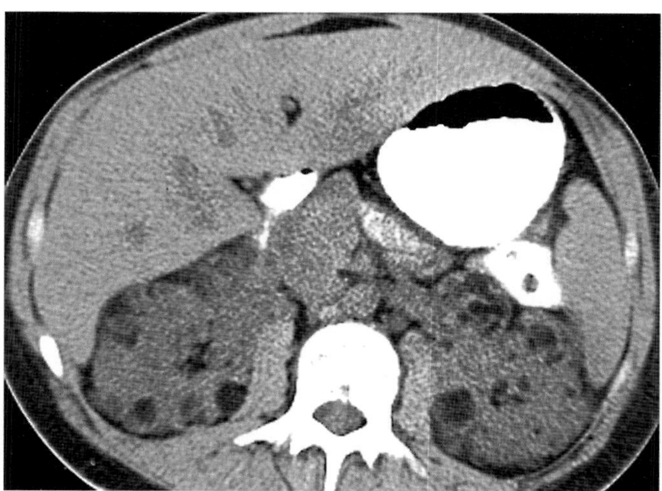

Figure 6-43 Angiomyolipomas in Tuberous Sclerosis
The patient is a 25-year-old female with TS and bilateral renal angiomyolipomas. Unenhanced axial CT scan demonstrates multiple fat-density bilateral renal masses typical of angiomyolipomas.

most common form of inherited cystic kidney disease. It is transmitted by an autosomal-dominant mode of inheritance, with 100% penetrance. Patients with this disease usually present in the third or fourth decades. Presentation varies, from manifestation of complications of the renal cystic disease including pain and hematuria with or without associated trauma to the kidney, stone disease, or renal insufficiency or renal failure, to rupture of the cerebral aneurysms that are associated with this disease.[54] In addition to bilateral renal cysts that are found in all individuals, 54% of individuals will also have cysts found in the liver and a few percent will have cysts of the pancreas. It remains controversial whether APCD is a risk factor for development of renal carcinoma.[55] On cross-sectional imaging exams, both kidneys will appear markedly enlarged and contain innumerable cysts that replace the majority of the renal parenchyma. The combination of large kidneys with near uniform replacement of the renal parenchyma by cysts is virtually pathognomonic of APCD. Some cysts can be complicated by internal hemorrhage (see Figure 6-44).

Acquired renal cystic disease: Acquired renal cystic disease (ARCD) is a well-known entity in which there is progressive development of multiple cysts in patients who have chronic renal failure. This is primarily seen in patients who are being treated with hemodialysis but can occur in patients on peritoneal dialysis and in some patients with renal insufficiency before dialysis is instituted.[56,57] The

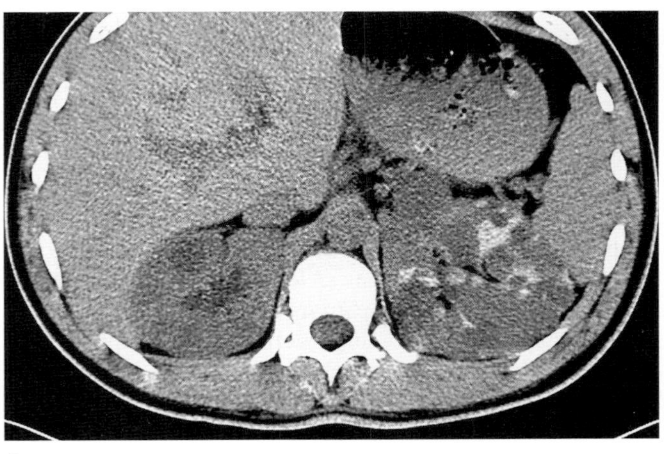

A

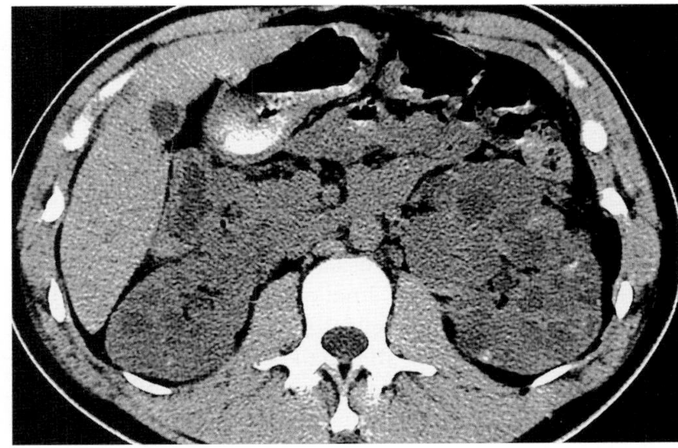

B

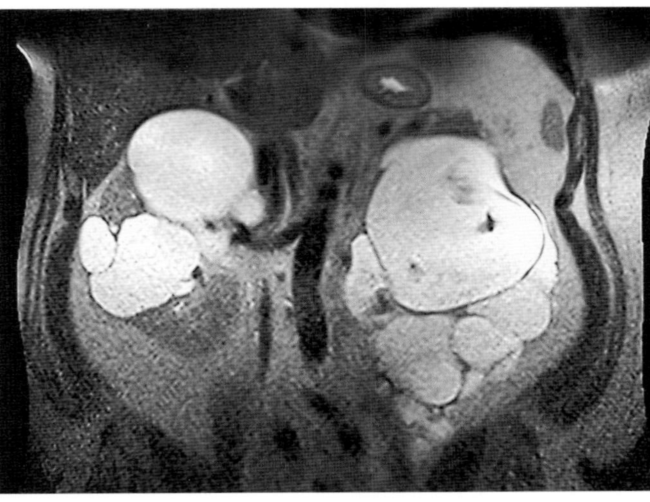

C

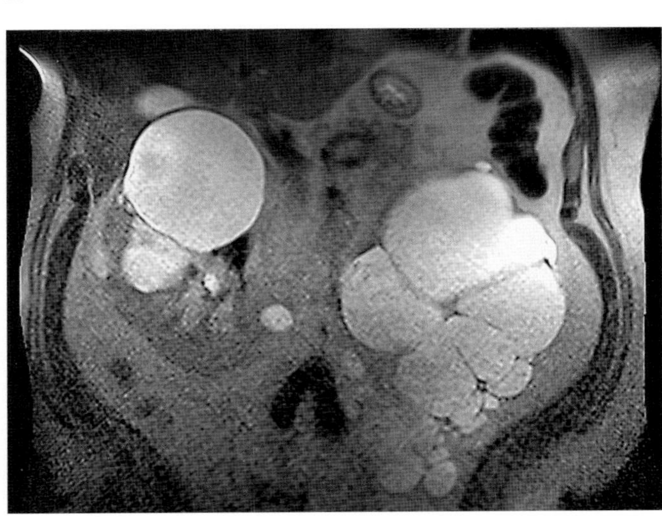

D

Figure 6-44 Autosomal Dominant Polycystic Kidney Disease (ADPKD) in 2 Patients
This 29-year-old man presented with left scrotal pain. **A** and **B**. Unenhanced CT images demonstrate enlarged kidneys that contain innumerable round, small low-attenuation regions characteristic of many small cysts. This appearance is essentially diagnostic of autosomal dominant polycystic kidney disease, an unsuspected finding in this patient. **C** and **D**. This second patient had chronic renal failure due to known polycystic kidneys. Coronal T2-weighted MRI examinations show the cysts to be numerous, massive in size, and nearly replacing the entire kidneys. This is the natural course of ADPKD and leads to progressive renal failure.

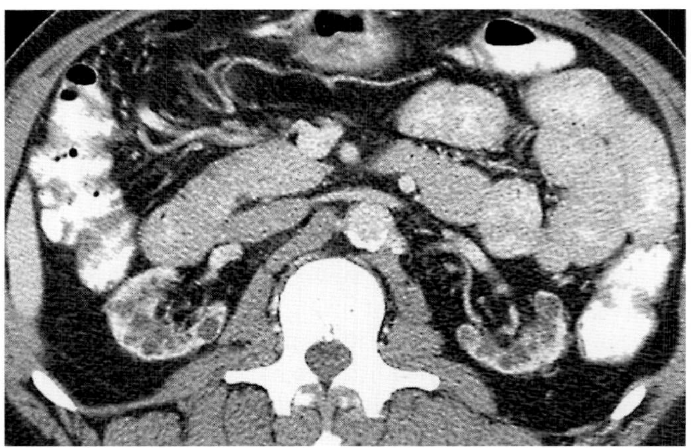

Figure 6-45 Acquired Renal Cystic Disease
The patient is a 51-year-old man with end-stage renal disease was receiving hemodialysis. Contrast-enhanced axial CT image demonstrates markedly atrophic kidneys containing innumerable tiny cysts.

cysts develop at a rate proportional to the duration of dialysis; after 3 years, 10% to 20% of patients have ARCD. The cysts in ARCD tend to regress after successful renal transplantation. The cysts are small, often contain dystrophic calcification, and commonly undergo hemorrhage. The kidneys of these patients are small because of chronic renal failure. The combination of diminutive size of these kidneys associated with many tiny cysts is highly suggestive of ARCD (see Figure 6-45).

Up to 7% of patients with ARCD will develop solid renal carcinomas. In general, these carcinomas are less aggressive than typical renal cancers.[58] Because the presence of dystrophic calcification often hinders examination with US, CT is the best imaging modality to examine the native kidneys to detect hemorrhage or solid renal neoplasms in patients with ARCD.

Tuberous sclerosis: TS complex is a rare, multisystem, genetic disease transmitted by autosomal dominant inheritance, with incomplete penetrance. Clinical features of the disease include mild to severe learning difficulties, including autism and mental retardation, seizures, dental pits, subungual fibromas, and characteristic skin lesions such as cutaneous angiofibromas (also called adenoma sebaceum), shagreen patches, ash leaf lesions. Imaging of the brain will often demonstrate cortical tubers (for which the disease is named), subependymal nodules, and rarely giant cell astrocytomas. In the abdomen, patients with TS can develop multiple renal angiomyolipomas and have an increased incidence of renal cysts.[59] These cysts are typically less than 3 cm in size and have a distinctive hyperplastic epithelium on light microscopy. However, they are indistinguishable from simple cortical cysts on radiologic imaging studies.[60]

Von hippel-lindau disease: Von Hippel-Lindau (VHL) disease is a genetically transmitted disorder consisting of CNS and retinal hemangioblastomas, renal carcinomas, pheochromocytomas, islet cell tumors of the pancreas, and cysts of various organs including the kidneys. Renal cysts develop in approximately 75% of patients with this disease and renal carcinomas occur in 25% to 45% of patients. The renal cysts in VHL are typically small, ranging in size from 0.5 to 3 cm, and demonstrate a range of appearances, from simple cysts to eccentric papillary solid projections into the lumen of the cyst, often representing a neoplasm developing in the cyst wall. Meticulous imaging technique, using thin-section CT or MRI, is best to detect the often tiny mural nodules in these cysts (see Figure 6-4). The number of cysts is variable in VHL.

DIFFUSE DISEASES OF THE KIDNEY

Diffuse disorders of the kidneys will most often be manifested as nephromegaly or renal atrophy.

Enlargement of the Kidneys

Diffuse enlargement of the kidneys will most often be the result of diffuse renal edema. Edema can be related to diffuse infection, that is, pyelonephritis, noninfectious causes such as acute glomerulonephritis or interstitial nephritis, acute renal cortical necrosis (ARCN), or vascular compromise. Renal edema due to urinary tract obstruction will also cause ipsilateral renal enlargement. Occasionally, infiltrative neoplastic processes such as lymphoma or leukemia may cause renal enlargement (Table 6-8).

Inflammatory causes of nephromegaly

The most common inflammatory condition of the kidney is pyelonephritis, which is also the most common cause of diffuse unilateral or bilateral renal enlargement. Diffuse acute glomerulonephritis or acute interstitial nephritis can also cause renal enlargement.

Table 6-8. Causes of Diffuse Uniform Kidney Enlargement

Acute Inflammation
Pyelonephritis
Glomerulonephritis
Interstitial nephritis
Acute tubular necrosis
Vascular insult
Acute renal artery occlusion
Acute renal vein thrombosis
Acute Obstruction
Neoplasms
Leukemia
Lymphoma

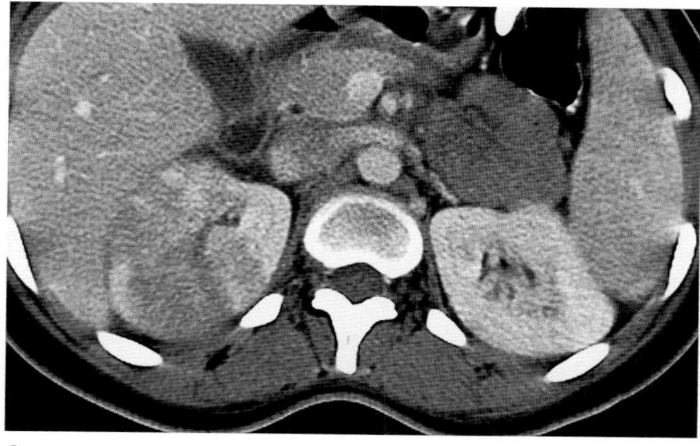

A

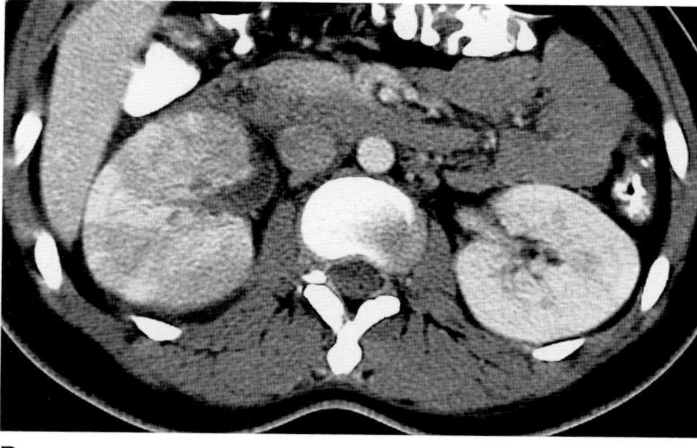

B

Figure 6-46 Pyelonephritis
This 20-year-old woman complained of nausea, vomiting, fevers, and right lower quadrant pain. **A** and **B.** Enhanced CT demonstrates an inhomogeneously enhancing right kidney. There are alternating bands of higher and lower attenuation, known as a striated nephrogram, a finding that is frequently seen in pyelonephritis. Note that the right kidney is enlarged. This is a result of renal edema and is a common feature of pyelonephritis.

Acute pyelonephritis: Acute pyelonephritis is a common disorder of the kidney most often a result of ascending infection in patients with bacterial cystitis. In many patients, the infected kidney will become diffusedly edematous leading to diffuse enlargement of the kidney that can be detected by CT, US, MRI, and IVU examinations (see Figure 6-46). Acute pyelonephritis is discussed most completely under the heading: **Kidney Disorders with a Specific Appearance.**

Glomerulonephritis and interstitial nephritis: Inflammatory diseases of the glomerulus (glomerulonephritis) and inflammatory diseases of the tubules and interstitium (interstitial nephritis) are common causes of renal failure. There are a large number of causes of glomerulonephritis and interstitial nephritis that are beyond the scope of this text. Imaging studies cannot reliably distinguish the types of glomerulonephritis and interstitial nephritis. In some cases of acute glomerulonephritis and interstitial nephritis, US, CT, MRI, and IVU will appear normal. However in many cases of these inflammatory disorders, the acutely inflamed kidneys will appear smoothly and symmetrically enlarged on imaging exams (see Figure 6-47). Ultrasound

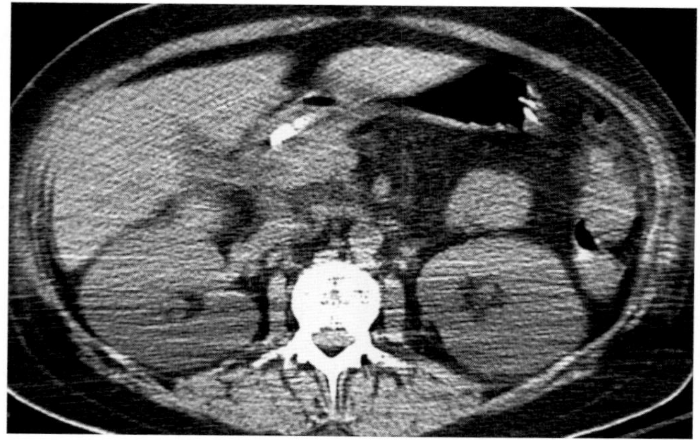

A

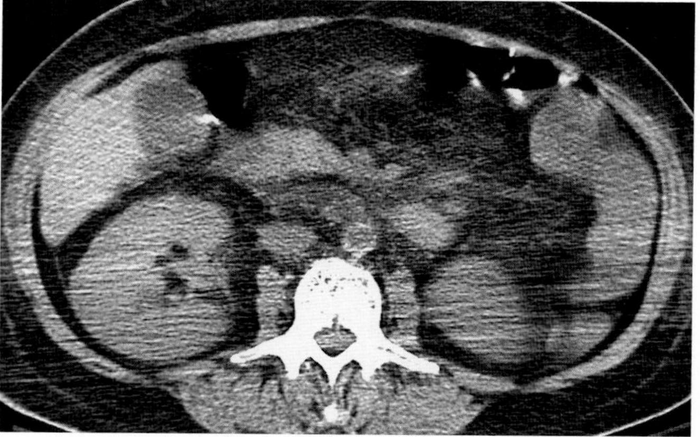

B

Figure 6-47 Nephromegaly due to Acute Renal Failure
This 45-year-old woman developed pneumococcal sepsis that caused disseminated intravascular coagulation (DIC), rhabdomyolysis, and resulted in acute renal failure. CT was performed to evaluate for a source of sepsis. **A** and **B.** Unenhanced CT shows uniform diffuse enlargement of both kidneys. Nephromegaly will usually be due to diffuse renal edema, in this case as a result of rhabdomyolysis-related acute renal failure. Note how the kidneys are slightly lower attenuation than the liver and paraspinal muscles, a finding that could be due to edema of the kidneys. (There is streak artifact through the kidneys. The patient was too ill to raise her arms above her head. The bones of the arms are dense and produce this streak artifact.)

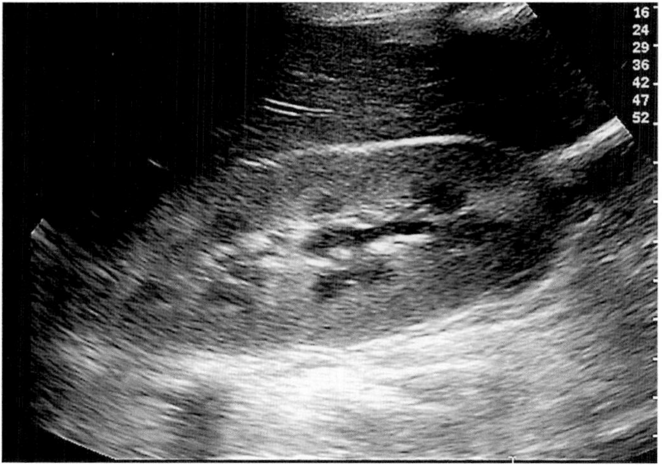

Figure 6-48 Acute Glomerulonephritis
Twenty-year-old woman with systemic lupus erythematosis and acute glomerulonephritis. Sagittal US image of the right kidney demonstrates an enlarged kidney with increased cortical echogenicity. The echogenicity of the renal parenchyma is greater than that of the adjacent liver. The left kidney, not shown, exhibited a similar appearance.

can in some cases assist in distinguishing glomerulonephritis from interstitial nephritis. In acute glomerulonephritis, US exams demonstrate either increased or decreased cortical echogenicity with sparing of the medulla (see Figure 6-48). In acute interstitial nephritis, US will demonstrate enlarged diffusely echogenic kidneys.[61] In most cases, IVU will demonstrate decreased opacification of the collecting systems in both conditions. Little has been written on CT findings of these entities.

Acute renal cortical necrosis: ARCN is a form of acute renal failure in which there is ischemic necrosis of the renal cortex with relative sparing of the renal medulla. ARCN can be due to a number of causes, including sepsis, burns, snake bites, toxins, transfusion reactions, and dehydration, but the majority of cases are associated with pregnancy, especially cases complicated by placental abruption, septic abortion, or placenta previa.[62] Initially, the kidneys are diffusely enlarged, and on intravenous contrast-enhanced CT, a characteristic peripheral zone of nonenhancement is seen in the kidneys (see Figure 6-49). With time, there is symmetrical shrinkage of the kidneys and in some cases development of diffuse cortical calcification. Calcification related to acute cortical necrosis is discussed later under the heading: **Calcifications in the Kidney Parenchyma: Nephrocalcinosis**.

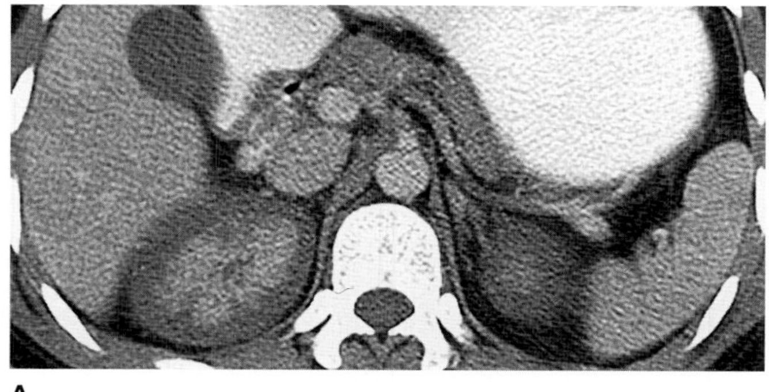

A

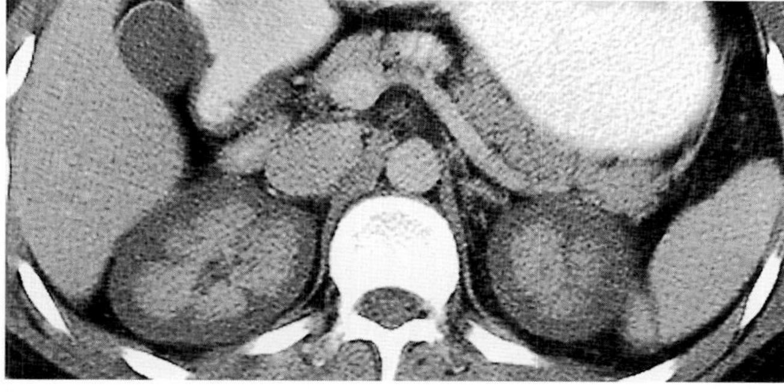

B

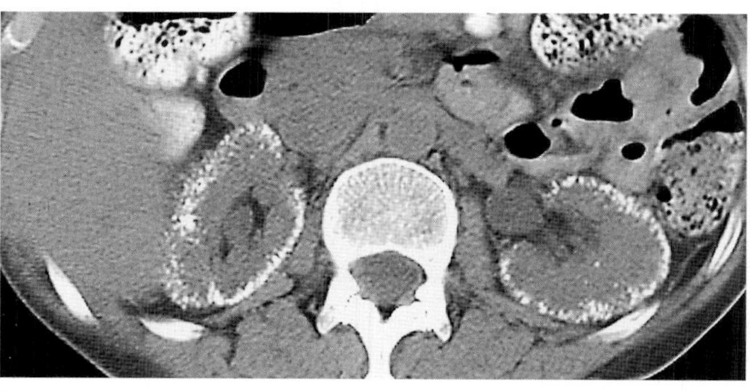

C

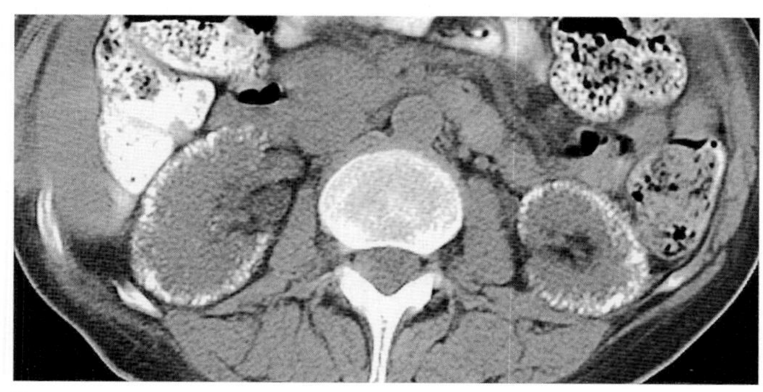

D

Figure 6-49 Acute Bilateral Renal Cortical Necrosis in 2 Patients
The first patient was a 22-year-old with acute abdominal pain. **A** and **B**. Axial CT images of an intravenous contrast-enhanced CT scan demonstrate characteristic peripheral cortical nonenhancement of both kidneys. The second patient was a 69-year-old woman being evaluated for weight loss. **C** and **D**. Unenhanced axial CT images demonstrate diffuse cortical calcifications, a characteristic result of prior acute cortical necrosis.

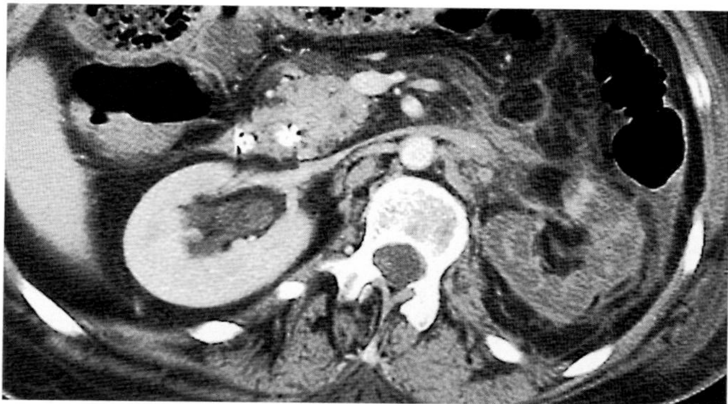

A

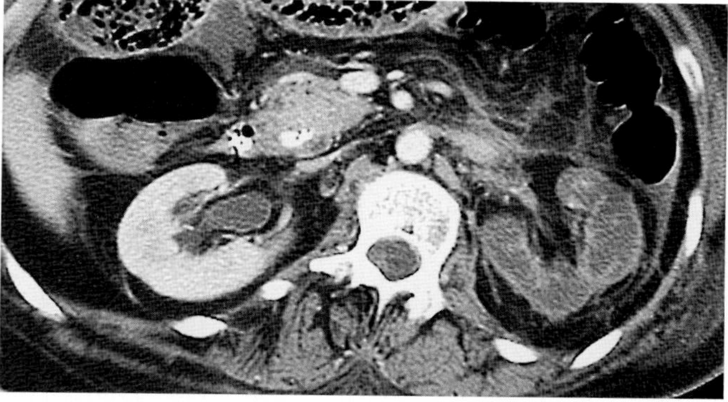

B

Figure 6-50 Traumatic Left Renal Artery Occlusion With Prominent Capsular Enhancement
The patient was a pedestrian hit by a train. **A** and **B.** Axial images from an intravenous contrast-enhanced CT scan performed after the patient underwent splenectomy demonstrate nonopacification of the proximal and mid left renal artery, global nonenhancement of the renal parenchyma except for a thin peripheral rim of enhancement, representing capsular collateral vessels.

Nephromegaly due to acute vascular insults

Acute occlusion of either the renal artery or RV can cause renal ischemia or infarction, leading to edema of the kidney.

Acute renal artery occlusion: With acute main renal artery occlusion, typically due to an embolus or traumatic arterial disruption, the kidney will increase in size due to edema, a finding that can be seen on any imaging study of the kidney. This is in contradistinction to occlusion of the renal artery due to severe atherosclerosis, which is a gradual process, and usually results in decrease in renal size due to atrophy. With an acute main renal artery occlusion, global renal infarction will also be manifested on contrast-enhanced CT and MRI as lack of contrast enhancement of the kidney except for a thin peripheral rim of enhancement, representing patent capsular vessels (see Figure 6-50).

Acute renal vein thrombosis: Glomerulonephritis is the most common cause of acute RVT. Other causes include: extension of renal carcinoma into the RV, extrinsic compression of the RV, clotting disorders, trauma, and dehydration. Contrast-enhanced CT is useful to detect RVT and to aid in determining the cause. Renal enlargement with decreased contrast opacification is seen, often with venous collaterals opacified. In general, MRI is considered even more accurate than CT in depicting the presence and extent of RVT and can be performed without contrast using gradient echo techniques in patients with contraindications to iodinated contrast and/or renal failure. Further, US may demonstrate an enlarged, hypoechoic kidney, and in some cases, image the thrombus (see Figure 6-51).

Nephromegaly due to ureteral obstruction

There is a constellation of imaging findings associated with acute ureteral obstruction, including nephromegaly. For further discussion of ureteral obstruction, please refer to Chapter 7.

Nephromegaly due to infiltrative tumor: lymphoma and leukemia

Diffuse infiltration of the kidneys with lymphoma is usually bilateral and seen in 20% of patients who have renal involvement with lymphoma. Because the lymphomatous tissue grows in the interstitium of the kidney, the renal contour is preserved. Diagnosis with imaging may be challenging; the use of intravenous contrast with CT is important. On CT examinations, the typical findings include heterogeneous enhancement of the kidneys, loss of the normal differential enhancement between the cortex and the medulla in the corticomedullary phase, and infiltration of the renal sinus fat (see Figure 6-52). Infiltrated kidneys demonstrate some compromise in function, but usually maintain sufficient function to remain clinically silent. Further, US findings of infiltrative renal lymphoma are often quite subtle and include globular enlargement of the kidneys with heterogeneous echotexture.[41,63]

Leukemia is the most common malignant cause of bilateral nephromegaly in children. Infiltration of the kidneys by leukemic cells as well as intrarenal hemorrhage and edema contribute to the bilateral renal enlargement, which can be marked.

Renal Atrophy

Chronic renal insufficiency or chronic renal failure will eventually result in decreased renal size, regardless of the cause. Some causes are listed (Table 6-9) (see Figure 6-53).

Unilateral renal atrophy can be a result of unilateral irradiation, vesicoureteral reflux, obstruction, or ischemia. Focal renal atrophy can occur following focal infarction or focal pyelonephritis. Small zones of atrophy may appear

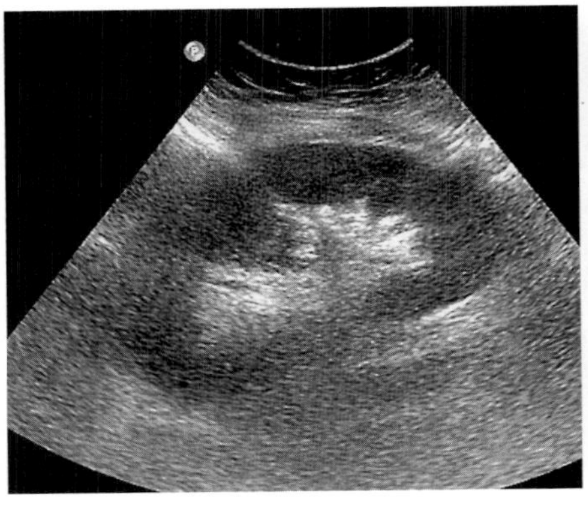

A

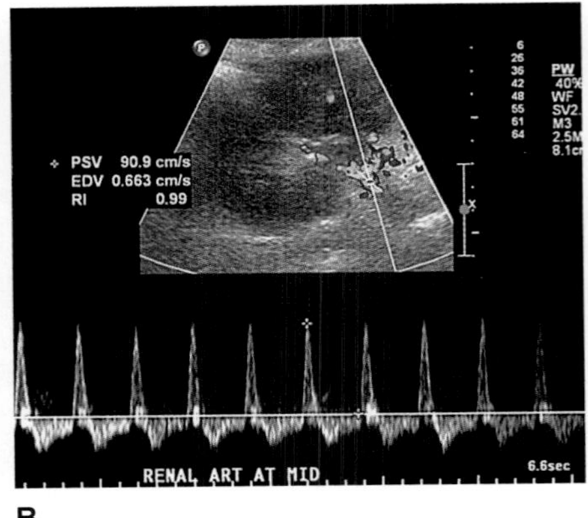

B

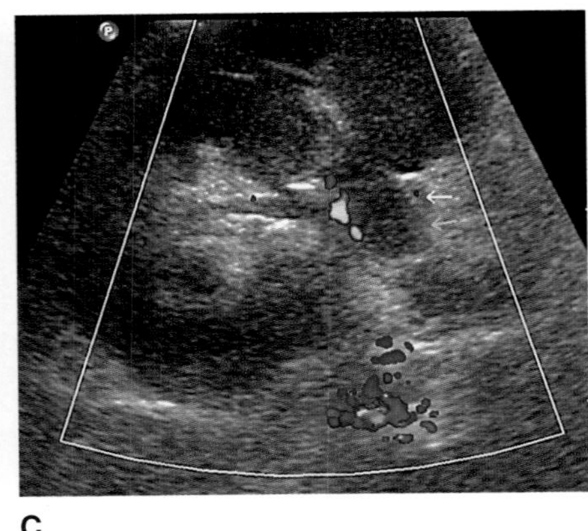

C

Figure 6-51 Acute Renal Vein Thrombosis in a Renal Transplant, US Examination
Static grayscale sagittal scan (**A**) demonstrates normal parenchymal echotexture of the transplant kidney. Spectral Doppler tracing of the main renal artery (**B**) demonstrates reversal of diastolic flow. Color Doppler examination of the RV (**C**) demonstrates no flow in the thrombosed vein (*arrows*).

as a focal depression of the surface of the kidney, whereas larger areas of atrophy may demonstrate zonal loss of cortical tissue (see Figure 6-54).

KIDNEY DISORDERS WITH A SPECIFIC APPEARANCE

Acute pyelonephritis, calcification of the kidney parenchyma, contrast nephropathy, and a variety of congenital disorders of the kidney have specific imaging appearances. These will be discussed here.

The Striated Nephrogram

The striated nephrogram represents alternating stripelike areas of normal and decreased contrast enhancement. This can be found in a focal region of the kidney or diffusely throughout 1 or both kidneys. The finding is most often associated with pyelonephritis, and it may be seen in other conditions. Berdon, in 1969, described striation in association with Tamm-Horsfall proteinuria, probably because of tubular obstruction by casts.[64] Bigongiari, in 1977, demonstrated with microradiography that the nephrographic striation visible on IVU in association with ureteric obstruction is produced by contrast accumulation in medullary rays, the bundles of renal tubules that form in the renal cortex and continue through the renal medulla. The striated nephrogram has also been described in RVT,[65] infantile polycystic disease,[66] and rhabdomyolysis.[67] Although the exact cause of the nephrographic striations in these conditions is not proven, a common explanation for the appearance is the presence of tubular stasis and urine hyperconcentration (see Figures 6-35 and 6-46).[68]

Imaging Notes 6-11. Causes of a Striated Nephrogram

- Acute pyelonephritis
- Tamm-Horsfall proteinuria
- Ureteric obstruction
- Renal vein thrombosis
- Autosomal recessive polycystic kidney disease
- Rhabdomyolysis

Acute pyelonephritis

Acute pyelonephritis is most often related to ascending infection following cystitis. Patients typically present with flank pain, fever, and pyuria. Radiologic imaging is not required for the diagnosis in most cases; however, radiologic imaging can be useful in evaluating patients who do not respond appropriately to standard antibiotic therapy. Pyelonephritis also can be revealed on imaging studies obtained to evaluate patients for whom an alternative diagnosis is suspected.

Results of imaging studies are normal in the majority of cases of acute uncomplicated pyelonephritis. The most comprehensive imaging test to demonstrate the presence and extent of pyelonephritis is CT. Scans performed prior to IV contrast administration can be normal or show renal enlargement, and can demonstrate associated abnormalities such as calculi and/or urinary tract obstruction. Intravenous contrast-enhanced scans depict pathology best when performed during the nephrographic phase. Enhanced CT typically demonstrates a striated nephrogram (see Figures 6-35 and 6-46). In acute pyelonephritis, the striations are due to tubular obstruction produced by inflammatory debris within the lumen, interstitial edema, and vasospasm.[69] With increasing degree of involvement, multiple wedge-shaped zones of decreased enhancement are seen. Fluid collections within the abnormal areas of parenchyma

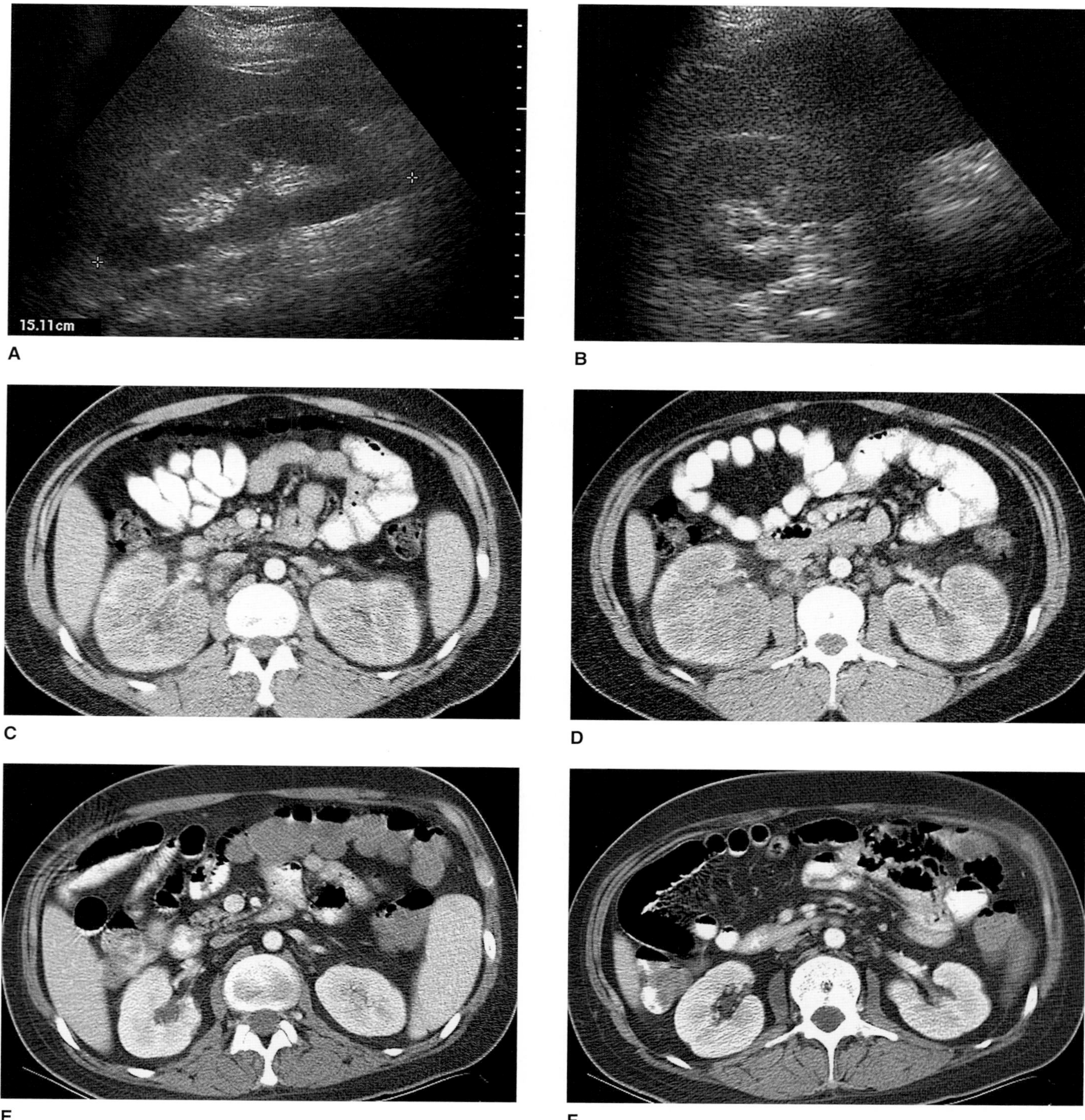

Figure 6-52 Bilateral Nephromegaly due to Lymphomatous Infiltration: Serial Imaging Studies
A renal US study showed an enlarged kidney in this 26-year-old man with a history of non-Hodgkin lymphoma. **A** and **B.** Sagittal and transverse US of right kidney, which measures more than 15 cm in length. Enlargement of the right kidney was noted on a right upper abdominal US to evaluate jaundice. A CT scan of the abdomen was then obtained. **C** and **D.** Images from an intravenous contrast-enhanced CT scan demonstrate diffusely infiltrating bilateral, poorly defined hypodense masses within enlarged kidneys, and enlarged retroperitoneal lymph nodes. **E** and **F.** Seven months after successful treatment for recurrent lymphoma, a repeat CT scan of the abdomen demonstrates that the renal masses have resolved, the kidneys are now normal in size, and the retroperitoneal lymph nodes have decreased in size.

Table 6-9. Causes of Renal Atrophy

Usually Bilateral
Chronic glomerulonephritis
Nephrosclerosis (hypertensive nephropathy)
Chronic interstitial nephritis
Usually Unilateral, but may be Bilateral
Radiation fibrosis
Chronic vesicoureteral reflux
Chronic obstruction
Chronic ischemia

indicate development of microabscesses. Other findings on CT in acute pyelonephritis include infiltration of the perinephric fat and thickening of Gerota fascia.

US in patients with acute pyelonephritis is normal or shows renal enlargement and diffusely hypoechoic renal parenchyma. Further, US is relatively insensitive when compared with contrast-enhanced CT in the evaluation of acute pyelonephritis, and can underestimate the degree of involvement. Abscess cavities typically appear as rounded areas of hypoechogenicity.

MRI also is able to depict the inflammatory process in acute pyelonephritis; an affected area will have low SI on T1-weighted images and increased SI on T2-weighted images, with a loss of normal corticomedullary differentiation. Moreover, MRI with intravenous gadolinium may demonstrate renal enlargement, perinephric stranding, focal areas of decreased enhancement, and a striated nephrogram similar to CT examinations. The lack of ionizing radiation makes MRI particularly suited for evaluating pregnant patients.

Calcifications in the Kidney Parenchyma: Nephrocalcinosis

Calcifications within the kidney can occur within the parenchyma (nephrocalcinosis) or within the renal collecting system (nephrolithiasis). Nephrolithiasis is discussed in Chapter 7. Nephrocalcinosis, the deposition of calcium within the renal parenchyma, is classified according to the area involved. The sites and patterns of calcification in nephrocalcinosis are well depicted on plain radiographs and US, although CT is more sensitive for detection of early manifestations. In addition, MRI is insensitive to the presence of calcification and will fail to detect many cases of nephrocalcinosis.

Medullary nephrocalcinosis

Calcification can uniformly involve the medulla or can preferentially involve the papillary tips. Uniform medullary nephrocalcinosis is most commonly due to hyperparathyroidism or distal renal tubular acidosis (type I) (see Figures 6-55 and 6-56). Nonuniform medullary nephrocalcinosis is most commonly due to medullary sponge kidney, a condition where calculi develop in the papillary tips of cystically dilated collecting ducts (see Figure 6-57).[70] Rarely, medullary nephrocalcinosis can be due to a variety of causes of hypercalcemia, some of which are listed in Table 6-10.

Cortical nephrocalcinosis

Deposition of calcium in the renal cortex, cortical nephrocalcinosis, is located in the periphery of the kidney. The most common causes of cortical nephrocalcinosis are chronic glomerulonephritis, acute cortical necrosis, and oxalosis (Table 6-11). In chronic glomerulonephritis, small, smooth kidneys are usually seen, which may

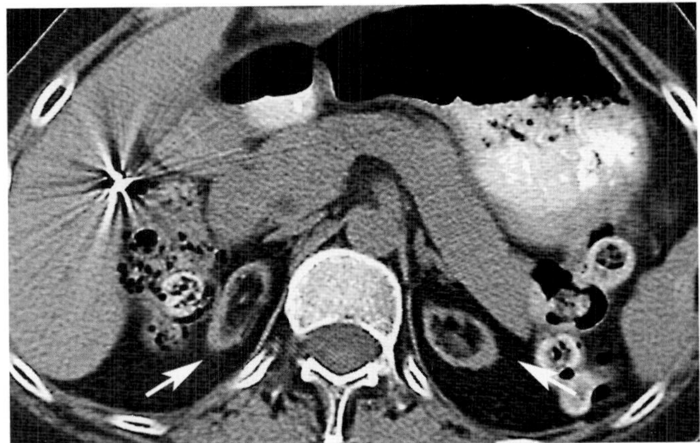

A

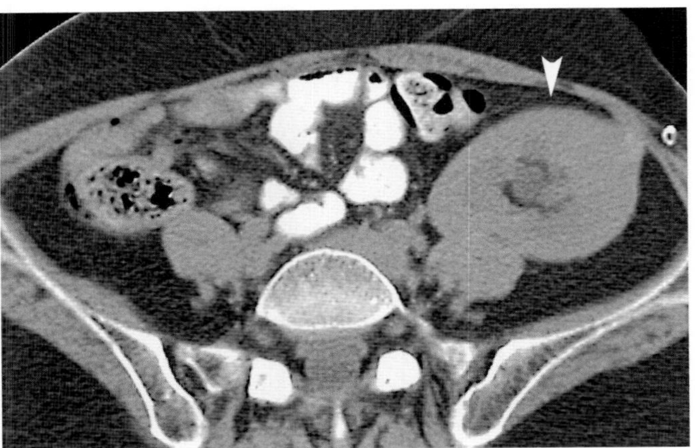

B

Figure 6-53 Atrophic Native Kidneys due to Systemic Lupus Erythematosus Nephropathy
This 46-year-old woman had received a kidney transplant for renal failure due to Systemic Lupus Erythematosus nephropathy.

A and **B.** Compare the size of the native kidneys (*arrows*) with the size of the renal transplant (*arrowhead*) in the left hemipelvis. Atrophy will usually indicate diminished renal function usually as a result of glomerulonephritis or interstitial nephritis.

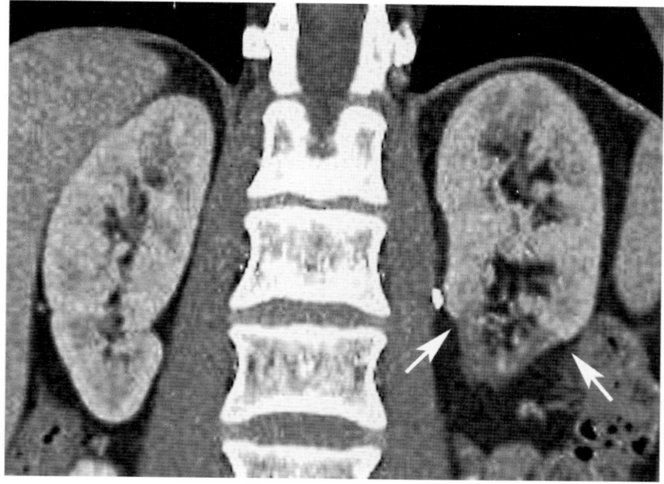

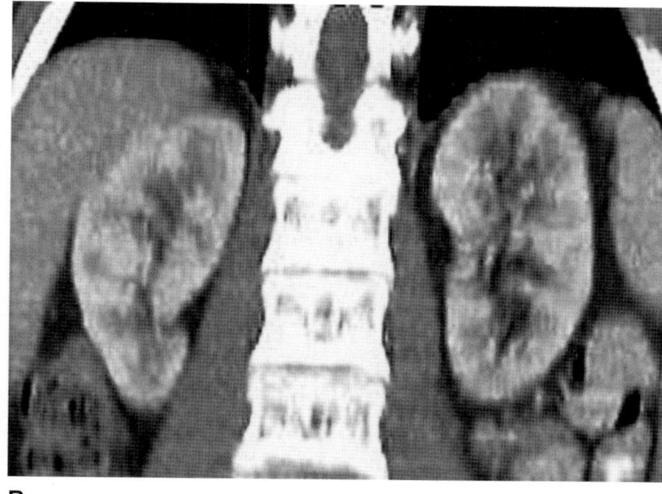

Figure 6-54 Chronic Focal Kidney Infarction
This 37-year-old man underwent retroperitoneal lymph node dissection for metastatic testicular cancer. Coronal reconstructions of contrast-enhanced CT scans obtained before and after the surgery. **A.** Three months after the surgery, there is a wedge shaped area of hypoattenuation (*arrows*) in the inferior pole of the left kidney that was not present on the (**B**) preoperative CT. Note that the lower pole renal parenchyma has diminished volume relative to the preoperative scan. These findings are typical of a localized atrophy of the kidney that occurs weeks to months after the vascular insult.

demonstrate cortical nephrocalcinosis. These findings can be seen in a host of other chronic renal diseases, and therefore imaging plays a limited role in the search for the underlying disease. ARCN, which can result from a number of causes (discussed in previous section), can result in various patterns of cortical calcification. The calcifications can outline the renal periphery, producing a "tramline" appearance, or can appear punctate or diffusely dense (see Figure 6-49). Nephrocalcinosis in patients with hyperoxaluria is caused by intratubular deposition of oxalate crystals in the proximal and distal convoluted tubules. Both primary and secondary hyperoxaluria can cause medullary or cortical and medullary nephrocalcinosis as well as nephrolithiasis (see Figure 6-58). Calcification can also occur in the cortex of a transplanted kidney as the result of chronic rejection.

Combined medullary and cortical nephrocalcinosis

In some cases, nephrocalcinosis can occur in both the cortex and medulla of the kidney. Conditions that commonly cause this are oxalosis and a variety of opportunistic infections in patients with acquired immunodeficiency syndrome (AIDS). Infections with *Pneumocystis carinii*, *Mycobacterium avium-intracellulare* (MAI), and cytomegalovirus in patients with AIDS can cause a stippled pattern of renal cortical calcification.

Contrast Nephropathy

Contrast-induced nephropathy (CN), an acute decline in renal function following the administration of iodinated intravenous contrast media (CM) in the absence of other causes, was recognized as early as the 1950s. Contrast-induced nephropathy is the third leading cause of new acute renal failure in hospitalized patients. Estimates of the incidence of CN based on prospective studies are extremely varied, from 0% to 22%.[71] Research studies typically define the abnormality as an increase in serum creatinine ≥25% or 50% above the baseline value. Risk factors for development of CN include baseline renal impairment, diabetes mellitus, higher administered doses of contrast media, reduced arterial volume (such as occurs with dehydration, congestive heart failure, major surgery, or cirrhosis), and concurrent use of potentially nephrotoxic drugs. Diabetic patients with preexisting renal insufficiency are particularly prone to irreversible CN. Although multiple myeloma is often reported as a risk factor for CN, a review of 7 retrospective studies of contrast media administration in patients with multiple myeloma failed to confirm an increased risk in these patients, in the absence of the aforementioned risk factors.[72] Patients with multiple myeloma who are to receive intravenous iodinated contrast should be well hydrated.

Many possible mechanisms for CN have been proposed, and the condition is felt by most investigators to be the result of multiple factors. Most research on this is focused on the hemodynamic and direct renal tubular toxic effect of iodinated contrast. Iodinated intravascular contrast causes initial renal arterial vasodilation followed by prolonged renal arterial vasoconstriction and decreased renal blood flow, likely resulting in some degree of renal ischemia, especially in vulnerable patients with underlying

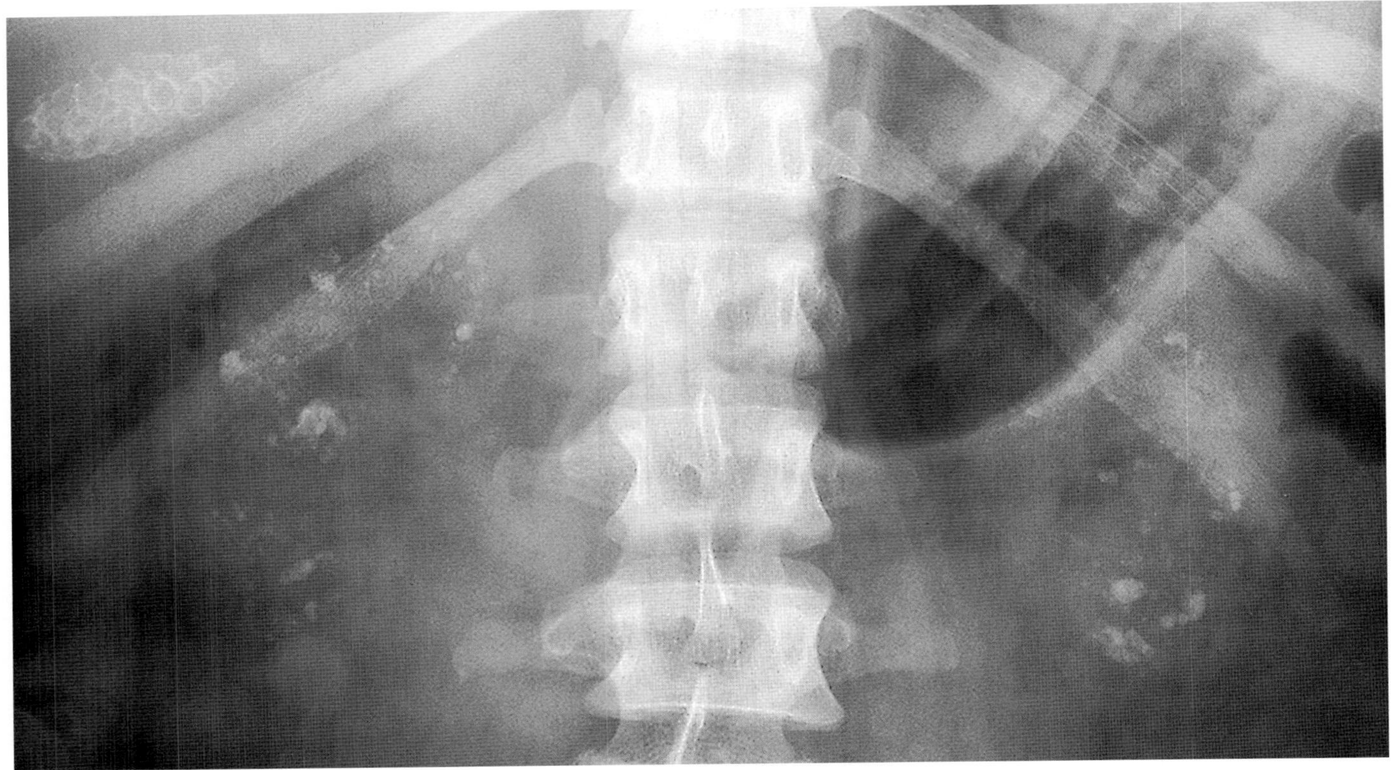

A

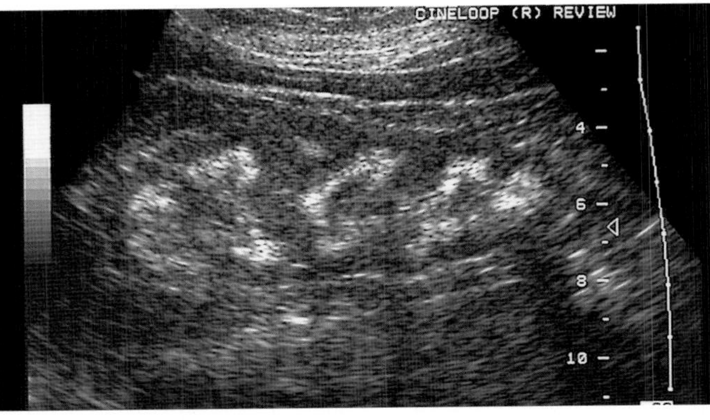

B

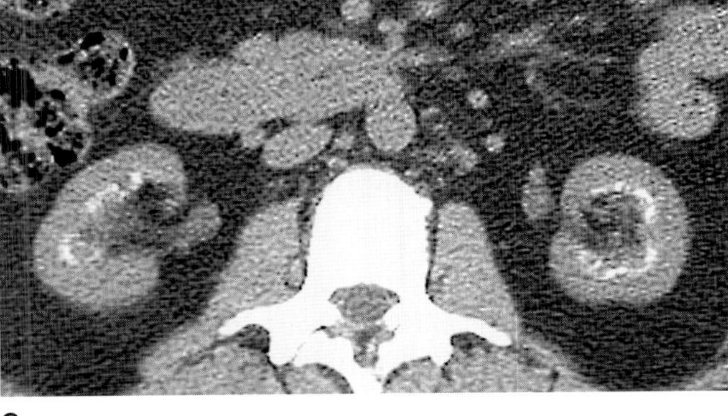

C

Figure 6-55 Medullary Nephrocalcinosis due to Renal Tubular Acidosis in 2 Patients
This 37-year-old woman had chronic renal failure due to renal tubular acidosis. **A.** Abdominal plain film demonstrates many small renal calcifications throughout the midportion of both kidneys. Although some of these could represent small renal calculi, most are present within the medulla of the kidney. **B.** Longitudinal US (same patient as A) of the left kidney demonstrates uniform echogenic foci, lining the renal medulla. Some demonstrate shadowing, especially in the lower pole. These findings are typical of medullary calcinosis. **C.** This 46-year-old man also had renal failure due to renal tubular acidosis. Axial CT image obtained without intravenous contrast administration demonstrates a uniform distribution of medullary calcifications in both kidneys.

microvascular disease. The iodinated contrast also has a direct toxic effect on renal tubular epithelium.

In the 1980s, CM formulations were introduced in which the iodine-containing benzene ring was nonionic, resulting in a marked decrease in osmolality (approximately 600 to 700 mOsm/kg water) as compared to then standard iodinated CM. These so-called "second-generation" CM are classified as low-osmolar CM (LOCM) and are the principal intravascular CM currently used for radiologic studies. Experimental and clinical studies have suggested that LOCM is associated with reduced nephrotoxicity compared with high-osmolar CM (HOCM) in high-risk patients.[73,74]

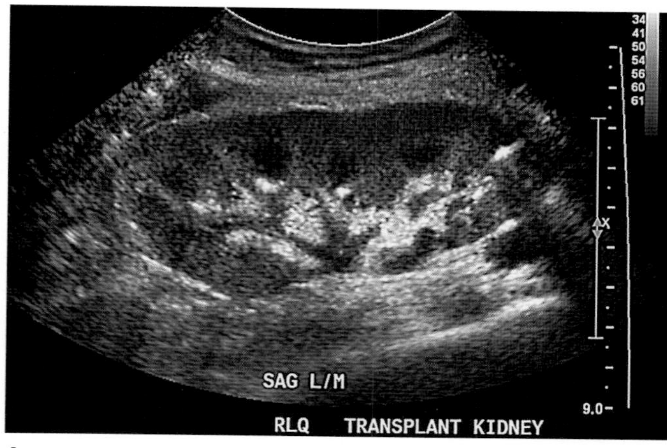

A

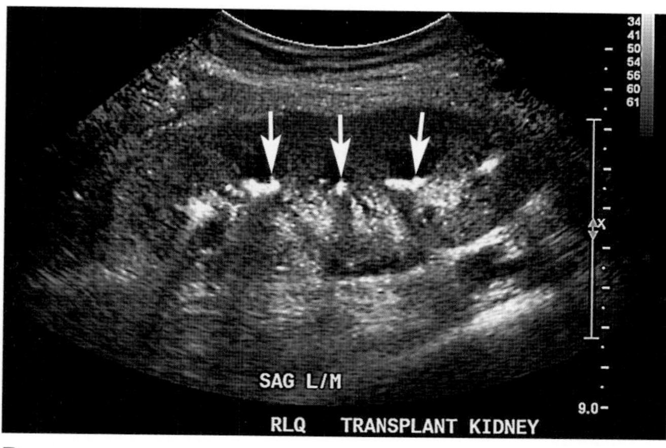

B

Figure 6-56 Nephrocalcinosis due to Rejection, in a Renal Transplant, US Study
This 72-year-old man had undergone a renal transplant 8 years prior to the study. He had a history of chronic transplant rejection, and presented for this US study with acute superimposed on chronic renal failure. Two sagittal US images of the renal transplant, (**A** and **B**), demonstrate echogenic shadowing foci distributed at the tips of the medullary pyramids (*arrows*), in keeping with medullary nephrocalcinosis.

Use of LOCM is also associated with a lower overall incidence of adverse effects, particularly non-life-threatening ones. However, risk of CN remains significant for patients with preexisting renal disease, especially for diabetic patients with renal impairment.

Patients with CN typically present with an acute rise in serum creatinine anywhere from 24 to 48 hours after the contrast study. Although in most cases serum creatinine returns to baseline value by 7 to 10 days, CN can occasionally be associated with significant adverse events, including renal failure requiring transient or permanent dialysis. Some degree of residual renal impairment has been reported in as many as 30% of patients, and there is some evidence that mortality may be increased in patients with CN.[75] Although a detailed discussion of proposed strategies for preventing CN is beyond the scope of this chapter, for patients at risk, adequate hydration is the most universally accepted measure to reduce the risk of nephrotoxicity. Other approaches, including administration of diuretics, vasoactive agents, and alternative contrast agents have been investigated.

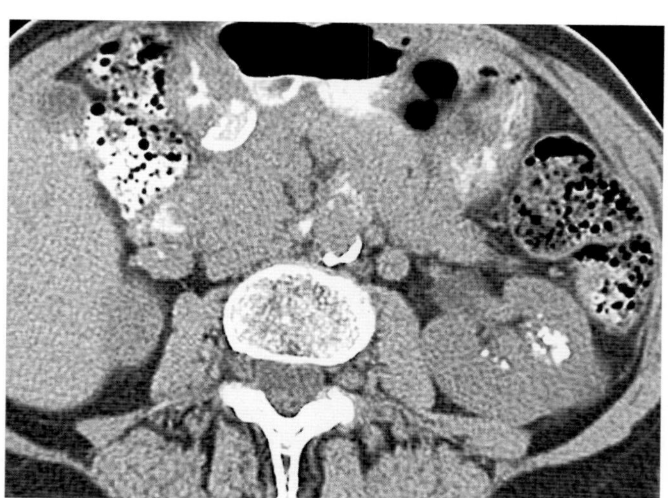

A

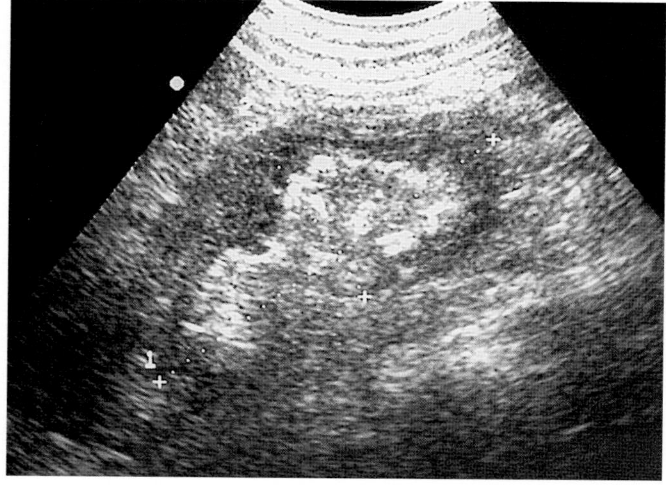

B

Figure 6-57 Medullary Sponge Kidney in 2 Patients
A. Axial CT image obtained without intravenous contrast administration demonstrates nonuniform distribution of tiny left renal calculi. **B.** Longitudinal US of the left kidney in a second patient demonstrates diffuse medullary echogenicity, typical of medullary nephrocalcinosis. Previous intravenous urogram (not shown) showed a papillary brush appearance typical of medullary sponge kidney.

Table 6-10. Common Causes of Medullary Nephrocalcinosis

Hyperparathyroidism
Renal tubular acidosis type 1 (distal)
Medullary sponge kidney
Hypercalcemia • malignancy • bone metastases • Cushing syndrome • milk-alkali syndrome • sarcoidosis • hypervitaminosis D
AIDS-associated infections (combined cortical and medullary nephrocalcinosis)

Although the patterns of renal enhancement in renal failure, including CN, were originally described as seen on IVU and plain films, the nephrographic abnormalities are visualized more conspicuously on CT. In both acute and chronic renal failure, the initial opacification of the renal cortex is decreased as compared to normal, and the washout is slower. With chronic renal failure the nephrogram is less dense than is seen in normal patients given the same contrast dose. In patients with acute renal failure, the densest opacification varies. A bilateral symmetrical prolonged dense nephrogram is usually the result of shock or acute tubular necrosis (ATN). If a contrast nephrogram without evidence of contrast excretion is seen on an imaging study timed for imaging during the excretion phase (such as an IVU or excretion phase CT study), the patient's vital signs should be assessed immediately. Although the mechanism is not well-understood, ATN can produce persistence of a high density contrast nephrogram for as long as several days following administration of intravenous contrast material. Therefore, the persistence of hyperattenuating kidneys beyond 24 hours following intravenous administration of iodinated contrasts should alert the radiologist to the presence of CN (see Figures 6-59 and 6-60).[68] A unilateral prolonged dense nephrogram is usually caused by acute ureteral obstruction, the so-called *obstructive nephrogram*. (This will be discussed in detail in Chapter 7.)

Table 6-11. Common Causes of Cortical Nephrocalcinosis

Renal cortical necrosis
Chronic glomerulonephritis
Renal transplant rejection
Chronic hypercalcemia
Oxalosis
AIDS-associated infections (combined cortical and medullary nephrocalcinosis)

Congenital Renal Anomalies

Congenital anomalies of the kidneys can be classified according to anomalies in number, size, position, or form.

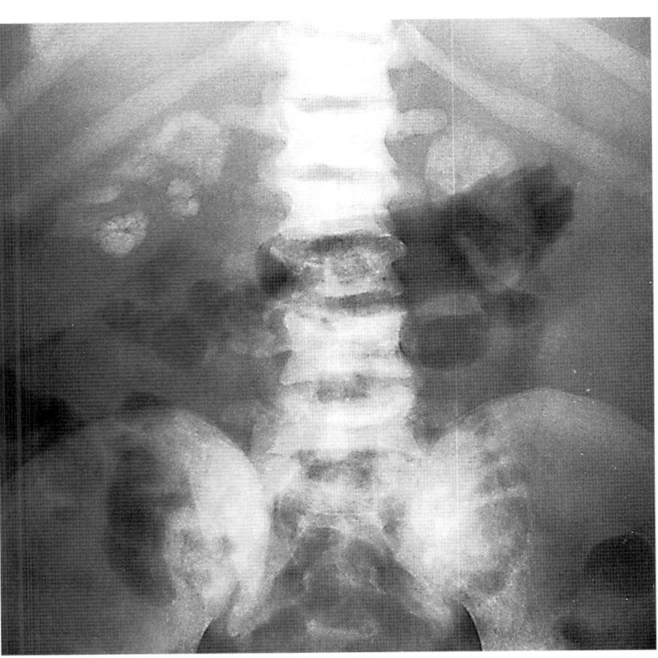

A

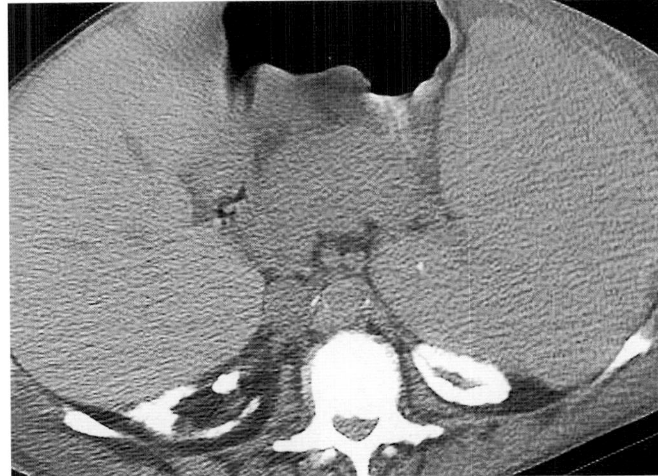

B

Figure 6-58 Oxalosis With Cortical Nephrocalcinosis
The patient is a 26-year-old female with congenital oxalosis, and failed liver and renal transplants. **A.** Abdominal plain film and (**B**) axial CT image demonstrate bilateral cortical nephrocalcinosis. Abnormally dense lumbosacral spine is also noted, due to renal osteodystrophy.

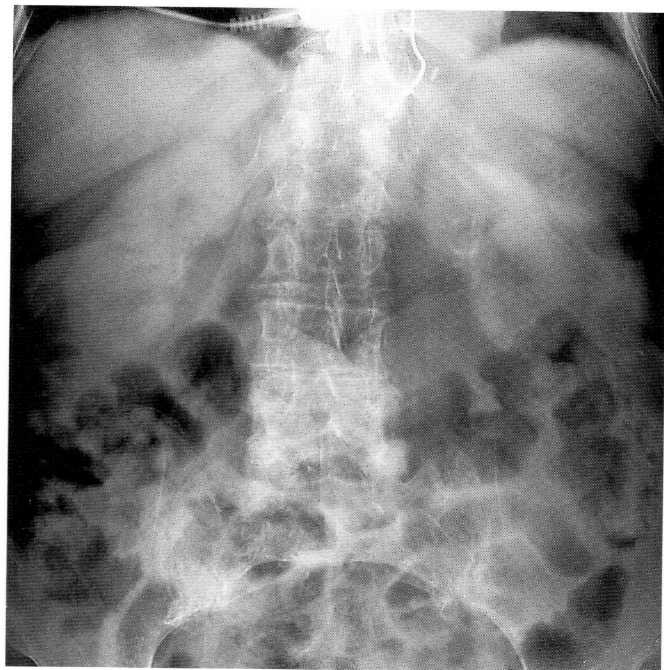

Figure 6-59 Plain-Film Demonstration of Contrast Nephropathy Abdominal plain film in an individual with abdominal pain shows clear demarcation of the kidneys that appear denser than the psoas muscles and other soft-tissue structures. The patient had received iodinated intravascular contrast for a coronary catheterization the day before and had rising serum creatinine; therefore, the findings are in keeping with contrast nephropathy. If the patient had just been injected with intravenous contrast, such an appearance, that is, bilateral dense nephrograms without evidence of renal excretion of contrast, could be produced by hypotension ("shock nephrogram"), as might occur during a serious anaphylactoid reaction to the administered contrast.

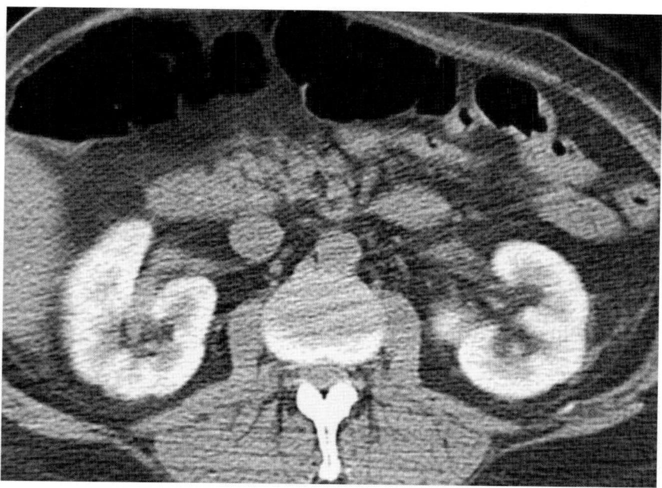

Figure 6-60 Dense Prolonged Nephrogram due to Acute Tubular Necrosis
Axial CT image at the level of the kidneys; no intravenous contrast was given for the study. The patient had received intravenous contrast for a CT scan the previous day.

Anomalies of number

Anomalies in renal number include supernumerary kidney, unilateral, and bilateral renal agenesis.

Supernumerary kidney: Supernumerary kidney, the presence of more than 2 kidneys, is extremely rare, with about 60 cases reported in the literature.[76] The supernumerary kidney can be drained by a bifid or by a separate ureter. When the ureters draining the supernumerary and usual kidney are separate, the supernumerary kidney almost always lies cranial to the usual kidney. When the ureter draining the supernumerary kidney and usual kidney are bifid, the supernumerary kidney nearly always lies below the usual kidney.

Unilateral agenesis: Agenesis of a kidney is defined as a kidney that fails to develop. Unilateral agenesis occurs in about 1 in 1000 of the general population. Most cases of renal agenesis are hereditary.[76] Renal agenesis is believed to occur as the result of failure of formation of the ureteral bud or due to a deficiency of the metanephric blastema. In the former, the ipsilateral ureter is absent and in the latter the ureter is present. With true agenesis, there is absence of the ureteral orifice, which can be seen at cystoscopy. The renal artery is absent and the ipsilateral adrenal gland is absent in 8% to 10% of cases. Compensatory hypertrophy of the contralateral kidney is almost always present.

Renal agenesis is associated with an increased incidence of Müllerian duct abnormalities that control the development of the female reproductive tract. These include uterovaginal atresia or uterovaginal duplication, unicornuate or bicornuate uterus, and absence or hypoplasia of the uterus.[76] Absence or aplasia of the vagina and uterus, termed Mayer-Rokitansky-Küster-Hauser syndrome, can be seen. In males with unilateral renal agenesis, there is often absence of the seminal vesicle or a seminal vesicle cyst (see Figure 6-61).

Bilateral renal agenesis: Bilateral renal agenesis, with an autopsy prevalence of 3.5 per 100 000 births, is incompatible with life and is found in males in 75% of cases. The condition is often detected in the antenatal period because of associated oligohydramnios. Neonates exhibit the characteristic Potter facies, with low-set ears and prominent supraorbital skin folds.

Anomalies of size

Renal hypoplasia is an unusual anomaly in which the kidney is at least 50% smaller than normal and contains a diminished number of calyces. This anomaly should be

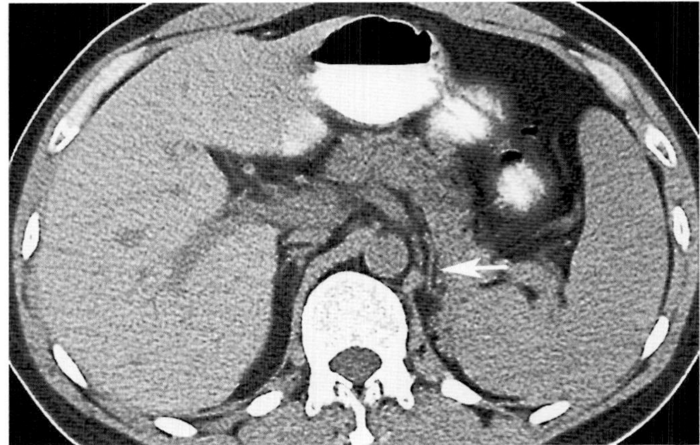

A

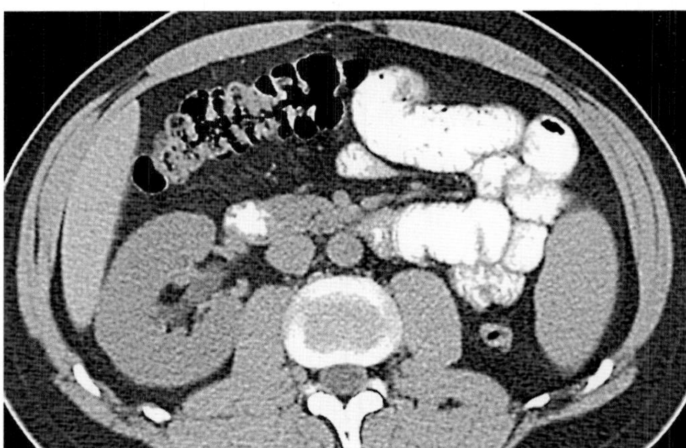

B

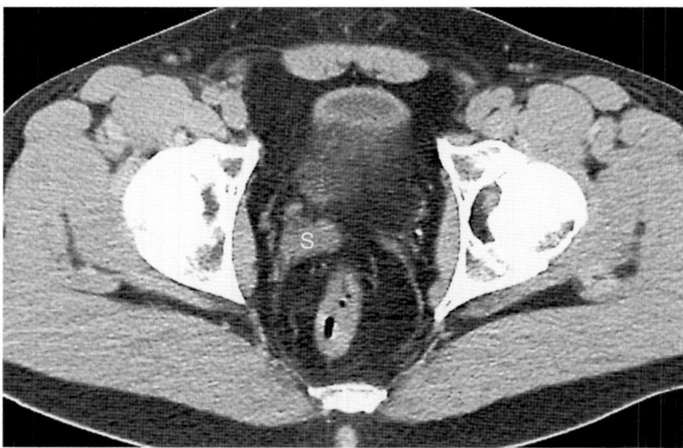

C

Figure 6-61 Left Renal Agenesis
Axial images from a CT scan of the abdomen and pelvis performed with only oral contrast demonstrates congenital absence of the left kidney in a 40-year-old man. **A.** The image through the uppermost portion of the abdomen demonstrates the pancreatic tail occupying the left renal fossa and the left adrenal gland in normal location (*arrow*). **B.** The left renal fossa is empty. **C.** Scan through the lower pelvis demonstrates absence of the left seminal vesicle, a commonly associated finding. S indicates normal right seminal vesicle.

distinguished from the majority of unilaterally small kidneys, which are decreased in size because of acquired conditions, including ischemia, reflux, or chronic obstruction, and contain a normal number of calyces.

Anomalies of position

Malrotation of a normally positioned kidney most often occurs as a result of failure of rotation of the kidney about its vertical axis. The renal pelvis will be located in an anterior (nonrotation) or anteromedial (partial malrotation) position. Rarely, the kidney may overrotate, with a laterally oriented renal pelvis.

The kidney initially develops opposite the level of the future S2 vertebra but at the conclusion of development is located at the L1-L2 level. Whether this change in position is truly due to ascent or to differential lengthening of the caudal part of the embryo is not agreed on. Renal ectopy is defined as a kidney with a congenitally abnormal position. The arterial blood supply to an ectopic kidney will always also arise from an ectopic site. The ureter to the ectopic kidney will have adjusted itself to the ectopic renal position, that is, it will be longer for a thoracic ectopic kidney and shorter for a pelvic kidney. This is in contradistinction to the ptotic kidney, which will have a normal ureteral length and a renal artery that arises from its normal site. Renal ectopia is classified according to the position of the affected kidney with respect to the location of its attendant ureter. Ipsilateral renal ectopia occurs when the kidney is on the same side of the body as the orifice of its attendant ureter, whereas contralateral, or crossed, ectopia occurs when the kidney is located on the side of the body opposite the orifice of its attendant ureter. Renal ectopias are further classified as cranial or caudal, depending on whether the ectopic kidney is located above or below the normal position. The most common site for an ectopic kidney is a pelvic kidney (see Figures 6-62 and 6-63). An intrathoracic kidney, a rare anomaly that is more common in males, occurs when the kidney has herniated superiorly through the lumbocostal triangle or the foramen of Bochdalek. Abdominal or iliac ectopia can be simple or crossed. The adrenal gland remains in its normal place but develops an elliptical shape, as is seen in renal agenesis.

Crossed ectopia with fusion is discussed below, in the next section. Crossed ectopia without fusion is rare and accounts for only 10% to 15% of all crossed ectopic kidneys. Crossed ectopia is theorized to originate from both the mesonephric ducts and the ureteral buds straying from their normal course during embryologic development. IVU can detect the anomaly, but in cases where surgery is planned for attendant conditions, cross-sectional imaging with US, or preferably CT, is useful to confirm that the 2 kidneys are separate. Bilateral crossed ectopia occurs when both kidneys have crossed to the opposite side but their attendant ureters insert on the normal side. A solitary crossed ectopic kidney is even more rare than crossed ectopia without fusion.

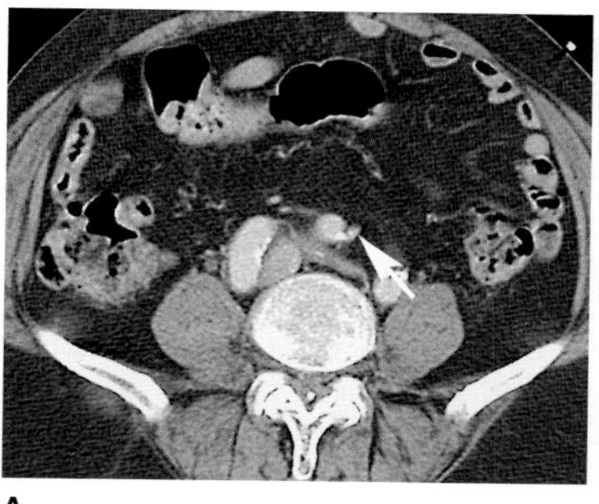
A

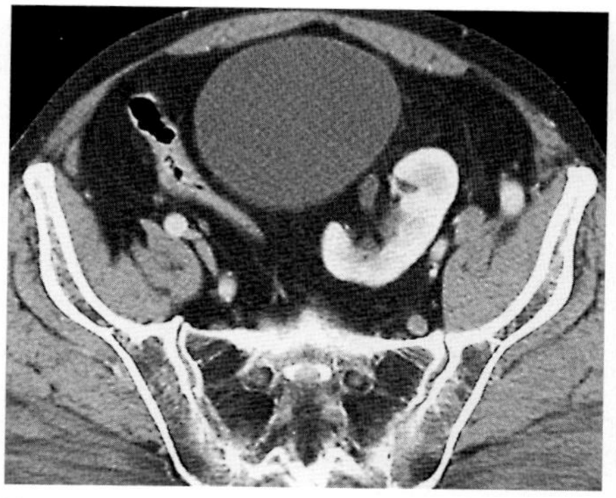
B

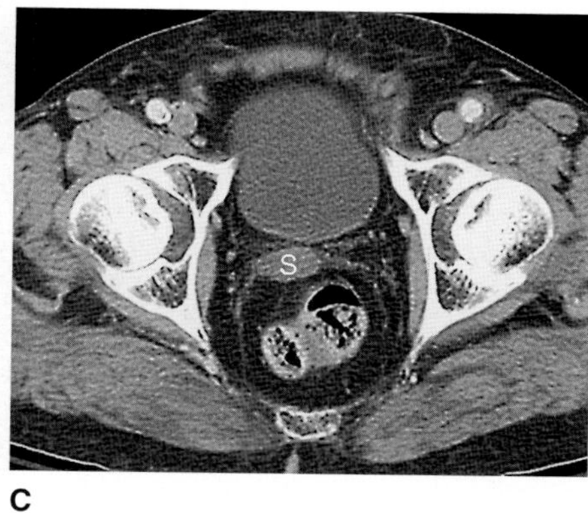

C

Figure 6-62 Pelvic kidney
A-C. The patient was a 67-year-old man who underwent an intravenous contrast-enhanced CT scan after a motor vehicle accident. A pelvic left kidney is demonstrated in axial image (B). Image (A) demonstrates the left renal artery originating from the left common iliac artery (*arrow*). The most caudal image (C) demonstrates absence of the left seminal vesicle, a finding commonly associated with congenital renal abnormalities. S indicates normal right seminal vesicle.

Ectopic kidneys are more likely to develop complications than are normally located kidneys, including susceptibility to injury, decreased function, ureteropelvic and ureterovesical junction obstruction, and calculus disease. Renal ectopia is associated with congenital abnormalities in other organ systems.

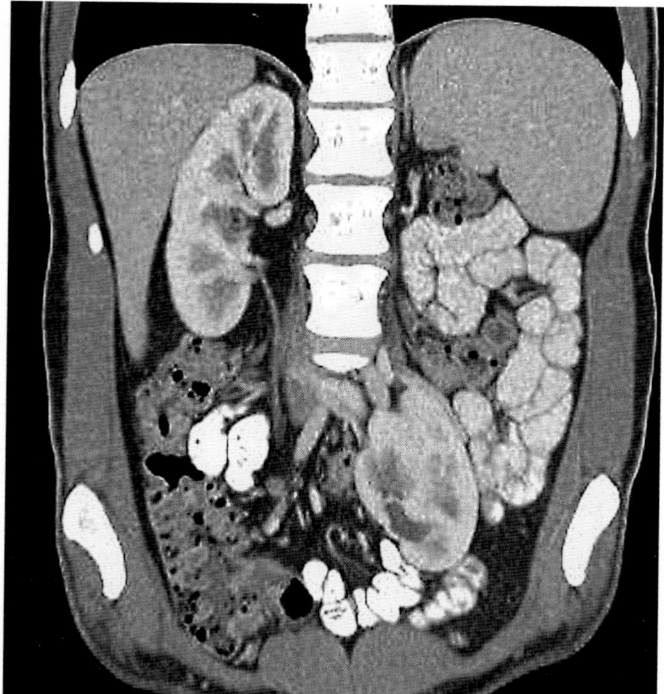

Figure 6-63 Ectopic Kidney
This 32-year-old woman complained of abdominal pain. Coronal image from a contrast-enhanced CT shows a pelvic position of the left kidney.

Anomalies of form

The 3 anomalies of kidney form are related to fusion of the 2 kidneys and are called horseshoe kidney, disc kidney, and crossed fused ectopia.

Horseshoe kidney: Horseshoe kidney is the most common renal anomaly, occurring in about 1 in 400 births. In this anomaly, the 2 kidneys are connected by an isthmus, with most of the parenchyma of each kidney located on either side. It is commonly believed that this fusion anomaly results from pressure on the lateral lower poles of the kidneys by the bilateral umbilical arteries, causing the kidneys to fuse as they ascend between the 2 vessels. However, the fact that at embryonic stage 15, prior to ascent, the kidneys grow very close together and practically touch one another, raises the possibility that fusion occurs at an earlier point in development.[76] The isthmus is composed of renal parenchyma or fibrous tissue. The isthmus, which is usually at the lower pole, is usually located anterior to the aorta and IVC.

Horseshoe kidneys are associated with a number of complications, neoplasms, and other congenital disorders. They are prone to injury, are often accompanied by varying degrees of ureteropelvic junction obstruction, and associated with calculus disease (see Figure 6-64). An increased incidence of Wilms tumor has been noted in children with a horseshoe kidney,[77] and patients with horseshoe kidney have an increased prevalence of primary renal carcinoid tumor.[78]

Imaging findings in patients with a horseshoe kidney include an abnormal axis for each kidney, with the lower poles more medially located with respect to the upper poles, a more caudal location than normal, and an anterior position of the renal pelves due to bilateral malrotation. Multiphase CT with 3-D reconstruction can be used to depict the complex anatomy associated with this anomaly.[79]

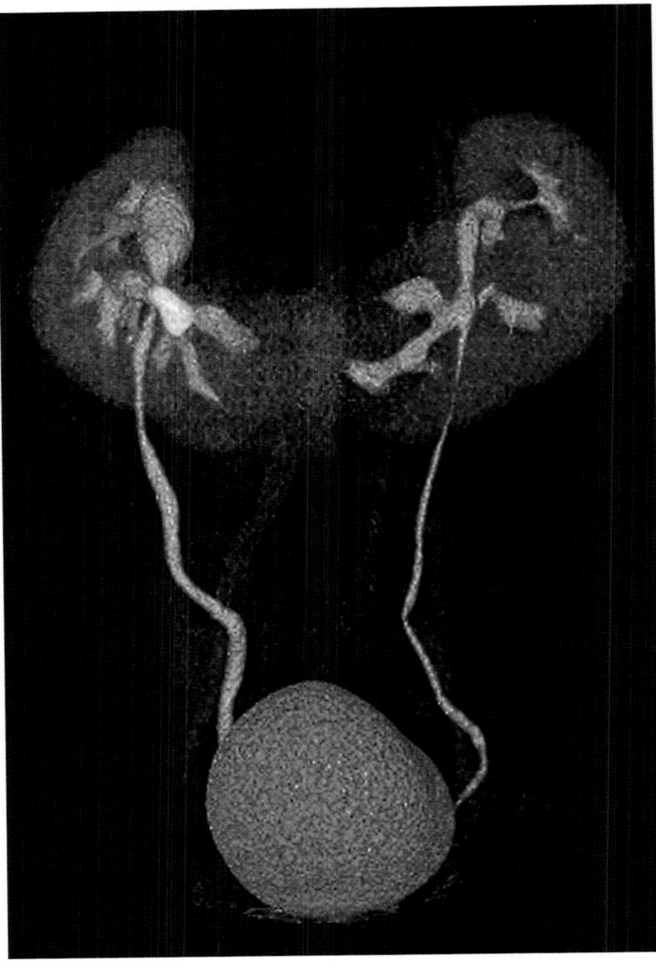

A

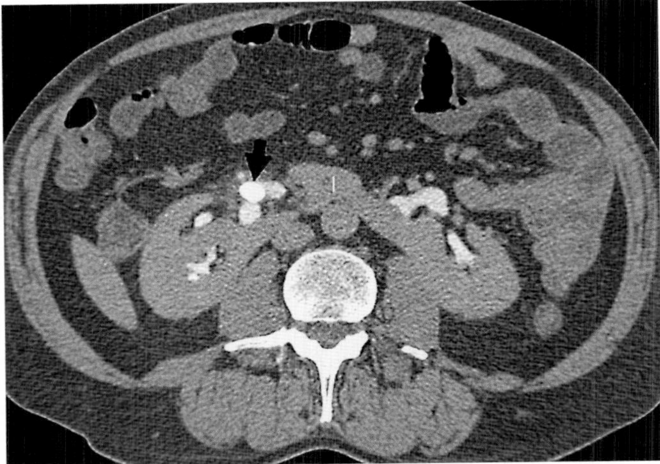

B

Figure 6-64 Horseshoe Kidney With a Calculus
A. Volume-rendered 3D image from a CT urogram demonstrates a calculus in the right renal unit. **B.** Axial image at the level of the isthmus (*labeled*), demonstrates the calculus (*arrow*). The wide window setting of the axial image (*wide grayscale*) allows differentiation of the high-density calculus from the less dense opacified collecting system of the kidney. I indicates isthmus.

Disc kidney: Another fusion anomaly is a disc, (also known as cake, or lump) kidney, a rare type of midline renal fusion where the kidney becomes a single disc, lying lower than the horseshoe kidney, often in the pelvis. The renal pelves are anteriorly located.

Crossed fused ectopia: In crossed fused ectopia, the kidney completely or near completely crosses the midline to the opposite side and fuses with the kidney on that side. The incidence is 1 in 1300 to 1 in 7600. It occurs in males more than females and is found on the right side 2 to 3 times more than on the left. There are a large number of types and classifications; many individual cases may not precisely fit predefined categories. Complications include high insertion of the ureter into the renal pelvis, resulting in an increased incidence of ureteropelvic junction obstruction, which may predispose to stone formation. Associated anomalies include many of those associated with horseshoe kidneys. IVU depicts the shape of the fused moiety, as well as the crossed ureter. Further, MRI or CT can depict the fused kidney and absent kidney on the opposite side (see Figure 6-65).

IMAGING OF THE KIDNEY AFTER RENAL SURGERY

The 4 common renal surgical procedures discussed herein are nephrectomy, nephroureterectomy, partial nephrectomy, and renal transplant.

Imaging Findings Following Nephrectomy

Radical nephrectomy became the established surgical treatment for localized kidney cancers, following Robson's publication of the landmark article in 1963[80] that described his results with the procedure and a second article[81] updating his experience in 88 patients, with only a 3% surgical mortality. Radical nephrectomy as originally defined by Robson involved surgical removal of all components within Gerota fascia, including the ipsilateral adrenal gland as well as the kidney. The adrenal gland was felt to be at risk for involvement with renal cell carcinoma because of its proximity to the kidney and potential pathways for spread of the kidney cancer, via vascular or lymphatic channels or local extension. Recent publications indicate that the incidence of solitary ipsilateral adrenal tumor involvement at time of surgery is much lower than previously thought, at 1% to 5%, and recommend against the standard practice of adrenalectomy with radical nephrectomy.[82] In Robson's era, before the advent of modern cross-sectional imaging, it is likely that the typical renal carcinomas that presented at later stages of growth were more often associated with ipsilateral adrenal involvement.

Postoperative complications after radical nephrectomy occur in approximately 20% of patients.[83] These may be systemic (cardiorespiratory, thrombophlebitis) or local, including manifestations of solid and hollow viscus

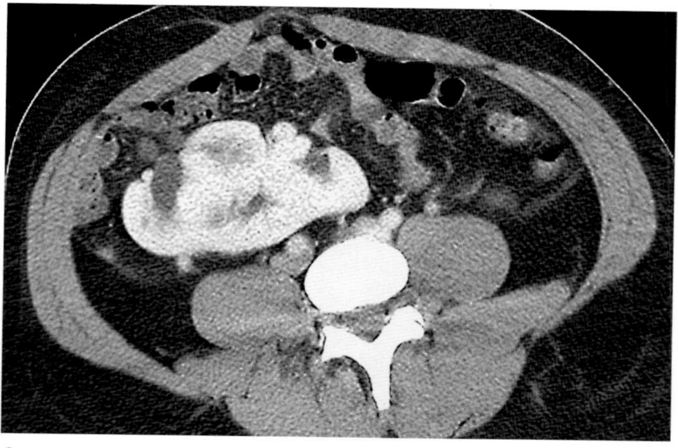

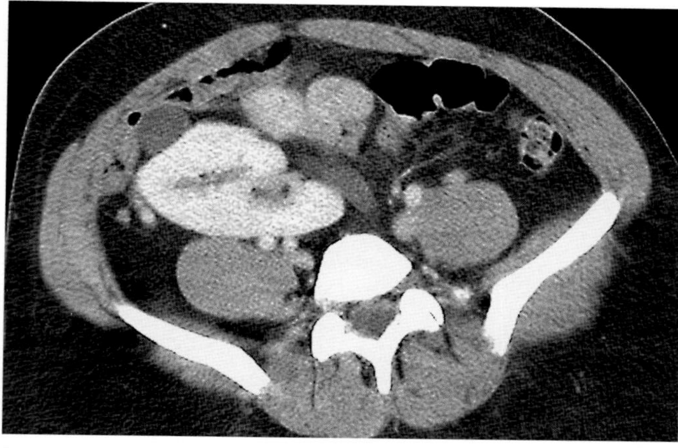

Figure 6-65 Crossed Fused Ectopia
A and **B**. Axial images of an intravenous contrast-enhanced CT scan demonstrate the fused kidney on the right side. The ureter of the fused left renal unit (B) will enter the bladder on the left side. The congenital abnormality was an incidental finding in this 42-year-old woman.

intraoperative injuries, pneumothorax, ileus, hemorrhage into the renal bed or due to adjacent organ trauma, accumulation of lymph or serous fluid in the nephrectomy bed, and infection. Computed tomographic scanning is useful to detect postoperative complications in the abdomen, and interventional radiology has a useful role in providing therapeutic percutaneous aspiration and drainage of postoperative collections.

Radical Nephroureterectomy

Radical nephroureterectomy involves, in addition to removal of the kidney, resection of the entire ureter, including the intramural portion and ureteral orifice. This surgical procedure is the standard treatment for upper urinary tract urothelial cancers, especially those that are large, high-grade, and invasive, or those that are large, multifocal or rapidly recurring medium-grade noninvasive tumors of the renal pelvis or proximal ureter.[84] The entire ureter is resected to avoid the significant risk of tumor recurrence in a remaining ureteral stump, which is at least 20% to 58%.[85] For further discussion on complications and radiologic imaging after radical nephroureterectomy, please refer to Chapter 7.

Imaging of the Kidney After Nephron-Sparing Surgery

Partial rather than radical nephrectomy as standard treatment for low-stage renal carcinoma began to gain acceptance during the 1990s, as published studies began to indicate that local recurrences are rare after partial nephrectomy for tumors less than 4 cm size, and that survival approaches 100%.[28] Today, partial nephrectomy is a widely accepted treatment for small renal cancers. Although partial nephrectomy is currently most often performed as an open procedure, laparoscopic partial nephrectomy, which is more technically challenging for the surgeon than the open procedure, has also been introduced to the surgical armamentarium.

Now that partial nephrectomy is performed frequently, the radiologist should be familiar with the varied normal postoperative appearances of the kidney on imaging studies after the procedure, and be able to recognize postoperative complications.[86] After resecting the tumor, the surgeon may pack perinephric fat into the surgical renal defect; this should not be mistaken for a fatty mass on postoperative imaging. Biologically absorbable hemostatic agents also can be used to help control intraoperative bleeding. These agents typically contain gas bubbles that should not be mistaken for gas within an abscess. Gas bubbles within bioabsorbable hemostatic agents usually appear in a fixed position, linearly arranged, and not associated with a fluid collection. During clamping of the renal hilar vessels, which is performed to optimize visualization of the tumor and surrounding tissue and create a bloodless operative field, arterial injury can occur and lead to postoperative infarction, hemorrhage, or pseudoaneurysm formation. For tumors that extend into the central renal parenchyma, calyceal entry can occur, either deliberately in order to obtain a clear tumor-free surgical margin or unintentionally. If the calyceal repair is not completely sealed, a urine leak can produce a postoperative fluid collection. Computed tomographic or MRI during the excretion phase is important to diagnose urine leaks that may be mistaken for other types of collections on routine nephrographic phase studies (see Figure 6-66). Local tumor recurrence is recognized as a briskly enhancing mass at the excision site, which, on subsequent scans shows interval enlargement rather than regression (see Figure 6-67).[87]

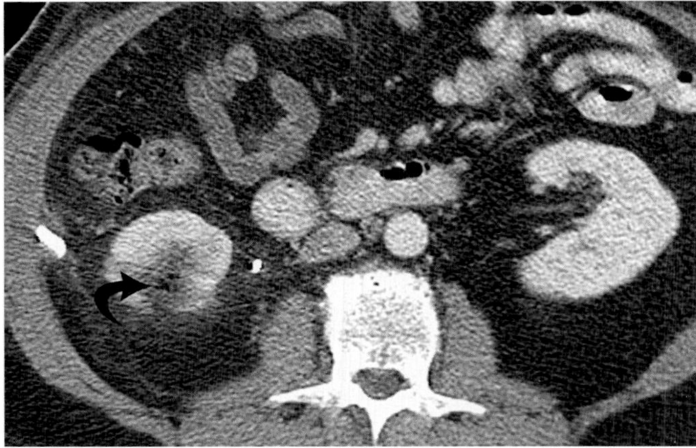
A

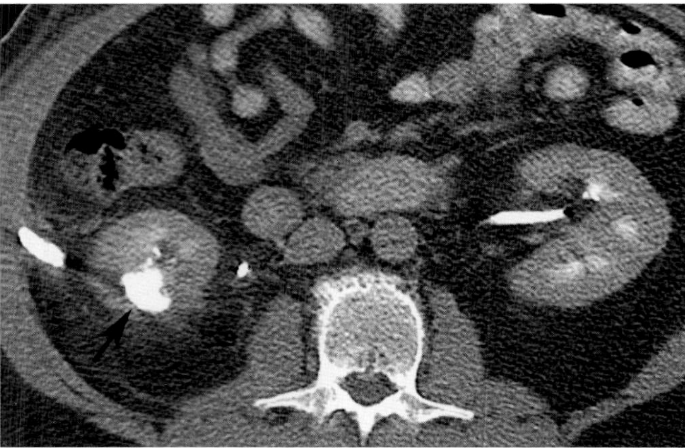
B

Figure 6-66 Urine Leak After Partial Nephrectomy
This patient had undergone partial nephrectomy 1 week prior for renal carcinoma. Axial CT images of an intravenous contrast-enhanced study performed during the nephrographic (**A**) and excretion (**B**) phases. The leak (*arrow*), seen as a collection of high-density excreted contrast, is only visible on excretion-phase image. The nephrographic-phase image shows a small amount of gas (*curved arrow*) at the site of resection.

Imaging of the Transplanted Kidney

For patients with end-stage renal failure, renal transplantation offers tremendous improvement of quality of life and long-term survival. The number of renal transplants performed every year in the U.S. has been steadily increasing, with over 16 000 in 2008. One-year patient survival rates in the U.S. are approximately 94% for cadaveric and 98% for living-donor kidney transplants, with 1-year allograft survival rates of 89% for cadaveric transplants and 95% for living kidney transplants.[88] Recent improvements in survival for organ transplant recipients can be attributed to improvements in surgical technique, advances in donor-recipient matching, and new immunosuppressive agents and regimens.[89] Reversible causes of transplant dysfunction must be promptly identified, as rapid intervention to treat complications optimizes chances for graft survival. Accurate diagnosis is best achieved by incorporation of clinical and laboratory data with findings on radiologic imaging studies, because different processes can exhibit similar findings on imaging. Meaningful interpretation of radiologic imaging studies of these patients requires both an understanding of the pathologic processes that can occur and an ability to recognize manifestations of these processes on imaging.

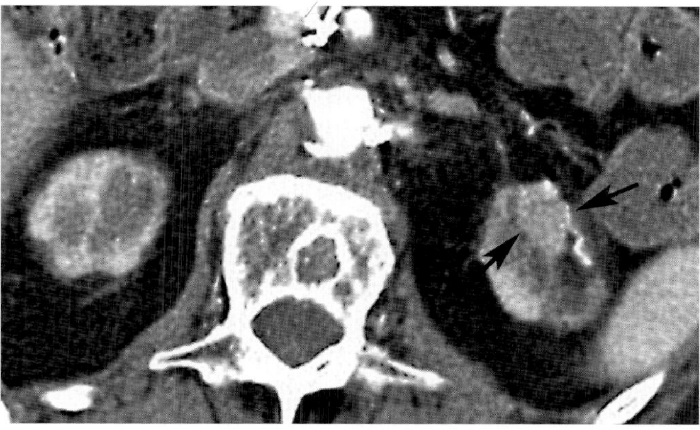

Figure 6-67 Local Tumor Recurrence After Partial Nephrectomy
This patient had undergone a prior partial nephrectomy for renal papillary carcinoma and a Whipple procedure for pancreatic adenocarcinoma. Axial CT image from an intravenous contrast-enhanced study demonstrates a focus of brisk enhancement adjacent to surgical suture material (*arrows*) in the left upper renal pole. This finding is indicative of local recurrence of the patient's renal carcinoma.

Surgical technique of renal transplantation

The transplant is usually positioned extraperitoneally into the right or left iliac fossa (see Figure 6-68). If both iliac fossae have had previous surgery, an intraperitoneal approach to the iliac vessels can be used. Cadaveric renal transplants are typically harvested with an intact main renal artery and an attached portion of the aorta, which is trimmed into an oval patch (Carrel patch). An end-to-side anastomosis is made to the recipient's common or external iliac artery. A living related donor transplant is harvested with only the main renal artery and anastomosed end-to-side to the recipient's common or external iliac artery, or less commonly, end-to-end to the recipient internal iliac artery. Multiple renal arteries are usually sutured to a common Carrel patch in cadaveric transplants or fashioned into a common stem in living related donor transplants.[90] The donor RV is anastomosed end-to-side to the recipient's common or external iliac vein. The transplant ureter is typically anastomosed to the dome of the recipient's urinary bladder (ureteroneocystostomy).

Complications of renal transplantation

Complications of renal transplantation can be categorized as anatomic complications, acute and chronic functional

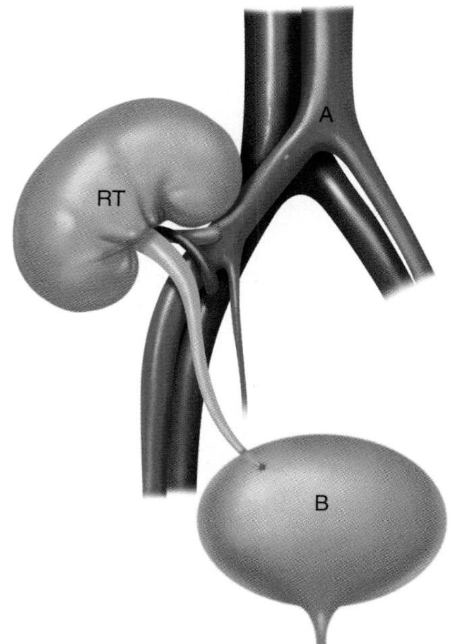

Figure 6-68 Anatomic Drawing of a Renal Transplant
In this drawing, a renal transplant in the right iliac fossa is depicted. The (donor) transplant renal artery is anastomosed to either the common iliac or external iliac artery, and the transplant RV is anastomosed to the common or external iliac vein. The ureter is connected to the dome of the bladder. RT indicates renal transplant; A, aorta; B, bladder.

complications, and posttransplant lymphoproliferative disorder (PTLD) (Table 6-12).

Anatomic complications of renal transplantation: Anatomic or structural complications of renal transplants include hematomas, seromas, lymphoceles, abscesses, urinomas, obstructive hydronephrosis, arterial or venous stenosis or thrombosis, and intrarenal arteriovenous fistulae and pseudoaneurysms. US is the mainstay for diagnosis of anatomic complications, as most of these conditions can be recognized by US. Many of these conditions can also be diagnosed by other cross-sectional imaging examinations.

Postoperative fluid collections: Small amounts of crescentic-shaped perinephric fluid are commonly seen after a renal transplant, reflecting postoperative hemorrhage or seroma. Signs of a clinically important fluid collection include rounded contour and lack of decrease in size over time. A collection under pressure can exert mass effect on the transplanted kidney and alter hemodynamics, producing a high-resistance spectral Doppler tracing of intrarenal arterial vessels near the collection. A fluid collection can also compress or kink the renal vascular pedicle, impairing inflow or outflow of blood to or from the transplant, compromising function (see Figure 6-69).

Hematoma: Because a peritransplant fluid collection demonstrated on US can be nonspecific in appearance, clinical

Table 6-12. Complications of Renal Transplantation

Functional Complications	*Usual Time of Occurrence After Transplantation*
Hyperacute rejection	Minutes to hours
Perioperative ischemic damage (ATN)	At time of transplant
Acute rejection	At least 4-5 d, most common during first 3 mo
Chronic rejection	Usually after a few months or years, develops slowly
Drug toxicity (usually immunosuppressive agents)	While on medication
Anatomic Complications	
Collections:	
Hematoma or seroma	Hours to days
Abscess	Several days to weeks
Lymphocele	4-6 wk
Urinoma	Within first 2 wk
Obstructive hydronephrosis	Days, months, years
Vascular:	
Renal arterial stenosis	Any time
Renal vein stenosis or thrombosis	Immediate postoperative period or later
Intrarenal arteriovenous fistulae and pseudoaneurysms	Any time, but typically the result of renal transplant biopsy
Posttransplantation Lymphoproliferative Disorder (PTLD)	Weeks to years

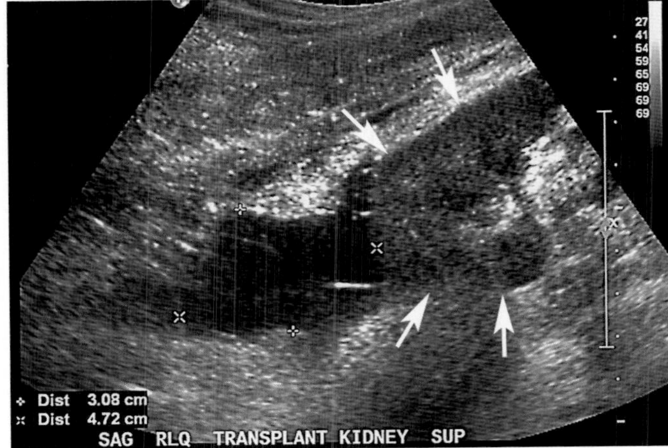

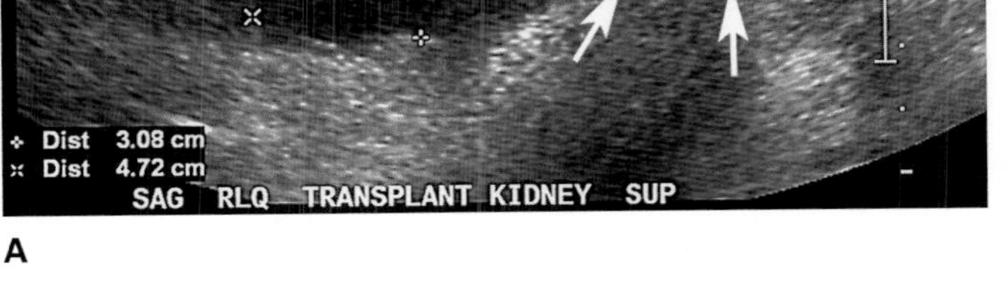

A

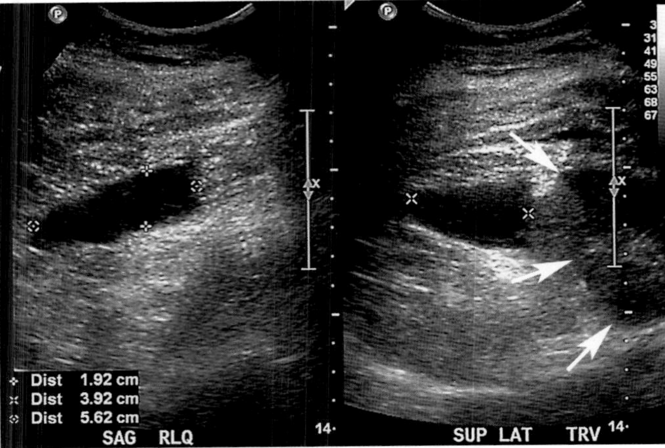

B

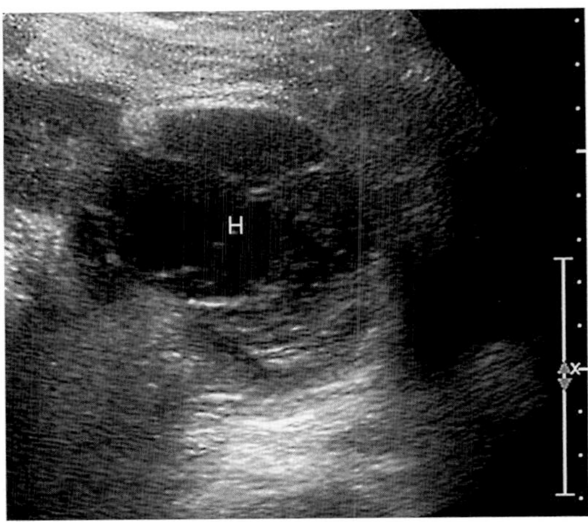

C

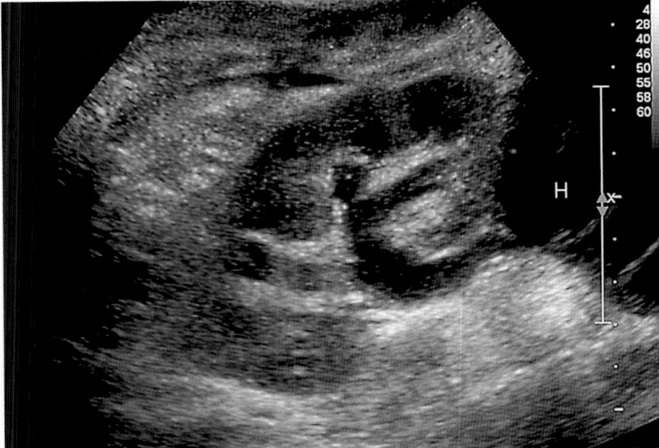

D

Figure 6-69 Post–Renal Transplant Hematoma on Serial US Examinations
This 58-year-old man had undergone placement of a renal transplant in the right lower abdomen. US performed immediately postoperatively (not shown) was normal. **A.** US obtained 3 days postoperatively demonstrates a fluid collection measuring approximately 3 × 4.7 cm at the superior margin of the transplant. Color Doppler examination (not shown) demonstrated the absence of flow within the collection, the vasculature appeared normal, and there was no hydronephrosis. **B.** US obtained 4 weeks later demonstrates decrease in size of the previously identified collection, measured near the upper pole of the transplant. **C.** However, at the inferomedial aspect of the transplant, a second, septated collection (labeled H) has developed compressing the transplant ureter. **D.** This new collection causes hydronephrosis of the transplant kidney. Percutaneous aspiration of the lower collection yielded serosanguinous fluid, which was catheter-drained, with lysis of the septations and relief of the hydronephrosis. Bacterial cultures of the fluid were negative. (Transplant margin is indicated by *white arrows* in A and B.)

and laboratory information should be considered when imaging studies are interpreted. Hematomas typically occur within the immediate postoperative period and US exams will usually reveal a fluid collection that contains internal echoes representing clots or layers of debris. With time, a hematoma will liquefy, becoming a complex cystic structure with internal septations and strands. Initially, CT will demonstrate fluid with higher attenuation than surrounding tissue on scans performed without intravenous contrast. In addition, MRI reveals tissue characteristics that correlate with the age of the hemorrhage (see Figure 6-69).

Abscess: In addition to hematoma, the presence of internal debris or gas should also raise the possibility of a renal or perinephric abscess (see Figure 6-70). The patient should be evaluated for clinical signs of infection. In many cases, CT will better demonstrate the extent of a pathologic collection that was initially diagnosed by US. This is especially useful when percutaneous drainage is being considered.

Lymphocele: Lymphocele is the most common peritransplant fluid collection, occurring in 1% to 15% of all patients who have received a renal transplant.[91] Lymphoceles are

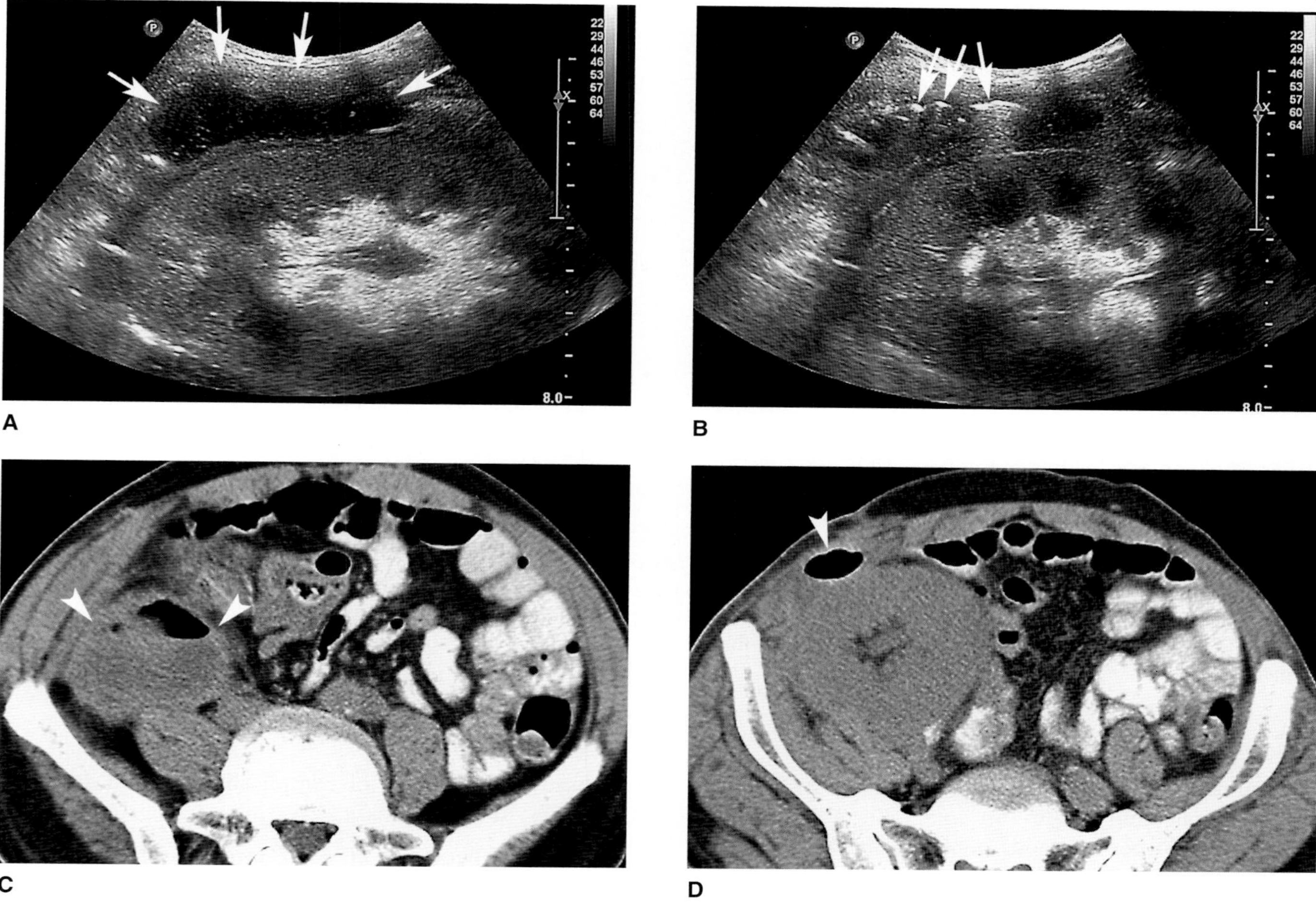

Figure 6-70 Peritransplant Gas-Containing Abscess
This 56-year-old man had undergone a renal transplant 13 weeks previously when he developed a complex fluid oozing from the surgical incision site. **A** and **B**. Sagittal images from an US examination demonstrate a fluid collection (*white arrows*). **C** and **D**. A CT scan performed with only oral contrast confirms the presence of the collection (*white arrowheads*) containing a gas-fluid level anterior and superior to the transplant. The collection was successfully treated with percutaneous catheter drainage.

usually detected 4 to 6 weeks after transplantation and are the result of intraoperative disruption of lymphatic channels near the vascular anastomoses.[89] In contrast with hematomas and abscesses, lymphoceles typically appear as well-defined, anechoic collections that can occasionally contain fine internal strands (see Figure 6-71). On CT, density measurements of lymphoceles range from 0 to 20 HU, often indistinguishable from urinomas on unenhanced scans. Although often without clinical relevance, in some cases, lymphoceles can compress the renal vascular pedicle or the transplant ureter and result in compromised function of the transplant.

Urinoma: Urinomas usually form within the first 2 weeks following surgery because of acute leaks from the ureteral anastomosis. US typically demonstrates a perinephric, anechoic fluid collection. On unenhanced CT, the collection will contain simple fluid. IVU or contrast-enhanced excretion-phase CT can demonstrate extravasation of contrast into the urinoma but is rarely performed on transplant patients because of the risk of CN. However, radionuclide examinations can be used to demonstrate accumulation of radiotracer activity within the collection, to confirm a diagnosis of a urinoma (see Figure 6-72). MRI can be helpful in demonstrating the protein-free nature of collection of urine.

Collecting system obstruction: Collecting system obstruction is unusual in renal transplants, occurring in less than 5% of patients. Transient dilation of the transplant collecting system due to edema of the ureteral anastomosis frequently occurs in the early postoperative period and is not clinically significant. Furthermore, the presence of a dilated transplant collecting system does not always indicate obstruction, as denervation of the collecting system produces decrease in tone and flaccidity, and reflux across the ureteroneocystostomy can produce dilation, especially when the bladder is distended. If, however, the serum

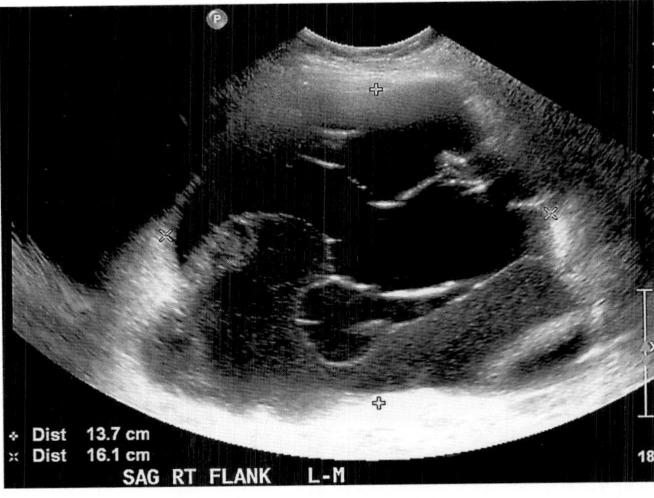

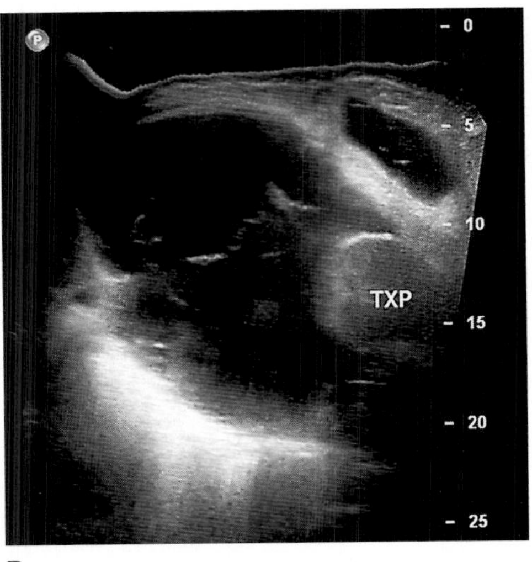

Figure 6-71 Peritransplant Lymphocele
The patient was a 43-year-old woman who had undergone a renal transplant 3 weeks ago, with severe right lower quadrant pain and no fever or voiding difficulty. **A.** Sagittal and (**B**) transverse US images demonstrate a sharply defined large septated collection in the right flank extending from just below the liver to the upper pole of the transplant (labeled TXP). Percutaneous aspiration yielded clear yellow fluid confirmed to represent lymph, and the collection was catheter-drained.

creatinine is rising in conjunction with the presence of a dilated collecting system, an antegrade pyelogram and placement of a percutaneous nephrostomy with a trial of drainage may be indicated to diagnose and treat a true ureteral obstruction.

The most frequent site of obstruction is at the ureterovesical anastomosis. Etiologies include strictures caused by either intraoperative injury or ischemia, or an intraluminal process such as a stone, blood clot, or sloughed papilla. Fine-needle antegrade pyelography is sometimes performed to diagnose transplant ureteral obstruction or leak. Percutaneous nephrostomy and ureteral stenting can be used for treatment of complications including leaks, strictures, or stone disease.[92,93]

Vascular complications of renal transplantation: Vascular complications of renal transplantation are seen in less than 10% of patients and are associated with a high morbidity and mortality. Complications include stenosis, compression, kinking, or thrombosis of the renal artery or vein, intrarenal arteriovenous fistulae, and pseudoaneurysms.

Renal artery stenosis: Renal transplant artery stenosis typically occurs within 1 to 2 cm of the anastomosis, and is usually caused by vessel wall ischemia as a result of surgical

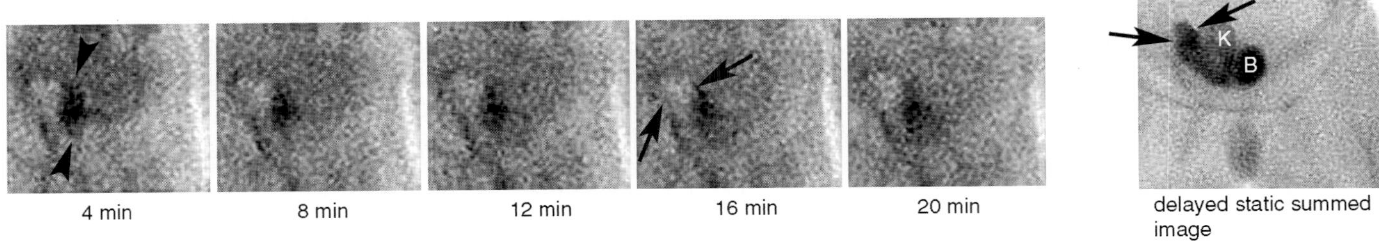

Figure 6-72 Peritransplant Urinoma on Nuclear Medicine Study
Tc99m-DTPA study of a renal transplant, in a patient 3½ weeks after renal transplant, placed in the right iliac fossa. Grayscale on images ranges from white (low activity) to black (high activity). Serial static images obtained at 4-minute intervals (each image summed over 30 s) demonstrate activity in the transplanted kidney and an oval-shaped region of photopenia to the right of the transplant (*arrows*). On the delayed static image, the previously photopenic area demonstrates increased activity, representing urine that has accumulated in the urinoma. The study demonstrates the importance of obtaining delayed imaging on radionuclide imaging studies when searching for urinoma. K indicates kidney; B, urinary bladder

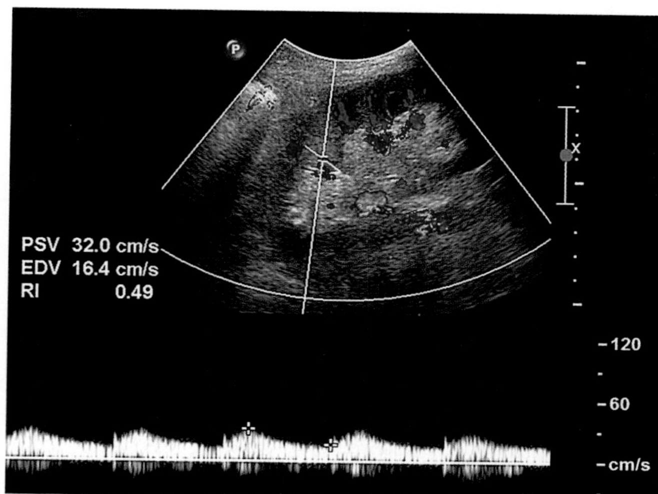

Figure 6-73 Renal Artery Stenosis in a Renal Transplant Color and spectral Doppler image from a US study of a renal transplant shows sampling of an intrarenal artery in a patient with stenosis of the transplant renal artery (not shown). The waveform demonstrates delayed upstroke, loss of the early systolic peak, and lower than normal resistive index due to increased diastolic flow relative to peak systolic velocity. This is the characteristic appearance of a "parvus tardus" waveform, which may occur as a consequence of the dampening effect of the upstream stenosis. Parvus tardus waveforms may also be the consequence of a more central stenosis, such as in the aorta, or due to aortic stenosis.

disruption of the vasa vasorum. Patients typically present with systemic hypertension or evidence of graft dysfunction. US of the intrarenal arteries demonstrate a tardus parvus waveform, characterized by a delayed upstroke in systole (acceleration time prolonged to >0.07 s), rounding of the systolic peak, and obliteration of the early systolic notch (see Figure 6-73). This finding should prompt investigation from the renal hilum to the iliac artery in search of a site of focal stenosis. A flow velocity >2 m/s with associated distal turbulence near the renal artery anastomosis is diagnostic of renal artery stenosis.[89] In addition, CT or MR angiography or conventional angiography can be used to confirm the diagnosis. When stenosis is identified early, treatment with percutaneous transluminal angioplasty has a high success rate.[94]

Renal artery thrombosis: Thrombosis of the main renal transplant artery is rare and usually due to an intraoperative technical problem. Color and power Doppler imaging shows absence of intrarenal arterial flow. However, absence of renal blood flow on Doppler exams can be seen in conditions other than arterial thrombosis, including hyperacute rejection and RVT. These conditions can be distinguished from arterial thromboses by 2 features: (1) demonstration of a patent main renal artery on grayscale imaging and (2) spectral Doppler exhibiting reversal of diastolic flow.[95]

Renal vein stenosis: Renal vein stenosis most commonly results from either perivascular fibrosis or compression of the vein by an adjacent fluid collection.

Renal vein thrombosis: Occlusive RVT occurs in up to 4% of renal transplants and typically occurs within the first postoperative week. Risk factors include intraoperative technical difficulties, hypovolemia, mechanical compression by adjacent fluid collections, and episodes of severe acute rejection. Spectral and color Doppler interrogation show absence of flow in the main RV (see Figure 6-51). The renal artery and segmental renal arteries may show reversal of diastolic flow. However, this is not a specific finding of RVT because reversal of diastolic flow in segmental renal arteries can be seen with conditions other than RVT, including severe rejection, pyelonephritis, large perinephric and subcapsular fluid collections, and drug toxicity. Failure to observe venous flow on persistent Doppler interrogation should raise suspicion of RVT.[89]

Arteriovenous malformation: Intraparenchymal arteriovenous malformations in most cases are a result of vascular trauma from percutaneous biopsy. Most are small and resolve spontaneously; however, rarely, they produce significant hemorrhage, and can require treatment with therapeutic embolization. Color Doppler examinations show a focal region of aliasing, with a flash of color caused by the vibration of surrounding tissues related to rapidly flowing blood through the fistula. Spectral Doppler shows low-resistance, high-velocity flow within the feeding artery, and turbulent pulsatile arterialized flow will be seen in the draining segmental vein.

Pseudoaneurysm: Arterial pseudoaneurysms can occur as the result of trauma from a percutaneous biopsy or can occur at the site of the arterial surgical anastomosis. On grayscale US exams, pseudoaneurysms can mimic a simple or complex cyst. However, color Doppler examinations will demonstrate a swirling flow pattern within the lesion, and spectral Doppler exams will demonstrates a central to-and-fro waveform (see Figure 6-74). Persistent or enlarging pseudoaneurysms can be treated with therapeutic embolization.

Acute and chronic functional complications:

Functional complications include hyperacute rejection, perioperative ischemia, ATN, acute rejection, drug toxicity (usually immunosuppressive agents), and chronic rejection. Unfortunately, unlike anatomic complications where imaging can play an important role in identifying the particular complication, the imaging findings of functional complications often overlap with each other

Hyperacute rejection: Hyperacute rejection occurs in the immediate perioperative period and is due to circulating antibodies against the transplanted organ. The diagnosis is usually made during or immediately following the surgical procedure, and imaging is seldom used for diagnosis.

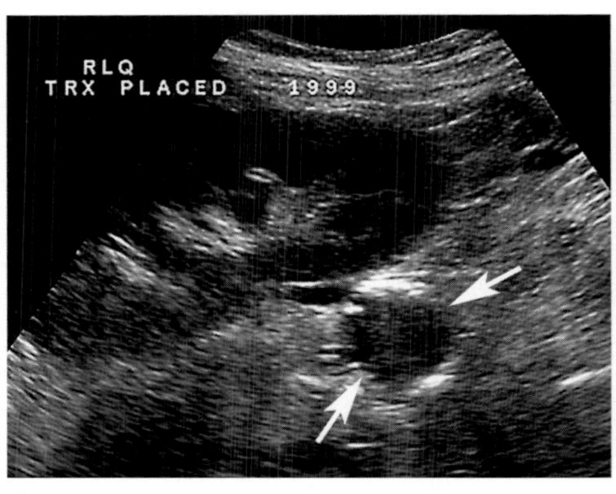

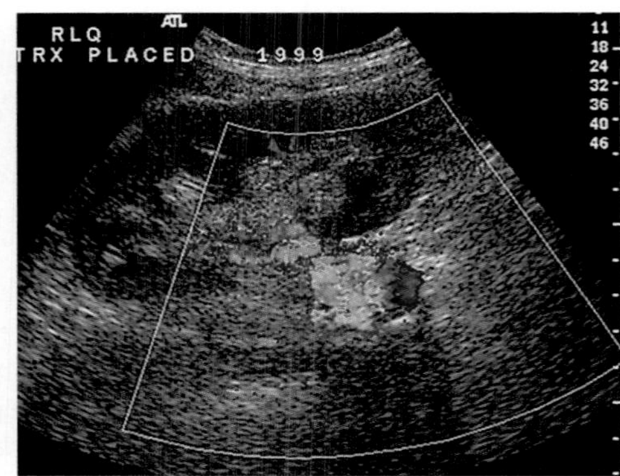

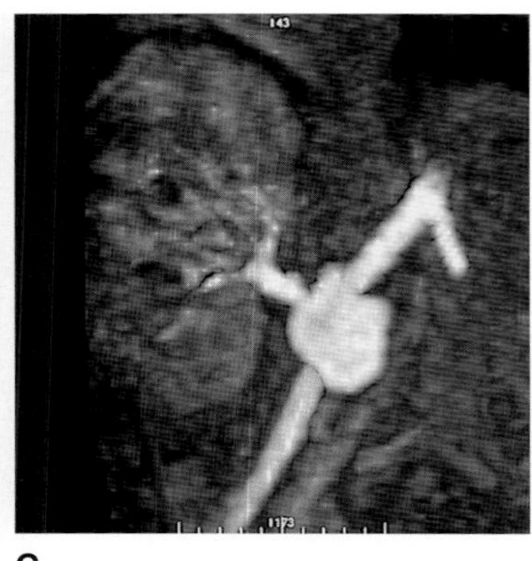

A B C

Figure 6-74 Renal Transplant Anastomotic Arterial Pseudoaneurysm
This 70-year-old man had received a renal transplant 10 years previously and was being evaluated for transplant dysfunction. **A.** Grayscale US image demonstrates a well-defined hypoechoic structure (*arrows*) at the arterial anastomosis. **B.** Color Doppler image shows rounded structure with "yin-yang" color flow pattern characteristic of a pseudoaneurysm. **C.** MRI coronal fat-saturated T1W postintravenous gadolinium MIP image at region of renal transplant artery anastomosis confirms the presence of a pseudoaneurysm.

Perioperative ischemia and acute tubular necrosis: During transportation of the transplanted kidney from the donor to the recipient, the transplanted kidney can become ischemic, resulting in ATN. The incidence of this transplantation-related ATN is proportional to the duration of ischemia. Most episodes of ATN will resolve spontaneously. ATN is present in most cadaveric grafts and most often resolves spontaneously over about 2 weeks. It is infrequently seen in patients who received transplants from living related donors, presumably because of the diminished cold ischemia time for these transplants.

Acute rejection: Acute rejection is a cellular-mediated immune phenomenon resulting in damage of the transplanted organ. This causes an edematous, swollen kidney, which histologically reveals a proliferation of monocytes, eosinophils, and plasma cells within the renal interstitium. Clinically, patients with acute rejection present with a rapid increase in serum creatinine, of 25% or more above the baseline level, over the course of 24 to 48 hours.

Cyclosporine toxicity: Cyclosporin A (CsA) is an immunosuppressant drug widely administered to post-allogeneic renal transplant patients to reduce the risk of organ rejection by decreasing the activity of the patient's immune system. Detailed description of the mechanism of action of CsA is beyond the scope of this chapter, but a major action is inhibition of lymphocytes, especially T lymphocytes, by a process that involves binding to cyclophilin, a cytosolic protein. The complex of CsA and cyclophilin inhibits calcineurin, a protein phosphatase responsible for dephosphorylation of the transcription factor NF-AT (nuclear factor of activated T-cells). CsA also inhibits lymphokine production and interleukin release.

Although CsA revolutionized transplantation medicine by improving short- and medium-term outcomes for solid organ transplantation, its success has been impeded by side effects including nephrotoxicity as well as other adverse effects including hypertension, hyperlipidemia, and induction of glucose intolerance. Recognition of these long-term side effects of CsA has led to development of alternate methods for assessing immunosuppressive drug absorption and levels, and new immunosuppressive treatments. Long-term follow-up studies will determine the safety and efficacy of these newer strategies.[96]

Chronic rejection: Chronic rejection can appear months to years after surgery, with a more insidious onset than acute rejection. Chronic rejection, a phenomenon that is not well understood, is associated with progressive azotemia and hypertension. The mechanisms for chronic rejection are believed to be multifactorial, including immunologic (cellular immunity and possibly antibody formation) and nonimmunologic (proliferative vascular lesions related to inflammation, similar in microscopic appearance to arteriosclerosis) processes.[97] Chronic rejection, along with antirejection drug nephrotoxicity and vasculopathy associated with hypertension, hyperlipidemia, and diabetes are factors that all can contribute to chronic allograft nephropathy.

Imaging findings in acute functional complications: Radionuclide renal examinations are commonly used to evaluate causes of graft dysfunction as indicated by a rising serum blood urea nitrogen and/or creatinine level.[98] ATN, acute rejection, and chronic rejection are the complications most commonly seen in referrals to nuclear medicine. For given findings on scintigraphic imaging, the differential diagnosis depends on correlation with the patient's clinical course, current treatment, and results of prior imaging tests, and therefore baseline studies obtained 1 to 2 days after transplantation are valuable.

Imaging Notes 6-12. Radionuclide Evaluation of Renal Transplant Dysfunction

Acute tubular necrosis (ATN):	First radionuclide exam with decreased function Delayed transit time is most prominent finding: • Delayed T-max • Delayed T-1/2 • High 20- to 3-min ratio
Acute Rejection:	First radionuclide exam normal, later exams decreased function
	Delayed accumulation on early, vascular phase, images: often, more so than with ATN
	Delayed transit time, as in ATN
Cyclosporine Toxicity:	Perfusion phase often normal
	Delayed clearance of radiotracer
	Difficult diagnosis, based on clinical findings and drug levels in addition to imaging.
Chronic Rejection:	Low uptake and normal parenchymal transit, with absent or minimal cortical retention.

Radionuclide measurements of renal function are categorized according to the 3 phases of the renogram, as described by Taplin.[99] The first phase, termed the vascular phase, corresponds to passage of a bolus of the tracer through the renal blood vessels after bolus administration and lasts for approximately 5 seconds. The second phase, the tubular phase, represents transit of excreted activity through the nephron to the pelvicaliceal system and lasts about 3 minutes. Lastly, the excretion phase corresponds to the drainage of the pelvicaliceal shown by recording renal activity for 20 minutes or longer. The excretion phase has been more precisely termed as the drainage phase, by Dubovsky et al.[98] The time from injection to peak activity is used to measure renal transit time. Sequential images and time-activity curves recorded at regions of interest are generated for each phase, with higher image frame rates used for the vascular phase. For the drainage phase, washout half-time is commonly used as a quantitative index. The ratio of background subtracted renal counts at 20 minutes to those at 3 minutes is often used as a measure of retained activity. Important long-established physiologic measurements for renal function include plasma clearance methods to determine glomerular filtration rate measured by inulin clearance, and the effective renal plasma flow measured by *para*-aminohippurate (PAH) clearance. Both of these tests may be performed from a blood sample obtained after an imaging dose of Tc-99m DTPA, I-131, or Tc-99m MAG_3 using standard techniques.

In ATN, the most predominant finding with tubular imaging agents (such as I-131 OIH and Tc-99m MAG) is delayed transit with delayed T-max, delayed T-1/2, and high 20- to 3-minute ratio. Blood flow and effective renal plasma flow are decreased, but these findings tend to be less marked than those of parenchymal retention. Although the imaging findings in acute rejection are similar to ATN, the time course is different. ATN would typically be present on the baseline postoperative study and improve in the ensuing 2 weeks, whereas acute rejection would be characterized by a decrease in function on serial examinations. In acute rejection, the vascular phase is also often delayed.

In chronic rejection, the transplanted kidney demonstrates cortical thinning, mild hydronephrosis. On radionuclide studies, the graft with chronic rejection shows low uptake and normal parenchymal transit with absent or minimal cortical retention.

Cyclosporine toxicity is a difficult diagnosis, usually made by exclusion made by correlating imaging findings with plasma cyclosporine levels. Radionuclide studies demonstrate prolonged rate of clearance, often with relatively normal perfusion.

Ultrasound examinations of graft dysfunction are generally nonspecific. On grayscale US, the relatively superficial location of most renal allografts allows easy visualization, but measurement of renal length may be somewhat limited by extension of the graft beyond the scanning sector, and the lack of normative data for comparison. Both cadaveric and living related donor kidneys can normally undergo significant enlargement, up to 40% in volume, after transplantation, with final size not reached until as long as 6 months.[100] Changes in cross-sectional surface area at the mid-kidney may be used to determine changes in allograft volume. Evaluation of renal parenchymal echogenicity on US is limited by lack of an adjacent reference organ such as liver.

In acute rejection, when present, findings consist of renal enlargement, with cortical swelling and increased or decreased echogenicity (see Figure 6-75). Loss of corticomedullary differentiation, prominence, and widening of the medullary pyramids, with increased or decreased

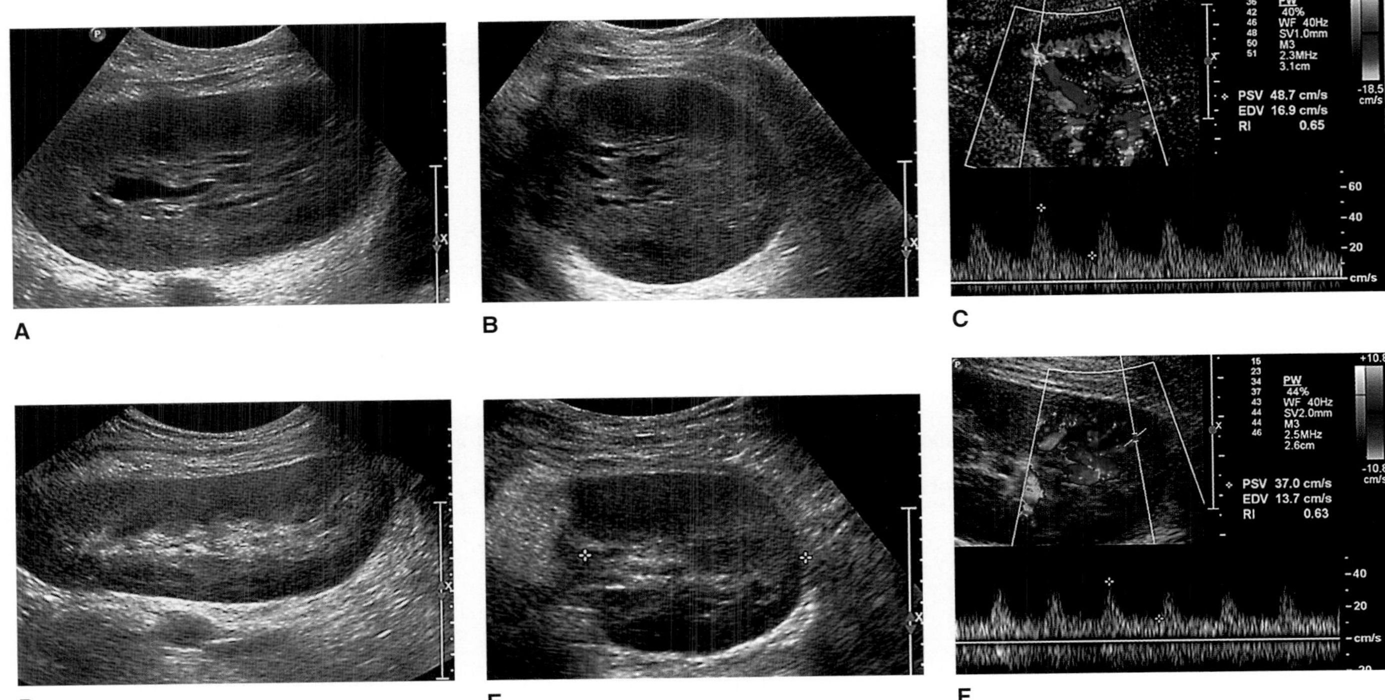

Figure 6-75 US of Acute on Chronic Rejection
The patient was the recipient of a deceased renal donor renal transplant 8 months before the US examination. The US study was obtained to evaluate rising serum creatinine. **A** and **B.** Grayscale images demonstrate a globular-shaped transplant kidney, with loss of corticomedullary differentiation and effacement of the central renal sinus fat. However, the RI of 0.65 (**C**) is normal, which illustrates the lack of reliability of the RI for diagnosis of AR. Biopsy of the transplant showed histologic findings in keeping with acute cellular rejection, superimposed on chronic rejection. **D-F.** The prior US study, obtained approximately 6 months before, demonstrated the transplant kidney to be of normal shape, with corticomedullary differentiation, and well-defined central renal sinus fat (D and E), and normal RI of 0.63 (F).

echogenicity, and urothelial thickening can also be seen, but these are all nonspecific signs and can be seen in patients who have acute rejection, ATN, infection, and cyclosporin toxicity, as well as vascular complications.[90] The swollen renal cortex can compress and narrow the central renal sinus fat echo. If a baseline sonogram is available, allograft enlargement, with a 10% or greater increase in surface area, has approximately 80% sensitivity and specificity for acute rejection.[100] In acute rejection, the intracapsular pressure of the swollen kidney rises, ultimately resulting in decreased vascular compliance. Early investigations suggested that the resistive index (RI), defined as the peak systolic velocity minus the lowest diastolic velocity divided by the peak systolic velocity, might be a useful indicator of acute rejection. Unfortunately, the RI is not a sensitive or specific indicator of acute rejection. During the early to mid stages of rejection, increased intrarenal pressure is counteracted by intrarenal regulatory mechanisms, such that the RI is rarely elevated. Only when acute rejection reaches severe levels does the RI typically become elevated. It should be noted that if a US scan performed in preparation for a renal biopsy shows an edematous, enlarged kidney with very high RIs, consideration should be given to postponing the biopsy, as puncturing the capsule of a transplant with increased renal pressure has a risk of transplant rupture. In addition, an elevated RI can be due to other causes, such as compression by an adjacent mass or fluid collection, compression effect by the US transducer, infection, ureteral obstruction, or ATN.[89] Power Doppler also lacks specificity in differentiating rejection from other functional causes of graft dysfunction. In ATN, grayscale US is reportedly often normal, but cortical swelling with prominence of the medullary pyramids, indistinguishable from acute rejection, also may be seen with significant frequency. Spectral Doppler studies may show an increase in the RI, although as noted above, this is nonspecific. In chronic rejection and chronic allograft nephropathy, cortical echogenicity is frequently increased, with cortical thinning and decreased size seen in later disease (see Figure 6-76). Doppler indices rarely show alteration in chronic rejection.[89]

Because of the inability of imaging to reliably diagnose the various causes of graft dysfunction, renal biopsy is often needed to establish the diagnosis.

Posttransplant lymphoproliferative disorder

PTLD represents the development of lymphoid collections as a complication of the immunosuppression

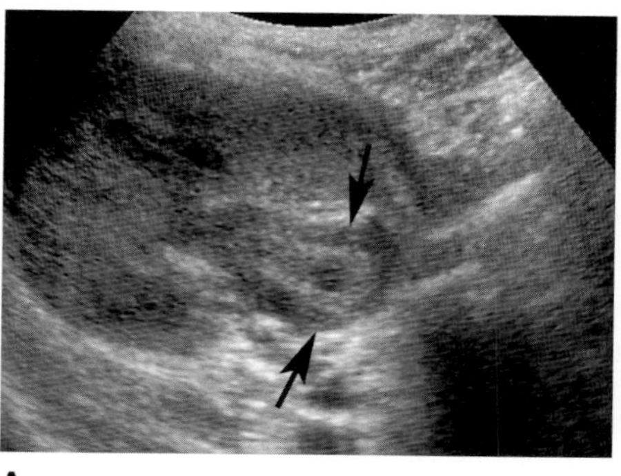
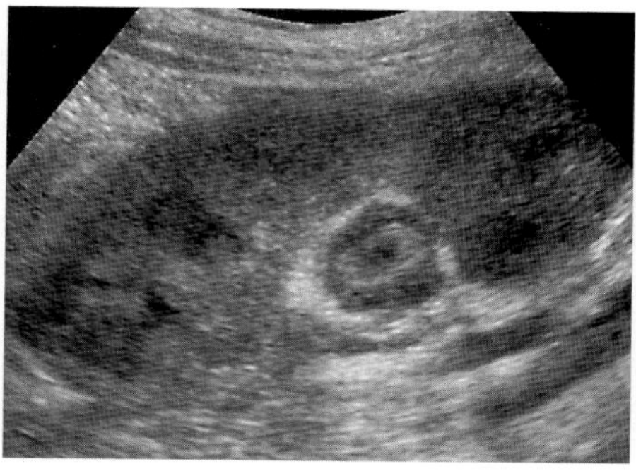
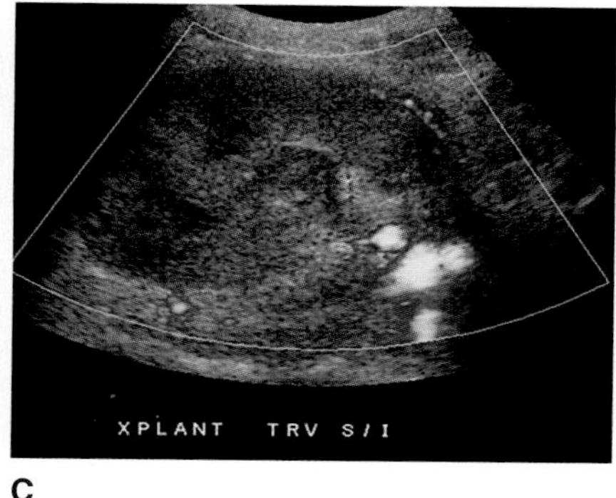

Figure 6-76 US Study of a Transplant with Chronic Rejection The patient was a 30-year-old woman who had received a renal transplant from a living related donor 2½ years previously. **A** and **B.** The kidney is echogenic, and there is marked thickening of the urothelium of the renal pelvis (*arrows*). **C.** Power Doppler examination shows almost no flow to the kidney. These findings are in keeping with end-stage chronic rejection.

necessary to maintain solid organ transplants. It has a frequency of 2% to 5% in patients who have received a renal transplant.[101] It is believed that the Epstein-Barr virus induces B cell proliferation that is unopposed by the pharmacologically suppressed T cells. The B cell proliferation ranges from a polymorphic form of premalignant hyperplasia to a monomorphic form, indistinguishable from lymphoma. Because patients with the premalignant form will often respond to treatment with decrease or cessation of immunosuppression alone, it is important to diagnose PTLD in its early polymorphic form. Untreated PTLD is usually fatal.

In addition, PTLD will most commonly cause intraabdominal disease. In a series by Pickhardt[101] of 51 patients who had undergone solid organ transplants, including 18 lung transplants, 15 kidney transplants, 10 heart transplants, and 8 liver transplants, abdominal involvement with PTLD occurred in 71%. Unlike most other lymphomas, the masses of PTLD typically involve extranodal sites, including the transplanted organ, liver, and bowel, and less commonly involve lymph nodes, seen in 81% of the patients with abdominal involvement in the Pickhardt series. Imaging manifestations include solitary or multiple, uniform hypoattenuating masses in the transplanted organ, liver, or other organs of the abdomen. Less commonly, the renal transplant will be diffusely enlarged by PTLD. A pancreas transplant can be involved as well, manifested by a focal mass or diffuse enlargement that can mimic pancreatitis.[89] Bowel involvement can be indicated by the presence of bowel wall thickening or bowel wall masses. Approximately 19% of patients will demonstrate abdominal or pelvic lymphadenopathy (see Figure 6-77).

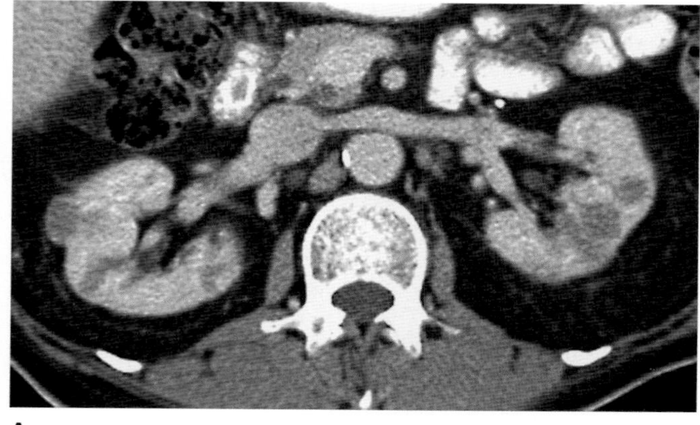
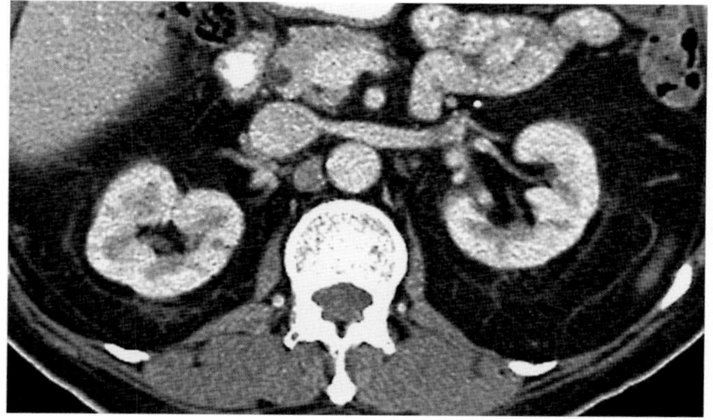

Figure 6-77 Posttransplant Lymphoproliferative Disorder (PTLD) Before and After Treatment This patient had previously undergone liver transplantation. **A.** Axial CT image from an intravenous contrast-enhanced study shows multiple low-density solid bilateral renal nodules. Diagnosis of PTLD was made on US-guided needle biopsy of 1 of the nodules. **B.** CT image 6 weeks after treatment with rituxan shows marked improvement of the lesions.

REFERENCES

1. Netter FH. Anatomy, structure, and embryology. In: Netter FH, ed. *The Ciba Collection of Medical Illustrations: CIBA Pharmaceutical*. West Caldwell, NJ: CIBA Pharmaceutical Co; 1987:2-35.
2. Hilton S, Papanicolaou N. The retroperitoneum: normal anatomy and benign and malignant retroperitoneal processes. In: Ramchandani P, ed. *RSNA Syllabus in Diagnostic Radiology: Genitourinary Radiology*. Philadelphia, PA: RSNA; 2006:145-146.
3. Platt J, Rubin J, Bowerman RA, Marn CS. The inability to detect kidney disease on the basis of echogenicity. *AJR Am J Roentgenol*. 1988;151:317-319.
4. Krestin GP. Genitourinary MR: kidneys and adrenal glands. *Eur Radiol*. 1999;9(9):1705-1714.
5. Choyke PL, Frank JA, Girton ME, et al. Dynamic Gd-DTPA-enhanced MR imaging of the kidney: experimental results. *Radiology*. 1989;170(3 pt 1):713-720.
6. Frank I, Blute ML, Cheville JC, Lohse CM, Weaver AL, Zincke H. Solid renal tumors: an analysis of pathological features related to tumor size [see comment]. *J Urol*. 2003;170(6 pt 1):2217-2220.
7. Kovacs G, Akhtar M, Beckwith BJ, et al. The Heidelberg classification of renal cell tumours. *J Pathol*. 1997;183(2):131-133.
8. Storkel S, Eble JN, Adlakha K, et al. Classification of renal cell carcinoma: Workgroup No. 1. Union Internationale Contre le Cancer (UICC) and the American Joint Committee on Cancer (AJCC). *Cancer*. 1997;80(5):987-989.
9. Kim JK, Kim TK, Ahn HJ, Kim CS, Kim K-R, Cho K-S. Differentiation of subtypes of renal cell carcinoma on helical CT scans. *AJR Am J Roentgenol*. 2002;178(6):1499-1506.
10. Renal tumors. In: Dunnick N, Sandler C, Newhouse J, Amis E Jr, eds. *Textbook of Uroradiology*. 4th ed. Philadelphia, PA: Lippincott Williams & Wilkins; 2008:135-164.
11. Motzer RJ, Bander NH, Nanus DM. Renal-cell carcinoma [see comment]. *N Engl J Med* 1996;335(12):865-875.
12. Fuhrman SA, Lasky LC, Limas C. Prognostic significance of morphologic parameters in renal cell carcinoma. *Am J Surg Pathol*. 1982;6(7):655-663.
13. Dyer R, DiSantis DJ, McClennan BL. Simplified imaging approach for evaluation of the solid renal mass in adults. *Radiology*. 2008;247(2):331-343.
14. Pahernik S, Ziegler S, Roos F, Melchior SW, Thuroff JW. Small renal tumors: correlation of clinical and pathological features with tumor size. *J Urol*. 2007;178(2):414-417; discussion 416-417.
15. Hsu RM, Chan DY, Siegelman SS. Small renal cell carcinomas: correlation of size with tumor stage, nuclear grade, and histologic subtype. *AJR Am J Roentgenol*. 2004;182(3):551-557.
16. Yuh BI, Cohan RH. Different phases of renal enhancement: role in detecting and characterizing renal masses during helical CT. *AJR Am J Roentgenol*. 1999;173(3):747-755.
17. Israel GM, Bosniak MA. How I do it: evaluating renal masses. *Radiology*. 2005;236(2):441-450.
18. Birnbaum BA, Maki DD, Chakraborty DP, Jacobs JE, Babb JS. Renal cyst pseudoenhancement: evaluation with an anthropomorphic body CT phantom. *Radiology*. 2002;225(1): 83-90.
19. Sun MRM, Ngo L, Genega EM, et al. Renal cell carcinoma: dynamic contrast-enhanced MR imaging for differentiation of tumor subtypes—correlation with pathologic findings. *Radiology*. 2009;250(3):793-802.
20. Ruppert-Kohlmayr AJ, Uggowitzer M, Meissnitzer T, Ruppert G. Differentiation of renal clear cell carcinoma and renal papillary carcinoma using quantitative CT enhancement parameters. *AJR Am J Roentgenol*. 2004;183(5):1387-1391.
21. Pedrosa I, Sun MR, Spencer M, et al. MR imaging of renal masses: correlation with findings at surgery and pathologic analysis. *Radiographics*. 2008;28(4):985-1003.
22. Outwater EK, Bhatia M, Siegelman ES, Burke MA, Mitchell DG. Lipid in renal clear cell carcinoma: detection on opposed-phase gradient-echo MR images [see comment]. *Radiology*. 1997;205(1):103-107.
23. Kidney. In: Greene F, Page D, Fleming I, et al., eds. *AJCC Cancer Staging Handbook*. 6th ed. New York: Springer-Verlag; 2002:355-360.
24. Catalano C, Fraioli F, Laghi A, et al. High-resolution multidetector CT in the preoperative evaluation of patients with renal cell carcinoma. *AJR Am J Roentgenol*. 2003;180(5):1271-1277.
25. Studer UE, Scherz S, Scheidegger J, et al. Enlargement of regional lymph nodes in renal cell carcinoma is often not due to metastases. *J Urol*. 1990;144(2 pt 1):243-245.
26. Nesbitt JC, Soltero ER, Dinney CP, et al. Surgical management of renal cell carcinoma with inferior vena cava tumor thrombus. *Ann Thorac Surg*. 1997;63(6):1592-1600.
27. Lawrentschuk N, Gani J, Riordan R, Esler S, Bolton DM. Multidetector computed tomography vs magnetic resonance imaging for defining the upper limit of tumour thrombus in renal cell carcinoma: a study and review. *BJU Int*. 2005;96(3):291-295.
28. Herr HW. Surgical management of renal tumors: a historical perspective. *Urol Clin North Am*. 2008;35(4):543-549; v.
29. Russo P, Huang W. The medical and oncological rationale for partial nephrectomy for the treatment of T1 renal cortical tumors. *Urol Clin North Am*. 2008;35(4):635-643; vii.
30. Lattouf J-B, Beri A, D'Ambros OFJ, Grull M, Leeb K, Janetschek G. Laparoscopic partial nephrectomy for hilar tumors: technique and results [see comment]. *Eur Urol*. 2008;54(2):409-416.
31. Wile GE, Leyendecker JR, Krehbiel KA, Dyer RB, Zagoria RJ. CT and MR imaging after imaging-guided thermal ablation of renal neoplasms. *Radiographics*. 2007;27(2):325-339; discussion 339-340.
32. Davenport MS, Caoili EM, Cohan RH, et al. MRI and CT characteristics of successfully ablated renal masses: imaging surveillance after radiofrequency ablation. *AJR Am J Roentgenol*. 2009;192(6):1571-1578.
33. Gervais DA, Arellano RS, McGovern FJ, McDougal WS, Mueller PR. Radiofrequency ablation of renal cell carcinoma: part 2, Lessons learned with ablation of 100 tumors. *AJR Am J Roentgenol*. 2005;185(1):72-80.
34. Prasad SR, Dalrymple NC, Surabhi VR. Cross-sectional imaging evaluation of renal masses. *Radiol Clin North Am*. 2008;46(1):95-111.
35. Davis CJ Jr, Barton JH, Sesterhenn IA, Mostofi FK. Metanephric adenoma. Clinicopathological study of fifty patients. *Am J Surg Pathol*. 1995;19(10):1101-1114.
36. Fielding JR, Visweswaran A, Silverman SG, Granter SR, Renshaw AA. CT and ultrasound features of metanephric adenoma in adults with pathologic correlation. *J Comput Assist Tomogr*. 1999;23(3):441-444.

37. Guinan P, Sobin LH, Algaba F, et al. TNM staging of renal cell carcinoma: Workgroup No. 3. Union International Contre le Cancer (UICC) and the American Joint Committee on Cancer (AJCC). *Cancer.* 1997;80(5):992-993.
38. Hornick JL, Fletcher CDM. PEComa: what do we know so far? *Histopathology.* 2006;48(1):75-82.
39. Rakowski SK, Winterkorn EB, Paul E, Steele DJR, Halpern EF, Thiele EA. Renal manifestations of tuberous sclerosis complex: Incidence, prognosis, and predictive factors. *Kidney Int.* 2006; 70(10):1777-1782.
40. Nelson CP, Sanda MG. Contemporary diagnosis and management of renal angiomyolipoma. *J Urol.* 2002; 168(4 pt 1):1315-1325.
41. Sheth S, Ali S, Fishman E. Imaging of renal lymphoma: patterns of disease with pathologic correlation. *Radiographics.* 2006;26(4):1151-1168.
42. Bailey JE, Roubidoux MA, Dunnick NR. Secondary renal neoplasms. *Abdom Imaging.* 1998;23(3):266-274.
43. McAninch J, Santucci R. Chapter 39—renal and ureteral trauma. In: Wein A, Kavoussi L, Novick A, Partin A, Peters C, eds. *Campbell-Walsh Urology.* 9th ed. Philadelphia, PA: Elsevier; 2007.
44. Mullinix AJ, Foley WD. Multidetector computed tomography and blunt thoracoabdominal trauma. *J Comput Assist Tomogr.* 2004;28(suppl 1):S20-S27.
45. Moore EE, Cogbill TH, Malangoni MA, et al. Organ injury scaling. *Surg Clin North Am.* 1995;75(2):293-303.
46. Santucci RA, Fisher MB. The literature increasingly supports expectant (conservative) management of renal trauma—a systematic review. *J Trauma.* 2005;59(2):493-503.
47. Harris AC, Zwirewich CV, Lyburn ID, Torreggiani WC, Marchinkow LO. CT findings in blunt renal trauma. *Radiographics.* 2001;21(Spec No):S201-S214.
48. Wong WS, Moss AA, Federle MP, Cochran ST, London SS. Renal infarction: CT diagnosis and correlation between CT findings and etiologies. *Radiology.* 1984;150(1):201-205.
49. Israel GM, Bosniak MA. An update of the Bosniak renal cyst classification system. *Urology.* 2005;66(3):484-488.
50. Kissane J. Congenital malformations. In: Jennette J, ed. *Heptinstall's Pathology of the Kidney.* 5th ed. Philadelphia, PA: Lippincott-Raven; 1998.
51. Tada S, Yamagishi J, Kobayashi H, Hata Y, Kobari T. The incidence of simple renal cyst by computed tomography. *Clin Radiol.* 1983;34(4):437-439.
52. Slywotzky CM, Bosniak MA. Localized cystic disease of the kidney. *AJR Am J Roentgenol.* 2001;176(4):843-849.
53. Freire M, Remer EM. Clinical and radiologic features of cystic renal masses. *AJR Am J Roentgenol.* 2009;192(5):1367-1372.
54. Grantham JJ. Clinical practice. Autosomal dominant polycystic kidney disease. *N Engl J Med.* 2008;359(14):1477-1485.
55. Keith DS, Torres VE, King BF, Zincki H, Farrow GM. Renal cell carcinoma in autosomal dominant polycystic kidney disease. *J Am Soc Nephrol.* 1994;4(9):1661-1669.
56. Park JH, Kim YO, Park JH, et al. Comparison of acquired cystic kidney disease between hemodialysis and continuous ambulatory peritoneal dialysis. *Korean J Intern Med.* 2000;15(1):51-55.
57. Hogg RJ. Acquired renal cystic disease in children prior to the start of dialysis. *Pediatr Nephrol.* 1992;6(2):176-178.
58. Grantham JJ, Levine E. Acquired cystic disease: replacing one kidney disease with another. *Kidney Int.* 1985;28(2):99-105.
59. Mitnick JS, Bosniak MA, Hilton S, Raghavendra BN, Subramanyam BR, Genieser NB. Cystic renal disease in tuberous sclerosis. *Radiology.* 1983;147(1):85-87.
60. Renal cystic disease. In: Dunnick N, Sandler C, Newhouse J, Amis E Jr, eds. *Textbook of Uroradiology.* 4th ed. Philadelphia, PA: Lippincott Williams & Wilkins; 2008:113-134.
61. Thurston W, Wilson S. The urinary tract. In: Rumack C, Wilson S, Charboneau J, eds. *Diagnostic Ultrasound.* 3rd ed. St. Louis, MO: Elsevier Mosby; 2005:381.
62. Renal Failure and Medical Disease. In: Dunnick N, Sandler C, Newhouse J, Amis E Jr, eds. *Textbook of Uroradiology.* 4th ed. Philadelphia, PA: Lippincott Williams & Wilkins; 2008:217-228.
63. Urban BA, Fishman EK. Renal lymphoma: CT patterns with emphasis on helical CT. *Radiographics.* 2000;20(1):197-212.
64. Berdon WE, Schwartz RH, Becker J, Baker DH. Tamm-Horsfall proteinuria. Its relationship to prolonged nephrogram in infants and children and to renal failure following intravenous urography in adults with multiple myeloma. *Radiology.* 1969;92(4):714-722.
65. Coel MN, Talner LB. Obstructive nephrogram due to renal vein thrombosis. *Radiology.* 1971;101(3):573-574.
66. Lieberman E, Salinas-Madrigal L, Gwinn JL, Brennan LP, Fine RN, Landing BH. Infantile polycystic disease of the kidneys and liver: clinical, pathological and radiological correlations and comparison with congenital hepatic fibrosis. *Medicine (Baltimore).* 1971;50(4):277-318.
67. Hunnam GR, Sherwood T. Striated nephrogram in rhabdomyolysis. *Br J Radiol.* 1985;58(691):682-683.
68. Saunders HS, Dyer RB, Shifrin RY, Scharling ES, Bechtold RE, Zagoria RJ. The CT nephrogram: implications for evaluation of urinary tract disease. *Radiographics.* 1995;15(5):1069-1085; discussion 1086-1088.
69. Craig WD, Wagner BJ, Travis MD. Pyelonephritis: radiologic-pathologic review. *Radiographics.* 2008;28(1):255-277; quiz 327-328.
70. Dyer RB, Chen MY, Zagoria RJ. Abnormal calcifications in the urinary tract. *Radiographics.* 1998;18(6):1405-1424.
71. Tublin ME, Murphy ME, Tessler FN. Current concepts in contrast media-induced nephropathy. *AJR Am J Roentgenol.* 1998;171(4):933-939.
72. McCarthy CS, Becker JA. Multiple myeloma and contrast media. *Radiology.* 1992;183(2):519-521.
73. Rudnick MR, Goldfarb S, Wexler L, et al. Nephrotoxicity of ionic and nonionic contrast media in 1196 patients: a randomized trial. The Iohexol Cooperative Study. *Kidney Int.* 1995;47(1):254-261.
74. Barrett BJ, Carlisle EJ. Metaanalysis of the relative nephrotoxicity of high- and low-osmolality iodinated contrast media. *Radiology.* 1993;188(1):171-178.
75. Murphy SW, Barrett BJ, Parfrey PS. Contrast nephropathy. *J Am Soc Nephrol.* 2000;11(1):177-182.
76. Nino-Murcia M, DeVries P, Friedland G. Congenital anomalies of the kidney. In: Pollack H, McClennan B, eds. *Clinical Urography.* 2nd ed. Philadelphia, PA: W.B. Saunders; 2000:702-734.
77. Neville H, Ritchey ML, Shamberger RC, Haase G, Perlman S, Yoshioka T. The occurrence of Wilms tumor in horseshoe kidneys: a report from the National Wilms Tumor Study Group (NWTSG). *J Pediatr Surg.* 2002;37(8):1134-1137.

78. McVey RJ, Banerjee SS, Eyden BP, Reeve RS, Harris M. Carcinoid tumor originating in a horseshoe kidney. *In Vivo.* 2002;16(3):197-199.
79. Lee CT, Hilton S, Russo P. Renal mass within a horseshoe kidney: preoperative evaluation with three-dimensional helical computed tomography. *Urology.* 2001;57(1):168.
80. Robson CJ. Radical nephrectomy for renal cell carcinoma. *J Urol.* 1963;89:37-42.
81. Robson CJ, Churchill BM, Anderson W. The results of radical nephrectomy for renal cell carcinoma. *J Urol.* 1969;101(3): 297-301.
82. O'Malley RL, Godoy G, Kanofsky JA, Taneja SS. The necessity of adrenalectomy at the time of radical nephrectomy: a systematic review. *J Urology.* 2009;181(5):2009-2017.
83. Swanson DA, Borges PM. Complications of transabdominal radical nephrectomy for renal cell carcinoma. *J Urol.* 1983; 129(4):704-707.
84. Flanigan R. Chapter 48—Urothelial tumors of the upper Urinary Tract. In: Wein A, Kavoussi L, Novick A, Partin A, Peters C, eds. *Campbell-Walsh Urology.* 9th ed. Philadelphia: W.B. Saunders, an imprint of Elsevier Inc; 2007.
85. Kakizoe T, Fujita J, Murase T, Matsumoto K, Kishi K. Transitional cell carcinoma of the bladder in patients with renal pelvic and ureteral cancer. *J Urol.* 1980;124(1):17-19.
86. Israel GM, Hecht E, Bosniak MA. CT and MR imaging of complications of partial nephrectomy. *Radiographics.* 2006; 26(5):1419-1429.
87. Lee MS, Oh YT, Han WK, et al. CT findings after nephron-sparing surgery of renal tumors. *AJR Am J Roentgenol.* 2007; 189(5):W264-W271.
88. U.S. Department of Health and Human Services, Health Resources and Service Administration, Organ Procurement and Transplantation Network (OPTN) website. 2009. http://optn.transplant.hrsa.gov/.
89. Pozniak M. US evaluation of the transplanted kidney. In: Ramchandani P, ed. *Genitourinary Radiology.* Oak Brook, IL: Radiological Society of North America; 2006:161-173.
90. Langer JE, Jones LP. Sonographic evaluation of the renal transplant. *Ultrasound Clin.* 2007;2(1):73-88.
91. Renal transplantation. In: Dunnick NR, Newhouse JH, Amis E Jr, eds. *Textbook of Uroradiology.* Philadelphia, PA: Lippincott Williams & Wilkins; 2008:229-245.
92. Bhagat VJ, Gordon RL, Osorio RW, et al. Ureteral obstructions and leaks after renal transplantation: outcome of percutaneous antegrade ureteral stent placement in 44 patients. *Radiology.* 1998;209(1):159-167.
93. Aytekin C, Boyvat F, Harman A, Ozyer U, Colak T, Haberal M. Percutaneous therapy of ureteral obstructions and leak after renal transplantation: long-term results. *Cardiovasc Intervent Radiol.* 2007;30(6):1178-1184.
94. Choyke P. Imaging the transplanted kidney. In: Pollack H, McClennan B, eds. *Clinical Urography.* Philadelphia, PA: W.B. Saunders; 2000:3111.
95. Muradali D, Wilson S. Organ transplantation. In: Rumack C, Wilson S, Charboneau J, eds. *Diagnostic Ultrasound.* St. Louis, MO: Elsevier Mosby; 2005:679.
96. Hesselink DA, Smak Gregoor PJH, Weimar W. The use of cyclosporine in renal transplantation. *Transplant Proc.* 2004; 36(2 suppl):99S-106S.
97. Kwun J, Knechtle SJ. Overcoming chronic rejection—can it B? *Transplantation.* 2009;88(8):955-961.
98. Dubovsky EV, Russell CD, Erbas B. Radionuclide evaluation of renal transplants. *Semin Nucl Med.* 1995;25(1):49-59.
99. Taplin GV. Kidney function and disease. In: Blahd WH, ed. *Nuclear Medicine.* 2nd ed. New York, NY: McGraw-Hill; 1971:382-386.
100. O'Neill WC, Baumgarten DA. Ultrasonography in renal transplantation. *Am J Kidney Dis.* 2002;39(4):663-678.
101. Pickhardt PJ, Siegel MJ. Posttransplantation lymphoproliferative disorder of the abdomen: CT evaluation in 51 patients. *Radiology.* 1999;213(1):73-78.

CHAPTER

Imaging of the Urinary System

Parvati Ramchandani, MD
Wallace T. Miller Jr., MD

Neoplastic and nonneoplastic pathology can cause focal or diffuse abnormalities in the collecting system, which can present as filling defects, mucosal abnormalities, or segmental narrowing on imaging studies.

ANATOMY AND HISTOLOGY OF THE URINARY SYSTEM

The pyelocalyceal systems and ureters together are referred to as the upper urinary tract. Uriniferous collecting tubules in the renal papillae pierce the papilla to open into the calyx, which then drains into the renal pelvis, the ureter, and the bladder. On average, there are 8 to 14 calyces in a kidney, but there can be fewer or more numerous calyces. In a kidney with fewer calyces, each calyx tends to be larger, as it drains a proportionally larger segment of the kidney and, conversely, each calyx tends to be smaller when there is more than the usual complement of calyces in a kidney. The renal collecting system and ureter is lined with a transitional cell epithelium that can have multiple layers; elastic connective tissue deep to the epithelium, known as the lamina propria; a muscular layer that is arranged in an inner longitudinal and outer circular muscle layers; and an outermost adventitial layer through which the vessels travel. Peristaltic activity of the muscle layer is important in the upper urinary tract, to actively drain urine into the urinary bladder. The bladder wall consists of the urothelial lining, which can be up to 7 cell layers in thickness, the submucosal connective tissue, which also contains smooth muscle fibers known as the lamina propria, and the muscular detrusor layer. Depth of invasion into the detrusor muscle is the most important factor in both the management and the prognosis of bladder neoplasms.

IMAGING MODALITIES IN THE EVALUATION OF THE URINARY SYSTEM

A variety of imaging modalities can be used to evaluate the urinary system. Most commonly this includes either intravenous urograms (IVU) or computed tomographic urograms (CTU) but less frequently, ultrasonography (US), standard CT and magnetic resonance imaging (MRI) can detect urothelial lesions.

Urography

Urography includes both intravenous urograms (IVUs) and CT urograms (CTUs). Intravenous urogram is also referred to as intravenous pyelogram (IVP) or excretory urogram. Both of these examinations opacify the urinary system through the excretion of intravenous contrast. In the case of IVU, the system is then imaged with x-rays of the abdomen and in the case of CTU the system is imaged with CT (see Figures 7-1 and 7-2). By filling and distending the urinary system, subtle mucosal masses, intraluminal abnormalities, and urinary strictures can be identified. CT urography has superseded IVU for evaluation of the urinary system for many indications over the past decade. In patients with hematuria, CTU confers the advantage that both the renal parenchyma and the urothelium can be evaluated with 1 study, as an IVU is relatively insensitive for detection of renal parenchymal masses. Further, CTU is also currently the first-line study for evaluating patients with suspected urothelial cancer, although no prospective study has been performed that compares the sensitivity of CTU versus IVU for detection of urothelial tumors, as discussed later. Moreover, CTU requires no bowel preparation for the patient, but a disadvantage is the radiation dose, which is several folds higher than for an IVU. A high-quality IVU study requires not only a vigorous bowel preparation but also a clear liquid diet for 12 hours preceding the study. On both an IVU and CTU, urothelial assessment is performed by looking for filling defects, luminal narrowing, and wall thickening.

Retrograde Pyelography

Retrograde pyelography requires the placement of a ureteral catheter by a urologist with cystoscopic guidance, followed by contrast injection. The study is performed if a patient cannot receive contrast because of renal insufficiency or adverse reaction to contrast, or there is a lesion detected on CTU or IVU that requires further evaluation. If a filling defect or other mucosal irregularity is seen, a brush biopsy can be performed with fluoroscopic guidance (see Figure 7-3).

Ultrasonography

US is of value in the assessment of a patient presenting with renal insufficiency and suspected urinary obstruction. It is also useful in the evaluation of renal and proximal ureteral calculi, although it is not as sensitive as noncontrast CT in detecting calculi smaller than 7 mm, particularly in obese patients. Calculi in the vicinity of the ureterovesical junction or in the urinary bladder can be detected by scanning through a full bladder or by transvaginal scanning in female patients. Large urothelial tumors in the renal pelvis or urinary bladder that project into the lumen may be visible on US (see Figure 7-4).

Computed Tomography

Scanning prior to administration of intravenous contrast is crucial to detect small calculi in the collecting system and ureters, as excreted contrast within the collecting system can obscure calculi (see Figure 7-5). It is important to have the bladder well distended to detect subtle wall thickening, a sign of early bladder tumors, because the normal underdistended bladder can appear to be thick walled. Focal enhancement in a distended bladder may be another

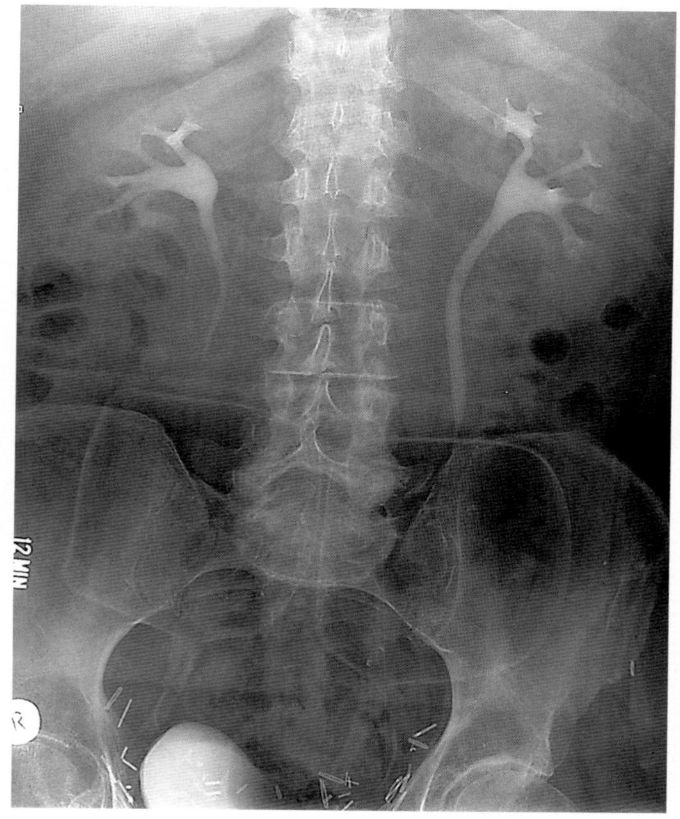

A

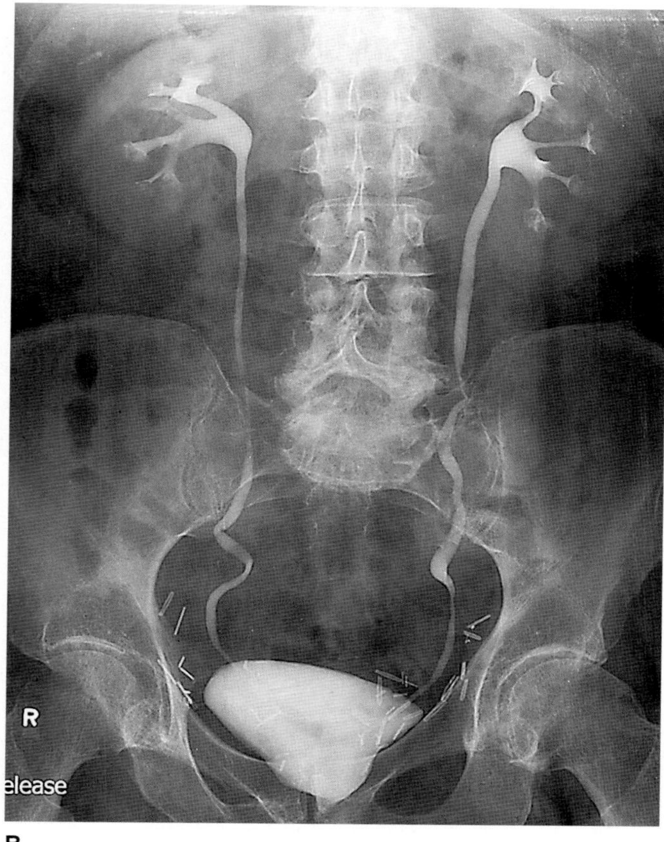

B

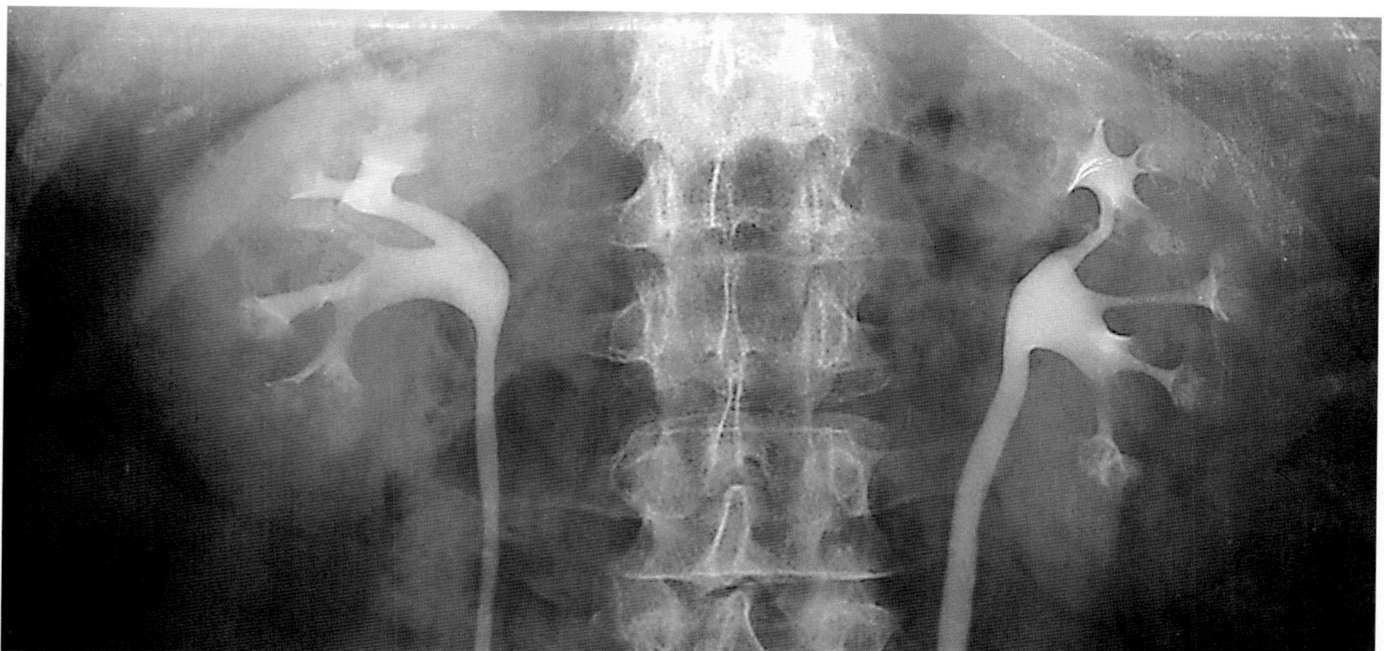

C

Figure 7-1 Normal Intravenous Urogram (IVU)
These are sequential images from an IVU on a 65-year-old man undergoing study for nonspecific flank pain. **A.** Image is obtained approximately 10 minutes after contrast injection. There is a compression belt across the pelvis, to allow distension of the collecting system for better evaluation. **B.** Image obtained after release of the compression demonstrates the ureters in their entirety. Notice the surgical clips in the pelvis from a previous radical prostatectomy for prostate cancer. **C.** Close-up to demonstrate the normal pyelocalyceal system. Notice the well-cupped calyces and the excellent depiction of the urothelium.

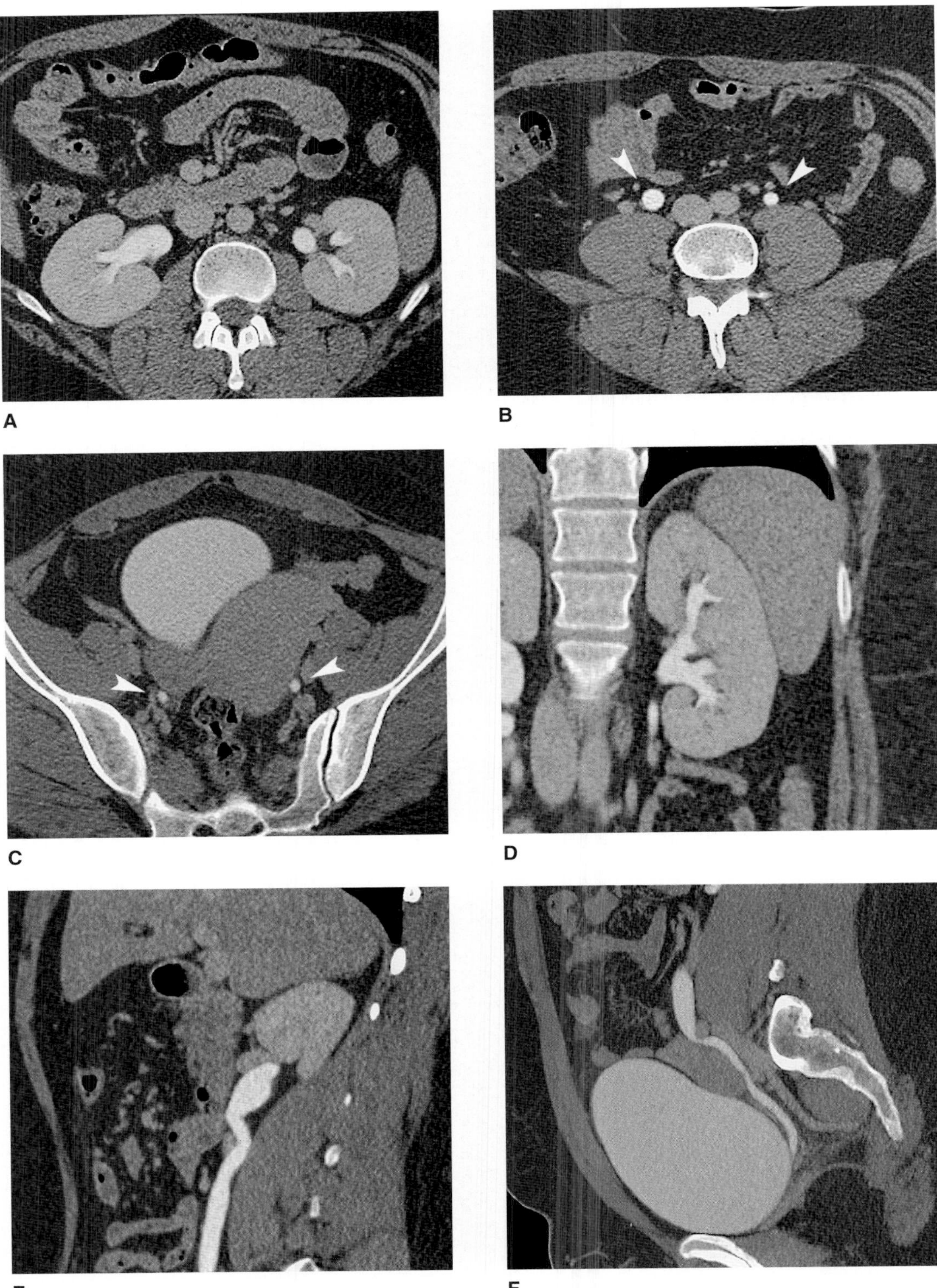

Figure 7-2 Normal CT Urogram
This 27-year-old woman had hematuria. **A-C.** Axial CT images from a CTU show excellent opacification of the renal pelvis and calices in (A) and the ureters (*arrowheads*) and urinary bladder in (C). These images are obtained several minutes (approximately 8-12 min) following the intravenous injection of contrast at the time when contrast is excreted. Intravenous furosemide and/or abdominal compression can be used to increase distention of the collecting system, both of which were used in this examination. **D-F.** Sagittal and coronal oblique maximum intensity projection images can demonstrate the collecting systems and ureters to greater effect. Occasionally, 3D reconstructions with either shaded surface display or maximum intensity projections can also be created although they add little to the diagnostic capabilities of the examination.

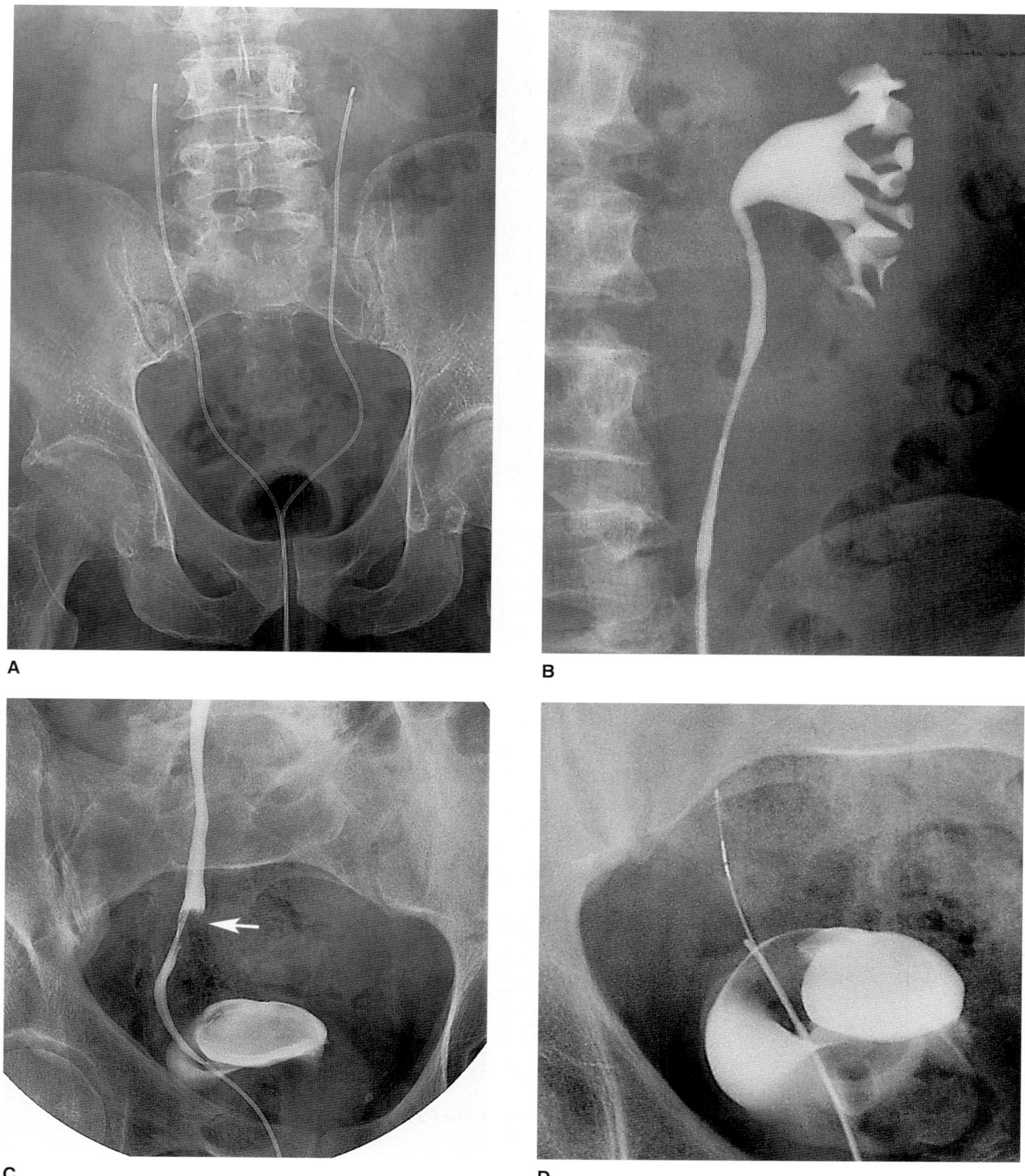

Figure 7-3 Retrograde Pyelography
A and **B.** This patient presented with microscopic hematuria. (A) Scout radiograph obtained after urologic insertion of retrograde catheters shows excellent positioning of the catheters in the proximal ureters. (B) Injection of contrast into the left ureteral catheter shows excellent delineation of the left collecting system and ureter. Compare the distention of the renal pelvis and calices with that seen in Figure 7-1. The greater distention of retrograde pyelography can improve detection of subtle urothelial abnormalities that can be more difficult to detect on a standard IVU where the collecting system is less distended. **C** and **D.** This patient presented with hematuria, and a small mass was identified in the right ureter on CTU (not shown). (C) Retrograde pyelogram confirms the presence of a focal shelflike narrowing (*arrow*) of the pelvic ureter, highly suspicious for a urothelial malignancy. (D) A brush biopsy wire has been inserted through the retrograde catheter and positioned at the location of the filling defect. Cytologic evaluation was positive for a urothelial carcinoma and the patient underwent surgical resection of the distal ureter.

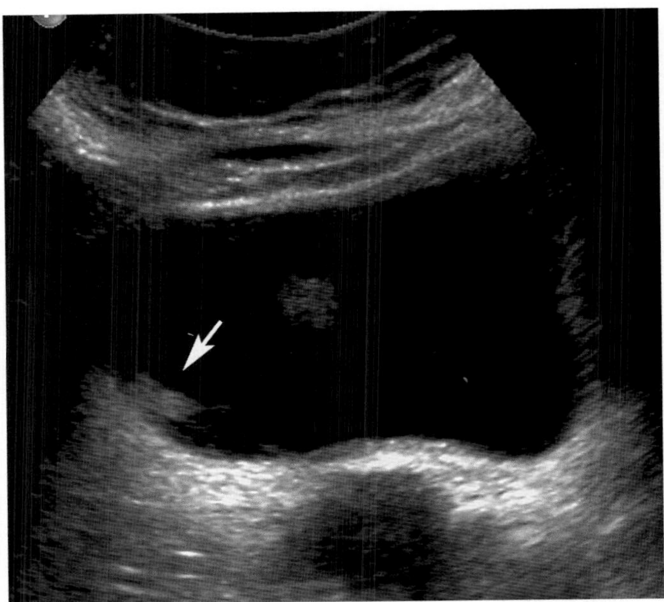

A

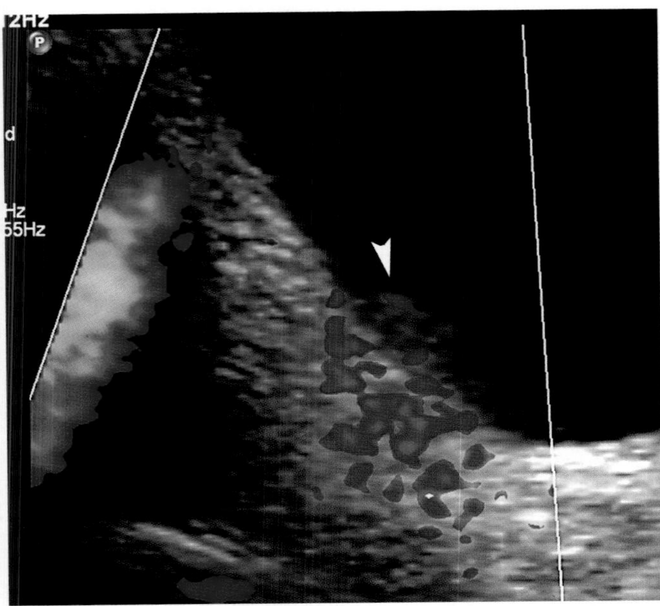

B

Figure 7-4 Bladder Sonogram
This 60-year-old woman presented with macroscopic hematuria. **A.** Transverse US of the distended urinary bladder with the patient in a left lateral decubitus position demonstrates an echogenic focus (*arrow*) adjacent to the posterior bladder wall. The lesion did not fall into the dependent portion of the bladder, suggesting that it represents a polyp. **B.** Color flow US shows flow (*arrowhead*) in the lesion, also indicating its polypoid nature. Biopsy of the lesion was diagnostic of a TCC.

sign of a bladder tumor. Detection of upper tract urothelial tumors is also improved when the collecting systems are distended with either infusion of saline or administration of intravenous furosemide.

Magnetic Resonance Imaging

MRI is limited in the detection of tumors in the upper urinary tract. It is useful in staging bladder tumors, as the layers of the bladder wall are better depicted on MRI than on CT. Although the detection of urinary tract calculi is difficult on MRI, they may be seen as low signal voids in a dilated and fluid-filled collecting system (see Figure 7-6).

FOCAL MASSES OR NODULES OF THE COLLECTING SYSTEM AND BLADDER

Focal masslike or nodular abnormalities of the urinary system in most cases will represent transitional cell carcinoma (TCC). However, rarely, they may be due to less common benign and malignant neoplasms. The unusual inflammatory process, ureteritis cystica, can also cause small focal nodular lesions in the wall of the ureter. Nonopaque uric acid calculi can be seen as filling defects in the opacified collecting system on an IVU or retrograde pyelogram, and CT confirmation is often required in such patients to confirm that the filling defect is related to a calculus and not a neoplasm. Blood clots within the collecting system are also seen as filling defects, but because of the presence of urokinase in the urine, they will dissolve in a few days to weeks and no longer be seen on imaging studies (see Figure 7-7).

Neoplasms

Neoplasms of the upper urinary tract (renal collecting system, renal pelvis, and ureter) and the urinary bladder can

Imaging Notes 7-1. Masslike Abnormalities in the Urinary System

- Urothelial cancer is the diagnosis of exclusion when a filling defect suggesting a mass is seen in the collecting system
- On an IVU or retrograde pyelogram, a radiolucent calculus may be seen as a filling defect, and CT or ultrasound confirmation is then required to confirm that a stone is present
- Blood clots can cause filling defects but should resolve on subsequent imaging done a few weeks later

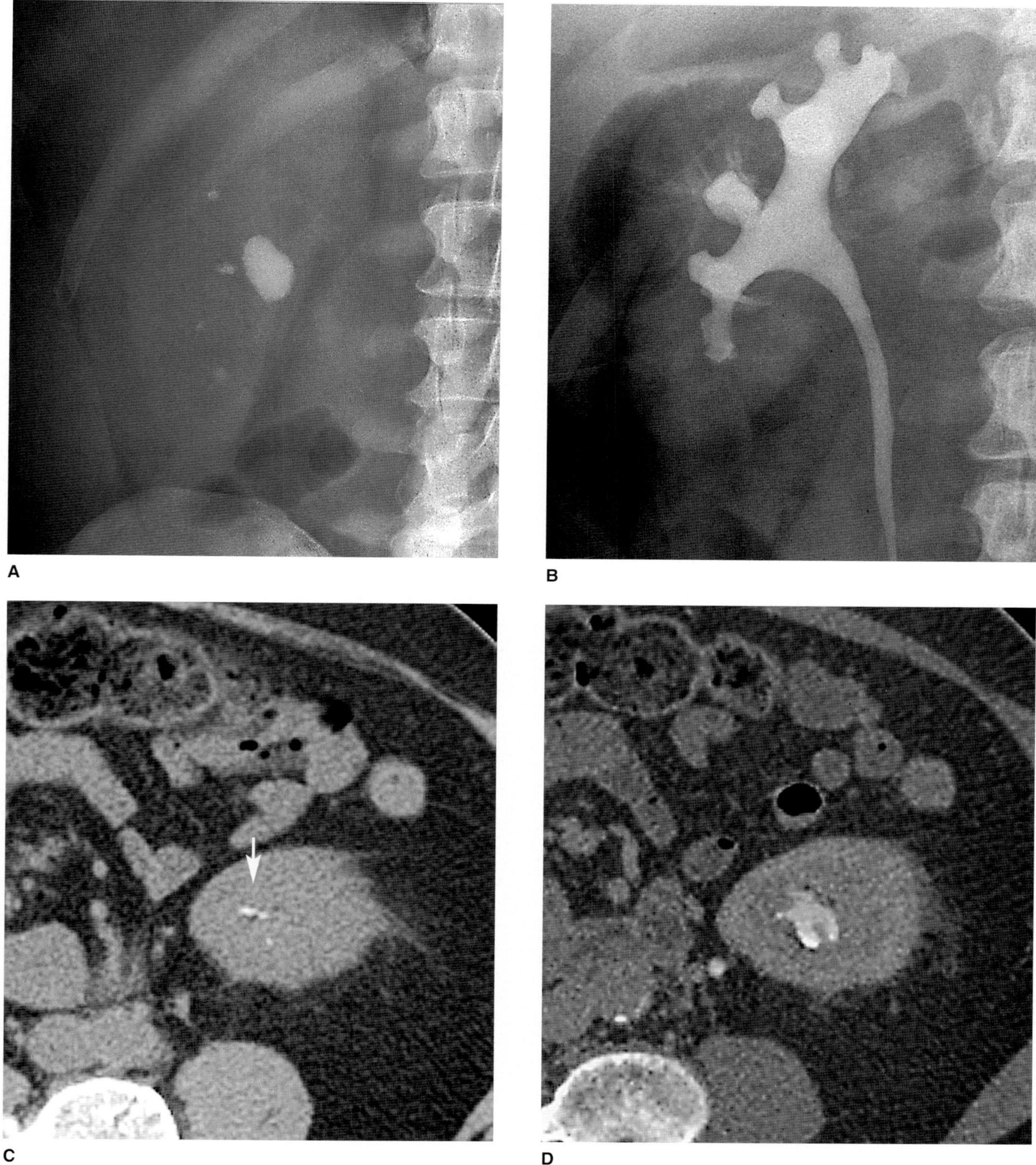

Figure 7-5 Stones Obscured by Contrast
A. Magnified image from the scout film of an IVU shows multiple small caliceal stones and 1 large pelvic stone in the right kidney collecting system. **B.** Image from the subsequent IVU shows the stones to be obscured by excreted intravenous contrast. **C.** Precontrast image from a CTU shows several punctate calcifications (*arrow*) in the lower pole of the left kidney. **D.** Urographic phase image at the same location shows the stones to be obscured by contrast in the collecting system.

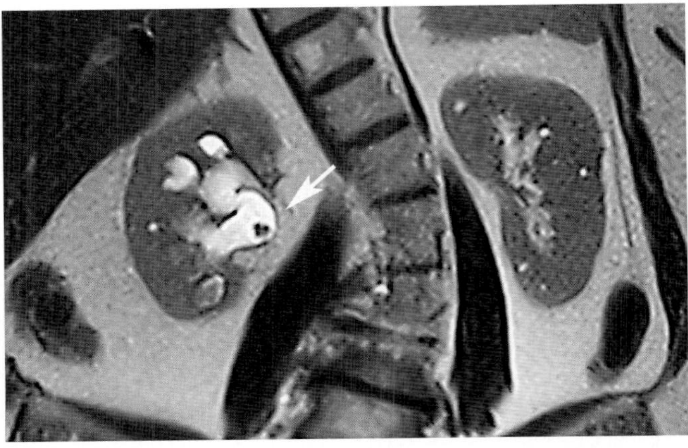

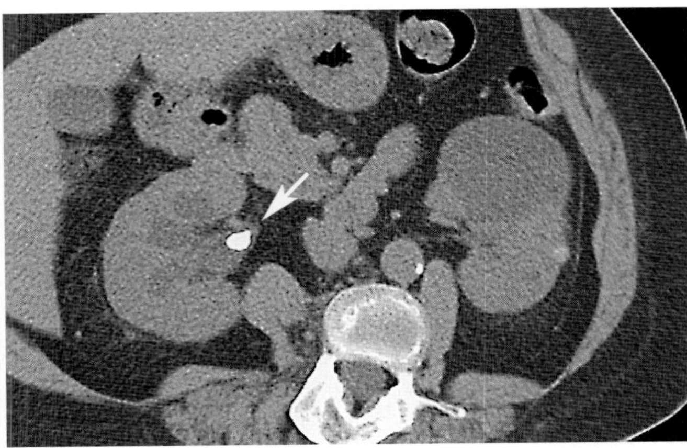

Figure 7-6 Renal Stones Demonstrated on MRI and CT
A. Coronal T2-weighted MRI sequence shows a small smooth filling defect (*arrow*) within the high signal urine of the right renal pelvis. This is likely to represent a renal calculus. **B.** Noncontrast CT confirms the presence of a calculus (*arrow*) in the right renal pelvis.

arise from the epithelium; the mesoderm; neural, vascular, and fibrous structures, or be secondary tumors due to hematogenous or local spread. Tumors arising from the epithelial lining (epithelial tumors) are the most common tumors in the urinary bladder and the collecting system and are referred to as urothelial tumors. Rare malignancies of the urinary tract include pheochromocytoma and small cell carcinoma of the bladder. Uncommon benign neoplasms include leiomyoma of the bladder wall and fibroepithelial polyp of the upper tracts.

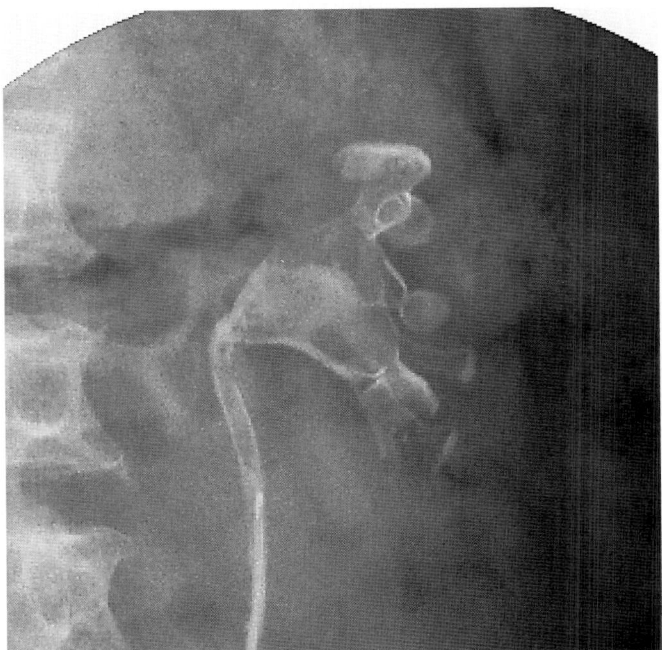

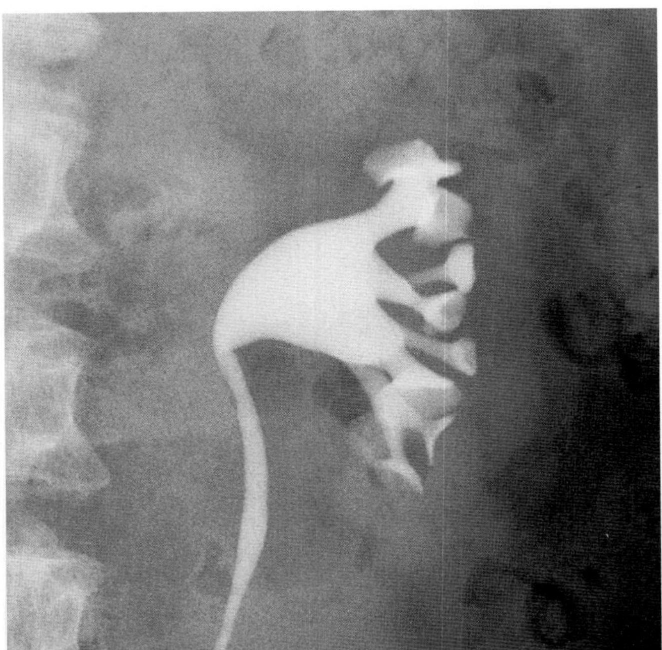

Figure 7-7 Blood Clots in the Collecting System
This 50-year-old patient presented with macroscopic hematuria. **A.** Retrograde pyelogram shows a filling defect that appears as a "cast" of the collecting system of the left kidney. The filling defect is outlined by a thin rim of contrast along the surface of the collecting system. **B.** Eight weeks later a follow-up retrograde pyelogram shows disappearance of the previous filling defect, confirming that it was a blood clot. The collecting system is normal in appearance with no urothelial abnormality.

Urothelial malignancies

Bladder cancer (urothelial malignancy of the bladder) is the most common neoplasm to affect the urinary system, with a peak incidence in the sixth and seventh decades of life. Men are affected 4 times more frequently than women. White patients have a higher incidence of bladder cancer than African American patients.[1,2] Patients usually present with either hematuria or symptoms of urinary frequency or dysuria. However, with the increasing use of cross-sectional imaging studies to evaluate all types of clinical problems, urothelial neoplasms can be found as an incidental mass on imaging being performed for another reason or may present with imaging evidence of urinary obstruction. Urothelial neoplasms are most commonly TCC, seen in 90% of cases. Other epithelial cancers of the urothelium include squamous cell carcinoma in 9% and adenocarcinoma in 1%.[3]

Histology: Transitional cell cancers are the most common tumors in the upper urinary tract and the bladder, with a characteristic propensity to be multifocal and to have a high rate of recurrence (see Figure 7-8). The bladder is affected 50 times more frequently than the upper urinary tract with

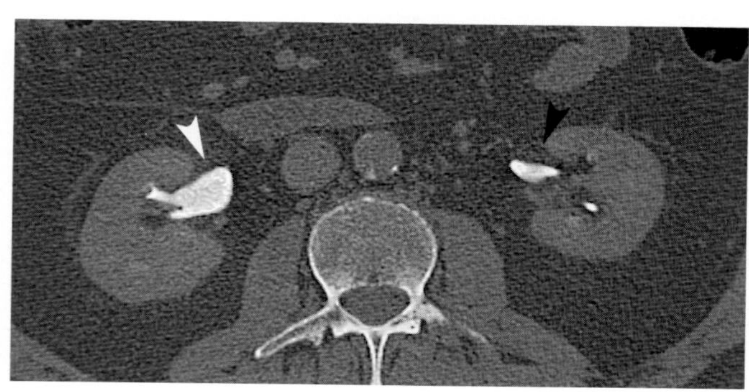

A

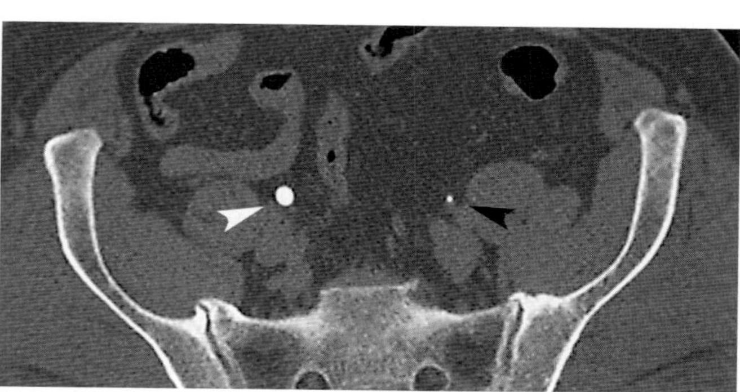

B

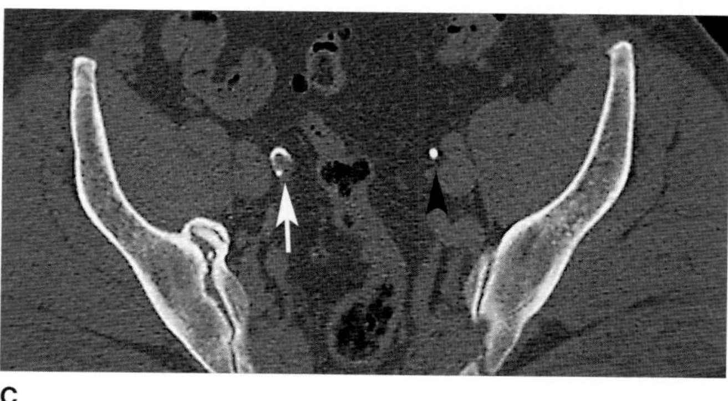

C

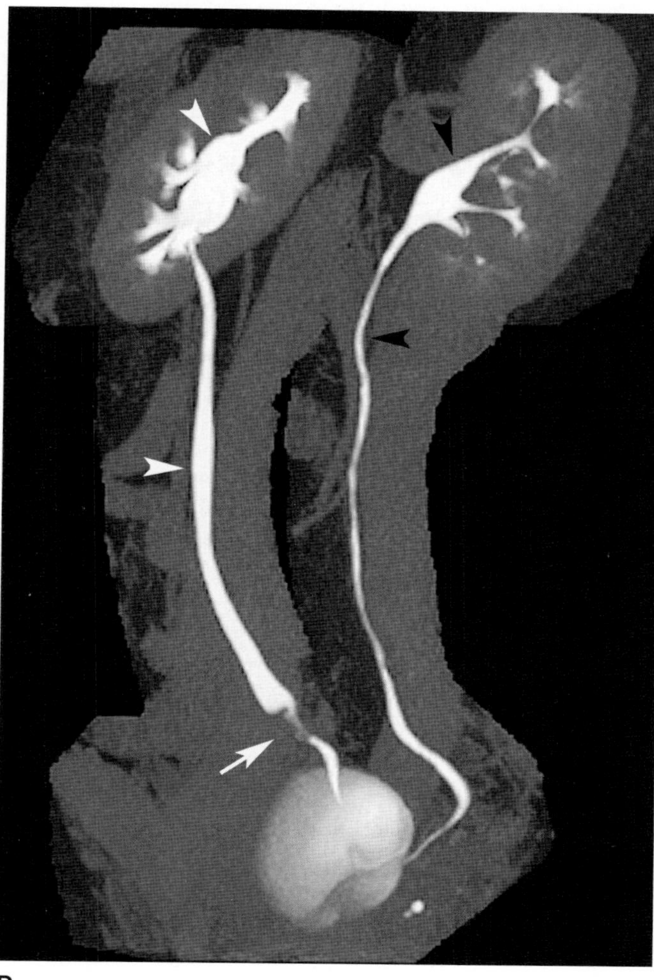

D

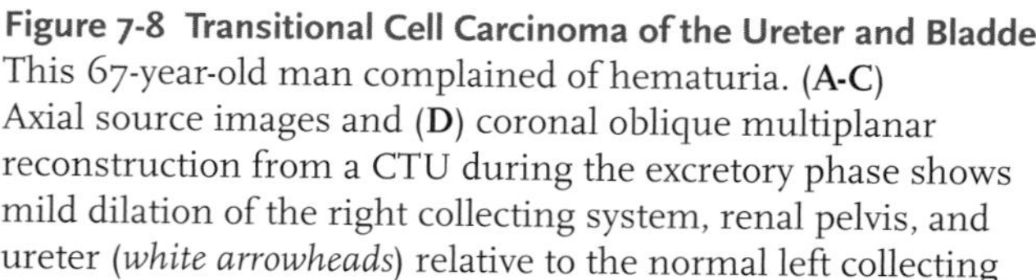

Figure 7-8 Transitional Cell Carcinoma of the Ureter and Bladder This 67-year-old man complained of hematuria. (**A-C**) Axial source images and (**D**) coronal oblique multiplanar reconstruction from a CTU during the excretory phase shows mild dilation of the right collecting system, renal pelvis, and ureter (*white arrowheads*) relative to the normal left collecting system, renal pelvis, and ureter (*black arrowheads*). In **C** there is a small filling defect (*arrow*) and in (D) there is a focal stricture (*arrow*) with a shelflike superior margin. This is a typical appearance of a ureteral cancer that was biopsy proven to represent a TCC.

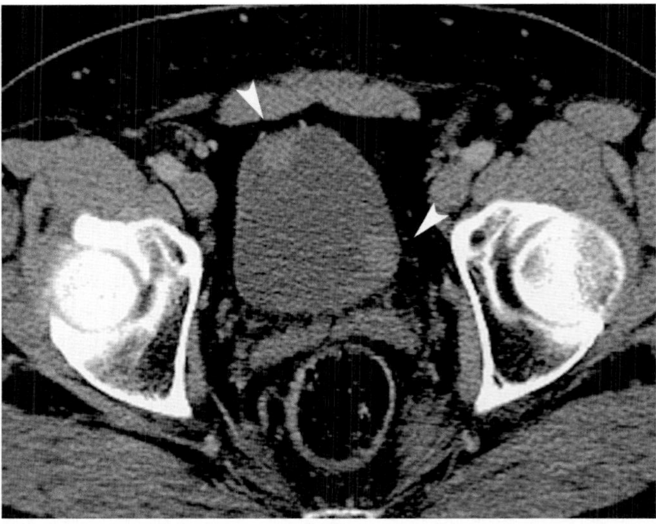

E

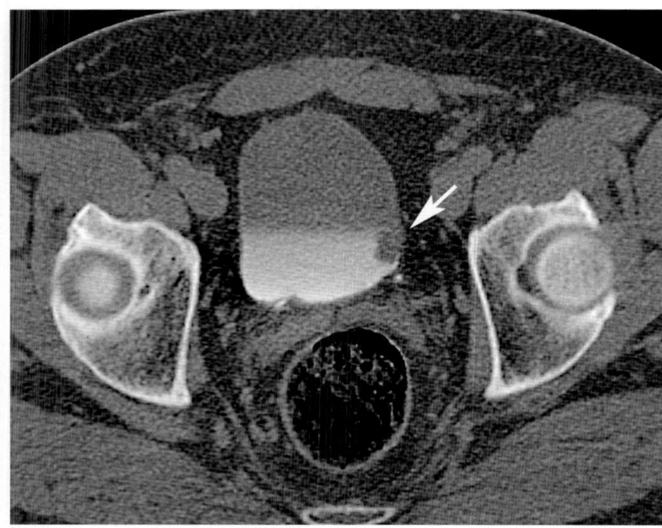

F

Figure 7-8 Transitional Cell Carcinoma of the Ureter and Bladder (*Continued*)
E. Contrast-enhanced image during the arterial phase of contrast shows 2 faint enhancing masses (*arrowheads*) projecting from the wall of the bladder into the bladder lumen. **F.** Excretory phase image at the same level shows contrast filling the posterior aspect of the bladder. The small mucosal mass on the left wall of the bladder is now seen as a filling defect in the contrast pool (*arrow*). The mass on the anterior wall is poorly visualized because it is surrounded by low-attenuation urine that has a similar attenuation to the mass. This is the typical appearance of small TCC of the bladder. For lesions located along the anterior wall of the bladder, a prone view in the excretory phase is often helpful in better delineating the anteriorly located tumors.

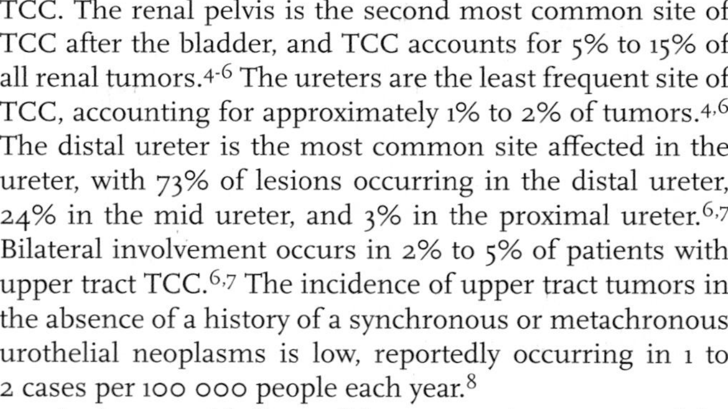

TCC. The renal pelvis is the second most common site of TCC after the bladder, and TCC accounts for 5% to 15% of all renal tumors.[4-6] The ureters are the least frequent site of TCC, accounting for approximately 1% to 2% of tumors.[4,6] The distal ureter is the most common site affected in the ureter, with 73% of lesions occurring in the distal ureter, 24% in the mid ureter, and 3% in the proximal ureter.[6,7] Bilateral involvement occurs in 2% to 5% of patients with upper tract TCC.[6,7] The incidence of upper tract tumors in the absence of a history of a synchronous or metachronous urothelial neoplasms is low, reportedly occurring in 1 to 2 cases per 100 000 people each year.[8]

As the uroepithelium of the upper urinary tract and the urinary bladder is similar, similar neoplasms occur throughout these structures and are referred to as "field neoplasms" or "field defects." Patients with bladder cancer are at a high risk for developing upper urinary tract TCC, which can occur in 2% to 4% of patients in a synchronous or metachronous fashion, whereas 40% of patients with upper tract tumors can develop TCC of the lower urinary tract.[6,7] When multiple, the lesions of TCC can arise in either a synchronous or metachronous fashion (see Figure 7-8). Therefore, patients with a previously diagnosed TCC will require routine surveillance imaging of the upper tracts and cystoscopy of the bladder to detect metachronous TCC.[9]

Squamous histology of urothelial neoplasms is largely confined to the bladder and is rare in the upper tracts. Squamous cell carcinomas (SCCs) are typically seen in association with chronic inflammation due to bladder stones, indwelling catheters, or infections such as that with *Schistosoma haematobium* (bilharziasis). The association between schistosomal infection and bladder carcinoma was first described in 1911, and it is due to exposure to freshwater snails in the rivers of North Africa. The parasite penetrates through the skin of the feet. Ova are deposited in the perivesical and lower periureteral venous plexus, where it causes bladder inflammation and bacterial coinfection. Malignancy, primarily SCC, ultimately develops as

Imaging Notes 7-2. Histology of Urothelial Malignancies

- The majority of urothelial malignancies are of transitional cell carcinoma histology and have tobacco smoking as a risk factor.
- Squamous histology is typically a complication of chronic inflammation due to
  - bladder calculi
  - indwelling catheters
  - recurrent/chronic infection
  - schistosomiasis
- Adenomatous histology is usually a tumor of urachal remnants and occurs at the anterior dome of the bladder or indicates invasion of the bladder from an extravesical malignancy.

a complication of chronic inflammation. Although most *Schistosoma*-related neoplasms are of squamous histology, there is also an increased risk of TCC and adenocarcinoma, in patients with bladder schistosomiasis, particularly in those who smoke. Schistosomiasis is discussed most completely under the heading **Bladder Wall Calcification** at the end of this chapter.

The large majority of urothelial adenocarcinomas arise from remnants of the urachus, the embryologic tube communicating between the bladder and the umbilicus. Adenocarcinoma is also seen with increased frequency in patients with cystitis glandularis, an idiopathic inflammatory condition of the pelvis seen predominantly in African American men that causes proliferation of pelvic fat and compression of the bladder and rectum. The congenital anomaly, bladder exstrophy, can also predispose to development of either SCC or adenocarcinomas of the bladder.

Etiology and risk factors: It is believed that noxious substances that are concentrated in the urine can act as carcinogens by inducing hyperplastic/metaplastic changes in the urothelium, and thus predispose patients exposed to such agents to the development of urothelial neoplasms.[4] Contact time with the urothelium appears to be an important factor in the probability of the development of cancer, accounting for the high incidence of urothelial tumors in the urinary bladder compared with the remainder of the upper urinary tract. Urinary stasis may also potentiate the development of urothelial neoplasms, such as with diverticula in the urinary bladder, or in patients with horseshoe kidneys where there is congenital ureteropelvic junction (UPJ) obstruction.[10] Exposure to carcinogens in tobacco smoke is the most common risk factor for the development of TCC, with heavy smokers of >40 pack-years being 5 times more likely to develop TCC compared with nonsmokers (see Table 7-1).[3]

Table 7-1. Risk Factors for the Development of Urothelial Malignancies

1. Toxic exposures a. **Tobacco smoke**[a] b. Aniline and azo dyes
2. Chronic irritation a. Bladder calculi b. Shistosomiasis hematobium infection
3. Medications a. Cyclophosphamide chemotherapy b. NSAID abuse (esp. phenacetin)
4. Congenital anomalies a. Bladder exstrophy b. Urachal remnants

[a]Risk factors in bold are common.

Other risk factors for development of urothelial neoplasms include industrial exposure to aniline and azo dyes, benzidine, and aromatic amines that were previously used in the manufacture of textiles, printing, and plastic manufacturing.[4] Chronic bladder irritation related to indwelling bladder catheters or certain urinary tract infections also has been linked to increased incidence of bladder urothelial malignancies, especially SCC.[11] *S haematobium* infection (bilharziasis) is endemic in many countries of Sub-Saharan Africa, and is associated with the development of SCCs, as well increasing the risk for development of other urothelial cancers, particularly in smokers.

Several medications can predispose to the development of urothelial malignancy. Cyclophosphamide (Cytoxan) is associated with a greatly increased risk of bladder Ca, with risk remaining for as long as 10 years after discontinuation of the drug.[12] Patients receiving cyclophosphamide can develop TCC, SCC, adenocarcinoma, fibrosarcoma, and also tumors in the pyelocalyceal system.

Analgesic abuse, especially phenacetin, has also been associated with an increased incidence of urothelial malignancies. Phenacetin, which is a component of compound analgesic agents—aspirin, phenacetin, and caffeine (APC tablets)—is associated with highly invasive TCC in renal pelvis. The drug availability has been severely restricted since 1979.[12] Analgesic nephropathy due to chronic ingestion of non-phenacetin nonsteroidal anti-inflammatory drugs, such as naproxen, aspirin, indomethacin, and paracetamol, has also been reported to confer a high risk of upper tract TCC in a renal transplant recipient population.[13] There is also a report of an over-the-counter Chinese herb for weight loss that is associated with the development of urothelial cancer.[14]

In Eastern Europe, there is an entity known as "Balkan nephropathy," which is an endemic degenerative interstitial nephropathy, which increases the risk of upper tract TCC 100- to 200-fold.[15]

Staging of bladder cancer: The bladder wall consists of a urothelial lining, which can be up to 7 cell layers in thickness, the submucosal connective tissue, which also contains smooth muscle fibers known as the lamina propria, and the muscular detrusor layer. Depth of invasion into the detrusor muscle is the most important factor in both the management and the prognosis. It follows, therefore,

Imaging Notes 7-3. Management of Bladder Neoplasms

- The most important factor in the management and prognosis of urothelial transitional cell carcinoma of the bladder is the depth of invasion of the tumor into the detrusor muscle.
- Superficial tumors can be resected with cystoscopy but deep muscle invasion requires cystectomy and urinary diversion.

that when a patient with bladder tumor is being evaluated and staged, the biopsy samples have to be deep enough to include the detrusor muscle for an accurate staging of the lesion.

The most widely used staging system is the TNM staging system (see Table 7-2).[16] T1 tumors are limited to the mucosa or subepithelial lamina propria. T2 tumors involve the superficial muscle (known as T2a tumors) or deep muscle (T2b). T3 tumors invade the perivesical tissues, either microscopically (T3a) or macroscopically (T3b). T4 tumors invade adjacent organs, such as the prostate or uterus, or extend to the pelvic side wall. N0 tumors have no nodal metastasis whereas higher N stages indicate nodal involvement. M1 disease indicates distant metastasis.[3,16]

Table 7-2. TNM Staging System for Bladder Carcinoma

Primary Tumor	
TX	Primary tumor cannot be assessed.
T0	No evidence of primary tumor.
Ta	Noninvasive papillary carcinoma.
Tis	Carcinoma in situ: "flat tumor."
T1	Tumor invades subepithelial connective tissue.
T2	Tumor invades muscularis propria.
pT2a	Tumor invades superficial muscularis propria (inner half).
pT2b	Tumor invades deep muscularis propria (outer half).
T3	Tumor invades perivesical tissue.
pT3a	Microscopically.
pT3b	Macroscopically (extravesical mass).
T4	Tumor invades any of the following: prostatic stroma, seminal vesicles, uterus, vagina, pelvic wall, abdominal wall.
T4a	Tumor invades prostatic stroma, uterus, vagina.
T4b	Tumor invades pelvic wall, abdominal wall.
Regional Lymph Nodes	
NX	Lymph nodes cannot be assessed.
N0	No lymph node metastasis.
N1	Single regional lymph node metastasis in the true pelvis (hypogastric, obturator, external iliac, or presacral lymph node).
N2	Multiple regional lymph node metastases in the true pelvis (hypogastric, obturator, external iliac, or presacral lymph node).
N3	Lymph node metastases to the common iliac lymph nodes.
Distant Metastasis	
M0	No distant metastasis.
M1	Distant metastasis.

Reproduced, with permission, from AJCC. Urinary bladder. In: Edge SB, Byrd DR, Compton CC, et al, eds. *AJCC Cancer Staging Manual*. 7th ed. New York, NY: Springer; 2010:497-505.

Superficial tumors account for 70% to 80% of urothelial malignancies of the bladder. They are limited to the mucosa or lamina propria, have a very low risk of metastasis but a strong propensity to recur, with 70% recurring within 3 years. Approximately 10% to 20% of recurrences will be found to have invasive disease.[7,17] Approximately 70% of superficial tumors are low-grade papillary carcinomas and approximately 30% are flat carcinomas in situ (CIS), which are of higher grade, have a greater propensity to recur, and are more likely to become muscle invasive. CIS cannot be detected on imaging and appear as "velvety" patches at cystoscopy. Muscle-invasive tumors involve the wall to a lesser or greater depth and can eventually invade the adjacent perivesical structures. Depth of invasion is the most important prognostic factor, with greater depth of invasion indicating increased risk of metastasis. Deeply invasive tumors have a poor prognosis, with only a 10% to 15% rate of cure.[7,17]

Lymphatic spread occurs initially to the regional nodes, including the perivesical, sacral, presacral, hypogastric, obturator, and external iliac groups. With progression, lymphatic involvement will spread to the common iliac chain and the para-aortic nodes.

Hematogenous metastasis can occur to the liver, lungs, bones, and adrenal glands. Prognosis for the patient worsens with advancing stage. The 5-year survival for superficial disease is 94% but only 6% for metastatic disease.

Staging of upper tract TCC: The TNM system is the most frequently used system for staging upper urinary tract tumors.[16] The staging systems are similar to that for bladder cancer, and imaging is very useful for detecting depth of tumor invasion and determining optimal management. With both renal pelvic and ureteral tumors, T1 tumors are those that are limited to the epithelium and subepithelial connective tissue and T2 tumors are those that invade the muscularis layer. T3 tumors of the renal pelvis extend into the peripelvic fat or renal parenchyma, whereas T3 tumors of the ureter extend beyond the muscularis into the periureteric fat. If imaging studies depict T3 disease, the most appropriate surgical treatment is surgical excision, so that the disease can be completely excised. T4 lesions extend into adjacent organs, or through the kidney into the perinephric fat. Nodal (N) and distant metastatic (M) disease are detailed (Table 7-3). Direct spread is common with upper tract TCC. Lymphatic extension is frequent because of the rich lymphatic drainage of the collecting system and ureter, with extension of disease to the

Table 7-3. Staging System for Urothelial Malignancy of the Renal Pelvis and Ureter

TX	Primary tumor cannot be assessed.
T0	No evidence of primary tumor.
Ta	Papillary noninvasive carcinoma.
Tis	Carcinoma in situ.
T1	Tumor invades subepithelial connective tissue.
T2	Tumor invades the muscularis.
T3	(For renal pelvis only) Tumor invades beyond muscularis into peripelvic fat or the renal parenchyma T3. (For ureter only) Tumor invades beyond muscularis into periureteric fat.
T4	Tumor invades adjacent organs, or through the kidney into the perinephric fat.
Regional Lymph Nodes	
NX	Regional lymph nodes cannot be assessed.
N0	No regional lymph node metastasis.
N1	Metastasis in a single lymph node, ≤2 cm in greatest dimension.
N2	Metastasis in a single lymph node, >2 cm but not >5 cm in greatest dimension; or multiple lymph nodes, none >5 cm in greatest dimension.
N3	Metastasis in a lymph node, >5 cm in greatest dimension.
Distant Metastasis	
M0	No distant metastasis.
M1	Distant metastasis.

Reproduced, with permission, from AJCC. Renal pelvis and ureter. In: Edge SB, Byrd DR, Compton CC, et al, eds. *AJCC Cancer Staging Manual*. 7th ed. New York, NY: Springer; 2010;491-496.

draining retroperitoneal lymph nodes. Hematogenous metastases and invasion of the renal vein and inferior vena cava are uncommon. T3 lesions of the renal pelvis have a more favorable prognosis than T3 lesions of the ureter, as the renal parenchyma acts as a barrier for direct spread. Invasive renal pelvic tumors infiltrate the renal sinus and parenchyma but typically preserve the reniform renal contour, a feature that distinguishes infiltrative urothelial cancer from renal cell carcinoma, which often causes a mass that deforms the renal contour (see Figure 6-5).

Clinical presentation and diagnosis: TCC has a peak incidence in the sixth and seventh decades of life and usually presents with either hematuria or with clinical symptoms and/or imaging evidence of urinary obstruction.

Cystoscopy and cystoscopically directed biopsy are the mainstays for the diagnosis and staging of bladder cancer. Biopsies should encompass all layers of the bladder wall for accurate staging, and the histopathologic evaluation is aimed at determining the cell type of the tumor as well as its grade and depth of invasion (Imaging Notes 7-3). The primary role of imaging currently in patients with invasive bladder cancer is to evaluate for perivesical and extravesical disease, and to look for upper tract involvement. When disease is suspected in the upper tract, further evaluation is performed with retrograde pyelograms and fluoroscopically guided brush biopsy of suspected malignancies or by uterteroscopy, depending on the institution.

Imaging findings in bladder cancer: The imaging evaluation of bladder malignancies is done primarily with CT or MRI examinations. Both IVU and US examinations can occasionally detect the primary bladder tumor, but they are not capable of accurately evaluating for extravesical spread, which is the primary function of imaging in the evaluation of bladder malignancies (see Figures 7-4 and 7-9).

The 2 main findings seen with urothelial malignancies of the bladder are focal or asymmetric bladder wall thickening, or an intraluminal mass or polyp (see Figures 7-8 and 7-9). Stippled calcifications can be seen on the surface of the tumor, and strongly suggest the diagnosis of a papillary neoplasm (see Figure 7-10). Although CT urography can demonstrate a bladder tumor, its role in the primary diagnosis of a suspected bladder tumor remains in evolution.[18] Further, CT is reported to have a sensitivity of 79% to 90% and specificity of 91% to 94% in detecting bladder carcinoma when cystoscopy is used as the gold standard.[19,20] In clinical practice, cross-sectional imaging studies are primarily utilized to stage a tumor rather than for primary detection of a bladder neoplasm. It is important to have the bladder well distended to detect subtle wall thickening, a sign of early bladder tumors, because the normal underdistended bladder can appear to be thick walled.

MRI is somewhat more accurate than CT for assessing the depth of tumor invasion into the bladder wall, as the layers of the bladder wall are somewhat better seen (see Figure 7-9). The bladder cancer lesions are isointense to detrusor muscle on T1-weighted sequences, slightly hyperintense relative to muscle on T2-weighted sequences, and demonstrate enhancement on dynamic postcontrast sequences.

Extravesical spread is indicated by the presence of soft-tissue nodules or fat stranding in the adjacent perivesical fat on both CT and MRI (see Figure 7-11). However, because imaging studies are often performed after a cystoscopic biopsy has already established the diagnosis, perivesical stranding can be seen as a result of the biopsy and can lead to overstaging of the malignancy if the interpreter is not careful to account for this factor. Accuracy in separating superficial from invasive disease in 1 series was 85%. Accuracy for differentiating organ confined versus

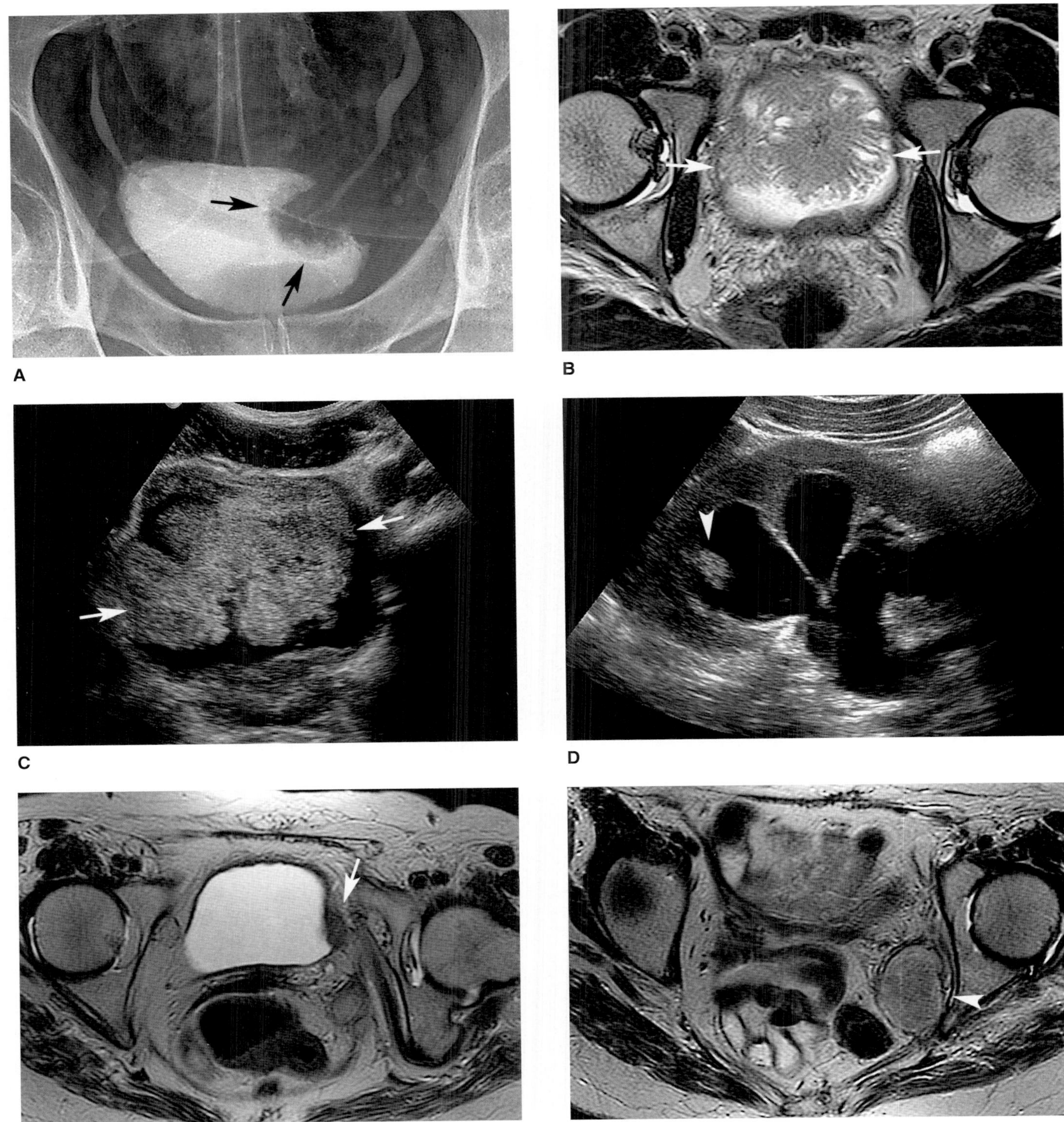

Figure 7-9 Transitional Cell Carcinoma (TCC) of Bladder in 3 Patients

This 70-year-old man presented with macroscopic hematuria. **A.** Image from an IVU shows a lobulated filing defect (*arrows*) displacing contrast from the left lateral wall of the urinary bladder, near the left ureteral orifice. Biopsy confirmed a diagnosis of TCC. **B-D.** This 35-year-old man presented with hematuria. (B) Axial T2-weighted image demonstrate a large frondlike mass (*arrows*) projecting into the lumen of the bladder from the anterior wall. This frondlike appearance is one of the appearances of TCC. (C) Transaxial US of the bladder shows a similar appearance to the mass (*arrows*). (D) Longitudinal US of the left kidney shows hydronephrosis and a small pedunculated nodule (*arrowhead*) in a superior calyx. This could represent debris or a blood clot but might indicate the presence of a metachronous upper tract primary. The hydronephrosis was due to obstruction of the distal left ureter by a second bladder primary TCC. **E** and **F.** T2-weighted, fat-saturated axial MRI images in a third patient demonstrate a focal region of bladder wall thickening (*arrow*) associated with a large left obturator lymph node (*arrowhead*). Focal wall thickening is another common appearance of bladder TCC. Lymph node metastasis will typically first involve the pelvic nodes, especially the obturator lymph nodes.

Imaging Notes 7-4. Evaluation of Bladder Cancer

Cross-sectional imaging in the evaluation of bladder cancer is done to determine intramuscular and extravesical spread of tumor:

1. Invasion of detrusor muscle (MR only)
   a. High T2 signal tumor within detrusor muscle
   b. Enhancing tumor within detrusor muscle
2. Invasion beyond the bladder wall
   a. Soft tissue nodules or fat stranding in the perivesical fat[a]
3. Lymphadenopathy
   a. Perivesical, sacral, presacral, hypogastric, obturator, and external iliac
4. Hematogenous metastasis
   a. Liver, lungs, bones, and adrenal glands

[a]Fat stranding can be caused by recent cystoscopic biopsy and can be a false-positive imaging finding for extravesical spread.

non–organ confined was 82%, primarily because of overstaging of inflammatory or reactive stranding.[21]

CT and MRI done with conventional techniques have similar rates of accuracy for pelvic nodal staging: 70% to 97% and 73% to 98%, respectively.[7] The role of advanced techniques such as dynamic contrast enhancement characteristics of lymph nodes or the use of MR lymphographic contrast agents such as ultra small particles of iron oxide remains the subject of study.

Cross-sectional imaging techniques, as well as conventional imaging, remain very valuable to evaluate bladder diverticula for the development of tumors, because cystoscopic evaluation of the interior of the diverticulum can be technically challenging. Tumors that occur within diverticula are more prone to early extravesical spread, as bladder diverticula are composed only of a mucosal layer and lack the detrusor as a barrier to the spread of the tumor.

Adenocarcinoma is a rare histology for a bladder primary malignancy and, if discovered, the imaging examination should be scrutinized to exclude an extravesical primary malignancy. The majority of primary bladder adenocarcinomas arise from remnants of the urachus. As a consequence, they are characteristically located on the anterior superior surface of the dome of the urinary bladder, and a mass in this location should suggest the potential for a urachal adenocarcinoma. These lesions may demonstrate calcification and can present at an advanced stage because the patients are often asymptomatic. An infected urachal diverticulum can simulate a primary adenocarcinoma. However, clinical features of infection such as fever and abdominal pain can be a clue to identifying an infected diverticulum. Frequently, biopsy is required to make a definitive distinction. Non–urachal-related adenocarcinomas are exceedingly rare and have an imaging appearance indistinguishable from the more common TCC.

SCCs have an imaging appearance indistinguishable from the more common TCC. However, these malignancies are typically seen in association with chronic inflammation

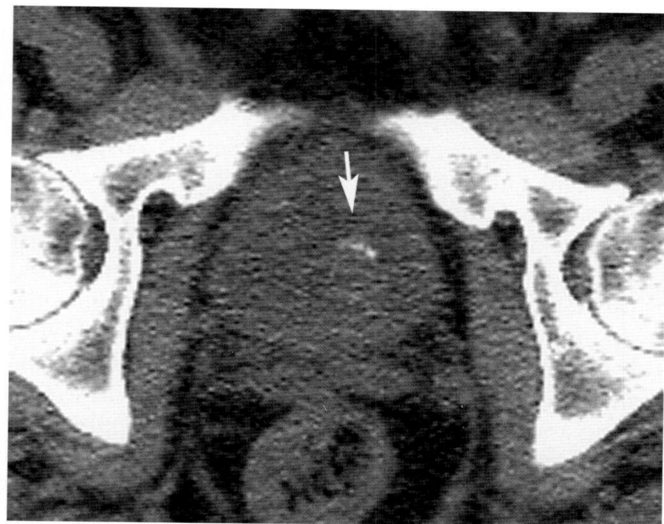
A

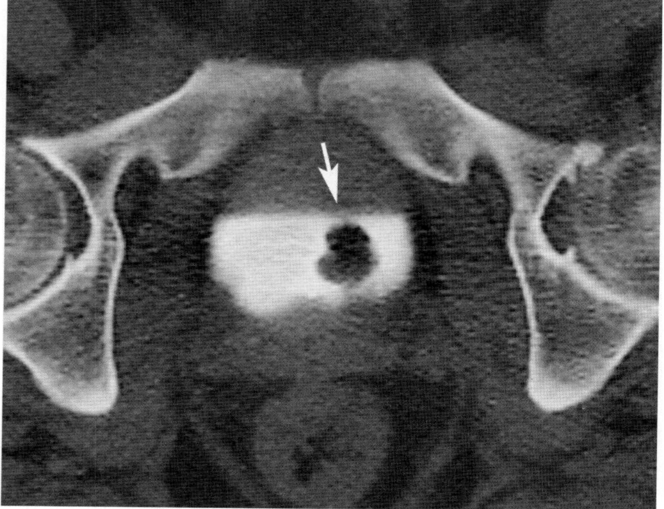
B

Figure 7-10 Calcified Bladder Cancer
This 62-year-old man presented with hematuria. **A.** Image from the unenhanced sequence of a CTU demonstrates a faint curvilinear calcification (*arrow*) within the bladder lumen that could represent a faintly calcified neoplasm. A calcified stone is less likely because the calcification is protruding into the lumen and is not settling into the dependent portion of the bladder, as expected with a stone. **B.** Urographic phase image confirms the presence of a polypoid mass (*arrow*), which was subsequently proven to represent a TCC.

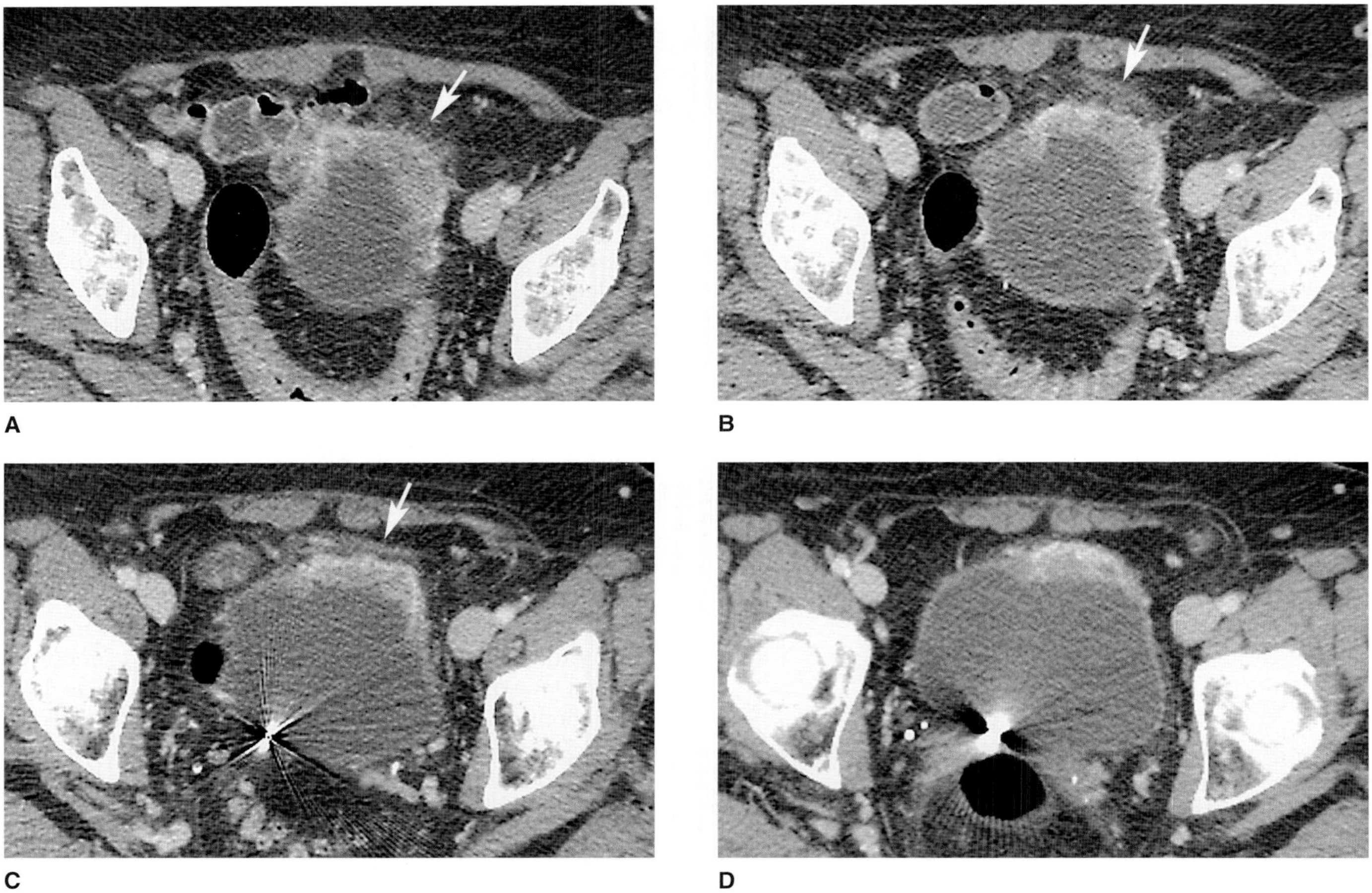

A

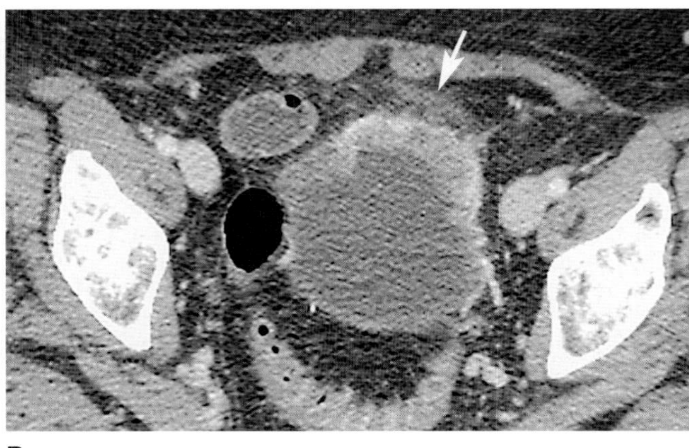

B

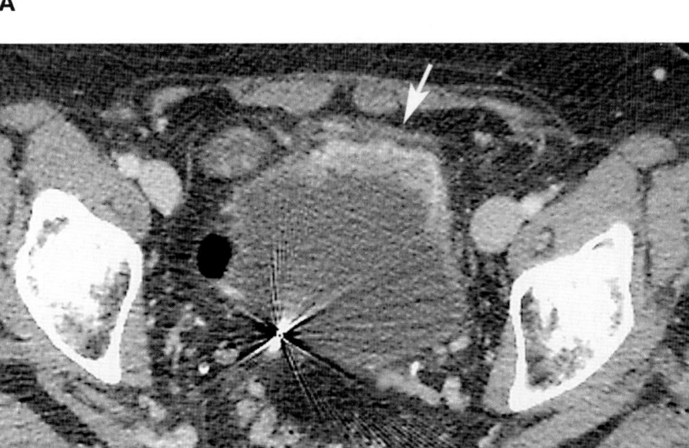

C

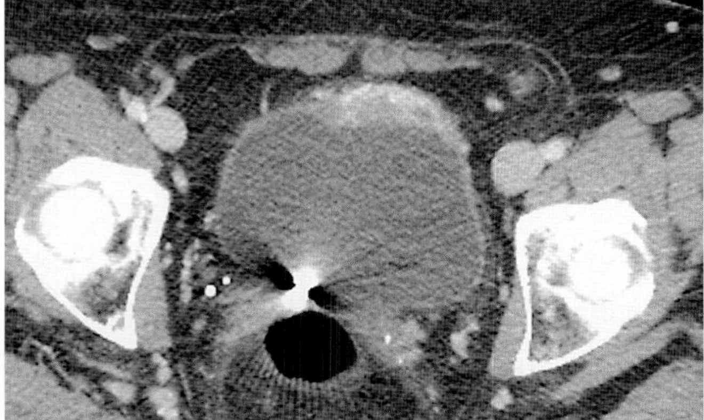

D

Figure 7-11 Perivesical Invasion by Transitional Cell Carcinoma (TCC)
This 67-year-old woman had hematuria. **A-D**. Contrast-enhanced CT shows extensive thickening (*arrows*) of the anterior wall and dome of the bladder, most likely representing a TCC of the bladder. Note the perivesical fat stranding. The margins between the bladder and perivesical fat are indistinct. These findings will usually indicate invasion of the perivesical fat, which was confirmed at cystectomy.

due to bladder stones, indwelling catheters, or infections such as *S haematobium* infection (bilharziasis). Thus, the presence of bladder stones, catheters, or bladder wall calcification, a manifestation of schistosomiasis, can be clues to a diagnosis of SCC. Typically, despite the heavy calcification of the bladder wall that is a feature of schistosomal infection, the bladder remains distensible and of normal volume.

Imaging features of upper tract urothelial malignancies: In contrast to bladder cancer, imaging is of paramount importance in the diagnosis as well as staging of upper tract urothelial tumors. Intravenous urography (IVU) has been largely supplanted by CTU for the evaluation of the upper urinary tracts in both newly diagnosed patients as well as for those undergoing surveillance for a history of urothelial cancer. The advantage of CTU is that diagnostic assessment and staging can be performed in one examination. The imaging findings on an IVU and retrograde pyelogram include filling defects, obstruction, and irregular areas of narrowing (see Figures 7-3 and 7-12).

Computed tomographic urography is currently the procedure of choice for the detection and staging of upper tract TCC, although no randomized prospective study comparing CT urography with excretory urography for sensitivity in detecting upper tract TCC has been published. With current techniques, a single CT examination allows for the evaluation of the urinary tract in multiple planes, as well as staging assessment for periureteric and renal infiltration, and the status of regional nodes and distant metastases (see Figure 7-13).

On noncontrast scans, stippled calcification may be seen on the surface of the tumor, similar to that in bladder TCC (see Figure 7-13). On arterial and nephrographic phase imaging, the lesions show some enhancement, and in the excretory phase, they are seen as filling defects, irregularly narrowed segments, or as focal wall thickening (see Figure 7-8). In 1 study, urothelial thickening was more predictive of tumor

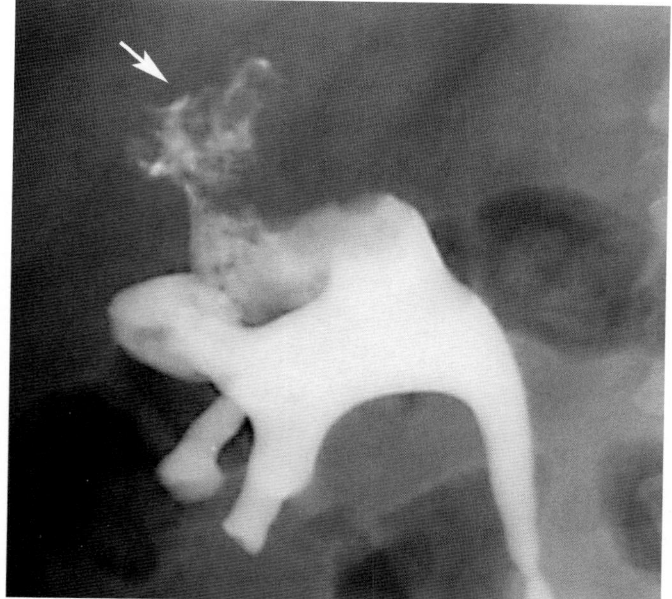

A

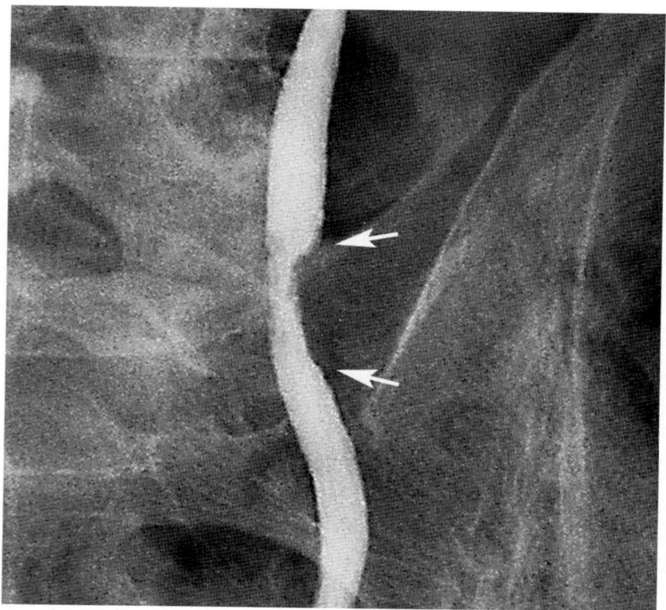

B

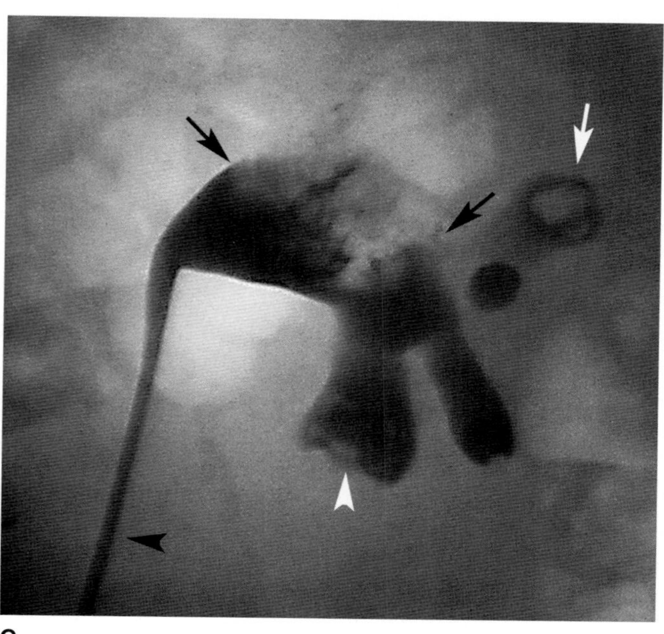

C

Figure 7-12 Imaging Manifestations of Upper Tract Urethelial Malignancies in 2 Patients
A and **B.** This 48-year-old man presented with a history of bladder cancer diagnosed 5 years previously. (A) Surveillance IVU shows a polypoid, multilobulated filling defect (*arrow*) in the upper pole calices, extending into the proximal renal pelvis. (B) Images of the left ureter shows a slightly irregular narrowing (*between arrows*) of the left ureter. These were shown to represent synchronous primary TCC. **C.** This 58-year-old man had microscopic hematuria. Retrograde pyelogram demonstrates a multilobulated filling defect (*delimited by the black arrows*) in the superior aspect of the renal pelvis. The upper pole calices do not fill with contrast because this mass has obstructed the connecting infundibuli. This is a typical appearance of a TCC. There is also a filling defect in the uppermost calyx (*white arrow*) that has a rounded appearance and is typical of a small air bubble that has been injected with the contrast. There is also a filiform filling defect in the inferior calyx that is probably a small blood clot (*white arrowhead*) but could be a second focus of TCC. The catheter (*black arrowhead*) from the retrograde pyelogram is seen in the ureter.

in the pelvicaliceal system than in the ureter, whereas filling defects were more predictive of a tumor in the ureter rather in the pelvicaliceal system.[8] Masses involving the calyces, infundibuli, UPJ, and ureters can cause obstruction and dilation of the collecting system proximal to the tumor. Ureteral lesions can completely occupy the lumen, such that only a thickened ureteral segment may be seen.

On MRI, TCC of the urinary tract are typically hypointense to isointense to the skeletal muscle on T2 images and hypointense to intermediate signal intensity on T1 images and show moderate enhancement in postcontrast images.[22-24]

When renal pelvic tumors are separated by a fat plane from the renal sinus, they can be classified as localized disease, and the treatment of choice in a patient with normal renal function is radical nephroureterectomy along with excision of a cuff of bladder. When tumors get larger and infiltrate the parenchyma, the reniform contour is maintained (see Figure 7-13). However, in extremely large lesions, the distinction between a large renal cell cancer and TCC can be difficult, as it is not possible to determine the origin of the mass (see Figure 7-13).

Although MRI is very valuable in the evaluation of the abdomen for metastatic disease and for assessment

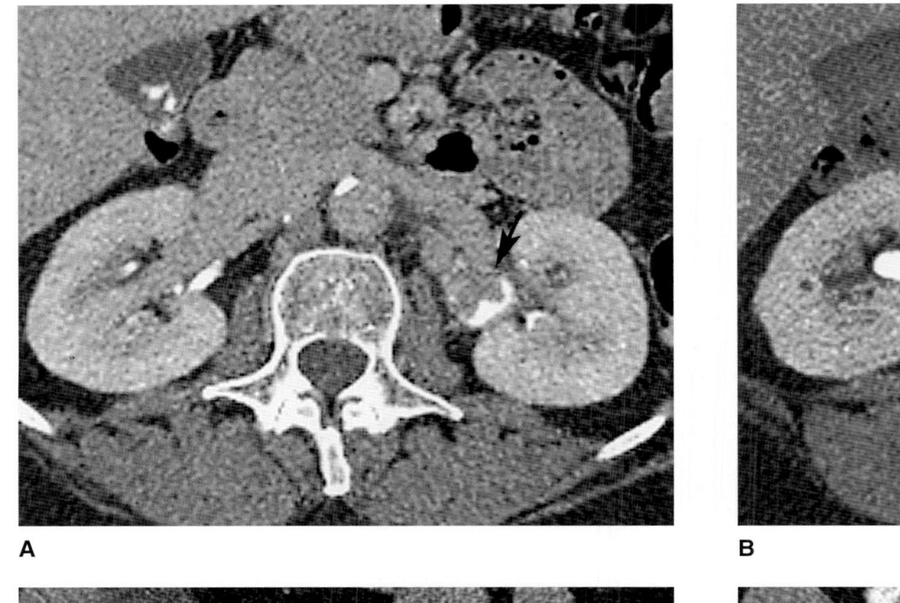

A

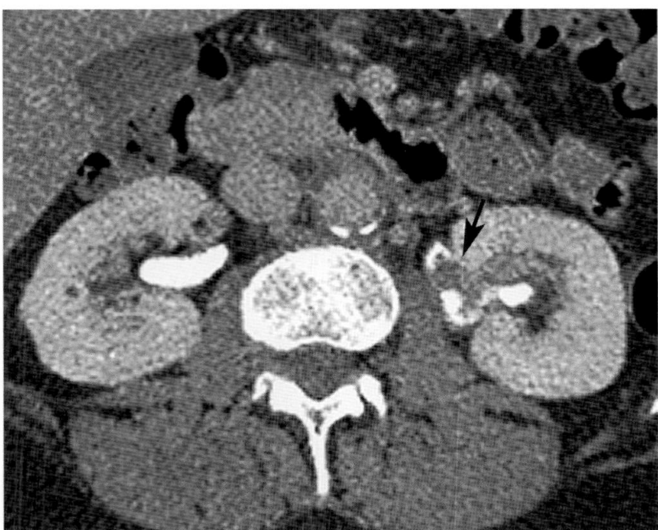

B

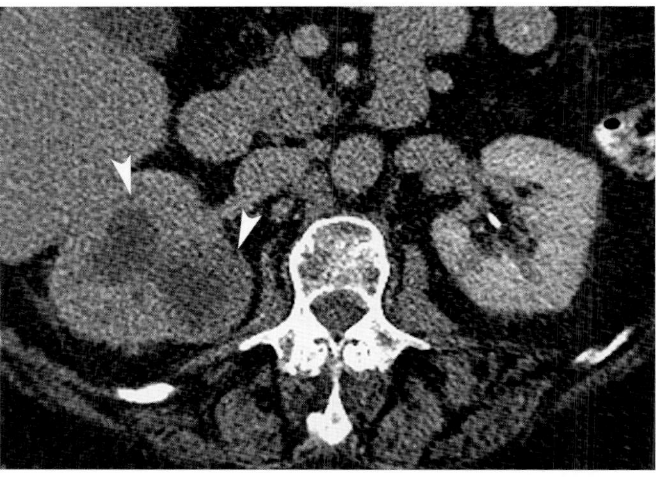

C

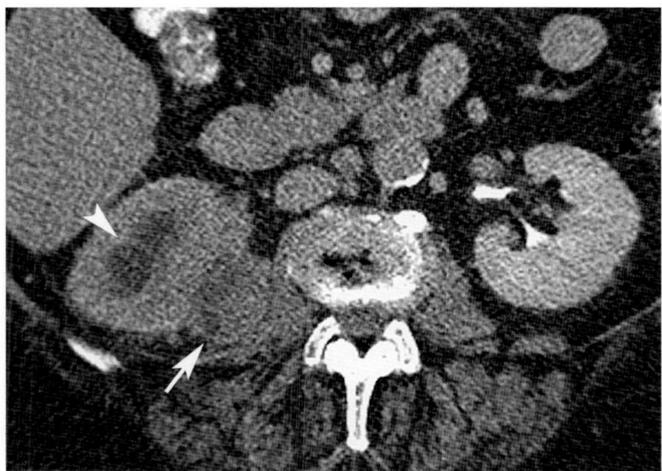

D

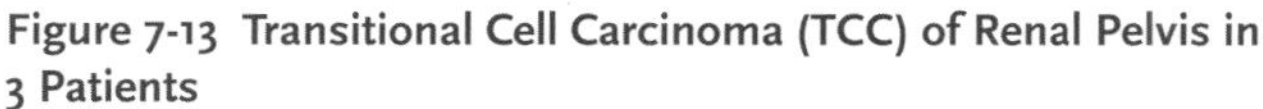

Figure 7-13 Transitional Cell Carcinoma (TCC) of Renal Pelvis in 3 Patients
A and **B**. This 55-year-old woman had hematuria and abdominal pain. Two images from a CTU show a lobulated filling defect (*black arrows*) within the left renal pelvis. This is a typical appearance of a medium-sized TCC of the renal pelvis. **C** and **D**. This 75-year-old woman had breast cancer. Excretory-phase images from an abdominal CT show a large lobulated mass filling the right renal pelvis (*white arrowheads*) and extending into the right proximal ureter (*white arrow*). There is no excretion of contrast into the right collecting system as the tumor is causing high-grade obstruction. Note the normal appearance of the left collecting system. Although this could represent a renal metastasis, the involvement of the collecting system and ureter is a characteristic trait of larger TCC and less common finding of metastases.

of lymphadenopathy, MR urography for evaluation of the collecting system is still in evolution. The significantly poorer spatial resolution of MR makes it inferior to CTU for assessment of upper tract urothelial lesions. If a patient cannot get intravenous contrast for a CTU or IVU, the procedure of choice is a retrograde pyeloureterogram.

Paraganglioma (pheochromocytoma) of the bladder

Paraganglioma (extra-adrenal pheochromocytoma) is a rare but well-recognized neoplasm of the urinary bladder because of the unique presentation of the tumor. Paragangliomas of the urinary bladder are believed to arise in the paraganglia of the autonomic nervous system, which are located submucosally either in (1) the dome or (2) the posterior wall, close to the trigone.[25,26] This characteristic location can be a clue to the diagnosis of bladder paragangliomas. These tumors secrete catecholamines and are a rare cause of systemic hypertension. The classic history is a triad of sustained hypertension, hematuria, and postmicturition syncope.[26] However, many patients will present throbbing headaches during micturition or isolated hematuria without other symptoms.[25]

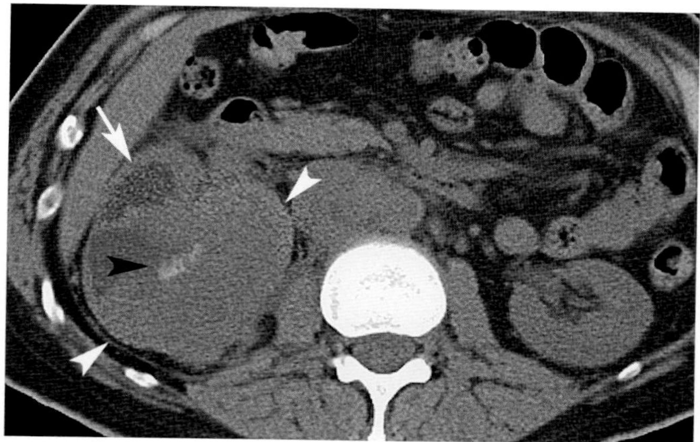

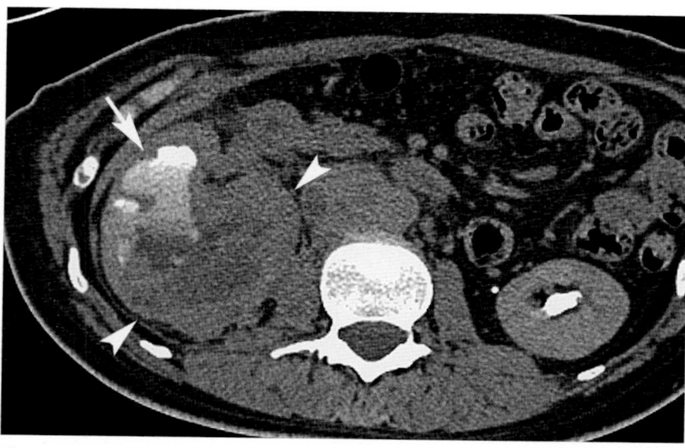

Figure 7-13 Transitional Cell Carcinoma (TCC) of Renal Pelvis in 3 Patients (*Continued*)
E and **F**. This 75-year-old man presented with back pain. (E) Precontrast and (F) excretory-phase images show a large mass (*white arrowheads*) which expands the kidney volume but does not cause a contour deformity. The mass has faint calcifications (*black arrowhead*) on the unenhanced image and causes obstruction and dilation of several calyces (*white arrows*). Note that the perinephric fat posterior to the mass is infiltrated—a sign that likely indicates extracapsular spread of malignancy. Biopsy was diagnostic of TCC in all 3 patients.

Reports of bladder paragangliomas suggest that they typically appear as sharply marginated masses within the wall of the bladder (see Figure 7-14).[26,27] Location in the dome or near the trigone can also be a clue to the diagnosis. On US, they can appear as a uniform echogenic mass.[26] Paragangliomas typically display intermediate signal intensity on T1-weighted images and high signal intensity on T2-weighted images, which is thought to be due to high intracellular water content and rich vascularity of the tumor.[26,27] Typically, there is intense enhancement of the tumor with the use of intravenous contrast (see Figure 7-14). If a pheochromocytoma is suspected, a definitive diagnosis can be made with ^{131}I-MIBG scintigraphy demonstration of uptake in the tumor.

Small cell carcinoma

Small-cell carcinoma of the bladder is a rare tumor, with only a few case reports in the English medical literature.[28,29] A multi-institutional review of 3778 patients with a primary malignancy of the urinary bladder demonstrated 18 cases (0.48%).[29] It often contains a mixture of small-cell carcinoma, TCC, and adenocarcinoma. Histologically and clinically, the tumor is similar to small-cell carcinoma of the lung.[28,29] Like with other urothelial-derived neoplasms, most patients present with hematuria. Small-cell carcinoma of bladder typically is an aggressive malignancy characterized by early systemic dissemination and death from metastatic disease. Imaging will usually show focal 2- to 10-cm bladder wall mass indistinguishable from advanced-stage TCC.[28,29] Hemorrhage and calcification of the mass can be seen. Most frequent sites of metastasis include regional lymph nodes, liver, skeleton, and peritoneum.[29]

Urachal carcinoma

The urachus is lined by transitional epithelium, which undergoes metaplasia to columnar epithelium in about one-third of subjects. The great majority of urachal cancers are adenocarcinomas, and up to 75% are mucin-producing adenocarcinomas. At CT, urachal adenocarcinoma is typically a midline supravesical mass that contains low-density mucin. Although calcification in urachal carcinoma is a rare plain film finding, it is seen in the majority of tumors examined with CT.[3] The calcification may show a peripheral curvilinear pattern, may be in coarse flecks, or may be punctate, the latter pattern being similar to that seen in mucinous adenocarcinoma of the bladder (see Figure 7-15).

Leiomyoma

Leiomyoma of the smooth muscle is the most common benign tumor in the urinary bladder and can rarely be discovered in the upper tract. It is reported to account for less than 1% of all bladder masses.[30] Histologically, the tumor is similar to the more common uterine fibroid. The reasons why some individuals develop leiomyomas of the urinary tract remains obscure. Many patients will be clinically asymptomatic, and the tumor is detected incidentally on physical examination or imaging examinations. When symptomatic, most bladder leiomyomas present with gross hematuria, pelvic pain, dysuria, or increased frequency.[31] Symptoms related to obstruction are rare but occasionally reported.

Most leiomyomas are less than 10 cm in diameter; however, sizes of a few millimeters to 30 cm have been reported. Lesions can (1) project into the lumen of the bladder (63%-83%), (2) project outward into the perivesical

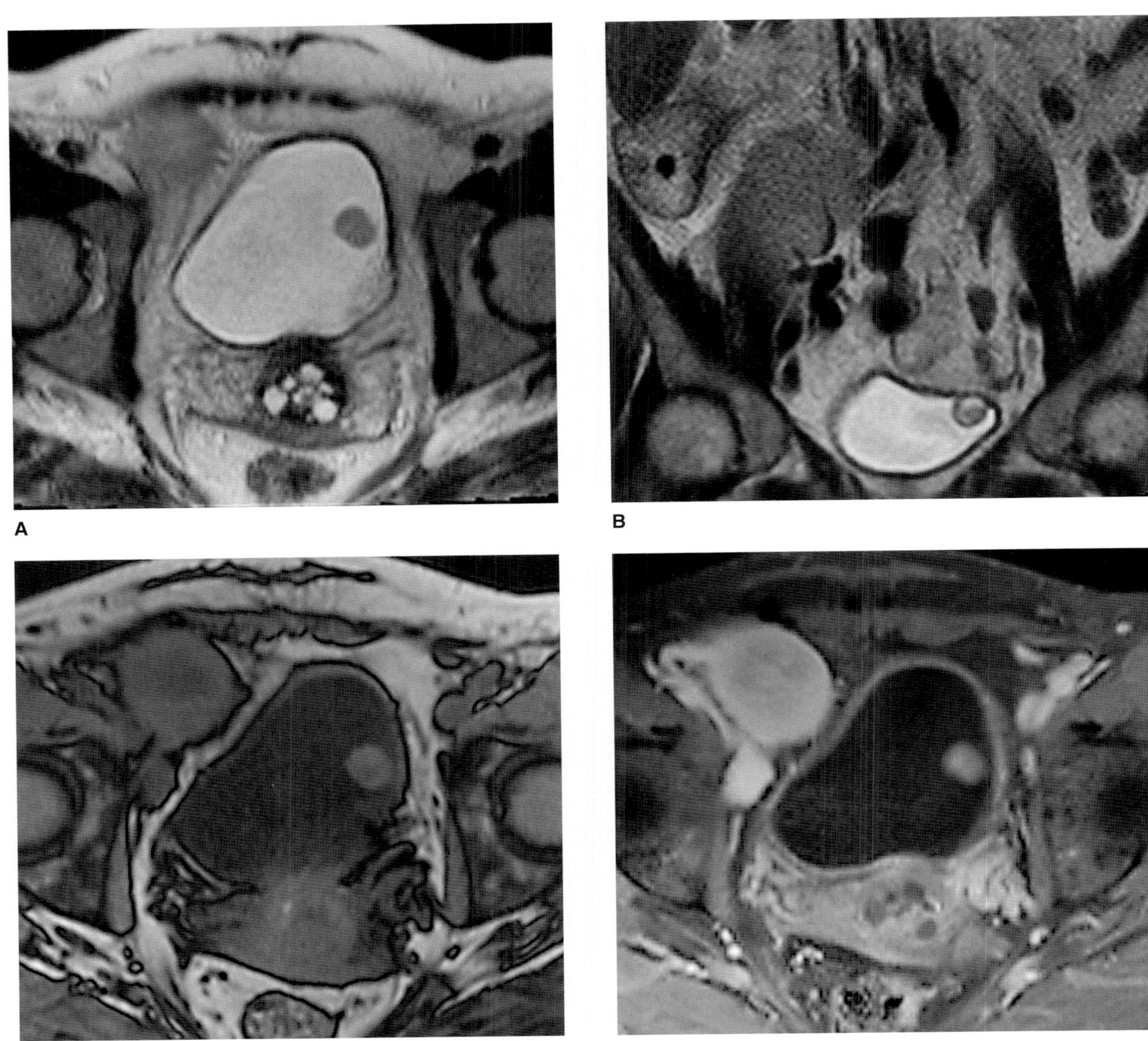

Figure 7-14 Paraganglioma of the Bladder
This 60-year-old man presented with hematuria. **A.** Axial and (**B**) coronal T2-weighted images demonstrate a small, oval, smoothly marginated polypoid mass projecting from the dome of the bladder. **C.** Precontrast and (**D**) postgadolinium enhanced T1-weighted images show the polyp to avidly enhance with contrast. Biopsy was diagnostic of a paraganglioma.

tissues (11%-30%), or (3) appear as an intramural mass (3%-7%). Typically, the lesions have a smooth contour, a feature suggesting their intramural location. On US, leiomyoma appears as a smooth hypoechoic solid mass, with varying degrees of internal echoes with a thin hyperechoic rim representing the bladder mucosa.[30] Images from CT examinations have shown a hypoattenuating, slightly heterogenous mass.[30] On MRI examinations, they are usually isointense to muscle on T1-weighted MRI and of low signal on T2-weighted MRI (see Figure 7-16).

Fibroepithelial polyp

Fibroepithelial polyp is the most common benign tumor of the upper urinary tract and occasionally can be found in the renal pelvis, urinary bladder, and urethra.[32-34]

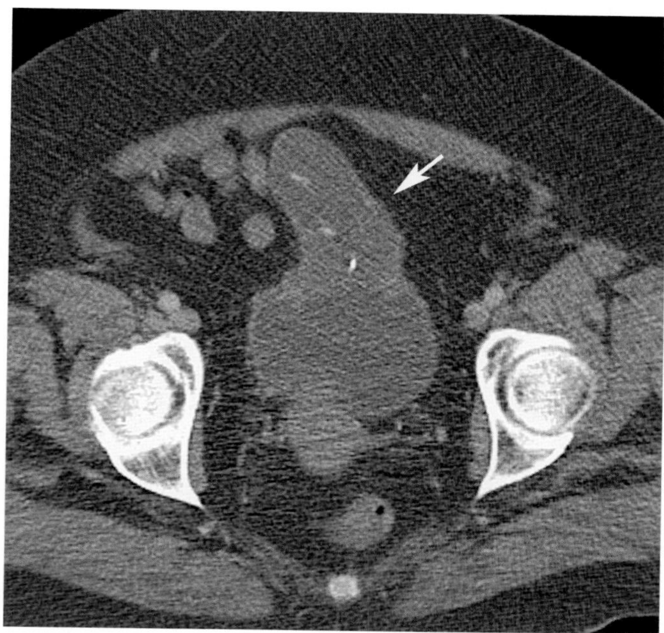

Figure 7-15 Urachal Adenocarcinoma
This 50-year-old woman presented with dysuria. Unenhanced CT demonstrates a heterogenous mass (*arrow*) projecting from the anterior wall of the bladder. This is the characteristic location of the urachus and, therefore, a urachal carcinoma should be high on the list of differential diagnosis. The calcification within the diverticular projection from the bladder is also a characteristic feature of adenocarcinomas. Surgical excision was consistent with an adenocarcinoma arising from the urachus.

Approximately 62% will arise in the proximal one-third of the ureter.[35] These are rare tumors, and a 63-year review of the Mayo Clinic registry demonstrated only 22 cases.[36] Fibroepithelial polyps are derived from the mesoderm and consist of hyperplastic fibroconnective tissue with a vascular stroma that is surrounded by transitional epithelium and represent a benign hamartoma.[37] In as much as a quarter of cases (6/22, 27%), multiple fibroepithelial polyps have been discovered in the same patient.[32]

They typically occur in younger patients, including children and young adults. The Mayo Clinic series had a mean age of 40 years. Patients typically present with hematuria and flank pain. Greater than half of patients (13/22, 59%) had a concurrent urinary disorder such as urolithiasis, ureteral stents, recurrent urinary tract infection, or UPJ obstruction in the Mayo Clinic study.[36] However, it is unclear whether this is a result of an association between polyps and urinary inflammation or that the presence of other disease makes it more likely that the fibroepithelial polyp is discovered.

On imaging, fibroepithelial polyps are polypoid lesions, with a mean diameter of 2 cm projecting into the lumen of the urinary tract.[36] They often demonstrate a long pedicle, and when involving the renal pelvis can extend into multiple calices producing a branching lesion with a similar shape to a staghorn calculus.[35] Fingerlike projections can be seen on the surface of the tumor (see Figure 7-17). At fluoroscopy during a retrograde pyelogram, the lesion may be seen to be mobile. One report of MRI of a fibrovascular polyp showed the mass to be hyperintense to the skeletal muscle on the T2-weighted images and hypointense on the T1-weighted images, with intense postcontrast enhancement, features are dissimilar to TCC of the urinary tract, which are hypointense to isointense to the skeletal muscle on T2 images, hypointense to intermediate signal intensity on T1 images, and show moderate enhancement in postcontrast images.[35]

Other benign neoplasms of the urinary tract

Other benign tumors that have been reported in the urinary tract include hemangiomas, papillomas, and inverted papillomas.[38] These have no special distinguishing features and are uncommon.

Metastasis

Secondary neoplastic involvement of the renal pelvis, ureters, and bladder is most often caused by direct extension of malignancy from adjacent organs.[39] This most commonly occurs with carcinoma of the bladder, prostate, cervix, and colon or due to retroperitoneal lymphoma.[39] Pelvic and retroperitoneal neoplasms can obstruct the renal pelvis and ureter, by encasing these structures. In most cases, this type of malignant involvement is obvious on imaging examinations.

Hematogenous metastasis to the renal pelvis, ureters, and bladder are uncommon.[40] The commonest primaries are those originating in the breast, but other primary sites have included stomach, melanoma, colon/rectum, uterus, cervix, prostate, bladder, lung, and pancreas.[39,41,42] Autopsy studies show that the majority of patients are asymptomatic; however, most that are discovered on imaging examinations present with urinary obstruction when involving the ureter.[39,40]

When involving the bladder, they will usually create 1 or multiple discrete masses or regions of wall thickening (see Figure 7-18).[41,42] When involving the ureter, the distal third is most commonly involved.[40] Metastasis to the ureters rarely cause a discrete mass lesion. In most cases, metastasis results in longitudinal spread of tumor in the submucosa of the ureter or perilymphatic tissues.[39] Breast cancer and stomach cancer can also cause peritumoral, periureteral fibrosis that can simulate the appearance of retroperitoneal fibrosis on imaging examinations.[39]

Case reports of bladder metastasis suggest that they most commonly appear as a unifocal or multifocal masses involving the wall of the bladder.[41-43] In some cases, these will be very discrete and represent an obvious mass and in others they will appear as focal nodular thickening of the wall. Rarely, metastasis can appear as diffuse wall thickening.[43-45]

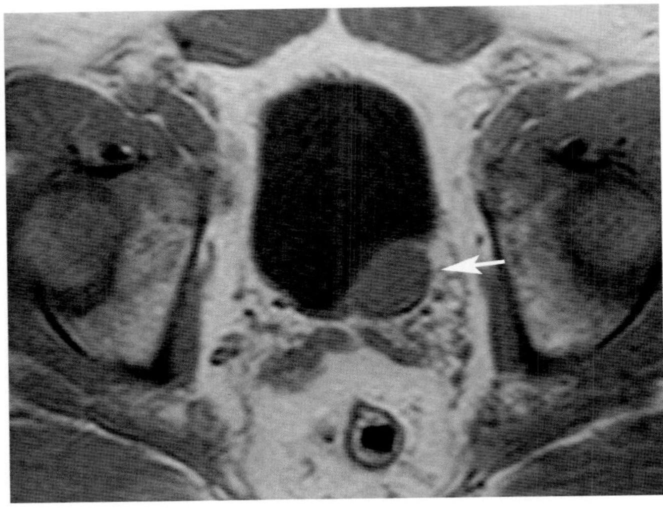

A

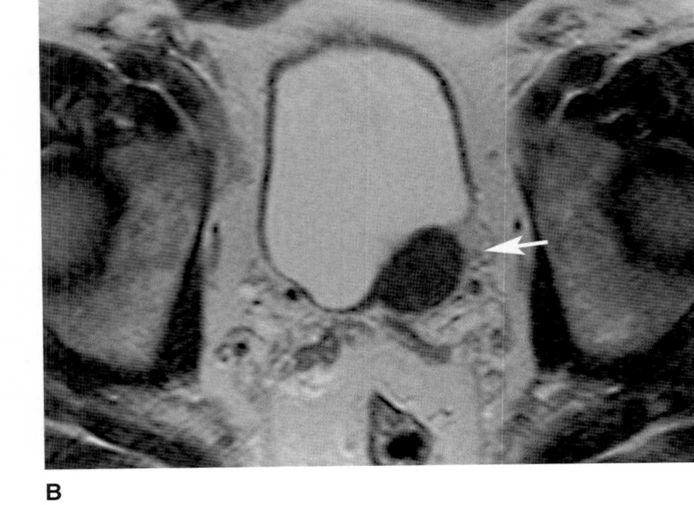

B

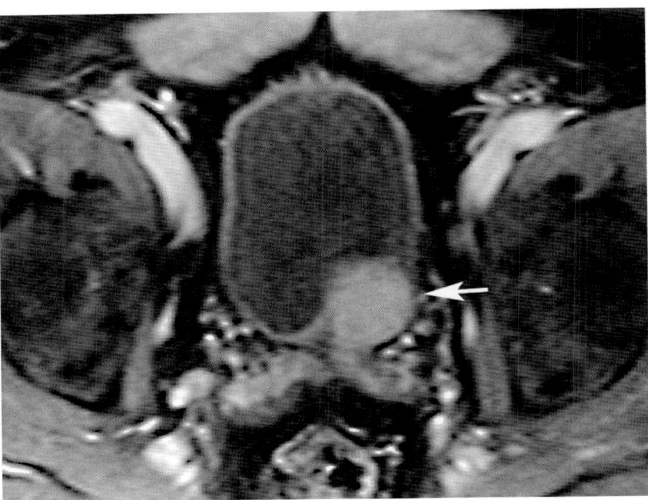

C

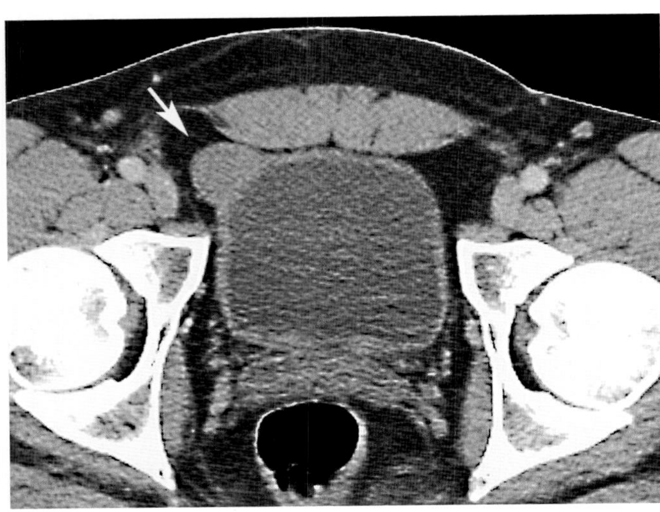

D

Figure 7-16 Bladder Leiomyoma in 2 Patients
A-C. This 55-year-old man presented with dysuria and hematuria. (A) Axial T1-weighted, (B) axial T2-weighted, and (C) axial T1 postgadolinium MRI images show a smoothly marginated mass (*arrows*) within the wall of the bladder. The signal intensities are those expected with muscle and notice that the bladder mass has the same signal intensity as the muscles in the pelvic side wall, making a leiomyoma the most likely imaging diagnosis. Further evaluation was diagnostic of a leiomyoma. **D.** This 43-year-old man presented with abdominal pain. Unenhanced axial CT shows a smoothly marginated, uniform attenuation, exophytic mass (*arrow*) projecting from the anterolateral wall of the bladder. This appearance is most consistent with a bladder leiomyoma but could also represent a paraganglioma (extra-adrenal pheochromocytoma). The lesion has remained stable for 4 years and a biopsy was nondiagnostic. This is presumed to represent a benign leiomyoma of the bladder wall.

Antegrade or retrograde urography in most cases of ureteral metastasis demonstrates unifocal or multifocal linear or corkscrew-like narrowing of the ureter, although occasionally a smooth round intraluminal filling defect can be identified.[39] In most cases, CT and MRI will also demonstrate features of ureteral obstruction such as proximal dilation. In approximately one-third of cases, ill-defined ureteral wall thickening will be demonstrated at the site of obstruction.[39] However, in many cases the metastasis will be difficult to appreciate and may only show increased attenuation or decreased signal intensity of the retroperitoneal fat and slight thickening of the renal fascia. A minority of cases will show obvious widespread retroperitoneal soft tissue nodules. Thus, in the majority of cases ureteral metastasis will have a very subtle or nonspecific imaging findings, and clinical history is required to arrive at the diagnosis.

Lymphoma

Lymphomas of the urinary system are uncommon. In most cases, they will represent secondary involvement of the urinary system from systemic lymphoma and will often be due

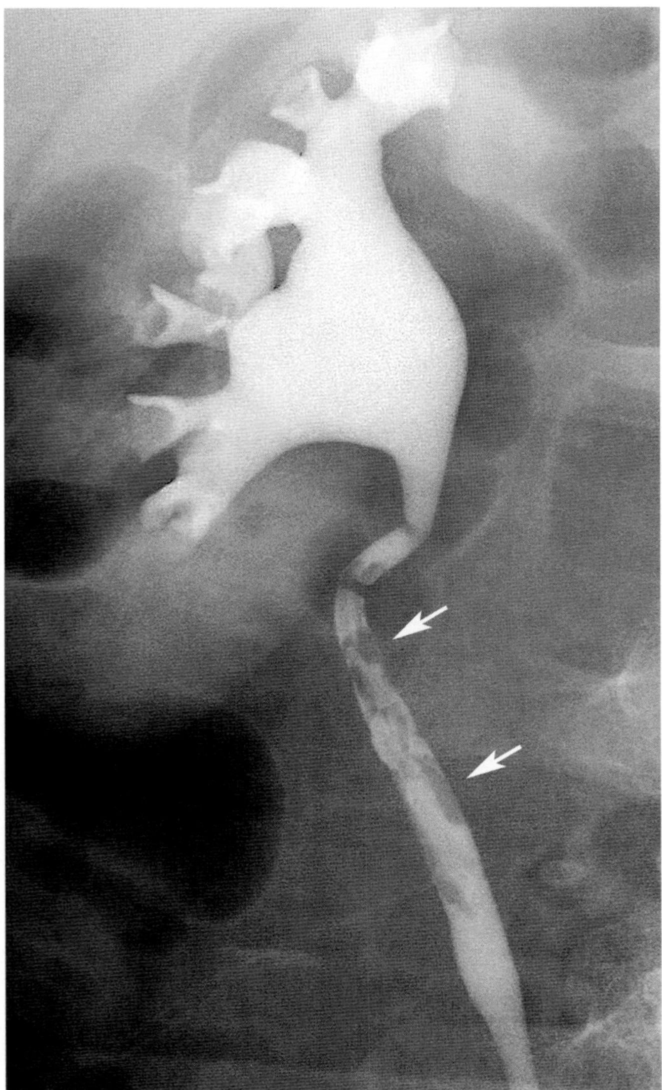

Figure 7-17 Fibroepithelial Polyp
This 36-year-old man presented with microscopic hematuria. Image from an IVU shows multiple filiform filling defects (*arrows*) within the proximal right ureter. This is the typical appearance of a fibroepithelial polyp, which was subsequently proven by ureteroscopically guided biopsy.

to direct invasion of a portion of the urinary system from an adjacent lymphomatous mass. However, rarely lymphoma can present as an isolated urinary system lesion.

As of 2007, there were 14 reported cases of primary lymphoma of the ureter.[46] Patients typically presented with either flank pain or asymptomatic hydronephrosis that was identified on imaging examinations. Diagnosis was typically made following surgical resection of the involved ureter. Three reports of abdominal MRI or CT demonstrated uniform enhancing thickening of the ureteral wall and hydronephrosis, without other findings.[46,47]

A 56-year review of the Mayo clinic tumor registry identified 36 cases of bladder lymphoma.[48] Patients with bladder lymphomas can be subdivided into 3 groups based on their clinical presentation. (1) Approximately 16% represent primary lymphoma isolated to the bladder wall.[48] These are typically low-grade MALT lymphomas and have an excellent long-term prognosis, typically with cure following surgical resection. (2) Approximately one-half of cases represent concurrent bladder involvement in a patient with systemic lymphoma (nonlocalized bladder lymphoma) and (3) approximately one-third of cases will represent recurrence of disease in a patient with previously diagnosed lymphoma (secondary lymphoma).[48] Necropsy studies show that approximately 10% to 20% of cases of systemic non-Hodgkin lymphoma can involve the bladder secondarily.[49,50] Nonlocalized and secondary bladder lymphomas can be of a wide variety of non-Hodgkin lymphoma and had a worse prognosis than primary bladder lymphoma with approximately 9-year median survival for nonlocalized cases and 0.6-year median survival for secondary cases.[48] The mean interval between diagnosis and secondary involvement of the bladder was 4.5 years (0.3-12 y).

Primary bladder lymphoma is 6.5 times more frequent in women than men and with mean age of 64 years old (20-85).[48,50] However nonlocalized and secondary bladder lymphoma are slightly more common in men. Presenting symptoms included urinary frequency, dysuria, hematuria, and lower abdominal and back pain, with approximately one-third presenting with ureteral obstruction.[48] Approximately 20% of patients will complain of longstanding chronic cystitis.

There are no reported imaging series of bladder lymphoma. However, pathologic and cystoscopic studies suggest that the lesions can be single or multiple rounded submucosal masses involving any portion of the bladder wall.[48] One case report showed a uniform attenuation mass smoothly expanding the wall of the bladder.[49] Two additional case reports demonstrated asymmetric, uniform attenuation (CT) and uniform echotexture (US), thickening of the bladder wall.[51] Extraurinary lymphomas can engulf the renal pelvis, ureters, or invade the bladder. Enlarged lymph nodes can cause extrinsic displacement and obstruction of the ureters.

Nonneoplastic Nodular Lesions of the Urinary System

Nonneoplastic focal and nodular lesions of the urinary bladder are uncommon, including pyeloureteritis cystica and cystitis glandularis (Table 7-4).

Pyeloureteritis cystica

Although originally attributed to chronic infection, pyeloureteritis cystica can also be seen in patients with other causes of urinary tract inflammation, including chronic nephrostomy catheters, ureteral stents, and long-standing urinary calculi.[52] Histologically, small epithelial-lined cysts (nests of von Brunn) can be found within the lamina propria. They represent detached buds of surface epithelium that have penetrated the wall of the ureter in response to chronic inflammation.[52] The cysts are usually persistent and

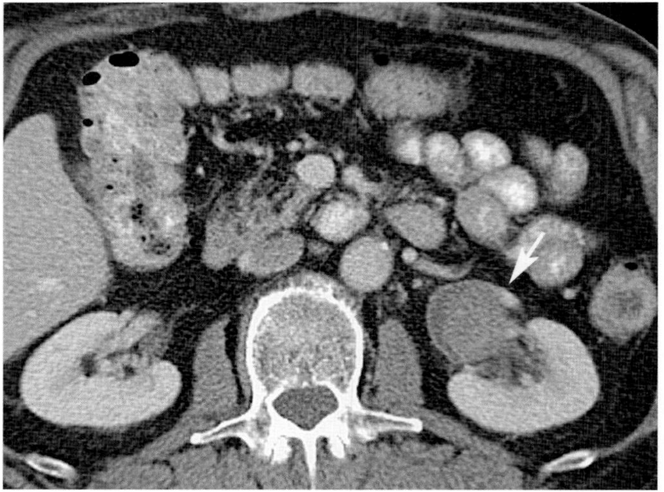
A

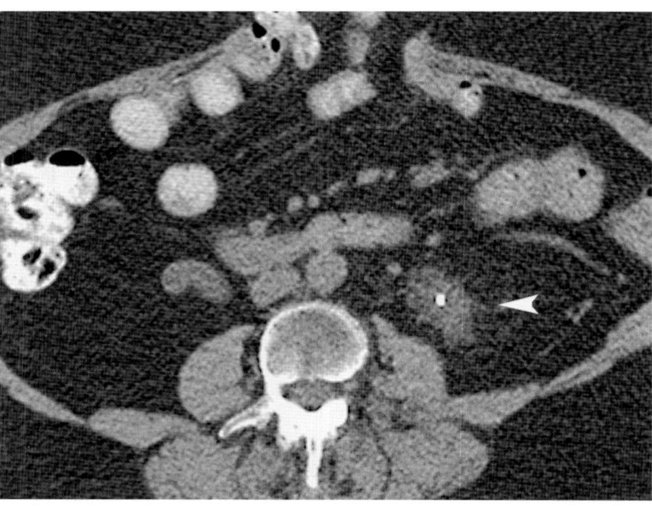
B

Figure 7-18 Metastasis to the Upper Tracts in 2 Patients
A. This 65-year-old man had malignant melanoma. Contrast-enhanced axial CT shows an enhancing soft tissue mass (*arrow*) in the left renal pelvis. This will most often represent a primary TCC of the kidney; however, in this clinical situation it could represent a metastasis. Brush biopsy was diagnostic of metastatic melanoma. Primary tumors that can metastasize to the urothelium include melanoma, breast cancer, and colon cancer. **B.** This 61-year-old woman with ovarian cancer developed azotemia. Noncontrast axial CT shows an irregular speculated mass (*arrowhead*) surrounding the left ureter. The high attenuation dot in the center of the mass is a left ureteral stent. The mass represents a metastasis from the patient's ovarian cancer to the periureteral lymphatics around the left ureter.

may increase in size over time. They are primarily found in the proximal one-third of the ureter. Cyst size is usually less than a centimeter in diameter and can protrude from the mucosal surface and rarely become pedunculated.[53] Most cases are clinically asymptomatic and discovered incidentally on imaging examinations. However, rarely patients can present with obstruction.[54]

Table 7-4. Causes of Focal Urothelial Lesions

A. Malignant neoplasms
1. **Transitional cell carcinoma**[a]
2. Squamous carcinoma
3. Paraganglioma (bladder)
4. Small cell carcinoma (bladder)
5. Metastasis
6. Lymphoma
B. Benign neoplasms
1. Leiomyoma (bladder)
2. Fibroepithelial polyp
3. Hemangioma
4. Papilloma
5. Inverted papilloma
C. Inflammatory lesions
1. Pyeloureteritis cystica
2. Cystitis glandularis
3. Inflammatory pseudotumor
4. Nephrogenic adenoma
D. Other conditions
1. Endometriosis

[a]Items in bold are common.

On antegrade and retrograde urograms, multiple, smooth, well-defined filling defects are a characteristic appearance (see Figure 7-19).[55,56] The smooth appearance and the multiplicity of the filling defects usually suggest the diagnosis, but in a patient with positive urine cytology and suspected upper tract urothelial neoplasm, ureteroscopy may be required to exclude a focal urothelial tumor. Pyeloureteritis cystica is difficult to detect on cross-sectional imaging examinations but may occasionally be seen on a high-quality CTU (see Figure 7-19).

Cystitis glandularis

The end result of chronic inflammation in the bladder can be the proliferation of solid nests of urothelial cells in the lamina propria beneath the surface urothelium, known as von Brunn nests. Continued chronic inflammation can lead to the Brunn nests developing into glandular structures, and the condition is then known as cystitis glandularis.[11,57-59] These changes can also be seen in patients with bladder exstrophy and pelvic lipomatosis. Cystitis glandularis may be a precursor to the development of adenocarcinoma of the bladder.

Cystitis glandularis is a common histologic diagnosis on bladder biopsies and involves the trigone of the urinary bladder most frequently. In more advanced cases, raised lesions in the bladder wall may be visible on imaging studies, as filling defects in the contrast-opacified urinary bladder, particularly in the region of the bladder base.

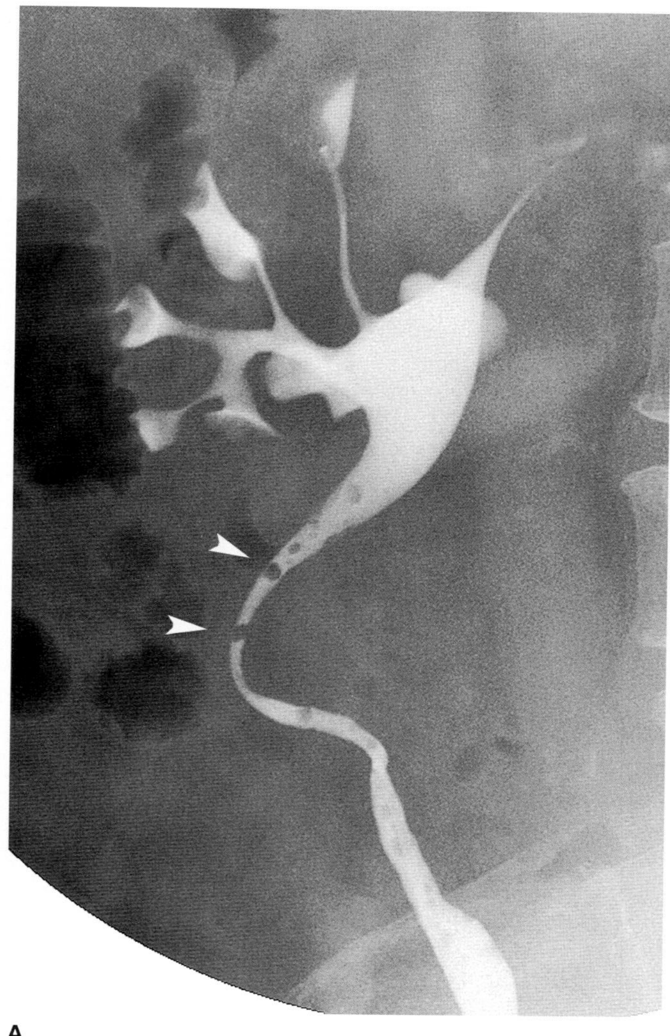

A

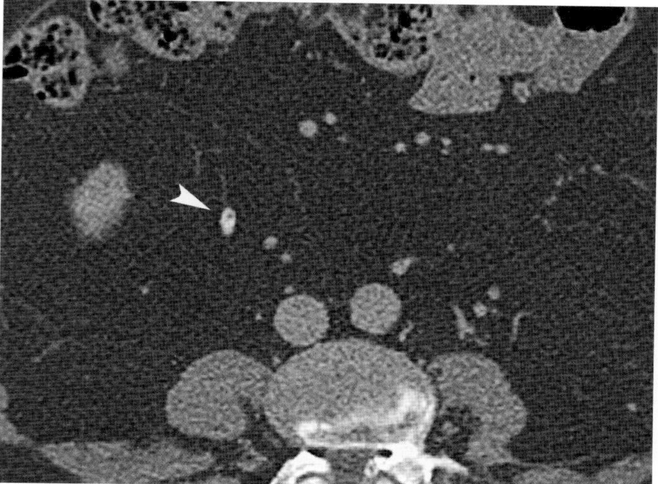

B

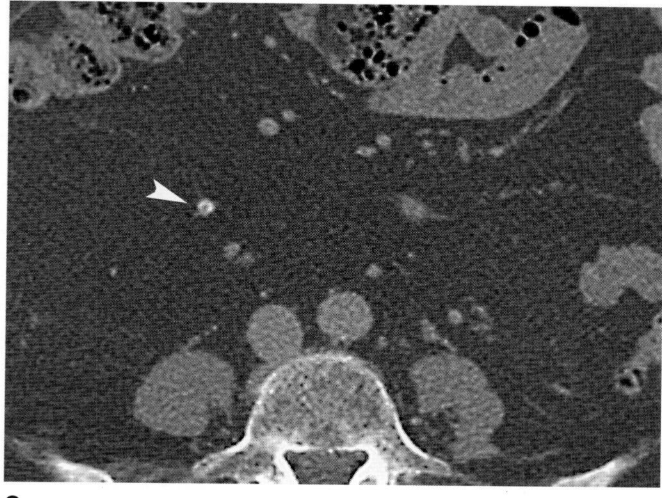

C

Figure 7-19 Ureteritis Cystica
This 60-year-old woman presented with hematuria. **A.** Frontal image from a retrograde pyelogram shows multiple smooth small oval defects within the right ureter (*arrowheads*). This is the typical picture of ureteritis cystica. **B** and **C.** Two images from a subsequent CTU show very faint filling defects (*arrowheads*) within the ureter. This is the CT manifestation of ureteritis cystica and is a very difficult diagnosis to make because of the small size of the lesions.

Other inflammatory masses of the urinary bladder

Other uncommon inflammatory masses that can involve the bladder include inflammatory pseudotumor, endometriosis, and nephrogenic adenoma.[60]

DIVERTICULA AND STRICTURES OF THE URINARY TRACT

Outpouchings of the urinary system occur in both the ureters (pseudodiverticulosis) and the bladder (bladder diverticula).

Ureteral Pseudodiverticulosis

Ureteral pseudodiverticulosis represents outpouchings of proliferated hyperplastic transitional epithelium into the loose subepithelial connective tissue that do not penetrate the muscularis propria of the ureter and are associated with chronic inflammatory changes.[61] Because the "diverticular"-like outpouchings do not contain all the layers of the ureteral wall, they are referred to as "pseudodiverticula." The etiology of pseudodiverticulosis is not known; however, there is a strong association between ureteral pseudodiverticulosis and carcinoma of the bladder, which has been reported in as many as 40% to 50% of patients but is believed to be approximately 25% of all cases.[62] This association has led to the recommendation that patients with ureteral pseudodiverticulosis be kept under surveillance for the development of bladder cancer.

Although any part of the ureter can be affected, ureteral pseudodiverticulosis is seen most commonly in the distal lumbar ureter and appear as tiny outpouchings

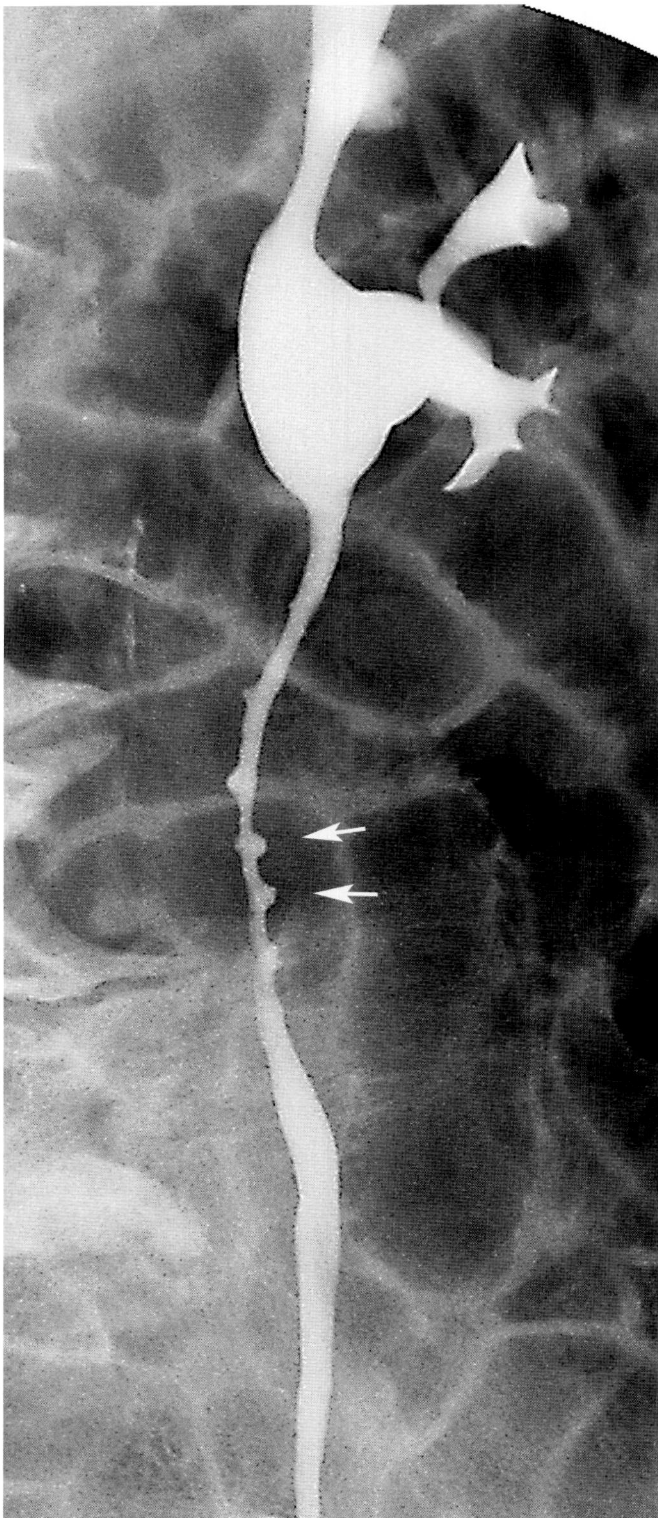

Figure 7-20 Ureteral Pseudodiverticulosis
This 70-year-old man presented with a history of bladder cancer. Image from a retrograde pyelogram shows several small outpouchings (*arrows*) from the lumen of the proximal ureter. This is the typical appearance of ureteral pseudodiverticulosis. The ureteral pseudodiverticula are best seen on a retrograde pyelogram because of the higher pressure of contrast injection, and difficult to identify on an intravenous urogram or a CTU.

of contrast from the lumen of the ureter on antegrade and retrograde pyelogram (see Figure 7-20).[62,63] The majority of cases are not detectable on CT examinations although rarely cases have been identified.[64] In greater than 90% of cases there are more than 1 pseudodiverticulum and in many cases the abnormality is bilateral.[63] Pseudodiverticulosis is best seen on retrograde pyelograms, likely due to the pressure of injection directly into the collecting system.[63] In the affected segment, the ureteral lumen can occasionally appear irregular, but pseudodiverticulosis should not produce obstruction. Luminal irregularity associated with pseudodiverticulosis and obstruction is worrisome for a concurrent urothelial neoplasm, which should be excluded with brush biopsies of the abnormal location. In approximately half of cases of associated malignancy (9/17 patients in one series), a filling defect can be detected within the urinary tract, usually within the bladder.[62] The finding of a filling defect had a 78% positive predictive value for the presence of an associated malignancy.

Bladder Diverticula

Most diverticula in the bladder are acquired abnormalities and are common in older men. The diverticula form because of herniation of the bladder mucosa and submucosa between hypertrophied muscle bundles of the bladder in patients with bladder outlet obstruction. Chronic bladder outlet obstruction is most often due to benign prostatic hyperplasia (BPH) and is the reason why bladder diverticula are most often found in this demographic group. Because diverticula contain no smooth muscle in the wall, urinary stasis is common in diverticula that have narrow necks connecting them to the bladder lumen. Stasis can lead to the development of stones within the diverticula and also results in a slightly higher incidence of bladder cancer in urinary bladder diverticula.[65,66]

On IVU and CTU diverticula will appear as contrast filled outpouchings projecting outward but in communication with the bladder lumen. On US, CT, and MRI examinations in which there is no contrast in the bladder, the diverticulum will appear as an oval projection from the surface of the bladder containing fluid (anechoic on US, low attenuation on CT, and high signal on T2-weighted MRI examinations) (see Figure 7-21). The interior of a bladder diverticulum should be smooth, with no filling defects. The presence of mucosal irregularity or filling defects should prompt a search for stones or urothelial tumors within the diverticulum.

Congenital diverticula contain all the layers of the bladder wall and are less commonly seen than acquired diverticula. They are usually seen in the pediatric population, with boys being more frequently affected. These diverticula are often located superolateral to the ureteral orifice and can distort the ureterovesical junction enough to cause ipsilateral vesicoureteral reflux (VUR) or, less commonly, ureteral obstruction.[67]

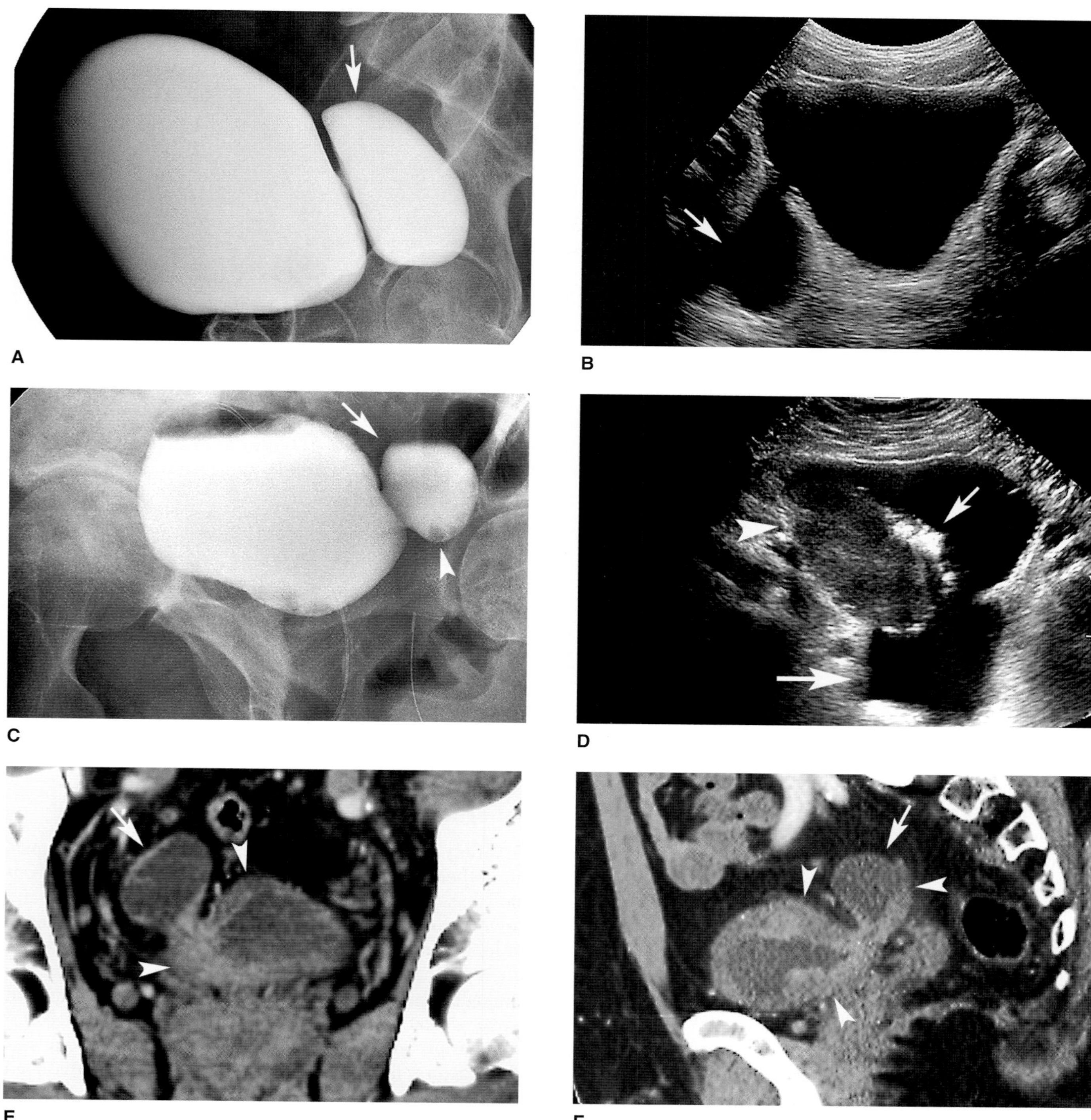

Figure 7-21 Bladder Diverticula and Complications in 5 Patients (**A**) Cystogram and (**B**) transverse US examination of the bladder in 2 separate patients show the typical appearance of a large bladder diverticula (*arrows*): a smooth-walled outpouching that communicates with the lumen of the bladder by a narrow neck. **C.** Cystogram in a third patient shows a similar-appearing diverticulum (*arrow*) extending from the posterior wall of the bladder. However, there are several small filling defects layering within the dependent portion of the diverticulum (*arrowhead*) indicating the presence of calculi. **D.** This fourth individual has a large diverticulum (*arrow*) projecting from the posterior wall of the bladder. Nevertheless, there is also a mixed echogenicity mass (*arrowhead*) projecting into the lumen of the bladder and diverticulum, representing a cancer complicating the diverticulum. There are bright echoes along the surface of the mass (*small arrow*) suggesting the presence of surface calcifications. **E** and **F.** Coronal and sagittal contrast-enhanced CT in a fifth patient shows a diverticulum (*arrow*) projecting from the right posterior wall of the bladder. Note the extensive, asymmetric thickening of the posterior wall of the diverticulum, which is contiguous with the thickening along the posterior and the lateral wall of the bladder (*arrowheads*), indicating spread of bladder carcinoma into the diverticulum.

Congenital urachal diverticula occur at the bladder dome and have been discussed in the section above.

Ureteral Strictures

Ureteral strictures can be subclassified as extrinsic or intrinsic and benign or malignant. Strictures are clinically significant because of their propensity to cause urinary obstruction. Urinary obstruction is discussed in detail under the subsequent heading: **Urinary obstruction**; however, we will discuss strictures briefly here.

Extrinsic strictures are those caused by constriction of the ureter by an extrinsic mass. In most cases, these will be due to direct extension of adjacent malignancies, especially cancers of the cervix, prostate, bladder, and colon. Occasionally, retroperitoneal lymphadenopathy, caused by metastatic cancer or lymphoma, can cause constriction of the ureter and urinary obstruction. Rarely, extrinsic constriction can be caused by the nonneoplastic condition of retroperitoneal fibrosis. With contrast urography, differentiation of extrinsic strictures from intrinsic strictures can be difficult. However, cross-sectional imaging will readily identify an extrinsic mass as the cause of stricture and obstruction and in many cases will indicate the source of the mass.

Intrinsic strictures are most often caused by TCC of the ureter, which has been discussed in detail under the previous heading: **Urothelial malignancies**. On contrast urography, malignant strictures related to TCC will characteristically have shelflike margins or an abrupt occlusion of the ureter. Cross-sectional imaging will show small eccentric or concentric mass involving the wall of the ureter or collecting system causing the narrowed ureteral lumen (see Figures 7-3, 7-8, and 7-12).

Benign intrinsic strictures can be congenital, iatrogenic, related to the prior passage of calculi, and postinflammatory.

Congenital strictures

UPJ anomalies can result in obstruction. Although usually diagnosed in children, adults may present with an undiagnosed UPJ obstruction. If the obstruction is severe with resultant obstruction and impaired contrast excretion, the anatomy will be difficult to demonstrate on a CTU or IVU, and a retrograde pyeloureterogram may be required. In such patients, it is important to demonstrate whether the UPJ is dependent in position relative to the renal pelvis, and evaluate for kinks that may suggest the presence of a crossing vessel that may be causing the obstruction. These observations are crucial in determining the management of the UPJ anomaly; a high riding UPJ may be treated with a surgical pyeloplasty whereas a dependent UPJ may be initially treated with endoscopic incision or balloon dilation (see Figure 7-22). If there is suspicion of a crossing vessel in association with the UPJ obstruction, confirmation of the renal vascular anatomy is obtained with CT or MR angiography.

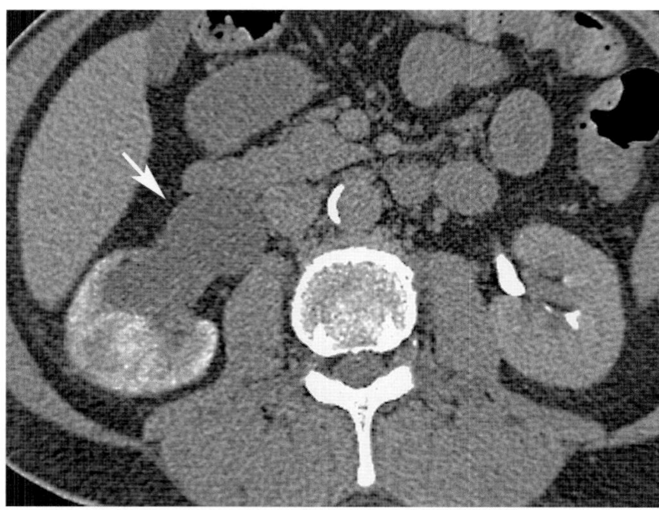

Figure 7-22 Congenital Ureteropelvic Junction (UPJ) Obstruction This 30-year-old man presented with right flank pain. Contrast-enhanced CT during the urographic phase demonstrates dilation of the right renal pelvis (*arrow*), which is extrarenal in position, a feature of congenital UPJ obstruction. Note the persistent nephrogram in the right kidney, compared to the left, attesting to the severity of obstruction—the cortex of the right kidney retains contrast whereas the left kidney attenuation is decreasing. Contrast is excreted from the left kidney but not from the right kidney. The distal right ureter (not shown) was normal in diameter. This combination of findings is characteristic of obstruction of the right kidney due to a congenital UPJ obstruction.

Iatrogenic strictures

A variety of surgical procedures performed by urologists and others can result in ureteral strictures. Urinary diversion has an anastomotic stricture rate of 1% to 8%, and ureteroscopy to remove ureteral stones has an incidence of less than 1%,[68-71] although the majority of benign strictures in the absence of urinary diversion are related to urologic endoscopic procedures. Factors associated with ureteroscopic-related stricture include (1) stone size, (2) stone impaction, and (3) proximal location and several surgical factors, including (1) large scope size, (2) prolonged case duration, (3) use of intracorporeal lithotripsy, and (4) perforation. Ureteral injury following pelvic and retroperitoneal surgery, particularly hysterectomy, can also result in ureteral stricture. A prospective study of 471 hysterectomies demonstrated a 1.7% incidence of ureteral injury, most of which were discovered at the time of surgery.[72] A single-center retrospective review of hysterectomies identified a 4.3% incidence of postoperative ureteral strictures.[73]

Most benign iatrogenic strictures will be identified based on the presence of urinary obstruction, a topic that will be discussed in detail later in this chapter. The strictures itself will usually appear as a smooth tapered narrowing of the ureter at the site of injury on antegrade and

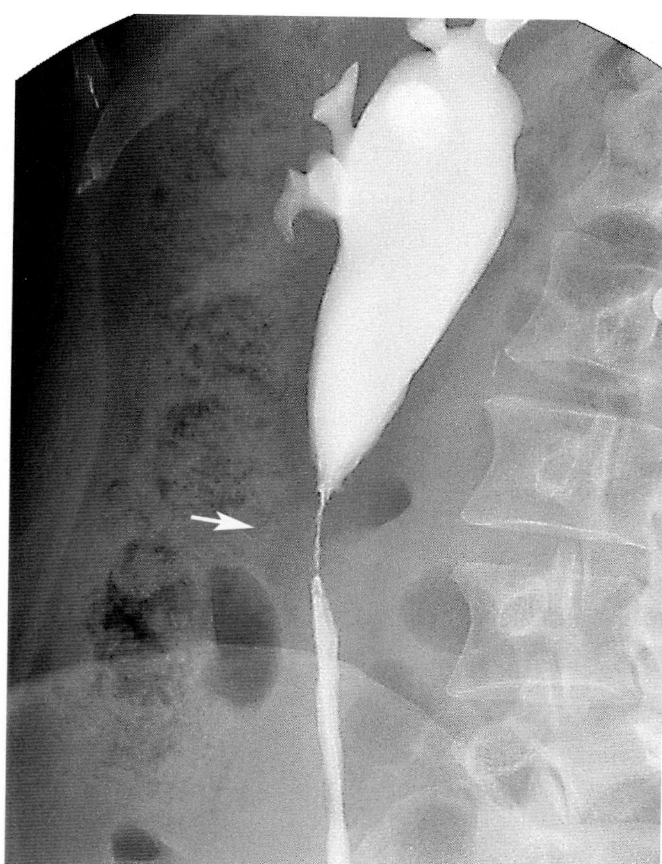

Figure 7-23 Postpyeloplasty Stricture
Retrograde pyelogram following surgical pyeloplasty for a congenital UPJ obstruction demonstrates a focal, smoothly tapered stricture (*arrow*) at the UPJ, representing a postsurgical stricture. The renal pelvis is extrarenal and therefore appears dilated. A ureteral stent was placed and the patient underwent another surgical repair after unsuccessful balloon dilation.

retrograde urograms (see Figure 7-23). On cross-sectional imaging, the narrowing will be confirmed and in nearly all cases, there will be absence of any soft-tissue lesion at the site of narrowing. The presence of a soft-tissue mass should raise the possibility of a neoplasm causing the stricture.

Strictures related to ureteral stones

In a review of 24 patients with chronically impacted ureteral stones, impacted for an average of 11 months, 24% of the patients developed postoperative ureteral strictures.[74]

Inflammatory strictures

In rare conditions such as malacoplakia, leukoplakia, amyloidosis, and squamous metaplasia, the ureter may show focal and irregular narrowing. The specific diagnosis of these rare conditions requires ureteroscopically guided biopsy.

Ureteral strictures can occur in granulomatous conditions such as tuberculosis and schistosomiasis; the ancillary radiologic findings of renal parenchymal disease in TB and mural calcification in the bladder in schistosomiasis can help to suggest the diagnosis (see Figure 7-24). Strictures with tuberculosis progress caudally from the kidney, whereas bilharzial strictures ascend from the ureterovesical junction. Inflammatory conditions in the retroperitoneum, such as retroperitoneal fibrosis, cause smooth extrinsic narrowing of the ureter, usually at the L2-L4 level. Although the diagnosis may be suggested on a retrograde pyelogram, correlation with CT or MRI is required to confirm the diagnosis. The ureters demonstrate smooth encasement, usually in the distal lumbar region (Table 7-5).

Tuberculosis

Genitourinary tuberculosis is the most common clinical site of extrapulmonary tuberculosis but remains uncommon and accounted for only 1.2% of tuberculosis reported to the New York Department of Health in 1999.[75] However, in the developing countries, as many as 15% to 20% of tuberculosis patients will have *Mycobacterium tuberculosis* recoverable in the urine.[75] Infection is spread hematogenously to the kidneys, lodging in the periglomerular capillaries. The development of disease depends on the immune status of the host, and spontaneous healing is the usual response. Microscopic cortical granulomas are pathologically identifiable in the kidneys and contain dormant bacilli that have the potential to reactivate years later, producing disease. Progressive disease or reactivation of dormant infection can lead to abscess formation in the papilla and lead to papillary necrosis.[73] Abscess cavities can communicate with the collecting system, resulting in direct extension of organisms to the urothelium of the collecting systems, ureters, and bladder.[73-79]

Infection of the papillary tips causes irregularity of the surfaces of the calices that can be seen on IVU.[75] Chronically, calcifications occur at the sites of infection, such that renal calcification is the most common manifestation of renal tuberculosis, occurring in approximately 24% of patients.[73,74] In severe cases, the kidney becomes small, scarred, hydronephrotic, and nonfunctioning, with multiple regions of calcification in the kidney—a finding called "autonephrectomy" or "putty kidney."[75,162] These calcifications often form sheets and appear to divide the kidney into multiple lobules surrounded by calcification.

With involvement of the papilla, the organism then has access to the urinary system. The walls of the collecting system and ureter become thickened, and strictures develop in approximately one-half of cases of renal tuberculosis (see Figure 7-24).[76] On IVU, the mucosal surface of the ureter can have a ragged irregular appearance.[75] Strictures characteristically occur at points of normal anatomic narrowing such as the infundibula, UPJ, across the pelvic brim, and at the vesicoureteral junction; strictures can occur at multiple sites (see Figure 7-24).[74] Infundibular stenosis will lead to caliceal dilation, whereas

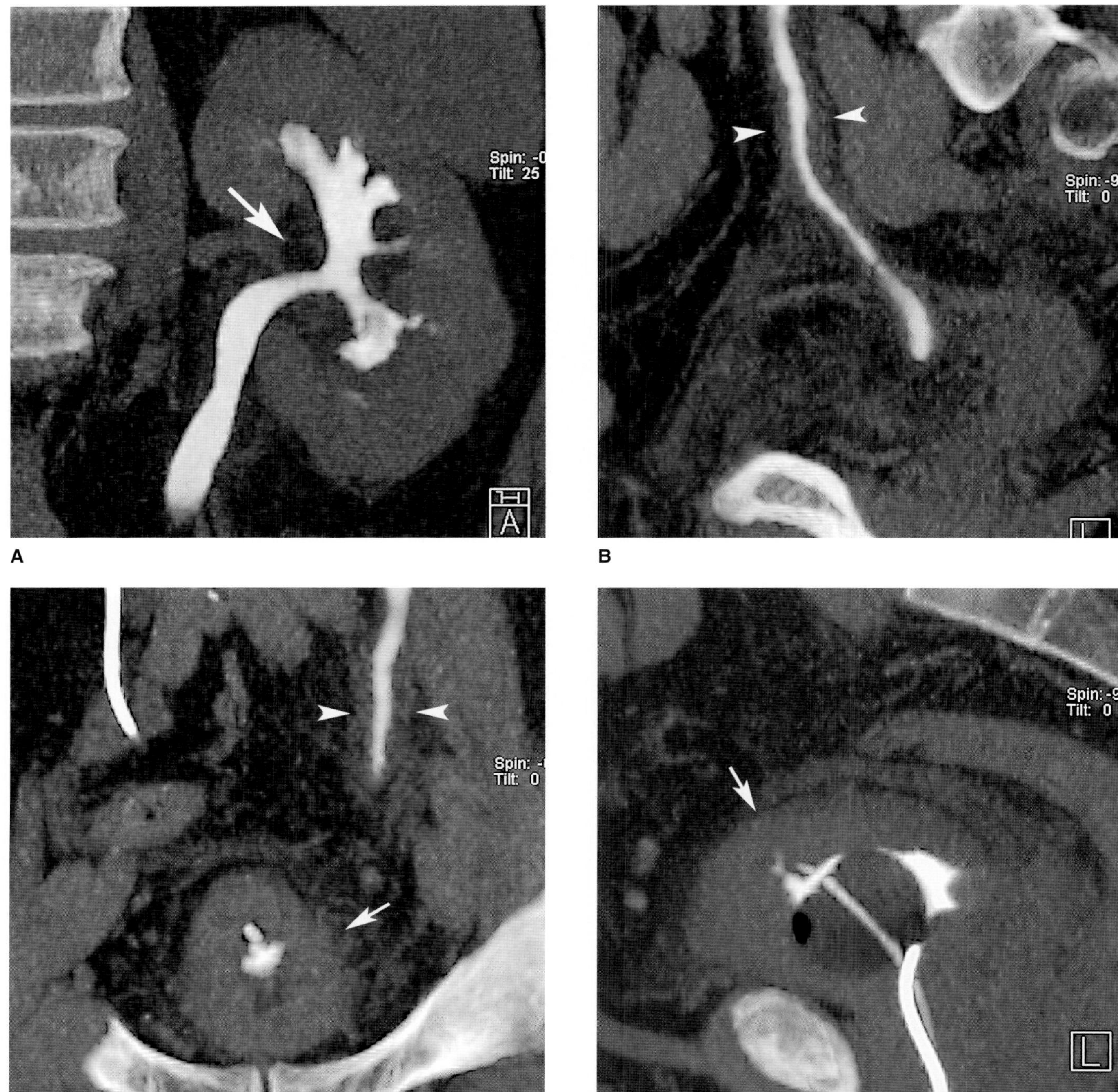

A B C D

Figure 7-24 Tuberculosis
This 61-year-old Greek immigrant had decreasing renal function. **A-D.** Maximum-intensity projection images from a CTU show diffuse thickening of the wall of the left ureter (*small arrowheads*) and bladder (*small arrow*). There is also stricturing of the left renal pelvis with mild clubbing of the calices.

ureteral strictures will lead to hydronephrosis and hydroureteronephrosis. Ureteral dilation may also in part be due to reflux as a result of tuberculous involvement of the bladder.[77] Granulomatous debris and strictures can lead to the formation of calculi in the collecting systems and the ureters.[75] In the end stages, the entire ureter can become calcified, so-called pipe-stem ureter.[73]

Tuberculosis also results in inflammatory thickening and then scarring of the bladder. There is diffuse wall thickening with a reduced bladder volume. Ulceration

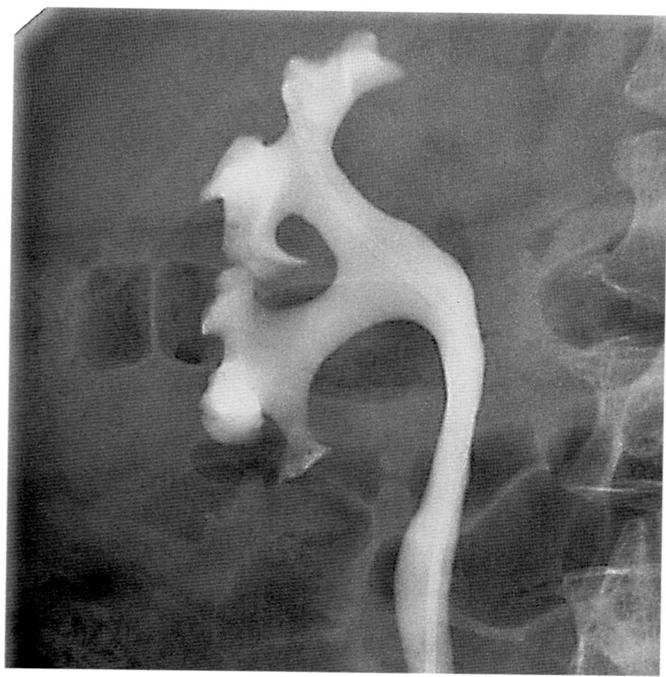

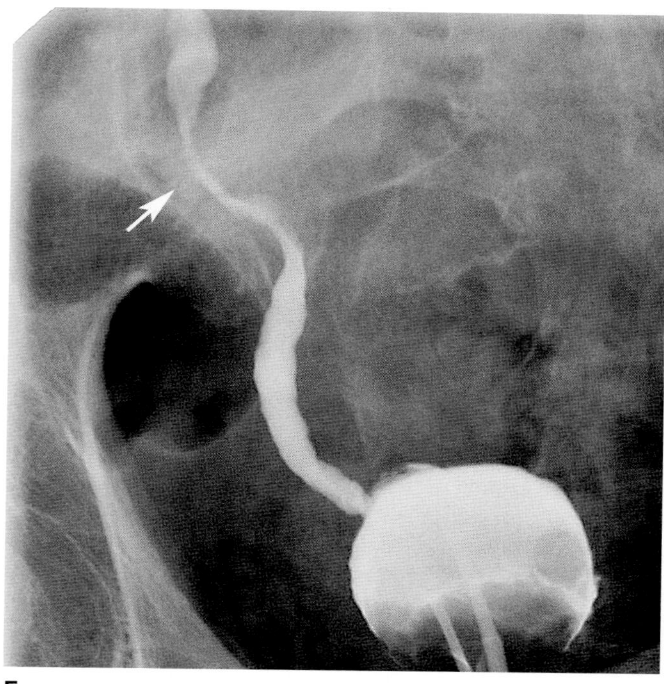

Figure 7-24 Tuberculosis (*Continued*)
E and **F**. Retrograde pyelogram shows similar mild clubbing of the right calices, a long tapered stricture of the pelvic ureter (*arrow*), and a nodular surface to the distal ureter and bladder. These findings are typical of urinary involvement by tuberculosis, which was subsequently proven by urine cultures.

of the wall and granulomatous filling defects can also be seen. In advanced disease, there is eventual scarring resulting in a small, irregular, calcified bladder. This appearance of the bladder is characteristic of tuberculosis but a similar finding can be seen in severe cyclophosphamide- and radiation-induced cystitis, although calcification is unusual in cystitis related to cyclophosphamide or radiation therapy. Schistosomiasis can cause bladder calcification but the wall is thin and the bladder remains normally distensible, an important distinguishing feature from a tuberculous bladder.

Other causes of benign strictures

Rare causes of benign strictures include radiation fibrosis, penetrating abdominal injuries with gunshot wounds, and/or iatrogenic trauma.

Table 7-5. Causes of Intrinsic Urinary Strictures

1. Urothelial malignancies a. **Transitional cell cancer**[a] b. Squamous cell cancer c. Other
2. **Congenital UPJ obstruction**
3. **Postsurgical**
4. Impacted stones
5. Tuberculosis
6. Schistosomiasis
7. Malacoplakia
8. Leukoplakia

[a]Items in bold are common.

URINARY TRACT TRAUMA

Trauma to the collecting system occurs most often in patients with severe blunt abdominal trauma and is nearly always associated with injury to the renal parenchyma that is discussed in Chapter 6. When deep lacerations are seen in the kidneys, imaging in the excretory phase is essential to exclude the presence of collecting system injury.[80-82] Penetrating trauma related to gunshot or stab wounds can also injure the kidneys and secondarily the collecting systems.

Most renal injuries that extend into the collecting system are managed conservatively, and urinary drainage or stenting are reserved for patients who develop complications from continued extravasation of urine; such complications consist mostly of infection of the urinomas.

UPJ injuries are a rare occurrence, seen in patients with severe abdominal trauma associated with rapid deceleration.[83] There can be tears or lacerations in the UPJ and in rare instances, the UPJ can be transected completely. UPJ injury should be suspected on a trauma CT scan when there is significant contrast extravasation in the absence of parenchymal lacerations of the kidneys. With complete transaction, there will be florid extravasation of contrast from the renal pelvis with no contrast opacification of the ureter.

Ureteral injuries are rare with blunt abdominal trauma, and are seen most frequently with either penetrating wounds, usually gunshot injuries, or iatrogenic injuries related to surgery in the pelvis.[84-86] Ureteral injury has been reported with all manner of surgeries including urologic, colorectal, vascular, and gynecologic surgery; the latter accounts for more than half of all iatrogenic ureteral injuries.[84] If the injuries are recognized intraoperatively, primary repair can be performed at the same time, but it is not uncommon for patients to present several weeks later with symptoms of urinary leakage, fever, or elevated serum creatinine levels, because of resorption of the urine leaking into the peritoneal cavity. When new ascites is seen on postoperative imaging studies, it is mandatory to tailor the studies to determine whether there is a collecting system injury; this most often requires that imaging be extended into the excretory phase to confirm the integrity of the collecting system.

Trauma to the urinary bladder is most frequently due to blunt trauma related to motor vehicle collisions, and associated pelvic fractures are seen in 80% of patients.[87] The most critical feature to evaluate is whether the injuries are intraperitoneal or extraperitoneal, as this distinction has an important bearing on the management of the patient. Extraperitoneal injuries are the more common injury and may be related to shearing of pelvic ligaments attached to the bladder, or to laceration of the bladder by bony spicules. On contrast examinations, this will appear as contrast extravasating into the perivesical soft tissues (see Figure 7-25). Intraperitoneal injuries can occur in the absence of pelvic fractures and are usually seen in severe blunt-force trauma to a distended urinary bladder.[88] The tear occurs at the

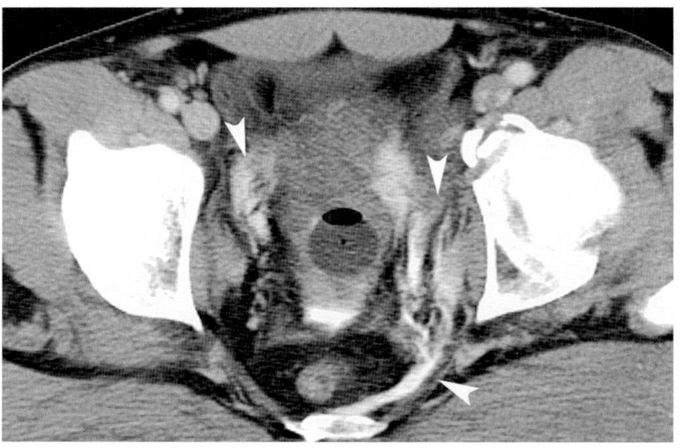

A

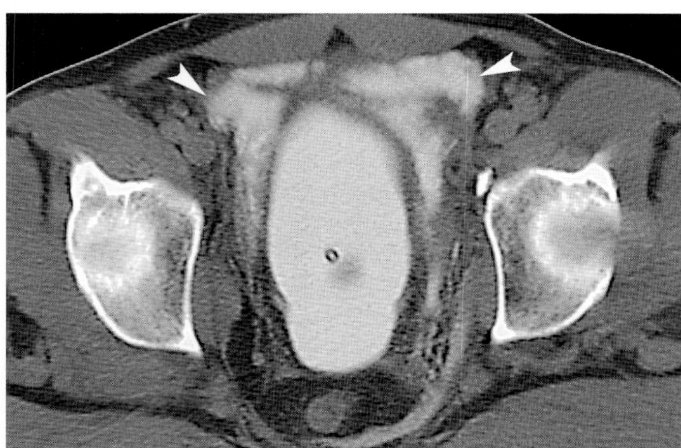

B

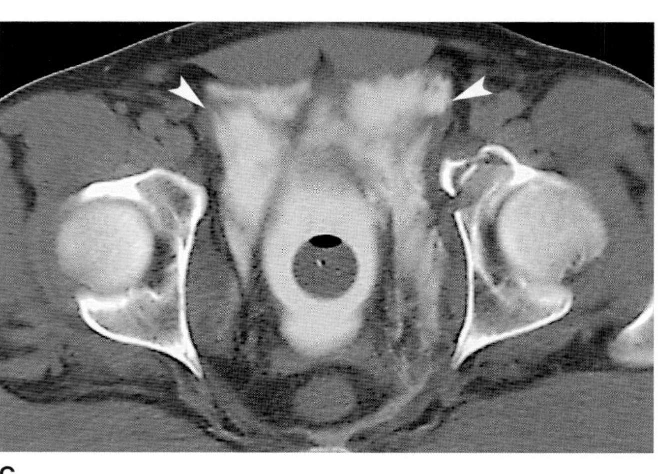

C

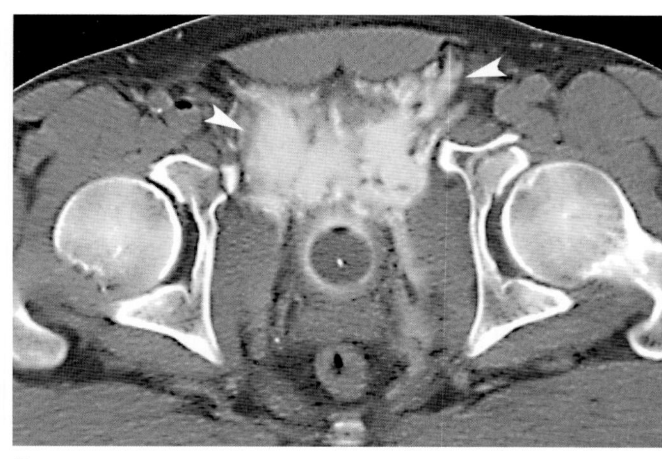

D

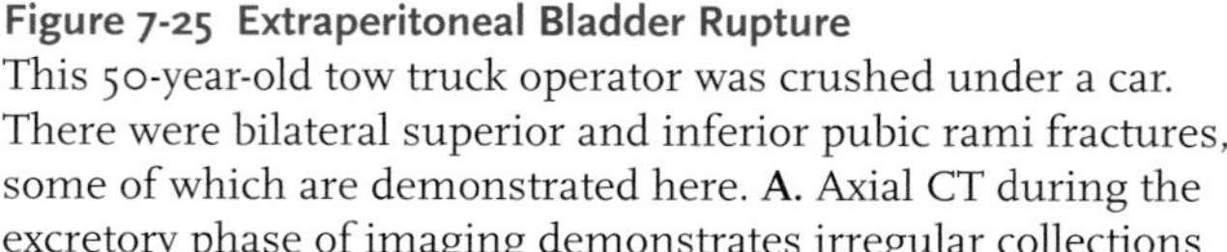

Figure 7-25 Extraperitoneal Bladder Rupture
This 50-year-old tow truck operator was crushed under a car. There were bilateral superior and inferior pubic rami fractures, some of which are demonstrated here. **A.** Axial CT during the excretory phase of imaging demonstrates irregular collections of contrast (*arrowheads*) in the pelvic soft tissues outside of the bladder. **B-D.** Axial CT images from a CT cystogram better show the extravesical contrast extravasation (*arrowheads*) in a molar tooth configuration. This is the typical appearance of an extraperitoneal rupture of the bladder.

bladder dome, which is the weakest portion of the urinary bladder and the urine leaks into the peritoneal cavity. Prior to contrast administration, ascites will be present on cross-sectional imaging examinations. Administration of contrast into the bladder will show extravasation of contrast into the peritoneum. In general, most extraperitoneal injuries will heal with conservative management with a bladder drainage catheter, whereas intraperitoneal injuries often require operative repair of the laceration.

Cystography performed with either conventional fluoroscopic control or CT cystography have equal sensitivity and high accuracy in demonstrating bladder injury. An important technical factor in performing such studies is to make sure the bladder is distended to the point where a detrusor contraction occurs. Small leaks will not be demonstrated if the bladder is not sufficiently distended.[88-92]

DIFFUSE ABNORMALITIES OF THE BLADDER, URETERS, AND COLLECTING SYSTEMS

Diffuse abnormalities of the urinary system include urinary obstruction and diffuse thickening of the bladder wall and diffuse thickening of the ureters.

Diffuse Dilation of the Ureters and Collecting Systems

Hydronephrosis indicates dilation of the renal collecting system and renal pelvis, whereas hydroureteronephrosis denotes dilation of the renal collecting system, renal pelvis, and ureter. Diffuse dilation is the only common diffuse abnormality of the urinary system. Like with the colon and other peristalsing tubal structures, dilation of the urothelial system usually indicates distal obstruction such as infundibular obstruction in the case of calyceal dilation, renal pelvis or UPJ obstruction in the case of a dilated pyelocalyceal system, and ureteral obstruction when the pyelocalyceal system and ureter are dilated. It is important to keep in mind that the finding of collecting system dilation does not necessarily indicate current obstruction; it can be a residual anatomic change related to previous obstruction. In an obstructed system, there is elongation of the smooth muscle of the pyelocalyceal system and ureter to accommodate the larger quantity of urine held in such a system. Even after relief of the obstruction, the anatomic changes will often not reverse because of permanent lengthening and loss of tone of the smooth muscle, and the collecting system may remain capacious and dilated in comparison to a system that has never been obstructed. It follows that in such patients, the diagnosis of superimposed acute obstruction can pose a considerable diagnostic challenge. This issue is frequently a problem for the right ureter of multigravid women. In late second and third trimesters of pregnancy, the ureter is obstructed as it crosses the pelvic brim by the enlarged uterus, and it is common to have moderate degrees of hydronephrosis in late pregnancy.

Imaging Notes 7-5. Hydroureteronephrosis

Hydroureteronephrosis is a result of urinary obstruction, vesicoureteral reflux, or prior obstruction or reflux.

This residual distensibility of the collecting system and ureter persists after delivery. In subsequent pregnancies, if the woman presents with flank pain, the finding of collecting system dilation is unhelpful in deciding whether the findings represent chronic findings or represent new acute on chronic obstruction. This will be addressed further in the section on acute renal colic.

The degree of collecting system and ureteral dilation is influenced by the severity and the duration of the obstructive process. In acute obstruction, the degree of dilation is typically very minimal; however, with chronic obstruction, urinary system dilation can be massive. Hydroureteronephrosis can also be seen with severe or persistent VUR, particularly in children.

Urinary obstruction

Obstruction to urinary flow results in progressive increase in urinary pressures leading to distention of the ureters, pelvis, and collecting system and can be an acute or chronic phenomenon.

Acute urinary obstruction: Acute urinary obstruction is most often secondary to urolithiasis and is a common problem in patients presenting to an acute care facility. The lifetime incidence of urolithiasis is estimated at 12%, and 2.3% of the population will experience renal colic in their lifetimes.[93] Patients typically present between 30 and 60 years of age and men are affected 3 times more often than women.[94,95] Patients typically present with acute renal colic. This is a severe pain that is waxing and waning or spasmodic, beginning abruptly in the flank and increasing rapidly, extending into the ipsilateral pelvis and labia or testicles. The pain can also be a steady and continuous discomfort that radiates to the lower abdomen and pelvis as the stone moves distally in the urinary tract. Urinalysis, to evaluate for microhematuria, is often the initial laboratory examination performed in patients who present with suspected renal colic. However, the presence or absence of microhematuria is not a reliable indicator of the urinary stone disease Hematuria is not detected in approximately 20% of patients who have documented urinary tract stones.[96] Detection of hematuria has been shown to be influenced by the timing of the urinalysis. In a retrospective study of more than 450 patients who had acute ureterolithiasis documented on CT, hematuria was present in 95% on day 1 but in only 65% to 68% on days 3 and 4.[96] Nausea and vomiting are common associated symptoms. Gross hematuria can be seen with stones lodged at the ureterovesical junction, with consequent irritation of the adjacent bladder, and can also be seen with large renal pelvic or bladder calculi.

Radiologic imaging plays a critical role in the evaluation and management of patients who have acute flank pain and suspected acute ureteral obstruction. Unenhanced helical CT is the diagnostic modality of choice and is both sensitive and specific for the diagnosis of urinary stone disease, with a reported sensitivity of 97% to 100% and specificity of 94% to 96%.[97,98] It can be performed rapidly without intravenous contrast, can identify and directly measure size of calculi, and can determine the degree of a possible associated urinary tract obstruction. False-negative CT results for stone detection range from 2% to 7% and are attributed largely to volume averaging and small stone size.[98,99] Smaller section widths result in a higher rate of urinary stone detection but add to the radiation dose burden of the patient. CT-section widths of 1.5 and 3.0 mm show no significant difference in the detection of urinary tract calculi, but 5.0-mm sections reveal significantly fewer urinary tract stones.[100]

Accurate determination of stone size is very important for clinical management, as spontaneous passage of ureteral stones is highly dependent on stone size. In 1 study, the mean diameter of stones that passed spontaneously was approximately 2.9 ± 2.0 mm whereas the mean diameter of stones for which conservative therapy failed was 7.9 ± 3.3 mm.[101] Stones that are 5 mm or less in diameter pass spontaneously in 68% of patients, whereas there is a 47% probability for spontaneous passage for stones between 5 and 10 mm in size.[102] Thus, there is a progressive decrease in the spontaneous passage rate as the size increases. Stones larger than 10 mm in diameter are unlikely to pass spontaneously. In general, CT scans provide more accurate estimates of size than abdominal radiographs in both the longitudinal and transverse axes, with the sizes being consistently greater on CT than on abdominal radiographs,[103,104] although these differences are not significant for stones between 2 and 13 mm in maximum diameter.

The imaging diagnosis of acute ureteral obstruction related to renal calculi is made by a combination of (1) identification of the stone within the ureter and (2) secondary signs of urinary tract obstruction. Secondary signs of acute obstruction include (1) hydronephrosis, (2)

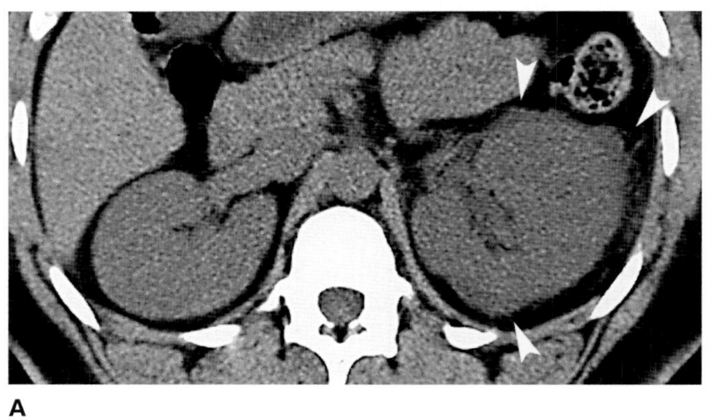

A

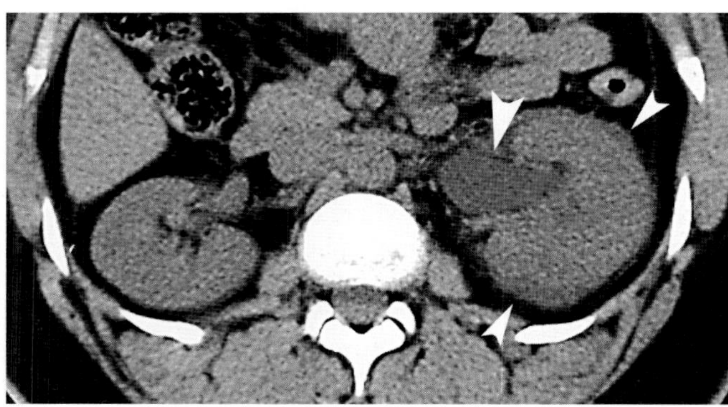

B

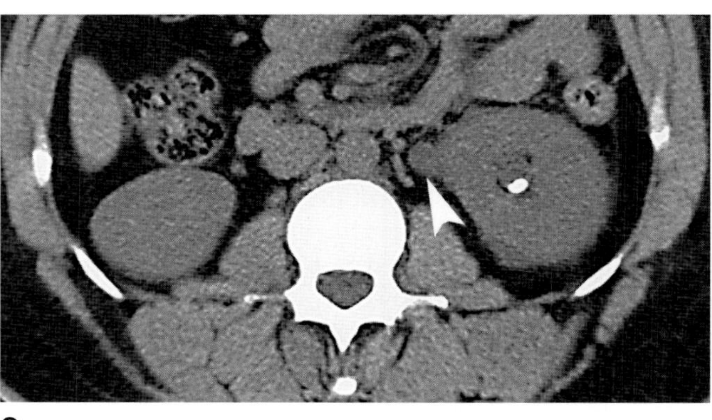

C

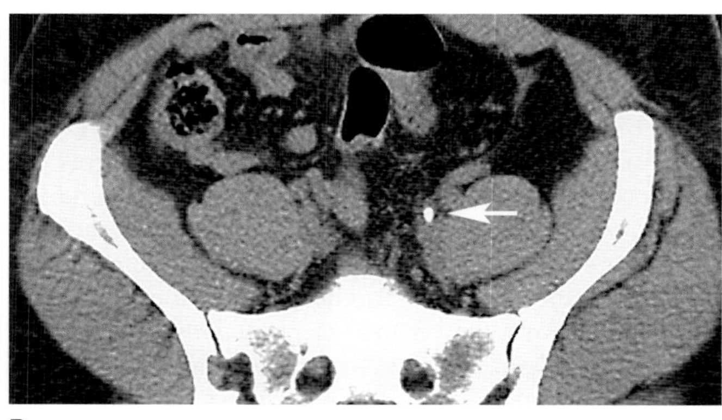

D

Figure 7-26 Acute Obstruction due to a Ureteral Calculus
This 39-year-old woman complained of left lower quadrant pain radiating to the left flank. **A-D.** Unenhanced CT shows the left kidney to be larger than the right and there is mild perinephric edema seen as irregularity of the contour of the left kidney (*small arrowheads*). There is also dilation of the left renal pelvis and ureter (*large arrowheads*). These are typical secondary findings of acute left renal obstruction. Careful review along the course of the left ureter demonstrated a small ureteral calculus (*arrow*) at the level of the pelvic brim. Did you notice the second stone in a lower pole calyx of the left kidney in image (C)?

Imaging Notes 7-6. CT/Urogram Findings of Acute Obstruction

Unenhanced CT
1. Lesion at the site of obstruction (stone, neoplasm)
2. Hydronephrosis or hydroureteronephrosis
3. Perinephric stranding
4. Periureteral stranding
5. Enlarged hypoattenuating ipsilateral kidney

Enhanced CT/urogram
1. Delayed nephrogram and pyelograms (excretion)
2. Increasingly dense nephrogram
3. Persistent column of contrast in ipsilateral ureter

perinephric stranding (edema), and (3) periureteral stranding (edema) (see Figure 7-26). In 1 report, these signs were seen in 69%, 65%, and 31.4% of patients with stones, respectively. All of these findings were absent in only 3.7% of patients who had ureteral calculi as a cause of their flank pain. The likelihood of the presence of these signs increases with increasing duration of pain, are usually not seen in the first 2 hours after the onset of pain, and develop fully about 8 hours after the onset of pain.[105,106]

Typically, there is mild hydroureteronephrosis of the affected collecting system, renal pelvis, and ureter. Careful comparison with the unaffected side will show the difference between obstructed and unobstructed renal pelvis and ureter. It is important not to mistake an extrarenal pelvis (a common normal variant) as hydronephrosis. The extrarenal position of the renal pelvis and the lack of intrarenal dilation is typical of an extrarenal pelvis and not hydronephrosis (see Figure 7-27). Mild increase in size of the obstructed kidney can occur with significant acute obstruction because of the urine retention. Stranding in the perinephric fat is likely related to decompression of the obstructed collecting system through small tears in the calyces, with urine leakage into the perinephric tissues and drainage through perirenal lymphatics (see Figure 7-26). Renal edema can be diagnosed when a density difference of 5 Hounsfield units (HUs) is seen between the 2 kidneys on unenhanced CT scans (see Figure 7-28).[107]

Absence of hydroureteronephrosis has the strongest negative predictive value for obstruction.[99] When hydroureteronephrosis is present but no urinary tract calculus can be identified, the differential diagnosis includes a recently passed stone, pyelonephritis, or a stone that is radiolucent or too small to detect.[99] Nearly all calculi are radiopaque on CT with the exception of concreted crystals of HIV protease inhibitors, which are not calculi in the true sense of the word. It is important to keep in mind that perinephric stranding and renal enlargement can be seen in cases of pyelonephritis without associated obstruction, thus emphasizing the need to correlate CT findings with clinical history.

Care must be taken in attributing perinephric stranding to urinary obstruction. Mild, symmetric, bilateral stranding is a common normal variant in older individuals. Unilateral asymmetric stranding will usually be a clue

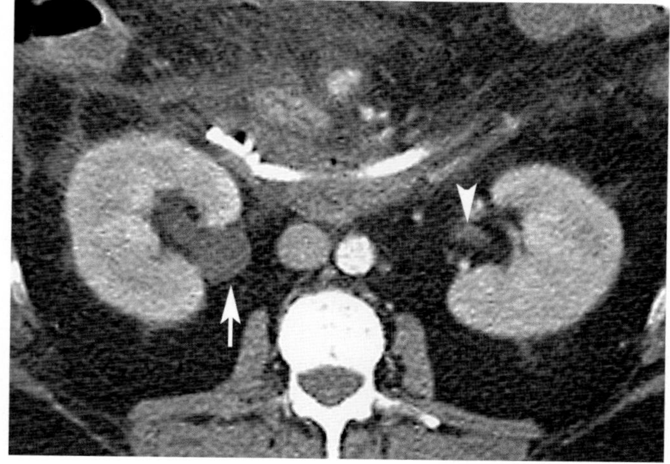
A

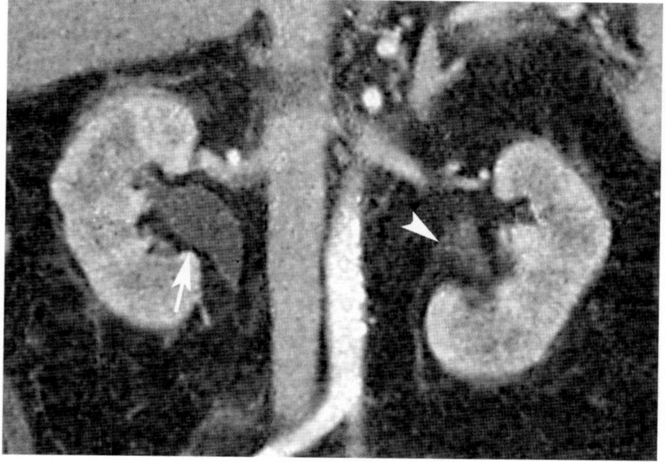
B

Figure 7-27 Extrarenal Pelvis
Contrast-enhanced CT in the (**A**) axial and (**B**) coronal planes shows the right renal pelvis (*arrows*) to be fuller than the left renal pelvis (*arrowheads*). However, there is symmetric enhancement of the 2 kidneys and there is no dilation of calices. This is the typical appearance of an extrarenal pelvis, a common normal variant. If the UPJ is poorly funneled with no tapering of the renal pelvis into the ureter, there will be UPJ obstruction. Congenital UPJ obstructions occur only when the renal pelvis is extrarenal, but an extrarenal pelvis usually has a normally funneled UPJ, as in this case.

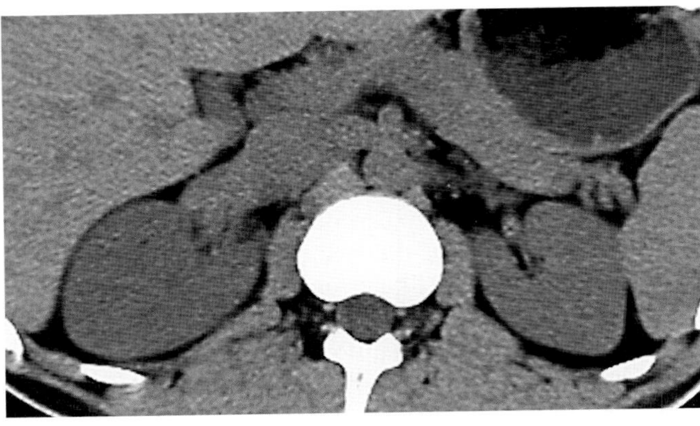

A

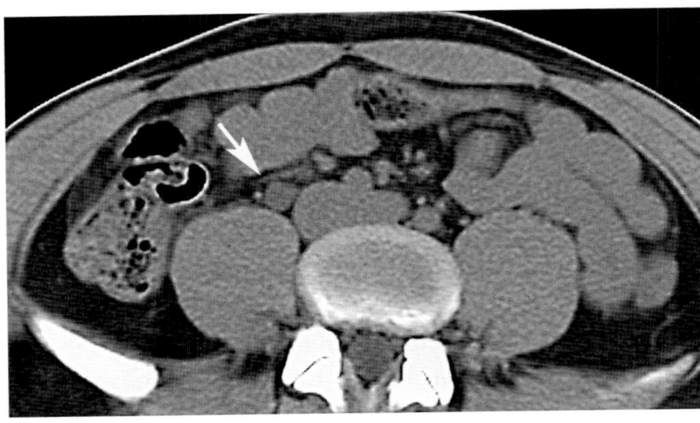

B

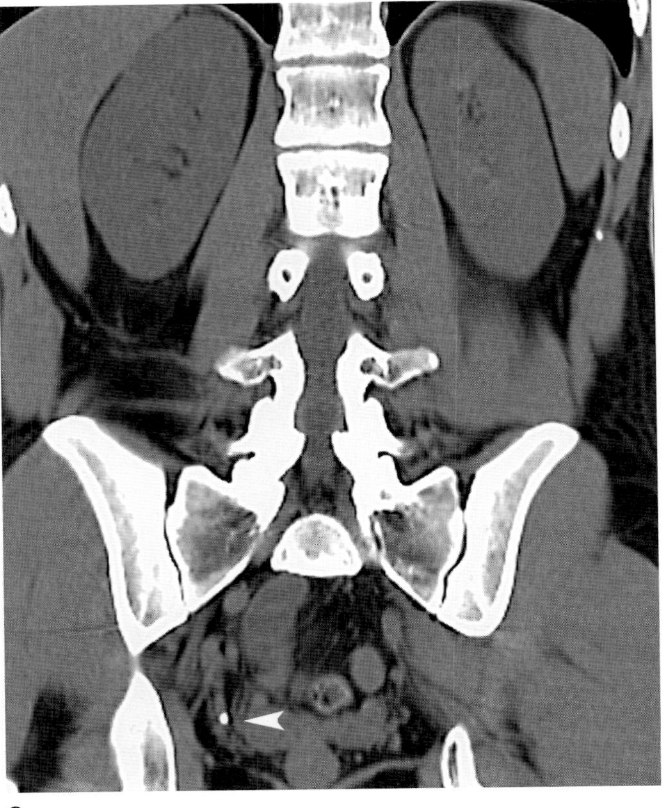

C

Figure 7-28 Obstructing Stone with Renal Edema
This patient presented with right lower quadrant pain. **A.** Unenhanced CT scan with narrow windows shows slight decreased attenuation of the right kidney relative to the left kidney, indicating right renal edema. **B.** Axial image a few centimeters lower shows the right ureter (*arrow*) is moderately dilated. **C.** Coronal reconstruction shows a small distal ureteral calculus (*arrowhead*).

to an abnormality in the affected kidney but can be a consequence of acute obstruction, pyelonephritis, renal vein occlusion, acute infarction, trauma, and other conditions.

Phleboliths are concentric calcifications in small pelvic veins. Distinguishing phleboliths from ureteral calculi can be problematic when interpreting a CT scan in a patient who has acute flank pain. An area of soft-tissue attenuation surrounding a suspected calcified ureteral calculus, referred to as a soft-tissue rim sign, may be seen on CT in 50% to 77% of ureteral calculi but is seen in only 0% to 8% of phleboliths;[108,109] reportedly, the specificity of the sign is 92%. The demonstration of this sign is dependent on the size of the calculus, being seen with 90% of stones smaller than 4 mm and absent with stones larger than 5 mm.[109] The absence of a soft tissue rim sign does not exclude the diagnosis of ureteral stone. The sign also is seen more often with distal ureteral stones than with proximal stones. Phleboliths may have an associated "tail" of soft-tissue attenuation (the so-called comet-tail sign) 65% of the time (see Figure 7-29).[109,110] A combination of these signs probably is the best aid in distinguishing phleboliths from ureteral calculi. The most reliable means of distinguishing ureteral calculi from phleboliths is to follow the course of the affected ureter. Calculi will be seen directly along the course of the ureter, whereas phleboliths will not be contiguous with the ureter. A radiolucent center may be useful for identifying phleboliths on an abdominal radiograph, but in a CT study of 120 phleboliths, 99% did not have a radiolucent center.[111] On occasion, in a symptomatic patient, there is no choice but to perform a contrast-enhanced CT scan in the excretory phase to distinguish a phlebolith from a ureteral calculus.

Another major advantage of CT in the management of patients with acute flank pain lies in its ability to detect causes of flank pain other than urinary stone disease. Alternative diagnoses span the spectrum of urinary tract pathology unrelated to stone disease, as well extraurinary pathology, and may be seen in 10% to 45% of patients.[94] The diagnosis of alternate pathologies is facilitated by the use of intravenous contrast.

If intravenous contrast is given, with significant urinary obstruction, there is a delay in the transit of contrast through the kidney. The homogeneous nephrographic phase is delayed, and there is delay in both contrast excretion and washout, because unopacified urine must be displaced before contrast can fill the renal tubules.

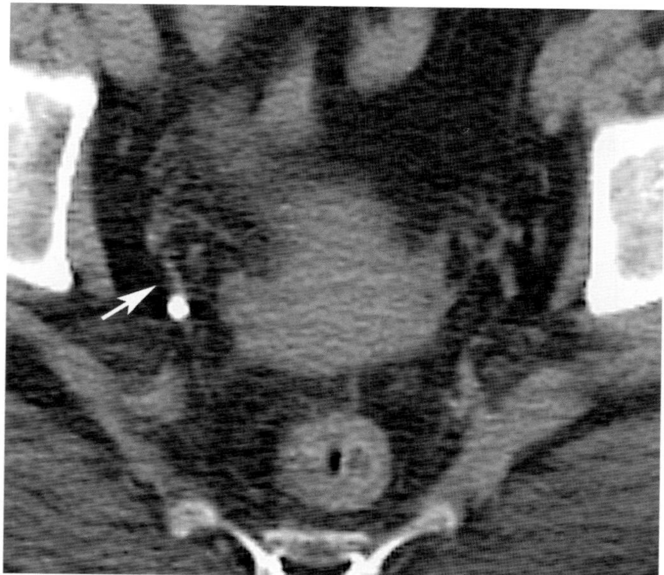

Figure 7-29 Comet Tail Sign
Unenhanced CT image demonstrates a small calcification in the right hemipelvis that could represent either a ureteral calculus or a phebolith. Note the small tail of soft tissue (*arrow*) attached to the calcification. This is a sign that is frequently associated with phebolіths.

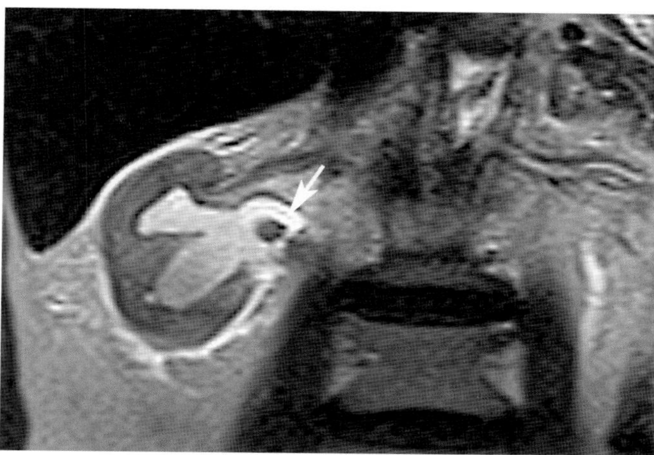

Figure 7-30 MRI of Acute Obstruction
This 25-year-old woman complained of abdominal pain. Coronal T2-weighted MRI image shows dilation of the calices and renal pelvis with a low-signal UPJ stone (*arrow*). There is also high-signal edema streaking the perinephric fat. These findings mimic those seen on CT and are the typical MRI features of acute obstruction due to a calculus.

Consequently, imaging soon after contrast administration will demonstrate normal enhancement of the unobstructed kidney and delayed enhancement of the obstructed kidney. After 10 to 15 minutes, the normal kidney will have excreted the majority of the filtered contrast and the attenuation of the kidney will decrease. However, the obstructed kidney will retain the contrast in the renal tubules and collecting ducts and so the attenuation of the kidney will progressively increase, a phenomenon known as an "increasingly dense or persistent nephrogram." There will also be delay in contrast opacification of the collecting system, renal pelvis, and ureter, a phenomenon known as a delayed pyelogram. Peristalsis will normally clear the ureters of contrast. Therefore, in the normal situation, the ureter will only be transiently filled with contrast and seen in a segmental fashion. An obstructed ureter remains filled with contrast and a persistent column of contrast will be seen within the ureter, far longer than in the normal unobstructed ureter.

All these signs were particularly important when IVU was the sole study used to diagnose acute ureteral obstruction. However, the unenhanced CT findings of obstruction described above correlate very well with findings of physiologically significant obstruction on an IVU, relegating IVU to a study of historical interest only in a patient presenting with acute flank pain.

Both US and MRI have been used to evaluate the patient who presents with acute flank pain. US often is used as the first imaging procedure in patients who should avoid radiation, such as pregnant women and children, but is much less sensitive than CT in depicting ureteral calculi, with a sensitivity of 61% compared to 96% for unenhanced CT.[112] The inability to detect small calculi makes MRI less useful in the setting of acute flank pain. Furthermore, urothelial lesions, blood clots, and debris can mimic calculi on MRI (see Figure 7-30).[113] Pregnant women with acute flank pain can pose a diagnostic challenge. Urinary calculus disease is common in pregnant women, and most women present in the second or third trimesters. Because of the overlying mineralized fetal skeleton, identifying a symptomatic ureteral calculus can be difficult on radiographs. Additionally, the exposures required to image the enlarged maternal abdomen with conventional radiography can increase the radiation dose to that of CT.[20] Thus, unenhanced CT may be the best technique to evaluate the symptomatic pregnant woman, as it is in the nonpregnant population (see Table 7-6).[114]

Chronic urinary obstruction: Unlike acute obstruction, it is rare for chronic obstruction to cause renal colic. As a consequence, chronic obstruction is typically clinically silent until late phases of obstruction. With prolonged obstruction, the elevated pressure in the ureters and collecting systems can be transmitted retrograde into the nephrons, resulting in a diminished glomerular filtration rate (GFR). Chronic unilateral obstruction is typically asymptomatic and the obstruction is detected incidentally on imaging examinations, which demonstrate an atrophic, hydronephrotic kidney. However, bilateral urinary obstruction is a cause of both acute and chronic renal failure. Serum creatinine and blood urea nitrogen will be elevated in such patients. Clinical symptoms of chronic obstruction are nonexistent or nonspecific findings associated with uremia such as weakness, peripheral edema, mental status changes, and

Table 7-6. Causes of Urinary Obstruction

A. Acute obstruction 1. **Calculus**[a] 2. Blood clot 3. Sloughed papilla from papillary necrosis 4. Mycetoma
B. Chronic obstruction 1. Neoplasm a. **Transitional cell carcinoma and other primary neoplasms** b. **Direct extension from extraurinary neoplasm** c. Lymphoma 2. **Postsurgical** 3. Posttraumatic 4. Crohn disease 5. Inflammatory processes a. Extrinsic inflammatory mass (TOA, diverticulitis) b. TB 6. Retroperitoneal fibrosis 7. Endometriosis 8. **Benign prostatic hyperplasia** 9. Neurogenic bladder 10. **Pregnancy** 11. Congenital a. Ureteropelvic junction (UPJ) obstruction b. Ureterovesical junction (UVJ) obstruction c. Posterior urethral valves d. Ectopic insertion of ureters e. Congenital megaureter

[a]Items in bold are common.

pallor. Prolonged obstruction also causes diminished renal blood flow and chronic ischemic damage to the affected kidney, which over time will cause renal atrophy.

Chronic obstruction is most often caused by pelvic neoplasms or BPH, but there are various other causes. Pregnancy will often cause mild chronic hydroureteronephrosis, especially of the right ureter and collecting system, particularly in late second and third trimesters. Imaging is the gold standard diagnostic tool for detection of urinary obstruction. When ureteral obstruction results in renal impairment, noncontrast CT appears to be the best imaging modality to identify calculus causes of obstruction whereas MR urography is superior for identifying noncalculous causes of obstruction.[115,116]

Chronic urinary obstruction will usually cause a greater degree of hydronephrosis or hydroureteronephrosis on imaging examinations. Chronic pressure on the walls of the ureters, pelvis, and collecting system results in slow progressive dilation. These findings will be demonstrated on all imaging examinations of the urinary system. The obstructed kidney will atrophy and in severe cases will cease to function. If contrast is administered, the obstructed kidney will have diminished opacity on IVPs, diminished attenuation on CT scans, and diminished intensity on MRI examinations. Nuclear scintigraphy will demonstrate diminished functioning of the obstructed kidney (see Figures 7-31 and 7-32). Perinephric and periureteral stranding (edema) is not a common feature in chronic obstruction.

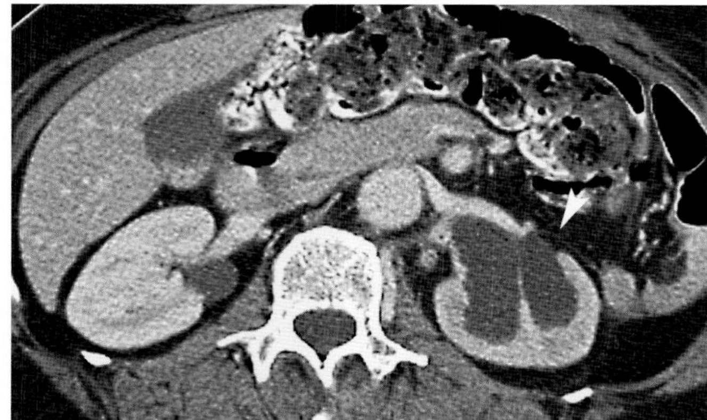

A

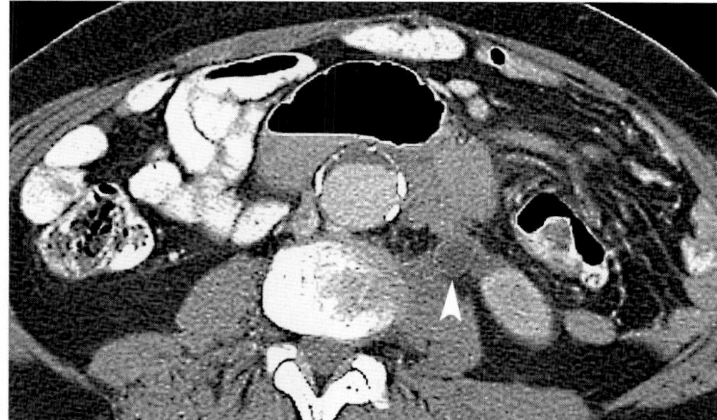

B

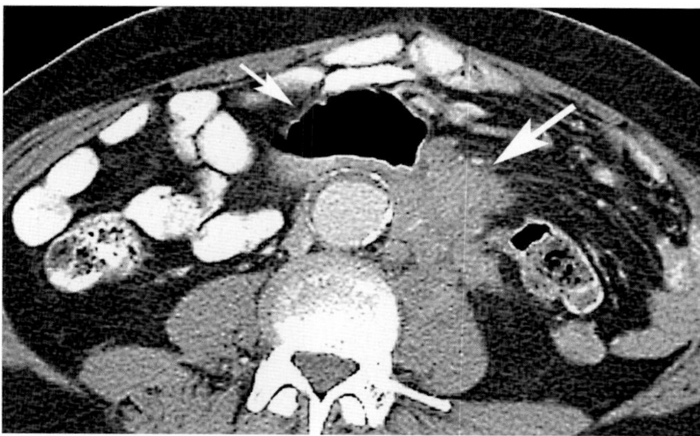

C

Figure 7-31 Ureteral Obstruction by Extrinsic Mass
This 60-year-old woman presented with weight loss. **A-C.** Contrast-enhanced CT images show a dilated left renal collecting system and ureter (*arrowheads*) caused by an irregular mass (*large arrow*) in the left retroperitoneum. This was shown to originate in the sigmoid colon and causes mild sigmoid colon dilation (*small arrow*).

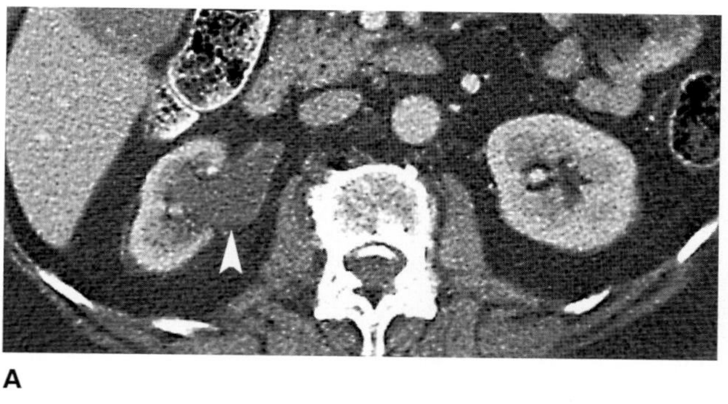
A

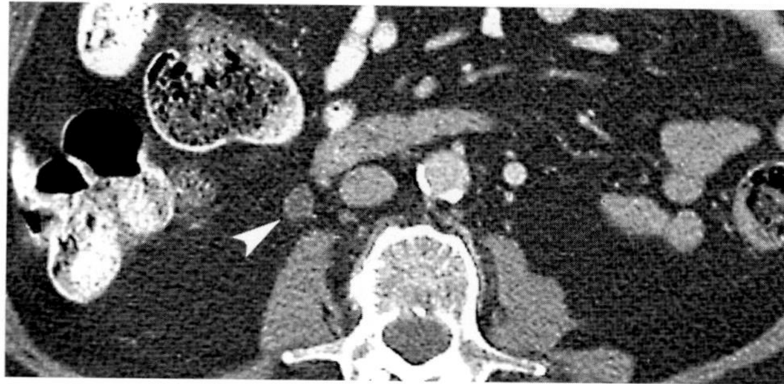
B

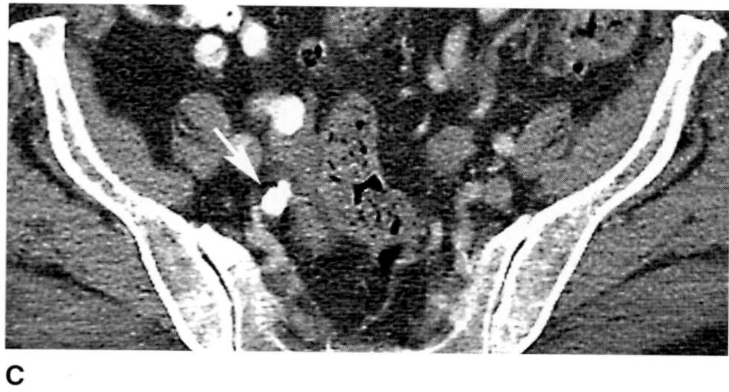
C

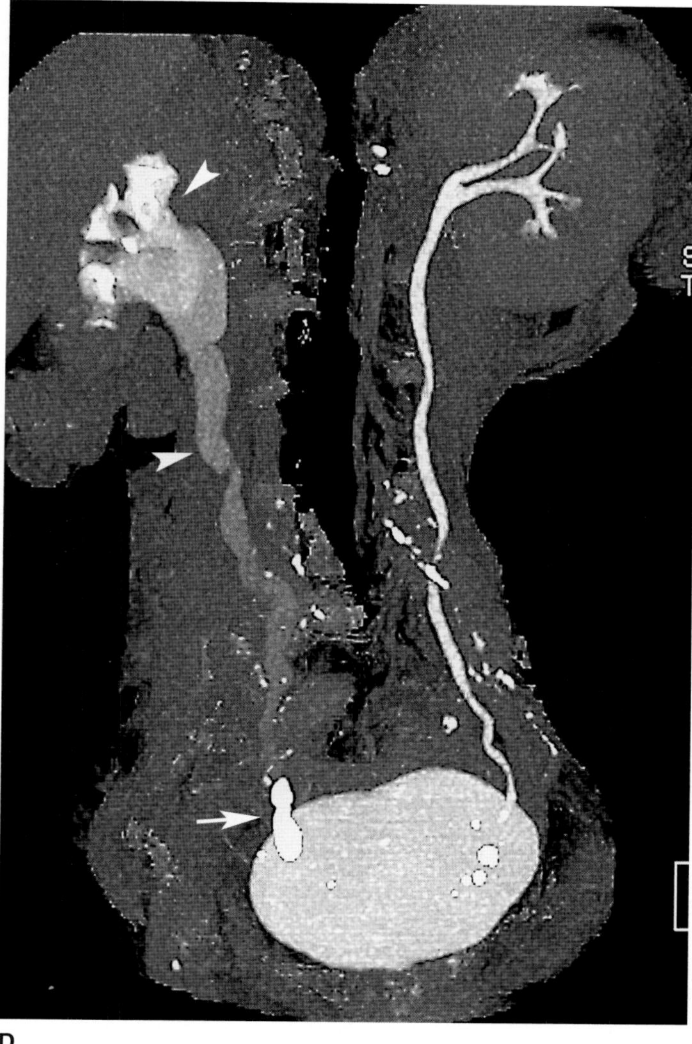
D

Figure 7-32 Chronic Ureteral Obstruction
This 79-year-old woman had weight loss and GI bleeding. **A-C.** Contrast-enhanced CT shows an atrophic right kidney and mild dilation of the right renal pelvis, collecting system, and right ureter (*arrowheads*) to the level of a large stone in the distal right ureter (*arrow*). The atrophy of the right kidney and the lack of perinephric and periureteral edema are characteristic of a chronic obstruction. **D.** These features are seen to better advantage on this MIP multiplanar reconstruction.

Patients with new onset renal failure will typically receive a renal US examination to determine whether urinary obstruction is the cause of renal failure. Depending on the degree of obstruction, the examination will demonstrate varying dilation of the renal collecting systems and pelves (see Figure 7-33). If obstruction is identified, then a noncontrast CT or MRI can be indicated to better evaluate the cause for chronic obstruction. (Iodinated CT contrast and gadolinium MRI contrast is often contraindicated in patients with renal failure.) These examinations will confirm bilateral hydronephrosis or hydroureteronephrosis and will often identify the underlying cause for obstruction. Although renal scintigraphy is useful to quantitate the relative functioning of the kidneys, it is less helpful in predicting recoverable function in a patient with severe obstruction.

Vesicoureteral reflux

VUR refers to the abnormal reflux of urine backward into the ureters from the bladder during voiding. In the normal individual, the ureter inserts diagonally through the wall of the bladder. With this configuration, contraction of the smooth muscle of the bladder wall results in constriction of the ureteral orifice, preventing reflux of urine into the ureters. However, in some individuals, the ureter inserts more perpendicularly into the bladder wall. With this configuration, bladder wall contraction fails to occlude the ureteral orifice and urine is forcefully refluxed into the ureter when intravesical pressure rises during voiding. The majority of cases of VUR represent this primary congenital failure of the natural passive one-way mechanism of

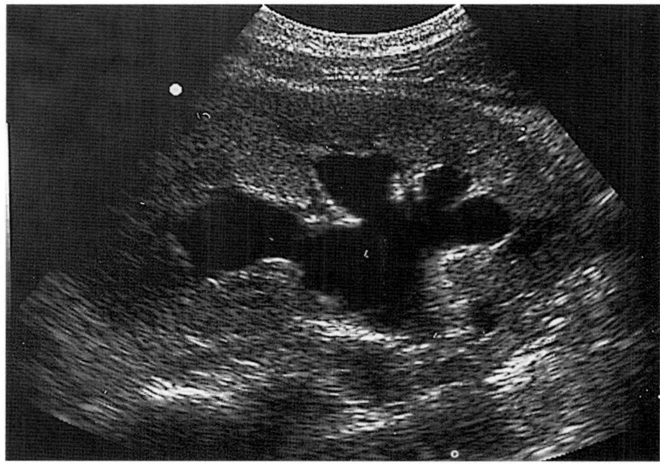

A

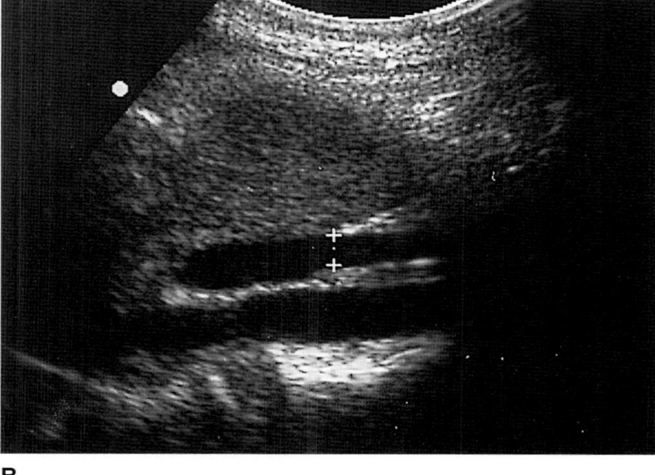

B

Figure 7-33 US of Chronic Obstruction Due to Cervical Cancer This 54-year-old woman with cervical cancer developed increasing blood urea nitrogen and creatinine. Longitudinal US of (**A**) the right kidney and (**B**) ureter show dilation of the collecting system and ureter. Findings in the left kidney and ureter were similar. This bilateral hydroureteronephrosis was due to invasion of the bladder trigone by cervical cancer.

the ureterovesical junction.[114,115] A minority of VUR cases, approximately 10%, occur secondary to other abnormalities of the ureteral insertion.[116,117] These include renal transplantation, ureterocele, ureteral duplication anomalies, and obstruction of the bladder outlet.

Congenital VUR typically occurs in infants and children and in most cases will resolve spontaneously as the child grows older. The younger the age of the patient and the lower the grade at presentation, the higher the chance of spontaneous resolution. It occurs more commonly in Caucasians, girls, and in those with a family history of VUR. In the majority of cases, VUR is asymptomatic and is clinically insignificant. However, when associated with urinary tract infections, VUR can result in extensive renal scarring and ultimately renal failure (reflux nephropathy). Other complications of renal scarring include systemic hypertension and growth impairment.[118] Reflux nephropathy is responsible for 30% to 50% of end-stage renal disease in pediatric patients and for 20% in adults.[119,120] Studies have shown that the children with VUR who present with a urinary tract infection and associated acute pyelonephritis are more likely to develop permanent renal cortical scarring than those children without VUR, with an odds ratio of 2.8.[118] Increasing grade of VUR and presence of bladder and bowel dysfunction are also risk factors for renal cortical scarring related to VUR.[118]

The severity of VUR is graded by how far the urine refluxes into the ureters and collecting system and the degree of ureteral and collecting system dilation (Table 7-7). Grading is performed by evaluating the extent of contrast reflux during voiding cystourethrogram (VCUG).[121] Studies have demonstrated that only grades 4 and 5 VUR are shown at VCUG with 100% reliability.[122] VUR can be intermittent and its severity can vary on sequential cystograms.[123,124] Studies using an US contrast agent have suggested that US examinations (cystosonography) can also be used to diagnose VUR with sensitivities and specificities similar to VCUG.[125] Once the diagnosis of VUR is made, follow-up to gauge the presence and severity can also be performed with radionuclide cystograms. In adults, reflux is usually an innocuous finding and can be seen in patients with indwelling catheters and those who have undergone recent bladder surgery.

Because evidence of renal scarring is the primary determinant of clinical outcomes due to VUR, and because medical and surgical interventions are predicated on the presence or absence of renal scarring, it is important to structurally and functionally evaluate the kidney for evidence of damage. US and DMSA radionuclide imaging are the suggested imaging studies of choice to evaluate for the presence of renal damage.[118] Changes of reflux nephropathy typically affect the poles of the kidney, particularly the upper

Table 7-7. International Classification of Vesicoureteral Reflux

- Grade I – reflux into nondilated ureter
- Grade II – reflux into the renal pelvis and calyces without dilation
- Grade III – mild/moderate dilation of the ureter, renal pelvis, and calyces with minimal blunting of the fornices
- Grade IV – dilation of the renal pelvis and calyces with moderate ureteral tortuosity
- Grade V – gross dilatation of the ureter, pelvis, and calyces; ureteral tortuosity; loss of papillary impressions

pole, with sparing of the interpolar region. On US and other cross-sectional imaging, this will appear as decreased thickness of the renal cortex and a focal depression of the contour of the kidney at the site of scarring.

Diffuse Thickening of the Bladder Wall

Thickening of the bladder wall can be seen on cross-sectional images. There are no precise criteria for a diagnosis of bladder wall thickening because the thickness of the bladder wall is greatly dependent on the degree of distention of the bladder. When collapsed, the bladder wall can be a few centimeters thick and be normal, whereas when fully distended should only be a few millimeters thick. Therefore, a diagnosis of bladder wall thickening is a subjective determination, based on clinical experience of the observer.[126]

Thickening of the bladder wall can be a result of (1) muscular hypertrophy of the wall, (2) malignant infiltration of the wall, or (3) wall inflammation and subsequent edema (Table 7-8). Muscular hypertrophy is the most common cause of diffuse bladder wall thickening and is a result of bladder outlet obstruction (see Figure 7-34). This accounted for 6/10 cases of diffuse bladder wall thickening in 1 series.[126] Bladder outlet obstruction is most often due to BPH but can be due to a variety of causes, which will be discussed more completely in the subsequent section of this chapter.

Table 7-8. Causes of Bladder Wall Thickening

A. Muscular hypertrophy
1. **Benign prostatic hyperplasia**[a]
2. Neurogenic bladder
3. Other causes of urethral obstruction
B. Malignant infiltration
1. **Transitional cell carcinoma**
2. Other urothelial malignancies
3. Lymphoma
4. Metastasis
C. Wall edema
1. Infectious cystitis
a. Bacterial
b. Tuberculosis
2. Chemotherapy
a. Cyclophosphamide
b. Other
3. Radiation therapy
4. Uncommon causes of cystitis
a. Eosinophilic cystitis
b. Malacoplakia
c. Systemic lupus erythematosis
d. Amyloidosis
5. Indwelling catheters and stents
6. Extrinsic inflammatory conditions
a. Crohn disease
b. Diverticulitis

[a]Causes in bold are common.

Imaging Notes 7-7. Bladder Wall Thickening

Diffuse bladder wall thickening is most often due to muscular hypertrophy as a result of obstruction due to BPH. Focal and asymmetric bladder wall thickening is most often due to malignant infiltration by TCC.

Malignant infiltration of the bladder wall will usually lead to asymmetric bladder wall thickening. In 1 series, 8/10 cases of asymmetric thickening were due to malignancy, most often TCC of the bladder (see Figures 7-9 and 7-11).[126] However, diffuse bladder wall thickening can rarely be a manifestation of malignancy and accounted for 1/10 cases in the series.[126] Although TCC is the most common malignant cause of bladder wall thickening, other malignant causes include other cell types of urothelial cancer, metastasis to the bladder, and lymphoma.[127-129]

Inflammation and edema are the least common cause of focal and diffuse bladder wall thickening, accounting for 2/10 focal and 1/10 diffuse cases in one series.[126] Inflammatory causes of diffuse bladder wall thickening include radiation- and chemotherapy-induced cystitis and infectious cystitis due to bacterial infections and tuberculosis. Rarely, thickening can be due to other inflammatory conditions including malacoplakia, systemic lupus erythematosus, eosinophilic cystitis, and amyloidosis.[58,130,131] Hemorrhagic cystitis related to previous radiation or chemotherapy, particularly with the use of cyclophosphamide, is a well-known cause of severe cystitis.[132-135] Patients usually present with gross hematuria, and clot retention is a common and serious clinical problem. Management of such patients is very difficult, and patients can have significant blood loss. Infectious causes of gross thickening are most strongly associated with tuberculosis of the bladder. Routine urinary tract infections are not usually imaged and are unlikely to demonstrate imaging abnormalities, but occasionally bacterial cystitis can result in bladder wall thickening (see Figure 7-35). Patients with indwelling catheters and stents can develop bladder wall thickening as a result of chronic irritation.

Bladder wall inflammation and subsequent thickening can also be due to involvement of the bladder from an inflammatory process outside of the bladder. This is best recognized as a complication of Crohn disease and diverticulitis.[58] This bladder wall thickening will often be an indicator of an inflammatory fistula from the bowel to the bladder. Enterovesical and colovesical fistulas are discussed in greater detail in a subsequent section titled: **Bladder Fistulae.**

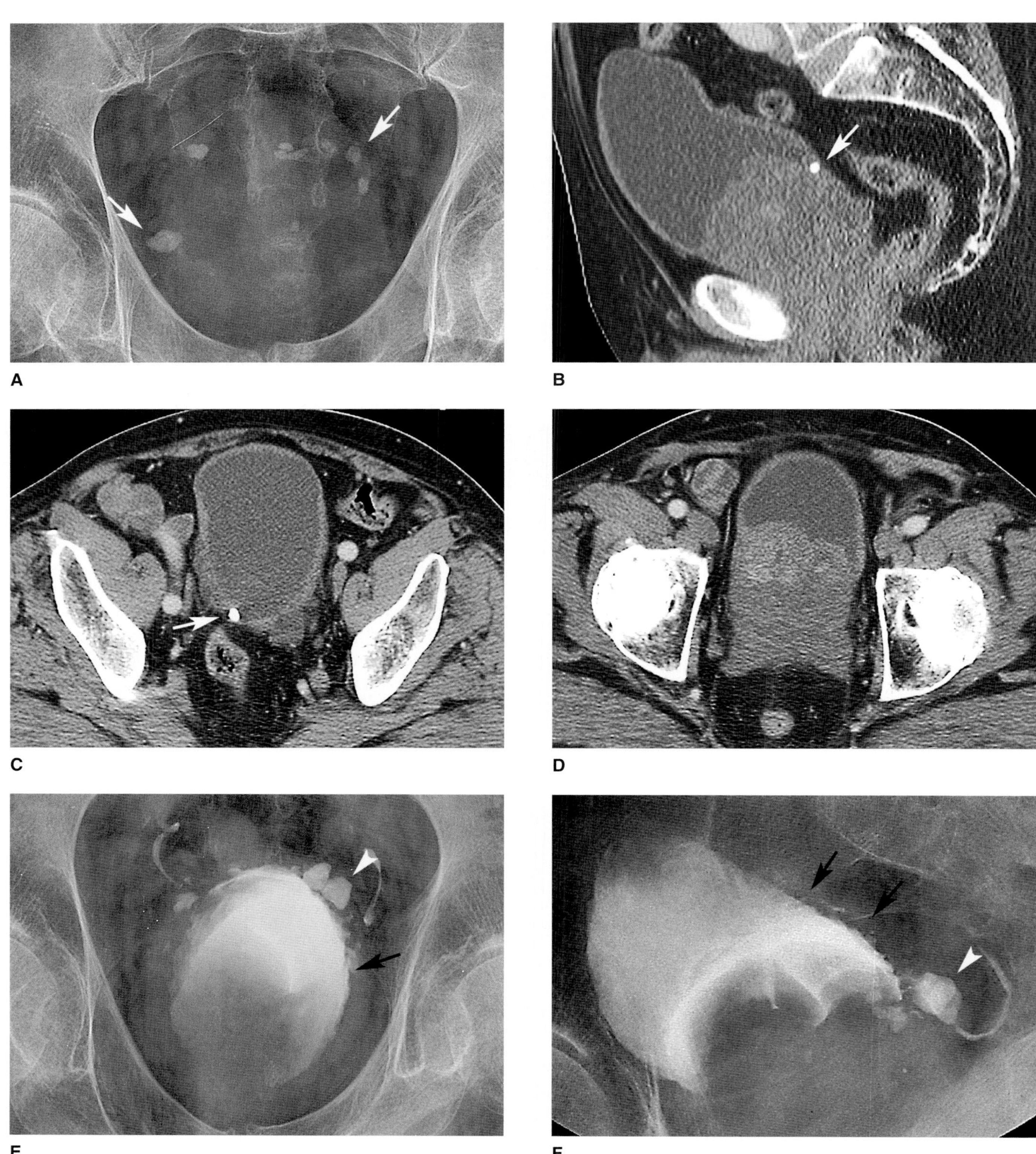

Figure 7-34 Bladder Changes Related to Benign Prostatic Hyperplasia (BPH)
This 68-year-old man had hematuria. **A.** Anteroposterior (AP) radiograph of the pelvis shows multiple oval calcifications (*white arrows*) overlying the region of the bladder and likely to represent bladder calculi. **B.** Sagittal reconstruction and (**C** and **D**) 2 axial images confirm the presence of bladder calculi (*white arrow*) and also show a massively enlarged prostate and diffuse bladder wall thickening. These findings are consistent with muscular hypertrophy of the bladder wall as a result of outlet obstruction due to BPH. (**E**) AP and (**F**) oblique views from an IVU show a large defect in the base of the bladder due to the enlarged prostate. There is also mild irregularity to the surface of the bladder (*black arrows*) typical of bladder trabeculation and multiple diverticula (*arrowheads*). These are the typical features of bladder outlet obstruction on contrast evaluations of the bladder.

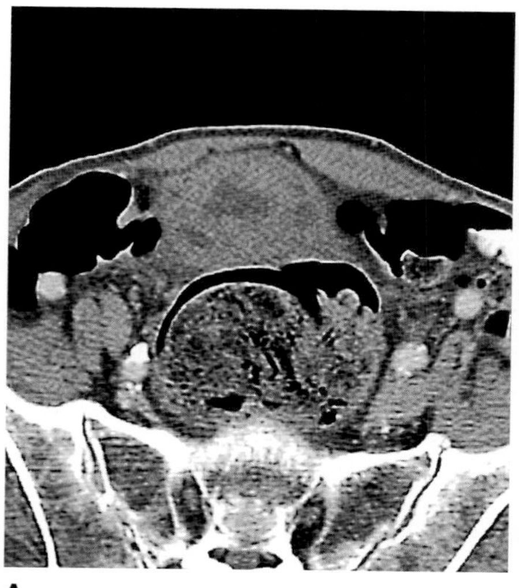
A

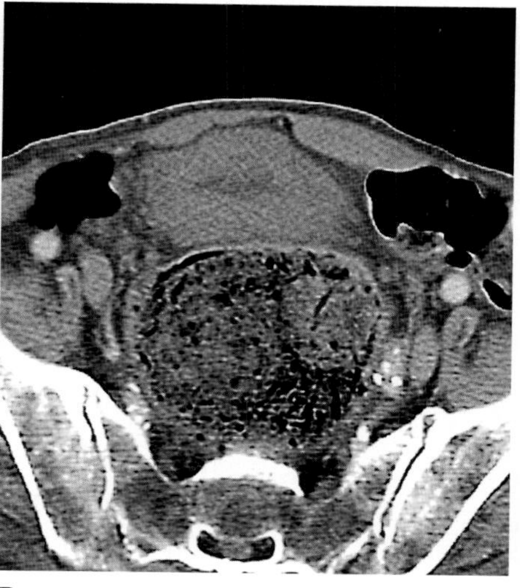
B

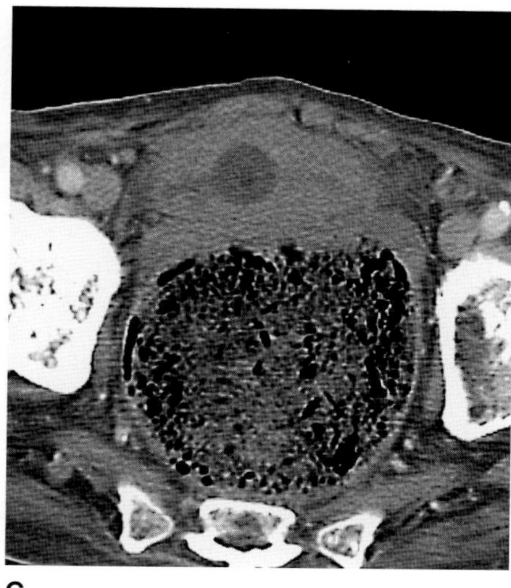
C

Figure 7-35 Corynebacterium Cystitis
This 91-year-old demented woman was persistently febrile. **A-C.** Unenhanced CT images demonstrate diffuse thickening of the wall of the bladder with small hypoattenuating regions in the bladder dome (A). In this setting, this is likely to indicate the presence of a cystitis. *Corynebacterium* species were cultured from the patient's urine.

Bladder outlet obstruction

Bladder outlet obstruction is a common problem, caused by compression or narrowing of bladder outflow channel at any location from the bladder neck to urethral meatus.

It is most often encountered in middle-aged and older men as a result of BPH.[136]

Typical presenting symptoms include hesitancy, sensation of incomplete bladder emptying, diminished urinary stream, postvoid urinary dribbling, urinary urgency, increased frequency of urination, nocturia, and occasional dysuria.[133]

The etiology of bladder outlet obstruction is often gender specific. As noted previously in men, bladder outlet obstruction is most often due to BPH. Young boys can present with bladder outlet obstruction because of congenital posterior urethral valves. Men are much more likely than women to develop urethral strictures.[133]

In women, bladder outlet obstruction is most often a complication of incontinence surgery, with an incidence of 2% to 22% of patients, depending on the surgical procedure.[134,137] Other causes of obstruction in women include[133] pelvic organ prolapse such as cystocele, rectocele, enterocele, and uterine procidentia. Extraurinary malignancies, such as uterine, ovarian, and cervical carcinoma, can also result in bladder outlet obstruction in women. Benign extraurinary masses, including vaginal cysts and Gartner duct cysts, can press on the urethra and result in obstruction. Rarely, urethral diverticula can cause bladder outlet obstruction.

Some causes that can be seen in either sex include rectal, bladder, and urethral carcinoma; bladder calculi; and neurogenic bladder due to a variety of causes such as multiple sclerosis.[133]

To maintain urine flow, the detrusor muscle bundles hypertrophy, leading initially to a trabeculated appearance of the bladder on cystograms, and eventually to formation of diverticula (see Figure 7-34). On cross-sectional imaging examinations, the wall of the bladder will often appear uniformly thickened. Occasionally, diverticula can also be identified (see Figure 7-34). The thickening of the bladder wall can also cause mild obstruction of the distal ureters as they travel through the bladder wall, with resultant mild hydronephrosis. The role of imaging in the evaluation of bladder outlet obstruction is to look for obstructing lesions, which can cause obstruction. Voiding cystourethrogram can also be used to directly visualize the urethra and identify strictures, diverticula, and other intrinsic causes of urethral obstruction.

Diffuse Thickening of the Ureteral Wall

This is usually seen in patients with indwelling ureteral stents but can rarely be caused by tuberculosis (see Figure 7-24). Most other neoplastic or inflammatory abnormalities in the ureter cause focal or localized abnormalities.

Pyelitis, ureteritis, and cystitis cystica

Ureteritis cystic was discussed in the previous section. Pyelitis cystica occurs in patients with long-term nephrostomy tubes and rarely in patients with large calculi in the upper tracts. Small filling defects will be seen in the pyelocalyceal system. If no calculi or stents are present, urothelial neoplasm is the diagnosis of exclusion.

Cystitis cystica is related to the presence of long-term Foley catheters or ureteral stents. Smooth filling defects may be seen in the bladder, particularly when the bladder is underdistended.

UNIQUE IMAGING FINDINGS IN THE URINARY SYSTEM

Imaging findings specific to the urinary system include calculi, calcifications within the structures of the urinary system, and fistulae from the urinary system to surrounding structures.

Upper Tract Urinary Calculi

Approximately 10% of the US population will have renal calculi detectable at some time during their life, the majority of which are clinically asymptomatic. Symptoms are usually the result of passage of a stone from the kidney to the bladder and include colicky back, flank, pelvic, and scrotal pain; nausea; vomiting; dysuria; and hematuria, as discussed above.

Urinary calculi are an aggregate of polycrystalline components (97.5%) on an organic mucoprotein or glycoprotein matrix (2.5%).[138] Two-thirds of stones are composed of a mixture of different crystalline structures. Single crystal (or pure) stones constitute only one-third of all urinary calculi. Some pure stones may have a characteristic radiographic appearance. Crystalline admixtures, on the other hand, are more commonly encountered in clinical practice and can have a variety of appearances.

Calcium phosphate calculi

Calcium phosphate (also known as apatite) is an important component of the stones that form in infected alkaline urine. Pure calcium phosphate stones are rare, often occur in association with primary hyperparathyroidism, and account for only 4% of all calcium phosphate stones. Other causes of calcium phosphate stones include renal tubular acidosis and sarcoidosis. The radiographic appearance of pure calcium phosphate stones is indistinguishable from pure calcium oxalate stones.

Magnesium ammonium phosphate hexahydrate (struvite) calculi or triple phosphate stones are typically branched in configuration and form a cast of the renal pelvis and 1 or more calyces and infundibuli. They occur in patients with chronic urinary tract infections. Concentric lamellations are a hallmark and are related to the deposition of poorly opaque struvite alternating with more opaque calcium components.

Calcium oxalate calculi

Calcium oxalate is a radiopaque crystal and 73% of all calculi contain more than 50% calcium oxalate, making it the most common constituent of urinary calculi. Calcium oxalate can occur in a pure form, but it is more frequently a component of mixed stones, and can be admixed with calcium phosphate, uric acid, and magnesium phosphate stones, imparting radiopacity to these less-radiodense constituents in patients with urinary tract infections.

Uric acid calculi

Hyperuricosuria due to excessive intake of purines, overproduction of uric acid due to endogenous purine metabolism, and myeloproliferative disorders such as acute leukemia are the primary causes of uric acid calculi. Foodstuffs rich in purine are largely those high in protein. Epidemiologic studies have demonstrated that purines from meat and fish increase the risk of developing gout, whereas purines from vegetables fail to change the risk, and dairy foods rich in purines appear to lower the risk of gout.[139,140] In Lesch-Nehan syndrome (juvenile gout), overproduction of purine results in hyperuricemia and the occurrence of multiple uric acid calculi. Patients are mentally retarded, prone to self-mutilation, with resultant amputation of fingertips and phalanges.

Persistent acidic urine enhances the crystallization of uric acid and in combination with low urine volumes, constitutes the major cause of uric acid calculi. Pure uric acid stones, which make up 41% of all uric acid calculi, are nonopaque on plain radiographs but are easily detectable on CT or US. However, because more than half of uric acid calculi have a coating of calcium salts, they can be variably radiopaque and therefore identifiable on plain films. When pure, these calculi tend to be small, smooth, and disk shaped. Large uric acid calculi are generally of mixed composition and may have a staghorn configuration. Gouty arthritis is seen in 21% of patients with gouty diathesis and uric acid stones.

Cystine stones

Cystinuria is an autosomal recessive disorder resulting in the failure to resorb the amino acids cysteine, ornithine, lysine, and arginine. Failure of resorption leads to an excessive concentration of this amino acid in the urine. In neutral or acidic urine, cystine may precipitate into the urine, forming crystals or stones in the kidneys, ureters, or bladder. Cystine stones are moderately opaque, although to a much less degree than calcium stones of the same size; the radiopacity has been attributed to the higher physical density and higher effective atomic number of cystine, and the presence of sulfur atoms within the stones.[138,141-143] The stones have a homogeneous, ground-glass opacity on abdominal radiographs and can be easily obscured on technically suboptimal examinations. Cystine stones are often large, multiple, and can be staghorn in configuration. The presence of staghorn calculi in children or young adults in the absence of infection should raise the suspicion of cystine stones.

Matrix stones

These are rare stones that are of a gelatinous or soft putty texture and can range in color from tan to red brown.[142]

They likely represent inspissated mucoproteins, which then organizes into a calculus with striations and laminations. Small amounts of crystals may deposit into the matrix and give them a gritty texture.

Matrix calculi occur in patients with a history of chronic urinary tract infections with Proteus species or coliform organisms. There is often a history of renal stone disease, renal surgery, urinary stasis, or obstruction and there is a female predilection in a ratio of 3:1.[142] These calculi are notorious for causing obstruction and for rapid regrowth.[144]

Matrix stones are nonopaque on plain radiographs but can demonstrate a rim of calcification or diffuse increased attenuation on unenhanced CT scan due to the minimal mineralization. However, matrix stones can be completely unmineralized and be of soft tissue attenuation on CT. They are seen as filling defects within the opacified collecting system. On US, matrix calculi are echogenic but may not cast an acoustic shadow because of the sparse calcification. They do not respond to ESWL as the soft gelatinous consistency of the stone is resistant to fragmentation and are best removed by percutaneous or endourologic means (Table 7-9).

Xanthine stones

These are extremely rare stones that result from an inborn error of metabolism in which there is a deficiency of the enzyme xanthine oxidase. This leads to production of xanthine and hypoxanthine as the end products of purine metabolism, rather than uric acid. The stones are usually small and radiolucent, but an admixture of calcium salts may confer radiopacity.

Stones can form as a result of supersaturation of crystal-forming salts in the urine and therefore maintenance of hydration will inhibit stone formation, but anatomic factors may also be responsible. Chronic stone formers have subepithelial calcific plaques composed of calcium phosphate that occur in the renal papillae and are known as Randall plaques. These plaques serve as nuclei for at least 15% of calcium oxalate stones; such stones are recognizable by the distinctive depression on the external surface of the stone that corresponds to the site of initial caliceal attachment of the stone and, a calcium phosphate nucleus is often found in the depression. If a papillary depression is seen at the base of a cone-shaped calculus, it is strongly indicative that the stone originated on a papillary tip and then grew in the calyx before breaking loose and becoming mobile in the collecting system. It is speculated that normal kidneys without infection or obstruction are unlikely to form stones in the absence of a calcium phosphate papillary nucleus. Randall plaques are usually visualized as slivers of calcification adjacent to the papillary tip on radiographs or CT scans and may be indistinguishable from small caliceal calculi that have already detached from the papilla and are free within the calyx.

Table 7-9. Causes of Urinary Calculi

1. Calcium stones (Ca oxalate, Ca phosphate, Ca urate) a. Hyperparathyroidism b. Renal tubular acidosis c. Sarcoidosis
2. Struvite stones (magnesium ammonium calcium phosphate) a. Chronic UTI (esp. *Proteus*, *Pseudomonas*, or *Klebsiella* species)
3. Uric acid stones a. Gout b. High purine intake (meat and fish) c. Hypermetabolic malignancies (esp. leukemia) d. Lesch-Nehan syndrome
4. Cysteine stones a. Metabolic defect in amino acid resorption b. Precipitation of some medications
5. Matrix stones a. Chronic UTI b. History of urologic surgery, urinary stasis or urinary obstruction
6. Xanthine stones a. Xanthine oxidase deficiency (inborn error of metabolism)

Imaging evaluation of urinary calculi

Imaging is the primary method for the diagnosis of renal, ureteral, and bladder calculi. Unenhanced CT is the gold standard for the diagnosis of urinary stones, with a sensitivity and specificity approaching 100%. However, renal calculi can be demonstrated on abdominal x-rays, intravenous urograms and other contrast studies of the urinary system, US, and MRI examinations with lower sensitivity and specificity. On abdominal x-rays, urinary calculi will appear as round or oval radiopacities overlying the expected course of the kidneys, ureter, or bladder. Struvite stone will typically have a lamellated appearance whereas cystine stones have a homogeneous ground-glass opacity and are less dense than calcium oxalate stones of comparable size (see Figure 7-36).

Abdominal radiography often is used as a first step in the radiologic workup of patients who have acute flank pain. Although 90% of urinary tract calculi are composed of calcium salts,[145] only 59% of urinary stones are visible on abdominal radiographs,[146] and appear as round or oval high-attenuation foci within the distribution of the renal collecting systems, ureter, or bladder. Small stones can be difficult to identify on abdominal radiographs, particularly in the presence of overlying bowel gas or fecal material. Seventy-nine percent of calculi larger than 5 mm and 95% of calculi with CT attenuation greater than 300 HU were detectable on conventional radiography in 1 study.[147] Stones composed purely of uric acid account for 5% to 10%

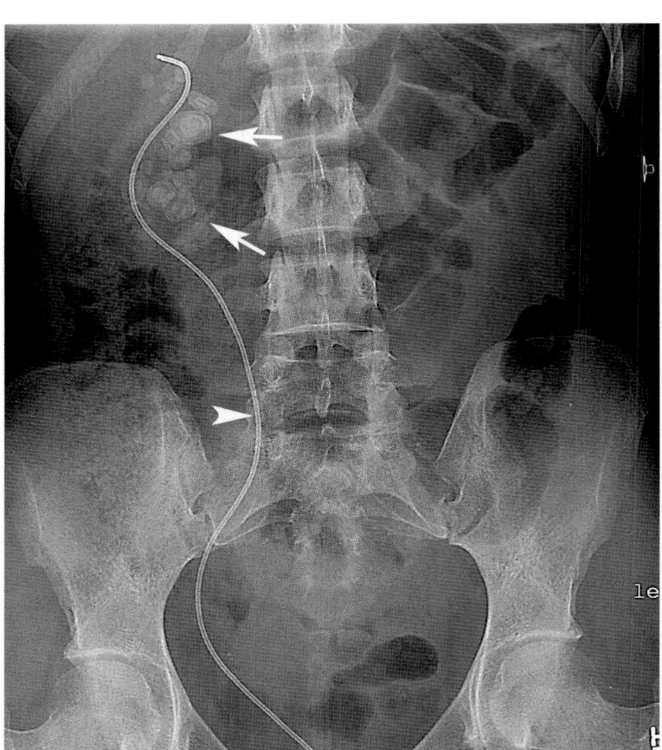

A

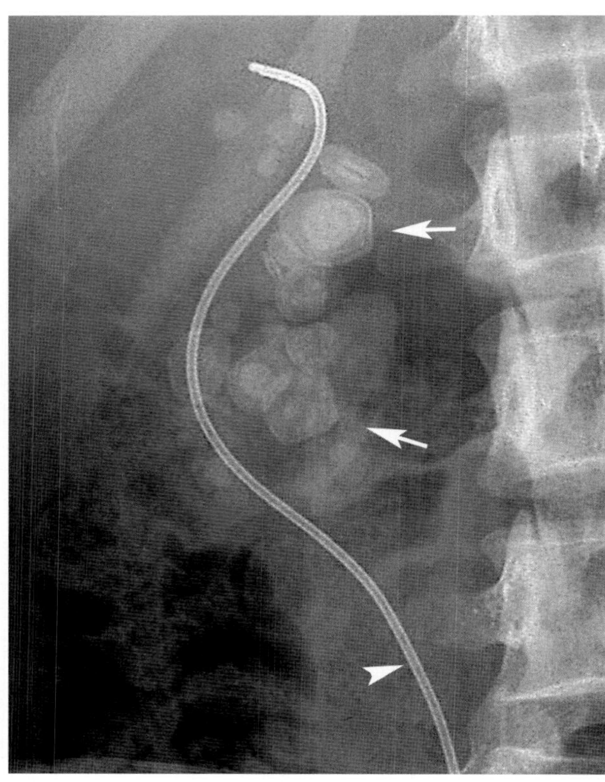

B

Figure 7-36 Struvite Kidney Stones
This 26-year-old woman had recurrent urinary tract infections. **A.** Anteroposterior view of the abdomen and (**B**) magnified view of right upper quadrant show multiple concentrically calcified renal calculi (*arrows*). This lamellated appearance indicates struvite stones, a type of renal calculus associated with recurrent urinary tract infections. There is also a retrograde ureteral catheter (*arrowheads*), which was placed for a retrograde pyelogram to delineate the anatomy of the collecting system (not shown).

of urinary calculi and may not be detectable on abdominal radiographs, regardless of size. Phleboliths can be impossible to distinguish from ureteral stones by abdominal radiography alone, although radiographic findings such as a central lucency or anatomic position may allow the differentiation of these structures from true ureteral calculi. Although phleboliths are most common in the pelvis, gonadal vein phleboliths can cause confusion in the abdomen when assessing for calculi in the lumbar ureter.

The scout film of an intravenous urogram will detect radiopaque urinary calculi. Most calculi are obscured by excreted contrast and may not be identifiable if their presence has not been confirmed on the scout films. Radiolucent calculi (pure uric acid stones) can be detected as a filling defect within the contrast-opacified collecting systems, ureter, or bladder.

As noted earlier, CT is the current gold standard in the imaging detection of urinary calculi. On CT examinations, they typically appear as uniform high attenuation round, oval, or branching structures in the expected distribution of the urinary system (see Figures 7-26, 7-28, 7-29, 7-32, and 7-37). The spatial resolution of CT is less than that of plain films and, therefore, fine detail such as lamellations that can be seen on abdominal films can be difficult to appreciate on CT and the stone can appear uniformly hyperattenuating. Using bone windows is often helpful in better evaluating the interior structure of a calculus.

The crystalline nature of urinary calculi causes them to be strong reflectors of ultrasound waves. They will appear as an echogenic focus within the distribution of the renal collecting systems, ureter, or bladder, with shadowing of the tissues deep to the stone (see Figure 7-37). Calculi as small as 0.5 mm can be detectable in optimal conditions. When stones are larger than 5 mm, US has been shown to have a sensitivity of 96% and specificity of nearly 100%.[148] Identification of ureteral jets within the urinary bladder lumen is helpful for assessing the presence of obstruction. One study showed an absent ureteral jet in 11 of 12 patients who had high-grade obstruction and in 3 of 11 patients who had low-grade obstruction.[149]

Urinary calculi contain relatively few hydrogen atoms when compared with other soft tissue. Therefore, most stones will appear as a signal void on MRI sequences and may be identifiable as a signal void only within a dilated collecting system (see Figure 7-30).

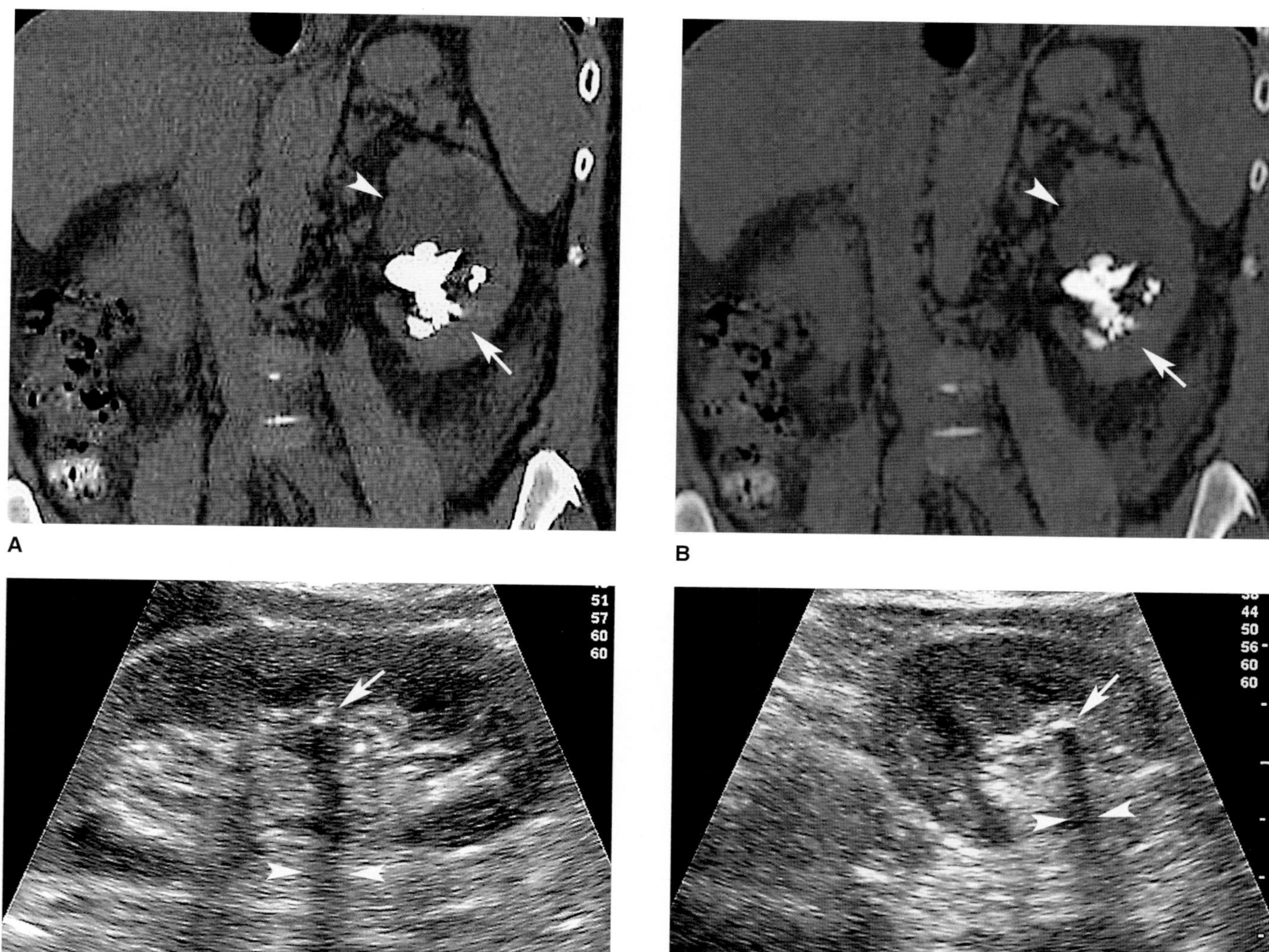

Figure 7-37 Renal Calculi
A and **B**. This 66-year-old man had abdominal pain. Coronal reconstructions from an unenhanced CT in (A) soft tissue and (B) bone windows show an incidentally discovered staghorn calculus (*arrows*) of the left kidney that causes obstruction and dilation of the upper pole collecting system (*arrowheads*).

C. Longitudinal and **(D)** transverse US images in this 72-year-old woman show a small echogenic focus (*arrows*) in the interpolar region of the left kidney at the junction of the cortex and the medulla. There is shadowing (*arrowheads*) deep to the echogenic focus, features typical of a small renal calculus.

Bladder Calculi

The majority of bladder calculi form in the urinary bladder because of urinary stasis. Unlike upper urinary tract calculi, they have relatively few causes. Primary bladder stones most commonly consist of ammonium acid urate and calcium oxalate, but many also contain calcium phosphate. Once bladder stones are removed and the urinary stasis is corrected, they hardly ever recur, unlike calculi, which form in the upper urinary tract and tend to be a recurrent and often a refractory clinical problem.

Bladder calculi can be classified as migrant calculi, primary idiopathic endemic calculi and secondary calculi, which include those stones related to urinary stasis and foreign bodies. All types of bladder calculi occur more commonly in males. They form because of elevated concentrations of urinary solutes (Table 7-10).

Migrant calculi

Migrant calculi form in the kidney, migrate down the ureter, and are retained in the bladder. Most calculi that pass spontaneously from the ureter to the bladder are less than 1 cm in diameter and, in adults, easily pass through the urethra. Migrant bladder calculi occur when there is a relatively small bladder outlet, as in children, or in the presence of concomitant bladder outlet obstruction. Stones that remain in the bladder can grow to a large size.

Table 7-10. Causes of Bladder Calculi

1. Migration from upper tracts (Migrant calculi)
2. Dietary phosphate deficiency (Primary idiopathic endemic calculi)
3. Secondary bladder calculi a. Urinary stasis/obstruction b. Chronic/recurrent infection c. Chronic/recurrent instrumentation d. Foreign body nidus e. Combinations of (a) through (d)

Primary idiopathic endemic calculi

Primary idiopathic endemic calculi occur in children and young adults and are believed to be due to dietary phosphate deficiency, with resultant low urine phosphate excretion and the formation of insoluble salts in the urine. This type of stone disease is extremely rare in developed countries but is still prevalent in underdeveloped areas.

Secondary bladder calculi

Secondary bladder calculi are those that occur as a result of anatomic or functional changes in the bladder, predisposing to stone formation, and include urinary stasis or obstruction, chronic or recurrent infection, instrumentation, and the presence of iatrogenic and accidental foreign bodies. In many instances, combinations of these factors lead to the development of urinary calculi.

Urinary stasis/obstruction: Bladder outlet obstruction is present in approximately 75% of adults with bladder calculi. In males, stasis is usually caused by bladder outflow obstruction due to BPH.[136] Obstruction leading to stone formation can also be due to urethral stricture, bladder neck hypertrophy, and neurogenic bladder. Females with large cystoceles are also at risk of developing bladder calculi.

Bladder stones form in approximately 40% of patients with schistosomiasis. Stones result from bladder neck fibrosis, which causes some degree of outlet obstruction. Superimposed bacterial infection is also frequently present. Schistosomiasis will be discussed in greater detail later in this chapter under the heading: **Bladder wall calcification.**

Uric acid is the most common type of stone associated with outlet obstruction. Less often, stones are composed of pure calcium oxalate or phosphate, cystine, calcium carbonate, or xanthine. No correlation between stone composition and the cause of obstruction has been identified.

Calculi related to infection: Bladder stones can be associated with urinary infection, most especially *Proteus mirabilis* (80%) and less frequently with *Pseudomonas*, *Klebsiella*, and *Streptococcus fecalis*.[4] All these organisms contain urease and can hydrolyze urea. Stones (magnesium ammonium phosphate and carbonate apatite) form when the urine becomes supersaturated with the crystals from such hydrolysis. Calcium oxalate, calcium phosphate, and uric acid crystalluria are also common in urinary infection. Thus, although magnesium ammonium phosphate and carbonate apatite stones (infection-induced or urease stones) are pathognomonic of infection, infection can also produce stones composed of calcium oxalate, calcium phosphate, or a mixture of both. Urease stones generally contain organic material (matrix), which is the result of proteinaceous and mucopolysaccharide debris from the inflamed urothelial lining of the ureter or bladder. These stones are frequently poorly mineralized and are often difficult to see radiographically. Persistent infection is common after surgical removal of urease stones, and unless infection is eradicated, such stones can recur. Eradication of infection can be difficult and may require long-term antimicrobial treatment, high fluid intake, and urease-inhibiting drugs such as hydroxyurea or acetohydroxamic acid (AHA).

Although infection can be the only cause of bladder stones, urinary stasis is often a coexistent lithogenic factor. This occurs in patients with bladder outlet obstruction and foreign bodies in the bladder, such as indwelling catheters, sutures, or foreign bodies self-introduced transurethrally.

Calculi related to instrumentation: Long-term bladder catheters often lead to bladder infection even if strict aseptic catheterization technique is used. Approximately 50% of catheter-associated stones are composed of struvite. The remainder are either mixtures of calcium oxalate and phosphate or pure calcium phosphate. Catheter-associated stones occur most often in patients with neurogenic bladder dysfunction and those in whom bladder stones have been incompletely removed. Encrustations can form either around the tip of the catheter or as eggshell crusts around the catheter balloon. These crusts fall off into the bladder and act as a nidus for further stone growth, which is characteristically crescentic in shape (see Figure 7-38). Intermittent clean self-catheterization may introduce pubic hairs (which act as nidi for stone formation) into the bladder.

Foreign body nidus calculi: Secondary bladder calculi can form around a foreign body in the bladder. Foley catheters act as foreign bodies, as has been discussed already. Other types of foreign body include a variety of objects introduced transurethrally, bone fragments from previous pelvic fractures, which penetrated the bladder wall, and foreign bodies relating to previous surgery, such as ureteric stents. Sutures or staples placed in the bladder wall can unintentionally be left exposed or may migrate through the bladder wall and penetrate the mucosa. Such foreign bodies act as nidi for formation of stones that are attached to the bladder wall, so-called hanging bladder stones. When calculi form on staples, the metallic staple is typically seen to lie eccentrically in the calculus (see Figure 7-39).

Clinical and imaging features of bladder calculi

Bladder calculi are often asymptomatic and discovered incidentally by imaging studies. Symptomatic calculi can

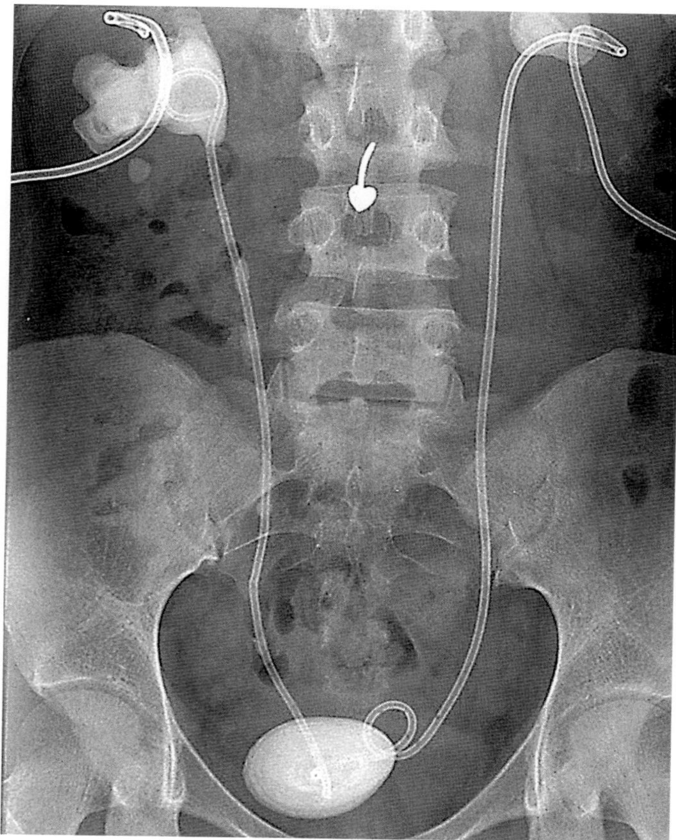

A

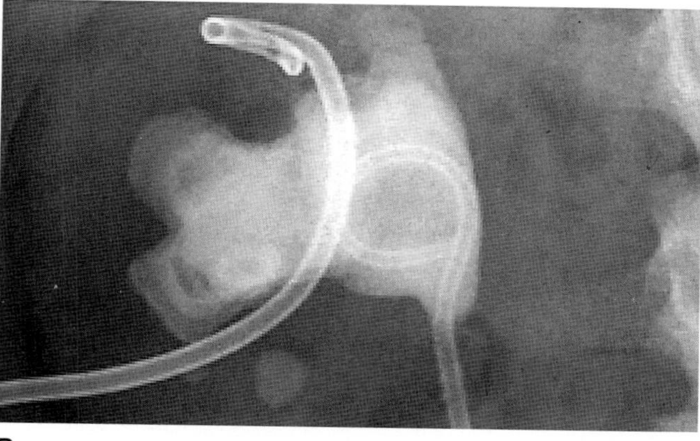

B

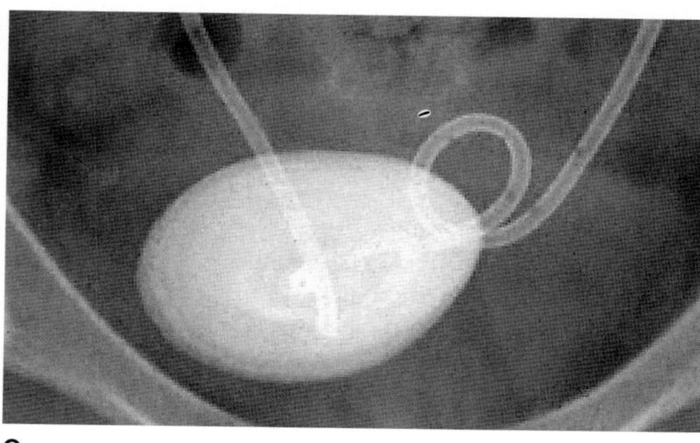

C

Figure 7-38 Encrusted Ureteral Stent
This 24-year-old woman presented with fever and back pain. Stents had been placed for stones disease 1 year ago. **A.** Abdominal radiograph and magnified views of the (**B**) right renal pelvis and (**C**) bladder regions show large lamellated calculi encrusting the pigtails of the right ureteral stent causing a staghorn calculus in the right kidney. Chronic indwelling foreign bodies including medical devices can act as a nidus for the development of calculi.

produce bladder pain, either a dull ache or a sudden sharp severe pain referred to the penis, buttocks, perineum, or scrotum. Interruption of micturition can occur because of a ball valve type of obstruction in the erect or seated position. Microscopic hematuria resulting from chronic irritation of the bladder mucosa is frequent but gross hematuria is uncommon. Infection-related stones are often associated with foul-smelling urine. Long-standing bladder calculi can produce sufficient edema of the ureteric orifices and secondary thickening of the bladder wall to obstruct the ureters.

Bladder stones can be quite small (only a few millimeters in size) or large enough to fill the bladder. They can be solitary or multiple, and have a variety of shapes: round, oval, square, multifaceted, or spiculated. Bladder stones vary from densely opaque through faintly opaque to radiolucent on conventional radiographs but nearly all will be detected by CT scans (see Figure 7-34). Pure uric acid stones, especially if small, are radiolucent and invisible on plain films. Larger uric acid calculi, either pure or adventitiously covered with small amounts of calcium salts, and pure struvite stones are faintly opaque.

On IVU and Cystography, densely opaque bladder calculi are well seen on plain films but may be completely obscured by excreted contrast medium in the bladder, because their density is similar. Oblique or lateral views may be necessary to prove that a pelvic calcification is intravesical and does not lie behind the bladder. This differentiation is often easier after micturition, when there is less contrast-laden urine in the bladder. Most calcified bladder stones are less dense than contrast medium and are seen as filling defects in the contrast-filled bladder. Oblique films may still be necessary to prove that a lucency lies inside the bladder, because bowel gas overlying the contrast-filled bladder may simulate an intravesical filling defect.

US is a sensitive method of detecting bladder calculi and is more sensitive in the detection of small calculi than either IVU or cystography. Calculi are seen in the urine-filled bladder as bright echogenicities, with acoustic shadowing posterior to them caused by a large proportion of the sound being absorbed by the calculus (see Figure 7-40). Their mobility can be shown by scanning the patient in the oblique or erect positions as well as supine. Bladder calculi can usually be distinguished from tumors, which are seen as fixed echogenicities not casting an acoustic shadow, and blood clots, which are mobile but do not cast an acoustic shadow.

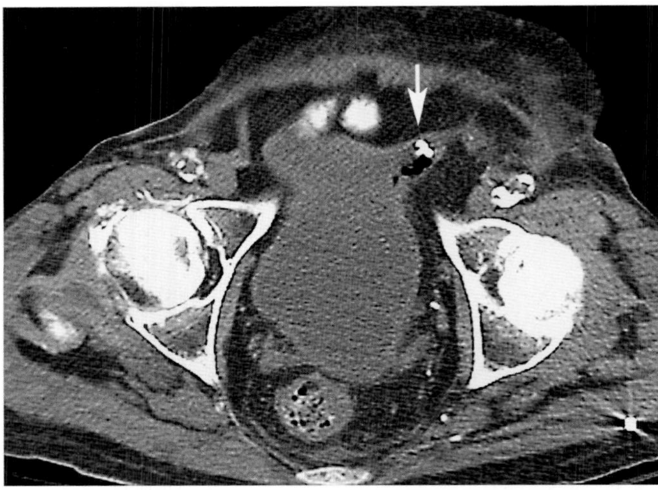

Figure 7-39 Hanging Bladder Calculus
This 60-year-old man had prior left renal transplant. The calcification in the left anterior bladder (*arrow*) wall likely developed at the anastomosis site of the transplant ureter to the bladder. When calculi are not located in the nondependent portion of the bladder, it raises the suspicion that they have formed on a foreign body such as a surgical clip or suture, which is exposed to the urine in the lumen of the bladder. If clips are appropriately submucosal in location, they should not cause calculus formation.

Bladder calculi are easily seen as dependent layering densities in the bladder on CT. If present within a diverticulum, the calculi will not migrate to a dependent position in the bladder (see Figure 7-40).

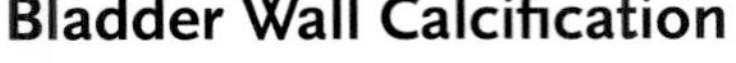

Bladder Wall Calcification

Bladder wall calcifications can be due to the infections schistosomiasis and tuberculosis and due to calcifications in epithelial neoplasms, either transitional cell or squamous cell carcinoma.

Schistosomiasis

Schistosomiasis (bilharziasis) is the most common cause of bladder wall calcification and is endemic in many parts of Africa and the Middle East. This parasite is carried by freshwater snails primarily found along the rivers of North Africa, especially the Nile, in countries such as Egypt, Sudan, Kenya, Uganda, and Senegal. The organism enters the human body through the skin, usually of the feet, and migrate to target organs, especially the liver and bladder. Bladder disease is caused when the adult female *S haematobium* lays her eggs in the bladder submucosa where they cause inflammation. Inflammation of the wall results in an increased incidence of bacterial coinfection and an increased risk of bladder malignancy. Most *Schistosoma*-related neoplasms are of squamous histology; however, there is also an increased risk of TCC and adenocarcinoma, in patients with bladder schistosomiasis, particularly in those who smoke. Chronic inflammation will ultimately result in fibrosis and calcification of the bladder wall. With extensive disease, calcification can affect the muscularis and adventitia as well as the submucosa.

Both abdominal radiographs and abdominal CT can detect the bladder wall calcifications found in patients with schistosomiasis (see Figure 7-41). With CT, it has been shown that the anterior bladder wall is affected first, although on plain films calcification is usually appreciated first at the bladder base. Calcification spreads around the

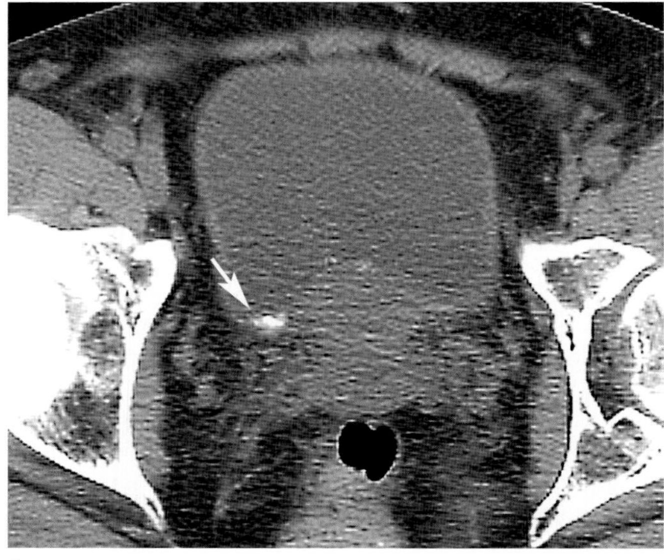

A

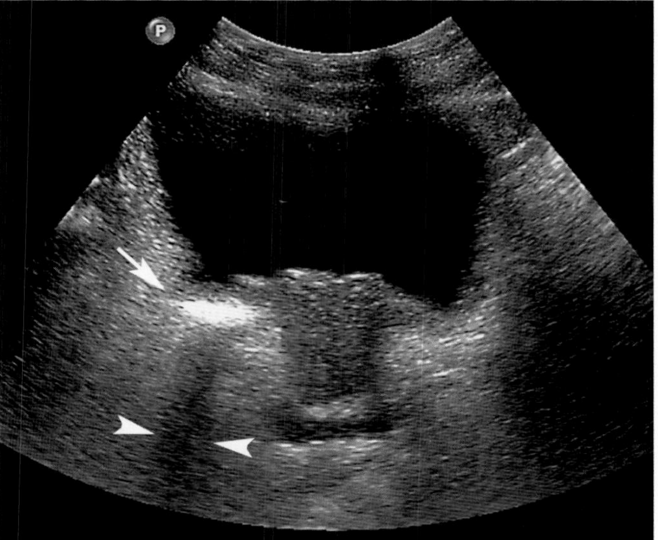

B

Figure 7-40 Bladder Calculi
This 60-year-old man had hematuria. **A.** Unenhanced CT and (**B**) transverse US of the bladder show a high-attenuation, echogenic focus (*arrows*) in the dependent portion of the bladder with shadowing (*arrowheads*) on the US examination. Features are typical of bladder calculi.

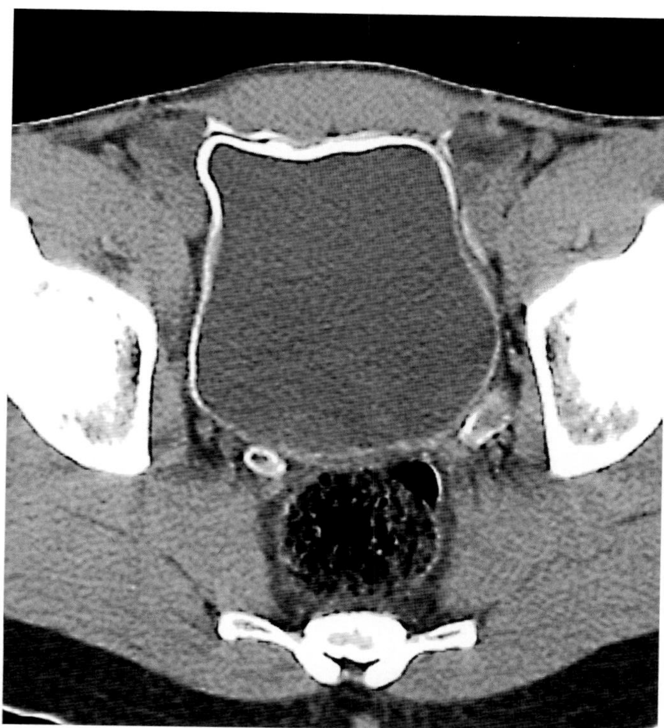

Figure 7-41 Schistosomiasis
This 40-year-old man from Mali presented with fever and malaise. There is thin continuous calcification of the entire bladder wall, and the bladder is well distended. The bladder remains thin walled and distensible in patients with schistosomiasis, despite the heavy calcification. TB and other granulomatous calcifications cause marked thickening of the bladder wall, and the bladder becomes nondistensible and small in size. Note calcification of the distal ureters as well.

wall of the bladder, leading to a ring-like appearance of the distended bladder on abdominal radiographs. Distensibility of the bladder is maintained and bladder capacity is normal. Calcification of the distal ureters is common, and the incidence of bladder calculi is increased.

Tuberculosis

Tuberculous calcification of the bladder is rare, and by the time it develops, there is usually extensive upper tract tuberculous involvement. Typically the bladder is fibrotic, contracted, and thick-walled, with multiple calcified granulomas, which are usually denser and more heterogeneous than the typical ring calcification in schistosomiasis. Calcification of the prostate, vas deferens, and epididymis can be associated.

Other causes of bladder wall calcification

Alkaline encrusting cystitis occurs when there is necrotic or ischemic bladder tissue, for example, following radiotherapy, and an alkaline urine, most commonly produced by a urease-producing bacterium such as *Proteus*. Calcium salts become encrusted on the bladder mucosa, and there can also be struvite or calcium phosphate stones.

Bladder necrosis with calcification can occur after systemic cyclophosphamide treatment and instillation of mitomycin C into the bladder.

Calculi form infrequently in a patent urachus or urachal diverticulum. They can be single or multiple, vary in shape from round to hourglass, and measure up to 4 cm. Most consist of calcium phosphate, calcium oxalate, and traces of struvite.

Bladder Fistulae

The most common type of fistula between the bowel and the urinary bladder is a colovesical fistula. Colovesical fistulae are most often due to diverticulitis of the colon, accounting for 50% to 70% of cases, and is typically located between the sigmoid colon and the urinary bladder.[150] Such fistulae are more common in men, possibly because the uterus protects from formation of these fistulae in women. An inflamed perforated diverticulum becomes adherent to the bladder and then leads to fistula formation. Colon cancer is a less common cause of colovesical fistulae.

Small bowel to bladder fistulae are less common than those from the colon. Inflammatory bowel disease such as Crohn disease usually causes an ileovesical fistula. Other rarer causes include fistulae arising from Meckel diverticulum, as a complication of appendicitis, and genitourinary coccidiomycosis and pelvic actinomycosis.[151]

Rectovesical fistulae are the least common enterovesical fistulae and are usually a complication of accidental trauma, recent surgery, or direct extension of a rectal malignancy.

Patients usually present with dysuria, bladder pain, increased frequency, pneumaturia, or fecaluria. Computed tomographic scanning is the most sensitive study for evaluating such patients. A loop of colon is usually adherent to the bladder, with an adjacent area of bladder wall thickening at the site of the fistula. Gas can be seen within the fistula track, or in the urinary bladder. Coronal and sagittal reformatted images are very useful in evaluation of such patients and an important supplement to axial images (see Figure 7-42). Barium enema and cystography are less sensitive studies in the evaluation of enterovesical fistulae but are occasionally used to show the fistula. After a negative barium enema, the voided urine can be centrifuged and a horizontal beam radiograph obtained to look for barium in the urine. This is known as a Bourne test and is sometimes useful in a problematic patient in whom the diagnosis cannot be established.[152]

Vesicovaginal fistulae are a frequent and a significant public health problem in developing countries. They are most often related to prolonged and obstructed labor, with pressure necrosis of the anterior vaginal wall and the posterior bladder wall. In the developed countries with modern obstetrical care, such fistulae are most often due to gynecologic surgery such as hysterectomy.[153] Patients present with urinary leakage through the vagina. Voiding cystourethrograms are performed to look for a vesicovaginal fistula, and if none is found, an upper tract study should also be performed to exclude a ureteral injury as a cause of the vaginal leakage of urine.

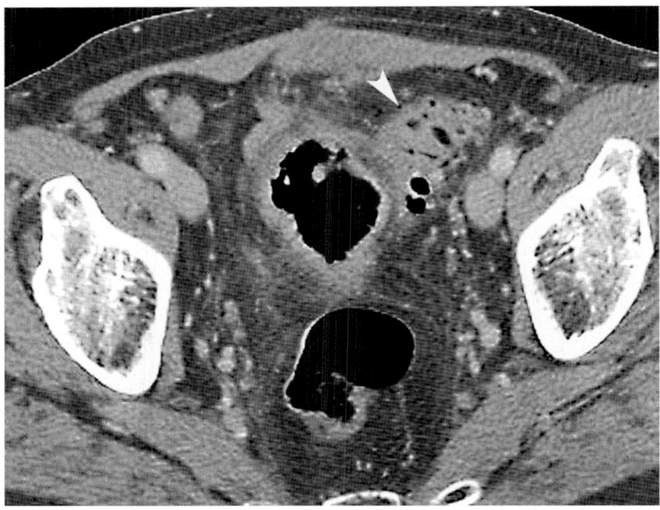

A

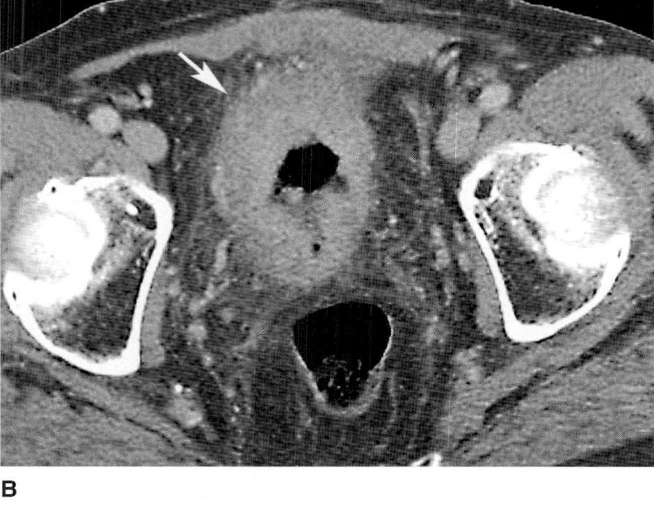

B

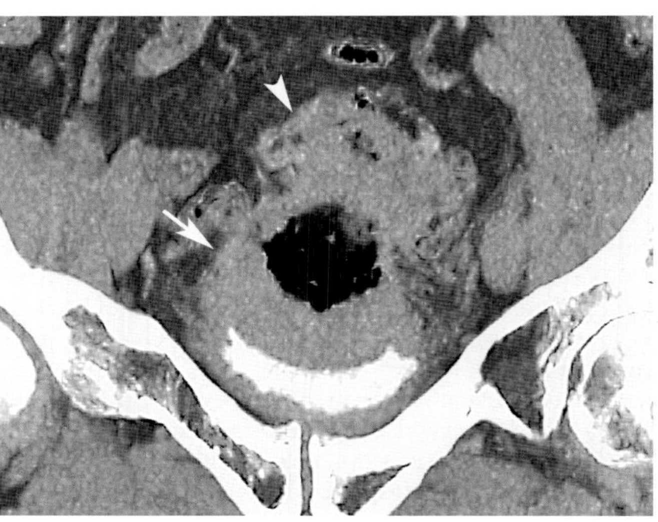

C

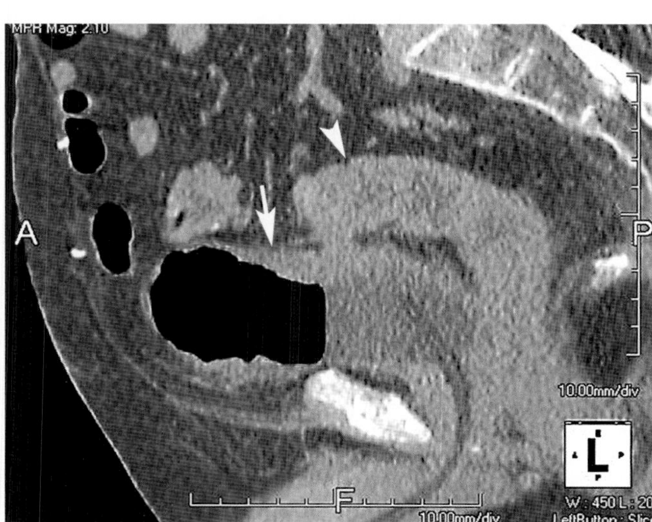

D

Figure 7-42 Colovesical Fistula
This 63-year-old man presented with complaints of passing gas through the urethra. Unenhanced CT performed in (**A** and **B**) the axial plane and (**C**) coronal and (**D**) sagittal reconstructions shows a grossly thickwalled bladder (*arrows*) that contains both gas and fluid. The rectosigmoid (*arrowheads*) is directly applied to the dome of the bladder without an intervening fat plane. These findings are highly suggestive of a colovesical fistula. Coronal and sagittal reconstructions are very useful additions to axial images when evaluating the bladder for fistulae.

Congenital Anomalies

Congenital anomalies of the urinary system include partial and complete duplication of the collecting systems and ureters and ureteroceles.

Duplication anomalies

Duplication anomalies are seen in 1 per 125 people. The prevalence is twice as high in females and unilateral duplication is 6 times more common than bilateral duplication.[154-157] The collecting systems can be duplicated on 1 or both sides, with 2 separate collecting systems that can drain into either 1 or 2 ureters. If the 2 ureters join before they open into the bladder, the duplication is considered to be partial. With complete duplication, the 2 ureters open independently into the urinary bladder. Most frequently, even with complete duplication, the 2 ureters insert into the normal position in the trigone of the urinary bladder, known as orthotopic insertion. However, in some cases ureteral insertion can be ectopic. The upper pole ureter is more likely to be ectopic in insertion, usually below the trigone and the UV junction, whereas the lower pole ureter inserts at the normal position in the trigone. When this occurs, the lower pole ureter is prone to reflux whereas the upper pole ureter is prone to obstruction. This is known as the Weigert-Meyer rule.[154-157]

Imaging Notes 7-8. The Weigert-Meyer Rule

Most patients with complete ureteral duplication have normal insertion of the ureter at the trigone of the bladder. However, when abnormally inserted, the ureters typically have the following insertion patterns and complication patterns dictated by the Weigert-Meyer rule:

Ureter	Insertion Site	Complication
Upper pole	Ectopic below trigone	Obstruction
Lower pole	Normal position	Reflux

Most patients with collecting system duplication are asymptomatic. With ureteral ectopy, girls may present with incontinence if the ureteral insertion is into the urethra or the vagina. Boys usually do not have incontinence as the ectopic ureter usually inserts above the external urinary sphincter and the abnormality may only be found incidentally, or if the obstruction causes infection.

Historically, IVU was very adept at demonstrating duplicated systems and the sites of ureteral insertion. However, more recently, MRI has been shown to be very useful in demonstrating the insertion site of the obstructed ectopic ureter and is usually the study of choice in the evaluation of a suspected ectopic ureter. If the ectopic ureter is not obstructed, CTU can also demonstrate the course and the insertion site of the 2 ureters (see Figure 7-43).

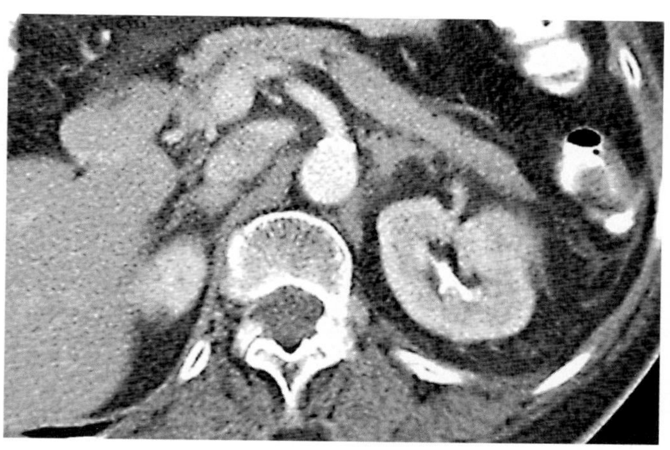

A

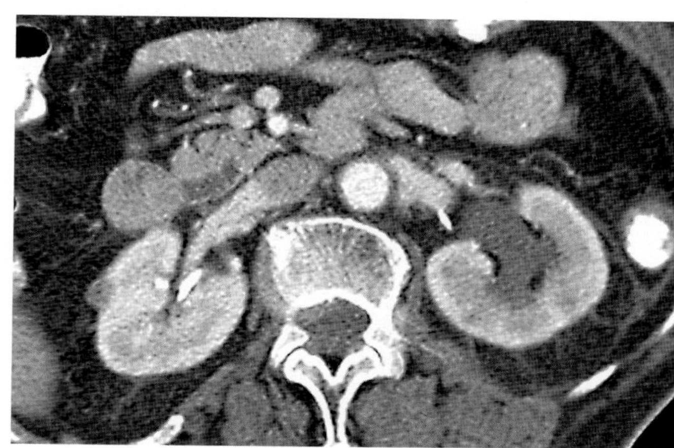

B

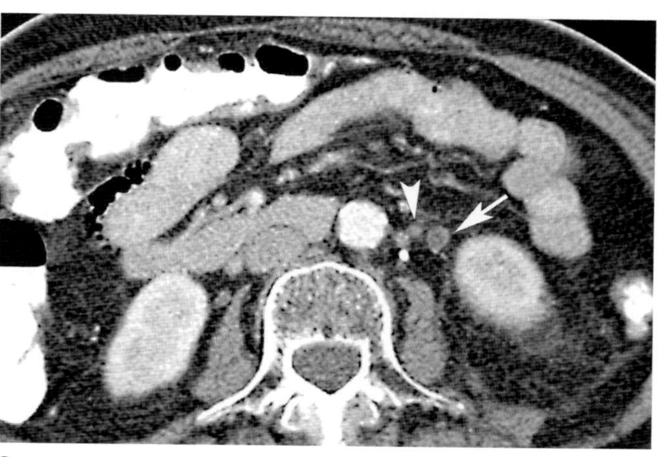

C

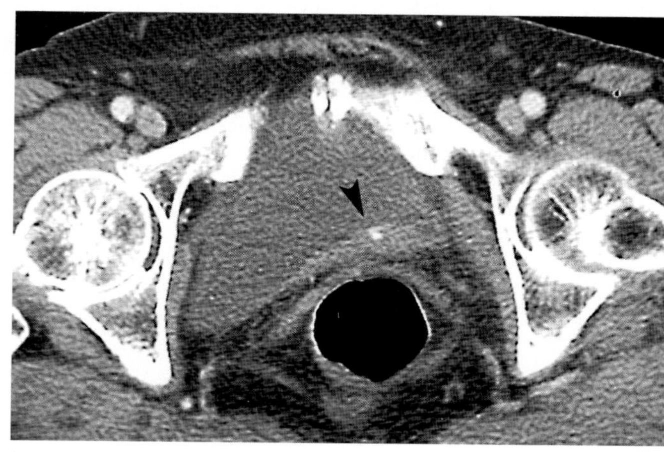

D

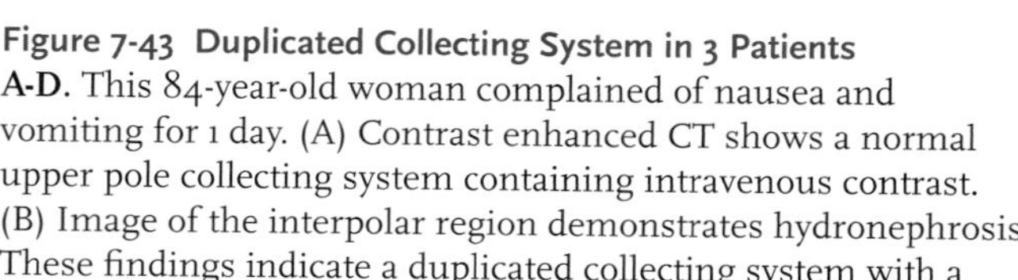

Figure 7-43 Duplicated Collecting System in 3 Patients
A-D. This 84-year-old woman complained of nausea and vomiting for 1 day. (A) Contrast enhanced CT shows a normal upper pole collecting system containing intravenous contrast. (B) Image of the interpolar region demonstrates hydronephrosis. These findings indicate a duplicated collecting system with a normal upper pole moiety and an obstructed lower pole moiety. (C) Careful observation demonstrates a dilated lower pole ureter (*white arrow*) and a normal upper pole ureter (*white arrowhead*). (D) Image through the pelvis shows a stone (*black arrowhead*) in the ureterovesicle junction as the cause of the lower pole obstruction.

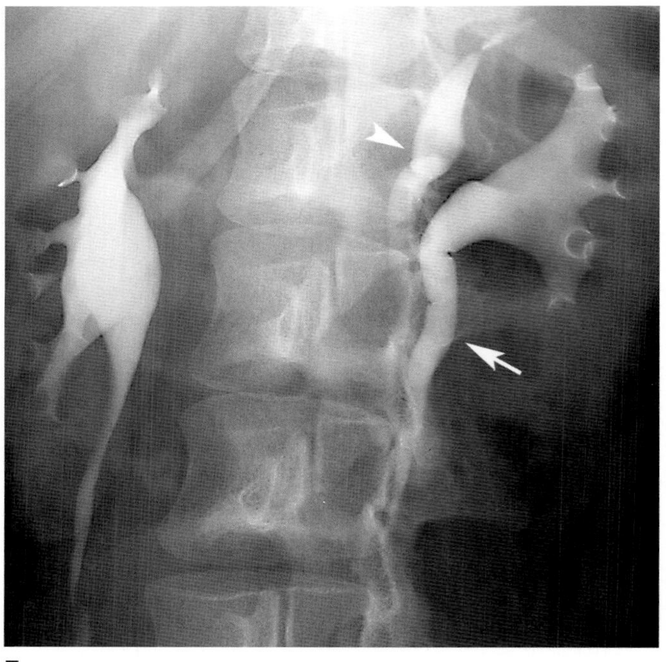

E

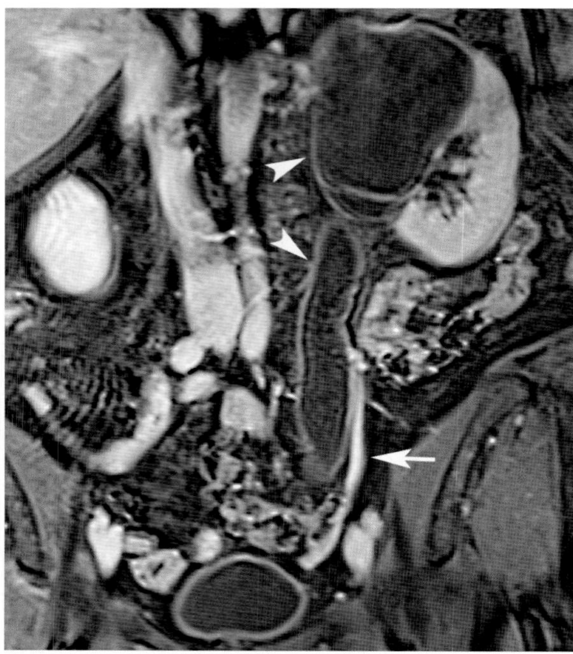

F

G

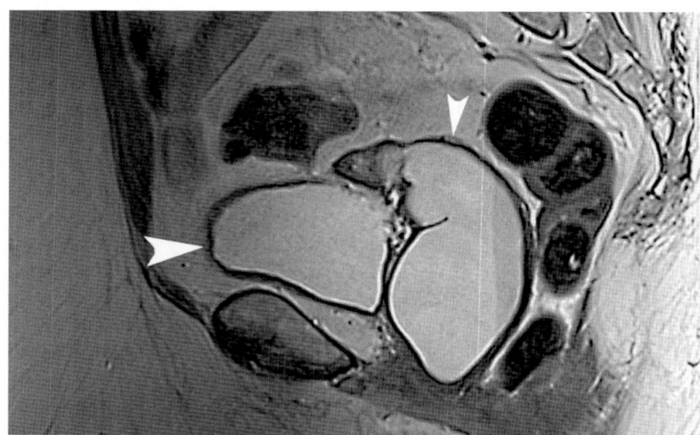

H

Figure 7-43 Duplicated Collecting System in 3 Patients (*Continued*) **E.** This 35-year-old woman had hematuria. Oblique image from an IVU shows 2 left ureters and collecting systems indicating a duplicated system with ad upper pole moiety (*arrowhead*) and a lower pole moiety (*arrow*). **F-H.** This 70-year-old woman had hematuria. (F) Coronal T2-weighted and (G and H) sagittal T1-weighted postgadolinium sequence images show a duplicated left collecting system with a normal lower pole ureter (*arrow*) and an obstructed upper pole (*arrowhead*). The distended end of the ureter, a ureterocele (*small arrowhead* in H) inserts ectopically below the bladder (*large arrowhead*) into the distal vagina.

Ureterocele

Ureterocele represents a focal dilation of the distal end of the ureter as it enters the urinary bladder. This is a congenital anomaly and can be an isolated finding or associated with other congenital anomalies of the urinary system, most commonly a duplicated collecting system. Ureteroceles can occur at the normal site of ureteral insertion at the trigone of the bladder (orthotopic ureterocele) or can insert ectopically into the urinary system at a location distal to the trigone, or into nonurinary structures including the seminal vesicles, vas deferens, or ejaculatory ducts in males or in the vagina, uterus, or Gartner duct in females.[155] Thus, 4 subgroups of ureteroceles can be identified based on whether they are associated with a single or duplicated system and whether they are orthotopically or ectopically inserted.[156] Orthotopic ureteroceles are most commonly associated with a single collecting system and ectopic ureteroceles are most commonly associated with a duplicated collecting system. Ureteroceles in ectopic systems are most commonly present in the upper pole collecting system that inserts in a position more distal to the normal ureteral orifice, although cranial ectopy has also been described.

It has been estimated that 1/100 000 individuals is born with a ureterocele.[157] They are more common in females and can be bilateral in a small percentage of cases. Ectopic ureteroceles are approximately 3 to 5 times more common than orthotopic ureteroceles.[158] It is believed that ureteroceles arise because of incomplete dissolution of Chwalla membrane, a developmental structure that separates the ureteral bud from the developing urogenital sinus. Incomplete dissolution leads to partial obstruction of the ureter and dilation of its distal segment. Occasionally, bladder cancer, stones, or tuberculosis can cause a stricture of the distal ureteral orifice, leading to obstruction and dilation of the distal ureter that resembles a ureterocele and is called a pseudoureterocele.[159]

In most cases, ureteroceles are asymptomatic and discovered during either prenatal screening or incidentally on imaging performed for other reasons. Occasionally, they can result in urinary tract infections, urinary retention, failure to thrive (infants), cyclic abdominal pain, urinary calculi, or obstructive voiding symptoms. Ureteroceles can be complicated by stones in 4% to 39% of cases.[160] Indications for surgical intervention include (1) recurrent urinary tract infections or flank pain, (2) evidence of deteriorating renal function due to obstruction, (3) stones complicating ureteroceles, and (4) symptomatic heterotopic ureteroceles in duplex collecting systems.[161]

On imaging examinations, a ureterocele will appear as a focal dilation of the distalmost aspect of the ureter. The normal ureter and ureterocele resemble a Cobra with the ureterocele representing the Cobra head (see Figure 7-44). The surface of a ureterocele should be very smooth and

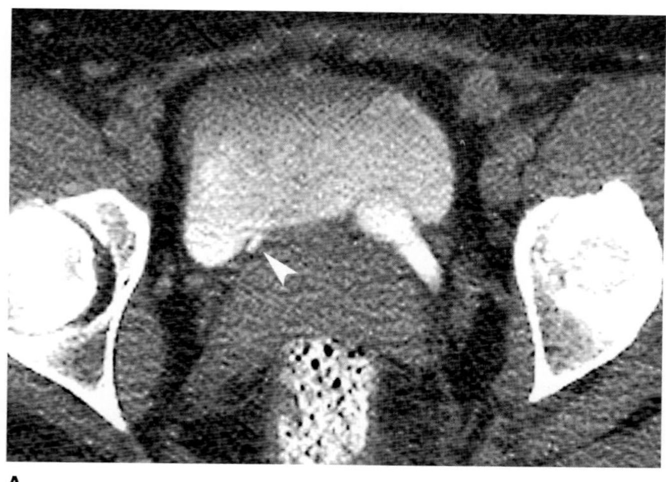
A

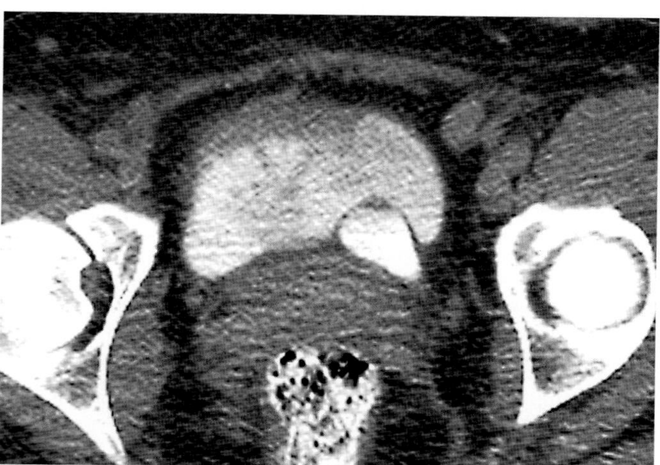
B

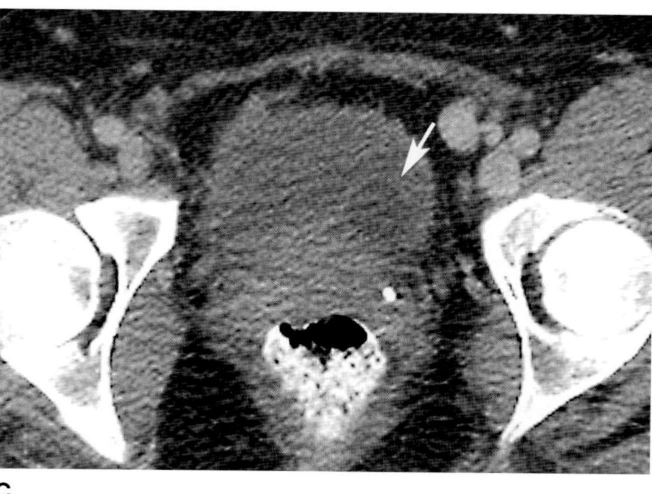
C

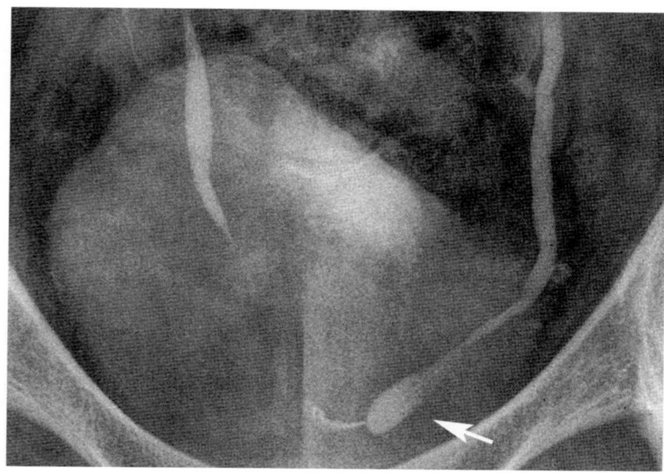
D

Figure 7-44 Orthotopic Ureterocele in 2 Patients
A-C. This 46-year-old woman had autoimmune hepatitis. **A** and **B.** Postcontrast CT images through the bladder demonstrate a club-shaped contrast collection in the expected location of the left ureteral orifice characteristic of a uterterocele. Note the normal right ureteral orifice (*arrowhead*). **C.** Precontrast CT image shows a faint oval structure (*arrow*), which is the ureterocele before its filling with contrast. **D.** This 56-year-old woman had pelvic surgery. Intravenous urogram shows focal, club-shaped dilation of the distal left ureter (*arrow*), typical of a ureterocele, an incidental finding.

regular. If there is irregularity, this can indicate the presence of a pseudoureterocele, and can indicate the presence of either a tumor or a stone at the UV junction, which should be excluded by cystoscopic inspection.[162,163]

REFERENCES

1. Fleshner N, Kondylis F. Demographics and epidemiology of urothelial cancer of urinary bladder. In: Droller M, ed. *Urothelial Tumors*. Hamilton, ON: Decker; 2004:1-16.
2. American Cancer Society. *Cancer facts & figures, 2008*. Atlanta, GA, 2008.
3. Fleshner N, Kondylis F. Demographics and epidemiology of urothelial cancer of urinary bladder. *Urothelial Tumors*. 2004:1-16.
4. Droller M. *Urothelial tumors*. ACS Atlas of Clinical Oncology Series; 2004.
5. Guinan P, Vogelzang NJ, Randazzo R, et al. Cancer Incidence and End Results Committee. *Urology*. 1992;40:393-399.
6. Tawfiek E, Bagley D. Upper-tract transitional cell carcinoma. *Urology*. 1997;50(3):321-329.
7. Vikram R, Sandler C, Ng C. Imaging and staging of transitional cell carcinoma: part 1, Lower urinary tract. *AJR Am J Roentgenol*. 2009;192:1481-1487.
8. Xu A, Ng CS, Kamat A, Grossman HB, Dinney C, Sandler CM. Significance of upper urinary tract urothelial thickening and filling defect seen on MDCT urography in patients with a history of urothelial neoplasms. *AJR Am J Roentgenol*. 2010; 195:959-965.
9. Maletic V, Cerovic S, Lazic M, Stojanovic M, Stevanovic P. Synchronous and multiple transitional cell carcinoma of the bladder and urachal cyst. *Int J Urol*. 2008;15(6):554-556.
10. Allen RCA, Schwartz BF. *Horseshoe Kidney*. 2012.
11. Mostofi FK, Thomson RV, Dean AL. Mucous adenocarcinoma of the urinary bladder. *Cancer*. 1955;8:741.
12. Colin P, Koenig P, Ouzzane A, et al. Environmental factors involved in carcinogenesis of urothelial cell carcinomas of the upper urinary tract. *BJU Int*. 2009;104(10):1436-1440.
13. Swindle P, Falk M, Rigby R, Petrie J, Hawley C, Nicol D. Transitional cell carcinoma in renal transplant recipients: the influence of compound analgesics. *Br J Urol*. 1998;81(2): 229-233.
14. Nortier J, Martinez M, Schmeiser H, et al. Urothelial carcinoma associated with the use of a Chinese herb (*Aristolochia fangchi*). *N Engl J Med*. 2000;342(23):1686-1692.
15. Stefanovic V, Radovanovic Z. Endemic nephropathy and associated urothelial cancer. *Natl Clin Pract Urol*. 2008;5: 105-112.
16. Greene F, Compton CC, Fritz AG, Shan JP, Winchester DP, eds. *AJCC Cancer Staging Atlas*. New York: Springer; 2006.
17. Bostwick D, Ramnani D, Cheng L. Diagnosis and grading of bladder cancer and associated lesion. *Urol Clin North Am*. 1999;26:493-507.
18. Cohan R, Caoili EM, Cowan NC, Weizer AZ, Ellis JH. MDCT urography: exploring a new paradigm for imaging of bladder cancer. *AJR Am J Roentgenol*. 2009;192:1501-1508.
19. Knox M, Cowan NC, Rivers-Bowerman MD, Turney BW. Evaluation of multidetector computed tomography urography and ultrasonography for diagnosing bladder cancer. *Clin Radiol*. 2008;63:1317-1325.
20. Sadow C, Silverman SG, O'Leary MP, Signorovitch JE. Bladder cancer detection with CT urography in an Academic Medical Center. *Radiology*. 2008;249:195-202.
21. Tekes A, Kamel I, Bluemke DA. Dynamic MR imaging of bladder cancer: Evaluation of staging accuracy. *AJR Am J Roentgenol*. 2005;184:121-127.
22. Browne RF, Meehan CP, Colville J, Power R, Torreggiani WC. Transitional cell carcinoma of the upper urinary tract: spectrum of imaging findings. *RadioGraphics*. 2005. 25:1609-1627.
23. Wong-You-Cheong JJ, Wagner BJ, Davis CJJ. Transitional cell carcinoma of the urinary tract: radiologic-pathologic correlation. *RadioGraphics*. 1998;18:123-142.
24. Obuchi M, Ishigami K, Takahashi K, et al. Gadolinium enhanced fat suppressed T1-weighted imaging for staging ureteral carcinoma: correlation with histopathology. *AJR Am J Roentgenol*. 2007;188:W256-W261.
25. Punekar S, Gulanikar A, Sobti MK, Sane SY, Pardanani DS. Pheochromocytoma of the urinary bladder (report of 2 cases with review of literature). *J Postgrad Med*. 1989;35:90.
26. Adeniji AO. Urinary bladder pheochromocytoma. *Appl Radiol*. 2009;38(6):39A-39C.
27. Warshawsky R, Bow SN, Waldbaum RS, Cintron J. Bladder pheochromocytoma with MR correlation. *J Comput Assist Tomogr*. 1989;13:714-716.
28. Ziari M, Sonpavde G, Shen S, Teh BS, Shu T, Lerner SP. Patients with unusual bladder malignancies and a rare cause of splenomegaly CASE 1. Small-cell carcinoma of the urinary bladder. *J Clin Oncol*. 2005;23(19):4458-4459.
29. Blomjous CE, Vos W, De Voogt HJ, Van der Valk P, Meijer CJ. Small cell carcinoma of the urinary bladder: a clinicopathologic, morphometric, immunohistochemical, and ultrastructural study of 18 cases. *Cancer*. 1989;64:1347-1357.
30. Singh O, Gupta SS, Hastir A. Laparoscopic enucleation of leiomyoma of the urinary bladder: a case report and review of the literature. *Urol J*. 2011;8:155-158.
31. Sakellariou P, Protopapas A, Kyritsis N, Voulgaris Z, Papaspirou E, Diakomanolis E. Intramural leiomyoma of the bladder. *Eur Radiol*. 2000;10:906-908.
32. Huppman A, Pawel B. Polyps and masses of the pediatric urinary bladder: a 21-year pathology review. *Pediatr Dev Pathol*. 2011;14(6):438-444.
33. Rodríguez Collar TL, Valdés Estévez B, López Marín L, Soranyer Horroutinel Scull R. Penile fibroepithelial polyp. Case report. *Arch Esp Urol*. 2010;63(4):309-312.
34. Williams TR, Wagner BJ, Corse WR, Vestevich JC. Fibroepithelial polyps of the urinary tract. *Abdom Imaging*. 2002;27:217-221.
35. Patheyar V, Venkatesh SK, Siew EP, Consiglieri DT, Putti T. MR imaging features of fibroepithelial ureteral polyp in a patient with duplicated upper urinary tract. *Singapore Med J*. 2011;52(3):E45-E47.
36. Childs MA, Umbreit EC, Krambeck AE, Sebo TJ, Patterson DE, Gettman MT. Fibroepithelial polyps of the ureter: a single-institutional experience. *J Endourol*. 2009;23(9):1415-1419.
37. Chen WF, Huang SC, Yu TJ, Chen WJ. Benign ureteral polyp as a cause of obstruction in a child. *Pediatr Surg Int*. 1994;9:436-437.
38. Genega EM, Porter CR. Urothelial neoplasms of the kidney and ureter. An epidemiologic, pathologic, and clinical review. *Am J Clin Pathol*. 2002;117(suppl):S36-S48.

39. Marincek B, Scheidegger JR, Studer UE, Kraft R. Metastatic disease of the ureter: patterns of tumoral spread and radiologic findings. *Abdom Imaging*. 1993. 18(1):88-94.
40. Richie JP, Kantoff PW. Neoplasms of the renal pelvis and ureter. In: Bast RJ, Kufe DW, Pollock RE, Weichselbaum RR, Holland JF, Frei E III, eds. *Holland-Frei Cancer Medicine*. 5th ed. Hamilton, ON: BC Decker; 2000: chap 106.
41. Wei-Ching L, Jeon-Hor C. Urinary bladder metastasis from breast cancer with heterogeneic expression of estrogen and progesterone receptors. *J Clin Oncol*. 2007;25(27):4308-4310.
42. Matsuhashi N, Yamaguchi K, Tamura T, Shimokawa K, Sugiyama Y, Adachi Y. Adenocarcinoma in bladder diverticulum, metastatic from gastric cancer. *World J Surg Oncol*. 2005;3:55.
43. Kim H, Kim SH, Hwang SI, Lee HJ, Han JK. Isolated bladder metastases from stomach cancer: CT demonstration. *Abdom Imaging*. 2001;26:333-335.
44. Ota T, Shinohara M, Kinoshita K, Sakoma T, Kitamura M, Maeda Y. Two cases of metastatic bladder cancers showing diffuse thickening of the bladder wall. *Jpn J Clin Oncol*. 1999; 29:314-316.
45. Leddy F, Peterson N, Ning T. Urogenital linitis plastica metastatic from stomach. *Urology*. 1992;39:464-467.
46. Kubota Y, Kawai A, Tsuchiya T, Kozima K, Yokoi S, Deguchi T. Bilateral primary malignant lymphoma of the ureter. *Int J Clin Oncol*. 2007;12(6):482-484.
47. Lebowitz JA, Rofsky NM, Weinreb JC, Friedmann P. Ureteral lymphoma: MRI demonstration. *Abdom Imaging*. 2007;20: 173-175.
48. Kempton CL, Kurtin PJ, Inwards DJ, Wollan P, Bostwick DG. Malignant lymphoma of the bladder: evidence from 36 cases that low-grade lymphoma of the MALT-type is the most common primary bladder lymphoma. *Am J Surg Pathol*. 1997;21(11):1324-1333.
49. Antunes AA, Nesrallah LJ, Srougi M. Non-Hodgkin lymphoma of the bladder. *Int Braz J Urol*. 2004;30:499-501.
50. Leite KRM, Bruschini H, Câmara-Lopes LH. Primary lymphoma of the bladder. *Int Braz J Urol*. 2004;30:37-39.
51. Amin R. Case report: primary non-Hodgkin's lymphoma of the bladder. *Br J Radiol*. 1995;68:1257-1260.
52. Shick JE. Pyeloureteritis cystica report of a case with spontaneous rupture of the ureter. *Radiology*. 1960;74:468-470.
53. Parker B, Patel B, Coffield K. Ureteritis cystica presenting as a retractile ureteral polyp. *J Urol*. 2002;168(1):195-196.
54. Ordon M, Ray AA, D'A Honey RJ. Ureteritis cystica: a rare cause of ureteral obstruction. *J. Endourol*. 2010;24(9): 1391-1393.
55. Petersen UE, Kvist E, Friis M, Krogh J. Ureteritis cystica. *Scan J Urol Nephrol*. 1991;25:1-4.
56. Rothschild JG, Wu G. Ureteritis cystica: a radiologic pathologic correlation. *J Clin Imaging Sci*. 2011;1:23.
57. Wiener D, Koss LG, Sablay B, Freed SZ. The prevalence and significance of Brunn's nests, cystitis cystica, and squamous metaplasia in normal bladders. *J Urol*. 1977;12:317.
58. Hochberg D, Motta J, Brodherson M. Cystitis glandularis. *Urology*. 1998;51:112-113.
59. Heyns C, De Kock ML, Kirsten PH, van Velden DJ. Pelvic lipomatosis associated with cystitis glandularis and adenocarcinoma of the bladder. *J Urol*. 1991;145:364-366.
60. Wong-You-Cheong J, Woodward PJ, Manning MA, Davis CJ. From the archives of the AFIP: inflammatory and nonneoplastic bladder masses: radiologic-pathologic correlation. *RadioGraphics*. 2006;26(6):1847-1868.
61. Cochran S, Waisman J, Barbaric Z. Radiographic and microscopic findings in multiple ureteral diverticula. *Radiology*. 1980;137:631-636.
62. Wasserman NF, Zhang G, Posalaky IP, Reddy PK. Ureteral pseudodiverticula: frequent association with uroepithelial malignancy. *AJR Am J Roentgenol*. 1991;157:69-72.
63. Wasserman NF, La Pointe S, Posalaky IP. Ureteral pseudodiverticulosis. *Radiology*. 1985;155:561-566.
64. Spalluto L, Woodfield C. Ureteral pseudodiverticulosis: a unique case diagnosed by multidetector computed tomography. *J Comput Assist Tomogr*. 2009;33(2):286-287.
65. Matta EJ, Kenney AJ, Barre GM, Vanlangendonck RM Jr. Intradiverticular bladder carcinoma. *RadioGraphics*. 2005; 25:1397-1403.
66. Melekos MD, Asbach HW, Barbalias GA. Vesical diverticula: etiology, diagnosis, tumorigenesis, and treatment. *Urology*. 1987;30:453-457.
67. Pieretti RV, Pieretti-Vanmarcke RV. Congenital bladder diverticula in children. *J Pediatr Surg*. 1999;34:468.
68. Karod J. Danella J, Mowad J. Routine radiologic surveillance for obstruction is not required in asymptomatic patients after ureteroscopy. *J Endourol*. 1999;13(6):433-436.
69. Schmidt J, Hawtrey CE, Flocks RH, Culp DA. Complications, results and problems of ileal conduit diversions. *J Urol*. 1973; 109:210-216.
70. Skinner D, Crawford E, Kaufman J. Complications of radical cystectomy for carcinoma of the bladder. *J Urol*. 1980;123: 640-643.
71. Chahal R, Sundaram SK, Iddenden R, Forman DF, Weston PM, Harrison SC. A study of the morbidity, mortality and long-term survival following radical cystectomy and radical radiotherapy in the treatment of invasive bladder cancer in Yorkshire. *Eur Urol*. 2003;43(3):246-257.
72. Vakili B, Chesson RR, Kyle BL, et al. The incidence of urinary tract injury during hysterectomy: a prospective analysis based on universal cystoscopy. *Am J Obstet Gynecol*. 2005;192(5): 1599-1604.
73. Hatch K, Parham G, Shingleton HM, Orr JW Jr, Austin JM Jr. Ureteral strictures and fistulae following radical hysterectomy. *Gynecol Oncol*. 1984;19(1):17-23.
74. Roberts W, Cadeddu JA, Micali S, Kavoussi LR, Moore RG. Ureteral stricture formation after removal of impacted calculi. *J Urol*. 1998;159(3):723-726.
75. Matos MJ, Bacelar MT, Pinto P, Ramos I. Genitourinary tuberculosis. *Eur J Radiol*. 2005;55:181-187.
76. Burrill J, Williams CJ, Bain G, Conder G, Hine AL, Misra RR. Tuberculosis: a radiologic review. *RadioGraphics*. 2007;27: 1255-1273.
77. Engin G, Acunas B, Acunas G, Tunaci M. Imaging of extrapulmonary tuberculosis. *RadioGraphics*. 2000;20(2):471-488.
78. Zissin R, Gayer G, Chowers M, Shapiro-Feinberg M, Kots E, Hertz M. Computerized tomography findings of abdominal tuberculosis: report of 19 cases. *Isr Med Assoc J*. 2001;3(6):414-418.
79. Leder R, Low V. Tuberculosis of the abdomen. *Radiol Clin North Am*. 1995;33:691-705.

80. Ramchandani P, Buckler P. Imaging of genitourinary trauma. *AJR Am J Roentgenol.* 2009;192(6):1514-1523.
81. Matthews L, Smith E, Spirnak J. Nonoperative treatment of major blunt renal lacerations with urinary extravasation. *J Urol.* 1997;157:2056-2058.
82. Santucci R, McAninch JW, Safir M, Mario LA, Service S, Segal MR. Validation of the American Association for the Surgery of Trauma Organ Injury Severity Scale for the kidney. *J Trauma.* 2001;50:195-200.
83. Kawashima A, Sandler CM, Corriere JN Jr, Rodgers BM, Goldman SM. Ureteropelvic junction injuries secondary to blunt abdominal trauma. *Radiology.* 1997;205:487-492.
84. Brandes S, Coburn M, Armenakas N, McAninch J. Diagnosis and management of ureteric injury: an evidence-based analysis. *BJU Int.* 2004;94:277-289.
85. Best C, Petrone P, Buscarini M, et al. Traumatic ureteral injuries: a single institution experience validating the American Association for the Surgery of Trauma-Organ Injury Scale grading scale. *J Urol.* 2005;173:1202-1205.
86. Selzman A, Spirnak J. Iatrogenic ureteral injuries: a 20-year experience in treating 165 injuries. *J Urol.* 1996;155:878-881.
87. Gomez R, Ceballos L, Coburn M, et al. Consensus statement on bladder injuries. *BJU Int.* 2004;94:27-32.
88. Sandler C, Goldman S, Kawashima A. Lower urinary tract trauma. *World J Urol.* 1998;16:69-75.
89. Quagliano P, Delair S, Malhotra A. Diagnosis of blunt bladder injury: a prospective comparative study of computed tomography cystography and conventional retrograde cystography. *J Trauma.* 2006;61:410-421.
90. Morey A, Iverson AJ, Swan A, et al. Bladder rupture after blunt trauma: guidelines for diagnostic imaging. *J Trauma.* 2001;51:683-686.
91. Chan D, Abujudeh HH, Cushing GL Jr, Novelline RA. CT cystography with multiplanar reformation for suspected bladder rupture: experience in 234 cases. *AJR Am J Roentgenol.* 2006;187:1296-1302.
92. Vaccaro J, Brody J. CT cystography in the evaluation of major bladder trauma. *RadioGraphics.* 2000;20:1373-1381.
93. Clark JY, Thompson IM, Optenberg SA. Economic impact of urolithiasis in the United States. *J Urol.* 1995;154(6): 2020-2024.
94. Jindal G, Ramchandani P. Acute flank pain secondary to urolithiasis: radiologic evaluation and alternate diagnoses. *Radiol Clin North Am.* 2007;45(3):395-410.
95. Pearle MS, Calhoun EA, Curhan GC. Urologic Diseases in America Project: urolithiasis. *J Urol.* 2005;173:848-857.
96. Kobayashi T, Nishizawa K, Mitsumori K, Ogura K. Impact of date of onset on the absence of hematuria in patients with acute renal colic. *J Urol.* 2003;170:1093-1096.
97. Chen MY, Zagoria RJ. Can noncontrast helical computed tomography replace intravenous urography for evaluation of patients with acute urinary tract colic. *J Emerg Med.* 1999;17:299-303.
98. Smith RC, Verga M, McCarthy S, Rosenfield AT. Diagnosis of acute flank pain: value of unenhanced helical CT. *AJR Am J Roentgenol.* 1996;166:97-101.
99. Fielding JR, Fox LA, Heller H, et al. Spiral CT in the evaluation of flank pain: overall accuracy and feature analysis. *J Comput Assist Tomogr.* 1997;21:635-638.
100. Memarsadeghi M, Heinz-Peer G, Helbich TH, et al. Unenhanced multi-detector row CT in patients suspected of having urinary stone disease: effect of section width on diagnosis. *Radiology.* 2005;235:530-536.
101. Takahashi N, Kawashima A, Ernst RD, et al. Ureterolithiasis: can clinical outcome be predicted with unenhanced helical CT? *Radiology.* 1998;208:97-102.
102. Preminger G, Tiselius HG, Assimos DG, et al.; EAU/AUA Nephrolithiasis Guideline Panel. EAU/AUA Nephrolithiasis Guideline Panel. 2007 guideline for the management of ureteral calculi. *J Urol.* 2007;178(6):2418-2434.
103. Olcott EW, Sommers FG, Napel S. Accuracy of detection and measurement of renal calculi: in vitro comparison of three-dimensional spiral CT, radiography, and nephrotomography. *Radiology.* 1997;204:19-25.
104. Parsons JK, Lancini V, Shetye K, Regan F, Potter SR, Jarrett TW. Urinary stone size: comparison of abdominal plain radiography and noncontrast CT measurements. *J Endourol.* 2003;17:725-728.
105. Katz DS, Lane MJ, Sommer FG. Unenhanced helical CT of ureteral stones: incidence of associated urinary tract findings. *AJR Am J Roentgenol.* 1996;166:1319-1322.
106. Varanelli MJ, Coll DM, Levine JA, Rosenfield AT, Smith RC. Relationship between duration of pain and secondary signs of obstruction of the urinary tract on unenhanced helical CT. *AJR Am J Roentgenol.* 2001;177:325-330.
107. Georgiades CS, Moore CJ, Smith DP. Differences of renal parenchymal attenuation for acutely obstructed and unobstructed kidneys on unenhanced helical CT: a useful secondary sign? *AJR Am J Roentgenol.* 2001;176(4):965-968.
108. Boridy IC, Kawashima A, Goldman SM, Sandler CM. Acute ureterolithiasis: nonenhanced helical CT findings of perinephric edema for prediction of degree of ureteral obstruction. *Radiology.* 1999;213:663-667.
109. Kawashima A, Sandler CM, Boridy IC, Takahashi N, Benson GS, Goldman SM. Unenhanced helical CT of ureterolithiasis: value of the tissue rim sign. *AJR Am J Roentgenol.* 1997;168:997-1000.
110. Boridy IC, Nikolaidis P, Kawashima A, Goldman SM, Sandler CM. Ureterolithiasis: value of the tail sign in differentiating phleboliths from ureteral calculi at nonenhanced helical CT. *Radiology.* 1999;211:619-621.
111. Traubici J, Neitlich JD, Smith RC. Distinguishing pelvic phleboliths from distal ureteral stones on routine unenhanced helical CT: is there a radiolucent center? *AJR Am J Roentgenol.* 1999;172:13-17.
112. Sheafor DH, Hertzberg BS, Freed KS, et al. Nonenhanced helical CT and US in the emergency evaluation of patients with renal colic: prospective comparison. *Radiology.* 2000; 217:792-797.
113. Sudah M, Vanninen R, Partanen K, Heino A, Vainio P, Ala-Opas M. MR urography in evaluation of acute flank pain: T2-weighted sequences and gadolinium-enhanced three-dimensional FLASH compared with urography—fast low-angle shot. *AJR Am J Roentgenol.* 2001;176:105-112.
114. Kenney PJ. CT evaluation of urinary lithiasis. *Radiol Clin North Am.* 2003;41:979-999.
115. Shokeir AA, El-Diasty T, Eassa W, et al. Diagnosis of ureteral obstruction in patients with compromised renal function: the role of noninvasive imaging modalities. *J Urol.* 2004;171: 2303-2306.

116. Shokeir AA, El-Diasty T, Eassa W, et al. Diagnosis of noncalcareous hydronephrosis: role of magnetic resonance urography and noncontrast computed tomography. *Urology.* 2004;63:225-229.
117. Smellie J, Normand I. Bacteriuria, reflux and renal scarring. *Arch Dis Child.* 1975;50:581-585.
118. Lebowitz R, Colodny A. Urinary tract infection in children. *Crit Rev Clin Radiol Nucl Med.* 1973;4:457-475.
119. Elder J, Peters CA, Arant BS Jr, et al. Pediatric Vesicoureteral Reflux Guidelines Panel summary report on the management of primary vesicoureteral reflux in children. *J Urol.* 1997;157:1846-1851.
120. Bisset GI, Strife J, Dunbar J. Urography and voiding cystourethrography: findings in girls with urinary tract infection. *AJR Am J Roentgenol.* 1987;148:479-482.
121. Peters C, Skoog SJ, Arant BS Jr, et al. Summary of the AUA guideline on management of primary vesicoureteral reflux in children. *J Urol.* 2010;184(3):1134-1144.
122. Bailey R. End-stage reflux nephropathy. *Nephron.* 1981;27: 302-306.
123. Gusmano R, Perfumo F. Worldwide demographic aspects of chronic renal failure in children. *Kidney Int.* 1993;43(suppl 41): S31-S35.
124. Fefferman N, Sabach AS, Rivera R, et al. The efficacy of digital fluoroscopic image capture in the evaluation of vesicoureteral reflux in children. *Pediatr Radiol.* 2009;39(11):1179-1187.
125. Jequier S, Jequier J. Reliability of voiding cystourethrography to detect reflux. *AJR Am J Roentgenol.* 1989;153:807-810.
126. Gelfand M, Strife J, Hertzberg V. Low-grade vesicoureteral reflux. Variability in grade on sequential radiographic and nuclear cystograms. *Clin Nucl Med.* 1991;16:243-246.
127. Paltiel H, Rupich R, Kiruluta H. Enhanced detection of vesicoureteral reflux in infants and children with use of cyclic voiding cystourethrography. *Radiology.* 1992;184:753-755.
128. Berrocal T, Gayá F, Arjonilla A, Lonergan GJ. Vesicoureteral reflux: diagnosis and grading with echo-enhanced cystosonography versus voiding cystourethrography. *Radiology.* 2001;221:359-365.
129. Caoili E, Cohan RH, Korobkin M, et al. Urinary tract abnormalities: initial experience with multi-detector row CT urography. *Radiology.* 2002;222(2):353-360.
130. Kim S, Choi YD, Nam JH, Kwon DD, Juhng SW, Choi C. Cytologic features of primary signet ring cell carcinoma of the bladder: a case report. *Acta Cytol.* 2009;53(3):309-312.
131. Oh K, Zang D. Primary non-Hodgkin's lymphoma of the bladder with bone marrow involvement. *Korean J Intern Med.* 2003;18(1):40-44.
132. Kim H, Kim SH, Hwang SI, Lee HJ, Han JK. Isolated bladder metastases from stomach cancer: CT demonstration. *Abdom Imaging.* 2001;26(3):333-335.
133. Kornu R, Oliver Q, Reimold A. Recognizing concomitant lupus enteritis and lupus cystitis. *J Clin Rheumatol.* 2008; 14(4):226-229.
134. Kawashima A, Alleman WG, Takahashi N, Kim B, King BF Jr, LeRoy AJ. Imaging evaluation of amyloidosis of the urinary tract and retroperitoneum. *Radiographics.* 2011;31(6):1569-1582.
135. Stillwell T, Benson RJ. Cyclophosphamide-induced hemorrhagic cystitis. A review of 100 patients. *Cancer.* 1988;61(3):451-457.
136. Dmochowski R. Bladder outlet obstruction: etiology and evaluation. *Rev Urol.* 2005;7(suppl 6):S3-S13.
137. Leach G, Dmochowski RR, Appell RA, et al. Female Stress Urinary Incontinence Clinical Guidelines Panel summary report on surgical management of female stress urinary incontinence. *J Urol.* 1997;158:875-880.
138. Coe F, Favus M. Nephrolithiasis. In: Isselbacher K, Braunwald E, Wilson JEA, eds. *Harrison's Principles of Internal Medicine.* 13th ed. New York, NY: McGraw-Hill;1994:1329.
139. Hu F, Rimm E, Smith-Warner SA, et al. Reproducibility and validity of dietary patterns assessed with a food frequency questionnaire. *Am J Clin Nutr.* 1999;69:243-249.
140. Feskanich D, Rimm EB, Giovannucci EL, et al. Reproducibility and validity of food intake measurements from a semiquantitative food frequency questionnaire. *J Am Diet Assoc.* 1993;93:790-796.
141. Brown RC, Loening SA, Ehrhardt JC. Cystine calculi are radiopaque. *AJR Am J Roentgenol.* 1980;135:565-567.
142. Stoller ML, Gupta M, Bolton D, Irby PB 3rd. Clinical correlates of the gross, radiographic, and histologic features of urinary matrix calculi. *J Endourol.* 1994;8:335-340.
143. Herring L. Observations on the analysis of ten thousand urinary calculi. *J Urol.* 1962;88:545-562.
144. Matthews LA, Spirnak PJ. A matrix calculus causing bilateral ureteral obstruction and acute renal failure. *J Urol.* 1995;154: 1125-1126.
145. Herring LC. Observations on the analysis of ten thousand urinary calculi. *J Urol.* 1962;88:545-562.
146. Levine JA, Neitlich J, Verga M, Dalrymple N, Smith RC. Ureteral calculi in patients with flank pain: correlation of plain radiography with unenhanced helical CT. *Radiology.* 1997;204(1):27-31.
147. Zagoria RJ, Khatod EG, Chen MYM. Abdominal radiography after CT reveals urinary calculi: a method to predict usefulness of abdominal radiography on the basis of size and CT attenuation of calculi. *AJR Am J Roentgenol.* 2001;176:1117-1122.
148. Middleton WD, Dodds WJ, Lawson TL, Foley WD. Renal calculi: sensitivity for detection with US. *Radiology.* 1988;167:239-244.
149. Burge HJ, Middleton WD, McClennan BL, Hildebolt CF. Ureteral jets in healthy subjects and in patients with unilateral ureteral calculi: comparison with color Doppler US. *Radiology.* 1991;180:437-442.
150. Garcea G, Majid I, Sutton CD, Pattenden CJ, Thomas WM. Diagnosis and management of colovesical fistulae; six-year experience of 90 consecutive cases. *Colorectal Dis.* 2006;8(4): 347-352.
151. Basler J, Schwartz BF. *Enterovesical Fistula.* 2009.
152. Amendola MA, Agha FP, Dent TL, Amendola BE, Shirazi KK. Detection of occult colovesical fistula by the Bourne test. *AJR Am J Roentgenol.* 1984;142(4):715-718.
153. Spurlock J, Chelmow D. *Vesicovaginal Fistula.* 2012.
154. Dalla PL, Bazzocchi M, Cressa C, Tommasini G. Radiological anatomy of the kidney revisited. *Br J Radiol.* 1990;753:680-690.
155. Glassberg KI, Braren V, Duckett JW, et al. Suggested terminology for duplex systems, ectopic ureters and ureteroceles. *J Urol.* 1984;132(6):1153-1154.
156. Park J. Normal and anomalous development of the urogenital system. In: Walsh P, Retik A, Vaughan EJ, et al., eds. *Campbell's Urology.* 8th ed. Philadelphia, PA: WB Saunders; 2002:1749-1750.

157. Schlussel R, Retik A. Ectopic ureter, ureterocele, and other anomalies of the ureter. In Walsh P, Retik A, Vaughan EJ, et al., eds. *Campbell's Urology*. 8th ed. Philadelphia, PA: WB Saunders; 2002:2038.

158. Fniedland G, Cunningham J. The elusive ectopic ureteroceles. *AJR Am J Roentgenol*. 1972;116:792-811.

159. Churchill B, Sheldon C, McLorie G. The ectopic ureterocele: a proposed practical classification based on renal unit jeopardy. *J Pediatr Surg*. 1992;27(4):497-500.

160. Pohl H, Joyce GF, Wise M, Cilento BG Jr. Vesicoureteral reflux and ureteroceles. *J Urol*. 2007;177(5):1659-1666.

161. Mandell J, Colodny AH, Lebowitz R, Bauer SB, Retik AB. Ureteroceles in infants and children. *J Urol*. 1980;123:921-926.

162. Lemaitre G, Desmidt J. Pseudo-ureterocele. *J Radiol*. 1980; 61:161-164.

163. Nash A, Knight M. Ureterocele calculi. *Br J Urol*. 1973;45: 404-407.

164. Singh I. Adult bilateral non-obstructing orthotopic ureteroceles with multiple calculi: endoscopic management with review of literature. *Int Urol Nephrol*. 2007;39:71-74.

165. Dyer RB, Chen M, Zagoria RJ. Classic signs in uroradiology. *RadioGraphics*. 2004;24:247-280.

166. Mitty HA, Schapira HE. Ureterocele and pseudoureterocele: cobra versus cancer. *J Urol*. 1977;117(5):557-561.

CHAPTER

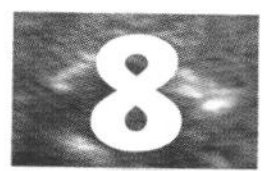

Imaging of the Adrenal

Nicholas Papanicolaou, MD, FACR
Susan Hilton, MD

ANATOMY, HISTOLOGY, AND ENDOCRINE FUNCTION

The adrenal glands, essential endocrine structures, are paired, small (4-6 g each) organs in the suprarenal retroperitoneum, each within its respective perinephric fascia. The surgical literature often describes the right gland as triangular or pyramidal in shape and the left one as elongated and crescentlike, each consisting of a body, a "medial" head, and a "lateral" tail. The imaging literature describes a body and 2 limbs, medial and lateral, in each gland.

Histologically, each adrenal is composed of a cortex and a medulla, both high in fat content but of vastly different biological functions. Most of the medulla is found in the head of the gland, and most of the cortex in the limbs. The cortex constitutes about 90% of the total gland volume, and forms 3 histologically distinct cellular zones under the adrenal capsule.[1] The zona glomerulosa, the most superficial one, secrets mineralocorticosteroid hormones (aldosterone); the zona fasciculata, the thickest one in the middle, secrets mostly glucocorticosteroids (cortisol); and, the zona reticularis, innermost layer, which produces estrogens, androgens, and some glucocorticosteroids. The cortex arises in mesenchymal cells located adjacent to the dorsal mesentery. The originally developed fetal cortex atrophies and is replaced by the adult cortex, which forms the above-mentioned 3 zones. The medulla is composed of neural crest components called chromaffin cells and is located underneath the adrenal cortex. The adrenal medulla is responsible for production and secretion of catecholamines (epinephrine, norepinephrine).[1] The adrenal glands are largest in size at birth, with a rapid decrease during the first several weeks of life. It should be noted that at birth the weight of the adrenal glands is about 0.2% of the total body weight (4 g each), about 20 times larger in relative terms compared to that in the adult human.[2]

A rich arterial supply to each adrenal gland is provided by 3 arteries. The superior adrenal artery arises in the inferior phrenic artery, a branch of the aorta. The middle adrenal artery arises directly from the aorta. Lastly, the inferior adrenal artery arises in the ipsilateral renal artery. At the level of each gland, the arterial supply takes the form of 50 to 60 thin branches, some of which form subcapsular plexuses and others go directly to the medulla. A single, central adrenal vein is formed by venous sinusoids in each gland. The right adrenal vein is short and drains directly into the cava. The left adrenal vein is longer and drains, often together with the left inferior phrenic vein, into the left renal vein opposite the left gonadal vein. Each central adrenal vein communicates with pericapsular veins, thus allowing for collateral drainage in case of venous thrombosis.[3]

Adrenal lymphatics drain directly into paracaval or paraaortic lymph nodes as well as into renal hilar lymphatics that drain into paracaval or paraaortic nodes. The innervation is autonomic and only to the medulla, in the form of sympathetic fibers from the T10-L1 spinal cord through the greater splanchnic nerve and celiac ganglia.[3]

Unilateral adrenal agenesis is encountered in about 10% of cases of renal agenesis.[4] Bilateral agenesis is incompatible with life. Fusion of the adrenals is rare, seen in cases of horseshoe kidney or renal ectopia.[5] The presence of accessory adrenal tissue ("adrenal rests") has been described in the vicinity of kidneys, gonads, and retroperitoneum, because of the proximity of the developing adrenal cortex to these organs and anatomic compartment. Of interest, in a series of consecutive autopsies, adrenal rests were present in 32% of cases, but only 16% of these rests contained both cortex and medulla.[6]

IMAGING MODALITIES IN ADRENAL GLAND DISEASES

Radiography and Urography

Plain radiographs have no role in investigating adrenal gland pathology. However, rarely, abdominal plain films will demonstrate a suprarenal soft-tissue attenuation mass or calcifications, indicating the presence of adrenal pathology. Like plain radiographs, intravenous (IV) urography does not have a role in the evaluation of adrenal diseases. However, if an adrenal mass is large enough, IV urography may demonstrate a deformity in the upper pole of the kidney or downward displacement of the kidney, indicating the presence of adrenal pathology.

Ultrasound Imaging

Ultrasonography (US) is an important tool in the search of suspected adrenal masses, especially in infants and children. However, the normal adrenal gland and many small adrenal lesions cannot be reliably identified by US. Scrotal sonography is useful in documenting adrenal rests within the testis.

CT and MRI Imaging

In most instances, computed tomography (CT) and magnetic resonance imaging (MRI) are the prime investigating imaging modalities for adrenal pathology. These modalities provide excellent visualization of the normal adrenal gland and can depict lesions as small as 5 mm in cross-sectional diameter. These modalities are also sensitive for the presence of mature fat and intracellular lipid, findings that can be used to distinguish between a variety of common adrenal pathologies.

On both CT and MRI, the normal adrenal gland appears an inverted "V" or inverted "Y" shape superior and medial to the kidney. On axial images, the right adrenal will be located between the right lobe of the liver and the crux of the diaphragm superior to the kidney. The left adrenal will be imbedded in the super adrenal fat just medial to the left crux of the diaphragm. On CT, the adrenal will have an intermediate attenuation surrounded by low-attenuation fat. On MRI, the adrenal will have an intermediate signal intensity, surrounded by high-intensity fat on both T1- and T2-weighted sequences (see Figure 8-1).

Adrenal Venography

Adrenal angiography and venography is used only sparingly in the evaluation of adrenal pathology. The most common use for adrenal venography is to guide venous blood sampling in certain patients evaluated for elevated cortisol or aldosterone levels.

NP-59 Imaging

The wide use of cholesterol by the adrenal cortex to synthesize its hormones led to the development of a radionuclide, the I-131 labeled 6-b-iodomethyl-19-norcholesterol (NP-59) as a specific agent for adrenal cortical imaging.[7] Treatment with potassium iodide 1 day before and 7 days after NP-59 administration is recommended to protect the

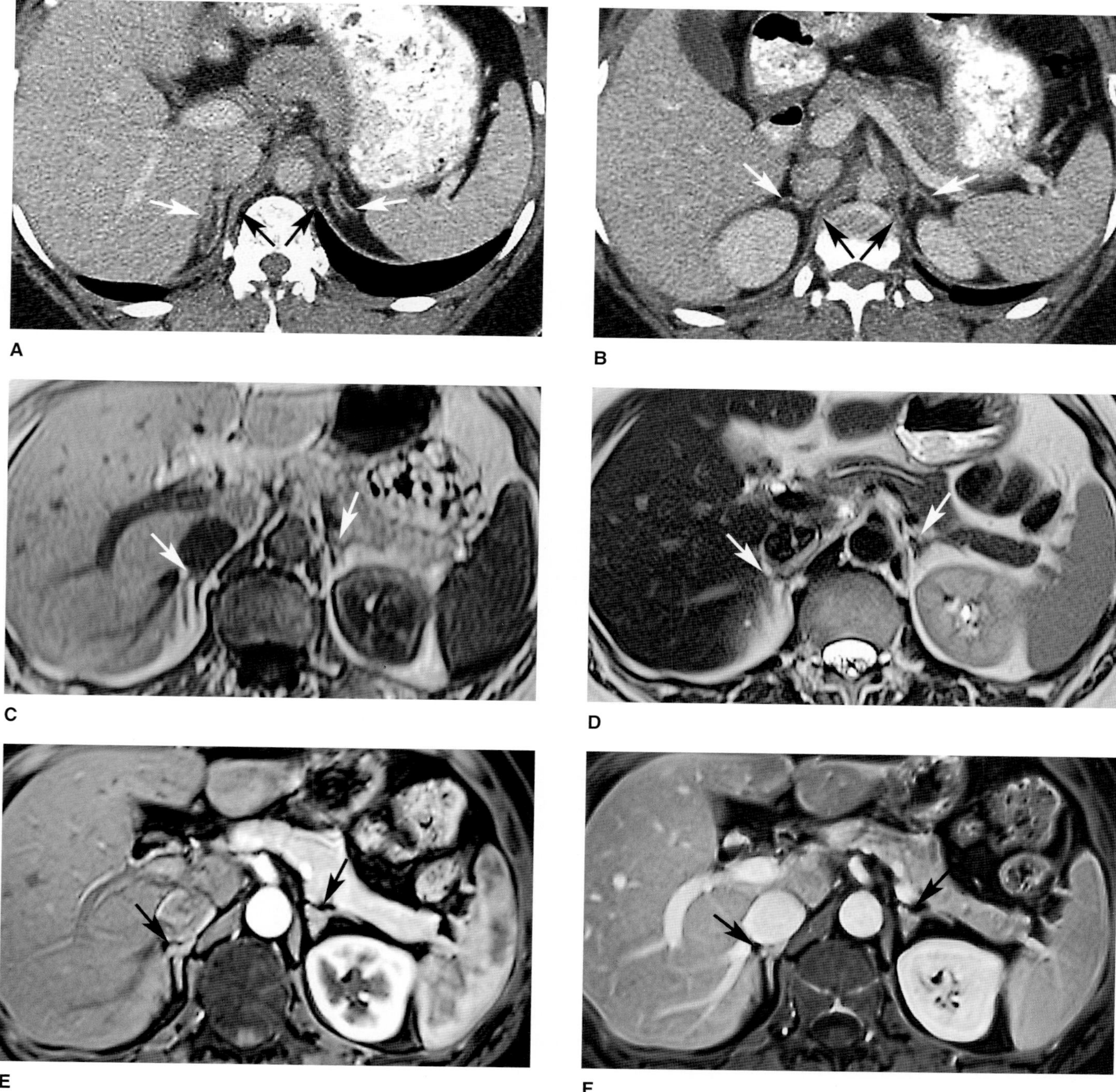

Figure 8-1 Normal Adrenal Gland
A-F. On both CT and MRI examinations, the normal adrenal glands appear as inverted V-shaped structures (*white arrows*) with 2 thin limbs. The right adrenal is imbedded in the fat between the liver laterally, the crux of the diaphragm (*black arrows*) medially. The left kidney is imbedded in the fat between the spleen, stomach, and pancreas laterally and the diaphragm crux (*black arrows*) medially. The adrenals are anterior and superior to the upper poles of the kidneys. Occasionally, only 1 of the limbs of the right adrenal can be seen, in which case, it appears as a thin linear structure between the liver and diaphragm crux. (A and B) On contrast-enhanced CT, they uniformly enhance (C-F) MRI in a second individual. On T1-weighted (C) and T2-weighted (D) images, the adrenal is an intermediate signal similar to muscle. With contrast enhancement, the gland uniformly and briskly enhances on both arterial-phase (E) and venous-phase (F) images.

thyroid gland. Imaging is performed 4 to 5 days post IV administration of NP-59, as the agent is slowly taken up and stored by the adrenal cortex, and background activity diminishes. Cushing syndrome due to unregulated adrenocorticotropic hormone (ACTH) production results in bilateral adrenal cortical uptake and visualization, whereas in cases of an autonomous adenoma, only the lesion is visualized, while there is no uptake at all by the remaining adrenal cortex. Drugs that increase plasma renin concentration (spironolactone, triamterene, amiloride, and others) given concurrently with NP-59, can induce early uptake of the radionuclide by the adrenal cortex of the contralateral normal gland in patients with adenomas, thus erroneously suggesting the diagnosis of bilateral adrenal hyperplasia.[8]

In patients with suspected primary aldosteronism, it is recommended that dexamethasone suppression is used concurrently with NP-59 scanning, in order to neutralize/suppress the influence of the pituitary ACTH and enhance the abnormally increased function of aldosterone-secreting cells in the adrenal cortex.[9] Dose and duration of dexamethasone are essential to improving the diagnostic yield of the scan. A daily dose of 4 mg dexamethasone for 7 days prior to and throughout imaging with NP-59 is recommended (see Figure 8-2).[8]

F18-FDG PET/CT Imaging

The introduction of routine PET imaging over the past decade has had a significant impact on the diagnosis and management of patients with oncologic and inflammatory processes. The normal adrenal glands display symmetric, low-level uptake similar to that of background blood pool.[10] Among the most common uses of PET/CT in oncologic patients is the whole body search and detection of potential malignant foci, including adrenal ones, before decisions on biopsy, further imaging, or treatment are made.[11,12]

^{18}F-fluorodeoxyglucose (FDG) positron emission tomography (PET) has also been shown to reliably discriminate between benign and malignant adrenal masses. Using a cutoff standardized uptake value (SUV) of 3.1, a large series of patients reported sensitivity, specificity, positive predictive and negative predicted values of 98.5%, 92%, 89.3%, and 98.9%, respectively, for PET alone, and 100%, 98%, 97%, and 100%, respectively, for PET/CT in separating benign from malignant lesions (see Figure 8-3).[13] Another study utilized an adrenal-to-liver ratio and recommended using 1.5 as a cutoff. At a ratio greater than 2, any adrenal lesion in patients with known carcinoma was malignant.[10] Using 1.5 as cutoff, there was a small overlap between benign and malignant lesions, because some necrotic malignant lesions may display low metabolic activity.[14] However, these malignancies could be distinguished from benign masses based on their CT appearance.

FOCAL LESIONS OF THE ADRENAL GLAND

A focal nodule or mass of the adrenal will usually represent a neoplasm of the gland. Rarely, an adrenal mass will represent acute renal hemorrhage.

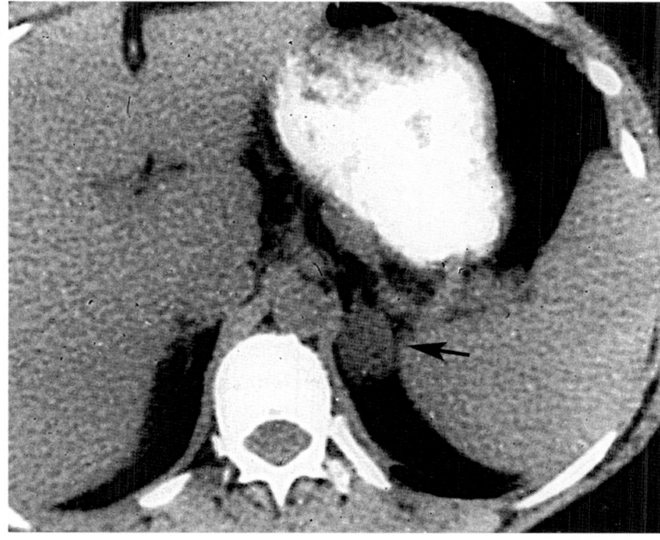

A

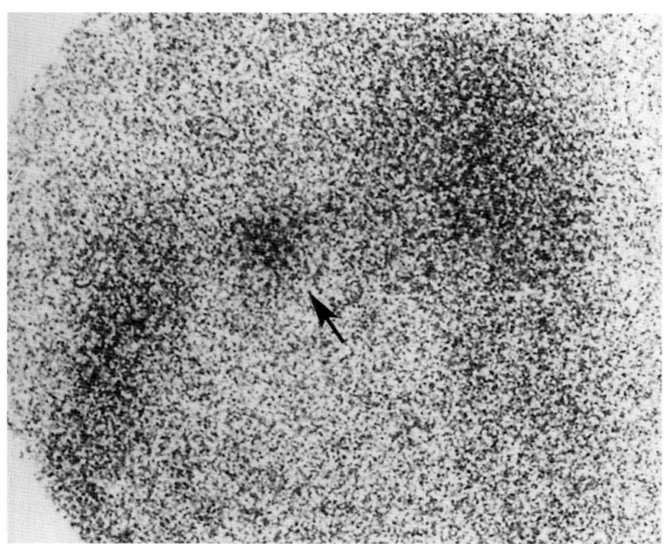

B

Figure 8-2 NP-59 Imaging
A. Unenhanced abdominal CT shows a small, low attenuation nodule (*arrow*) in the left adrenal gland, consistent with an adenoma in this patient with primary aldosteronism (Conn syndrome). **B.** I-131 NP-59 radionuclide scintigram (patient positioned prone) confirms focal uptake of the radionuclide by the adenoma (*arrow*). Additional areas of increased uptake represent the liver (*right*) and spleen (*left*), a normal finding.

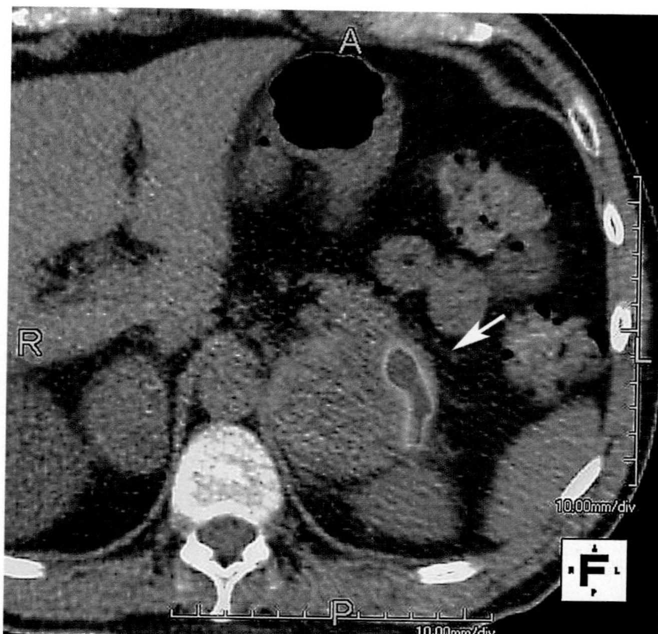

Figure 8-3 FDG PET Image of Adrenal Metastasis
This 64-year-old man had lung cancer. Fused image from a PET-CT shows a heterogeneously metabolically active, 4.3-cm left adrenal mass with an SUV of 10. In this clinical setting, these features are consistent with an adrenal metastasis.

Table 8-1. Neoplasms of the Adrenal

A. Neoplasms of the Adrenal Cortex
1. **Adrenal Adenoma**[a]
a. **Nonfunctioning**
b. Functioning
2. Adrenal Cortical Carcinoma
a. Nonfunctioning
b. Functioning
B. Neoplasms of the Adrenal Medulla
1. Pheochromocytoma
C. Other Neoplasms
1. **Metastasis**
2. Lymphoma
3. Myelolipoma
4. Hemangioma

[a]Items in bold are common.

Adrenal Neoplasms

The cells of the adrenal cortex can give rise to the common benign neoplasm, adrenal adenoma, or the rare adrenal cortical carcinoma. The adrenal medulla, like the sympathetic ganglia, develops from cells originating in the neural crest. These neuroendocrine cells give rise to tumors that form a spectrum of benign (ganglioneuroma, pheochromocytoma) and malignant lesions (neuroblastoma, pheochromocytoma).[15] The least differentiated, therefore most malignant, tumors manifest themselves in infancy and childhood and the less aggressive and/or benign tumors affect older children and adults (pheochromocytomas are usually benign). The adrenal is a common site of metastatic disease, and adrenal metastases are among the most common adrenal neoplasms. Myelolipoma, lymphoma, and hemangioma of the adrenal may also be encountered (Table 8-1).

Adrenal adenoma

Adrenal adenomas are benign tumors of the adrenal cortex, have no known malignant potential, and are the most common adrenal lesions. They have been reported in 1.4% to 8.7% of postmortem examinations, depending on the criteria used.[16-19] Their incidence is even higher among elderly patients, or patients with hypertension or diabetes mellitus.[18,19] Adenomas are detected on survey abdominal CT examinations in at least 1% of patients.[20,21]

The majority of adrenal adenomas are discovered incidentally during cross-sectional imaging examinations performed for reasons unrelated to the presence of the adenoma. In a small percentage, adenomas are found during the evaluation for 1 of several hormonally mediated syndromes, including Cushing syndrome, primary aldosteronism (Conn syndrome), and some virilization and feminization syndromes. These are discussed most completely later in this chapter under the heading: **Other Imaging and Clinical Features of Adrenal Diseases.**

Imaging characteristics of adrenal adenomas: Although some larger adenomas can be identified by sonograph, the small size of most adenomas renders the modality less effective than CT and MRI. CT and MRI are the modalities of choice for imaging the patient suspected of having a hyperfunctioning adenoma.[16,22] Lesions as small as 5 to 10 mm in the largest dimension can be detected. The sensitivity of CT detection of adrenal adenomas is estimated in excess of 85% for patients with hyperaldosteronism.[23]

Both hyperfunctioning and nonhyperfunctioning adrenal adenomas have similar imaging appearances and appear as round- or oval-shaped masses that usually measure 2 to 5 cm in the largest dimension, although lesions as small as 1 cm or less can also be demonstrated (see Figures 1-8 and 8-4).[24] Thin slice images (2- to 3-mm-thin slices at similar increments) are routinely obtained through the adrenal glands and are recommended to identify smaller lesions. In patients with nonhyperfunctioning adenomas, the remainder of the adrenal gland will appear normal. However, with hyperfunctioning adenomas producing

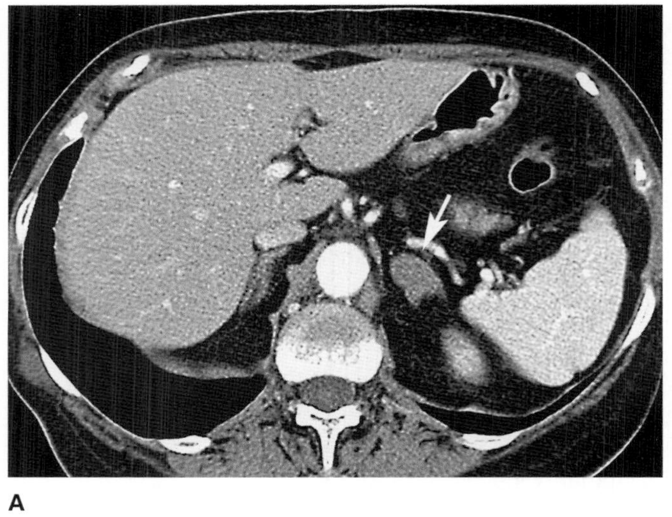
A

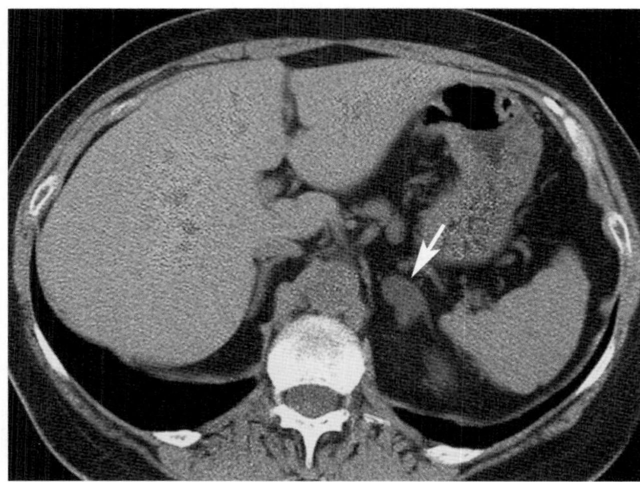
B

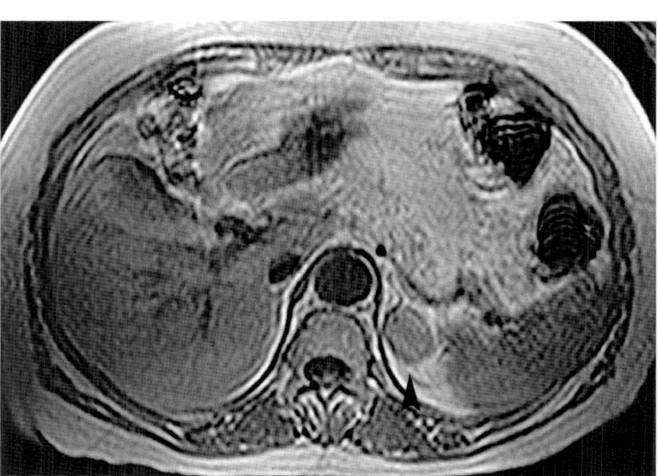
C

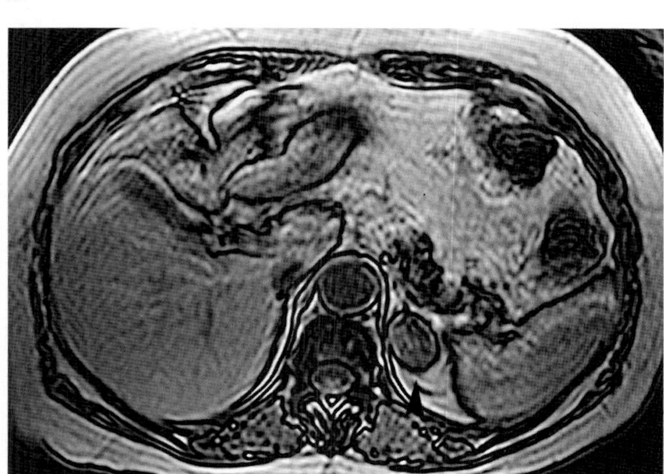
D

Figure 8-4 Lipid-Rich Adrenal Adenoma in 2 Patients
A and **B**. This 57-year-old man had a recently diagnosed lung cancer. (A) Enhanced CT as part of the workup of his lung cancer demonstrates a 2-cm nodule (*arrow*) in the left adrenal gland that measured 40 HU. This lesion could represent either an adrenal metastasis or an incidental adrenal adenoma. (B) Unenhanced CT scan obtained several days later shows the left adrenal nodule (*arrow*) to appear lower attenuation than the liver, spleen, and muscles. The nodule measured 3 HU, diagnostic of an adrenal adenoma. **C** and **D**. This 65-year-old man had an adrenal mass discovered on a CT scan performed for unrelated reasons. (C) T1 in-phase and (D) T1 out-of-phase images through the left adrenal mass (*arrowheads*) are performed. Note how the abdominal organs in D appear to be etched in black. This is a result of the canceling effects of water protons in the organ and lipid protons in the surrounding fat and identifies this as an out-of-phase image where the signal from water protons and lipid protons are subtracted. This artifact is absent from C because the signal from water and lipid protons are summated. Note how the signal from the center of the left adrenal mass (*arrowheads*) decreases from C to D. This is diagnostic of an adrenal adenoma.

cortisol, the remainder of the ipsilateral adrenal gland and the contralateral adrenal may become atrophic, because the levels of the circulating ACTH are very low. Aldosterone-producing adenomas are smaller than those secreting cortisol, and therefore more difficult to detect. The average size of such a nodule is about 1.8 cm.[25]

Most adenomas contain large amounts of intracellular lipid; thus, many of them display attenuations near to or slightly above that of water on unenhanced CT scans.[26] These adenomas are also known as lipid-rich, and constitute about 70% of all adenomas.[27] If a threshold of 10 Hounsfield units (HU) or less is applied, the unenhanced CT has a specificity of 98% in diagnosing a lipid-rich adenoma (see Figures 1-8 and 8-4).[28]

MRI can also be used to identify intracellular lipid in adrenal adenomas with the use of chemical shift imaging[29,30] and has been shown to be more sensitive for the detection of intracellular lipid than unenhanced CT.[31] The protons in fat and water molecules have different resonance frequency rates, because fat protons are more

Imaging Notes 8-1. Diagnosis of Adrenal Adenoma

Uniform, round, or oval nodule with any of the following characteristics

1. Unenhanced CT attenuation <10 HU
2. Loss of signal on out-of-phase T1 MRI
3. Pre-enhancement and postenhancement CT with % enhancement washout >60%
4. Enhanced CT % relative washout >40%

shielded from the external magnetic field than water protons and as a result resonate at a slower frequency. T1-weighted chemical shift imaging allows 2 sets of sequences to be acquired, an in-phase sequence and an opposed-phase sequence. In the in-phase sequence, the signal from water and lipid protons is added in each voxel and in the opposed-phase sequence, the signal from lipid protons is subtracted from water protons in each voxel. Tissues with voxels containing both lipid and water have signal loss (ie, appear darker) on opposed-phase images. Using the chemical shift technique, the sensitivity and specificity for differentiating adenomas from metastases ranges from 81% to 100% and 94% to 100%, respectively (see Figures 1-8 and 8-4).[29,30,32-36] Approximately 30% of adenomas are relatively lipid-poor by CT examinations, and their attenuation on unenhanced CT is >10 HU and up to 20% of adenomas are relatively lipid poor by MRI examinations using chemical shift techniques. In this situation, additional imaging, specifically a dynamic contrast enhancement CT examination, is necessary for adequate characterization of adrenal adenomas. Post IV contrast administration, adrenal adenomas invariably enhance, sometimes to 80 HU or more. Although the degree of enhancement may not differ from that of other adrenal tumors, adenomas are unique, in that, they display rapid washout of the contrast medium compared to adrenal metastases on delayed, 10- to 15-minute post IV contrast injection CT imaging.[37-40] This phenomenon has been used to distinguish between lipid-poor adenomas and adrenal malignancies, especially adrenal metastases.

Two measurements can be obtained, the absolute and relative enhancement washout (AEW and REW), depending on whether or not an unenhanced CT series is available. The AEW is calculated based on the formula: AEW = $(E - D)/(E - U) \times 100$, where E stands for attenuation value after enhancement, D stands for the delayed attenuation enhancement of the lesion (10 or 15 minutes), and U for the unenhanced attenuation value. A 60% washout at 15 min results in 88% sensitivity and 96% specificity for the diagnosis of an adenoma.[16] The REW, used when unenhanced images are not available, is calculated using the formula: REW = $(E - D)/E \times 100$. A 40% REW results in 96% sensitivity and 100% specificity for the diagnosis of an adenoma.[16] Of note, lipid-rich and lipid-poor adenomas display near identical washout measurements.[41] These attenuation measurements pre and post IV contrast enhancement, including the washout estimates, are powerful diagnostic imaging tools in making the distinction between 2 common adrenal lesions, the benign adenomas and malignant metastases, very often obviating the need for biopsy (see Figure 8-5).

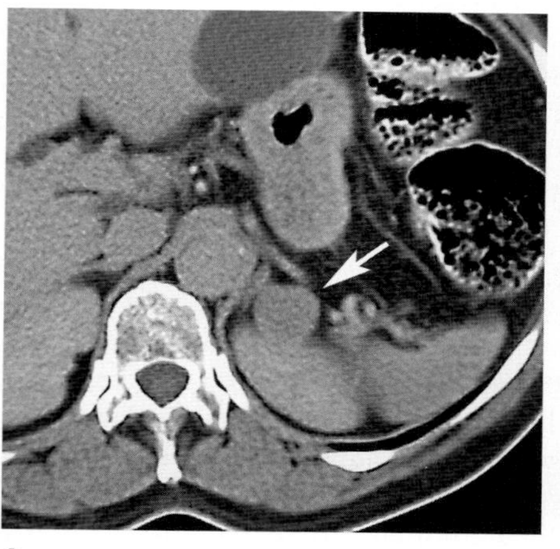
A

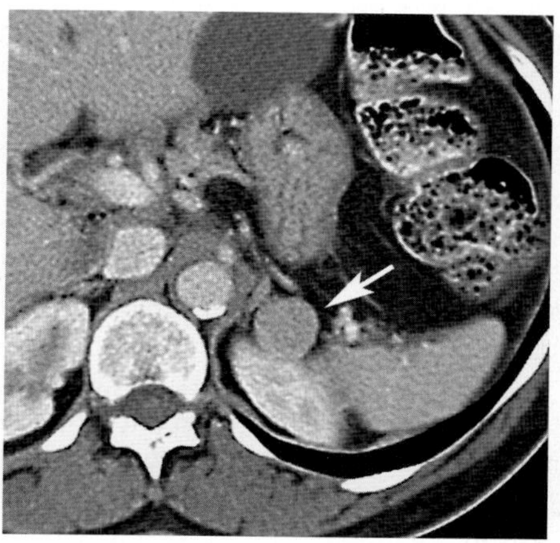
B

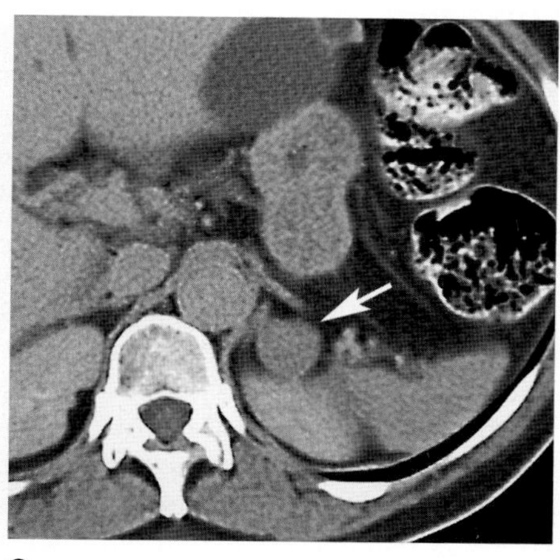
C

Figure 8-5 Lipid-Poor Adenoma
This 62-year-old woman was diagnosed with lung cancer. **A.** Unenhanced CT image shows a 1.5-cm nodule (*arrow*) in the left adrenal that measured 23 HU. This is an indeterminate adrenal lesion that could represent either an adenoma or metastasis. Images obtained 60 seconds after contrast administration (**B**) and 15 minutes after contrast administration (**C**) show the nodule (*arrows*) to measure 80 HU and 40 HU. This gives a washout of 70%, identifying the nodule as a lipid-poor adenoma.

Imaging Notes 8-2. Washout Calculations for Adrenal Adenomas

Absolute enhancement washout: $AEW = (E - D)/(E - U) \times 100$
Relative enhancement washout: $REW = (E - D)/E \times 100$

E – attenuation value after enhancement

D – delayed attenuation enhancement after 10 or 15 min

U – unenhanced attenuation value

Reproduced, with permission, from Caoili EM, Korobkin M, Francis IR, et al. Adrenal masses: characterization with combined unenhanced and delayed enhanced CT. *Radiology*. 2002;222:629-633

A very small percentage of pathologically proven adrenal adenomas deviates from the typical homogeneous, oval or round nodule. On occasion, adenomas can be large, irregular in contour, heterogeneous, and can contain hemorrhagic material or calcifications.[42] Washout calculations cannot be applied for such lesions. Depending on their size, appearance, and clinical context, percutaneous biopsy or excision is often necessary.

Adrenocortical carcinoma

Adrenocortical carcinoma is a rare malignant neoplasm derived from the cortex of the adrenal gland that accounts for approximately 0.2% of all cancer deaths. These tumors are usually large infiltrating masses at presentation and have a very poor prognosis. Only 30% of cases will be confined to the adrenal gland at initial diagnosis.[43] The majority of adrenal cortical carcinomas are hormonally active and secrete a variety of substances, including cortisol, androgens, estrogens, or aldosterone, and in approximately 60% of cases, the presentation will be due to endocrine-related syndromes, most commonly Cushing syndrome but also including virilization, adrenogenital syndrome, precocious puberty, feminization, hyperaldosteronism, and Conn (primary aldosteronism) syndrome.[44,45] Nonfunctioning tumors are discovered at a later stage, typically with symptoms of abdominal pain, a palpable upper abdominal mass, or with symptoms related to metastases. Adrenocortical carcinoma affects women more often, though nonfunctioning tumors are more prevalent in men. Although very rare among children, adrenocortical carcinoma can be seen in some cases of the Beckwith-Wiedemann syndrome, which is usually associated with Wilms tumor or hepatoblastoma, or in association with hemihypertrophy (also referred to as hemihyperplasia).[46] The TNM staging system for adrenal cortical carcinoma is outlined (Table 8-2).

Table 8-2. TNM Staging System for Adrenal Cortical Carcinoma

• Tumor	
▪ T1 - Tumor confined to adrenal gland and less than 5 cm	
▪ T2 - Tumor confined to adrenal gland and greater than 5 cm	
▪ T3 - Tumor invasion into periadrenal fat	
▪ T4 - Tumor invasion of adjacent organs	
• Node	
▪ N0 - Negative lymph nodes	
▪ N1 - Positive lymph nodes	
• Metastases	
▪ M0 - No metastases	
▪ M1 - Distant metastases	
Stage I	T1, N0, M0
Stage II	T2, N0, M0
Stage III	T3, N0, M0 or T1-2, N1, M0
Stage IV	Any T, N, M1, or T3-4, N1, M0

Reproduced, with permission, from Norton JA. Adrenal tumors. In: DeVita VT Jr, Hellman S, Rosenberg SA, eds. *Cancer: Principles and Practice of Oncology*. 7th ed. Philadelphia, PA: Lippincott Williams & Wilkins;2005:1528-1539.

Size is an important imaging feature among adrenal lesions. Most primary masses <3 cm are benign, whereas most masses >6 cm are malignant.[47] Nonfunctioning adrenal cortical carcinoma typically presents as a large suprarenal mass with an average cross-sectional diameter of 12 cm. CT typically shows a large, heterogeneous, suprarenal mass, with areas of central hypoattenuation indicating necrosis, scattered calcifications, and high-attenuation regions indicating hemorrhage (see Figure 8-6).[16,48] On MRI, adrenal cortical carcinoma is typically T1-weighted hypointense and T2-weighted hyperintense compared to the liver.[16,48-51] Like adrenal adenomas, adrenal cortical carcinoma has increased intracellular lipid content. Chemical shift imaging can be applied to detect the high intracellular lipid content of the tumor by showing signal drop on opposed-phase images compared to in-phase images. Adrenal cortical carcinoma will often invade adjacent tissues, obliterating the tissue planes between the mass and adjacent fat and other organs. As a result of this large size and the propensity to invade adjacent tissues, it can be difficult to distinguish adrenal cortical carcinoma from exophytic renal cell carcinomas, other malignant adrenal mass, such as metastasis or lymphoma, and retroperitoneal sarcomas (see Figure 8-6). Multiplanar, isotropic reconstruction of axial CT images and the direct multiplanar capabilities of US and MRI makes determination of the origin of the tumor easier.[49] The tumor is often hypovascular, a feature that may help distinguish adrenal

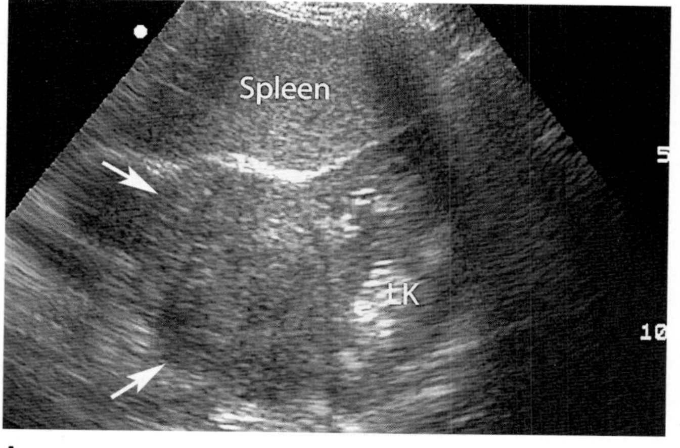

A

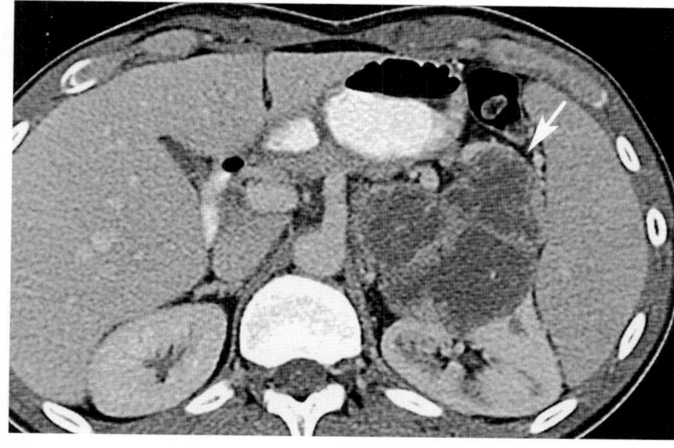

B

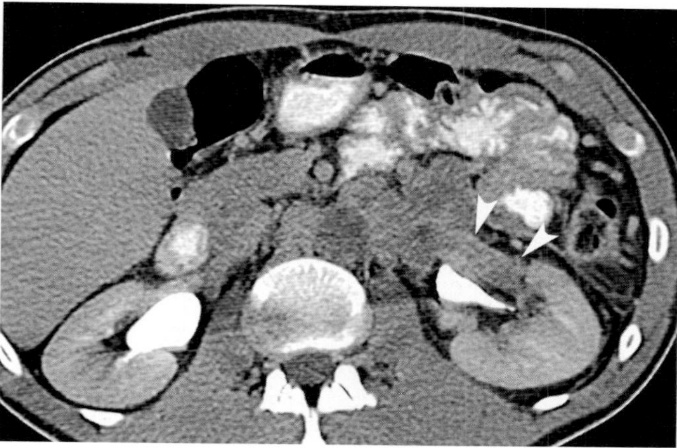

C

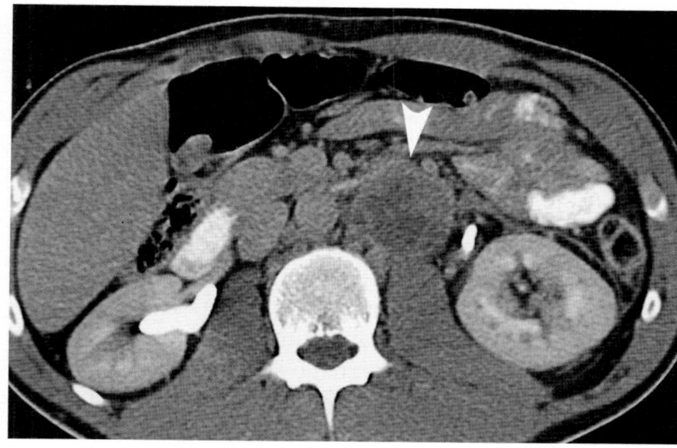

D

Figure 8-6 Adrenal Cortical Carcinoma
This 31-year-old man presented with left testicular swelling from a varicocele. **A.** US of the left retroperitoneum demonstrates a large heterogenous mass (*arrows*) superior to the left kidney. **B-D.** Contrast-enhanced CT confirms the presence of a heterogeneously enhancing left suprarenal mass (*arrow* in B), which has invaded the left renal vein (*small arrowheads* in C) and causes left para-aortic adenopathy (*large arrowhead* in D). This appearance is most likely to represent an adrenal cortical carcinoma or upper-pole renal cell carcinoma. Subsequent needle biopsy was diagnostic of an adrenal cortical carcinoma.

cortical carcinoma from the normally hypervascular renal cell carcinoma. Adrenal cortical carcinoma also has a propensity for intravascular invasion into the renal vein or inferior vena cava.

Pheochromocytoma

Pheochromocytoma is the most common neoplasm of the adrenal medulla. The tumor typically presents in the third and fourth decades of life and affects male and female patients equally. The neoplasm is derived from the chromaffin cells of the adrenal medulla. Histologically identical neoplasms occur at sites of other chromaffin cells, including the sympathetic chain and para-aortic bodies, such as the organ of Zuckerkandl and the carotid body.[52] When ectopic, these neoplasms are called paragangliomas. Approximately 98% of these tumors arise in the abdomen and 2% in the neck/thorax.

Most pheochromocytomas/paragangliomas occur sporadically. However, they have also been associated with a wide variety of syndromes, including (1) von Hippel-Lindau disease (VHL), (2) neurofibromatosis type 1, (3) multiple endocrine neoplasia (MEN 2) syndrome, (4) Carney syndrome or triad (also pulmonary chondromas and gastric stromal tumors), (5) tuberous sclerosis, and (6) Sturge-Weber disease. A rare, familial type of pheochromocytoma has also been described as an autosomal dominant trait, often leading to presentation in younger patients. The incidence of pheochromocytoma is approximately 5% to 15% of VHL patients, approximately 1% of neurofibromatosis patients, and approximately 25% of Carney syndrome patients.[53]

The rule of 10% is an often sited maxim concerning pheochromocytomas such that among sporadic pheochromocytomas, approximately 10% will be bilateral, 10% will occur at ectopic sites, and 10% will be malignant. Patients with MEN 2 and the familial variety of pheochromocytoma have an even higher incidence of multiplicity and bilaterality. Some studies have identified ectopia in as many as 25% of sporadic pheochromocytomas,[54] most of them in the organ of Zuckerkandl or near the adrenals, however, sites of disease can be wide ranging. In patients with Carney triad, most lesions are functioning, ectopic paragangliomas.[53] Paragangliomas are more often malignant and, therefore, more likely to metastasize than pheochromocytomas.

Catecholamine secretion is the hallmark of pheochromocytomas/paragangliomas and are estimated to be the cause of high blood pressure in 0.1% to 0.5% of patients with newly diagnosed hypertension.[55] Rarely, potentially lethal hypertensive crises can occur as a result of catecholamine secretion by these neoplasms. Hypertensive crisis can be elicited unexpectedly during induction of anesthesia, during pregnancy or surgery, and rarely have been described after intravascular administration of ionic contrast media,[56] and can be clinically problematic, because the presence of a pheochromocytoma usually is not suspected or known, and its diagnosis not established until after 1 or several hypertensive crises take place. Hypertensive crisis typically presents with headache, hypertension, and palpitations. Other symptoms include excessive sweating, visual disturbance, tremor, nausea, vomiting, and nonspecific thoracic or abdominal pain. In many instances, the symptoms can be paroxysmal or infrequent. Rarely, patients can present with cerebral hemorrhage or myocardial infarction. A small percentage of pheochromocytomas will be detected accidentally on abdominal CT or MRI performed for unrelated reasons.

In the presence of symptoms compatible with a pheochromocytoma, patients should undergo appropriate screening for the disease. The most commonly used tests are assays that detect and estimate levels of free catecholamines (epinephrine and norepinephrine) or their metabolites (metanephrine and vanillylmandelic acid) in plasma or 24-hour urine samples.[57,58] Measurements of total urine metanephrine are up to 95% accurate, especially in patients with sustained hypertension. In some cases, a timed urine collection within short periods of time after an attack may be the best test for measuring metanephrine levels.

The treatment of choice in a patient with clinical and biochemical evidence of pheochromocytoma and an adrenal mass is adrenalectomy. Patients at risk of developing multiple and bilateral pheochromocytomas (MEN 2 or familial types), who present with a unilateral adrenal mass, should undergo excision of the involved adrenal, and placed on surveillance for other tumors in the adrenals or elsewhere. If bilateral adrenal masses are found, one could consider, if technically feasible, cortex-sparing adrenalectomy to avoid the relatively high risk of acute adrenal insufficiency and chronic corticosteroid replacement therapy.[59] Patients with pheochromocytomas need careful follow-up because of the risk of residual or recurrent tumor and metastatic disease. Patients with nonresectable malignant or metastatic tumors can be conservatively treated for long periods of time. Bone lesions often respond to radiation and soft-tissue masses can be partially controlled by chemotherapy, including administration of I-131 metaiodobenzylguanidine (MIBG).[60,61]

Localization and imaging of pheochromocytomas: The most appropriate imaging modalities include MIBG scintigraphy, CT, and MRI.

Metaiodobenzylguanidine (MIBG), a derivative of guanethidine, is a very suitable radionuclide agent for the localization of adrenergic tissues. The radioactive element is either I-131 or I-123. Radioactive MIBG is given IV, after the thyroid gland has been blocked with iodides to inhibit glandular uptake of free radioactive iodine and whole body scans are generated. MIBG is an excellent imaging modality, with an accuracy of 90% or better in detecting pheochromocytomas (see Figure 8-7).[62] If the primary is

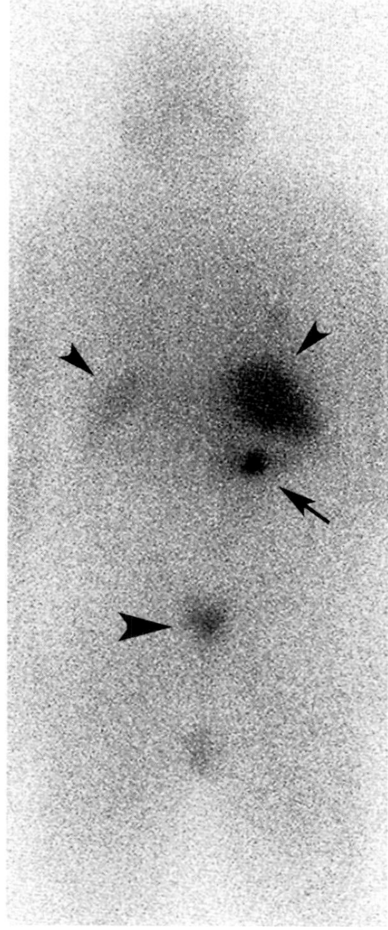

Figure 8-7 Pheochromocytoma
Metaiodobenzylguanidine scan performed from the back of this 75-year-old man shows normal activity in the liver and spleen (*small arrowheads*) and the bladder (*large arrowhead*). There is also a focal area of increased activity medial to the liver (*arrow*), typical of a right adrenal pheochromocytoma.

malignant, MIBG can detect sites of metastases. The radionuclide can also be used to deliver therapeutic radiation doses to metastatic lesions throughout the body.[60]

In general, CT and MRI have been shown to be accurate in the detection of pheochromocytomas and are more widely available and easier to perform than MIBG scans.[63-65] On cross-sectional imaging, pheochromocytoma typically appears as a large lesion, 4 to 5 cm in largest dimension mass. In addition, CT will often demonstrate regions of necrosis and/or hemorrhage as low-attenuation or high-attenuation foci, respectively. Calcifications occur uncommonly.

Pheochromocytomas typically appear T1 hypointense and T2 hyperintense on MR spin echo imaging. The hyperintensity on T2-weighted images is so intense that it is often compared with a "light bulb" (see Figure 8-8). Like CT, larger tumors will often contain central necrosis and hemorrhage giving the mass an inhomogeneous appearance with the typical features of fluid and blood (see Figure 8-8). Unfortunately, the MRI appearance of a pheochromocytoma is not specific, and there is a considerable overlap, in up to one-third of cases, between a pheochromocytoma and other adrenal neoplasms, such as adrenocortical carcinoma.[66]

The viable portions of the neoplasm will usually briskly enhance following contrast administration on both CT and MRI examinations (see Figure 8-8). In the past, there had been concern for potential hypertensive crisis following use of intravascular ionic contrast media, and patients have received α- and β-adrenergic receptor blockade prior to IV contrast administration. This practice does not appear to be necessary with the use of nonionic agents, and is now abandoned.[56,67]

Neuroblastoma, ganglioneuroblastoma, and ganglioneuroma

The other common type of tumors arising in the adrenal medulla is the **neuroblastoma** and its counterparts, the more differentiated and less malignant **ganglioneuroblastoma**, as well as the benign **ganglioneuroma**. Neuroblastoma is the most common solid abdominal neoplasm in childhood, ranking behind leukemia, lymphoma, and CNS tumors, but ahead of Wilms tumor or rhabdomyosarcoma.

Most tumors arise in patients 2 to 3 years old but have been observed in infants and adults also. Its propensity to infiltrate the bone marrow can make it easy to confuse with leukemia. The majority of tumors secrete catecholamines and their metabolites, as a result of their derivation from neuroendocrine cells similar to those found in a pheochromocytoma.[68]

Signs and symptoms are dependent on the location of the mass. Most patients with masses that arise in the adrenal present with a palpebral abdominal mass. Other symptoms include abdominal pain or back pain, constipation, fever, weight loss, and other constitutional symptoms.

About one-third of neuroblastomas are found in the adrenal glands. Enlargement of the liver, bone pain, or anemia secondary to bone marrow replacement indicate tumor spread.

A widely used, though not universally accepted, staging classification has been proposed by Evans, D'Angio, and Randolph (see Table 8-3).[69] An alternative to the above clinical staging system is one proposed by the International Neuroblastoma Risk Group (INRG), a system that stratifies risk prior to treatment, based on the experience of a very large international cohort of patients with the disease. The INRG system analyzed the statistical and clinical significance of 13 potential prognostic factors (eg, stage, age, histology, grade of tumor differentiation, status of the MYCN oncogene, chromosomal components) and created survival curves using event-free survival periods as the primary end point.[70]

Plain radiographs of the abdomen can show a flank mass or posterior mediastinal mass. Stippled calcifications are present on up to 30% of radiographs.

Neuroblastomas are typically detected in utero or during infancy or young childhood.[71] Imaging studies have shown that approximately two-thirds occur in an intra-abdominal location, most in the region of the adrenal glands, with 15% to 35% occurring as an intrathoracic paraspinal mass.[72,73] Rarely, they can appear at a wide variety of other sites.

Fetal sonograms have increasingly identified neuroblastomas. US of infants is also frequently used to evaluate for the presence of a suspected abdominal mass. On US, neuroblastomas typically appear as a cystic, hyperechoic, or mixed cystic and solid mass in a suprarenal location.[74,75] However, masses have been identified in multiple locations throughout the fetus, including the thorax and brain. Small tumors are homogeneous and hyperechoic, whereas larger ones are usually heterogeneous with intraparenchymal calcification that appear as small regions of shadowing within the mass.[74,75]

On CT, neuroblastomas typically appear as large soft-tissue masses with punctate areas of calcification.[76] The mass typically crosses the midline and encases or displaces the major surrounding vascular structures (see Figure 8-9).

MRI is also commonly used, because of its lack of radiation, and ability to perform multiplanar whole body imaging for detection of metastases. Masses typically are large, measuring as much as 16 cm in the largest dimension, although lesions as small as 2 cm can be detected and are of decreased signal intensity compared to muscle on T1-weighted images and increased signal intensity on T2-weighted images.[72,77] In the majority of cases, signal intensity can be heterogeneous on both T1- and T2-weighted sequences, and in a few cases, homogeneous. Calcifications are seen as punctate, low-signal foci within the mass. Invasion of the neural foramina, vascular encasement, and bone marrow invasion is seen in a significant number of patients.[72,77]

Further, MIBG scans are an important complementary imaging modality in patients with neuroblastoma,

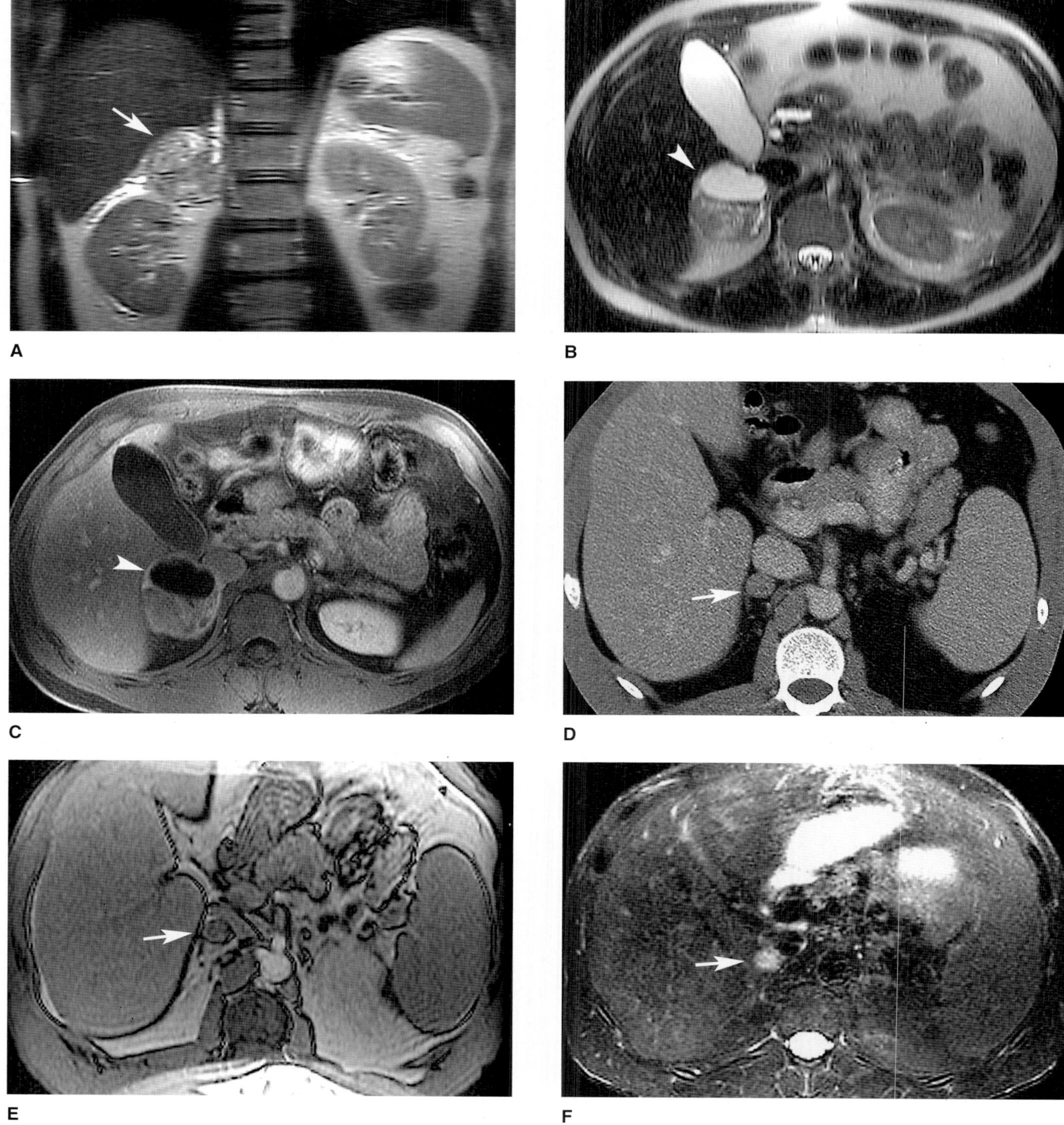

Figure 8-8 Pheochromocytoma in 2 Patients
A-C. This 45-year-old man presented with seizures and systemic hypertension. (A) Coronal T2-weighted MRI image shows a heterogeneous mass (*arrow*) superior to the right kidney in the expected location of the right adrenal. (B) T2-weighted axial image and (C) T1 postcontrast axial image confirm the heterogeneity of the mass. The anterior portion of the mass (*arrowheads*) is hyperintense on the T2-weighted image and nonenhancing, indicating a cystic region in the mass, probably because of necrosis. The solid portions of the mass enhance with contrast. These are a feature of an aggressive adrenal neoplasm. Biopsy was diagnostic of a high-grade malignant pheochromocytoma. **D-F**. This 48-year-old man was being evaluated for testicular carcinoma. (D) Contrast-enhanced CT shows a uniformly enhancing, 1.5-cm, solid nodule (*arrow*) in the right adrenal gland. Most likely differential was either an adenoma or metastasis. (E) Opposed-phase T1-weighted MRI sequence shows no signal loss in the nodule (*arrow*). (F) T2-weighted sequence shows uniform high signal in the nodule (*arrow*). These features are atypical for both an adrenal adenoma and for adrenal metastasis but are often features of small pheochromocytomas. Adrenal biopsy was diagnostic of a benign pheochromocytoma.

Table 8-3. Evans, D'Angio, and Randolph Staging System for Adrenal Cortical Carcinoma

Stage I	Tumor confined to organ of origin (rare, cured by surgery)
Stage II	Tumor extends beyond organ of origin, does not cross the midline, but may involve ipsilateral lymph nodes (65% 5-year survival)
Stage III	Tumor crosses midline, and may involve contralateral or ipsilateral lymph nodes (30% 5-year survival)
Stage IV	Distant metastases (common, liver, bones, bone marrow, etc <5% survival)
Stage IVS	Younger patients with stage I or II primary tumor and liver/skin metastases, but no bone involvement (reasonably good prognosis)

especially in the detection of metastatic disease. In a study of 28 children with histologically proven neuroblastoma who underwent concurrent MIBG, CT, and US examinations, MIBG scans proved the most sensitive for identifying the location of primary and metastatic tumors. Of 63 lesions, MIBG detected 86%, CT 67%, and US 49% of lesions.[78]

Metastases to the adrenal gland

The adrenal glands are among the most common location for metastatic disease, after the lungs, liver, and bones.[79] The primary malignancies most likely to metastasize to the adrenals are lung, breast, melanoma, and kidney, although many more neoplasms can also metastasize there, such as gastrointestinal primaries (esophagus, stomach, pancreas, and colon), hepatocellular carcinoma, uterine tumors, and sarcomas.[80] It has long been known that adrenal metastases are relatively common at autopsy series of patients with various malignancies, most of them microscopic.[81,82] In such instances, the adrenals will have a normal appearance on cross-sectional imaging, such as CT, MRI, or US.

In many cases, the adrenal lesions are frequently seen simultaneously with metastases to other organs. In such cases, correct identification of the adrenal metastases does not affect staging and treatment. If the adrenal lesion(s) is the only potential and critical metastasis found at a staging CT, additional imaging can be successful in excluding a benign lesion, such as an adenoma, or other adrenal pathology. Percutaneous or laparoscopic biopsy remains an option in selected cases, when necessary.[83] In other cases, a gradual increase in the size of a small or subtle adrenal lesion on follow-up CT or MRI over time strongly suggests a metastatic lesion. Likewise, a decrease in size of an adrenal mass following successful chemotherapy of the primary tumor strongly suggests metastasis.

With few exceptions, appearances of metastasis are nonspecific, with considerable overlap between primary and metastatic adrenal malignancies. The common benign adrenal masses, adenoma and myelolipoma, can be specifically identified based on their imaging characteristics. Also, metastases are much more common than primary adrenal malignancies.

Metastases to the adrenals can be unilateral or bilateral, and can measure from a few millimeters to several centimeters in diameter. With bilateral adrenal involvement, a patient can develop adrenal insufficiency, the symptoms of which may be difficult to distinguish from those of the underlying malignancy. Small metastases typically appear

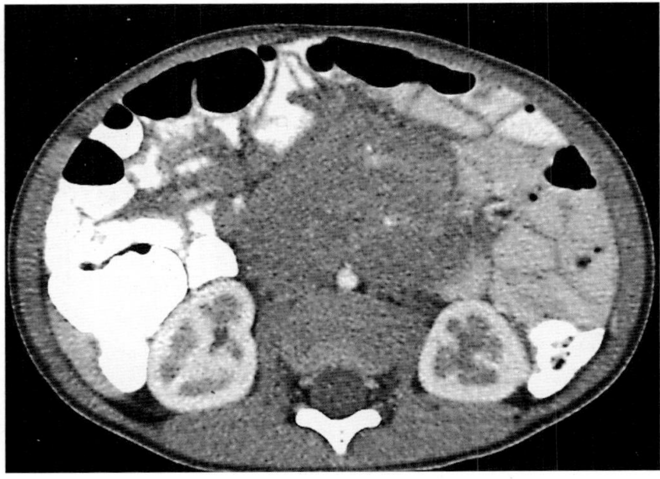

A

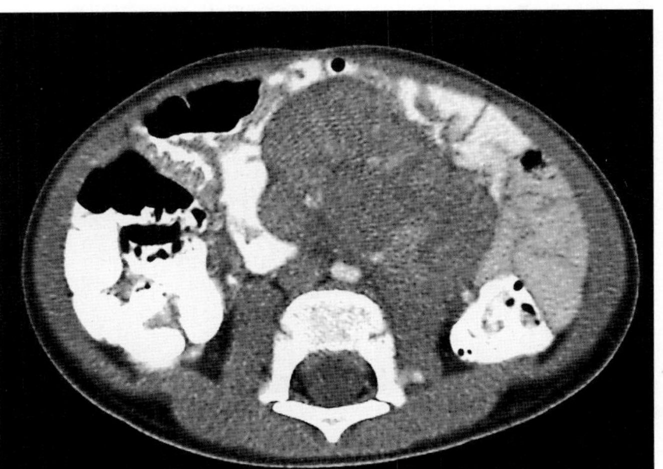

B

Figure 8-9 Neuroblastoma
This 2-year-old child presented with an abdominal mass. **A** and **B**. Contrast-enhanced CT demonstrates a large inhomogeneously enhancing midline mass with small punctate areas of calcification, typical of a neuroblastoma. Biopsy confirmed a diagnosis of neuroblastoma.

as soft-tissue attenuation lesions. As metastases enlarge, they often become heterogeneous with central necrosis and/or tumoral hemorrhage. On CT examinations, this will typically appear as regions of decreased attenuation in the central aspects of the mass. On MRI examinations, cystic degeneration usually presents as low signal intensity on T1-weighted and high signal intensity on T2-weighted images. Hemorrhage on MRI can have a variety of signal characteristics depending on the state of hemoglobin within the hemorrhage (see Figure 8-10). Rarely, metastatic disease can be of low attenuation on CT, mimicking an adrenal cyst; this is particularly true of squamous cell carcinomas.[84] Melanoma to the adrenal gland causes solid or cystic lesions with nonspecific CT appearance. However, it can appear hyperintense on T1-weighted MR images, because of the paramagnetic effect of the melanin pigments.[85]

Because both adenomas and metastases are relatively common lesions, CT (unenhanced or washout techniques) or MRI (in- and opposed-phase GRE T1 imaging) are commonly used to separate the two. Even among patients with known extraadrenal primary neoplasms, an adrenal lesion is metastatic in only 25% to 50% of cases.[86,87] Rarely, an adrenal mass may represent a "collision tumor," a coincidental combination of metastasis and adenoma in the same gland. Chemical-shift MRI is best suited to distinguish the 2 components of the adrenal mass.[88]

In addition, PET and PET-CT are commonly used to look for the presence of metastasis and, on occasion, will detect adrenal metastasis (see Figure 8-3). As noted earlier, 18-F FDG PET has also been shown to reliably discriminate between benign and malignant adrenal masses, including adrenal metastases. A cutoff SUV value of 3.1 has a sensitivity, specificity, positive predictive, and

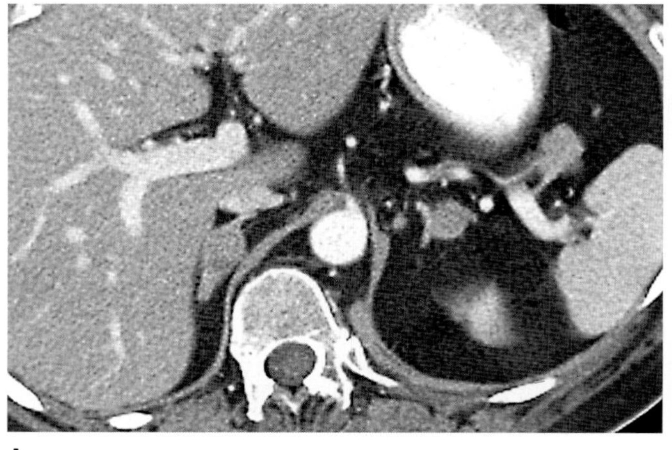

A

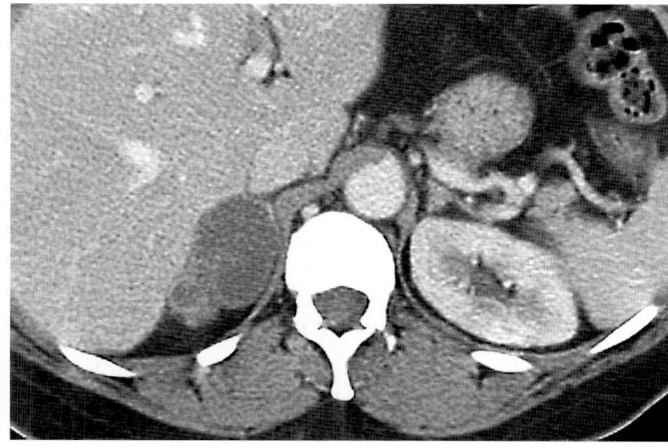

B

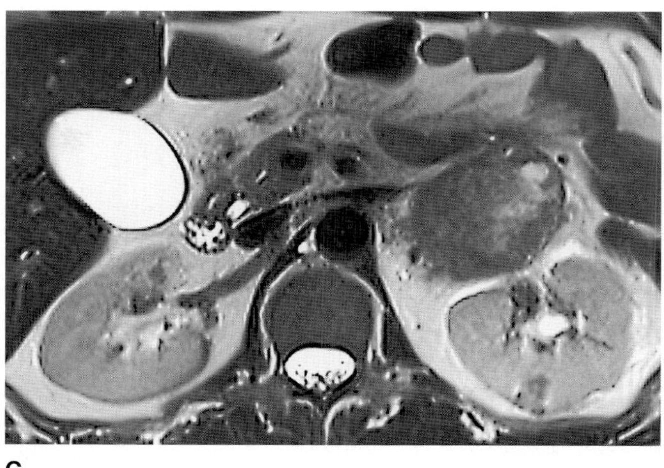

C

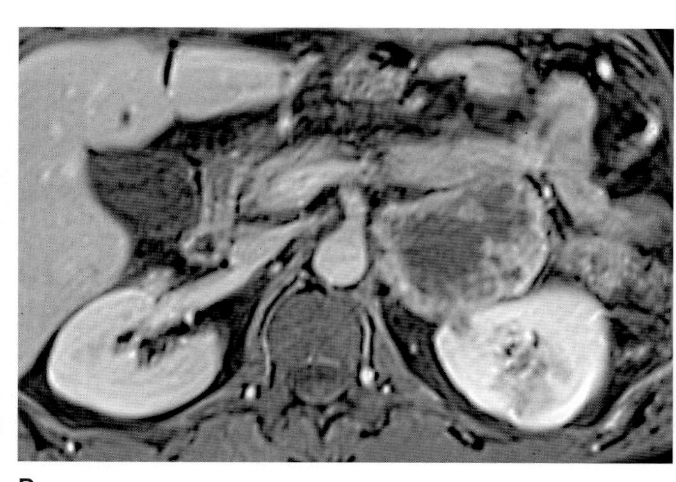

D

Figure 8-10 Adrenal Metastasis in 3 Patients
The patients in **A** and **B** both had lung cancer and the patient in **C** and **D** had renal cell carcinoma. (A) Contrast-enhanced CT shows 2 small, solid, enhancing masses, 1 in each adrenal. The imaging appearance is consistent with either metastasis or adenomas; however, they were not present on a CT of 6 months earlier and represent small metastasis. (B) Contrast-enhanced CT shows a 3-cm, slightly heterogenous, rim-enhancing, centrally hypoattenuating mass typical of larger metastasis with central necrosis. (C) T2-weighted and (D) T1-weighted postgadolinium images show a large heterogenous rim-enhancing mass in the left adrenal typical of a centrally necrotic metastasis.

negative predicted values of 98.5%, 92%, 89.3%, and 98.9%, respectively, for PET alone, and 100%, 98%, 97%, and 100%, respectively, for PET/CT, in separating benign from malignant lesions.[13]

Adrenal lymphoma

Lymphoma of the adrenal gland is uncommon, and non-Hodgkin lymphoma is the most common subtype. The literature reports a 4% incidence of adrenal involvement in patients with non-Hodgkin lymphoma.[89] Adrenal lymphoma can be bilateral in 50% of the cases and is usually associated with retroperitoneal adenopathy or other sites of disease.[90] At autopsy, about one-quarter of patients with lymphoma develop adrenal involvement.[89-91] In most cases, the adrenal gland is involved by direct extension from contiguous nodal disease in the retroperitoneum. Less commonly, adrenal lymphoma can appear as a discrete adrenal mass, either as part of widespread disease or, rarely, as primary lymphoma, without other macroscopic sites of involvement.[92] In some instances, adrenal parenchymal replacement by tumor can be extensive enough that the patients may suffer from adrenal insufficiency.[93]

On cross-sectional imaging, adrenal lymphoma often appears as a homogeneous adrenal mass that is indistinguishable from lipid poor adenomas, metastases, and some primary adrenal tumors.[16,22] On sonography, adrenal lymphoma typically appears hypoechoic and homogeneous, similar to the usual features of lymphoma at other sites in the body.[94] On unenhanced CT, most adrenal lymphomas appear as homogeneous, soft-tissue attenuation lesions. Post IV contrast administration, the masses are hypovascular, and display mild enhancement. Central necrosis is uncommon, but can be seen in large, rapidly growing lesions. Calcifications are rare, and when found are typically in response to treatment.[95] The MRI findings are nonspecific, appearing as uniformly low signal masses on T1-weighted images and high signal masses on T2-weighted images (see Figure 8-11).[96]

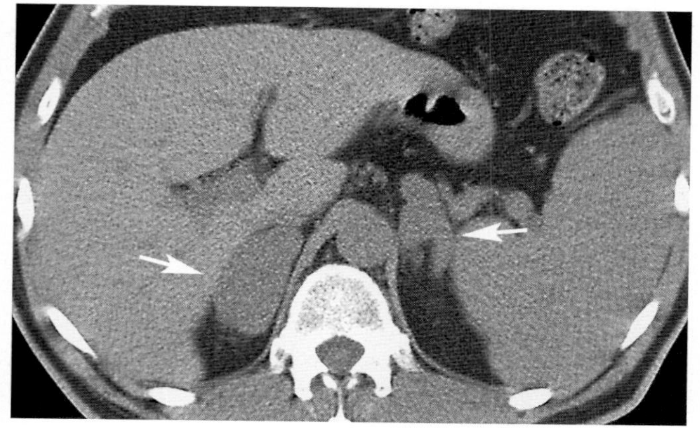
A

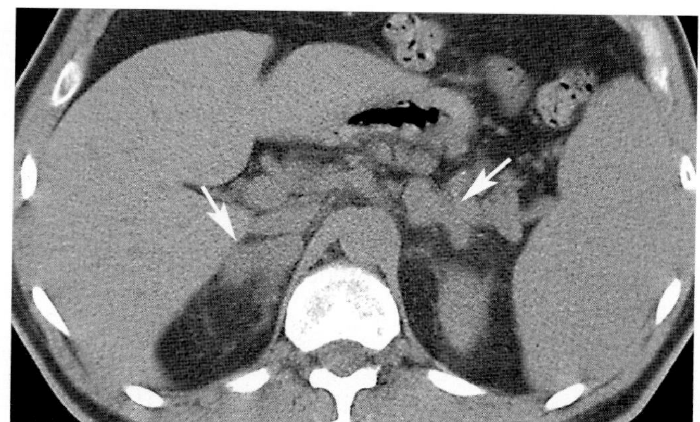
B

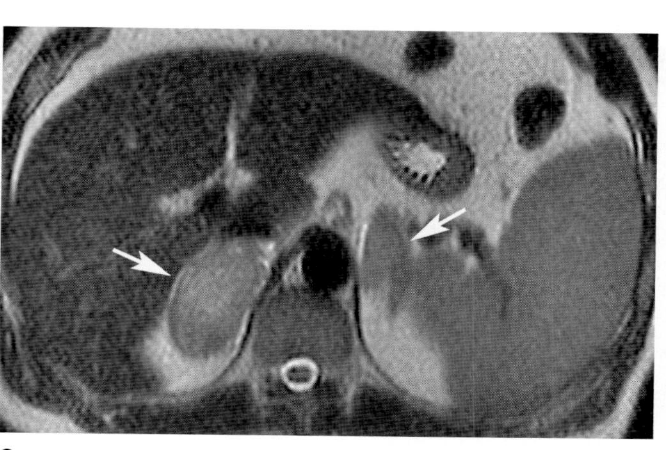
C

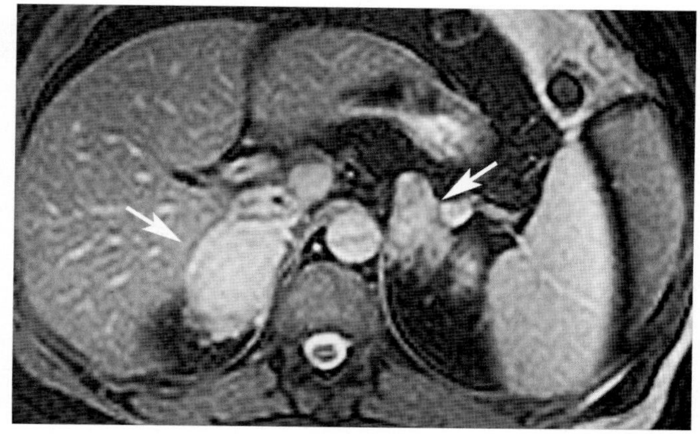
D

Figure 8-11 Adrenal Lymphoma
This 61-year-old woman presented with anorexia, weight loss, and adrenal insufficiency. (**A** and **B**) Unenhanced CT shows diffuse uniform attenuation, enlargement of the adrenal glands bilaterally (*arrows*) that forms a mass in the right adrenal. (**C**) T2-weighted and (**D**) T1-weighted postgadolinium sequences show the mass to be uniform signal intensity and to enhance uniformly. Biopsy was diagnostic of a large B-cell lymphoma. Note the mild splenomegaly, a potential clue to the ultimate diagnosis.

On follow-up imaging, adrenal lymphoma is expected to respond in a fashion similar to the other sites of disease. If the adrenal lesion does not respond concordantly with other sites of disease, further investigation for alternative diagnoses is warranted.

Adrenal myelolipoma

Adrenal myelolipoma is a discrete, nonfunctioning, benign lesion made of mature adipose cells and hematopoietic cellular elements, such as erythrocytes, megakaryocytes, lymphocytes, and myelocytes. Myelolipomas can vary considerably in size. In a series of 59 cases, the mean size was 11 cm; one-fifth of the lesions displayed chunky calcifications, and 10% of them presented with spontaneous hemorrhage.[97,98] The larger the size of a lesion, the more likely it is to present with hemorrhage. Myelolipomas occur equally in men and women and are more common in the fifth and sixth decades of life. They are usually unilateral, although bilateral lesions have been reported.[97,98] Adrenal myelolipomas should not be considered as sites of extramedullary hematopoiesis, because the latter does not contain fatty components.

Myelolipomas are almost always found incidentally in patients imaged by US, CT, or MRI for other reasons.[97,99] On rare occasions, a large myelolipoma may cause symptoms by virtue of its size or if it results in significant hemorrhage.

On sonography, the fatty elements of the lesion appear hyperechoic (see Figure 8-12). Calcifications, when present, appear as focal brightly hyperechoic foci with shadowing. Separation from an adjacent renal angiomyolipoma can be challenging.

On CT, macroscopic fat is detected in all lesions diagnosed as myelolipomas (see Figures 1-5 and 8-12). The proportion of fatty versus hematopoietic elements varies from lesion to lesion. The hematopoietic component is of soft-tissue attenuation, and enhances post IV contrast administration. Recent hemorrhage presents as soft-tissue attenuation collection in the suprarenal area, causing the lesion to be poorly defined and creating considerable stranding in the perinephric and posterior paranephric or retroperitoneal fat. Calcifications are easily depicted.[100] Large myelolipomas may be difficult to differentiate from retroperitoneal liposarcomas on CT. Angiography can be of help by identifying the origin of the vascular supply to the ipsilateral adrenal and, in the case of a myelolipoma, to the mass itself.[101]

On MRI, the fatty elements are hyperintense on T1-weighted imaging, a nonspecific finding that can be seen in any hemorrhagic mass. To make the diagnosis of a myelolipoma, fat-suppression T1-weighted techniques are obtained and compared to regular T1-weighted images. If the lesion exhibits signal loss on fat suppression, the presence of macroscopic fat is proven, and the diagnosis is established. Using the same fat suppression sequences, tumoral hemorrhage, bright on regular T1-weighted images, can also be detected, based on its lack of signal change post suppression, as compared to macroscopic fat. Use of chemical shift is also helpful, if the myelolipoma is of soft-tissue attenuation on CT, without discrete amounts of macroscopic fat. A drop in signal intensity on opposed-phase T1-weighted imaging, as in the case of adenomas, will indicate the presence of intracellular fat.[99,102]

Imaging Notes 8-3. Imaging Features of Adrenal Neoplasms

Neoplasm	Size	Necrosis	Characteristic Features
Adenoma	usually <3 cm	never	intracellular lipid rapid washout
Metastasis	any size	occasional	slow washout
Cortical carcinoma	usually >3 cm	frequent	slow washout
Pheochromocytoma	usually >3 cm	occasional	hyperintense T2 MRI 131I-MIBG+
Neuroblastoma	usually >3 cm	rare	punctate calcifications 131I-MIBG+
Myelolipoma	any size	never	macroscopic fat
Hemangioma	usually >3 cm	never	phleboliths punctate calcifications globular enhancement
Lymphoma	usually > 3cm	rare	retroperitoneal mass engulfing adrenal

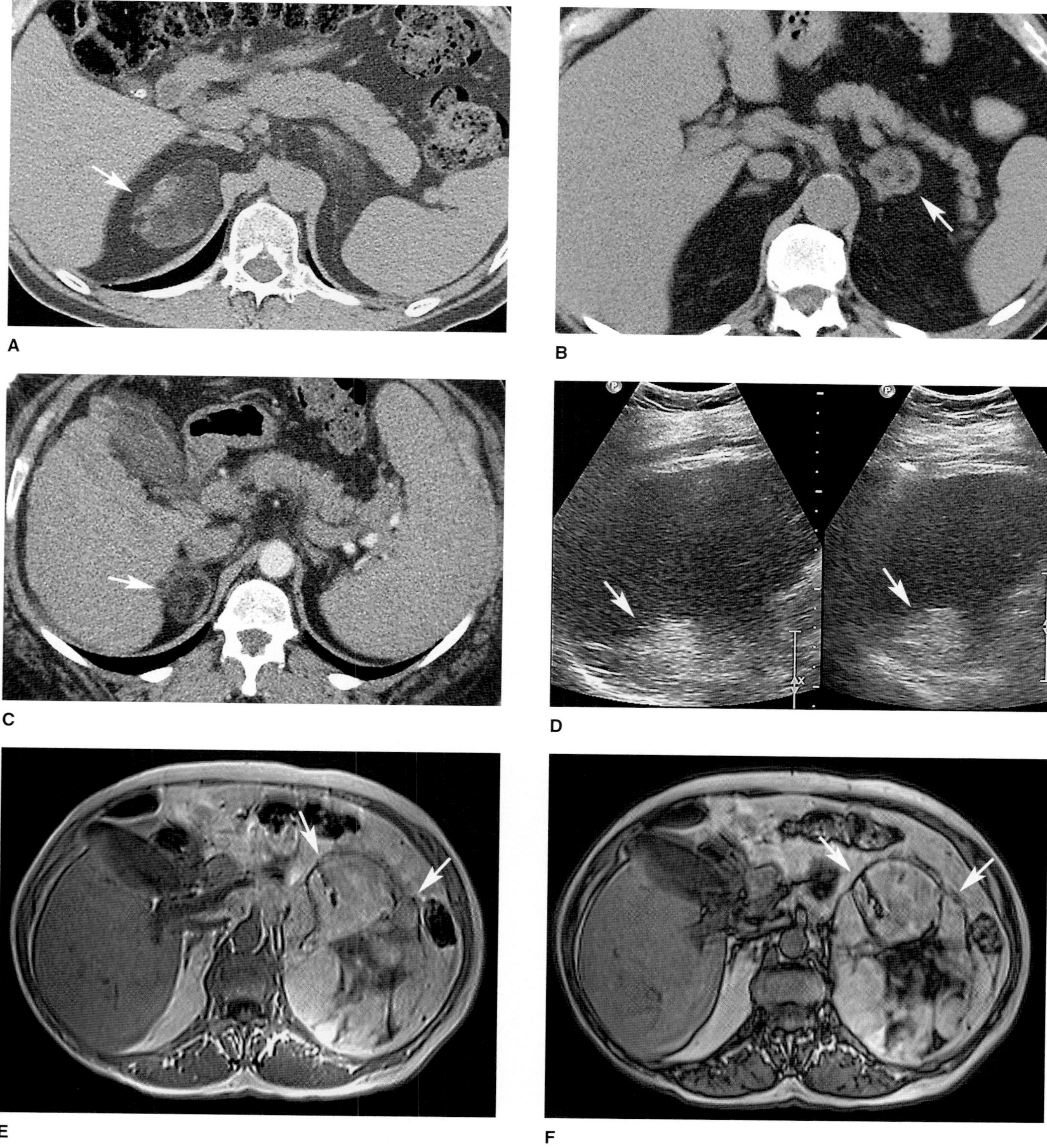

Figure 8-12 Myelolipoma in 4 Patients
These 4 patients were being evaluated for reasons other than adrenal pathology. **A-C.** Unenhanced CT in each patient demonstrates a mixed solid and fat attenuation mass (*arrows*) in the expected location of the adrenal glands. Note the variable amount of fat in the lesions. **D.** US of the patient in (C) shows a heterogeneously echogenic mass (*arrows*) posterior to the liver and above the kidney, features typical of an adrenal myelolipoma. **E.** In phase T1-weighted image and (**F**) opposed phase T1-weighted image in a fourth patient shows a large predominantly fatty mass (*arrows*) in the left retroperitoneum. This could possibly represent a well differentiated liposarcoma but biopsy showed a myelolipoma.

Adrenal hemangioma

Hemangioma of the adrenal is extremely uncommon, with only a few reported cases.[103] Similar to hemangiomas elsewhere in the body, the uncommon adrenal hemangioma is a benign, nonfunctioning lesion consisting of dilated, tubular spaces lined by endothelium and filled with blood. The presence of phleboliths in a soft-tissue attenuation adrenal lesion is common and helps in making the diagnosis. Some believe that the incidence of adrenal hemangiomas may be higher than generally reported. It is hypothesized that repeat hemorrhage, thrombosis, and calcifications within hemangiomas result in an appearance similar to that of hemorrhagic adrenal cysts.

Adrenal hemangiomas are seen more commonly in women and typically present between the ages of 50 and 70 years. The majority are larger than 10 cm at presentation.[104] Most lesions are incidentally discovered. However, rarely an adrenal hemangioma can attain such a large size, such that mass effect or spontaneous hemorrhage render the lesion symptomatic and result in its detection.[105]

On US examinations, adrenal hemangiomas appear as a heterogeneously echogenic suprarenal mass. Diffused irregular anechoic areas with hyperechoic septa are seen throughout the lesion typical of cavernous hemangiomas in any location.[106]

On CT, adrenal hemangioma appears as a heterogeneous, smoothly marginated, relatively low attenuation soft-tissue mass containing speckled and coarse calcifications from prior hemorrhage and ring calcifications representing phleboliths.[104,107] Occasionally, hemangiomas can contain intralesional macroscopic fat that can be detected by CT and MRI.[104]

MRI shows low signal intensity on T1-weighted images and high signal on T2-weighted images.[104] In some cases, multiple internal septations can be seen on the T2-weighted images, representing the walls of the vascular channels.

Post IV contrast administration, heterogeneous enhancement is observed on both CT and MRI. The classic nodular, interrupted, peripheral enhancement described in hepatic hemangiomas has also been described in case reports of adrenal hemangiomas.[104,108,109] Slow, venous filling has been described on angiography.

Large lesions resembling an adrenal hemangioma can rarely represent hemangiosarcomas that will require surgical resection.

Nonneoplastic Causes of Adrenal Nodules and Masses

Adrenal hemorrhage is a common nonneoplastic cause of an adrenal nodule or mass.

Adrenal hemorrhage

Unilateral and bilateral adrenal hemorrhage is a rare event that can be observed at any age. Causes include blunt and penetrating trauma, coagulopathy, and physiologic stress such as sepsis or neonatal asphyxia (Table 8-4).

Table 8-4. Causes of Adrenal Hemorrhage

1. Trauma a. Blunt b. Penetrating
2. Coagulopathy
3. Physiologic stress a. Neonatal asphyxia b. Sepsis c. Burns d. Hypotension

Neonatal adrenal hemorrhage is the most common cause of an adrenal mass in the newborn. The condition is overwhelmingly unilateral, >90% of cases, and more common in male infants. The etiology is often uncertain, but there is an association with traumatic delivery, especially in the breech presentation, and maternal diabetes.[110,111] The clinical picture varies from an asymptomatic abdominal mass, prolonged neonatal jaundice second to breakdown of hemoglobin, to dramatic hypotension and shock, in case of massive bleeding. Imaging is mostly obtained by sonography, though noncontrast CT or MRI are helpful to distinguish simple hemorrhage from one that coincides with or is due to a neuroblastoma. Serial imaging will demonstrate eventual involution of the mass; in some cases, circular or angular calcifications may develop several months later.

In the adult, adrenal hemorrhage is uncommon and can be associated with sepsis, burns, stress, blunt trauma, or hypotension. The hematologic disorders, thrombocytopenia, disseminated intravascular coagulation, therapeutic anticoagulation, antiphospholipid antibody syndrome, and systemic lupus erythematosus, have been associated with adrenal hemorrhage. Trauma is also a known cause of adrenal hemorrhage, where it can be bilateral in up to 20% of cases.[112] Bilateral hemorrhage can lead to clinical adrenal insufficiency (Addison disease), often several weeks following the incident.[113]

Adrenal hemorrhage is unilateral in approximately 80% of cases, the majority of which involve the right adrenal.[114] One theory suggests that acute elevations in intra-abdominal pressure are transmitted into the inferior vena cava and cause elevations in adrenal venous pressures. Because the right adrenal vein is shorter than the left adrenal vein, greater pressures are transmitted to the right than the left adrenal gland.

Adrenal hematoma typically appears as a suprarenal, round, or oval mass on cross-sectional imaging examinations (see Figure 8-13). In many cases, it can be indistinctly marginated with stranding of the suprarenal, retroperitoneal fat. On CT, an acute hematoma will appear

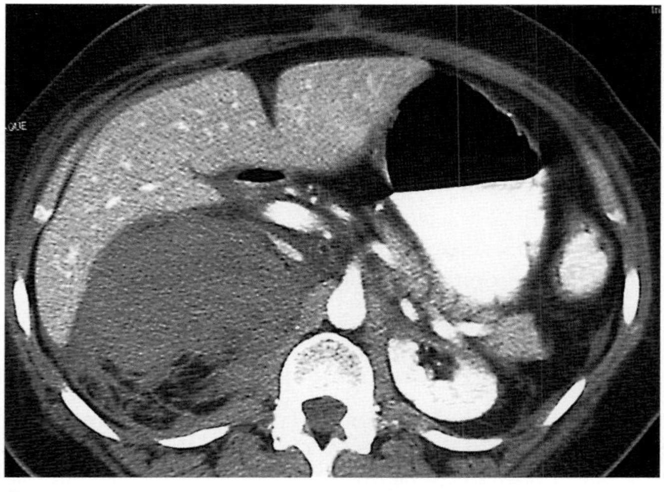

A

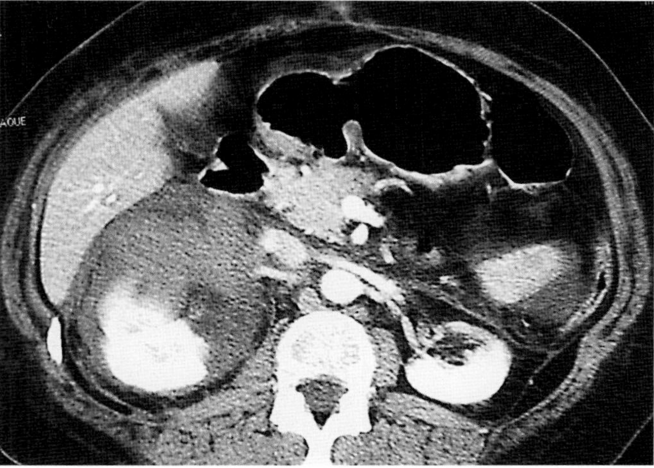

B

Figure 8-13 Spontaneous Adrenal Hemorrhage
This 43-year-old woman underwent lobectomy for lung cancer. In the postoperative period, she was found to have an acute drop in serum hemoglobin. **A** and **B**. Enhanced CT demonstrates an inhomogeneous mass in the retroperitoneum just superior to the right kidney with stranding of the adjacent retroperitoneal fat. Notice how portions of the mass, especially in B, appear hyperattenuating relative to skeletal muscle. This mass was not present on the preoperative CT and is consistent with spontaneous adrenal hemorrhage.

as hyperattenuating (value >50 HU), whereas subacute hematoma often is equal in attenuation to that of soft tissue (35-40 HU) (see Figure 8-14). Chronically, the hematoma will often liquefy and appear as a complex cystic mass. (See the subsequent section entitled **Pseudocysts.**) Calcifications can eventually form months later. Further, MRI is best suited to detect the presence of blood byproducts. Subacute hemorrhage appears as a high-signal-intensity process on both T1- and T2-weighted scans, because of the paramagnetic effect of methemoglobin.[115] Later on, a dark ring can be seen surrounding the hematoma because of formation of hemosiderin or ferritin.[115,116] The hematoma usually liquefies and slowly resolves over time (see Figure 1-10).

Cystic-Appearing Adrenal Nodules and Masses

Adrenal cysts are an uncommon finding with an incidence on autopsy studies of 0.064% to 0.18%.[117] In the past, they have been associated with abdominal or flank pain, gastrointestinal symptoms as a result of mass effect on adjacent abdominal structures, or as a palpable abdominal mass. However, currently, many adrenal cystic masses are discovered incidentally on cross-sectional imaging studies performed for reasons unrelated to the mass.[117] A study from the Mayo Clinic reviewed 41 excised adrenal cystic lesions: 66% were symptomatic, typically with pain or gastrointestinal symptoms, and 33% were incidental.[118] However, because most asymptomatic, incidentally discovered adrenal cysts are not surgically resected, the incidence of symptomatic cysts is probably overrepresented in this series. They are more common among women and can be bilateral in about 10% of cases.[119]

Histologically, adrenal cysts can be divided into 4 groups: pseudocysts, endothelial cysts, epithelial cysts, and parasitic cysts. There is some debate in the literature whether pseudocysts or endothelial cysts are most common. The incidence of pseudocysts among series ranges from 39% to 78% of cases and the incidence of endothelial cysts ranges from 20% to 45% of cases.[118,119-121] Epithelial

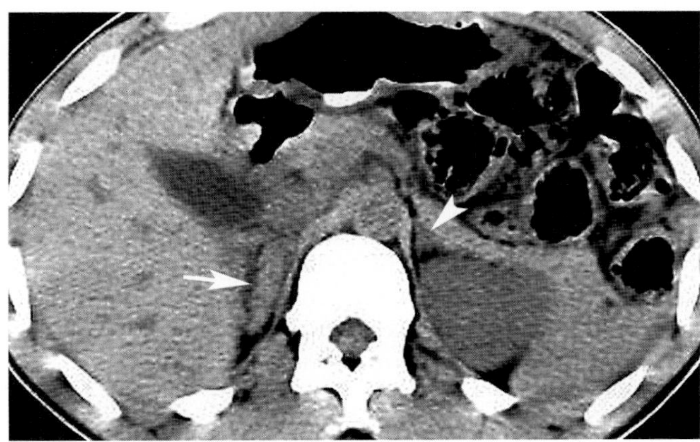

Figure 8-14 Posttraumatic Adrenal Hemorrhage
This 26-year-old man was struck in the right upper quadrant during a soccer game. The right adrenal gland (*arrow*) is diffusely thickened and hyperattenuating but the left adrenal gland (*arrowhead*) is normal appearing. These findings are indicative of hemorrhage into the right adrenal as a result of the trauma.

Table 8-5. Causes of Adrenal Cysts

1. Prior hemorrhage (pseudocysts)
2. Endothelial cysts a. Blood vessel ectasia (angiomatous cyst) b. Lymphatic ectasia (lymphangiomatous cyst)
3. Epithelial cyst (true cyst)
4. Paracytic cyst a. Echinococcal infection b. Leishmaniasis

and paracystic cysts account for less than 15% of adrenal cysts (Table 8-5).

Pseudocysts and cystic neoplasms

Pseudocysts usually are the result of hemorrhage into normal adrenal tissue and occasionally may be due to hemorrhage into an adrenal tumor. Histologically, they are typically large unilocular cysts, with walls composed of dense, fibrous connective tissue, without an endothelial layer. The walls range from 1 to 5 mm in thickness, and can contain islands of adrenal cortical tissue in up to 19% of cases.[117]

According to 2 studies, approximately 7% of pseudocysts develop from necrosis within adrenal neoplasms, including adenomas, hemangiomas, pheochromocytomas, adrenal cortical carcinomas, and malignant hemangioendotheliomas.[117,121]

Rarely, adrenal hematomas can become secondarily infected to create adrenal abscesses. This has most often been reported in neonates.[122]

Endothelial cysts

Endothelial cysts, often called "simple cysts," are cysts characterized by smooth, flattened endothelial lining, and filled with clear or milky fluid.[117] They can be subcategorized into lymphangiomatous and angiomatous cysts. Lymphangiomatous cysts arise from ectasia of lymphatic vessels in adrenal glands or cystic degeneration of a hamartoma. Angiomatous cysts are thought to arise from ectasia of blood vessels or may form after repeated episodes of hemorrhage in adrenal hemangiomas.[117]

Epithelial cysts

Epithelial cysts, or "true cysts," contain a smooth, flattened epithelial lining. Epithelial-lined cysts are subdivided into 3 groups based on pathogenesis: (1) glandular or retention cysts, which develop because of inclusion of displaced tissue from nonadrenal tissue during fetal development; (2) cystic adenomas; and (3) embryonal cysts.

Parasitic cysts

Most parasitic adrenal cysts are a result of echinococcal infection but rarely can be due to leishmaniasis.[117] However, less than 0.5% of all patients with echinococcal infection will have adrenal involvement. Eosinophilia is noted in 20% of parasitic infections. Many patients may be clinically asymptomatic; however, complications include hemorrhage and shock (anaphylaxis) from a ruptured adrenal cyst or compression on the liver and infrahepatic vessels.[117]

Imaging features of adrenal cysts

Most cysts are small, although large ones up to 10 cm in diameter have been reported. Occasionally, adrenal cysts can be identified on chest or abdominal radiographs as thin, peripherally (rim) calcified lesions to the right or left of the spine in the upper abdomen (see Figure 8-15).[123,124] Rim calcifications are relatively common among adrenal cysts and are located either in the wall or septa.[124,125] The majority of calcified cysts likely represent pseudocysts from prior adrenal hematomas.

Noncalcified cysts have imaging features consistent with other cysts anywhere in the body. Endothelial and epithelial cysts typically are unilateral, thin-walled, smooth-bordered, round or oval masses with pure cystic internal structure.[126] Lymphangiomatous variants of endothelial cysts can contain internal septa.[127] On CT, they will have an attenuation usually less than 20 HU. On MRI, they appear as intermediate signal intensity on T1-weighted sequences and high signal on T2-weighted sequences, without soft-tissue components. The contents of adrenal cysts do not enhance after IV contrast injection.[126,127] This is the important feature of the cyst that differentiates it from a lipid-rich adenoma, which has a fluidlike low attenuation on unenhanced CT, but clearly enhances, if IV contrast material is given.

Imaging of pseudocysts will typically demonstrate a cystic mass with walls ranging from 1 to 5 mm thick. The contents of the cysts can appear as simple fluid in approximately one-half of patients (anechoic on US, 0-20 HU on CT, and hyperintense on T2-weighed MRI) or can contain internal debris or septations in the remaining (see Figure 8-15).[128] Features of blood products can be seen with MRI examinations. Calcification of the wall or septum is moderately common.[128] The presence of wall thickening or nodularity, especially if the nodule(s) enhance, in a cystic adrenal lesion on cross-sectional imaging is of concern for a necrotic tumor, such as a pheochromocytoma or adrenal cortical carcinoma. One report of 7 pathologically proven benign pseudocysts showed that the solid-appearing elements in pseudocysts did not enhance on CT images following IV contrast administration.[128]

Echinococcal cysts can have a variety of appearances. Typically, they demonstrate one of several imaging features that are characteristic of echinococcal cysts.[103] Most

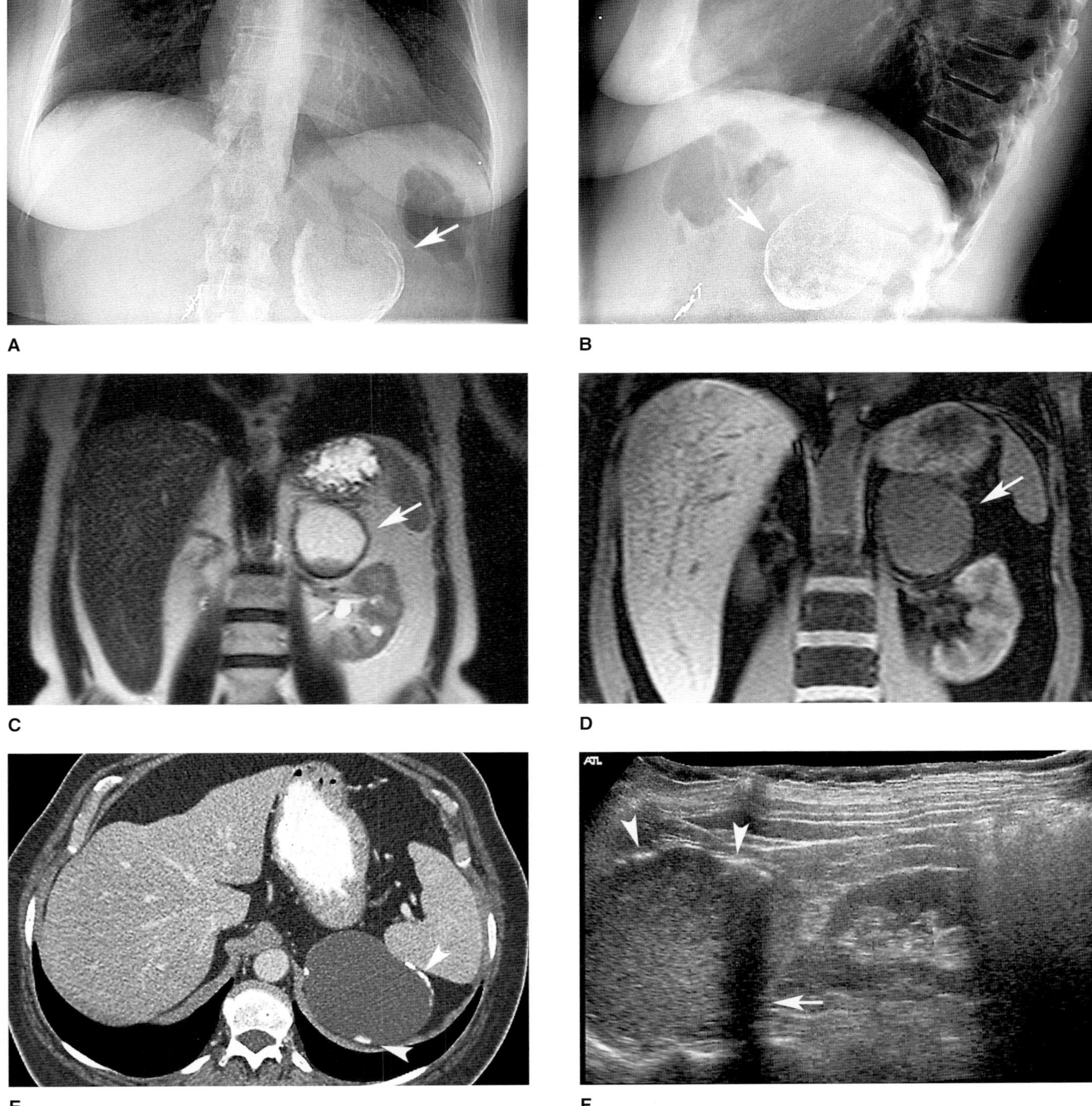

Figure 8-15 Calcified Pseudocyst in 2 Patients
A-D. This 50-year-old woman had breast cancer. Magnified images from (A) posteroanterior and (B) lateral chest radiograph shows a rim calcified mass (*arrows*) in the left retroperitoneum. In most cases, this will represent a calcified cyst in the adrenal, pancreas, or kidney. (C) Coronal T2-weighted and (D) coronal T1-weighted postgadolinium MRI images show an adrenal mass (*arrows*) that is high signal on T2-weighted sequences and does not enhance following gadolinium administration. There is debris seen in the dependent portion of the cyst in C. These findings are consistent with a proteinaceous adrenal cyst, most likely a pseudocyst from prior hemorrhage. **E** and **F**. This 62-year-old woman was being evaluated for pulmonary nodules. (E) Contrast-enhanced CT shows a fluid attenuation mass with small focal regions of peripheral calcification (*arrowheads*) in the expected location of the adrenal. (F) Ultrasonographic examination show the mass to contain multiple internal echoes, with linear peripheral echogenic foci (*arrowheads*) representing the rim calcification. Note the shadowing (*arrow*) due to one of the calcifications. These features are characteristic of a benign, complicated adrenal cyst, probably a pseudocyst.

typical of these is a dominant cystic mass containing multiple smaller daughter cysts that line the internal wall of the dominant cyst. Occasionally, fine calcifications, called "hydatid sand" are found in the dependent portion of the cyst. With death of the organism, the internal membranes can become detached from the wall of the cyst and float within the central contents of the cyst, a finding called the "water lily sign." Some echinococcal cysts appear as unilocular cysts that are indistinguishable from other simple adrenal cysts.

Percutaneous aspiration of adrenal cyst fluid may occasionally be used in case of inconclusive imaging, such as large, suprarenal cystic lesions of unclear origin. Fluid analysis may reveal the presence of adrenal cortical hormones or precursors, indicating adrenal origin.[125]

BILATERAL ENLARGEMENT OF THE ADRENAL GLAND

Bilateral enlargement of the adrenal gland can be due to adrenal hyperplasia and granulomatous infections of the adrenal gland. In some cases, bilateral adrenal metastases or hemorrhage will cause bilateral adrenal masses.

Adrenal Hyperplasia

Adrenal hyperplasia represents a nonmalignant proliferation of normal adrenal cortical cells and nearly always involves both adrenal glands. Histologically, this can result from proliferation of any 1 of the 3 layers of the adrenal cortex, the zona glomerulosa, which produces aldosterone; the zona fasciculata, which produces cortisol; and the zona reticularis, which produces androstenedione.

Adrenal hyperplasia is most clearly associated with syndromes of increased adrenocortical hormone production: Cushing syndrome (increased cortisol production), primary aldosteronism (increased aldosterone production), and adrenogenital syndrome (increased androstenedione production also called congenital adrenal hyperplasia).[129,130] In some cases, adrenal hyperplasia can occur without apparent alterations in serum hormone levels and, despite the enlarged gland, the patient is asymptomatic.[131-133] Acute stress will result in diminished size of the adrenal glands, as they use up their stores of cholesterol and cholesterol-derived hormones. However, chronic stress can result in hyperplasia of the gland (Table 8-6).

Table 8-6. Causes of Adrenal Hyperplasia

A. Associated with hyperfunctioning of the gland
1. Cushing syndrome
    a. ACTH-secreting pituitary adenoma
    b. ACTH-secreting nonpituitary tumor
        i. Bronchogenic carcinoma
        ii. Thymoma
        iii. Bronchial carcinoid
        iv. Pheochromocytoma
        v. Neuroendocrine tumor of the pancreas
2. Primary aldosteronism
3. Congenital adrenal hyperplasia (adrenogenital syndrome)
4. Chronic physiologic stress

B. Without hyperfunctioning of the gland (usually nodular hyperplasia)

Morphologically, adrenal hyperplasia can take 1 of 2 macroscopic pathologic and 3 imaging appearances. (1) In some cases, there is uniform proliferation of cortical tissue, resulting in uniform enlargement of the glands bilaterally. On cross-sectional imaging, this will often appear as uniform thickening of the limbs of both adrenals (see Figure 8-16). It will appear hyperenhancing following IV administration of iodinated CT contrast or gadolinium-based MRI contrast agents. This appearance is strongly associated with the syndromes of hormone imbalance. (2) In other situations, the proliferation is asymmetric, resulting in multinodular thickening of the glands, called nodular adrenal hyperplasia. In nodular adrenal hyperplasia, the nodules are small and multiple, distributed throughout both glands. Nodular hyperplasia has been associated with systemic hypertension, and can otherwise be clinically asymptomatic, without associated hormonal imbalances.[132,133] On cross-sectional imaging, this will appear as multiple, small, typically less-than-5-mm, nodules distributed through both adrenal glands (see Figure 8-17). (3) In some cases, the adrenal gland may be of normal thickness on cross-sectional imaging, despite pathologic evidence of hyperplasia. In this latter case, NP-59 scintigraphy may correctly identify cases of adrenal hyperplasia by detecting increased bilateral adrenal uptake.

Granulomatous Infections of the Adrenal Gland

Both tuberculosis and histoplasmosis can develop disseminated infection throughout the adrenal gland resulting in a multinodular enlargement of the gland.

Tuberculosis

A 28-year autopsy review of tuberculosis in Hong Kong demonstrated 6% incidence of adrenal involvement, the sixth most common site after the lungs, liver, spleen, kidneys, and bones.[134] In the same series, 13% of patients with adrenal involvement developed Addison disease, and bilateral involvement at autopsy was seen in 69% of cases. The adrenals were approximately 40% enlarged over the normal gland at autopsy evaluation. In most

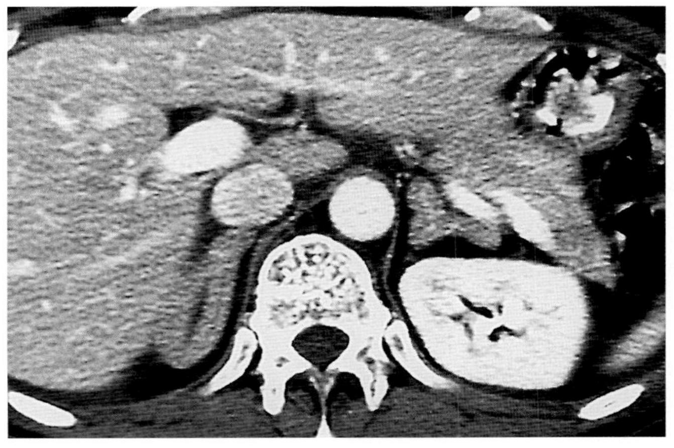
A

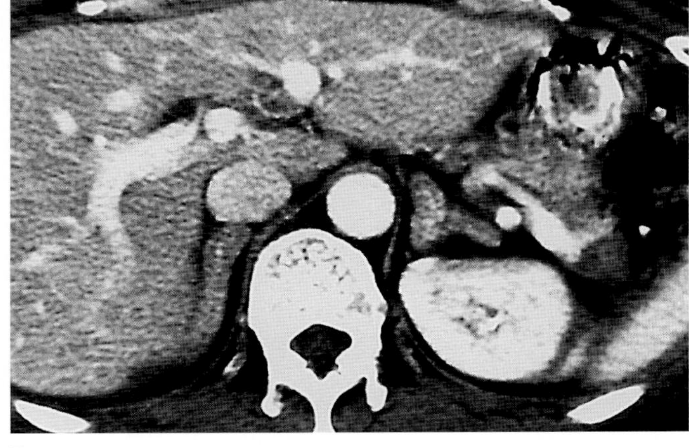
B

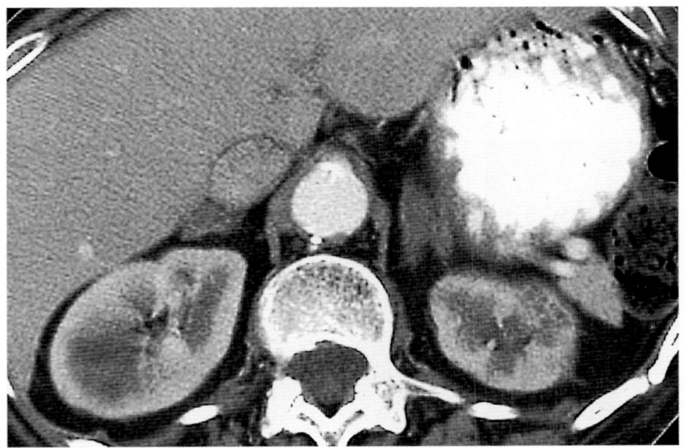
C

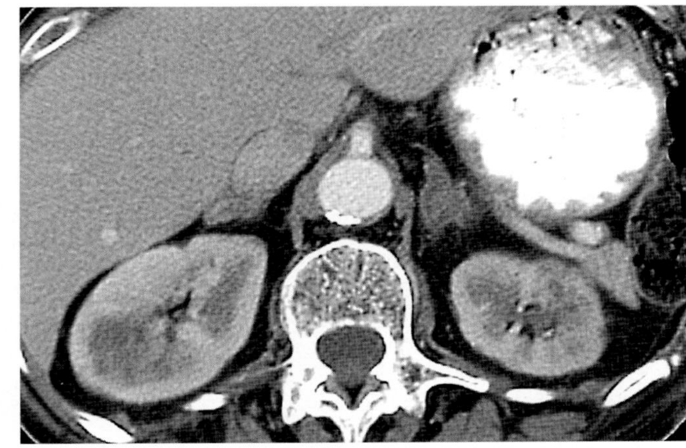
D

Figure 8-16 Adrenal Hyperplasia in 2 Patients
A and **B**. This 55-year-old man had a brain mass. Computed tomographic images through the adrenal glands demonstrate diffuse uniform enlargement of the cortex of the adrenals bilaterally, characteristic of adrenal hyperplasia. Notice how the cortex of the adrenals enhances more intensely than the adrenal medulla. Further biochemical and clinical analysis confirmed a diagnosis of Cushing syndrome. **C** and **D**. This 70-year-old woman had a primary lung cancer. Contrast-enhanced CT shows diffuse uniform enlargement of the adrenals bilaterally. The cause was never evaluated. It is likely that she had hyperplasia due to ectopic production of ACTH by the lung cancer but it is possible that the hyperplasia was a response to chronic stress of a metastatic malignancy.

cases, adrenal disease is clinically undetected at the time of infection and discovery of adrenal involvement is identified by imaging examinations months and years after the initial infection.

If detected during the acute phase of infection, usually during the evaluation for Addison disease, adrenal tuberculosis will demonstrate bilaterally enlarged adrenals in approximately 90% of cases (see Figure 8-18).[135] In approximately half of cases, multiple small hypoattenuating lesions enlarging the adrenal gland or bilateral adrenal masses were identified.[134,135] The chronic manifestation of adrenal tuberculosis is atrophy and calcification of the gland.[136] Calcifications are commonly bilateral, and can appear as small punctate or larger, chunky calcifications within an atrophied gland.[137]

Histoplasmosis

Histoplasma capsulatum is a ubiquitous dimorphic saprophyte that is endemic in the southern parts of North America but can be found worldwide.[138] It naturally occurs in soil rich in bird and bat droppings.[138] In the soil, it exists as a mycelium, but in tissue, it forms small budding cells. In most individuals, it causes a self-limited flulike illness. However, in some individuals, especially those who are immunocompromised, it can cause a severe disseminated illness. Adrenal involvement is often asymptomatic but can occasionally cause adrenal insufficiency.[138-142]

The cross-sectional imaging features of adrenal histoplasmosis vary depending on the stage of the disease.

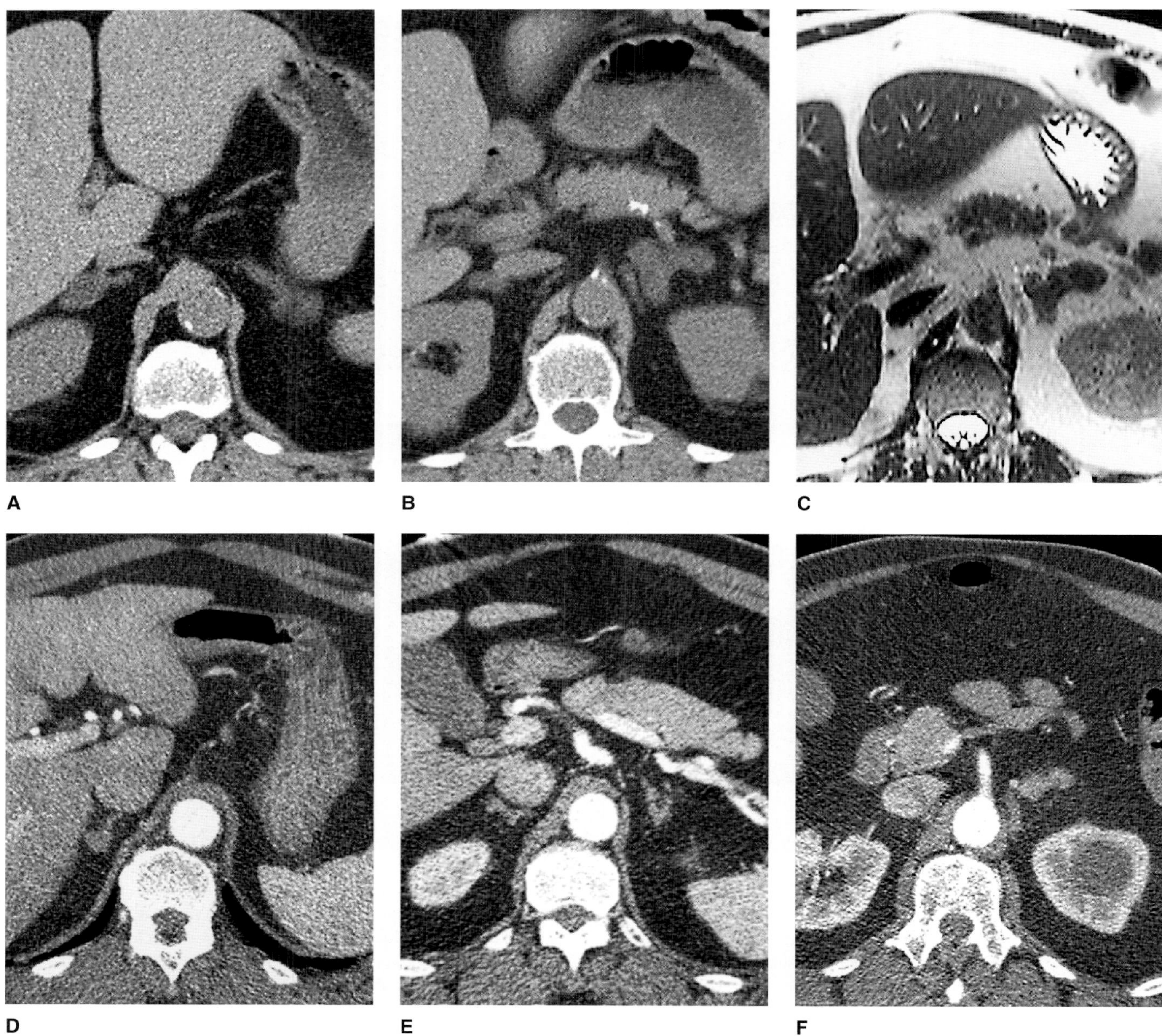

Figure 8-17 Nodular Adrenal Hyperplasia in 2 Patients
A-C. This 68-year-old man had prostate cancer and poorly controlled systemic hypertension. (A and B) Unenhanced CT shows some areas of nodular enlargement and some areas of relatively normal adrenal gland thickness. The nodular areas are slightly decreased attenuation. (C) T2-weighted MRI shows the same nodular thickening and show that the nodules are slightly lower signal compared with other thickened portions of the gland. **D-F**. This 59-year-old man had colon cancer and benign essential hypertension. Contrast-enhanced images show multinodular thickening of the adrenal gland. These cases are pathologically unproven but likely represent nodular adrenal hyperplasia.

At the acute phase of infection, imaging will typically demonstrate nodular or masslike enlargement of both adrenal glands. The enlargement can be solid appearing or contain multiple cystic regions that are hypoechoic on US and hypoattenuating on CT.[138-142] The lesions can be homogeneously or heterogeneously enhancing, and when heterogenous, they will often rim enhance around hypoechoic regions. In the healing phase, 1 or multiple calcifications are demonstrated.

Bilateral Adrenal Metastases

Adrenal metastases are frequently bilateral in distribution. In most cases, it is obvious that they represent bilateral

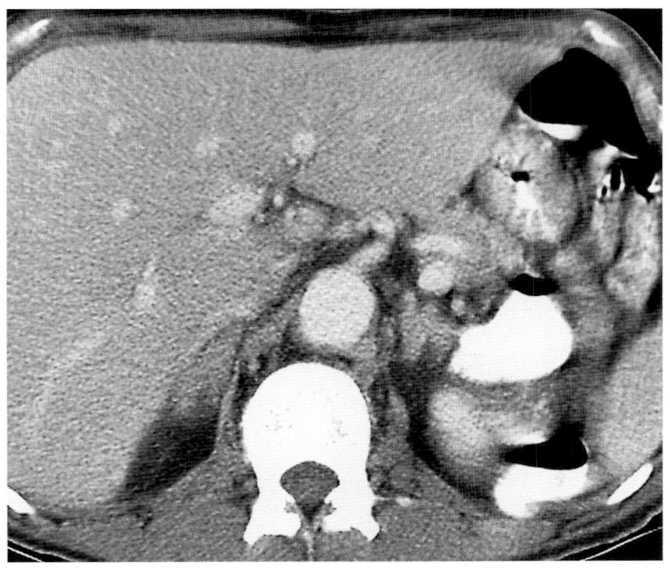

Figure 8-18 Adrenal Disease in Tuberculosis
This 59-year-old man had known active tuberculosis and had persistent fevers. There is mild diffuse enlargement of the adrenal glands bilaterally, the most common adrenal manifestation of patients with tuberculosis. This can represent either adrenal involvement by tuberculosis or represent hyperplasia due to the stress of chronic infection.

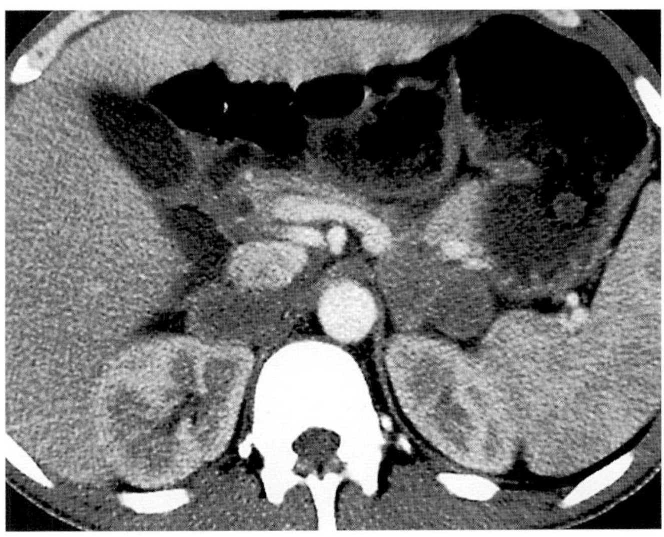

Figure 8-19 Bilateral Adrenal Metastasis
This 49-year-old man had lung cancer. Contrast-enhanced CT shows nodular enlargement of the adrenals bilaterally. This appearance has been seen in patients with tuberculosis and adrenal metastasis but would be unusually large for adrenal hyperplasia. In this clinical setting, these findings are most consistent with bilateral metastasis.

adrenal masses rather than hyperplasia of the gland (see Figure 8-19).

OTHER IMAGING AND CLINICAL FEATURES OF ADRENAL DISEASES

Adrenal imaging is occasionally performed to evaluate for the cause of one of a few hormonal syndromes associated with adrenal pathology: Cushing syndrome, primary hyperaldosteronism, and feminization or virilization syndromes. This is an important topic that will be discussed here. The only imaging characteristic of adrenal lesions that are not adrenal masses or diffuse enlargement, is the presence of adrenal calcification, which will also be discussed here.

Hormonal Syndromes Associated with Adrenal Pathology

Cushing syndrome

Cushing syndrome is a syndrome of hirsutism, amenorrhea, truncal obesity, weakness, hypertension, and hyperglycemia and is a result of sustained high level of serum cortisol. In approximately 25% of cases, Cushing syndrome is caused by an autonomous (non–ACTH dependent), cortisol-secreting adrenal adenoma or adenocarcinoma. Approximately 75% of cases of Cushing syndrome are due to excessive ACTH stimulation, which causes hyperplasia of the adrenal cortex. Causes of excess ACTH include pituitary adenomas (Cushing disease) and nonpituitary neoplasms that secrete ACTH, including bronchogenic carcinoma, thymoma, bronchial carcinoid, pheochromocytoma, and islet cell tumor of the pancreas.[129,143,144] Among patients with ACTH dependent Cushing syndrome, females outpace males by a 3:1 margin.

Patients with Cushing syndrome will frequently undergo CT or MRI of the brain to search for a pituitary adenoma, and abdominal CT or MRI to evaluate for adrenal characteristics of the syndrome. Occasionally, CT of the thorax and abdomen will be performed to search for nonpituitary ACTH-secreting neoplasms.

Evaluation of the adrenal glands will frequently point to the cause of Cushing syndrome. In approximately one-quarter of patients, a unilateral nodule or mass will be identified, indicating the presence of a hyperfunctioning adrenal adenoma or adrenal cortical carcinoma.[24,49] The remaining parts of the involved adrenal gland, as well as the uninvolved, contralateral adrenal are atrophic, because the levels of the circulating ACTH are very low. Most patients with ACTH-dependent Cushing syndrome will demonstrate CT or MRI evidence of bilateral adrenal hyperplasia (see Figure 8-16).[129] In some patients with ACTH dependent Cushing syndrome, the adrenal glands may appear normal. However, in patients with Cushing syndrome, the absence of a unilateral adrenal mass points to bilateral adrenal hyperplasia, even if the glands appear normal on cross-sectional imaging. Occasionally, multiple small nodules will

Imaging Notes 8-4. Imaging Features of Cushing's Syndrome

Adrenal	Pituitary	Other Site	Cause
<3-cm nodule	normal	normal	cortisol-secreting adrenal adenoma
>3-cm mass	normal	normal	cortisol-secreting cortical carcinoma or cortisol-secreting large adrenal adenoma
Hyperplasia or normal	nodule/mass	normal	ACTH-secreting pituitary adenoma
Hyperplasia or normal	normal	lung nodule	ACTH-secreting bronchogenic carcinoma or ACTH-secreting carcinoid tumor
Hyperplasia or normal	normal	anterior mediastinal mass	ACTH-secreting thymoma
Hyperplasia or normal	normal	lung nodule	ACTH-secreting bronchogenic carcinoma
Hyperplasia or normal	normal	pancreas mass	ACTH-secreting neuroendocrine carcinoma

be found in the adrenal glands in a patient with Cushing disease. In this situation, it can be difficult to determine whether the elevated cortisol is due to adrenal hyperplasia or whether one of the nodules represents an autonomous hyperfunctioning adrenal adenoma. Furthermore, occasionally patients with bilateral adrenal hyperplasia will also have a CT- or MRI-detected non hyperfunctioning adenoma, which can be mistaken as a functional, unilateral adenoma. In confusing cases, a combination of CT or MR with radionuclide NP-59 scintigraphy may lead to the correct diagnosis in many patients.[8] Cushing syndrome due to unregulated ACTH production results in bilateral adrenal cortical uptake and visualization, whereas in cases of an autonomous adenoma, only the lesion is visualized, while there is no uptake at all by the remaining adrenal cortex. In rare instances, adrenal venous blood sampling will be needed to identify the unilateral or bilateral source of excess cortisol.[8]

Rare types of bilateral hyperplasia in Cushing syndrome, such as massive macronodular and primary pigmented nodular hyperplasia, need to be differentiated from the common nodular hyperplasia. They are associated with low ACTH levels, lack of an adenoma, and adrenal enlargement on CT; the autonomous cortisol production in these cases can only be treated by bilateral adrenalectomies.

Primary aldosteronism (Conn syndrome)

Aldosterone is a mineralocorticoid responsible for the regulation of blood pressure. This process occurs through rennin-angiotensin-aldosterone feedback loop. When blood volume is low, juxtaglomerular cells in the kidneys secrete renin, which stimulates the production of angiotensin I which is then converted to angiotensin II. Angiotensin II has 2 major effects, constriction of blood vessels, resulting in increased blood pressure, and stimulation of the adrenal cortex to produce the hormone aldosterone. Aldosterone causes the renal tubules to increase the reabsorption of sodium and water into the blood, increasing blood volume, which also increases blood pressure. Elevated blood volume results in a decrease in renin and subsequent decrease in aldosterone.

Hyperaldosteronism can be caused by direct elevation in aldosterone (primary aldosteronism) or by elevations in renin and angiotensin, leading to secondary increases in aldosterone (secondary aldosteronism). Decreased renin levels indicate primary rather than secondary aldosteronism.[129] Approximately 90% of cases of primary aldosteronism are a result of either bilateral adrenal hyperplasia or an aldosterone-secreting adrenal adenoma. Less common causes include unilateral adrenal hyperplasia, aldosterone-secreting adrenal cortical carcinoma, and, rarely, disorders of the renin-angiotensin system.[131,145-147] Adenomas are more often detected in women, whereas adrenal hyperplasia is more often detected in men. Recognition of Conn syndrome (primary aldosteronism due to an adrenal adenoma) as a cause of systemic hypertension is an important diagnosis because resection of the adenoma will lead to curing of systemic hypertension.[129]

Patients typically present with systemic hypertension, which is caused by elevations in serum sodium. Primary aldosteronism is now recognized to be the most common form of secondary hypertension although it still accounts for <1% of cases of systemic hypertension.[129,147] Patients can also present with muscle weakness, myalgias, tetany, and ECG abnormalities, which are a result of hypokalemia.

Imaging Notes 8-5. Imaging Features of Primary Hyperaldosteronism

Adrenal	Cause
<3-cm nodule	aldosterone-secreting adrenal adenoma
>3-cm mass	aldosterone-secreting cortical carcinoma or aldosterone-secreting large adrenal adenoma
Bilateral hyperplasia	idiopathic bilateral hyperplasia
Unilateral hyperplasia	idiopathic unilateral hyperplasia

As in Cushing syndrome, adrenal imaging plays an important role in identifying the cause of primary aldosteronism. Cross-sectional imaging can show a unilateral mass or bilateral adrenal hyperplasia. In confusing cases, scintigraphy with NP-59 can add further functional information (Imaging Notes 8-5).

With the exception of bilateral adrenal hyperplasia, patients with primary aldosteronism will undergo surgical excision of the offending lesion.

Feminization syndromes

Feminization caused by adrenal tumors is rare. Both adrenal adenomas and cortical carcinomas have been associated with feminization, with most cases due to malignant tumors. Clinically, the presenting manifestations are precocious puberty in females and gynecomastia in males. In general, CT or MRI is the appropriate imaging modality for the depiction of the responsible adrenal lesions.[148,149]

Virilization Syndromes

Virilization syndromes in women and children can be caused by a variety of underlying conditions of the ovary, adrenals, and pituitary. Adrenal causes include congenital adrenal hyperplasia, adrenocortical carcinoma, and rare testosterone-secreting adenomas. Ovarian causes of female virilization, such as polycystic ovaries, and rare tumors, such as arrhenoblastomas, can be differentiated from adrenal causes by measuring the 17-ketosteroids in the urine, which is elevated in cases of adrenal pathology only. Pelvic US, CT, and/or MRI can be used to identify macroscopic pathology of the adrenal, ovary, or pituitary. I-131 NP-59 with dexamethasone suppression can also be used to detect adrenal and, sometimes, rare ovarian or testicular neoplasms causing virilization.[150,151]

Congenital adrenal hyperplasia (adrenogenital syndrome): Congenital adrenal hyperplasia (CAH), sometimes referred to as adrenogenital syndrome, is due to ACTH-driven overproduction of adrenal sex hormones. This term encompasses a number of autosomal recessive inborn errors of metabolism caused by enzymatic deficiencies that interfere with adrenal cortical hormone production. These defects usually lead to elevated ACTH, when cortisol levels are diminished, and/or increased production of renin and angiotensin, when aldosterone levels are low.

Currently, in the United States and many other countries, every child born is screened for CAH at birth. The test searches for elevated 17-hydroxyprogesterone (17-OHP), which enables the early detection of CAH. Newborns detected early can be treated appropriately so they can live a relatively normal life.[152]

The most common inborn error in patients with CAH is the 21-hydroxylase deficiency, which results in impaired production of both cortisol and aldosterone, and elevated ACTH and renin. Hypertension and salt wasting are common in these patients.[130] Elevations in ACTH also cause elevations in adrenal androgens, which can cause virilization of the patient.

Much less common is the 11-β-hydroxylase deficiency, which affects the latter part of the cortisol synthesis. As a result, the inactive precursor 11-deoxycortisol and the weak mineralocorticoid 11-deoxycorticosterone accumulate in large amounts, the latter causing hypertension despite normal aldosterone and renin values. Adrenal androgens are again elevated because of the excess ACTH secretion, which can cause virilism in children and female patients.

The treatment of the various types of CAH typically includes replacement of the missing hormones and supplements of sex hormones as needed, in an effort to normalize body growth by delaying precocious puberty or early bone maturation.

Congenital adrenal hyperplasia results in marked enlargement of the adrenal glands and can also cause the development of hormonally responsive testicular masses. Adrenal enlargement is most often evaluated by sonography, which will usually easily detect bilateral enlargement in affected infants.[153] Testicular masses represent clusters of endocrine tissue that, under prolonged ACTH stimulation, hypertrophy. These lesions, often bilateral, are a cause of benign testicular masses and can be demonstrated by sonography or MRI.[154]

Adrenal Calcification

Adrenal calcification is most often a result of prior hemorrhage but can also be due to prior granulomatous infection, as a manifestation of adrenal cysts, or associated with some adrenal tumors. Some patients with Addison disease can also demonstrate adrenal calcification (Table 8-7).

Table 8-7. Causes of Adrenal Calcification

Causes
1. Prior adrenal hemorrhage
2. Prior granulomatous infection a. Tuberculosis b. Histoplasmosis
3. Addison disease (probably due to prior tuberculosis)
4. Wolman disease
5. Calcified neoplasms a. Myelolipoma b. Neuroblastoma c. Other less commonly calcified neoplasms i. Metastasis ii. Adenoma iii. Cortical carcinoma iv. Pheochromocytoma v. Hemangioma

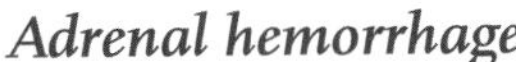

Adrenal hemorrhage

It is generally believed that hemorrhage is the most common cause of adrenal calcifications. This topic has been discussed previously.

Calcification related to prior hemorrhage can take 1 of 2 morphologic appearances. If there is total reabsorption of the hematoma, the calcification can take on the shape of a shrunken and densely calcified small adrenal gland. If the hematoma is not completely reabsorbed, a nonenhancing pseudocyst with peripheral or septal calcification remains (see Figure 8-20).[155]

Granulomatous disease of the adrenal

Granulomatous disease is by far the most common infectious process affecting the adrenals. Tuberculosis and histoplasmosis commonly result in adrenal calcifications.[137,156] Less often, blastomycosis and cryptococcosis can also cause adrenal calcification. Calcifications as a result of these granulomatous infections are indistinguishable from one another and are most often 1 or several small punctate lesions within an atrophied gland.[137,155] Occasionally, they can appear as larger masslike calcifications (see Figure 8-20).

Addison disease

Addison disease or adrenal insufficiency is a rare, chronic endocrine disorder where the adrenal glands do not produce sufficient steroid hormones (glucocorticoids and, often, mineralocorticoids). There is a variety of causes including congenital adrenal dysgenesis, impaired steroid creation due to a variety of metabolic disorders, and most commonly, adrenal destruction or replacement. Adrenal destruction is most commonly due to autoimmune disorders, but can be due to adrenal infections, especially tuberculosis, bilateral adrenal

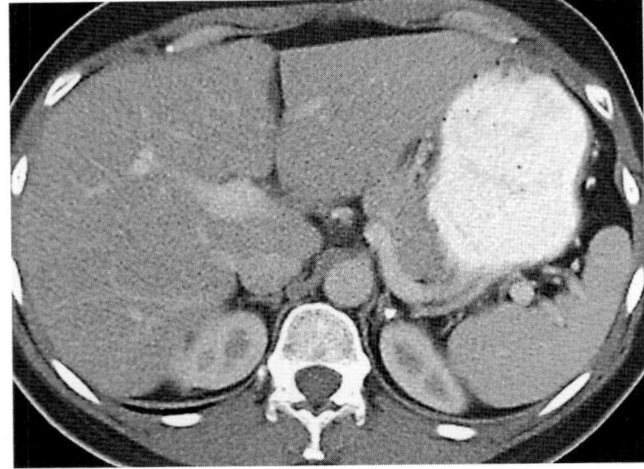

A

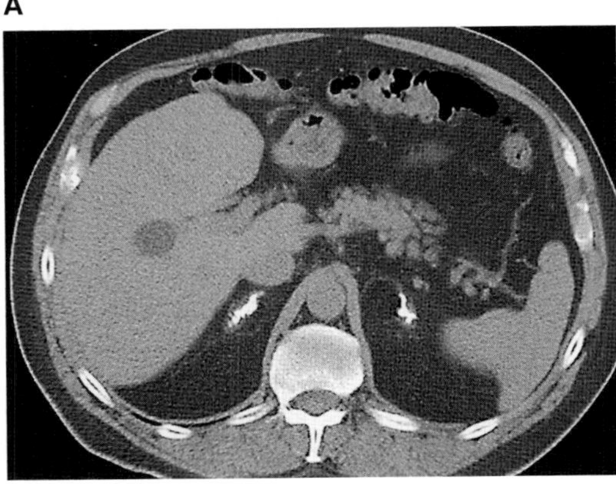

B

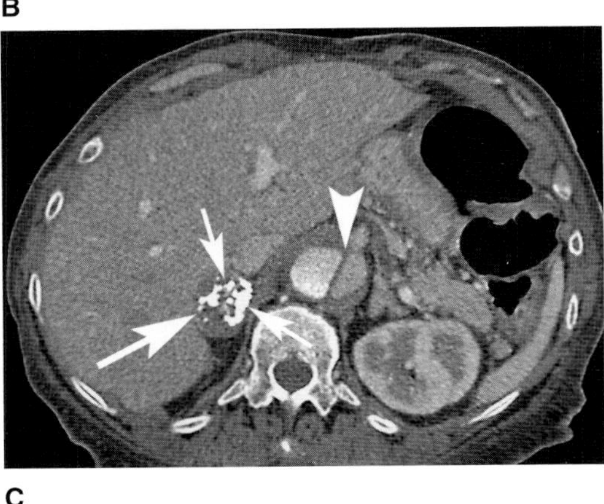

C

Figure 8-20 Adrenal Calcifications in 3 Patients
A. This 40-year-old woman had a lung biopsy demonstrating pulmonary Langerhans cell histiocytosis and also multiple pulmonary granulomas as a result of a previous infection. Enhanced CT shows a punctate calcification in the left adrenal consistent with the patient's history of a granulomatous infection. **B.** This 68-year-old man had transitional cell carcinoma. Unenhanced CT shows linear calcifications in the adrenals bilaterally, likely because of prior granulomatous disease or bilateral adrenal hemorrhage. **C.** This 59-year-old woman had tearing chest pain. Enhanced CT image demonstrates an intimal flap (*arrowhead*) separating the true and false lumens of an aortic dissection. An incidental mass (*large arrow*) containing multiple irregular calcifications (*small arrows*) is also found in the right adrenal gland. This could represent either an old calcified hematoma or a calcified, lipid-poor myelolipoma. The etiology if this lesion was never pathologically confirmed.

hemorrhage, and bilateral adrenal metastases. Historically, one-third of cases have been due to adrenal tuberculosis.[134] However, with the declining incidence of tuberculosis, it has become a less common cause of Addison disease.

Patients with Addison disease typically present with headache, orthostatic hypotension, nausea, vomiting, weight loss, malaise, decreased appetite muscle weakness, muscle pains, and mucocutaneous pigmentation.[134] Serologic studies will demonstrate hyponatremia, hyperkalemia, and diminished levels of cortisol.

Probably because of the association of Addison disease with adrenal tuberculosis, calcified, irregular, thick-walled adrenal lesions can be seen in some cases of adrenal insufficiency.[157,158] In 1 study of 31 patients with Addison disease and pathologic confirmation, adrenal calcifications were only seen in patients with adrenal tuberculosis.[159]

Wolman disease

Wolman disease is a rare autosomal recessive inborn error of metabolism in which foam cells containing cholesterol and triglycerides infiltrate the abdominal organs.[155] The disease is usually fatal by 6 months of age, and patients often present with abdominal enlargement due to hepatosplenomegaly. Computed tomographic examinations can demonstrate diffuse bilateral adrenal gland calcification, within a normally shaped gland.

Calcified cysts

As noted earlier, calcification of adrenal cysts is common. In most cases, the calcification will be linear or curvilinear and line the walls and/or septa of the cyst (see Figure 8-15).

Calcified neoplasms

Calcification within certain adrenal neoplasms is moderately common. The most commonly calcified neoplasm in children is the neuroblastoma, which typically demonstrates multiple small punctate calcifications within a large retroperitoneal or thoracic mass. The most commonly calcified mass in adults is the myelolipoma that will characteristically demonstrate moderate chunky calcifications within a larger soft tissue and fatty mass. Other adrenal neoplasms that have been shown to contain calcifications include adenomas, metastasis, cortical carcinomas, pheochromocytomas, and hemangiomas.[155,156] Confusion with benign causes of adrenal calcification is very rare because in virtually all cases, the calcification will be imbedded within a larger mass, whereas benign calcifications are seen either in isolation or as linear or curvilinear calcifications typical of adrenal cysts.

PROCEDURES ASSOCIATED WITH ADRENAL DISEASES

Procedures associated with adrenal diseases include percutaneous biopsy and, possibly, percutaneous adrenal ablation.

Percutaneous, Image-Guided Adrenal Biopsy

With recent advances in medical imaging (CT, MRI, and PET), the vast majority of adrenal lesions can be accurately and noninvasively characterized, so that the need for tissue sampling has become a rarity.[160] In the era prior to CT and MRI diagnosis of adrenal adenoma based on imaging characteristics, more than half of adrenal lesions that were biopsied were histologically proven adenomas even in patients with known malignancies.[87,160] Nowadays, biopsy of these adrenal incidentalomas has been largely abandoned.[161] This unnecessary and potentially harmful statistic has been markedly decreased, and indications for percutaneous sampling of the adrenals have evolved to reflect current needs and recommendations.[83]

The main indication for adrenal biopsy is among patients with proven or suspected malignancy, and adrenal lesion(s) that does not fulfill the imaging criteria for adenoma or other benign lesion. In the majority of cases, these will represent metastasis in a patient with a known extraadrenal malignancy but occasionally will represent a primary adrenal malignancy. Among the many patients with a known primary neoplasm and an incompletely characterized adrenal mass, a biopsy is indicated, if the result helps to determine the stage of the tumor and, thus, influence treatment decisions. The classic example is the patient with a known extraadrenal primary neoplasm, and a solitary, indeterminate adrenal lesion. However, if an adrenal lesion is found in a patient with many other metastases, no benefit is derived from its biopsy.

Although suspected pheochromocytomas have been biopsied percutaneously without reported morbidity, it is warranted to obtain a 24-hour urine specimen for catecholamines and byproducts, or I-123 MIBG scintigraphy prior to biopsy, if clinical symptoms raise concern for a pheochromocytoma.[83] Complications that may be avoided include potentially dangerous hypertensive crisis or significant retroperitoneal hemorrhage.[160,162]

REFERENCES

1. Neelon FA. Physiology of the adrenal gland. In: Pollack HM, McClennan BL, eds. *Clinical Urography*. 2nd ed. Philadelphia, PA: WB Saunders; 2000:2707-2713.
2. Bronsheim M, Tzidony D, Dimant M, Hajos J, Jaeger M, Blumenfeld Z. Transvaginal ultrasonographic measurements of the fetal adrenals at 12 to 17 weeks gestation. *Am J Obstet Gynecol*. 1993;169:1205-1210.
3. Mitty H, Parsons RB. Adrenal embryology, anatomy, and imaging techniques. In: Pollack HM, McClennan BL, eds. *Clinical Urography*. 2nd ed. Philadelphia, PA: WB Saunders; 2000:2691-2706.
4. Peterson RO. *Urologic Pathology*. Philadelphia, PA: JB Lippincott; 1987.
5. Burton EM, Strange ME, Edmonds DB. Sonography of the circum-renal and horseshoe adrenal gland in the newborn. *Pediatr Radiol*. 1993;23(5):262-265.

6. Graham LS. Celiac accessory adrenal glands. *Cancer.* 1953;6: 149-154.
7. Rose DS, Shreve P, Gross MD, et al. Scintigraphic localization of adrenal disease. In: Pollack HM, McClennan BL, eds. *Clinical Urography*. Philadelphia, PA: WB Saunders; 2000:2780-2782.
8. Gross MD, Shapiro B, Grekin RJ, et al. The scintigraphic localization of the adrenal lesion in primary aldosteronism. *Am J Med.* 1984;77:839-842.
9. Conn JW, Cohen EL, Herwig KR. The dexamethasone-modified adrenal scintiscan in hyporeninemic aldosteronism (tumor vs hyperplasia): a comparison with adrenal venography and adrenal aldosterone. *J Clin Lab Med.* 1976;88:841-856.
10. Mosley CK, Schuster DM. Practical PET/CT of the abdomen. In: Wahl RL, ed. *Clinical PET and PET/CT Imaging, Categorical Course in Diagnostic Radiology*, 93rd Scientific Assembly and Annual Meeting of the Radiological Society of North America. Oak Brook, IL: Radiological Society of North America; 2007:77.
11. Yun M, Kim W, Alnafisi N, et al. 18-F-FDG PET in characterizing adrenal lesions detected on CT or MRI. *J Nucl Med.* 2001;42:1795-1799.
12. Kumar R, Xiu Y, Yu JQ, et al. 18F-FDG PET in evaluation of adrenal lesions in patients with lung cancer. *J Nucl Med.* 2004;45:2058-2062.
13. Metser U, Miller E, Lerman H, et al. 18-F-FDG PET/CT in the evaluation of adrenal masses. *J Nucl Med.* 2007;47:32-37.
14. Blake MA, Slattery JM, Kaltra MK, et al. Adrenal Lesions: characterization with fused PET/CT image in patients with proved or suspected malignancy-initial experience. *Radiology.* 2006;238:970-977.
15. Stowens D. Neurolastoma and related tumors. *Arch Pathol.* 1957;63:451-459.
16. Dunnick NR, Korobkin M. Imaging adrenal incidentalomas. *AJR Am J Roentgenol.* 2002;179:559-568.
17. Commons RR, Callaway CP. Adenomas of the adrenal cortex. *Arch Intern Med.* 1948. 81:37-41.
18. Kokko JP, Brown TC, Berman MM. Adrenal adenoma and hypertension. *Lancet.* 1967;1:468-470.
19. Hedeland H, Oestberg G, Hoekfelt B. On the prevalence of adrenocortical adenoma in an autopsy material in relation to hypertension and diabetes. *Acta Med Scand.* 1968;184:211-214.
20. Aso Y, Homma Y. A survey of incidental adrenal tumors in Japan. *J Urol.* 1992;147:1478-1481.
21. Song JH, Chaudhry FS, Mayo-Smith WW. The incidental adrenal mass on CT: prevalence of adrenal disease in 1,049 consecutive adrenal masses in patients with no known malignancy. *AJR Am J Roentgenol.* 2008;190(5):1163-1168.
22. Mayo-Smith WW, Boland GW, Noto RB, Lee MJ. State-of-the-art adrenal imaging. *Radiographics.* 2001;21:995-1012.
23. Ikeda DM, Francis IR, Glazer GM, Amendola MA, Gross MD, Aisen AM. The detection of adrenal tumors and hyperplasia in patients with primary aldosteronism: comparison of scintigraphy, CT, and MR imaging. *AJR Am J Roentgenol.* 1989;153:301-306.
24. Dunnick NR. Adrenal imaging. *AJR Am J Roentgenol.* 1990;154:927-936.
25. Young WF Jr, Hogan MJ, Klee GG, Grant CS, van Heerden JA. Primary aldosteronism: diagnosis and treatment. *Mayo Clinic Proc.* 1990;65:96-110.
26. Korobkin M, Giordano TJ, Brodeur FJ, et al. Adrenal adenomas: relationship between histologic lipid and CT and MR findings. *Radiology.* 1996;200:743-747.
27. Boland GW, Lee MJ, Gazelle GS, Halpern EF, McNicholas MM, Mueller PR. Characterization of adrenal masses using unenhanced CT: an analysis of the CT literature. *AJR Am J Roentgenol.* 1998;171:201-204.
28. Lee MJ, Hahn PF, Papanicolaou N, et al. Benign and malignant adrenal masses: CT distinction with attenuation coefficients, size, and observer analysis. *Radiology.* 1991;179:415-418.
29. Mitchell DG, Crovello M, Matteucci T, Petersen RO, Miettinen MM. Benign adrenocortical masses: diagnosis with chemical shift MR imaging. *Radiology.* 1992;185:345-351.
30. Bilbey JH, McLoughlin RF, Kurkjian PS, et al. MR imaging of adrenal masses: volume of chemical-shift imaging for distinguishing adenomas from other tumors. *AJR Am J Roentgenol.* 1995;164:637-642.
31. Israel GM, Korobkin M, Wang C, Hecht EN, Krinsky GA. Comparison of unenhanced CT and chemical shift MR imaging in evaluating lipid rich adenomas. *AJR Am J Roentgenol.* 2004;183:215-219.
32. Outwater EK, Siegelman ES, Radecki PD, Piccoli CW, Mitchell DG. Benign adrenocortical masses: diagnosis with chemical shift MR imaging. *AJR Am J Roentgenol.* 1992;185:345-351.
33. Korobkin M, Lombardi TJ, Aisen AM, et al. Characterization of adrenal masses with chemical shift and gadolinium-enhanced MR imaging. *Radiology.* 1995;197:411-418.
34. Mayo-Smith WW, Lee MJ, McNicholas MM, Hahn PF, Boland GW, Saini S. Characterization of adrenal masses (<5 cm) by use of chemical shift MR imaging: observer performance versus quantitative measures. *AJR Am J Roentgenol.* 1995;165:91-95.
35. Tsushima Y, Ishizaka H, Matsumoto M. Adrenal masses: differentiation with chemical-shift, fast low-angle shot MR imaging. *Radiology.* 1993;186:705-709.
36. Heinz-Peer G, Hönigschnabl S, Schneider B, Niederle B, Kaserer K, Lechner G. Characterization of adrenal masses using MR imaging with histopathologic correlation. *AJR Am J Roentgenol.* 1999;173: 15-22.
37. Korobkin M, Brodeur FJ, Francis IR, Quint LE, Dunnick NR, Londy F. CT time-attenuation washout curves of adrenal adenomas and nonadenomas. *AJR Am J Roentgenol.* 1998;170:747-752.
38. Szolar DH, Kammerhuber FH. Adrenal adenomas and nonadenomas: assessment of washout of delayed contrast-enhanced CT. *Radiology.* 1998;207:369-375.
39. Caoili EM, Korobkin M, Francis IR, et al. Adrenal masses: characterization with combined unenhanced and delayed enhanced CT. *Radiology.* 2002;222:629-633.
40. Sangwaiya MJ, Boland GW, Cronin CG, Blake MA, Halpern EF, Hahn PF. Incidental adrenal lesions: accuracy of characterization with contrast-enhanced washout multidetector CT—10-minute delayed imaging protocol revisited in a large patient cohort. *Radiology.* 2010;256:504-510.
41. Caoili EM, Korobkin M, Francis IR, Cohan RH, Dunnick NR. Delayed enhanced CT of lipid poor adenomas. *AJR Am J Roentgenol.* 2000;175:1411-1415.
42. Newhouse JH, Heffess CS, Wagner BJ, Imray TJ, Adair CF, Davidson AJ. Large degenerated adrenal adenomas: radiologic-pathologic correlation. *Radiology.* 1999;210:385-391.

43. Norton JA. Adrenal tumors. *Cancer: Principles and Practice of Oncology*. Philadelphia, PA: Lippincott Williams & Wilkins; 2005:1528-1539.
44. Luton JP, Cerdas S, Billaudm L. Clinical features of adrenocortical carcinoma, prognostic factors, and the effect of mitotane therapy. *N Engl J Med*. 1990;322:1195-1201.
45. Lipsett MB, Hertz R, Ross GT. Clinical and pathophysiologic aspects of adrenocortical carcinoma. *Am J Med*. 1963;35: 374-383.
46. Kay R, Schumacher OP, Tank ES. Adrenocortical carcinoma in children. *J Urol*. 1983;130:1130-1132.
47. Fassnacht M, Kenn W, Allolio B. Adrenal tumors: how to establish malignancy? *J Endocrinol Invest*. 2004;27:387-399.
48. Fishman EK, Deutch BM, Hartman DS, Goldman SM, Zerhouni EA, Siegelman SS. Primary adrenocortical carcinoma: CT evaluation with clinical correlation. *AJR Am J Roentgenol*. 1987;148:531-535.
49. Mayo-Smith WM, Lee MJ, McNicholas MM, Hahn PF, Boland GW, Saini S. Characterization of adrenal masses (<5 cm) by use of chemical shift MR imaging: observer performance versus quantitative measures. *AJR Am J Roentgenol*. 1995;168:91-95.
50. Chezmar JL, Robbins SM, Nelson RC, Steinberg HV, Torres WE, Bernardino ME. Adrenal masses: characterization using MR imaging. *Radiology*. 1988;166:357-359.
51. Schlund JF, Kenney PJ, Brown ED, Ascher SM, Brown JJ, Semelka RC. Adrenocortical carcinoma: MR imaging appearance with current techniques. *J Magn Reson Imaging*. 1995;5:171-174.
52. Francis IR, Gross MD, Shapiro B, Korobkin M, Quint LE. Integrated adrenal imaging. *Radiology*. 1992;184:1-13.
53. Francis IR, Korobkin M. Pheochromocytoma. *Clinical Urography*, 2nd ed. Philadelphia, PA: WB Saunders; 2000:2753.
54. Madani R, Al-Hashmi M, Bliss R, Lennard TW. Ectopic pheochromocytoma: Does the rule of tens apply? *World J Surg*. 2007;31:849-854.
55. Goldfien A. Adrenal medulla. In: Greenspan FS, Baxter TD, eds. *Basic Endocrinology*. 4th ed. E. Norwalk, CT: Appleton & Lange; 1994: 370.
56. Raisanen J, Shapiro B, Glazer GM, Desai S, Sisson JC. Plasma catecholamines in pheochromocytoma: effects of urographic contrast media. *AJR Am J Roentgenol*. 1984;143:43-46.
57. Lenders J, Pacak K, Walther M, et al. Biochemical diagnosis of pheochromocytoma: which test is best? *J Am Med Assoc*. 2002;31:849-854.
58. Ilias I, Pacak K. Current approaches and recommended algorithm for the diagnostic localization of pheochromocytoma. *J Clin Endocrinol Metab*. 2004;89:479-491.
59. Yip L, Lee JE, Shapiro SE, et al. Surgical management of hereditary pheochromocytoma. *J Am Coll Surg*. 2004;198: 525-534.
60. Havekes B, Lai EW, Corssmit EP, Romijn JA, Timmers HJ, Pacak K. Detection and treatment of pheochromocytomas and paragangliomas: current standing of MIBG scintigraphy and future role of PET imaging. *Q J Nucl Med Mol Imaging*. 2008;52:419-429.
61. Shapiro B, Copp JE, Sisson JC, Eyre PL, Wallis J, Beierwaltes WH. Iodine-131 metaiodobenzylguanidine for the locating of suspected pheochromocytoma: experience in 400 cases. *J Nucl Med*. 1985;26:576-585.
62. Ilias I, Divgi C, Pacak K. Current role of metaiodobenzylguanidine in the diagnosis of pheochromocytoma and medullary thyroid cancer. *Semin Nucl Med*. 2011;41:364-368.
63. Miyajima A, Nakashima J, Baba S, Tachibana M, Nakamura K, Murai M. Clinical experience with incidentally discovered pheochromocytoma. *J Urol*. 1997;157:1566-1568.
64. Varghese JC, Hahn PF, Papanicolaou N, Mayo-Smith WW, Gaa JA, Lee MJ. MR differentiation of pheochromocytoma from other adrenal lesions based on qualitative analysis of T2 relaxation times. *Clin Radiol*. 1997;52:603-606.
65. Krebs TL, Wagner BJ. MR imaging of the adrenal gland: radiologic-pathologic correlation. *Radiographics*. 1998;18: 1425-1440.
66. Francis IR, Korobkin M. Pheochromocytoma. In: Pollack HM, McClennan BL, eds. *Clinical Urography*, 2nd ed. Philadelphia, PA: WB Saunders; 2000:2757.
67. Bessell-Browne R, O'Malley ME. CT of pheochromocytoma and paraganglioma: risk of adverse events with IV administration of nonionic contrast material. *AJR Am J Roentgenol*. 2007;188:970-974.
68. Bosniak MA. Neoplasms of the adrenal medulla. In: Pollack HM, McClennan BL, eds. *Clinical Urography*. 2nd ed. Philadelphia, PA: WB Saunders; 2000:2748.
69. Evans AE. Staging and treatment of neuroblastoma. *Cancer*. 1980;45:1799-1802.
70. Monclair T, Brodeur GM, Ambros PF, et al. The International Neuroblastoma Risk Group (INRG) staging system: an INRG Task Force report. *J Clin Oncol*. 2009;27:298-303.
71. Forman HP, Leonidas JC, Berdon WE, Slovis TL, Wood BP, Samudrala R. Congenital neuroblastoma: evaluation with multimodality imaging. *Radiology*. 1990;175:365-368.
72. Sofka CM, Semelka RC, Kelekis NL, et al. Magnetic resonance imaging of neuroblastoma using current techniques. *Magn Reson Imaging*. 1999;17(2):193-198.
73. Merten DF, Gold SH. Radiologic staging of thoracoabdominal tumors in childhood. *Radiol Clin North Am*. 1994;32:133-149.
74. Grando A, Monteggía V, Gandara C, Ruano R, Bunduki V, Zugaib M. Prenatal sonographic diagnosis of adrenal neuroblastoma. *J Clin Ultrasound*. 2001. 29:250-253.
75. Baunin C, Rubie H, Robert A, et al. Diagnostique anténatal d'un neuroblastome. *Pédiatrie*. 1991;45:601.
76. Peretz GS, Lam AH. Neuroblastoma from Wilms tumor by computed tomography. *J Comput Assist Tomogr*. 1985;9(5): 889-893.
77. Dietrich RB, Kangarloo H, Lenarsky C, Feig SA. Neuroblastoma: the role of MR imaging. *AJR Am J Roentgenol*. 1987;148:937-942.
78. Lastoria S, Maurea S, Caracò C, et al. Iodine-131 metaiodobenzylguanidine scintigraphy for localization of lesions in children with neuroblastoma: comparison with computed tomography and ultrasonography. *Eur J Nucl Med*. 1993;20(12):1161-1167.
79. Katz RI, Shirkoda A. Diagnostic approach to incidental adrenal nodules in the cancer patient. *Cancer*. 1985;55:1995-2000.
80. Glomset DA. The incidence of metastasis of malignant tumors to the adrenals. *Am J Med*. 1938;32:74-85.
81. Abrams HL, Spiro R, Goldstein N. Metastases in carcinoma: analysis of 1000 autopsied cases. *Cancer*. 19503:74-85.
82. Pagan JJ. Computed tomography and percutaneous needle biopsy in their diagnosis. *Cancer*. 1984;53:1055-1060.

83. Young WFJ. The incidentally discovered adrenal mass. *N Engl J Med.* 2007;356:601-610.
84. Welch TJ, Sheedy PF 2nd, Stephens DH, Johnson CM, Swensen SJ. Percutaneous adrenal biopsy: review of a 10-year experience. *Radiology.* 1994;193:341-344.
85. Atlas SW, Braffman BH, LoBrutto R, Elder DE, Herlyn D. Human malignant melanomas with varying degrees of melanin content in nude mice: MR imaging, histopathology, and electron paramagnetic resonance. *J Comput Assist Tomogr.* 1990;14:547-554.
86. Bernardino ME, Walther MM, Phillips VM, et al. CT-guided adrenal biopsy: accuracy, safety, and indications. *AJR Am J Roentgenol.* 1985;144:67-69.
87. Silverman SG, Mueller PR, Pinkney LP, Koenker RM, Seltzer SE. Predicitve value of image-guided adrenal biopsy: analysis of results in 101 biopsies. *Radiology.* 1993;187:715-718.
88. Schwartz LH, Macari M, Huvos AG, Panicek DM. Collision tumors of the adrenal gland: demonstration and characterization at MR imaging. *Radiology.* 1996;201:757-760.
89. Glazer HS, Lee JK, Balfe DM, Mauro MA, Griffith R, Sagel SS. Non-Hodgkin lymphoma: computed tomographic demonstration of unusual extranodal involvement. *Radiology.* 1983;149:211-217.
90. Feldberg MAM, Hendriks MJ, Klinkhamer AC. Massive bilateral non-Hodgkin's lymphomas of the adrenals. *Urol Radiol.* 1986;8:85-88.
91. Pauling MR, and Williamson BRJ. Adrenal involvement in non-Hodgkin lymphoma. *AJR Am J Roentgenol.* 1983;141: 303-305.
92. Curry NS, Chung CJ, Potts W, Bissada N. Isolated lymphoma of genitourinary tract and adrenals. *Am J Med.* 1993;78:711-714.
93. Shea TC, Spark R, Kane B, Lange RF. Non-Hodgkin's lymphoma limited to the adrenal gland with adrenal insufficiency. *Am J Med.* 1985;15:135-139.
94. Vicks BS, Perusek M, Johnson J, Tio F. Primary adrenal lymphoma: CT and sonographic appearances. *J Clin Ultrasound.* 1987;15:135-139.
95. Alvarez-Castells A, Pedraza S, Tallada N, Castella E, Gifre L, Torrents C. CT of primary bilateral adrenal lymphoma. *J Comput Assist Tomogr.* 1993;17: 408-409.
96. Lee FT Jr, Thornbury JR, Grist TM, Kelcz F. MR imaging of adrenal lymphoma. *Abdom Imaging.* 1993;18:95-96.
97. Kenney PJ, Wagner BJ, Rao P, Heffess CS. CT and pathologic features. *Radiology.* 1998;208(87-95).
98. Goldman HB, Howard RC, Patterson AL. Spontaneous retroperitoneal hemorrhage from a giant adrenal myelolipoma. *J Urol.* 1996;155:639.
99. Cyran KM, Kenney PJ, Memel DS, Yacoub I. Adrenal myelolipoma. *AJR Am J Roentgenol.* 1996;166:395-400.
100. Rofsky NM, Bosniak MA, Megibow AJ, Schlossberg P. Adrenal myelolipomas: CT appearance with tiny amounts of fat and punctate calcification. *Urol Radiol.* 1989;11:148-151.
101. Tsukaguchi I, Sato K, Ohara S, Kadowaki T, Shin T, Kotoh K. Adrenal myelolipoma: report of a case with CT and angiographic evaluation. *Urol Radiol.* 1989;5:47-49.
102. Israel GM. MRI of the kidneys and adrenal glands. In: Ho VB, Kransdorf MJ, Reinhold C, eds. *Body MRI: Categorical Course Syllabus.* Leesburg, VA: American Roentgen Ray Society; 2006:91-102.
103. Otal P, Escourrou G, Mazerolles C, et al. Imaging features of uncommon adrenal masses with histopathologic correlation. *RadioGraphics.* 1999;19: 569-581.
104. Termote B, Verswijvel G, Palmers Y. Fat containing adrenal cavernous haemangioma: CT and MRI findings. *JBR-BTR.* 2007;90:516-518.
105. Vergas AD. Adrenal hemangioma. *Urology.* 1980;16:389-390.
106. Xu H-X, Liu G-J. Huge cavernous hemangioma of the adrenal gland: sonographic, computed tomographic, and magnetic resonance imaging findings. *J Ultrasound Med.* 2003;22: 523-526.
107. Lee WJ, Weinreb J, Kumari S, Phillips G, Pochaczevsky R, Pillari G. Adrenal hemangioma. *J Comput Assist Tomogr.* 1982;6:389-394.
108. Rieber AB, Brambs HJ. CT and MRI of adrenal hemangioma. A case report. *Acta Radiol.* 1995;36:659-661.
109. Hamrick-Turner JE, Abbitt PL, Allen BC, Fowler JE Jr, Cranston PE, Harrison RB. Adrenal hemangioma: MR findings with pathologic correlation. *J Comput Assist Tomogr.* 1993;17:503-505.
110. Sarnaik AP, Sanfilippo DJ, Slovis TL. Ultrasound diagnosis of adrenal hemorrhage in meningococcemia. *Pediatr Radiol.* 1988;18:427.
111. Khuri FJ, Alton DJ, Hardy BE, Cook GT, Churchill BM. Adrenal hemorrhage in neonates: report of 5 cases and review of the literature. *J Urol.* 1980;124:684-687.
112. Burks DW, Mirvis SE, Shanmuganathan K. Acute adrenal injury after blunt abdominal trauma: CT findings. *AJR Am J Roentgenol.*, 1980;158:503-507.
113. Wolverson MK, Kannengieser H. CT of bilateral adrenal hemorrhage with acute adrenal insufficiency in the adult. *AJR Am J Roentgenol.* 1984;142:311-314.
114. Murphy BJ, Casillas J, Yrizarry JM. Traumatic adrenal hemorrhage: radiologic findings. *Radiology.* 1988;169:701-703.
115. Kawashima A, Sandler CM, Ernst RD, et al. Imaging of nontraumatic hemorrhage of the adrenal gland. *Radiographics.* 1999;19:949-963.
116. Hahn PF, Saini S, Stark DD, Papanicolaou N, Ferrucci JT Jr. Intraabdominal hematoma: the concentric-ring sign in MR imaging. *AJR Am J Roentgenol.* 1987;148:115-119.
117. Wedmid A, Palese M. Diagnosis and treatment of the adrenal cyst. *Curr Urol Rep.* 2010;11:44-50.
118. Erickson LA, Lloyd RV, Hartman R, Thompson G. Cystic adrenal neoplasms. *Cancer.* 2004;101:1537-1544.
119. Abeshouse GA, Goldstein RB, Abeshouse BS. Adrenal cysts: review of the literature and report of three cases. *J Urol.* 1959;81:711-719.
120. Kearney GP, Mahoney EM. Adrenal cysts. *Urol Clin North Am.* 1977;4:273-283.
121. Neri LM, Nance FC. Management of adrenal cysts. *Am Surg.* 1999;65:151-163.
122. Atkinson GOJ, Kodroff MB, Gay BBJ, Ricketts RR. Adrenal abscess in the neonate. *Radiology.* 1985;155:101-104.
123. Wahl HR. Adrenal cysts. *Am J Med.* 1951;27:758-759.
124. Rozenblit A, Morehouse HT, Amis ES. Cystic adrenal lesions: CT features. *Radiology.* 1996;201:541-548.
125. Tung GA, Pfister RC, Papanicolaou N, Yoder IC. Adrenal cysts: imaging and percutaneous aspiration. *Radiology.* 1989;173: 107-110.

126. Sanal HT, Kocaoglu M, Yildirim D, et al. Imaging features of benign adrenal cysts. *Eur J Radiol.* 2006;60:465-469.

127. Guo YK, Yang ZG, Li Y, et al. Uncommon adrenal masses: CT and MRI features with histopathologic correlation. *Eur J Radiol.* 2007;62:359-370.

128. Wang LJ, Wong Y-C, Chen C-J, Chu S-H. Imaging spectrum of adrenal pseudocysts on CT. *Eur J Radiol.* 2003;13:531-535.

129. Dunnick NR. Hyperfunctioning lesions of the adrenal cortex. In: Pollack HM, McClennan BL, eds. *Clinical Urography.* 2nd ed. Philadelphia, PA: WB Saunders; 2000:2714.

130. White PC, New MI, Dupont B. Congenital adrenal hyperplasia. *N Engl J Med.* 1987;316:1519-1524.

131. Buurman H, Saeger W. Abnormalities in incidentally removed adrenal glands. *Endocr Pathol.* 2006;17(3):277-282.

132. Saeger W, Reinhard K, Reinhard C. Hyperplastic and tumorous lesions of the adrenals in an unselected autopsy series. *Endocr Pathol.* 1998;9(3):235-239.

133. Reinhard C, Saeger W, Schubert B. Adrenocortical nodules in post-mortem series. Development, functional significance, and differentiation from adenomas. *Gen Diagn Pathol.* 1996; 141(3-4):203-208.

134. Lam K-Y, Lo C-Y. A critical examination of adrenal tuberculosis and a 28-year autopsy experience of active tuberculosis. *Clin Endocrinol.* 2001;54(5):633-639.

135. Guo YK, Yang ZG, Li Y, et al. Addison's disease due to adrenal tuberculosis: contrast-enhanced CT features and clinical duration correlation. *Eur J Radiol.* 2006;62:126-131.

136. Buxi TBS, Vohra RB, Sujatha MD, Byotra SP, Mukherji S, Daniel M. CT in adrenal enlargement due to tuberculosis: a review of literature with five new cases. *Clin Imaging.* 1992;16(2):102-108.

137. Yılmaz T, Sever A, Gür S, Killi RM, Elmas N. CT findings of abdominal tuberculosis in 12 patients. *Comput Med Imaging Graph.* 2002;26(5):321-325.

138. Kumar N, Singh S, Govil S. Adrenal histoplasmosis: clinical presentation and imaging features in nine cases. *Abdom Imaging.* 2003;28:703-708.

139. Jagat J, Mukherjee ML, Villa LT, Lee KO. Bilateral adrenal masses due to histoplasmosis. *J Clin Endocrinol Metab.* 2005;90(12):6725-6726.

140. Subramanian S, Abraham OC, Rupali P, Zachariah A, Mathews MS, Mathai D. Disseminated histoplasmosis. *J Assoc Physicians India.* 2005;28:703-708.

141. Roubsanthisuk W, Sriussadaporn S, Vawesorn N, et al. Primary adrenal insufficiency caused by disseminated histoplasmosis: report of two cases. *Endocr Pract.* 2002;8:237-241.

142. Rozenblit AM, Kim A, Tuvia J, Wenig BM. Adrenal histoplasmosis manifested as Addison's disease: unusual CT features with magnetic resonance imaging correlation. *Clin Radiol.* 2001;56:682-684.

143. Nieman LK, Ilias I. Evaluation and treatment of Cushing's syndrome. *Am J Med.* 2005;118:1340-1346.

144. Doppman JL, Nieman LK, Miller DL, et al. Ectopic adrenocorticotropic hormone syndrome: localization studies in 28 patients. *Radiology.* 1989;172:115-124.

145. Blevins LSJ, Wand GS. Primary aldosteronism: an endocrine perspective. *Radiology.* 1992;184:677-682.

146. Irony I, Kater CE, Biglieri EG, Shackleton CH. Correctable subsets of primary aldosteronism: primary adrenal hyperplasia and renin responsive adenoma. *Am J Med.* 1990;3:576-582.

147. Young WF. Primary aldosteronism: renaissance of a syndrome. *Clin Endocrinol.* 2007;66(5):607.

148. Howard CP, Takahashi H, Hayles AB. Feminizing adrenal adenoma in a boy. *Mayo Clin Proc.* 1977;52:354-357.

149. deAsis DN, Samaan NA. Feminizing adrenocortical carcinoma with Cushing's syndrome and pseudohyperparathyroidism. *Arch Intern Med.* 1978;138:301-303.

150. Gross MD, Freitas JE, Swanson DP, Woodbury MC, Schteingart DE, Beierwaltes WH. Dexamethasone suppression adrenal scintigraphy in hyperandrogenism. *J Nucl Med.* 1984;22:12-17.

151. Gross MD, Shapiro B, Thrall JH, Freitas JE, Beierwaltes WH. The scintigraphic imaging of endocrine organs. *Endocr Rev.* 1984;5:221-225.

152. Pang S, Shook MK. Current status of neonatal screening for CAH. *Curr Opin Pediatr.* 1997;9:419-423.

153. Sivit CJ, Hung W, Taylor GA, Catena LM, Brown-Jones C, Kushner DC. Sonography in neonatal congenital adrenal hyperplasia. *AJR Am J Roentgenol.* 1991;156:141-143.

154. Vanzulli A, DelMaschio A, Paesano P, et al. Testicular masses in association with adrenogenital syndrome. *Radiology.* 1992;183:425-429.

155. Hindman N, Israel GM. Adrenal gland and adrenal mass calcification. *Eur J Radiol.* 2005;15:1163-1167.

156. Kenney PJ, Stanley RJ. Calcified adrenal masses. *Urol Radiol.* 1987;9(1):9-15.

157. Wilms GE, Baert AL, Kint EJ, Pringot JH, Goddeeris PG. Computed tomographic findings in bilateral adrenal tuberculosis. *Radiology.* 1983;146:729-730.

158. Radin DR. Disseminated histoplasmosis: abdominal CT findings in 16 patients. *AJR Am J Roentgenol.* 1991;157:955-958.

159. Vita JA, Silverberg SJ, Goland RS, Austin JH, Knowlton AI. Clinical clues to the cause of Addison's disease. *Am J Med.* 1985;78(3):461-466.

160. Paulsen SD, Nghiem HN, Korobkin M, Caoili EM, Higgins EJ. Changing role of imaging-guided percutaneous biopsy of adrenal masses: evaluation of 50 adrenal biopsies. *AJR Am J Roentgenol.* 2004;182:1033-1037.

161. Mazzaglia PJ, Monchik JM. Limited value of adrenal biopsy in the evaluation of adrenal neoplasm. *Arch Surg.* 2009;144:465-470.

162. McCorkell SJ, Niles NL. Fine-needle aspiration of catecholamine-producing adrenal masses: a possibly fatal mistake. *AJR Am J Roentgenol.* 1985;145:113-114.

CHAPTER

Imaging of the Uterus and Cervix

Skip M. Alderson, MD
Drew A. Torigian, MD, MA
Wallace T. Miller Jr., MD

NORMAL UTERUS AND CERVIX

Anatomy

The uterus is the female reproductive organ where the embryo and fetus develop during pregnancy. In that role, the uterus undergoes morphologic changes in a cyclic fashion in response to hormonal fluctuations during a woman's menstrual cycle. The uterus can be thought of as being composed of 2 parts—the body and the cervix. The body forms the upper portion of the uterus and the cervix forms the smaller cylindrical lower portion that communicates with the upper vagina. The fundus is considered to be that part of the body that is superior to the ostia of the fallopian tubes. Finally, the isthmus is the inferior narrower portion of the uterus that is continuous with the cervix. The uterine wall is composed of 3 layers—serosa (the most superficial), myometrium, and endometrium (the deepest). The myometrium can be divided into an inner myometrium (junctional zone) and outer myometrium. The serosal surface is the peritoneum reflected on the uterus. The peritoneal cavity extends posterior to the uterus as the rectouterine pouch or pouch of Douglas and anteriorly as the vesicouterine pouch.

Morphologic Changes

The uterus and cervix normally change over the lifetime of a woman under the influence of fluctuating hormonal levels. At birth, the uterus is tubular with an average length of 3.4 cm and fundal width of 1.2 cm, and the cervical width averages 1.4 cm.[1] Shortly after birth, because of the decreasing effect of maternal hormones, the uterus shrinks and the body and fundus are approximately equal in size to that of the cervix.[2] After 7 years of age and continuing through puberty, the uterus enlarges and assumes an adult configuration, with the uterus being larger than the cervix.[1] In the adult, the uterine dimensions vary with parity. The nulliparous uterus averages 3 cm × 5 cm × 7 cm (anteroposterior dimension × width × length).[3] The multiparous uterus is typically larger in all dimensions.[3] After menopause, the uterus gradually atrophies and ultimately assumes a prepubertal size and configuration.

Not only does the overall size and shape of the uterus change with age, but so does the endometrial thickness. Knowledge of the age-appropriate endometrial thickness is vital in avoiding misdiagnosis. Endometrial growth is hormonally controlled. As such, at birth and shortly thereafter, the endometrium can usually be seen as it is under the influence of circulating maternal hormones.[1] In prepubertal girls, the endometrium is sometimes seen as a thin layer. During a woman's fertile years, typically between the early teenage years and the age of 50, the endometrium mirrors the cyclical hormonal changes with each menstrual cycle. Immediately after the cessation of menses, the endometrium is at its thinnest, measuring only 2 to 3 mm.[3] Under the predominant influence of estrogen, the endometrium will thicken during the proliferative phase to a thickness of about 8 mm.[3] Finally, during the secretory phase, progesterone is the dominant circulating hormone and the endometrium thickens further, sometimes reaching a thickness of 15 mm or more.[3] At the end of the secretory phase, menstrual bleeding begins and the cycle repeats. With menopause, the female hormonal levels drop and the endometrium thins accordingly. Depending on the source cited, the normal postmenopausal endometrium thickness is 4 or 5 mm and should be uniform without focal thickening.

Normal Imaging Appearances

Ultrasonography

Ultrasonography (US) is the primary modality used to image the female pelvis, particularly when evaluation of the uterus and cervix is desired. Transabdominal and transvaginal probes are available and are typically complementary. When imaging transabdominally, it is best to scan through a full urinary bladder as this serves as an acoustic window. In the majority of cases, the endometrium can be seen as a discrete hyperechoic structure deep to the myometrium.[3] When fluid is present in the endometrial canal, the endometrium on each side of the fluid should be measured individually and summed, excluding the fluid from the overall endometrial thickness. A small amount of fluid in the endometrial canal is usually a normal finding.[3] In addition, US can occasionally resolve the junctional zone, or inner myometrium, from the outer myometrium as a zone of hypoechogenicity interposed between the hyperechoic endometrium and intermediately echogenic outer myometrium.[3] For the most part, however, the myometrial echotexture is uniform (see Figure 9-1). The serosal layer is not typically identified as a discrete layer. Prominent serosal veins are commonly seen. Although the cervix also has a zonal anatomy comprising the endocervix and ectocervix, these are not easily discernible sonographically.

Magnetic resonance imaging

Magnetic resonance imaging (MRI) provides the most detailed and accurate imaging evaluation of the uterus and cervix. However, because of the cost and limited availability, MRI is usually reserved for cases in which the US findings

A

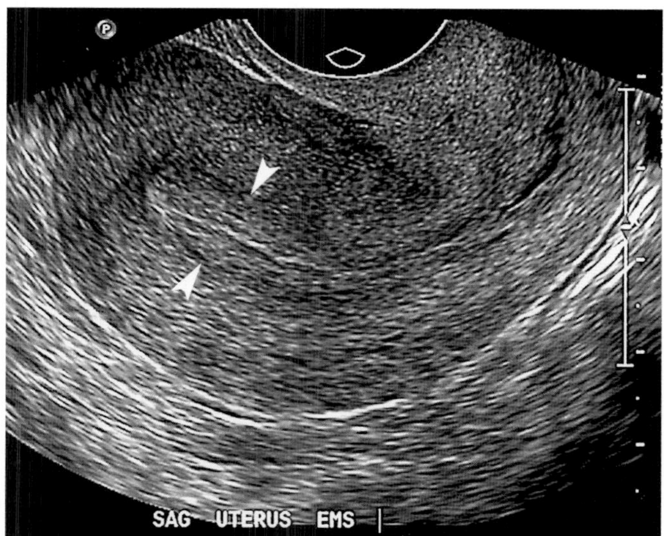

B

Figure 9-1 Normal US of the Uterus and Cervix
A. Transabdominal and (**B**) transvaginal views of the uterus. Although the endometrium and inner and outer myometrium are not easily resolved transabdominally, the different layers are well visualized transvaginally. The endometrium (*arrowheads*) appears as a thin band of greater echogenicity in the central uterus.

are unclear, the US examination is technically limited, or when more precise tissue characterization is necessary. MRI is also frequently used to stage cervical and endometrial neoplasms. Additionally, MRI can be used to follow patients after certain procedures such as uterine artery embolization (UAE), when changes beyond lesion size (eg, necrosis, hemorrhage, enhancement pattern) are helpful in assessing treatment response. The protocol for a routine MRI examination usually includes axial T1-weighted images and axial, sagittal, and fat-suppressed coronal T2-weighted images. Imaging after intravenous (IV) contrast administration is often performed, but is not always necessary. If contrast is to be administered, fat-suppressed T1-weighted image in the axial plane before and after contrast administration are obtained with identical parameters. Sagittal and coronal planes of imaging after contrast administration may be obtained as well. If MRI is being performed to evaluate for a congenital anomaly, 3-plane T2-weighted images should be obtained with respect to the long axis of the uterus, thereby providing visualization of the outer uterine contour to best advantage. Most diagnoses are made on the T2-weighted image because the high soft-tissue contrast resolution provides more structural information than the other sequences in most cases. One notable exception to this general rule is the diagnosis of hematocolpos and hematometros, which are best depicted on T1-weighted images, and typically manifest as fluid with high signal intensity (SI) on T1-weighted images due to subacute hemorrhage.

On T1-weighted images, the individual layers of the uterus and cervix are not well differentiated and appear as relatively homogeneous structures of intermediate SI relative to skeletal muscle. However, on T2-weighted images, the uterus has a trilaminar appearance with discrete visualization of the endometrium, junctional zone, and outer myometrium.[4] The endometrium is rich in glandular tissue and as a result is uniformly high SI on T2-weighted images.[4] Because the endometrium is highly vascular, it brightly enhances following IV contrast administration.[4] The junctional zone, or inner myometrium, is much more readily seen on MRI than with US and should measure less than 12 mm and have homogeneous SI that is less than that of the adjacent endometrium and outer myometrium on T2-weighted images.[4] Small foci of increased SI in the junctional zone are abnormal and usually represent ectopic endometrial glands in the setting of adenomyosis. The outer myometrium has intermediate to slightly high SI on T2-weighted images relative to skeletal muscle (see Figure 9-2). As on US, the serosal layer is not well seen as a distinct layer. However, slow flow in serosal veins will often present as high SI on gradient echo images. The zonal anatomy of the cervix consists of a high-SI endocervix that is continuous with the endometrium and a low-SI ectocervix that is continuous with the myometrium on T2-weighted images.

Computed tomography

Computed tomography (CT) is not the preferred modality for evaluating the uterus and cervix because of its inherently lower tissue contrast compared with US and MRI. However, because CT is commonly used to evaluate the abdomen and pelvis, the normal appearance of the uterus and cervix should be understood. Likewise, knowledge of the limitations of CT in diagnosing pathologic conditions of the uterus and cervix is important to avoid overdiagnosis and misdiagnosis. Normally, the uterus and cervix will appear as uniform smoothly marginated soft tissue attenuation structures (see Figure 9-3). The endometrial cavity may be of lower attenuation than the myometrium. After IV contrast administration, the endometrium typically avidly enhances and is of higher attenuation than the enhancing myometrium, although the distinct layers are not always discernible. Occasionally, the junctional zone and outer myometrium may have differential enhancement and, therefore, may be distinguishable from each other.[5]

Hysterosalpingography

At hysterosalpingography (HSG), the opacified endometrial cavity appears as an inverted triangle, with the base in the cranial location and the apex in the caudal location.[6] Contrast homogeneously opacifies the endometrial cavity, which should have sharply defined borders. The fallopian tubes are thin and smooth in contour, and are slightly dilated in their ampullary segments. Contrast should freely spill out from the fimbriated ends into the peritoneal cavity (see Figure 9-4).

Positron emission tomography

As might be expected, the standardized uptake value (SUV) of the endometrium on [^{18}F]-2-fluoro-2-deoxy-2-d-glucose (FDG) positron emission tomographic (PET) studies varies with age, menopausal status, and phase of the menstrual cycle.[7] A study of normal healthy volunteers showed that FDG uptake in the endometrium is highest at midcycle during the late follicular to early luteal phases and during the first 3 days of menses.[7] The mechanism of uptake during menses is not certain, but may be related to subendometrial uterine peristalsis and tends to localize to the central cavity.[7] Non–menstrual-related endometrial uptake, on the other hand, is more likely to localize to the uterine wall.[7] Fluorodeoxyglucose uptake was not observed during the early follicular or late luteal phases.[7] In the same study, no physiologic activity was seen at any time in the uterus of any of the postmenopausal volunteers.[7] Therefore, increased endometrial uptake in postmenopausal women should be considered as suspicious for uterine pathology until proven otherwise and warrants further evaluation.

FOCAL UTERINE ABNORMALITIES

Focal lesions within the uterus can be centered within the myometrium or endometrium.

Focal Myometrial Masses

Focal myometrial masses will represent uterine leiomyomas in the vast majority of cases. Less commonly, they can

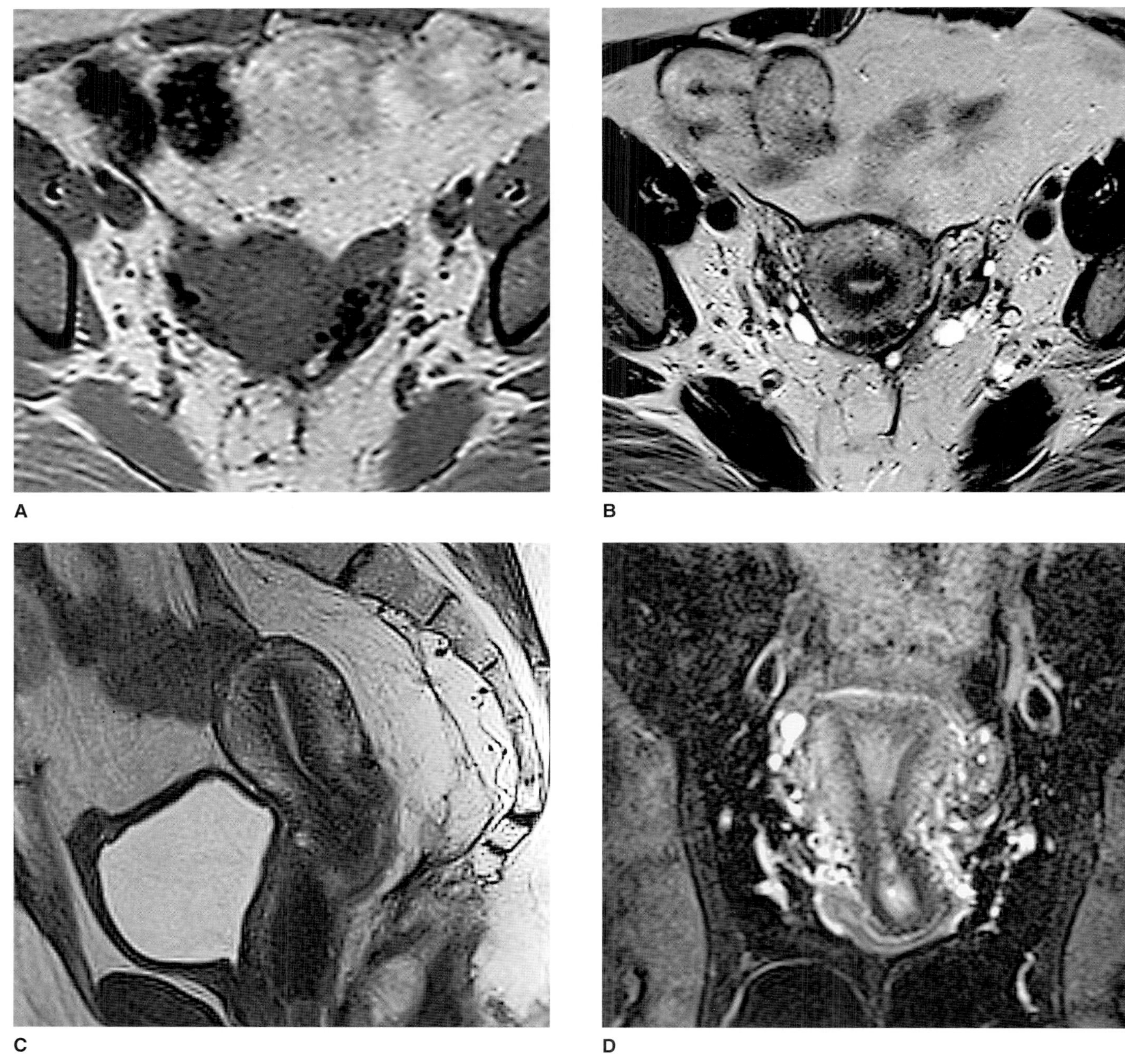

Figure 9-2 Normal MRI of the Uterus and Cervix
MRI of the female pelvis at 1.5 Tesla. **A**. The uterus is uniform in SI on the T1-weighted image. **B-C**. However, a trilaminar appearance is readily appreciated on the axial (B) and sagittal (C) T2-weighted images as well as the coronal STIR (**D**). The endometrium has high SI, whereas the inner myometrium is low in SI. The outer myometrium is intermediate in SI.

be caused by uterine sarcomas, adenomyosis, or transient uterine contractions (Table 9-1).

Uterine leiomyoma

Leiomyomas, also known as fibroids, are the most common tumor of the female genitourinary tract and will affect up to 30% to 40% of women over the age of 35.[8,9] African Americans are affected more frequently than Caucasians.[3] They represent benign neoplasms composed predominantly of smooth muscle cells separated by variable amounts of fibrous connective tissue and are surrounded by a pseudocapsule. Leiomyomas are hormonally responsive and, as a result, are not typically present prior to menarche, can demonstrate dramatic growth during pregnancy

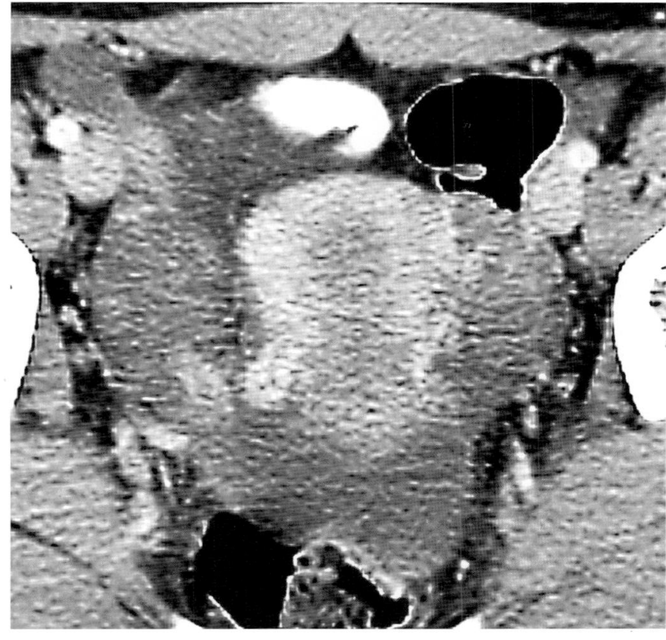

A

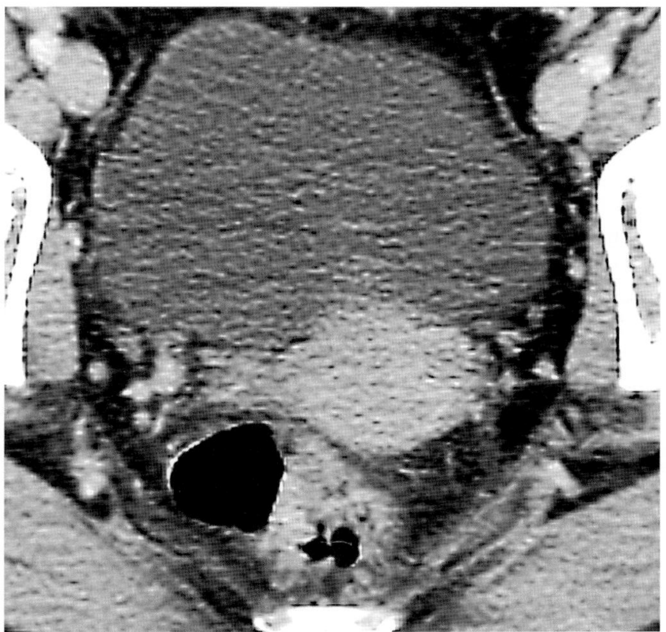

B

Figure 9-3 CT of Normal Uterus and Cervix
A and **B**. Axial contrast-enhanced CT of the uterus in 2 different patients show the variable appearance of the normal uterus at CT. In some cases, the uterus will appear uniform attenuation throughout as in (B). In other situations, especially during the later phases of the menstrual cycle, the endometrium can appear hypoenhancing, as in (A), a finding that should not be interpreted as representing pathology.

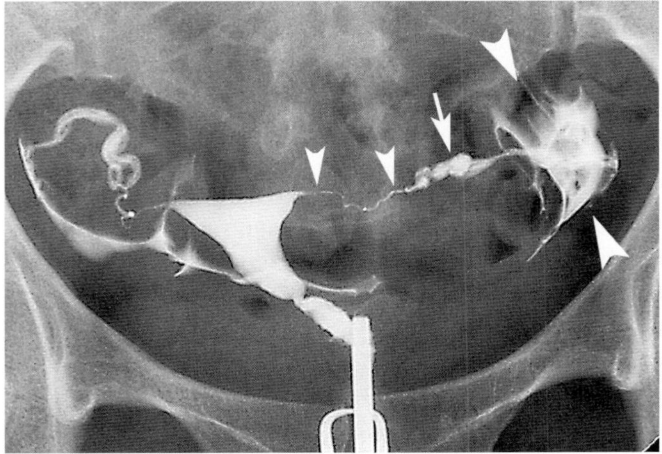

Figure 9-4 Normal Hysterosalpingogram
Anteroposterior image of the uterus during a hysterosalpingogram shows a triangular collection of contrast with smooth contours representing the normal uterine cavity. The fallopian tubes appear as smooth cork-screw tubular structures extending from the cornua bilaterally. The isthmic portions (*small arrowheads*) of the tubes are very narrow and appear as pencil-thin lines that widen into the ampullary and infundibular portions (*arrow*) of the tubes. At the fimbria, contrast spills into the peritoneum creating wispy, amorphous collections of contrast (*large arrowheads*).

or during estrogen therapy, and will often regress after menopause. Unopposed estrogen is the dominant factor driving leiomyoma growth.[10]

Most patients, nearly 80%, with uterine leiomyomas will be asymptomatic. When symptomatic, patients will most often present with heavy menstrual bleeding, a palpable pelvic mass, pelvic fullness, chronic or cyclical pelvic pain, constipation, or infertility.[11] Fibroids will occasionally present with acute pelvic pain, particularly in the setting of an exophytic fibroid that has torsed.[12] More unusual

Table 9-1. Causes of a Focal Myometrial Mass

1. Uterine leiomyoma (fibroid)
2. Uterine sarcoma a. Carcinosarcoma (mixed müllerian tumor) b. Leiomyosarcoma c. Endometrial stromal sarcoma
3. Adenomyosis a. Focal adenomyosis b. Adenomyoma
4. Transient uterine contractions

presentations include hydronephrosis as a result of local mass effect on the ureters or as a vaginal mass secondary to prolapse. A pelvic mass may or may not be felt during bimanual physical examination.

Leiomyomas are classified with regard to their location within the uterus—fundal, body, or cervical—as well as their location within the uterine wall—intracavitary, submucosal, intramural, or subserosal, as location may be related to the presence or absence of symptoms and may also influence potential treatment options. The majority of leiomyomas are intramural and clinically asymptomatic.[13] Patients with intramural lesions are less likely to present with abnormal bleeding because the lesions have little or no contact with the endometrium. On the other hand, submucosal leiomyomas are the least frequent type, accounting for only 5% of cases, but are more commonly symptomatic.[13] As previously stated, subserosal fibroids can occasionally torse, especially if connected to the uterus by a narrow pedicle. Fibroids may also cause pelvic pain as a result of degeneration as the tumors outgrow their blood supply or lose their hormonal stimulation. Various types of degeneration have been described with histology demonstrating hemorrhage, necrosis, calcification, and myxoid changes.[10] Rarely, these benign tumors will invade the uterine or ovarian veins and extend into the inferior vena cava, sometimes reaching the right heart and pulmonary arteries, as a rare condition termed IV leiomyomatosis.[14]

Further, US and MRI are the primary modalities used to establish the diagnosis of a leiomyoma and to characterize its size and location. A study that directly compared MRI and US with hysterectomy specimens demonstrated that both techniques were highly accurate for diagnosing the presence of leiomyomas (MRI: sensitivity 99%, specificity 86%; US: sensitivity 99%, specificity 91%) and for determining tumor size.[15] Not surprisingly, MRI has been shown to be more accurate in depicting fibroid location, especially in large or myomatous uteri. This is related to the high tissue contrast resolution inherent to MRI, the larger field of view, and operator independence. Another study reported MRI to be more accurate than both US and HSG in identifying the presence and location of leiomyomas in infertile women prior to myomectomy.[16] On average, MRI missed 1 leiomyoma for every 2 or 3 patients and US missed more than 1 leiomyoma per patient. Nevertheless, most patients are initially evaluated with pelvic US because of its cost advantage, availability, and overall accuracy. If the US findings are equivocal, MRI is often performed.

Usually, US will reveal leiomyomas as hypoechoic masses in the uterus; they less often appear isoechoic or hyperechoic (see Figure 9-5).[3] Smaller leiomyomas usually have a uniform echotexture, but larger ones are frequently more heterogeneous due to cystic or myxoid degeneration or necrosis.[3] These tumors will contain smaller anechoic foci reflecting their cystic components. Calcification within fibroids appears similar to calcification elsewhere as a hyperechoic focus with posterior acoustic shadowing (see Figure 9-6). In some cases, the mass will only be inferred because of enlargement or contour deformity of the uterus. Exophytic fibroids can appear as adnexal masses and may be confused with ovarian lesions, but demonstration of a stalk or connection to the uterus is the key to a correct diagnosis. In most cases, leiomyomas will have prominent peripheral flow with little or no central flow on color Doppler US.[13]

Uterine leiomyomas are easily seen with routine MRI of the pelvis; IV contrast is not needed to make the diagnosis but can be helpful in certain situations. On T1-weighted images, leiomyomas typically have homogeneous intermediate SI relative to normal myometrium. On T2-weighted images, they typically appear as well-circumscribed masses of homogeneously low SI compared with that of the surrounding myometrium (see Figure 9-5).[17] Degenerated leiomyomas can have a variable MRI appearance.[17] Leiomyomas with cystic or myxoid degeneration will demonstrate high SI that approaches that of simple fluid on T2-weighted images. The cystic regions will not enhance, whereas myxoid regions will enhance with gadolinium-based contrast agents (see Figure 9-7). Necrotic tumors will also demonstrate variable imaging features on T1- and T2-weighted images that reflect the various stages of hemorrhage evolution. Fatty degeneration is revealed as high SI on T1-weighted images similar to macroscopic fat elsewhere in the pelvis with loss of SI on fat-suppressed T1-weighted images (see Figure 9-8). Some leiomyomas will exhibit a high-SI rim on T2-weighted images because of a pseudocapsule of edema, dilated lymphatic vessels, or dilated veins.[4] In the absence of metastatic disease, there are no well-established imaging criteria to distinguish leiomyomas from leiomyosarcomas. In general, leiomyosarcomas are much less common than leiomyomas and will generally have irregular margins, be larger in size, and more heterogeneous in SI. Although not necessary to make the diagnosis of uterine leiomyomas, IV contrast material can provide information about the lesion's vascularity. This is helpful if UAE is being considered for treatment, as tumors will little or no enhancement tend to respond poorly, whereas those

Imaging Notes 9-1. Distinguishing Leiomyomas and Leiomyosarcomas

There are no reliable imaging findings that distinguish the common benign uterine leiomyoma from the rare malignant leiomyosarcoma. Leiomyosarcoma should be considered when a uterine mass is large and has a heterogeneous appearance with irregular margins. Lymph node enlargement, distant metastases, and peritoneal carcinomatosis may also be seen with leiomyosarcomas. Uterine masses that continue to grow despite technically successful uterine artery embolization should be viewed with suspicion.

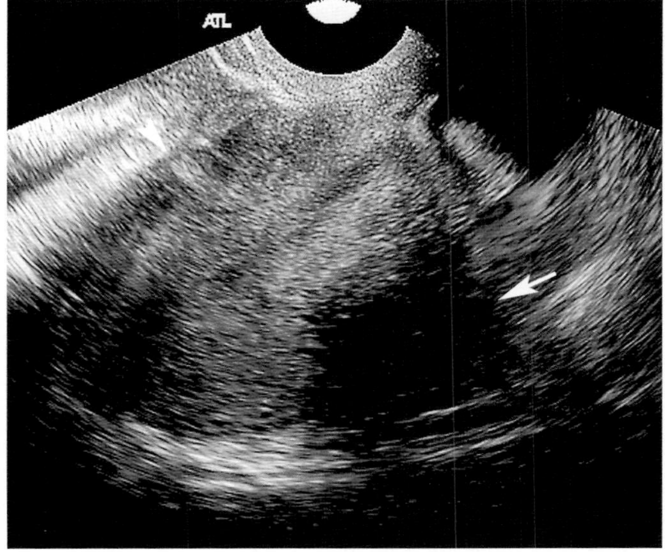

A

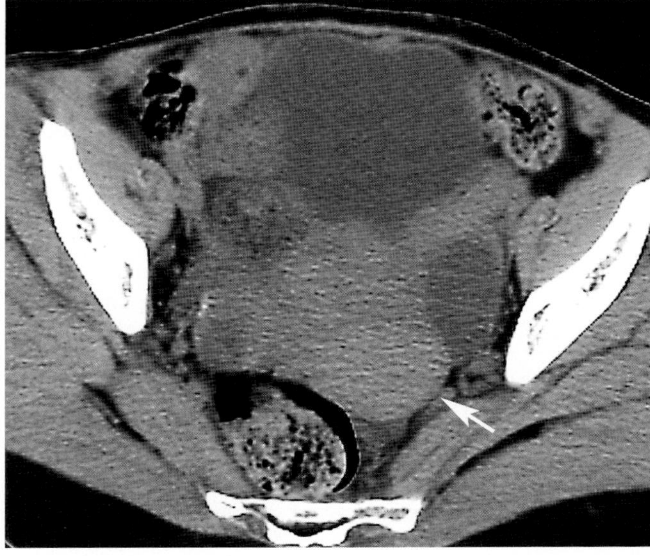

B

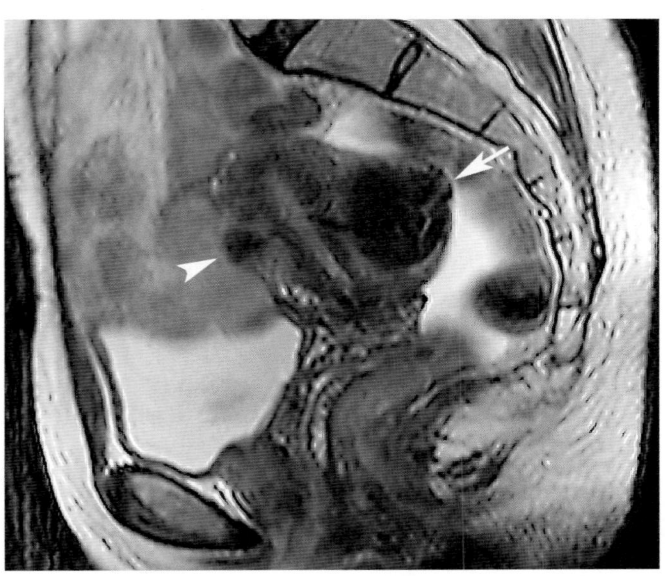

C

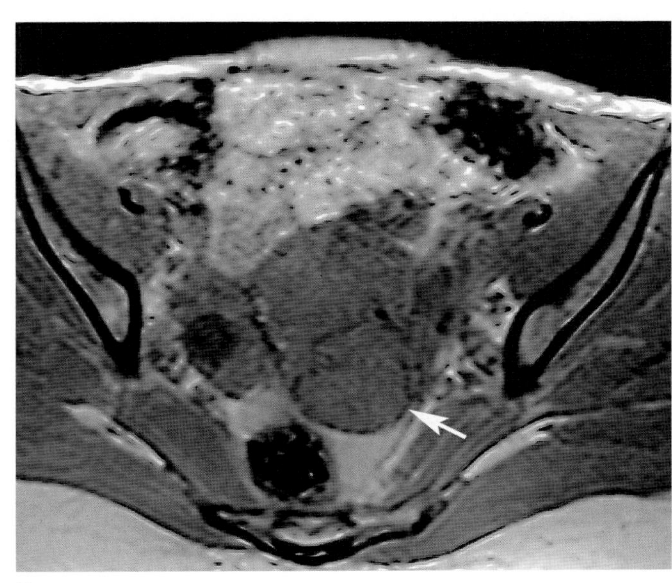

D

Figure 9-5 Uterine Fibroids
A 44-year-old woman with pelvic pain. **A.** Sagittal view of the uterus from TVUS demonstrates a hypoechoic shadowing mass in the posterior aspect of the uterine body. **B.** Unenhanced CT shows a contour deformity (*arrow*) of the uterus indicating the presence of a fibroid. **C.** Sagittal T2-weighted image demonstrates the fibroid as a round hypointense mass. A smaller fibroid not appreciated on the US or CT is present on the anterior wall (*arrowhead*). **D.** Axial T1-weighted image shows a contour deformity (*arrow*) along the posterior aspect of the uterus, which is all that can be seen of the uterine fibroid on this pulse sequence.

lesions with avid enhancement have better outcomes.[4] Similarly, tumors with high SI on T1-weighted images due to hemorrhagic or fatty degeneration are less likely to decrease in size after UAE; surgical treatment options may better serve these women.[4] Following successful UAE, contrast-enhanced MRI can demonstrate decrease in fibroid size and enhancement.

In most cases, uterine leiomyomas will not be detected on abdominal plain film radiography, as there is no intrinsic contrast with the surrounding uterus and other soft tissues. As such, radiographs are not routinely used when fibroids are suspected. Nonetheless, leiomyomas may be seen incidentally on radiographs performed for other reasons. Very large masses can occasionally be seen as a nonspecific soft tissue density pelvic mass displacing air-filled loops of bowel. In older patients, degenerated fibroids are frequently calcified, and radiographs will reveal coarse calcifications in the pelvis (see Figure 9-9).

Imaging Notes 9-2. Imaging Features Predicting Poor Response to Uterine Artery Embolization for Uterine Fibroids

1. Minimal or no contrast enhancement. Fibroids that do not enhance are effectively devascularized, and further devascularization by embolization may be of little benefit.
2. Fibroids with high signal intensity on T1-weighted images (indicating hemorrhagic necrosis or fatty degeneration).

Submucosal fibroids may be identified on HSG as filling defects, often with a smooth contour (see Figure 9-7).[6] Large tumors may distort the endometrial canal. These filling defects are best appreciated on the early filling images, as their conspicuity may decrease as the endometrial canal becomes further distended with contrast.

CT is the least sensitive of the cross-sectional imaging modalities for the evaluation of uterine fibroids. However, uterine fibroids are commonly encountered on CT studies obtained for other reasons. They can be suspected if the uterus appears enlarged or has a contour deformity (see Figure 9-5). In some cases, they will appear as discrete soft-tissue masses associated with the uterus (see Figure 9-10).[12]

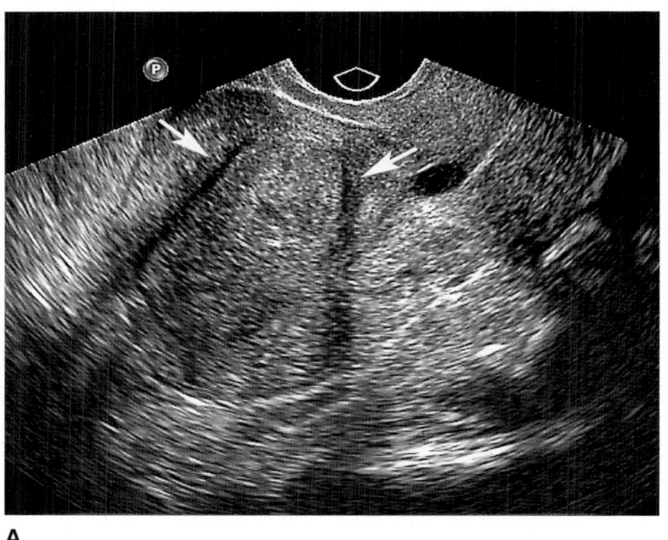

A

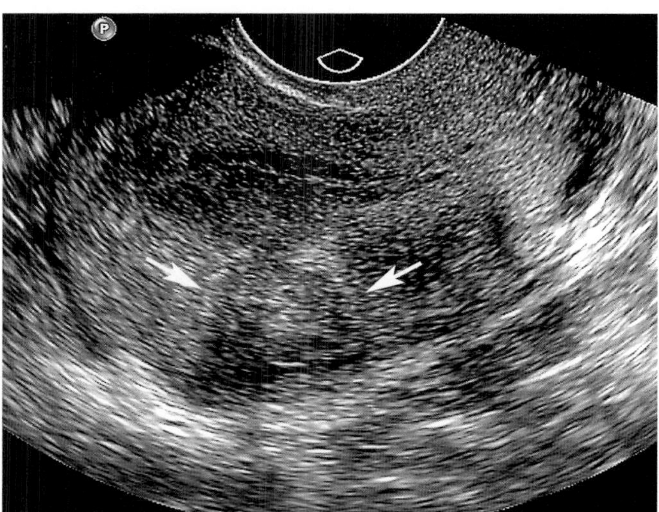

B

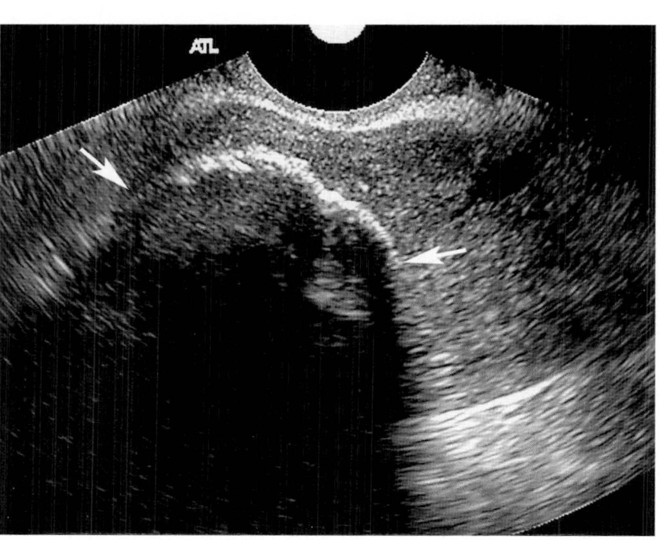

C

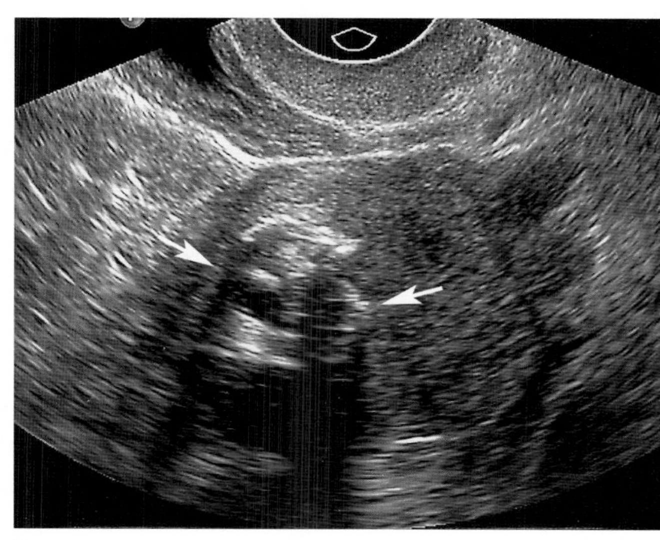

D

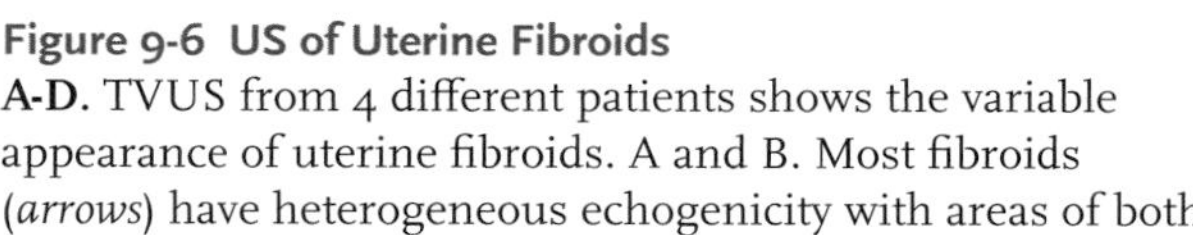

Figure 9-6 US of Uterine Fibroids
A-D. TVUS from 4 different patients shows the variable appearance of uterine fibroids. A and B. Most fibroids (*arrows*) have heterogeneous echogenicity with areas of both hyperechogenicity and hypoechogenicity. C and D. Calcification within degenerated fibroids results in hyperechoic foci (*arrows*) with intense posterior acoustic shadowing.

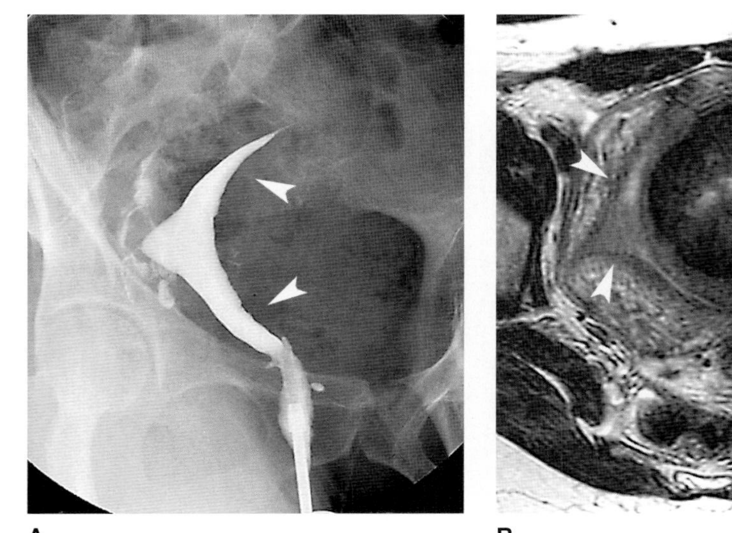
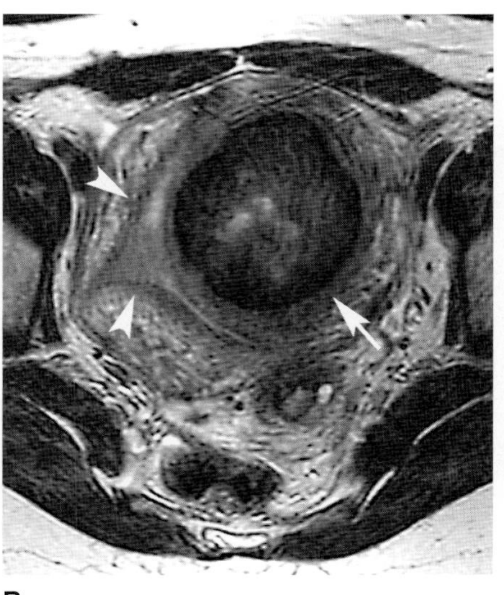
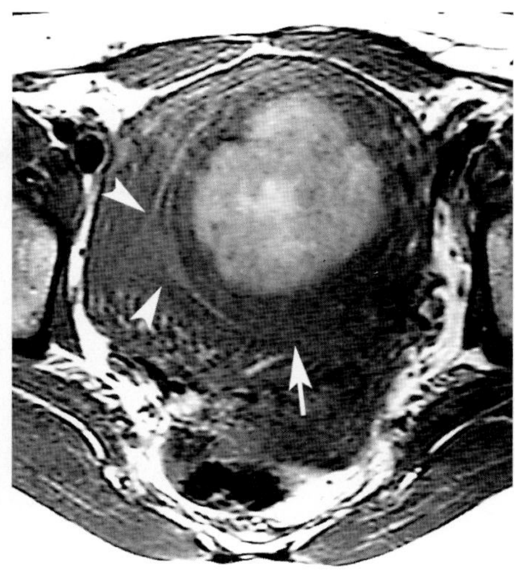

A B C

Figure 9-7 Submucosal Fibroid with Myxoid Degeneration **A.** Hysterosalpingogram shows a large smooth filling defect along the left side of the uterus, displacing it to the right (*arrowheads*). **B.** Axial T2-weighted image and (**C**) T1-weighted image with gadolinium contrast confirm the presence of a submucosal fibroid (*arrow*) displacing the endometrial canal (*arrowheads*). Note that the fibroid has high central T2 signal, which enhances—features indicating myxoid degeneration.

Calcification within degenerated fibroids is easily seen. Similarly, cystic or myxoid degeneration or central necrosis will often appear as regions of low attenuation.[12] Following IV contrast administration, leiomyomas can appear hypoattenuating, isoattenuating, or hyperattenuating relative to the normal myometrium. Small tumors will appear homogeneous, but larger masses will often appear heterogeneous as a result of degeneration or necrosis.

Uterine fibroids are frequently seen incidentally on FDG-PET studies that are obtained in women for other indications. Initial reports suggested that leiomyomas could be differentiated from leiomyosarcomas on the basis of FDG uptake, the former having no or little uptake and the latter being FDG avid. However, other reports have demonstrated FDG uptake in fibroids, thus limiting the ability of FDG-PET to distinguish these tumors.[9] Focal uptake within fibroids is observed more often in premenopausal women than postmenopausal women (10% vs 1%), perhaps related to hormonal influences on glucose metabolism. In this study, it was also observed that more than half of those fibroids with focal FDG uptake had SI on T2-weighted images that was equal to or higher than the adjacent myometrium.[9] This may be secondary to increased cellularity, as fibroids with higher T2-weighted SI are typically thought to be more cellular and contain less collagen. Finally, SUV levels can fluctuate with time, so increasing or newly appearing activity does not necessarily indicate malignant transformation.

Uterine sarcomas

Uterine sarcomas are considerably less common than other uterine cancers, representing approximately 3% to 5% of all uterine malignancies.[8] Sarcomas arise from mesenchymal elements in the endometrium or myometrium and, as a result, are a histologically diverse group of tumors. The 3 most common uterine sarcomas, in order of frequency, are carcinosarcoma (formerly malignant mixed müllerian tumor), leiomyosarcoma, and endometrial stromal sarcoma.[8] Other types are extremely rare. While the vast majority of leiomyosarcomas arise de novo within the myometrium, around 1% or less arise from the malignant degeneration of a leiomyoma.[18] In the absence of metastatic disease, leiomyomas and leiomyosarcomas are differentiated pathologically, based on the number of mitotic figures and the presence or absence of cellular atypia. A smooth muscle tumor of uncertain malignant potential (STUMP) is a smooth muscle tumor whose metastatic potential lies between that of a leiomyoma and a leiomyosarcoma. In general, uterine sarcomas affect women between the ages of 40 and 60 years and most commonly present with abnormal vaginal bleeding or a pelvic mass. The most significant risk factors appear to be a history of prior pelvic radiation and long-term tamoxifen use.[8] Unfortunately, the diagnosis of a uterine sarcoma is most commonly made pathologically at the time of surgery, often for presumed fibroids.

The imaging appearance of uterine sarcomas depends on the tumor type, invasiveness, and presence or absence of hemorrhage or necrosis. Tumor spread via direct extension, lymphatic drainage, or peritoneal or hematogenous dissemination can be identified.[18] In general, sarcomas appear as large masses that have a heterogeneous appearance with irregular margins. The endometrial canal can become distended with tumor, glandular secretions, or blood. The tumor can be seen to invade the myometrium

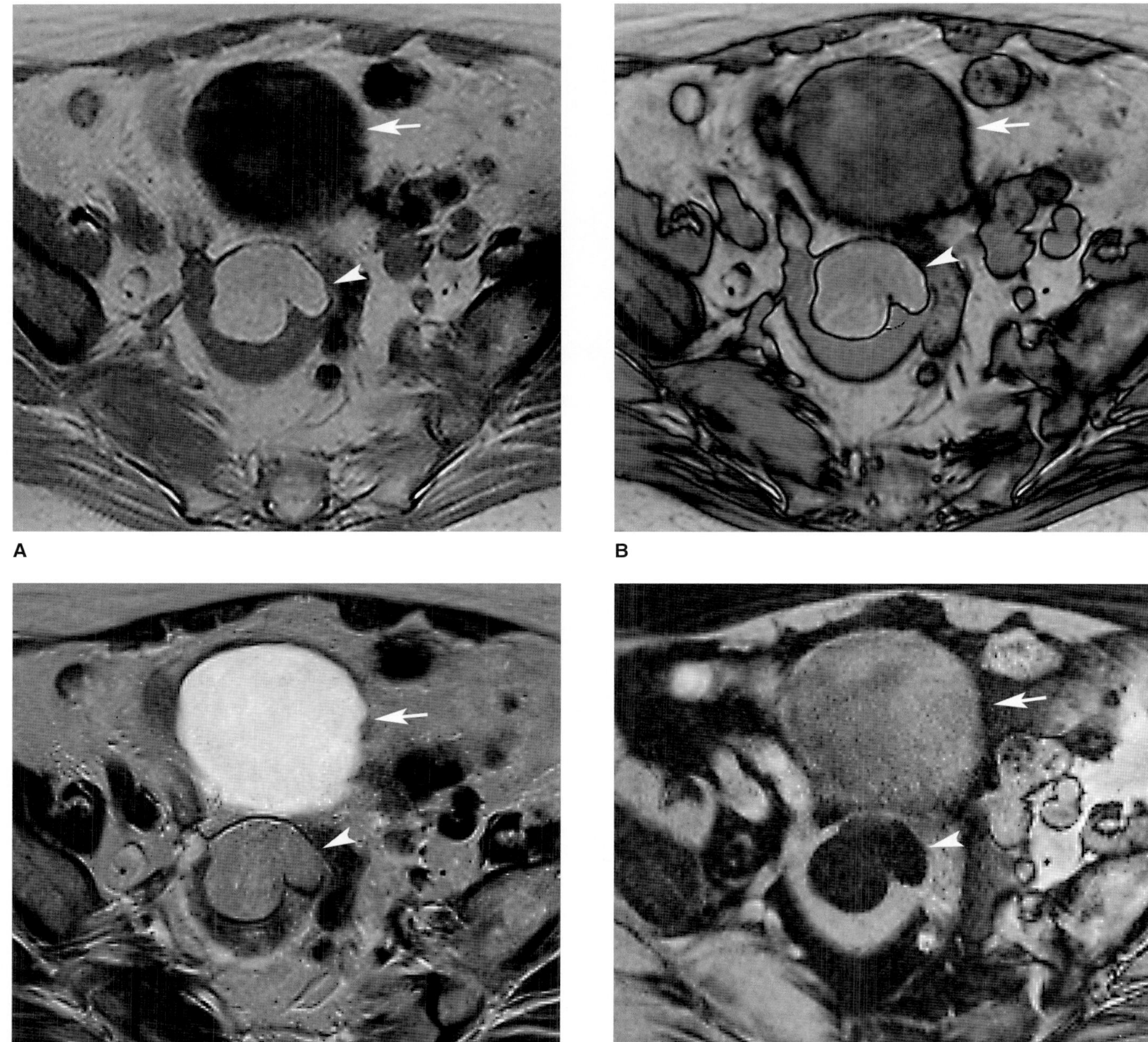

Figure 9-8 Fibroid with Fatty Degeneration
Axial (**A**) in-phase T1-weighted, (**B**) out-of-phase T1-weighted, (**C**) T2-weighted, and (**D**) T2-weighted fat suppressed images demonstrate a lobulated mass (*arrowheads*) in the anterior body of the uterus. The mass has SI which follows that of the abdominal fat on all sequences, has a peripheral etching artifact (indicating a fat-water interface) in (B), and loses SI after application of fat suppression (D). This represents fatty degeneration of a uterine fibroid and is also called a "lipoleiomyoma." The T1 hypointense and T2 hyperintense structure (*arrows*) anterior to the uterus is the urinary bladder.

or parametrium. Pelvic lymphadenopathy, ascites, or peritoneal metastases can often be seen. MRI is the study of choice to define extent of tumor and to characterize it as malignant. The appearance varies with the type of sarcoma, but generally appears as a homogeneous or heterogeneous mass on T1-weighted images with SI similar to that of the myometrium. Intratumoral hemorrhage will be shown as regions of high SI on T1-weighted images. Unlike fibroids, which

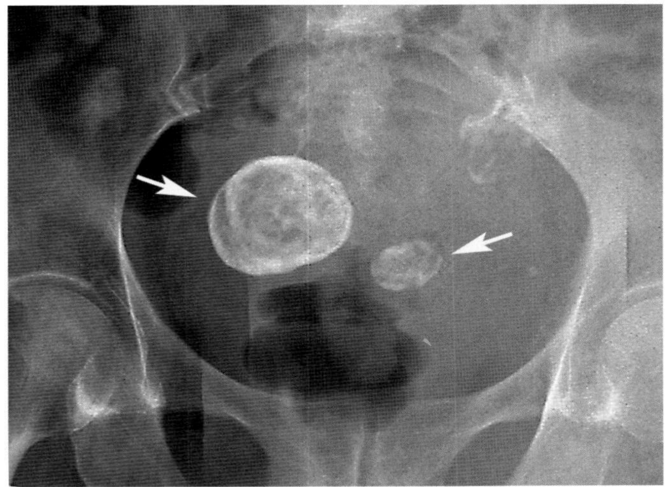

Figure 9-9 Calcified Uterine Fibroids
Anteroposterior radiograph of the pelvis shows 2 calcified masses (*arrows*) within the central pelvis. This is a typical appearance of calcified uterine fibroids.

are typically well circumscribed and of homogeneous low SI on T2-weighted images, sarcomas tend to be larger and have irregular margins with a more heterogeneous appearance with areas of low, intermediate, and high SI. The tumor margins can be seen to interrupt the low-SI junctional zone or grossly penetrate the serosal surface. Contrast-enhanced T1-weighted images will also show a heterogeneous appearance related to the presence of necrosis (see Figure 9-11).

Focal adenomyosis and adenomyoma

Adenomyosis is a disorder where endometrial glands and stroma are ectopically located within the myometrium of the uterus. Since adenomyosis typically presents as a diffuse imaging abnormality, it is discussed most completely in the subsequent section titled "Diffuse Abnormalities of the Uterus." However, in some cases it can cause either an indistinct focal abnormality or a discrete focal mass in the uterus and will be discussed briefly here.

Imaging findings reflect the ectopic endometrial glands and associated muscular hypertrophy that are seen in pathologic specimens of adenomyosis. Sonographically, adenomyosis typically appears as diffuse ill-defined areas of heterogeneous echotexture and hypoechogenicity. However, less commonly, adenomyosis will appear as a single or multiple regions of heterogeneous echotexture and hypoechogenicity. Focal adenomyosis can be confused with uterine fibroids; however, unlike leiomyomas, which are usually devoid of central color flow, Doppler imaging of focal adenomyosis will demonstrate normal vessels coursing through the areas of adenomyosis. Furthermore, adenomyosis often has little mass effect on the endometrium and seldom results in a uterine contour deformity, unlike uterine fibroids.

Imaging Notes 9-3. Features Differentiating Focal Adenomyosis from Uterine Fibroids on US Examinations

Feature	Adenomyosis	Fibroid
Margin	indistinct	distinct
Blood flow	present	absent
Contour deformity	absent	often present

Adenomyomas represent discrete masses of ectopic endometrial glands surrounded by myometrial hypertrophy and are difficult to distinguish from focal adenomyosis and uterine fibroids. Some adenomyomas will appear as focal low-SI masses on T2-weighted images, similar in appearance to fibroids but with internal foci of high SI similar to adenomyosis (see Figure 9-12). These combined features will be indicative of the presence of an adenomyoma. When the internal high T2-weighted image SI is not present, adenomyomas are not easily distinguished from uterine fibroids.

Transient uterine contraction

Transient uterine contractions are normal in both the gravid and non-gravid uterus and can be seen while imaging the pelvis. The contractions are most commonly seen on T2-weighted images and appear as focal or diffuse low-SI masses that may distort the endometrium (see Figure 9-13).[21,25] The imaging appearance can be indistinguishable from that of focal adenomyosis or fibroids. The key to the correct diagnosis is recognition of the transient nature of the abnormality, which does not persist on subsequent acquisitions. Similarly, uterine contractions resemble fibroids by US and appear as a circumscribed hypoechoic mass. The gray-scales appearances may be indistinguishable with the exception that the contraction is seen to move or resolve with time. Color Doppler can help differentiate the 2 entities, as fibroids typically have peripheral, but no

Imaging Notes 9-4. Distinguishing Adenomyomas from Fibroids on MRI

An adenomyoma can be indistinguishable from a uterine fibroid on MRI examinations, as both may appear as focal circumscribed masses with low signal intensity on T2WI. However, the presence of internal foci of high T2WI signal intensity, similar to adenomyosis, will indicate the diagnosis of an adenomyoma.

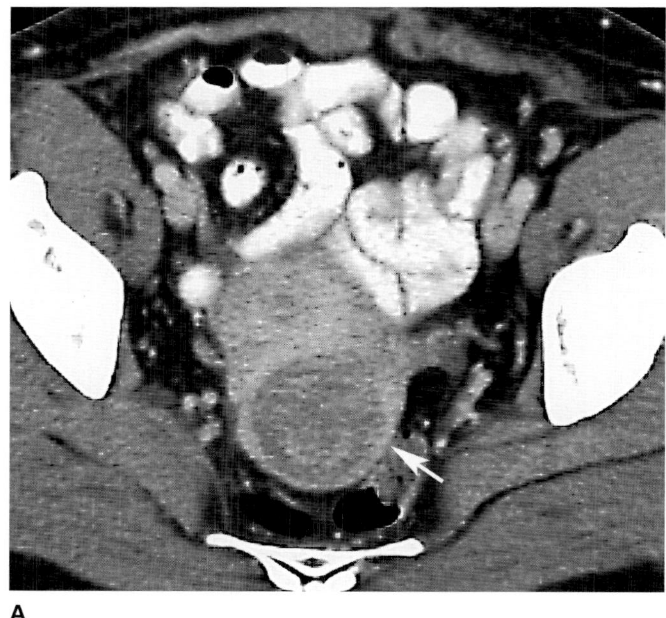

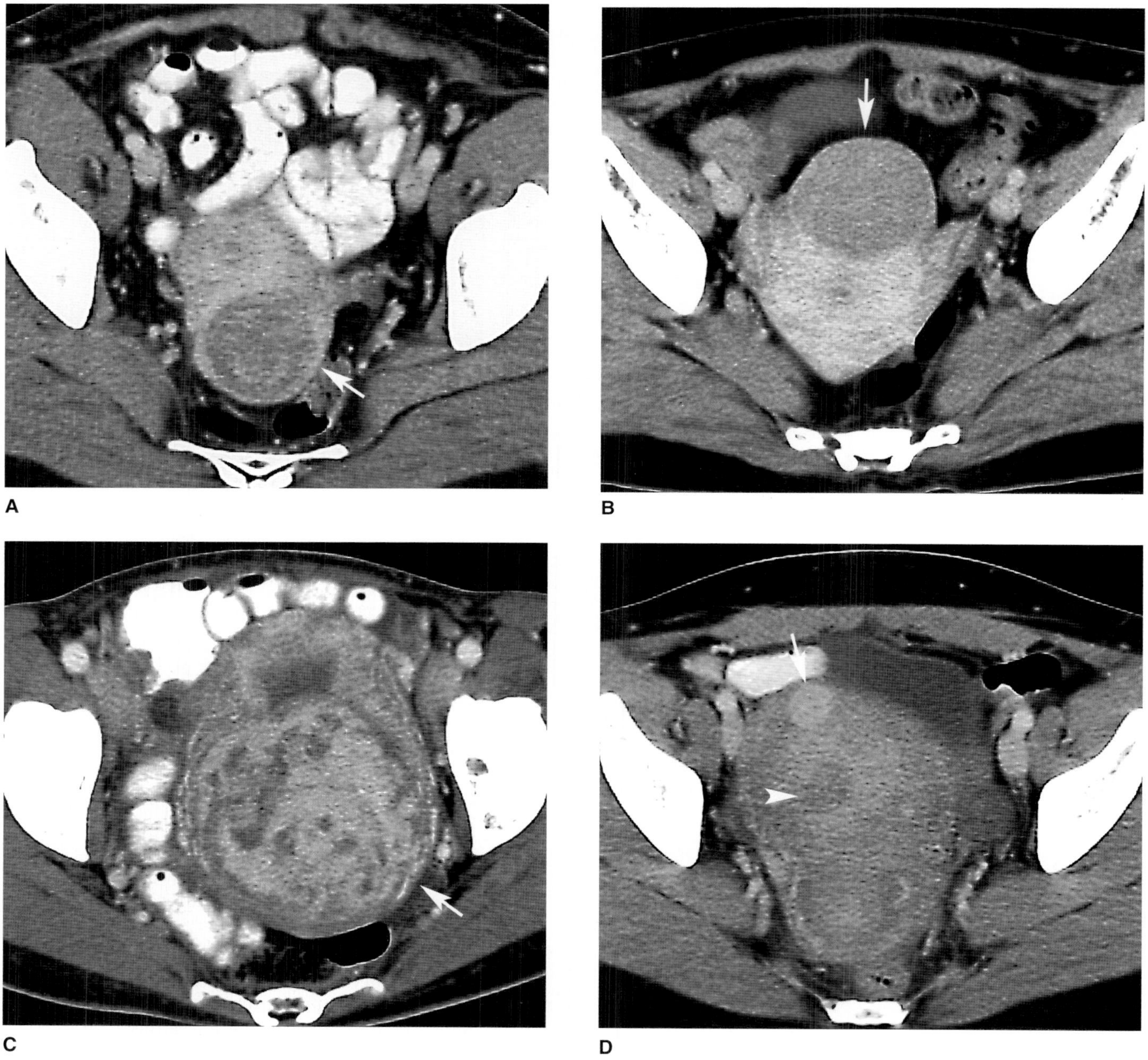

A

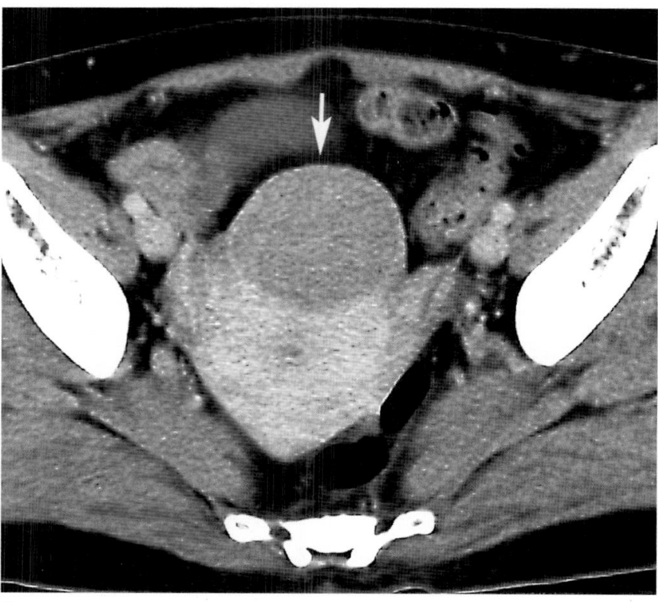

B

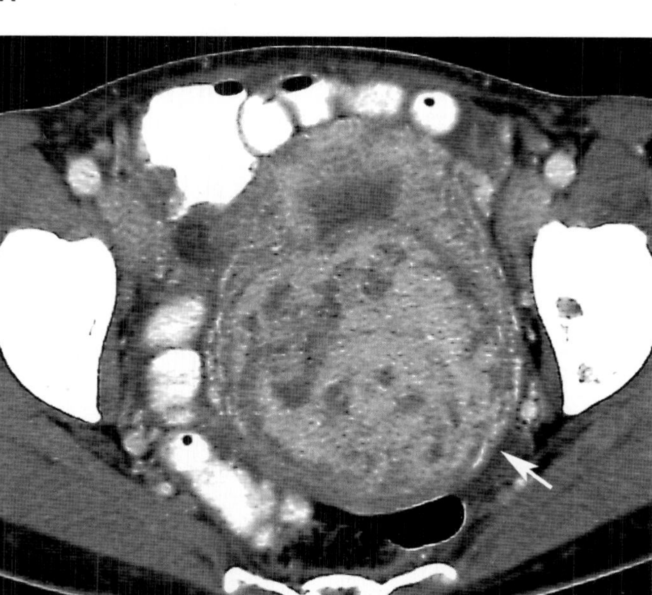

C

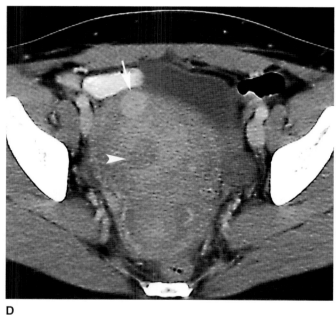

D

Figure 9-10 CT of Uterine Fibroids
Contrast-enhanced CT scans (**A-D**) of 4 separate patients demonstrate discrete uterine masses (*arrows*) in the subserosal (A and B), submucosal (C), and intramural (*arrowhead* in D) locations. The masses are variably hypoattenuating, hyperattenuating, or isoattenuating relative to the myometrium, demonstrating the variable appearance of uterine fibroids. The large fibroid in (C) is more heterogeneous in appearance.

central, flow and uterine contractions usually have color flow throughout the area of myometrial thickening.[66] The contractions can persist for up to 30 to 45 minutes.

Focal Endometrial Masses

Polyps, endometrial hyperplasia, and endometrial carcinoma will most often appear as diffuse endometrial thickening on US, MRI, and CT examinations of the uterus and

Imaging Notes 9-5. Transient Uterine Contractions

Transient uterine contractions can mimic focal masses on imaging exams. They are frequently mistaken for fibroids, as they appear as focal hypoechoic masses on US and low-signal-intensity masses on T2WI. The key to the correct diagnosis is recognition that the finding is transient.

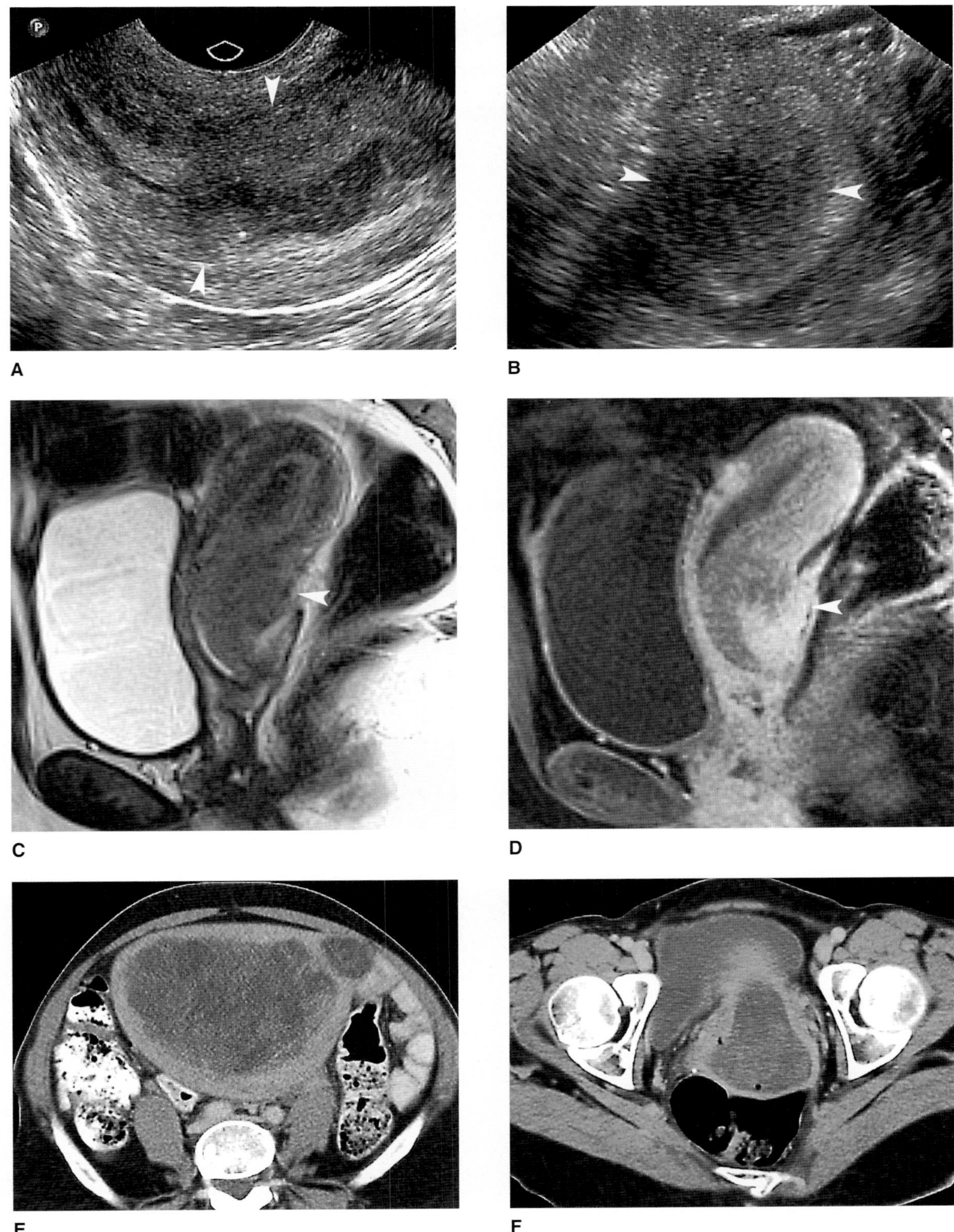

Figure 9-11 Uterine Sarcomas
A. Sagittal and (**B**) coronal TVUS of the uterus demonstrates a heterogeneous, indistinctly marginated mass (*arrowheads*) in the posterior wall and lower uterine segment of the uterus. Note the irregular shape of the lower uterine canal. **C.** Corresponding T2-weighted image and (**D**) fat-suppressed postcontrast T1-weighted image confirm the presence of an irregular mass with indistinct margins. These findings raise the possibility of a uterine sarcoma, which was confirmed at surgical biopsy and resection. **E** and **F.** Contrast-enhanced CT images in a different patient demonstrate an inhomogeneously enhancing mass within the uterus that extends into the endocervical canal. This could represent a large endometrial carcinoma. However, surgical biopsy was diagnostic of a high-grade uterine sarcoma.

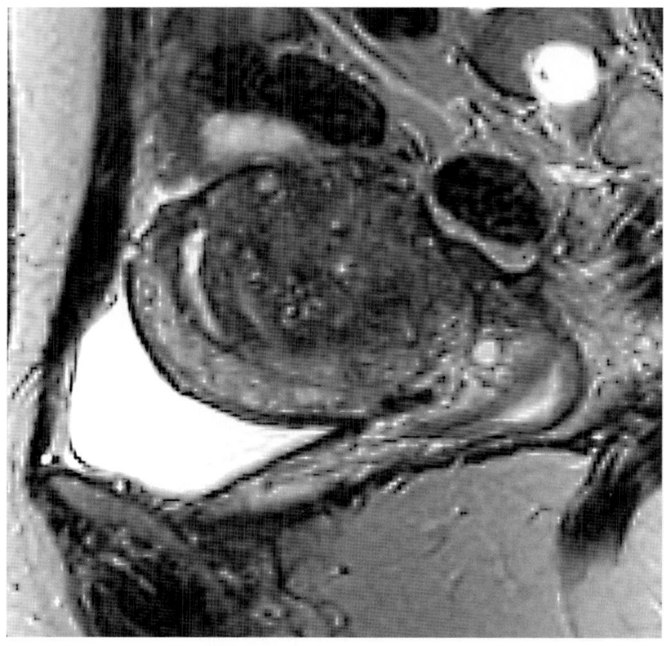

A

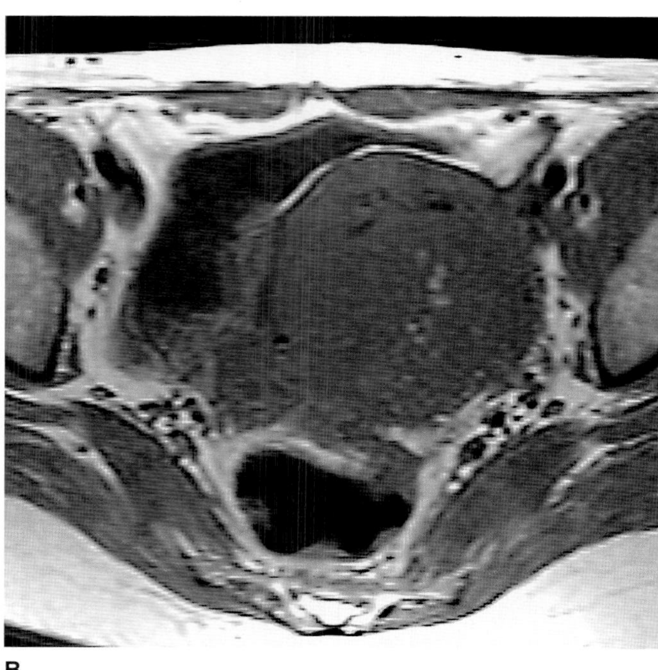

B

Figure 9-12 Adenomyoma
A. Sagittal T2-weighted image and (**B**) axial T1-weighted image demonstrate a focal myometrial mass in the posterior body of the uterus. In most cases, masses in this location will represent leiomyomas. However, this mass contains multiple foci of high T1 and T2 SI indicating the presence of hemorrhage products and endometrial glands. This combination of findings is indicative of an adenomyoma.

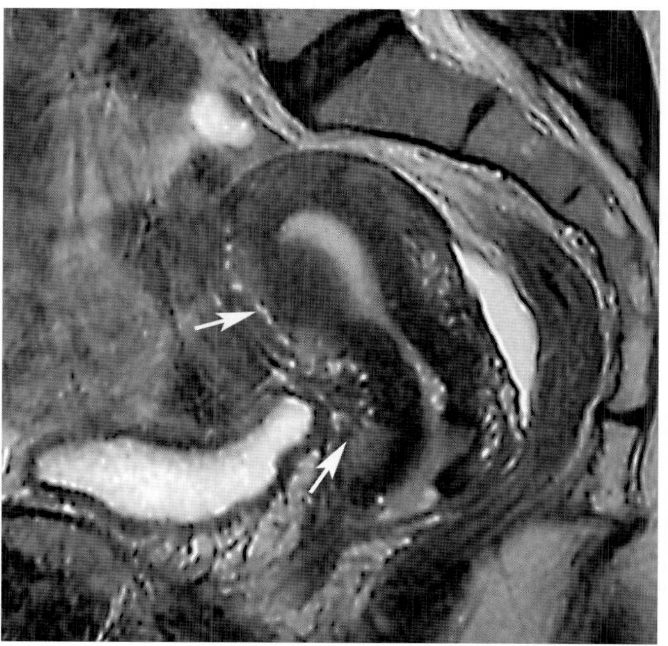

A

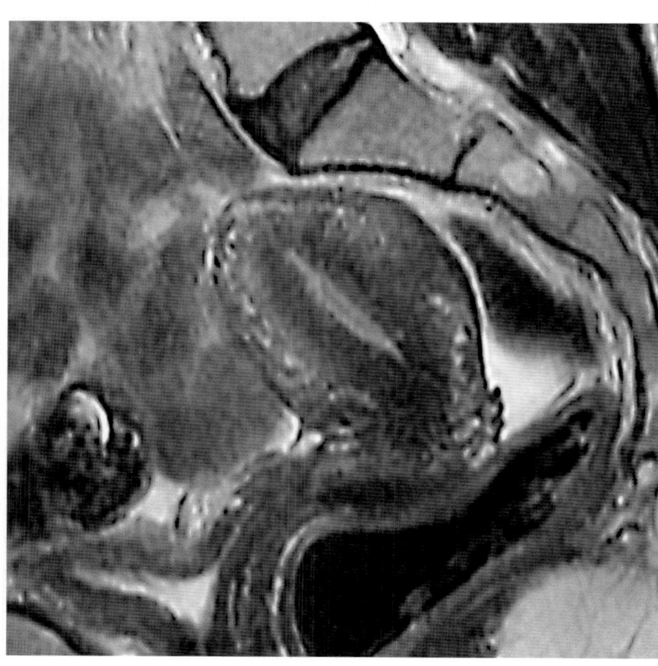

B

Figure 9-13 Transient Uterine Contraction Appearing as Myometrial Masses
A. Sagittal T2-weighted image shows several lobular mass–like low-SI areas within the anterior uterine body. **B.** Sagittal T2-weighted image taken 6 months later shows absence of the masses that represented transient uterine contractions.

are discussed in the next section under the heading: **Diffuse Endometrial Thickening**. However, fluid present within the endometrial cavity may outline these lesions and they can appear as discrete endometrial masses. Submucosal leiomyomas and uterine sarcomas can also project into the endometrial cavity producing an apparent focal endometrial mass.

DIFFUSE ABNORMALITIES OF THE UTERUS

Diffuse abnormalities of the uterus include diffuse endometrial thickening and diffuse abnormalities of the myometrium.

Diffuse Endometrial Thickening

The normal premenopausal endometrium thickens in response to circulating hormones and in a menstruating woman, the thickness of the endometrium is usually not an important finding. However, in postmenopausal women, endometrial thickening, defined as an endometrial thickness greater than 5 mm, is an abnormal finding. In most cases, postmenopausal endometrial thickening will be discovered during an US examination as part of the evaluation for postmenopausal bleeding. Vaginal bleeding in post menopausal woman is most often secondary to endometrial atrophy (~75%), endometrial polyps, endometrial hyperplasia, and endometrial carcinoma (Table 9-2).[2,26] Owing to the risk of endometrial carcinoma and because imaging cannot always reliably differentiate endometrial hyperplasia, polyps, and carcinoma, detection of an abnormal postmenopausal endometrium requires further evaluation. A 2001 consensus statement by a panel of experts from the Society of Radiologists in Ultrasound has proposed that tissue sampling or saline-infused sonohysterography should be performed when transvaginal US (TVUS) in a woman with postmenopausal bleeding demonstrates a focal endometrial abnormality, diffuse endometrial thickening greater than 5 mm, or when the entire endometrium is not adequately visualized.[27]

Endometrial hyperplasia

Endometrial hyperplasia represents a spectrum of proliferative lesions of the endometrium ranging from benign to premalignant to malignant, resulting from the abnormal proliferation of the endometrial glands and supporting stroma.[2] Several classification schemes have been proposed for the different endometrial hyperplasias, all of which attempt to delineate those conditions with malignant potential from those that are uniformly benign. Unfortunately, from an imaging standpoint, these lesions are morphologically similar and cannot be reliably differentiated. Determination of malignant potential, which in turn guides management, falls under the domain of the pathologist.

Endometrial hyperplasia most commonly affects women in their perimenopausal and postmenopausal years and presents with irregular and heavy vaginal bleeding.[28] Hyperplasia results from the unopposed action of estrogen on the endometrium; progesterone has the opposite effect and inhibits endometrial growth.[26,29] Thus, conditions that expose the endometrium to higher than normal levels of estrogen (endogenous or exogenous) place women at risk for the development of endometrial hyperplasia. These conditions include obesity, diabetes mellitus, hypertension, nulliparity, hormone replacement therapy, anovulatory cycles, polycystic ovarian disease, and estrogen-producing tumors (eg, granulosa cell tumors, ovarian thecomas).[28,30] Women with hyperplasia with atypia will have concomitant endometrial carcinoma 30% to 40% of the time.[26]

US and MRI are the imaging modalities best able to reveal the endometrial proliferation. By both modalities, endometrial hyperplasia typically appears as homogeneous diffuse thickening of the endometrium (see Figure 9-14). In many cases, the endometrium will measure 10 mm or more.[2] Cystic spaces, representing dilated glands, may also been seen within the areas of thickening.[28] The echotexture is usually homogeneous but can occasionally be heterogeneous with areas of hyperechogenicity and hypoechogenicity. As a result of its lower contrast resolution, CT is not the modality of choice in evaluating endometrial hyperplasia. However, women with endometrial hyperplasia can be imaged by CT for other reasons. In this situation, endometrial hyperplasia will most often appear as homogeneous endometrial thickening (see Figure 9-15). Occasionally, focal hyperplasia results in a focal endometrial mass, which appears similar to an endometrial polyp, endometrial carcinoma, or submucosal fibroid (Table 9-3).[2,26,30]

Table 9-2. Causes of Postmenopausal Bleeding

1. Endometrial atrophy
2. Endometrial hyperplasia
3. Endometrial polyp
4. Endometrial carcinoma

Endometrial polyp

Endometrial polyps are benign localized hyperplastic overgrowths of endometrial glands and stroma.[26] Polyps are second to endometrial atrophy in causing postmenopausal bleeding.[26] Premenopausal women may present with abnormal vaginal bleeding or infertility. Polyps are most often solitary but can be multiple in approximately 20% of cases.[2,26,31] They are most often pedunculated via a thin fibrovascular stalk, but occasionally are sessile with a broad-based attachment to the endometrium.[2,26,31] Rarely, endometrial polyps are histologically classified as adenomyomatous and contain hypertrophic smooth muscle and

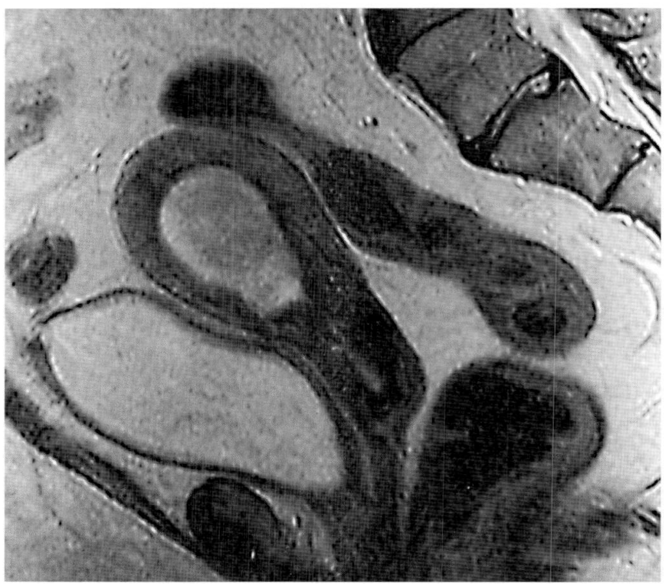

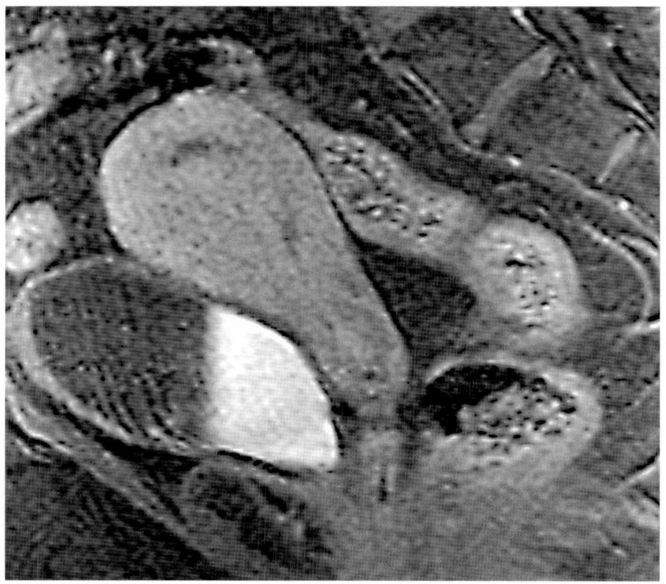

Figure 9-14 Endometrial Hyperplasia
A 38-year-old woman with history of infertility and polycystic ovary syndrome and family history of endometrial carcinoma. **A.** Sagittal T2-weighted image and (**B**) sagittal fat-suppressed postcontrast T1-weighted image demonstrate a diffusely thickened and uniformly enhancing endometrium. This is a nonspecific finding that could be due to endometrial hyperplasia, polyp, or carcinoma. Biopsy was diagnostic of endometrial hyperplasia.

endometrial glands. Foci of hyperplasia or carcinoma are found histologically within polyps about 1% of the time.[2,31,32]

Polyps are generally found in women undergoing pelvic US for postmenopausal bleeding, but can also be identified on MRI. Polyps typically appear as diffuse or focal endometrial thickening (see Figure 9-16).[26,31] The polyp can be seen as a discrete mass when endometrial fluid is present.[26,31] Saline-infused sonohysterography, which purposefully provides endometrial fluid, is the optimum study to delineate endometrial polyps as well-circumscribed smooth uniformly echogenic intracavitary masses (see Figure 9-17). Small cystic spaces may be seen in the polyps, representing dilated glands.[2,30] The endometrial-myometrial interface should be normal. This can be an important distinguishing feature between polyps and invasive endometrial carcinoma where the endometrial-myometrial interface is disrupted. With color Doppler US, vessels in the stalk can be identified (see Figure 9-17).[30] As expected, saline-infused sonohysterography outperforms routine TVUS with greater sensitivity (93% vs 65%) and specificity (94% vs 76%).[26]

Similarly, polyps are revealed on T2-weighted image MRI as intermediate- to high-SI sessile or pedunculated masses surrounded by higher SI fluid or endometrium (see Figure 9-17).[33] Small foci of high T2-weighted image SI within the polyp correspond to the cystic glands.

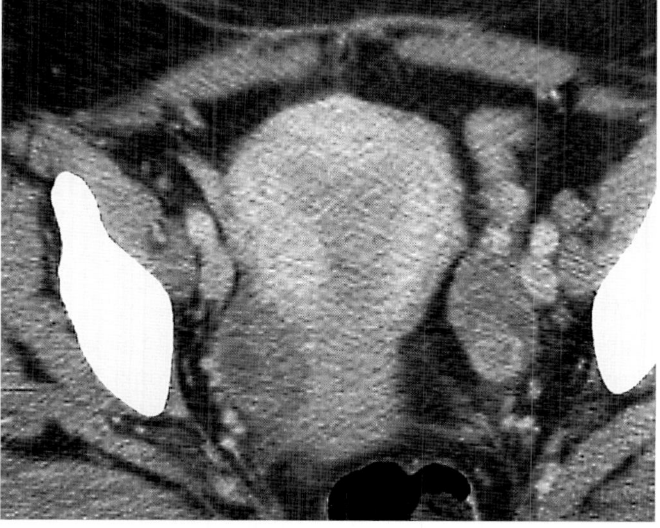

Figure 9-15 Endometrial Hyperplasia on CT
A 43-year-old woman with abdominal pain. Contrast-enhanced CT of the uterus demonstrates diffuse thickened endometrium. The endometrium is homogeneously enhancing. Complete workup, including endometrial biopsy, revealed endometrial hyperplasia.

Table 9-3. Causes of a Focal Endometrial Mass

1. Endometrial polyp
2. Endometrial hyperplasia
3. Endometrial carcinoma
4. Submucosal fibroid

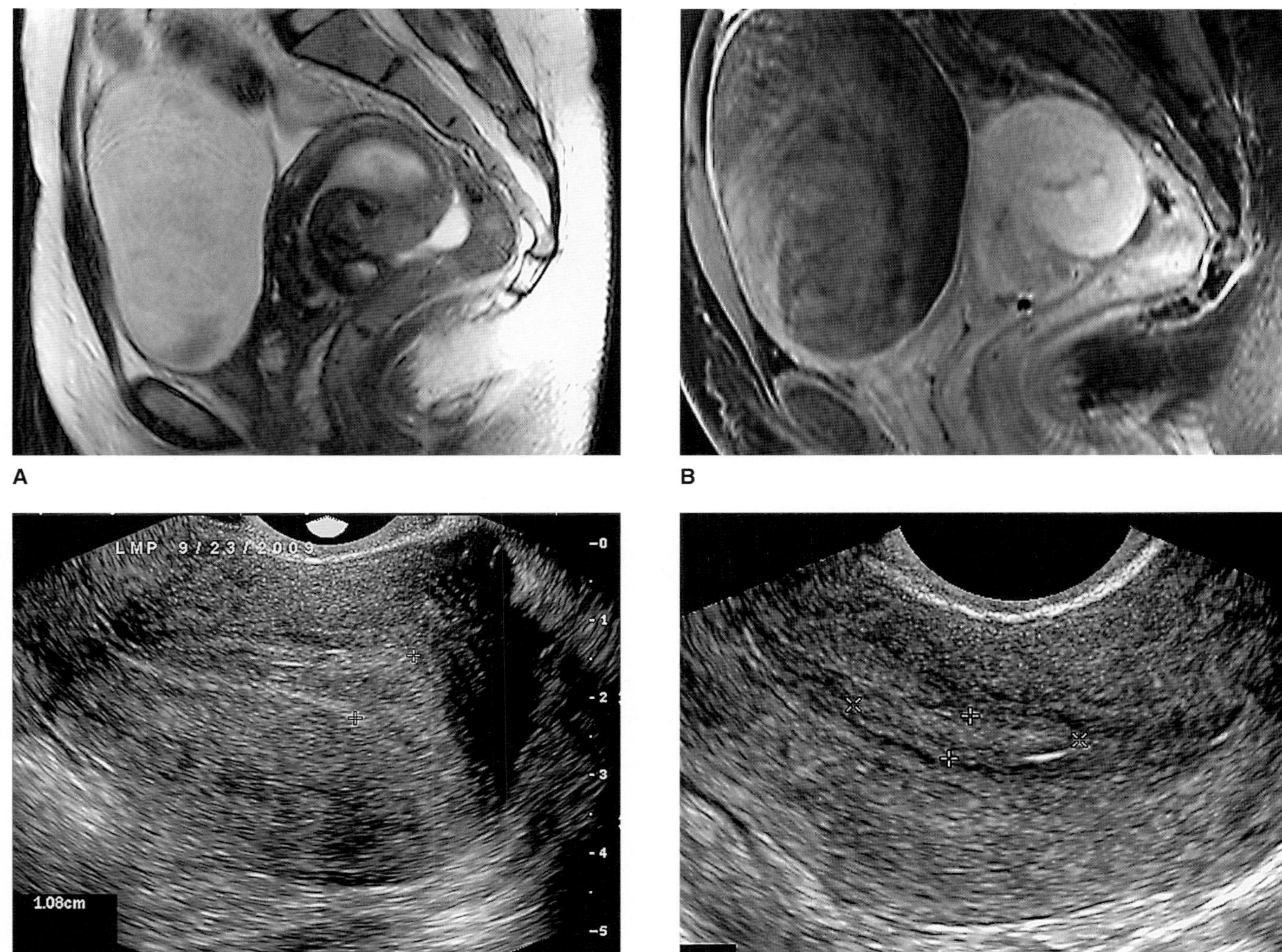

Figure 9-16 Endometrial Polyp Appearing as Diffuse Thickening A 25-year-old woman with history of infertility. **A.** Sagittal T2-weighted image and (**B**) sagittal fat-suppressed postcontrast T1-weighted image show uniformly enhancing diffuse endometrial thickening. **C.** Sagittal TVUS shows uniform endometrial thickening. In most menstruating women, this will represent the normal proliferative endometrium. **D.** A second sagittal TVUS view suggests the presence of a discrete structure within the endometrial canal. The pathologic specimen was characteristic of a polyp.

The fibrovascular core may appear as a central stripe of low SI on T2-weighted images within the stalk of the polyp.[33] The sensitivity and specificity of MRI are reported as 79% and 89%, respectively.[33] In some cases, endometrial polyps will appear as uniform thickening of the endometrial stripe indistinguishable from endometrial hyperplasia or carcinoma (see Figure 9-16). One study showed that accuracy was not high enough to obviate need for biopsy.[33]

Endometrial polyps are not reliably detected or characterized by CT. The endometrium may appear normal if the polyp is small or may present as focal or diffuse endometrial thickening.

Polyps appear as nonspecific smooth filling defects in the contrast pool at HSG, similar in appearance to intracavitary fibroids and some focal endometrial cancers (see Figure 9-16).[6] The reported sensitivity of HSG varies between 50% and 98%.[6]

Endometrial carcinoma

Endometrial carcinoma is the most common gynecologic malignancy in the United States and the fourth most common cause of cancer in women, accounting for an estimated 6% of new cancer diagnoses in 2008.[34] The average estimated lifetime risk is 1 in 41.[34] Interestingly, the incidence has declined about 0.8% per year since 1998.[35] It is estimated that 40,100 women will be diagnosed with endometrial cancer in 2008 and 7,470 will die.[35] The median age at diagnosis is 61 years, with 90% of cases occurring over 50 years of age.[27,36] Eighty percent of cases occur after menopause.[36]

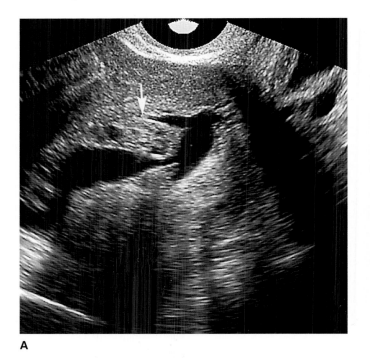

A

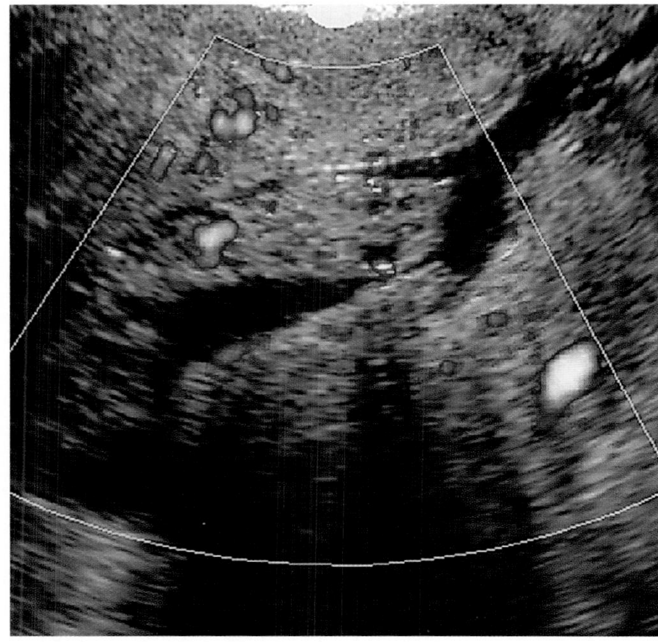

B

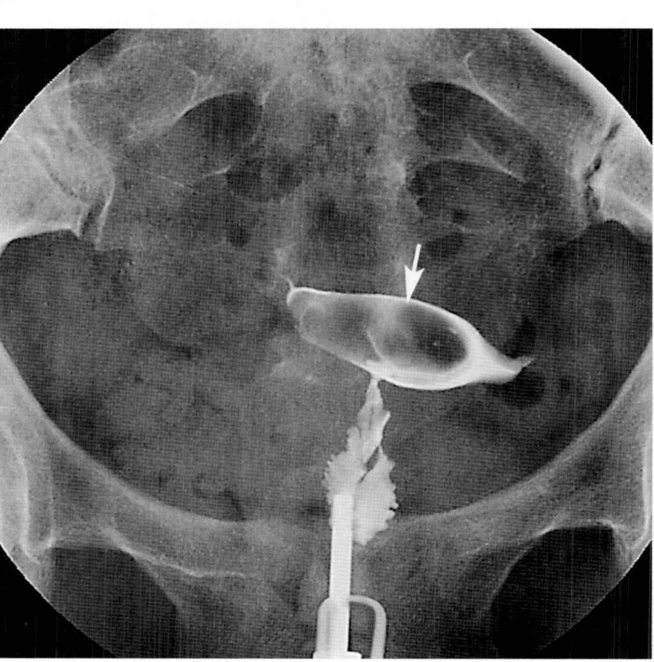

C

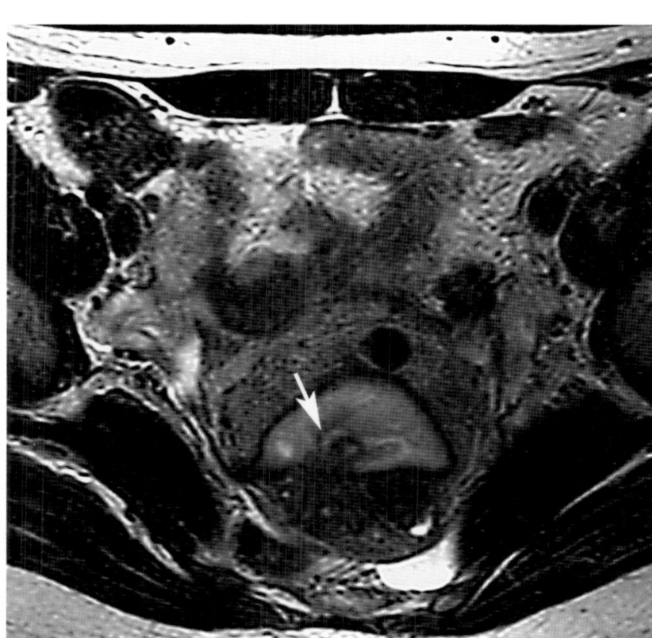

D

Figure 9-17 Endometrial Polyp
Three women with history of vaginal bleeding. **A.** Sagittal image from a saline-infused sonohysterogram demonstrates a polypoid mass (*arrow*) projecting into the fluid-filled endometrial canal. Small cystic spaces are commonly seen in polyps. **B.** Power Doppler shows blood flow within the mass as well as a prominent central vessel. **C.** Hysterosalpingogram in a different patient shows a sausage-shaped filling defect (*arrow*) within the endometrial canal. Contrast surrounds most of the mass, except for a small region along the right lateral wall of the endometrium. These findings are typical of an intrauterine polyp. **D.** Axial T2-weighted image in a third patient shows a small polypoid lesion (*arrow*) against the background of the high-SI endometrium. Focal thickening of the junctional zone with foci of high T2 SI in the posterior wall is indicative of focal adenomyosis.

Risk factors are similar to those for endometrial hyperplasia, with risk related to continuous endogenous or exogenous estrogen stimulation. These include obesity, anovulatory cycles, nulliparity, cirrhosis, estrogen-producing tumors, diabetes mellitus, and tamoxifen therapy.[36,37] The majority of cases have a precursor lesion such as hyperplasia with atypia or endometrial intraepithelial neoplasm.[36] About 10% of endometrial carcinomas do not result from excess estrogen stimulation and are more frequently aggressive with a poorer prognosis.[36]

Endometrial carcinoma has traditionally been classified into 3 types—type I, type II, and type III.[36] The different types affect different demographics, have different histologic subtypes, and carry different prognoses. Type I is the most common type and typically occurs in younger, obese, Caucasian women and is related to estrogen stimulation. These patients tend to have well-differentiated low-grade tumors, with endometrioid as the most common subtype, which frequently arise in a background of hyperplasia. These lesions are superficially invasive with rare extrauterine spread, resulting in an excellent prognosis.[36] Type II accounts for about 10% of cases and typically occurs in thin, multiparous, African American women.[36] These patients often develop poorly differentiated tumors with deep myometrial invasion and have a high incidence of metastasis to pelvic lymph nodes and other sites. Type II cancers are more frequently of the papillary serous or clear-cell histologies and carry a worse prognosis. Finally, type III disease is hereditary and may have a familial association or occur in the setting of Lynch II syndrome.

The majority of patients with endometrial carcinoma will present with abnormal vaginal bleeding; however, only between 4% and 10% of cases of postmenopausal bleeding will be due to endometrial carcinoma.[26,30,37] About 25% of patients will be perimenopausal and the abnormal bleeding pattern may be more difficult to recognize. Bleeding frequently prompts patients to present early and approximately 75% of women are diagnosed with stage I disease.[37] Prognosis depends on the stage of disease and is determined surgically, most frequently with total hysterectomy, bilateral salpingo-oophorectomy, pelvic washings, and pelvic and para-aortic lymphadenectomy.[38,39]

Factors that appear to predict survival include depth of myometrial invasion, histologic subtype, degree of histologic differentiation, lymph node status, and tumor stage.[37,39] The degree of myometrial invasion is one of the most reliable prognostic indicators, with superficially invasive cancers having a better prognosis than deeply invasive cancers. Not surprisingly, well-differentiated tumors typically have lesser degrees of myometrial invasion than poorly differentiated tumors and thus have a better prognosis. As noted previously, the endometrioid subtype has improved survival relative to papillary serous and clear-cell variants. Endometrial cancer is most often staged according to the criteria put forth by the International Federation of Obstetrics and Gynecology (FIGO) (Table 9-4).[37,39] Stage I disease is limited to the uterine corpus and is divided into Ia, Ib, and Ic. Stage Ia tumors are confined to the endometrium, whereas stage Ib and Ic tumors invade <50% and ≥50% the thickness of the myometrium, respectively. Direct invasion of the cervix confers a diagnosis of stage II disease and increases mortality. Invasion of the vagina, adnexa, or pelvic or para-aortic lymph node metastasis indicates stage III disease. With stage IV disease, more advanced tumors demonstrate direct invasion of the bladder or bowel wall and distant metastases including peritoneal implants, hematogenous metastases, and intra-abdominal or inguinal lymph node metastases.

On US, endometrial carcinoma will often appear as irregular endometrial thickening with areas of heterogeneous echotexture (see Figure 9-18).[26,30,39] The margins of the endometrial mass are frequently ill-defined. The findings are not specific and can overlap with those of endometrial polyps and hyperplasia. A more specific finding of carcinoma is interruption of the endometrial-myometrial interface; this indicates invasive disease and should not be seen with polyps or hyperplasia.[2,26,30,39] A small volume of fluid in the endometrial canal or homogeneous thickening of the endometrium are findings that are less likely to indicate endometrial carcinoma and will usually indicate other endometrial pathologies. In 2 studies of postmenopausal bleeding, endometrial cancers had an average endometrial stripe thickness of 18.2 ± 6.2 mm and 21.1 ± 11.8 mm and in no case was the thickness less than 5 mm.[40,41] In postmenopausal women with vaginal bleeding, various endometrial thicknesses have been proposed as thresholds that should prompt endometrial biopsy. Many sources propose that an endometrial thickness greater than 4 mm should prompt histologic evaluation. In 1 series, this criterion had an 87.3% positive predictive value for endometrial pathology and a 100% negative predictive value for endometrial carcinoma.[41] Use of the 4-mm criterion can reduce the number of uterine curettages by 70%. As the threshold increases, sensitivity is traded for specificity and small cancers may be missed. One study showed a 0.6% prevalence rate of endometrial cancer when the endometrial thickness

Imaging Notes 9-6. Imaging Findings Favoring Endometrial Carcinoma over Other Endometrial Pathologies

1. Excessive thickening of the endometrial stripe
2. Absence of endometrial fluid
3. Heterogeneous echotexture/signal intensity of the endometrial stripe
4. Indistinct margins of the endometrial mass
5. Invasion of the myometrium with loss of the endometrial-myometrial interface

Table 9-4. TNM[a] and FIGO[b] Staging of Endometrial Carcinoma with Corresponding MRI Findings

TNM	FIGO Stage	Description	MRI Findings
TX		Primary tumor cannot be assessed	
T0		Primary tumor cannot be identified	None
Tis	0	Carcinoma in situ	None
T1	I	Confined to uterine corpus	Tumor confined to uterine corpus
T1a	Ia	Confined to the endometrium without myometrial invasion	Diffusely or focally thickened endometrium with abnormal SI; junctional zone intact
T1b	Ib	Myometrial invasion <50%	Abnormal SI of tumor interrupts low-SI junctional zone with <50% myometrial invasion; irregularity of the endometrial-myometrial interface
T1c	Ic	Myometrial invasion ≥50%	Abnormal SI of tumor interrupts low-SI junctional zone with ≥50% myometrial invasion; irregularity of the endometrial-myometrial interface
T2	II IIa IIb	Extension into cervix but not beyond the uterus Cervical extension limited to endocervix Extension into the cervical stroma	Tumor extends from uterine corpus into cervix Widening of the endocervical canal and internal os; low-SI cervical stroma intact Abnormal SI of tumor interrupts low-SI cervical stroma
T3	III	Regional extension beyond the uterus but not outside the true pelvis (excludes invasion of the rectum or bladder)	Tumor extends beyond the uterus
T3a	IIIa	Extension to serosa and/or adnexa and/or positive peritoneal cytology	Abnormal SI of tumor extends beyond outer uterine contour
T3b	IIIb	Vaginal involvement (via direct extension or metastasis)	Interruption of the low-SI vaginal wall
N1	IIIc	Metastases to pelvic and/or para-aortic lymph nodes	Enlarged regional lymph nodes >1 cm in short axis
T4	IV IVa	Extension out of the true pelvis and/or invasion of the rectal or bladder mucosa Invasion of the rectal or bladder mucosa	Tumor extends beyond true pelvis or into rectal and/or bladder mucosa Loss of normal tissue planes and interruption of low-SI rectal or bladder wall
M1	IVb	Distant metastases, including abdominal (excluding para-aortic) and inguinal lymph node metastases	Metastases in distant organ(s) and/or abdominal or inguinal lymphadenopathy; ascites, peritoneal thickening, nodularity, or enhancement
N-Regional Lymph nodes			
NX		Regional lymph nodes cannot be assessed	
N0		No regional lymph node metastases	
N1		Regional lymph node metastases to pelvic and/or para-aortic nodes	
M-Distant Metastases			
MX		Distant metastases cannot be assessed	
M0		No distant metastases	
M1		Distant metastases, including abdominal (excluding para-aortic) and inguinal lymph node metastases	

[a]Data from Rubin P, Hansen JT. *TNM Staging Atlas*. Philadelphia, PA: Lippincott Williams & Wilkins; 2008.

[b]Data from Staging Classifications and Clinical Practice Guidelines for Gynaecological Cancer, FIGO Committee on Gynecologic Oncology; 2000.

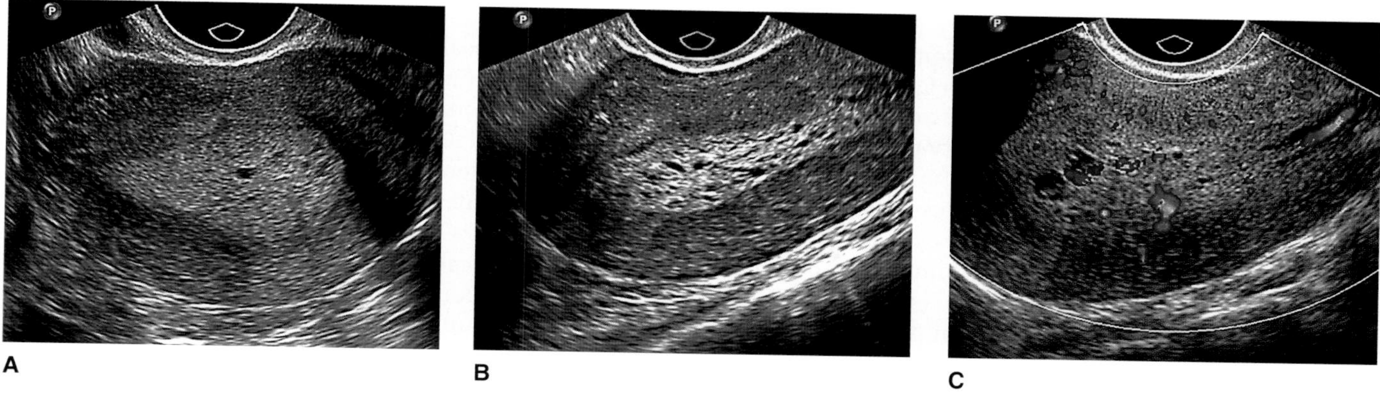

Figure 9-18 US of Endometrial Carcinoma
A 66-year-old woman with postmenopausal bleeding. **A.** Coronal and (**B**) sagittal ultrasound images of the uterus demonstrate massive endometrial thickening. **C.** Color Doppler image shows blood flow within the endometrium. Although this could represent endometrial hyperplasia, the possibility of an endometrial carcinoma should be excluded. Endometrial biopsy was diagnostic of endometrial carcinoma.

was 4 mm or less.[42] Color Doppler US has been reported to add value in differentiating benign and malignant disease, as malignancy demonstrates lower resistive indices related to angiogenesis. However, there is much overlap of flow impedances from benign and malignant diseases, and so the use of Doppler US in characterizing endometrial masses remains controversial.[2,28,39]

In general, MRI is the most accurate modality for the staging of endometrial carcinoma, with staging accuracy reported in the 83% to 92% range.[37,39] In addition, MRI has been shown to be 87% sensitive and 91% specific for myometrial invasion, 80% sensitive and 96% specific for cervical invasion, and 50% sensitive and 95% specific for nodal metastases.[39] The tumor typically appears as a thickened endometrial stripe. On T2-weighted images, this will usually appear as heterogeneous SI greater than that of the myometrium; isointensity or hypointensity compared to the myometrium is less frequently encountered.[2,37,39] On T1-weighted images, the tumor usually appears isointense to the myometrium and endometrium but is occasionally hypointense.[2,37] Myometrial invasion can be excluded when the low-SI junctional zone is intact, while irregularity of the endometrial-myometrial interface is suggestive of invasion (see Figure 9-19).[2,37] The junctional zone may be difficult

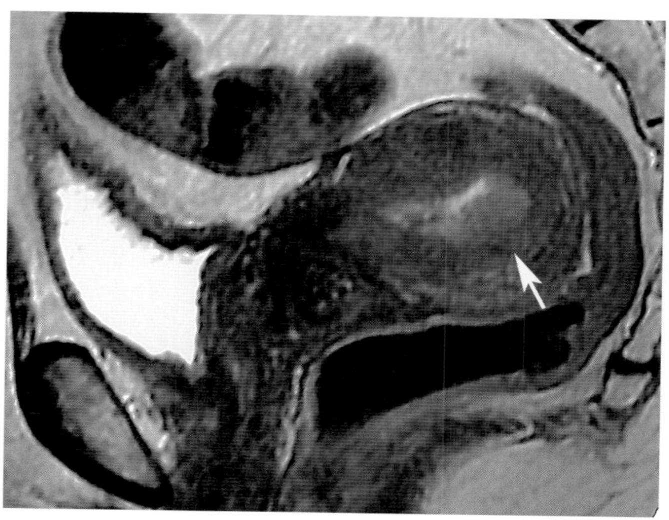

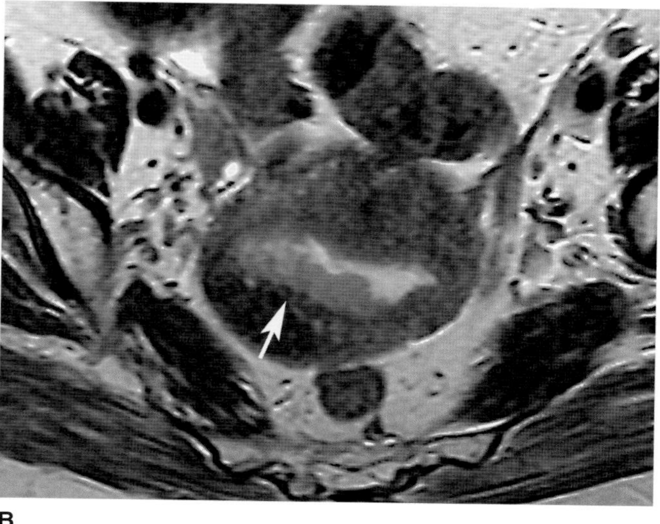

Figure 9-19 Endometrial Carcinoma without Invasion of Myometrium
A 65-year-old woman with postmenopausal bleeding. **A.** Sagittal and (**B**) axial T2-weighted image demonstrate focal thickening of the posterior wall of the endometrium (*arrows*) with a small amount of high-SI fluid in the endometrial canal. Note the sharply defined border between the mass and junctional zone suggesting the absence of myometrial invasion. Surgical resection was diagnostic of a noninvasive high-grade endometrial carcinoma with papillary serous and endometrioid features.

to visualize in older patients secondary to atrophy, distortion by tumor, or in the setting of concomitant adenomyosis. Dynamic contrast-enhanced T1-weighted images are particularly helpful in demonstrating myometrial invasion and have a significantly higher accuracy than T2-weighted images in staging disease (91% vs 83%).[29] After contrast administration, tumor will enhance less avidly than the myometrium, thereby providing contrast between the tissues (see Figure 9-20).[2,37,39,43] Determining the presence or absence of myometrial invasion is important as those patients with deep myometrial invasion (invasion ≥50% of the myometrial thickness) are at increased risk for pelvic and retroperitoneal nodal metastases compared to those with superficial (invasion <50% of the myometrial thickness) or no myometrial invasion.[39] Thus, knowledge of the presence and depth of myometrial invasion may guide the surgeon's extent of nodal dissection. Stage I disease is confined to the uterus, whereas cervical invasion signifies stage II disease.[39] Cervical invasion is revealed as widening of the endocervical canal (superficial extension, ie, stage IIa) or interruption of the low-SI cervical stroma (extension beyond the uterus, ie, stage IIb).[37] Tumor extending

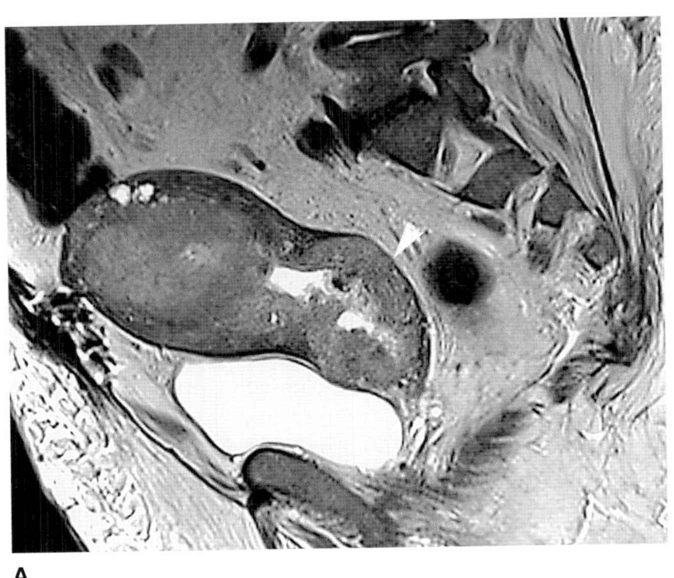

A

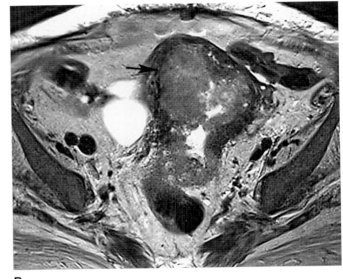

B

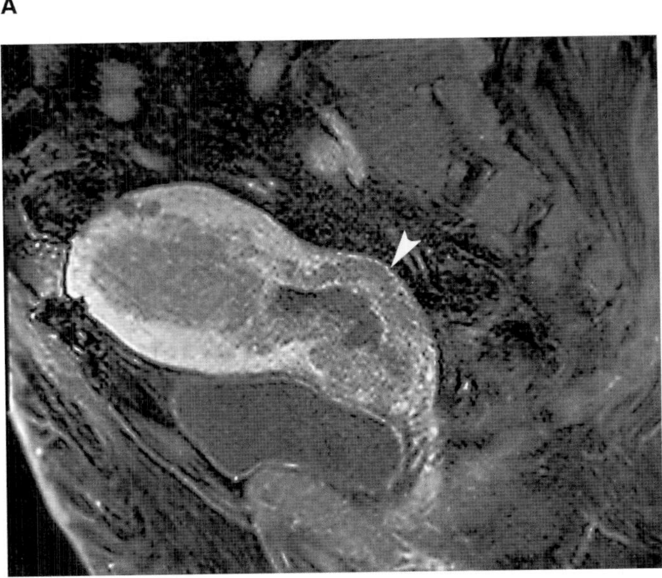

C

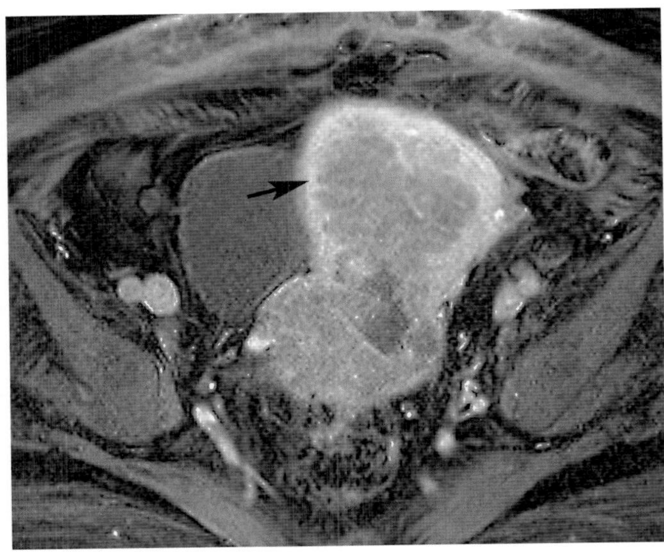

D

Figure 9-20 Endometrial Carcinoma with Deep Myometrial Invasion and Invasion of the Cervix
A 69-year-old woman with postmenopausal bleeding. **A.** Sagittal and (**B**) axial T2-weighted images and (**C**) sagittal and (**D**) axial fat-suppressed postcontrast T1-weighted images show a large inhomogeneous hypovascular mass (*arrows* in B and D) that invades more than 50% of the thickness of the myometrium and nearly completely replaces the cervix (*arrowheads* in A and C). On the T2-weighted image, notice the loss of the normal low-SI junctional zone and cervical stroma.

beyond the outer myometrium into the adnexa or vagina or the presence of pelvic and/or para-aortic lymphadenopathy (lymph node size >1 cm in the short axis) indicates stage III disease.[37] The prevalence of malignant lymphadenopathy for noninvasive and superficially invasive tumors is approximately 3% but is as high as 40% for tumors with deep invasion.[38] Finally, stage IV disease is present when there is tumor extension out of the true pelvis or into the urinary bladder or rectum. Bladder or rectal invasion is seen as focal loss of normal tissue planes and loss of the normal low-SI wall of these structures on T2-weighted images. Peritoneal carcinomatosis is also indicative of stage IV disease.[37]

CT in patients with endometrial carcinoma will often demonstrate an enlarged uterus. In about two-thirds of cases, a discrete mass that is lower in attenuation than the myometrium can be detected in the region of the endometrium (see Figure 9-21). However, in the remainder of cases, the tumor cannot be seen separately from the normal uterus because of limited tissue contrast.[39] The ability of CT to accurately stage endometrial carcinoma is limited.[39] The sensitivity and specificity of CT in determining depth of myometrial invasion are 83% and 42%, respectively.[39] The sensitivity and specificity for depicting cervical invasion are 25% and 70%, respectively.[39] Nevertheless, CT is useful in assessing for advanced disease as it may demonstrate lymphadenopathy, distant metastases, or peritoneal carcinomatosis. Bladder and bowel invasion can also be identified.

Further, FDG-PET provides complementary functional information to the structural information provided by CT and MRI. The sensitivity in overall lesion detection is higher with PET combined with MRI or CT than PET, MRI, or CT alone and may facilitate management in certain cases.[44,45] Several studies have shown that FDG-PET should not routinely replace operative staging because of the limited sensitivity in the 50% to 67% range. However, FDG-PET has been shown to be highly accurate in assessing women suspected of recurrent disease after treatment (see Figure 9-22).[46] Additionally, FDG-PET has been shown to alter management decisions in nearly half of cases by appropriately upstaging or downstaging disease and detecting recurrent disease.[45,46]

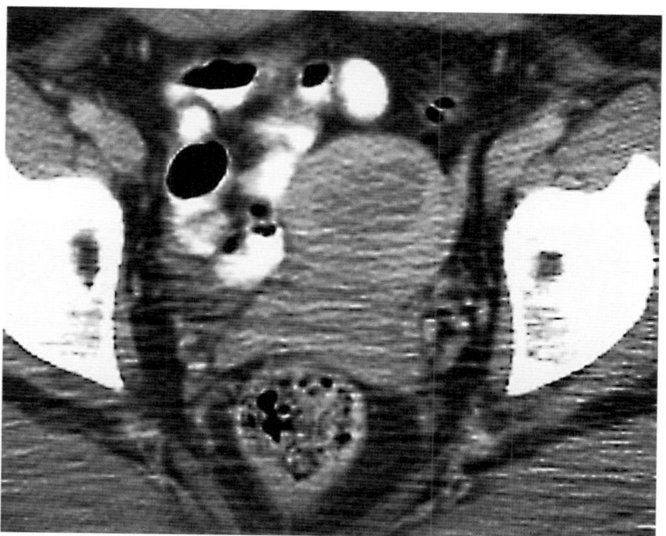

Figure 9-21 Endometrial Carcinoma
A 53-year-old woman with vaginal bleeding. Enhanced CT image demonstrates an ill-defined low attenuation region in the endometrial canal. In a premenopausal woman, this could represent the normal secretory phase of the endometrium. However, in a postmenopausal woman, this is an abnormal finding and could indicate a submucosal fibroid, endometrial polyp, endometrial hyperplasia, or endometrial carcinoma. Endometrial curettage yielded endometrial carcinoma.

Endometrial sarcoma

Uterine sarcomas are uncommon representing approximately 3% to 5% of all uterine malignancies and can arise from mesenchymal elements in the endometrium or myometrium.[8] The imaging appearance of uterine sarcomas depends on the tumor type, invasiveness, and presence or absence of hemorrhage or necrosis but typically appear as large heterogenous intrauterine masses with irregular margins. In some cases, the endometrial canal can become distended with tumor, glandular secretions, or blood and appear as a primary endometrial mass that can be confused with endometrial carcinoma (see Figure 9-23). Endometrial sarcoma is discussed most completely in the previous section titled **Focal Myometrial Masses**.

Tamoxifen-induced changes

Tamoxifen citrate is an orally administered antiestrogen agent that binds to estrogen receptors and is most commonly used for breast cancer prophylaxis. In postmenopausal women with estrogen receptor positive breast cancer, tamoxifen use has been shown to improve disease-free and overall survival as well as decrease the incidence of contralateral breast cancer.[49] Estrogen receptor negative and premenopausal women also benefit from the medication.[49] While tamoxifen has antiestrogen effects on breast tissue, it is a weak estrogen agonist in postmenopausal endometrial tissue.[49] As a result, tamoxifen use is associated with an increased incidence of several endometrial pathologies including polyps, hyperplasia (without and with atypia), carcinoma, and carcinosarcoma.[32,49] An estimated 50% of women taking tamoxifen will develop an endometrial abnormality within 6 to 36 months with risk related to duration of treatment and cumulative dose.[32,49] Nonetheless, there is no consensus on the appropriate clinical and imaging surveillance of these patients. Moreover, endometrial abnormalities may or may not cause symptoms, the most common being abnormal vaginal bleeding. Most women at least undergo an annual pelvic examination and pelvic US; some also undergo annual endometrial

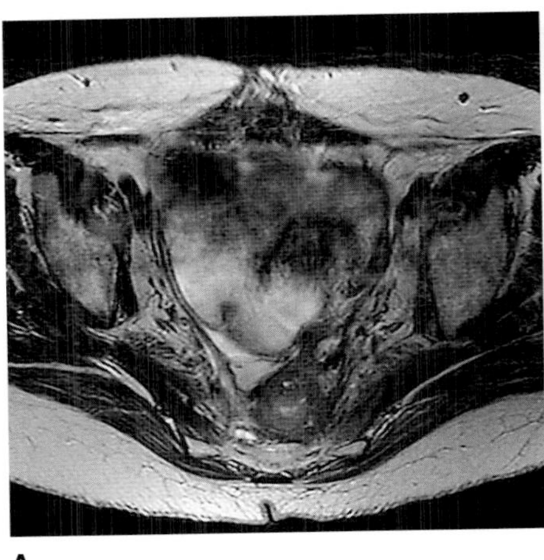

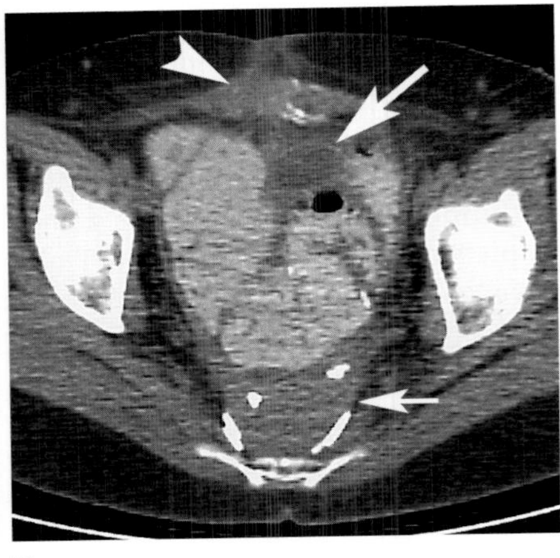

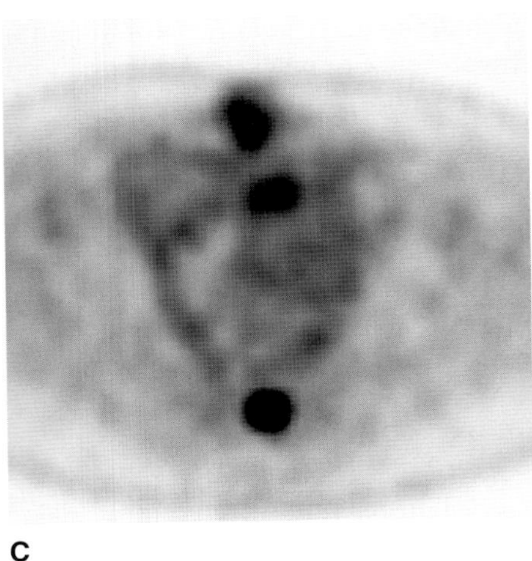

Figure 9-22 Recurrent Endometrial Carcinoma Depicted by PET-CT
A 74-year-old woman with endometrial cancer previously treated nonsurgically. **A.** Axial T2-weighted image of the pelvis shows posttreatment changes as well as a soft-tissue mass in the anterior pelvis. The uterus was atrophic but otherwise considered normal. **B.** Unenhanced CT image from a PET-CT study shows a low-attenuation mass in the anterior pelvis (*large arrow*) and presacral soft-tissue thickening, and stranding in the anterior abdominal wall (*arrowhead*). These findings are nonspecific but could represent posttreatment inflammation/scarring or recurrent malignancy. **C.** PET image from the same examination shows increased uptake in all 3 locations consistent with recurrent malignancy.

biopsy. The normal endometrial thickness in tamoxifen-treated women is controversial, on average measuring 9 to 13 mm.[49] Given the high risk of malignancy, sonohysterography has been recommended as the next step for women who have endometrial thickness greater than 4 mm on TVUS (49). Additionally, symptomatic women should undergo prompt evaluation.

The most common imaging finding is homogeneous endometrial thickening with or without endometrial/subendometrial cysts (see Figure 9-24).[49] The cysts pathologically correspond to cystic spaces lined by atrophic endometrium within a dense fibrous stroma.[49] The exact location of the cysts has been debated to be within the endometrium or at the endometrial-myometrial junction. The other endometrial abnormalities generally appear similar in untreated and tamoxifen-treated women, but there are some differences. For example, endometrial polyps are typically larger in size in tamoxifen-treated women, averaging 5 cm compared with 0.5 to 3 cm in untreated women (see Figure 9-24).[49] A higher rate of malignant transformation

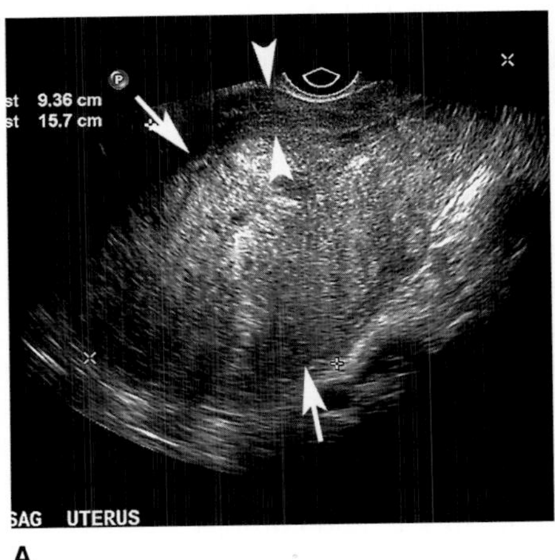

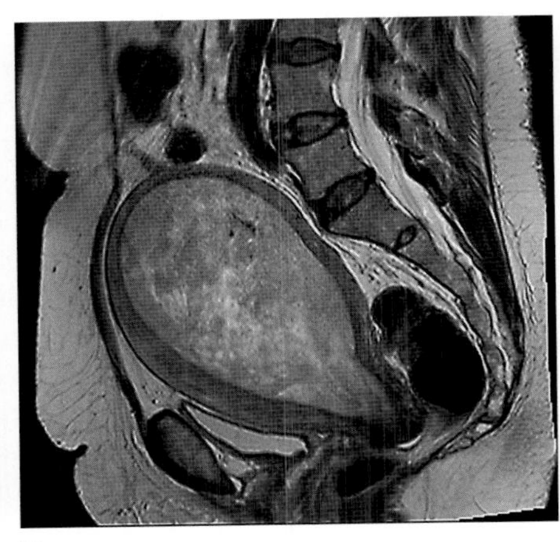

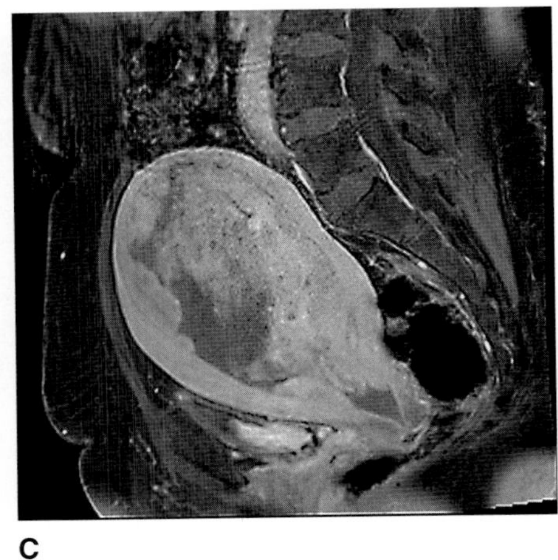

Figure 9-23 Carcinosarcoma
A 58-year-old woman with postmenopausal bleeding. **A.** Longitudinal view of the uterus from a transvaginal US shows a large inhomogeneous intrauterine mass. Note the borders of the mass (*arrows*) are distinct from the uterine wall (*arrowheads*). **B.** Sagittal T2-weighted image and (**C**) T1-weighted image postgadolinium contrast images confirm the presence of a large inhomogeneously enhancing intrauterine mass. This was thought to represent an endometrial carcinoma although surgical biopsy was diagnostic of a carcinosarcoma (mixed müllerian tumor).

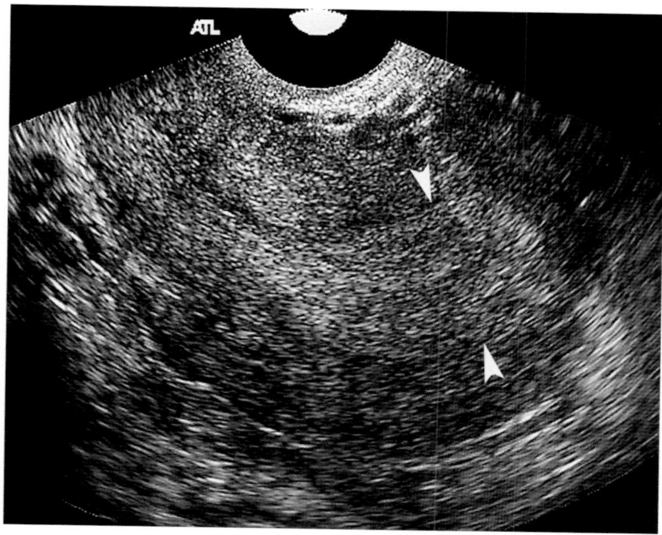

A

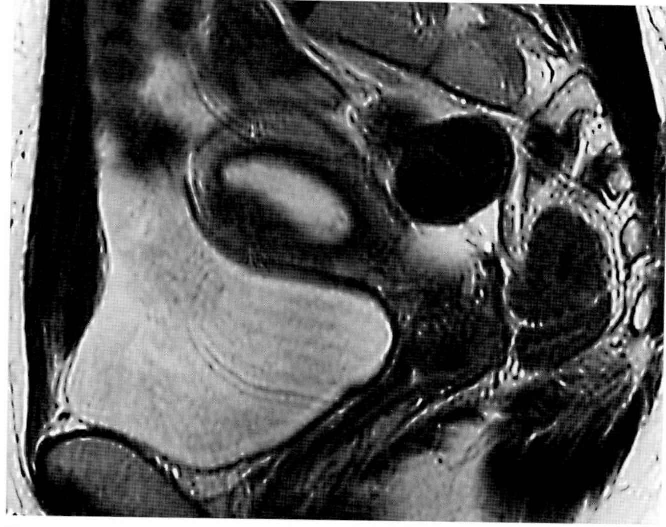

B

Figure 9-24 Tamoxifen-Induced Endometrial Thickening Two women receiving tamoxifen therapy for breast cancer. **A.** Sagittal TVUS and (**B**) sagittal T2-weighted image show extensive uniform endometrial thickening (*arrowheads*) typical of endometrial hyperplasia because of the hormonal effects of tamoxifen.

of endometrial polyps has also been observed pathologically in tamoxifen-treated women.[32] Early reports indicated that tamoxifen-related endometrial carcinomas were more aggressive than those in the general population, but this was disproved in subsequent studies.[32,49] The imaging appearances of the various pathologies are covered elsewhere in this chapter.

Diffuse Myometrial Abnormalities

Diffuse myometrial abnormalities include the abnormal infiltration of the muscle by endometrial tissue, termed *adenomyosis,* and diffuse enlargement of the muscle due to infection and inflammation.

Adenomyosis

Adenomyosis is a relatively common nonneoplastic disorder that is diagnosed histologically by the presence of endometrial glands and stroma ectopically located within the myometrium.[19] Hypertrophy of the surrounding smooth muscle is also present. The reported prevalence varies but has been reported in up to 30% to 60% of hysterectomy specimens.[20] Adenomyosis usually affects women in their late reproductive years presenting with menorrhagia, dysmenorrhea, or metrorrhagia.[21] Pelvic examination can reveal an enlarged soft tender uterus. Nearly all affected women are multiparous. The condition can also be asymptomatic in about one-third of patients and is found only by imaging or on pathologic examination. The frequency and severity of symptoms correlates with the extent and depth of penetration. Coexistent uterine pathology is often present, the most common entities including leiomyomas, endometrial polyps, endometrial hyperplasia, and endometrial adenocarcinoma.[22]

On gross inspection, the uterus is often enlarged and globular in appearance. Macroscopic cysts, sometimes filled with blood, can be present.[22] Microscopically, the ectopic endometrial glands are scattered in the myometrium and surrounded by hypertrophic smooth muscle. The ectopic endometrial glands can involve the myometrium diffusely or focally.[22] Occasionally, the ectopic endometrial glands, stroma, and myometrium aggregate into a nodular circumscribed mass called an adenomyoma. (This has been discussed previously under the heading **Focal Myometrial Masses.**) Adenomyomas can be found either within the myometrium or endometrium.

The clinical diagnosis of adenomyosis is suspected in middle-aged multiparous women with an appropriate history. However, the clinical diagnosis is missed in as much as 75% of patients or made inappropriately in as many as approximately 35% of patients.[22] Given the low accuracy of the clinical examination for the presence of adenomyosis, imaging plays an essential role in the diagnosis of this disorder. In general, US and MRI are the most accurate imaging modalities in diagnosing adenomyosis and are often helpful in confirming clinical suspicion. The reported sensitivity and specificity of TVUS range between 53% and 89% and between 50% and 99%, respectively.[23] A transvaginal approach allows a more accurate diagnosis than transabdominal imaging. In a review that pooled data from 3 studies directly comparing MRI and TVUS, MRI seemed to perform slightly better.[23] Diagnostic accuracy of both modalities decreases in the setting of concomitant fibroids, with sensitivity of US and

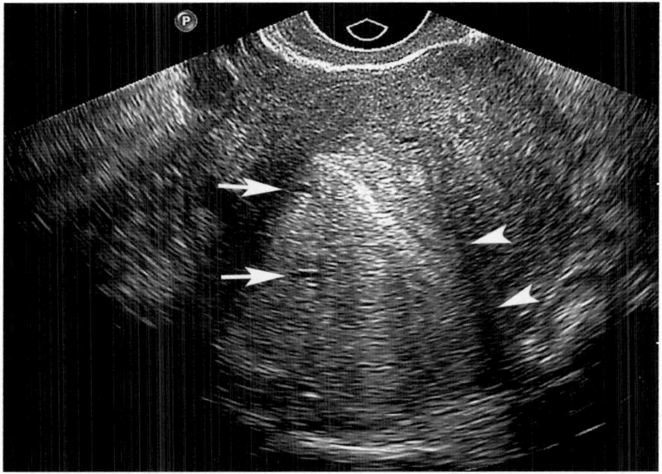

A

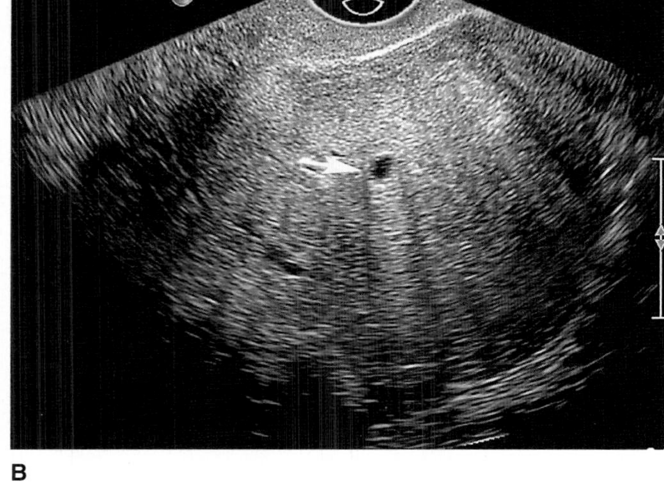

B

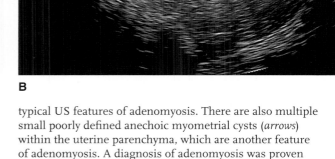

Figure 9-25 Diffuse Adenomyosis
A 49-year-old woman with history of ovarian carcinoma (not shown). **A** and **B.** Two longitudinal views of the uterus from a transvaginal examination show a heterogeneous echotexture to the myometrium with many regions of linear refractive shadowing (*arrowheads*) through the myometrium. These are typical US features of adenomyosis. There are also multiple small poorly defined anechoic myometrial cysts (*arrows*) within the uterine parenchyma, which are another feature of adenomyosis. A diagnosis of adenomyosis was proven following transabdominal hysterectomy with bilateral salpingo-oophorectomy.

MRI falling to 33% and 67%, respectively.[24] Though less sensitive, CT can also detect the pathologic changes of adenomyosis.[5]

The primary imaging findings reflect the ectopic endometrial glands and associated muscular hypertrophy. Sonographically, adenomyosis typically appears as diffuse ill-defined areas of heterogeneous echotexture and hypoechogenicity (see Figure 9-25).[19,24] The areas of decreased echogenicity correspond to the muscular hypertrophy and the heterogeneous areas correspond to the ectopic endometrial glands.[19] The margins are often poorly circumscribed and appear to blend with unaffected areas. Linear refractive shadowing originating from the myometrium is a characteristic feature of adenomyosis (see Figure 9-25). A more specific finding of adenomyosis is the presence of small anechoic spaces or myometrial cysts, which represent foci of hemorrhage or distended endometrial glands.[19,24] These cysts are small and irregularly marginated, which can make it difficult to appreciate their presence (see Figure 9-25). With Doppler imaging, normal vessels can be seen coursing through areas of adenomyosis. This is in contradistinction to leiomyomas, which are usually devoid of central color flow.[19] Adenomyosis often has little mass effect and seldom results in a uterine contour deformity, findings that can help differentiate it from uterine fibroids.[19]

The most reliable method of diagnosing adenomyosis is MRI, primarily through the evaluation of T2-weighted images. It reveals the muscular hypertrophy as low-SI thickening of the junctional zone.[5,19] Normal junctional zone thickness should not be greater than 12 mm and appears as a low-SI band between the high-SI endometrium and intermediate-SI outer myometrium. Thickening of the junctional zone (≥12 mm) is abnormal and indicative of adenomyosis and may be diffuse or focal depending on the distribution of adenomyosis (see Figure 9-26). Within the thickened junctional zone, small high-SI foci represent ectopic endometrial glands (see Figure 9-27).[19] Small myometrial cysts also can be seen, occasionally demonstrating high SI on T1-weighted images secondary to hemorrhagic fluid content.[21]

When the junctional zone can be identified separately from the outer myometrium and endometrium, the diagnosis of adenomyosis can be made on enhanced CT. The uterus is enlarged and the junctional zone may be diffusely or focally thickened with attenuation between that of the endometrium and outer myometrium.[5] The myometrial cysts are usually too small to accurately characterize based on attenuation measurements, but appear as foci of low attenuation in the thickened junctional zone. Occasionally, inhomogeneous enhancement of the myometrium can be a finding indicating the presence of adenomyosis (see Figure 9-26).

Adenomyosis may be seen on HSG that are usually performed in women in the workup of infertility. If the ectopic endometrial glands maintain a connection to the endometrial cavity, contrast instilled into the endometrial canal will opacify the ectopic glands.[6] The result is an irregular contour of the endometrial canal with small diverticula or outpouchings (see Figure 9-28). When the glands do not communicate with the canal, adenomyosis is usually not apparent on HSG and the study appears normal.

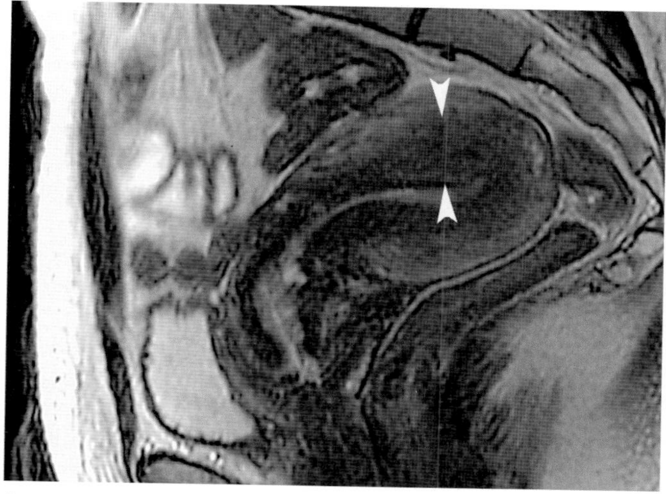

A

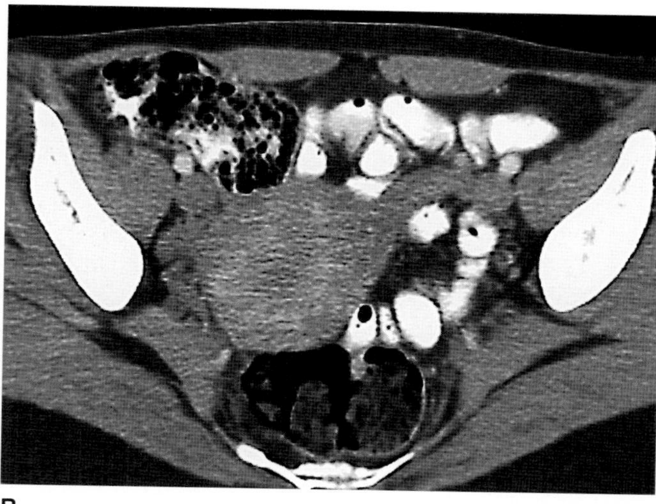

B

Figure 9-26 Adenomyosis
A 48-year-old woman with heavy menstrual bleeding. **A.** Sagittal T2-weighted image demonstrate diffuse thickening of the junctional zone (*arrowheads*) of the uterus. Compare the width and distinctness of the junctional zone in this patient with the zone in **Figure 9-2 Normal MRI of the Uterus and Cervix.** This appearance is diagnostic of uterine adenomyosis. **B.** CT scan in the same patient shows inhomogeneous enhancement of the uterine myometrium. Although subtle, this can be a CT finding of adenomyosis.

Less commonly, adenomyosis will appear as a focal myometrial abnormality rather than a diffuse process. Single or multiple regions of heterogeneous echotexture and hypoechogenicity may be seen with US. Adenomyomas, discrete masses of ectopic endometrial glands with surrounding hypertrophic myometrium, will also appear as a focal uterine abnormality. These features of adenomyosis have been discussed in the section titled **Focal Myometrial Abnormalities**.

Endometritis

Endometritis most commonly occurs in the postpartum period, but can also be seen in conjunction with cervical stenosis, after instrumentation, or in association with salpingitis and tubo-ovarian abscess in the setting of pelvic inflammatory disease.[10,12] In the postpartum period, endometritis presents after cesarean section with fever, an enlarged tender uterus, and vaginal discharge.[47] It is the

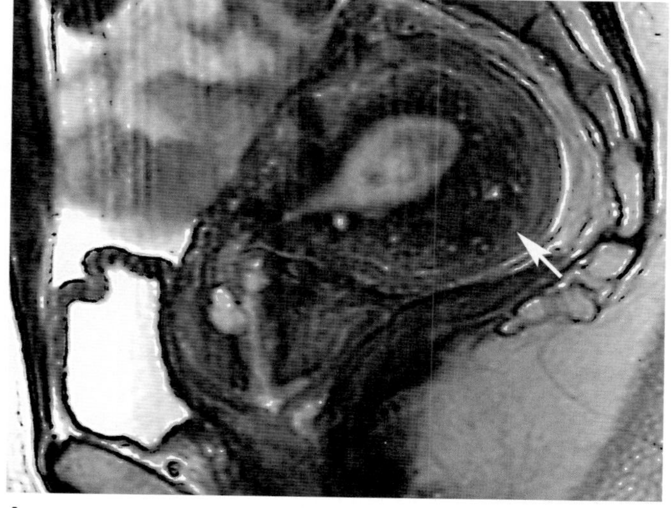

A

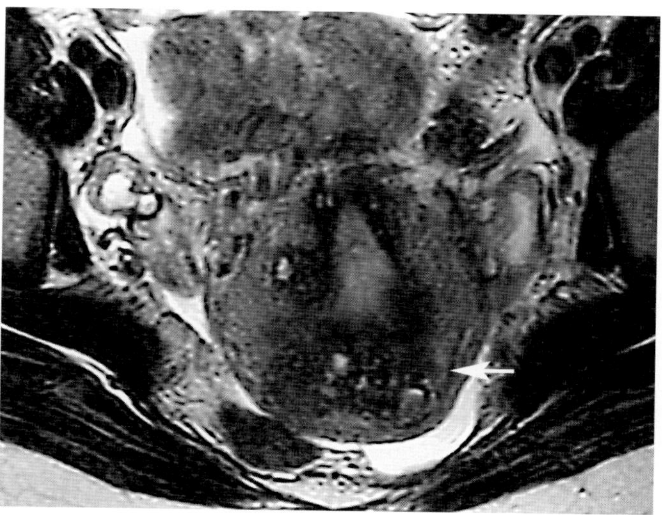

B

Figure 9-27 Focal Adenomyosis with Myometrial Cysts
A. Sagittal and (**B**) axial T2-weighted images demonstrate focal thickening of the posterior aspect of the junctional zone (*arrows*) typical of adenomyosis. Note the multiple small hyperintense myometrial cystic foci representing ectopic endometrial glands, a characteristic feature of adenomyosis.

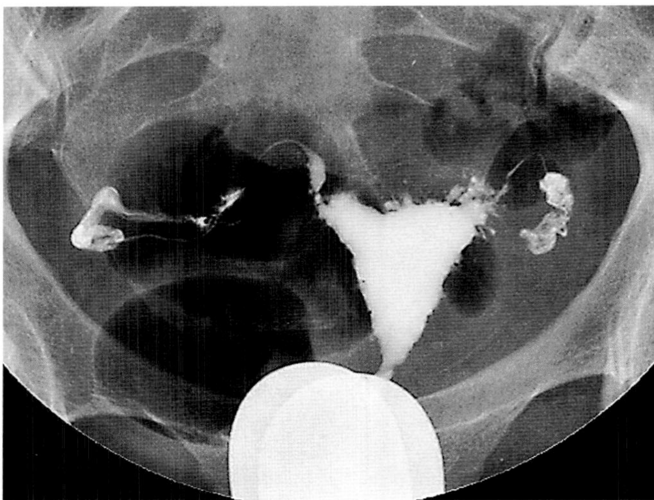

Figure 9-28 Uterine Diverticula Indicating Adenomyosis
A 41-year-old woman with history of multiple spontaneous abortions and infertility. Hysterosalpingogram reveals multiple small diverticula projecting from the uterine cavity. This appearance is diagnostic of uterine adenomyosis.

most common cause of postpartum fever with a reported prevalence of 3.8%.[47] Women who deliver vaginally are affected much less frequently.[48] Initial management is usually based on clinical assessment, as the imaging findings of endometritis and the normal postpartum uterus overlap.[2,47]

In general, US and CT are the most common modalities employed when imaging is necessary, often because of persistent fever or poor treatment response. Typically, endometritis will appear as diffuse enlargement of the uterus. Imaging can also demonstrate findings indicating diffuse uterine edema such as decreased echogenicity on US examinations and decreased attenuation on CT studies (see Figure 9-29). Following contrast enhancement, endometritis will often demonstrate prominent endometrial enhancement.[48] The normal endometrial stripe thickness after delivery is no greater than 15 mm. Unfortunately, in the normal postpartum state, the uterus often appears diffusely enlarged and can contain a small volume of fluid or blood in the endometrial canal, findings that can be similar to endometritis.[2,47] A small amount of gas can also be present in up to 21% of normal postpartum women, sometimes remaining for several weeks and the endometrium can be heterogeneously thickened and can be difficult to distinguish from retained products of conception.[47] Endometritis can lead to myometrial or pelvic abscesses, which appear similar to abscesses elsewhere in the body. Ovarian or pelvic vein thrombosis, retained products of conception, pelvic hematoma, and pelvic abscess can present with similar symptoms and should be included in the clinical differential diagnosis of endometritis.

CERVICAL LESIONS

Aside from nabothian cysts, the majority of lesions involving the cervix are neoplastic in etiology. Benign cervical masses include leiomyomas and polyps. A variety of primary and secondary malignant masses may involve the cervix, including cervical carcinoma, adenoma malignum, and other tumors (Table 9-5).

Nabothian Cyst

Nabothian cysts result from the dilation of endocervical glands and are common incidental findings on imaging studies performed for other reasons.[53] They have no clinical significance. They may be seen as single or multiple clustered cysts and may be simple or have hemorrhagic or proteinaceous fluid contents. These benign cysts are usually superficial and close to the endocervical canal, but may be located deeper within the cervix.[54] In most cases, they appear as a simple cyst on all modalities: round or oval, thin or imperceptible wall and anechoic on US, fluid in attenuation on CT, and very high in SI on T2-weighted images on MRI (see Figure 9-30). However, in some cases, the fluid contents are not simple and can demonstrate increased echogenicity on US, increased attenuation on CT, and variably increased SI on T1-weighted image and variably decreased SI on T2-weighted image on MRI images. The cysts can be clustered together to appear as a multicystic mass (see Figure 9-31). Nabothian cysts do not enhance after IV contrast administration, helping to differentiate deep nabothian cysts from adenoma malignum, the latter of which frequently contains solid-enhancing components.[54]

Cervical Leiomyoma

Cervical leiomyomas are pathologically identical to those that occur in the uterine corpus, but are less common and account for <10% of fibroids.[54] Patients may present with a palpable abnormality, abnormal vaginal bleeding, or bladder or bowel symptoms related to mass effect on these structures.[53,54] Submucosal fibroids may extend into the cervical canal or vagina and present as a pelvic mass.[53] Occasionally, cervical leiomyomas result in dystocia if the birth canal is obstructed.[54] The imaging appearance of cervical leiomyoma is similar to those that occur in the uterine corpus and is described in a separate section (see Figure 9-32).

Adenoma Malignum

Also known as minimal-deviation adenocarcinoma, adenoma malignum is a well-differentiated subtype of mucinous adenocarcinoma of the cervix that arises from the endocervical glands.[54,55] The neoplastic glands are only minimally deviated from normal and may be misdiagnosed as normal.[55] This subtype is uncommon and accounts for about 3% of cervical adenocarcinomas and about 0.15% to

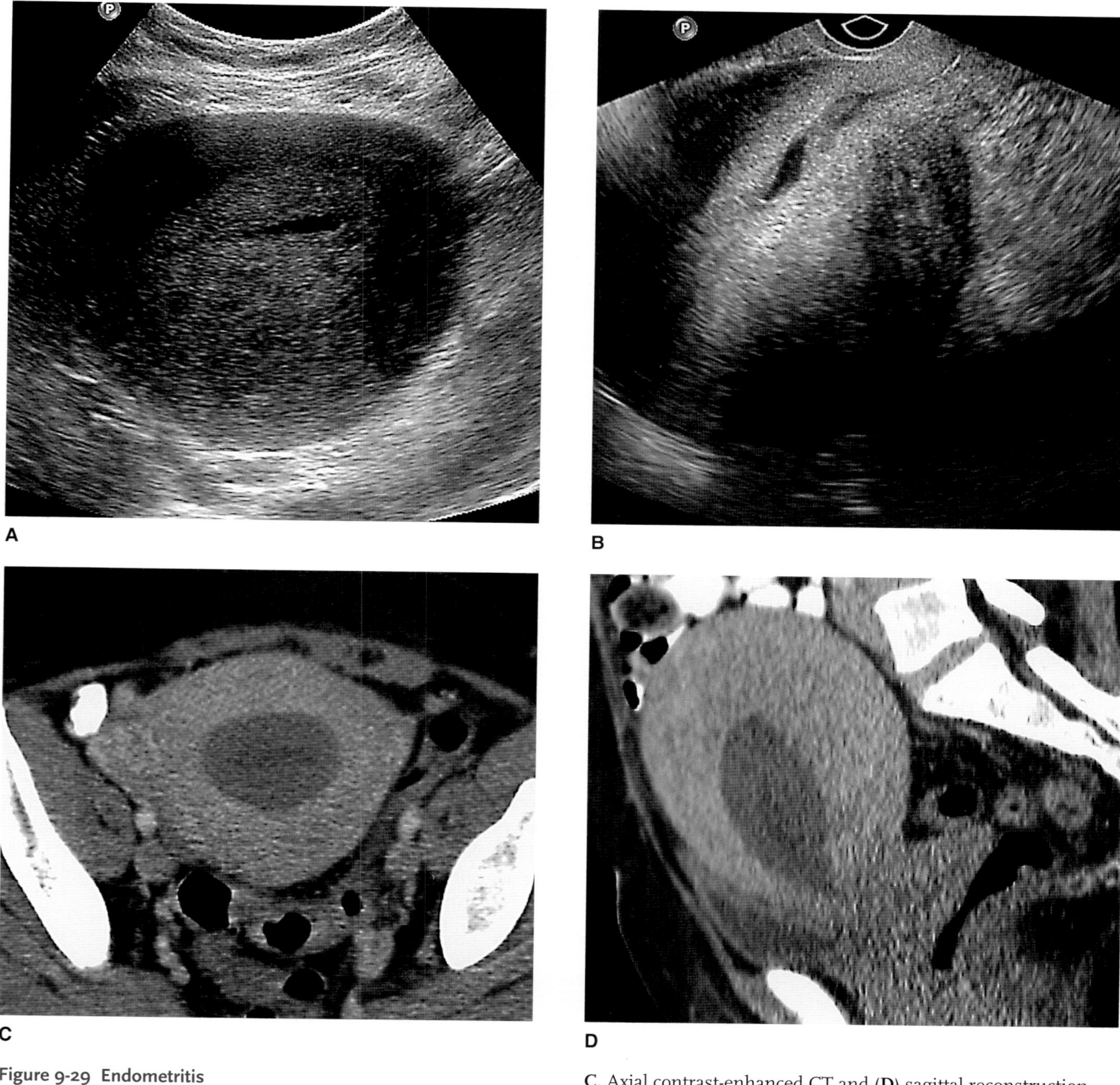

Figure 9-29 Endometritis
A 48-year-old woman with history of recent dilation and curettage for a thickened endometrial stripe now presents with progressive fever and lower abdominal pain. **A.** Transverse and (**B**) longitudinal views of the uterus from a transvaginal US examination show a diffusely enlarged, hypoechoic uterus. **C.** Axial contrast-enhanced CT and (**D**) sagittal reconstruction of the uterus also show a diffusely enlarged uterus with low attenuation material in the endometrial canal similar to the US. These findings indicated diffuse uterine edema and in this clinical setting are diagnostic of endometritis.

0.45% of all cervical malignancies.[56] Watery vaginal discharge is the classic presenting symptom of this lesion.[53] Abnormal vaginal bleeding may or may not be present. The tumor may grow within the cervix and may not be apparent on physical examination.[57] Adenoma malignum is associated with Peutz-Jeghers syndrome, which is characterized by mucocutaneous pigmentation and gastrointestinal hamartomatous polyps.[53,54] Prognosis is typically poor secondary to early peritoneal and distant spread as well as a traditionally poor response to radiation and chemotherapy.[53,54,56]

Adenoma malignum appears as a nodular or annular multicystic mass that extends from the endocervical glands

Table 9-5. Causes of a Cervical Mass

1. Nabothian Cysts
2. Neoplasms a. Cervical Leiomyoma b. Squamous carcinoma c. Adenoma malignum d. Other malignancies i. lymphoma ii. primary malignant melanoma iii. rhabdomyosarcoma iv. small cell carcinoma v. metastasis (urinary bladder, colon, ovary)
3. Cervical polyp

to the deep cervical stroma.[54] Cysts may vary in size ranging from microscopic to approximately 2 cm; most cysts, however, are less than 1 cm in size.[57] In addition, US and CT may be able to identify the lesion, but differentiation from nabothian cysts is problematic. Although imperfect, MRI is the imaging modality of choice to make this diagnosis. The cystic components are generally hyperintense on T2-weighted images and isointense or slightly hyperintense on T1-weighted images, reflecting mucinous fluid contents.[54,55,57] The intervening septations have low SI on T2-weighted image. Enhancing solid components are also frequently present, which helps to distinguish this entity from nabothian cysts and endocervical glandular hyperplasia (neither of which has solid-enhancing components).[54,55,57] Additionally, adenoma malignum tends to have a vague hazy interface with the surrounding stroma, whereas nabothian cysts are more clearly delineated. Nevertheless, the MRI finding of a multicystic cervical mass is not specific for adenoma malignum, and benign entities such as endocervical hyperplasia and deep nabothian cysts may have an identical appearance.

Cervical Cancer

Cervical cancer is the third most common gynecologic malignancy in the United States.[58] An estimated 11,070 new cases will be diagnosed in 2008 with a lifetime risk of 1 in 145.[35] In 2008, there will be an estimated 3,870 deaths from cervical cancer with African Americans twice as likely to die as Caucasians.[34,35] Most women are asymptomatic, but can present with abnormal vaginal bleeding.[35] Cervical cancer is most commonly the result of infection by certain types of the human papillomavirus (HPV) and less commonly occurs in women not infected by HPV.[35] Risk factors for acquiring HPV include unprotected sex and sex at an early age or with multiple partners.[35] Long-term use of oral contraceptives and cigarette smoking also increases a woman's risk of developing cervical cancer.[35] Overall, 1- and 5-year survival rates are 88% and 72%, respectively.[35] If the tumor is local, 5-year survival is ~92%.[35] Eighty-five percent to 90% of cervical cancers are squamous cell carcinomas, whereas adenocarcinoma comprises the remaining 10% to 15%.

Cervical cancer is most commonly detected via Papanicolaou smear or during a gynecologic physical examination. However, occasionally, it will be initially detected on cross-sectional imaging examinations performed for other reasons. If large enough, cervical cancers are seen as cervical masses sonographically (see Figure 9-33). Because of its limited tissue contrast, US may not reveal the tumor or may be unable to provide accurate staging information. However, occasionally, the mass can be seen as a hypoechoic mass within the substance of the cervix (see Figure 9-34).

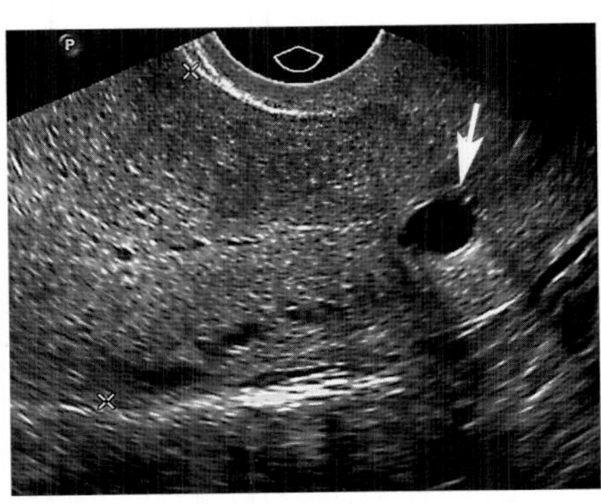

A

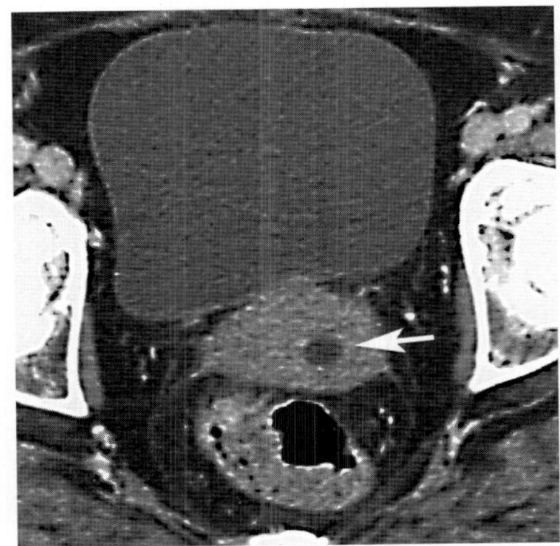

B

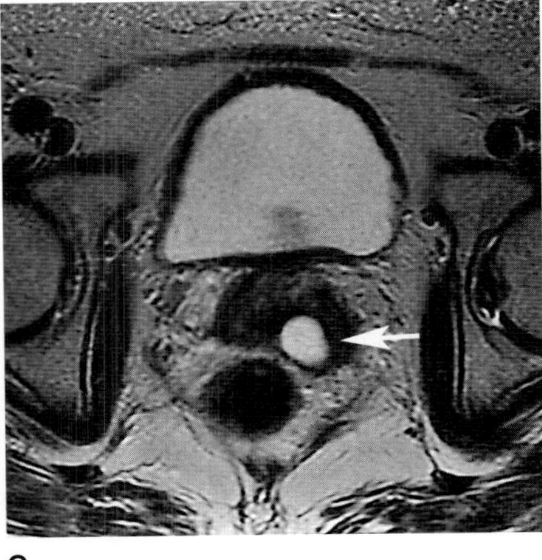

C

Figure 9-30 Nabothian Cyst
A. Longitudinal US, (**B**) contrast-enhanced CT, and (**C**) T2-weighted MRI image show the imaging characteristics of a simple cyst (*arrows*) involving the submucosal portion of the cervix. This is the typical appearance of a nabothian cyst.

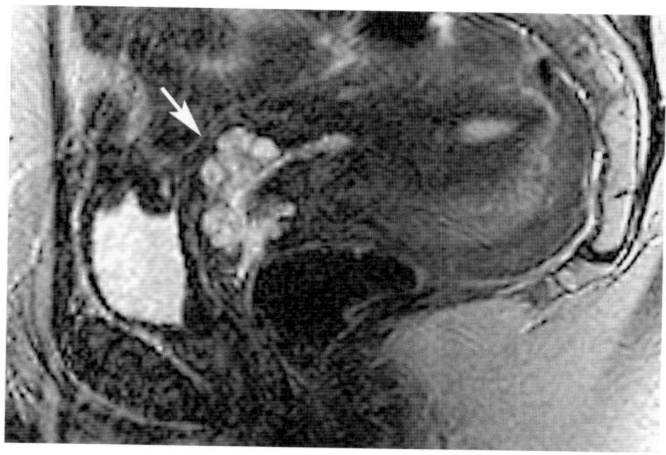
A

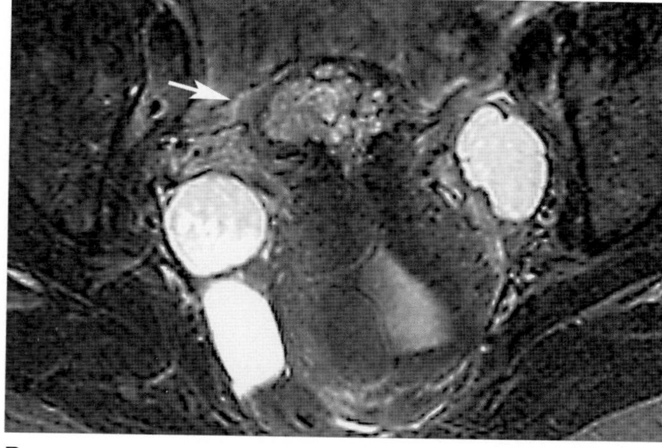
B

Figure 9-31 Complex Nabothian Cyst
A 46-year-old woman undergoing evaluation for a complex left ovarian cyst. **A.** Sagittal and (**B**) axial T2-weighted image MRI images show a complex multicystic mass (*arrows*) in the cervix. This could represent the rare malignancy, adenoma malignum, or an atypical appearance of the more common nabothian cyst. Histologic evaluation confirmed a diagnosis of a nabothian cyst.

Hydronephrosis due to involvement of the ureters is easily demonstrated. Further, CT may demonstrate a soft-tissue mass that may contain areas of heterogeneous attenuation secondary to necrosis (see Figure 9-33). Invasion of the parametrium may be seen as soft-tissue extension into the parametrial fat, irregular cervical margins, or obliteration of the parametrial fat (see Figure 9-35). Hydronephrosis and nodal and distant metastases and peritoneal spread may be seen with advanced disease.

Once discovered, most cervical cancers are staged using a clinical assessment devised by FIGO (Table 9-6).[58] FIGO staging includes examination under anesthesia, chest

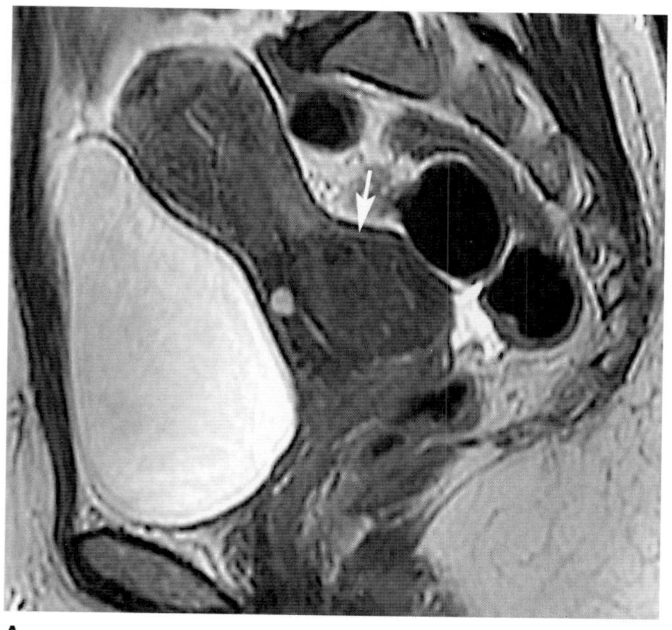
A

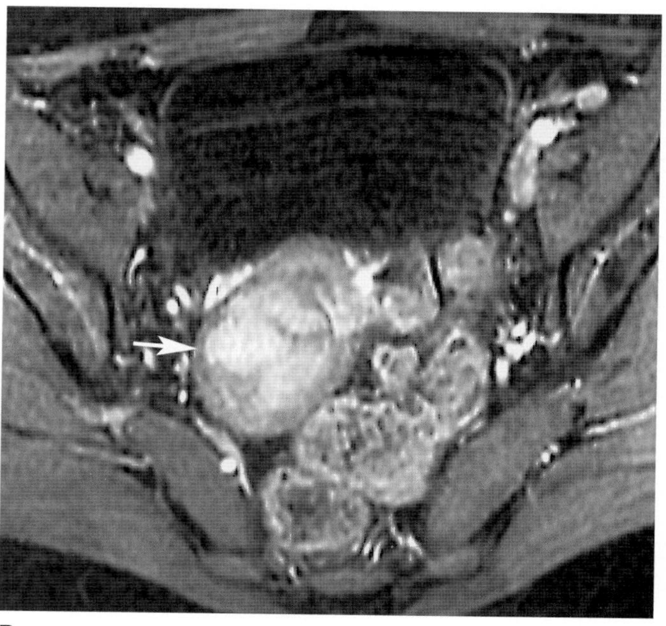
B

Figure 9-32 Cervical Leiomyoma
A. Sagittal T2-weighted and (**B**) axial T1-weighted postgadolinium contrast images demonstrate a focal, well-circumscribed mass (*arrow*) with low T2 SI and enhancement involving the posterior aspect of the cervix. This has similar imaging features to a uterine leiomyoma and represents a cervical leiomyoma. There is also a small cyst in the anterior cervix characteristic of a nabothian cyst.

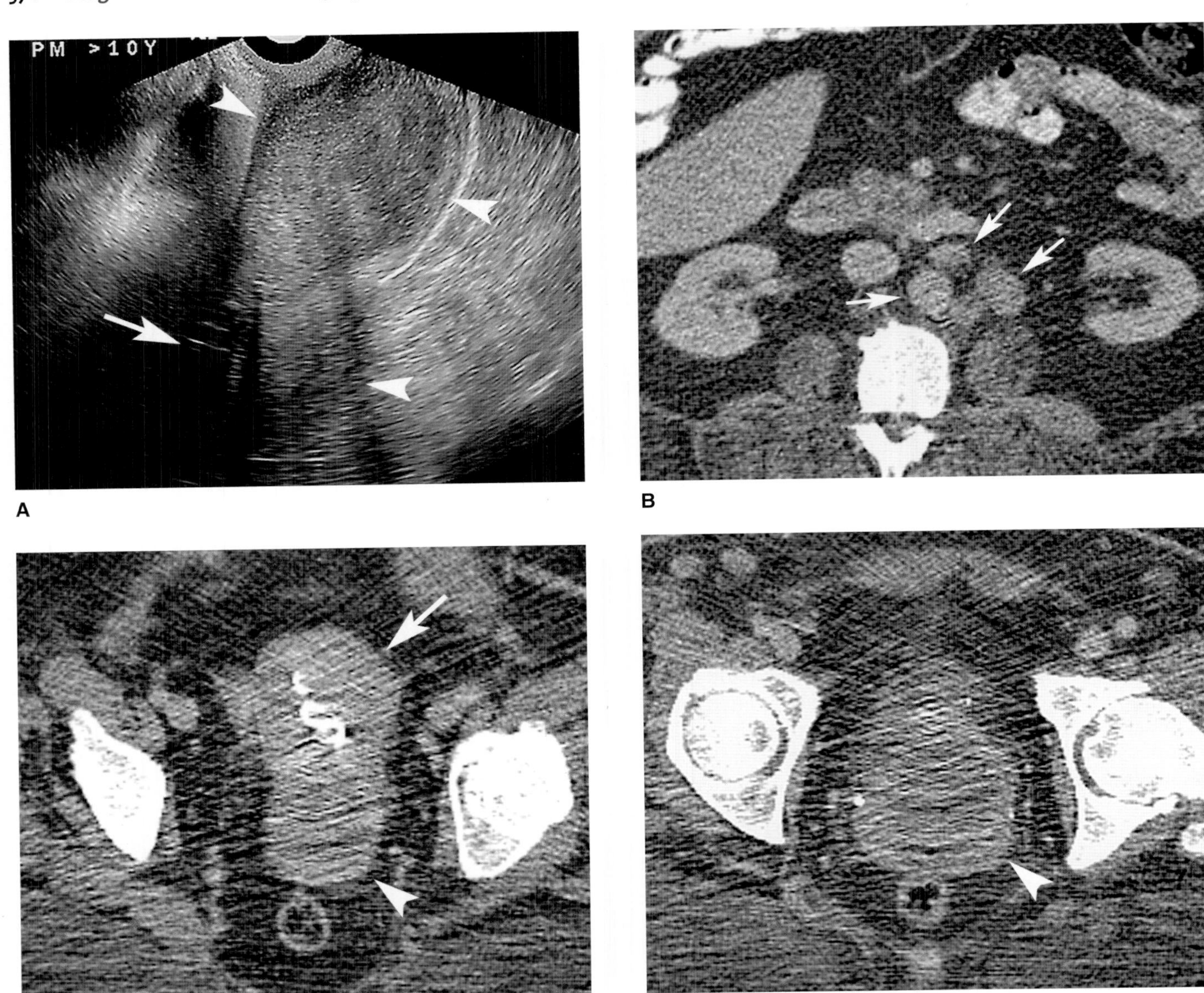

Figure 9-33 Cervical Cancer with Metastatic Lymphadenopathy A 64-year-old woman had an US examination to evaluate the position of a long indwelling intrauterine device (IUD). **A.** Longitudinal transvaginal US shows a large heterogeneous cervical mass (*arrowheads*) below the main body of the uterus (*arrows*). **B-D.** Contrast-enhanced CT confirms the presence of a large cervical mass (*arrowheads*) below the IUD-containing uterus (*large arrow*). The fat planes surrounding the cervical mass are sharp, suggesting that the mass has not invaded beyond the cervix into the parametrium. However, multiple enlarged retroperitoneal lymph nodes (*small arrows*) are seen in the upper abdomen at the level of the kidneys, indicating the presence of nodal metastasis.

radiography, an IV pyelogram, cystoscopy, a barium enema, and proctoscopy. Overall, MRI and FIGO had similar staging accuracy of 81% and 79%, respectively.[54] However, in patients with stage IIa or higher disease, the accuracy of MRI and FIGO staging were 74% and 53%, respectively.[54] Because stage IIa and lower disease is treated surgically and stage IIb and higher disease is treated with chemotherapy and radiation, accurate staging is necessary for appropriate treatment planning. Although clinical staging based on the FIGO criteria remain the gold standard, MRI is frequently performed as part of the initial workup in patients with a new diagnosis of cervical cancer. Further, MRI can accurately measure tumor size to within 5 mm compared to that determined by histologic staging of the surgical specimen.[54] The accuracy of MRI for assessment of parametrial, vaginal, and pelvic sidewall invasion is reported to be 88%, 93%, and 95%, respectively.[54] T2-weighted images are the most useful sequences for assessment of

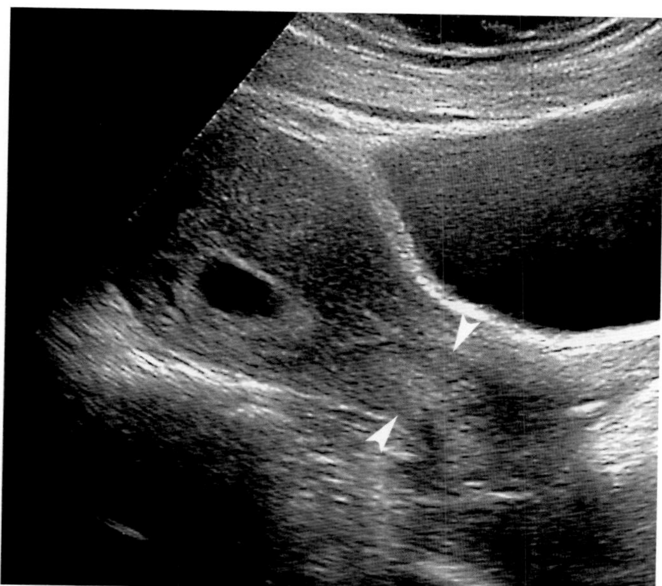

Figure 9-34 Cervical Cancer Confined to the Cervix
A 33-year-old woman undergoing evaluation for early pregnancy. The examination shows a small intrauterine sac indicative of an early pregnancy. There is also an irregularly marginated hyperechoic mass (*arrowheads*) in the posterior wall of the cervix.

tumor size, parametrial and vaginal invasion, and regional lymphadenopathy.

In stage I disease, the cancer is confined to the cervix and is subdivided by the size and extent of the tumor (Table 9-6). Stage Ia disease is microinvasive disease that is generally not seen on imaging examinations.[58] Occasionally, increased SI on T2-weighted images will be present in the cervix related to prior biopsy and should not be confused with the presence of tumor. Stage Ib1 disease will usually be detectable by MRI, measures less than 4 cm, and is confined to the cervix (see Figure 9-34). If trachelectomy is being considered, the length of the cervix and the distance between the tumor and internal os should be described. Stage Ib2 disease is larger than 4 cm, but remains confined to the cervix. As in stage Ib1 disease, tumor does not extend beyond the low-SI ring of the inner cervical stroma on T2-weighted images.

Stage II disease is defined as superficial invasion of the vagina and/or parametrial tissues.[58] Stage IIa disease is present when there is tumor extension into the upper two-thirds of the vagina.[58] In this stage, MRI reveals disruption of the low-SI wall of the upper vagina on T2-weighted images.[53,58] Stage IIb disease is present when there is tumor extension into the parametrium. Parametrial invasion is present when there is extension of tumor through both the low-SI inner cervical stroma and the intermediate-SI outer cervical stroma on T2-weighted images.[53,58] Additionally, irregularity of the cervical-fat interface, encasement of the parametrial vessels, or thickening and nodularity of the uterine ligaments can be seen (see Figure 9-35). Tumors of stage IIb and higher are treated with chemoradiation rather than surgery.[53,58]

Stage III disease is characterized by deep invasion of the vagina and/or parametrial tissues.[53,58] Stage IIIa disease is characterized by invasion of the tumor into the lower one-third of the vagina.[53,58] On T2-weighted images, interruption of the low-SI vaginal wall is seen.[53,58] Stage IIIb disease is similar to stage IIb but with involvement of the pelvic sidewall musculature or hydronephrosis or a nonfunctioning kidney due to ureteral involvement.[53,58]

Stage IV disease is defined as direct invasion of other nonvaginal pelvic organs or as distant metastasis.[53,58] Stage IVa disease is present when the cancer invades the bladder wall or rectal wall mucosa.[53,58] This stage is diagnosed by MRI when there is interruption or thickening of the low-SI rectal or bladder wall on T2-weighted images.[53,58] Stage IVb disease is present when there are distant metastases. Para-aortic and inguinal lymph node metastases, but not pelvic lymph node metastasis, are considered as stage IVb disease (see Figure 9-33).[53,58] Sites of distant metastasis include the liver, bone, lung, and peritoneum.

Although not included in the FIGO staging system, the status of the pelvic and para-aortic lymph nodes carries significant prognostic implications.[54] For example, disease-free survival at 3 years for those with stage Ib or IIa disease was 100% and 67% in the absence and presence of positive lymph nodes, respectively.[54] Patients with advanced disease (stage IIb to IVa) had 3-year disease-free survival rates of 56% and 24% in the absence and presence of positive lymph nodes, respectively.[54] Parametrial and paracervical nodes are typically the sentinel nodal groups and the initial sites of nodal metastases. Unfortunately, however, MRI and CT are not accurate in the diagnosis of lymph node metastasis. Utilizing a size criterion of a short axis measurement ≥1 cm as indicating presence of metastasis, the sensitivity of MRI is only 60%.[43] An insensitive but specific finding of metastatic lymphadenopathy is the presence of central necrosis.[59] One potentially useful technique for lymph node evaluation is administration of ultrasmall superparamagnetic iron oxide particles. Normal lymph nodes take up the particles and subsequently lose SI because of the susceptibility effects of iron oxide.[43] Lymph node metastases do not take up the particles and, therefore, do not lose SI after iron particle administration.

In general, FDG-PET/CT has been shown to be quite sensitive and specific in identifying metastatic nodes (see Figure 9-35).[60] False-negative results may be related to micrometastases in lymph nodes smaller than 5 mm for which FDG-PET is less sensitive.[61,62] FDG-PET is also very sensitive and specific in identifying distant metastases with false positives usually the result of infectious or inflammatory conditions or other primary malignancies.[61,62] Additional uses of FDG-PET in the management of cervical

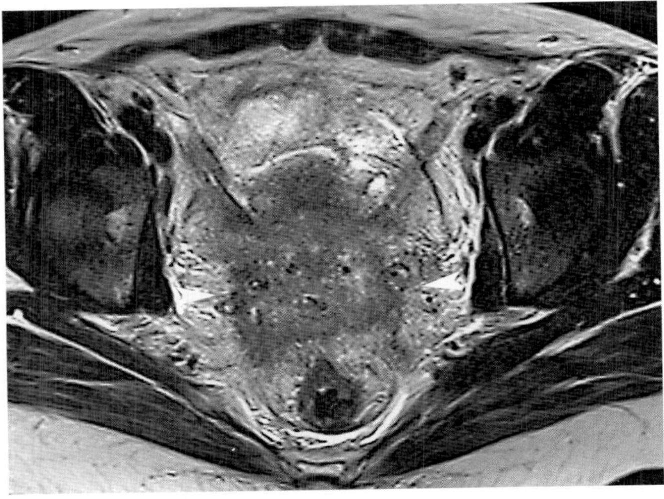

A

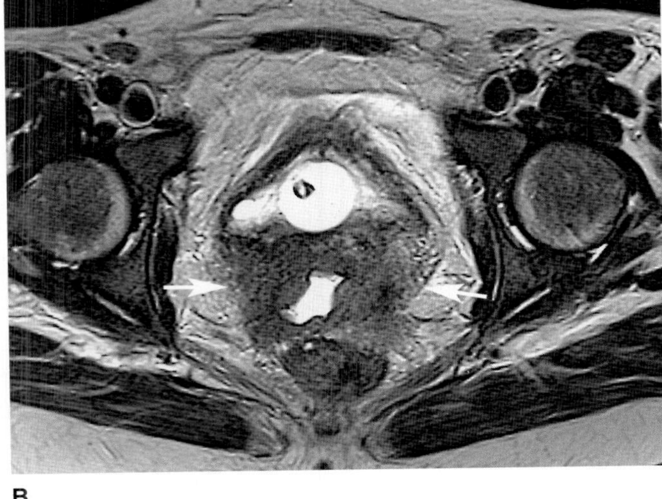

B

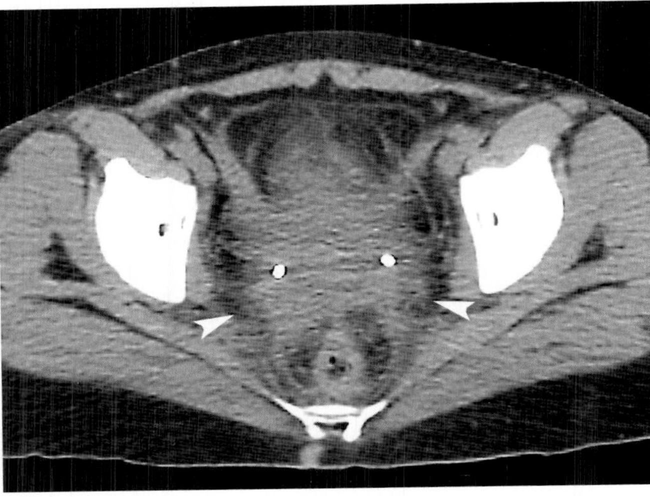

C

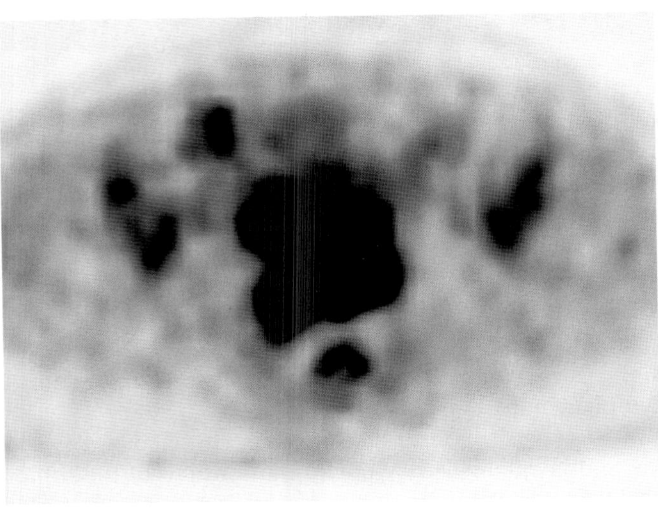

D

Figure 9-35 Cervical Cancer with Parametrial and Vaginal Invasion A 34-year-old woman with history of menorrhagia presented with abdominal pain and heavy vaginal bleeding. **A** and **B.** Axial T2-weighted image demonstrate a large heterogeneous mass replacing the cervix (*arrowheads*) and invading the proximal vagina (*arrow*). Note how indistinct the margins of the mass are relative to the surrounding pelvic fat, indicating invasion of the parametrial fat. **C.** Unenhanced CT image from a PET-CT also shows a large indistinctly marginated mass (*arrowheads*) replacing the cervix and invading the surrounding fat. **D.** PET image at the same level shows intense activity in the mass but also within multiple osseous and peritoneal metastases that were difficult to appreciate on the anatomic images.

cancer include radiation therapy planning, assessment of response to radiation therapy and neoadjuvant chemotherapy, and detection of recurrent or persistent disease.

Other Cervical Malignancies

Rarely, a cervical mass will represent a malignancy other than cervical cancer or adenoma malignum. These include lymphoma, primary malignant melanoma, adenoid cystic carcinoma, rhabdomyosarcoma, small cell carcinoma, and metastasis. Metastases to the cervix most commonly originate in the urinary bladder, colon, or ovary.

UNIQUE UTERINE AND CERVICAL ABNORMALITIES: CONGENITAL ANOMALIES

Congenital anomalies of the uterus are not uncommon, with prevalence estimates in the 0.2% to 5% range.[64] The true prevalence of these abnormalities is difficult to measure as many women are asymptomatic and do not undergo imaging assessment.[64] Those who present for evaluation frequently complain of pelvic pain or palpable abnormality if there is obstruction of the uterine outflow, infertility, or pregnancy loss.[64] Women with infertility have a higher

Table 9-6. TNM[a] and FIGO[b] Staging of Cervical Carcinoma with Corresponding MRI Findings

TNM	FIGO Stage	Description	MRI Findings
TX		Primary tumor cannot be assessed	None
T0		Primary tumor cannot be identified	None
Tis	0	Carcinoma in situ	None
T1	I	Tumor confined to cervix	
T1a	Ia	Microinvasive disease	None
T1a1	Ia1	Stromal invasion ≤3 mm in depth and ≤7 mm in horizontal spread	None
T1a2	Ia2	Stromal invasion >3 and ≤5 mm in depth and ≤7 mm in horizontal spread	None; may see high T2 SI related to biopsy
T1b	Ib	Clinically invasive disease (>5 mm)	High-SI tumor surrounded by intact low-SI stromal ring
T1b1	Ib1	Clinically visible lesion ≤4 cm	High-SI tumor surrounded by intact low-SI stromal ring
T1b2	Ib2	Clinically visible lesion >4 cm	High-SI tumor surrounded by intact low-SI stromal ring
T2a	IIa	Invasion beyond the uterus but not to the lower third of the vagina; no parametrial invasion	Disruption of the low-SI wall of the upper two-thirds of the vagina by high-SI tumor
T2b	IIb	Parametrial invasion not extending to the pelvic sidewall	Disruption of the low-SI cervical stroma by high-SI tumor; irregularity of the cervix-parametrial fat interface; parametrial vessel encasement; nodularity of uterine ligaments
T3a	IIIa	Invasion to the lower one-third of the vagina without extension to the pelvic sidewall	Disruption of the low-SI wall by high-SI tumor to the lower one-third of the vagina
T3b	IIIb	Invasion to the pelvic sidewall or tumor causes hydronephrosis or a nonfunctioning kidney	Tumor extending into parametrium to within 3 mm of the pelvic sidewall; hydroureter or hydronephrosis
T4	Iva	Invasion of the rectal or bladder mucosa or extension out of the true pelvis	Disruption of the low-SI rectal or bladder wall
M1	IVb	Distant metastases including para-aortic and inguinal lymph node metastases	Variable depending on site of involvement
N-Regional Lymph nodes			
NX		Regional lymph nodes cannot be assessed	
N0		No regional lymph node metastases	
N1		Regional lymph node metastases to pelvic and/or para-aortic nodes	
M-Distant Metastases			
MX		Distant metastases cannot be assessed	
M0		No distant metastases	
M1		Distant metastases	

[a]Data from Rubin P, Hansen JT. *TNM Staging Atlas*. Philadelphia, PA: Lippincott Williams & Wilkins; 2008.
[b]Data from Staging Classifications and Clinical Practice Guidelines for Gynaecological Cancer, FIGO Committee on Gynecologic Oncology; 2000.

incidence (7%-10%) of uterine anomalies than those without infertility, and those with recurrent pregnancy loss have an even higher incidence (30%-40%).[64]

The American Society of Reproductive Medicine (formerly the American Fertility Society) classification of uterine anomalies was last revised in 1988 and is the most widely accepted system forming the basis for practice for most clinicians. Seven classes of uterine anomalies are outlined in the classification according to etiology.

Understanding of the various congenital anomalies begins with a basic review of embryology. The uterus, cervix, and upper two-thirds of the vagina form during the sixth through twelfth weeks of gestation from the müllerian or paramesonephric ducts.[64] The paired ducts undergo lateral fusion in a caudal-to-cranial fashion. The cranial portions of the ducts do not fuse and become the fallopian tubes, while the fused caudal portion undergoes vertical fusion with the urogenital sinus, which is responsible for the lower one-third of the vagina. The müllerian ducts then undergo canalization and the shared central wall of the fused ducts is reabsorbed, thereby creating a single cavity in the uterus and vagina.[64] Disruption or failure of this process results in an anomalous configuration (Table 9-7). The embryologic origins of the müllerian ducts are in proximity to the metanephric ducts that develop to form the kidneys. As a result, anomalous development of one is frequently associated with anomalous development of the other. Approximately 40% to 50% of congenital renal anomalies are associated with uterine malformation, whereas 30% to 40% of uterine anomalies have an associated renal malformation.[64]

Class I anomalies result from failure of development of the normal müllerian ducts.[64] The result is agenesis or hypoplasia of the vagina, cervix, fundus, fallopian tubes, or a combination thereof. Patients most frequently present with primary amenorrhea in adolescence. Uterine agenesis, also known as Mayer-Rokitansky-Küster-Hauser syndrome, includes congenital absence of the uterus and upper vagina with normal ovaries and fallopian tubes.

Table 9-7. Müllerian Duct Developmental Error and Resulting Uterine Anomaly

Failure of development of one or both ducts	Uterine agenesis Uterine hypoplasia Unicornuate uterus (with or without a rudimentary horn)
Failure of canalization of the ducts	Unicornuate uterus with a rudimentary without an endometrial cavity
Failure of lateral fusion of the ducts	Uterus didelphys Bicornuate uterus
Failure of reabsorption after lateral fusion	Septate uterus (complete and partial) Arcuate uterus

Class II anomalies are caused by agenesis or hypoplasia of one of the paramesonephric ducts and result in a unicornuate uterus.[64] A unicornuate uterus is banana-shaped and may have a rudimentary horn if the abnormal duct partially forms. Rudimentary horns may or may not canalize and those that do canalize may or may not communicate with the uterus. Importantly, women who have unicornuate uteri with noncommunicating rudimentary horns are at risk of developing endometriosis as antegrade menstruation cannot occur and endometrial tissue is expelled in a retrograde fashion.[17,64] In this situation, the rudimentary horn will often be surgically resected to prevent this complication. Unicornuate uteri are associated with the highest rate of pregnancy loss.[17] T2-weighted images demonstrate normal zonal anatomy (see Figure 9-36).

Class III anomalies are caused by failure of lateral fusion of the müllerian ducts.[64] The result is a uterus didelphys with 2 completely separate uteri, each with its own cervix, possibly with 2 vaginas. This anomalous configuration is the least associated with infertility (aside from the arcuate configuration).[17] If there is obstruction of uterine outflow by underdevelopment of the cervix or vagina, patients may present with pelvic pain or mass related to hematocolpos. Two uterine horns and cervices with normal zonal anatomy are seen on T2-weighted images (see Figure 9-37).

Class IV anomalies occur when there is partial lateral fusion of the müllerian ducts.[64] Because lateral fusion proceeds in the caudal to cranial direction, the bicornuate uterus has a single cervix with 2 separate uterine horns. There is a cleft between the unfused uterine horns creating a concave outer contour greater than 1 cm deep.[17] This configuration has been described as a heart-shaped uterus and is an important feature that distinguishes the bicornuate from the septate uterus. These patients are typically asymptomatic, but have a higher incidence of spontaneous abortion. Diagnostic imaging criteria include an intercornual distance of at least 4 cm, concavity of the outer fundal contour by at least 1 cm, and an intercornual angle of greater than 60° (see Figure 9-38).[17,65]

Class V anomalies result from failure of or incomplete resorption of the central septum that had formed as the result of complete lateral fusion.[64] The septum may be a combination of fibrous tissue and muscle and its size depends on the degree of failure of resorption. The septum may extend from the fundus to the cervix (septate) or only partially from the fundus to the cervix (subseptate). Because lateral fusion is complete, the outer uterine contour is often convex or flat, but may have a concavity of less than 1 cm (as opposed to a bicornuate uterus).[17] An intercornual distance of less than 4 cm and an intercornual angle of <60° are also imaging features of a septate uterus.[17] Fibrous septa demonstrate low SI on T2-weighted images, whereas muscular septa have intermediate SI (see Figure 9-39).[17] Septate uteri are the most commonly identified anomaly in women evaluated for

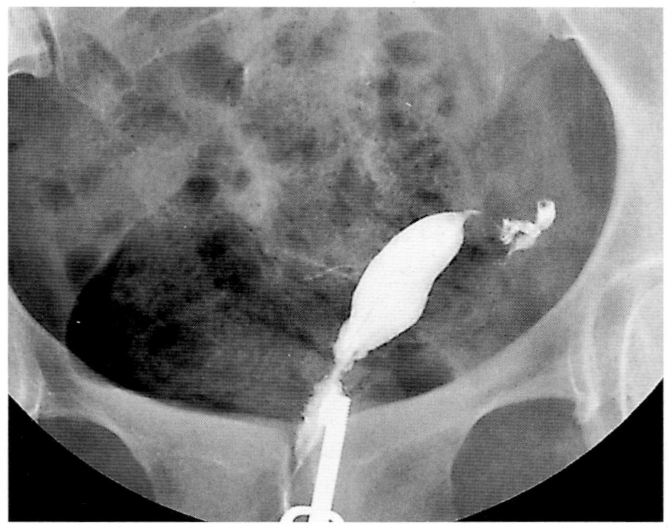

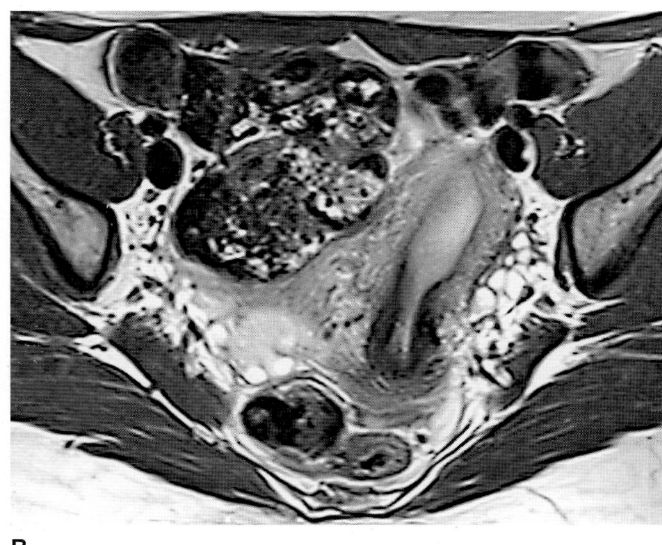

A B

Figure 9-36 Unicornuate Uterus
A 29-year-old woman with history of infertility. **A.** Hysterosalpingogram shows a single left fallopian tube and a uterus with a sausage-shaped endometrial cavity, rather than the usual triangular configuration—findings suggesting a unicornuate uterus. **B.** T2-weighted image shows a small sausage-shaped uterus typical of a unicornuate uterus.

repeated abortions.[17] Hysteroscopic metroplasty to resect the septum is reported to improve fertility and fetal survival.[11]

Class VI comprises an arcuate configuration of the uterus with a slight indentation of the fundal endometrial canal with a normal external contour.[64] This shape is on a continuum with the septate uterus, but the septum is resorbed to less than 1 cm from the fundus. An arcuate uterus is considered to be a normal variant by many and has no or little effect on fertility (see Figure 9-40).[64,65]

Class VII anomalies are a group of malformations related to the intrauterine exposure to diethylstilbestrol, a synthetic estrogen used in the 1940s to 1970s to prevent spontaneous abortion. Anomalous configurations include a T-shaped uterus, uterine hypoplasia, and irregular

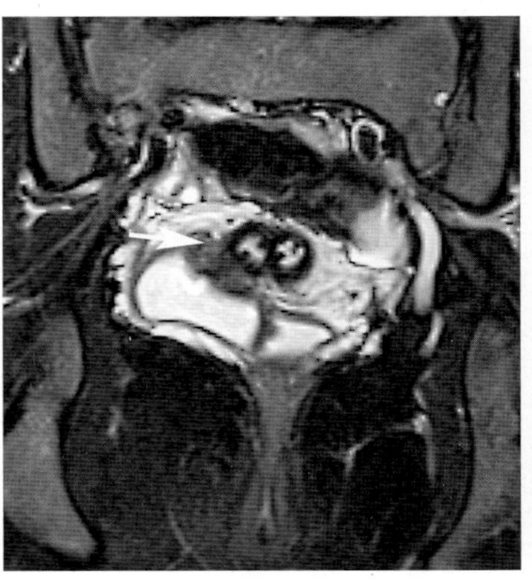

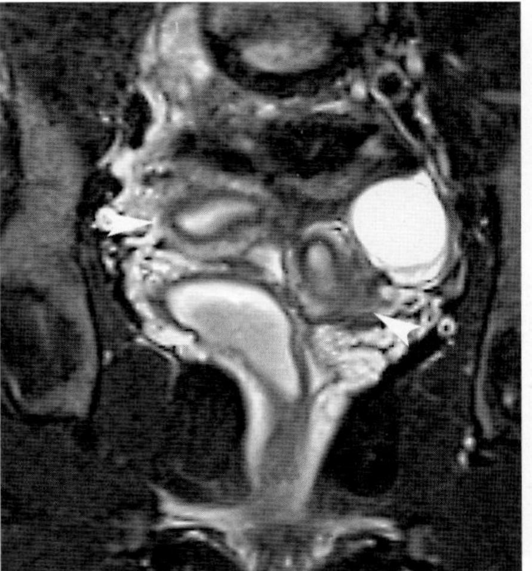

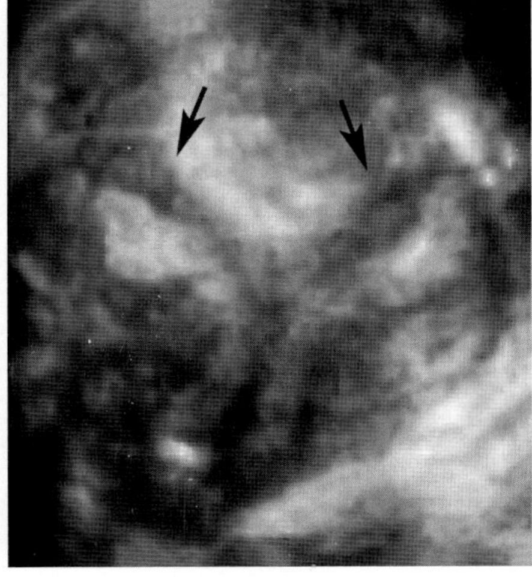

A B C

Figure 9-37 Uterus Didelphys
A 15-year-old woman presented with continuous vaginal drainage between menses. **A** and **B.** Coronal T2-weighted image demonstrate paired cervices (*white arrows*) and paired uteri (*arrowheads*) characteristic of uterus didelphys. **C.** Coronal 3-D US image shows the complete division of uteri and cervices to better advantage.

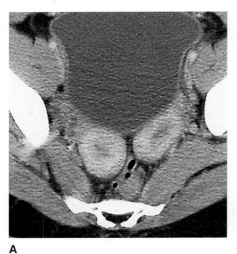

A

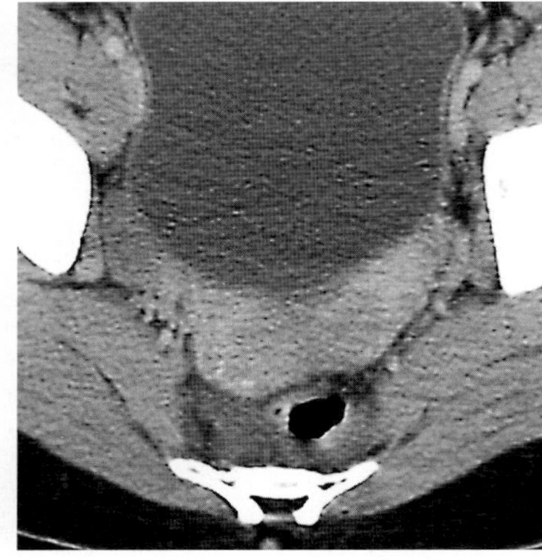

B

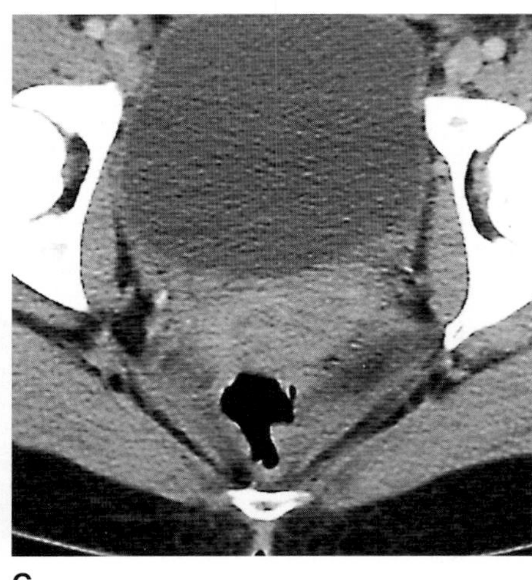

C

Figure 9-38 Bicornuate Uterus
A 21-year-old woman presents with abdominal pain. **A-C.** Contrast-enhanced CT demonstrates 2 separate uterine horns that merge to form a single cervix. This is the typical appearance of a bicornuate uterus.

constrictions (see Figure 9-41).[17] Diethylstilbestrol-related anomalies are associated with an increased risk of spontaneous abortion, preterm delivery, and ectopic pregnancy.[17] The areas of constriction are shown as localized thickening of the junctional zone on T2-weighted images.

Diagnosis of congenital uterine anomalies had traditionally been made by HSG with laparoscopy and hysteroscopy. In general, HSG reveals filling defects that may suggest a septate or bicornuate uterus. The outer uterine contour, however, is not delineated, and therefore it is not possible to reliably distinguish a septate uterus from a bicornuate uterus. Measurement of the intercornual angle may be helpful, with an angle >75° to 105° suggesting a bicornuate uterus and <75° suggesting a septate uterus.[64,65] A unicornuate uterus

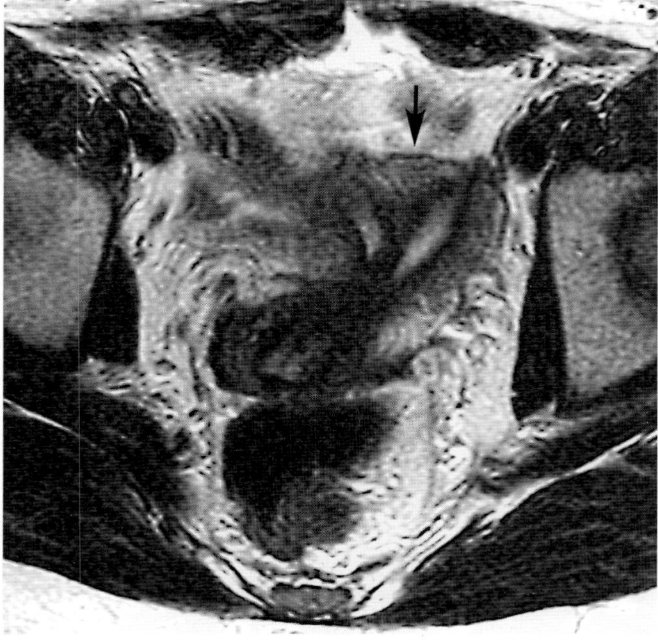

A

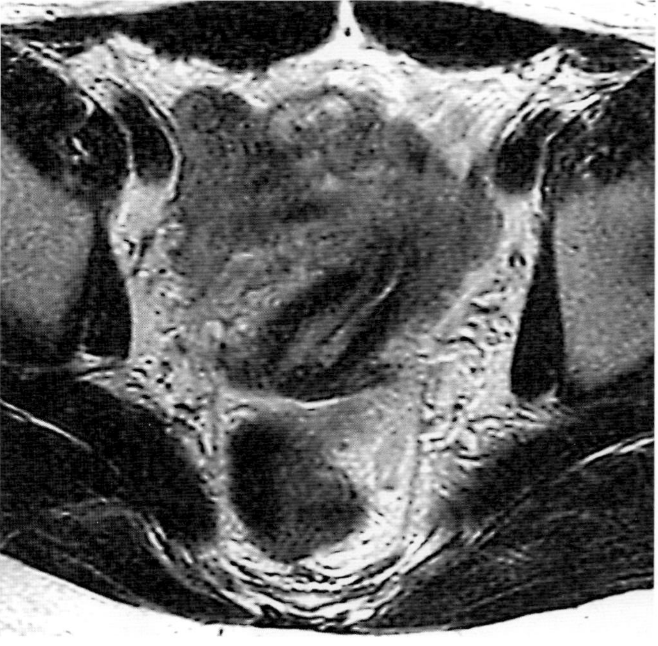

B

Figure 9-39 Septate Uterus
A 24-year-old woman with abnormal uterine configuration on US and pelvic pain. **A** and **B.** T2-weighted image demonstrate the superior border of the uterus (*arrow*) to be flat with a continuous myometrium from one horn to the next. However, the endometrial canal is divided into 2 segments by a low-SI fibrous septum extending to the cervix. These features are diagnostic of a septate uterus.

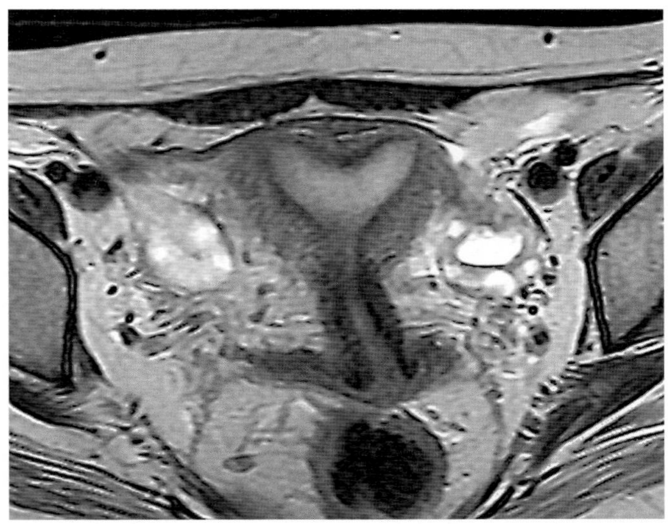

Figure 9-40 Arcuate Uterus
A 16-year-old woman with a complex ovarian cyst seen on a US study. Axial T2-weighted image shows slight indentation of the fundal endometrial canal but with a normal external contour. This is typical of an arcuate uterus.

appears as a deviated small endometrial canal with a single fallopian tube. If an apparent unicornuate uterus is identified, a second cervix must also be considered, as unilateral contrast injection of a uterus didelphys will simulate a unicornuate configuration. It is also important to know that a noncommunicating rudimentary horn of a unicornuate uterus will not be identified by HSG. One review of the literature comparing HSG to hysteroscopy reported a weighted mean sensitivity and specificity of HSG of 78% and 90%, respectively. However, differentiation between classes of anomalies was poor.[64] Women suspected of having a congenital malformation frequently underwent confirmatory laparoscopy.

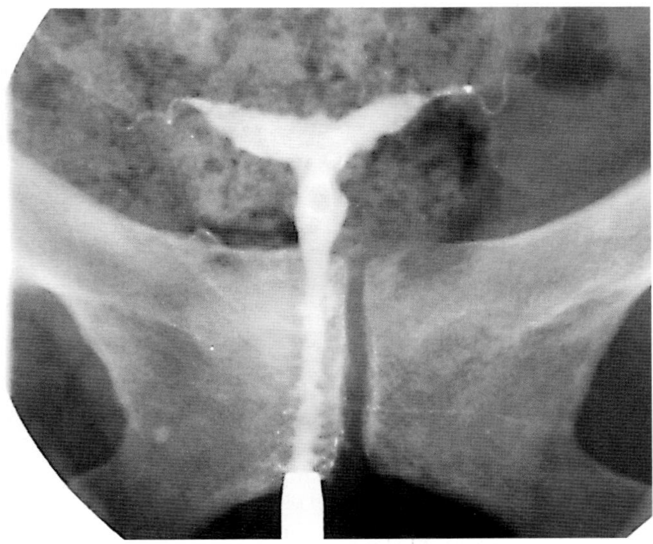

Figure 9-41 T-Shaped Uterus (Class VII Anomaly)
A 40-year-old woman with infertility and history of intrauterine diethylstilbestrol (DES) exposure. Hysterosalpingogram shows a T-shaped, rather than the normal V-shaped, configuration of the uterine canal. This is a known malformation related to intrauterine DES exposure.

In general, MRI and US are now offered as more accurate and less invasive techniques in evaluating women suspected of having uterine anomalies. Further, MRI examinations should include evaluation of the kidneys for associated abnormalities. In addition, the planes of acquisition should be adjusted to the long axis of the uterus to visualize the uterine contours to best advantage. T2-weighted images reveal the zonal anatomy of the uterus, and T1-weighted images are helpful in characterizing hemorrhage in the endometrial canal and adnexae. Enhanced images are not required routinely.

Transvaginal US with both 2-D and 3-D probes may aid in classifying uterine anomalies. The hyperechoic endometrium is often seen to split or separate near the fundus in cases of septate and bicornuate uteri. In general, 3-D US can show the outer uterine contour better than 2-D US, making the distinction between septate and bicornuate easier.[64] Saline-infused sonohysterography is the US equivalent of the HSG, but has been reported as superior to HSG.[64]

POSTPROCEDURE FINDINGS FOLLOWING CERVICAL AND UTERINE INTERVENTIONS

Intrauterine Adhesions (Asherman Syndrome)

Intrauterine adhesions, commonly known as Asherman Syndrome, typically form following traumatic insult to the endometrium, most frequently from uterine curettage, hysteroscopy, or after abortion.[11,50] Fibrous bands form from the uterine walls in areas of traumatized endometrium and result in distortion and obliteration of the cavity and sometimes of the internal cervical os.[50] In addition, dense myometrial adhesions and a thin sclerotic endometrium without adhesions may form.[50] Synechiae may ultimately lead to mechanical obstruction of the uterus. Patients report secondary amenorrhea or hypomenorrhea as well as infertility.

Intrauterine adhesions are revealed as filling defects in the uterus at HSG (see Figure 9-42).[6] Care must be taken to differentiate the filling defects due to adhesions from those of air bubbles, endometrial polyps, or leiomyomas. If the patient has a sclerotic endometrium with few adhesions, HSG will frequently be normal.[50]

Conventional transabdominal and transvaginal US are often limited in identifying intrauterine adhesions, especially when no fluid or blood is present in the endometrial canal to outline the synechiae.[50] In high-risk patients, however, TVUS may be more accurate.[51] Saline-infused sonohysterography, however, may be able to directly demonstrate the fibrous bands and delineate their extent and

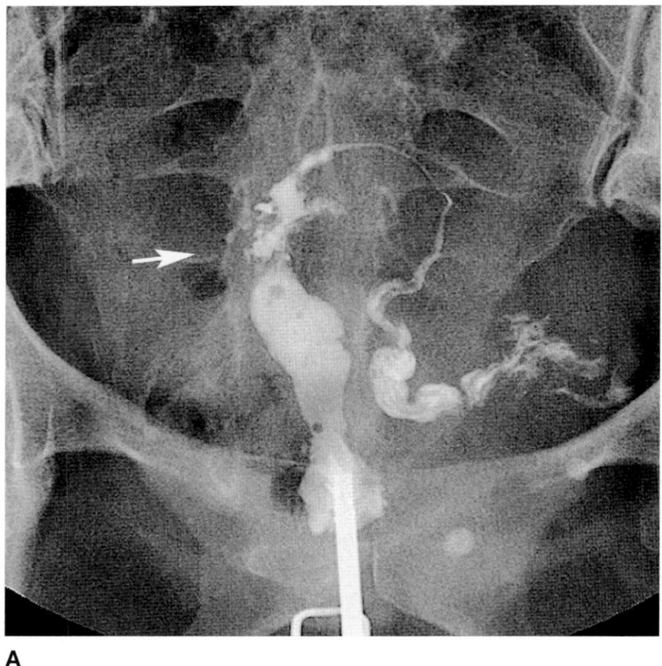
A

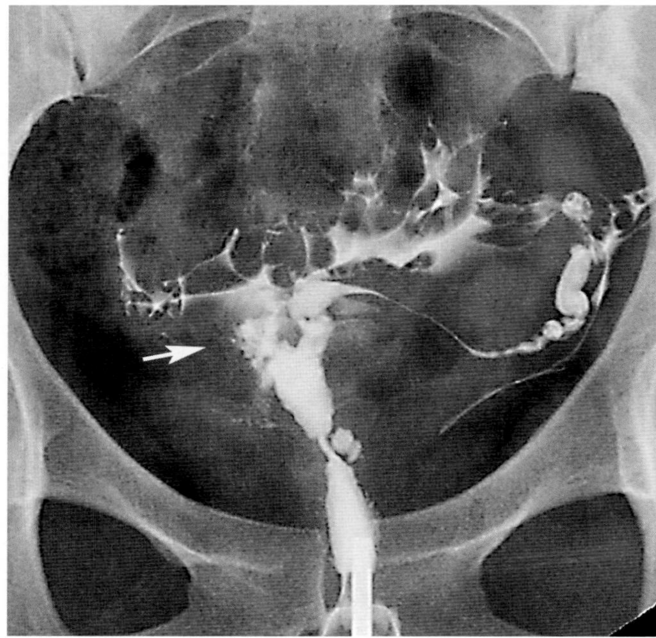
B

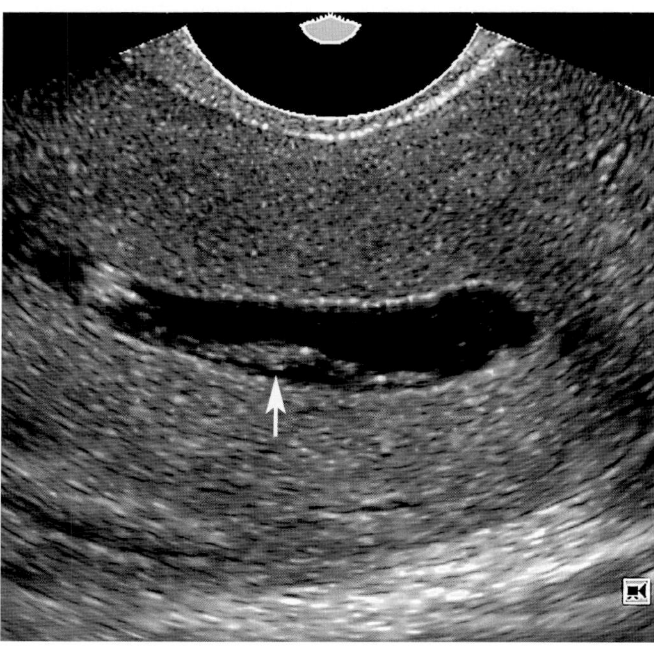
C

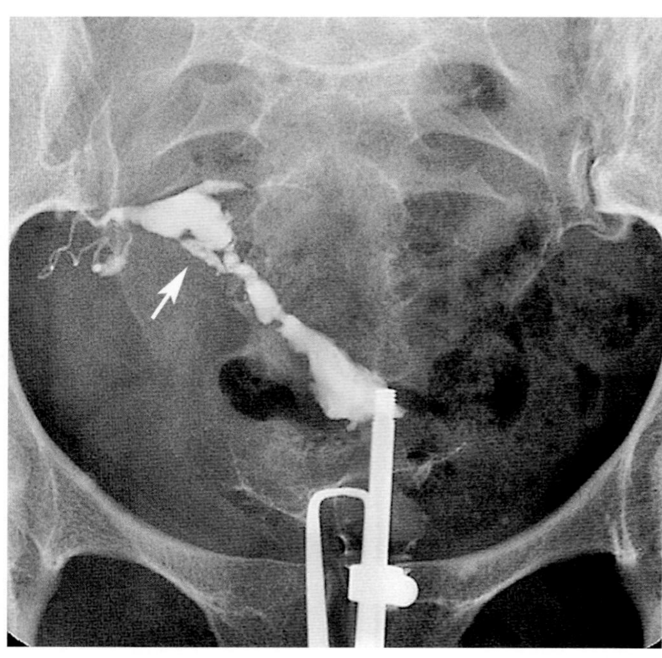
D

Figure 9-42 Intrauterine Adhesions in 2 Patients
A and **B.** A 34-year-old woman with infertility. (A) Early phase of the hysterosalpingogram demonstrates an irregular shape to the superior aspect of the uterine cavity. (B) Later phase image shows multiple intrauterine filling defects and an irregular surface to the uterine cavity indicating the presence of multiple intrauterine adhesions. **C** and **D.** A 48-year-old woman with history of endometriosis and prior hysteroscopically removed fibroids. (C) Sonohysterogram demonstrates threadlike echogenic foci (*arrow*) within the uterine cavity indicating adhesions. (D) Hysterosalpingogram reveals threadlike intrauterine defects (*arrow*) typical of adhesions.

location (see Figure 9-42). Sonohysterography combined with HSG have a reported sensitivity of 75% and positive predictive value of 42.9% (compared to hysteroscopy).[50]

The adhesions are well demonstrated on T2-weighted images as low-SI bands crossing the endometrial canal and causing distortion and/or obliteration of the endometrial cavity.[52] The normally high endometrial SI on T2-weighted image is absent (see Figure 9-43).

In some cases, the presence of intrauterine or cervical adhesions can be inferred by the retention of menstrual

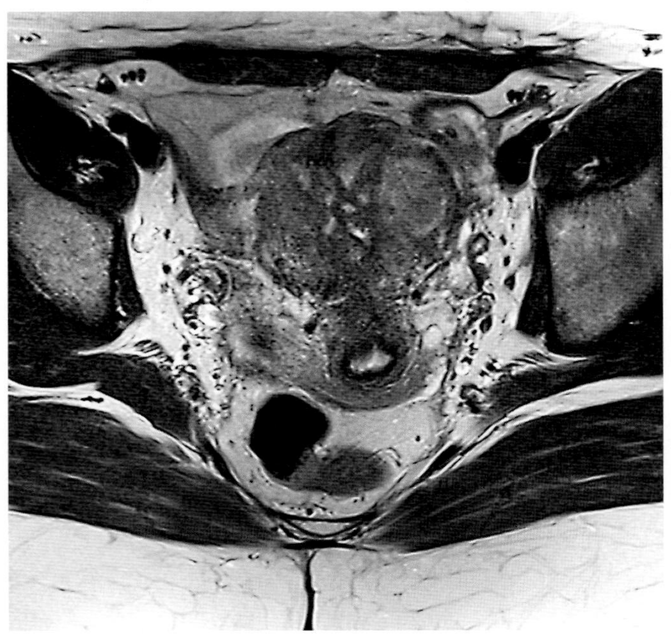

A

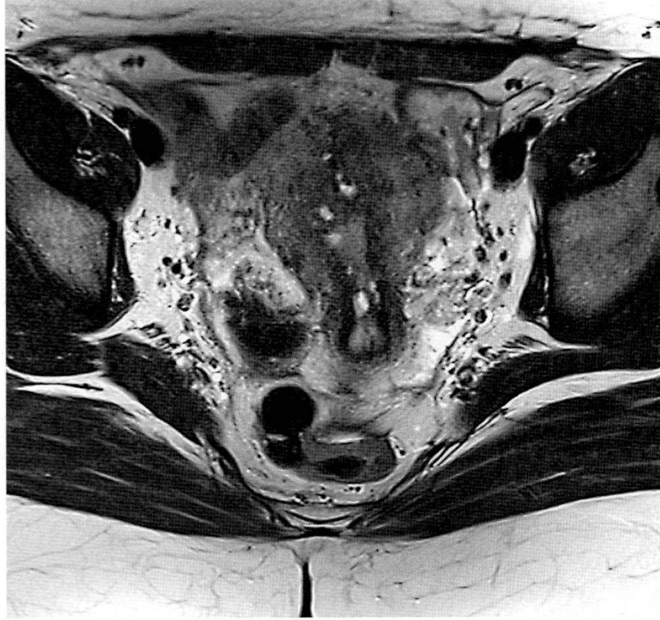

B

Figure 9-43 MRI of Intrauterine Adhesions
A 34-year-old woman with history of infertility and uterine fibroids subsequently removed by hysteroscopy. **A** and **B.** Postoperative axial T2-weighted image through the uterus and cervix demonstrate multiple low-SI bands within the endometrial canal and associated distortion of the endometrial canal, consistent with endometrial adhesions related to the prior surgery.

blood products within the uterine cavity. Further, US, CT, and MRI examinations will demonstrate complex fluid collections within the intrauterine cavity that show the characteristic imaging features of blood products.

Imaging Findings and Complications of Hysterectomy and Pelvic Radiation Therapy

In general, CT and MRI are useful to evaluate the pelvis postoperatively to identify tumor recurrence as well as treatment complications. Women with carcinoma in situ or microinvasive cervical cancer who are treated with cervical conization may have a defect in the cervix or a smaller-than-usual cervical portio.[53]

Those with stage Ib and IIa cervical cancer are usually treated with abdominal radical hysterectomy, including excision of the upper third of the vagina, parametrial and paravaginal tissues, and sacrouterine ligaments.[63] Pelvic node dissection is usually performed, but external beam and intracavitary radiation sometimes replace nodal dissection.[63] After hysterectomy, the vaginal cuff should appear as linear soft tissue on CT or as linear low SI on T2-weighted images.[63]

More advanced cervical cancer is not amenable to surgical resection and is frequently treated with chemoradiation therapy. After radiation therapy, positive responses are associated with decreasing size and SI of the tumor as well as reconstitution of the cervical zonal anatomy.[63]

Tumor recurrence most commonly occurs in the pelvis within the cervix, vaginal cuff, parametrium, or pelvic sidewall. Recurrent cervical carcinoma frequently presents as a new or enlarging mass that has increased SI on T2-weighted images.[63] Recurrent tumor may also be detected on CT as a mass that has less avid enhancement than the cervix.[63] If recurrence occurs in the preserved cervix, obstruction of the uterine outflow may lead to hematometras. Similar to primary tumors, recurrences may invade the bladder or rectum or may result in hydronephrosis. Recurrent tumor sometimes presents as a cystic mass that needs to be differentiated from a postoperative fluid collection. Recurrent tumor should be suspected if the finding is made 6 months or more after the surgery.[63] In general, FDG-PET/CT is accurate in detecting recurrent disease and is often helpful in differentiating tumor recurrence from treatment-related changes.[31]

Complications following surgery include abscess, ureteral fistula, hemorrhage, and lymphocele formation.[63] After radiation therapy, complications include rectovesical fistula, radiation colitis or enteritis, ureteral and bowel strictures, and sacral insufficiency fracture.[63] CT is most commonly used in evaluating these posttreatment changes, but barium studies and IV or CT urograms may also be useful.

Imaging Findings and Complications of Uterine Artery Embolization

Uterine artery embolization is an endovascular procedure that is most commonly performed for the treatment of symptomatic fibroids and adenomyosis. On occasion, UAE may be performed emergently, usually in the setting of postpartum hemorrhage. When performed for the treatment of uterine fibroids, MRI is often utilized to monitor treatment response. Additionally, although UAE is considered safe, the procedure is associated with a short-term complication rate of approximately 8.5% and a serious complication rate of 1.25%.[66] When procedural complications are suspected, CT and MRI often play crucial roles in their identification.

Routine follow-up is commonly performed with MRI. Expected findings after successful embolization include a decrease in tumor size, a decrease in or lack of enhancement, coagulative or hemorrhagic tumor necrosis, and occlusion of the uterine arteries (see Figure 9-44).[66,67] Hemorrhage within the fibroid is revealed as high SI on T1-weighted image and high attenuation on unenhanced CT. Treated (and untreated) fibroids may become calcified, identified as foci of susceptibility on MRI.

In the acute setting, CT is frequently the initial study obtained when procedural complications are suspected.

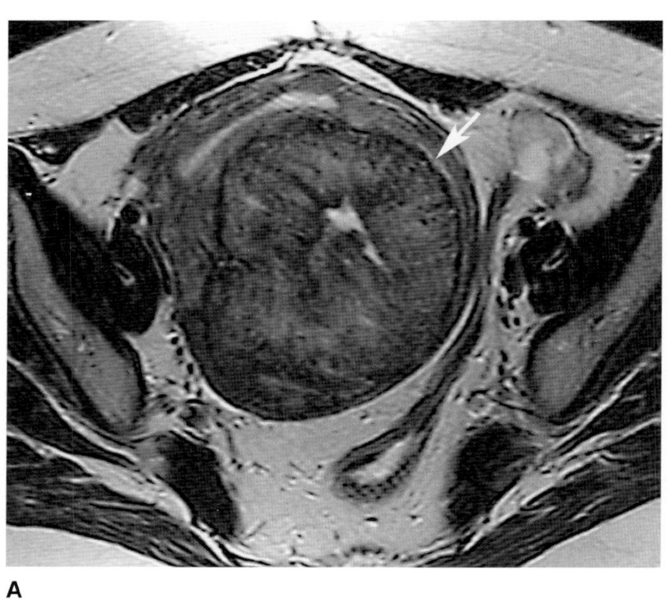

A

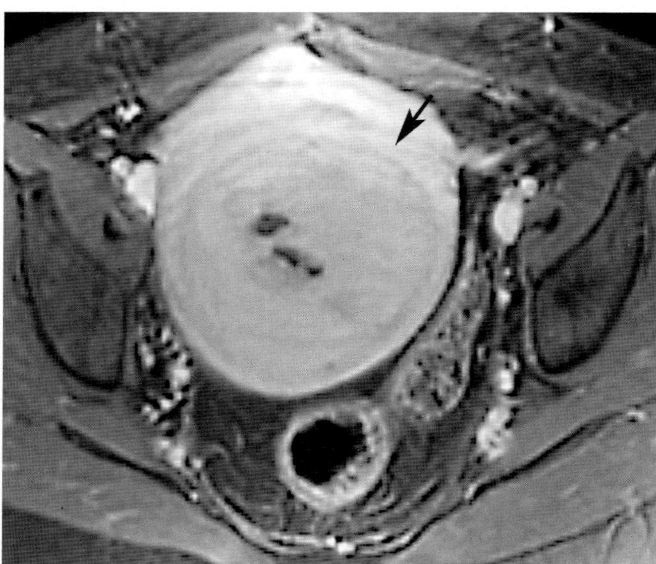

B

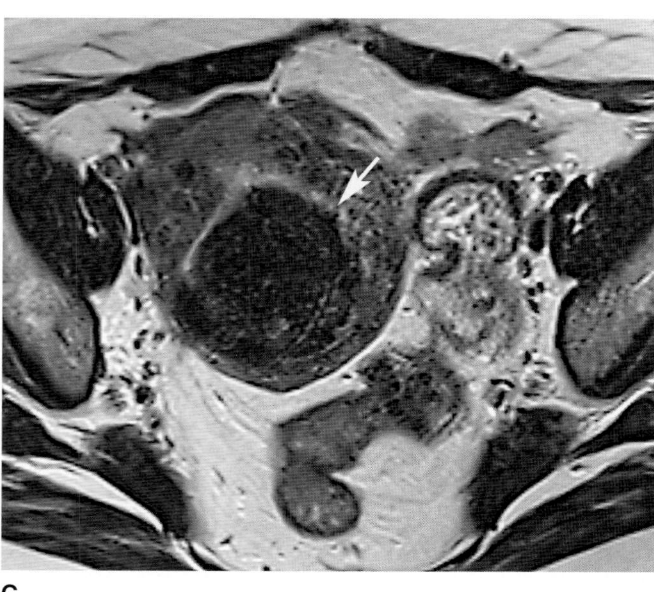

C

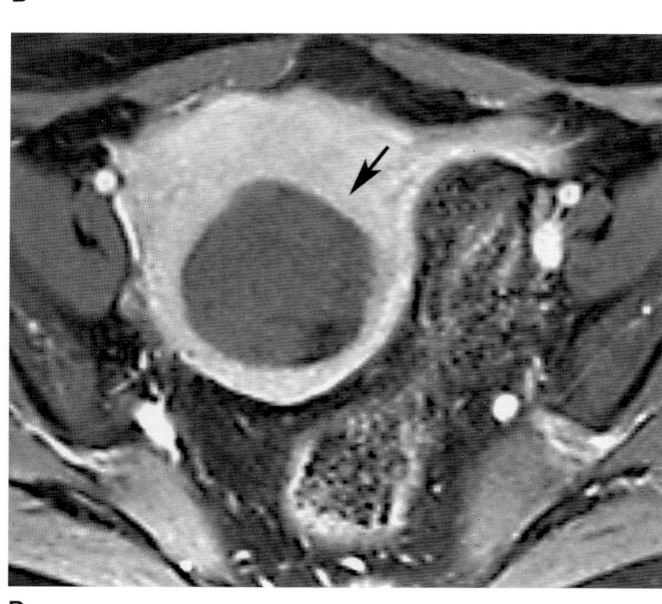

D

Figure 9-44 Uterine Artery Embolization for Uterine Fibroids A 42-year-old woman with history of menorrhagia. **A.** T2-weighted image and (**B**) postgadolinium contrast T1-weighted image demonstrate a large enhancing intracavitary leiomyoma (*arrows*). **C.** T2-weighted image and (**D**) postgadolinium contrast T1-weighted image obtained after UAE show decreased size and enhancement of the uterine leiomyoma (*arrows*). Low SI of fibroid on the T2-weighted image indicates presence of coagulative necrosis and/or fibrosis.

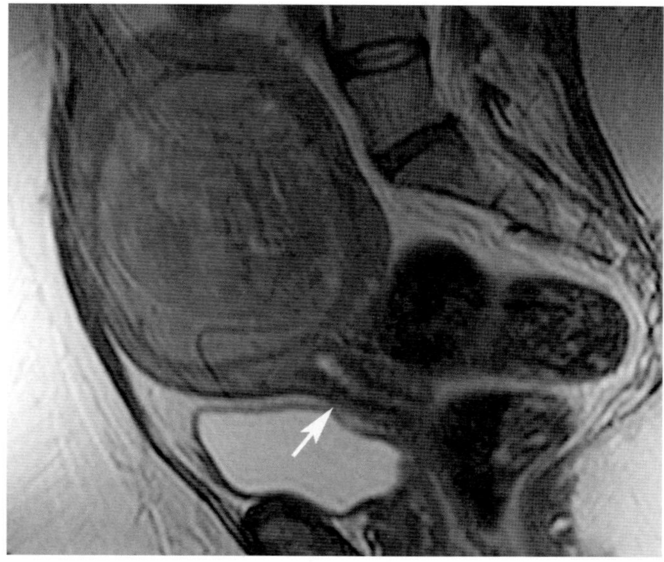

A

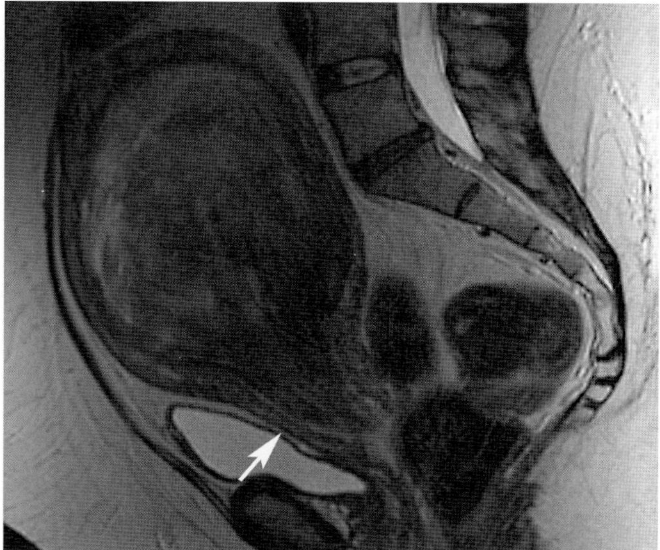

B

Figure 9-45 Spontaneous Vaginal Expulsion of an Intrauterine Fibroid after UAE
A 48-year-old woman with fever and pelvic pain following uterine artery embolization. **A.** Sagittal T2-weighted image shows a large intracavitary fibroid with a closed internal cervical os (*arrow*). **B.** Sagittal T2-weighted image performed after UAE shows movement of the fibroid into the cervix with expansion of the internal cervical os (*arrow*), indicating spontaneous expulsion of the tumor.

Further, CT is best for identifying fluid or gas collections, hemorrhage, and vascular complications. In addition, MRI may reveal these complications as well as allow for a more sensitive evaluation of the myometrium and fibroids. After embolization, fibroids that are in contact with the endometrium are at risk of undergoing spontaneous vaginal expulsion.[66,67] This is seen on MRI as an infarcted nonenhancing fibroid with high T1-weighted image and low T2-weighted image SI that expands the uterine and cervical canals (see Figure 9-45). Hysteroscopic resection may be required if the fibroid fails to pass spontaneously, there is heavy bleeding or infection, or the fibroid remains attached to the myometrium. Subserosal fibroids with a narrow stalk (<2 cm) are at risk of losing their connection to the uterus and becoming intraperitoneal, thereby raising the risk of pain and infection.[67]

Following UAE, many patients report increasing pelvic pain, vaginal discharge, and fever. These signs and symptoms are nonspecific and most often due to postembolization syndrome, but need to be differentiated from a procedure-related infection.[67] These patients are often imaged, and gas may be seen within the myometrium or fibroids. Intrafibroid gas may be seen as a normal finding after UAE and does not necessarily indicate the presence of infection or pyomyoma. Gas in a linear or branching distribution is less worrisome than that which is globular or in a fluid collection.[66,67] Other MRI and CT findings of endometritis include an enlarged uterus and hematoma. Uterine infarction is a rare life-threatening complication manifested as increased myometrial SI on T2-weighted images and lack of myometrial enhancement; antibiotic therapy and hysterectomy are generally required to prevent sepsis.[66,67]

If devascularization is incomplete or there is recanalization of the uterine arteries, fibroids may regrow or recur, with most symptomatic recurrences occurring after 2 years.[66] On occasion, during imaging follow-up after a technically successful UAE, the presumed fibroid does not undergo the anticipated changes, but rather grows or shows continued enhancement and has intermediately high T2-weighted image SI. In such situations, the radiologist should consider malignant degeneration or inadvertent embolization of a uterine sarcoma.

REFERENCES

1. Siegel MJ. Pediatric gynecologic sonography. *Radiology.* 1991; 179:593-600.
2. Nalaboff KM, Pellerito JS, Ben-Levi E. Imaging the endometrium: disease and normal variants. *Radiographics.* 2001;21:1409-1424.
3. Middleton WD, Kurtz AB, Barbara SH. Pelvis and Uterus. In: *Ultrasound: The Requisites.* 2nd ed. St Louis, MO: Mosby; 2004: 530-586.
4. Siegelman ES. MRI of the female pelvis. In: *Body MRI.* Philadelphia, PA: Elsevier Saunders; 2005:269-342.
5. Woodfield CA, Siegelman ES, Coleman BG, Torigian DA. CT features of adenomyosis. *Eur J Radiol.* 2009;72(3):464-469.
6. Simpson WL, Beitia LG, Mester J. Hysterosalpingography: a reemerging study. *Radiographics.* 2006;26:419-431.
7. Nishizawa S, Inubushi M, Okada H. Physiological ^{18}F-FDG uptake in the ovaries and uterus of healthy female volunteers. *Eur J Nucl Med Mol Imaging.* 2005;32:549-556.

8. Lin JF, Slomovitz BM. Uterine sarcoma 2008. *Curr Oncol Rep.* 2008;10:512-518.
9. Nishizawa S, Inubushi M, Kido A, et al. Incidence and characteristics of uterine leiomyomas with FDG uptake. *Ann Nucl Med.* 2008;22:803-810.
10. Potter AW, Chandrasekhar CA. US and CT evaluation of acute pelvic pain of gynecologic origin in nonpregnant premenopausal patients. *Radiographics.* 2008;28:1645-1659.
11. Taylor E, Gomel V. The uterus and fertility. *Fertil Steril.* 2008; 89:1-16.
12. Bennett GL, Slywotzky CM, Giovanniello G. Gynecologic causes of acute pelvic pain: spectrum of CT findings. *Radiographics.* 2002;22:785-801.
13. McLucas B. Diagnosis, imaging and anatomical classification of uterine fibroids. *Best Pract Res Clin Obstet Gynaecol.* 2008;22: 627-642.
14. Chen BB, Chen CA, Liu KL. Leiomyomatosis with extension to the left gluteal muscle, inferior vena cava, and right atrium. *Am J Roentgenol.* 2006;187:W546-W547.
15. Dueholm M, Lundorf E, Hansen E, et al. Accuracy of magnetic resonance imaging and transvaginal ultrasonography in the diagnosis, mapping, and measurement of uterine myomas. *Am J Obstet Gynecol.* 2002;186:409-415.
16. Dudiak CM, Turner DA, Patel SK, et al. Uterine leiomyomas in the infertile patient: preoperative localization with MR imaging versus US and hysterosalpingography. *Radiology.* 1988;167: 627-630.
17. Imaoka I, Wada A, Matsuo M, et al. MR imaging of disorders associated with female infertility: use in diagnosis, treatment, and management. *Radiographics.* 2003;23:1401-1421.
18. Rha SE, Byun JY, Jung SE, et al. CT and MRI of uterine sarcomas and their mimickers. *Am J Roentgenol.* 2003;181:1369-1374.
19. Reinhold C, Tafazoli F, Mehio A, et al. Uterine adenomyosis: endovaginal US and MR imaging features with histopathologic correlation. *Radiographics.* 1999;19:S147-S160.
20. Kitawaki J. Adenomyosis: the pathophysiology of an oestrogen-dependent disease. *Best Pract Res Clin Obstet Gynaecol.* 2006; 20:493-502.
21. Tamai K, Togashi K, Ito T, et al. MR imaging findings of adenomyosis: correlation with histopathologic features and diagnostic pitfalls. *Radiographics.* 2005;25:21-40.
22. Bergeron C, Amant F, Ferenczy A. Pathology and physiopathology of adenomyosis. *Best Pract Res Clin Obstet Gynaecol.* 2006;20:511-521.
23. Dueholm M. Transvaginal ultrasound for diagnosis of adenomyosis: a review. *Best Pract Res Clin Obstet Gynaecol.* 2006;20:569-582.
24. Dueholm M, Lundorf E. Transvaginal ultrasound or MRI for diagnosis of adenomyosis. *Curr Opin Obstet Gynecol.* 2007; 19:505-512.
25. Holloway BJ, Lopez C, Balogun M. Technical report: a simple and reliable way to recognize the transient myometrial contraction—a common pitfall in MRI of the pelvis. *Clin Radiol.* 2007;62:596-599.
26. Davidson KG, Dubinsky TJ. Ultrasonographic evaluation of the endometrium in postmenopausal vaginal bleeding. *Radiol Clin North Am.* 2003;41:769-780.
27. Goldstein RB, Bree RL, Benson CB, et al. Evaluation of the woman with postmenopausal bleeding: Society of Radiologists in Ultrasound-Sponsored Consensus Conference statement. *J Ultrasound Med.* 2001;20:1025-1036.
28. Mogavero G, Sheth S, Hamper UM. Endovaginal sonography of the nongravid uterus. *Radiographics.* 1993;13:969-981.
29. Sivridis E, Giatromanolaki A. The endometrial hyperplasias revisited. *Virchows Arch.* 2008;453:223-231.
30. Davis PC, O'Neill MJ, Yoder IC, et al. Sonohysterographic findings of endometrial and subendometrial conditions. *Radiographics.* 2002;22:803-816.
31. Kitajima K, Murakami K, Yamasaki E, et al. Performance of FDG-PET/CT for diagnosis of recurrent uterine cervical cancer. *Eur Radiol.* 2008;18:2040-2047.
32. Cohen I. Endometrial pathologies associated with postmenopausal tamoxifen treatment. *Gynecol Oncol.* 2004;94:256-266.
33. Grasel RP, Outwater EK, Siegelman ES, et al. Endometrial polyps: MR imaging features and distinction from endometrial carcinoma. *Radiology.* 2000;214:47-52.
34. American Cancer Society. *Cancer Statistics 2008.* Atlanta GA: American Cancer Society; 2008.
35. American Cancer Society. *Cancer Facts & Figures 2008.* Atlanta, GA: American Cancer Society; 2008.
36. Sorosky JI. Endometrial cancer. *Obstet Gynecol.* 2008;111:436-447.
37. Manfredi R, Gui B, Maresca G, et al. Endometrial cancer: magnetic resonance imaging. *Abdom Imaging.* 2005;30:626-636.
38. Kitajima K, Murakami K, Yamasaki E, et al. Accuracy of 18F-FDG PET/CT in detecting pelvic and paraaortic lymph node metastasis in patients with endometrial cancer. *Am J Roentgenol.* 2008;190:1652-1658.
39. Akin O, Mironov S, Pandit-Taskar N, et al. Imaging of uterine cancer. *Radiol Clin North Am.* 2007;45:167-182.
40. Karlsson B, Granberg S, Wikland M, et al. Transvaginal ultrasonography of the endometrium in women with postmenopausal bleeding—a Nordic multicenter study. *Am J Obstet Gynecol.* 1995;172:1488-1494.
41. Granberg S, Wikland M, Karlsson B, et al. Endometrial thickness as measured by endovaginal ultrasonography for identifying endometrial abnormality. *Am J Obstet Gynecol.* 1991;164:47-52.
42. Dubinsky TJ. Value of sonography in the diagnosis of abnormal vaginal bleeding. *J Clin Ultrasound.* 2004;32:348-353.
43. Kinkel K. Pitfalls in staging uterine neoplasm with imaging: a review. *Abdom Imaging.* 2006;31:164-173.
44. Park JY, Kim EN, Kim DY, et al. Comparison of the validity of magnetic resonance imaging and positron emission tomography/computed tomography in the preoperative evaluation of patients with uterine corpus cancer. *Gynecol Oncol.* 2008;108:486-492.
45. Chao A, Chang TC, Ng KK, et al. ^{18}F-FDG PET in the management of endometrial cancer. *Eur J Nucl Med Mol Imaging.* 2006;33:36-44.
46. Kitajima K, Murakami K, Yamasaki E, et al. Performance of FDG-PET/CT in the diagnosis of recurrent endometrial cancer. *Ann Nucl Med.* 2008;22:103-109.
47. Vandermeer FQ, Wong-You-Cheong JJ. Imaging of acute pelvic pain. *Clin Obstet Gynecol.* 2009;52:2-20.
48. Menias CO, Elsayes KM, Peterson CM, et al. CT of pregnancy-related complications. *Emerg Radiol.* 2007;13:299-306.
49. Ascher SM, Imaoka I, Lage JM. Tamoxifen-induced uterine abnormalities: the role of imaging. *Radiology.* 2000;214:29-38.

50. Berman JM. Intrauterine adhesions. *Semin Reprod Med.* 2008; 26:349-355.
51. Fedele L, Bianchi S, Dorta M, et al. Intrauterine adhesions: detection with transvaginal US. *Radiology.* 1996;199:757-759.
52. Bacelar AC, Wilcock D, Powell M, et al. The value of MRI in the assessment of traumatic intra-uterine adhesions (Asherman's syndrome). *Clin Radiol.* 1995;50:80-83.
53. Okamoto Y, Tanaka YO, Nishida M, et al. MR imaging of the uterine cervix: imaging-pathologic correlation. *Radiographics.* 2003;23:425-245.
54. Rezvani M, Shaaban A. Imaging of cervical pathology. *Clin Obstet Gynecol.* 2009;52:94-111.
55. Itoh K, Toki T, Shiohara S, et al. A comparative analysis of cross sectional imaging techniques in minimal deviation adenocarcinoma of the uterine cervix. *Br J Obstet Gynaec.* 2000;107:1158-1163.
56. Sugiyama K, Takehara Y. MR findings of pseudoneoplastic lesions in the uterine cervix mimicking adenoma malignum. *Br J Radiol.* 2007;80:878-883.
57. Doi T, Yamashita Y, Yasunaga T, et al. Adenoma malignum: MR imaging and pathologic study. *Radiology.* 1997;204:39-42.
58. Smith GE, Gormly KL. Magnetic resonance imaging in the staging of cervical carcinoma: a pictorial review. *J Med Imaging Radiat Oncol.* 2008;52:427-433.
59. Follen M, Levenback CF, Iyer RB, et al. Imaging in cervical cancer. *Cancer.* 2003;98(9 suppl):2028-2038.
60. Loft A, Berthelsen AK, Roed H, et al. The diagnostic value of PET/CT scanning in patients with cervical cancer: a prospective study. *Gynecol Oncol.* 2007;106:29-34.
61. Sironi S, Buda A, Picchio M, et al. Lymph node metastasis in patients with clinical early-stage cervical cancer: detection with integrated FDG PET/CT. *Radiology.* 2006;238:272-279.
62. Wright JD, Dehdashti F, Herzog TJ, et al. Preoperative lymph node staging of early-stage cervical carcinoma by [^{18}F]-fluoro-2-deoxy-D-glucose-positron emission tomography. *Cancer.* 2005;104:2484-2491.
63. Jeong YY, Kang HK, Chung TW, et al. Uterine cervical carcinoma after therapy: CT and MR imaging findings. *Radiographics.* 2003;23:969-981.
64. Puscheck EE, Cohen L. Congenital malformations of the uterus: the role of ultrasound. *Semin Reprod Med.* 2008;26:223-231.
65. Saravelos SH, Cocksedge KA, Li TC. Prevalence and diagnosis of congenital uterine anomalies in women with reproductive failure: a critical appraisal. *Hum Reprod Update.* 2008;14:415-429.
66. Kitamura Y, Ascher SM, Cooper C, et al. Imaging manifestations of complications associated with uterine artery embolization. *Radiographics.* 2005;25:S119-S132.
67. Verma SK, Gonsalves CF, Baltarowich OH, et al. Spectrum of imaging findings on MRI and CT after uterine artery embolization. *Abdom Imaging.* 2010;35:118-128.

CHAPTER 10

Imaging of the Ovary and Fallopian Tubes

Jill Langer, MD

Ultrasonography (US), especially transvaginal ultrasonography (TVUS), has become the primary imaging technique for the evaluation of the ovary and fallopian tube, particularly in symptomatic patients. Magnetic resonance imaging (MRI) is often used to investigate indeterminate US findings, whereas computed tomography (CT) is the primary modality used for gynecologic malignancy staging. However, adnexal lesions are commonly imaged during pelvic US and CT performed on women of all ages, particularly those with acute pelvic pain. Although the vast majority of adnexal lesions are benign in nature, the detection of an adnexal mass raises concern for a potential ovarian neoplasm, particularly in the postmenopausal patient. It is important for those interpreting images to be able to recognize those features that strongly predict that an adnexal lesion is benign as well as those that predict a malignancy in order to direct the management of the patient.

ANATOMY

On imaging exams, the adnexa refer to the ovary, fallopian tube, and supporting connective tissue structures. The ovaries are most commonly located in the ovarian fossa of the lower pelvis, anterior and medial to the external iliac artery.[1,2] However, because of the varying laxity of their supporting ligaments, ovarian position is variable and influenced by uterine size, degree of filling of the urinary bladder, and distention of the rectosigmoid colon. Ovaries may be located in the upper pelvis or lower abdomen, particularly in the presence of a large ovarian or extra-ovarian mass. The ovary of an adult woman is approximately 2.5 to 5 cm long, 1.5 to 3 cm in width, and 1 to 2 cm thick. The size of the ovary is typically reported by volume, calculated by the formula for a prolate ellipse (0.523 × length × width × thickness). Normal volumes are 3.0 mL (range 0.2-9 mL) before menarche, 9.8 mL (range 2.5-21.9 mL) for menstruating women, and 5.8 mL (range 1.2-14.1 mL) for postmenopausal women.[3]

The ovary contains millions of microscopic primordial or immature follicles, several of which will enlarge on a continual basis. In the first half of a normal menstrual cycle, follicles grow to 2 to 9 mm, becoming visible by high-resolution imaging. The ovarian stroma has a central medullary component and an outer cortex in which most developing follicles are noted, a feature that helps to define the appearance of normal ovaries, particularly on TVUS and MRI (see Figure 10-1).[4-6] Ovarian follicles may or may not be detected by CT depending on the size of the follicles, the phase of contrast enhancement and the slice thickness.[1,8,9]

The normal fallopian tube extends laterally from the upper lateral margin of the uterus to the ipsilateral ovary and in adults, it is approximately 9 to 11 cm long and 1 to 4 mm wide. It is composed of 4 segments (from medial to lateral): the 1-cm intramural segment (composed of

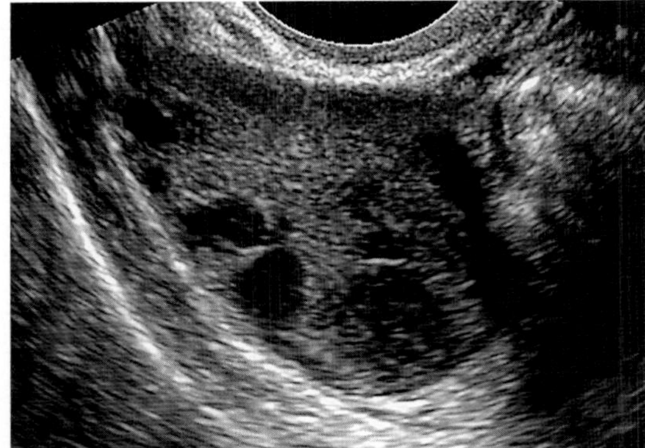

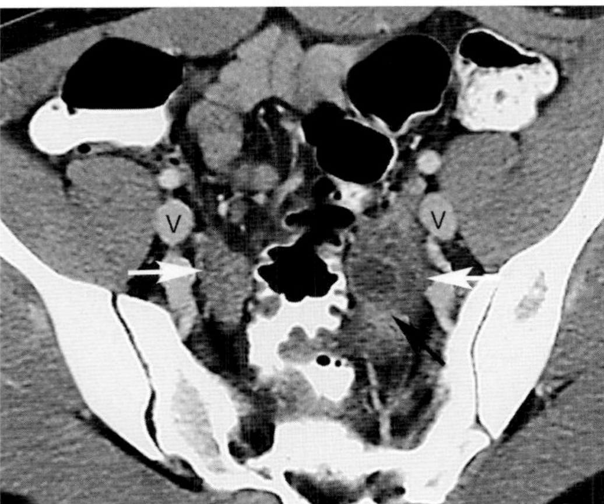

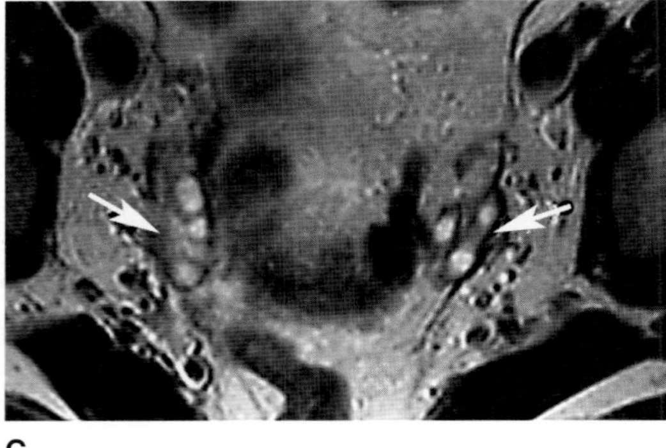

Figure 10-1 Normal Ovary With Follicles
A. On transvaginal pelvic US, the adult ovary will appear as an ovoid soft-tissue structure, most commonly adjacent to the pelvic sidewall. Follicles appear as small cystic structures with thin walls and sharply defined borders, containing anechoic or minimally complicated fluid. **B.** Contrast-enhanced axial CT image of the pelvis shows multiple faint small regions of low-attenuating representing ovarian follicles (*white arrows*). A larger 2-cm dominant follicle or corpus luteum (*black arrow*) is seen in the left ovary in this patient scanned at midcycle. The ovaries are located in the ovarian fossa, adjacent to the external iliac vessels (v = external iliac vein). **C.** T2-weighted axial MRI of the pelvis shows multiple small high-signal-intensity cystic lesions, predominantly in the periphery of each ovary (*white arrows*), representing follicles.

Imaging Notes 10-1. Normal Ovaries

The identification of normal, fluid-filled follicles is the principal finding that defines the appearance of normal ovaries.

uterine and interstitial portions); the narrow, 2- to 3-cm long isthmus; the ampulla, which comprises the majority of the length on the tube; and the infundibulum, which is composed of 25 irregular fimbriae that overhang the ovary.[7] Throughout its extrauterine course, the tube lies within a peritoneal fold along the superior margin of the broad ligament, called the mesosalpinx. The wall of the tube consists of longitudinal folds and mucosal rugae, which increase in number and complexity from the medial to the lateral aspect of the tube. The normal decompressed fallopian tube is not well visualized by imaging unless outlined by large amount of pelvic fluid (see Figure 10-2).[1,7]

Adnexal masses are primarily distinguished on the basis of whether they cause a purely or minimally complex cystic lesion, a more complicated cystic lesion, or a solid lesion on imaging exams.

CYSTIC ADENEXAL MASSES

Cystic adnexal masses can be due to a variety of causes. Most commonly, they will represent a physiologic ovarian cyst such as a dominant follicle, corpus luteum, or

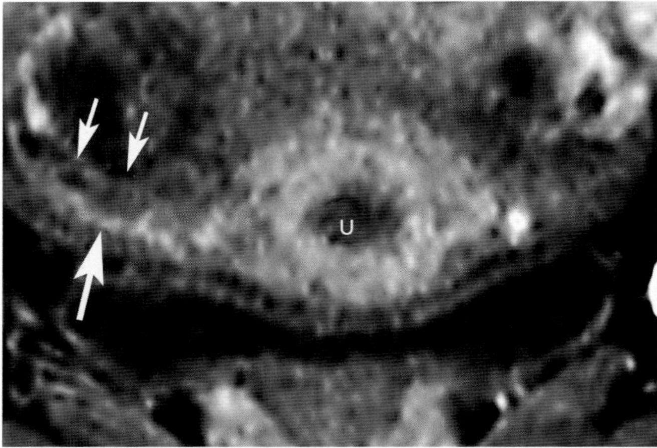

Figure 10-2 Normal Fallopian Tube
Magnified reformatted high-resolution coronal contrast-enhanced CT image shows a normal right fallopian tube (*small arrows*) within the mesosalpinx. Additionally, an enhancing vessel (*large arrow*) is visible within the mesosalpinx, likely an ovarian artery branch of the uterine artery providing blood supply to the ovary. The uterine cavity (U) is seen as a hypoechoic region at the center of the uterus.

Table 10-1. Causes of Cystic Adnexal Mass

Causes
1. Physiologic ovarian cysts a. Follicular cysts b. Corpus luteum cysts c. Hemorrhagic cysts d. Postmenopausal simple cysts e. Abnormal creation of physiologic cysts i. Polycystic ovarian syndrome ii. Hyperstimulated ovaries
2. Cystic ovarian neoplasms a. Germ cell neoplasms i. Teratoma/teratocarcinoma b. Epithelial neoplasms i. Serous cystadenoma and cystadenocarcinoma ii. Mucinous cystadenoma and cystadenocarcinoma iii. Endometrioid carcinoma iv. Clear cell carcinoma
3. Endometrioma
4. Mesothelial cysts
5. Peritoneal inclusion cysts
6. Dilatation of the fallopian tube a. Hydrosalpinx b. Hematosalpinx c. Pyosalpinx or tubo-ovarian abscess
7. Fallopian tube carcinoma
8. Ectopic pregnancy

hemorrhagic cyst. Less commonly, they will represent an ovarian neoplasm, endometrioma, mesothelial cyst, peritoneal inclusion cyst, fluid-filled fallopian tube, or ectopic pregnancy (Table 10-1).

Physiologic Ovarian Cysts

Most cystic ovarian lesions detected in premenopausal patients represent normal physiologic lesions, including the developing follicle, follicular cyst, and corpus luteum.[1,4-6,8,9] In some cases, follicular cysts or the corpus luteum will develop internal hemorrhage and are called "hemorrhagic cysts." In 2 situations, polycystic ovarian syndrome and ovarian hyperstimulation syndrome, abnormal hormonal physiology results in the production of an abnormal number of cysts in the ovaries.

Follicular maturation and follicular cysts

In response to follicle-stimulating hormone (FSH), 1 or more of the enlarging immature follicles will become the dominant follicle, growing to a diameter of approximately 20 to 25 mm and then rupture at ovulation, releasing the oocyte. Developing follicles typically appear as a sharply marginated, simple-appearing cyst.[2] The pre-ovulatory dominant follicle can have a slightly complicated appearance, with the oocyte and its supporting structures (the cumulus oophorus) visible as a curvilinear septation with the follicle on TVUS (see Figure 10-3).[2] In a small number of women, a mature follicle will fail to ovulate and continue to enlarge into the next menstrual cycle, appearing as a simple or minimally complicated cyst.[2,4] A recent consensus statement noted that in women of reproductive age, entirely simple appearing cysts are almost always benign.[10] Simple ovarian cysts under 3 cm can be considered a normal finding, those between 3 and 5 cm do not need follow-up, those between 5 and 7 cm should be followed yearly,

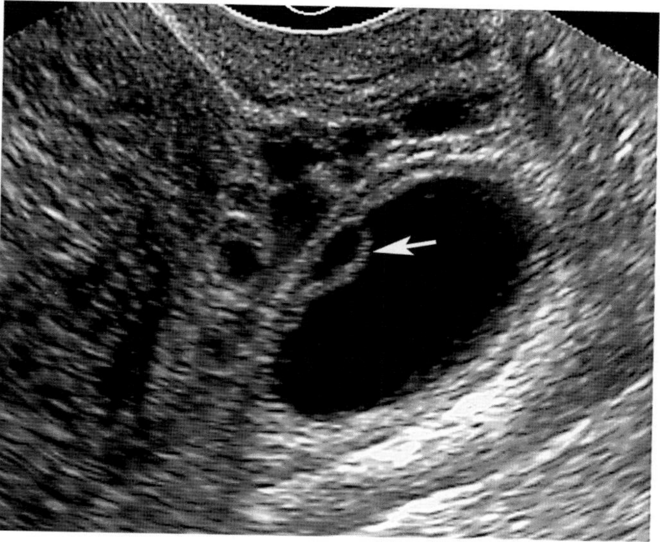

Figure 10-3 Dominant Follicle
A sagittal transvaginal US image of the left ovary of 24-year-old woman obtained in the preovulatory phase of the menstrual cycle shows a dominant follicle measuring 21 mm. This follicle contains a curvilinear protrusion into the follicle (*arrow*) indicative of the cumulus oophorus and its surrounding complement of granulosa cells separating just prior to ovulation.

Imaging Notes 10-2. Simple Cysts in Menstruating Women

The vast majority of simple or minimally complicated cystic masses noted in the ovaries of menstruating-age women are physiologic cysts. If there is concern for a neoplasm, it is best to perform a follow-up ultrasound examination after one or two menstrual cycles because many lesions will resolve spontaneously.

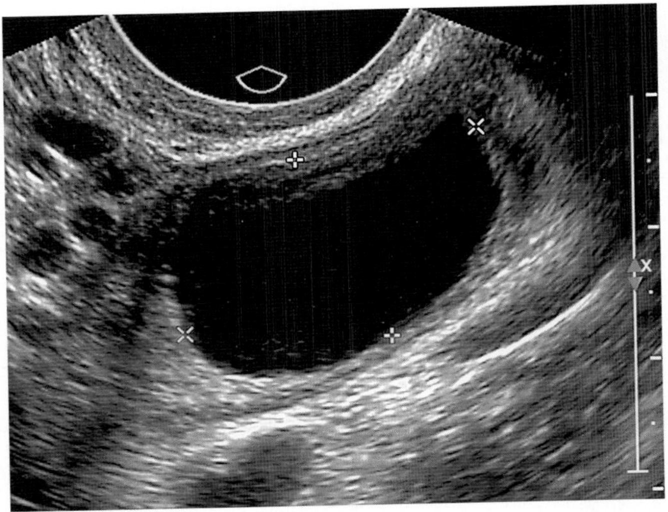
A

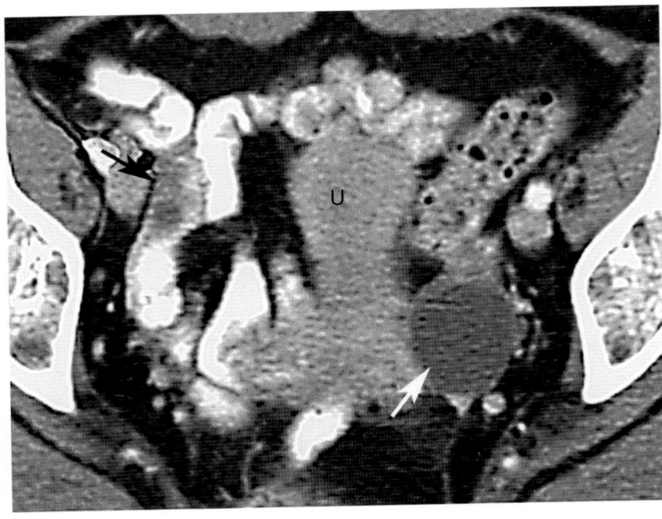

B

Figure 10-4. Follicular Cyst in 2 Patients
A. Transvaginal pelvic US, in this 27-year-old patient with irregular menstrual cycles, shows a 4.2-cm simple right ovarian cyst. This has sharply defined, thin walls without mural nodules and contains anechoic fluid. This lesion resolved on follow-up US 6 weeks later and was likely a follicular cyst. **B.** Axial CT image in a different patient imaged just after mid cycle shows a simple, thin-walled ovarian cyst in the left ovary (*white arrow*) measuring 3.2 cm, likely a physiologic or follicular cyst. A low-attenuating small follicle is also seen in the right ovary (*black arrow*) (U = uterus).

and those over 7 cm require further evaluation either by MR or by surgical removal.[10] For reproductive-age women with minimally complicated cystic lesions, such as those with thin septations or minimal wall irregularity, repeating the ultrasound exam after one or two menstrual cycles is recommended to assess for possible involution of an atypical follicular cyst (see Figure 10-4).[4,10,11]

Corpus luteum

Following ovulation, the remnant of the ruptured follicle forms an important physiologic structure, the corpus luteum. The corpus luteum secretes progesterone, which is essential for establishing and maintaining an early pregnancy. It evolves from the remnant of the mature follicle through a process of cellular hypertrophy and increased vascularization of the cyst wall.[12,13] Typically, the corpus luteum is less than 3.0 cm in maximal dimension, reflecting its origin as a follicle, but may be as large as 6 cm and is seen in the latter half of the menstrual cycle and in the first few weeks of early pregnancy. A corpus luteum is typically unilocular but will have a thicker and more irregular or partially collapsed wall than a follicular cyst (see Figure 10-5). It will often contain complex fluid, reflecting blood products and lymph that filled follicle at the time of rupture.[2,13] On MRI, the wall of the corpus luteum can exhibit slightly increased intensity on T1-weighted images, and low intensity on T2-weighted images (see Figure 10-5).[5,6,14] The wall may show avid enhancement on MRI and CT, reflecting the increased vascularity of the thick luteinized cell layer but is usually less than 3 mm in thickness.[6,8,9,15] The corpus luteum can rupture, producing free fluid adjacent to the ovary and dependently within the cul-de-sac region of the pelvis (see Figure 10-5).[8,9,15]

Hemorrhagic cysts

Bleeding into a follicular cyst or corpus luteum can happen at any time during the menstrual cycle and results in a hemorrhagic cyst. Patients typically present with the abrupt onset of acute pelvic pain. Less commonly, the patient is asymptomatic.

On imaging exams, hemorrhagic cysts can have a variable appearance depending on the stage of clot formation, lysis, and retraction. On US, hemorrhagic cysts often contain interdigitating strands of fibrin, a characteristic appearance referred to as fish weave or reticular pattern (see Figure 10-6).[4,13,16,17] These strands differ from true septations, which are commonly present in cystic ovarian neoplasms, by their thin size (under 1 mm), their lack of vascularity, and their poor reflectivity of sound, making them only faintly visible. Retracting clot within a hemorrhagic cyst should not be mistaken for a solid component of a cystic neoplasm. Retracting clot will have concave or straight margins at its fluid interface and will typically appear less echogenic than the cyst wall on TVUS. The soft-tissue mural nodules detected in an ovarian neoplasm are of equal or much greater echogenicity than the wall and have convex margins at the fluid interface (see Figure 10-6).[4,16,17] In addition, retracting clot will fail to show vascular flow on Doppler exam or enhancement by CT or MRI.[5,6,14] On CT, a

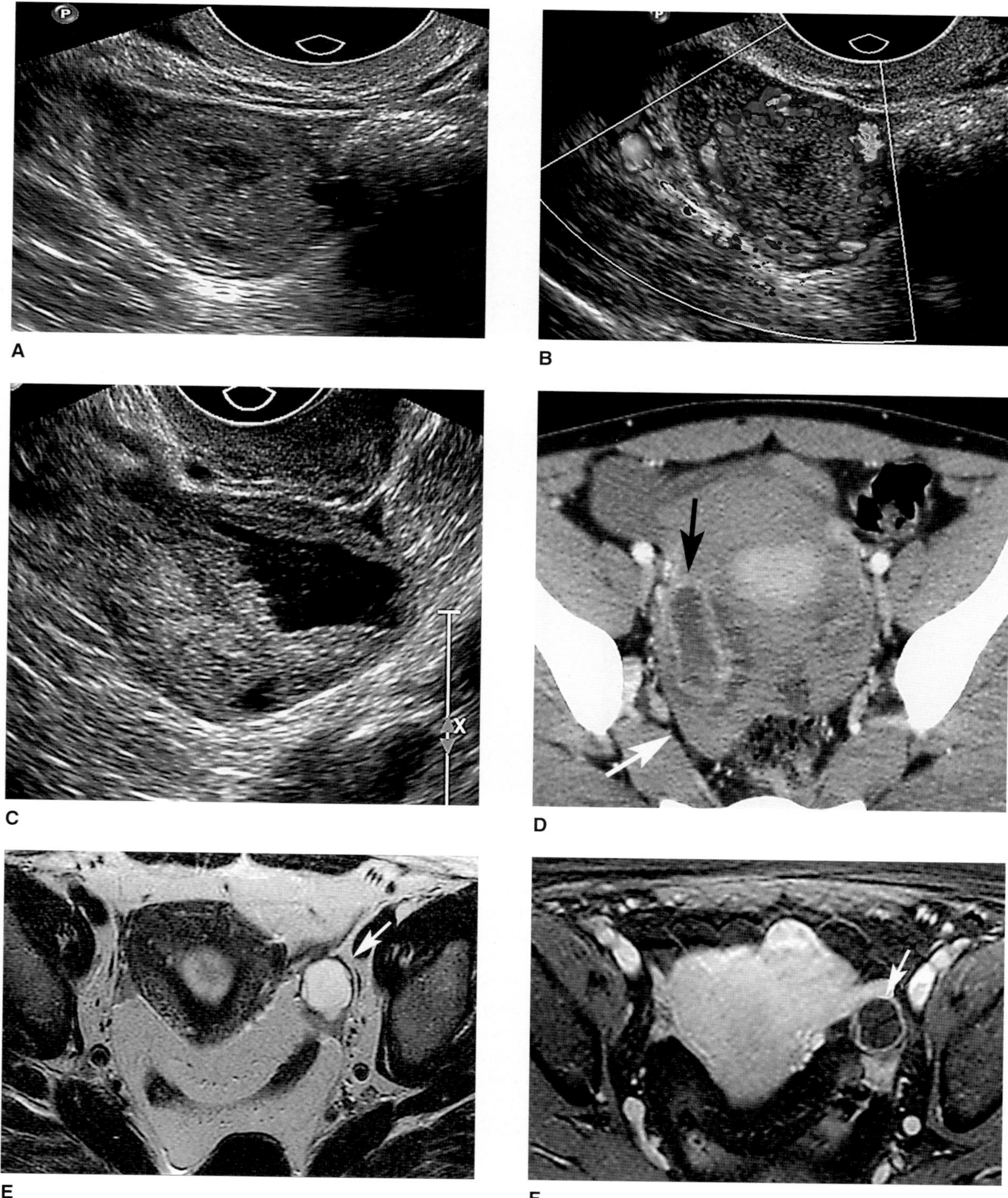

Figure 10-5 Corpus Luteum in 4 Patients
Grayscale (**A**) and Color Doppler image (**B**) of a corpus luteum cyst shows a nearly solid-appearing corpus luteum. The echogenic material within the cyst is fluid containing acute hemorrhage. Note how on color Doppler examination, only the wall has vascular flow and the cyst contents are avascular. **C.** Transvaginal pelvic US image, in a second patient, shows a cyst with a thick and echogenic wall, which is crenulated, characteristic of a corpus luteum in the process of involution in the later phase of the menstrual cycle. **D.** Axial CT image, in a third patient, shows a corpus luteum (*black arrow*) in the right ovary that has a thick enhancing wall with a region of discontinuity along its posterior margin because of partial rupture. High-attenuation fluid is also noted in the cul de sac (*white arrow*) indicating hemoperitoneum. **E.** An axial T2-weighted MRI in a fourth patient shows a left ovarian cyst (*arrow*) that has high signal central fluid and a low signal wall. **F.** Axial T1-weighted contrast-enhanced MRI of the patient in (E) shows avid wall enhancement of the corpus luteum (*arrow*), reflecting the increased vascularity of the thick luteinized cell layer, and low-signal central fluid.

A

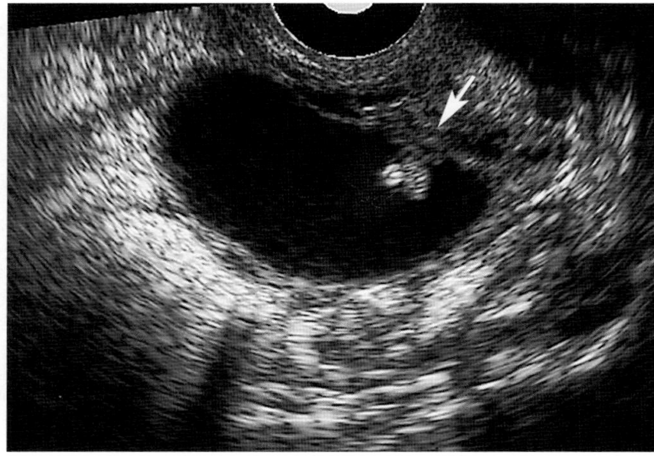

B

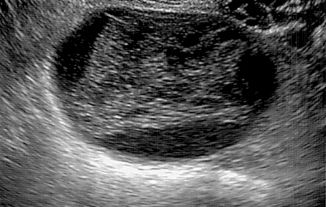

C

D

Figure 10-6 US of Hemorrhagic Cysts in 3 Patients
Hemorrhagic cysts may have a variety of appearances on sonography reflecting the acuity of the hemorrhage and the degree of clot lysis and retraction. **A.** A transvaginal US examination shows a 5.5-cm complex cystic mass with a reticular pattern of central echoes that was incidentally imaged in this 26-year-old patient. **B.** A transvaginal examination performed 6 weeks later shows interval decrease in the size of the cystic lesion, now measuring less than 3 cm. A solid component (*arrow*) that had no flow on color Doppler examination (not shown) is now present along the wall of the cyst secondary to the retracting clot. Retracting thrombus within a hemorrhagic cyst can mimic soft-tissue mural nodules seen in cystic neoplasms. In this case, the interval decrease in lesion size and the new appearance of this avascular nodule in the short interval between scans allows the diagnosis of an involuting hemorrhagic cyst. **C.** This hemorrhagic cyst in a second patient demonstrates a central region of echoes that has a straight margin typical of retracting internal clot. **D.** Transvaginal US in a third patient shows a complex cystic lesion (*inner set of electronic calipers*) with more heterogeneous internal echogenicity, but no internal flow (not shown) in this patient with acute pelvic pain. This lesion resolved on follow-up US examination and likely represented a hemorrhagic cyst imaged in the acute stage.

hemorrhagic cyst appears as a unilocular cyst with an internal attenuation of 25 to 100 Hounsfield units (HU). Fluid-fluid levels and hemoperitoneum can be noted after rupture.[8,9] Rarely, massive rupture can occur with significant hemoperitoneum (see Figure 10-7). On MRI, a hemorrhagic ovarian cyst will have high signal on T1 weighting, similar to findings seen in an endometrioma (see Figure 10-7).[6] Since hemorrhagic cysts will resolve

Imaging Notes 10-3. Hemorrhagic Cyst

The characteristic sonographic features of a hemorrhagic cyst, including the straight borders of retracting clot and the reticular pattern of interdigitating strands of fibrin, allow differentiation from an ovarian neoplasm.

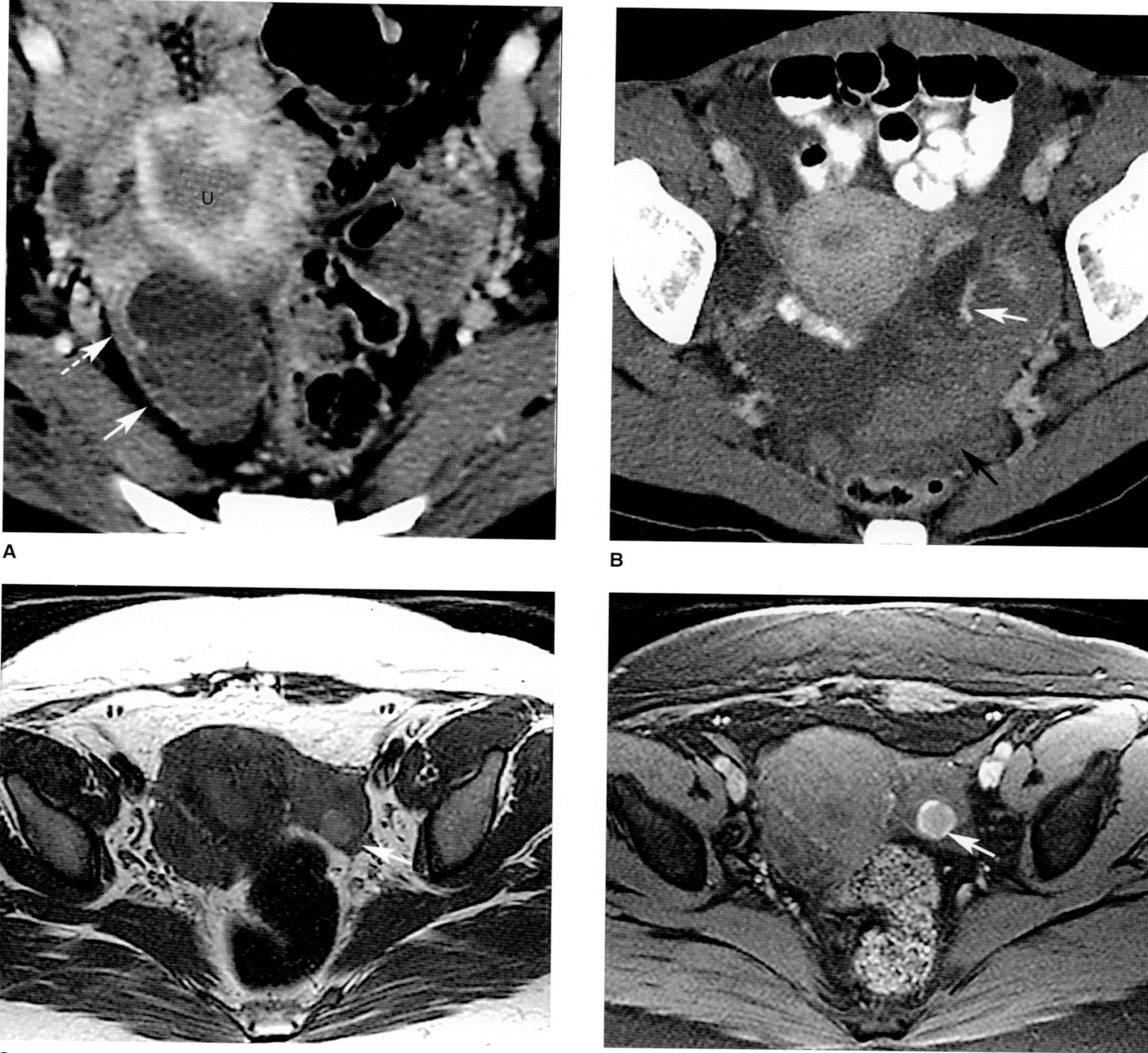

Figure 10-7 Hemorrhagic Cysts on CT and MRI
A. Contrast-enhanced CT shows a hemorrhagic cyst in the right ovary that has a region of fluid attenuation (*dashed arrow*) as well as a region of higher attenuation (*solid arrow*) representing hemorrhagic fluid (U = uterus). **B.** Contrast-enhanced CT in a second patient with pelvic pain and hypotension shows a hemorrhagic cyst in the left adnexa with active extravasation (*white arrow*) of intravenous contrast with a moderate amount of high-attenuation hemoperitoneum (*black arrow*). Occasionally, rupture of a follicular or hemorrhagic cyst may cause a significant hemoperitoneum and require surgical intervention. **C.** Axial T1-weighted image in a third patient shows a high-attenuating 1-cm lesion in the left ovary (*arrow*) of this 25-year-old patient. On T1-weighted imaging, the high signal could represent either complicated fluid, such as hemorrhagic fluid, or a fat-containing lesion. **D.** On this fat-saturated T1-weighted image, the subcutaneous fat loses signal, whereas the cyst (*arrow*) remains high in signal, consistent with a hemorrhagic cyst.

spontaneously, follow-up sonography in 6 to 12 weeks can be recommended if hemorrhagic cyst is considered as a possible diagnosis for a complex adnexal lesion in a pre-menopausal patient.[4,10]

Postmenopausal simple cysts

Although the postmenopausal pelvis was thought to be hormonally quiescent, simple ovarian cysts are detected in 10 to 15% of all postmenopausal women undergoing transvaginal sonography.[18-20] Folliculogenesis ceases after menopause but sporadic ovulatory events may still occur in menopause, especially in the first 5 years.[10] Simple cysts under 1 cm are therefore considered clinically unimportant and do not need follow-up.[10] Simple cysts over 1 cm and less than 7 cm are unlikely to be malignant and should be followed up by yearly pelvic sonography (see Figure 10-8).[10] An enlarging lesion could represent a neoplasm and should be removed.[18,19] Simple-appearing cystic masses greater than 7 cm in postmenopausal women usually undergo surgical excision. The risk of malignancy of simple-appearing cysts evaluated by transvaginal ultrasound is estimated to be 0.7% for premenopasual women and 1.6% for postmenopausal women.[21,22] A vast majority of malignant neoplasms that appear as simple cysts by imaging are found to have tiny mural nodules on pathology and most are over 7.5 cm in diameter.

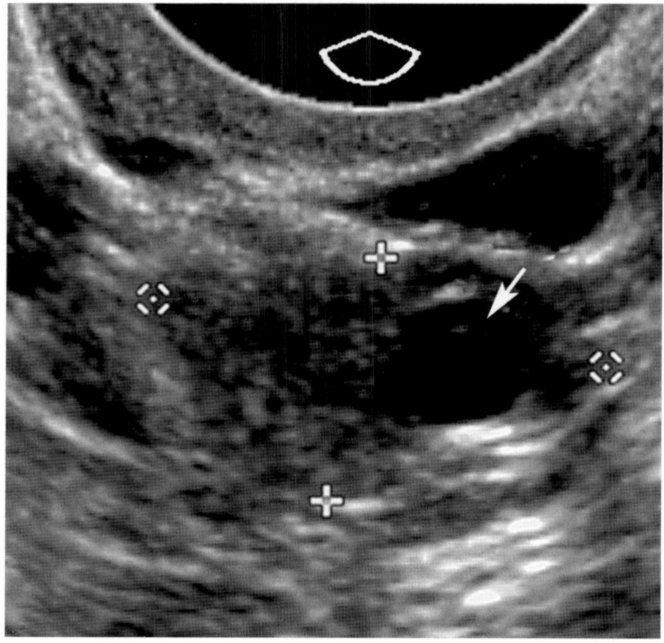

Figure 10-8 Postmenopausal Ovarian Cyst
Transvaginal sonography shows an 8-mm simple cyst (*arrow*) detected incidentally in this postmenopausal patient. Note the small size of the postmenopausal ovary. A simple-appearing cyst of this size can be managed conservatively.

Abnormal creation of physiologic cysts

The normal creation and dissolution of physiologic cysts is a cyclical process in the ovary in response to fluctuations in sex-related hormones. Abnormalities in the quantities of sex hormones can result in the overproduction of physiologic cysts. This phenomenon is seen in 3 situations: polycystic ovarian syndrome, ovarian hyperstimulation syndrome, and hyperreactio luteinalis.

Polycystic ovarian syndrome: Polycystic ovarian syndrome (PCOS) is a common endocrine disorder of unknown cause that affects approximately 5% women of reproductive age and is a leading cause of infertility. PCOS is very varied in its clinical presentation, with signs and symptoms that include oligomenorrhea, hirsutism, acne, male pattern baldness, and metabolic alterations such as obesity and insulin resistance.[23] Laboratory examinations demonstrate excessive amounts of androgenic hormones. A consensus conference held in 2003 established criteria for the diagnosis of PCOS as the presence of 2 of the following 3 criteria: (1) oligomenorrhea or anovulation; (2) hyperandrogenism; (3) imaging evidence of polycystic ovaries—in patients in whom other endocrine disorders, such as androgen-secreting tumors, congenital adrenal hyperplasia, and Cushing syndrome, have been excluded.[23,24]

Polycystic ovaries are defined as ovaries containing 12 or more immature follicles, each measuring 2 to 9 mm in diameter and/or an ovarian volume of more than 10 cm^3 in the absence of a dominant cyst or corpus luteum.[24] A single ovary with these characteristics is sufficient to fulfill the imaging criteria and unilateral presentation can be seen in up to 35% of patients with PCOS.[24,25] Other common US features of PCOS are a spherical shape of the ovary and prominent central echogenic stroma tissue (see Figure 10-9).[24] It is important to note that ovaries with these same imaging characteristics may also be seen in patients without PCOS, for example, during puberty and in women recovering from hypothalamic amenorrhea. Women with polycystic ovaries on US who do not have the clinical or biochemical stigmata of PCOS should not be considered as having the syndrome. However, it has been noted that when women who have polycystic ovaries without clinical PCOS undergo hormonal stimulation for

Imaging Notes 10-4. Polycystic Ovaries

The imaging features of polycystic ovaries are either
1. ovaries containing 12 or more follicles, each measuring 2 to 9 mm in diameter *or*
2. an increased ovarian volume of more than 10 cm^3

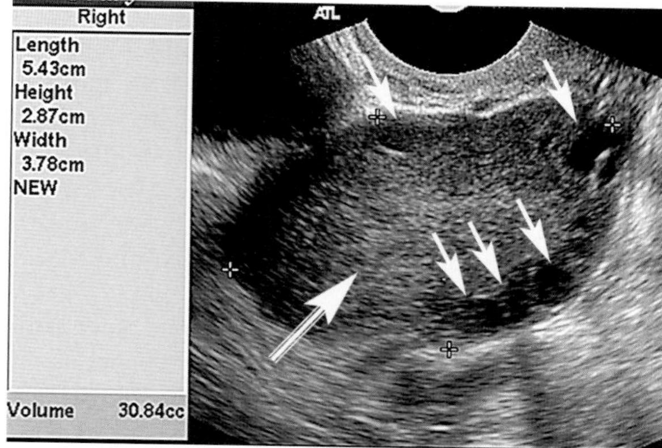

A

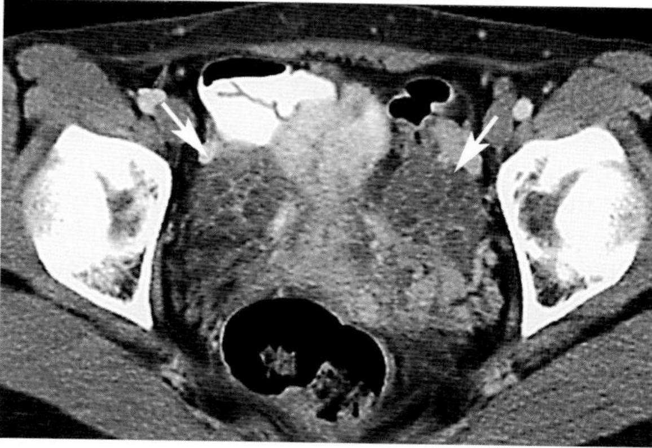

B

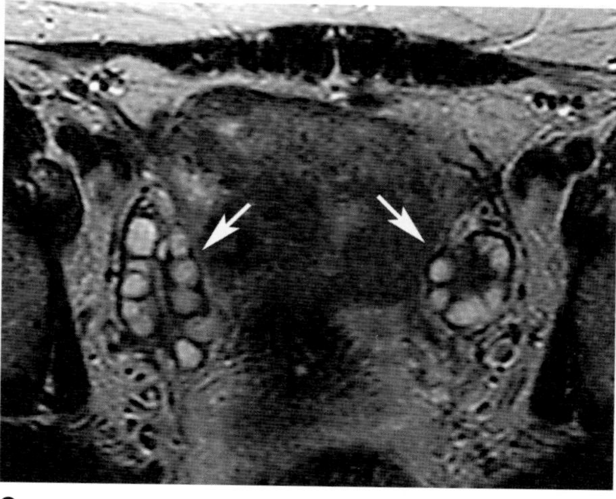

C

Figure 10-9 Polycystic Ovaries in 2 Patients
A. Transvaginal US image shows an enlarged ovary (calculated volume of 30.84 mL) with a prominent central echogenic stroma (*stripped arrow*) and multiple peripheral immature follicles (*small arrows*). More than 20 immature follicles were noted in this ovary, and the left ovary (not shown) had a similar appearance. **B.** Contrast-enhanced CT image shows the ovaries (*arrows*) to be enlarged, rounded, and to have multiple follicles in another PCOS patient. **C.** T2-weighted MRIs shows enlarged ovaries (*arrows*) with increased central dark stroma and multiple, small peripheral follicles of uniform size in the periphery in a different PCOS patient.

in vitro fertilization, they have the same increased risk of developing hyperstimulation syndrome as women with documented PCOS.[23]

Hyperstimulated ovaries: Increased human chorionic gonadotropin (hCG) serum levels or increased sensitivity to normal levels can cause marked enlargement of the ovaries and production of multiple physiologic cysts, called theca lutein cysts.[26] When the elevated serum hCG level occurs during ovulation induction performed for treatment for infertility, the condition is called *ovarian hyperstimulation syndrome.* If associated with a normal pregnancy, multiple gestations, or gestational trophoblastic disease, the condition is termed *hyperreactio luteinalis.* Ovarian hyperstimulation syndrome tends to present in the first trimester and is associated with ascites and pleural effusions. Hyperreactio luteinalis tends to have a more indolent course and presents later in pregnancy. In both conditions, the ovaries are markedly enlarged, with multiple simple and/or hemorrhagic cysts. On US, the central echogenic stoma extends from the central aspect of the ovary peripherally and is stretched by the multiple cysts producing a characteristic "spoke wheel" appearance (see Figure 10-10).[27,28]

Cystic Ovarian and Adnexal Lesions

Approximately 80% of ovarian tumors that occur in adult women are benign, 10% to 15% are primary ovarian malignancies, and 5% are due to ovarian metastases.[29-32] The majority of ovarian neoplasms that are found in younger woman are benign. The incidence of malignancy increases dramatically around the time of menopause and continues to rise with aging such that approximately 40% of tumors in postmenopausal women are malignant.[29] Primary ovarian tumors are classified based on their tissue origin as germ cell tumors, epithelial tumors, or sex cord-stromal tumors. The neoplasms that are predominantly cystic in appearance are discussed here. Solid ovarian neoplasms are discussed later in the chapter.

Germ cell neoplasms

Teratomas: Germ cell tumors arise from the oocyte and are the second most common ovarian neoplasm. The vast majority of germ cell tumors are benign mature teratomas, which accounts for 20% of all ovarian tumors in adults, 50% of all ovarian tumors in children and is the most common tumor in women less than 45 years of age.[33]

They are often incidentally detected, but can be symptomatic if complicated by torsion, infection, or rupture. Bilateral lesions are noted in 15% to 25% of patients. Teratomas comprise a number of histologic types of tumors, all of which contain mature or immature tissues of germ cell origin. The most common of these tumors is the mature cystic teratoma, also known as a dermoid cyst. Mature cystic teratoma typically contains mature tissues of ectodermal (skin, hair follicles, and sebaceous or

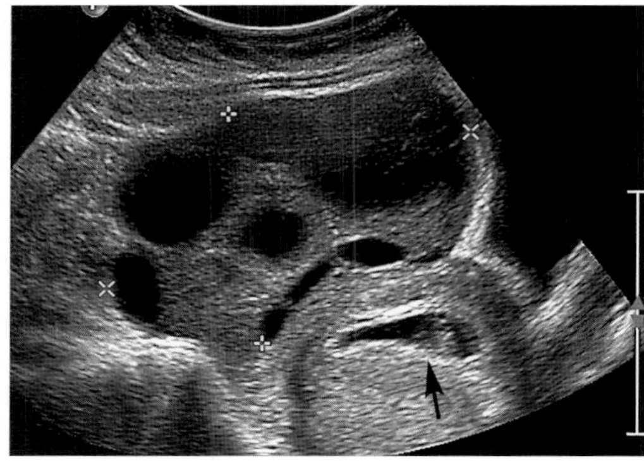

A

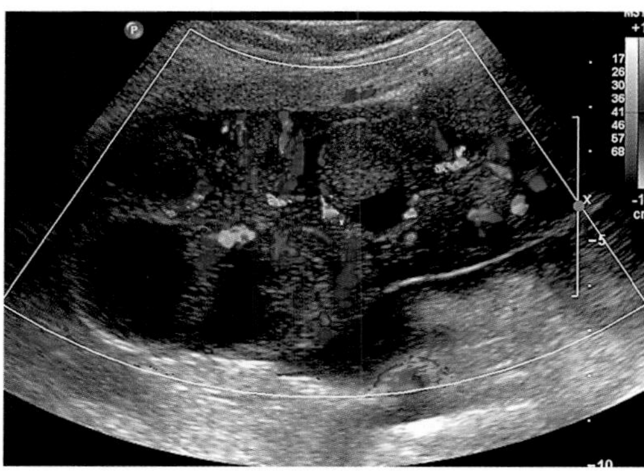

B

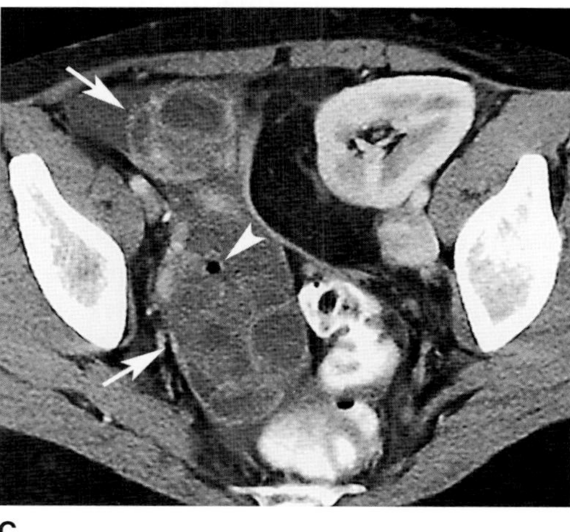

C

Figure 10-10 Hyperstimulated Ovaries
A. Transabdominal US image shows an enlarged ovary with multiple cysts (*outlined by calipers*) just above the gravid uterus (*arrow*) in this patient with elevated hCG levels and ovarian hyperstimulation syndrome (OHSS) in the early first trimester of pregnancy after ovulation induction. **B.** Color Doppler shows the typical "spoke wheel" pattern of flow within the ovarian parenchyma, which is stretched around the multiple theca lutein cysts. This flow pattern allows differentiation from a multilocular cystic mass or ovarian torsion as potential etiologies for an enlarged ovary. **C.** CT scan in a different patient receiving fertility therapy demonstrates ovaries (*arrows*) with multiple enlarged follicular cysts, typical of OHSS. There is a small dot of air (*arrowhead*) in 1 ovary because of recent follicular harvest. There is also a transplant kidney in the left iliac fossa.

sweat glands), mesodermal (muscle, fat), and endodermal (mucinous or ciliated epithelium) origin. Many dermoids contain a soft-tissue excrescence containing hair called the dermoid plug or Rokitansky nodule in which calcified elements representing bone or tooth fragments are also commonly noted. In monodermal teratomas, one of these tissue types, for example, thyroid tissue in struma ovarii and neuroectodermal tissue in carcinoid tumor, predominates.[33,34]

Mature cystic teratomas have a broad spectrum of appearances ranging from nearly entirely cystic lesion, to a mixed cystic and solid, fat-containing lesion, to a noncystic lesion composed almost entirely of fat. On US, the Rokitansky nodule appears as a highly echogenic mural nodule with distal acoustic shadowing and is called "the tip of the iceberg sign."[33-35] Other US features characteristic of dermoids include regional or diffuse bright echoes caused by sebaceous material, hyperechoic lines and dots or the "dermoid mesh" corresponding to strands of hair, floating fat globules, and a fat-fluid level (see Figure 10-11).[4,36,37] Despite the wide variety of appearances, the identification of these characteristic US features allows a highly confident diagnosis of a dermoid and at the same time a relatively confident exclusion of malignancy.[4,38,39]

Macroscopic fat is present in more than 97% of mature cystic teratomas and is specific for a germ cell neoplasm.[33] On MRI, the fat component will appear bright on T1-weighted imaging and intermediate gray signal on T2-weighted imaging. By using fat suppression techniques, a drop in signal intensity of the bright component as compared with the conventional T1-weighted imaging confirms the presence of fat (see Figure 10-12).[5,14,33] In addition, the fat in dermoids results in chemical shift artifact at the fat-fluid interface, which appears as bright or dark bands along the frequency encoding direction (see Figure 10-13).[14]

On CT, the fat component will appear as markedly low attenuation areas within the mass and measure less than –60 HU (see Figure 10-12).[33,40] Because ovarian teratomas can contain tooth and/or bone tissues, these calcified structures can be seen by abdominal plain films. They will typically appear as a small dense focus of calcification that loosely resembles a tooth or small bone localized within the pelvis (see Figure 10-14).[33] The tooth and bone fragments are most easily appreciated by CT and appear as nonspecific low-signal-intensity regions on MRI.[33]

Imaging Notes 10-5. Mature Fat in Ovarian Masses

The presence of fat in an ovarian lesion as detected by CT or MRI is diagnostic of a germ cell tumor, the vast majority of which will be a benign mature cystic teratoma (dermoid cyst).

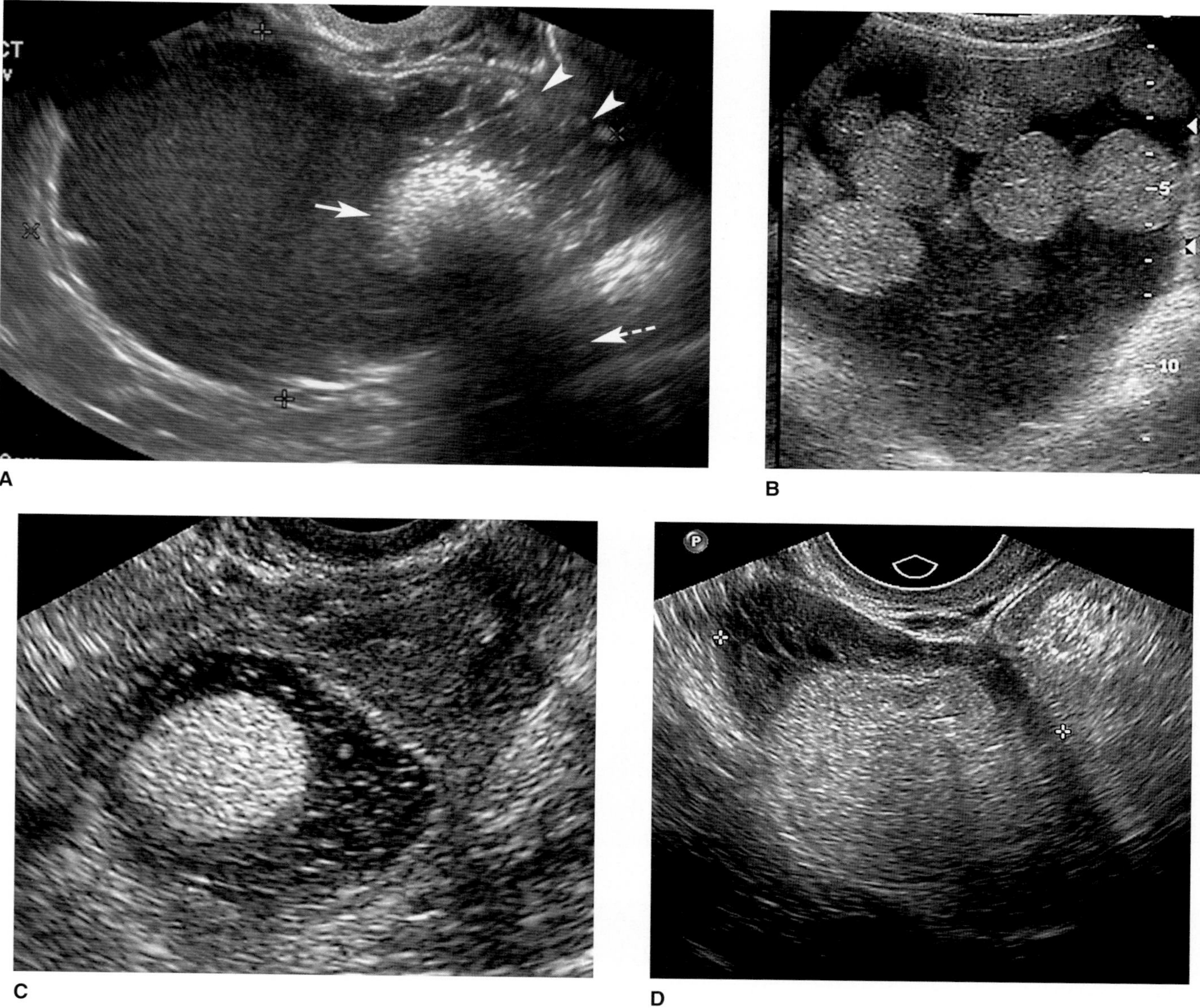

Figure 10-11 Mature Cystic Teratoma in 4 Patients
A. This 10-cm complex cystic ovarian lesion contains a central highly echogenic nodule (*white arrow*) which represents the dermoid plug. The hair and sebaceous material within this plug causes distal acoustic shadowing (*dashed arrow*) deep to the mid aspect of the nodule, which has been called the "tip of the iceberg sign." Hyperechoic lines and dots, called the dermoid mesh, are also noted (*arrowheads*). **B.** Transabdominal examination in another patient shows a 10-cm lesion with multiple fat globules, a less common but highly specific appearance of a mature cystic teratoma. **C.** Transvaginal US in a different patient shows a complex cystic lesion with a hyperechoic solid component without shadowing and hyperechoic lines and dots (dermoid mesh). **D.** Transvaginal US in a different patient demonstrates a highly echogenic solid lesion within the ovary (*outlined by calipers*).

In its pure form, mature teratoma is always benign, but rarely malignant transformation of the squamous lining can occur. The presence of a large and irregular soft-tissue component, penetration or invasion of the capsule by the soft-tissue component, and pelvic ascites are features of malignant transformation (see Figure 10-15).[33,41]

Immature teratoma, a malignant form of germ cell tumor, is a relatively rare tumor found in children and young adults. This tumor contains varying amounts of immature or embryonic elements, with the grade of the tumor correlating with the proportion of immature tissue. These lesions maybe predominantly cystic and contain calcifications and fat similar to mature cystic teratomas. However, the cystic component is simple fluid rather than sebaceous fluid and its fatty content is usually scant and occurs in punctate foci throughout the solid component. Calcifications also tend to be punctate and scattered rather than large and within the Rokitansky nodule. Many lesions

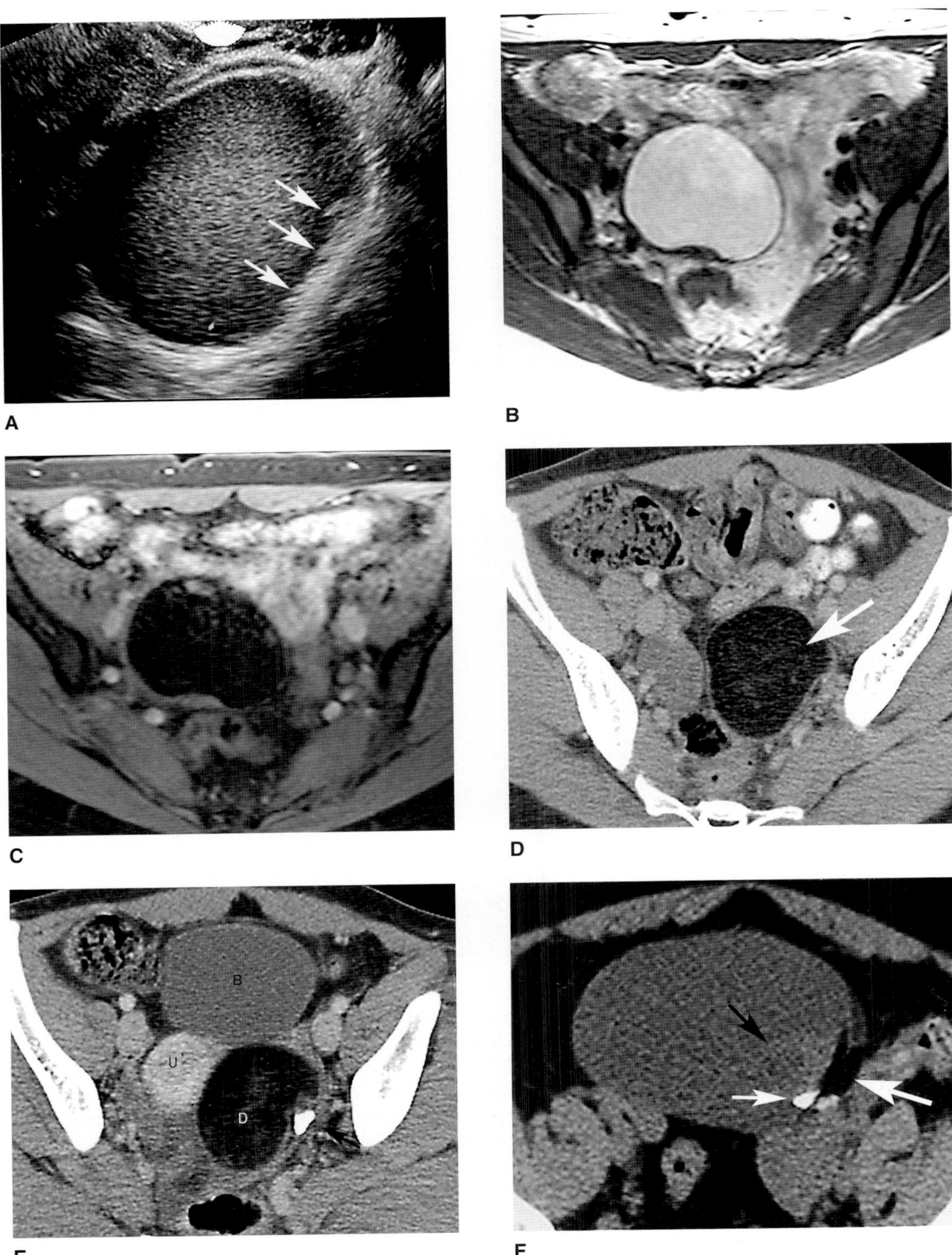

Figure 10-12 Mature Cystic Teratoma in 4 Patients
A. Transvaginal US image of the right ovary in this 50-year-old patient shows a 6-cm cystic lesion with homogeneous echoes and wall irregularity (*arrows*). The appearance is nonspecific and could be related to a hemorrhagic cyst, endometrioma, or a cystic ovarian neoplasm. **B.** T1-weighted axial MRI shows the lesion to have bright internal signal and a small region of wall thickening posteriorly. **C.** T1-weighted fat-saturated image shows marked loss of signal, indicating that the lesion contains fat consistent with a predominantly cystic, fat-containing mature cystic teratoma. **D.** Axial CT image of the pelvis in a second patient shows a nearly entirely fat-containing left ovarian mass (*arrow*) consistent with a mature cystic teratoma in this 42-year-old woman. **E.** A mature cystic teratoma in a third patient with dermoid plug containing a tooth or bone fragment (*arrow*) is seen in this 23-year-old patient. **F.** This mature cystic teratoma, in a fourth patient, is predominantly cystic with a dermoid plug that contains fat (*large white arrow*), a calcification (*small white arrow*), and soft-tissue elements (*black arrow*).

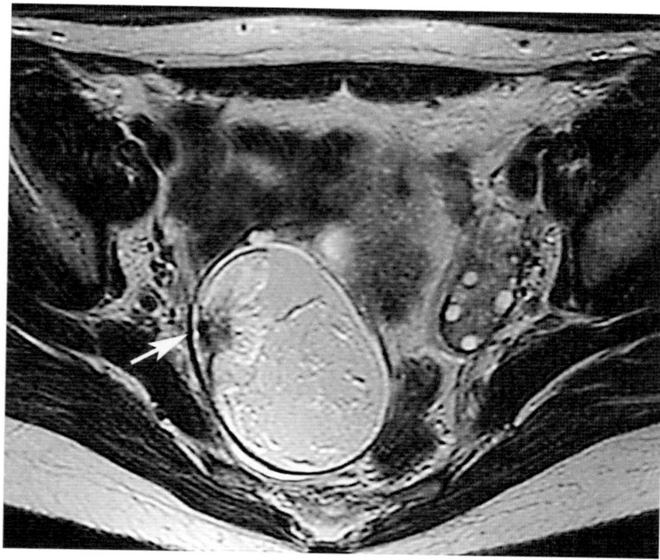

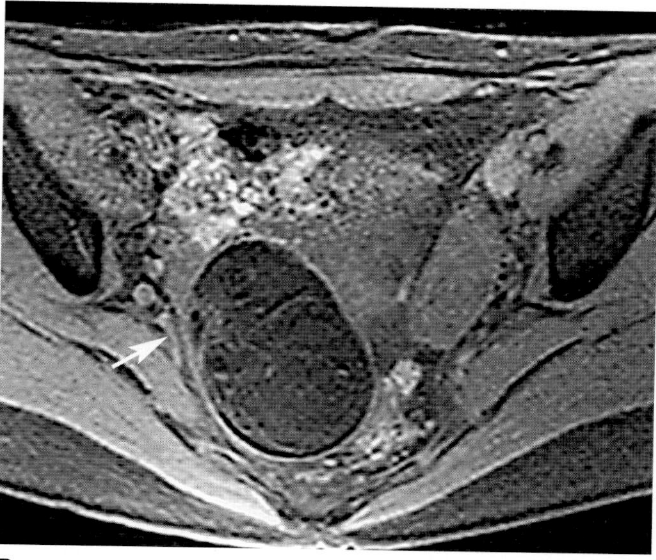

Figure 10-13 Mature Cystic Teratoma
A. Axial T2-weighted MRI nicely shows the dermoid plug (*arrow*) in this mature cystic teratoma. The darker portions of the plug correspond to calcified components of the plug such as bony elements and teeth. The fat-containing cystic fluid is intermediate in signal, similar to the subcutaneous fat. **B.** A fat-saturated T1-weighted image shows the characteristic loss of signal of the cystic component. Note the dark line just inside the bright line around the periphery of the lesion along the lateral aspect of the lesion, which shifts to just outside the white line along the medial aspect. This is caused by the chemical shift artifact that occurs secondary to a difference in the rotational frequency of fat molecules relative to water molecules during MRI. It is noted along the periphery of the dermoid cyst, where fat-containing pixels are adjacent to water (soft tissue)–containing pixels.

are predominantly solid or have large solid soft-tissue elements with microcystic spaces, which correspond to respiratory epithelium on histology (see Figure 10-15).[42] The other germ cell tumors, dysgerminoma, endodermal sinus tumor, choriocarcinoma, and embryonal cell carcinoma are usually predominantly solid lesions and are discussed under the heading **Solid Adnexal Masses.**

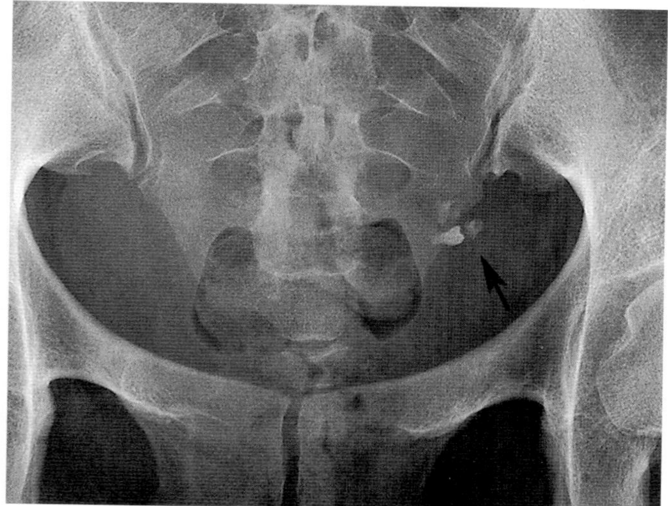

Figure 10-14 Mature Cystic Teratoma
A plain film of the pelvis shows multiple tooth fragments (*arrow*) in this patient with a mature cystic teratoma.

Epithelial neoplasms

Epithelial tumors account for 60% of all ovarian neoplasms, but more than 85% of all malignancies, and derive from serous, mucinous, or endometrioid epithelium.[30,31,43] Serous and mucinous histologies typically cause cystic masses and will be discussed under this heading.

Serous cystadenoma and cystadenocarcinoma: Serous lesions are the most common histologic subtype of epithelial tumor and are the most common type of ovarian carcinoma. About 60% of serous tumors are benign cystadenomas, 25% are malignant cystadenocarcinomas, and 15% are classified as lesions of low malignant potential (LMP).[53] LMP lesions, also called borderline tumors, are true malignancies but tend to have minimal invasion on histologic analysis. They tend to affect younger women and present with early stage I disease and, therefore, carry a better prognosis than ovarian malignancies of higher grade. Serous cystadenomas and LMP tumors tend to be predominantly cystic lesions with simple or minimally complicated fluid, thin or nodular septations, and small papillary mural projections that represent proliferating neoplastic epithelium growing over a stromal vascular core (see Figure 10-16).[43-46] Identification of vascular flow or enhancement in these papillary projections and

Imaging Notes 10-6. Vascular Papillary Projections in Cystic Ovarian Masses

> The detection of vascularity within papillary projections of an ovarian lesion is an important finding that differentiates cystic neoplasms from hemorrhagic functional cysts that can contain solid-appearing avascular debris and thrombus. The size of the nodule and level of vascularity also correlates with an increased risk of malignancy and the aggressiveness of the tumor.

larger mural nodules are the best predictors of an epithelial neoplasm, and their size often correlates with the risk of malignancy as well as the aggressiveness of the tumor (see Figure 10-16).[45,46] Accordingly, malignant serous cystadenocarcinomas usually are more complex, appearing with irregular septations and larger papillary projections and mural nodules than their benign counterparts (see Figure 10-17).

Mucinous cystadenoma and cystadenocarcinoma: Approximately 20% to 25% of ovarian tumors are mucinous in origin; 80% of mucinous lesions are benign, 10% are malignant, and 10% are tumors of LMP.[43-46] Mucinous tumors are usually multiloculated masses, with each locule containing differing amount of mucin. This phenomenon produces a mosaic imaging pattern that has been likened to "stained glass" (see Figure 10-18).[14] Serous tumors are more likely to be bilateral than mucinous tumors (20% vs 5%) and when malignant are more likely to present with evidence of metastatic disease such as ascites or peritoneal implants.[46,47]

Endometrioid and clear cell carcinoma: Endometrioid and clear cell carcinoma are less common epithelial ovarian neoplasms that account for 17.5% and 7.4% of ovarian carcinomas, respectively, and occur with greater frequency in patients with endometriosis.[30,48,49] These lesions have a variable imaging appearance, including predominantly cystic with mural nodules, multiloculated cystic, and predominantly solid lesions. Clear cell carcinomas typically appear as a large cystic lesion with solid protrusions of varying size similar to serous epithelial neoplasms and should also be suspected when a large solid nodule is noted in an endometrioma (see Figure 10-19).[30,29]

Imaging is not always able to reliably distinguish benign cystic ovarian lesions from malignant ones, but in experienced hands, US and MRI can predict malignancy with more than 90% accuracy.[14,38,39,50,51] In general, the presence of solid elements, excluding the markedly hyperechoic and fat-containing solid elements typical of dermoids and the presence of central vascularity are the

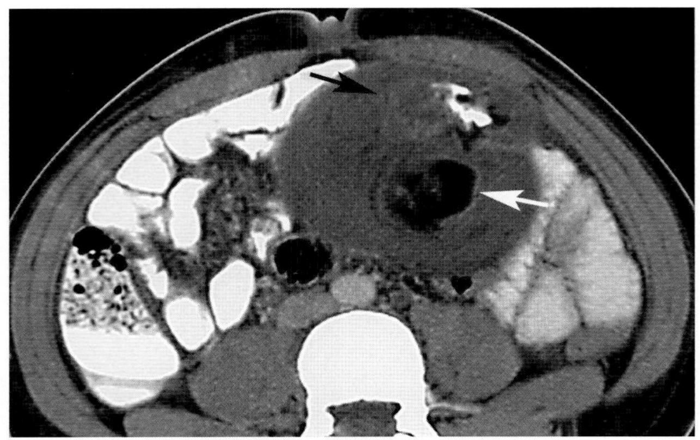

A

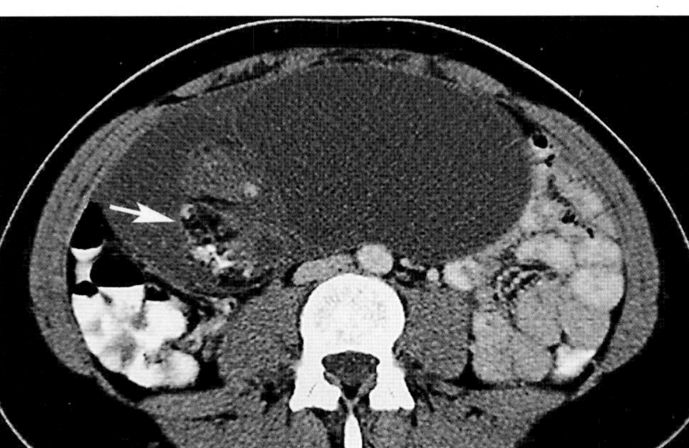

B

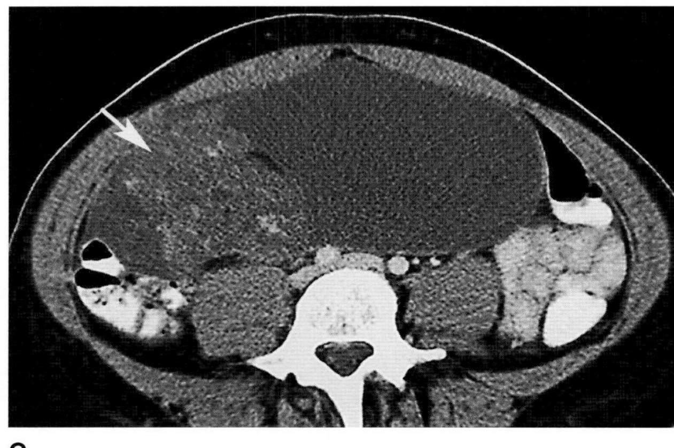

C

Figure 10-15 Malignant and Immature Teratomas in 2 Patients
A. A contrast-enhanced axial CT image of the pelvis shows a fat-containing lesion (*white arrow*) that has an irregular, solid component (*black arrow*) and is filled with complex fluid. The large size, irregular shape, and displacement of the plug to the central aspect of the lesion raised suspicion that this mature cystic teratoma had undergone malignant degeneration. **B.** and **C.** A contrast-enhanced axial CT image of the pelvis in this 18-year-old patient shows a 15-cm cystic lesion with a soft-tissue component that contains irregular regions of fat (*arrow*) and dystrophic calcifications. (C) CT image at a level below that in (A) shows the large enhancing soft-tissue component (*arrow*) of this lesion that proved to be an immature teratoma on resection.

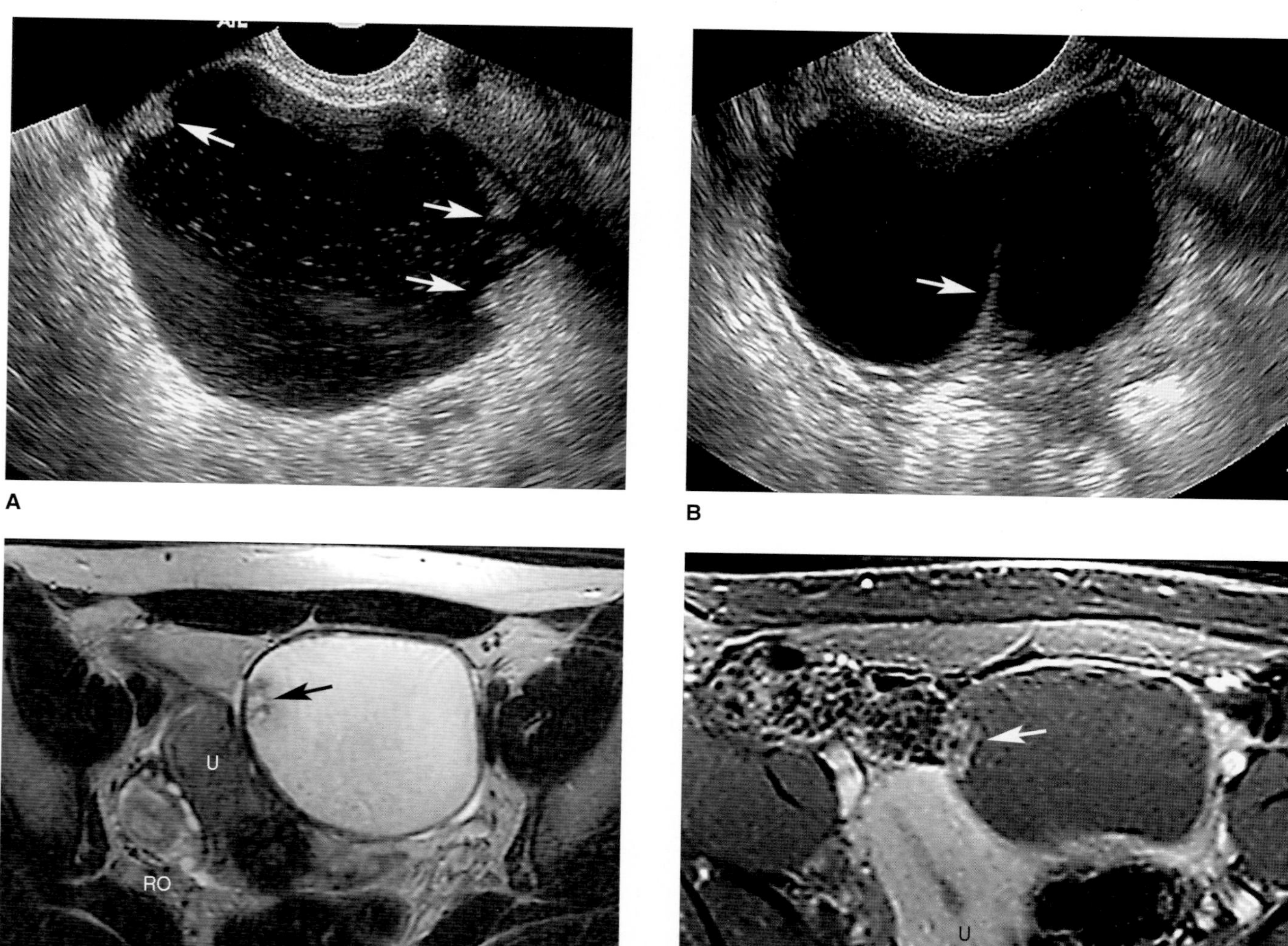

Figure 10-16 Serous Cystadenoma in 3 Patients
A. Transvaginal US shows several mural nodules (*arrows*) and slightly complicated fluid, seen as fine internal echoes within this 5-cm serous cystadenoma in a 48-year-old patient. These small nodules were not seen on the transabdominal scan (not shown). The complexity of cystic lesions is often best evaluated by transvaginal US. **B.** This 6-cm serous cystadenoma in a second patient contains a thickened septation (*arrow*). **C.** T2-weighted axial image shows an 8-cm cystic lesion with a mural nodule (*arrow*) in a third patient (RO = right ovary; U = uterus). **D.** T1-weighted fat-saturated image obtained after the administration of gadolinium shows enhancement of the mural nodule (*arrow*)—a feature that indicates a neoplasm (U = uterus).

best predictors that a complex cystic lesion is an ovarian malignancy on US.[4,38] On MRI, wall thickness of greater than 3 mm, and septation thickness of greater than 3 mm are correlated with malignancy.[14] Ancillary findings such as ascites, adenopathy, and peritoneal implants also are strong predicators of malignancy (see Figure 10-20).[4,38,52] Larger and more complicated ovarian masses will usually be removed via laparotomy, in order to adequately remove the neoplasm and search for peritoneal implants. However, a persistent minimally complicated cystic ovarian mass can usually be removed laparoscopically because many are benign, and if malignant, the risk of an invasive carcinoma is low.[53]

Extra-Ovarian Cystic Lesions

Approximately 10% to 15% of cystic pelvic lesions that are surgically removed because they are suspected as arising from the ovary are actually extraovarian in origin.[4,53] Because the differential diagnosis and management of extraovarian lesions is quite different than ovarian lesions, it is quite important to consider the possibility

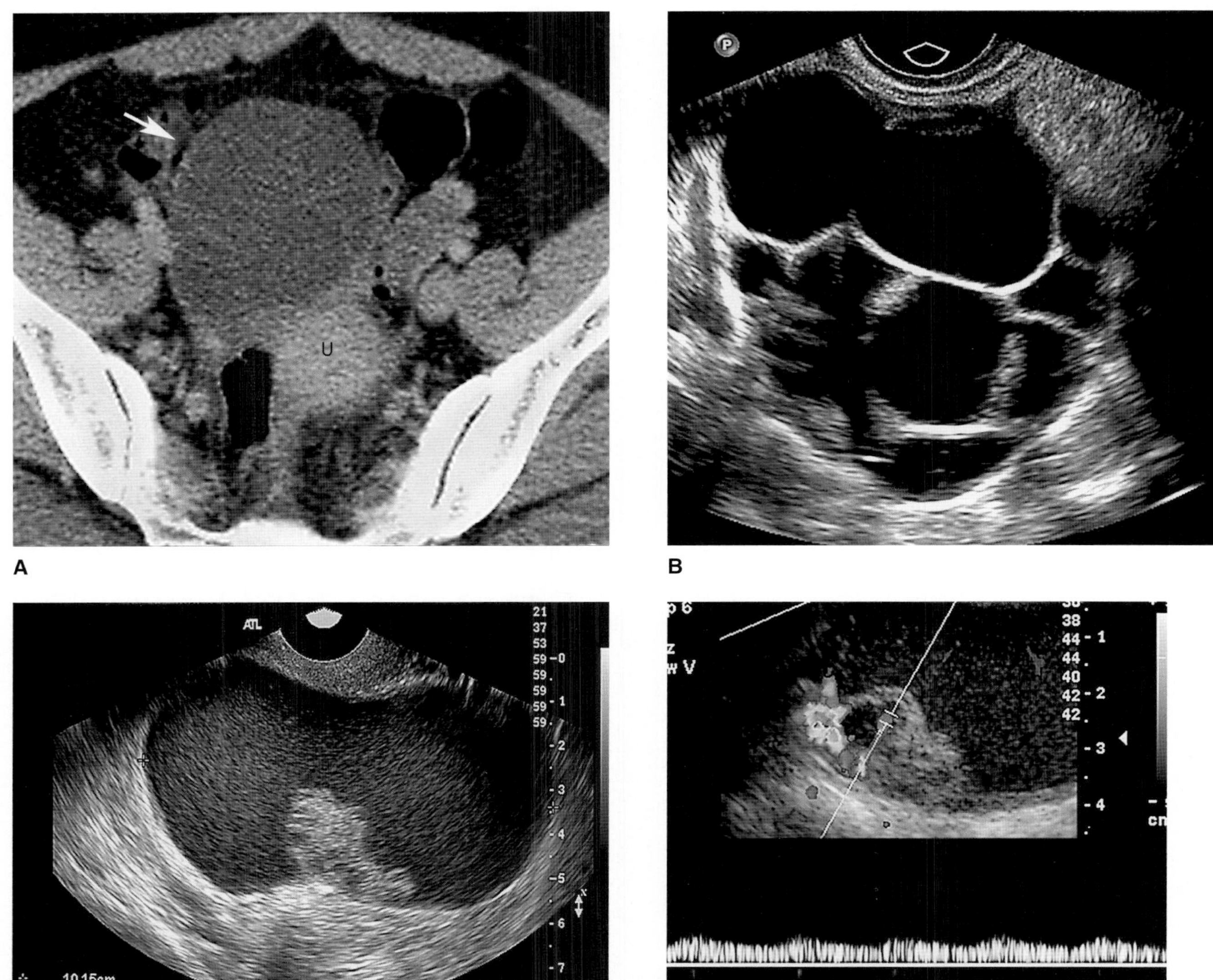

Figure 10-17 Serous Cystadenocarcinoma in 2 Patients
A. Contrast-enhanced axial CT images shows a 7-cm cystic right adnexal lesion (*arrow*) with faintly visible septations (U = uterus). **B.** The multiple thick septations are much better appreciated on this transvaginal US image. The lesion proved to be a borderline serous cystadenocarcinoma. **C.** Transvaginal US, in a second patient, shows 10.15-cm adnexal lesion with complex fluid and large mural nodule. **D.** Color Doppler examination of the patient in (C) shows marked flow within the solid component of this cystic lesion, a key finding of cystic neoplasms. Surgical resection was diagnostic of a serous cystadenocarcinoma.

that an adnexal lesion that is discovered by imaging may not be arising from the ovary. Identifying normal follicle-containing ovarian parenchyma surrounding a mass, "the ovarian crescent sign" is helpful to document an ovarian origin of a lesion, whereas identification of a separate and distinct ipsilateral ovary indicates that the mass does not arise from the ovary (see Figure 10-21).[54,55] The most commonly encountered cystic extraovarian lesions are almost always benign and include endometriomas, paraovarian or paratubal mesothelial cysts, peritoneal inclusion cysts, and dilated fallopian tubes (Table 10-2).

Endometrioma

Endometriosis, the implantation of ectopic endometrial tissue, affects an estimated 10% of premenopausal women. As much as 80% of ectopic endometrial tissue implants on the ovary and when large enough is detectable by imaging as an endometrioma.[56] Enlarging endometriomas can destroy portions of the ovary as the normal ovary is stretched and distorted by the growing lesion. Endometrioma rupture results in the release of hemorrhagic material into the peritoneum causing adhesions and fibrosis of the bowel and fallopian tubes.

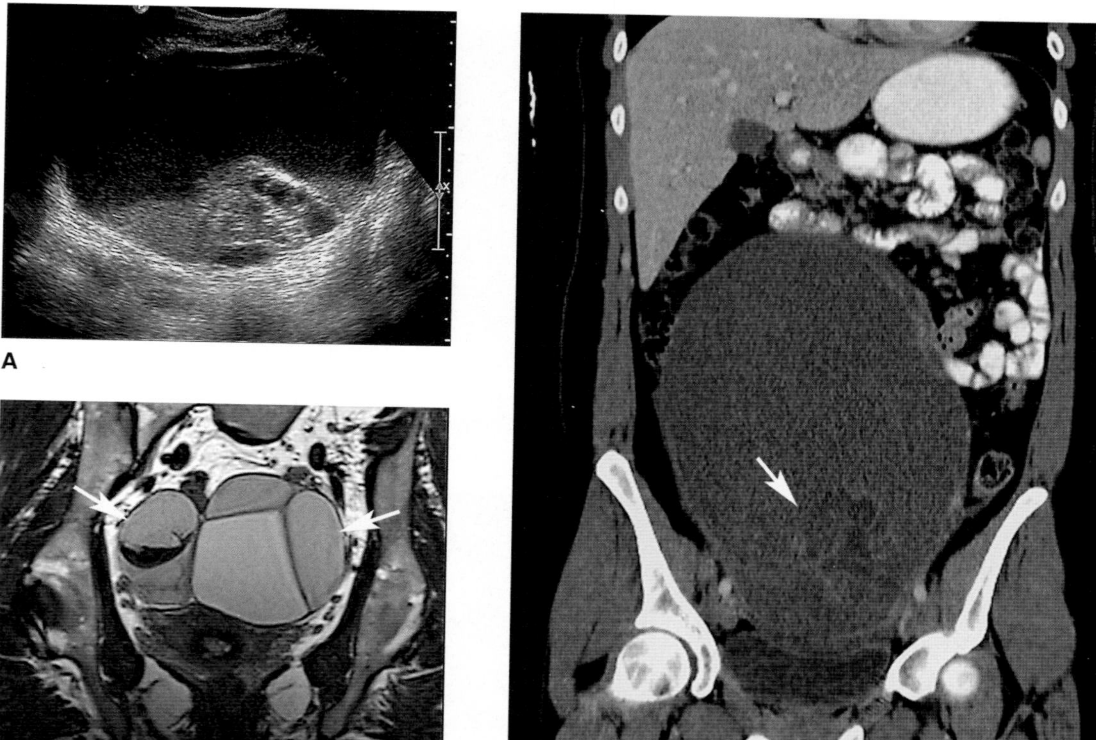

Figure 10-18 Mucinous Cystadenoma in 3 Patients
A. Sagittal image of this 12-cm mucinous cystadenoma shows a complicated cystic lesion that has layering mucinous fluid of higher echogenicity as well as a multilocular solid component. **B.** A coronal T2-weighted MRI shows bilateral mucinous cystadenomas (*arrows*) in a different patient. The varying amounts of mucin cause the various locules within these lesions to have varying intensities, a pattern that has been likened to stained glass. **C.** Coronal reformatted CT in another patient shows an 18-cm predominantly cystic mucinous cystadenoma that has an inferior multilocular component containing low-density mucinous fluid (*arrow*).

Endometriomas are complex cystic lesions that have a variety of imaging appearances. On US, the majority of lesions will appear as a homogenous cystic mass with low-level echoes and good through sound transmission without internal vascular flow.[57-59] This finding has been called the "ground glass" appearance (see Figure 10-22). Some endometriomas will demonstrate hyperechoic foci within the wall of a cystic lesion, which are thought to be due to cholesterol deposition from chronic cellular degeneration and are considered highly suggestive of an endometrioma.[57] Some endometriomas will appear multilocular with nonnodular septations and wall nodularity.[58] This type of appearance may be difficult to distinguish from a neoplasm.

MRI is the most sensitive and specific imaging technique for characterizing ovarian endometriomas and has the greatest sensitivity of all imaging modalities for detecting nonovarian cystic and fibrotic peritoneal implants.[59-61] Further, MRI has a sensitivity of 68% to 90%, and a specificity of 83% to 98% for the diagnosis of endometriosis.[60] The most specific MRI findings of endometriomas are multiple cystic masses, often bilateral, of high signal on T1-weighted images and low signal on

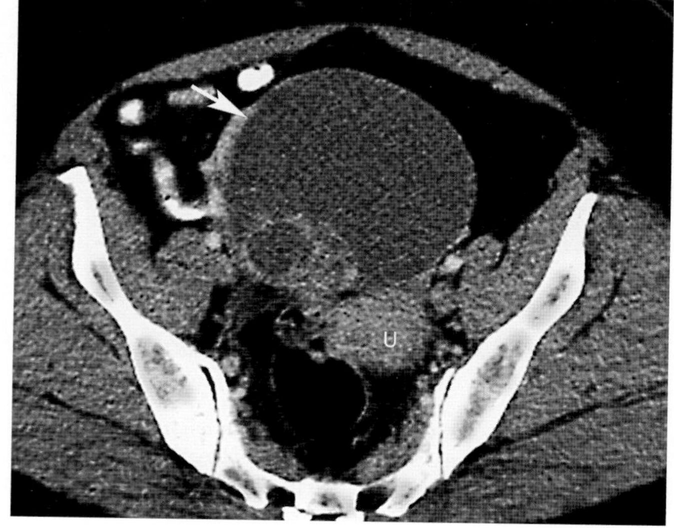

Figure 10-19 Clear Cell Carcinoma
Contrast-enhanced CT image of the pelvis in a 34-year-old patient shows a cystic neoplasm with a heterogeneous solid component that proved to be a clear cell carcinoma (U = uterus).

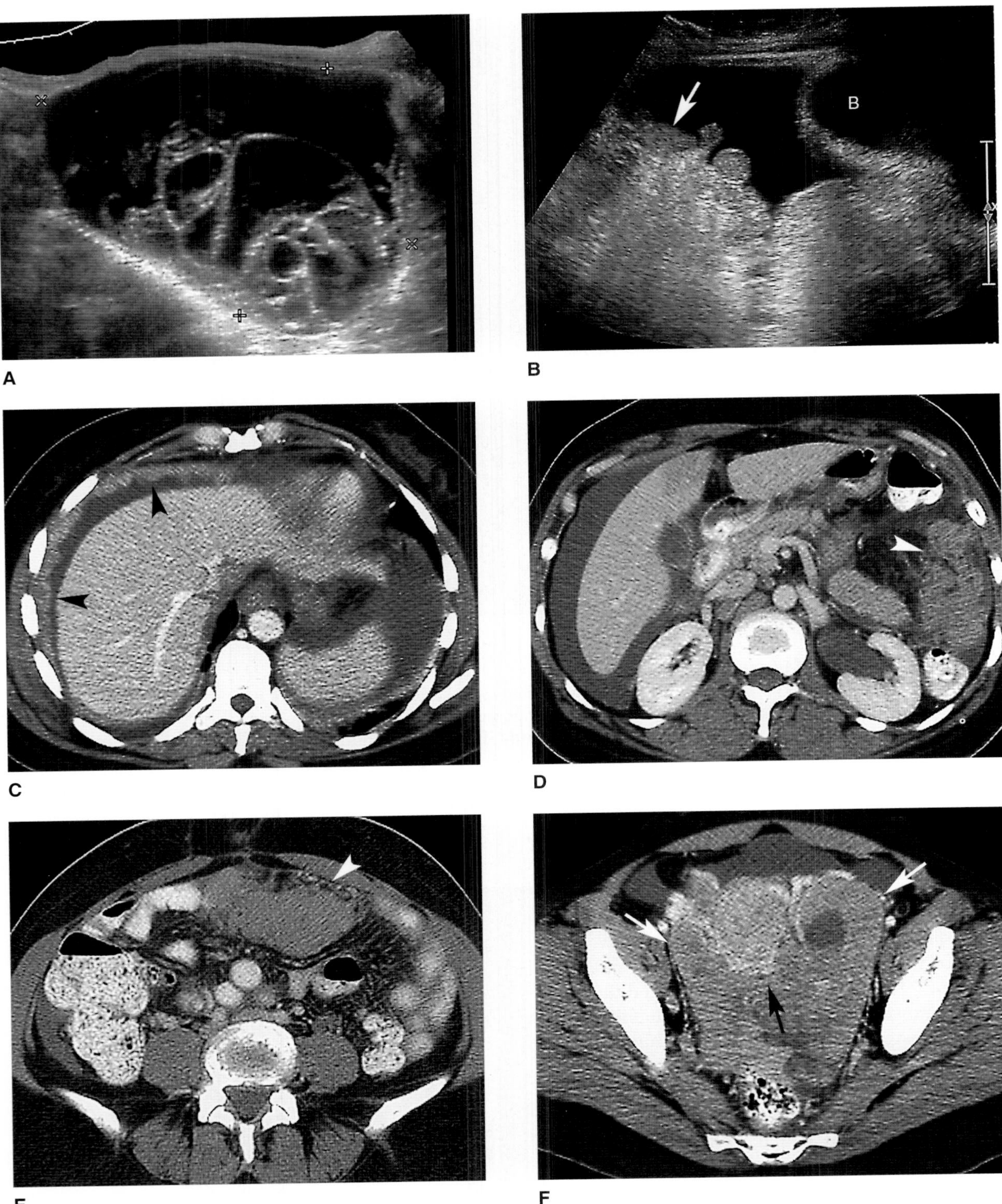

Figure 10-20 Metastatic Serous Cystadenocarcinoma in 2 Patients
A. This 14-cm complex cystic lesion (*outlined by calipers*) demonstrates thick and irregular septations, features highly suspect for a neoplasm. **B.** The identification of soft-tissue peritoneal metastatic implants (*arrow*) on the surface of the bowel, well outlined by pelvic ascites just above the urinary bladder, is a strong predicator of a malignancy (B = bladder). **C-F.** Contrast-enhanced CT in a 46-year-old woman with abdominal distention demonstrates nodular thickening of the right hemidiaphragm (*black arrowheads*) in (C), omental soft-tissue masses (*white arrowheads*) in (D and E), ascites in all images, and bilateral predominantly solid adnexal masses (*white arrows*) on either side of the uterus (*black arrow*) in (F). This combination of findings is typical of advanced peritoneal metastasis from an ovarian epithelial malignancy, in this case bilateral mucinous cystadenocarcinoma. There is also left hydronephrosis in (D) due to ureteral obstruction by the pelvic masses.

Imaging Notes 10-7. Endometrioma

MRI has the highest sensitivity and specificity for the diagnosis of endometriomas due to the ability of MRI to detect blood products of varying ages.

Imaging Features of Endometriomas

US	• Homogenous cystic mass with low-level internal echoes ("ground glass" cyst) • Hyperechogenic cholesterol foci in the wall of the cyst • Less commonly septations, wall nodularity, internal solid-appearing clots
MRI	• Cystic mass with high-signal T1-weighted, low-signal T2-weighted (occasionally high-signal T2-weighted if recent hemorrhage.) • High T1-weighted signal persists on fat-suppressed images • Shading: range of low signal intensities within cyst on T2 weighting

T2-weighted images. Endometriomas retain high signal on fat-suppressed T1-weighted imaging, a differentiating feature from a fat-containing mature cystic teratoma (see Figure 10-22).[60-62] Many endometriomas will demonstrate shading: a range of low signal intensities on T2-weighted images.[62] Some will demonstrate low signal intensity within the cyst wall on T2-weighted images. Occasionally, an endometrioma can have high signal on both T1- and T2-weighted images, likely reflecting recent hemorrhage

Imaging Notes 10-8. Peritoneal Inclusion Cysts

Cystic adnexal lesions that appear to surround the ovary and have geometric borders are likely peritoneal inclusion cysts.

into the lesion.[6,60] Wall enhancement due to granulation tissue may also be noted. Endometriomas larger than 1 cm are routinely imaged by MR, but lesions may not be easily detected.[56]

The CT appearance of an endometrioma is variable and includes solid and cystic heterogeneous adnexal masses of varying attenuation.[8,9]

Mesothelial cysts

Paraovarian and paratubal cysts arise in the broad ligament as derivatives of mesothelial or perimesothelial structures. They are most common in premenopausal women but have been shown to occur in women of all ages.[55,63-66] These lesions appear as simple cysts, often adjacent to but separate from the ipsilateral ovary (see Figures 10-21 and 10-23). Rarely, they may be complicated by bleeding, rupture, torsion, or infection and can appear more complex. Often, paratubal and paraovarian cysts are small and incidentally noted on imaging exams obtained for other reasons; however, larger lesions can be palpable. Paraovarian tumors are uncommon but should be considered if a mural nodule or septations are noted in an extraovarian cystic lesion.[67,68]

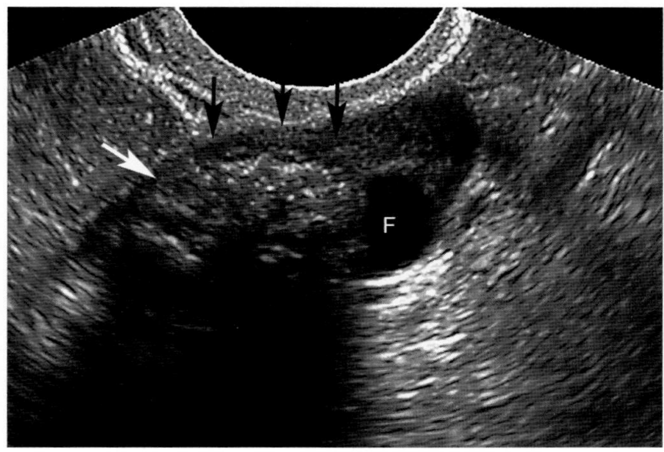

A

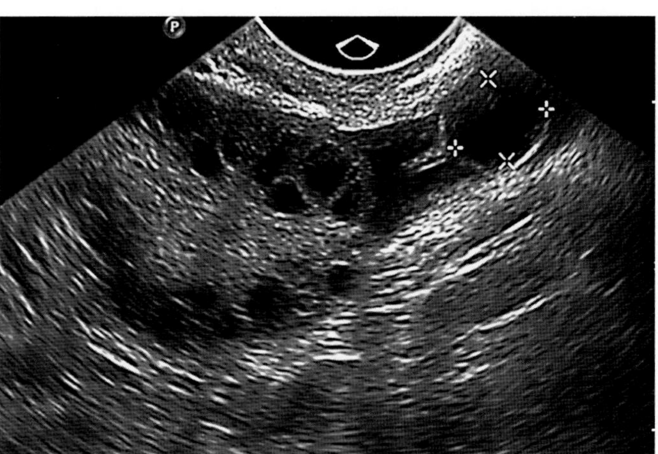

B

Figure 10-21 Ovarian Crescent Sign
A. Transvaginal US image shows a densely calcified lesion (*white arrow*). The ovarian parenchyma, identified by the follicle, can be seen to extend along the surface (*black arrows*) and surround the mass, indicating an intraovarian location of the lesion (F = follicle). **B.** This paraovarian cyst (outlined by calipers) is seen separately from the adjacent ipsilateral ovary, indicating an extraovarian lesion. Note that the adjacent ovary is polycystic in appearance in this patient with PCOS.

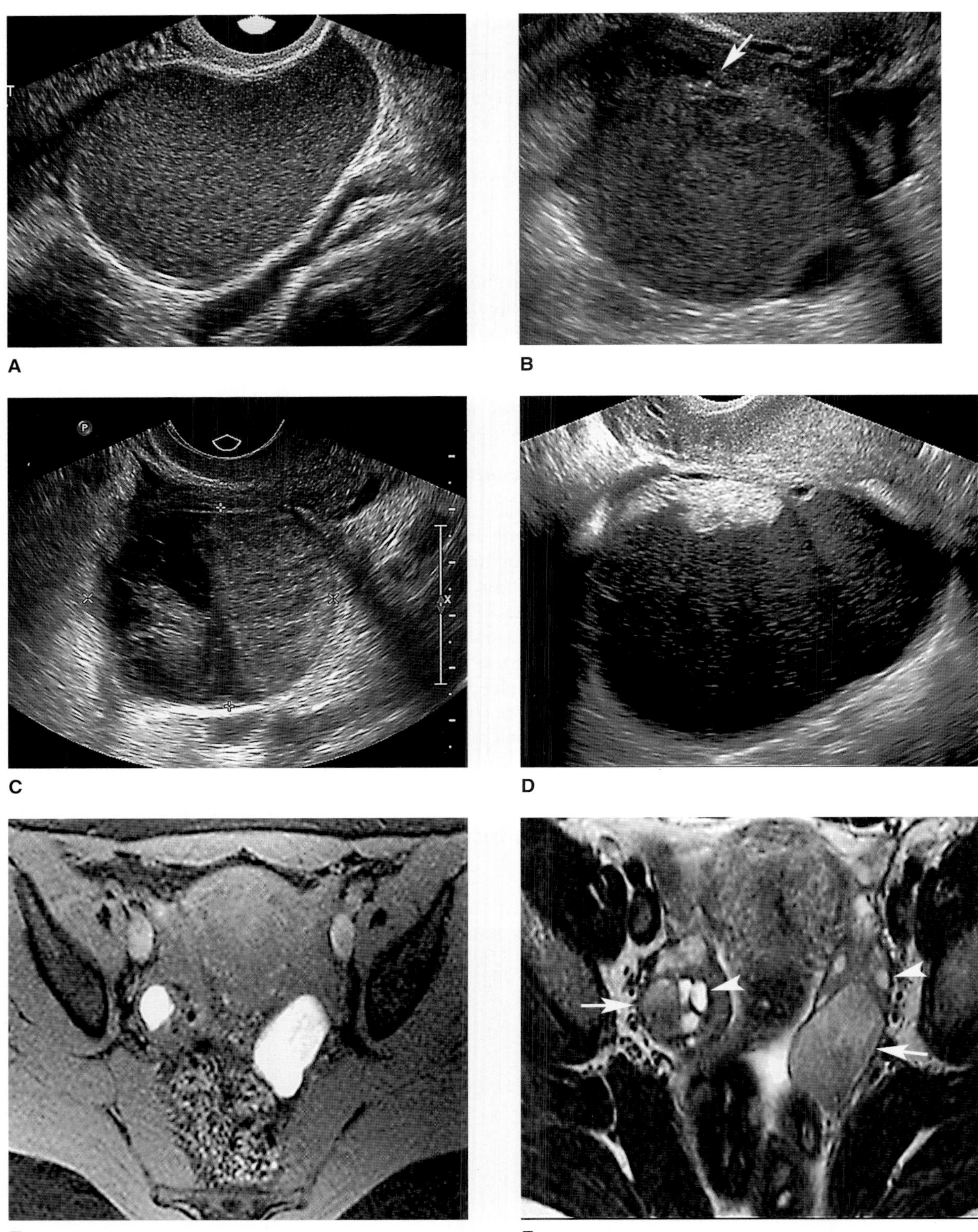

Figure 10-22 Endometriomas on US and MRI
Endometriomas have a variety of appearances on sonography. **A.** Homogeneous low-level echoes, called the "ground glass" appearance. **B.** A solid mural nodule with hyperechoic foci (*arrow*), thought to be related to cholesterol and other breakdown products. **C.** Mixed cystic and solid elements, without vascular flow (not shown). Endometriomas periodically hemorrhage into themselves and may have an appearance that overlaps with a hemorrhagic cyst. **D.** Echogenic fluid with an echogenic mural thrombus. This appearance is nonspecific and overlaps with cystic neoplasms, especially mature cystic teratomas. **E.** Axial T1-weighted fat-saturated MRI and (**F**) axial T2-weighted MRI show bilateral lesions with high signal on T1 and varying low signal on T2 (*white arrows*) as compared to the bright-signal ovarian follicles (*arrowheads*), because of blood products of varying ages, a signal intensity change referred to as shading.

Table 10-2. Extraovarian Cystic Pelvic Masses

1. Mesothelial (paraovarian or paratubal) cyst
2. Peritoneal inclusion cyst
3. Dilated fallopian tube a. Hydrosalpinx b. Hematosalpinx c. Pyosalpinx/tubo-ovarian abscess

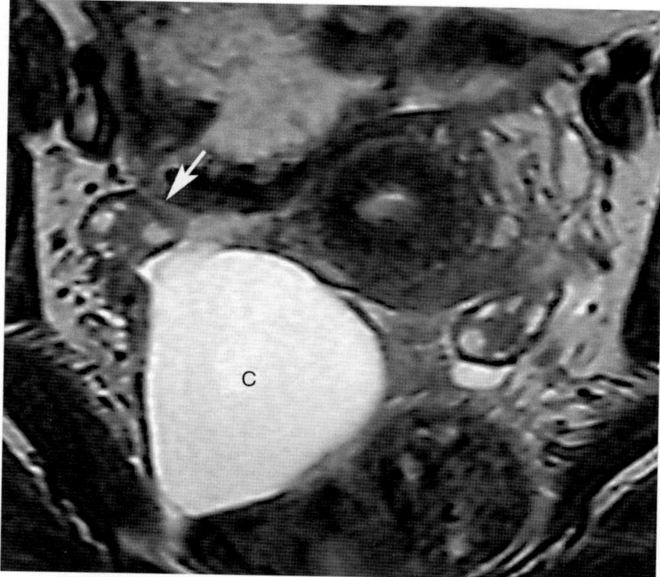

Figure 10-23 Paraovarian Cyst MRI
T2-weighted axial MRI shows a high-signal cyst adjacent to but separate from the right ovary (*arrow*) (C = cyst).

Peritoneal inclusion cysts

Peritoneal inclusion cysts (PICs) occur when ovulatory fluid produced by the normal ovary is unable to be absorbed by the peritoneum secondary to scarring from prior pelvic surgery, pelvic inflammatory disease, and/or endometriosis.[69-71] Over time, the trapped fluid forms a loculated collection surrounding the ovary, bounded by peritoneal adhesions (see Figure 10-23). The key to the diagnosis of a peritoneal inclusion cyst is recognition of a normal-appearing ovary within the PIC, called the "ovary in the cyst" sign, and the geometric shape conforming to the anatomic boundaries of the pelvis (see Figure 10-24). On US, PICs may be anechoic or contain a few internal septations. With extensive adhesions, the septations may be thicker and irregular and even have low-resistance vascular flow mimicking a cystic or multilocular neoplasm (see Figure 10-24).[71,72]

Dilation of the fallopian tube

A distended fallopian tube develops when the distal aspect of the fallopian becomes occluded and the tube fills with serous fluid (hydrosalpinx), blood (hematosalpinx), or infected material (pyosalpinx).

Hydrosalpinx: Hydrosalpinx can occur as an isolated finding or as 1 component of a complex adnexal lesion that has caused distal tubal occlusion. The most common cause of hydrosalpinx is scarring from prior pelvic inflammatory disease. Other causes include endometriosis, peritubal adhesions from a previous pelvic surgery, particularly hysterectomy, tubal cancer, and tubal pregnancy (Table 10-3).[7,73-75] Symptoms of hydrosalpinx vary. Some patients experience recurrent lower abdominal pain or pelvic pain; others are asymptomatic. Because tubal function is impeded, infertility is common in patients with unilateral or bilateral hydrosalpinges.

The classic appearance of an uncomplicated hydrosalpinx is a tubular, sausage-shaped structure positioned between the uterus and the ovary.[7,73] However, portions of the tube, particularly the ampullary segment, may become markedly dilated, reaching more than 10 cm in diameter, causing the tube to assume a folded configuration, mimicking a multilocular or septated cystic adnexal mass. Unless the normal ipsilateral ovary can be confidently identified, the appearance may raise concern for an ovarian neoplasm. On US, scanning in multiple planes may be helpful in elucidating the tubular configuration of a hydrosalpinx by noting that the fluid-containing compartments can be connected and that suspected septations were simulated by the walls of the distended tube (see Figure 10-25).[73,74] An indentation in the opposing walls of a cystic adnexal mass, "the waist sign," has been shown to be the best predictor of a hydrosalpinx (see Figure 10-25).[75] If there has been previous inflammation, the mucosal lining of the tube may appear as polypoid protrusions into the lumen of the tube, producing the so-called cog-wheel or beads-on-a-string appearance (see Figure 10-25).[73,75] The multiplanar capability of MR and reconstructed CT images may be helpful to differentiate from a multilocular cystic ovarian mass (see Figure 10-25).[76]

Hematosalpinx: In the nonpregnant female patient, a hematosalpinx is most commonly seen in patients with endometriosis. Often, endometrial implants on the serosa of the tube cause repeated bouts of hemorrhage and

Imaging Notes 10-9. Hydrosalpinx

Features of a hydrosalpinx include a tubular configuration, multiple polypoid-appearing thickened folds, and diametrically opposed inward scalloping of the adjacent walls of the tube.

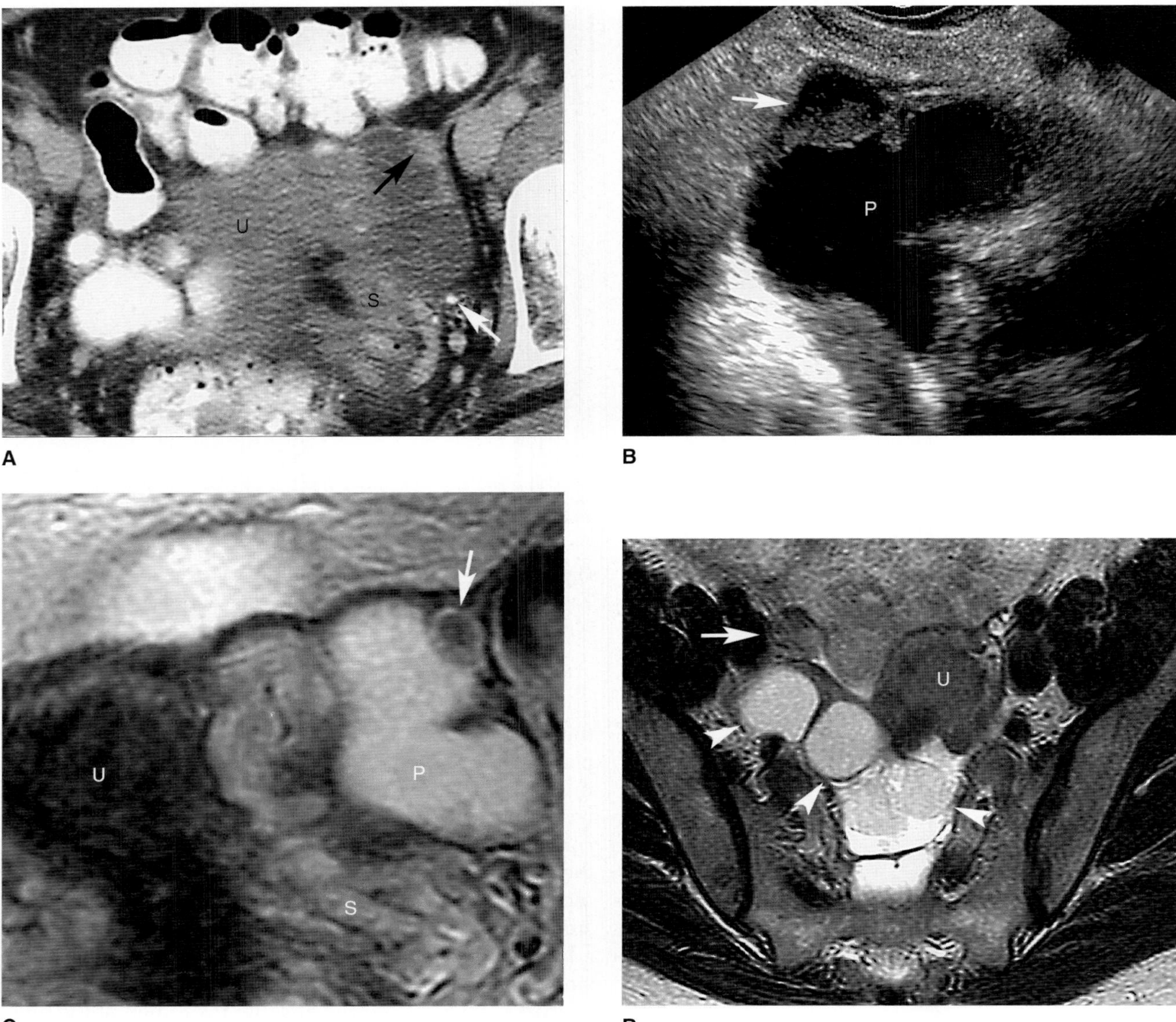

Figure 10-24 Peritoneal Inclusion Cyst
A. Axial CT image in a 56-year-old perimenopausal patient with multiple bouts of sigmoid diverticulitis showed a complex cystic left adnexal mass (*white arrow*). The enhancing structure in the lateral aspect of the lesion (*black arrow*) was not recognized to represent the left ovary (U = uterus; S = sigmoid colon). **B.** Sagittal transabdominal US image shows the left ovary (*arrow*) adjacent but separate from the peritoneal inclusion cyst (P = peritoneal inclusion cyst). **C.** Axial T2-weighted MRI also depicts the left ovary (*arrow*) adjacent but separate from the peritoneal inclusion cyst (P = peritoneal inclusion cyst; U = uterus; S = sigmoid colon). **D.** T2-weighted axial MRI in a second patient shows a multiloculated peritoneal inclusion cyst (*arrowheads*) adjacent to but separate from the right ovary (*arrow*) (U = uterus).

fibrosis, with resultant formation of peritubal adhesions and simple hydrosalpinx. A less common type of tubal endometriosis is intraluminal, which results in hematosalpinx and, in certain patients, may be the only imaging finding indicative of endometriosis.[7,56] Hematosalpinx can also be noted in adnexal or isolated tubal torsion, in patients with an obstructing tubal tumor and from retrograde menstrual flow in patients with hematometrocolpos. On US, low-level echoes or layering material may be seen within the tubal fluid. On MRI, hyperintense tubal fluid seen on

Table 10- 3. Causes of Fallopian Tube Obstruction

1. Peritubal adhesions a. Pelvic inflammatory disease (PID) b. Prior pelvic surgery
2. Endometriosis
3. Fallopian tube carcinoma
4. Prior ectopic pregnancy

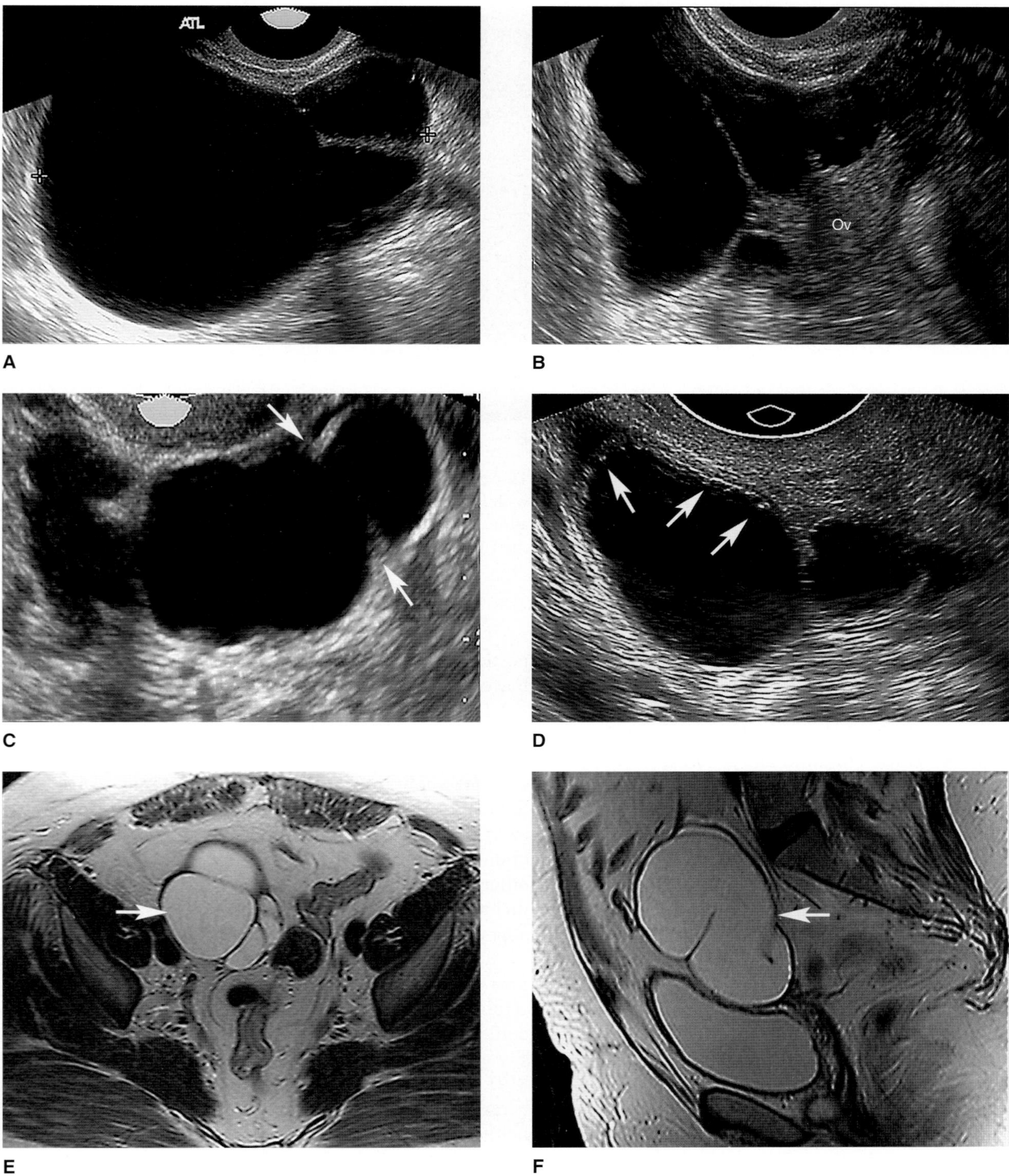

Figure 10-25 Hydrosalpinx in 5 Patients
A. Coronal transvaginal US image shows what appears to be a multilocular, cystic adnexal lesion (*outlined by calipers*). **B.** Oblique sagittal images show a normal ovary and an adjacent dilated fallopian tube. The perpendicular orientation of the tube with respect to the imaging plane in (A) imaged adjacent portions of the dilated fallopian tube, simulated a cystic mass (Ov = ovary). **C.** US of a second patient shows a hydrosalpinx that demonstrates inward indentations (*arrows*) of its opposing walls, called the waist sign. This finding is the best predictor that a cystic adnexal lesion is a hydrosalpinx. **D.** This hydrosalpinx in a third patient demonstrates thickening of the endosalpingeal folds, called the cog wheel sign, which appears as small, evenly spaced nodularity of the mucosal surface of the tube. **E.** Axial T2 and (**F**) paramedian sagittal T2-weighted images in a fifth patient. Image (E) shows a complex cystic right adnexal lesion (*arrow*). A normal right ovary was not seen. (F) Paramedian sagittal T2-weighted image of the right adnexa shows the tubular configuration of this hydrosalpinx (*arrow*).

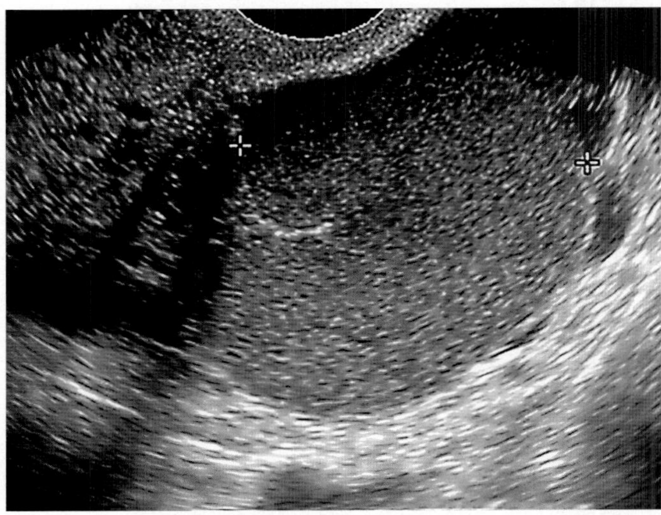

A

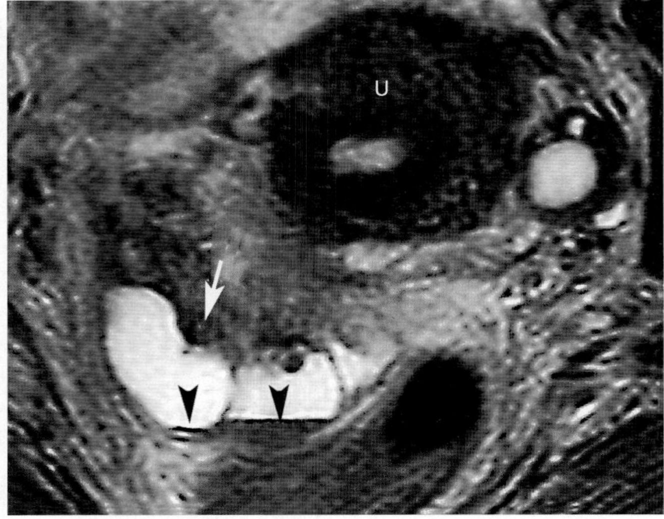

B

Figure 10-26 Hematosalpinx in 2 Patients
A. A thin-walled distended fallopian tube fluid (marked by calipers) with echogenic, hemorrhagic fluid, similar to that seen in ovarian endometriomas, proved to be a hematosalpinx in this 36-year-old patient with known endometriosis. **B.** A T2-weighted axial MRI shows a dilated fallopian tube (*arrow*) with hematocrit levels (*arrowheads*) in this patient with right adnexal torsion (U = uterus). (See Figure 10-37F for images of the right ovary.)

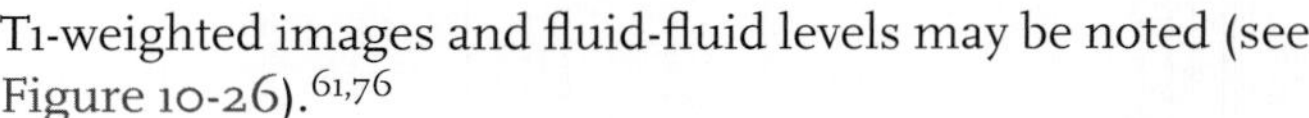

T1-weighted images and fluid-fluid levels may be noted (see Figure 10-26).[61,76]

Pelvic inflammatory disease, pyosalpinx, and tubo-ovarian abscess: Pelvic inflammatory disease (PID) refers to sexually transmitted infections of the upper female genital tract, including endometritis, salpingitis, oophoritis, peritonitis, and/or tubo-ovarian abscess (TOA). It has been estimated that approximately 10% to 15% of American women have had at least 1 episode of PID. Tubal inflammatory disease plays a role in 30% of women with infertility and 50% of ectopic pregnancies.[77,78] Although the early changes of PID are subtle and nonspecific, the hallmark findings of tubal and peritubal inflammation are present in more severe cases.

On US, the tubal wall appears thickened, measuring more than 5 mm and there is often increased blood flow on color Doppler imaging. If the lumen of the tube becomes occluded, the tube will fill with a purulent exudate, which appears as complicated fluid with echoes, fluid-debris levels, or, rarely, gas-fluid levels. The inflammatory process can spread to the ovary, producing a tubo-ovarian complex.[73,78] At this stage, the infected ovary is adherent to the fallopian tube and can appear swollen with irregular complicated cystic regions and indistinct margins, but with identifiable ovarian parenchyma. A tubo-ovarian abscess is diagnosed when there is complete breakdown of the ovarian and tubal architecture into a nondescript inflammatory mass without recognizable structures (see Figure 10-27).[78] PID is almost always a bilateral inflammatory process, but 1 side may be more severely affected. In severe cases, the inflammatory process may spread to involve the cul-de-sac and upper portions of the abdomen. Hydroureteronephrosis and bowel wall thickening can also develop.

Cross-sectional imaging is not necessarily needed but is often obtained when the symptoms are more generalized and PID is not suspected on a clinical basis. In general, CT may show mild inflammatory stranding, a distended fallopian tube, or 1 or more pelvic abscesses (see Figure 10-27).[8,9,79] Though the clinical and imaging findings are often specific for the diagnosis of PID, there are several other common conditions in the differential diagnosis including peritonitis from another source such as ruptures, appendicitis, or ruptured endometrioma.

On both CT and MRI, both hydrosalpinx and pyosalpinx appear as a dilated, fluid-filled tubular structure. With acute pyosalpinx, the wall of the tube may be thickened and demonstrate enhancement. The density and signal intensity of the fluid within the tube is variable on both CT and MRI but tends to be more heterogeneous when an underlying pyosalpinx is present (see Figure 10-27). However, neither CT nor MRI can reliably distinguish between a hydrosalpinx and pyosalpinx.[7,73]

Ectopic pregnancy

An ectopic pregnancy is defined as any pregnancy that occurs outside the uterine cavity. Pregnancies in the fallopian tube account for approximately 97% of all ectopic pregnancies, with 55% of these occurring in the ampullary segment, 25% in the isthmus, 17% in the fimbria, and 3% in the interstitial portion of the tube. The remaining 3% of ectopic pregnancies implant in the cervix, ovary, or the abdominal cavity, listed in decreasing order of frequency.[80,81] Predisposing factors include a history of pelvic

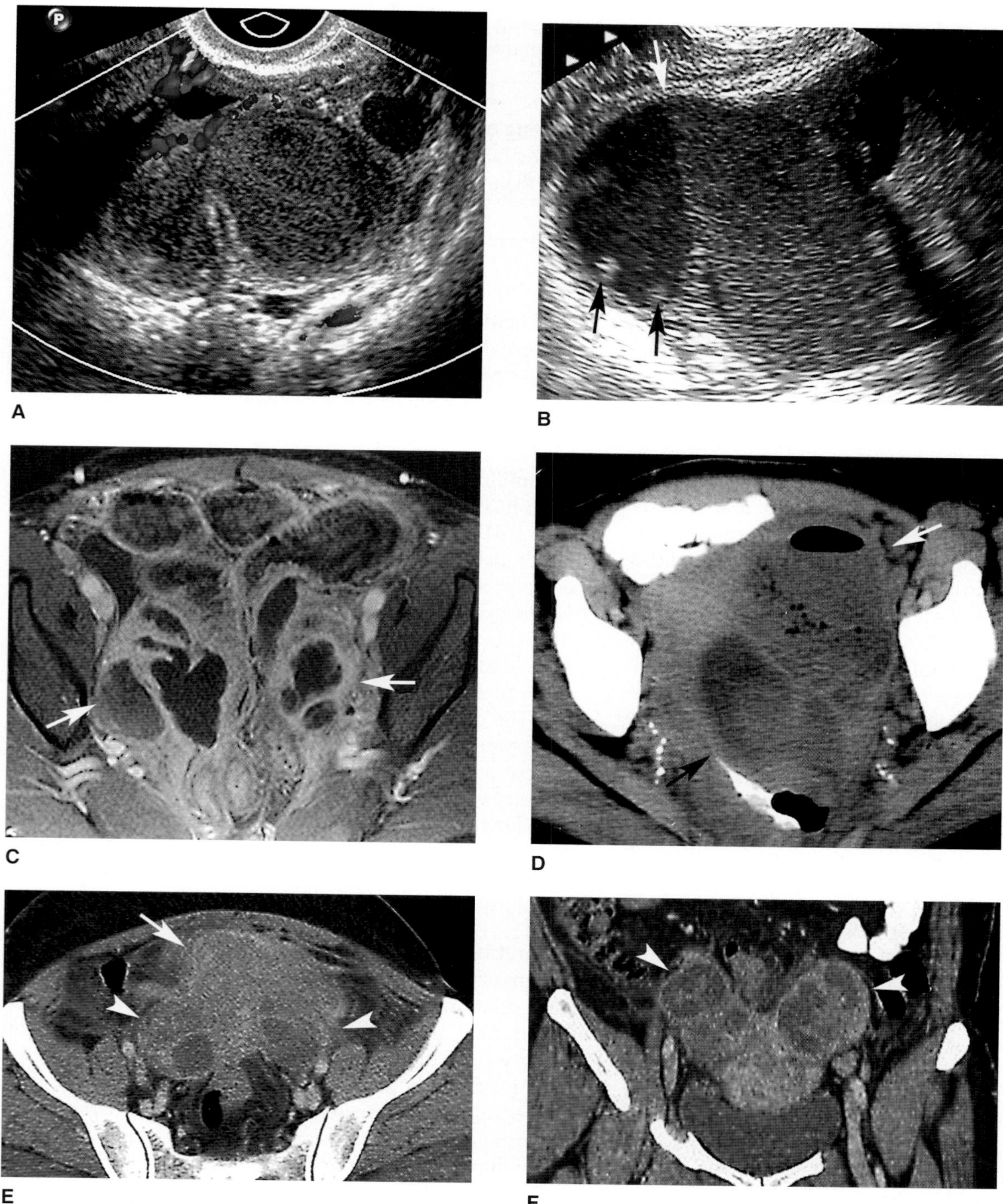

Figure 10-27 Pyosalpinx and PID in 5 Patients
A. Transvaginal US image of a pyosalpinx shows a dilated fallopian tube containing complex fluid. The tube is thick-walled with increased vascular flow, findings that are the hallmarks of acute salpingitis. **B.** A fluid-complex fluid level is seen in this pyosalpinx in a second patient that also demonstrates thickening of the endosalpingeal folds (*arrows*). **C.** A contrast-enhanced axial T1-weighted MRI of the pelvis shows markedly thickened fallopian tubes bilaterally (*arrows*) with extensive enhancement of the fallopian tube walls and internal heterogeneous fluid in this 36-year-old patient with multiple episodes of PID. **D.** A contrast-enhanced axial CT image in a fourth patient with severe PID shows a debris-filled fallopian tube (*black arrow*) and a gas-containing abscess in the left adnexa in this patient with a tubo-ovarian abscess. **E.** Contrast-enhanced CT in a fifth patient shows bilateral complex cystic adnexal masses (*arrowheads*) on either side of a low-attenuation, edematous uterus findings consistent with bilateral TOA. Note that the fat planes appear blurred, a finding that usually indicates adjacent inflammation. **F.** Coronal reconstruction in the same patient as (E) shows the tubular nature of the bilateral TOA (*arrowheads*) to better advantage. Note how the cystic regions appear to form a convoluted tube winding backwards and forwards.

Table 10-4. Predisposing Factors for Ectopic Pregnancy

1. Pelvic inflammatory disease
2. Tubal surgery
3. Prior ectopic pregnancy
4. Assisted reproduction
5. Endometriosis
6. Intrauterine contraceptive devise usage
7. Current smoking
8. Congenital exposure to diethylstilbestrol

inflammatory disease, tubal surgery, prior ectopic pregnancy, assisted reproduction, endometriosis, intrauterine contraceptive device usage, current smoking, and in utero exposure to diethylstilbestrol (Table 10-4).[82] Because many ectopic pregnancies occur in patients without identified risk factors, many clinicians have a low threshold for evaluating all women with a positive pregnancy test by pelvic US.[80,83]

Determining the presence or absence of an intrauterine pregnancy is a very important first step in the US evaluation of a patient with a positive pregnancy test. Because the coexistence of an intrauterine pregnancy with an ectopic pregnancy (heterotopic pregnancy) is relatively rare, with a frequency of 1 to 4000 to 1 in 30 000 in the general population, US detection of an intrauterine pregnancy makes the possibility of an ectopic pregnancy as the etiology of the patient's symptoms extremely unlikely (see Figure 10-28).[80,83] However, in patients undergoing assisted reproduction, heterotopic pregnancy occurs in as many as 1 in 100 patients making the presence of an intrauterine pregnancy less helpful to exclude a coexisting ectopic pregnancy.[80]

Visualization of an extrauterine gestational sac containing a living embryo is diagnostic of an ectopic pregnancy; however, this finding is noted in only 26% of patients who undergo US (see Figure 10-28).[84-86] More commonly, the diagnosis of an ectopic pregnancy is made with high probability when there is no evidence of an intrauterine pregnancy in combination with 1 or more adnexal abnormalities.[80,83,84-86] In the setting of evaluation for an ectopic pregnancy, the finding of any nonovarian adnexal mass carries a positive predictive value of 96.3% for the diagnosis of ectopic pregnancy.[84-88] The adnexal mass represents the ectopic gestational sac or its remnants, often in association with hematosalpinx (see Figure 10-28). The absence of an abnormal adnexal findings does not exclude the diagnosis of ectopic pregnancy; normal-appearing adnexa can be noted in up to 25% of patients evaluated.[83,84] Correlation with quantitative β–human chorionic gonadotropin (β-hCG) levels is necessary when neither an intrauterine pregnancy nor findings suspect for an ectopic pregnancy are noted. If the β-hCG level is under the discriminatory level, which is 1500 mIU/mL in most laboratories, the patient may have either an early, nonvisualized intrauterine pregnancy, or an ectopic pregnancy. Serial quantitative β-hCG and repeat US is necessary until a definitive diagnosis is made.[83] If the β-hCG is above the discriminatory level, the patient is considered at high risk for a nonvisualized ectopic pregnancy, in the absence of a recent spontaneous abortion.

Imaging Notes 10-10. Intrauterine Gestation and Ectopic Pregnancy

> In patients without a history of assisted reproduction, the identification of a normal intrauterine pregnancy nearly excludes the diagnosis of an ectopic pregnancy.

Imaging Notes 10-11. Adenexal Mass and Ectopic Pregnancy

> In the setting of evaluation for an ectopic pregnancy, the finding of any nonovarian adnexal mass or complex free pelvic fluid carries a 96.3% positive predictive value for the diagnosis of ectopic pregnancy.

The detection of complex fluid in the cul-de-sac due to hemoperitoneum is an important clue to the diagnosis of ectopic pregnancy. It may be the only abnormal finding in up to 15% of patients and has a positive predictive value of 93% for an ectopic pregnancy in the appropriate clinical situation.[84,89] In general, in a patient with a positive β-hCG, the greater the quantity of fluid and the more complex the fluid, the more likely the patient is to have an ectopic pregnancy.[83,88]

Interstitial (cornual) ectopic pregnancy: An interstitial pregnancy occurs as a result of abnormal implantation of the gestational sac in the most proximal portion of the fallopian tube, the portion that is contained within the muscular wall of the uterus. Although interstitial pregnancies account for only 2% to 4% of all ectopic gestations, they cause a disproportionately high incidence of hemoperitoneum and shock, and the mortality rate is approximately twice that of other types of ectopic pregnancies because of the rich vascular supply of this region of the uterus compared with the tube.[90,91] Patients with prior salpingectomy are at particularly increased risk for interstitial pregnancies.

When a gestational sac is noted to be in an eccentric location, with a thin rim, under 5 mm, or no rim of surrounding myometrial tissue, an interstitial pregnancy should be considered.[80,90] An interstitial pregnancy is seen to lie outside of the endometrial canal rather than within it; often there is a bulge to the outer contour of the uterus at the site of implantation. An additional more sensitive and specific sign of interstitial pregnancy is the "interstitial line" sign. This represents the linear echogenic edge of the endometrium extending to the edge of the interstitial pregnancy (see Figure 10-29).[90]

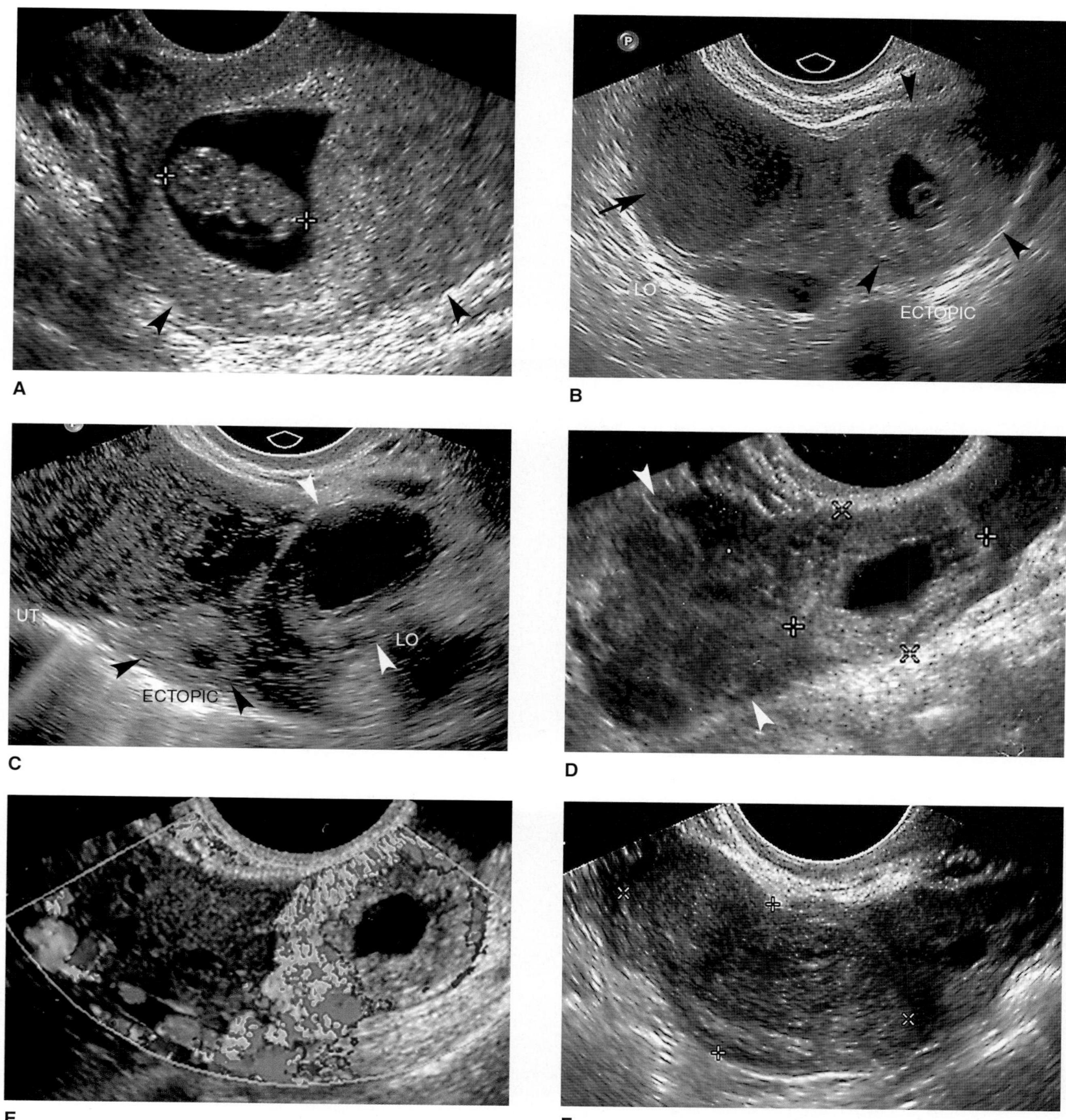

Figure 10-28 US Features of Ectopic Pregnancy Compared With a Normal Intrauterine Pregnancy
A. Transvaginal US image shows a gestational sac with an embryo (outlined by calipers) surrounded by the normal uterine wall (*arrowheads*) in this patient with 9 weeks of amenorrhea and vaginal bleeding. Demonstration of a normal IUP significantly lowers the risk of an ectopic pregnancy, especially in patients with a history of assisted fertilization. **B.** Transvaginal US image in a second patient shows a thick-rimmed cystic mass containing a yolk sack in the tissues adjacent to the left ovary (LO = left ovary). This is a live ectopic pregnancy. Note the complex cyst in the left ovary typical of a corpus luteum. **C.** Transvaginal US image in a third patient shows an ectopic gestational sac (*black arrowheads*) with a thick rim in the left adnexa, adjacent to the left ovary (*white arrowheads*) and outside of the uterus (LO = left ovary; UT = uterus). **D.** Transvaginal US image in a fourth patient demonstrates an extrauterine gestational sac (*marked by calipers*) with a surrounding hematosalpinx (*arrowheads*). **E.** Color Doppler of the same patient as in (D) shows marked vascular flow in the echogenic rim, a finding typical of the chorionic tissue surrounding the ectopic gestational sac. **F.** A solid, somewhat tubular mass (marked by calipers) representing a hematosalpinx and was the only clue to the diagnosis of an ectopic pregnancy in this patient.

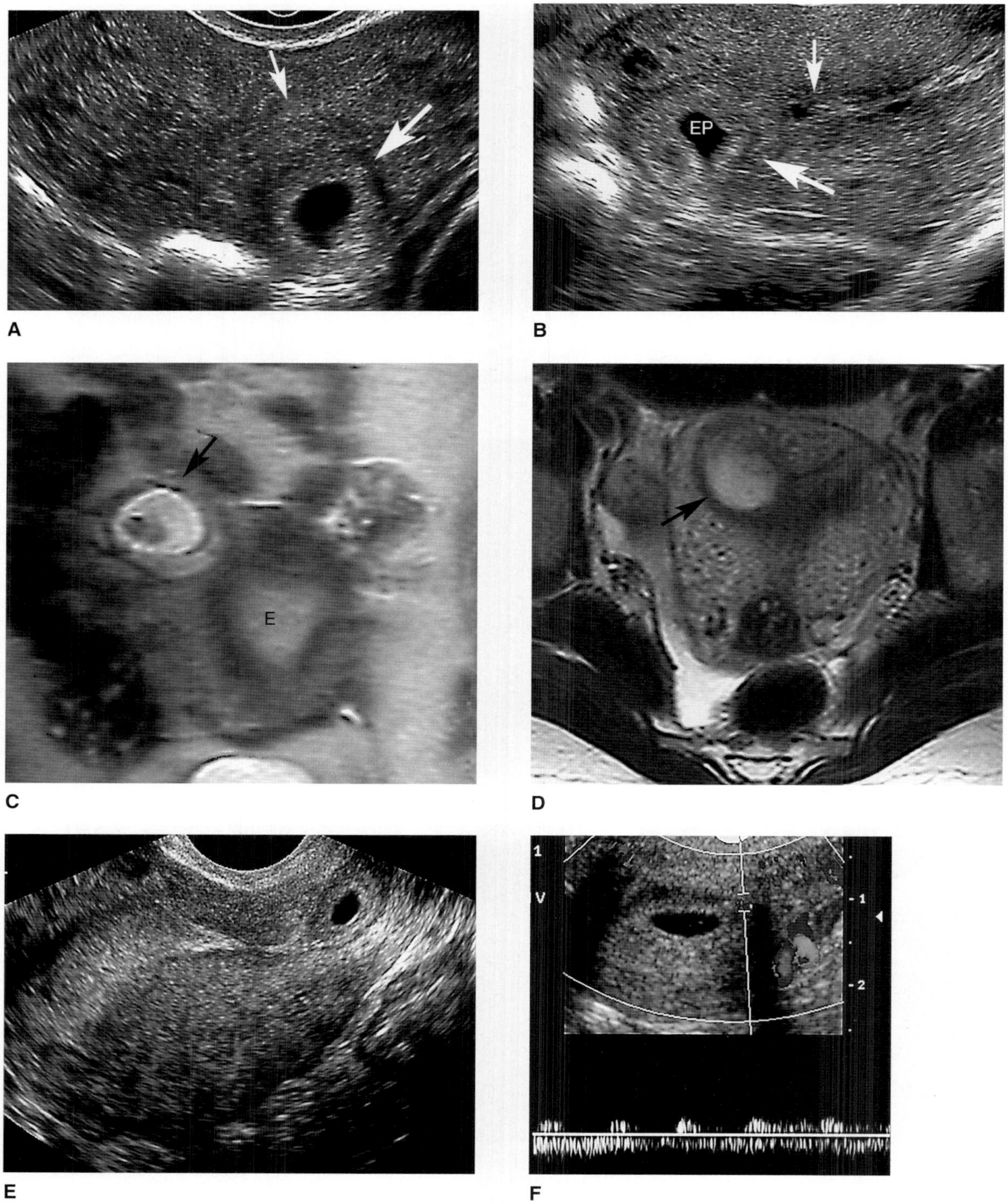

Figure 10-29 Unusual Locations for Ectopic Pregnancy

A. Transvaginal US image shows an ectopic pregnancy (*long arrow*) in the interstitial portion of the uterus, remote from the endometrium (*short arrow*). **B.** Sagittal image in a second patient shows an interstitial ectopic pregnancy just beyond the endometrial cavity (*short arrow*). A thin line representing the mucosa within the interstitial portion of the tube (*long arrow*) extends to the interstitial ectopic pregnancy. This finding is called the "interstitial line sign" (EP = ectopic pregnancy). **C.** Coronal T2-weighted MRI in a third patient shows an interstitial ectopic pregnancy (*arrow*) in the right cornual region of the uterus (E = endometrial canal). **D.** Coronal T2-weighted MRI in a fourth patient thought to have a possible interstitial pregnancy due to an eccentrically located gestational sac (not shown) shows an intrauterine pregnancy (*arrow*) in the right horn of a subseptate uterus. **E.** Transvaginal US image shows a well-formed gestational sac in the cervix. **F.** Coronal color Doppler transvaginal image of the patient in (E) shows vascular flow in the peritrophoblastic tissue surrounding the sac, a finding that favors a cervical implantation rather than gestational sac passing through the cervix in the progress of a spontaneous abortion.

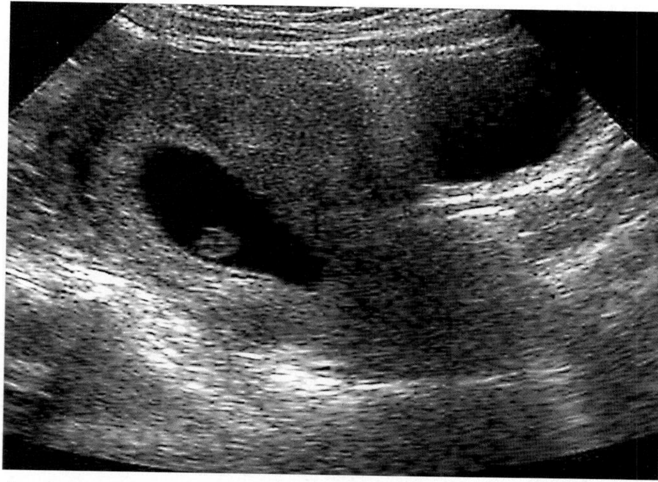
A

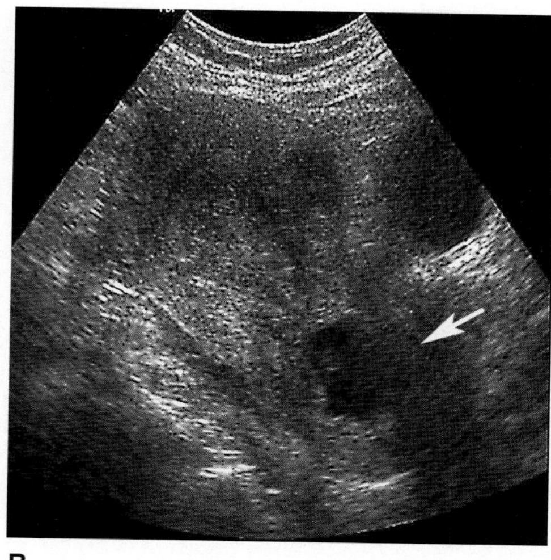
B

Figure 10-30 Spontaneous Abortion in Progress
A. Transabdominal image shows an intrauterine gestational sac in the lower portion of the endometrial canal in this patient with vaginal bleeding and pelvic pain. **B.** An image from an examination performed a few minutes later shows that the sac (*arrow*) has passed into the cervix, consistent with a spontaneous abortion in progress.

However, an eccentric location of a normal intrauterine gestational sac can also be secondary to uterine contractions, a gestation in 1 horn of a bicornuate uterus, and a myomatous uterus with distortion of the uterine canal. Three-dimensional US and MRI may be helpful in differentiating an interstitial pregnancy from an eccentric intrauterine pregnancy secondary to uterine anomalies and uterine fibroids when conventional US is indeterminate (see Figure 10-29).[92,93]

Extratubal ectopic pregnancy: Extratubal ectopic pregnancies such as cervical, ovarian, and intra-abdominal ectopic pregnancy are rare but can be life-threatening.[80,94,95] A true cervical implantation needs to be differentiated from the more common occurrence of a gestational sac passing into the cervix during a spontaneous abortion in progress. The gestational sac of a cervical ectopic pregnancy is usually round or oval, is more likely to contain a viable embryo or yolk sac, and may demonstrate peritrophoblastic flow on color Doppler exam (see Figure 10-29).[80,81] An aborting gestational sac is more likely to be irregularly shaped, to lack a viable embryo, and may slide within the endocervical canal when gentle pressure is applied with a transvaginal probe (see Figure 10-30).[80,81]

SOLID ADENEXAL MASSES

Most solid or predominantly solid adnexal masses are malignant.[4,14,38] The differential diagnosis of solid ovarian masses includes germ cell tumors, sex-cord stromal tumors, epithelial ovarian tumors other than serous and mucinous subtypes, metastatic disease to the ovary, and ovarian torsion (Table 10-5).

Solid Ovarian Neoplasms

As noted previously, primary ovarian tumors are classified based on their tissue origin as germ cell tumors, epithelial tumors, or sex cord-stromal tumors.

Solid germ cell neoplasms

The vast majority of solid germ cell tumors are malignant, but rarely a benign mature cystic teratoma can present as a solid lesion. Germ cell neoplasms account for less than 5% malignant ovarian tumors, with the majority occurring

Table 10-5. Causes of Solid Adnexal Mass

1. Solid ovarian neoplasms
a. Solid germ cell neoplasms
i. Dysgerminoma
ii. Endodermal sinus tumor (yolk sac tumor)
iii. Embryonal cell carcinoma
iv. Choriocarcinoma
v. Mixed germ cell tumor
b. Solid epithelial neoplasms
i. Endometrioid cancer
ii. Clear cell carcinoma
c. Sex-cord stromal tumors
i. Fibroma, thecoma, and fibrothecoma
ii. Granulosa cell tumors
iii. Sertoli-Leydig cell tumors
d. Metastatic disease to the ovary
2. Adnexal torsion

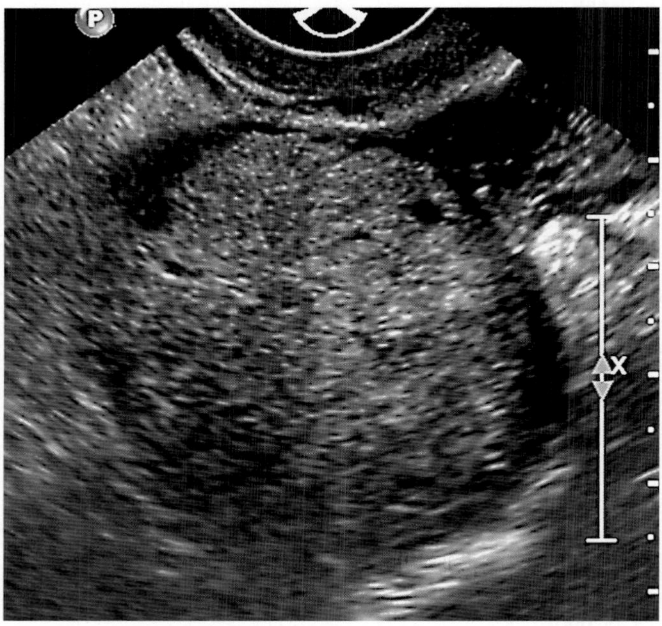

A

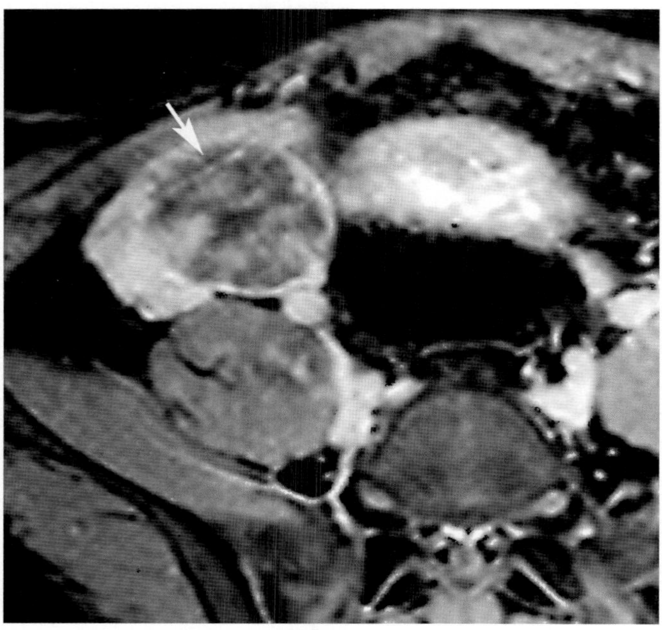

B

Figure 10-31 Dysgerminoma
A. Transvaginal US shows a 6-cm solid mass in the right ovary of this 18-year-old patient with pelvic pain. **B.** Contrast-enhanced axial fat-suppressed T1-weighted MRI shows heterogeneous enhancement within the tumor (*arrow*).

in young adults and children.[96,97] Often these lesions are discovered as a palpable mass, or because they produce pain from torsion. Dysgerminoma is the most common germ cell malignancy accounting for 1% to 2% of all ovarian cancers.[97,98] It is composed of germ cells that have not differentiated and is histologically similar to a seminoma of the testicle. About 5% of these lesions contain syncytiotrophoblastic cells and secrete hCG. Dysgerminomas typically appear as large, multilobulated solid lesions (see Figure 10-31).[30,96-98] Endodermal sinus or yolk sac tumor is the second most common malignant germ cell tumor and tends to be a rapidly growing and highly aggressive malignancy. a-Fetoprotein (AFP) levels are often elevated in these patients. The tumor is often quite large when diagnosed often and appears as a mixed cystic and solid lesion, often with ascites and peritoneal metastases.[96] Other malignant germ cell tumors include choriocarcinoma and embryonal cell carcinomas; however, it is more common for these malignancies to be present in mixed germ cell tumors, which are tumors that contain elements of more than 1 of the germ cell line, rather than in a pure form. They have a variety of appearances but are most often large, heterogeneous, predominantly solid masses when diagnosed.[96]

Solid epithelial neoplasms

Serous and mucinous epithelial neoplasms are 2 of the most common tumors of the ovary. The benign cystadenomas and cystadenocarcinomas of low malignant potential are predominantly cystic in appearance and have been discussed previously under the heading of Cystic Adnexal Masses. Malignant serous tumors range from mixed cystic and solid to entirely solid in appearance and may have punctate calcifications. Bilateral tumors occur in more than 60% of cases, and extension of the tumor to the pelvic organs or peritoneum may be evident on imaging (see Figure 10-32).[43] Endometrioid cancer can have a variable imaging appearance, including predominantly cystic with mural nodules, multiloculated cystic, and predominantly solid lesions. Bilateral involvement is seen in 30% to 50% of patients with endometrioid carcinoma, and synchronous endometrial hyperplasia or carcinoma is noted in 15% to 30% of women (see Figure 10-33).[30]

Sex-cord stromal tumors

Tumors of the connective tissues and supporting cells of the ovary are the least common neoplasms of the ovary. They account for approximately 8% of all ovarian neoplasms and occur in all age groups.[99] These are most often fibromas but also include thecomas, fibrothecomas, granulosa cell tumors, and Sertoli-Leydig cell tumors.

Fibroma, thecoma and fibrothecoma: There are 2 notable exceptions to the rule that a solid adnexal lesion is highly likely to be malignant: ovarian fibromas/thecomas and exophytic uterine leiomyomas.[4] Fibromas, thecomas, and fibrothecomas are related tumors of the ovarian stroma that are predominantly benign. The lesions are composed of fibroblasts and densely packed collagenous connective

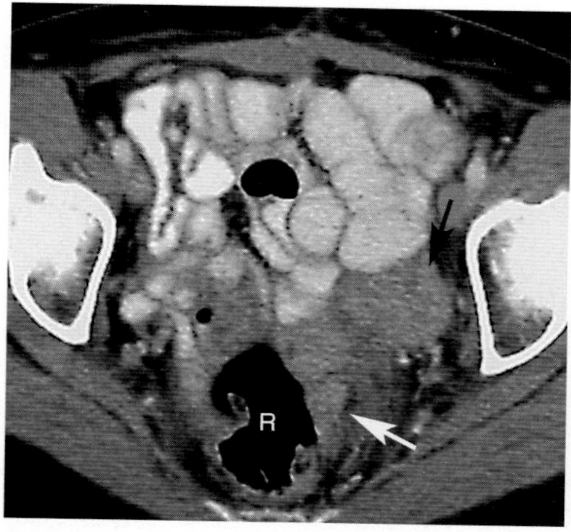

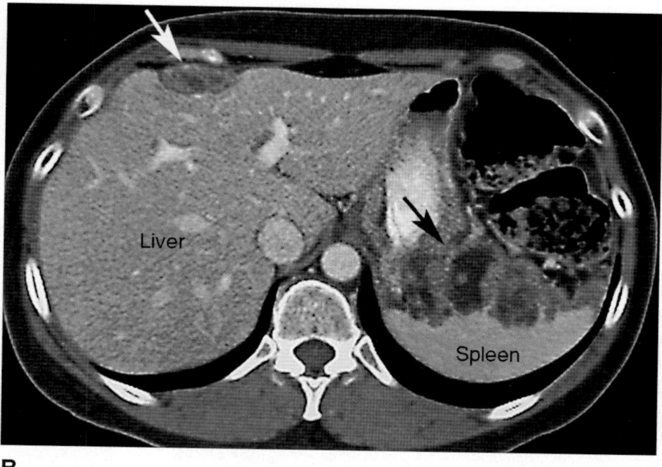

Figure 10-32 Solid Ovarian Carcinoma
A. A contrast-enhanced CT image of the pelvis shows a 4-cm solid serous ovarian carcinoma (*black arrow*) that extends to the surface of the rectum (R = rectum). **B.** Images of the upper abdomen show peritoneal implants on the surface of the liver (*white arrow*) and the spleen (*black arrow*).

tissue and have minor histologic differences but clinically behave similarly. Ultrasonographic examinations will demonstrate a round or oval mass with uniform internal echoes (see Figure 10-34).[4,100] The density of the connective tissue in these tumors is so great that it often causes complete attenuation of the sound beam, a feature not typical of other solid ovarian masses.[4,100] On MRI, these lesions will have dark signal on both T1- and T2-weighted images, a typical appearance of fibrous tissues anywhere, and weak

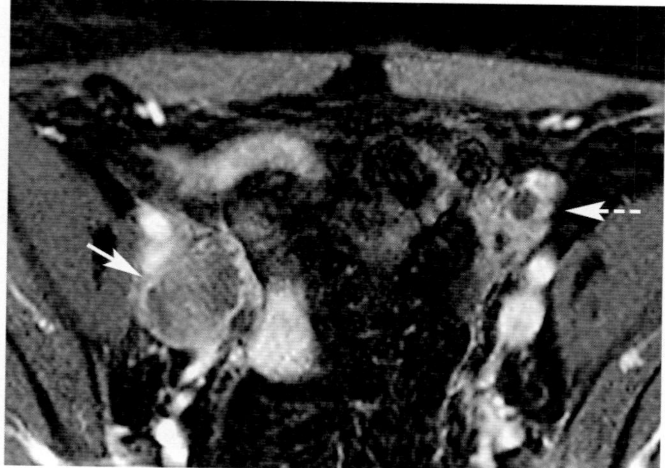

Figure 10-33 Endometrioid Carcinoma
A contrast-enhanced fat-suppressed T1-weighted image of the pelvis in a patient with known endometriosis shows an enhancing right adnexal mass (*arrow*) that proved to be an endometrioid carcinoma. Dashed arrow indicates the left ovary.

enhancement, because of the minimal blood flow in these tumors (see Figure 10-34).[101] The major differential diagnosis for an ovarian fibroma is an exophytic subserosal myoma of the uterus. Identification of a uterine bridge of tissue connecting the lesion to either the uterus or the adjacent normal ipsilateral ovary helps to distinguish a pedunculated myoma from a solid ovarian mass (see Figure 10-35).[4,102] On MRI, identification of vascular flow voids between the lesion and the adjacent myometrium, indicating that the blood flow to the mass originates in the uterus, is a clue that the mass represents a uterine fibroid and not an ovarian fibroma. However, this feature is only reliably present on large masses, particularly those larger than 7 cm.[102]

Granulosa cell tumors: Granulosa cell tumors account for 1% to 2% of all ovarian neoplasms and is the most common estrogen-secreting tumor. Most tumors follow a benign course but about 10% behave as s low-grade malignancy.[30,103] The adult type accounts for 95% of all granulosa cell tumors and occurs predominantly in perimenopausal and postmenopausal women. The estrogenic effects of the lesion may cause vaginal bleeding from endometrial hyperplasia, polyps, or carcinoma. Imaging findings vary

---

Imaging Notes 10-12. Exophytic Myoma Mimicking an Ovarian Mass

> Most solid ovarian masses are malignant in nature. However, a solid exophytic myoma may simulate a solid ovarian mass in cases in which the normal ipsilateral ovary is not visualized.

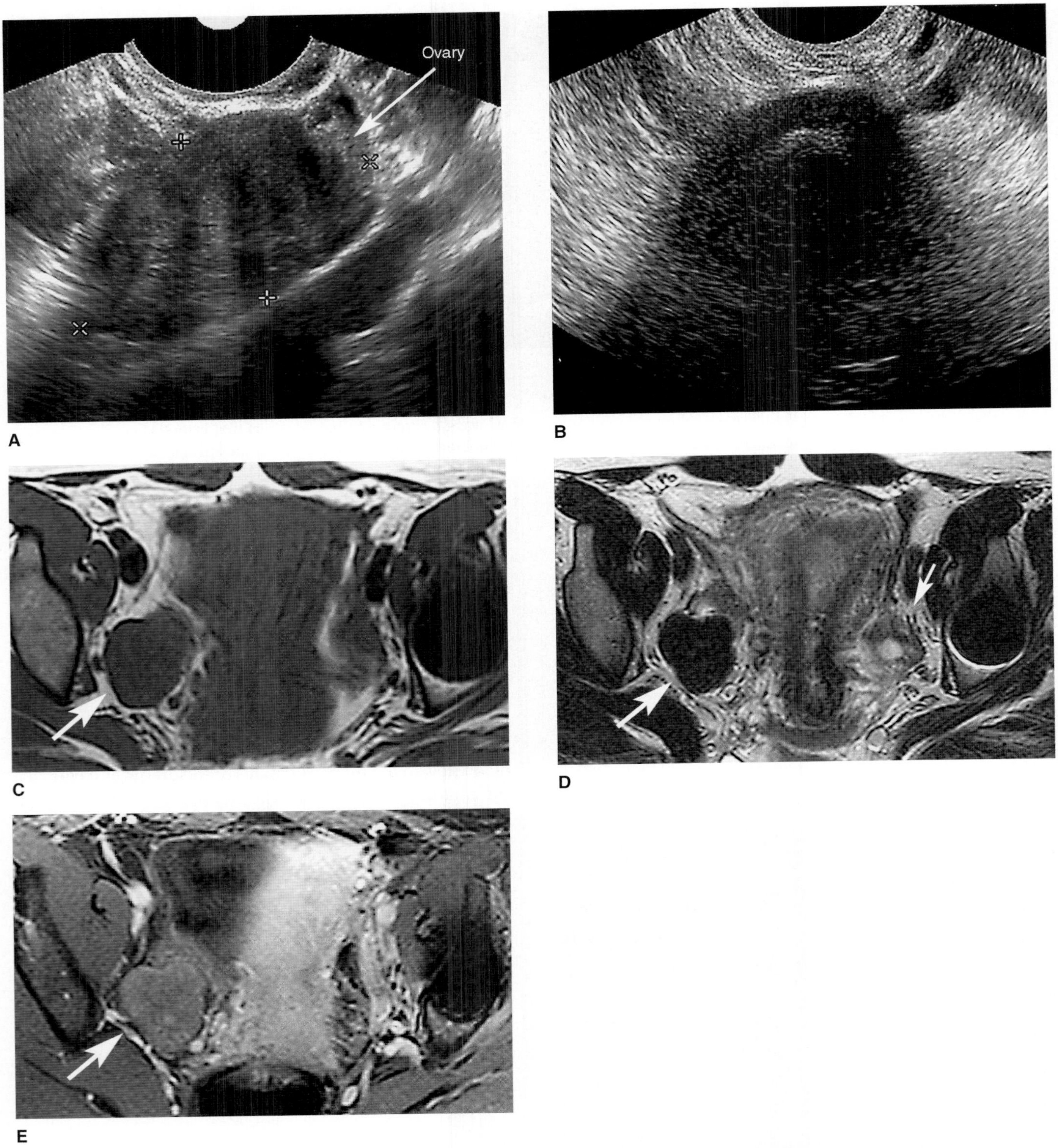

A

B

C

D

E

Figure 10-34 Ovarian Fibroma in 3 Patients
A. Transvaginal US shows a 6-cm solid homogeneous mass arising from the left ovary. This is a typical US appearance of an ovarian fibroma. **B.** Transvaginal US image, in a second patient shows complete drop out of sound in the expected location of the right ovary. Some fibromas can be so dense that they absorb all of the sound and create shadowing deep to the mass. **C.** Axial T1-weighted, (**D**) axial T2-weighted, and (**E**) axial T1 postgadolinium images in a third patient shows a solid, homogeneously low-signal-intensity right ovarian mass (*large arrow*), which has well-defined, lobulated borders and shows relatively homogeneous enhancement following the administration of gadolinium. These findings are typical of ovarian fibromas. Compare the fibromas with the normal left ovary (*small arrow*) in (D).

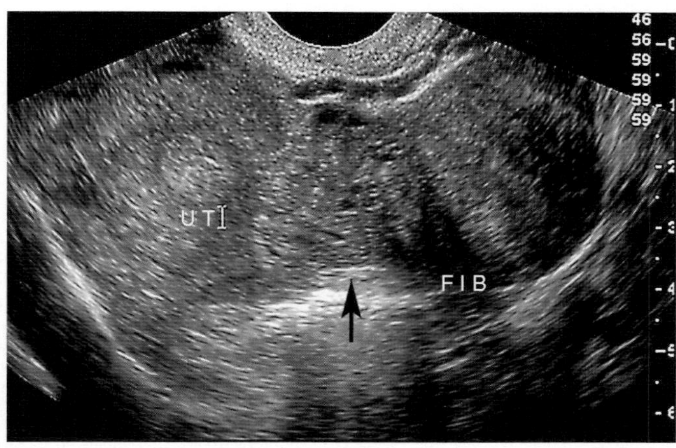

A

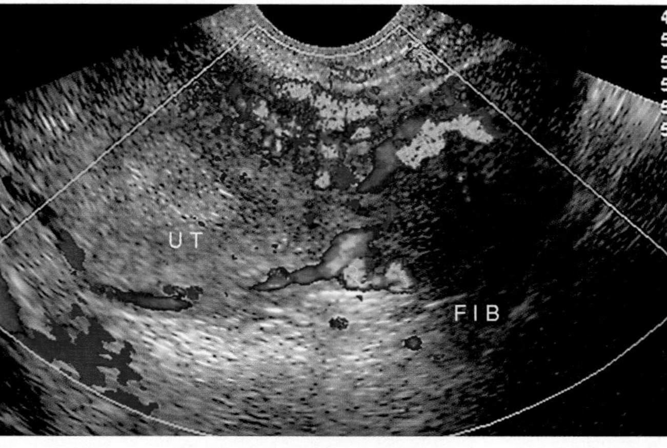

B

Figure 10-35 Pedunculated Fibroid Mimicking an Ovarian Fibroma
A. Coronal transvaginal US shows a bridge of connecting myometrial tissue (*black arrow*) between the uterus and a solid left adnexal mass (UT = uterus; FIB = fibroid). Identification of this connection allows a diagnosis of an exophytic fibroid and differentiation from other solid adnexal masses. **B.** Color Doppler image shows uterine vessels extending from the body of the uterus to the exophytic fibroid.

from solid lesions with various degrees of hemorrhage and fibrotic change, to multilocular masses to predominantly cystic tumors.

Sertoli-leydig cell tumors: Sertoli-Leydig cell tumors occur in young women and are considered a low-grade malignancy. These tumors account for 0.5% of all tumors and are the most common virilizing tumor. They are typically well-defined, enhancing solid lesions with intratumoral cysts.[30,99]

Metastatic disease to the ovary

The ovaries are the most common site of metastatic tumors in the female genital tract. Approximately 15% of all ovarian malignant tumors are metastatic, and most commonly are noted in patients with gastrointestinal tract malignancies, breast carcinoma, melanoma, and widely disseminated lymphoma.[4,30,104,105] The metastases show a wide range of imaging appearances, ranging from complex cystic lesions to solid lesions. Some clues to the diagnosis include the presence of bilateral lesions in 60% to 80% of patients and the retention of sharp margins and the oval shape of the ovary.[104] Metastatic disease should be strongly considered when bilateral solid ovarian masses are noted and may be the initial presentation of an extraovarian primary malignancy (see Figure 10-36).[105]

Adnexal Torsion

Adnexal torsion is caused by complete or partial rotation of the adnexa along its vascular pedicle, resulting in varying degrees of arterial, venous, and/or lymphatic obstruction. Most commonly, both the ovary and the fallopian tube are torsed; less commonly, just the ovary or fallopian tube is torsed.[106,107] Patients present with acute onset of severe pelvic pain localizing to the affected adnexa, often with anorexia, nausea, and vomiting. Less commonly, the pain may be intermittent, reflecting intermittent episodes of incomplete torsion. Early diagnosis and surgical intervention may make it possible to untwist the pedicle and conserve the normal ovarian parenchyma; adnexectomy is necessary if the ovary has been infarcted.[108]

Adnexal torsion occurs predominantly in the first 3 decades of life. Predisposing factors, such as an ipsilateral functional cyst or neoplasm, can be found in 50% to 81% of cases.[106,107] The most common tumor associated with ovarian torsion is a mature cystic teratoma (dermoid cyst) accounting for between 3.5% and 16.1% of all cases.[106] Other risk factors include the gravid state, ovarian hyperstimulation due to infertility treatment, and heavy lifting. Risk factors for tubal torsion include preexisting hydrosalpinx, prior tubal ligation, and paratubal cysts or neoplasm.[67,73]

The spectrum of radiographic findings of adnexal torsion reflects the degree and duration of vascular compromise to the adnexa and the presence or absence of an underlying lesion. In cases of incomplete torsion, an entity known as massive ovarian edema may develop.[108] The ovary becomes enlarged, often more than 10 times its normal volume and may have multiple small, peripheral fluid-filled spaces representing transudation of fluid into subcortical follicles (see Figure 10-37). If there has been a sufficient period of ischemia, the ovary may have complex cystic regions or a more solid appearance,

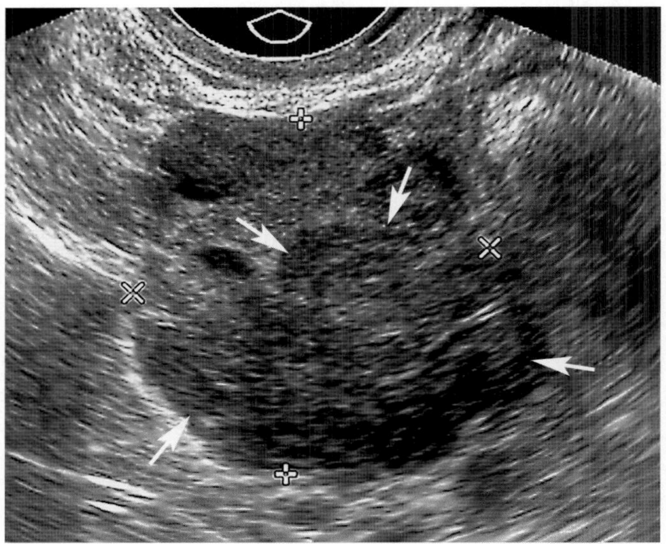

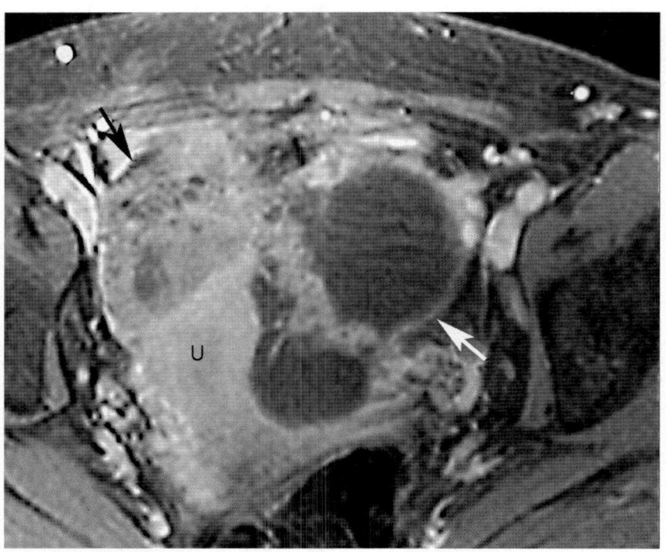

Figure 10-36 Ovarian Metastases
A. Transvaginal US shows a solid lesion (*arrows*) infiltrating into the inferior aspect of the left ovary (outlined by calipers) indicating ovarian involvement of lymphoma in this 21-year-old woman. **B.** Axial T1-weighted fat-suppressed MRI shows bilateral ovarian metastases in this 62-year-old women with colon carcinoma. The right ovarian metastasis (*black arrow*) is more solid in appearance, whereas the left ovarian metastasis is mixed cystic and solid. Note that both lesions are sharply marginated and the oval shape of the ovaries is relatively well preserved (U = uterus).

secondary to ischemic necrosis and internal hemorrhage (see Figure 10-37).[108,109]

Most torsed ovaries demonstrate abnormal flow patterns on color Doppler US. However, variation in the completeness of the obstruction of the vascular supply has led to a variety of reported flow patterns in cases of adnexal torsion, including several reports of normal flow in affected ovaries.[108,109] The abnormally twisted vascular pedicle, known as the "whirlpool sign," can be identified by US in up to 88% of cases (see Figure 10-37).[110,111] An atypical location of the torsed ovary, above the fundus of the uterus or crossing the midline to lie close to the contralateral ovary, are important ancillary findings. Often simple or complex cul-de-sac fluid is noted.

In general, CT and MRI are superior to US at identifying the general configuration of the twisted adnexal structures and in the detection of hemorrhagic infarction of the ovary and/or tube.[88,91-94] On CT scans, infiltration of the periadnexal fat, deviation of the uterus to the involved side, and misplacement of the torsed adnexa in the pelvis to the contralateral side or to the midline is noted in 40% of patients (see Figure 10-37).[112] If there has been ischemic necrosis, CT will demonstrate hemorrhage into the ovary or tube as high attenuation exceeding 50 HU on noncontrast scans. On MRI examinations, high signal on fat-suppressed T1-weighted images suggests hemorrhage or vascular congestion. The most specific CT and MRI findings of adnexal torsion are identification of the twisted vascular pedicle and wall thickening of the fallopian tube secondary to congestion and edema, a finding noted in 84% of cases (see Figure 10-37).[112-114] In cases of torsion secondary to an underlying cystic lesion of the ovary, smooth wall thickening of the lesion is noted in 75% of patients. When eccentric wall thickening of greater than 10 mm is present, hemorrhagic infarction or underlying malignancy should be suspected.[113]

Imaging Notes 10-13. Ovarian Torsion

On sonography, ovarian torsion is best diagnosed by observing the grayscale features of ovarian enlargement and edema, abnormal position of the ovary, and twisting of the vascular pedicle rather than by assessing the presence or absence of intraovarian blood flow.

Fallopian Tube Carcinoma

Primary fallopian tube cancers are extremely rare, accounting for 0.3% to 1.1% of all gynecologic malignancies, and typically occur in postmenopausal patients.[115-117] Patients will typically present with vaginal bleeding, pelvic pain, and watery vaginal discharge. The tumor will most commonly have serous adenocarcinoma histology but can also have endometrioid or transitional cell carcinoma histology.

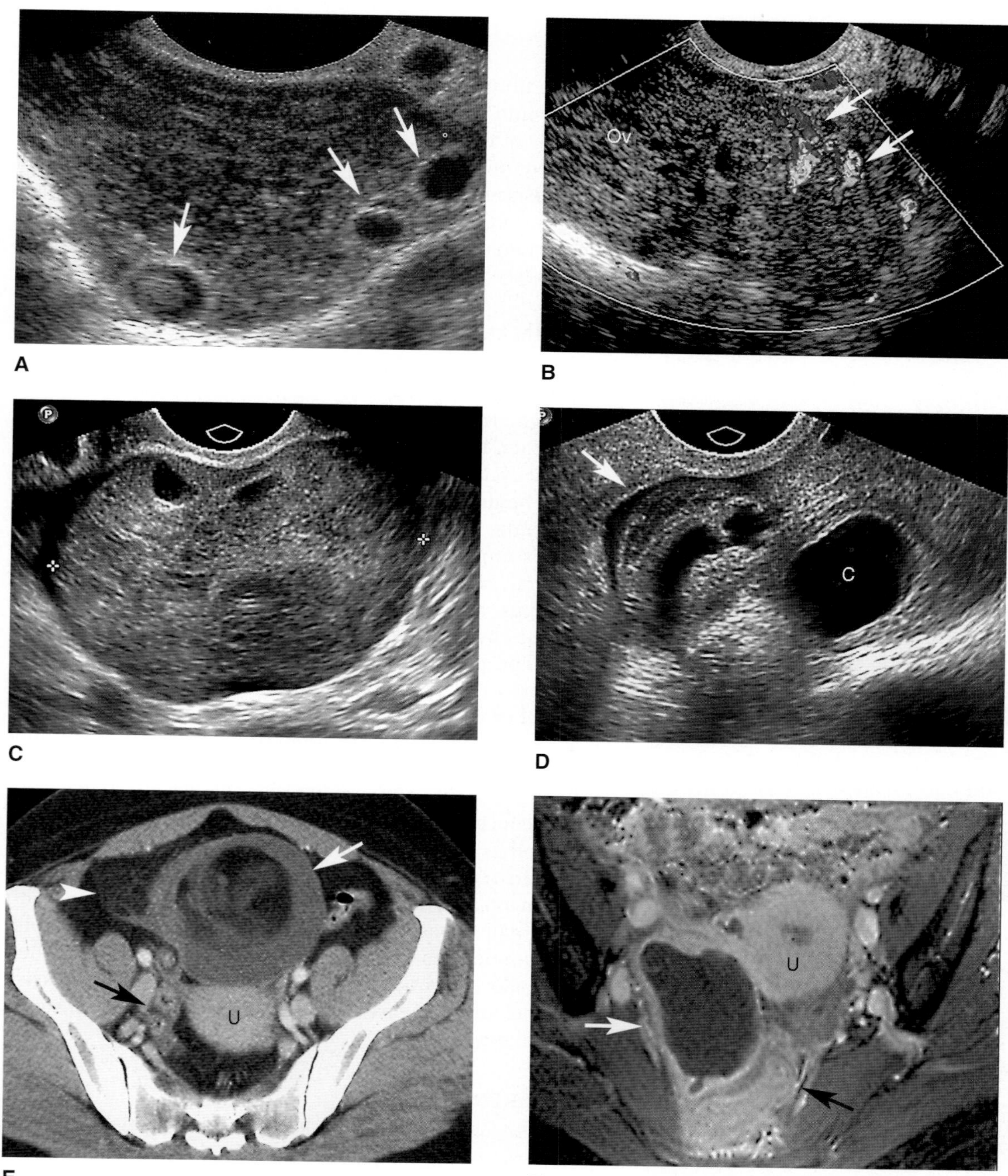

Figure 10-37 Imaging Features of Ovarian Torsion in 5 Patients
A. Transvaginal US shows a markedly enlarged ovary, more than 10 times its normal size, with prominent peripheral cystic spaces (*arrows*) in this patient with adnexal torsion. This represents extensive edema due to the torsion. **B.** Color Doppler coronal transvaginal image of the left adnexa in a second patient shows twisting of the vessels of the left mesosalpinx (*arrows*) adjacent to an edematous left ovary (Ov = ovary). This is known as the "whirlpool sign" and is a finding diagnostic of ovarian torsion. **C.** Transvaginal US in a third patient shows a markedly enlarged heterogeneous ovary secondary to ischemia from torsion. **D.** A coronal image in the same patient as in (C) shows the edematous and ischemic fallopian tube (*arrow*) surrounded by a small amount of free fluid. A cystic space is seen in the periphery of the ovary that represents a region of cystic degeneration or underlying physiologic cyst within the ovary (C = cystic space). **E.** Contrast-enhanced axial CT image in a fourth patient shows a right mature cystic teratoma (*white arrow*) that has torsed and is located in the midline of the pelvis anterior to the uterine fundus. The lesion shows high attenuation and smooth wall thickening due to hemorrhage. There is stranding of the mesentery (*arrowhead*) and the twisted vessels of the right mesosalpinx are visible (*black arrow*) (U = uterus). **F.** A gadolinium-enhanced T1-weighted fat-suppressed image in a fifth patient shows a right ovary (*white arrow*) that has undergone ischemic infarction because of adnexal torsion. Only the thin rim of ovarian parenchyma enhances. The torsed and edematous mesosalpinx (*black arrow*) is seen below the right ovary. This patient also had a hematosalpinx, which is shown in Figure 10-26 (U = uterus).

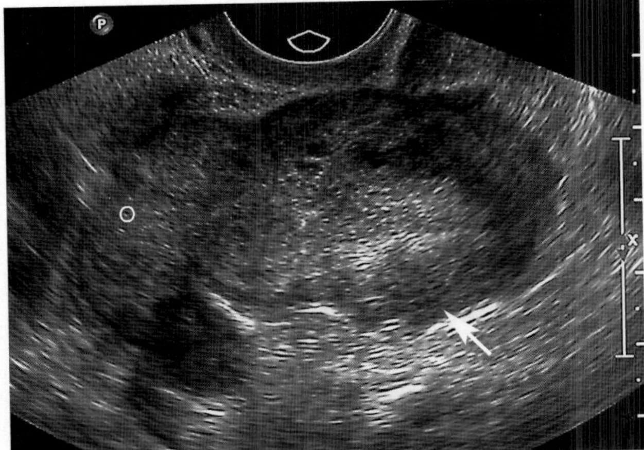

A

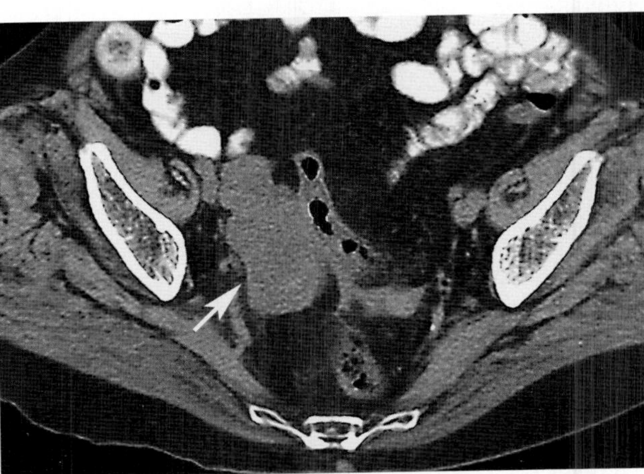

B

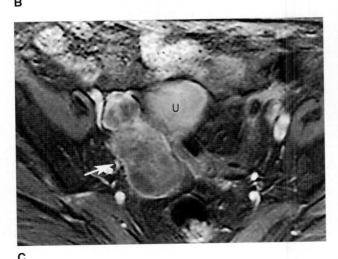

C

Figure 10-38 Fallopian Tube Carcinoma
A. Transvaginal US image in this 67-year-old patient with pelvic pain showed a solid, somewhat tubular mass (*arrow*) adjacent to the right ovary, suggesting a primary fallopian tube tumor (O = ovary). **B.** Image from a non–contrast-enhanced CT shows the mass (*white arrow*). **C.** Axial T1-weighted fat-suppressed MRI shows heterogeneous enhancement of the tumor (U = uterus). Surgical excision was diagnostic of a carcinoma of the fallopian tube.

Most tumors arise in the ampullary portion of the tube, grow into the lumen, and occlude the more proximal segments of the tube. In most cases, the tumor will appear as a predominantly solid mass, with small regions of cystic necrosis and hemorrhage. However, because tubal dilation is also present, the imaging appearance of fallopian tube carcinoma is of a complex mixed cystic and solid adnexal mass (see Figure 10-38).[73,74,115-117]

SUMMARY

Adnexal lesions are commonly seen on pelvic imaging, and fortunately the vast majority of these lesions are benign. Many are physiologic ovarian cysts developing and then regressing during the course of 1 or a few menstrual cycles. Several complex cystic ovarian lesions, such as a hemorrhagic cyst, endometrioma, or mature cystic teratoma, will have a typical US appearance that allows a presumptive diagnosis with a high level of accuracy. In general, MRI can be used to investigate indeterminate US findings, adding specificity for the diagnosis of endometriomas by demonstrating signal intensity consistent with blood products of varying ages and intralesional fat within mature cystic teratomas. Identification of the normal ipsilateral ovary is an important key to the diagnosis of cystic adnexal lesions that are nonovarian in origin, including dilated fallopian tubes, paraovarian cysts, and peritoneal inclusion cysts. Although imaging features of benign cystic neoplasms overlap with low-grade ovarian carcinoma and other nonneoplastic lesions, the ability of imaging to demonstrate the absence of features seen in most aggressive neoplasms may allow the patient to be managed with minimally invasive surgery when the lesion persists. Solid ovarian lesions are usually malignant; however, when MRI allows characterization of a lesion as a nonaggressive fibrous tumor, the patient may be a candidate for conservative management.

REFERENCES

1. Saksouk FA, Johnson SA. Recognition of the ovaries and ovarian origin of pelvic masses with CT. *Radiographics.* 2004;24:S133-S146.
2. Ritchie WGM. Sonographic evaluation of normal and induced ovulation. *Radiology.* 1986;161:1-10.
3. Cohen HL, Tice HM, Mandel FS. Ovarian volumes measured by US: bigger than we think. *Radiology.* 1990;177:189-192.
4. Brown DL. A practical approach to the ultrasound characterization of adnexal masses. *Ultrasound Q.* 2007;23: 87-105.
5. Pretorius ES, Outwater EK, Hunt JL, Siegelman ES. Magnetic resonance imaging of the ovary. *Topics Magn Reson Imaging.* 2001;21:131-146.
6. Tamai K, Koyama T, Saga T, et al. MR features of physiologic and benign conditions of the ovary. *Eur Radiol.* 2006;16:2700-2711.
7. Kim M, Rha SE, Oh SN, et al. MR imaging findings of hydrosalpinx: a comprehensive review. *Radiographics.* 2009;29:495-507.

8. Potter AW, Chandrasekhar CA. US and CT evaluation of acute pelvic pain of gynecologic origin in non-pregnant pre-menopausal patients. *Radiographics.* 2008;28:1645-1659.
9. Bennett GL, Slywotzky CM, Giovanna G. Gynecologic causes of acute pelvic pain: spectrum of CT findings. *Radiographics.* 2002;22:785-801.
10. Levine D, Brown DL, Andreotti RF et al. Management of asymptomatic ovarian and other adnexal cysts imaged at US: Society of Radiologists in Ultrasound Consensus Conference Statement. *Radiology.* 2010;256:943-954.
11. Timor-Tritsch IE, Goldstein SR. The complexity of a "complex mass" and the simplicity of a "simple cyst." *J Ultrasound Med.* 2005;24:255-258.
12. Baerwald AR, Adams GP, Pierson RA. Form and function of the corpus luteum during the human menstrual cycle. *Ultrasound Obstet Gynecol.* 2005;25:498-507.
13. Swire MN, Castro-Aragon L, Levine D. Various sonographic appearances of the hemorrhagic corpus luteum. *Ultrasound Q.* 2004;20:45-58.
14. Imaoka I, Wada A, Kaji Y, et al. Developing an MR imaging strategy for diagnosis of ovarian masses. *Radiographics.* 2006;26:1431-1448.
15. Borders RJ, Breiman RS, Yeh BM, Qayyum A, Coakley FV. Computed tomography of corpus luteal cysts. *J Comput Assist Tomogr.* 2004;28:340-342.
16. Patel MD, Felstein VA, Filly RA. The likelihood ratio of sonographic findings for the diagnosis of hemorrhagic ovarian cysts. *J Ultrasound Med.* 2005;24:607-614.
17. Jain KA. Sonographic spectrum of hemorrhagic ovarian cysts. *J Ultrasound Med.* 2002;21:879-886.
18. Levine D, Gosink BB, Wolf SI, Feldesman MR, Pretorius DH. Simple adnexal cysts: the natural history in postmenopausal women. *Radiology* 1991;184:653-659.
19. Conway C, Zalud I, Dilena M, et al. Simple cyst in the postmenopausal patient: detection and management. *J Ultrasound Med.* 1998;17:369-372.
20. McDonald JM, Modesitt SC. The incidental postmenopausal adnexal mass. *Clin Obstet Gynecol.* 2006;49:506-516.
21. Ekerhovd E, Wienerroith H, Staudach A, Granberg S. Preoperative assessment of unilocular adnexal cysts by transvaginal ultrasonography: a comparison between ultrasonographic morphologic imaging and histopathologic diagnosis. *Am J Obstet Gynecol.* 2001;184:48-54.
22. Modesitt SC, Pavlik EJ, Ueland FR, et al. Risk of malignancy in unilocular ovarian cystic tumor less than 10 centimeters in diameter. *Obstet Gynecol.* 2003;102:594-599.
23. Ehrmann DA. Polycystic ovary syndrome. *N Engl J Med.* 2005;352:1223-1237.
24. Balen A, Laven JSE, Tan S, Dewailly D. Ultrasound assessment of the polycystic ovary: international consensus definitions. *Hum Reprod Update.* 2003;9:505-514.
25. Battaglia C, Regnani G, Primvera M, Salvatori M, Volpe A. Polycystic ovary syndrome: it is always bilateral? *Ultrasound Obstet Gynecol.* 1999;14:183-187.
26. Haimvov-Kochman R, Yanai N, Yagel S, Amsalem H, Lavy Y, Hurwitz A. Spontaneous ovarian hyperstimulation syndrome and hyperreactio luteinalis are entities in a continuum. *Ultrasound Obstet Gynecol.* 2004;24:L675-L678.
27. Chiang G, Levine D. Imaging of adnexal masses in pregnancy. *J Ultrasound Med.* 2004;23:805-819.
28. Bromley B, Benacerraf B. Adnexal masses during pregnancy: accuracy of sonographic diagnosis and outcome. *J Ultrasound Med.* 1997;16:447-452.
29. Koonings PP, Campbell K, Mishell DR Jr, Grimes DA. Relative frequency of primary ovarian neoplasms: a 10-year review. *Obstet Gynecol.* 1989;74:921-926.
30. Jung SE, Lee JM, Rha SE, Byun JY, Jung JI, Hahn ST. CT and MR imaging of ovarian tumors with emphasis on differential diagnosis. *Radiographics.* 2002;22:1305-1325.
31. Jeong YY, Outwater EK, Kang HK. Imaging evaluation of ovarian masses. *Radiographics.* 20:1445-1470, 2000.
32. Ghossain MA, Buy JN, Ligneres C, et al. Epithelial tumors of the ovary: comparison of MR and CT findings. *Radiology.* 1991;181:863-870.
33. Outwater EK, Siegelman ES, Hunt JL. Ovarian teratomas: tumor types and imaging characteristics. *Radiographics.* 2001;21:475-490.
34. Patel MD, Feldstein VA, Lipson SD, et al. Cystic teratomas of the ovary: diagnostic value of sonography. *AJR Am J Roentgenol.* 1998;171:1061-1065.
35. Mais V, Guerriero S, Ajossa S, Angiolucci M, Paoletti AM, Melis GB. Transvaginal ultrasonography in the diagnosis of cystic teratoma. *Obstet Gynecol.* 1995;85:48-52.
36. Rathod K, Kale H, Narlawar R, et al. Unusual "floating balls" appearance of an ovarian cystic teratoma: sonographic and CT findings. *J Clin Ultrasound.* 2001;29:41-43.
37. Kim HC, Kim SH, Lee HJ, et al. Fluid-fluid levels in ovarian teratomas. *Abdom Imaging.* 2002;27:100-105.
38. Brown DL, Doubilet PM, Miller FH, et al. Benign and malignant ovarian masses: selection of the most discriminating gray-scale and Doppler sonographic features. *Radiology.* 1998;208:103-110.
39. Jermy K, Luis C, Bourne T. The characterization of common ovarian cysts in premenopausal women. *Ultrasound Obstet Gynecol.* 2001;17:140-144.
40. Buy JN, Ghossain MA, Moss AA, et al. Cystic teratoma of the ovary: CT detection. *Radiology.* 1989;171:697-701.
41. Kido A, Tohashi K, Konishi I, et al. Dermoid cysts of the ovary with malignant transformation: MR appearance. *AJR Am J Roentgenol.* 1999;172:445-449.
42. Yamaoka T, Toagashi K, Koyama T, et al. Immature teratoma of the ovary: correlation of MR imaging and pathologic findings. *Eur Radiol.* 2003;13:313-319.
43. Buy JN, Ghossain MA, Sciot C, et al. Epithelial tumors of the ovary: CT findings and correlation with US. *Radiology.* 1991;178:811-818.
44. Pasqual MA, Tresserra F, Grases PJ, Labastida R, Dexeus S. Borderline cystic tumors of the ovary: gray-scale and color Doppler findings. *J Clin Ultrasound.* 2002;30:76-82.
45. Outwater EK, Huang AB, Dunton CJ, Talerman A, Capuzzi DM. Papillary projections in ovarian neoplasms: appearance on MRI. *J Magn Reson Imaging.* 1997;7:689-695.
46. Wagner BJ, Buck JL, Seidman JD, McCabe KM. Ovarian epithelial neoplasms: radiologic-pathologic correlation. *Radiographics.* 1994;14:1351-1374.
47. Kurtz AB, Tsimikas JV, Tempany CM, et al. Diagnosis and staging or ovarian cancer: comparative values of Doppler and conventional US, CT and MR imaging correlate with

surgery and histopathologic analysis—report of the Radiology Diagnostic Oncology Group. *Radiology.* 1999;212:19-27.

48. Tanaka YO, Yoshizako T, Nishida M, Yamaguchi M, Sugimura K, Itai Y. Ovarian carcinoma in patients with endometriosis. MR imaging findings. *AJR Am J Roentgenol.* 2000;175: 1423-1430.
49. Matsuoka Y, Ohtomo k, Araki T, Kojima K, Yoshikawa W, Fuwa S. MR imaging of clear cell carcinoma of the ovary. *Eur Radiol.* 2001;11:946-951.
50. Guerriero S, Ajossa S, Garau N, et al. Ultrasonography and color Doppler-based triage for adnexal masses to provide the most appropriate surgical approach. *Am J Obstet Gynecol.* 2005;192:402-406.
51. Timmerman D, Schwarzler P, Collins WP, et al. Subjective assessment of adnexal masses with the use of ultrasonography: an analysis of interobserver variability and experience. *Ultrasound Obstet Gynecol.* 1999:13:11-16.
52. Hricak H, Chen M, Coakley FV, et al. Complex adnexal masses: detection and characterization with MR imaging—multivariate analysis. *Radiology.* 2000;214:39-46.
53. Canis M, Botchorshvilli R, Manhes H, et al. Management of adnexal masses. *Semin Surg Oncol.* 2000;19:28-35.
54. Hillaby K, Aslam N, Salim R, et al. The value of the detection of normal ovarian tissue ("the ovarian crescent sign") in the differential diagnosis of adnexal masses. *Ultrasound Obstet Gynecol.* 2004;23:63-67.
55. Kim JS, Woo SK, Suh SJ, et al. Sonographic diagnosis of paraovarian cysts: value of detecting a separate ipsilateral ovary. *AJR Am J Roentgenol.* 1995;164:1441-1444.
56. Woodward PJ, Sohaey R, Mezzetti TP. Endometriosis: radiographic-pathologic correlation. *Radiographics.* 2001;21:193-216.
57. Patel MD, Feldstein VA, Chen DC, Lipson SD, Filly RA. Endometriomas: diagnostic performance of US. *Radiology.* 1999;210:739-745.
58. Bhatt S, Kocakoc E, Dogra VS. Endometriosis: sonographic spectrum. *Ultrasound Q.* 2006;22:273-280.
59. Moore J, Copley S, Morris J, Lindsell D, Golding S, Kennedy S. A systematic review of the accuracy of ultrasound in the diagnosis of endometriosis. *Ultrasound Obstet Gynecol.* 2002;20:630-634.
60. Outwater E, Schiebler M, Owen RS, Schnall MD. Characterization of hemorrhagic adnexal lesions with MR imaging: blinded reader study. *Radiology.* 1993;186:489-494.
61. Gougoutas CA, Siegelman ES, Hunt J. Pelvic endometriosis: various manifestations and MR imaging findings. *AJR Am J Roentgenol.* 2000;175:353-358.
62. Togashi K, Nishimura K, Kimura I, et al. Endometrial cysts: diagnosis with MR imaging. *Radiology.* 1991;180:73-78.
63. Barloon TJ, Brown BP, Abu-Yousef MM, Warnock NG. Paraovarian and paratubal cysts: preoperative diagnosis using transabdominal and transvaginal sonography. *J Clin Ultrasound.* 1996;24:117-122.
64. Savelli L, Ghi T, De Iaco P, et al. Paraovarian/paratubal cysts: comparison of transvaginal sonographic and pathological findings to establish diagnostic criteria. *Ultrasound Obstet Gynecol.* 2006;28:330-334.
65. Athey PA, Cooper NB. Sonographic features of parovarian cysts. *AJR Am J Roentgenol.* 1985;144:83-86.
66. Kishimototo K, Ito K, Awaya H, Matsunaga N, Outwater EK, Siegelman ES. Paraovarian cyst: MR imaging features. *Abdom Imaging.* 2002;27:685-689.
67. Alpern MB, Sandler MA, Madrazo BL. Sonographic features of parovarian cysts and their complications. *AJR Am J Roentgenol.* 1984;143:157-160.
68. Korbin CD, Brown DL, Welch WR. Paraovarian cystadenomas and cystadenofibromas: sonographic characteristics in 14 cases. *Radiology.* 1998;208:459-462.
69. Sohaey R, Gardner T, Woodward PJ, Peterson CM. Sonographic diagnosis of peritoneal inclusion cysts. *J Ultrasound Med.* 1995;14:913-917.
70. Kim JS, Lee HJ, Woo S, Lee TS. Peritoneal inclusions cysts and their relationship to the ovaries: evaluation with sonography. *Radiology.* 1997;204:481-484.
71. Guerriero S, Ajossa S, Mais V, et al. Role of transvaginal sonography in the diagnosis of peritoneal inclusion cysts. *J Ultrasound Med.* 2004;23:1193-1200.
72. Kurachi H, Murakami T, Nakamura H, et al. Imaging of peritoneal pseudocysts; value of MR imaging compared with sonography and CT. *AJR Am J Roentgenol.* 1993;161:589-591.
73. Rowling SE, Ramchandani P. Imaging of the fallopian tube. *Semin Roentgen.* 1996;31:299-311.
74. Benjaminov O, Atri M. Sonography of the abnormal fallopian tube. *AJR Am J Roentgenol.* 2004;183:737-742.
75. Patel MD, Acord DL, Young SW. Likelihood ratio of sonographic findings in discriminating hydrosalpinx from other adnexal masses. *AJR Am J Roentgenol.* 2006;186: 1033-1038.
76. Outwater EK, Siegelman ES, Chiowanich P. Dilated fallopian tubes: MR imaging characteristics. *Radiology.* 1998;208: 463-469.
77. Horrow MM. Ultrasound of pelvic inflammatory disease. *Ultrasound Q.* 2004;20(4):171-179.
78. Timor-Tritsch IE, Lerner JP, Monteagudo KE, Heller DS. Transvaginal sonographic markers of tubal inflammatory disease. *Ultrasound Obstet Gynecol.* 1998;12:56-66.
79. Sam JW, Jacobs JE, Birnbaum BA. Spectrum of CT findings in acute pyogenic pelvic inflammatory disease. *Radiographics.* 2002;22:1327-1334.
80. Levine D. Ectopic pregnancy. *Radiology.* 2007;245:385-397.
81. Dogra V, Paspulati RM, Bhatt S. First trimester bleeding evaluation. *Ultrasound Q.* 2005;21:69-85.
82. Ankum WM, Mol BW, Van de Veen F, Bossuyt PM. Risk factors for ectopic pregnancy: a meta-analysis. *Fertil Steril.* 1996;65:1093-1099.
83. Braffman BH, Coleman BG, Ramchandani, et al. Emergency department screening for ectopic pregnancy: a prospective US study. *Radiology.* 1994;190:797-802.
84. Nyberg DA, Mack LA, Jeffrey RB Jr, et al. Endovaginal sonographic evaluation of ectopic pregnancy: a prospective study. *AJR Am J Roentgenol.* 1987;149:1181-1186.
85. Brown DL, Doubilet PM. Transvaginal sonography for diagnosing ectopic pregnancy: positivity criteria and performance characteristics. *J Ultrasound Med.* 1994;13:259-266.
86. Atri M, Leduc C, Gillett P, et al. Role of endovaginal sonography in the diagnosis and management of ectopic pregnancy. *Radiographics.* 1996;16:755-774.

87. Atri M, deStempel J, Bret P. Accuracy of transvaginal ultrasound for detection of hematosalpinx in ectopic pregnancy. *J Clin Ultrasound.* 1992;20:255-261.
88. Nyberg DA, Hughes MP, Mack LA, et al. Extrauterine findings of ectopic pregnancy on transvaginal US: importance of echogenic fluid. *Radiology.* 1991;178:823-826.
89. Frates MC, Brown DL, Doubilet PM, Hornstein MD. Tubal rupture in patients with ectopic pregnancy: diagnosis with transvaginal ultrasound. *Radiology.* 1994;191:769-772.
90. Ackerman T, Levi C, Dashefsky S, Hold S, Lindsay D. Interstitial line: sonographic finding in interstitial (cornual) ectopic pregnancy. *Radiology.* 1993;189:83-87.
91. Chen GD, Lin MT, Lee MS. Diagnosis of interstitial pregnancy with sonography. *J Clin Ultrasound.* 1994;22:439-442.
92. Izquierdo LA, Nicholas MC. Three-dimensional transvaginal sonography of interstitial pregnancy. *J Clin Ultrasound.* 2003;31:484-487.
93. Tamai K, Koyama T, Togashi K. MR features of ectopic pregnancy. *Eur Radiol.* 2007;17:3236-3246.
94. Doubilet PM, Benson CB, Frates MC, et al. Sonographically guided minimally invasive treatment of unusual ectopic pregnancies. *J Ultrasound Med.* 2004;23:359-370.
95. Frates MC, Benson CB, Doubilet PM, et al. Cervical ectopic pregnancy: results of conservative treatment. *Radiology.* 1994;191:773-775.
96. Brammer HM III, Buck JL, Hayes WS, Sheth S, Tavassoli FA. Malignant germ cell tumors of the ovary: radiologic-pathologic correlation. *Radiographics.* 1990;10:715-724.
97. Kim SH, Kang SB. Ovarian dysgerminoma: color Doppler ultrasonographic findings and comparison with CT and MR imaging findings. *J Ultrasound Med.* 1995;14:843-848.
98. Tanaka YO, Kurosaki Y, Nishida M, et al. Ovarian dysgerminoma: MR and CT appearance. *J Comput Assist Tomogr.* 1994;18:442-448.
99. Outwater EK, Wagner BJ, Mannion C, McLarney JK, Kim B. Sex cord-stromal and steroid cell tumors of the ovary. *Radiographics.* 1998;18:1523-1546.
100. Athey PA, Malone RS. Sonography of ovarian fibromas/thecomas. *J Ultrasound Med.* 1987;8:431-436.
101. Troiano RN, Lazzarini KM, Scoutt LM, Langer RC, Flynn SD, McCarthy S. Fibroma and fibrothecoma of the ovary: MR imaging findings. *Radiology.* 1997;204:795-798.
102. Kim SH, Sim JS, Seong CK. Interface vessels on color/power Doppler US and MRI: a clue to differentiate subserosal uterine myomas from extrauterine tumors. *J Comput Assist Tomogr.* 2001;25:36-42.
103. Morikawa K, Hatabu H, Togashi K, Kataoka ML, Mori T, Konishi J. Granulosa cell tumor of the ovary: MR findings. *J Comput Assist Tomogr.* 1997;21:1001-1004.
104. Ha HK, Baek SY, Kim SH, Kim HH, Chung EC, Yeon KM. Krukenberg's tumor of the ovary: MR imaging features. *AJR Am J Roentgenol.* 1995;164:1435-1439.
105. Brown DL, Zou KH, Tempany CM, et al. Primary versus secondary ovarian malignancy: imaging findings of adnexal masses in the radiology diagnostic oncology group study. *Radiology.* 2001;219:213-218.
106. Nichols DH, Julian PJ. Torsion of the adnexa. *Clin Obstet Gynecol.* 1985;28:375-380.
107. Hibbard LT. Adnexal torsion. *Am J Obstet Gynecol.* 1985;152:456-461.
108. Albayram F, Hamper UM. Ovarian and adnexal torsion; Spectrum of sonographic findings with pathologic correlation. *J Ultrasound Med.* 2001;20:1083-1089.
109. Baumgartel PB, Fleisher AC, Cullinan JA, Bluth RF. Color Doppler sonography of tubal torsion. *Ultrasound Obstet Gynecol.* 1996;7:367-370.
110. Vijayaraghavan SB. Sonographic whirlpool sign in ovarian torsion. *J Ultrasound Med.* 2004;23:1643-1649.
111. Lee EJ, Kwon HC, Joo HJ, Suh JH, Fleischer AC. Diagnosis of ovarian torsion with color Doppler sonography: depiction of twisted vascular pedicle. *J Ultrasound Med.* 1998;17:83-89.
112. Hiller N, Appelbaum L, Simanovsky N, Lev-Sagi A, Aharoni D, Tamar S. CT features of adnexal torsion. *AJR Am J Roentgenol.* 2007;189:124-129.
113. Rha SE, Byun JY, Jung SE, et al. CT and MR imaging features of adnexal torsion. *Radiographics.* 2002;22:283-294.
114. Chiou SY, Lev-Toaff AS, Masuda E, Feld RI, Bergin D. Adnexal torsion: new clinical and imaging observations by sonography, computed tomography, and magnetic resonance imaging. *J Ultrasound Med.* 2007;26:1289-1301.
115. Kurjak A, Kupesic S, Jacobs I. Preoperative diagnosis of the primary fallopian tube carcinoma by three-dimensional static and power Doppler sonography. *Ultrasound Obstet Gynecol.* 2000;15:246-251.
116. Ko M, Jeng C, Chen S, Tzeng C. Sonographic appearance of fallopian tube carcinoma. *J Clin Ultrasound.* 2005;33:372-374.
117. Kawakami S, Togashi K, Kimura I, et al. Primary malignant tumor of the fallopian tube: appearance at CT and MR imaging. *Radiology.* 1993;186:503-508.

CHAPTER

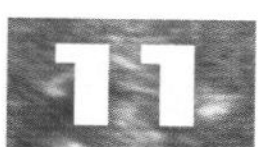

Imaging of the Prostate and Seminal Vesicles

Lisa P. Jones, MD, PhD
Jill Langer, MD
Parvati Ramchandani, MD

THE NORMAL PROSTATE AND SEMINAL VESICLES

Anatomy

The prostate gland is located inferior to the urinary bladder surrounding the urethra, with the widest portion superiorly referred to as the base and the tapered inferior portion referred to as the apex (see Figure 11-1). The prostate is divided histologically into 4 zones: the transition and central zones, which together are often referred to as the central gland, the peripheral zone located posterior and lateral to the central gland and around the apical urethra, and the nonglandular fibromuscular stroma anteriorly. The transition, central, and peripheral zones comprise 5%, 20%, and 70% to 80% of the prostatic glandular tissue, respectively.[1] The transition zone is located anteriorly

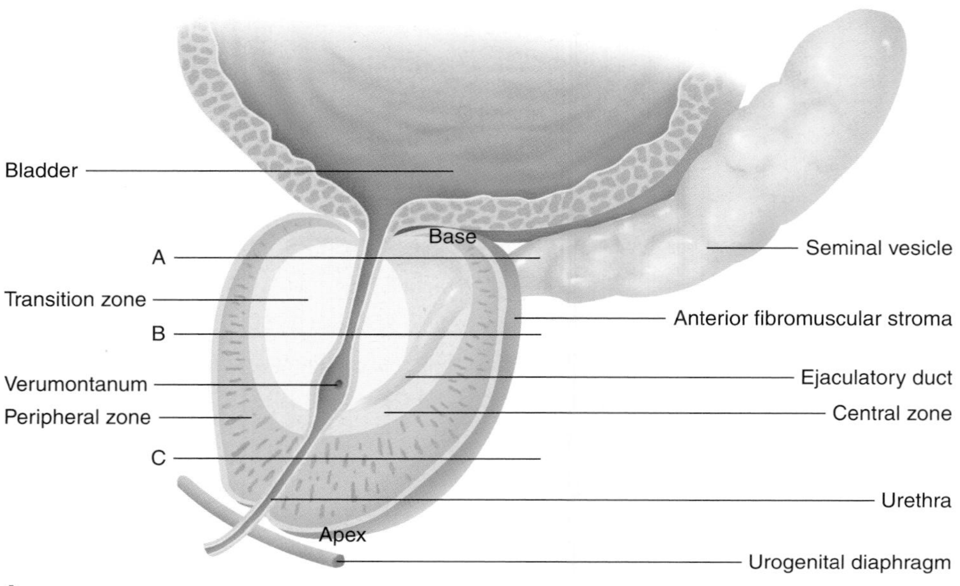

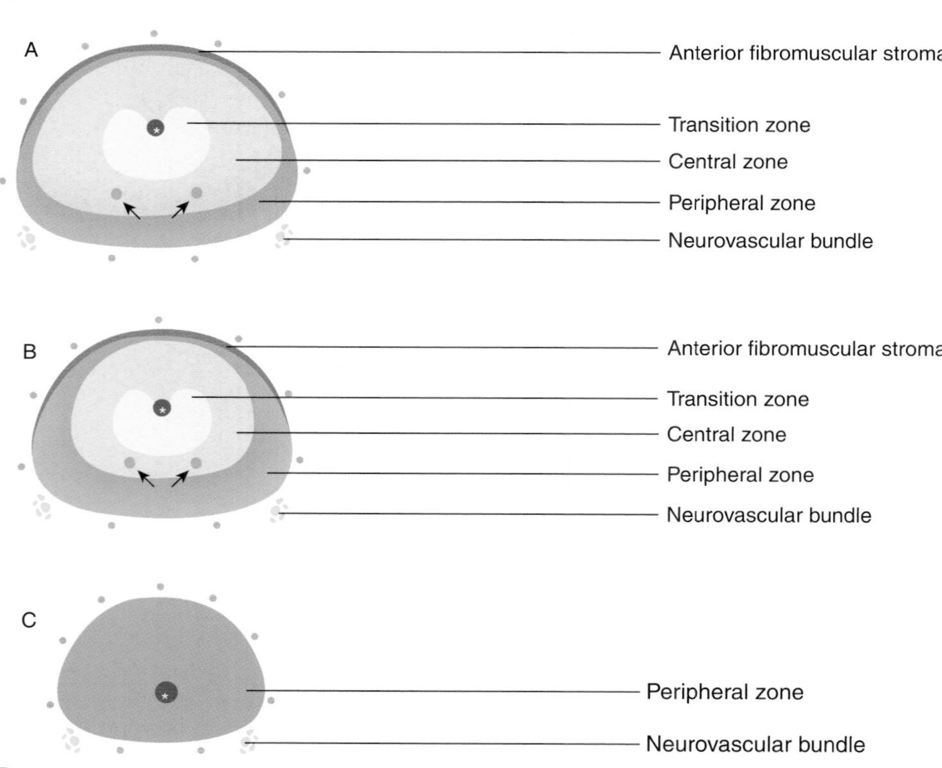

Figure 11-1 Prostate Anatomy and Diagram
A. Drawing shows sagittal view of prostate anatomy. **B.** Prostate anatomy. Drawings show axial views of prostate near level of base A, middle portion B, and apex C of gland corresponding to lines labeled A, B, and C in (A). Asterisks indicate urethra; short arrows indicate ejaculatory ducts in (B). Reproduced from Kundra V, Silverman PM, Matin SF, Choi H. Imaging in oncology from the University of Texas M.D. Anderson Cancer Center: diagnosis, staging, and surveillance of prostate cancer. *Am J Roentgenol.* 2007;189:830-844, with permission.

and laterally to the urethra and the central zone is located posteriorly and superiorly between the peripheral zone and the urethra, surrounding the ejaculatory ducts. The prostate is invested by fibrous connective tissue that is well developed posteriorly and posterolaterally, which has historically been termed "the capsule," although some argue that true capsule is not present histologically.[2] The central gland and the peripheral zone are separated by a plane of tissue. This plane of tissue has been referred to as the "surgical capsule" or "pseudocapsule" but is of little clinical import. The neurovascular bundles are located at the 5- and 7-o'clock positions, posterolaterally, in the region of the rectoprostatic angles. The neurovascular bundles send penetrating branches into the prostate in the region of the base and apex that disrupt the integrity of the prostatic capsule, providing potential routes for tumor spread.[3]

The normal volume/dimension of the prostate is 20 to 30 mL in young men.[4] As a rough estimate, a single transverse diameter below 4 cm is generally associated with a normal size, whereas a diameter greater than 5 cm suggests enlargement of the gland. The seminal vesicles and vas deferentia are located posterior and superior to the base of the prostate. The seminal vesicles are approximately 3 cm in length and 1.5 to 2 cm in width on average. The excretory duct of the seminal vesicle joins the terminal vas deferentia to form the ejaculatory ducts that drain into the urethra in the region of the verumontanum. The prostate is derived from the urogenital sinus, whereas the seminal vesicles, vas deferentia, epididymis, and ejaculatory ducts are derived from the mesonephric ducts (Wolffian ducts) that also give rise to the collecting system and ureter. The paramesonephric ducts (Mullerian duct) give rise to the prostatic utricle and the appendix testis.[5]

Indications for Imaging

The most common indications for imaging of the prostate and seminal vesicles are infertility, hematospermia, elevated prostate-specific antigen (PSA), outlet obstruction, and suspected prostatitis/prostate abscess.

Imaging Modalities

Transrectal ultrasonography (US) and endorectal magnetic resonance imaging (MRI) provide the best anatomic depiction of the prostate and are the imaging modalities of choice. Transrectal ultrasound has the advantages of low cost, portability, and widespread availability and permits real-time imaging. Common applications for transrectal ultrasonography (TRUS) include estimation of volume, assessing for acute disease such as prostatitis or prostatic abscess, and in the initial evaluation for etiologies of infertility to detect cysts or stones. However, the primary use of US is to guide procedures such as radiofrequency transducer placement for radiotherapy, brachytherapy seed placement, cryoablation, abscess drainage, and random core biopsies for detection of prostate cancer.

Endorectal MRI provides superior anatomic detail and soft-tissue contrast, compared with US. Currently, endorectal MRI shows promise as tool for prostate cancer staging. Neither MRI nor US is sufficiently sensitive to screen for prostate carcinoma, although recent studies have shown that MRI may contribute significant incremental value to both digital rectal examination (DRE) and TRUS-guided biopsy ($P < .01$ for each) in detection of cancer and may be indicated if cancer is suspected despite negative TRUS and biopsy findings.[6]

The MRI protocol typically includes large field-of-view images along with small field-of-view endorectal coil axial T1-, axial T2-, coronal T2-, and sagittal T2-weighted images. The US examination consists of axial and sagittal views of the prostate as well as measurements of the prostate in 3 dimensions and measurement of the seminal vesicles.

Imaging Appearance

The central gland and peripheral zone can be differentiated by MRI and US; however, the zonal components of the central gland cannot be distinguished. On US, the peripheral zone is homogeneous and hyperechogenic relative to the central gland, which is heterogenous. The urethra is seen as a shadowing curvilinear structure traversing the central gland on sagittal images (see Figure 11-2).

On MRI, the appearance of the prostate depends on the type of sequence. On T1-weighted images, the zonal anatomy is not evident and the prostate has a homogenous intensity. However, on T2-weighted images, the glandular rich peripheral zone is hyperintense relative to the central gland and the central gland is typically heterogeneous, whereas the peripheral zone is relatively homogenous aside from reticulation related to connective tissue septa. The central gland and the peripheral zone are separated by the low-T2-signal "surgical" capsule. The peripheral zone is separated from the extraprostatic tissues by a low-T2-signal "true" capsule (see Figure 11-3).

The zonal anatomy of the prostate is poorly depicted by computed tomography (CT). The prostate appears as an intermediate-attenuation oval soft-tissue structure just caudal to the base of the bladder. On early postcontrast images, sometimes the central gland and peripheral zone may be distinguished because of heterogenicity and slightly greater enhancement of the central gland (see Figure 11-4).

On US, the seminal vesicles vary in echogenicity depending on the complexity of the fluid, but most commonly are hypoechogenic or close to anechoic (see Figure 11-2). On MRI, the seminal vesicles appear as paired structures above the prostate composed of multiple lobules that contain relatively simple fluid (low T1, high T2 signal). The vas deferens are paired thick-walled tubular structures that travel medial to the seminal vesicles before joining with the excretory duct to form the ejaculatory ducts, which sometimes may be seen as tiny low-T2-signal structures in

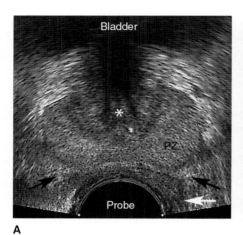

A

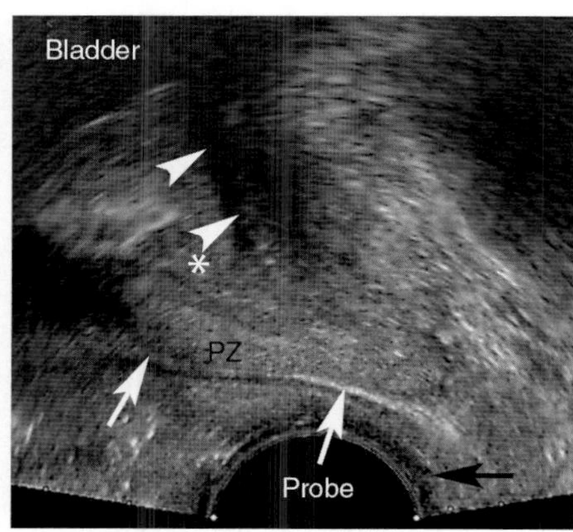

B

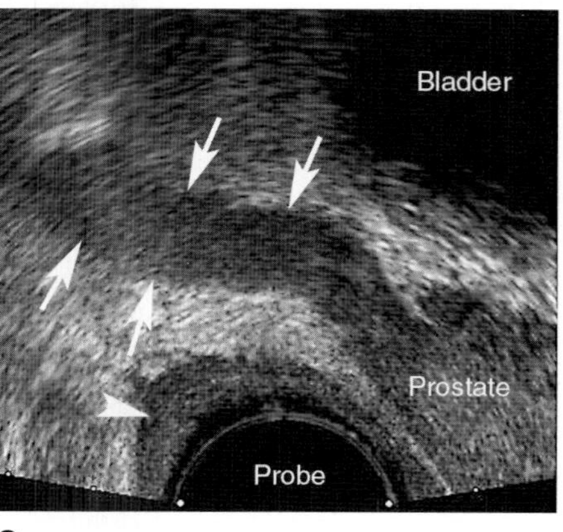

C

Figure 11-2 Normal Transrectal Ultrasound Appearance of Prostate
A. Axial image showing the hyperechogenic peripheral zone and the heterogenous central gland with the urethra (*asterisk*). PZ = peripheral zone. Note the rectoprostatic angles (*black arrows*) and the rectal wall (*white arrow*). **B.** Sagittal transrectal sonographic image showing PZ, urethra (*arrowheads*), posterior border of the prostate (*white arrows*), and rectal wall (*black arrow*). **C.** Oblique image of the right seminal vesicle (*arrows*), note the rectal wall (*arrowhead*).

the posterior aspect of the central gland (see Figure 11-3). On CT, the seminal vesicles appears as paired hypodense structures with internal lobulation superior and posterior to the prostate (see Figure 11-4).

FOCAL PROSTATE LESIONS

Focal lesions of the prostate can be divided into solid-appearing and cystic lesions.

Solid-Appearing Focal Prostate Lesions

Etiologies for a solid-appearing, focal abnormality include prostate cancer, adenomatous nodules, rare other neoplasms, bacterial and granulomatous prostatitis, infarct, phlegmon, iatrogenic, fibrosis/atrophy, and hemorrhage (Table 11-1). The relative likelihood of the different processes depends on location. In the central gland, benign prostatic hyperplasia (BPH) is most common, with other top considerations including prostate cancer, arising from the transition zone, hemorrhage, and secondary involvement of the prostate by either urethral carcinoma or primary bladder carcinoma. In the peripheral zone, the most likely etiologies are prostate cancer, postbiopsy hemorrhage, and prostatitis. Some of the same processes that result in focal lesions may also produce a diffuse abnormality that will be discussed later.

On MRI, most solid lesions will appear as areas of decreased T2 signal. On CT, most prostate lesions are poorly visualized, although subtle areas of increased or decreased attenuation or enhancement may be present. On US, the most common appearance of a lesion is an area of decreased echogenicity, with or without associated changes in vascularity on color Doppler. Clinical correlation with tumor markers (eg, PSA) and possible biopsy is typically necessary to render a specific diagnosis. Individual disease processes are now discussed in more detail.

Imaging Notes 11-1. Location Dependence of the Most Common Prostate Lesions

- BPH most commonly occurs in the transition zone (which is part of the "central gland"), but is relatively infrequent in the peripheral zone
- Adenocarcinoma occurs most frequently in the peripheral zone (70%), and less commonly in the central gland.

Neoplasms

Neoplasms are common focal lesions of the prostate, usually representing prostate adenocarcinoma, which is often referred to more simply as "prostate cancer". However, the prostate may be affected by a variety of other benign and malignant primary neoplasm, as will be detailed below.

Prostate adenocarcinoma

Adenocarcinoma of the prostate arises from the prostate acini and accounts for 95% of prostate malignancies.[1] Prostate adenocarcinoma is the second most common cancer in American men after skin cancer and is second only to lung cancer as a cause of cancer deaths in men, with a lifetime risk for developing prostate cancer of 1/6 for

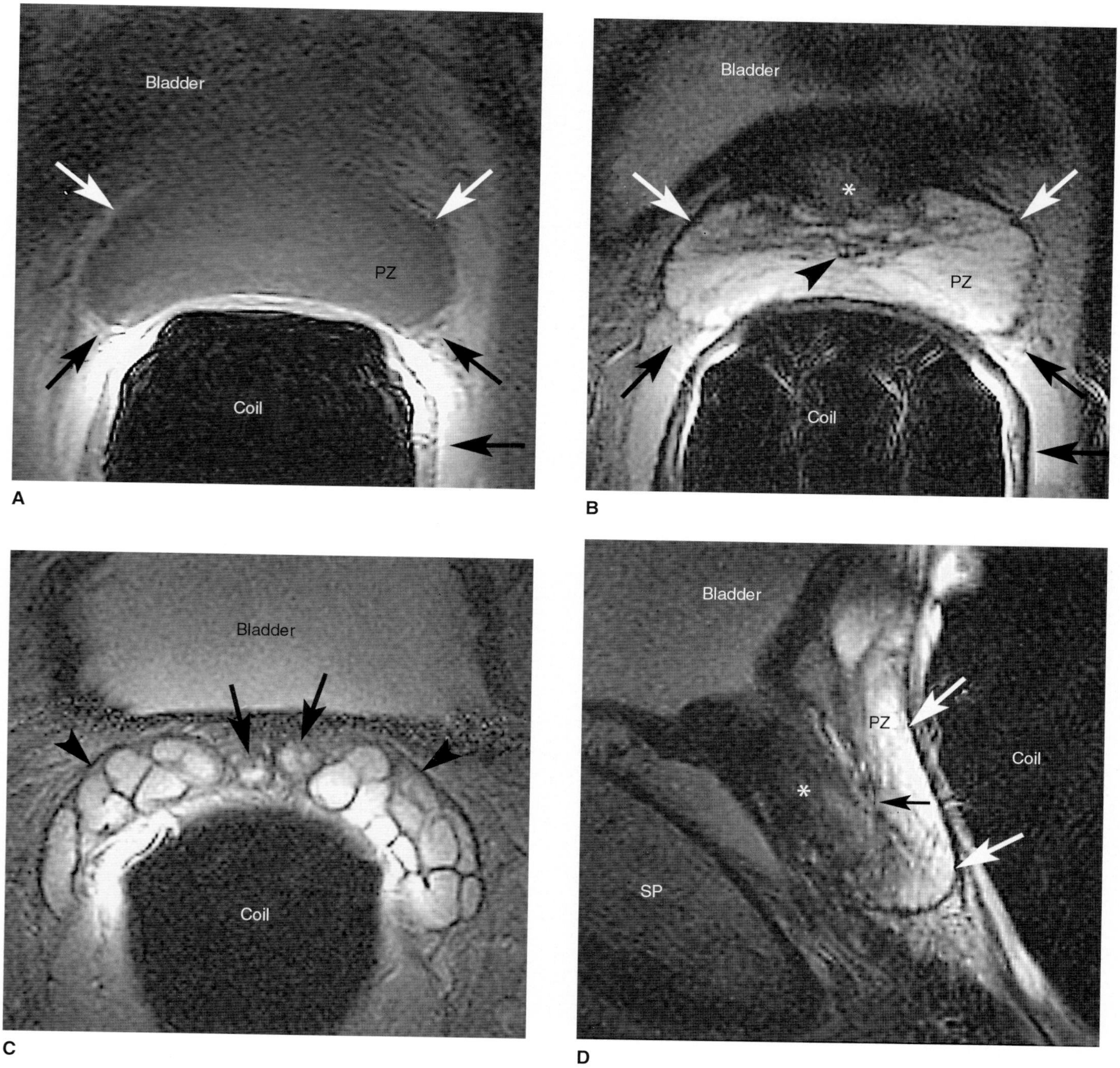

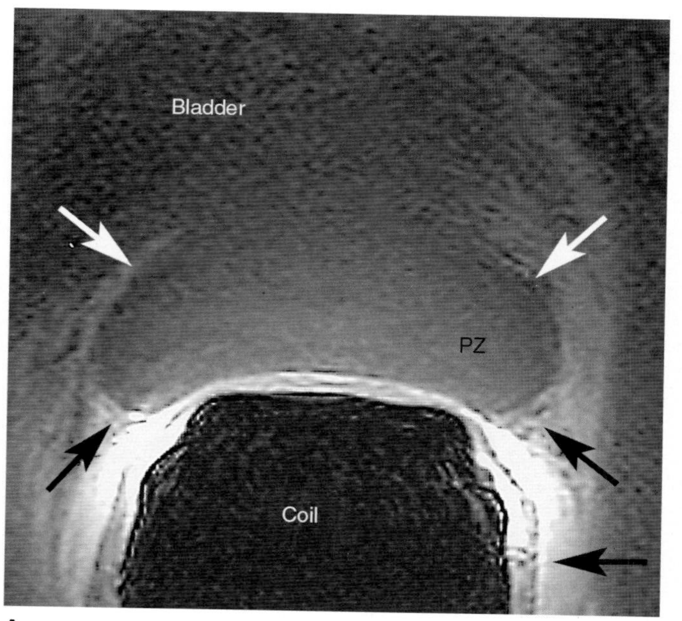

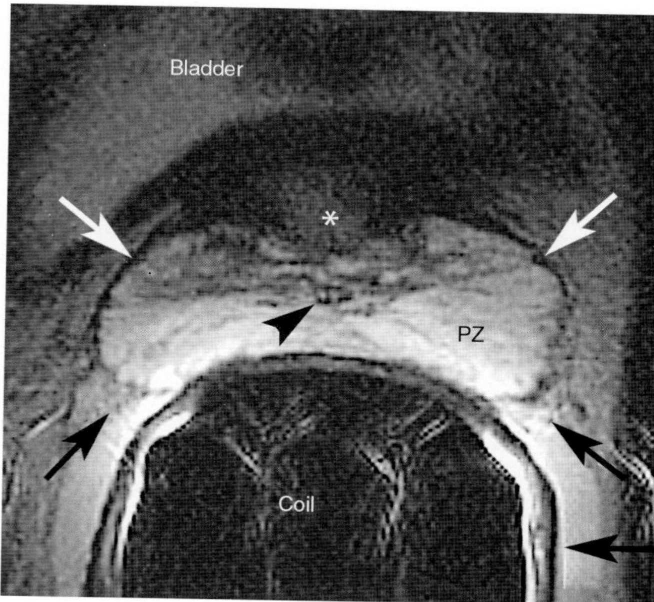

C

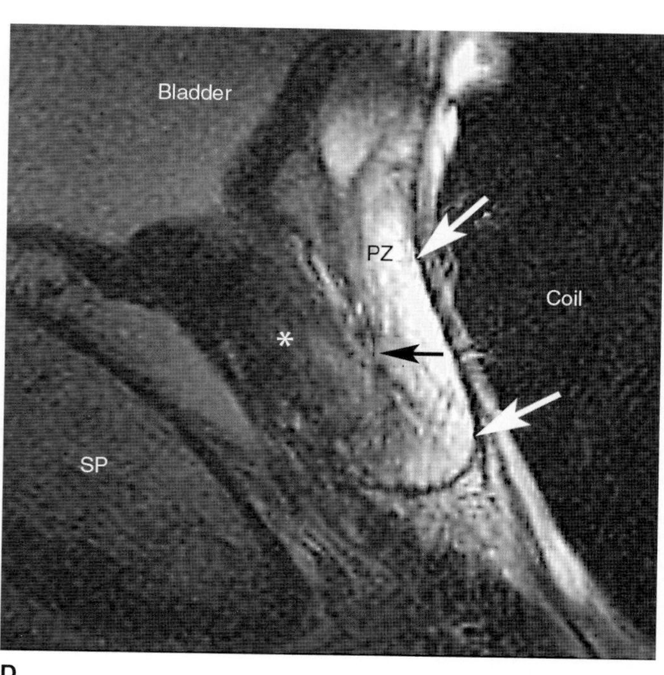

Figure 11-3 Normal MRI Anatomy of the Prostate
A. Axial T1-weighted image through the midprostate. Note that the central gland and peripheral zone have similar intermediate signal intensity. The bladder is collapsed and the rectum is distended by the endorectal coil balloon. The neurovascular bundles are seen as a small structure at the rectoprostatic angles surrounded by high-signal periprostatic fat (*black arrows*). The rectal wall is seen surrounding the coil (*short black arrow*). Coil = coil balloon. **B.** Axial T2-weighted image at the same level as **A** showing the hyperintense peripheral zone with collagenous reticulation. Note that on T2-weighted sequences, the central gland is distinct from the peripheral zone. There is a thin black line surrounding the peripheral zone that represents the prostatic capsule (*white arrows*). Note the ejaculatory ducts (*arrowhead*), neurovascular bundles (*black arrows*), region of urethra (*asterisk*), and rectal wall (*short black arrow*). **C.** Axial T2-weighted image above the level of **B** shows the seminal vesicles (*arrowheads*) and ampullary portion of the vas deferens (*arrows*) as well as the fluid-filled bladder. **D.** Sagittal image close to the midline showing peripheral zone (PZ) and central gland (*asterisk*) as well as the low-signal "surgical capsule" (*black arrow*) and the prostatic capsule (*white arrows*). SP = symphysis pubis.

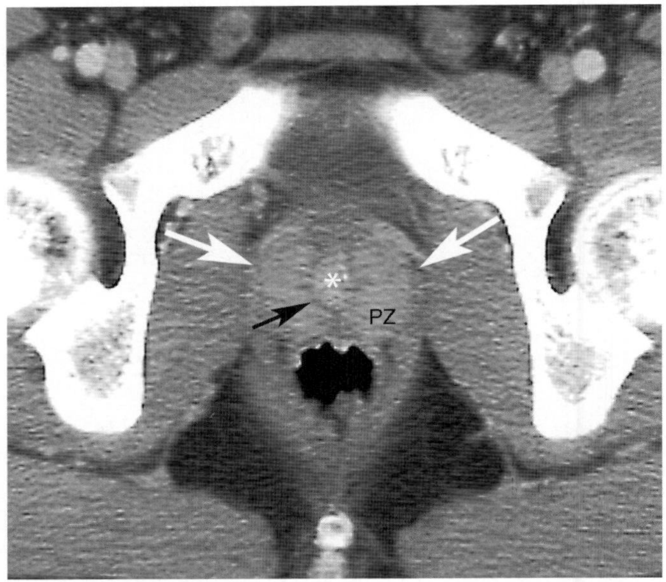

A

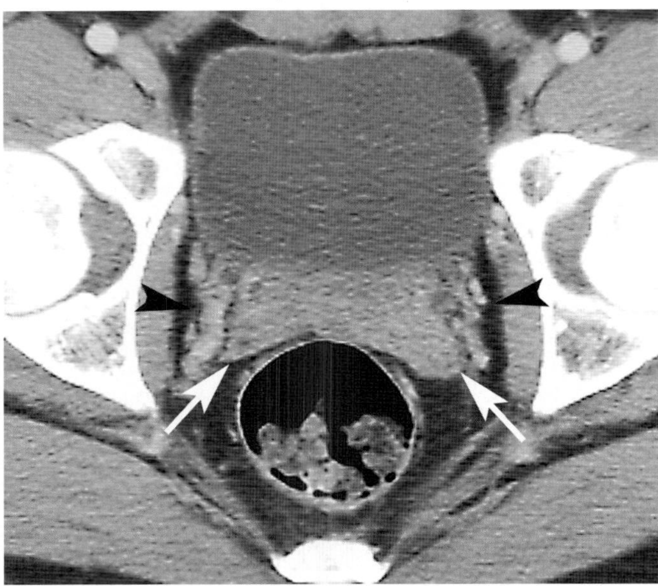

B

Figure 11-4 Normal CT of the Prostate
A. Axial enhanced image with narrow windows through the midprostate (*arrows*) delineates the peripheral zone (PZ), central gland, and urethra (*asterisk*) and surgical capsule (*thin black arrows*). **B.** Axial enhanced CT image through the pelvis just above (A) shows the seminal vesicles (*white arrows*) and periprostatic venous plexus (*black arrows*).

American males. It is estimated that 186,000 men will be diagnosed with prostate cancer and that 28,600 deaths will occur in 2008.[7]

Clinical features: Prostate cancer is usually asymptomatic. However, involvement of the neurovascular bundles can cause erectile dysfunction, narrowing and invasion of the urethra can cause bladder outlet obstruction, and involvement of the ejaculatory ducts or seminal vesicles can cause hematospermia. Occasionally, patients will present with symptoms related to metastatic disease such as bone pain.

Table 11-1. Focal Solid-appearing Prostate Lesions

1. Neoplasms a. Prostate adenocarcinoma b. Tumors other than prostate adenocarcinoma c. Adenomatous nodules (BPH)
2. Prostatitis a. Infections i. Bacterial prostatitis/phlegmon ii. Granulomatous prostatitis b. Idiopathic (majority)
3. Hemorrhage
4. Focal fibrosis or infarction

Prostate cancer screening, although widely practiced, remains controversial. While it is clear that the screening efforts in the past decade have resulted in a downward stage migration with a resultant increase in the incidence of early stage prostate cancer, this has not yet been shown to contribute to a decrease in prostate specific mortality.[8-10] Nonetheless, the American Cancer Society and the American Urological Association advocate annual PSA testing and DRE for men older than age 50. In men with a positive family history of prostate cancer or African American race, the recommendation is to begin screening at age 40 because of an increased risk of prostate cancer in these groups.

Digital rectal examination has been estimated to have a sensitivity of 59% and a specificity of 94% for detecting prostate cancer with a positive predictive value (PPV) ranging from 5% to 38%. In addition, PSA testing permits detection of prostate cancer at an earlier stage. In tumors detected with PSA screening, approximately 60% to 80% of tumors are organ confined, compared with 20% to 40% with DRE alone. Unfortunately, PSA, a glycoprotein produced by prostate epithelial cells, is a nonspecific marker. Prostate cancer tends to increase PSA more than benign conditions; however, there remains significant overlap in the serum PSA levels between individuals with prostate cancer and those with prostatitis, BPH, prior recent prostate biopsy, prior Bacillus Calmette-Guérin (BCG) treatment, ejaculation obstruction, and acute urinary obstruction.

The optimal PSA cutoff to balance sensitivity and specificity continues to be under investigation. Most consider biopsy for men when the PSA level reaches 4 ng/mL, although lower thresholds have been advocated for younger men where BPH is less common. This cutoff is imperfect. The PPV for detection of prostate carcinoma on biopsy for a PSA of 4 to 10 ng/mL, is estimated to be approximately 22% compared with a PPV of 67% for a PSA of >10 ng/mL.[10] Sensitivity estimates range from 70% to 80% to as low as 20% to 30% with a cutoff of 4.[11]

Pathologic diagnosis is based on TRUS-guided biopsies, which are performed according to a random pattern unless a focal abnormality is detected during the US. The sensitivity depends on the number of biopsies performed and the size of the gland, but it is in the range of 95% for 10 biopsies.[12]

Staging and prognosis: Once the diagnosis of prostate adenocarcinoma has been established, the grade and stage of the tumor are evaluated, as these are the most important factors in determining prognosis and treatment. Histologic evaluation of prostate cancer is based on the Gleason grading system, which involves identifying the predominate histologic pattern and secondary histologic pattern, each of which is assigned a grade from 1 to 5. These numbers are summed to give a score, a number between 2 and 10. Scores less than 6 have a good prognosis, whereas scores 8 to 10 have a worse prognosis, with higher recurrence risk and higher stage at presentation.[3] Tumors that are very poorly differentiated, scores 9 and 10, can have a normal serum PSA level and are often metastatic at presentation.

Staging of prostate cancer commonly employs the TNM system, which describes the local extent of tumor (T), lymph node involvement (N), and presence of distant metastasis (M) (Table 11-2). Staging can be based on either clinical or pathologic criteria.

One of the most important distinctions from a treatment perspective is differentiating organ confined (T1, T2) from non–organ-confined disease (T3, T4), because patients with non–organ-confined disease are not optimal candidates for surgery, as will be discussed later. A tumor is considered T3 if it invades the periprostatic tissues or involves the seminal vesicles but is not extensive enough to be considered T4. Extension into the periprostatic tissues (T3a) typically occurs posteriorly and posterolaterally where the neurovascular bundles penetrate the capsule.[13] Seminal vesicle invasion (T3b) can occur through several routes. In some cases, the tumor may invade the periseminal vesicle soft tissues first, prior to invasion of the seminal vesicles. In other cases, the tumor will invade the seminal vesicles directly through the base of the prostate. The tumor can also invade the seminal vesicles through the ejaculatory ducts. Hematogenous metastases to the seminal vesicles may occur, but are rare.[2] Invasion of the muscular wall of the seminal vesicle is associated with a significantly worse prognosis than involvement of other periprostatic tissues.[14] A tumor is considered T4 if it has spread to involve the bladder neck, external sphincter, rectum, levator ani muscles, and/or pelvic side wall (Table 11-2).[2]

The most frequent sites of metastatic prostate cancer are lymph nodes and bones. The regional lymph nodes are located in the true pelvis and include obturator, external and internal iliac and sacral groups (lateral, presacral, or promontory) and involvement in these locations is considered N1. Involvement of lymph nodes outside the confines of the true pelvis are considered distant metastases (M1a), and include common iliac, deep and superficial inguinal, aortic, retroperitoneal lymph nodes, as well as left supra-diaphragmatic nodes.[15] Nodal spread is not necessarily contiguous, as para-aortic lymph nodes may be involved up to 50% of the time without pelvic lymphadenopathy because of hematogenous dissemination.[3]

Bone metastases (M1b) occur initially to the pelvis, spine, ribs, and femoral heads often via the periprostatic venous plexus of Santorini that communicates with the paravertebral venous plexus of Batson. Prostate cancer in the vast majority of cases results in sclerotic bone metastasis. Other sites of metastatic disease (M1c) can occur with advanced disease, including lung, liver, and adrenal gland in decreasing order of frequency on autopsy studies.[2] However, these are rare sites of involvement and should lead to consideration of the possibility of either atypical or high-grade prostate cancer or another primary, especially if bone metastases are not present. Overall, the incidence of metastatic disease is extremely low in patients with T1-T2 tumor, serum PSA less than 20 ng/mL, and Gleason score lower than 8.[3]

The prognosis and treatment of prostate cancer depends on the stage of the tumor. Most men with organ-confined disease or focal "capsular penetration" can expect a cure and, therefore, are the optimal candidates for surgery.[16] In fact, in some patients with very low risk disease (T1, low grade), watchful waiting is a management option, because some detected tumors can be clinically insignificant. By contrast, the presence of established extraprostatic disease is a predictor for disease progression after prostatectomy. For example, only 25% of patients with seminal vesicle invasion are biochemically progression free 10 years after prostatectomy[2] and

Imaging Notes 11-2. Important Imaging Features of Prostate Cancer

1. Evaluate for local spread
   a. Periprostatic tissues, not including the seminal vesicles (T3a)
   b. Seminal vesicle invasion (T3b)
   c. Adjacent organs: bladder, external sphincter, rectum, pelvic sidewall (T4)
2. Identify regional lymphadenopathy
   a. Pelvic lymphadenopathy (N1)
   b. Distant lymphadenopathy (M1a)
3. Search for hematogenous metastasis
   a. Most commonly bone (M1b)
   b. Lung, liver, adrenal (M1c)

Table 11-2. TMN System of Staging Prostate Cancer (Clinical)

T1	Clinically inapparent tumor neither palpable nor visible by imaging
T1a	Tumor incidental histologic finding in 5% or less of tissue resected (post TURP)
T1b	Tumor incidental histologic finding in more than 5% of tissue resected (post TURP)
T1c	Tumor identified by needle biopsy (because of elevated PSA)
T2	Tumor is palpable on DRE or visible by imaging
T2a	Tumor involves half of one lobe or less
T2b	Tumor involves more than half of one lobe but not both lobes
T2c	Tumor involves both lobes
T3	Tumor extends through the prostate capsule
T3a	Extracapsular extension (unilateral or bilateral)
T3b	Tumor invades seminal vesicles
T4	Tumor is fixed or invades adjacent structures other than seminal vesicles, including bladder neck, external sphincter, rectum levator muscles, and/or pelvic side wall
N0	No regional lymph node metastasis
N1	Regional lymph node metastasis
M0	No distant metastasis
M1 M1a	Distant metastasis Nonregional lymph nodes(s)
M1b	Bones
M1c	Other sites(s) with or without bone disease

Stage I	T1a	N0	M0	G1[a]
Stage II	T1a	N0	M0	G2, 3-4
	T1b	N0	M0	Any G
	T1c	N0	M0	Any G
	T1	N0	M0	Any G
	T2	N0	M0	Any G
Stage III	T3	N0	M0	Any G
Stage IV	T4	N0	M0	Any G
	Any T	N1	M0	Any G
	Any T	Any N	M1	Any G

[a]G: Tumor grade is assessed as follows:

- G1: Well-differentiated (slight anaplasia) Gleason 2-4
- G2: Moderately differentiated (moderate anaplasia) Gleason 5-6
- G3-4: Poorly differentiated/undifferentiated (marked anaplasia) Gleason 7-10

Reproduced, with permission, from the AJCC Cancer Staging Manual, 7th Edition (2010) published by Springer-Verlag New York, Inc.

patients with lymph node involvement at the time of surgery are never free of progression. Therefore, in these patients, surgery is generally not performed and therapy is usually based on a combination of radiation, either brachytherapy or external beam radiation, and hormonal therapy. The addition of hormonal therapy has been shown to improve 5-year survival when compared with radiation alone. In patients with distant metastasis, hormonal therapy is the mainstay of treatment; however, tumors often become androgen independent after a few years and escape hormonal control.[3]

Imaging modalities: MRI, CT, and US have different roles in the evaluation of prostate cancer. In general, MRI, because of its superior soft-tissue contrast, offers the most accurate imaging means for determining extent and location of prostate cancer and, therefore, is the preferred imaging examination for the local staging. By contrast, CT is often the modality of choice to evaluate for metastatic disease (lymphadenopathy and osseous metastases) because of its lower cost, larger area of anatomic coverage, and better spatial resolution relative to MRI. US, unlike either MRI or CT, has the advantage of real-time imaging, and consequently is used primarily as a method of directing prostate procedures, such as biopsies, brachytherapy seed placement, or abscess aspiration.

Imaging appearance

Ultrasonography: Prostate carcinoma has a variable appearance on US examinations: the majority, approximately 75%, appear hypoechogenic relative to the peripheral zone (see Figure 11-5). Unfortunately, the PPV of a hypoechogenic lesion in the peripheral zone is at best 40% to 50%[17] because a variety of nonmalignant lesions can appear similarly hypoechogenic, including transducer artifact, focal prostatitis, hematoma, and BPH nodules. Most of the remainder of prostate carcinomas, approximately 25%, appear isoechogenic[18] and a very few, 1% to 5%, appear hyperechogenic. It has been suggested that hyperechogenicity reflects the presence of stromal fibrosis or a desmoplastic response. No difference in the biologic activity of different echogenicity cancers has been observed. Prostate cancer can also be associated with secondary findings, including increased vascularity within the lesion on color Doppler and capsular bulging. These findings may aid in identification of isoechogenic lesions. Transrectal US has been used for local staging of prostate cancer in some studies but the added value is uncertain.[19]

Imaging Notes 11-3. Prostate Cancer

70% of prostate cancers will originate in the peripheral zone
MRI: Low signal lesion within the high signal peripheral zone
US: Hypoechgenic focus within the hyperechogenic peripheral zone

Findings that can suggest extraprostatic extension include bulging or irregularity of the surface of the capsule adjacent to a lesion, obliteration of the rectoprostatic angle and disruption of the capsular surface. Seminal vesicle invasion can be suspected if there is a hypoechogenic lesion at the base of the prostate with contiguous solid tissue in the seminal vesicle, solid hypoechoic masses in the seminal vesicles, or asymmetry.[6]

Magnetic resonance imaging: Although MRI is typically not performed for tumor detection, the primary tumor is often visible on MRI. The accuracy based on T2- and T1-weighted images is approximately 60% to 80% for localizing prostate cancer, with a PPV on the order of 50%.[20-24] Currently, dynamic contrast enhancement, MR spectroscopy, and diffusion MRI are areas of active research and may improve accuracy.[3,6,11,25]

Seventy percent of adenocarcinomas occur in the peripheral zone, typically appearing as a T2 hypointense/T1 isointense lesion that effaces the normal collagenous network of the peripheral zone (see Figures 11-5 and 11-6). In the majority of cases, these tumors will be detected by DREs and/or US-guided prostate biopsies.

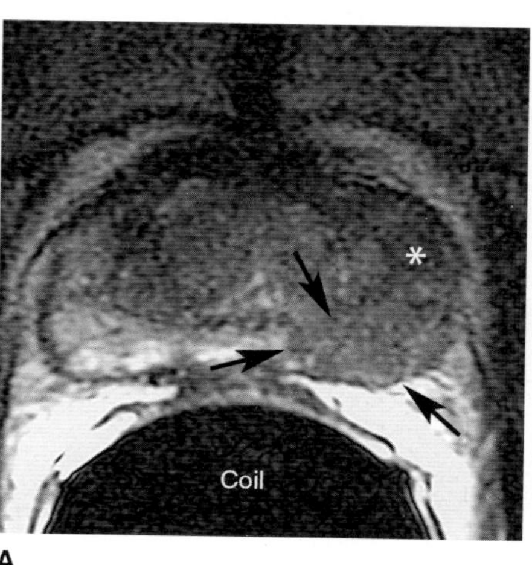

A

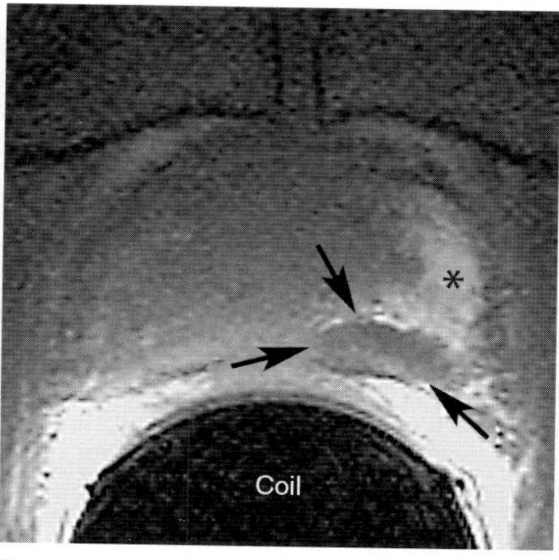

B

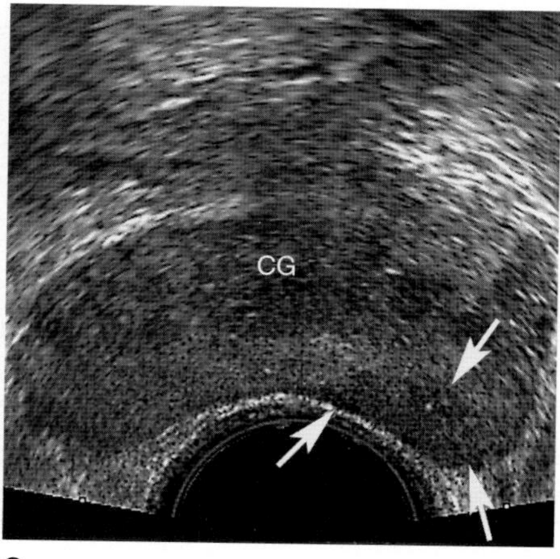

C

Figure 11-5 Prostate Carcinoma by US and MRI
A. Axial T2-weighted image showing hemorrhage (*asterisk*) in the peripheral zone obscuring the margins of the tumor nodule (*arrows*). **B.** Axial T1-weighted image showing the "MR exclusion principle" with the tumor nodule (*arrows*), outlined by hemorrhage (*asterisk*). Note that tumor shows low signal on T1-weighted images by contrast to blood, which is high signal. **C.** Axial TRUS image showing corresponding hypoechogenic nodule (*arrows*). CG = central gland.

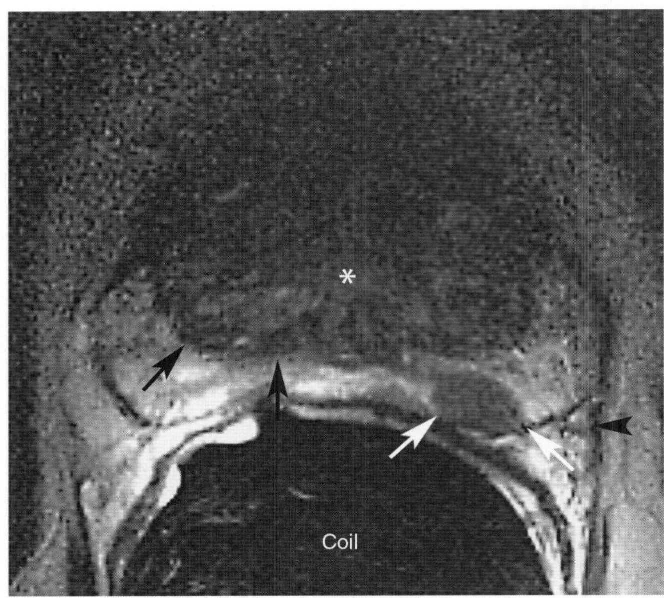

A

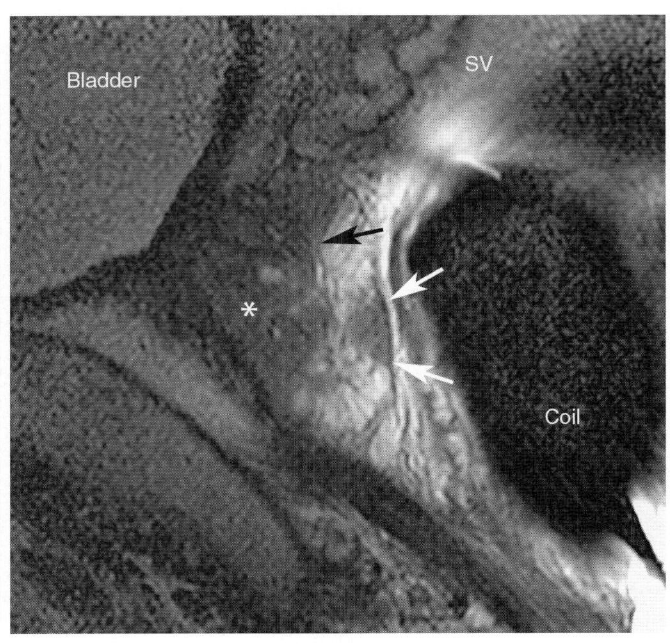

B

Figure 11-6 Confined Prostate Carcinoma by MRI
A and **B.** Axial and sagittal T2-weighted images showing low-signal tumor nodule (*white arrows*) abutting the low-signal prostatic capsule near the neurovascular bundle (*arrowhead* in A). Note the enlargement of the central gland (*asterisk*) due to BPH with low-signal "surgical capsule" separating the central gland from the peripheral zone (*black arrow*).

Thirty percent of adenocarcinomas occur in the central gland, usually arising from the transition zone. These tumors are more difficult to detect clinically and can be missed by both DRE and by conventional biopsies that primarily sample the peripheral zone.[26] This is a situation where MRI of the prostate may play an important role. Although historically, transition zone tumors have been considered difficult to detect on MRI and US because of background heterogeneity related to BPH, 2 recent studies have shown promising results for MRI detection of transition zone carcinomas. A study by Akin et al reported a sensitivity and specificity of 75% to 80% and 78% to 87%, respectively, and a study by Li et al reported an accuracy of 73% for the detection of prostate cancer in the central gland on endorectal MRI examinations.[26,27] The criteria for tumor included (1) homogenous low-T2-signal region in the central gland, (2) poorly defined lesion margins, (3) lack of a low-signal rim (a rim is commonly seen in adenomatous nodules), (4) interruption of the surgical pseudocapsule, (5) urethral or anterior fibromuscular stromal invasion, or (6) lenticular shape (see Figure 11-7).[27] Therefore, in the setting of a rising PSA despite negative biopsies, the possibility of a transition zone carcinoma should be considered and either endorectal prostate MRI and/or transition zone/anterior biopsies should be considered to detect these tumors.[21]

Although histologically identical to the tumors that occur in the peripheral zone, transition zone tumors show differing clinical features, including higher mean PSA levels (31 vs 11 ng/mL), higher tumor volumes (11.2 vs 5 mL), lower Gleason scores (6.2 vs 7.4), and higher percentage of organ-confined tumor (67%-89% vs 41%-56%), as well as tendency for extracapsular tumor to occur anteriorly.[28]

MRI also shows some promise as a tool for increasing the accuracy of staging. Clinical staging often underestimates the extent of tumor. In 1 study, seminal vesicle invasion was found in up to 15% of prostatectomy specimens.[29] Because spread of tumor beyond the prostate is usually best

Imaging Notes 11-4. Features That May Help to Distinguish Central Gland Prostate Carcinoma From Changes Related to BPH

Central gland cancer	Adenomatous Nodule
Homogeneous low T2 signal	Heterogenous T2 signal
Poorly defined margins	Sharply defined margins
No low-signal rim	Low-signal rim surrounding nodule
Interruption of the surgical capsule	No interruption of the surgical capsule
Lenticular shape	Round or oval

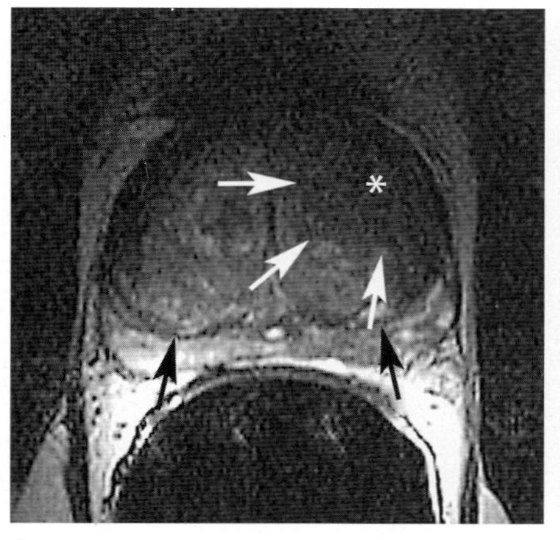

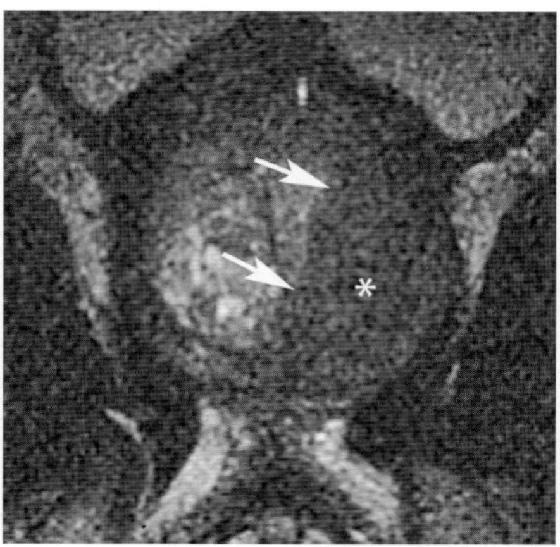

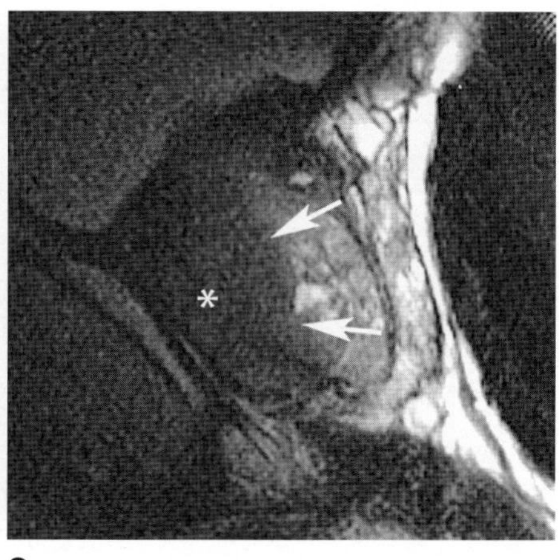

Figure 11-7 Transition Zone Adenocarcinoma
A. Seventy one-year-old with PSA of 41 and Gleason 8 tumor on core biopsy. Axial (A), coronal (B) and sagittal (C) T2-weighted images showing homogenous area of low signal intensity replacing the normal heterogenous central gland, representing tumor (indicated by *, outlined by white arrows). Note heterogeneity and enlargement of the central gland due to BPH with low signal "surgical capsule" (*black arrows* in A).

managed nonsurgically, preoperative detection of extracapsular spread, such as spread to the seminal vesicles, can improve treatment planning. To this end, several models utilizing clinical parameters including DRE, PSA levels, and Gleason scores have been developed to estimate the risk of extraprostatic spread.[30,31] Recently, endorectal MRI has been shown to have incremental value over these models[32,33] for predicting organ-confined disease. This effect is most pronounced in patients who are classified as intermediate or high risk for disease progression. Patients are considered to be intermediate risk if they are clinical stage T1-2, with Gleason score 7 and/or PSA 10.1 to 20 ng/mL and are considered high-risk with clinical stage of T3-4 or a Gleason score > 7, or a PSA > 20 ng/mL.

One of the most important qualities of endorectal prostate MRI is its ability to detect extraprostatic extension of tumor, which it does with greater than 90% specificity, if stringent criteria are applied. These criteria include the presence of irregular bulging of the prostate with disruption of the low-signal capsule and/or tumor infiltration of the periprostatic fat. Manifestations of periprostatic tumor infiltration include asymmetry of the neurovascular bundles, obliteration of the rectoprostatic angle or tumor signal in the periprostatic fat (see Figure 11-8). Less specific signs include tumor-capsule interface of >1 cm or a smooth bulge.[3,20,34,35] Seminal vesicle invasion can be predicted with high accuracy by the presence of tumor at the prostate base that extends beyond the capsule in combination with low signal intensity within a seminal vesicle that has lost its normal architecture (see Figure 11-9).[36] The differential diagnosis for low signal in the seminal vesicles will be discussed in a subsequent section.

MRI can also reveal locally advanced (T4 disease). Contiguous organ invasion is indicated by loss of intervening fat planes and tumor signal within the organ. If tumor invasion is extensive, it can result in a bladder mass and ureteral obstruction, mimicking a bladder primary (see Figure 11-10). Similarly, rectal invasion by prostate carcinoma can mimic rectal carcinoma (see Figure 11-11). In both cases, PSA and other tumor markers may be helpful, although ultimately biopsy may be required for diagnosis.

Computed tomography: Typically, the primary tumor is poorly visualized by CT, although occasionally the tumor may be seen as a hyperenhancing area in the prostate on early postcontrast images. However, CT may reveal complications associated with locally advanced prostate cancer, such as rectal invasion or bladder invasion with or without hydronephrosis, and may reveal signs of metastatic disease (see Figures 11-10 through 11-13).

Other prostate neoplasms

Histologic types other than adenocarcinoma account for approximately 5% of prostate neoplasms. Correct diagnosis

Imaging Notes 11-5. Features of Extracapsular Spread of Prostate Carcinoma

1. Irregular bulging of the prostate
2. Disruption of the prostate capsular line
3. Tumor signal in the periprostatic tissues
   a. Asymmetry of the neurovascular bundles
   b. Obliteration of the rectoprostatic angle
   c. Low signal tumor within the periprostatic fat

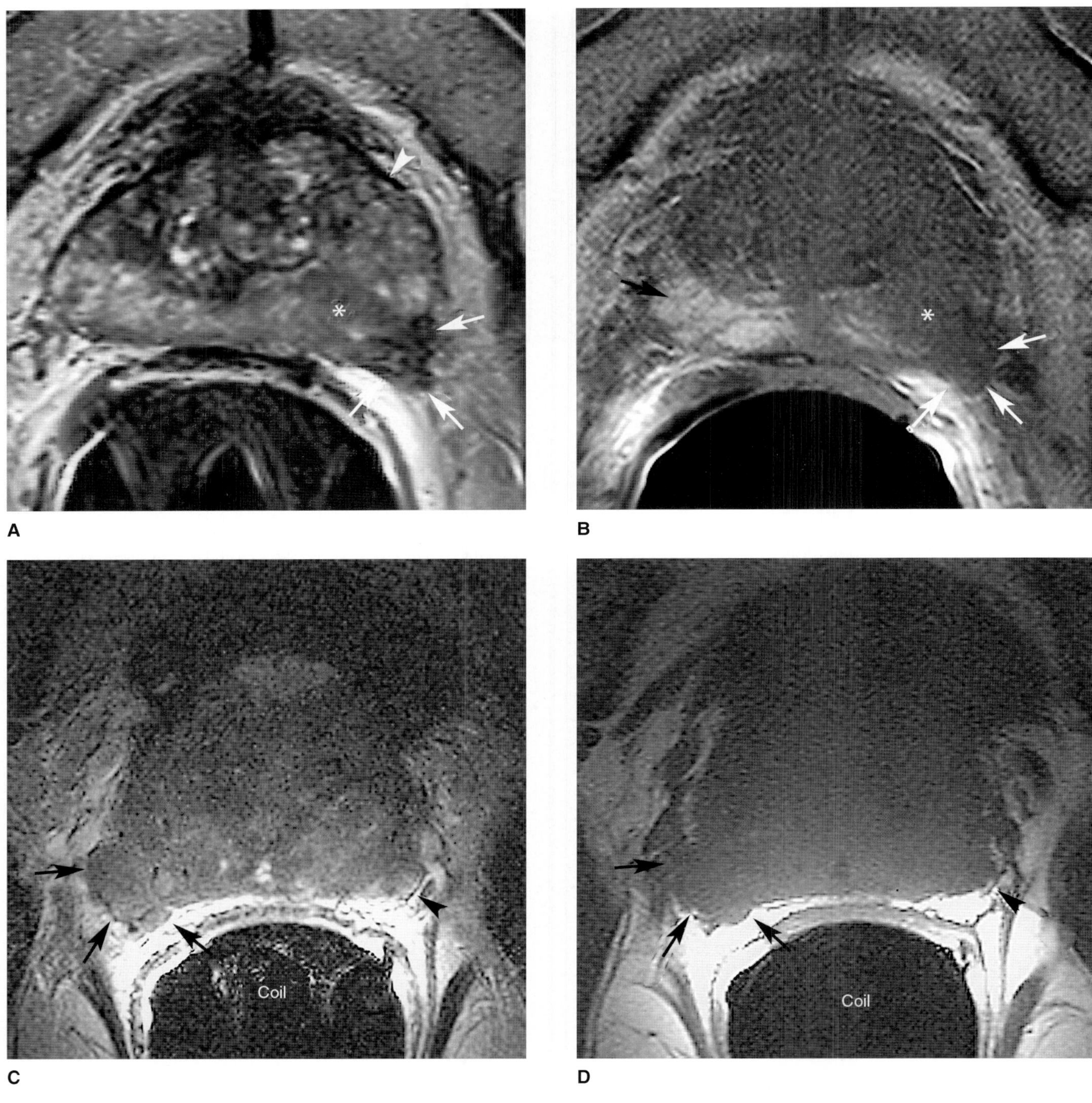

Figure 11-8 Examples of Extracapsular Extension
Axial T2-weighted (**A**) and axial T1-weighted (**B**) images showing tumor (*asterisk*) in the left basilar peripheral zone surrounded by high signal hemorrhage (*black arrow* in B), with macroscopic tumor in the left rectoprostatic angle in the region of the neurovascular bundle (*white arrows*). Note the normal prostatic capsule anteriorly (*arrowhead* in A). *asterisk* = tumor. **C** and **D.** A 48-year-old with Gleason 9 prostate cancer. Axial T2-weighted (C) and T1-weighted (D) images showing prostate diffusely infiltrated by tumor with irregular bulging in the region of the right (*arrows*) and left (*arrowhead*) neurovascular bundles.

is important for prognosis and treatment. Unusual prostatic neoplasms may be divided into (1) epithelial neoplasms, (2) neuroendocrine tumors (small cell carcinoma), (3) nonepithelial stromal neoplasms, and (4) secondary tumors, including metastases, direct invasion by adjacent tumors, leukemia, and lymphoma. For a complete discussion, the interested reader is referred to several excellent review articles.[37-41]

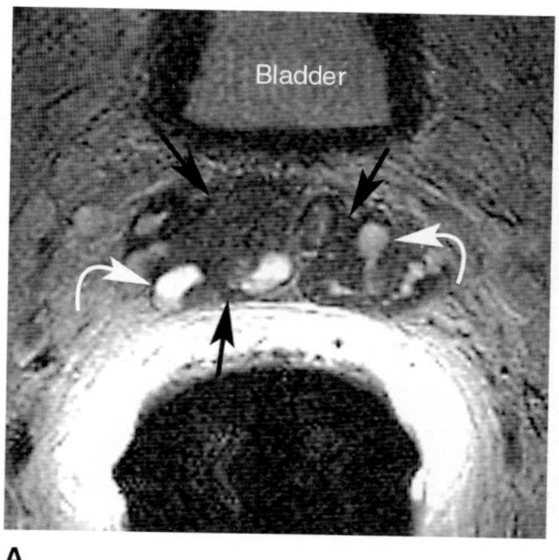

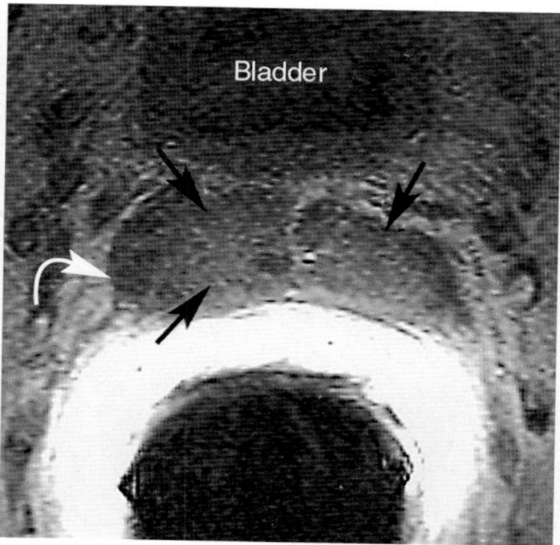

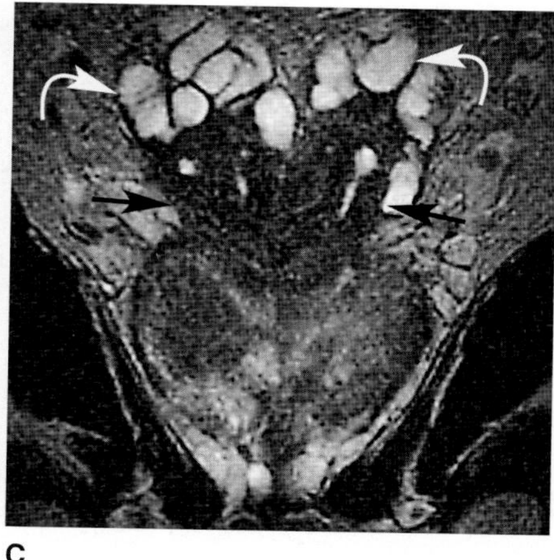

Figure 11-9 Seminal Vesicle Invasion by Prostate Carcinoma
Sixty seven-year-old with PSA of 5 and Gleason 9 adenocarcinoma on biopsy. **A** and **B.** Axial T2-weighted (A) and axial T1-weighted (B) images at the level of the seminal vesicles reveals hypointense soft tissue due to tumor infiltrating the medial seminal vesicles (*arrows*) with residual normal seminal vesicle laterally (*curved arrows*). **C.** Coronal T2-weighted image showing tumor (*arrows*) infiltrating into both seminal vesicles (*curved arrows*).

Other malignant epithelial neoplasms: Malignant epithelial neoplasms (other than conventional adenocarcinoma) include several histologic variants, including (1) ductal carcinoma, (2) primary transitional carcinoma, (3) squamous carcinoma, and (4) mucinous adenocarcinoma. The majority of these cannot be reliably distinguished from adenocarcinoma based on imaging appearance, but there are some suggestive clinical features, as discussed below.[37-41]

Ductal carcinoma can arise from the central ducts or the peripheral ducts. When it arises in the central ducts,

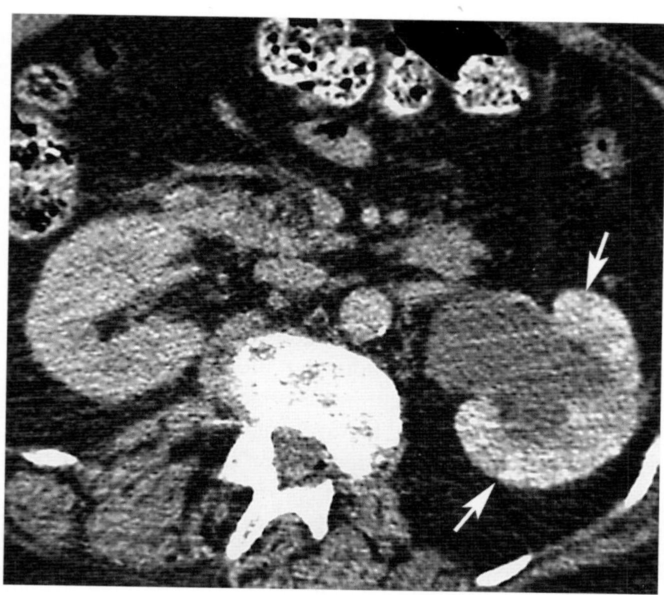

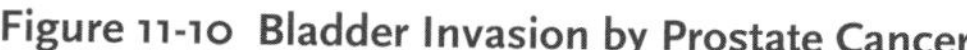

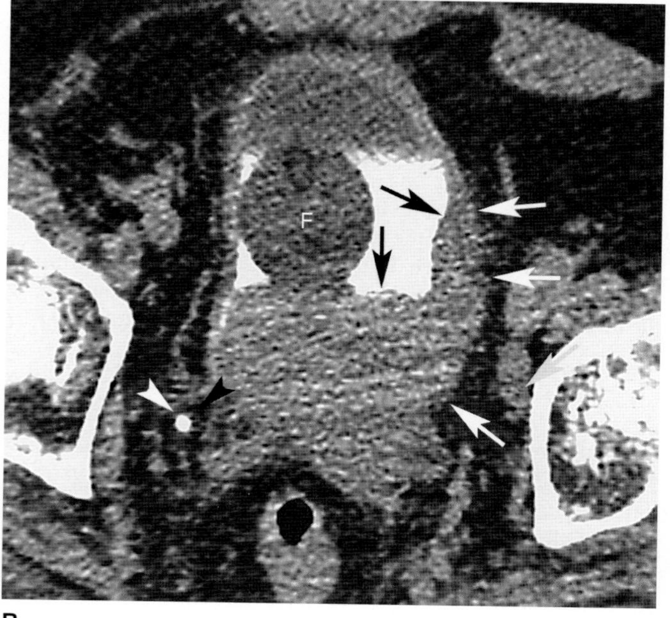

Figure 11-10 Bladder Invasion by Prostate Cancer
A. Axial excretory-phase CT image showing left hydronephrosis, absent excretion, and delayed nephrogram due to involvement of the left ureterovesical junction by tumor. **B.** Axial excretory phase CT image of the pelvis demonstrating irregular bladder wall thickening involving the region of the left ureterovesicle junction (*white* and *black arrows*), which was initially interpreted as a transitional cell carcinoma of the bladder. However, the patient was found to have markedly elevated PSA and prostate cancer by biopsy, and the wall thickening was due to invasion by prostate cancer. F = Foley balloon. Arrowhead points to right ureter.

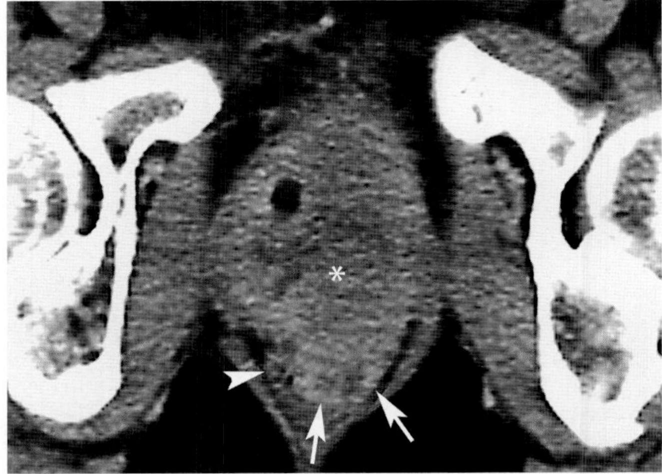

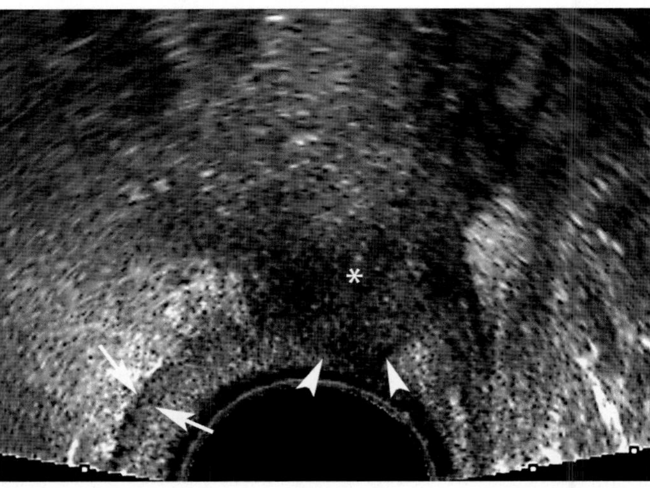

Figure 11-11 Rectal Invasion by Prostate Cancer
A. Axial image through the level of the prostate shows heterogeneously enhancing tumor (*asterisk*) with extracapsular tumor (*arrows*) invading the anterior rectal wall (*arrowhead*). Note the Foley catheter in place. **B.** Transrectal US image showing tumor (*asterisk*) invading the anterior rectal wall (*arrowheads*). Compare the invaded wall with the normal rectal wall on the right (*arrows*).

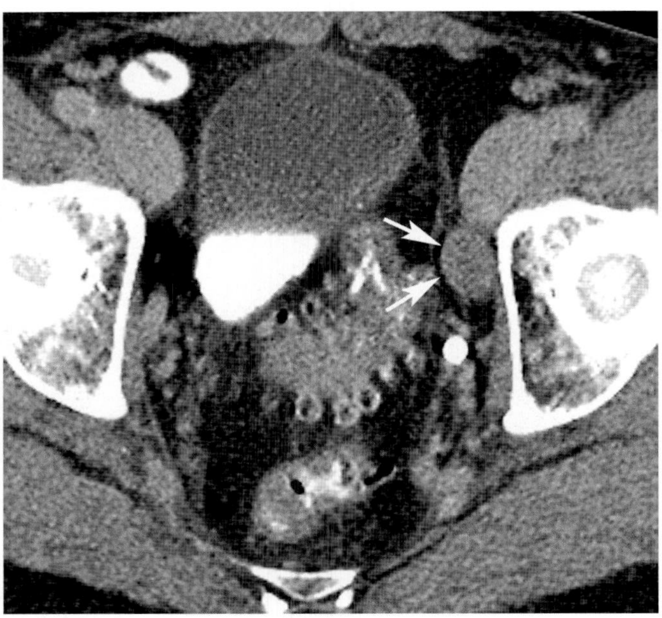

Figure 11-12 Metastatic Lymphadenopathy from Prostate Cancer
Axial excretory-phase CT image through the pelvis demonstrating an enlarged heterogenous left external iliac lymph node (*arrows*) in a patient with Gleason 8 tumor and PSA of 20.

it can grow as a polypoid lesion in the urethra and cause obstructive symptoms and hematuria, mimicking urothelial neoplasm. On the other hand, peripheral duct tumors usually clinically mimic conventional prostatic adenocarcinoma.[2] Ductal carcinoma tends to be higher grade, to have a worse prognosis, and to be less hormonally responsive than adenocarcinoma of the prostate. However, spread occurs in a similar manner to adenocarcinoma. The imaging appearance is for the most part nonspecific, although there are a few case reports of ductal carcinomas presenting with cystic or hemorrhagic components.[42,43]

Transitional cell carcinoma (TCC) is the second most common epithelial neoplasm of the prostate but accounts for less than 3% of prostatic tumors in adults. Although growing within the prostate, TCC of the prostate represents a tumor of the prostatic urethra. They are differentiated from prostate cancer by normal PSA, tumor cells negative for PSA and PAP on histology, and lack of response to hormonal therapy. When transitional histology is discovered on prostate biopsy, the primary differential diagnosis revolves around whether the tumor is a primary malignancy of the prostate or represents secondary involvement from a TCC bladder primary (see Figure 11-14). These are treated with cystoprostatectomy when localized.

Rarely, carcinomas of the prostate will have **squamous differentiation**. Squamous carcinoma demonstrates aggressive behavior and androgen independence. In 20% to 50% of patients, squamous carcinoma will be a complication of previous irradiation for prostate adenocarcinoma. Other suggestive clinical features include normal PSA, history of schistosomiasis infection, or the presence of lytic bone metastases (see Figure 11-15).

Mucinous adenocarcinoma is a rare variant of epithelial prostate malignancies accounting for less than 1% to 2% of tumors. It is defined as an adenocarcinoma in which at least 25% of the volume of the tumor consists of extracellular mucin in the absence of an extraprostatic mucinous primary tumor of origin.[37] The tumor tends to be of higher grade than conventional adenocarcinoma and therefore is typically more aggressive.[38,44] The large mucin content of the tumor can be a clue to the diagnosis, because the T2 MRI signal intensity of these tumors approaches that

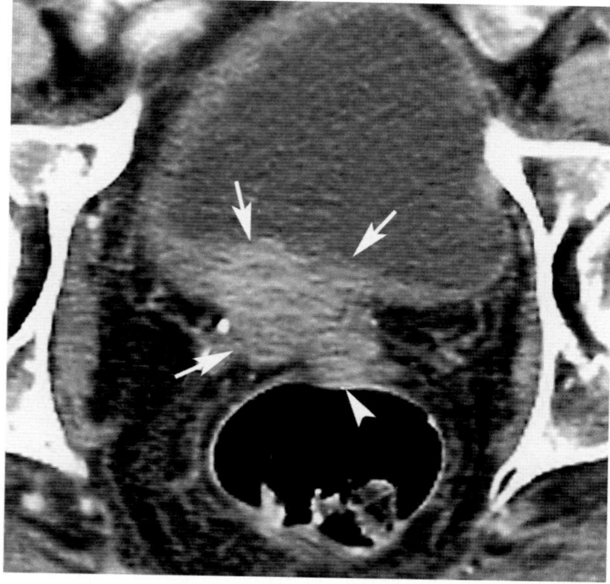

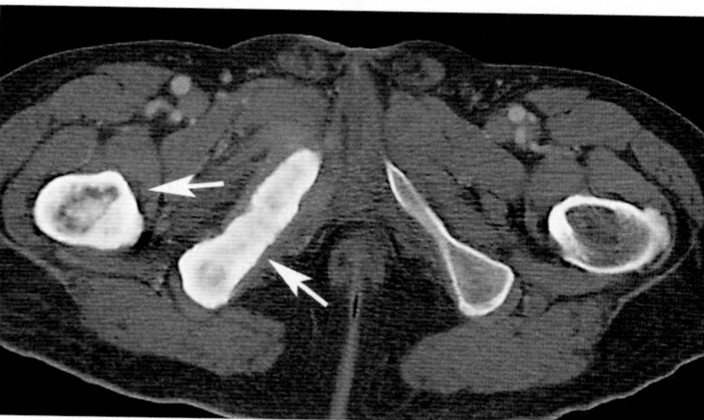

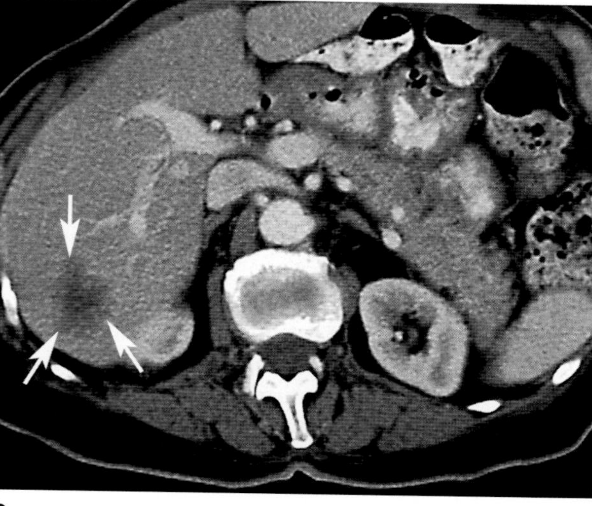

Figure 11-13 Distant Metastatic Disease from Prostate Cancer
A. Axial enhanced CT image showing tumor (*arrows*) invading the urinary bladder and abutting the rectum (*arrowhead*). **B.** Axial bone window CT image through the pelvis showing sclerotic areas in the right proximal femur and right ischium due to osteoblastic metastases (*arrows*). **C.** Axial enhanced CT image at the level of the liver showing a liver metastasis (*arrows*).

of fluid (see Figure 11-16). This imaging appearance can be similar to that of glandular-rich adenomatous nodules or other multiloculated lesions of the prostate that will be discussed later.

Small cell carcinoma: Small cell carcinoma of the prostate is distinguished by rapid progression, early visceral metastases (including liver, bones, lung, CNS), poor response to androgen ablation therapy, relatively low PSA, and lytic more often than blastic metastases (see Figure 11-17).[45] Because of the presence of neuroendocrine cells, paraneoplastic syndromes may be present, including Cushing syndrome, hypercalcemia, thyrotoxicosis, ADH production, and Eaton-Lambert syndrome.[40,46]

Sarcomas and other nonepithelial neoplasms: Most nonepithelial tumors of the prostate are sarcomas. The 2 most common sarcomas are rhabdomyosarcoma and leiomyosarcoma.

Rhabdomyosarcoma is the most common sarcoma of the prostate. It is primarily seen in children. It is a very aggressive tumor characterized by rapid growth, such that invasion of the periprostatic tissues and bulky lymphadenopathy are commonly present at time of diagnosis.[47] The site of origin may be difficult to distinguish when the tumor is locally advanced. The primary sites of metastases are the liver, lung, and skeleton.[47] The differential diagnosis in children includes neuroblastoma, primitive neuroectodermal tumor, lymphoma, and Ewing tumor.[41]

Leiomyosarcoma is the second most common prostate sarcoma and is seen primarily in adults, with a mean of 61 years in a report of 23 cases.[48] On imaging, leiomyosarcoma is differentiated from adenocarcinoma by large size, with a mean cross-sectional diameter of 9 cm[48] and a different mode of spread (see Figure 11-18). Metastatic disease occurs most commonly to the lung, in approximately 30% of patients, followed by metastasis to bone and liver. Regional lymph node spread is less common, occurring in only about 10% of patients.[38] The most important predictors of survival are negative surgical margins and the absence of metastatic disease. Early diagnosis with resection offers the best chance for cure.[49]

Other nonepithelial neoplasms of the prostate also include leiomyoma, solitary fibrous tumor, stromal tumors of uncertain malignant potential (STUMP), and stromal sarcoma of the prostate.[50-52]

Secondary involvement of the prostate by extraprostatic neoplasms: Approximately, 1.2% of prostatic malignancies are due to secondary involvement of the prostate by direct invasion of contiguous malignancies or hematogenous metastasis. Direct invasion can occur with tumors of the bladder, rectum, urethra, and periprostatic tissues (see Figure 11-19). Hematogenous metastases are most commonly from malignant melanoma or lung cancer.[41] In most cases, secondary involvement can be identified by (1) history of another type of tumor, (2) epicenter of

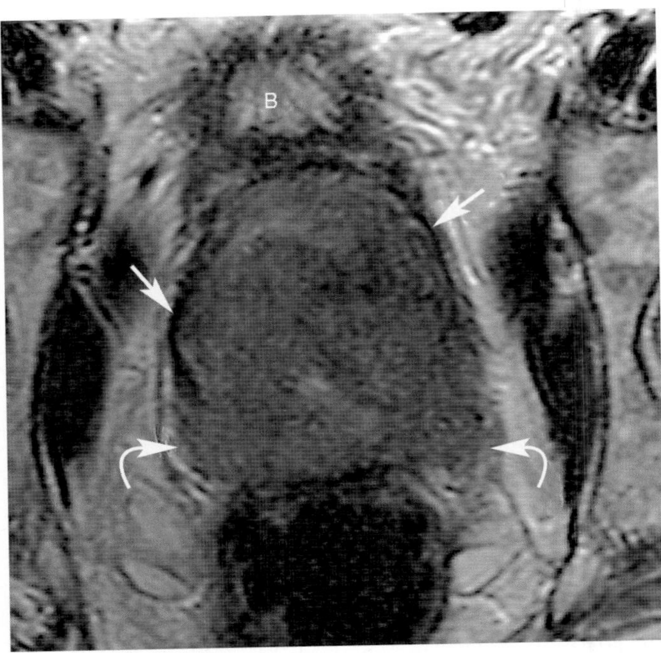

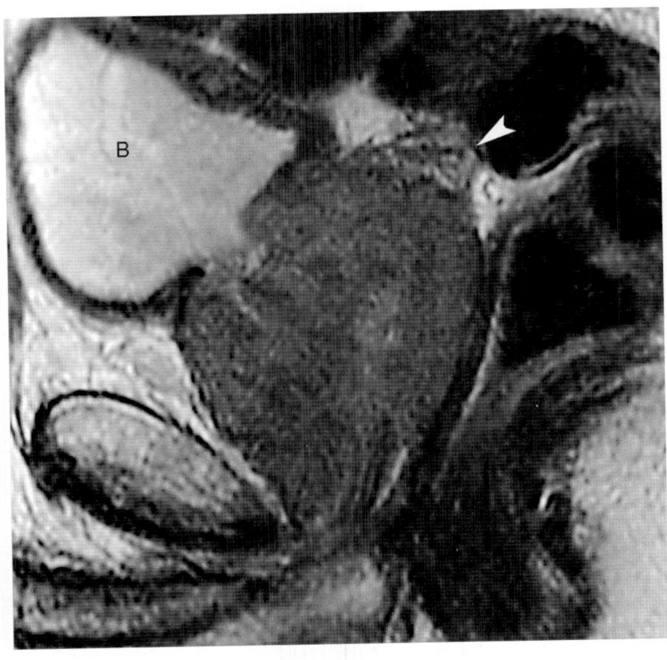

Figure 11-14 Transitional Cell Carcinoma of the Prostate
Axial T2 (**A**) and sagittal (**B**) T2-weighted image showing diffuse replacement of the prostate by tumor with loss of the normal internal structure. Note that the prostatic capsule (*straight arrows*) is disrupted posteriorly where there is extracapsular extension (*curved arrows*). PSA was normal at 1.7 ng/mL, which would be atypical for conventional prostatic adenocarcinoma and suggests an atypical histology. Arrowhead indicates the seminal vesicles in (B). The normal bladder (B) is seen anterior and superior to the prostate.

mass located in an organ other than the prostate, (3) tumor markers (eg, PSA), and (4) different pattern of metastases (eg lytic bone metastases or early visceral metastases). However, occasionally biopsy may be required.

Lymphoma of the prostate: Lymphoma of the prostate is a rare phenomenon, usually due to non-Hodgkin lymphoma rather than Hodgkin disease. Prostatic lymphoma can occur as either primary extranodal lymphoma, in approximately 35% of cases, or as a site of secondary involvement, in approximately 65% of cases.[53] Histology of primary lymphoma of the prostate is usually diffuse large B-cell lymphoma and has an age of presentation similar to that of prostate adenocarcinoma with an average age of 62 years.[53,54] In primary lymphoma of the prosate, most patients present with obstructive urinary symptoms and an abnormal digital rectal examination and systemic symptoms are rare. As with most other tumors of the prostate, either primary or secondary lymphoma will typically appear hypoechoic on US exams relative to normal prostate and isointense on T1-weighted and hypointense on T2-weighted images relative to the peripheral zone. Clues to the correct diagnosis include a history of lymphoma, normal PSA, avid ^{18}F-fluorodeoxyglucose (FDG) uptake, and distribution/pattern of disease involvement atypical for prostate adenocarcinoma. For example, visceral involvement, lytic metastases, or lymphadenopathy in the chest without abdominal pelvic lymphadenopathy (see Figure 11-20).

Benign Prostatic Hyperplasia

Benign prostatic hyperplasia usually involves the transition zone of the prostate, resulting in diffuse enlargement and heterogeneity of the central gland and, therefore, will be more fully discussed under: **Diffuse Abnormalities of the Prostate** (see Figure 11-21). However, occasionally hyperplastic nodules may extend into the peripheral zone, or appear as discrete focal nodules in the central gland. Imaging features that may help differentiate BPH nodules from prostate adenocarcinoma include the presence of mixed signal within the nodule because of the presence of glandular and stromal elements, well-defined margins, and visible pseudocapsules.[26] The imaging features differentiating transition zone prostate adenocarcinoma from BPH have already been previously discussed (see under heading: **Prostate adenocarcinoma**).

Postbiopsy Hemorrhage

Small focal regions of hemorrhage as a result of transrectal biopsies of the prostate are a common phenomenon and are frequently identified on imaging. In 1 study, postbiopsy hemorrhage was detected in 49% patients who underwent

Imaging Notes 11-6. Distinguishing Features of Prostate Malignancies

Unusual Prostatic Neoplasms	Features
Epithelial tumors other than adenocarcinoma: TCC, SCC, mucinous, ductal, other	Atypical pattern of spread, for example, lytic metastases from SCC, aggressive behavior Mucinous is T2 hyperintense
Malignant nonepithelial tumors: rhabdomyosarcoma (kids), leiomyosarcoma (adults), other rare sarcomas	Large size
Other: small cell carcinoma of the prostate (most common), carcinoid, carcinosarcoma, melanoma, germ cell tumor	Small cell carcinoma: paraneoplastic syndromes, atypical pattern of spread with early visceral involvement
Secondary tumors: lymphoma, direct invasion from contiguous tumor (urethral, urinary bladder, Cowper duct), metastases (melanoma, lung, pancreas, stomach, penis, larynx)	Lymphoma: PET +, normal PSA, LAN in atypical distribution, other visceral involvement, history of lymphoma Mets: tumor markers, metastases elsewhere
Other epithelial tumors: leiomyoma, neurofibroma, paraganglioma, pheochromocytoma, hemangioma, angiomyxoma, Stromal tumor of uncertain malignant potential (STUMP)	Leiomyoma: normal PSA, well circumscribed, likely still will require biopsy to prove B9

Modified from Khan, 1999.

MRI more than 21 days after transrectal biopsy.[55] In some cases postbiopsy changes persisted for as long as 4½ months. Postbiopsy hemorrhage often results in areas of decreased T2 signal within the peripheral zone because of the presence of intracellular methemoglobin. This finding can resemble prostate carcinoma on T2-weighted images; however, unlike prostate cancer, these regions typically are associated with increased T1 signal and tend not to disrupt the normal peripheral zone architecture.

In addition, hemorrhage tends to preferentially distribute in normal peripheral zone excluding areas of tumor, because of the anticoagulant properties of the citrate, which is present in lower quantities in tumor. Therefore, on T1-weighted images, tumor nodules may be surrounded by T1 hyperintense hemorrhage, which has been termed the "MR

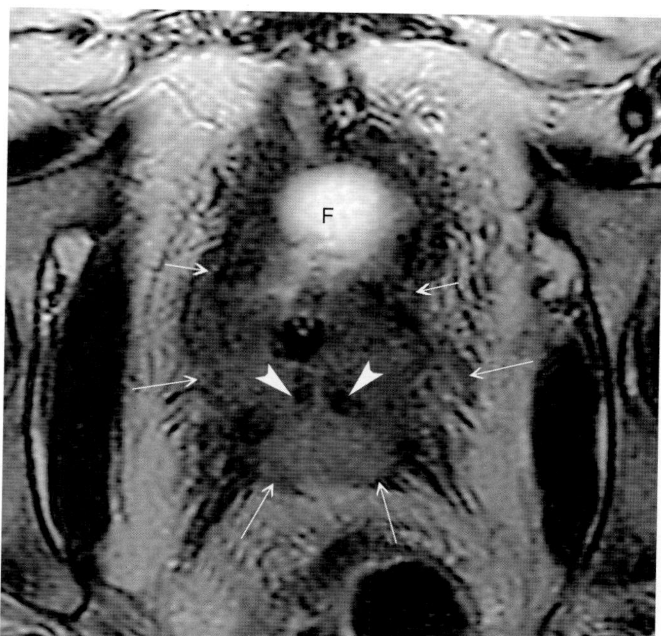

A

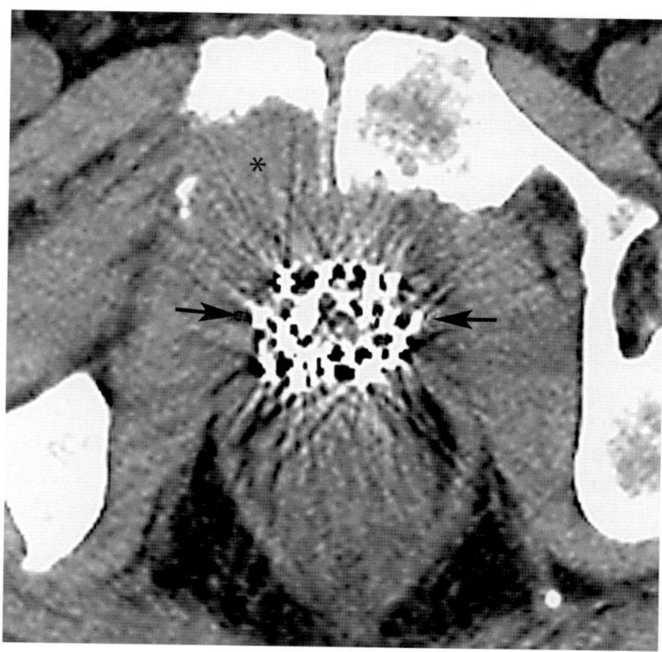

B

Figure 11-15 Squamous Cell Carcinoma
A 63-year-old with history of brachytherapy for prostate cancer with PSA less than 1 and biopsy revealing squamous cell carcinoma. **A.** Axial T2-weighted images show an infiltrating mass (*outlined by long arrows*) involving posterior wall of the urinary bladder (*short arrows*) and base of prostate, surrounding the vas deferens (*arrowheads*) and seminal vesicles. A suprapubic catheter (F) is also present. **B.** Axial CT shows radiation seeds (*arrows*) and lytic bony metastasis (*asterisk*).

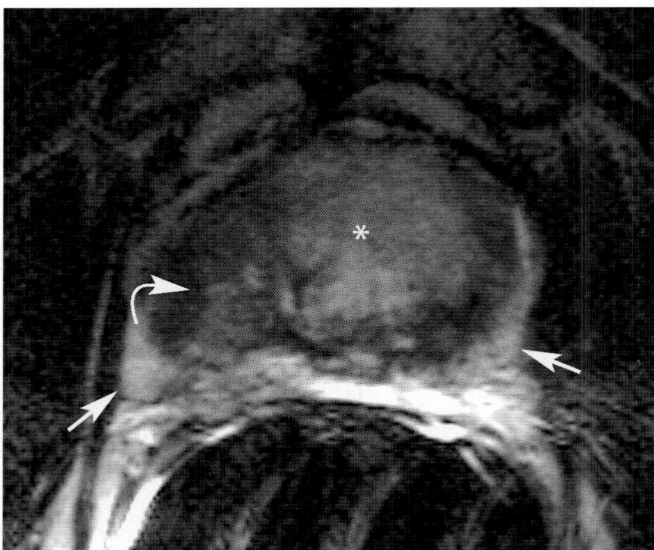

Figure 11-16 Mucinous Adenocarcinoma of the Prostate
This 73-year-old with PSA measuring 1.1 had prostate biopsy revealing mucinous adenocarcinoma (PSAP and PSA negative). Axial T2-weighted image demonstrates T2-hyperintense area (*asterisk*) in the central gland, with ill-defined borders replacing the normal architecture in the central gland (*curved arrow*). Note the area is almost as hyperintense as the peripheral zone, a finding suggestive of mucinous histology. The T2-hyperintense appearance can also be seen with a glandular-rich BPH nodule; however, glandular-rich BPH nodules typically are more heterogenous and have well-defined borders unlike the current case. (See Figure 11-32, for example of glandular right BPH nodules.)

exclusion sign" (see Figures 11-5 and 11-22).[56] Although hemorrhage typically does not produce mass effect, occasionally postbiopsy hematomas can simulate a nodule. However, the clinical history of recent prostate biopsies and the high signal on T1-weighted images indicating the presence of blood products are helpful signs differentiating hematoma from prostate cancer and/or extracapsular spread of cancer.

Chronic Prostatitis

Chronic prostatitis can be a cause of focal or multifocal abnormalities within the prostate gland. By contrast, acute prostatitis usually results in diffuse enlargement of the gland on all cross-sectional imaging studies and will be discussed later under the heading: **Diffuse Prostate Enlargement**.

The most common etiology for chronic prostatitis is sterile inflammation of the gland that is called "chronic abacterial prostatitis." Other causes include granulomatous inflammation of the gland, termed "granulomatous prostatitis," and repeated/chronic bacterial infection, termed "chronic bacterial prostatitis." In most cases, chronic bacterial prostatitis is caused by the same bacterial infections that cause acute bacterial prostatitis. In the United States, granulomatous prostatitis is most commonly due to the instillation of BCG into the bladder as treatment for superficial bladder cancer. (1) Other causes of granulomatous prostatitis include infection with mycobacterium tuberculosis, brucellosis, treponema palladium, parasites (schistosomiasis, echinococcus), and fungi (coccidiomycosis, blastomycosis, histoplasmosis, cryptococcus) and viruses (herpes zoster).[57] Noninfective etiologies of granulomatous prostatitis include iatrogenic causes (postsurgical), systemic diseases such as sarcoidosis and Wegener's disease (2%-7%) (41), foreign body reaction, and idiopathic (Table 11-3).[58] Chronic prostatitis can be asymptomatic at presentation or can present with a variety of symptoms, including pelvic or perineal pain, dysuria, hematuria, postejaculatory pain, hematospermia, and/or infertility.

Chronic prostatitis has a varied appearance on cross-sectional imaging. Most commonly, it manifests as geographic non–contour-deforming areas of decreased echogenicity on US (possibly with increased flow on color Doppler) or decreased T2 signal on MRI. However, occasionally chronic prostatitis can present as a focal, mass-like lesion,[59] which is indistinguishable from neoplasm by imaging, but may be suspected based on clinical features such as young age, normal PSA, and typical symptoms (see Figure 11-23). Chronic prostatitis can also cause prostatic calcifications, which appear as echogenic foci with posterior acoustic shadowing on US and as hypointense foci on T1- and T2-weighted images on MRI. Abnormalities of the seminal vesicles are relatively common and may include atrophy[60] or septal thickening related to chronic seminal vesiculitis or dilation related to ejaculatory duct stenosis or calculi.[58] Unlike acute bacterial prostatitis, there is little or no associated inflammatory change in the periprostatic fat.

Chemotherapy and Radiation Treatment Effect

Hormonal and radiation therapy also may result in decreased signal within the peripheral zone and seminal vesicles, which is usually diffuse but may be heterogeneous.[61] Clues that abnormal signal represents treatment effect include (1) small size of prostate, (2) presence of brachytherapy seeds or radiofrequency transducers, and (3) clinical history of hormonal or radiation therapy.

Other Focal Prostate Lesions

Other focal hypoechoic and/or hypointense lesions within the peripheral zone that can mimic prostate cancer include volume averaging of the high central zone (see Figure 11-24).[62] Periurethral collagen related to incontinence treatment status postprostatectomy may mimic an abnormal-appearing prostate but is further discussed elsewhere.

Summary of Solid-appearing Focal Prostate Lesions

It is useful to consider prostatic lesions according to their location, in either the central gland or the peripheral zone.

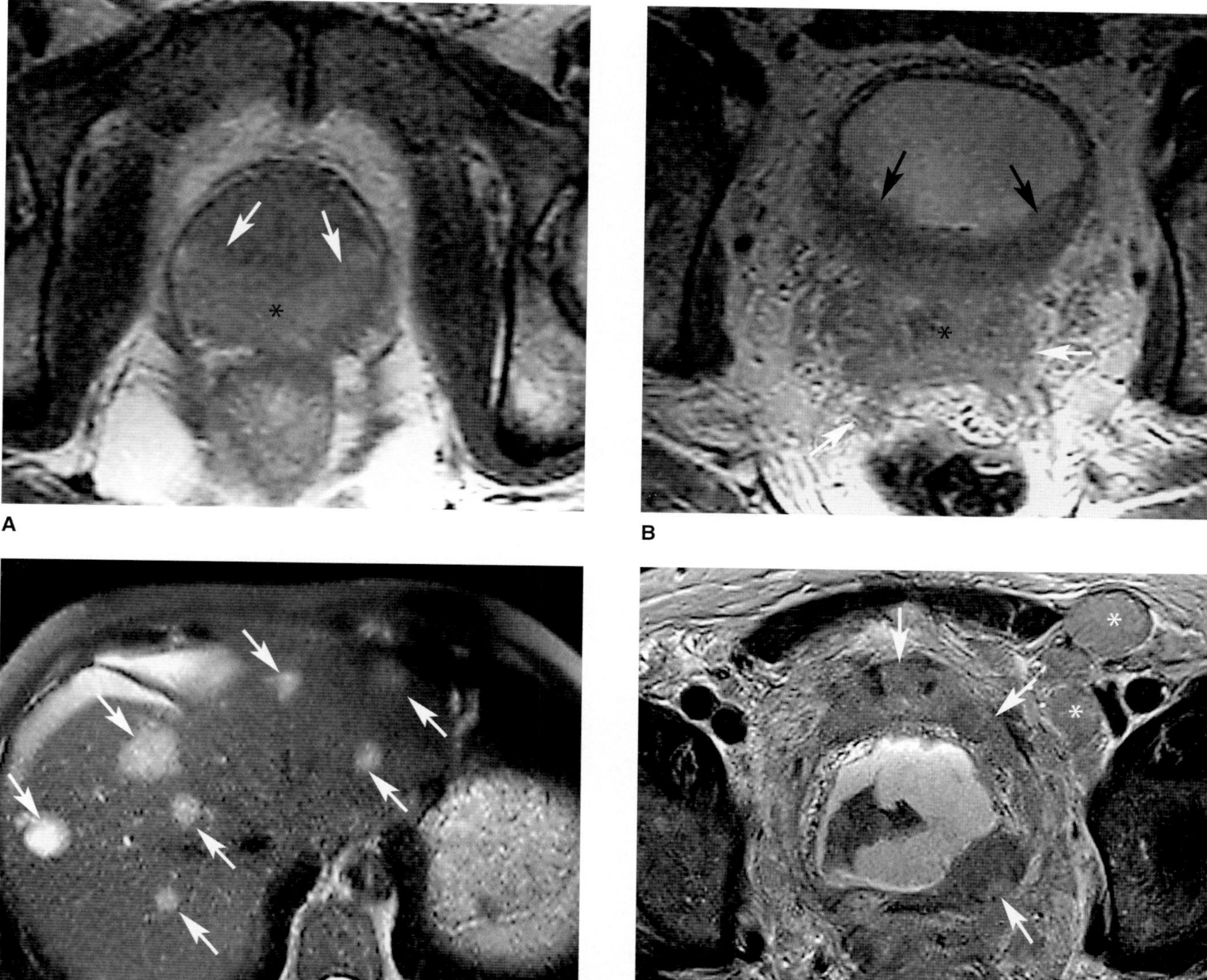

Figure 11-17 Small Cell Carcinoma of the Prostate
A-D. A 64-year-old, presented with hematuria and 2-3 weeks of left lower quadrant pain (PSA 1.9). (A) Axial T2-weighted images at the level of the midprostate showing low-signal tumor throughout the gland (*asterisk*) with effacement of normal boundary (*arrows*) between the central gland and peripheral zone. (B) Axial T2 image superior to (A) at the base of the prostate demonstrating tumor (*asterisk*) invading the urinary bladder, which demonstrates irregular thickening (*black arrows*) and infiltrating the periprostatic fat posteriorly (*white arrows*). (C) Axial fat-saturated T2-weighted image through the level of the liver showing multiple lesions typical of metastases (*arrows*); no bone metastases were present. This atypical pattern of metastatic disease is a feature of small-cell carcinoma of the prostate. (D) Axial T2-weighted image from a follow-up MRI 8 months later showing rapid progression of disease despite therapy reflecting the typically aggressive behavior of small cell carcinoma, with diffuse mural involvement of the urinary bladder by tumor (*arrows*), infiltration of the perirectal fat (*arrowhead*), and progressive lymphadenopathy (*asterisk*). Heterogeneous signal in the lumen of the urinary bladder was shown to be clot on other sequences.

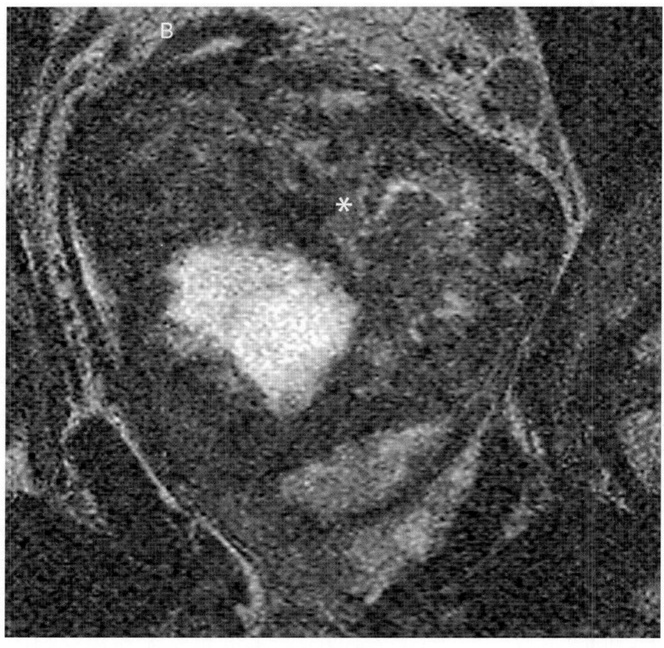

A

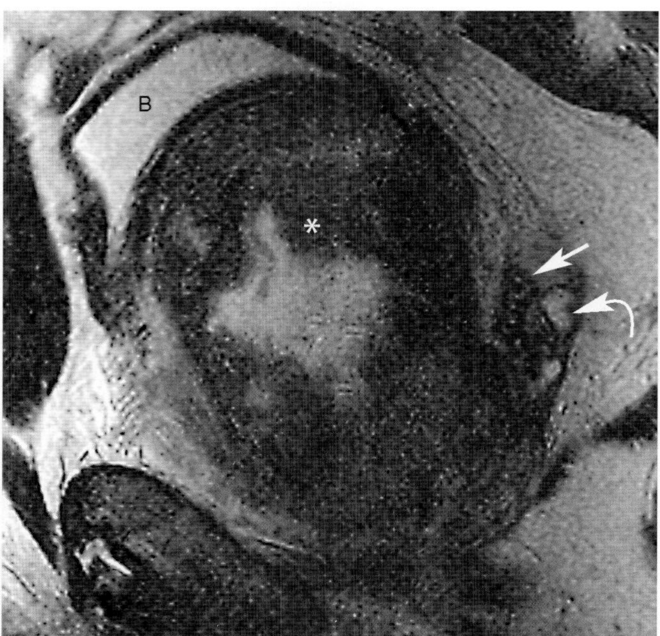

B

Figure 11-18 Prostate Leiomyosarcoma
This 48-year-old man complained of dysuria, decreased urinary stream, and difficulty voiding. **A** and **B**. Coronal and sagittal T2-weighted images show a very large partially necrotic prostatic mass (*asterisk*), which compresses the bladder (B). Note the vas deferens (*straight arrow*) and the seminal vesicle (*curved arrow*) in (B). Prostate carcinoma is usually not this large. BPH may have a similar appearance (see Figure 11-18 C and D) but does not demonstrate central necrosis, which is a feature suggestive of more aggressive histology.

In the central gland, by far, the most likely etiology of a focal lesion is a hyperplastic nodule; however, 20% of adenocarcinomas arise in the central gland and, therefore, tumor should be considered if a lesion has ill-defined margins, infiltrative growth, homogeneous signal, extracapsular extension, or if there are other findings to indicate malignancy (elevated PSA, evidence of metastatic disease).

In the peripheral zone, tumor is more common than in the central gland but must be distinguished from the wide variety of other benign conditions that may result in a focal abnormality, including BPH, prostatitis, postbiopsy hemorrhage, fibrosis, infarction. Imaging features concerning for a malignant lesion include disruption of prostatic architecture, the presence of mass effect (capsular bulge), extraprostatic extension, and metastatic disease. Clinical features supporting a diagnosis of adenocarcinoma include older age and abnormally elevated and/or rising PSA. Unusual prostatic neoplasms are often indistinguishable from adenocarcinoma but sometimes might be suspected based on a number of factors, including: unusual patterns of metastatic disease (eg, visceral organ involvement, lytic bone lesions), normal PSA, history of lymphoma or other primary tumor, unusual age group (eg, rhabdomyosarcoma in children), or large size (sarcoma). Regarding benign lesions, only hemorrhage may be specifically identified based on the characteristic T1 hyperintense appearance of blood on MRI with a history of prior biopsy. Chronic prostatitis, on the other hand, may have identical signal to a localized prostate cancer. However, chronic prostatitis might be suggested if a lesion has no mass effect, does not disrupt the architecture of the peripheral zone, and is found in the setting of a normal PSA in a young age group. BPH nodules usually have mixed signal due to glandular and stromal components (in contrast to tumor that is typically homogeneous) and usually have well-defined borders. Changes related to treatment (chemotherapy, radiation therapy, collagen injections) may be suggested by the appropriate history and normal PSA. Although the features described here may hint at diagnosis, there is still extensive overlap in both the imaging appearance and clinical presentation of malignancy and benign lesions (except perhaps in the case of hemorrhage), and therefore biopsy is often necessary to establish a specific diagnosis.

Cystic Lesions of the Prostate

Cystic lesions are masses composed primarily of fluid-containing spaces. The appearance of a cystic lesion depends on its complexity (eg, the presence of solid components, septations) as well as the composition of the fluid (eg, proteinaceous, hemorrhagic, or simple). Cysts are considered simple if they satisfy the following criteria: fluid signal (low T1, high T2 on MRI, anechoic on US, and between 0 and 20 HU on CT), thin or imperceptible wall,

Imaging Notes 11-7. Imaging Features of Solid Prostate Nodules

Focal Solid-appearing Lesion in the Prostate	Helpful Features
Prostate adenocarcinoma	Low T1, Low T2; elevated PSA; ± METS
Other tumor (see below for details)	Likely will require biopsy for diagnosis
Prostatitis	Low T1, Low T2 Acute: pain, tenderness, fever, leukocytosis, phlegmon can look SOLID Chronic: may be indistinguishable from prostate adenocarcinoma; less of a tendency to disrupt normal reticular architecture, can be sterile or due to recurrent infection or atypical infections
Hemorrhage	High T1, Low T2; T1 signal tend to outline the tumor "MRI exclusion principle"
Seeds	Low T1, low T2; punctate; bloom on in phase sequences
BPH nodule	Usually more heterogenous than tumor, but may be indistinguishable and require biopsy
Treatment change (radiation, hormonal therapy)	Low T1, low T2 diffusely in small prostate; similar changes in seminal vesicles; history
Infarct	Low T1, low T2, no specific features
Mimic: Periurethral collagen injections	Low T1, low T2; history of prostatectomy and incontinence, normal PSA. Main Differential diagnosis (diff dx) is local recurrence

no internal structure, and no internal vascularity. On US, an additional feature of a cyst is the presence of "through transmission," which refers to an apparent increased brightness of the echoes deep to a structure because of a less than expected beam attenuation (as occurs with fluid). Cystic lesions not satisfying these criteria are considered complex, possibly because of infection, hemorrhage, or neoplasm. Manifestations of complex cysts include debris (which may appear as particulate fluid or echogenic material on US or as heterogenous signal or debris on MRI or CT), wall thickening, septations, and solid components. On all 3 cross-sectional imaging studies, enhancing soft-tissue components are a feature concerning for neoplasm.

The differential diagnosis for cystic lesions in and around the prostate can be divided into 3 categories: (1) intraprostatic cystic lesions, (2) extraprostatic cysts, and (3) cyst mimics (Table 11-4). Extraprostatic cysts will be discussed under the heading: **Disorders of the Seminal Vesicle and Periprostatic Tissues**.

Intraprostatic Cysts

Prostatic cysts are commonly subdivided according to location either close to the midline (referred to from here on as simply "midline") of off-midline. Of these, midline intraprostatic cysts are more common, occurring in up to 7.8% of asymptomatic men.[63] Midline cysts include prostatic utricle cysts, müllerian duct cysts, ejaculatory duct cysts, cystic tumors/BPH, and abscesses. Off-midline cysts include BPH nodules with cystic change, retention cysts, abscesses, and cystic tumors.[64] These entities will now be separately discussed.

Congenital cysts

Most congenital cysts are utricular and müllerian duct cysts.[5,64] Although ejaculatory duct cysts may also be congenital, they are discussed with acquired cysts. Müllerian and utricle cysts can be very difficult to differentiate from each other, although there are some differences that may suggest one diagnosis or the other.

Utricle cysts: The prostatic utricle is a midline blind pouch near the verumontanum that communicates with the urethra via an opening just superior to the ejaculatory ducts, It typically measures only a few millimeters in size. When the utricle is dilated, it is referred to as a "utricle cyst." Utricle cysts are the most common congenital intraprostatic cyst. They may be detected early in life because of the association of these cysts with a variety of genitourinary abnormalities, including hypospadia, cryptorchidism, and unilateral renal agenesis.[41] Interestingly, in patients with hypospadias, the size of the utricle appears to correlate with the severity of the hypospadias.[41] Aside from their association with genitourinary abnormalities, utricular cysts are usually clinically inapparent but occasionally, utricle cysts may present with irritative urinary tract symptoms, suprapubic pain, hematuria, infertility, or with postvoid dribbling (because of the communication with the urethra).[64]

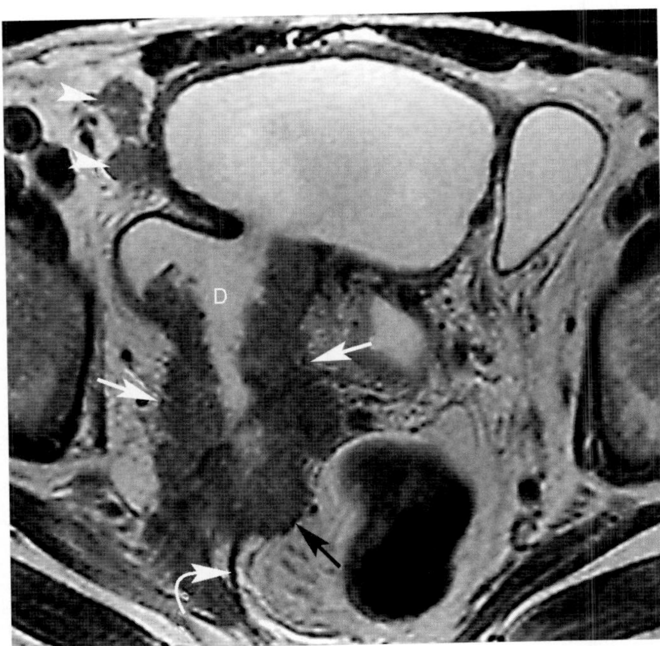

A

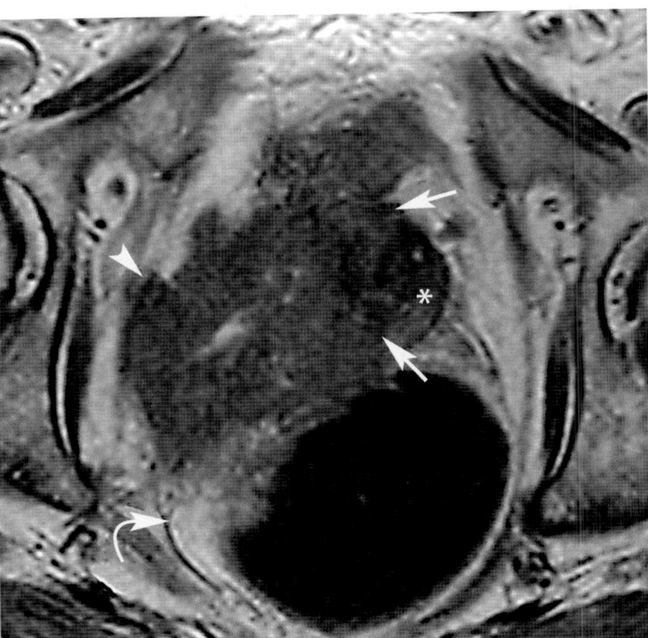

B

Figure 11-19 Direct Invasion of the Prostate by Bladder Carcinoma A 79-year-old man with invasion of the prostate by squamous cell carcinoma arising in a diverticulum. **A.** Axial T2-weighted image at the level of the bladder showing invasive squamous cell carcinoma (*white straight arrows*) arising in a right lateral bladder diverticulum (D) with malignant lymphadenopathy (*arrowheads*) and extramural tumor invading the mesorectal fascial (tumor indicated by *black arrow*, fascia indicated by *curved white arrow*). **B.** Axial T2-weighted image at the level of the prostate shows infiltrative tumor (*arrowhead*) with replacement of the right side of the prostate. The boundary of the tumor with the residual more normal left prostate (*asterisk*) is indicated by *arrows*. Note the tumor extends to and probably through the mesorectal fascia (indicated by curved *white arrow*).

On imaging, uncomplicated utricle cysts are simple-appearing pear-shaped, midline cysts that arise at the level of the verumontanum and communicate with the urethra, usually measuring 4 to 6 mm at the blind end and extending 8 to 10 mm in length.[64] They can contain sperm, and typically are small enough that they do not extend above the prostate gland (see Figure 11-25). Complications of utricle cysts that may be identified by imaging include stones, secondary infection, internal hemorrhage, tumor (clear cell, squamous, or endometrioid histology), and ejaculatory duct obstruction. Superinfection and/or hemorrhage may be suggested by the presence of complex fluid, debris, septations, and wall thickening, whereas the presence of an enhancing solid component to the cystic lesions is suspect for carcinoma. Ejaculatory duct obstruction may be inferred from dilation of the ejaculatory duct and of the seminal vesicles, and can be a cause of infertility.

Müllerian duct cysts: Müllerian cysts are congenital cysts that arise from cephalic remnants of the müllerian duct.[41] They most commonly appear as midline cysts arising from the region of the verumontanum and mimic the more common utricular cyst (see Figure 11-26). However, in contrast to utricle cysts, which are always midline, some müllerian duct cysts will be found lateral to the midline. Müllerian cysts are also typically larger than utricular cysts and may extend above the base of prostate. Unlike utricle cysts, müllerian cysts never contain sperm, and usually do not communicate with the urethra. Like utricular cysts, müllerian duct cysts are typically asymptomatic but can occasionally present with dysuria, burning, hematuria, or infertility and may rarely be complicated by infection, internal hemorrhage, or carcinomatous degeneration. Müllerian cysts more commonly contain stones than other prostatic cysts.

Acquired noninfectious/nonneoplastic parenchymal cysts

The glandular and tubular structures surrounding the prostate can become obstructed leading to dilation of the tubules proximal to the obstruction. Both ejaculatory duct cysts and retention cysts can be due to this type of process. Cysts can also result from acinar atrophy.

Ejaculatory duct cysts: Ejaculatory duct cysts are a result of congenital or acquired obstruction of the ejaculatory duct. Rarely, ejaculatory duct "cysts" represent diverticula of the duct.[5,64] Ejaculatory duct cysts occur along the expected course of the ejaculatory ducts and, therefore, are midline when they occur at the level of the verumontanum and just lateral to the midline when they occur at the prostatic base (see Figure 11-27). When large, these may extend above the level of the prostate and simulate müllerian cysts but usually contain sperm on aspiration. The appearance varies depending on the presence of protein/hemorrhage related to prior infection. There may be associated dilation of the

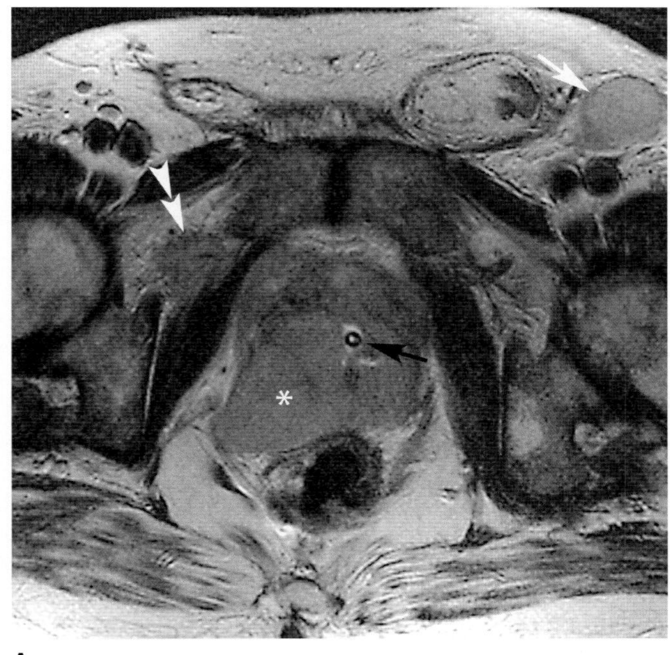

A

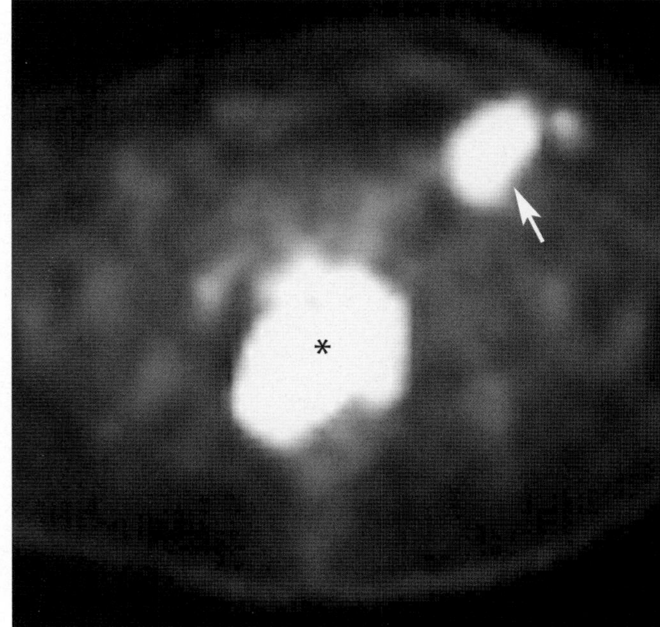

B

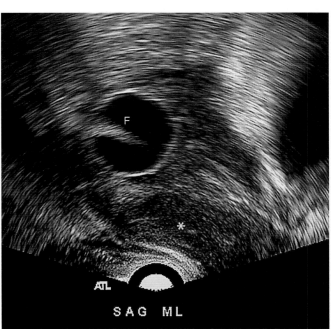

C

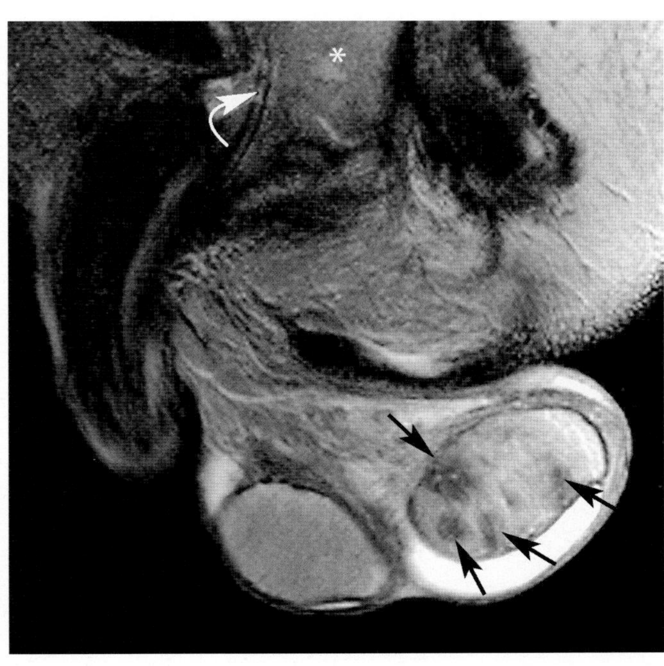

D

Figure 11-20 B-cell Lymphoma of the Prostate
A 74-year-old man who presented with bladder outlet obstruction and was found to have B-cell lymphoma on TURP. **A** and **B.** Axial T2-weighted image through the pelvis (A) and corresponding PET image at close to the same level (B) showing avid FDG uptake in the region of the prostate (*asterisk*) and left inguinal lymph nodes (*arrow*); the MRI image also shows a Foley catheter (*black arrow*). Multiple FDG-avid foci were also seen in the testicles and in other pelvic lymph nodes (*double arrowhead* in A). No bony lesions were seen. The pattern of lymphadenopathy, absence of bone lesions, presence of testicular lesions, and uptake on PET are atypical for prostate cancer and suggest another diagnosis, in this case, lymphoma. **C.** Sagittal transrectal sonographic image showing Foley catheter in place (F) and diffusely decreased echogenicity in the prostate (*asterisk*), which was hypervascular on color Doppler (not shown). **D.** Sagittal T2-weighted image through the right testicle showing multiple lesions (*arrows*) that were FDG avid, in keeping with lymphoma. Partially visualized is the prostatic lymphoma (*asterisk*) and the Foley catheter (*curved arrow*).

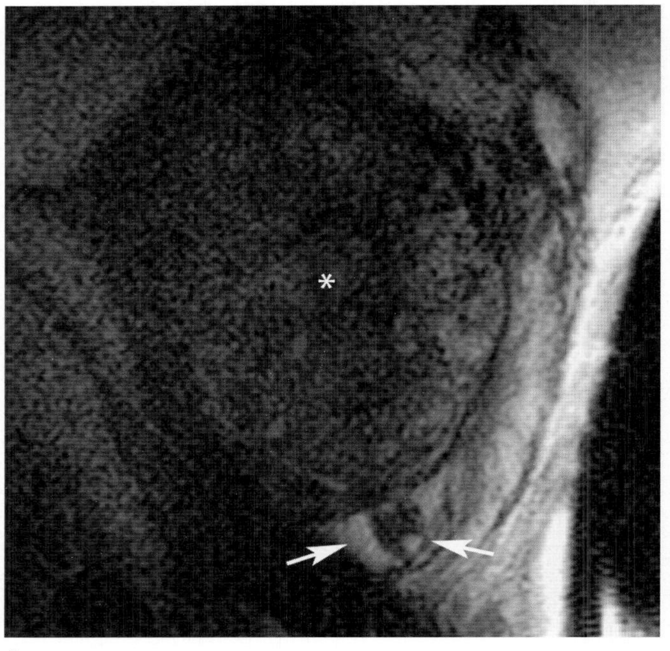

A

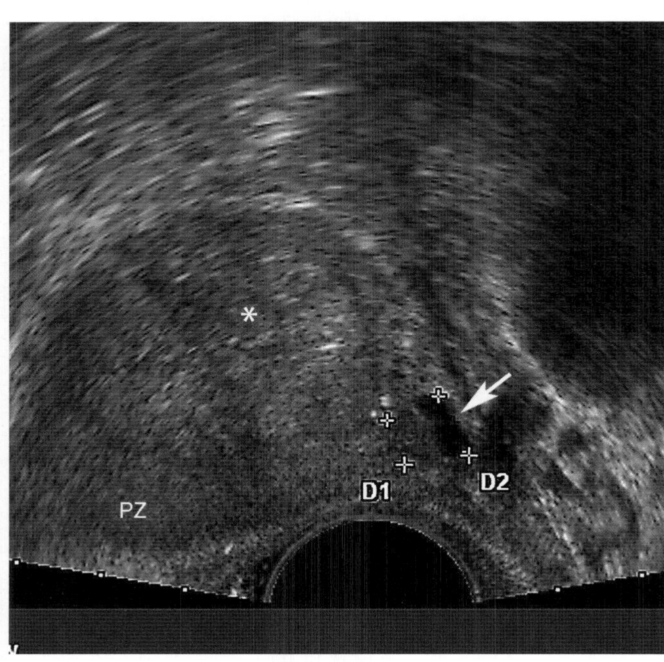

B

Figure 11-21 BPH in the Peripheral Zone
A. Sagittal T2-weighted image shows a mixed signal nodule in the apical peripheral zone (*arrows*) that was benign on histology, likely an exophytic BPH nodule protruding into the peripheral zone from the enlarged central gland (*asterisk*). **B.** Sagittal TRUS image showing mixed cystic and solid nodule in the apical peripheral zone corresponding to the nodule in (A). Cystic components are common in BPH and rare with tumor. PZ = peripheral zone.

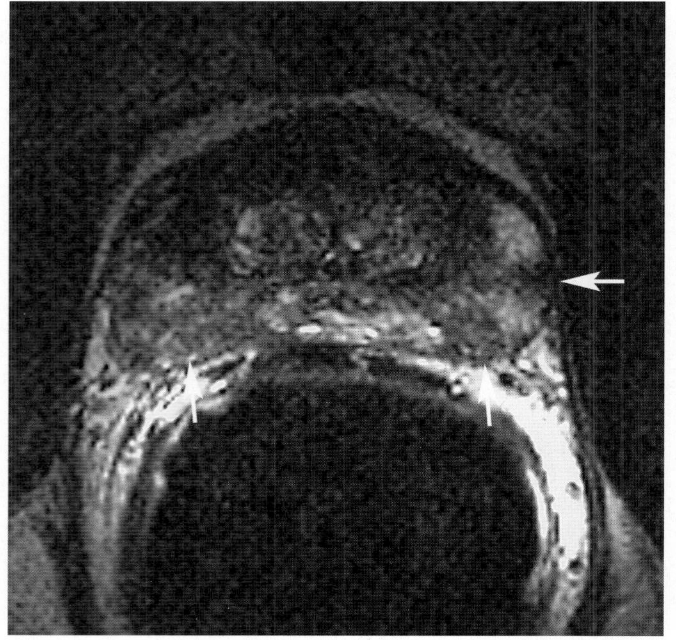

A

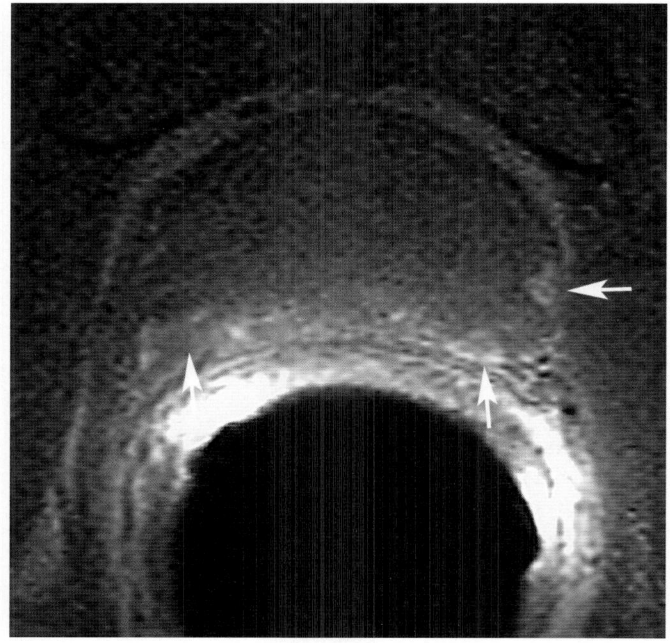

B

Figure 11-22 Postbiopsy Hemorrhage
A and **B.** Patchy postbiopsy hemorrhage. Axial T2-weighted (A) and axial T1-weighted image (B). On the axial T2-weighted image, the hemorrhage appears as low-signal areas (A, *arrows*) and corresponds to high signal foci on the T1-weighted image (B, *arrows*). Tumor would be expected to be low signal on the T1-weighted images (see Figure 11-5).

Table 11-3. Causes of Prostatitis

1. Acute
   a. Bacterial prostatitis
      i. *Escherichia coli*/other gram-negative rods
      ii. Enterococcus
      iii. Staphylococcus
2. Chronic
   a. Abacterial (sterile) prostatitis
   b. Bacterial prostatitis[a]
   c. Granulomatous prostatitis
      i. BCG bladder instillation
      ii. TB
      iii. Fungal infections
         Coccidiomycosis
         Blastomycosis
         Histoplasmosis
         Cryptococcus
      iv. Brucellosis
      v. *Treponema pallidum*
      vi. Parasites
         Schistosomiasis
         Echinococcus
      vii. Herpes simplex
      viii. Sarcoidosis
      ix. Wegener granulomatosis
      x. Post biopsy
      xi. Idiopathic

[a]Same organisms as acute bacterial prostatitis.

ipsilateral seminal vesicle. Sometimes, ejaculatory duct stones may be identified as the cause of the obstruction. Clinically, patients may have ejaculatory pain, infertility, hematospermia, and perineal pain.

Retention cysts/cystic atrophy: Retention cysts result from obstruction of prostatic glandular elements[64] and may occur anywhere in the prostate, including the peripheral zone. These are usually simple cysts measuring 1 to 2 cm in size. However, retention of secretions or acinar atrophy with cyst formation may also lead to areas of duct ectasia (microcysts), which appears as a "spongy" area in the lateral peripheral zone or transition zone. Atrophy with cyst formation may also appear as a multicystic nodule composed of tiny cysts.[65]

Cystic lesions associated with prostatitis

Patients with prostatitis can develop 2 cystic complications: abscess in patients with acute prostatitis and "cavitary" prostatitis in patients with chronic prostatitis.

Prostatic abscesses: Abscesses develop in approximately 0.5% to 2.5% of patients hospitalized for prostatitis.[57,58] Urinary pathogens such as coliform bacteria account for most abscesses. Atypical organisms may be found in immunosuppressed patients and in those at risk for hematogenous seeding of the prostate, such as patients with endocarditis or catheter-related infections. Risk factors for development of an abscess include diabetes mellitus, chronic renal dialysis, immunosuppression, chronic urinary catheterization, and recent urethral manipulation. Clinically, prostatic abscess is difficult to distinguish from prostatitis but may be suggested by poor response to antibiotic therapy. The diagnosis may be confirmed by TRUS-guided aspiration.

On all cross-sectional imaging modalities, prostatic abscess appears as a complex irregular, often multiseptated, fluid collection (see Figure 11-28). Frequently, CT or MRI will demonstrate inflammatory stranding in the periprostatic tissues. In some patients the prostatic abscess can extend into the periprostatic tissues including the

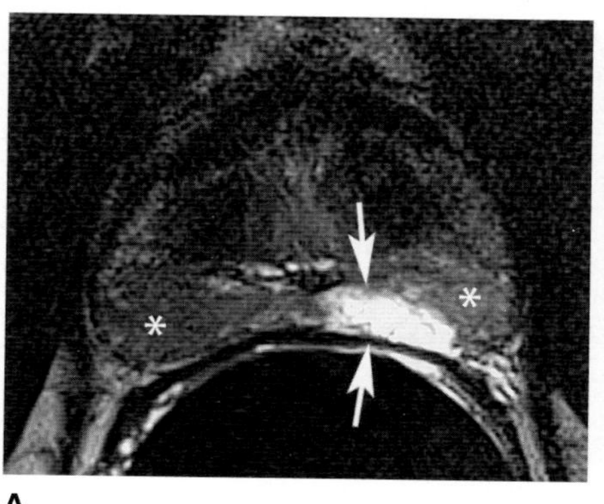

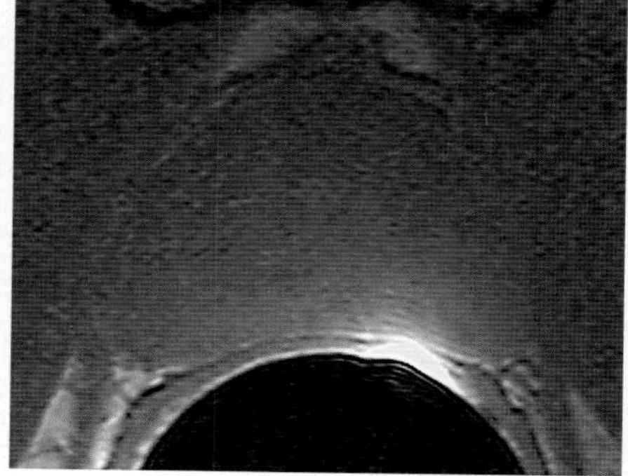

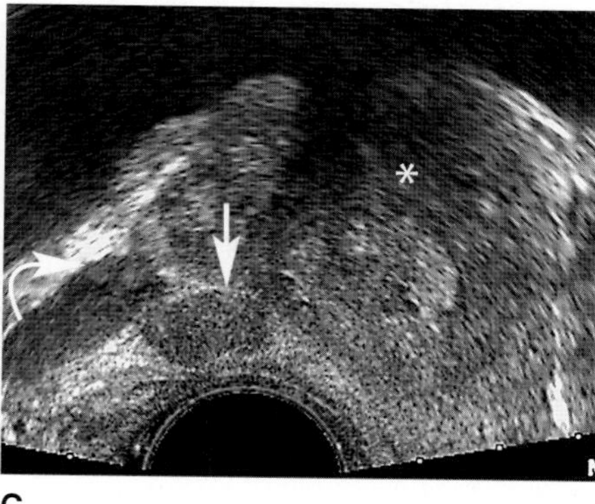

Figure 11-23 Chronic Examples of Prostatitis
A and **B.** Chronic prostatitis on MRI in a 40-year-old with pelvic pain, PSA measuring <1. Axial T2-weighted image (A) shows multiple foci of low signal in the peripheral zone (*asterisk*, compare to normal peripheral zone indicated by *arrows*) with isointense signal to prostate on T1-weighted images (B). These signal characteristics are identical to tumor; however, chronic prostatitis might be suggested based on clinical factors as well as by relative lack of mass effect, patchy appearance, and relative preservation of collagenous network. **C.** Prostatitis on US. Sagittal TRUS image demonstrates a hypoechogenic nodule (*straight arrow*) with hypervascularity on color Doppler (not shown), indistinguishable from prostate carcinoma; this was chronic prostatitis on biopsy. Note BPH (*asterisk*) and seminal vesicle (*curved arrow*).

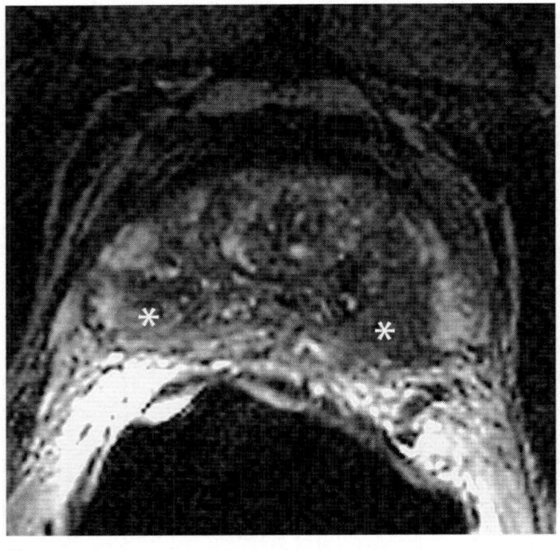
A

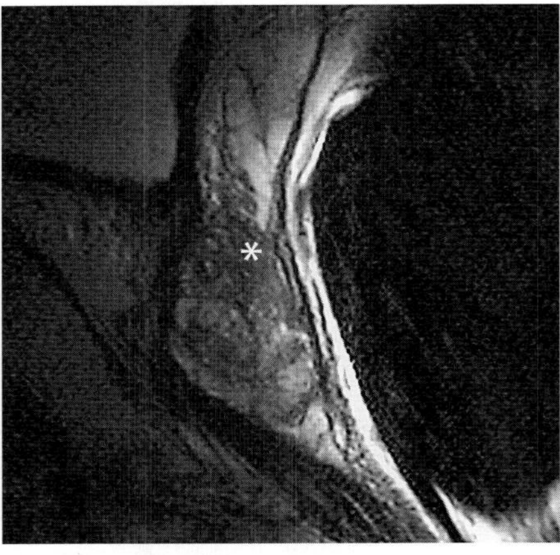
B

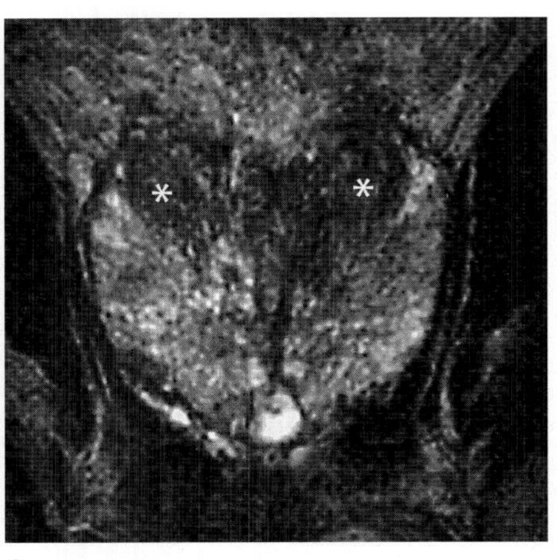
C

Figure 11-24 Volume Averaging Mimicking Prostate Cancer **A.** Axial T2-weighted image demonstrating low-signal areas (*asterisk*) in the region of the base, producing an appearance similar to prostate cancer. **B** and **C.** Sagittal (B) T2-weighted image shows that these areas (*asterisk*) correspond to normal tissue subjacent to the seminal vesicles. This tissue can also be recognized by a characteristic appearance on coronal T2-weighted images as symmetric low-signal areas (*asterisk*) at the base. Cross-referencing in this way can prevent misinterpretation as tumor.

seminal vesicles. Rarely, prostatic abscesses will contain gas. Peripheral hyperemia can be present that is seen as increased vascularity in the periprostatic tissues on color Doppler US and rim enhancement on CT and MRI. The important distinguishing features between prostatic abscesses and other cystic lesions are (1) clinical symptoms of infection, (2) presence of inflammatory stranding, and (3) rim enhancement. Abscesses greater than 1.5 cm typically required drainage, which can be performed under TRUS guidance, with a success rate of more than 80% in conjunction with antibiotics.[58]

Table 11-4. Differential Diagnosis Cystic Prostate Lesions

A. Intraprostatic cystic lesions
1. Müllerian duct cysts and prostatic utricle cysts
2. Ejaculatory duct cysts
3. Prostatic retention cysts
4. Cystic degeneration of benign prostatic hypertrophy
5. Cysts associated with tumors
6. Infectious, inflammatory, and parasitic cysts
7. Ejaculatory duct diverticulum
B. Periprostatic cystic lesions
1. Seminal vesicle cysts
2. Cysts of the vas deferens
3. Cowper gland cysts
4. Cystic neoplasms
5. Collections (abscess, hematoma)
C. Entities that may mimic prostatic and periprostatic cystic lesions
1. Defect from transurethral resection of the prostate
2. Hydroureter and ectopic insertion of the ureter
3. Bladder diverticulum
4. Prominent seminal vesicles

Modified from Curran S, Akin O, Agildere AM. Endorectal MRI of prostatic and periprostatic cystic lesions and their mimics. *AJR Am J Roentgenol.* 2007 May;188(5):1373-1379.

Cavitary prostatitis: Some patients with chronic prostatitis will develop the complication known as cavitary prostatitis. Chronic prostatitis can result in fibrosis and constriction of the intraprostatic ducts that can result in acinar dilation and breakdown of interacinar tissue, ultimately leading to the formation of small cavities. The imaging appearance of cavitary prostatitis has been described as a "swiss cheese prostate" because of the presence of multiple cysts of varying sizes throughout the prostate gland. Cystic change in the setting of BPH can have a similar appearance, but a clinical history of chronic prostatitis would support a diagnosis of cavitary prostatitis.[64]

Cystic neoplasms

Cystic neoplasms of the prostate are very rare. They can occur because of cystic degeneration or necrosis of an otherwise solid neoplasm or because the tumor

Imaging Notes 11-8. Features Suggesting Prostatic Abscess

Prostatic cyst with the following features:
1. Clinical symptoms suggesting infection
2. Rim enhancement
3. Periprostatic fat stranding
4. Gas within the cyst

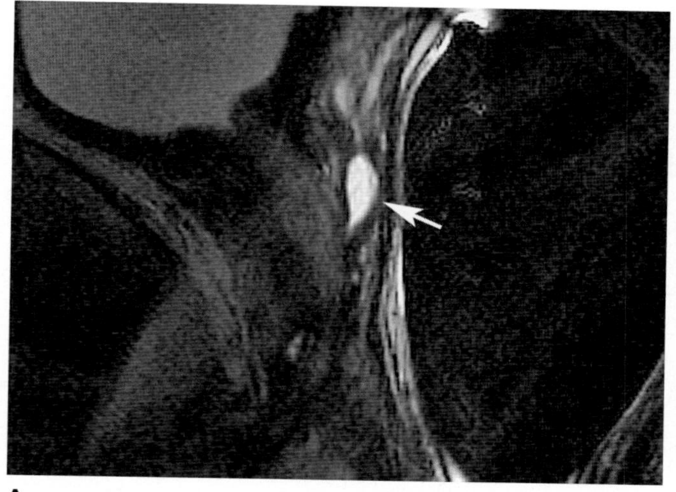

A

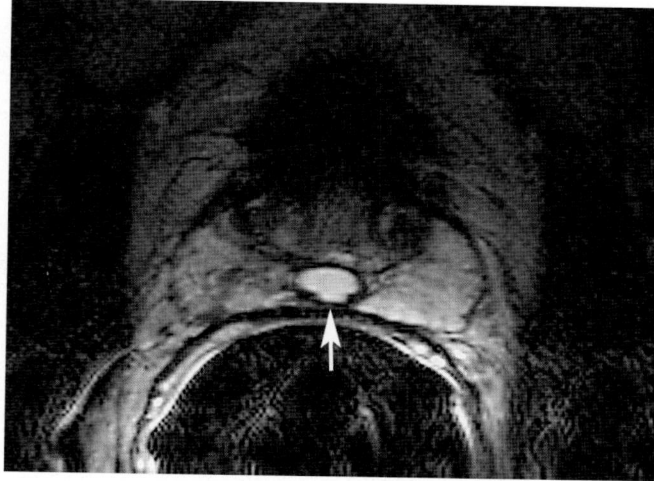

B

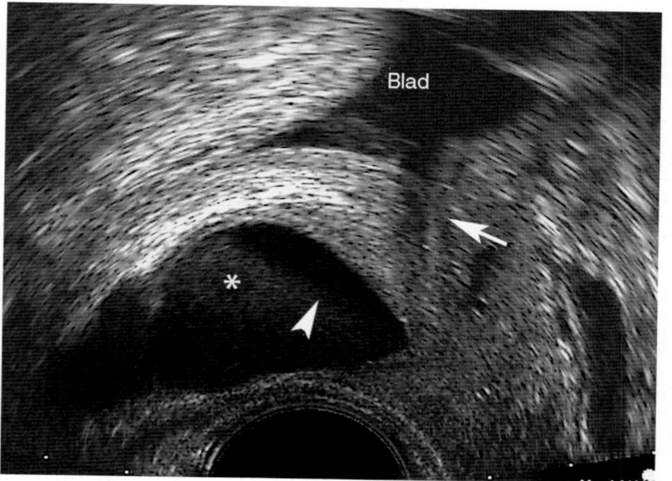

C

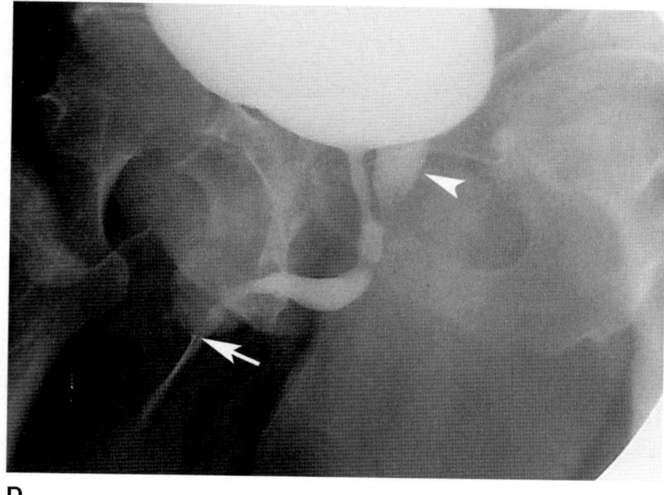

D

Figure 11-25 Utricle Cyst
A and B. Utricle cyst on MRI. Sagittal (A) and axial (B) T2-weighted images show intraprostatic midline cyst extending from region of verumontaum, consistent with a utricle cyst. **C.** Utricle cyst on US in a different patient. Sagittal TRUS showing a large utricle cyst (*asterisk*) containing debris (*arrowhead*); note urethra (*arrow*) anteriorly. **D.** Utricle cyst on voiding cystourethrogram. Fluoroscopic image from a voiding cysoturethrogram in a patient with hypospadias (*arrow*, note inferior location of meatus) showing a large pear-shaped contrast collection (*arrowhead*) communicating with the urethra (*arrow*), in keeping with a utricle cyst. Hypospadias is associated with utricle cysts.

itself is composed of or arises from a "true" cyst (see Figure 11-29).[43,66] Neoplasms that are associated with "true" cysts include the benign multilocular cystadenoma and the malignant papillary cystadenocarcinoma.[67-70]

Benign prostatic hyperplasia with cystic degeneration

Cystic degeneration of the nodules of BPH is the most commonly observed cystic lesion of the prostate.[64] Multiple cystically degenerated BPH nodules are frequently seen in the same individual. They can occur anywhere in the transition zone and therefore can be midline or off-midline and usually appear as multilocular nodule sharply delineated from normal parenchyma by a pseudocapsule.[65] These cysts can contain hemorrhagic fluid because of infarction and necrosis of the hyperplastic nodules (see Figure 11-30).[64]

Other rare cystic lesions of the prostate

Other rare causes of intraprostatic cysts include parasitic cysts (echinococcal or bilharziasis), dermoid cysts, and the phyllodes variant of atypical prostatic hyperplasia.[5]

Lesions that mimic cysts of the prostate

Mucinous adenocarcinoma and glandular-rich BPH nodules can appear as very hyperintense lesions on T2-weighted MRI sequences because of the presence of mucin in the

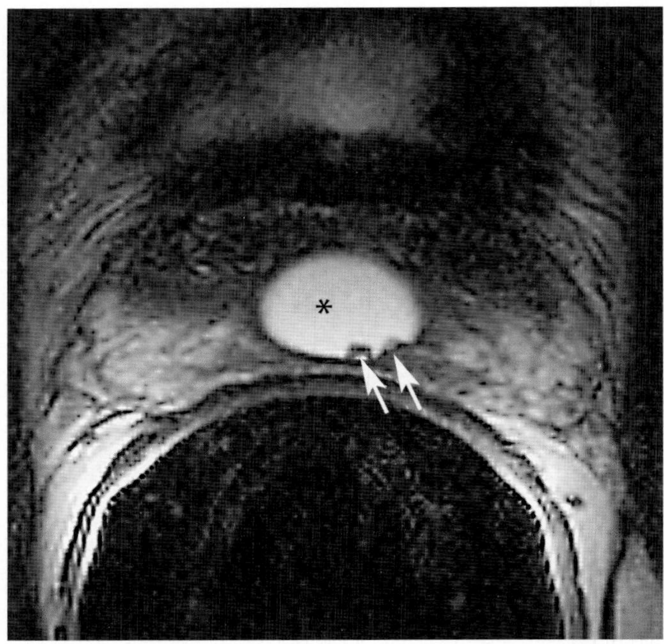

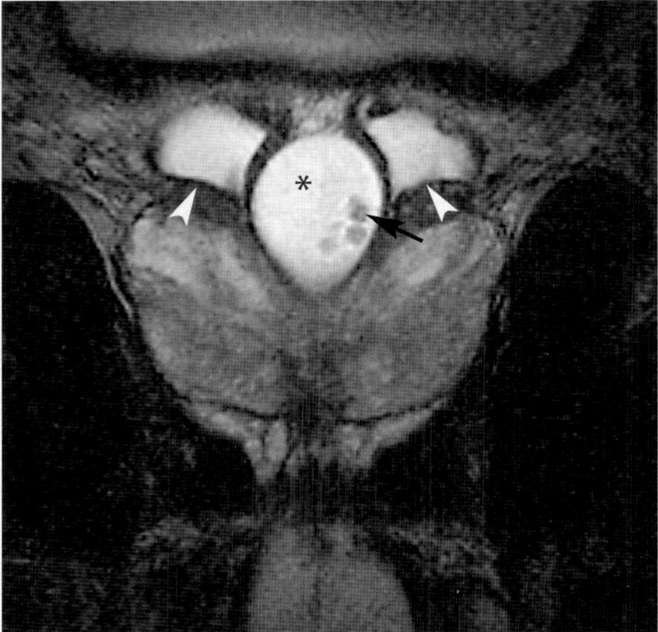

Figure 11-26 Müllerian Cyst
Axial (**A**) and coronal (**B**) T2-weighted images showing midline cystic pear-shaped structure (*asterisk*) extending outside the prostate and containing low-signal foci in a dependent location (*arrows*) reflecting calculi. Note the dilation of the ejaculatory duct/excretory ducts (*arrowhead*) suggestive of partial obstruction due to mass effect from the cyst.

tumor and glandular-rich components in the BPH nodule. In cross section, the defect of a TURP can appear as a central cystic area within the prostate.

Mucinous adenocarcinoma: Mucinous adenocarcinoma is a rare variant of prostate adenocarcinoma accounting for less than 2% of tumors. It is defined as a tumor in which at least 25% of the volume of the tumor consists of extracellular mucin and there is no extraprostatic site of tumor that could metastasize to the prostate gland.[37] Mucinous adenocarcinoma tends to be of higher grade than conventional adenocarcinomas and is typically a more aggressive malignancy.[38,44] On T2-weighted MRI sequences, the mucin content of the tumor causes the signal intensity of these tumors to approach that of fluid and can mimic a multiloculated lesion of the prostate (see Figure 11-31).[71] Although US or intravenous contrast can confirm that the lesion is noncystic, biopsy may be necessary to distinguish the lesion from glandular-rich BPH.

Glandular-rich hyperplastic nodules: Nodules associated with BPH have a variable imaging appearance depending on the distribution of stromal and glandular components. Nodules that are glandular rich will be very T2 hyperintense on MRI and, therefore, may demonstrate signal intensity approaching that of fluid (see Figure 11-32). The presence of a well-defined pseudocapsule is suggestive of a BPH nodule as opposed to a mucinous tumor, which is more likely to have infiltrative margins.

Transurethral prostatectomy defect: Transurethral resection of the prostate is commonly performed to treat obstructive symptoms related to BPH. In the procedure, periurethral glandular tissue is removed through the

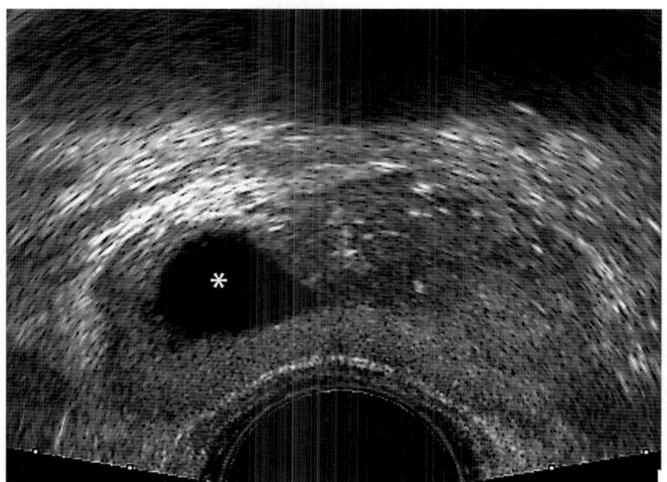

Figure 11-27 Ejaculatory Duct Cyst
Axial transrectal image through the prostate showing an eccentrically located cystic structure (*asterisk*) in the expected region of the right ejaculatory duct. This was not present on MRI (not shown) 2 years ago, and is in keeping with an acquired, as opposed to congenital, cyst.

Imaging Notes 11-9. Distinguishing Features of Prostatic Cysts

Cyst Type	Distinguishing Features
Utricular cyst[a]	Midline, usually small, originates near verumontanum, intraprostatic, communicates with urethra, association with congenital abnormalities, may contain sperm
Mullerian cyst[a]	Midline to off midline, originates near verumontanum, variable in size but usually larger than utricle cyst, may extend above base of prostate, doesn't communicate with urethra, stones more common than utricle cysts, usually no associated congenital anomalies
Ejaculatory duct cyst[a]	Paramedian but may appear almost midline, variable in size with possible extraprostatic extension, may contain sperm, may be associated with seminal vesicle dilation
Retention cysts	May occur anywhere but usually off midline, usually small (1-2 cm), no sperm on aspiration, no communication with genitourinary tract
Cystic BPH	Usually central gland, associated with BPH nodules
Abscess	Off midline, variable size, complex cystic lesion with irregular borders; may demonstrate gas, peripheral hypervascularity, periprostatic inflammatory change; pus on aspiration
Cavitary prostatis	Multiple small cystic lesions, "Swiss cheese" prostate
Necrotic prostate carcinoma	Any location, complex cystic lesion with solid tissue components, usually relatively small
Multilocular cystadenoma, cystadenocarcinoma	Large size, often with extraprostatic extension, multiloculated cystic mass
Mimics of cystic lesions (T2 hyperintense on MRI), glandular-rich BPH and mucinous variant prostate carcinoma	Enhance with contrast or internal vascularity or solid appearance on ultrasound (mucinous or glandular lesions); TURP defect—characteristic appearance of irregular widening of region of urethra on sagittal or coronal images

[a]Usually simple appearing unless complicated by infection, hemorrhage or rarely by neoplasm.

urethra, producing a characteristic defect in the central gland that communicates with the bladder superiorly and is contiguous with the urethra inferiorly. On longitudinal images, this will appear as widening of the prostatic urethra. However, on transaxial images, the TURP defect will appear as an oval fluid collection in the central portion of the gland, just inferior to the base of the bladder (see Figure 11-33).

DIFFUSE ENLARGEMENT OF THE PROSTATE

Diffusely enlarged prostate gland may be due to BPH, prostatitis, or diffuse tumor.

Benign Prostatic Hyperplasia

Benign prostatic hyperplasia ("benign prostatic hypertrophy") is due to hyperplasia, not "hypertrophy," of the stromal and epithelial elements of the prostate, predominately in the periurethral transition zone. This process is thought to be androgen dependent and leads to enlargement of the transition zone via the development of hyperplastic nodules. These lesions range from nodules composed primarily of fibromuscular stroma to nodules that are primarily composed of glandular elements.[1] The total prostate volume increases from approximately 25 mL for men in their 30s to 35 to 45 mL for men in their 70s, and the transition zone volume increases from 15 to 25 mL for similarly aged men.[72] Up to 4% of men older than age 70 have prostates greater than 100 mL.[73] The development of BPH nodules can lead to compression and obstruction of the urethra. Interestingly, there is no direct correlation between size of the prostate and the degree of obstruction.

Imaging Notes 11-10. Diffuse Enlargement of the Prostate

Disorder	Helpful Features
BPH	Marked heterogenous enlargement of central gland; normal PZ architecture
Acute prostatitis	Pain, fever, leukocytosis; resolution with therapy
Tumor	Homogenous enlargement with irregular border; disruption of architecture; positive tumor markers (eg, PSA); metastases or local invasion

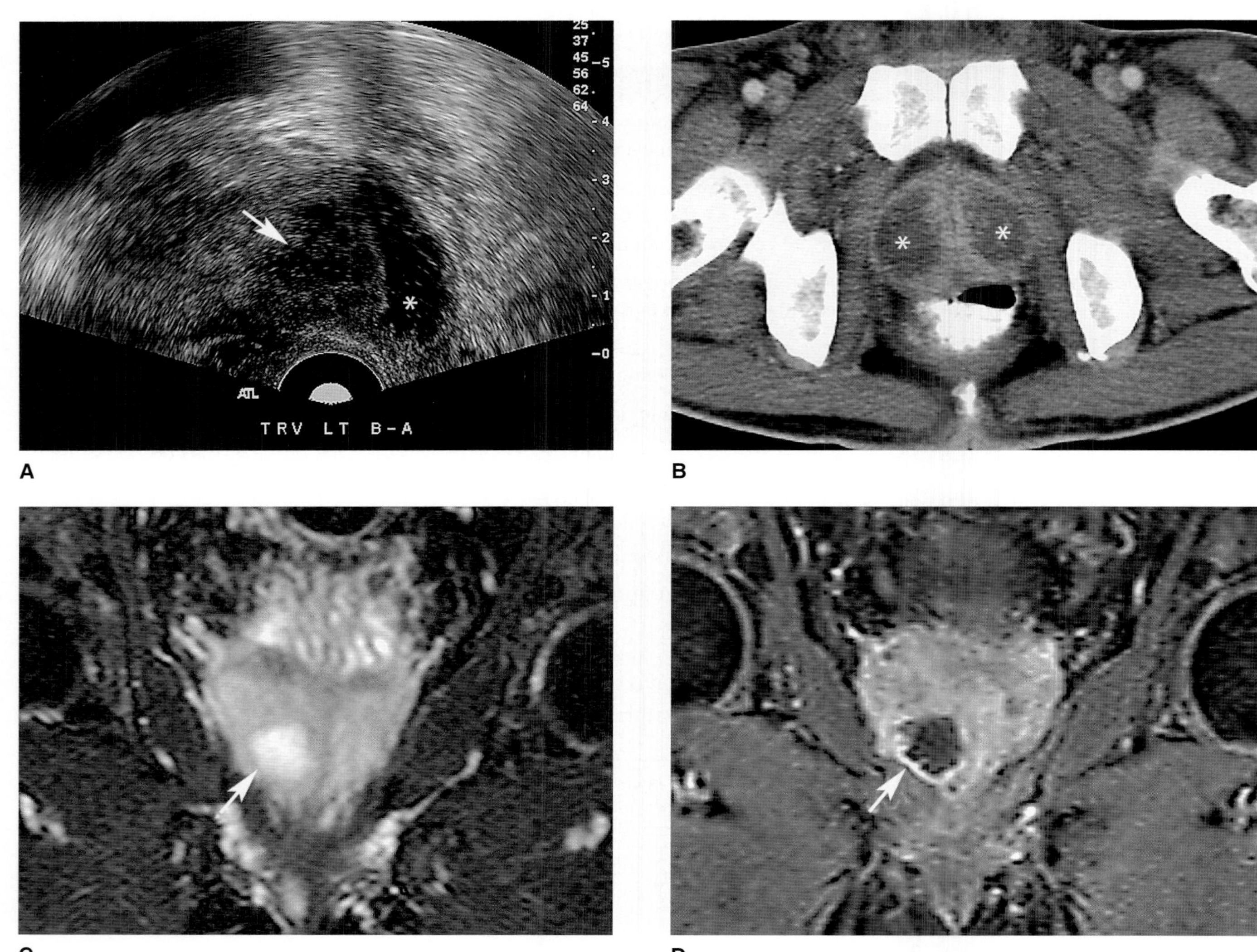

Figure 11-28 Prostate Abscesses
A. Acute abscess and prostatitis on US. Transrectal axial sonographic image demonstrates a vague irregular hypoechogenic region involving the left peripheral zone and central gland (*arrow*) that was hyperemic on color Doppler (not shown) reflecting prostatitis. There is also an irregular complex cystic area (*asterisk*) representing a prostatic abscess. **B.** Prostate abscesses on CT in a patient with *Klebsiella pneumoniae* infection. Axial enhanced CT image at the level of the prostate demonstrate low density rim enhancing areas (*asterisk*) in the prostate in keeping with abscesses due to septic emboli. **C** and **D.** Abscess on MRI, thought to be due to BCG therapy. Coronal T2-weighted (C) and coronal fat-saturated postgadolinium T1-weighted (D) images show a thick rim-enhancing fluid signal collection (*arrow*) in the right prostatic apex that developed following BCG therapy for bladder cancer.

The incidence of BPH increases with age and is generally not present below the age of 30, occurs in up to 50% of men between the ages of 51 and 60 and up to 88% of men older than age 80.[73] As a consequence, the incidence of obstructive symptoms due to BPH increases with age, affecting approximately 20% of men in their 40s and approximately 50% to 60% of men in their 70s.[72] Symptoms include decreased force of urinary stream, hesitancy, straining, nocturia, and urinary retention. If the degree of obstruction is severe, the patient may present with hydronephrosis and azotemia.

With BPH, there is enlargement of the central gland due to variable amounts of glandular and stromal elements in adenomatous nodules. On imaging, this appears as a multinodular central gland with heterogenous signal on MRI, heterogenous echotexture on US, and heterogeneous attenuation on CT (see Figure 11-34). Occasionally, BPH nodules will extend into the peripheral zone.[74] Imaging features that may help differentiate BPH nodules from prostate adenocarcinoma include the presence of mixed signal because of the presence of glandular and stromal elements and visible pseudocapsules.[26] With progressive

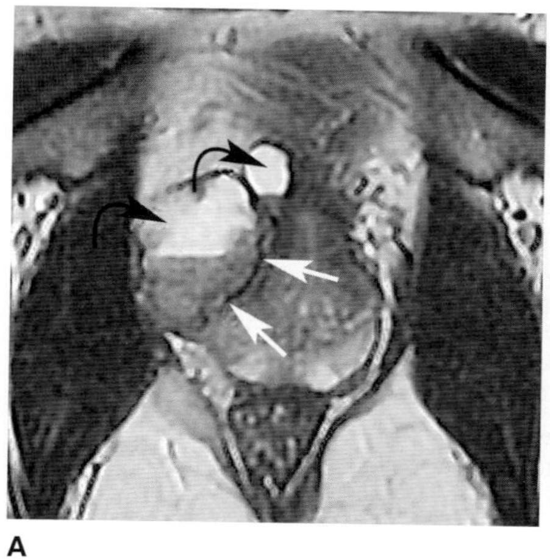

A

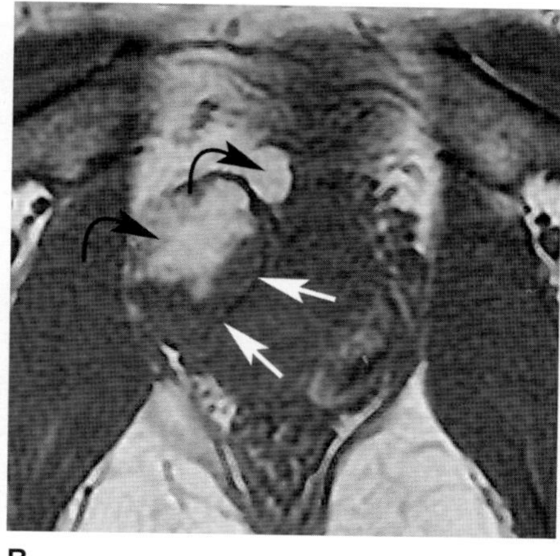

B

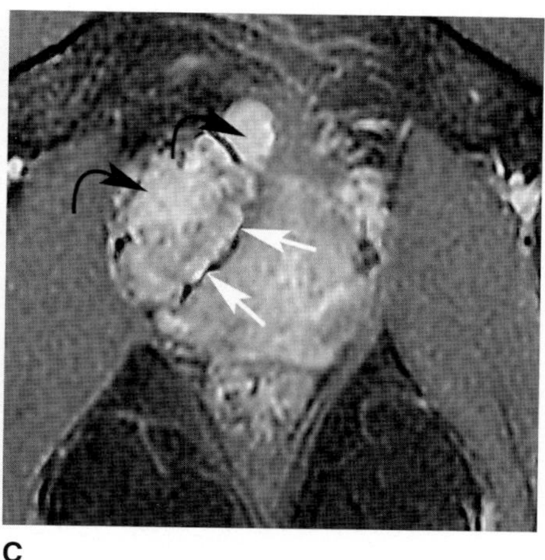

C

Figure 11-29 Cystic Malignancy of the Prostate
Gleason 9 tumor in a patient with PSA measuring 0.3, thought to be either ductal or transitional by histology. Axial T2-weighted (**A**), axial T1-weighted (**B**), and axial fat-saturated axial T1-weighted postgadolinium (**C**) sequences showing a mass with areas of cystic degeneration (*curved arrows*) with hyperintense T1 signal indicative of hemorrhage or protein, as well as peripheral solid-enhancing components (*straight arrows*).

enlargement of the central gland, the peripheral zone becomes compressed. A cleavage plane between the central gland and the peripheral zone becomes more visible and is termed the "surgical capsule" (or pseudocapsule). When BPH is identified, secondary findings related to urodynamically significant outlet obstruction may be present, including bladder wall thickening, trabeculation, saccules, diverticula, bladder stones, and hydronephrosis.

The enlarged prostate may protrude into the bladder base. At first glance, this might mimic a primary tumor of the urinary bladder; however, further inspection will reveal continuity of the "bladder mass" with the prostate, in keeping with prostatic origin.

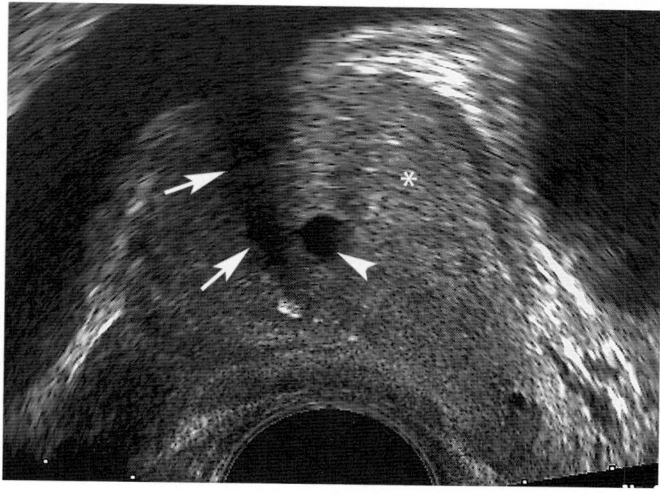

Figure 11-30 Cystic Change in BPH
Sagittal TRUS shows a subcentimeter anechoic space (*arrowhead*) in the central gland (*asterisk*) representing either cystic degeneration of a BPH nodule or a retention cyst; note the posterior bowing of the urethra (*arrows*), which is a finding seen with BPH.

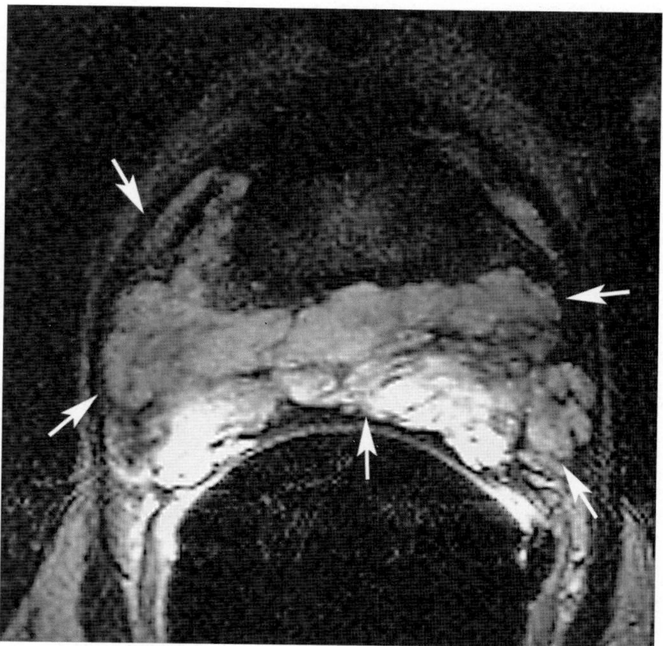

Figure 11-31 Mucinous Adenocarcinoma of the Prostate
A 75-year-old, PSA not available, with poorly differentiated tumor on biopsy. Axial T2-weighted image demonstrates a mass (*arrows*) with signal intensity approaching fluid, infiltrating much of the peripheral zone, and extending into the central gland. In this case, the high T2 signal of the mass is most in keeping with mucin in a mucinous adenocarcinoma, as opposed to representing fluid.

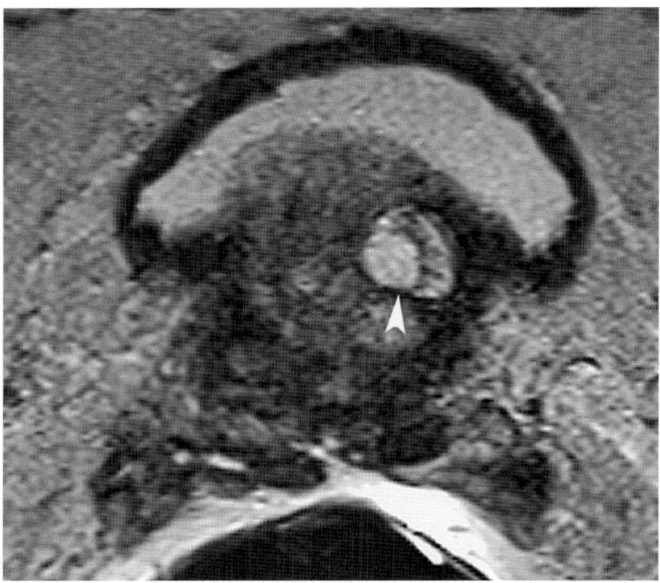

Figure 11-32 Glandular-Rich Hyperplastic Nodule
Axial T2-weighted image demonstrating a BPH nodule (*arrowhead*) that is predominately hyperintense on T2-weighted images, which could reflect either cystic change or a predominately glandular component to the nodule.

Acute Bacterial Prostatitis

Prostatitis is the most common urologic diagnosis in men younger than 50 years and the third most common urologic diagnosis in men older than 50 years, after benign prostatic hyperplasia and prostate cancer. Acute bacterial prostatitis is usually due to an ascending infection, with reflux of infected material into the prostate from either the ejaculatory ducts or the urethra.[1,57,58,75] Less commonly, seeding of the prostate may occur from lymphohematogenous routes. Prostatitis can also result from iatrogenic causes such as catheterization, biopsy, cystoscopy, surgical manipulation of the urethra or prostate, and other procedures. Most cases of acute prostatitis are caused by the bacteria responsible for urinary tract infections, including *Escherichia coli*, other gram-negative rods, enterococci, and staphylococci. Clinically, acute bacterial prostatitis presents with fever, chills, and dysuria, with a tender, warm boggy prostate on physical examination. Imaging is not necessary for establishing the diagnosis, which is based on the clinical features and urine culture, but may be helpful in identifying abscesses in those who fail to improve with antibiotic therapy.

On imaging, the prostate shows features of acute inflammation, including prostatic enlargement, increased vascularity, and surrounding inflammatory changes that

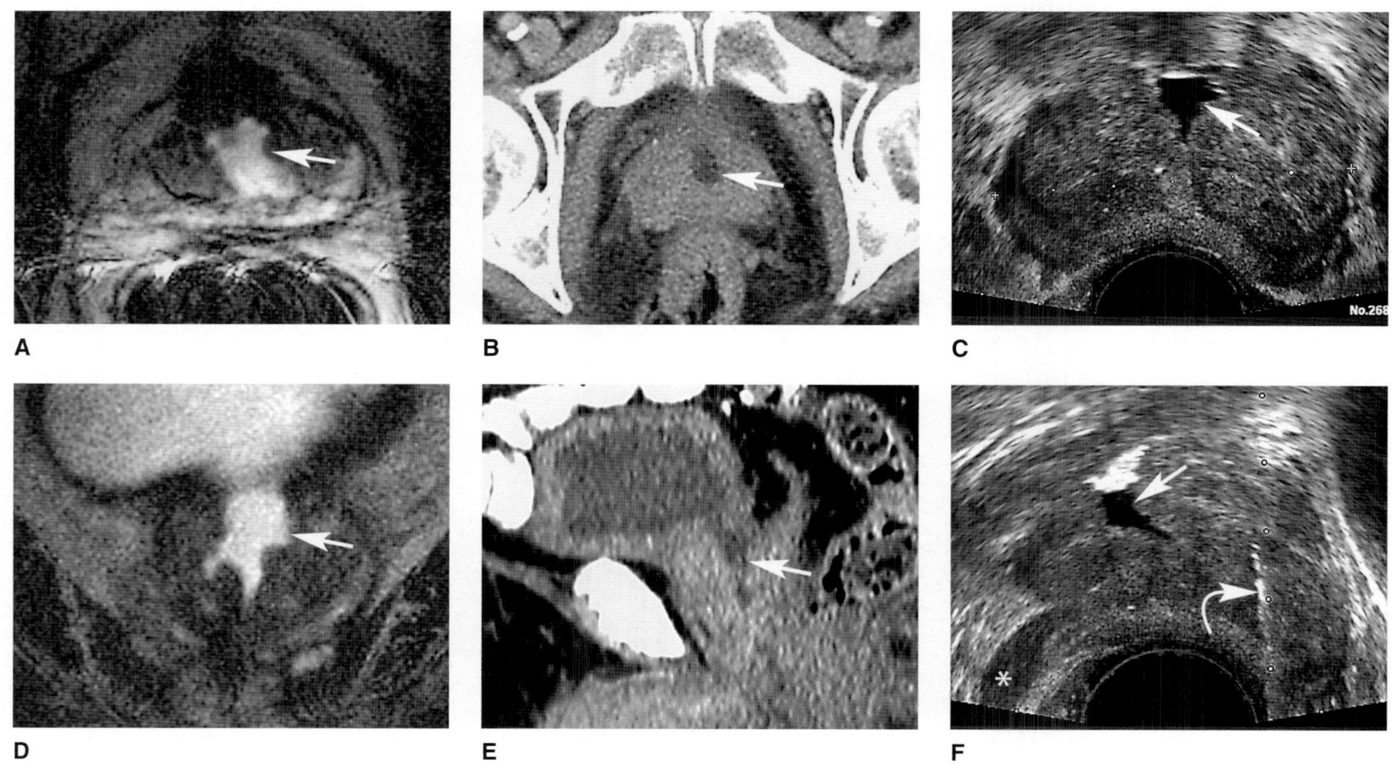

Figure 11-33 TURP Defect
A-C. Axial T2-weighted MRI (A), axial CT (B), and axial TRUS (C) images through the prostate demonstrating a fluid-filled area in the central aspect of the prostate (*arrow*), mimicking a cystic lesion. **D-F.** Coronal T2-weighted MRI (D), sagittal CT (E), and sagittal TRUS (F) images demonstrate the apparent "cystic" area, representing focal irregular widening of the urethra because of prior transurethral resection of the prostate (*arrow*). Note biopsy needle (*curved arrow*) and seminal vesicle (*asterisk*) in (F).

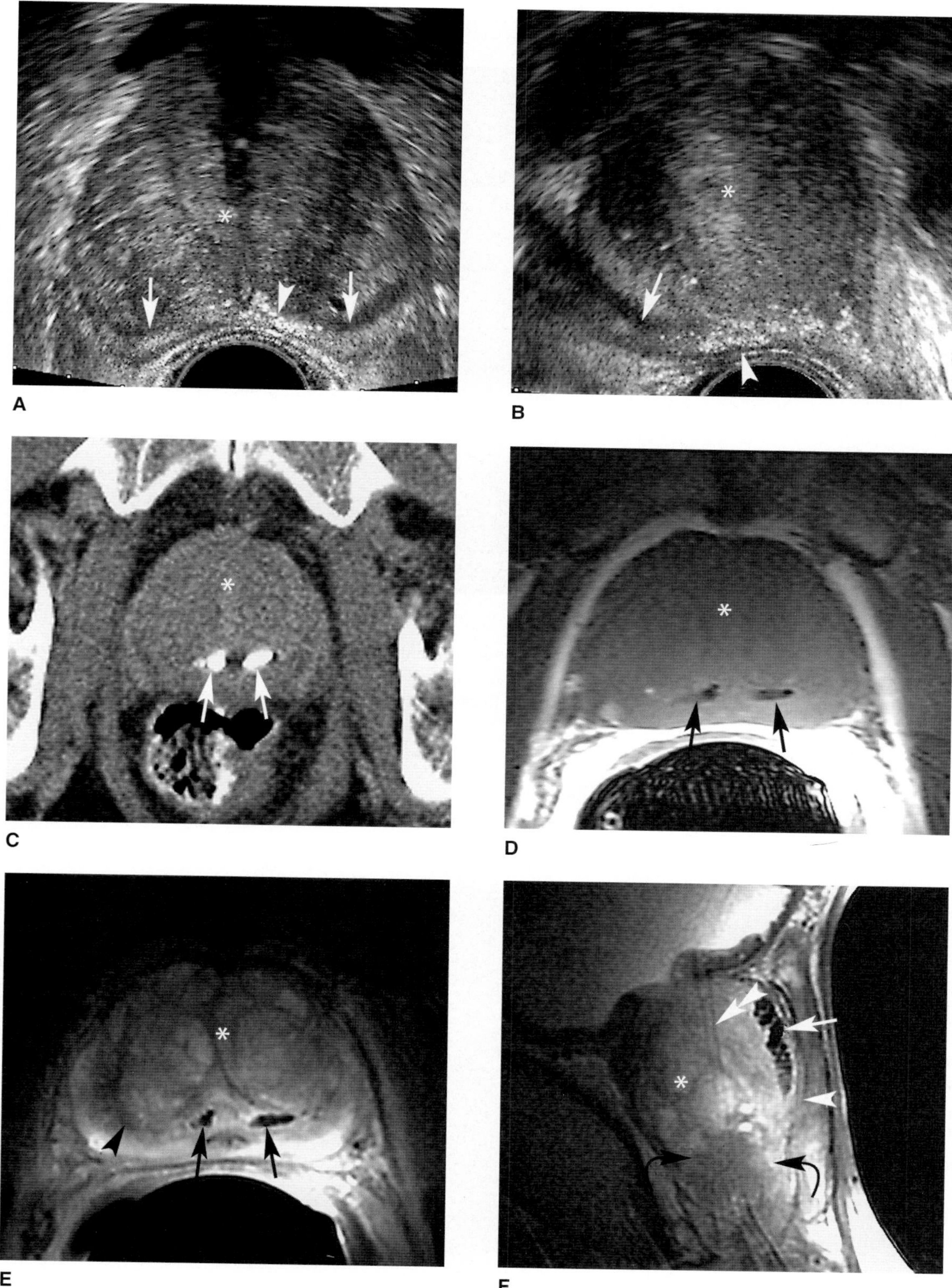

Figure 11-34 Benign Prostatic Hyperplasia (BPH)
A and **B.** BPH on US. Axial (A) and sagittal (B) TRUS images through the prostate demonstrating marked enlargement of the central gland (*asterisk* in all images) with compression of the peripheral zone. Note "surgical capsule" between the peripheral zone and central gland (*arrows*). Calcifications are present in the peripheral zone, likely from prior inflammation (*arrowheads*). **C-F.** BPH on MRI and CT in a separate patient. BPH is poorly visualized by CT scan (C) and by axial T1-weighted images (D) except as prostatic enlargement. Calcifications along the surgical capsule typical of corpora amylacea appear hyperdense on CT and low signal on MRI (*black arrows* in (D and E) and *white arrow* in (F)). Benign prostatic hyperplasia is well depicted on axial (E) and sagittal (F) T2-weighted images appearing as heterogenous enlargement of the central gland separated from the peripheral zone by the "surgical capsule" (*arrowhead*). Low signal tumor (*curved arrows* in F) is seen as loss of the normal heterogeneity of the central gland. Note mild posterior bowing of urethra (*double arrowhead*)

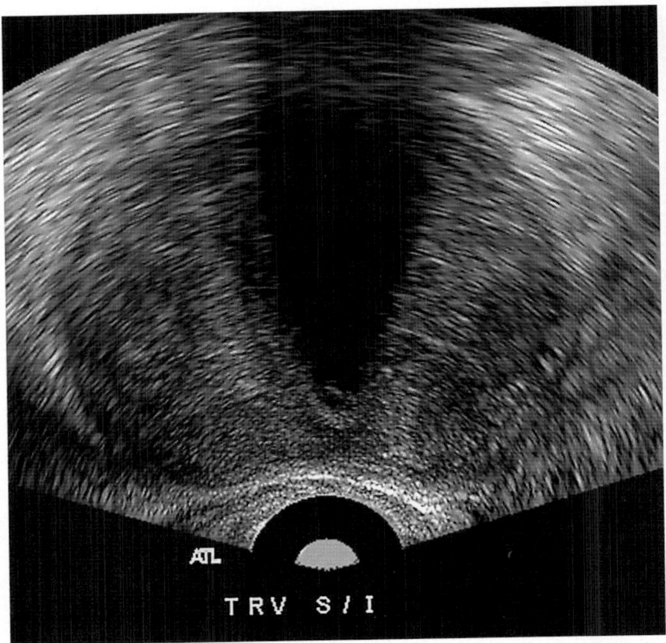

A

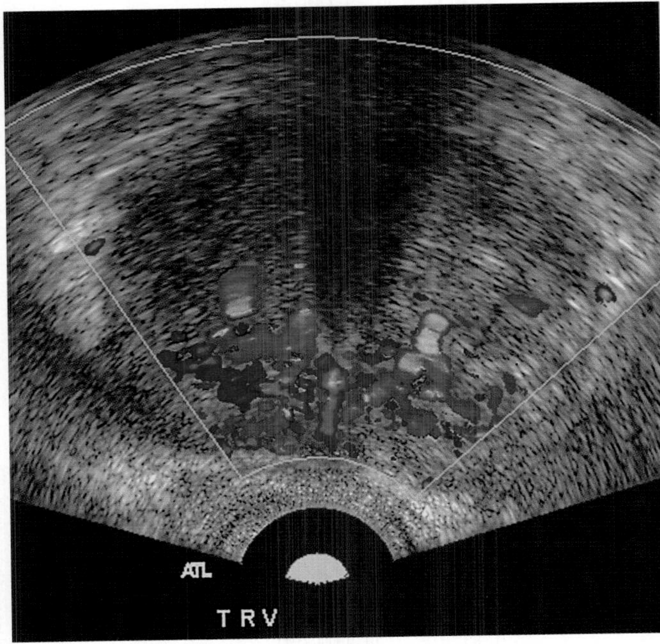

B

Figure 11-35 Acute Prostatitis
Transrectal US axial grayscale (**A**) and color Doppler (**B**) images of the prostate showing hypervascular hypoechoic enlarged prostate with poor differentiation of the peripheral zone and central gland. Compare this to the other examples in this chapter with BPH where there is preservation of normal prostatic architecture.

may involve the periprostatic fat and seminal vesicles.[57,58] On grayscale TRUS, the prostate is tender, rounded in configuration, and demonstrates loss of differentiation between the central gland and peripheral zone because of decreased echogenicity of the edematous peripheral zone (see Figure 11-35). Small focal hypoechoic areas may represent microabscesses or areas of more focal congestion and suppuration. Markedly increased vascularity is typical of acute bacterial prostatitis and is usually most pronounced around the seminal vesicles and ejaculatory ducts. In general, MRI and CT are rarely used in the setting of acute prostatitis but show analogous findings, with an enlarged, hypervascular gland with diffusely abnormal peripheral zone signal (MRI) associated with periprostatic inflammatory change.

Chronic prostatitis has been discussed under the heading: **Solid Focal Prostate Lesions**.

Diffuse Prostate Carcinoma

Most prostate malignancies will appear as a focal mass on US and MRI examinations of the prostate. However, occasionally tumor will diffusely infiltrate the prostate. In this situation, the prostate usually is enlarged and there is usually loss of normal tissue architecture, including obliteration of the normal distinction between the peripheral zone and central gland, as may be seen on MRI and US (see Figures 11-14 and 11-36). Because of the relatively poor tissue

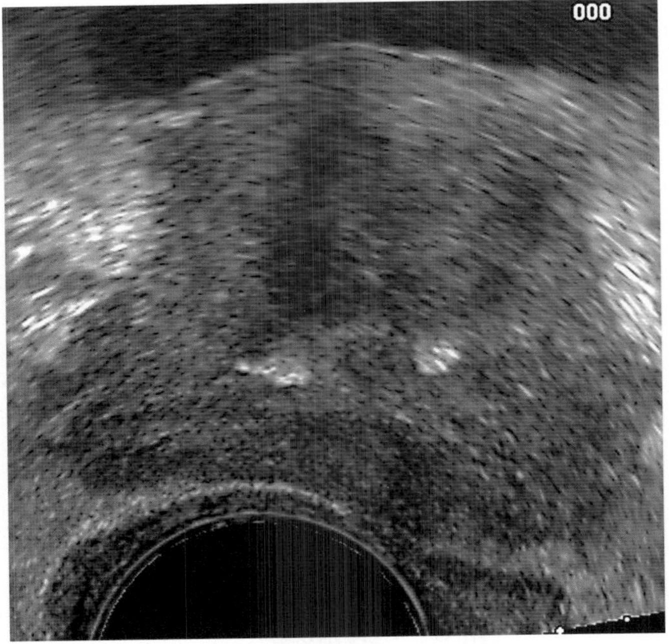

Figure 11-36 Diffuse Prostate Adenocarcinoma
Transrectal US axial image demonstrates diffuse enlargement and infiltration of prostate similar to diffuse prostatitis in Figure 11-35. In this case, this represented diffuse infiltration of the prostate by adenocarcinoma.

contrast on CT compared with MRI, diffuse tumor may appear only as enlargement of the prostate. However, other findings detectable by CT may point to malignancy, including tumor infiltration of the periprostatic tissues/local organ invasion, lymphadenopathy, and metastatic disease.

Prostate Lymphoma

Prostate lymphoma can present as diffuse prostatic enlargement (see Figure 11-37). Prostate lymphoma is discussed more completely under the heading: **Solid-Appearing Focal Prostate Lesions.**

DIFFUSELY ABNORMAL SMALL PROSTATE AND MIMICS

A small prostate in an older man may be from radiation or chemotherapy for prostate cancer. Occasionally, what appears to be a small prostate represents residual glandular tissue or malignancy following prostatectomy, or collagen injections for incontinence following prostatectomy.

Imaging Notes 11-11. Small-Appearing Prostate with Diffuse Signal Abnormality

Cause	Helpful Features
Posttreatment change	History of prostate cancer and treatment with hormone/ radiation therapy; presence of brachytherapy seed or RF markers, marrow changes from radiation
Periurethral collagen injections	History of postprostatectomy incontinence; undetectable PSA
Local recurrence	History of prostatectomy, elevated PSA
Residual prostate tissue	History of prostatectomy or TURP

Prostatic Atrophy

The most common causes of prostate atrophy are radiation therapy, either external beam radiation or brachytherapy, and/or hormonal therapy for prostate cancer (see Figure 11-38). On MRI, atrophy appears as a small gland with overall decreased T2 signal resulting in diminished contrast between the peripheral zone and the central gland. On US, the prostate appears diffusely decreased in echogenicity. The normal contour and architecture of the prostate is usually preserved. Other imaging clues to the diagnosis include radiation change, fatty replacement of the marrow in the osseous pelvis, or visualization of brachytherapy seeds.

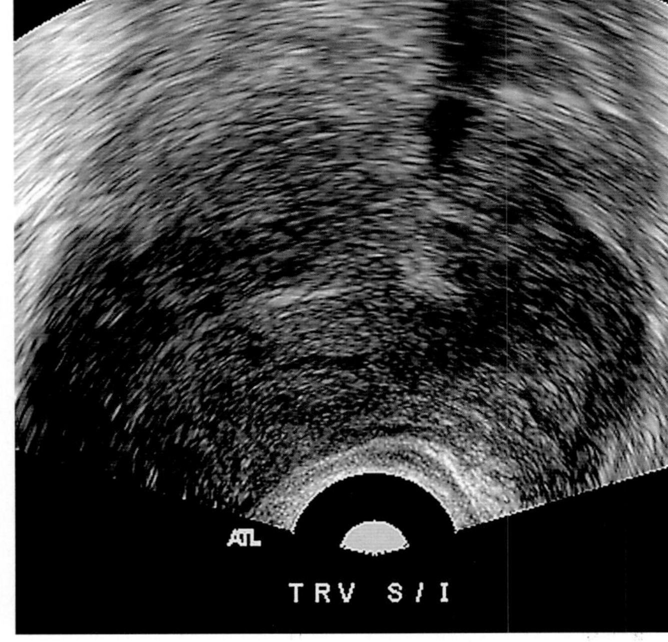

A

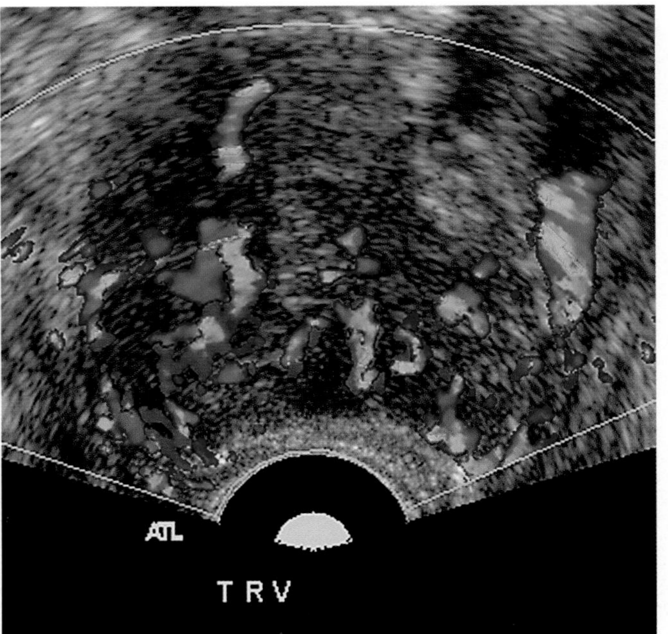

B

Figure 11-37 Diffuse Prostate Lymphoma
Transrectal US axial grayscale (**A**) and color Doppler (**B**) images demonstrates diffuse enlargement and infiltration of prostate similar to Figures 11-35 and 11-36. However, in this case the patient had no signs of infection, and biopsy revealed diffuse infiltration with lymphoma.

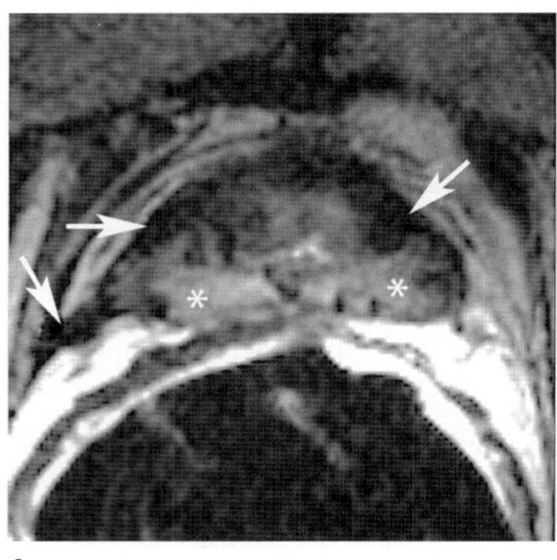

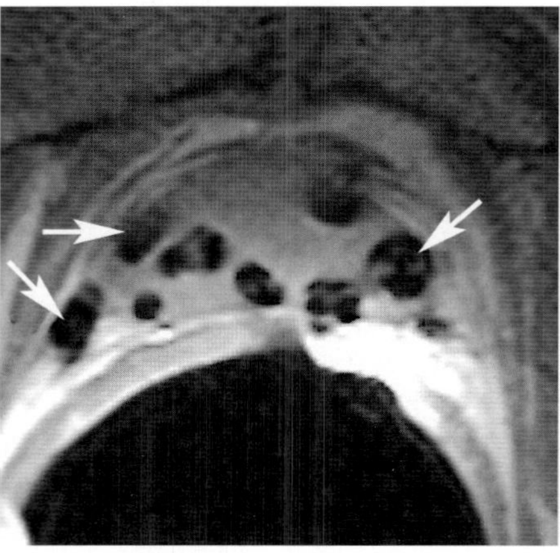

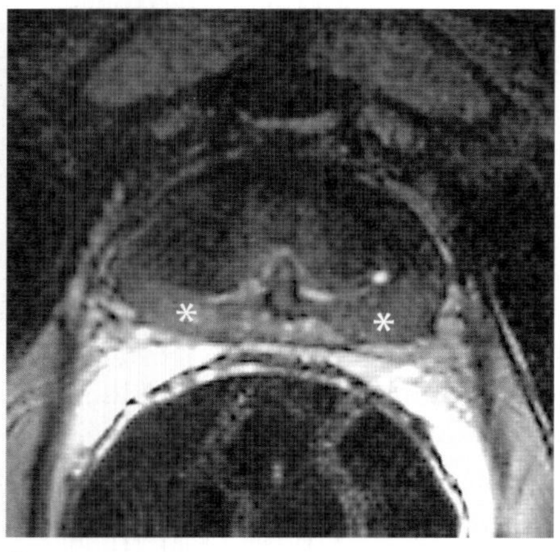

A B C

Figure 11-38 Prostate Atrophy due to Radiotherapy and Chemotherapy
A and **B.** Postradiation therapy changes in the peripheral zone. Note small prostate size and diffusely low T2 signal in the peripheral zone (*asterisk*) as seen on (A) axial T2-weighted sequences, in this case because of brachytherapy. The seeds are seen as signal voids on the (B) axial T1-weighted and axial T2-weighted sequence (*arrows*). **C.** Posttreatment changes in the peripheral zone. Axial T2-weighted image showing small prostate with diffusely decreased signal in the peripheral zone (*asterisk*) due to hormonal therapy; a similar appearance could also be produced by external beam radiation therapy.

Prostate Atrophy Mimic: Residual Prostate Tissue

In some cases, prostatectomy is incomplete and residual tissue is identified in the prostatectomy bed. Features suggesting this diagnosis include eccentric periurethral soft tissue with irregular margins, postsurgical changes (eg surgical clips), and history of prior prostatectomy. Imaging is unable to reliably distinguish benign residual tissue from recurrent and/or residual malignancy. Correlation with PSA as well as biopsy is often necessary (see Figure 11-39).

Prostate Atrophy Mimic: Periurethral Collagen Injection

Periurethral collagen injection is not infrequently performed for the treatment of postprostatectomy incontinence. The collagen appears as multiple periurethral nodules, which

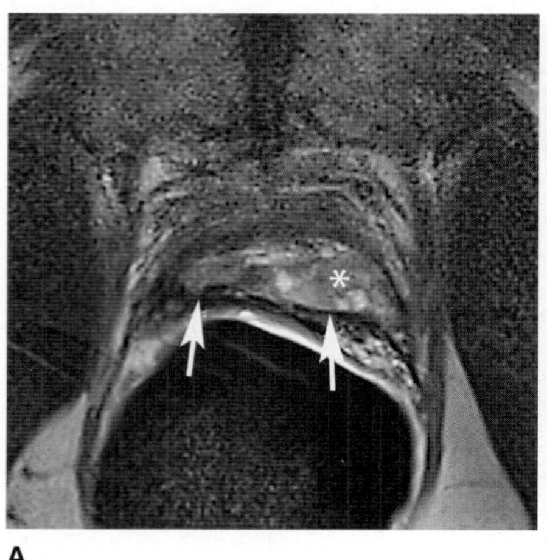

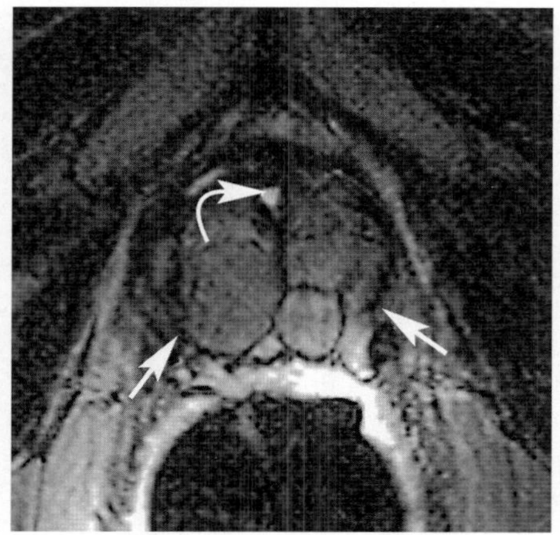

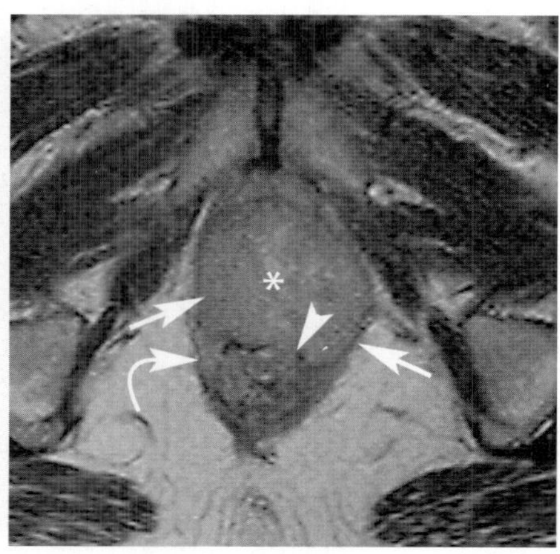

A B C

Figure 11-39 Prostate Atrophy Mimics
A. Axial T2-weighted image following robotic prostatectomy shows low signal scar (*arrows*) and soft tissue in the region of the anastomosis (*asterisk*) most in keeping with residual prostate tissue. **B.** Periurethral collagen. Axial T2-weighted image showing soft-tissue nodularity (*arrows*) surrounding the urethra (*curved arrow*) a patient with a history of collagen injections for postprostatectomy incontinence. In the absence of the appropriate history, the appearance can be mistaken for tumor recurrence. **C.** Recurrent tumor. Irregular soft tissue in the prostatectomy bed (*asterisk*), which on the axial T2-weighted image has irregular margins (*straight arrows*) and contacts the rectum (*arrowhead*). Curved arrow points to levator ani.

on MRI are low signal on T1- and T2-weighted images but usually higher in T2 signal than muscle.[76] This appearance is unlikely to be confused with prostatic atrophy where the prostate is small but demonstrates normal prostatic architecture and contour. However, recurrent tumor may have an identical appearance and should be suspected in the setting of rising PSA or in the absence of a history of collagen injections. In equivocal cases, TRUS-guided biopsy may be performed; contrast-enhanced study also may be helpful as tumor should enhance and collagen should not (see Figure 11-39).

PERIPROSTATIC CYSTIC LESIONS

There are a variety of causes of periprostatic cysts to be discussed

Seminal Vesicle Cysts

Seminal vesicle cysts can be *congenital* or *acquired*. Congenital cysts are present at birth and are typically asymptomatic but can become symptomatic in young adulthood, probably as a result of sexual activity. Congenital seminal vesicle cysts are associated with urinary tract anomalies including renal agenesis, renal maldevelopment, and ectopic insertion of the ureter. Other associations with seminal vesicle cysts include autosomal dominant kidney disease (44%-60%), (in which case the cysts are typically bilateral), hemivertebra, absence of the testes and absence of the vas deferens.[77,78]

The most common urinary tract abnormality associated with seminal vesical cysts is ipsilateral renal agenesis, occurring in approximately two-thirds of patients.[79] This association can be explained by their embryologic origin. The ureteral bud arises from the distal mesonephric duct and is responsible for inducing differentiation of the metanephric blastema into the kidney. The mesonephric duct differentiates into the appendix of the epididymis, paradidymis, epididymis, vas deferens, ejaculatory duct, seminal vesicle, and hemitrigone.[80] Maldevelopment of the distal mesonephric duct results in both faulty ureteral budding and atresia of the ejaculatory duct, causing seminal vesicle cysts and ipsilateral renal agenesis.

An abnormally cephalic origin of the ureteral bud from the mesonephric duct results in ectopic ureteral insertion into derivatives of the mesonephric duct, most commonly the prostatic urethra and the seminal vesicle.[80] Ectopic insertion of the ureter into the seminal vesicle usually results in both cystic dilation of the seminal vesicle and maldevelopment of the ipsilateral kidney.

Acquired seminal vesicle cysts are due to acquired obstruction of the ejaculatory duct, most commonly due to prostatitis or stones, and less likely from neoplasm, BPH or prior surgery. Acquired cysts tend to occur in older adults and are more commonly bilateral when compared to congenital cysts.

Seminal vesicle cysts are often asymptomatic but can also present with a wide variety of symptoms, including pain, dysuria, hematuria, urinary tract infections, epididymitis, and prostatitis. Less commonly, they may be associated with hematospermia, infertility, and if large, symptoms associated with mass effect. Seminal vesicle cysts usually contain sperm if aspirated.

Imaging demonstrates an eccentrically located retrovesical cystic mass superior to the prostate that is contiguous with the seminal vesicle (see Figure 11-40). If hemorrhage or protein is present, the mass may appear soft-tissue density on CT, show complex fluid signal on MRI, and contain debris/particulate fluid on US. Seminal vesicle cysts will typically opacify on vasovesiculography.

Seminal Vesicle Dilation

The seminal vesicles are approximately 3 cm in length and 1.5 cm in width on average. On all imaging modalities, the seminal vesicles are considered dilated if they measure >1.5 cm in diameter (see Figure 11-41). Typically, the multilobulated appearance of the seminal vesicles (as seen on MRI and US, but not well seen by CT) is preserved; however, in some cases, there may be loss of the normal convolutions.[81] Seminal vesicle dilation can be a result of normal aging or due to normal variations in the frequency of sexual intercourse[81] but may also be a consequence of ejaculatory duct obstruction due to chronic inflammation, stones, or congenital cysts. Findings that may point to ejaculatory duct obstruction as a cause of enlarged seminal vesicles include dilation of the ejaculatory ducts (measuring >2 mm), or of the vas deferens, or visualization of causes of obstruction such as stones, midline cysts, or chronic prostatitis. Seminal vesicle stones and hemorrhagic material in the seminal vesicle can also be seen in the setting of dilation. In equivocal cases, more definitive evaluation for ejaculatory duct obstruction can be obtained by invasive procedures, including TRUS-guided seminal vesicle puncture, vesiculography, and chromotubation.[58]

Müllerian, Ejaculatory Duct and Utricle Cysts

When large, ejaculatory duct and müllerian duct cysts (discussed in more depth previously) extend out of the prostate and may be off midline, but may be distinguished from seminal vesicle cysts by the presence of separate normal seminal vesicle (see Figure 11-42).

Cowper Gland Cyst

Cowper gland cysts may be congenital or acquired. When acquired, they are usually due to trauma or infection. They are differentiated from other cysts by their characteristic location adjacent to the bulbomembranous portion of the posterior urethra either posterolaterally or posteriorly (see Figure 11-42).[81] Small cysts are usually asymptomatic.

Periprostatic Abscess

Prostatic abscesses can extend into the periprostatic tissues to involve the seminal vesicles, but should be readily

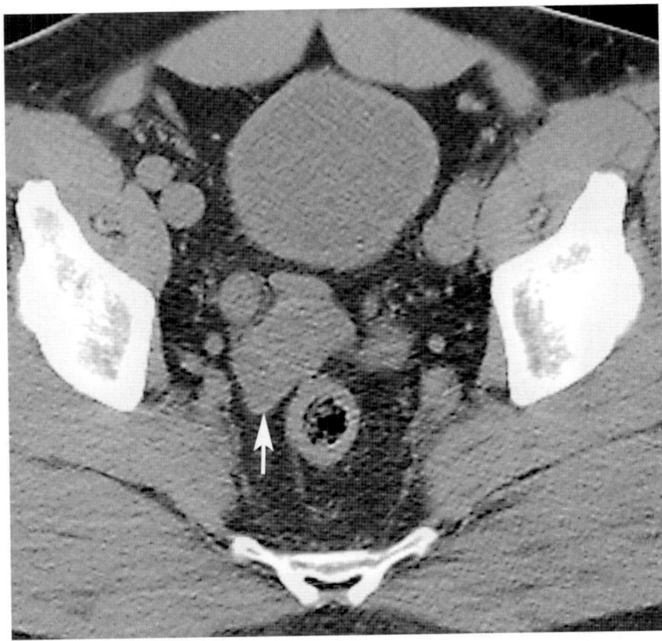
A

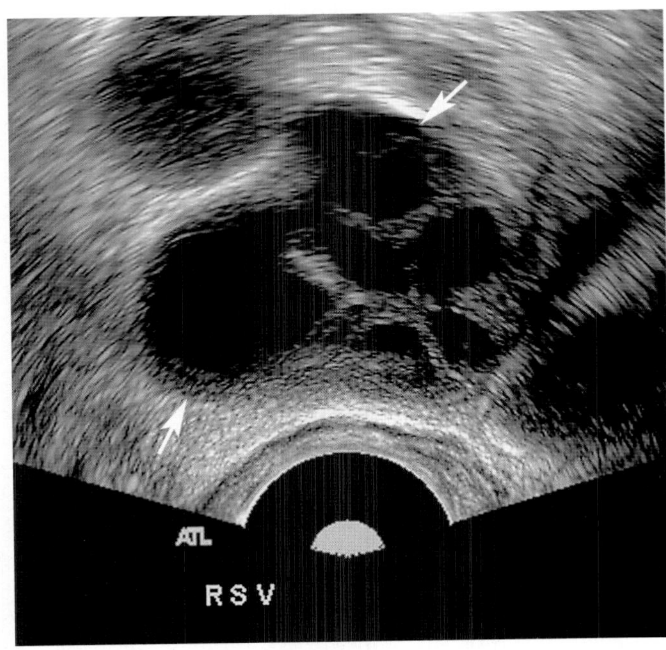

B

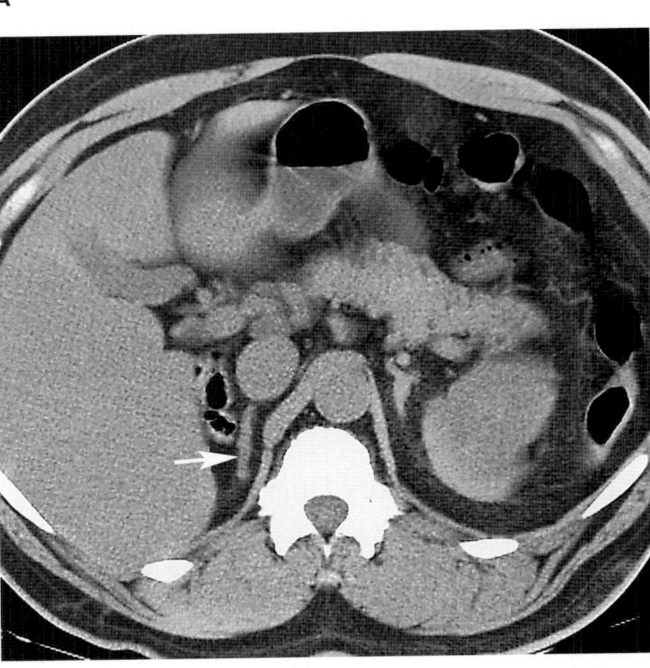
C

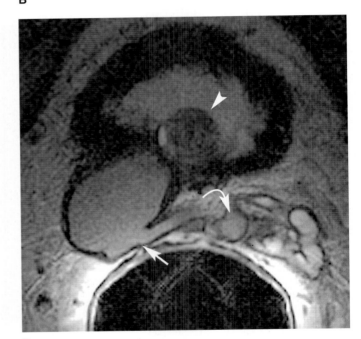

D

Figure 11-40 Seminal Vesicle Cyst
A and **B.** Axial unenhanced CT image (A) through the pelvis and TRUS image (B) showing a lobulated fluid density structure (*arrows*) in the expected region of the seminal vesicle in keeping with a seminal vesicle cyst. **C.** Axial unenhanced image at the level of the kidneys demonstrating "flattened" appearance of the adrenal gland (*arrow*) in the setting of ipsilateral renal agenesis. **D.** Axial T2-weighted image in a different patient with right renal ageneisis (not shown) demonstrating a cyst (*straight arrow*) communicating with the right seminal vesicle (*curved arrow*). Note central gland hypertrophy partially visualized (*arrowhead*). Although ejaculatory duct cysts and müllerian cysts may extend out of the prostate, they do not communicate with the seminal vesicle.

differentiated from other periprostatic cysts by the clinical scenario and by imaging findings associated with abscesses such as rim enhancement, gas within the cyst, and perilesional inflammatory fat stranding (see Figure 11-42).

Postbiopsy Hematoma

Postbiopsy hematomas can also occur in the periprostatic tissues. In most cases, there will be a clinical history of prostate biopsy. MRI examinations will demonstrate signal

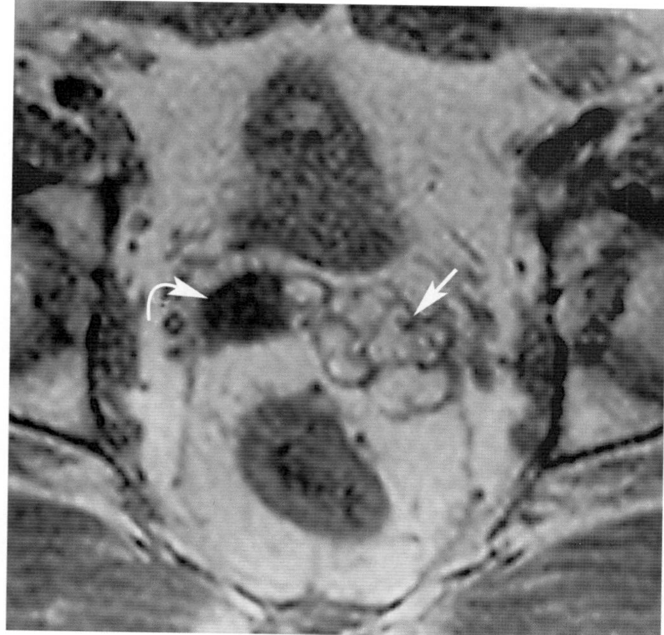

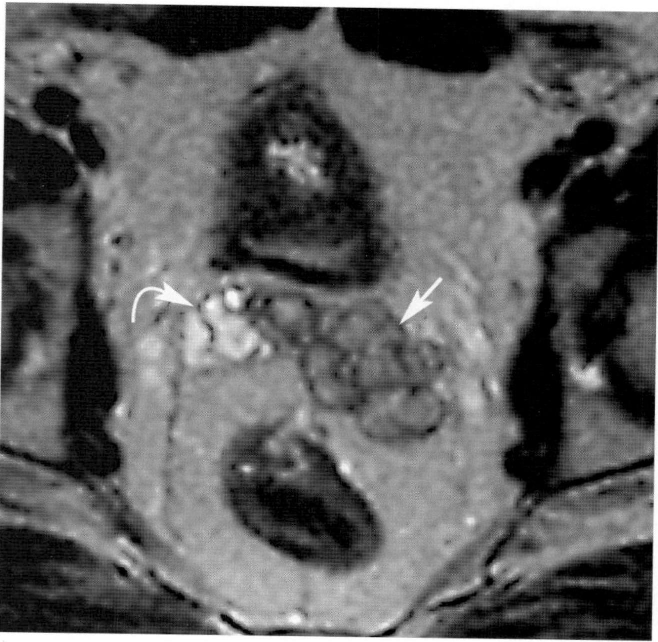

Figure 11-41 Cystic Dilation of the Seminal Vesicle
Axial T1-weighted (**A**) and axial T2-weighted images (**B**) in a patient with dysplastic left kidney (not shown) demonstrating cystic enlargement of the left seminal vesicle (*straight arrow*), which contains T1 hyperintense fluid indicative of proteinaceous or hemorrhagic content. Note normal right seminal vesicle (*curved arrow*).

characteristics of subacute blood, including hyperintense signal on T1-weighted MRI.

Other Periprostatic Fluid-Filled Lesions

Ureteroceles, hydronephrotic kidneys, and bladder diverticula can result in a fluid-filled structure in the retrovesical space but can be differentiated on the basis of other features.[79] An ectopic ureterocele is associated with ipsilateral collecting system duplication. A hydronephrotic pelvic kidney will be associated with absence of an ipsilateral orthotopic kidney, reniform shape, and the branching appearance of a dilated collecting system. Bladder diverticula will be adjacent to the bladder and will usually demonstrate communication with the urine in the bladder. Other rare periprostatic cystic lesions include peritoneal inclusion cysts, teratomas, and lymphangiomas.[82,83]

UNIQUE PROSTATE, SEMINAL VESICLE, AND PERIPROSTATIC LESIONS

Prostatic Calcifications

Calcifications within the substance of the prostate are a common phenomenon. They may be endogenous (develop within prostatic acini) or exogenous (derived from urine)[84] (Table 11-5).

The most common prostatic calcification is due to endogenous calcification of corpora amylacea. Corpora amylacea are lamellated bodies composed of the mucoproteins in the prostatic secretions and sloughed epithelial cells. Corpora amylacea are usually found in the acini of the peripheral zone or central zone, most commonly along the surgical capsule (see Figure 11-43).[84] Calcification of these bodies occurs slowly over time and they usually are incidentally found in the aging prostate with no clinical significance.

Endogenous calcification can be associated with pathologic conditions. For example, calcifications occurring in the apical peripheral zone inferior to the verumontanum, or diffuse "blocklike" regional nonshadowing areas

Table 11-5. Causes of Prostatic or Periprostatic Calcification

A. Normal aging
1. BPH
2. Corpora amylacea
B. Inflammation
1. Chronic prostatitis (bacterial or abacterial)
2. Granulomatous disease (e.g. TB)
3. Prior radiation
C. Other
1. Stasis of secretions due to obstruction
2. Systemic conditions (hypercalcemia)
3. Exogenous calcifications (calculus in urethra or in urethral diverticulum)

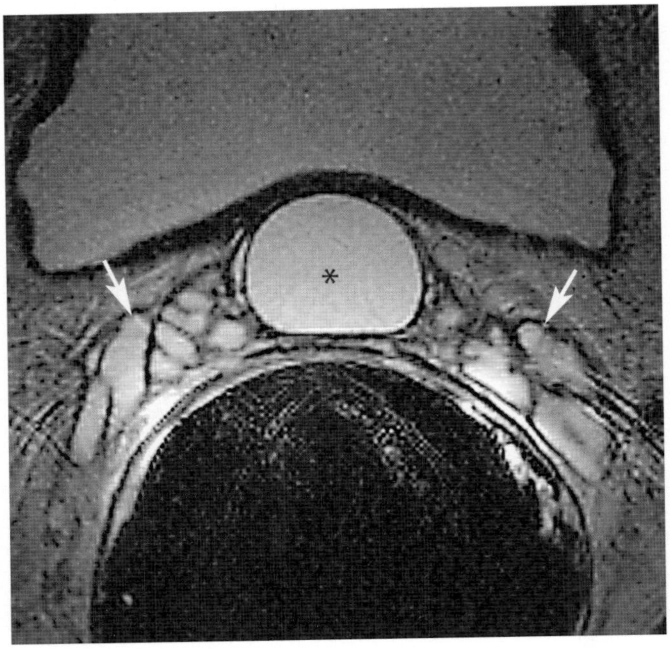

A

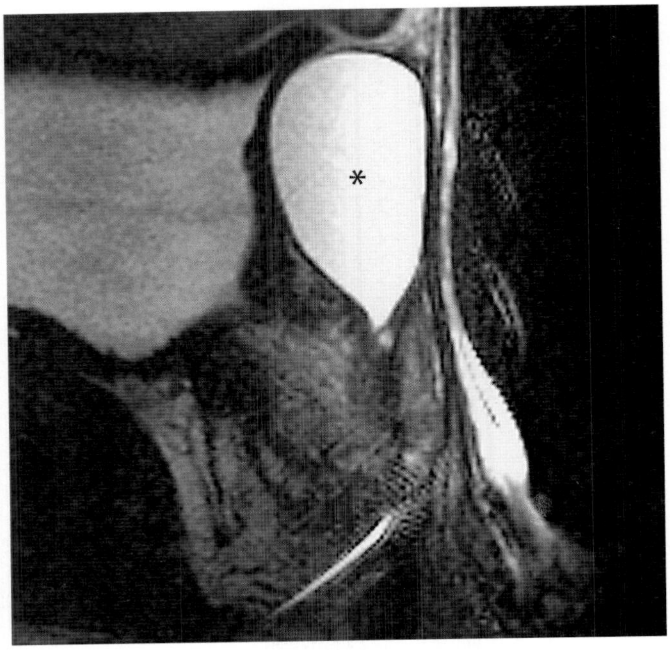

B

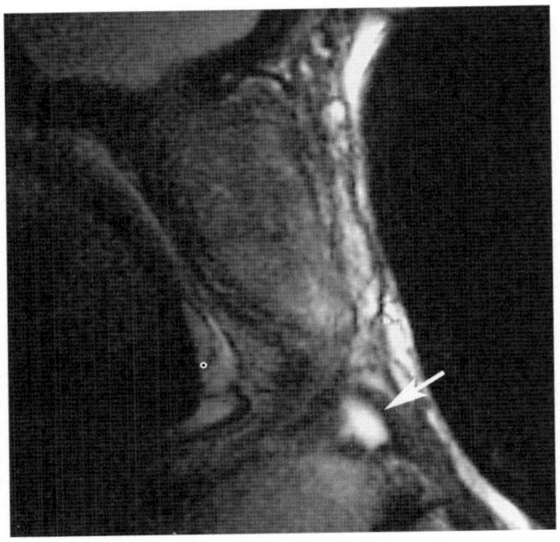

C

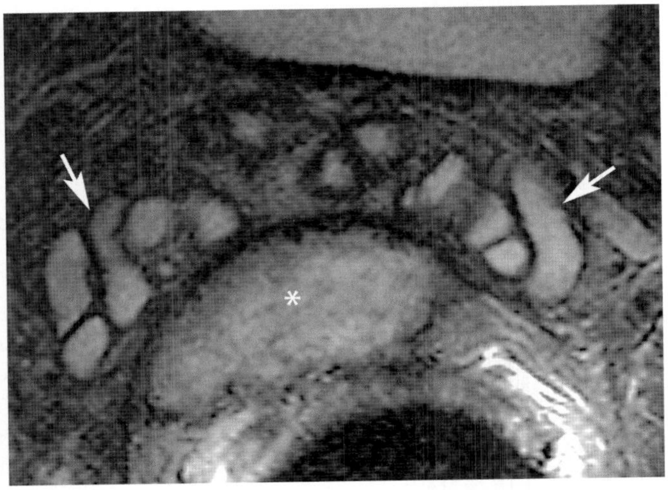

D

Figure 11-42 Other Periprostatic Cystic Lesions
A and **B.** Axial T2-weighted image (A) demonstrates a cystic structure (*asterisk*) in the vicinity of the seminal vesicles. Based on the axial images, the major differential considerations would be seminal vesicle cyst, ejaculatory duct cyst, and müllerian cyst. Sagittal T2-weighted image (B) shows the cyst (*asterisk*) to be separate from the seminal vesicles with a pear shape and neck approaching the urethra, and appearance most in keeping with a müllerian cyst. **C.** Probable Cowper gland cyst. Sagittal T2-weighted image showing a cystic periurethral structure (*arrow*) in the region of the urogenital diaphragm (in the expected location of Cowper glands), most likely a retention cyst. **D.** Postbiopsy abscess. Axial T2-weighted image demonstrates at thick-walled collection (*asterisk*) posterior to the seminal vesicles (*arrows*) post biopsy, in keeping with an abscess that resolved over time.

of calcification, are suggestive of chronic prostatitis (see Figure 11-43).[57] Relatively extensive calcification throughout the prostate has been described due to tuberculosis prostatitis.[85] Other causes of endogenous calcifications include dystrophic calcifications related to BPH, calcification related to metabolic disorders such as hypercalcemia, vitamin D intoxication and ochronosis, and calcifications related to stasis of secretions as may occur by obstruction of prostatic ducts by strictures, hyperplasia, or less likely, cancer.[84]

Ejaculatory duct calcifications simulate intraprostatic calcifications but may be identified by their characteristic paramedian location (see Figure 11-43). These are discussed in more detail in the subsequent section: **Calcifications of the ejaculatory duct**.

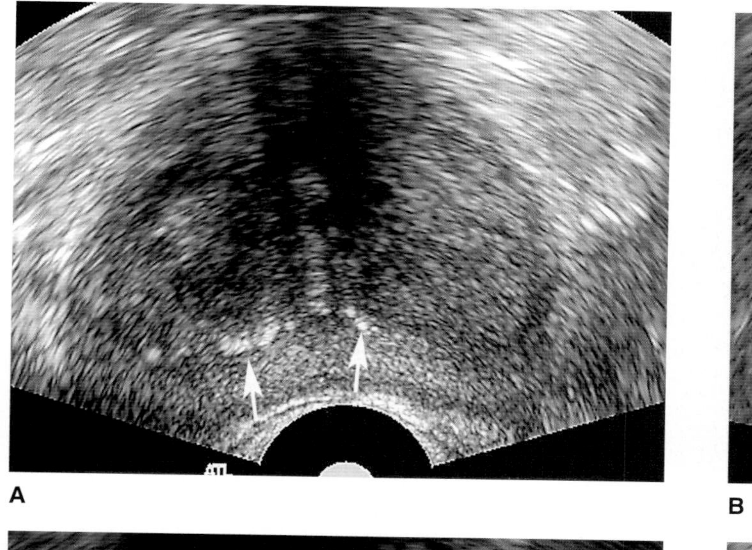

A

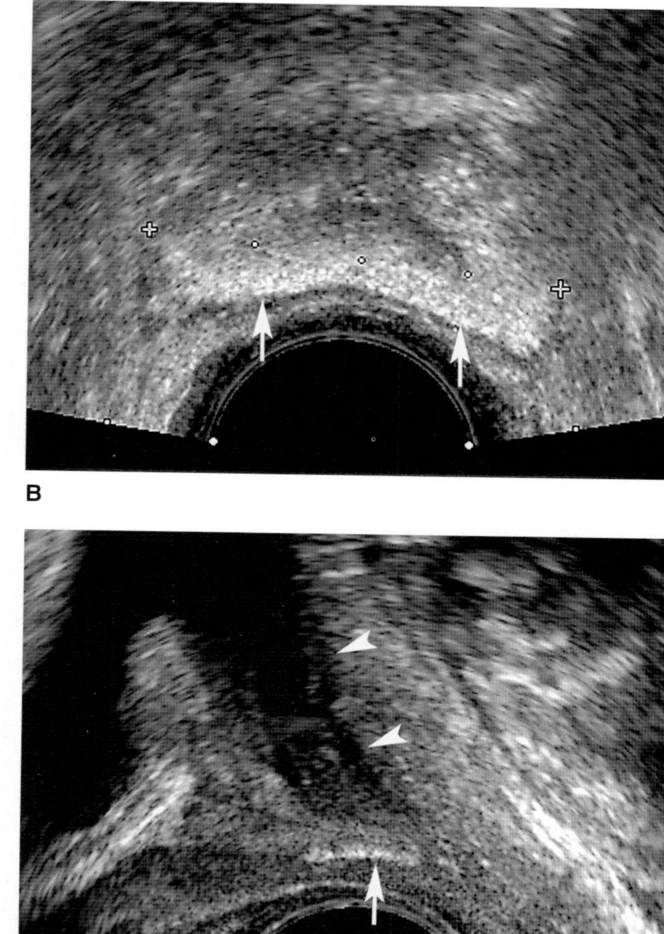

B

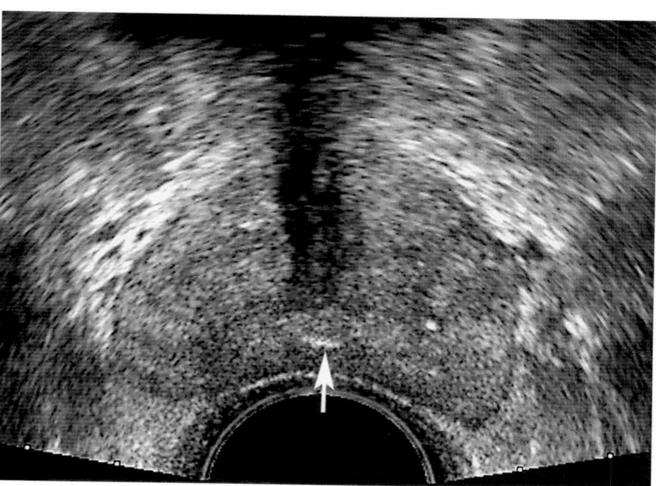

C

D

Figure 11-43 Prostate Calcifications
A. Corpora amylacea. Echogenic foci (*arrows*) along the surgical capsule are typical in location for corpora amylacea, an incidental finding in the aging prostate. **B.** Peripheral zone calcifications. Axial TRUS images showing fine nonshadowing diffuse peripheral zone calcifications (*arrows*), a pattern typical of chronic prostatitis. **C** and **D.** Ejaculatory duct calcifications. Axial (C) and sagittal (D) TRUS images showing punctate calcification near the midline of the prostate on the axial image (C, *arrow*), which are in the typical distribution of the ejaculatory duct on the sagittal image (D, *arrows*). Calcifications in and about the ejaculatory ducts may be sequela of or cause of ejaculatory duct stenosis, which may result in upstream dilation of the seminal vesicles or ejaculatory ducts. Arrowheads point to the urethra.

Exogenous calcification can also be due to migrated urinary bladder calculi lodged in the prostatic urethra or periurethral calculi in a urethra diverticula.

Calcifications appear as echogenic foci with or without posterior acoustic shadowing on US, as hyperdense foci on CT, and as signal voids on both T1- and T2-weighted MRI sequences (see Figures 11-34 and 11-43). Brachytherapy seeds can mimic calcification but may be differentiated based on regular pattern and history, as well as the presence of ring down on US, susceptibility artifact on MRI, and density greater than calcium on CT (see Figures 11-15, 11-38, and 11-44).

Calcifications of Other Male Reproductive Structures

Calcifications can also be found in the vas deferens and ejaculatory duct.

Calcifications of the Vas Deferens

Calcification of the vas deferens can be seen on abdominal plain films and abdominal CT. They appear as curvilinear tubular calcifications extending upward from the central pelvis toward the lateral pelvis (see Figure 11-45). The most

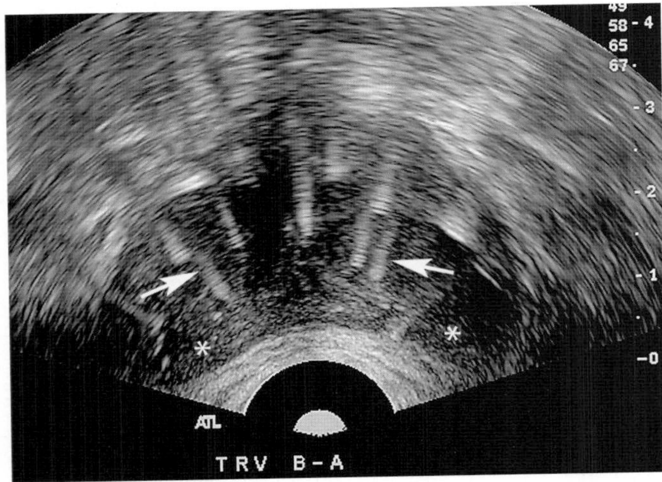

Figure 11-44 Radiation Seeds
Brachytherapy seeds. Axial TRUS image showing multiple echogenic foci (*arrows*) with ringdown artifact typical of metal, in keeping with brachytherapy seeds. Note diffusely decreased signal in the peripheral zone (*asterisk*) reflecting treatment effect.

common causes are aging and diabetes mellitus but vas deferens calcifications can also be a result of tuberculous or other infections (gonorrhea, syphilis, schistosomiasis, and chronic urinary tract infections). When calcification occurs as a result of aging or diabetes, there is bilaterally symmetric calcification of the muscular elements of the vas deferens without luminal narrowing. It is believed that the calcifications occur at a greater frequency and younger age in the setting of diabetes mellitus. Inflammatory and infectious calcifications develop intraluminally and are more frequently unilateral, segmental, and/or irregular.

Calcifications of the Ejaculatory Duct

Calcifications around the ejaculatory duct as well as calcification within the ejaculatory duct (ED lithiasis) are findings that are seen more commonly in hypofertile men when compared with men with normal fertility.[58] Ejaculatory duct calcifications are identified by the characteristic paramedian location (see Figure 11-43). When these calcifications are detected, other imaging findings suggestive of ejaculatory duct obstruction (dilated ejaculatory ducts, dilated seminal vesicles, seminal vesicle, and/or vas deferens lithiasis) should be sought.

Abnormal Low T2 Signal in the Seminal Vesicles on MRI Exams

On T2-weighted MRI sequences, the seminal vesicles normally appear as bow-tie-shaped convolutions of tubules that typically measure <5 mm in diameter and have low T2 signal walls and central high T2 signal intensity fluid.[81] Therefore, focal or diffuse low T2 signal within the seminal vesicles is a marker for pathology. Causes of low T2 signal include invasion of the seminal vesicles by prostatic tumor, intratubular hemorrhage, proteinaceous fluid, amyloid deposition within the seminal vesicles, sequela or hormonal therapy, or very rarely primary tumor of the seminal vesicles or other tumor.

Seminal vesicle invasion

Invasion of the seminal vesicles by prostate carcinoma is the most clinically important cause for low T2 signal in the seminal vesicles. Invasion by prostate cancer should be suspected if there is disruption of the normal seminal vesicle architecture and if there is contiguous tumor between the seminal vesicle and the base of the prostate

Imaging Notes 11-12. Differentiating Features of Low T2 Signal in the Seminal Vesicles

Cause	Imaging Features	Clinical Features
Hemorrhage	High signal on T1-weighted images, normal lobular architecture	History of biopsy or hematospermia
Seminal vesiclitis	Normal lobular architecture, debris, adjacent inflammatory changes, findings of prostatitis	No history of tumor
Amyloid	Atrophy, preservation of normal lobular architecture	Older individual
Hormonal/radiation therapy	Atrophy, normal architecture	History of hormonal or radiation therapy
Invasion by prostate cancer	Loss of normal seminal vesicle architecture, contiguous tumor at prostatic base	Elevated PSA, history of prostate adenocarcinoma
Primary seminal vesicle tumor	Loss or normal seminal vesicle architecture, tumor in periglandular fat	Symptoms related to invasion of adjacent structures, elevated CA-125 for primary seminal vesicle carcinoma

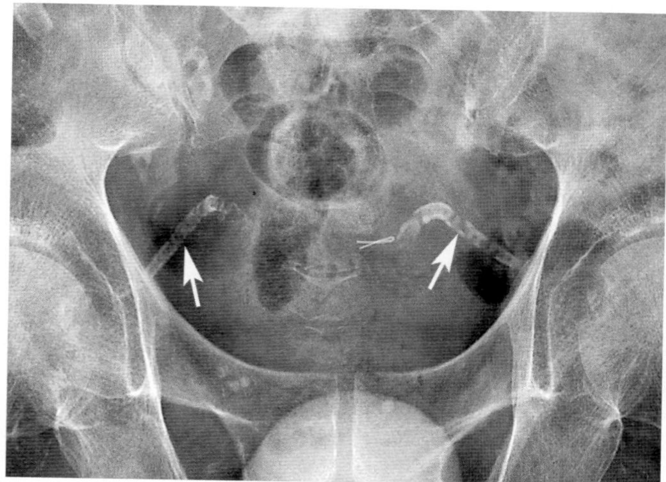

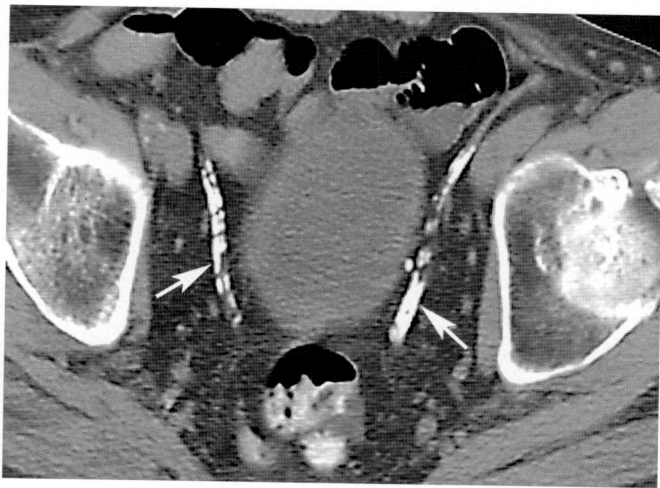

Figure 11-45 Vas Deferens Calcifications
A. Pelvic radiographic demonstrating tubular radiodensities (*arrows*) with the characteristic appearance of vas deferens calcifications, a finding commonly present in the setting of diabetes. **B.** Axial CT image in the same patient illustrating the extensive vas deferens calcifications (*arrows*).

(see Figure 11-46). If the imaging appearance is indeterminate, and it is important to diagnose the presence of seminal vesicle invasion, TRUS-guided biopsies of the seminal vesicles may be performed, which has a reported accuracy of 91% in 1 series.[86] The seminal vesicles may also be secondarily involved by tumors from the urinary bladder and rectum, as well as metastases from distant primaries in the form of peritoneal carcinomatosis.

Other seminal vesicle tumors

Primary seminal vesicle carcinoma is very rare, with fewer than 100 cases reported in the literature, in adults of all ages.[87] Symptoms may include hematospermia, hematuria, and outlet obstruction but usually are absent in early disease. On imaging, in the rare situation where the tumor is small or organ confined, soft-tissue enlargement of the seminal vesicle or a rectovesical mass may suggest the diagnosis (see Figure 11-46). However, most seminal vesicle carcinomas present at an advanced stage with invasion of adjacent organs, such as the prostate or urinary bladder, and therefore may be confused with adenocarcinomas arising from these structures. Normal PSA, normal carcinoembryonic antigen, and elevated CA125 as may occur with seminal vesicle carcinoma are clinical clues that may point to the diagnosis.[87]

Other tumors of the seminal vesicles are exceedingly rare but include secondary involvement by lymphoma or other rare neoplasms such as leiomyosarcoma, angiosarcoma, müllerian adenosarcoma–like tumor, carcinoid, seminoma, and cystosarcoma phyllodes (see Figure 11-46).[77]

Seminal vesicle hemorrhage

Seminal vesicle hemorrhage is the imaging correlate of hematospermia and a frequent cause of low T2 signal in the seminal vesicle. The most common cause of hematospermia is prior prostate biopsy. Most other cases of hematospermia are idiopathic, up to 79% in 1 report, followed by benign causes such as prostatitis, seminal vesiculitis, prostate calculi, and BPH, along with some rare etiologies, including prostate and bladder carcinomas.[81,88] In young men, bladder and prostate tumors are only, very rarely, an etiology of hematospermia and therefore hematospermia may be managed conservatively. However, in 1 report, 14% of older patients with hematospermia were diagnosed with prostate cancer, and, therefore, screening for prostate cancer may be prudent when a man aged >40 is diagnosed with hematospermia.[81,89] Blood products within the seminal vesicle are usually in the subacute phase of evolution at the time of imaging and typically will appear as high signal on T1-weighted images and variable signal on T2-weighted images (see Figure 11-47). The high T1 signal is a clue differentiating seminal vesicle hemorrhage from the other causes of low T2 signal in the seminal vesicles, which are typically low in T1 signal.

Seminal vesiculitis

Seminal vesiculitis typically is due to extension from bacterial prostatitis; although in endemic countries, tuberculosis and schistosomiasis are other causes. In its subacute to chronic phase, it can also result in proteinaceous or hemorrhagic debris within the seminal vesicle, leading to low T2 signal. The inflammation and debris can result in dilation and cystic change or conversely, atrophy of the seminal vesicle. The seminal vesicle wall can be thickened, and there can also be findings of chronic prostatitis. In the acute phase, other findings such as hyperemia, inflammatory stranding, and abscesses may also be present (see Figure 11-47).[77]

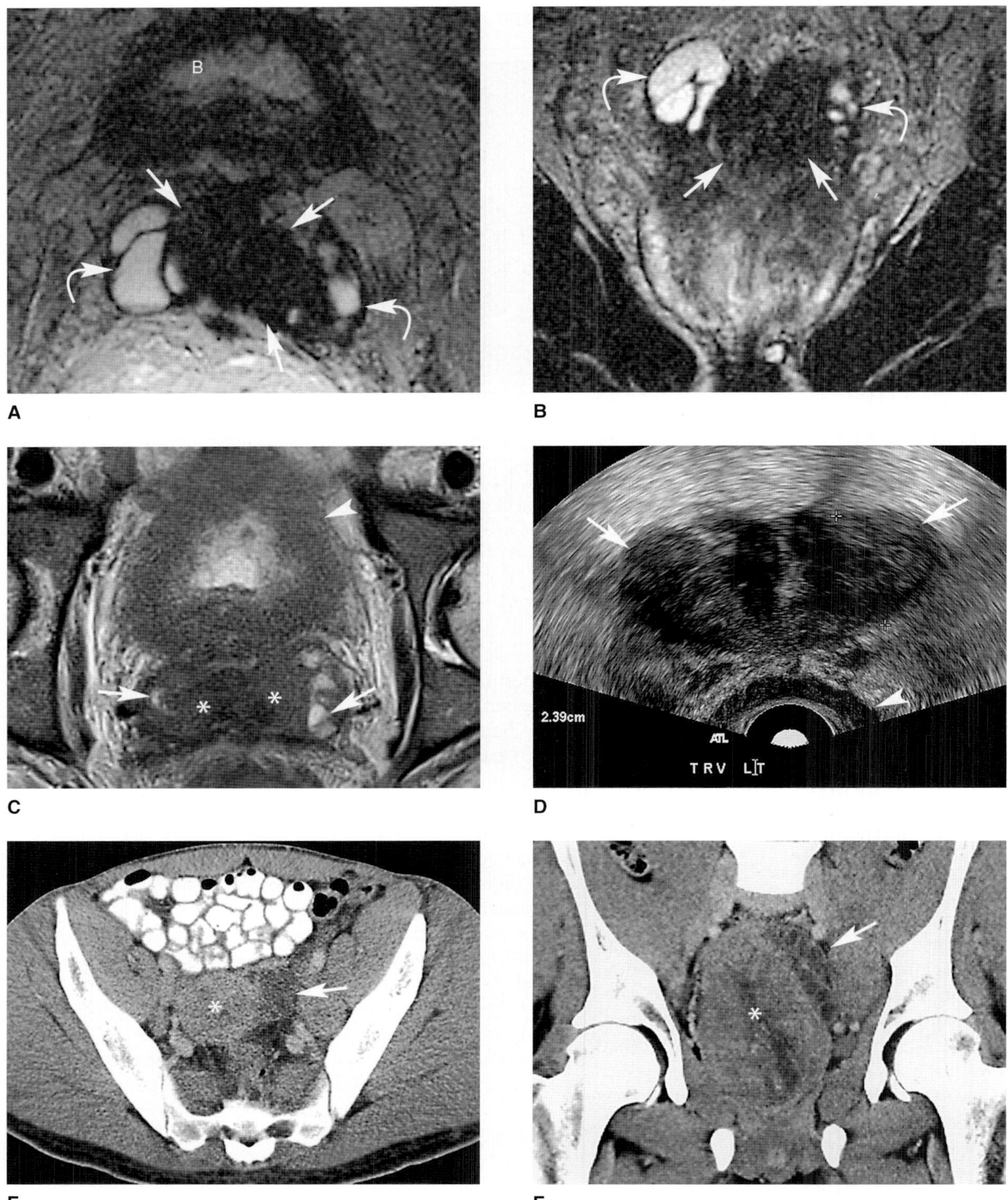

Figure 11-46 Neoplastic Involvement of the Seminal Vesicles in 3 Patients

Neoplastic involvement can be suspected if there is irregular soft-tissue enlargement or infiltration of the seminal vesicles, in combination with history of malignancy. **A** and **B.** Seminal vesicle invasion from prostate cancer. (A) Axial and (B) coronal T2-weighted images demonstrating low signal soft tissue (*straight arrows*) infiltrating the medial seminal vesicles with loss of normal lobular architecture (*curved arrows* indicating preserved seminal vesicles), in keeping with seminal vesicle invasion from prostate cancer. **C** and **D.** Seminal vesicle lymphoma in a patient with aggressive enteropathy-associated T-cell lymphoma. (C) Axial T2-weighted image shows soft-tissue replacement (*asterisk*) of most of the seminal vesicles (*arrow*) that was FDG avid, which would be atypical for prostate carcinoma. Note soft-tissue thickening of urinary bladder (*arrowhead*), also proven to be lymphoma. (D) On US, the seminal vesicles demonstrate enlargement, decreased echogenicity, and loss of normal architecture (*arrows*). Rectal wall was also diffusely thickened (*arrowhead*). **E** and **F.** Seminal vesicle carcinoma. Axial (E) and coronal (F) images from enhanced CT in a young male shows large mass (*asterisk*) centered in the right seminal vesicle with extension into of the prostate and left seminal vesicle; note the left seminal vesicle is partially spared (*arrow*). Biopsy was most consistent with primary seminal vesicle carcinoma.

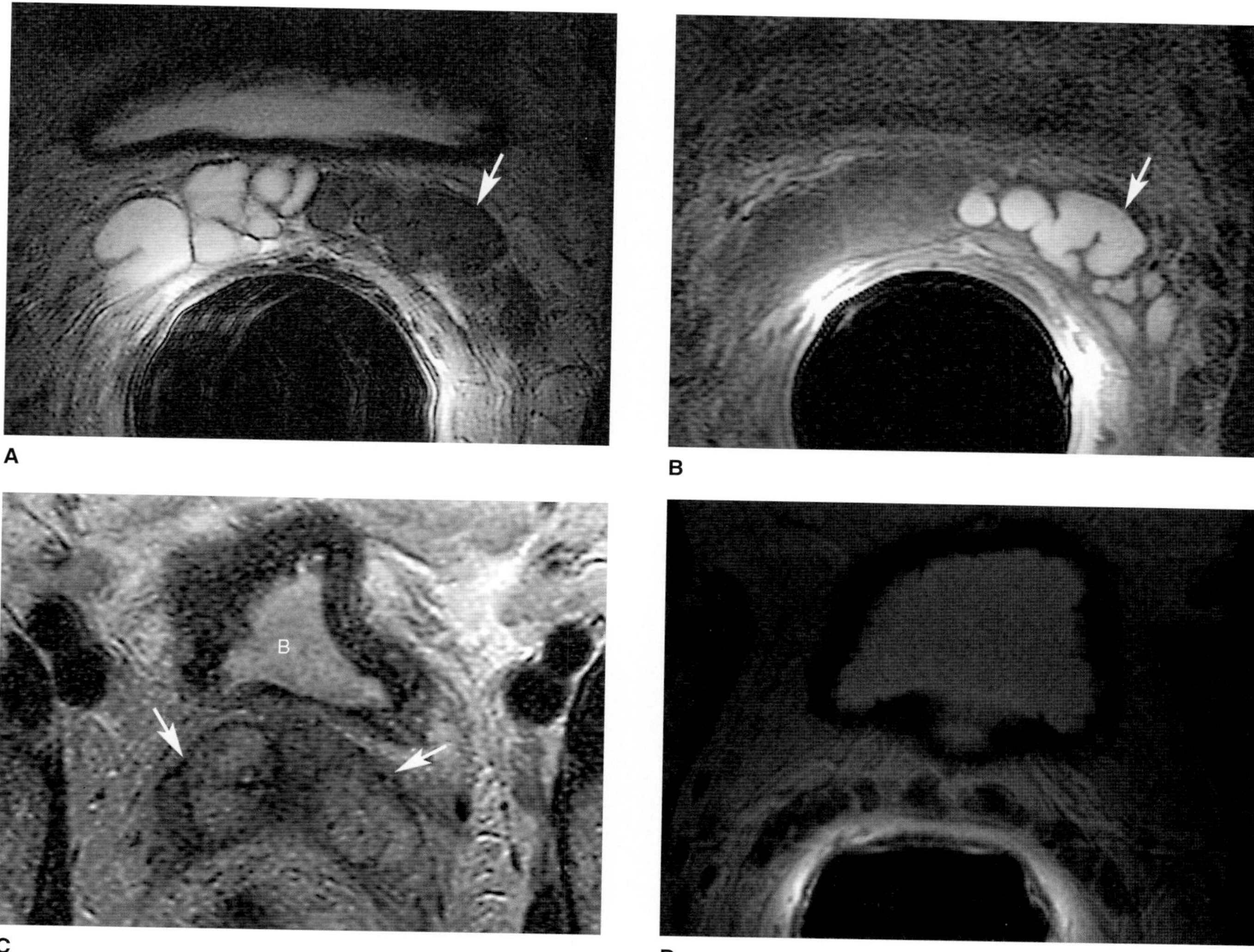

Figure 11-47 Non-neoplastic Low T2 Signal in the Seminal Vesicles **A** and **B**. Postbiopsy hemorrhage. Axial T2-weighted image (A) shows low signal (*arrow*) diffusely throughout the left seminal vesicle with preservation of the lobular architecture, which on an axial T1-weighted image (B) corresponds to high signal (*arrow*), in keeping with hemorrhage. **C**. Acute seminal vesiculitis. Axial T2-weighted image demonstrates low signal throughout both seminal vesicles (*arrows*) compared to the signal intensity of urine in the bladder (B). **D**. Presumed amyloid. Axial T2-weighted image in an older gentleman shows diffusely low-signal retracted seminal vesicles with preservation of lobular architecture; this appearance is most consistent with amyloid or end-stage fibrosis of the seminal vesicles from prior inflammation. Treatment effect (due to radiation or hormonal therapy for prostate cancer) may result in a similar appearance.

Amyloidosis

Senile seminal vesicle amyloidosis, which occurs in up to 17% of men older than age 50, is another benign cause of low signal in the seminal vesicles. This phenomenon can be mistaken for invasion of the seminal vesicle by prostate carcinoma.[83] Atrophy of the seminal vesicle and preservation of normal lobular pattern can be a clue to the nonneoplastic etiology: seminal vesicle amyloidosis.

Iatrogenic

Hormonal and/or radiation therapy commonly leads to low T2 signal and atrophy of the seminal vesicles. This can have an imaging appearance similar to seminal vesicle amyloidosis. However, the diagnosis of hormonal/radiation therapy as the cause of the signal abnormality is based on clinical history of ongoing or prior therapy.

Seminal vesicle calculi

Calcifications can occur in the seminal vesicles, usually as sequel of prior infection or inflammation. Uremia, hyperparathyroidism, and diabetes are other uncommon causes. The calcifications appear as intraluminal low-signal-intensity foci on T2-weighted images (see Figure 11-48).

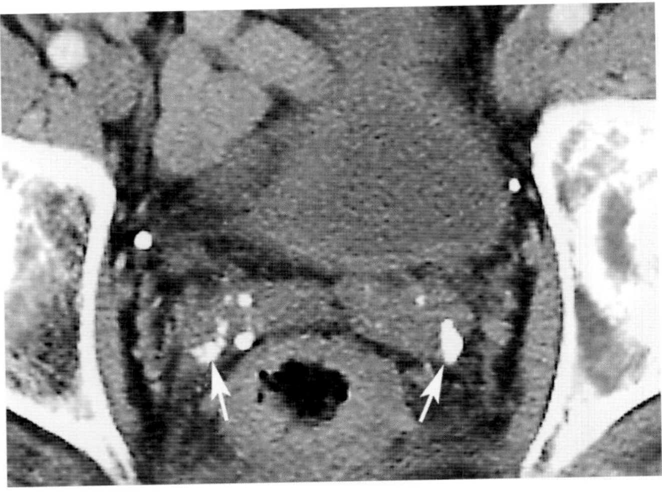

A

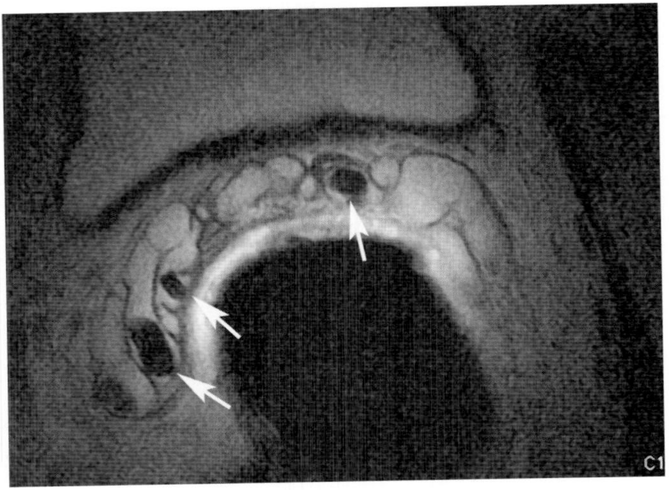

B

Figure 11-48 Seminal Vesicle Calculi
A. Axial image from an enhanced CT scan showing hyperdense foci within the seminal vesicles (*arrows*) in keeping with calcifications. **B.** Axial T2-weighted image demonstrates low T2 signal rounded structures within the seminal vesicles (*arrows*) representing seminal vesicle calculi.

Congenital Anomalies of the Prostate, Seminal Vesicles, and Related Structures

Agenesis of vas deferens is present in 1% to 7% of otherwise normal males.[60] Bilateral vas deferens agenesis is present in 99% of those with cystic fibrosis, and two-thirds of those with bilateral agenesis have mutations in the cystic fibrosis transporter gene. In cystic fibrosis, agenesis is postulated to be a result of luminal blockage of the vas deferens and seminal vesicles by thick secretions. There is usually associated seminal vesicle agenesis; however, the kidneys are usually normal in cystic fibrosis since the blockage is believed to occur after 7 weeks in gestation.[79] Other associated findings include prominence of the rete testis and the epididymal head as well as decreased T2 signal in the peripheral zone of the prostate on MRI.[90] When bilateral, agenesis results in infertility despite normal testicular spermatogenesis.

Agenesis can also be due to an early insult to the mesonephric duct during embryogenesis. If an embryologic

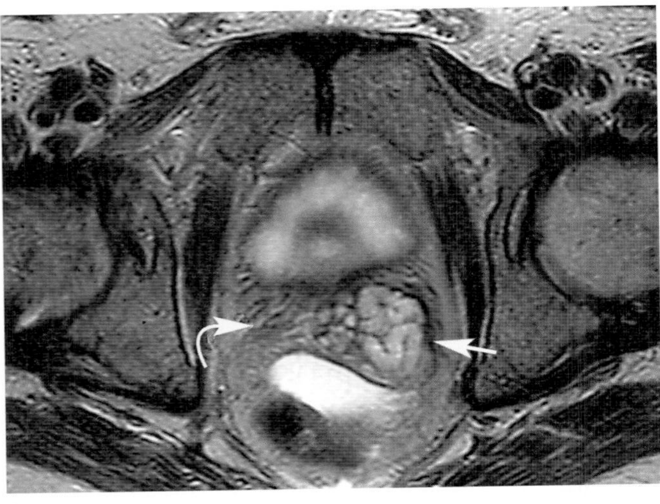

A

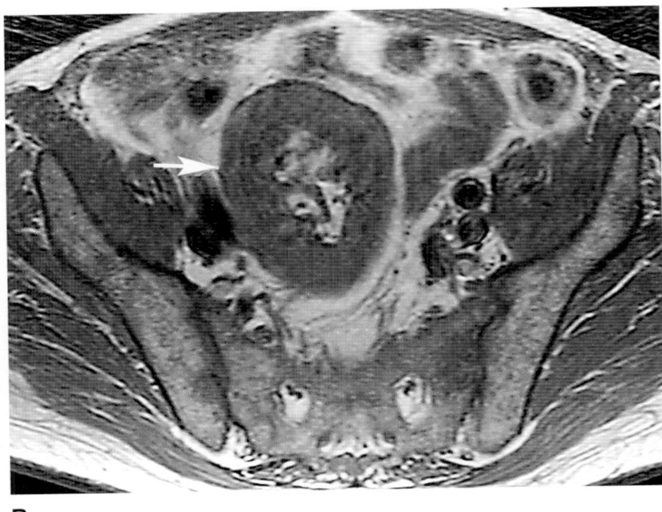

B

Figure 11-49 Agenesis of the Seminal Vesicle
A. Axial T2-weighted image shows a normal left seminal vesicle (*straight arrow*), with no right seminal vesicle present in the expected location (*curved arrow*). **B.** Axial T1-weighted image more superiorly in the pelvis shows pelvic kidney (*arrow*) ipsilateral to the side of the seminal vesicle agenesis.

insult occurs before the seventh week of gestation, when the ureteric bud arises from the mesonephric duct, seminal vesicle agenesis will result and is reported in 45% of cases of bilateral vas deferens agenesis and up to 86% of cases of unilateral agenesis.[77] Seminal vesicle agenesis is commonly associated with renal agenesis, which occurs in 79% of cases. However, in 9% of cases there is an ipsilateral normal kidney (see Figure 11-49).[77]

FINDINGS RELATED TO SURGICAL AND MEDICAL INTERVENTION IN THE PROSTATE

The mainstays of therapy for prostate cancer include radical prostatectomy, brachytherapy seed placement, external beam radiation, and hormonal therapy.

Normal Postoperative Findings

Radical prostatectomy involves removal of the prostate and seminal vesicles with creation of an anastomosis between the bladder neck and membranous urethra and preservation of the neurovascular bundles if possible to preserve potency. A lymphadenectomy is commonly also performed. MRI can be obtained following prostatectomy if there is an abnormal digital rectal examination or if there is a rise in the PSA. This is not an uncommon situation as biochemical failure occurs following prostatectomy in 10% to 53%, most occurring in the first 5 years following surgery.[91]

The normal appearance of the prostatectomy bed is illustrated (see Figure 11-50). Findings that may be visualized in the surgical bed include fibrosis, surgical clips, seminal vesicle remnants, residual prostatic tissue, postoperative chronic collections, periurethral collagen, and tumor recurrence.[92] Fibrosis is manifested as low T1/T2 signal in the region of the anastomosis as well as in the rectovesical region, which demonstrates minimal if any enhancement. Surgical clips can be identified based on the susceptibility artifact they produce. In 1 study, seminal vesicle remnants were reported in 20%, where they were bilateral in 80% and complete seminal vesicles were found in 30%.[93] In 53%, these appeared as convoluted fluid-filled remnants, and in the remainder, as low-signal masses. In the same study, an additional 38% of patients demonstrated low-signal masses in the lateral postprostatectomy fossa suggestive of fibrotic tips. Although such low-signal masses can mimic recurrence, the irregular convoluted appearance should suggest the diagnosis of residual seminal vesicles.

Periurethral collagen, which is injected to treat incontinence, appears as intermediate- to low-signal masses near the anastomosis (see Figures 11-39 and 11-51). Collagen typically may be differentiated from tumor based on history, normal PSA, and lack of enhancement following gadolinium, as discussed in previous sections.

Residual prostatic tissue can rarely be visualized following prostatectomy (see Figure 11-39). The imaging appearance of residual tissue cannot be reliably distinguished from tumor recurrence.

Postoperative collections should demonstrate features of either simple or complex fluid, with rim enhancement only, and typically should resolve over time.

Local recurrence most commonly appears as a soft-tissue nodule that is similar to hyperintense relative to muscle on T2-weighted images (see Figure 11-52). This overlaps in appearance with benign processes such as fibrosis or inflammatory tissue. Recently, 2 studies[91,94] have demonstrated improved accuracy for identifying local recurrence using a dynamic contrast-enhanced protocol with tumor differentiated from benign processes by the presence of early enhancement. A sensitivity and specificity up to 88% (69%-98%), and 100% (84%-100%) was reported in 1 of the studies.[94] In spite of these promising results, in equivocal cases, biopsy may still be necessary. Magnetic resonance spectroscopy and diffusion weighted sequences are evolving techniques technique, under investigation, which may be helpful in distinguishing residual tissue from local recurrence but is beyond the scope of this chapter.[95]

Following radiation therapy and hormonal therapy, the prostate decreases in size and there is fibrosis and loss of hydration of the prostate and seminal vesicles, resulting in decreased signal on T2-weighted images (see Figure 11-38).

If radiation therapy was performed using brachytherapy, then multiple low-signal seeds will be visualized that result in susceptibility artifact on MRI, echogenic foci on US, and high-attenuation foci on CT (see Figures 11-15, 11-38, and 11-44). Imaging can be used to evaluate for satisfactory placement of radiation seeds.

Complications of Treatment of Prostate Cancer

Complications are discussed in excellent review by Yablon et al, the contents of which are summarized here.[96] Complications of radical prostatectomy can be divided into intraoperative, perioperative, and long-term complications. Intraoperative complications include rectal injury (1%) and ureteral injury (0.05%-1.6% of cases). Rectal injury not recognized at the time of surgery may present in the postoperative period as a fistula to the urethra, skin, and urinary bladder. Ureteral injuries can result in leak with urinoma or urinary obstruction.

Perioperative complications include anastomotic leak, collections, and catheter-related stricture and fistula. Anastomotic leak typically occurs posterolaterally, where it is difficult to achieve tension-free sutures because of poor surgical access. On voiding cystourethrogram, anastomotic leaks have indistinct, amorphous contours in contrast to plication defects, which appear as well-defined outpouchings (see Figure 11-53). Anastomotic leak is treated by catheter drainage until resolution. Potential postoperative

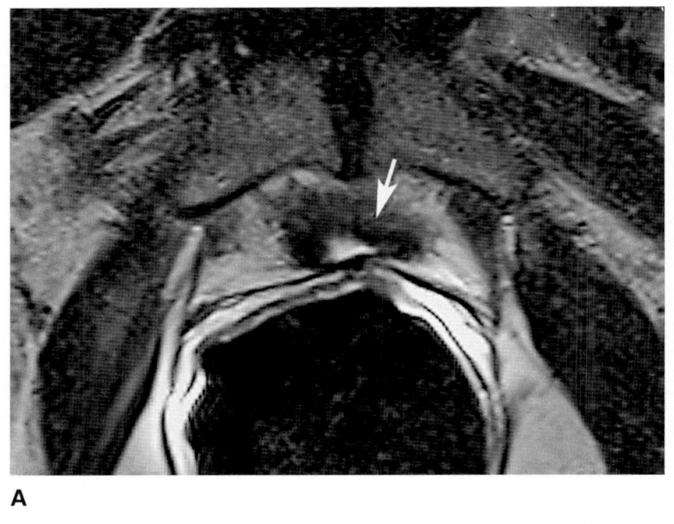

A

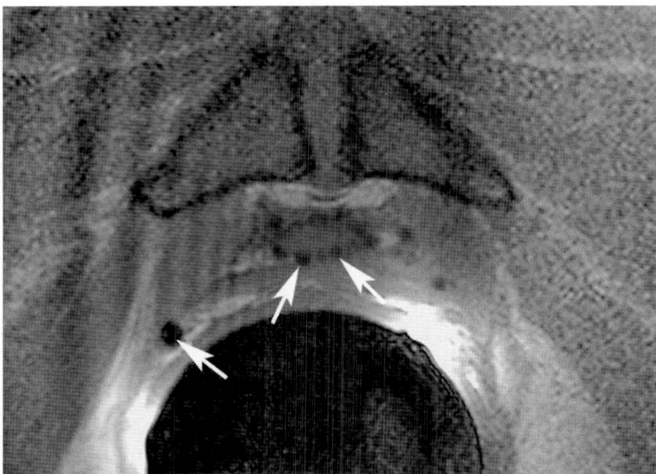

B

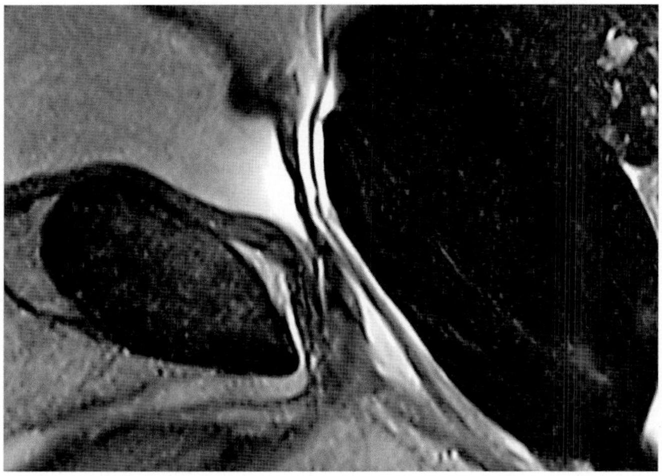

C

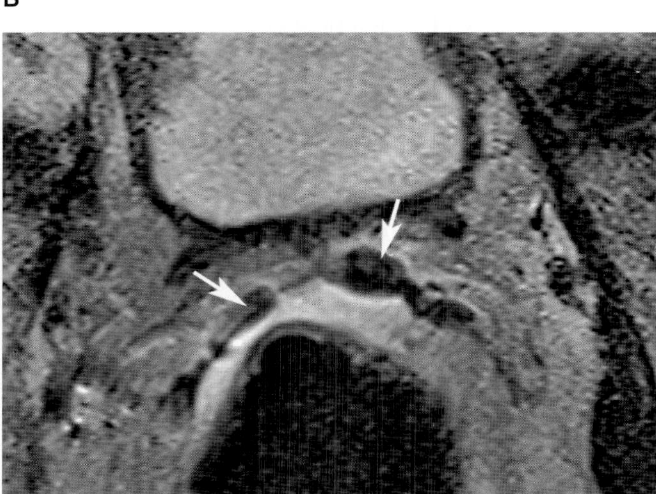

D

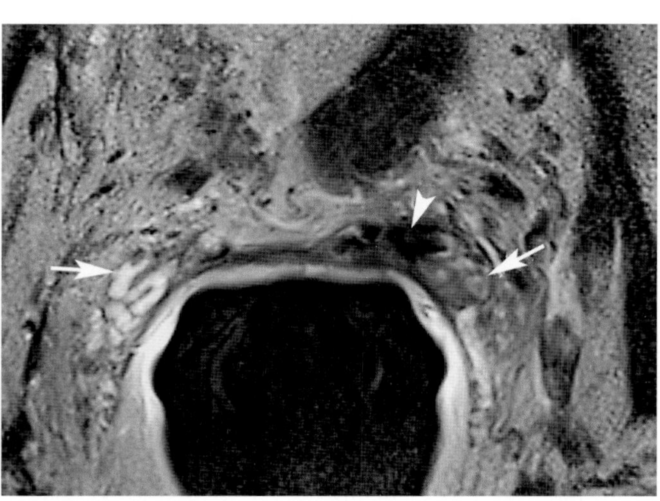

E

Figure 11-50 Normal Postprostatectomy Appearance
A. Axial T2-weighted image showing region of the vesicourethral anastomosis (*arrow*) with central fluid signal. Note absence of soft-tissue nodularity. **B.** Axial T1-weighted image at the same level as (A) showing foci of low signal (*arrows*) reflecting susceptibility artifact from microscopic amounts of metal. **C.** Sagittal T2-weighted image demonstrating normal appearance of the region of the anastomosis with funneled appearance to the bladder neck. **D.** Axial T2-weighted images at the level of the seminal vesicles demonstrating low signal areas representing a combination of signal voids due to surgical clips (*arrows*) and postsurgical fibrosis. **E.** Axial T2-weighted image in a separate patient demonstrating residual seminal vesicle tips (*arrows*) and signal voids due to surgical clips (*arrowhead*).

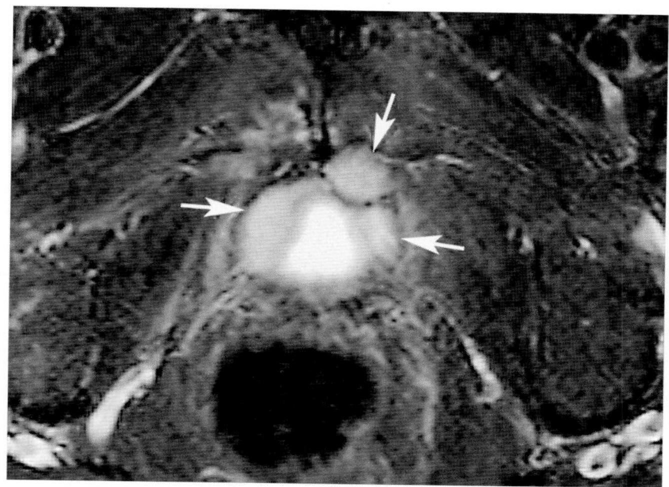

A

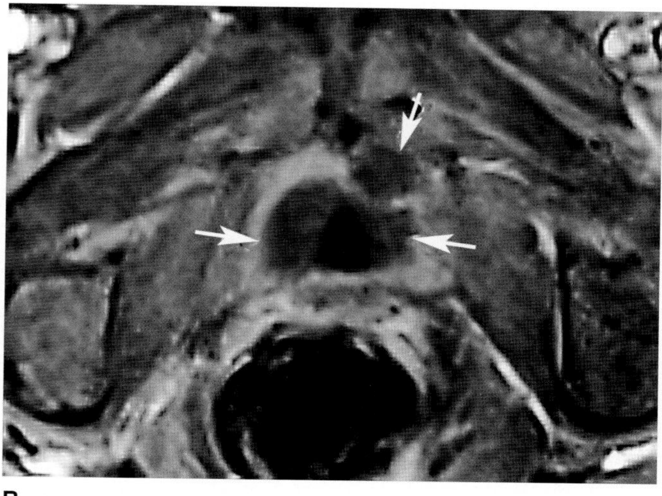

B

Figure 11-51 Periurethral Collagen Injections
A and **B**. Periurethral collagen. Axial T2-weighted sequence (A) demonstrating soft-tissue nodules (*arrows*) around the anastomosis, which demonstrate no internal enhancement on (B) axial T1-weighted fat saturated postgadolinium images, in keeping with periurethral collagen in this patient with longstanding history of incontinence that eventually required placement of an artificial urethral sphincter.

collections include abscess, hematoma, and lymphocele. Of these, lymphocele is common, occurring in up to 60% who undergo open lymphadenectomy. Most lymphoceles are asymptomatic and small, but treatment, typically with drainage, with or without sclerosis, may be necessary if the lymphocele is > 5 cm, compresses important structures, becomes infected, or is associated with pain. Fistula to adjacent structures such as the rectum is an uncommon complication.

Long-term complications include anastomotic strictures, incontinence, erectile dysfunction, and tumor recurrence. A recent study has reported an incidence of anastomotic strictures of 4.8%, which may be due to surgical technique or postoperative fibrosis. These can be treated with transurethral balloon dilation, which is effective in 60% of cases initially but has unknown long-term duration. Incontinence is the most distressing complication, and is common. Total incontinence is reported in up to 17% of men, and stress incontinence is reported in up to 35% of men. Treatment options include injection of a periurethral bulking agent such as collagen, and placement of a total artificial urethral sphincter (AUS). An AUS consists of a cuff placed around the proximal bulbar urethra, which is connected via tubing traveling in the subcutaneous tissues to a sphincter control pump placed in the scrotum (see Figure 11-54). Complications related to the AUS include urethral atrophy beneath the cuff, cuff erosion kinked tubing, pump malfunction, pump migration, and infection. Erectile dysfunction occurs in 10% to 90% and may be treated medically, or by placement of a penile prosthesis. Tumor recurrence has already been discussed.

Common complications of radiation therapy include urinary complications such as cystitis, urethritis, voiding dysfunction, stress urinary incontinence (up to 12% in patients with prior TURP), as well as other complications such as proctitis, urinary fistula, sinus tract formation, radiation-induced osteitis, and erectile dysfunction.

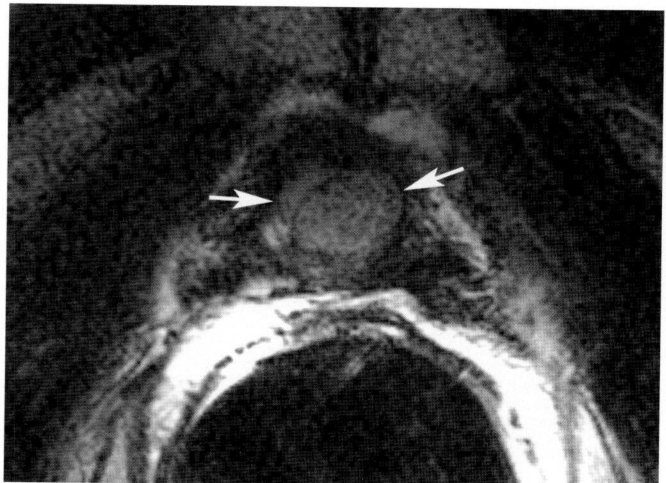

Figure 11-52 Local Recurrence of Prostate Cancer
Axial T2-weighted image in a patient with rising PSA showing soft-tissue nodularity (*arrows*) that is higher in signal than fibrosis, in keeping with locally recurrent tumor. Compare with Figure 11-51. Unlike periurethral collagen, recurrent tumor would be expected to enhance and the patient would not have a history of collagen injections.

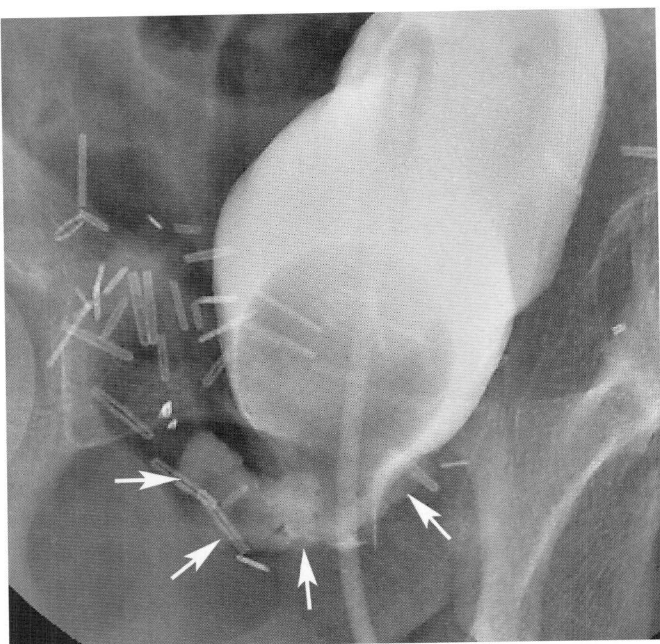

A

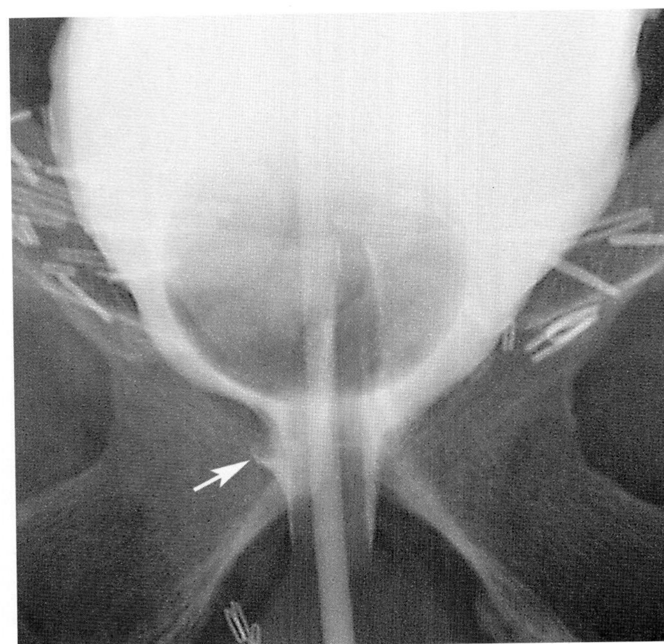

B

Figure 11-53 Anastomotic Leak versus Plication Defect
A. Image from a voiding cysoturethrogram in a patient approximately 10 days following radical prostatectomy shows multiple surgical clips in the pelvis and a Foley balloon in the bladder. There is amorphous contrast material (*arrows*) surrounding the region of the vesicourethral anastomosis that progressively increased in size during the course of the examination, in keeping with moderate to large anastomotic leaks. The Foley catheter was left in place to allow for further healing. **B.** Imaging from a voiding cysoturethrogram from a separate patient 2 weeks following radical prostatectomy shows a Foley balloon in place and multiple pelvic surgical clips. There is a tiny well-defined outpouching of contrast from the right aspect of the anastomosis that did not change over the course of the examination, reflecting a plication defect (*arrow*).

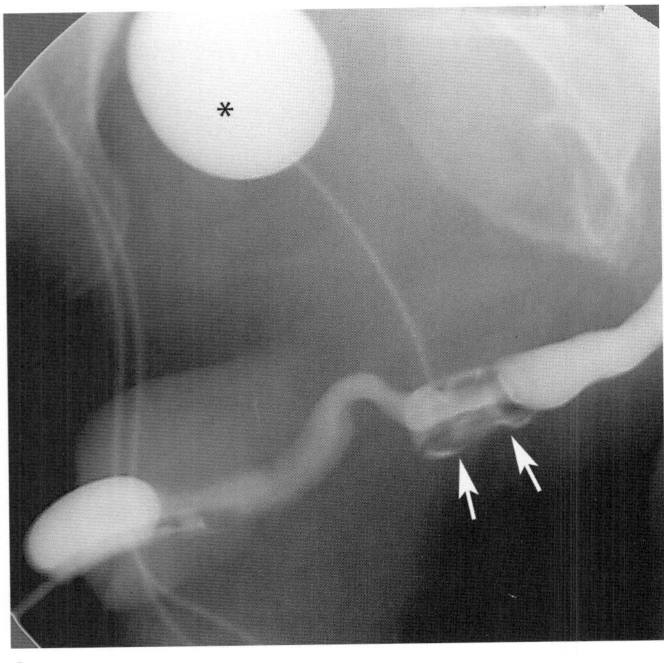

A

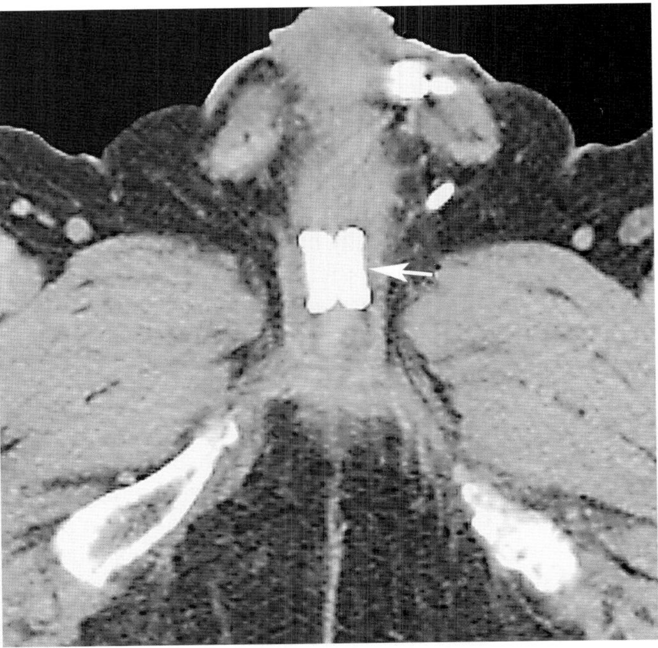

B

Figure 11-54 Artificial Urethral Sphincter
A. Image from a retrograde urethrogram show a device (*arrows*) in the region of the midbulbar urethra that is attached to a reservoir (*asterisk*). This is the characteristic appearance of an artificial urethral sphincter. **B.** Axial CT image from the same patient shows the appearance of a urethral sphincter as a hyperdense structure in the region of the bulbar urethra (*arrow*).

REFERENCES

1. Kumar V, Abbas AK, Fausto N, Robbins SL, Cotran RS. *Robbins and Cotran Pathologic Basis of Disease*. Philadelphia, PA: Elsevier Saunders; 2005:1050-1056.
2. Epstein JI. Chapter 91—Pathology of prostatic neoplasia. In: Wein AJ, Kavoussi LR, Novick AC, Partin AW, Peters CA, eds. *Campbell-Walsh Urology*. 9th ed. Philadelphia, PA: WB Saunders; 2007.
3. Kundra V, Silverman PM, Matin SF, Choi H. Imaging in oncology from the University of Texas M.D. Anderson Cancer Center: diagnosis, staging, and surveillance of prostate cancer. *AJR Am J Roentgenol*. 2007;189:830-844.
4. Halpern EJ. Prostate and seminal vesicle measurements. In: Goldberg BB, McGahan JP, eds. *Atlas of Ultrasound Measurements*. Philadelphia, PA: Mosby Elsevier; 2006: 370-374.
5. Curran S, Akin O, Agildere AM, Zhang J, Hricak H, Rademaker J. Endorectal MRI of prostatic and periprostatic cystic lesions and their mimics. *AJR Am J Roentgenol*. 2007;188:1373-1379.
6. Hricak H, Choyke PL, Eberhardt SC, Leibel SA, Scardino PT. Imaging prostate cancer: a multidisciplinary perspective. *Radiology*. 2007;243:28-53.
7. Jemal A, Siegel R, Ward E, et al. Cancer statistics, 2008. *CA Cancer J Clin*. 2008;58:71-96.
8. Scardino P. Update: NCCN prostate cancer clinical practice guidelines. *J Natl Compr Canc Netw*. 2005;3(suppl 1):S29-S33.
9. Kawachi MH, Bahnson RR, Barry M, Carroll PR, Carter HB, Catalona WJ, Epstein JI, Etzioni RB, Hemstreet GP 3rd, Howe RJ, Kopin JD, Lange PH, Lilja H, Mohler J, Moul J, Nadler RB, Patterson S, Pollack A, Presti JC, Stroup AM, Urban DA, Wake R, Wei JT; National Comprehensive Cancer Network. NCCN clinical practice guidelines in oncology: prostate cancer early detection. *J Natl Compr Canc Netw*. 2007 Aug;5(7):714-736.
10. Carter HB, Allaf ME, Partin AW. Chapter 94—Diagnosis and staging of prostate cancer. In: Wein AJ, Kavoussi LR, Novick AC, Partin AW, Peters CA, eds. *Campbell-Walsh Urology*. 9th ed. Philadelphia, PA: WB Saunders; 2007.
11. Claus FG, Hricak H, Hattery RR. Pretreatment Evaluation of Prostate Cancer: Role of MR Imaging and 1H MR Spectroscopy. *Radiographics*. 2004;24:S167-S180.
12. Ramey JR, Halpern EJ, Gomella LG. Chapter 92—Ultrasonography and biopsy of the prostate. In: Wein AJ, Kavoussi LR, Novick AC, Partin AW, Peters CA, eds. *Campbell-Walsh Urology*. 9th ed. Philadelphia, PA: WB Saunders; 2007.
13. McNeal JE, Villers AA, Redwine EA, Freiha FS, Stamey TA. Capsular penetration in prostate cancer. Significance for natural history and treatment. *Am J Surg Pathol*. 1990;14:240-247.
14. Epstein JI, Carmichael M, Walsh PC. Adenocarcinoma of the prostate invading the seminal vesicle: definition and relation of tumor volume, grade and margins of resection to prognosis. *J Urol*. 1993;149:1040-1045.
15. Green FL, Page DL, Fleming ID, et al. *AJCC Cancer Staging Handbook*. 6th ed. New York: Springer-Verlag; 2002.
16. Potter SR, Partin AW. Prostate cancer: detection, staging, and treatment of localized disease. *Semin Roentgenol*. 1999;34:269-283.
17. Lee F, Torp-Pedersen S, Littrup PJ, et al. Hypoechoic lesions of the prostate: clinical relevance of tumor size, digital rectal examination, and prostate-specific antigen. *Radiology*. 1989;170:29-32.
18. Dahnert WF, Hamper UM, Eggleston JC, Walsh PC, Sanders RC. Prostatic evaluation by transrectal sonography with histopathologic correlation: the echopenic appearance of early carcinoma. *Radiology*. 1986;158:97-102.
19. Yu KK, Hricak H. Imaging prostate cancer. *Radiol Clin North Am*. 2000;38:59-85, viii.
20. Graser A, Heuck A, Sommer B, et al. Per-sextant localization and staging of prostate cancer: correlation of imaging findings with whole-mount step section histopathology. *AJR Am J Roentgenol*. 2007;188:84-90.
21. Beyersdorff D, Taupitz M, Winkelmann B, et al. Patients with a history of elevated prostate-specific antigen levels and negative transrectal US-guided quadrant or sextant biopsy results: value of MR imaging. *Radiology*. 2002;224:701-706.
22. Ikonen S, Karkkainen P, Kivisaari L, et al. Magnetic resonance imaging of clinically localized prostatic cancer. *J Urol*. 1998;159: 915-919.
23. Futterer JJ, Heijmink SWTPJ, Scheenen TWJ, et al. Prostate cancer localization with dynamic contrast-enhanced MR imaging and proton MR spectroscopic imaging. *Radiology*. 2006;241:449-458.
24. Nakashima J, Tanimoto A, Imai Y, et al. Endorectal MRI for prediction of tumor site, tumor size, and local extension of prostate cancer. *Urology*. 2004;64:101-105.
25. Choi YJ, Kim JK, Kim N, Kim KW, Choi EK, Cho K-S. Functional MR imaging of prostate cancer. *Radiographics*. 2007;27:63-75.
26. Akin O, Sala E, Moskowitz CS, et al. Transition zone prostate cancers: features, detection, localization, and staging at endorectal MR imaging. *Radiology*. 2006;239:784-792.
27. Li H, Sugimura K, Kaji Y, et al. Conventional MRI capabilities in the diagnosis of prostate cancer in the transition zone. *AJR Am J Roentgenol*. 2006;186:729-742.
28. Noguchi M, Stamey TA, Neal JE, Yemoto CE. An analysis of 148 consecutive transition zone cancers: clinical and histological characteristics. *J Urol*. 2000;163:1751-1755.
29. Linzer DG, Stock RG, Stone NN, Ratnow R, Ianuzzi C, Unger P. Seminal vesicle biopsy: accuracy and implications for staging of prostate cancer. *Urology*. 1996;48:757-761.
30. Partin AW, Kattan MW, Subong EN, et al. Combination of prostate-specific antigen, clinical stage, and Gleason score to predict pathological stage of localized prostate cancer. A multi-institutional update. *J Am Med Assoc*. 1997;277:1445-1451.
31. D'Amico AV, Whittington R, Malkowicz SB, et al. Predicting prostate specific antigen outcome preoperatively in the prostate specific antigen era. *J Urol*. 2001;166:2185-2188.
32. Wang L, Hricak H, Kattan MW, et al. Prediction of seminal vesicle invasion in prostate cancer: incremental value of adding endorectal MR imaging to the Kattan nomogram. *Radiology*. 2006;242:182-188.
33. Wang L, Hricak H, Kattan MW, Chen H-N, Scardino PT, Kuroiwa K. Prediction of organ-confined prostate cancer: incremental value of MR Imaging and MR spectroscopic imaging to staging nomograms. *Radiology*. 2005;238:597-603.
34. Yu KK, Hricak H, Alagappan R, Chernoff DM, Bacchetti P, Zaloudek CJ. Detection of extracapsular extension of prostate carcinoma with endorectal and phased-array coil MR imaging: multivariate feature analysis. *Radiology*. 1997;202:697-702.
35. Cornud F, Flam T, Chauveinc L, et al. Extraprostatic spread of clinically localized prostate cancer: factors predictive of pT3 tumor and of positive endorectal MR imaging examination results. *Radiology*. 2002;224:203-210.

36. Sala E, Akin O, Moskowitz CS, et al. Endorectal MR Imaging in the evaluation of seminal vesicle invasion: diagnostic accuracy and multivariate feature analysis. *Radiology.* 2006;238:929-937.

37. Grignon DJ. Unusual subtypes of prostate cancer. *Mod Pathol.* 2004;17:316-327.

38. Varghese SL, Grossfeld GD. The prostatic gland: malignancies other than adenocarcinomas. *Radiol Clin North Am.* 2000;38: 179-202.

39. Chang JM, Lee HJ, Lee SE, et al. Unusual tumours involving the prostate: radiological-pathological findings. *Br J Radiol.* 2008;81:907-915.

40. Mazzucchelli R, Lopez-Beltran A, Cheng L, Scarpelli M, Kirkali Z, Montironi R. Rare and unusual histological variants of prostatic carcinoma: clinical significance. *BJU Int.* 2008;102:1369-1374.

41. Khan A, Ramchandani P. Unusual and uncommon prostatic lesions. *Semin Roentgenol.* 1999;34:350-363.

42. Kajiwara M, Mutaguchi K, Usui T. Ductal carcinoma of the prostate with multilocular cystic formation [in Japanese]. *Hinyokika Kiyo.* 2002;48:557-560.

43. Zini L, Villers A, Leroy X, Ballereau C, Lemaitre L, Biserte J. Cystic prostate cancer: a clinical entity of ductal carcinoma [in French]. *Prog Urol.* 2004;14:411-413.

44. Saito S, Iwaki H. Mucin-producing carcinoma of the prostate: review of 88 cases. *Urology.* 1999;54:141-144.

45. Schwartz LH, LaTrenta LR, Bonaccio E, Kelly WK, Scher HI, Panicek DM. Small cell and anaplastic prostate cancer: correlation between CT findings and prostate-specific antigen level. *Radiology.* 1998;208:735-738.

46. Abbas F, Civantos F, Benedetto P, Soloway MS. Small cell carcinoma of the bladder and prostate. *Urology.* 1995;46:617-630.

47. Lazar EB, Whitman GJ, Chew FS. Embryonal rhabdomyosarcoma of the prostate. *AJR Am J Roentgenol.* 1996;166:72.

48. Cheville JC, Dundore PA, Nascimento AG, et al. Leiomyosarcoma of the prostate. Report of 23 cases. *Cancer.* 1995;76:1422-1427.

49. Sexton WJ, Lance RE, Reyes AO, Pisters PW, Tu SM, Pisters LL. Adult prostate sarcoma: the M. D. Anderson Cancer Center Experience. *J Urol.* 2001;166:521-525.

50. Hansel DE, Herawi M, Montgomery E, Epstein JI. Spindle cell lesions of the adult prostate. *Mod Pathol.* 2007;20:148-158.

51. Kaufman JJ, Berneike RR. Leiomyoma of the prostate. *J Urol.* 1951;65:297-310.

52. Kitajima K, Kaji Y, Imanaka K, Hayashi M, Kuwata Y, Sugimura K. MR imaging findings of pure prostatic leiomyoma: a report of two cases. *J Comput Assist Tomogr.* 2006;30:910-912.

53. Bostwick DG, Iczkowski KA, Amin MB, Discigil G, Osborne B. Malignant lymphoma involving the prostate: report of 62 cases. *Cancer.* 1998;83:732-738.

54. Bostwick DG, Mann RB. Malignant lymphomas involving the prostate. A study of 13 cases. *Cancer.* 1985;56:2932-2938.

55. White S, Hricak H, Forstner R, et al. Prostate cancer: effect of postbiopsy hemorrhage on interpretation of MR images. *Radiology.* 1995;195:385-390.

56. Tamada T, Sone T, Jo Y, et al. Prostate cancer: relationships between postbiopsy hemorrhage and tumor detectability at MR *diagnosis. Radiology.* 2008;248:531-539.

57. Wasserman NF. Prostatitis: clinical presentations and transrectal ultrasound findings. *Semin Roentgenol.* 1999;34:325-337.

58. Langer JE, Cornud F. Inflammatory disorders of the prostate and the distal genital tract. *Radiol Clin North Am.* 2006;44: 665-677, vii.

59. Shukla-Dave A, Hricak H, Eberhardt SC, et al. Chronic prostatitis: MR imaging and 1H MR spectroscopic imaging findings—initial observations. *Radiology.* 2004;231:717-724.

60. Parsons RB, Fisher AM, Bar-Chama N, Mitty HA. MR imaging in male infertility. *Radiographics.* 1997;17:627-637.

61. Schiebler ML, Schnall MD, Pollack HM, et al. Current role of MR imaging in the staging of adenocarcinoma of the prostate. *Radiology.* 1993;189:339-352.

62. Wang L, Zhang J, Schwartz LH, et al. Incremental value of multiplanar cross-referencing for prostate cancer staging with endorectal MRI. *AJR Am J Roentgenol.* 2007;188:99-104.

63. Ishikawa M, Okabe H, Oya T, et al. Midline prostatic cysts in healthy men: incidence and transabdominal sonographic findings. *AJR Am J Roentgenol.* 2003;181:1669-1672.

64. Nghiem HT, Kellman GM, Sandberg SA, Craig BM. Cystic lesions of the prostate. *Radiographics.* 1990;10: 635-650. [published erratum appears in *Radiographics.* 1990;10(5):963]

65. Galosi AB, Montironi R, Fabiani A, Lacetera V, Galle G, Muzzonigro G. Cystic lesions of the prostate gland: an ultrasound classification with pathological correlation. *J Urol.* 2009;181:647-657.

66. Tsujimoto Y, Satoh M, Takada T, et al. Papillary cystadenocarcinoma of the prostate: a case report [in Japanese]. *Hinyokika Kiyo.* 2007;53:67-70.

67. Rusch D, Moinzadeh A, Hamawy K, Larsen C. Giant multilocular cystadenoma of the prostate. *AJR Am J Roentgenol.* 2002;179:1477-1479.

68. Allen EA, Brinker DA, Coppola D, Diaz JI, Epstein JI. Multilocular prostatic cystadenoma with high-grade prostatic intraepithelial neoplasia. *Urology.* 2003;61:644.

69. Ishida K, Kubota Y, Takada T, et al. A case of prostate cancer with cyst formation [in Japanese]. *Hinyokika Kiyo.* 2003;49:235-237.

70. Tuziak T, Spiess PE, Abrahams NA, Wrona A, Tu SM, Czerniak B. Multilocular cystadenoma and cystadenocarcinoma of the prostate. *Urol Oncol.* 2007;25:19-25.

71. Outwater E, Schiebler ML, Tomaszewski JE, Schnall MD, Kressel HY. Mucinous carcinomas involving the prostate: atypical findings at MR imaging. *J Magn Reson Imaging.* 1992;2:597-600.

72. Roehrborn CG, Mcconnell JD. Chapter 86—benign prostatic hyperplasia: etiology, pathophysiology, epidemiology, and natural history. In: Wein AJ, Kavoussi LR, Novick AC, Partin AW, Peters CA, eds. *Campbell-Walsh Urology.* 9th ed. Philadelphia, PA: WB Saunders; 2007.

73. Berry SJ, Coffey DS, Walsh PC, Ewing LL. The development of human benign prostatic hyperplasia with age. *J Urol.* 1984;132: 474-479.

74. Lovett K, Rifkin MD, McCue PA, Choi H. MR imaging characteristics of noncancerous lesions of the prostate. *J Magn Reson Imaging.* 1992;2:35-39.

75. Potter SR, Partin AW. Prostatitis syndromes and benign prostatic hyperplasia. *Semin Roentgenol.* 1999;34:256-268.

76. Maki DD, Banner MP, Ramchandani P, Stolpen A, Rovner ES, Wein AJ. Injected periurethral collagen for postprostatectomy urinary incontinence: MR and CT appearance. *Abdom Imaging.* 2000;25:658-662.

77. Kim B, Kawashima A, Ryu J-A, Takahashi N, Hartman RP, King BF Jr. Imaging of the seminal vesicle and vas deferens. *Radiographics.* 2009;29:1105-1121.

78. Patel B, Gujral S, Jefferson K, Evans S, Persad R. Seminal vesicle cysts and associated anomalies. *BJU Int.* 2002;90:265-271.

79. Arora SS, Breiman RS, Webb EM, Westphalen AC, Yeh BM, Coakley FV. CT and MRI of congenital anomalies of the seminal vesicles. *AJR Am J Roentgenol.* 2007;189:130-135.

80. Livingston L, Larsen CR. Seminal vesicle cyst with ipsilateral renal agenesis. *AJR Am J Roentgenol.* 2000;175:177-180.

81. Torigian DA, Ramchandani P. Hematospermia: imaging findings. Abdom Imaging 2007;32:29-49.

82. Hatano K, Tsujimoto Y, Ichimaru N, Miyagawa Y, Nonomura N, Okuyama A. Rare case of aggressive angiomyxoma presenting as a retrovesical tumor. *Int J Urol.* 2006;13:1012-1014.

83. Ramchandani P, Schnall MD, LiVolsi VA, Tomaszewski JE, Pollack HM. Senile amyloidosis of the seminal vesicles mimicking metastatic spread of prostatic carcinoma on MR images. *AJR Am J Roentgenol.* 1993;161:99-100.

84. Dahnert WF. Prostatic Calcifications. In: Resnick M, Watanabe H, Karr JP, eds. *Diagnostic Ultrasound of the Prostate.* New York: Elsevier Science; 1989:178-182.

85. Jung YY, Kim JK, Cho K-S. Genitourinary tuberculosis: comprehensive cross-sectional imaging. *AJR Am J Roentgenol.* 2005;184:143-150.

86. Wymenga LF, Duisterwinkel FJ, Groenier K, Mensink HJ. Ultrasound-guided seminal vesicle biopsies in prostate cancer. *Prostate Cancer Prostatic Dis.* 2000;3:100-106.

87. Thiel R, Effert P. Primary adenocarcinoma of the seminal vesicles. *J Urol.* 2002;168:1891-1896.

88. Jinza S, Noguchi K, Hosaka M. Retrospective study of 107 patients with hematospermia [in Japanese]. *Hinyokika Kiyo.* 1997;43:103-107.

89. Han M, Brannigan RE, Antenor JA, Roehl KA, Catalona WJ. Association of hemospermia with prostate cancer. *J Urol.* 2004;172:2189-2192.

90. Simpson WL Jr, Rausch DR. Imaging of male infertility: pictorial review. *AJR Am J Roentgenol.* 2009;192:S98-S107.

91. Cirillo S, Petracchini M, Scotti L, et al. Endorectal magnetic resonance imaging at 1.5 Tesla to assess local recurrence following radical prostatectomy using T2-weighted and contrast-enhanced imaging. *Eur Radiol.* 2009;19:761-769.

92. Allen SD, Thompson A, Sohaib SA. The normal post-surgical anatomy of the male pelvis following radical prostatectomy as assessed by magnetic resonance imaging. *Eur Radiol.* 2008;18: 1281-1291.

93. Sella T, Schwartz LH, Hricak H. Retained seminal vesicles after radical prostatectomy: frequency, MRI characteristics, and clinical relevance. *AJR Am J Roentgenol.* 2006;186:539-546.

94. Casciani E, Polettini E, Carmenini E, et al. Endorectal and dynamic contrast-enhanced MRI for detection of local recurrence after radical prostatectomy. *AJR Am J Roentgenol.* 2008;190:1187-1192.

95. Pucar D, Shukla-Dave A, Hricak H, et al. Prostate cancer: correlation of MR imaging and MR spectroscopy with pathologic findings after radiation therapy—initial experience. *Radiology.* 2005;236:545-553.

96. Yablon CM, Banner MP, Ramchandani P, Rovner ES. Complications of prostate cancer treatment: spectrum of imaging findings. *Radiographics.* 2004;24:S181-S194.

CHAPTER

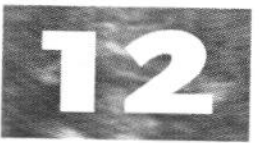

Imaging of the Scrotum and Penis

Lisa P. Jones, MD, PhD
Jason N. Itri, MD, PhD
Jill Langer, MD
Parvati Ramchandani, MD

THE NORMAL SCROTUM

Anatomy

The scrotum is a multilayered sac divided by a midline septum, with each half containing a testis, epididymis, and intrascrotal portion of the spermatic cord. The tunica vaginalis is a pouch of serous membrane derived from the processus vaginalis that is reflected on the internal surface of the scrotum, the parietal layer, and covers the surface of the testis and the epididymis, the visceral layer. Only the posterior aspect of the testis, which is the site of attachment, is not covered by the tunica vaginalis. The parietal and the visceral layers are normally separated by a few milliliters of fluid.

The testes are symmetric ovoid organs covered by a fibrous layer called the tunica albuginea. The tunica dives into the testicle forming the mediastinum testis. Septa arising from the mediastinum divide the testis into 250 to 400 lobules, each containing 1 to 3 seminiferous tubules, spermatocytes that give rise to sperm, Leydig cells that produce testosterone, and supporting Sertoli cells.[1] The seminiferous tubules become the tubuli recti, which drain into dilated spaces in the mediastinum called the rete testis. The rete testis drain through 10 to 15 efferent ductules into the ductus epididymis, a 6- to 8-cm tubule that courses through the epididymis, and curves acutely in the region of the tail to become the ductus deferens.[2] The epididymis lies along the posterolateral aspect of the testis and is composed of a head, body, and tail. The head (globus major) is located at the superior pole, whereas the tail (globus minor) is located along the inferior pole. The testes contain four appendages: the appendix testis, appendix epididymis, the paradidymis, and vas aberrans. The appendix testis is a paramesonephric duct remnant, whereas the other appendages are mesonephric duct remnants. The appendix testis and appendix epididymis can occasionally be detected by ultrasonography (US) and magnetic resonance imaging (MRI) examinations and will usually appear as small, <5-mm ovoid structures in the region of the upper pole of testis.[2] The paradidymis and vas aberrans are usually not visualized by imaging examinations (see Figure 12-1).

The adult size of the testis is in the range of 3 to 5 cm in length and 2 to 3 cm in anteroposterior and transverse dimension, with a volume in the range of 15 to 20 mL. Slight asymmetry in volume is normal. Testicular size varies with age and sexual development. Before age 12, the volume is 1 to 2 mL and increases with puberty. Testicular volume decreases in elderly men. The epididymis measures 6 cm in length, with the head measuring 5 to 12 mm, the body measuring 2 to 4 mm, and the tail measuring 2 to 5 mm. The scrotal wall, from the tunica vaginalis to the skin surface, measures 2 to 8 mm with the range due to variable contraction of the cremaster muscle.[3]

There are 3 arteries within the spermatic cord, supplying the scrotum and contents. These are the testicular artery, which is a branch of the abdominal aorta, the deferential artery, which is a branch of the superior vesicle artery, and the cremaster artery, which is a branch of the inferior epigastric artery. The epididymal artery, which is a branch of the testicular artery, and the cremaster and deferential arteries, supply the epididymis, vas deferens, and the paratesticular tissues. The testicle is supplied by the testicular artery, which enters the tunica albuginea forming capsular arteries, which in turn give rise to centripetal arteries that penetrate into the testis toward the mediastinum. In 50% of normal testis, there is a transmediastinal artery that courses from the mediastinum to supply capsular arteries. This artery is usually accompanied by a

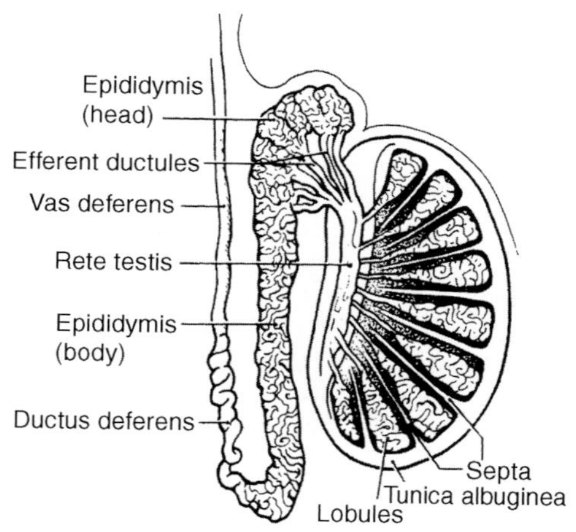

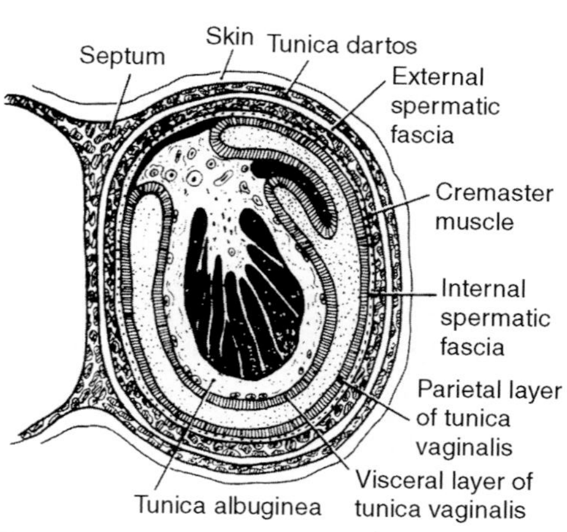

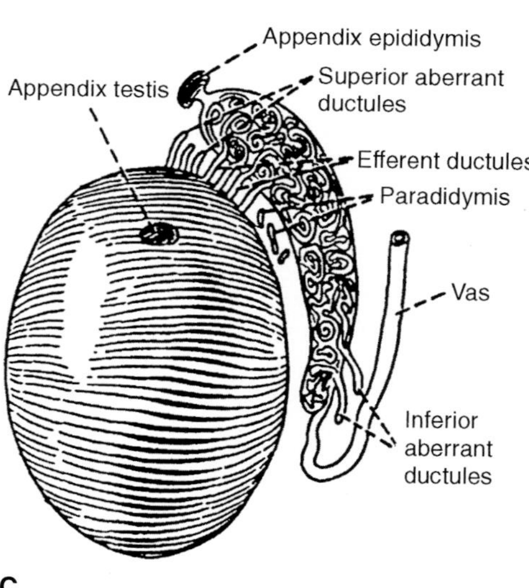

Figure 12-1 Normal Anatomy of the Testis
The normal anatomy of the scrotum is detailed in these 3 diagrams. (Part A: Reprinted with permission from Akbar SA, Sayyed TA, Jafri SZ, et al. Multimodality imaging of paratesticular neoplasms and their rare mimics. *Radiographics.* 2003;23(6):1461-1476; Part B: Reprinted with permission from McClennan P: Clinical Urography, vol 2. New York, NY: Elsevier, 2000; and Part C: Reprinted with permission from Rolnick D, Kawanoue S, Szanto P, et al. Anatomical incidence of testicular appendages. *J Urol.* 1968;100(6):755-756.)

large vein. The scrotal skin is supplied by branches of the pudendal artery. The venous drainage of the testis is via the pampiniform plexus to gonadal veins, which drain to the inferior vena cava (IVC) on the right and to the left renal vein on the left.

Ultrasonographic Appearance

The testicles are ovoid structures that should have a homogeneous, symmetric echotexture, and similar size (see Figure 12-2). The mediastinum testis is identifiable as a hyperechogenic linear region along the posterior testicle. The tunica albuginea may be difficult to visualize in the absence of a hydrocele, but when seen usually appears as a thin layer along the surface of the testis. The epididymis is usually isoechoic to slightly hypoechoic relative to the testicle and is seen along the posterolateral surface of the testicle, with a triangular head at the superior pole that tapers to a smaller linear structure inferiorly. The head of the epididymis is usually isoechogenic to testis while the tail is usually slightly hypoechogenic.[2] A small amount of fluid is normally present in the tunica vaginalis surrounding the testes.

On color Doppler, both the testicles and epididymis demonstrate symmetric flow. On spectral Doppler, intratesticular arteries demonstrate a low-resistance waveform with a mean resistive index of 0.62 with a range of 0.48 to 0.75. The resistive index of arteries in the epididymis ranges from 0.46 to 0.68 (see Figure 12-3).[2,9]

MRI Appearance

The normal testis is low- to intermediate-signal on T1-weighted images and high-signal on T2-weighted images relative to skeletal muscle (see Figure 12-4). The tunica albuginea is seen as a low-signal rim around each testicle. The mediastinum testis usually appears as a band of low signal. Occasionally, intralobular septa may be seen as linear low-T2-signal structures radiating to the mediastinum testis. The epididymal head is hypointense to the testis but hyperintense to muscle on T2-weighted images and is isointense to testis on T1-weighted images. T2-weighted images are useful for depicting solid intratesticular masses, which are usually low-signal relative to the testis. T1-weighted images are useful for detecting substances such as fat or hemorrhage.[5] Gadolinium can occasionally be helpful in differentiating a benign cystic lesion from a cystic neoplasm or to assess testicular perfusion.

FOCAL TESTICULAR DISORDERS

Solid-Appearing Intratesticular Lesion or Mass

One of the primary indications for scrotal imaging is to determine if a palpable abnormality is intratesticular or

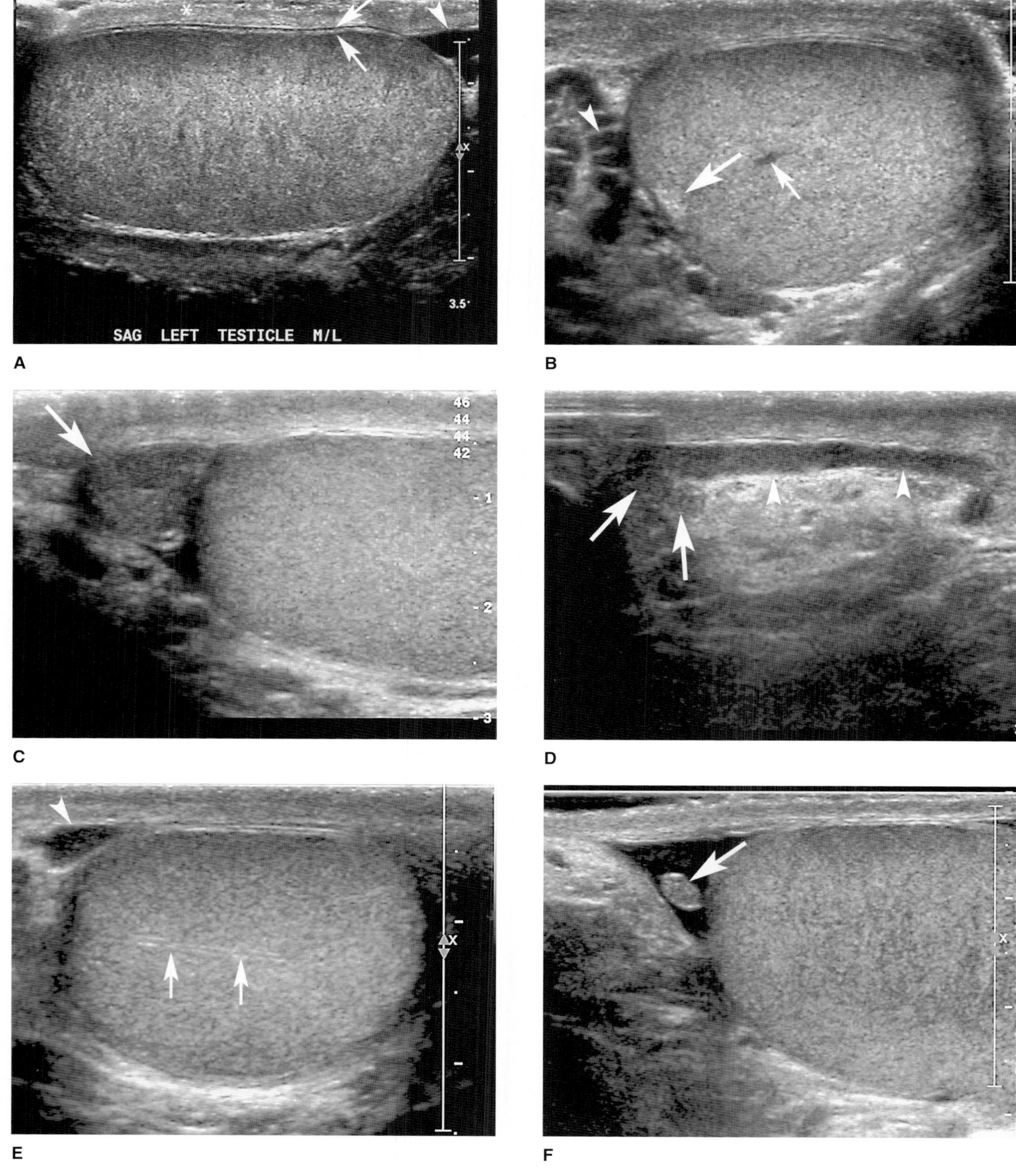

Figure 12-2 Normal Sonogram of the Scrotum
A. Sagittal image through the testicle demonstrates homogenous echotexture. Tunica albuginea indicated by *thin arrows*; *asterisk* shows normal thickness of scrotal wall, *arrowhead* indicates small amount of physiologic fluid. **B.** Transverse grayscale image through the testicle illustrates the mediastinum testis (*larger arrow*), transmediastinal vessel (*small arrow*), and normal veins of the pampiniform plexus (*arrowhead*). **C.** Sagittal image of the scrotum shows the epididymis as a triangular structure slightly hypoechoic to adjacent testicle (*arrow*). **D.** Sagittal image of the scrotum illustrates the head (*arrows*) and body and tail (*arrowheads*) of the epididymis. **E.** Transverse grayscale image shows a transmediastinal vessel (*arrows*) and the epididymal body in transverse (*arrowhead*). **F.** Image showing the appendix testis (*arrow*).

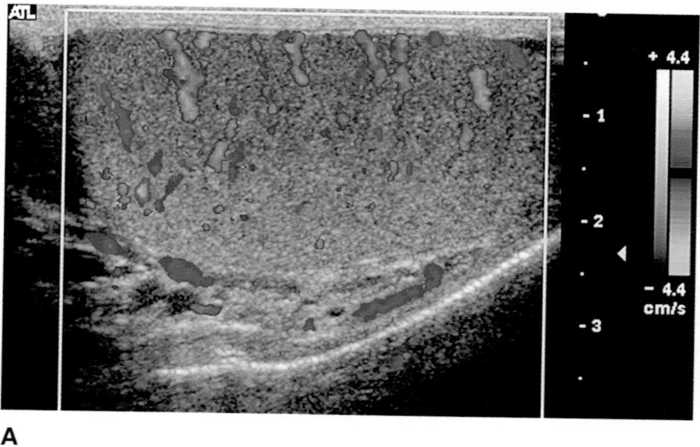

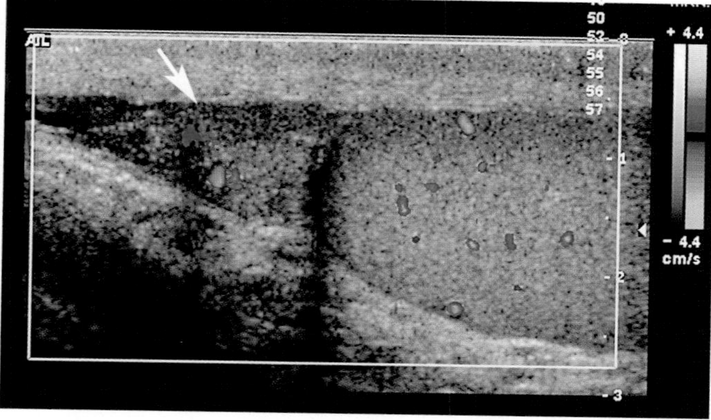

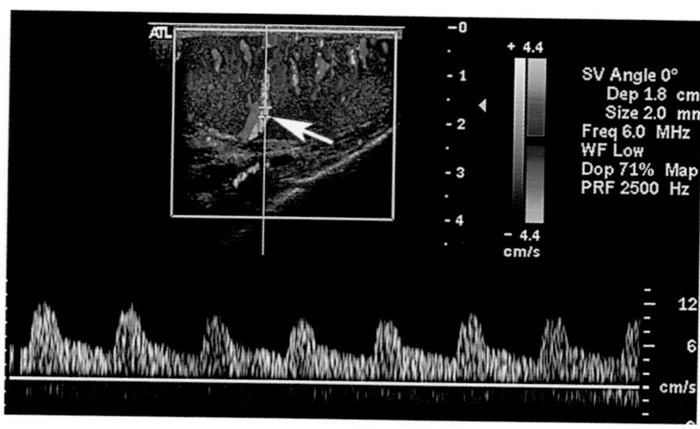

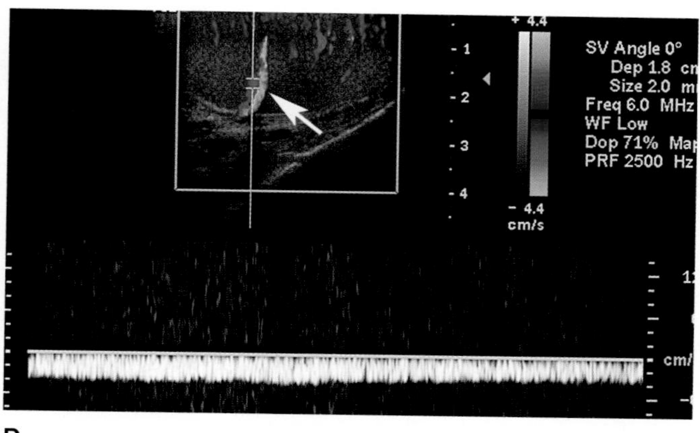

Figure 12-3 Normal Doppler Evaluation of the Testicle
A and **B**. Color Doppler images demonstrate normal testicular and epididymal (*arrow*) blood flow. The vascularity of the testicles should be symmetric. Color Doppler parameters should be optimized to detect slow flow. Spectral Doppler evaluation shows normal low-resistance arterial flow (**C**) and normal venous flow (**D**) on sampling of intratesticular vessels (*arrows*).

extratesticular, as most intratesticular masses in adults are malignant whereas most extratesticular masses are benign (Table 12-1).

Germ cell neoplasms

Primary testicular tumors account for only approximately 1% of all malignant neoplasms in men but are the most common cancer in 25- to 35-year-old men.[5] Ninety percent to 95% of these are derived from germs cells. Risk factors for germ cell tumors include cryptorchidism, Klinefelter syndrome, and testicular feminization syndrome as well as intersex syndromes, family history, and prior diagnosis of testicular tumor.[6,7] Patients present with a painless testicular mass in approximately 70% of cases, but can present with acute scrotal pain (10%), following trauma (10%), or with symptoms related to metastatic disease (10%).[1]

Intratubular germ cell neoplasia is thought to be the precursor of most germ cell tumors, although not clearly implicated as a precursor lesion of pediatric yolk sac tumors and teratomas, or of adult spermatocytic seminoma.[6] Nonetheless, it is considered to be the testicular equivalent of carcinoma in situ. Fifty percent of patients with intratubular germ cell neoplasia will develop an invasive tumor in 5 years. The prevailing theory of development is that these abnormal cells progress either along a unipotential gonadal line and form seminoma or along a totipotential cell line and form nonseminomatous tumors. The totipotential cells can remain largely undifferentiated (embryonal carcinoma) or develop toward embryonic differentiation (teratoma) or extraembryonic differentiation (yolk sac tumors, choriocarcinoma). Because these cells can develop along several pathways at once, multiple histologic types often occur together, yielding a mixed germ cell tumor. For clinical purposes, germ cell tumors are divided into 2 groups: seminomatous and nonseminomatous germ cell tumors (NSGCT), as will be discussed in subsequent sections on the individual germ cell neoplasms following a discussion of common features of testicular carcinoma[7] (Table 12-2).

Metastases from testicular germ cell tumors can spread by both lymphatic and hematogenous routes. Most germ cell tumors spread first via the lymphatics. Since lymphatic drainage follows the testicular veins, spread usually

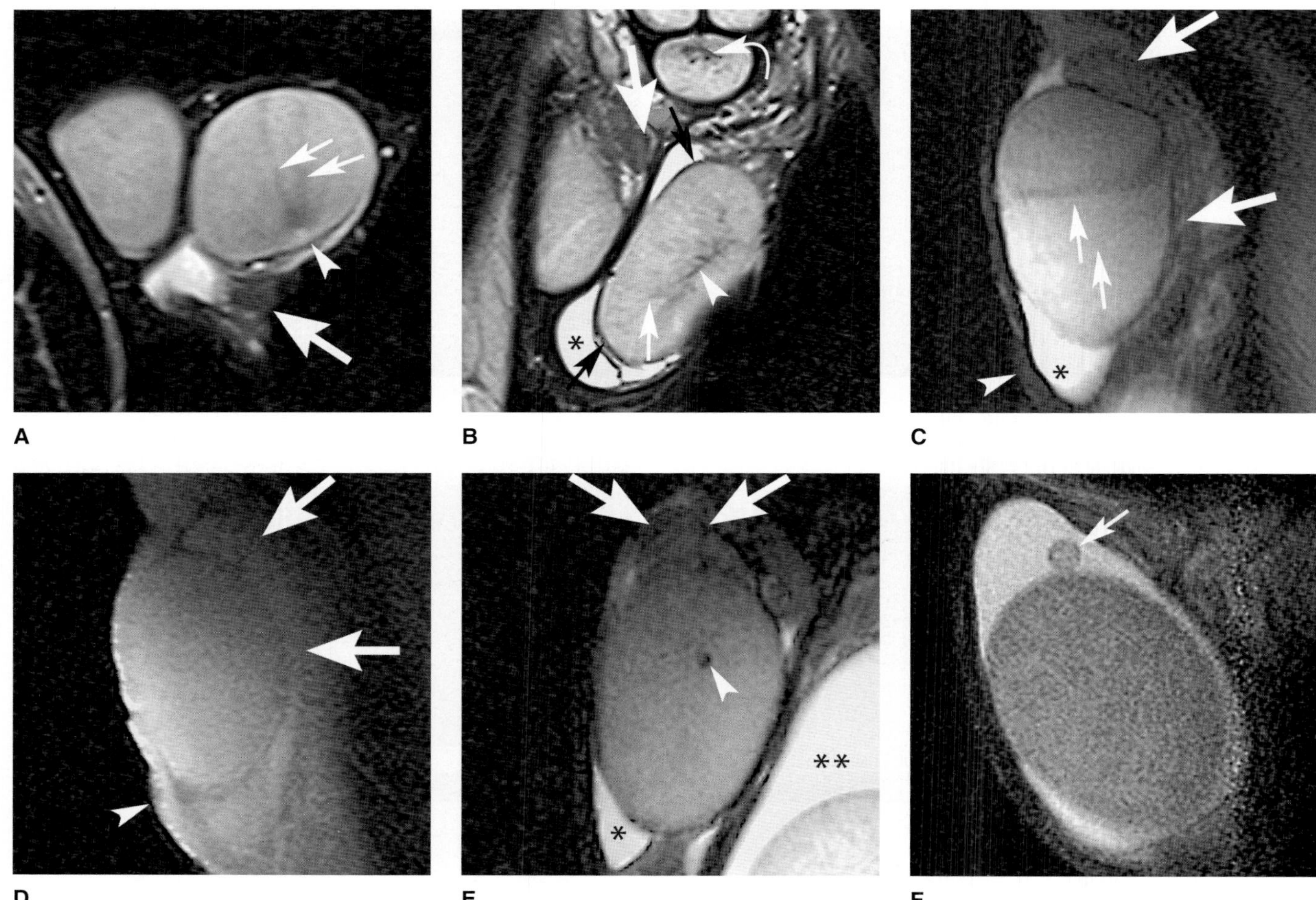

Figure 12-4 Normal MRI of the Scrotum
A. Axial and (B) coronal T2-weighted images show the normal T2 hypointense lobular septa (*thin white arrows*) converging on the mediastinum testis (*arrowhead*). The images also show a portion of the epididymis (*thick arrow*), which is T2 hypointense relative to the testis. The tunica albuginea appears as a thin T2 hypointense line around the testis (*black arrows* in B); note also the urethra (*curved arrow* in B) in the corpora spongiosum. Physiologic fluid is present around the testis (*asterisk*). C. Sagittal T2 and (D) sagittal fat-saturated postcontrast T1 images demonstrate the epididymis (*fat arrows*) as a low-signal structure along the posterior aspect of the epididymis, which is mildly hyperenhancing relative to normal testicular parenchymal. Note the lobular septa (*thin white arrows* in C) and the scrotal wall (*arrowheads*). E. Coronal T2-weighted image show a low T2 signal structure (*arrowhead*) in the testis corresponding to a vessel. Note also the epididymal head (*thick arrows*) and a small hydrocele (*asterisk*). Partially visualized is a larger left hydrocele (*2 asterisks*) in this patient with left epididymo-orchitis. F. Sagittal T2-weighted image demonstrating the appendix testis (*arrow*).

occurs first to retroperitoneal lymph nodes, skipping the pelvic lymph node chains. For the right testis, spread initially occurs to interaortocaval chain at the second lumbar vertebral body, and to precaval, right paracaval, and retrocaval nodes.[7,8] For the left testis, spread initially is to left para-aortic nodes in an area bounded by the renal vein, aorta, ureter, and inferior mesenteric artery and to preaortic nodes.[7,8] Some crossover of lymphatic involvement can occur in a right-to-left fashion. Left-to-right crossover is rare.[1] As the volume of tumor increases, eventually spread can occur from the first-echelon nodes to the common, internal, and external iliac nodes.

There are 2 situations when the classic pattern of spread does not occur and there is early involvement of the pelvic lymph nodes chains. First, tumor invasion of

Imaging Notes 12-1. Lymphatic spread

- **Lymphatic metastasis** from testicular germ cell neoplasms occur first to the retroperitoneal nodal chains, skipping the pelvic nodal chains, occurring on the right to the interaortocaval chain at the second lumbar vertebral and on the left, to the left para-aortic lymph node in the region of the left renal vein. This is because lymphatic drainage of the testis follows the testicular vein.
- **Hematogenous metastases** are usually a late finding, with the exception of choriocarcinoma, and usually occur in the lung, liver, brain, and bone.

Table 12-1. Causes of Unilateral Testicular Lesions

1. Neoplasms
   a. Germ cell neoplasms
      i. Seminomatous germ cell tumors
      ii. Nonseminomatous germ cell tumors (NSGCT)
   b. Sex-cord stromal neoplasms
      i. Leydig cell tumors
      ii. Sertoli cell tumors
      iii. Other stromal neoplasms
   c. Other neoplasms
      i. Epidermoid cyst
      ii. Lymphoma
      iii. Leukemia
      iv. Testicular metastasis
2. Orchitis
   i. Bacterial
   ii. Granulomatous
3. Abscess
4. Hematoma
5. Splenogonadal fusion
6. Testicular sarcoidosis
7. Congenital adrenal rests
8. Mimics
   i. Complex cysts
   ii. Adenomatoid tumor of the tunica albuginea

paratesticular tissues such as the epididymis or the scrotal wall, both of which have different lymphatic drainage than the testis, can lead to direct spread to the external iliac nodes or inguinal lymph nodes, respectively.[7] Second, prior scrotal surgery can disrupt the expected patterns of spread, thereby leading to early metastases to the inguinal or pelvic lymph nodes chains. For this reason, a transscrotal surgical approach is contraindicated and orchiectomy is performed through an inguinal approach.[8]

Hematogenous spread usually occurs late with the exception of choriocarcinoma where it is the primary mode of spread. The most common hematogenous site of spread is the lung, followed by liver, brain, and bone.[7] Brain metastases are more common with choriocarcinoma than with other histologies. Other unusual sites of disease, such as peritoneum, kidney, and spleen, are more frequently observed at the time of relapse in patients than at the time of initial diagnosis.

Table 12-2. Testicular Germ Cell Tumors

- Seminomatous types
  - Seminoma
    - Spermatocystic seminoma
    - Anaplastic
- Nonseminomatous germ cell tumors
  - Mixed germ cell neoplasm
  - Teratoma
  - Embryonal carcinoma
  - Yolk sac tumor
  - Choriocarcinoma

There are numerous staging systems in current use. One of the most commonly used is the TNM (tumor, node, metastasis) classification set forth by the American Joint Committee on Cancer. In clinical practice, patients are often classified as having low-stage or advanced-stage disease. In low-stage disease, the tumor is confined to the testis, epididymis, or spermatic cord (T1-T3) and mild to moderate adenopathy (N1 and N2) can also be present. Advanced-stage disease includes tumors that invade the scrotal wall (T4), significant retroperitoneal adenopathy (N3), or visceral metastases (M1).

Seminomatous germ cell tumors: Seminomas are the most common type of germ cell tumor, accounting for 40% to 50% of germ cell tumors. They are composed of a relatively uniform population of cells that resemble primordial germ cells or early gonocytes.[6] They usually present in patients 30 to 50 years in age, which is older on average than patients with NSGCT. A history of cryptorchidism is present in 10% to 15% of cases.[9] Approximately 15% of seminomas will be associated with elevation of serum beta–human chorionic gonadotropin (β-hCG) because of the presence of syncytiotrophoblasts. However, serum β-hCG levels are typically lower in seminomas than in NSGCTs.[6] Serum α-fetoprotein levels are normal in pure seminoma, and the presence of an elevated serum α-fetoprotein level indicates that the tumor is an NSGCT.

Testicular seminoma has the best prognosis of all the germ cell tumors because it is very radiosensitive and chemosensitive and tends to remain localized for extended periods of time. Approximately 70% of seminomas are confined to the scrotum at diagnosis, with 20% presenting with retroperitoneal metastases and 5% presenting with extranodal disease[9] compared with 40% confinement to the scrotum for NSGCT.[6] Treatment usually is radiation therapy for low-stage tumors and a combination of chemotherapy and radiation therapy for more advanced tumors. The cure rate of low-stage disease approaches 98%, and even patients with metastatic disease can be cured in 90% cases.[10]

On ultrasound examinations (US), most seminomas appear as homogenous hypoechogenic masses, reflecting the relative uniformity of the cellular population comprising the tumor (see Figure 12-5). However, larger tumors may be heterogeneous, with 10% of seminomas containing small cystic areas, corresponding to dilated rete testis caused by tumor-related occlusion of tubules.[9] Seminomas can sometimes infiltrate and replace the entire testicle,[6] in which case a diffuse texture change will be seen (see **Neoplasms causing diffuse testicular abnormality** later in this chapter). Multinodular appearing

Imaging Notes 12-2. Staging

TNM Stage	Description
Primary tumor (pT)	
pTX	Primary tumor cannot be assessed (radical orchidectomy not performed)
pT0	No evidence of primary tumor
pTis	Intratubular germ cell neoplasia
pT1	Tumor is limited to testis and epididymis without vascular or lymphatic invasion without involvement of the tunica vaginalis
pT2	Tumor is limited to testis and epididymis with vascular or lymphatic invasion with involvement of tunica vaginalis
pT3	Tumor invades spermatic cord with or without vascular or lymphatic invasion
pT4	Tumor invades scrotum with or without vascular or lymphatic invasion
Regional lymph nodes (N)	
Clinical involvement	
NX	Regional nodes cannot be assessed
N0	No regional lymph node metastasis
N1	One or multiple lymph nodes all ≤2 cm in greatest dimension
N2	One or multiple lymph nodes, with the largest having a maximal diameter between 2 and 5 cm.
N3	Lymph node diameter >5 cm in greatest dimension
Pathologic involvement	
pN0	No regional lymph node metastases
pN1	One or multiple lymph node metastasis with diameter ≤2 cm and 5 or fewer positive nodes
pN2	One or multiple lymph nodes with the largest having a maximal diameter between 2 and 5 cm, more than 5 nodes positive, with none >5 cm, or evidence of extranodal extension of tumor
pN3	Metastasis with a lymph node mass >5 cm in greatest dimension
Distant metastases (M)	
MX	Distant metastasis cannot be assessed
M0	No distant metastasis
M1a	Nonregional lymph node or pulmonary metastasis
M1b	Distant metastasis other than to nonregional lymph nodes and lungs
Serum tumor markers (S)	
SX	Tumor marker studies not available or not performed
S0	Tumor marker levels within normal limits
S1	LDH <1.5 × normal; β-hCG <5000 IU/L; and α-fetoprotein <1000 ng/mL
S2	LDH 1.5-10 × normal; β-hCG 5000-50 000 IU/L; or α-fetoprotein 1000-10 000 ng/mL
S3	LDH >10 × normal; β-hCG >50 000 IU/L; or α-fetoprotein >10 000 ng/mL

Abbreviation: LDH, lactate dehydrogenase.
Adapted from AJCC:Cancer staging book.[158]

seminomas also occur but in most cases the nodules are in continuity with one another, as part of the same tumor, rather than representing separate synchronous tumors in a truly multifocal neoplasm.[9] Bilateral seminoma is rare, and is usually due to asynchronous tumors.[7] Seminomas are typically confined by the tunica albuginea and rarely extend to paratesticular structures. Therefore, gross invasion of the spermatic cord or tunica albuginea should prompt consideration of another tumor type, particularly lymphoma, which also tends to be relatively homogenous and hypoechoic.

On MRI, seminomas characteristically appear isointense on T1-weighted images and predominantly low-signal-intensity on T2-weighted images relative to testicular parenchyma. Following contrast material administration, septa within the seminoma typically enhance to a greater

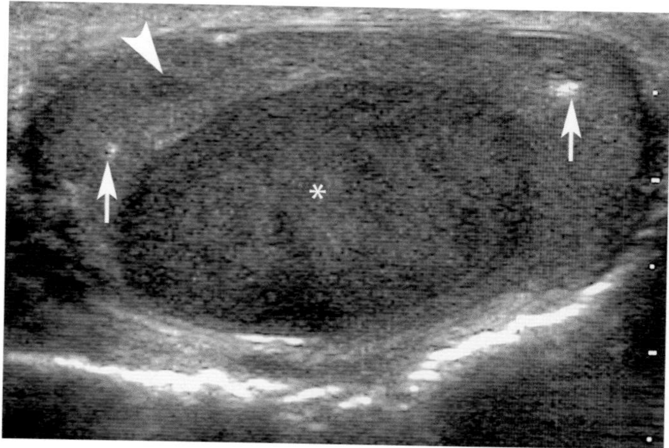

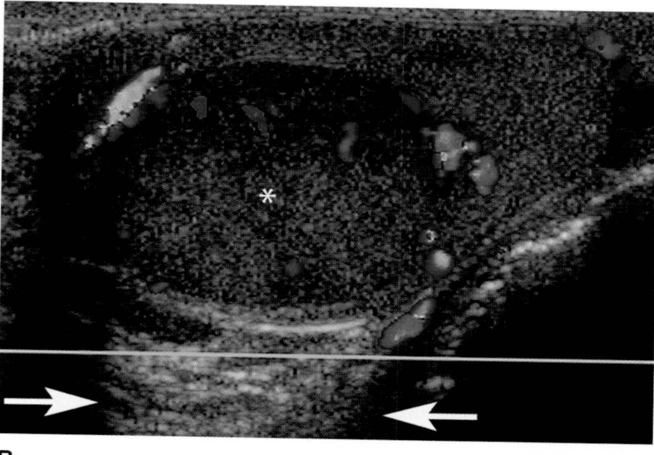

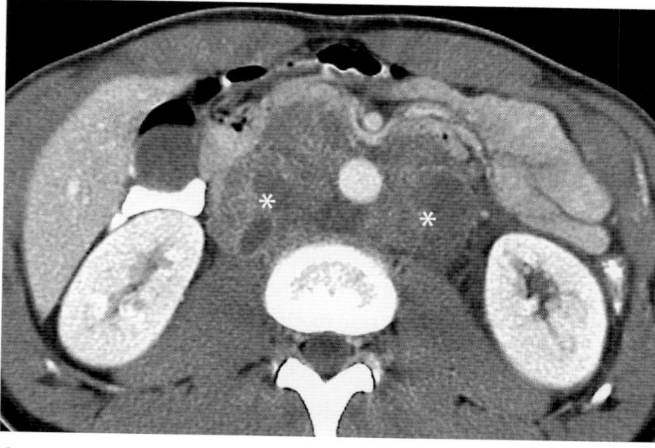

Figure 12-5 Seminoma With Retroperitoneal Metastases
A and **B**. Grayscale (A) and (B) color Doppler images of the testis demonstrate the presence of a relatively uniform hypoechoic intratesticular mass (*asterisk*) with through transmission (*arrows* in **B**). Although through transmission typically is a feature of a cyst, it can be seen in tumors characterized by a uniform population of cells, such as seminoma and lymphoma. The presence of color flow within the lesion excludes the possibility that this represents a complex cyst. Note dystrophic testicular calcifications (*small arrows* in A) and a second hypoechoic focus (*arrowhead*), also likely representing tumor. **C**. Axial image from an enhanced CT scan demonstrate aortocaval and left para-aortic bulky lymphadenopathy originating in the region of the left renal hilum and extending inferiorly (*asterisk*). IVC is difficult to visualize in C due to invasion.

degree than the tumor itself (see Figure 12-6).[11] Similar to the US examination, the tumor is usually confined to the testicle, without extension into the surrounding tissues.

Spermatocytic seminoma: Spermatocytic seminoma should be differentiated from seminoma, which is a histologically and clinically distinct neoplasm. Unlike seminoma, spermatocytic seminoma does not arise from intratubular germ cell neoplasia. Affected individuals with spermatocystic seminoma are generally over the age of 65 years, whereas seminomas typically affect middle-aged men. Spermatocystic seminoma is a slow-growing tumor that rarely, if ever, produces metastases. In general, the prognosis for spermatocystic seminoma is excellent. The tumor appears similar to, but tends to be larger than, classic seminoma, but otherwise is indistinguishable from seminoma on the basis of imaging appearance.[6]

Nonseminomatous germ cell tumors (NSGCT): NSGCTs arise from a totipotent germ cell, which can remain undifferentiated, resembling embryonic stem cells, as in the case of embryonal carcinoma, or can differentiate into various lineages generating yolk sac tumors, choriocarcinomas, and teratomas. Further, NSGCTs can either be composed of 1 histologic pattern or can be composed of multiple germ cell components, in which case they are referred to as a mixed germ cell neoplasm. Despite the histologic diversity of NSGCTs, the general therapeutic approach is similar among the different pathologic subtypes, and differs from that for seminoma.

In general, NSGCTs are more biologically aggressive than seminoma, with nodal or other metastatic involvement at presentation in 60% to 75%. Additionally, NSGCTs are less radiosensitive than seminomas and are treated with various combinations of chemotherapy and lymphadenectomy, rather than radiotherapy.[8] Consequently, the prognosis for NSGCT is not quite as good as for seminoma, but cure is still achievable in up to 80% even in the setting of metastatic disease and lymphadenopathy.[10]

Interestingly, unlike most other types of tumors, nonseminomatous germ cell tumor metastases can have histologic characteristics that are different from those of the primary testicular tumor, reflecting the totipotential nature of the germ cells. This can have implications for treatment.[7] For example, an enlarging retroperitoneal mass following treatment can indicate development of mature teratoma in

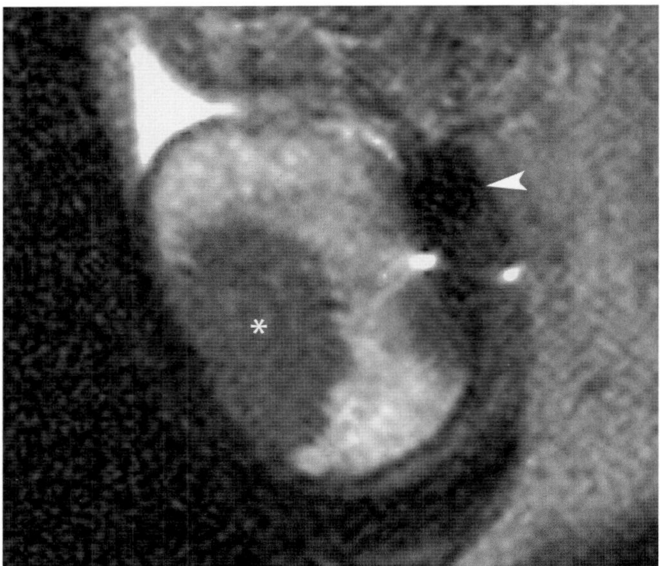

A

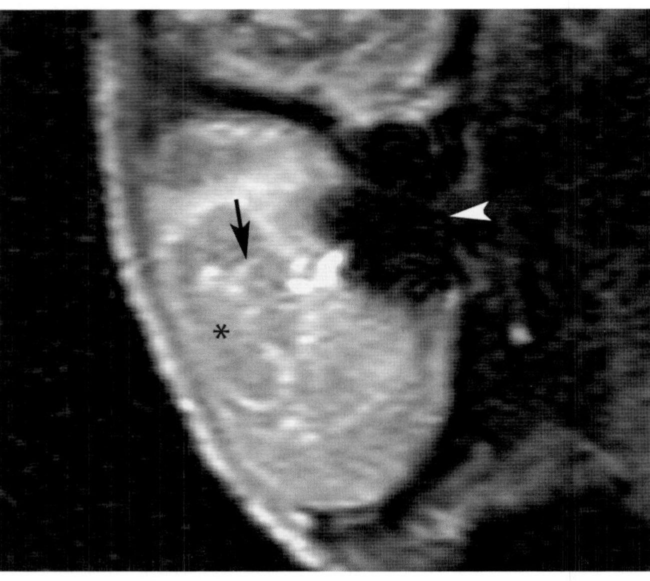

B

Figure 12-6 MRI of Seminoma
Sagittal T2-weighted (**A**) and postgadolinium fat-saturated T1-weighted sequences (**B**) demonstrate the presence of a homogenous low-T2-signal intratesticular mass (*asterisk*) with enhancing septa (*arrow*), which is suggestive but not specific for seminoma. Arrowhead points to a signal void due to susceptibility artifact from metal.

the metastatic lymphadenopathy even if mature teratoma was not present in the primary tumor. This is referred to as "growing teratoma syndrome" and is important to differentiate from relapse,[12] as the preferred treatment approach is surgical, since mature teratoma is generally poorly responsive to chemoradiation. Treatment for mature teratoma is aimed at reducing potential morbidity associated with local invasion as well as reducing the risk of dedifferentiation into a malignant histology. The diagnosis of "growing teratoma syndrome" should be suspected if tumor markers are negative in the setting of enlarging cystic components in a retroperitoneal mass, and/or if the mass is not hypermetabolic on positron emission tomography (PET) scan.[13] Persistence of disease at one or several foci despite regression at other foci can also be an indicator of "growing teratoma syndrome."

Mixed germ cell neoplasm is the most common type of NSGCT. Embryonal histology is the most common element occurring in up to 87%, with teratoma occurring in 50%, yolk sac elements in up to 44%, and choriocarcinoma in only 8% to 16%.[1,7,9] Compared with seminoma, mixed germ cell neoplasms occur in younger men (average age of 30, compared with 40 for seminoma), tend to present at a more advanced stage, and are associated with elevated tumor markers in 80%, either β-hCG (due to the choriocarcinoma component) or α-fetoprotein (due to yolk sac and rarely due to teratoma component) or both. Lactate dehydrogenase can also be elevated, and though not specific for testicular carcinoma does correlate with the bulk of the disease and is used in staging. The sonographic and MRI appearance of mixed germ cell tumors reflects the heterogeneous composition of these neoplasms. On US, they often have an inhomogeneous echotexture (71%), irregular or ill-defined margins (45%), echogenic foci (35%), and cystic components (61%) (see Figures 12-7 and 12-8). The cystic components can reflect true cysts due to teratoma, dilated rete testis, or areas of necrosis. Echogenic foci represent areas of hemorrhage, calcification, or fibrosis. Similarly, MRI usually reveals poorly marginated tumors that are inhomogeneous. In addition, MRI can identify the presence of fat indicative of a teratomatous component as a T1 hyperintense area that loses signal with fat suppression or as an area that loses signal on out-of-phase T1-weighted sequences because of the presence of lipid and water in the same voxel.[11]

Embryonal carcinoma accounts for 3% of tumors and tends to occur in men in their 30s.[7] The tumor cells often stain with both β-hCG and α-fetoprotein.[6] These tumor markers are elevated in 60% to 70% of cases of embryonal carcinoma. Further, US and MRI examinations typically demonstrate a small irregular mass with inhomogeneous echotexture and heterogeneous T1 and T2 signal, which contain cystic spaces in 20%.[7] Embryonal carcinoma is, on average, smaller but more aggressive than seminoma. It is reported to invade the tunica albuginea in up to 20% to 25% of cases, which can be seen as distortion of the testicular contour on imaging examinations.[9]

Teratoma refers to a tumor composed of various cellular elements reminiscent of normal derivatives of more than 1 germ layer and can be categorized as mature or immature. Pure teratoma is relatively common in children and infants, second only to yolk sac tumors in frequency, but in adults constitutes only 2% to 3% of testicular neoplasms.

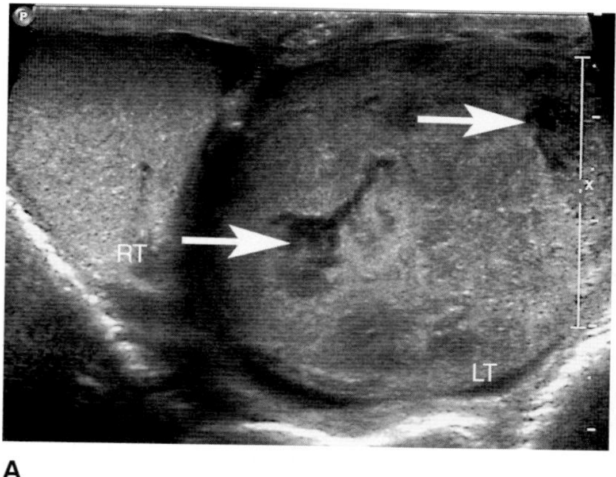

A

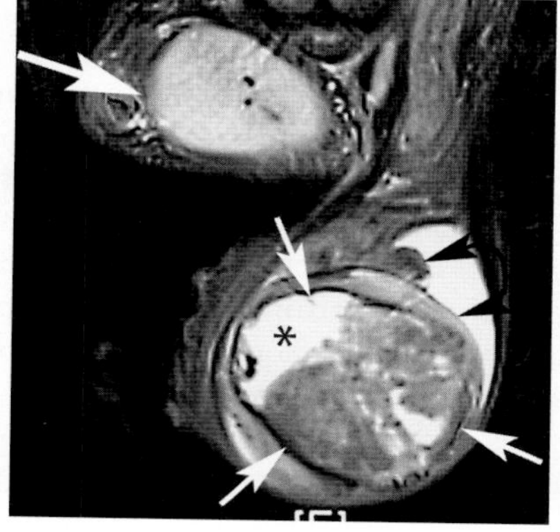
B

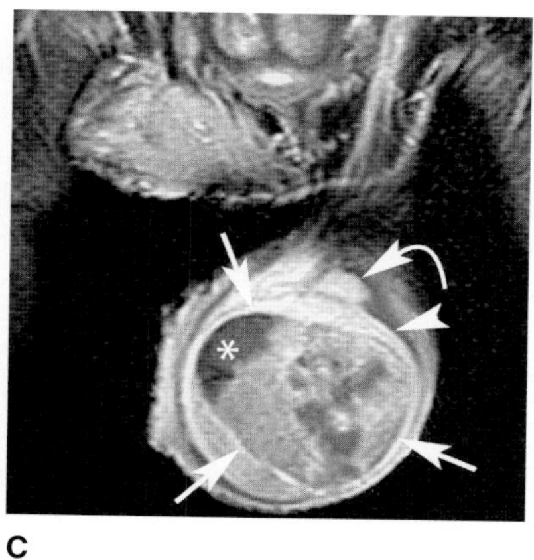
C

Figure 12-7 Nonseminomatous Germ Cell Tumor
A. This transverse US image demonstrates a large heterogeneous intratesticular mass with areas of necrosis (*arrows*), enlarging the left testis. **B.** Coronal T2-weighted and (**C**) postgadolinium T1-weighted images demonstrate a heterogenous mass (*small arrows*) in the left testicle with areas of necrosis (*asterisk*). Note the rind of normal testicle superiorly (*arrowhead*). Note also the epididymis (*curved arrows*) and the normal right testicle (*larger white arrow* in B). Surgical excision demonstrated a nonseminomatous germ cell tumor composed of 80% seminoma and 20% embryonal tumor.

However, teratomatous elements are commonly found in mixed germ cell tumors. α-Fetoprotein is elevated in 38% and β-hCG in 25% of cases of pure teratoma.[9] In children, both mature and immature teratomas typically have a benign behavior. However, in the postpubertal male teratomas are usually aggressive tumors and are treated as malignant regardless of whether the elements appear histologically mature or immature. Both mature and immature teratomas can metastasize, and the metastases can contain nonteratomatous elements.[7] On US examinations, these tumors tend to be very large and markedly inhomogeneous, frequently containing echogenic foci that represent calcification, cartilage, immature bone, and fibrosis. Cystic components are more commonly seen in teratomas than in other NSGCTs.[1] On MRI, the presence of fat is suggestive of teratomatous elements.

Yolk sac tumors, also known as endodermal sinus tumors, are the most common germ cell tumor in children where the prognosis is excellent. In adults, the pure form is rare; however, the presence of yolk sac elements in mixed tumors is common and is associated with a worse prognosis.[1] Yolk sac tumors produce α-fetoprotein, which is elevated in 90% of tumors.[6,9] Imaging features are nonspecific, especially in children where the only findings may be testicular enlargement without a well-defined mass. In adults, treatment does not differ from other NSGCTs;

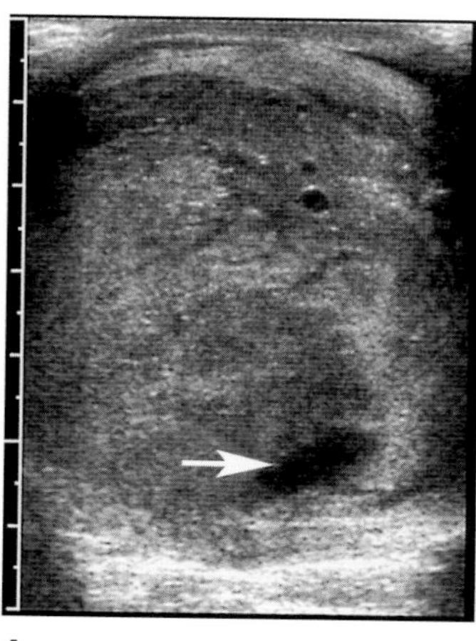
A

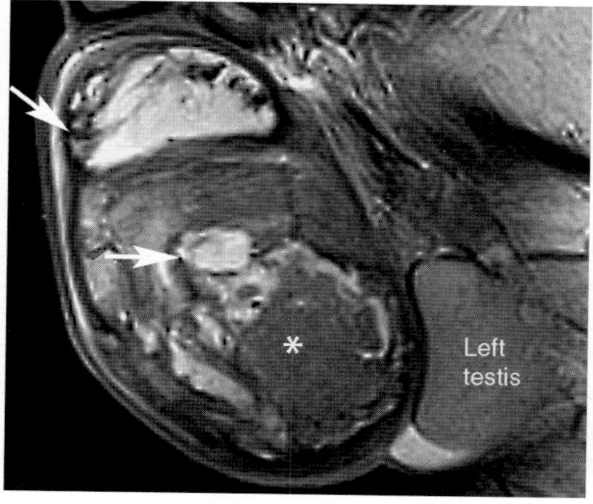

B

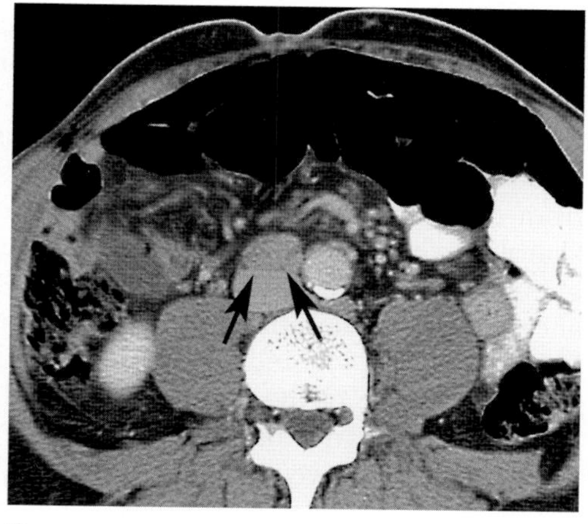
C

Figure 12-8 Mixed Germ Cell Tumor
A. Transverse US image shows replacement of the right testis by a heterogenous mass with necrotic areas (*arrow*). **B.** Sagittal T2-weighted image shows similar findings to A with arrows indicating fluid signal areas in keeping with necrosis and solid areas of tumor invasion (*asterisk*). **C.** Axial enhanced CT image through the retroperitoneum shows a single abnormal precaval lymph (*arrows*) node likely to represent nodal metastasis.

however, in children, if the tumor is confined and the α-fetoprotein is not elevated, treatment may consist only of orchiectomy followed by observation, with use of chemotherapy only if relapse occurs.[7]

Choriocarcinoma is a highly malignant neoplasm that, in its pure form, accounts for only 0.3% of testicular germ cell tumors. It typically develops in patients in the second and third decades of life; human chorionic gonadotropin is usually elevated and it causes gynecomastia in 10% of cases.[7] Hematogenous metastases occur early and are frequently hemorrhagic, with common sites including lung, liver, gastrointestinal tract, and brain. Pure choriocarcinoma has the worst prognosis of all germ cell tumors, with death usually occurring within 1 year of diagnosis. Patients with mixed germ cell tumors with choriocarcinoma fare better than those with pure choriocarcinoma tumors, but a very high level of human chorionic gonadotropin (>50,000 IU/L) portends a poor prognosis, with a 5-year survival rate of 48%.[7] On US and MRI, the primary tumor is usually hemorrhagic resulting in a mixed cystic and solid appearance.

Other testicular tumors

Other testicular tumors include Leydig cell tumor, Sertoli tumors, epidermoid cysts, lymphoma, leukemia, and other rare neoplasms.

Leydig cell tumors: Non–germ cell sex-cord stromal tumors account for 4% of all testicular tumors. Leydig cell tumors are the most common tumor in this group, accounting for 3% of all testicular tumors, mostly occurring in young children 3 to 6 years of age and in adults in the third to fifth decades of life. There is a reported association with Klinefelter syndrome.[1] Approximately 30% of patients will have an endocrinopathy secondary to secretion of androgens or estrogens by the tumor.[7] The endocrinopathy can manifest as isosexual pseudoprecocity in children, and as gynecomastia or impotence in adults.[1] Approximately 10% of Leydig cell tumors are malignant. Malignant tumors typically occur in the elderly and do not have preceding symptoms or endocrinopathy.

The appearance of Leydig cell tumors is varied. In 1 older surgical study of 40 cases, the tumors ranged in size from 0.5 to 10 cm with a mean of 3 cm, and were mostly sharply circumscribed except for 7 that had infiltrative margins. However, a relatively recent report of the US appearance of 10 cases described the tumors as ranging in size from 0.4 to 3 cm with most less than 1 cm. This same report found that none of the lesions were calcified, 90% were hypoechogenic, and that 88% showed peripheral hypervascularity.[15] However, other imaging appearances have also been reported, including hyperechogenic tumors and tumors with diffusely increased vascularity. Few reports exist about the MRI appearance. In a review of 3 cases of Leydig cell tumor, it was found that marked enhancement of the tumor may favor a diagnosis of Leydig cell histology over conventional germ cell neoplasm (see Figure 12-9).[16]

Sertoli cell tumors: Sertoli cell tumors are the next most common sex cord stromal tumor, accounting 1% of testicular tumors, and like Leydig cell tumors, are benign in approximately 90% of cases. Unlike Leydig cell tumors, sufficient hormone production to result in clinical endocrinopathy is rare. Most often the tumors appear as small, unilateral, and well-circumscribed, but otherwise nonspecific, masses. However, a subtype, the large cell calcifying Sertoli tumor, presents as multiple bilateral calcified masses.

Other stromal tumors of the testis: Other rare sex-cord stromal tumors include granulosa cell tumors, fibroma-thecomas, and mixed sex-cord stromal tumors (see Figure 12-10). Gonadoblastoma is a special tumor that also contains sex-cord-stromal elements but is distinguished by the presence of germ cells. Gonadoblastoma typically occurs in the setting of gonadal dysgenesis and intersex syndromes.[7] These tumors are very rare, and the imaging appearance has not been well characterized in the radiology literature.

Epidermoid cyst: Epidermoid cysts are benign intratesticular masses with no malignant potential, constituting approximately 1% of testicular tumors. Like germ cell tumors, they usually present as painless palpable testicular masses. However, unlike germ cell tumors, epidermoid cysts can be treated with enucleation rather than orchiectomy because they are benign. Pathologically, they are cystic cavities with a fibrous wall at least partially lined with stratified squamous epithelium, and containing desquamated keratinized epithelium and keratin debris.[7]

Despite their cystic character, on US, epidermoid cysts are typically well-circumscribed masses measuring from 1 to 3 cm in diameter that appear solid, without through transmission (see Figure 12-11). This is a result of the complex content. The exact US appearance depends on the maturation, compactness, and quantity of keratin within the cyst, and consequently the internal echogenicity of the lesion varies from hypoechogenic with a few low-level internal echoes to hyperechogenic. Despite this variability, several US patterns have been described that are suggestive of an epidermoid. Of these, the most characteristic is the **"onion-ring" appearance**, in which there are alternating hyperechoic and hypoechoic layers representing layers of compact keratin and loosely dispersed desquamated squamous epithelium (see Figure 12-12).[1] Another typical pattern is the **"target" appearance**, in which there is a central focus of increased echogenicity, representing an aggregate of keratin, surrounded by a hypoechoic region. Other epidermoids appear as hypoechoic masses with a hyperechoic or calcified rim. As expected with a cyst, there is no flow within epidermoid on Doppler evaluation.

On MRI, epidermoid cysts also appear as sharply marginated nonenhancing masses, typically with a low-T2-signal wall and T2 hyperintense contents (representing the keratin). In some cases, epidermoids may demonstrate

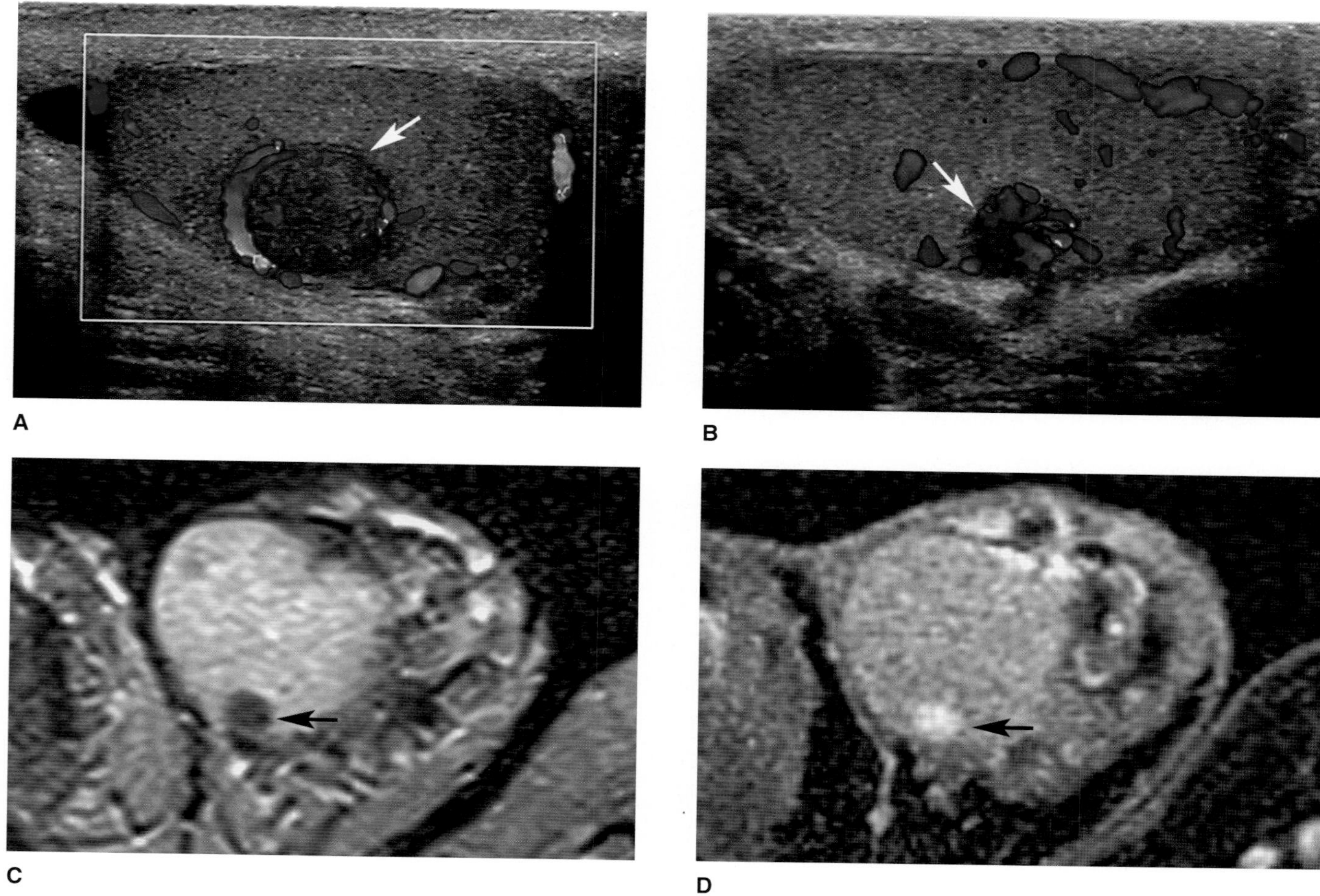

Figure 12-9 Leydig Cell Tumor in 3 Patients
A. Color Doppler US image shows a relatively homogenous, hypoechoic mass (*arrow*) with peripheral flow. **B**. Color Doppler image in a different patient demonstrates diffuse vascularity throughout a small hypoechoic mass (*arrow*). **C**. T2-weighted and (**D**) T1-weighted postgadolinium axial images show a hyperenhancing mass (*arrows*). All 3 masses represented Leydig cell tumors at surgical excision.

a lamellated "onion ring"–type pattern on T2-weighted sequences or a "target" appearance (low-signal rim, hyperintense middle, and low-signal central focus), analogous to the US (see Figure 12-12). However, in other cases, the MRI signal characteristics are those of a nonspecific complex cyst (see Figure 12-11). Theoretically, the presence of lipid within an epidermoid might be detected on MRI as signal loss on out-of-phase images; however, this has not yet been reported.

Note that although the onion ring appearance is characteristic of epidermoid, it is not pathognomonic as the appearance has also been reported with 2 cases of teratoma.[15] Nonetheless, an onion ring appearance in association with negative tumor markers is still highly suggestive of epidermoid. In such cases, enucleation rather than orchiectomy may be considered, with the final surgical procedure determined by the pathologic diagnosis.

Lymphoma: Non-Hodgkin's lymphoma accounts for 1% to 7% of all testicular tumors.[18] The testicle may be the primary and only site of lymphoma. However, more commonly, lymphomatous involvement of the testicle is a manifestation of more generalized disease, either as a presenting site (which, in 10% of patients may be the only area of disease initially) or as a secondary site, and/or site of recurrence in patients with established lymphoma.[19] Testicular lymphoma carries a poor prognosis with a 5-year survival rate of about 12% and a median survival time of less than 12 months.[18,20] Clinically, testicular lymphoma is distinct from germ cell tumors in 2 major ways. First, it occurs in an older population, accounting for 50% of testicular neoplasms in men older than age 60 years.[1] Second, although most patients present with painless testicular enlargement, in up to 25%, systemic symptoms, including weight loss, fever, and anorexia, have been reported as the initial complaint.[7]

On imaging, lymphoma often resembles seminoma, appearing as focal or diffuse homogeneous lesions that are hypoechoic on US and T2 hypointense on MRI, reflecting a uniform cell population and infiltrative nondestructive growth.[18,20] Imaging features favoring lymphoma over

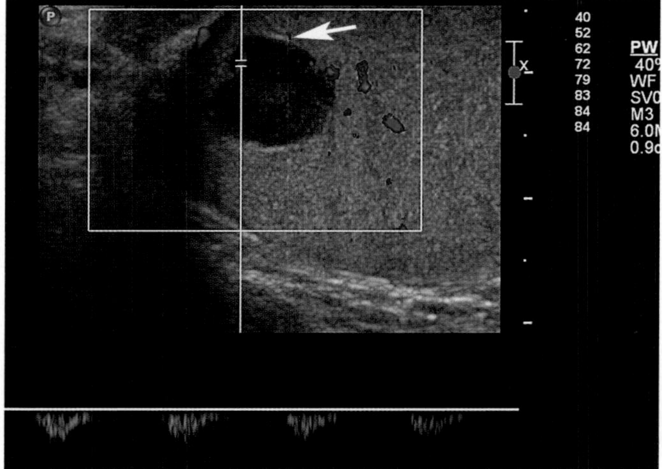

A

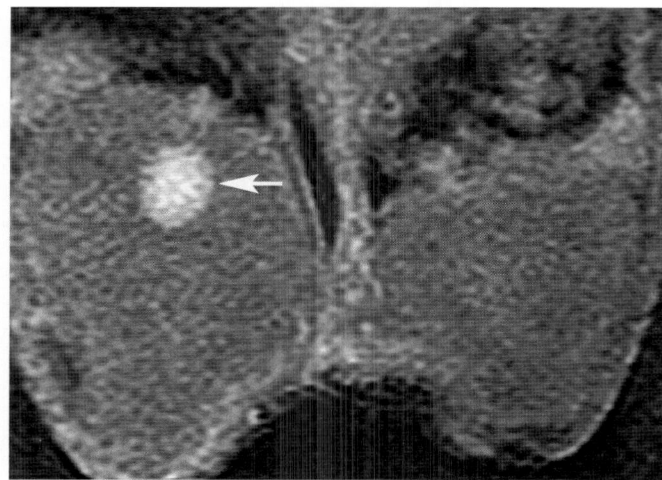

B

Figure 12-10 Low-grade Spindle Cell Neoplasms
A. Color and spectral Doppler image demonstrates a hypoechoic lesion with an echogenic border (*arrow*) and slight through transmission. The gray-scale appearance could indicate either a uniform solid mass or a complex cyst. However, arterial flow is documented on spectral Doppler indicating that this is a solid mass. **B.** Coronal postcontrast image confirms this is a solid mass showing avid enhancement (*arrow*), a feature that raises the possibility of a stromal neoplasm. The mass was isointense to testicle on precontrast images and low signal relative to testicle on T2-weighted images (not shown). Surgical biopsy was diagnostic of a low-grade spindle cell neoplasm.

seminoma include (1) direct invasion of the epididymis and the spermatic cord; (2) indistinct as opposed to lobulated, well-defined margins; (3) preservation of normal testicular contour; and (4) bilateral testicular involvement.[1,18,20] The imaging appearance in combination with the patient's age at presentation, symptoms, and medical history may allow the interpreter to make the appropriate diagnosis of lymphoma.

Leukemia: Primary leukemia of the testis is very rare. However, secondary leukemic involvement of the testis is common, occurring in up to 65% of men with acute leukemia and up to 35% of men with chronic leukemia in autopsy series.[1] Clinically detectable disease is less common, reported in 1 study to be present in 8% of children with acute leukemia.[21] The testis is a common location for recurrence because the blood–testis barrier allows leukemic cells to be "hidden" during chemotherapy such that the testis serves as a "sanctuary site." Consequently, testicular involvement by leukemia is often found during bone marrow remission. The US appearance is similar to that of lymphoma. The diagnosis may be suspected in a child in bone marrow remission for leukemia who presents with a painless enlarging testis.[22]

Imaging Notes 12-3. Distinguishing Features Between Testicular Lymphoma and Seminoma

Lymphoma	Seminoma
Extension into the epididymis/spermatic cord	Confined to testis
Indistinct margins	Lobulated, well-defined margins
Normal testicular contour	Distortion testicular contour
Can be bilateral	Unilateral
Systemic symptoms	Local symptoms/ no symptoms

Testicular metastasis: Testicular metastases are uncommon, occurring in <1% of those with an extrascrotal primary solid neoplasm. Possible routes of spread include retrograde venous or lymphatic spread, hematogenous spread, and direct tumor invasion.[23] Retrograde venous or lymphatic spread is usually due to other genitourinary neoplasms such as bladder, prostate, or renal carcinomas. Occasionally, tumors with para-aortic lymphadenopathy can also spread via a retrograde fashion into the testis. Hematogenous spread is most often a result of bronchogenic carcinoma or melanoma. The most common primary sources are prostate tumors (35%), lung tumors (19%), malignant melanoma (9%), colon tumors (9%), and kidney tumors (7%).[1] The best diagnostic clue is the history of a known primary with tendency to metastasize to the testicles; however, such a history is present in only 37% of patients at the time of diagnosis of the testicular mass. The

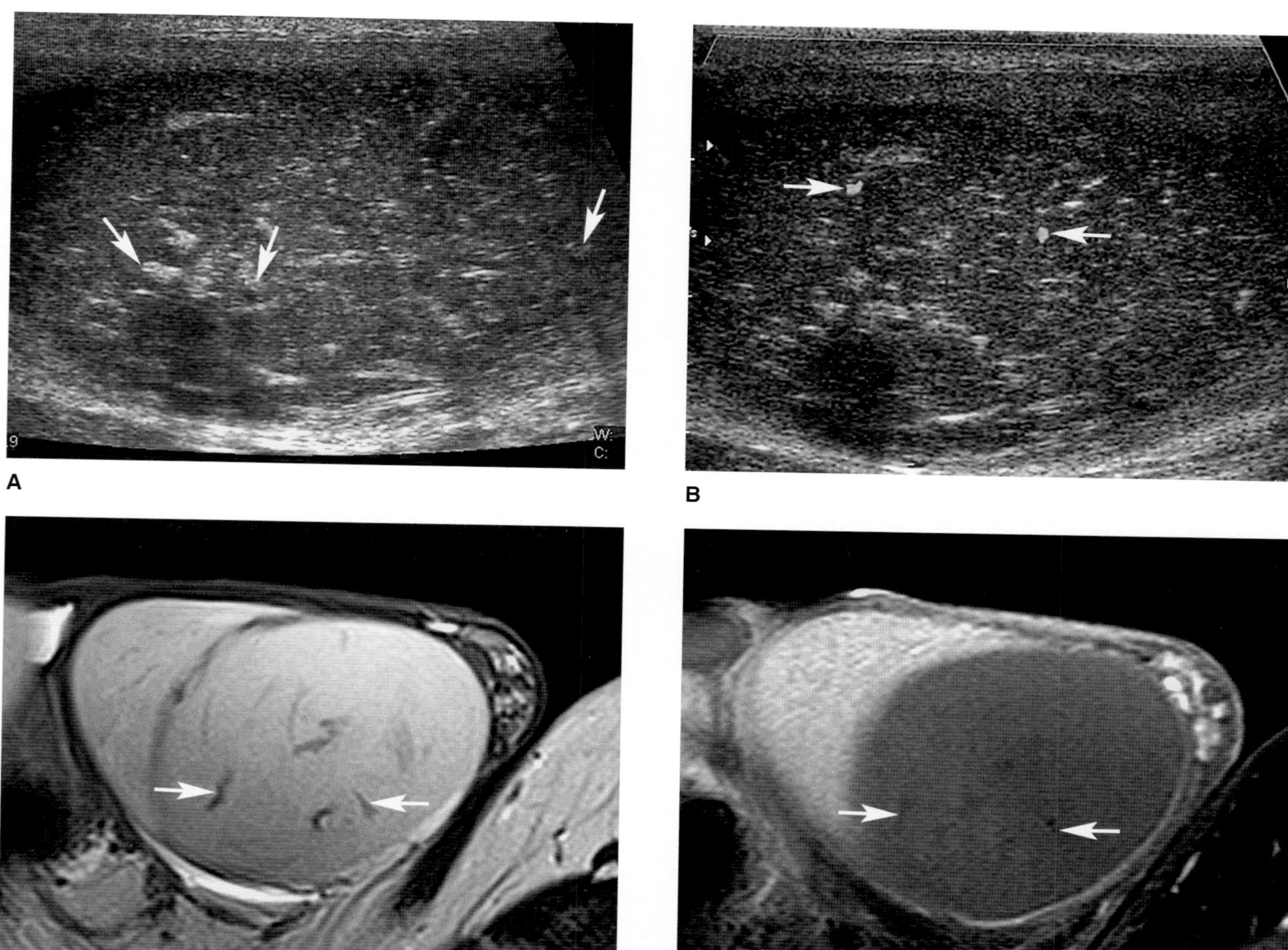

Figure 12-11 Epidermoid Cyst of the Testis
A. Sagittal grayscale image demonstrates a hypoechoic well circumscribed mass containing numerous echogenic foci, some of which demonstrate posterior acoustic shadowing (*arrows*), indicative of calcifications. The US appearance is suggestive of a solid mass. **B**. Color Doppler image shows flecks (*arrows*) of mixed color (admixed red and blue), which is suggestive of "twinkle" artifact from calcifications as opposed to real flow. Thus, the lesion could represent a complex cyst. **C**. Axial T2 and (**D**) postcontrast T1-weighted images show a well-circumscribed nonenhancing mass with internal foci of low signal (*arrows*) corresponding to the calcifications identified on US. The lack of enhancement suggests that this represents a complex cyst. Excision demonstrated an epidermoid cyst.

presence of metastatic disease elsewhere may also point to the diagnosis.

Other rare testicular neoplasms: Other rare intratesticular tumors include plasmocytomas, mesenchymal tumors, intratesticular adenomatoid tumor, and adenocarcinoma of the rete testes, none of which demonstrate specific findings.

Orchitis and epididymo-orchitis

Orchitis is usually associated with epididymitis and can be caused by bacterial, mycobacterial, fungal, and protozoal organisms. The imaging appearance of orchitis in some cases is influenced by the causative organism.

Bacterial orchitis: Pyogenic bacterial orchitis is discussed most completely under the heading: **Diffusely Enlarged Testicle with Abnormal Echogenicity or Signal Intensity**, subheading **Orchitis and epididymo-orchitis**. In most cases, US evaluation of patients with bacterial orchitis will demonstrate a diffusely enlarged testicle with heterogeneous echotexture. However, occasionally orchitis can result in a focal abnormality within the testis. When orchitis appears as a focal lesion, it can be difficult to differentiate from a

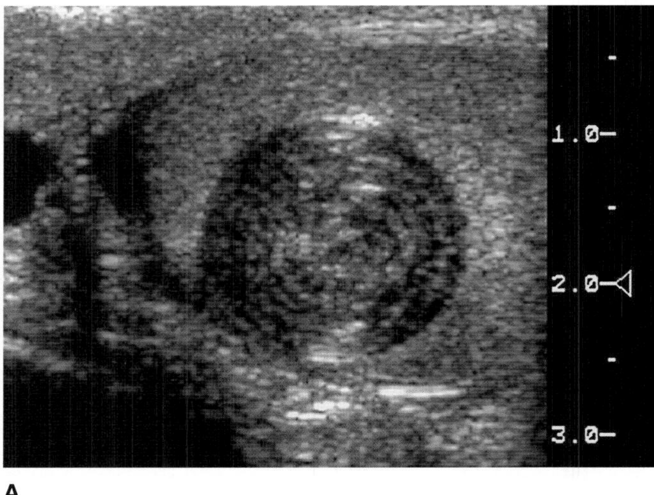

A

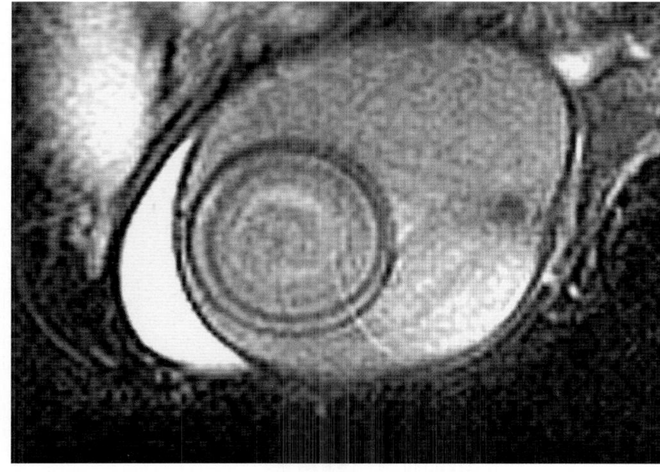

B

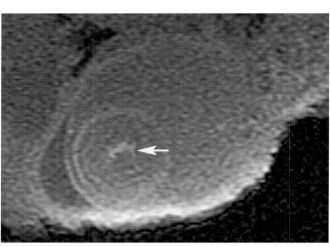

C

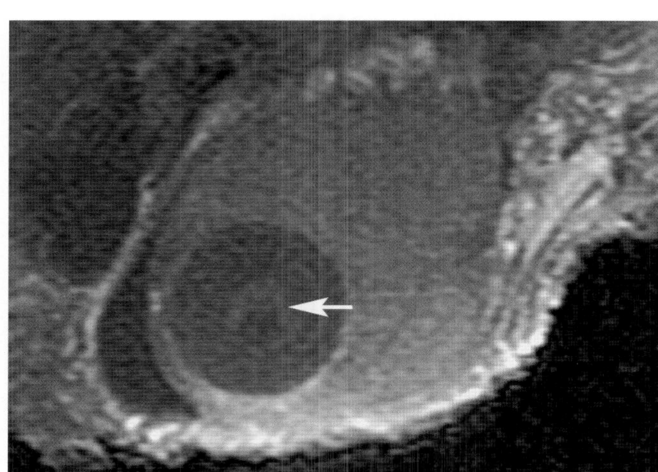

D

Figure 12-12 Onion-Ring Appearance of Testicular Epidermoid **A**. Grayscale US image demonstrates a well-circumscribed hypoechoic lesion characterized by a lamellated appearance, which showed no flow on color Doppler (not shown) (**B**) T2-weighted and (**C**) T1-weighted pre-contrast and (**D**) T1-weighted postgadolinium fat saturated T1-weighted images show a lesion with a "onion-ring" appearance, which does not enhance with contrast. Note that the T1 hyperintense area in the center of the lesion (*arrows* in **C** and **D**) is also hyperintense precontrast, representing proteinaceous material. This is the characteristic appearance of a testicular epidermoid cyst.

neoplasm of the testis. Evidence of epididymitis, hydrocele, skin thickening, and clinical findings of infection support a diagnosis of epididymo-orchitis rather than a neoplasm. However, follow-up to resolution is generally recommended.

Tuberculous orchitis and other granulomatous orchitis: Although occasionally idiopathic, granulomatous orchitis is usually a result of infection from a variety of organisms, including tuberculosis, Bacillus Calmette-Guérin (BCG, because of prior intravesical BCG therapy for bladder cancer), syphilis, fungi, and parasites. Tuberculous orchitis is most common. The remainder of the discussion concerns tuberculous orchitis, as the prototype of a granulomatous infection.

Imaging Notes 12-4. Features More Common in Focal Orchitis than Testicular Neoplasm

1. Concurrent epididymitis (hypervascular, enlarged and/or hypoechoic epididymis)
2. Concurrent hydrocele
3. Skin thickening
4. Clinical presentation with scrotal pain and fever
5. Imaging resolution following antibiotic therapy

Several patterns of tuberculous orchitis have been described. These include (1) focal mass, (2) nodular enlarged heterogeneously hypoechoic testis, (3) diffusely enlarged homogeneously hypoechoic testis, (4) diffusely enlarged heterogeneously hypoechoic testis, and (5) presence of multiple small hypoechoic nodules (miliary pattern) (see Figure 12-13).[24] Of these, the miliary pattern has been suggested to be characteristic of tuberculous orchitis.[25,26] With the other patterns of tuberculous orchitis, the differential diagnosis depends to some degree on the degree of associated epididymal involvement.

Most tuberculous infections of the scrotum tend to involve the epididymis first, and to a much greater extent than the testis, a feature that favors infection/inflammation over tumor.[7] In this situation, the main differential considerations are pyogenic epididymo-orchitis and sarcoid. Unlike pyogenic epididymo-orchitis, tuberculous infections tend to produce heterogeneous, hypoechogenic enlargement of the epididymis with linear or spotty peripheral vascularity, as opposed to hypervascular homogeneous enlargement. Other findings that can suggest a tuberculous infection as opposed to pyogenic infection include scrotal calcifications, sinus tracts, failure to resolve with conventional antibiotic therapy, subacute presentation, and evidence of granulomatous infection in other organs.[26] Sarcoid can be indistinguishable from tuberculosis by imaging; however, clinical findings or imaging findings of sarcoid elsewhere may point to a diagnosis of sarcoid.

If epididymal involvement is less than the testicular involvement, one of the main differential considerations would be lymphoma. In this situation, differentiating between tuberculous orchitis and lymphoma can be difficult; however, features favoring lymphoma include a history of lymphoma and direct extension of the testicular mass into the epididymis, as opposed to separate lesions in the epididymis and testis.

Rarely, tuberculous orchitis can present as a mass isolated to the testis, without epididymal involvement (see Figure 12-13). In this situation, the main differential consideration is a testicular neoplasm. In 1 report, tuberculous inflammation was found to be less likely to result in distortion of the testicular contour compared with tumor, which may be a clue to the diagnosis.[25] However, in most cases, isolated masslike tuberculosis orchitis will be indistinguishable from tumor based on scrotal imaging, and diagnosis will require correlation with other clinical and imaging findings, and possibly tissue sampling.

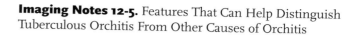

Imaging Notes 12-5. Features That Can Help Distinguish Tuberculous Orchitis From Other Causes of Orchitis

1. Diffuse bilateral hypoechoic nodules (miliary pattern)
2. Presence of scrotal calcifications, sinus tracts, and abscesses
3. Heterogeneous hypoechoic enlargement of the epididymis
4. Evidence of tuberculosis in other tissues of the body
5. Subacute/chronic presentation

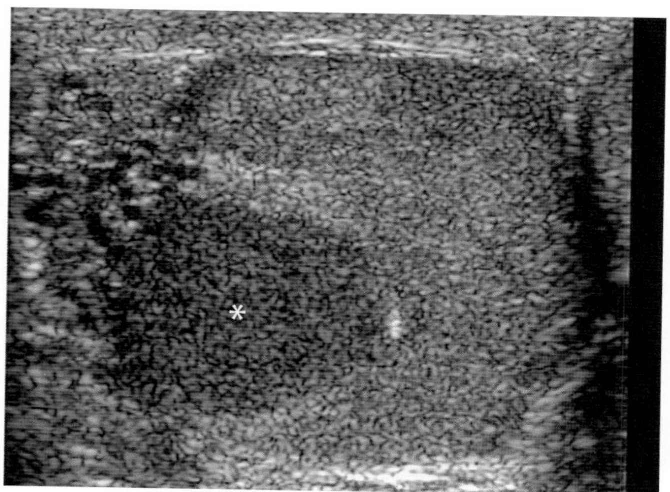

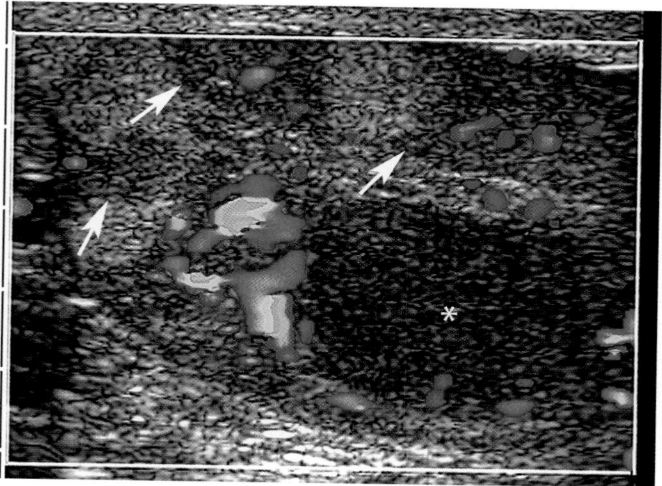

Figure 12-13 Chronic Granulomatous Orchitis
A. Transverse grayscale image shows a uniformly hypoechoic mass (*asterisk*) within the testicle. **B.** Color Doppler sagittal image shows paucity of flow in the lesion (*asterisk*) with increased peripheral flow within the testis. There are also several adjacent hypoechoic areas (*arrows*). Differential diagnosis would include testicular neoplasms and focal orchitis. Orchiectomy revealed chronic granulomatous orchitis.

Abscess

Intratesticular abscess usually develops secondary to pyogenic epididymo-orchitis, but has also been reported as a complication of trauma and infarction.[1] In addition, testicular abscess may occur as a consequence of systemic infections such as mumps, small pox, typhoid, scarlet fever, and tuberculosis.[19] On US, complex cystic lesions such as abscesses may be solid-appearing due to the presence of multiple internal echoes related to the presence of complex fluid and debris. Imaging clues favoring abscess include paucity of internal vascularity, hypervascular rim, other US findings of epididymo-orchitis, as well resolution on follow-up.[1]

Hematoma

Hematomas of the testis almost invariably are iatrogenic or posttraumatic. On US, the appearance of a hematoma varies with age. Acute hematoma usually appears echogenic and solid, evolving into a hypoechogenic mass with septa and loculation before becoming mostly cystic in after 1 to 2 weeks (see Figure 12-14).[27] No internal vascularity is detectable by color Doppler in hematomas. A history of trauma can suggest the diagnosis. However, since 10% to 15% of tumors are found incidentally during imaging after an episode of trauma, follow-up is generally advised to ensure resolution/decrease in size.[28] In equivocal cases, MRI may be able to confirm a diagnosis of hematoma by revealing a non-enhancing lesion with signal intensity characteristic of hemorrhage. Hemorrhage varies in signal depending on age. Acute blood appears T1 isointense/T2 hypointense due to deoxyhemoglobin, subacute blood is T1 hyperintense/T2 variable due to intracellular and extracellular methemoglobin, and a chronic hematoma can have a low-signal-intensity rim secondary to hemosiderin deposition.[27]

The various manifestations of testicular trauma are discussed most completely under **Diffuse Testicular Disorders**, subheading **Trauma and Testicular Rupture.**

Splenogonadal fusion

Splenogonadal fusion refers to a rare malformation in which accessory splenic tissue is present in the scrotum. (discussed in more detail under **Other Paratesticular Masses**).[29] Occasionally, the accessory spleen can be fused with, and inseparable from, the testis. As a consequence, it can be mistaken for a neoplasm arising from the peripheral testicle, which may lead to unnecessary orchiectomy. An important clue to the diagnosis of splenogonadal fusion is a color Doppler pattern with central flow and peripheral branching, which is in contrast to most neoplasms, where the flow usually has a disorganized pattern. If the diagnosis of splenogonadal fusion is suspected preoperatively, a 99mTc-sulphur colloid scan demonstrating activity in the scrotum is diagnostic of the disorder.

Testicular sarcoidosis

Testicular sarcoidosis rarely presents as a solitary lesion, more typically appearing multiple, small, bilateral masses.[7] When solitary, differentiation from primary testicular malignancy may be problematic. (Sarcoidosis is discussed most completely under the heading **Other Paratesticular Masses.**)

Other causes of solid appearing testicular lesion

Several other entities may mimic a solid testicular mass, including complex cysts, intratesticular varicocele, other intratesticular vascular malformations, adrenal rests, autoimmune vasculitis, and focal fibrosis. Intratesticular varicoceles can usually be differentiated from other intratesticular masses by the tubular, serpiginous appearance of the lesion. Adrenal rests typically appear as solid bilateral intratesticular masses; however, occasionally they will appear as a unilateral mass. (Adrenal rests are discussed most completely under the heading **Bilateral Testicular Masses** later in this chapter.) Testicular fibrosis usually appears as multiple, geographic regions of altered echogenicity on US or signal abnormality

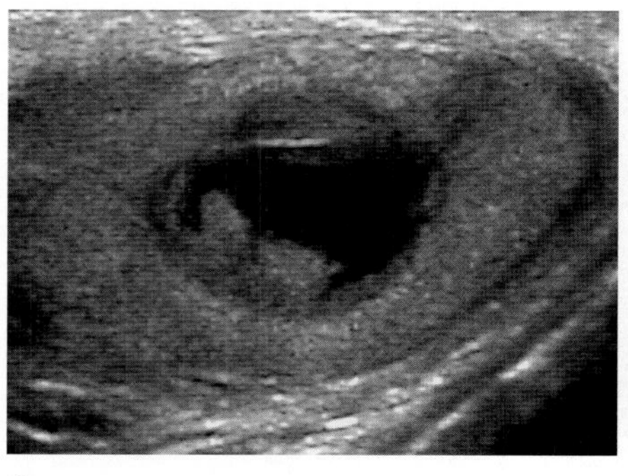
A

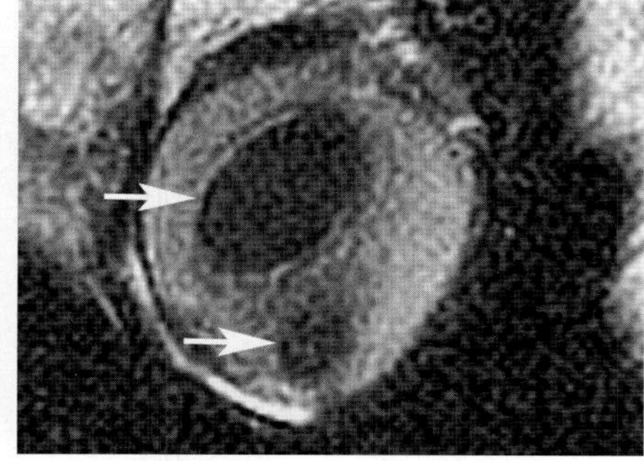
B

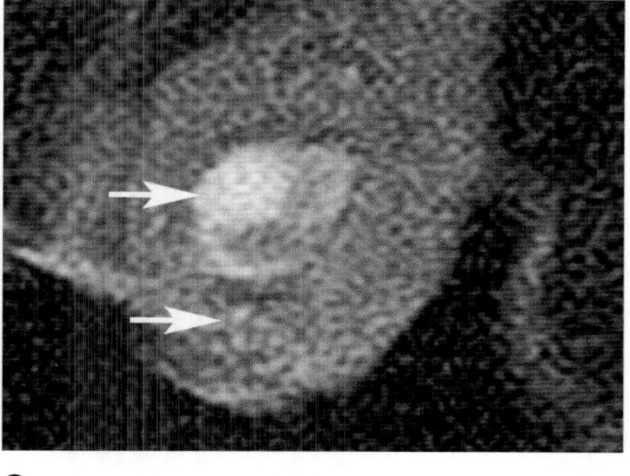
C

Figure 12-14 Testicular Hematoma
This young man had received a direct blow to the testicle. **A.** Sagittal grayscale sonographic image shows a mixed cystic and solid mass. No color was detectable with color or power Doppler in the mass. **B.** Coronal T2 and (**C**) fat-saturated T1-weighted images show T2 hypointense areas (*arrows* in **B**) that are T1 hyperintense (*arrows* in **C**), signal characteristics typical of blood products. The masses did not enhance following gadolinium. These findings are all consistent with a testicular hematoma.

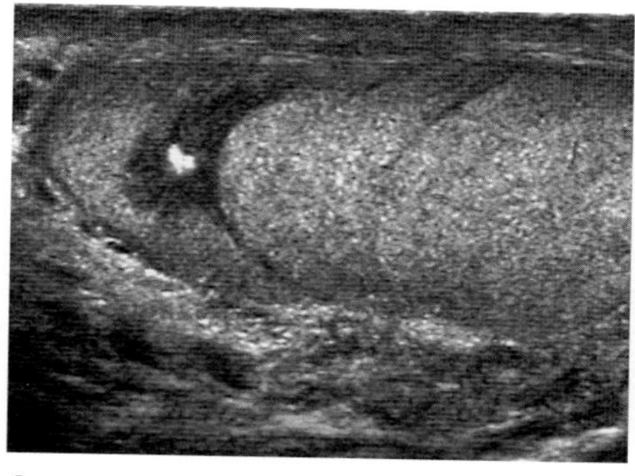

A

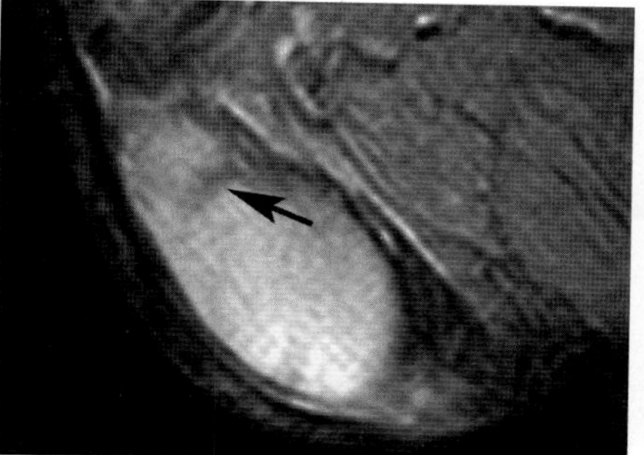

B

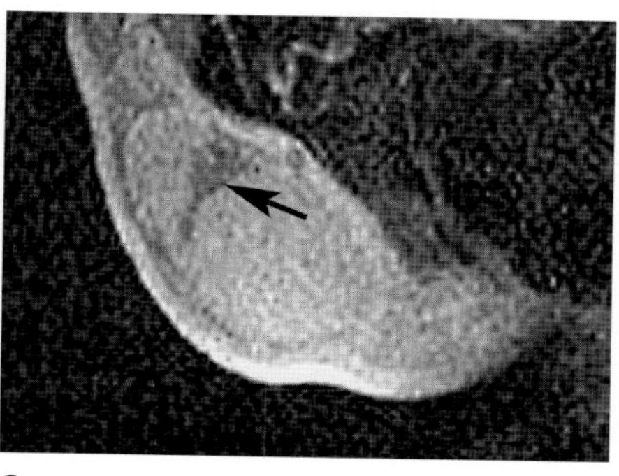

C

Figure 12-15 Focal Fibrosis
A. Sagittal grayscale image demonstrates a focal irregularly shaped hypoechoic lesion with a calcification. **B**. Sagittal T2-weighted and (**C**) postgadolinium images demonstrate a geographic area of decreased T2 signal (*arrows*) with no appreciable enhancement postgadolinium and capsular retraction. This was stable on follow-up examinations and is most consistent with an area of focal fibrosis from a prior insult.

on MRI; however, occasionally it can appear as a solitary focal testicular lesion (see Figure 12-15). Clues to the diagnosis include preservation of normal testicular architecture and, in chronic lesions, the presence of capsular retraction indicative of volume loss. (Testicular fibrosis is discussed most completely under the heading: **Geographic Testicular Lesions.**)

Geographic Testicular Lesions

In most cases, nonround or geographic testicular lesions will represent a benign disorder, typically infarction, orchitis, testicular fibrosis, or a US artifact called the "two-tone testicle" (Table 12-3).

Imaging Notes 12-6. Differentiating Features of Solid-Appearing Intratesticular Lesions

Mass	Differentiating Features
Germ cell neoplasm Seminoma NSGCT	Tumor markers; retroperitoneal lymphadenopathy Homogeneous mass Heterogeneous mass calcifications, hemorrhage, cysts
Stromal neoplasm	Gynecomastia, other endocrinopathy
Lymphoma/leukemia	History of lymphoma/leukemia, infiltration of the epididymis/spermatic cord (lymphoma), homogeneous
Epidermoid	"Onion ring," rim calcification, no flow on color Doppler
Metastasis	History of extratesticular primary, multiple testicular masses
Abscess	Other findings of EO (epididymorchitis), resolution over time
Focal orchitis	Other findings of EO, resolution with time
Infarct	Geographic, hypovascular, involutes
Atrophy/fibrosis	Geographic, hypovascular, if chronic, capsular retraction
Hematoma	Other findings of trauma, involution over time
Granulomatous orchitis (sarcoid, infectious)	Presence of epididymal involvement; clinical findings suggesting TB (eg, history of HIV, +PPD) or sarcoid (eg, elevated serum ACE); imaging findings of TB or sarcoid elsewhere
Splenogonadal fusion	Flow pattern on color Doppler, associated with other congenital anomalies
Mimic (vascular malformation)	Spectral Doppler shows venous flow that increases with Valsalva
Mimic (complex cyst)	No flow; through transmission
Mimic (tunical mass)	Peripheral epicenter

Table 12-3. Causes of Geographic Testicular Lesions

1. Infiltrative neoplasms
2. Inflammatory/postinflammatory conditions a. Orchitis b. Testicular fibrosis/atrophy
3. Infarction
4. Artifact: the 2-tone testicle

Neoplasm

It is rare for a neoplasm to appear as a regional nonmasslike testicular abnormality. However, uncommonly, tumors such as lymphoma or seminoma can have an infiltrative growth pattern resulting in a geographic-appearing abnormality. In such cases, sometimes the diagnosis of an infiltrative neoplasm may be suspected if there is disruption of the normal testicular architecture or mass effect. Failure of resolution of the abnormality on follow-up examinations and elevated tumor markers would also suggest a diagnosis of an infiltrative tumor rather than an inflammatory lesion.

Orchitis and epididymo-orchitis

Orchitis usually appears as diffuse hyperemia, enlargement, and decreased echogenicity of the testis. However, it can present as a focal abnormality, which may be masslike (as discussed in a previous section), or may appear as a geographic area of altered echogenicity on US or signal abnormality on MRI. In such cases, the abnormal area usually appears hypoechoic on US and hyperintense on T2-weighted sequences because of the presence of edema, but sometimes the area of orchitis can appear echogenic on US and heterogeneous in signal intensity on MRI sequences due to the presence of hemorrhage. Unlike testicular infarction, the geographic abnormality is typically hypervascular (see Figure 12-16). Associated findings of tenderness, enlarged hyperemic epididymis, hydrocele, and skin thickening support a diagnosis of orchitis. However, sonographic follow-up may be necessary to confirm resolution and exclude tumor. Orchitis is discussed most completely under the heading: **Diffusely Enlarged Testicle with Abnormal Echogenicity or Signal Intensity**, subheading **Orchitis and epididymo-orchitis**.

Testicular fibrosis/atrophy

In most cases, testicular fibrosis will appear as multiple, irregularly margined areas of decreased echogenicity within the substance of the testicle(s). However, testicular fibrosis can appear as a single lesion within the testis (see Figure 12-17). When this occurs, the lesion typically involves a geographic region of the testis without mass effect. Unlike orchitis or infarction, the testicular blood flow in patients with regional fibrosis is often normal appearing within the affected region. Atrophy is more fully discussed under **Bilateral Testicular Masses**, subheading **Bilateral inflammatory or postinflammatory masses**.

Segmental infarction

Segmental infarction is an uncommon entity with a variety of causes, most commonly epididymo-orchitis, torsion-detorsion, accidental or surgical trauma, and rarely vasculitis, and hematologic disorders. Infarction in the setting of severe epididymo-orchitis is a result of impaired testicular blood flow due to severe inflammation and edema. Regional infarction as a result of torsion-detorsion

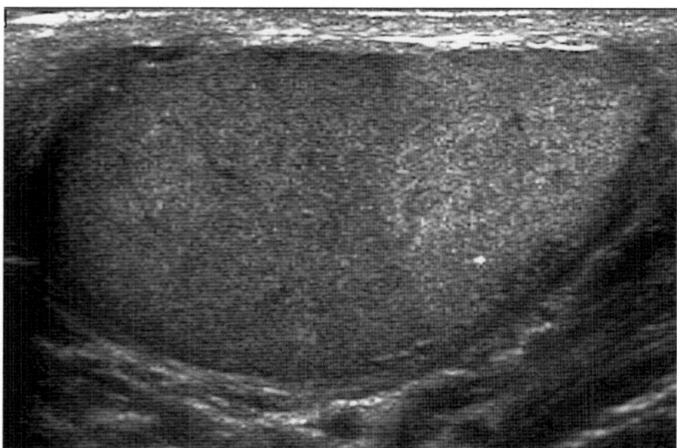

A

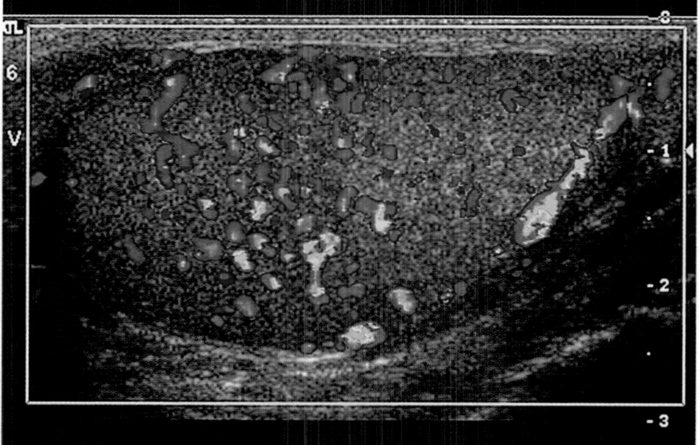

B

Figure 12-16 Focal Geographic Orchitis
A. Grayscale and (**B**) color Doppler images demonstrate geographic decreased echogenicity involving the upper pole of the testis (note the linear border) with increased vascularity. These findings resolved on follow-up imaging and are indicative of focal orchitis.

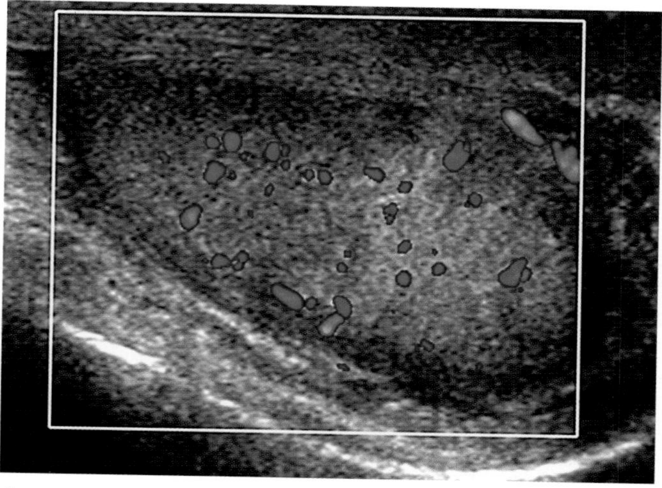

A

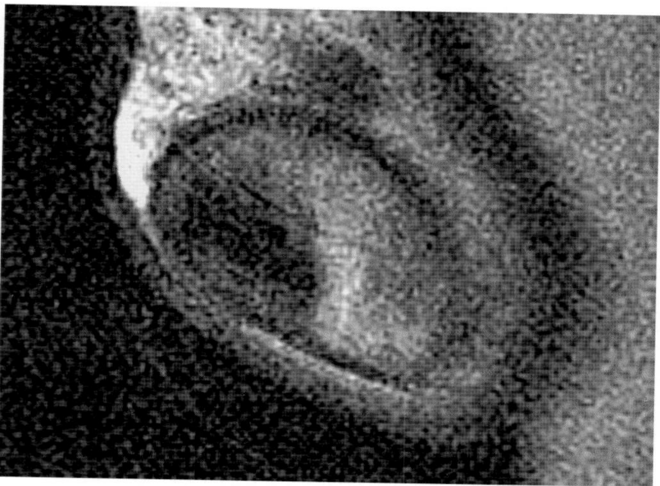

B

Figure 12-17 Geographic Fibrosis
This 80-year-old man had a history of recurrent episodes of epididymo-orchitis. **A.** Color Doppler image demonstrates geographic decreased echogenicity of the upper pole of the testis (note linear border) with normal to decreased vascularity. **B.** Sagittal T2 weighted image demonstrates a geographic hypointense area in the upper pole of the testis. These findings are in keeping with an area of fibrosis or scarring from prior episodes of infection.

classically involves the upper pole of the testis and is associated with a horizontal position of the testis.[28] In addition to accidental trauma, segmental infarction has been reported following varicocelectomy and herniorrhaphy.[32] With these surgical procedures, the ischemia is a result of direct injury to testicular artery or vein or extrinsic compression of these blood vessels by an inguinal canal hematoma.[30] Small vessel diseases and hematologic disorders that have been reported to cause testicular infarction include diabetes mellitus, sickle cell disease, Henoch-Schönlein purpura, Wegener granulomatosis, polyarteritis nodosa, polycythemia, and protein S deficiency.[30,32] In approximately 80% of cases, segmental infarction of the testis affects the upper hemisphere of the testicle.[32] This upper pole predilection may be due to variable deficiency or absence of anterior epididymal artery, which normally provides collateral flow to the upper pole capsular artery.[32]

On US examinations, segmental testicular infarction typically appears as a hypoechoic, geographic region of the testis with decreased vascularity (see Figure 12-18). If the US appearance is not sufficiently diagnostic, then MRI can aid in diagnosis by demonstrating a wedge-shaped lesion without mass effect with vertex toward the mediastinum and rim enhancement postcontrast. In most cases, the lesion is low signal on T2-weighted images.[32] In some cases, MRI will demonstrate areas of intralesional hemorrhage, seen as areas of T1 hyperintensity within the lesions.

Artifact: the two-tone testicle

Shadowing from the mediastinum testis or from a transmediastinal vessel can result in apparent decreased echogenicity of a segment of the testicle, known as the "two-tone testicle."[29] The area of decreased echogenicity will not persist with different transducer angulations, confirming the artifactual origin of the apparent lesion.

Bilateral Testicular Lesions

Bilateral testicular masses are uncommon but can be caused by a variety neoplastic, inflammatory, and other unusual conditions (Table 12-4).

Imaging Notes 12-7. Differentiating Features of Geographic Testicular Lesions

Geographic Lesions	Differentiating Features
Infarct	Lack of mass effect, decreased vascularity
Orchitis	Increased vascularity, findings of epididymitis
Atrophy	Lack of mass effect, normal vascularity
Infiltrating tumor	Mass effect, disruption of normal testicular flow, increased vascularity
Two-tone testis	Artifact, goes away with changes in transducer position

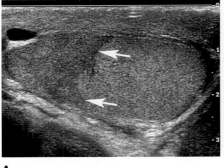

A

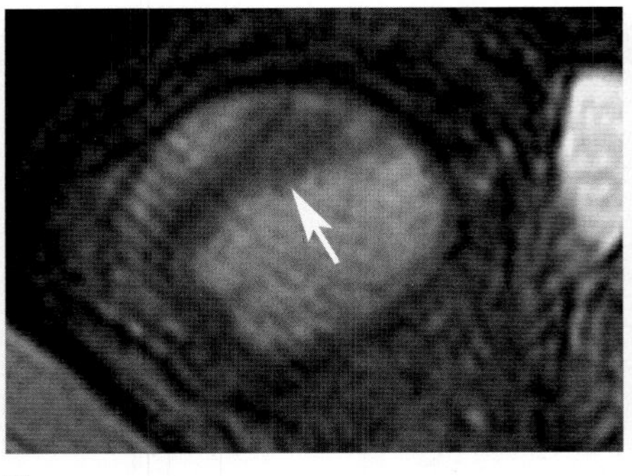

B

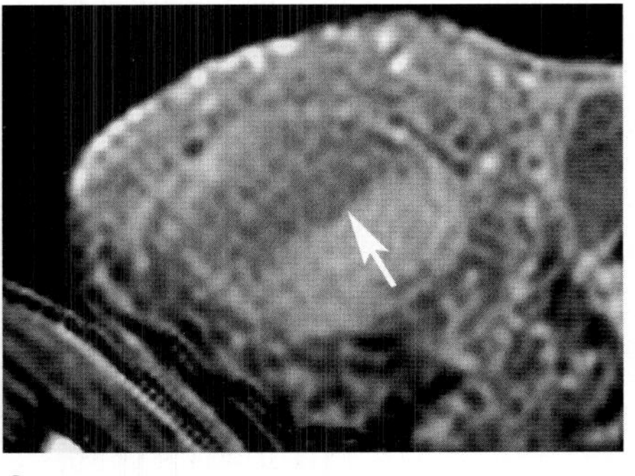

C

Figure 12-18 Segmental Testicular Infarction
This 58-year-old man had undergone vasectomy and surgical repair of right groin muscle injury that involved "repositioning" of the spermatic cord. **A**. Grayscale US image demonstrates geographic decreased echogenicity (*arrows*) of the upper pole with volume loss. **B**. Axial T2 and (**C**) postgadolinium T1-weighted fat saturated images demonstrate a geographic region of nonenhancement with low T2 signal (*arrows*). Given the clinical history, this geographic lesion is most consistent with a chronic segmental infarction.

Bilateral neoplasms

Bilateral testicular neoplasms are most often due to lymphoma, leukemia, or metastasis but can rarely be due to synchronous primary neoplasms.

Lymphoma and leukemia: Lymphoma is the most common bilateral testicular neoplasm, demonstrating synchronous involvement of the contralateral testis in up to 19% of cases. Leukemia is the second most common bilateral neoplasm.[20] Lymphoma typically occurs in men aged 50 or older, whereas leukemia of the testis is typical found in boys during bone marrow remission, because of persistence of disease in the testicle, where the blood–testis barrier limits the efficacy of chemotherapeutic agents. Lymphoma and leukemia have a similar sonographic appearance, presenting as either a homogeneous hypoechogenic enlarged testis or as uniformly hypoechogenic mass lesions within the testes (see Figure 12-19). (Lymphoma and leukemia of the scrotum are discussed most completely under the heading **Focal Testicular Disorders**, subheading **Other testicular tumors**.)

Table 12-4. Causes of Bilateral Testicular Lesions

1. Neoplasms a. Lymphoma b. Leukemia c. Metastasis d. Synchronous primary testicular neoplasms (rare)
2. Inflammatory or post inflammatory conditions a. Tuberculous orchitis b. Sarcoidosis c. Testicular fibrosis
3. Other unusual conditions a. Leydig cell hyperplasia b. Congenital adrenal rests

Metastases: Metastases to the testis usually are unilateral. However, bilateral metastases have been reported with a frequency of 8% in a recent series.[33]

Bilateral primary testicular neoplasms: Germ cell tumors are reported to be bilateral at presentation in about 1%.[34] Synchronous germ cell neoplasms account for approximately 10% of all bilateral neoplasms. Most synchronous germ cell tumors have an identical histologic diagnosis. (see Figure 12-20).[35]

Bilateral inflammatory or postinflammatory lesions

The systemic inflammatory conditions of tuberculosis and sarcoidosis can occasionally result in bilateral testicular lesions. Testicular fibrosis often appears as bilateral testicular lesions.

Tuberculous orchitis: In most cases, tuberculous orchitis involves a single testicle.[25] However, occasionally tuberculosis can appear as multiple very small hypoechoic lesions in both testes, representing a "miliary pattern," which has been suggested to be virtually diagnostic of tuberculous orchitis.[24,25,77] Granulomatous orchitis is discussed most completely under the heading: **Solid-Appearing Intratesticular Nodule or Mass**, subheading: **Orchitis and epididymo-orchitis**.

Sarcoidosis: Of those individuals with sarcoidosis of the genital tract, 70% will have involvement of the epididymis. Most of the remainder will have disease isolated to the

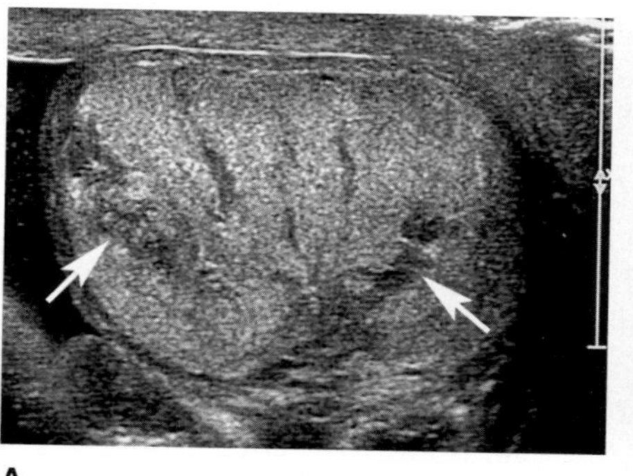

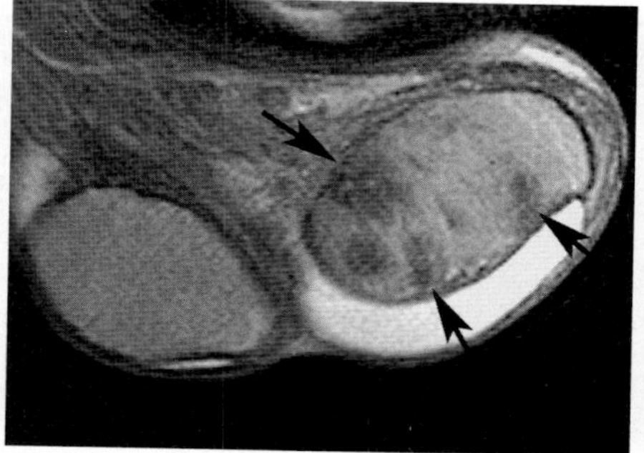

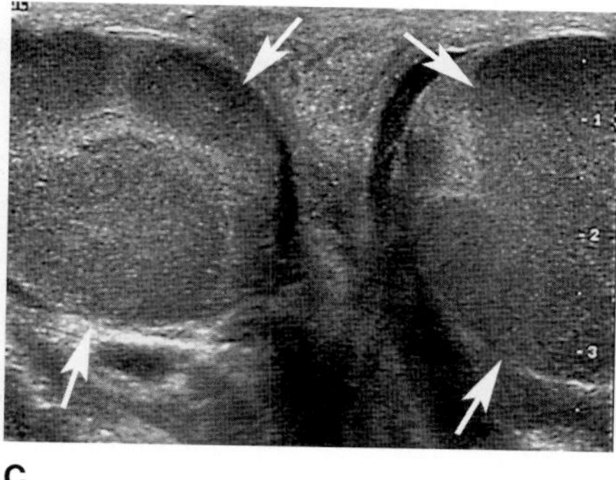

Figure 12-19 Testicular Lymphoma
This patient had a history of extratesticular lymphoma. **A.** Grayscale US and (**B**) T2-weighted MRI images demonstrate multiple lesions in the testicles (*indicated with arrows*) some of which were FDG avid (PET not shown). Similar, but fewer in number, lesions were present in the other testicle. **C.** Transverse grayscale image through the testicles of a different patient with lymphoma shows multiple bilateral homogenous masses (*some indicated with arrows*) that were hypervascular on color Doppler representing testicular involvement by lymphoma.

testis. Testicular lesions can be solitary, but they are more often reported to be multiple, small to medium, bilateral masses (see Figure 12-21).[7,36] On ultrasound, the lesions are usually hypoechoic, but occasionally may contain echogenic areas representing calcifications.[23] The lesions also tend to demonstrate more defined margins as compared with leukemic/lymphomatous infiltrates.[36] Other clues to the diagnosis include a history of sarcoid, African American race, elevated serum angiotensin-converting enzyme (ACE) levels, negative tumor markers, and in some cases response to steroid therapy. MRI of testicular sarcoid typically reveals T2 hypointense enhancing lesions that are indistinguishable from neoplasm. (Sarcoidosis of the scrotum is discussed most completely under the heading **Extratesticular Disorders**, subheading **Diffuse Enlarged Epididymis.**)

Testicular fibrosis/atrophy: Testicular fibrosis is the result of a previous insult to the testis resulting in scarring. This process can be found to affect 1 or both testes and is typically found in older patients. There are a variety of predisposing conditions for testicular fibrosis. Testicular fibrosis is discussed most completely in the subsequent section in this chapter entitled **Diffusely Enlarged Testicle with Abnormal Echogenicity or Signal Intensity**. Testicular fibrosis often appears as multiple geographic, elongated, or

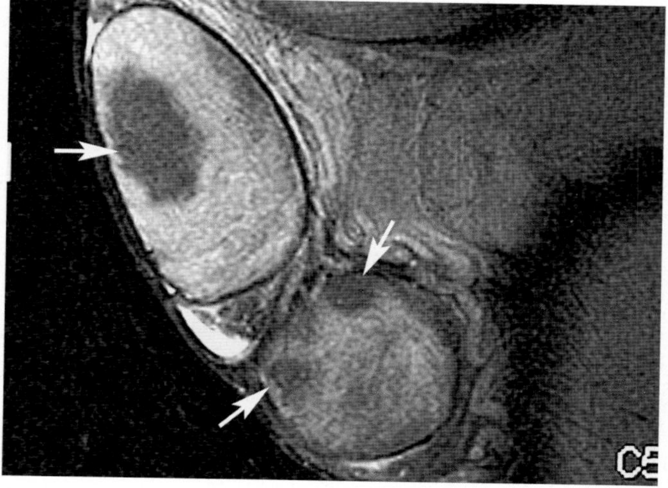

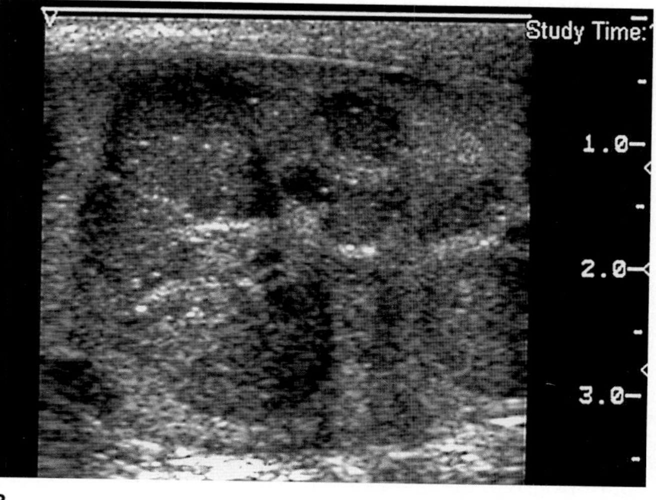

Figure 12-20 Multifocal Seminoma in 2 Patients
A. Sagittal T2-weighted image demonstrates bilateral testicular masses (*arrows*). **B.** Ultrasonographic image in another patient shows multiple right testicular lesions. The left testicle (not shown) appeared normal. In both patients, surgical biopsy was diagnostic of multifocal seminoma.

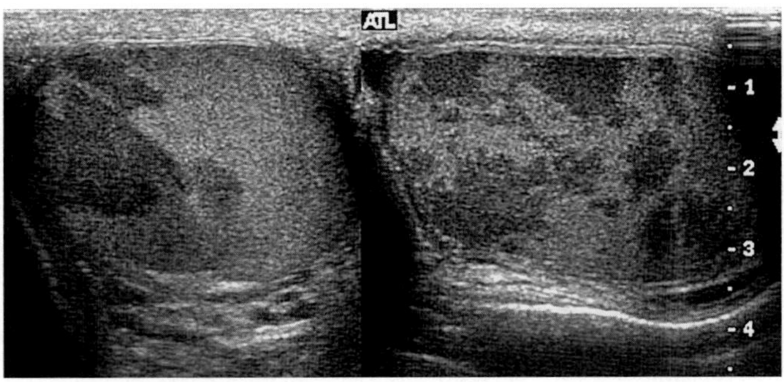

Figure 12-21 Testicular Sarcoidosis
Transverse sonographic image through the testicles demonstrates multiple hypoechoic lesions of various sizes throughout both testicles. The patient had pulmonary sarcoidosis and no history of lymphoproliferative disorder, infection, or prior testicular insult, and was without clinical progression over 3 years. These lesions are thought to represent testicular sarcoidosis but have not been biopsied.

triangular regions of decreased echogenicity in a testis (see Figure 12-22). In most cases, on US, the hypoechoic lesions lack mass effect and will have normal blood flow similar to the normal portions of the testis. The MRI appearance has not been extensively reported in the literature, but testicular atrophy/fibrosis usually appears as hypoenhancing geographic nonmasslike areas of low T2 signal, which can be associated with capsular retraction and do not produce disruption of testicular architecture.

Other unusual causes of bilateral testicular lesions

Two unusual conditions can result in bilateral testicular lesions: Leydig cell hyperplasia and congenital adrenal rests.

Leydig cell hyperplasia: Leydig cell hyperplasia is a rare benign condition usually without symptoms that is characterized pathologically by hyperplastic Leydig cells infiltrating between the seminiferous tubules forming nodules ranging in size from 1 to 6 mm in both testicles. It is thought to be due to chronic Leydig cell stimulation, which may be from increased serum luteinizing hormone (LH) or from elevated human chorionic gonadotropin, which is structurally similar to LH. Known causes of Leydig cell hyperplasia include cryptorchidism; congenital adrenal hyperplasia; hCG production by germ cell tumors, especially choriocarcinoma; pituitary abnormalities; Klinefelter syndrome; exogenous hCG therapy; and antiandrogen therapy for prostate cancer. Leydig cell hyperplasia has also been associated with cachexia and chronic diseases such as tuberculosis, syphilis, and alcoholism.[37] On US, typically several small (<5 mm) hypoechogenic lesions are seen bilaterally throughout the testes (see Figure 12-23). However, the lesions of Leydig cell hyperplasia have also been reported to appear hyperechogenic in some patients.[37] On MRI, Leydig cell hyperplasia appears as small T2-hypointense foci that may demonstrate mild enhancement postcontrast.

Congenital adrenal rests: Testicular adrenal rests represent hyperplasia of ectopic adrenal tissue in response to markedly elevated levels of adrenocorticotropic hormone (ACTH). Causes of testicular adrenal rests include congenital adrenal hyperplasia, usually because of 21-hydroxylase deficiency, Addison disease, and Cushing syndrome. Adrenal rests are most commonly recognized in the setting of congenital adrenal hyperplasia, where they have been detected in up to 8% of patients. Adrenal rests are bilateral in 83% to 100% of cases, medium sized, often oblong in shape, produce minimal disruption of testicular structure, and are usually located eccentrically in the

Imaging Notes 12-8. Differentiating Features of Bilateral Testicular Masses

Bilateral Testicular Masses	Differentiating Features
Leydig cell hyperplasia	Small, history of predisposing conditions
Sarcoid	No clear distinguishing features but tend to be better defined than lesions of lymphoma; African American race; extratesticular findings of sarcoid
Congenital Adrenal rests	History of congenital adrenal hyperplasia; Elevated ACTH, oblong, little disruption of testicular architecture, near mediastinum testis, spokelike vascularity, regression with steroid treatment, elevated cortisol in testicular veins
Secondary malignancy (leukemia/ lymphoma most common)	History of lymphoma, greater involvement of testis than epididymis (if epididymis is involved)
Granulomatous infections (TB)	Findings of TB elsewhere, usually have involvement of epididymis; miliary testicular pattern is characteristic
Testicular fibrosis	Geographic regions without abnormal vascularity in small to normal-sized testicles usually in older individuals; history of subfertility or hypogonadism

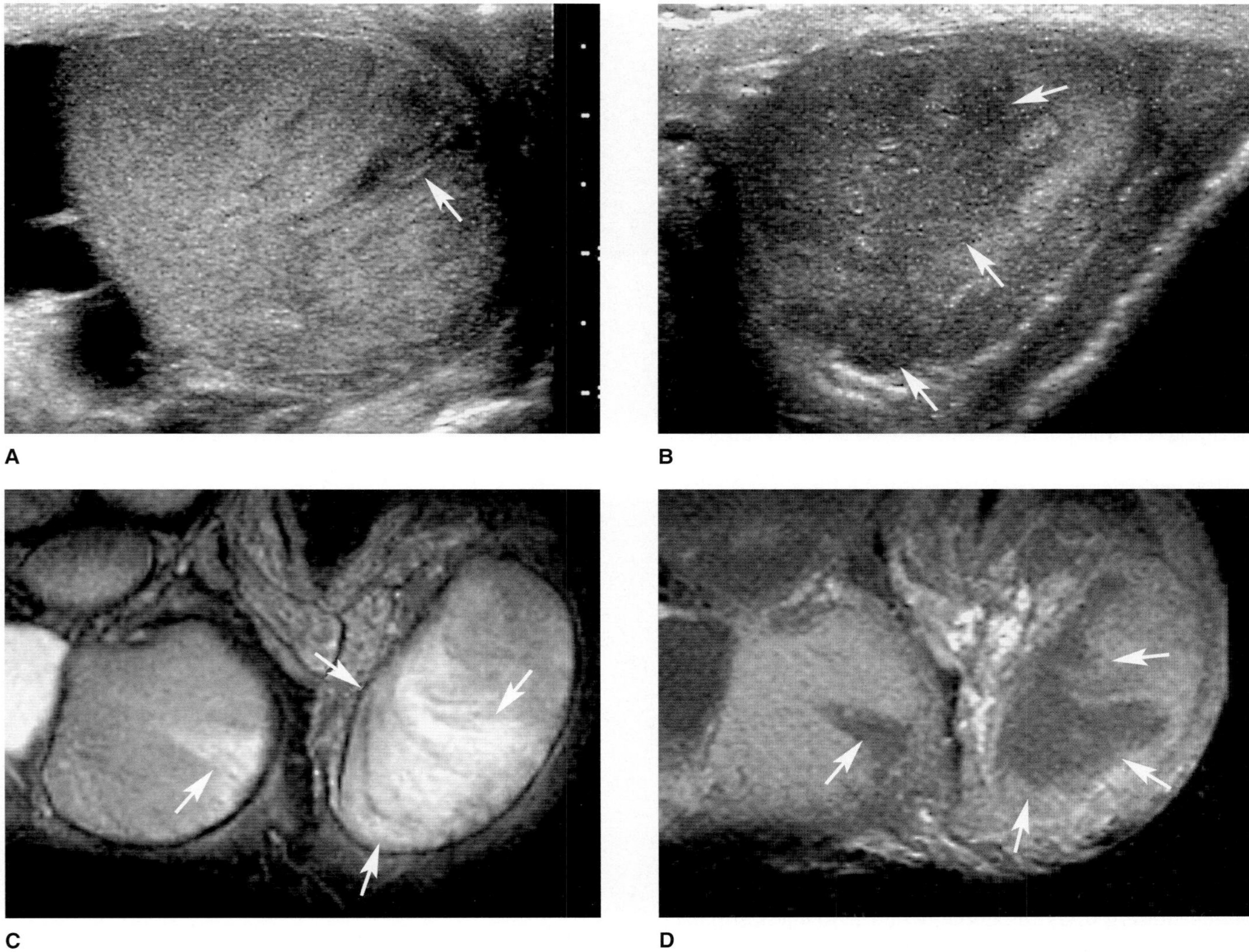

Figure 12-22 Bilateral Atrophy
Transverse grayscale images through the (**A**) right and (**B**) left testicles demonstrate patchy areas of decreased echogenicity without mass effect (*arrows*). **C**. Coronal T2 and (**D**) postgadolinium fat-saturated T1-weighted images demonstrate corresponding hypovascular T2-hyperintense areas (*arrows*) most consistent with atrophy as a sequela of prior insult. In this example, the abnormal areas are T2 hyperintense, but more commonly the areas are T2 hypointense as shown in Figures 12-15 and 12-17.

region of the mediastinum testis (86%) (see Figure 12-24). On US, the lesions are usually hypoechogenic, although some series have reported that the lesions can occasionally be hyperechogenic with shadowing.[38] On color Doppler, a pattern of multiple vessels radiating toward a central point in the mass giving a spokelike appearance was described in 11 of 18 patients, in 1 study.[39] The MRI appearance has not been extensively studied, but the lesions tend to be T2 hypointense, slightly T1 hyperintense (thought to be related to lipid content), and enhancing.[40] Theoretically, the lesions might show dropout of signal on out-of-phase images similar to adrenal adenomas, a finding that has been reported for adrenal rest tissue in a paraovarian location but not yet reported for testicular adrenal rests.[41] If there is a question about the diagnosis, testicular vein sampling may show elevated cortisol levels when compared with peripheral blood levels.[7] Steroid treatment directed at reducing ACTH usually results in stabilization or regression of the masses.

Cystic Testicular Lesions

Cystic masses are, by definition, fluid containing. These may be either simple cysts or complex cysts. For a cystic lesion to be simple, it must be unilocular, contain simple fluid, have a thin imperceptible wall, and have no internal structure. Complex cystic lesions are those that do not satisfy the criteria for a simple cyst, either because they

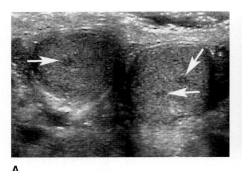

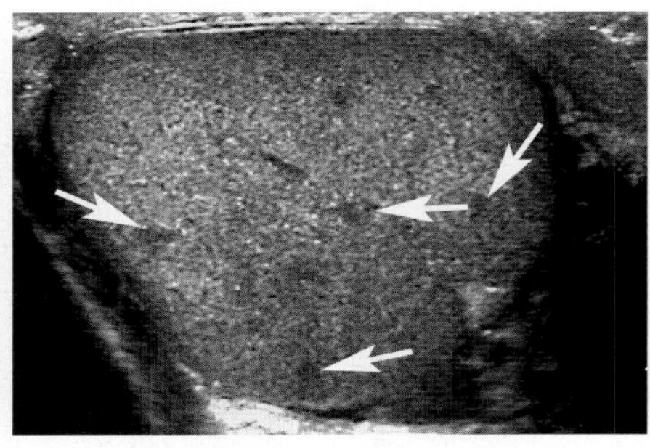

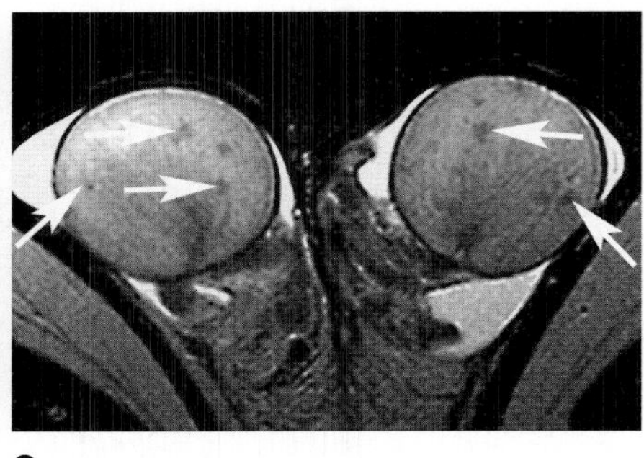

A B C

Figure 12-23 Leydig Cell Hyperplasia in 2 Patients
A. This patient had Klinefelter syndrome. Ultrasonographic image of both testicles demonstrates multiple, scattered <5-mm hypoechoic foci (*arrows*) in both testicles characteristic of Leydig cell hyperplasia. **B.** Transverse grayscale US image of the right testis and (**C**) axial T2-weighted MRI image through both testicles in a second patient demonstrate multiple tiny lesions (*arrows*) that were stable over time. In the absence of an alternative explanation such as sarcoidosis or granulomatous disease, these most likely represent Leydig cell hyperplasia.

contain complex fluid (proteinaceous or hemorrhagic) or because they manifest features such as a thickened or nodular wall, septations, multiple loculations, or solid components (Table 12-5).

Simple testicular cysts

Simple testicular cysts are benign "leave-alone" lesions and include tunica albuginea cysts and testicular cysts.

Tunica albuginea cyst: Cysts of the tunica albuginea are believed to be of mesothelial origin and are lined by nonciliated cuboidal cells. These usually range in size from 2 to 5 mm and most commonly are discovered as an incidental finding or as the etiology of a palpable lump. The median age of presentation is 40 years. US usually reveals a small simple subcapsular unilocular cyst without solid components, most commonly along the upper anterior or lateral aspects of the testicle (see Figure 12-25). Tunica albuginea cysts can occasionally calcify and be complex or multilocular.[27,44]

Testicular cyst: In contrast to tunica albuginea cysts, intratesticular cysts are generally not palpable, even when large.[27,44] Microscopically, the cyst wall is lined by cuboid to low columnar epithelium.[42] Proposed etiologies include prior inflammation, surgery, or trauma. Testicular cysts are incidentally detected in up to 10% of patients undergoing scrotal sonography, usually in men older than age 40.[43] They typically range in size from 2 to 20 mm, are solitary, and are most often located near the mediastinum testis although they can be located anywhere in the testis. On US, testicular cysts are usually simple cysts characterized by anechoic center, imperceptible wall, and through transmission (see Figure 12-26). Rarely, testicular cysts can contain internal echoes reflecting the presence of complex fluid. Ipsilateral spermatoceles are frequently present.

Complex testicular cysts

Unlike simple cysts, the differential diagnosis for complex cystic lesions includes both benign and malignant

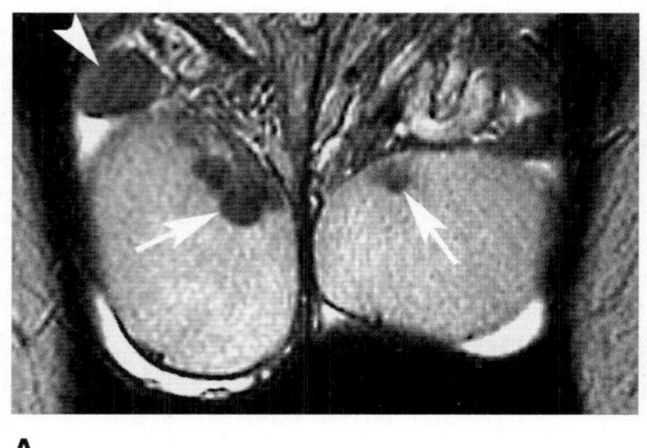

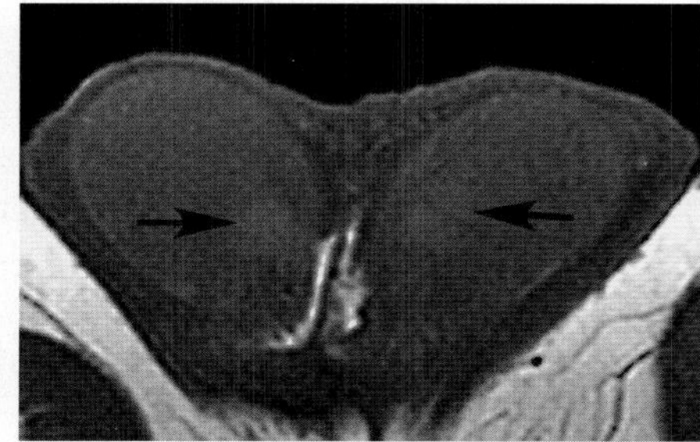

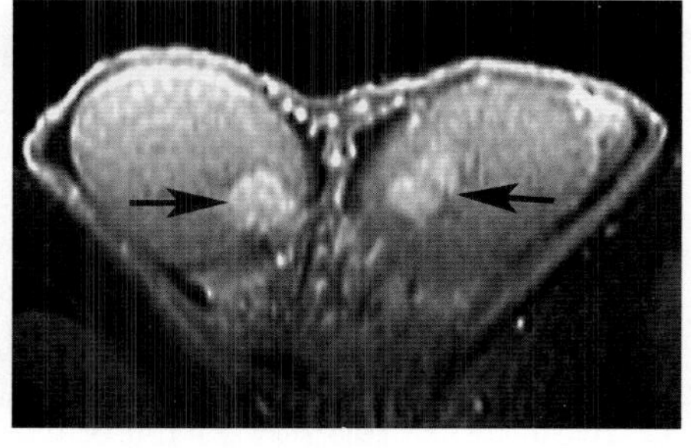

A B C

Figure 12-24 Congenital Adrenal Rests
This 23-year-old man had a history of congenital adrenal hyperplasia. **A.** Coronal T2-weighted, (**B**) axial T1-weighted, and (**C**) postcontrast fat-saturated T1-weighted MRI sequences demonstrate bilateral oblong enhancing nodular lesions (*arrows*) in the region of the mediastinum testis with slight T1 hyperintensity. These features are typical of congenital adrenal rests. *Arrowhead* in A indicates the right epididymis.

Table 12-5. Cystic Appearing Testicular Lesions

1. Cysts associated with neoplasms a. Cystic neoplasm i. Cysts associated with germ cell tumors (especially teratoma) ii. Epidermoid cyst (usually appears solid) iii. Cystadenoma/cystadenocarcinoma of the rete testis (very, very rare) b. Necrotic neoplasm c. Obstruction of the rete testis by neoplasm
2. Abscess
3. Hematoma
4. Other cystic lesions a. Tunica albuginea cyst b. Testicular cyst c. Tubular ectasia of the rete testis d. Cystic dysplasia of the testis (very rare)
5. Cyst mimics a. Intratesticular varicocele b. lymphoma

etiologies. However, usually, malignant lesions can be differentiated from benign lesions by the presence of solid components.

Cysts associated with germ cell neoplasms: A germ cell neoplasm can appear to be cystic or have cystic components for a variety of reasons. In some cases the neoplasm forms cysts, as in the case for some teratomas and less commonly in granulosa tumor. In other cases, cystic areas occur because of intratumoral hemorrhage or necrosis. Finally, tumor-related occlusion of the rete testis can secondarily produce cysts. The most common germ cell tumor to appear cystic is a teratoma. However, cystic areas have been reported in up to 60% of NSGCT and up to 10% of seminomas. In the case of seminomas, the cystic areas are usually due to tumor-related occlusion of the rete testis and are small.

Neoplasm-related cysts can usually be differentiated from other types of cysts by the presence of solid components within the mass. Solid components usually contain flow on Doppler evaluation.[42] However, sometimes flow cannot be detected sonographically in the solid components, either because of technical limitations or because the tumor is hypovascular. In such cases, MRI can help to reveal the presence of solid enhancing tumor components (see Figure 12-27).

Epidermoid cyst: Epidermoid cysts are cystic cavities containing desquamated keratinized epithelium and keratin debris, with a fibrous wall that is at least partially lined with stratified squamous epithelium.[7] Epidermoids typically appear solid on US, often with a characteristic "onion-ring" imaging appearance that is discussed more completely under the heading: **Solid-Appearing Intratesticular Nodule or Mass**. However, occasionally, epidermoids may appear as a nonspecific complex cystic mass characterized by low-level internal echoes, absent internal vascularity, and through

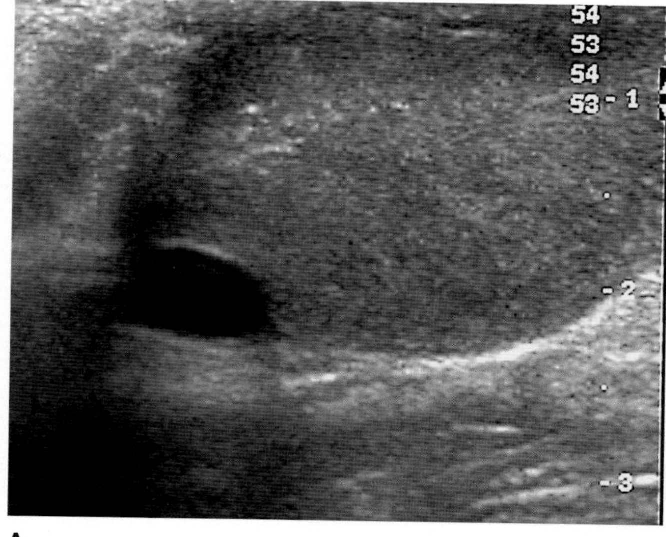

A

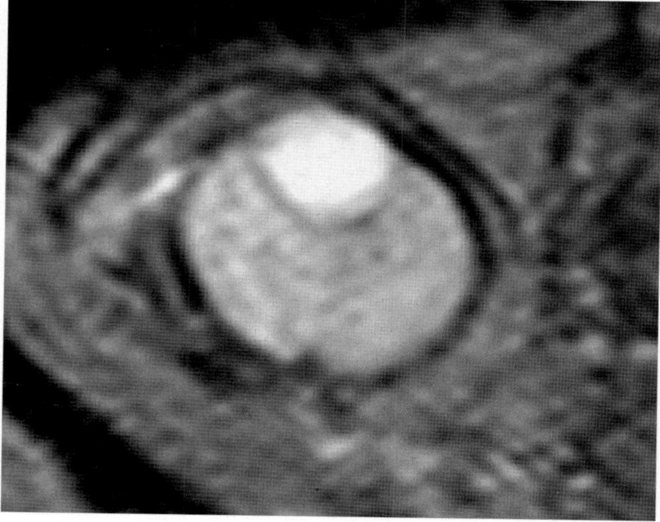

B

Figure 12-25 Tunica Albuginea Cyst
A. Transverse sonographic image demonstrates an anechoic lesion centered in the region of the tunica albuginea with a well-defined wall and through transmission. These are characteristic US features of a tunica albuginea cyst. **B.** T2-weighted image in a different patient shows a peripheral lesion isointense to fluid without enhancement (not shown). These are characteristic MRI features of a tunica albuginea cyst.

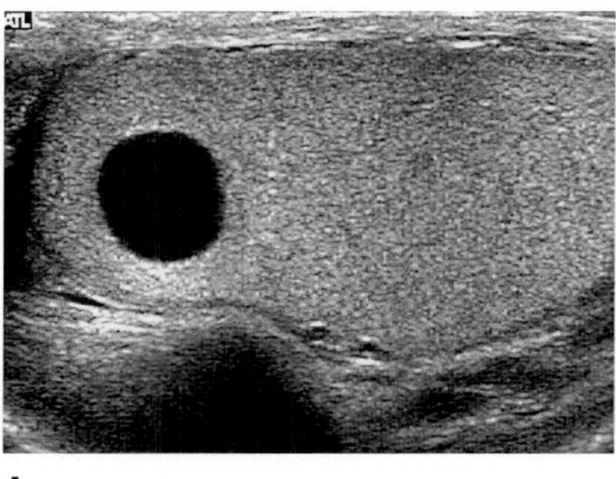

A

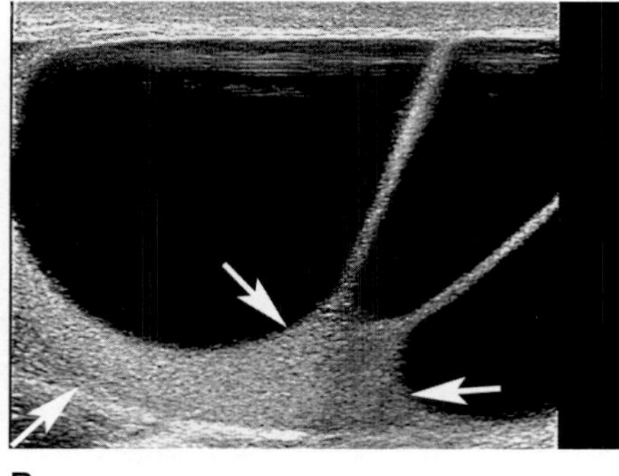

B

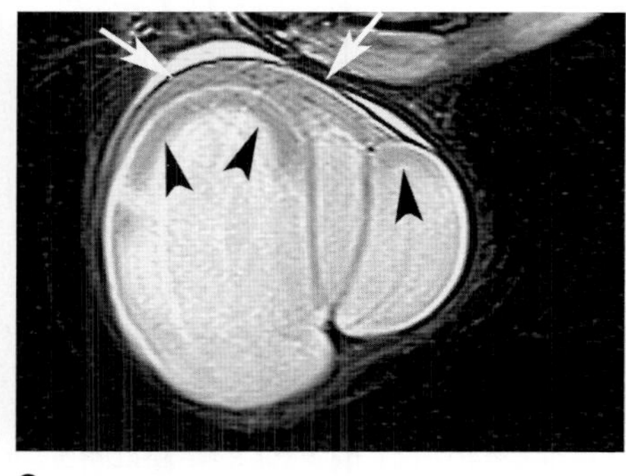

C

Figure 12-26 Testicular Cysts
A. Sagittal grayscale image demonstrates an intratesticular mass in the upper pole with the features of a simple cyst, including a well-defined wall, through transmission, lack of internal echoes, and no flow on color Doppler. B. Grayscale and (C) T2-weighted images demonstrate 3 adjacent anechoic masses on ultrasound that appear on MRI as fluid signal nonenhancing masses surrounded partially by a claw of testicular parenchyma (*arrows*), in keeping with intratesticular cysts. Note that the intervening tissue between the cysts might mimic septations in a multilocular cystic mass, but the lobular configuration and beak of tissue between the cysts suggests otherwise. Note the apparent low signal in the superior aspect of the cysts (*black arrowhead*). This most likely represents artifactual loss of signal related to intracystic motion of fluid.

transmission on US. Epidermoids with this appearance can be difficult to distinguish sonographically from a neoplasm. MRI is helpful in this situation as epidermoid should appear as a *nonenhancing* mass that may contain complex fluid (lower in T2 signal and higher in T1 signal than simple fluid), whereas neoplasm should have *enhancing* components. Note that although abscess and hematoma can resemble epidermoid on both MRI and US, history and other imaging findings of infection or trauma usually distinguishes these entities from epidermoid.

Infectious cysts: testicular abscess: Abscess is usually found as a complication of epididymo-orchitis, although it can also complicate infarction, torsion, trauma, or necrotic tumor among other things.[19] On US, an abscess usually demonstrates shaggy irregular walls, low-level internal echoes, hypervascular margins, and lack of internal vascularity. On MRI, a testicular abscess typically appears as a rim-enhancing T2-hyperintense lesion. A diagnosis of abscess may be supported by the presence of other findings of infection, including epididymitis, as well as by resolution with time, and negative tumor markers.

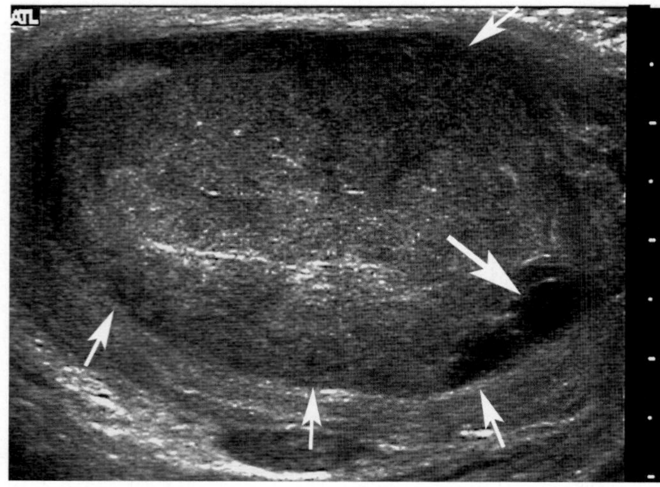

A

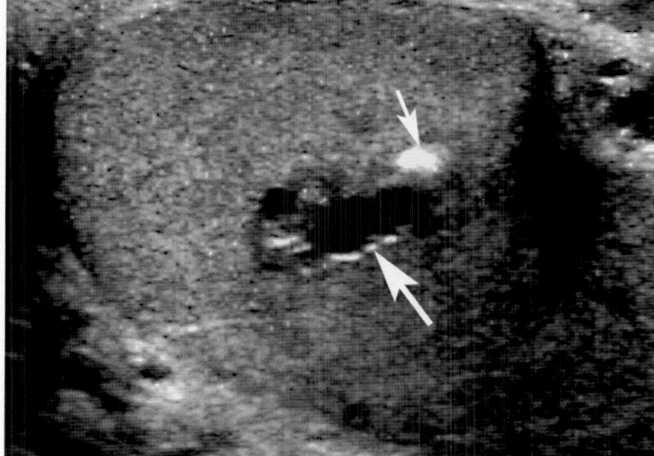

B

Figure 12-27 Cysts Associated With Neoplasms
A. Grayscale US image demonstrates a few small cystic spaces (*large arrow*) at the periphery of a large solid mass (*small arrows*). The excised tumor was proven to represent a seminoma.

B. Grayscale US image shows a mass with cystic spaces (*large arrow*) and calcifications (*small arrow*) in a patient with marked retroperitoneal lymphadenopathy. Pathology revealed a 0.5 cm mature teratoma.

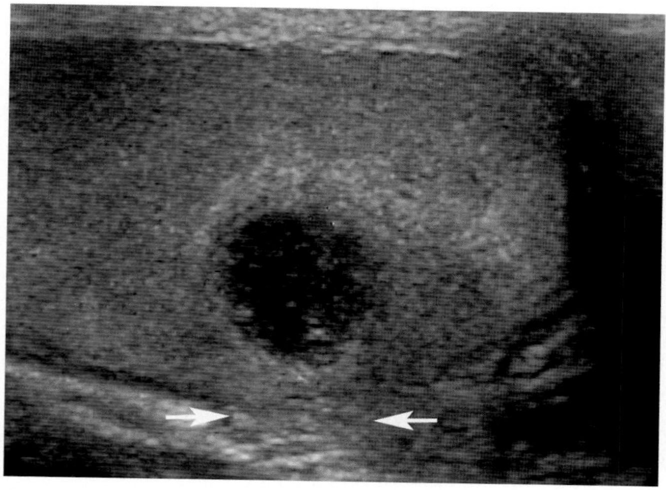

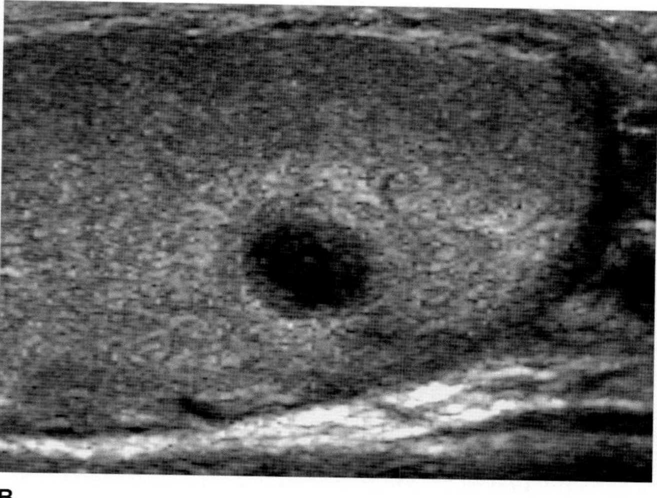

Figure 12-28 Evolving Hematoma
A. Grayscale image about a week after trauma demonstrates a hypoechoic lesion with through transmission. **B.** Follow-up examination a month later demonstrates interval decrease in size most in keeping with a hematoma.

Traumatic cysts: hematoma: Subacute-chronic intratesticular hematomas that have undergone liquefaction can appear as a complex cystic mass, which can be difficult to distinguish from a neoplasm (see Figure 12-28). At MRI, the presence of blood products and absence of enhancement may be helpful in establishing a diagnosis of hematoma in equivocal cases. Improvement with sonographic follow-up and normal tumor markers would also be reassuring. Testicular hematomas have been discussed most extensively under the heading: **Solid-Appearing Intratesticular Nodule or Mass**.

Tubular ectasia of the rete testis: Tubular ectasia of the rete testis is a benign condition that results from partial or complete obliteration of the efferent ducts or ducts of the epididymis. When these structures become obstructed, the rete testis becomes cystically dilated. Tubular ectasia of the rete testis typically occurs in men older than age 55 years. The process is bilateral in 29% to 69% of cases, but is usually asymmetric.[44] There are associated epididymal cysts or spermatoceles in up to 80% of cases.[42] The imaging appearance of tubular ectasia of the rete testis is characteristic. On US, tubular ectasia of the rete testis appears as an elongated region of cystic spaces in the region of the mediastinum testis without solid components or calcifications, and on MRI it appears as a nonenhancing low T1/high T2 signal area in the expected location of the mediastinum testis (see Figure 12-29). There is 1 neoplasm (cystadenoma or cystadenocarcinoma, discussed next) which can mimic the appearance of tubular ectasia of the rete testis, but it is extremely rare.

Neoplasms mimicking ectasia of the rete testis: The neoplasms most likely to produce an appearance similar to tubular ectasia of the rete testis are the very rare adenocarcinoma and cystadenoma of the rete testis.[46,47] Cystadenocarcinoma may be differentiated from tubular ectasia of the rete testis by the presence of solid elements within the cystic mass.[45] There is only 1 case report of the imaging appearance of testicular cystadenoma, which did not describe solid nodular components. However, in that report, cystadenoma could be differentiated from severe tubular ectasia, by the multitude of septations, number of cystic components, extratesticular extension, and a focal conglomeration of the cysts.[45,47]

Cystic dysplasia of the testis: Cystic dysplasia is a rare congenital malformation that is thought to be due to defective communication between efferent ductules and the tubules of the rete testis. Most cases are diagnosed in infancy or childhood, by contrast to tubular ectasia of the rete testes, which is found in older men. On US, cystic dysplasia appears as multiple cystic lesions extending out from the mediastinum into the parenchyma of the testicle. The cysts may enlarge the testicle. An association with renal agenesis and dysplasia has been described.[48]

Mimics of testicular cystic lesions

Varicoceles and testicular lymphoma can occasionally be confused with testicular cysts.

Intratesticular varicocele: Intratesticular varicocele represents a benign enlargement of intratesticular veins.[49,50] It has been reported in 1% to 2% of those referred for scrotal US, and when found is bilateral in about one-quarter of patients.[49] Pathogenesis has not been established but is thought to be similar to that for extratesticular varicocele, where either obstruction of the gonadal vein or

Imaging Notes 12-9. Differentiating Features of Cystic Testicular Masses

Cystic Testicular Lesion	Differentiating Features
Testicular cyst/ tunica albuginea cyst	Simple, no solid components, negative tumor markers
Epidermoid cyst	Avascular, more common to have "onion-ring" appearance or "rim calcification" than appear cystic; when appears as a complex cyst may need to confirm lack of enhancement with MRI, –TuMa
Cystic dilation of the rete testis	Multiple cysts of varying sizes in the region of the mediastinum testis, older men, often bilateral
Cystic dysplasia	Usually diagnosed in infancy, associated with renal agenesis/ dysplasia
Cystic tumor/ cysts associated with tumor	Solid components, +TuMa
Lymphoma (cyst mimic)	Lack of a well-defined wall, + internal vascularity, history of lymphoma
Intratesticular varicocele	Tubular structures that demonstrate augmented venous flow with Valsalva
Abscess	Complex fluid collection, rim hypervascularity, associated findings epididymitis; resolves with time, –TuMa
Hematoma	Complex fluid collection, other findings of trauma; characteristic MRI appearance of blood, resolves with time, –TuMa

Note: TuMa refers to Tumor Markers.

incompetence of the valves of the gonadal vein predisposes patients to distention of the intrascrotal veins. Intratesticular varicoceles occur in conjunction with extratesticular varicocele in 44% to 86% of cases.[50] The clinical significance of intratesticular varicocele has yet to be established, although some believe that it (1) can cause pain due to stretching of the tunica albuginea and (2) that there may be an association with testicular atrophy and infertility.

The grayscale sonographic appearance of a intratesticular varicocele is similar to that of a extratesticular varicocele, except the multiple anechoic, serpiginous, tubular structures representing dilated vessels, are located within the testicle as opposed to in the paratesticular tissues. As with a conventional varicocele, color and spectral Doppler evaluation of these dilated vessels demonstrates venous flow that increases during Valsalva maneuver (see Figure 12-30). Occasionally, an intratesticular varicocele can have a rounded appearance mimicking a solid mass. However, augmentation of flow during Valsalva maneuver should reveal the vascular nature of the lesion.[50] Other vascular abnormalities such as pseudoaneurysm and arteriovenous fistula may also be found in the testicle but are exceptionally rare and not further discussed here.

Lymphoma: On ultrasound, lymphoma is often very hypoechoic and, because of its uniform composition, can be associated with through transmission, thereby potentially mimicking a complex cyst on grayscale images. However, unlike a cyst, lymphomatous lesions typically do not have a well-defined wall. Furthermore, in some cases, flow can be detected in lymphoma on color Doppler, suggesting solid composition. In cases that are equivocal by ultrasound, MRI may be able to differentiate lymphoma from a complex cyst by revealing the presence of diffuse solid enhancement throughout the lesion.

DIFFUSE TESTICULAR DISORDERS

Diffuse abnormalities of the testicle can either be due to diffuse enlargement and/or altered echogenicity or signal intensity, or may manifest as diffusely increased blood flow within the testicle.

Diffusely Enlarged Testicle with Abnormal Echogenicity or Signal Intensity

Diffuse testicular abnormality may be caused by acute conditions, including testicular infarction, infection, and trauma as well as by nonacute conditions such as neoplasms and atrophy (Table 12-6).

Testicular infarction

Testicular infarction is most often caused by testicular torsion but can be a consequence of a variety of disorders.

Spermatic cord torsion: US plays a very important role in differentiating spermatic cord torsion, which is a surgical emergency, from other etiologies of acute scrotum such as epididymo-orchitis, torsion of the appendix testis, trauma, neoplasms, and inguinal pathology such as incarcerated hernia. In testicular torsion, venous obstruction occurs first, followed by arterial obstruction. This results in testicular ischemia, the degree of which depends on the extent of torsion, which ranges from 180 to 720 degrees.[1] There are 2 types of torsion, extravaginal and intravaginal. Extravaginal torsion occurs exclusively in newborns due to torsion outside the tunica vaginalis. The testicle is typically infarcted and necrotic at birth. Intravaginal torsion occurs within the tunica vaginalis and is more common, typically

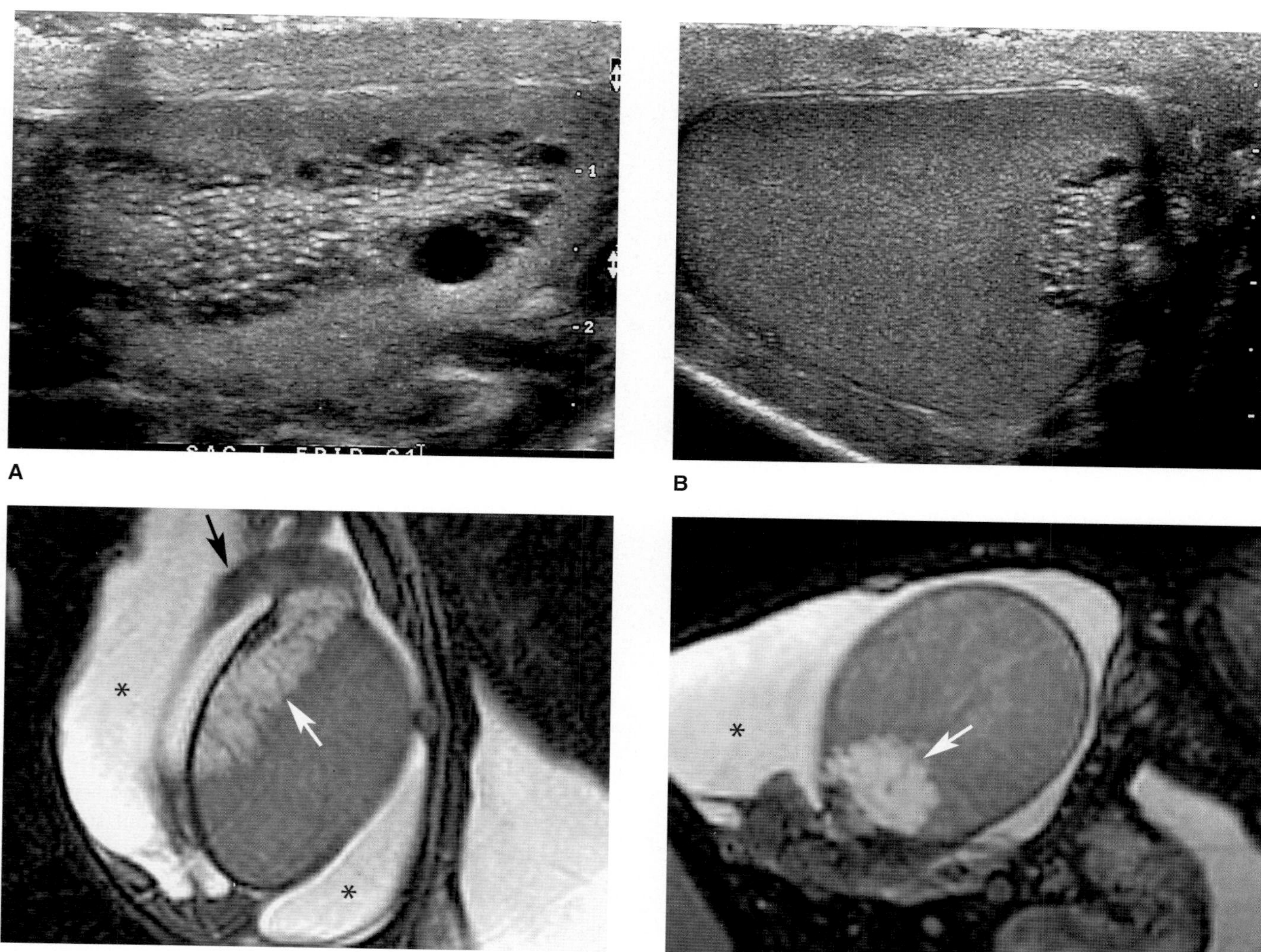

Figure 12-29 Tubular Ectasia of the Rete Testis in 2 Patients
A. Longitudinal and (B) transverse grayscale US images demonstrate innumerable small cystic spaces in the region of the mediastinum testis. Several epididymal cysts were also present (not shown). C. Coronal and (D) axial T2-weighted images in a different patient from A and B shows T2 hyperintense confluent cystic structures in the region of the mediastinum testis (*white arrows*). Note hydrocele (*asterisk*) and epididymis (*black arrow* in A). This demonstrates the typical imaging appearance of tubular ectasia of the rete testis on ultrasound and MRI.

occurring around the time of puberty.[19] Intravaginal torsion is predisposed to by the "bell-clapper deformity" in which the tunica vaginalis completely encircles the epididymis, distal spermatic cord, and testis rather than attaching to the posterolateral aspect of the testis. This deformity leaves the testis free to swing and rotate within the tunica vaginalis like a bell-clapper.[1] The bell-clapper deformity usually involves both testicles and had been reported to occur in up to 12% of individuals in 1 autopsy series.[51]

Torsion presents with acute-onset severe scrotal pain followed by nausea, vomiting, and low-grade fever. Physical examination usually reveals a swollen, tender hemiscrotum with an absent cremaster reflex, and pain that is not relieved with elevation of the scrotum. The majority of studies have shown that most testicles remain viable if the testis is detorsed within 6 hours of presentation; hence early diagnosis is critical to testicular salvage. After 24 hours, the probability of testicular viability is very low, although viability has been documented for testicles torsed for as long as 5 days.[52] Treatment is surgical detorsion with bilateral orchiopexy to prevent recurrence of the torsion.

Grayscale US findings vary with the duration and degree of rotation of the spermatic cord. Early in the course of torsion, the testicle is uniform in echogenicity, a finding that is predictive of testicular viability (see Figure 12-31).[52] With increasing duration of torsion, the testicle becomes enlarged and hypoechogenic, and by 24 hours often develops a heterogeneous echotexture due to vascular congestion, hemorrhage, and infarction (see Figure 12-32). If torsion is

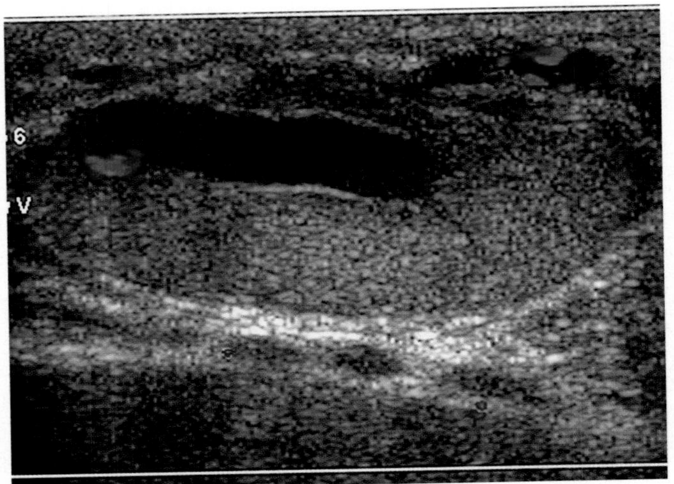

A

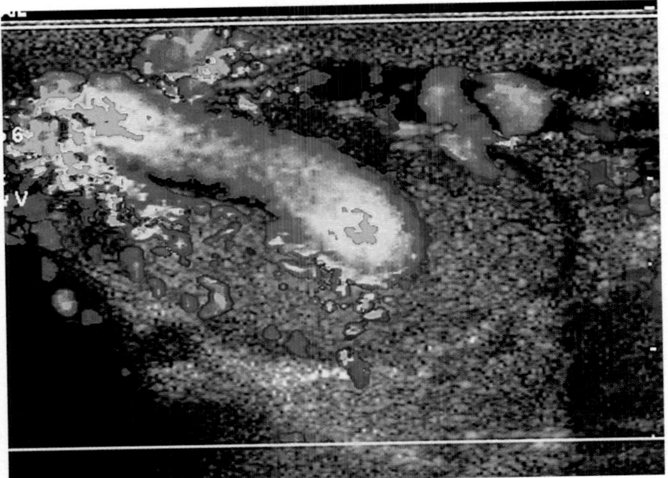

B

Figure 12-30 Intratesticular Varicocele
Color Doppler images (**A**) without and (**B**) with Valsalva maneuver demonstrate an anechoic tubular intratesticular structure at rest (A), which fills in with color on Valsalva maneuver (B) typical of an intratesticular varicocele.

missed, the infarcted testicle eventually becomes atrophic.[28] A small hydrocele and an enlarged edematous epididymis due to involvement of the epididymal blood supply can also be present. Evaluation of the spermatic cord may reveal a "cord knot or twist" that appears as a lobulated extratesticular mass with concentric layers due to coiling/spiraling of the vessels (see Figure 12-31). This phenomenon produces a "target" or "doughnut" appearance on grayscale US images. If the transducer is moved perpendicular to the axis of the torsion mass, swirling of the spermatic cord structures will be seen, which has been termed the "whirlpool" sign.[53] The presence of a "cord knot" or "whirlpool sign" is very specific for torsion.[53] Spermatic cord edema can also be present and is seen as enlargement of the vascular structures in the cord and increased echogenicity of the fat.[53]

Color and spectral Doppler imaging is imperative to timely diagnosis of torsion, as the gray appearance of the testicle and epididymis is nonspecific, overlapping with other causes of acute scrotal pain, such as epididymoorchitis, and furthermore, the torsion knot, while a specific finding, may be difficult to demonstrate. In the setting of high-grade torsion, color and spectral Doppler examinations reveal absent or markedly decreased blood flow to the testicle, which differentiates torsion from epididymo-orchitis, in which testicular blood flow is increased. In lesser degrees of torsion (<540 degrees), some flow, especially arterial flow, can be present in the testicle but such flow is generally diminished relative to the contralateral testis

Table 12-6. Causes of a Diffusely Abnormal Testis

1. Testicular torsion
2. Orchitis
3. Testicular fibrosis/atrophy
4. Neoplasm
5. Trauma
6. Testicular prosthesis

Imaging Notes 12-10. Imaging Features of Testicular Torsion

Testicle	Size	Echogenicity	Blood Flow
Early <6 h	normal	normal	decreased/absent[a]
Mid >6 h	enlarged	homogeneously hypoechoic	decreased/absent
Late > 24 h	enlarged	heterogeneous	absent
Spermatic cord Spermatic cord knot with "target," "donut," or "whorled" appearance			
Other findings Hydrocele Spermatic cord edema Enlarged epididymis with decreased flow			
Pitfalls Blood flow can be normal in partial or early torsion, or increased if there is torsion-detorsion			

[a]Findings in bold are indicative of testicular ischemia-torsion.

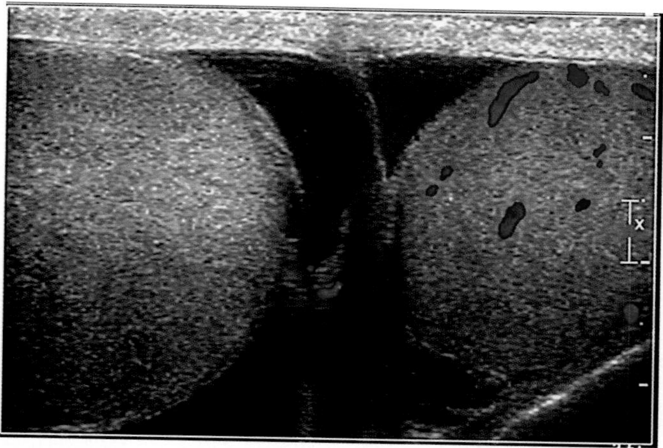

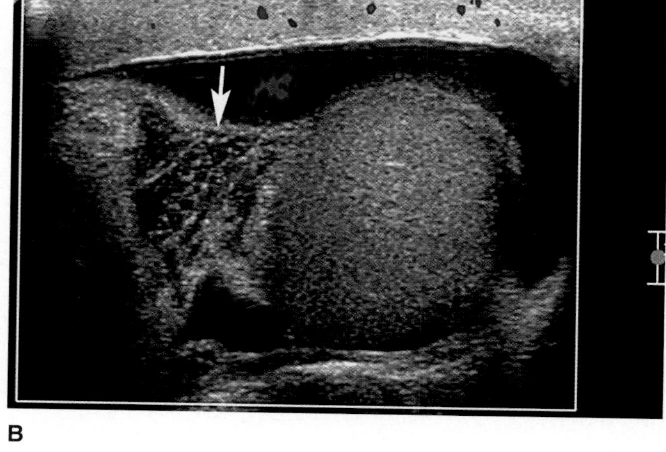

Figure 12-31 Early Spermatic Cord Torsion
This patient presented with acute-onset right scrotal pain. **A.** Color Doppler image reveals a paucity of flow in an enlarged right testicle as well as a hydrocele seen as anechoic fluid surrounding the testicle. These findings are indicative of testicular torsion. The relatively homogeneous echotexture of the testicle is a predictor of viability. **B.** Color Doppler image demonstrates an extratesticular hypovascular mass with a suggestion of swirling, reflecting an edematous twisted spermatic cord (*arrow*), adding further confidence to the diagnosis of testicular torsion.

or demonstrates abnormal features on spectral Doppler such as diminished or absent diastolic flow or abnormal resistive indices.[19,54] Doppler evaluation has been reported to have an overall accuracy of 97%, with a sensitivity of 86% for testicular torsion.[55] Despite the high accuracy, it is important to recognize that Doppler imaging may demonstrate normal testicular blood flow in some patients with surgically proven torsion, presumably because of partial or early torsion. Additionally, in the setting of transient torsion (also known as intermittent torsion), US can reveal increased testicular blood flow due to reperfusion, if the evaluation is performed immediately following detorsion. This can simulate epididymo-orchitis; however, the absence of symptoms at the time of examination as well as a history of intermittent sharp pain should point to the correct diagnosis. False-positive examinations, in which the apparent decrease in testicular blood flow is artifactual, are very rare. However, false positives can occur, due to inadequate optimization of Doppler parameters for the detection of slow flow, or due to asymmetric beam attenuation related to structures superficial to the testis (thickened scrotal wall, hematoma, hernia-containing bowel), or due to the difficulty in detecting blood flow in small testicles in the pediatric population.

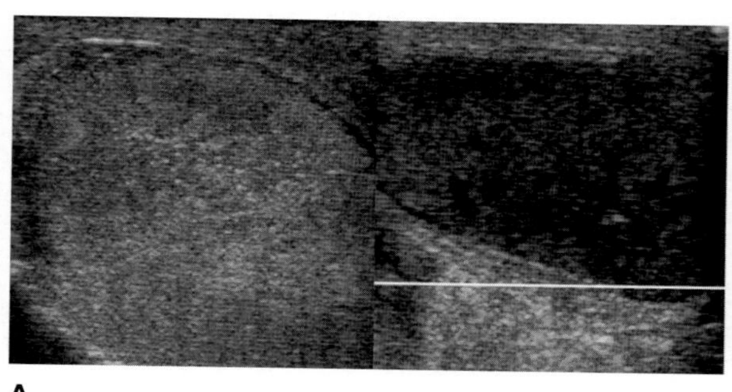

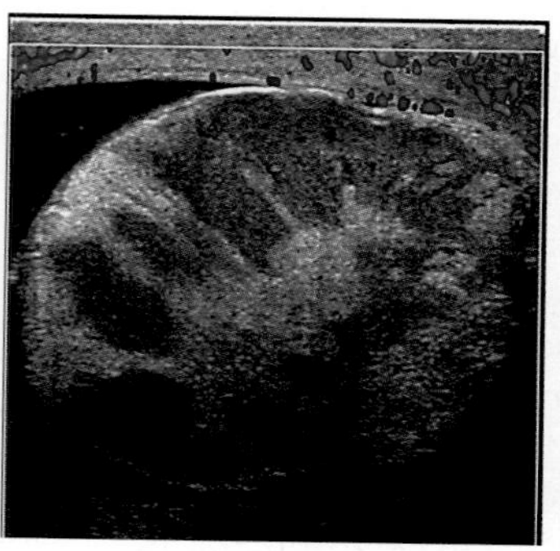

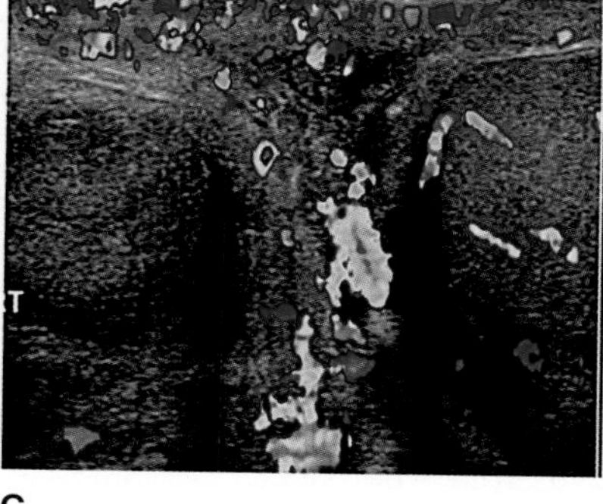

Figure 12-32 Late Torsion With Testicular Infarction in 3 Patients
The patient in **A** presented with acute-onset left scrotal pain. **A.** Grayscale image of the left testicle at presentation (left) and a few days later (right) shows decrease in size and echogenicity of the testis over time (compare right to left) due to evolving infarction. The patient in **B** presented with history of 3 days of testicular pain. **B.** Color Doppler image shows an enlarged heterogenous avascular testis in keeping with infarction. **C.** Color Doppler image in a third patient shows a heterogenous, avascular right testicle. Note increased reactive vascularity of the paratesticular tissues. The heterogenous echotexture of these testicles (B and C) is reflective of testicular infarction and non-viability.

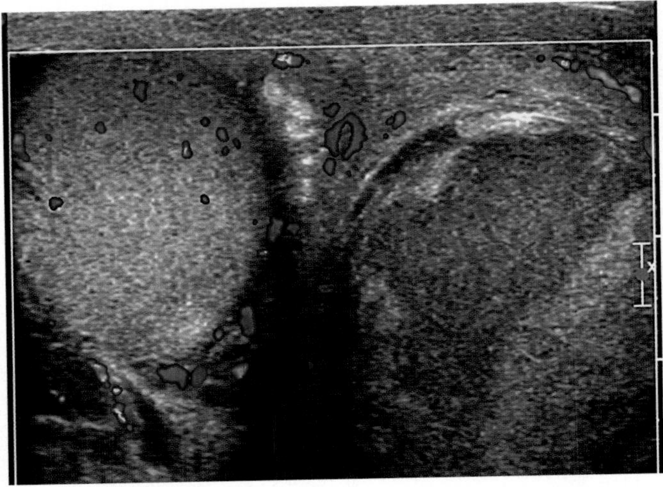

A

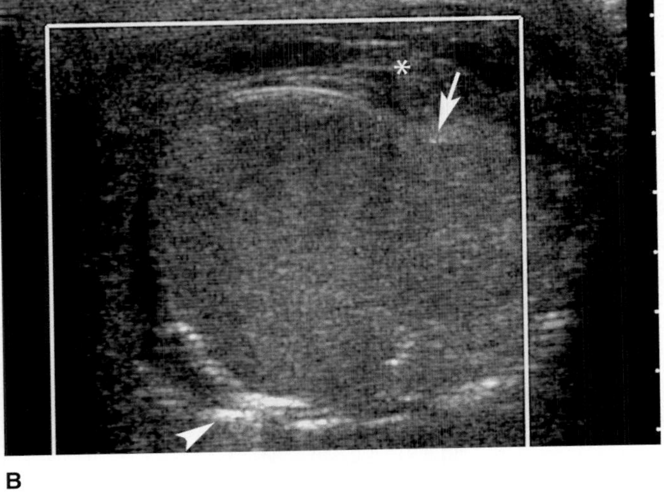

B

Figure 12-33 Other Causes of Testicular Infarction
A. History of hernia repair. Color Doppler image shows a heterogenous enlarged avascular testicle (right side of image) due to infarction following hernia repair, probably due to spermatic cord compromise during the surgery. **B.** Different patient. This man had penetrating injury to the scrotum. Color Doppler image demonstrates an avascular heterogenous testicle with lobulated contour due to tunical disruption (*arrow*), as well as intrascrotal gas (bright foci, *arrowhead*), and a paratesticular hematoma (*asterisk*), reflecting sequela of penetrating injury to the scrotum and spermatic cord. The absence of blood flow indicates infarction of the testicle as a result of the trauma.

The epididymis and cord knot usually demonstrate decreased flow early in torsion; however, if the diagnosis of testicular infarction is delayed, there can be hyperemia of the epididymis and other paratesticular tissues, a finding that should not be mistaken for epididymitis (see Figure 12-32).

As a result of the urgency of the diagnosis and the high sensitivity and specificity of US for the diagnosis of torsion, MRI is not used in the diagnosis of suspected torsion.

Other causes for testicular ischemia or infarction: Other disorders can compromise testicular blood flow, mimicking torsion. (See Regional Infarction, under Geographic Testicular Lesions) (see Figure 12-33). Of these, the most common are severe epididymo-orchitis, trauma, and inguinal hernia repair. Inguinal hernia repair is reported to cause testicular atrophy in 0.03% to 0.5% following primary inguinal hernia repair and between 0.8% and 5% for recurrent inguinal hernia repair, presumably because of ischemia or infarction related to compromise of the spermatic cord vessels.[31] Other very rare causes of testicular ischemia/infarction include a vasculitis such as polyarteritis nodosa, hematologic disorders such as polycythemia and sickle cell disease, and hypercoagulable states.[19,32] Compression of the testicle by a hydrocele or hematoma may also reduce testicular blood flow, but the degree of compromise is usually not severe.

Orchitis and epididymo-orchitis

Orchitis usually is a complication of acute pyogenic bacterial epididymitis. (Epididymitis is discussed in detail under the heading: **Diffusely Thickened Epididymis**, subheading: **Acute epididymitis and epididymo-orchitis.**) Bacteria spread from the epididymis into the testis in 20% to 40% of cases of acute epididymitis, resulting in "epididymo-orchitis."[1] In adolescents, epididymo-orchitis is usually due to sexually transmitted bacteria, such as *Chlamydia trachomatis* and *Neisseria gonorrhoeae*, whereas in men older than age 45, most cases are due to urinary coliforms such as *Escherichia coli* and *Proteus mirabilis*. Regardless of the specific organism, patients typically present acutely with fever and severe scrotal pain. The imaging appearance is variable depending on the severity of the infection. When acute bacterial orchitis is mild, US typically reveals a unilateral, diffusely enlarged, hyperemic testicle that is relatively homogeneous in echotexture, aside from a mildly "striated" appearance with thin linear hypoechogenic bands radiating outward from the mediastinum testis (see Figure 12-34). When infection becomes more severe, the testicle may become progressively more abnormal in grayscale appearance because of ischemia, abscess formation, and hemorrhage, resulting in heterogeneous echotexture and overall decreased echogenicity (see Figure 12-35). In extreme cases, testicular infarction can occur, resulting in absent vascularity, mimicking infarction due to torsion. On MRI, mild orchitis is manifested with testicular enlargement, often with mildly inhomogeneous enhancement and inhomogeneous signal (see Figure 12-36). As with US, more severe infection leads to more heterogeneous signal.[4] Other imaging findings associated with epididymo-orchitis include diffuse enlargement and hyperemia of the epididymis, skin thickening, and hydrocele, which support a diagnosis of infection, in the appropriate clinical setting.

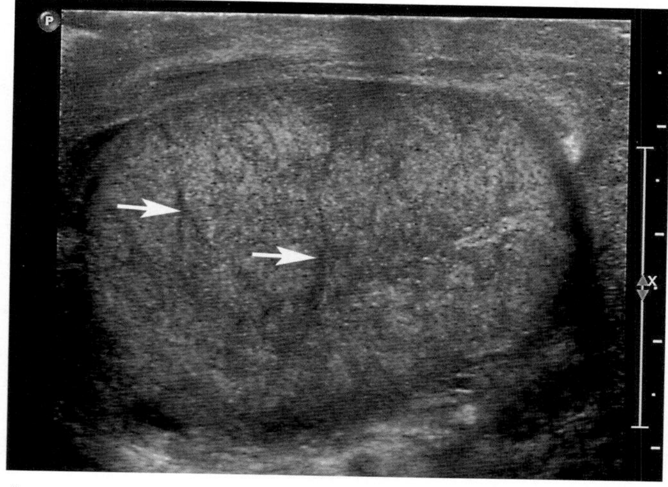

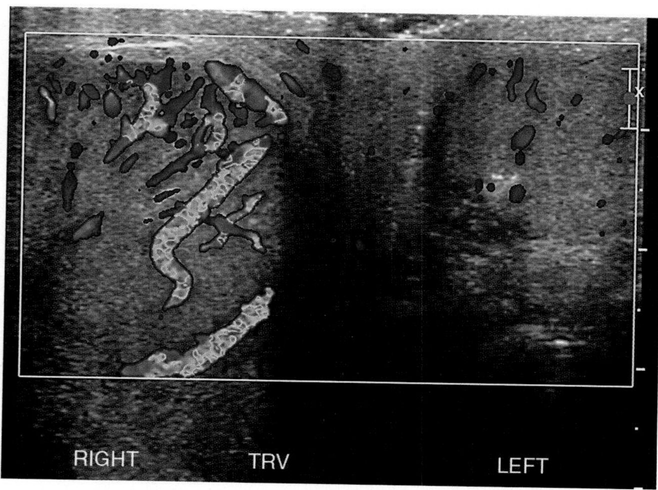

Figure 12-34 Orchitis
A. Sagittal grayscale image of the right testis shows testicular enlargement and faint hypoechoic bands (*arrows*) producing a "striated" appearance to the testicle. This pattern can be seen with testicular edema from any cause, or with testicular atrophy and very rarely lymphoma. **B**. Transverse color Doppler image shows increased blood flow in the right testis compared with the left, in keeping with orchitis.

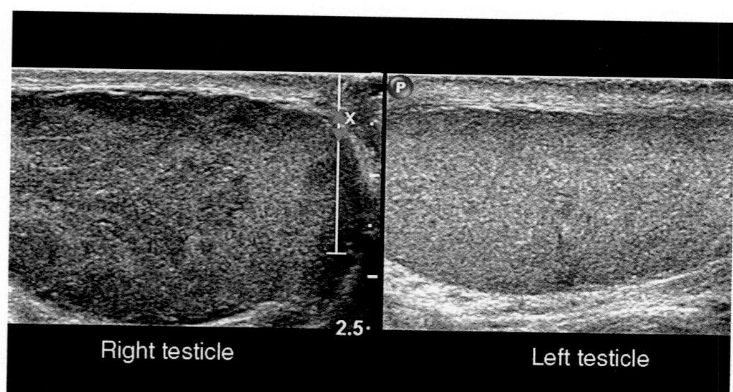

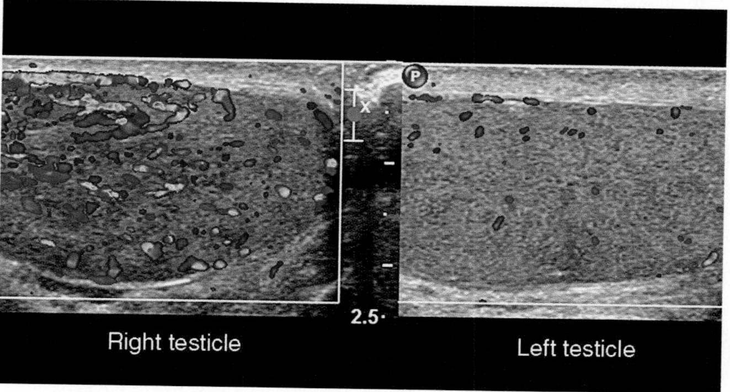

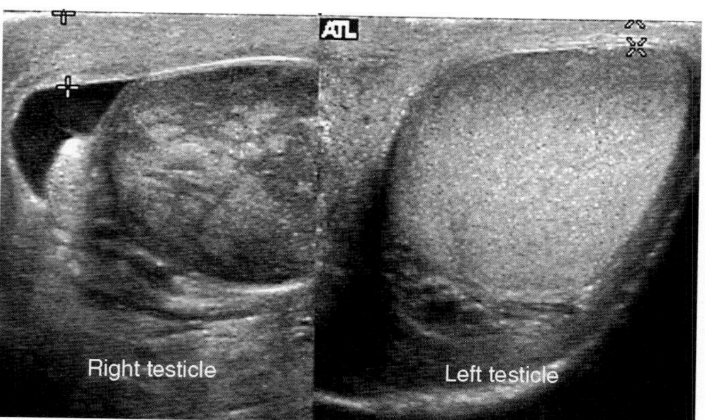

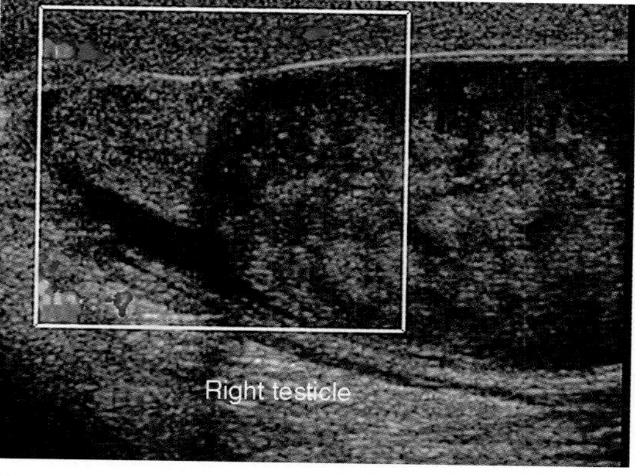

Figure 12-35 Epididymo-orchitis Versus Torsion
A. Grayscale and (**B**) color Doppler images in a patient with right testicular pain shows a heterogenous, **hypervascular** right testicle, in keeping with orchitis. **C**. Grayscale and (**D**) color Doppler images in a patient with right testicular pain demonstrates a heterogeneous, **hypovascular** right testicle and epididymis, indicating a diagnosis of infarction due to torsion. Note the similarity in the clinical presentation and grayscale imaging appearance of orchitis and testicular torsion. In many cases, the only discriminating feature between orchitis and testicular torsion is the difference in testicular blood flow.

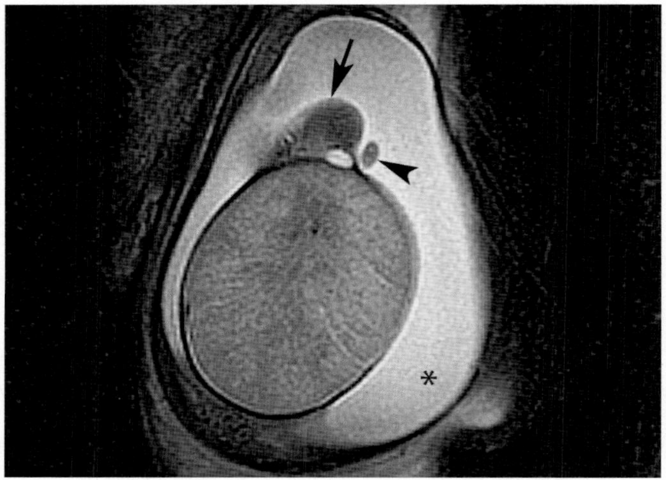

A

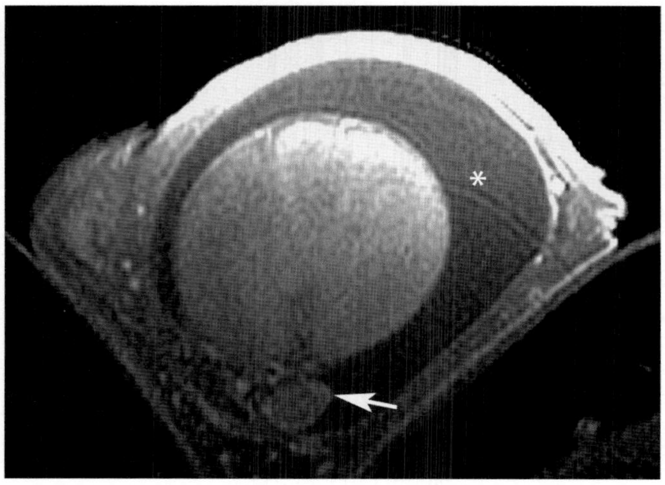

B

Figure 12-36 MRI of Orchitis
A. Coronal T2 and (**B**) axial postgadolinium fat-saturated T1-weighted images demonstrate an enlarged striated heterogeneously enhancing testicle with an associated hydrocele (*asterisk*) characteristic of orchitis. The epididymis (*arrow*) and appendix testis (*arrowhead*) can be seen.

Other causes of orchitis include granulomatous infections, viral infections, trauma, and vasculitis. In many cases, granulomatous orchitis can be differentiated from bacterial orchitis based on subacute presentation as well as imaging features discussed under the heading: **Solid-Appearing Intratesticular Nodule or Mass**, subheading **Orchitis and epididymo-orchitis.**[24] Viral orchitis is most commonly due to mumps and occurs in 20% to 30% of postpubertal patients infected with the mumps virus. Symptoms of orchitis usually manifest 4 to 6 days after the onset of mumps parotitis but can occur without parotid involvement. Mumps orchitis is bilateral in 30% of cases and usually does not affect the epididymis. These features can help distinguish mumps orchitis from pyogenic orchitis.[2] Other rare causes of orchitis included trauma and systemic vasculitis such as polyarteritis nodosa or Behçet disease, as well as infection with the HIV and cocksackie B viruses.

Trauma and testicular rupture

Trauma to the testis is one of the most common testicular disorders, but accounts for <1% of all trauma-related injuries. The peak incidence occurs in the age range of 10 to 30 years. Blunt trauma is the most common mechanism of injury, with athletic injury accounting for 50% and motor vehicle accident for 9% to 17% of cases. Less common mechanisms of injury include penetrating trauma, postsurgical injury, and thermal injury (burn). The right testis is injured more frequently than the left, probably because of its greater propensity to be trapped against the pubis or inner thigh. Patients with scrotal trauma usually present emergently and rapid diagnosis is important to guide treatment and to prevent complications.[56]

In the setting of testicular trauma, the testicular echogenicity can be focally or diffusely abnormal because of a variety of conditions, including contusion, hematoma, fracture, ischemia, infarction, and testicular rupture.[1,28,56]

The most important of these conditions to recognize is testicular rupture. In testicular rupture, there is hemorrhage and extrusion of the testicular contents into the scrotal sac. Testicular rupture is a surgical emergency because if the condition is untreated for greater than 72 hours, 56% of patients require orchiectomy for a non-salvagable testicle and the remainder run an increased risk of developing sperm antibodies that can render the patient infertile.[28] Of patients who receive surgical therapy within 72 hours, there is an 80% salvage rate. The imaging diagnosis of testicular rupture can be difficult, with a reported accuracy varying from 56% to 94%.[56] Discontinuity of the tunica albuginea is the only specific finding of testicular rupture but this is not always readily identified. Other findings suggesting rupture include an ill-defined testicular contour or protrusion of testicular contents beyond the normal contour of the testis (implying a gap in the tunica albuginea) in combination with diffusely heterogeneous testicular echotexture due to areas of hemorrhage and ischemia (see Figure 12-37). The combination of heterogeneous testicle and loss of normal contour has been reported to have a sensitivity and specificity of 100% and 93.5%, respectively for testicular rupture.[56] MRI usually is not obtained in the setting of rupture but might show disruption of the low-signal tunica albuginea with hematoma. One potential pitfall for testicular rupture is testicular deformity from prior orchiopexy (see Figure 12-38). However, postsurgical change is typically bilateral, asymptomatic, and associated with a history of cryptorchidism, whereas testicular rupture is associated with pain, a history of trauma, and intrascrotal hemorrhage.

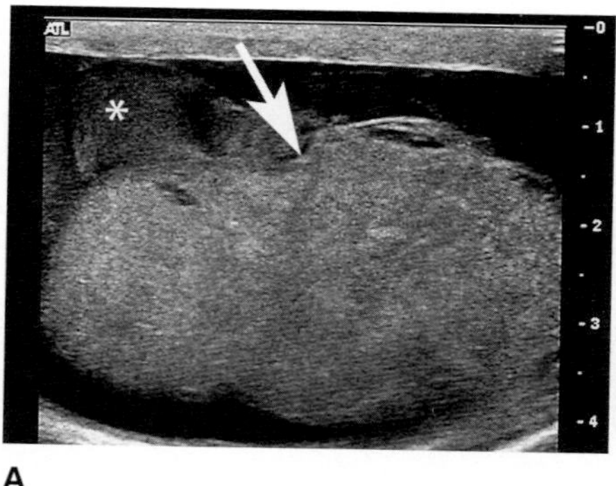

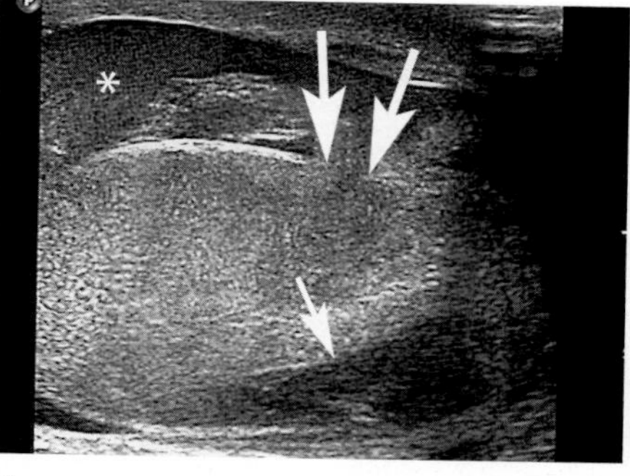

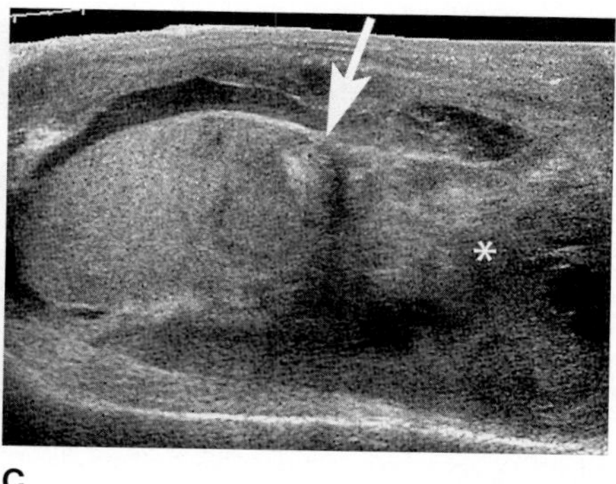

Figure 12-37 Testicular Rupture in Several Different Patients A to C. Longitudinal grayscale images of 3 different patients demonstrating disruption of the tunica albuginea (*arrows*) with gross deformity of the testis. Note adjacent hematoma and hematocele (*asterisk*). Small arrow points to intratesticular hematoma in B. Also note the surrounding skin thickening in patient in C.

In contrast to rupture, most other testicular injuries (testicular fracture and testicular hematoma) are managed without surgical intervention unless associated with areas of ischemia or infarction.[1] Testicular fracture appears as a linear hypoechogenic band that represents a break in the normal testicular architecture and is differentiated from rupture by intact tunica albuginea and smooth testicular contour (see Figure 12-39). Areas of testicular devascularization related to fracture or rupture are identified based on focal decreased or absent vascular signal in the testicular parenchyma on color and spectral Doppler evaluation. Although a testicular hematoma also appears as an area of absent blood flow on color Doppler, it can usually be differentiated from testicular infarction by greater disruption of testicular architecture and by the presence of a testicular mass (see Figure 12-39). Hematomas are initially echogenic and subsequently become more complex, containing cystic and solid-appearing components. Extratesticular findings of trauma include hydrocele or hematocele, traumatic epididymitis, skin thickening, scrotal hematoma, and spermatic cord hematoma (see Figures 12-37 and 12-40). If there has been penetrating injury, intrascrotal gas can be present. Patients with spermatic cord hematoma should have testicular blood flow evaluated to exclude compromise as a result of compression or injury of the spermatic cord blood vessels.

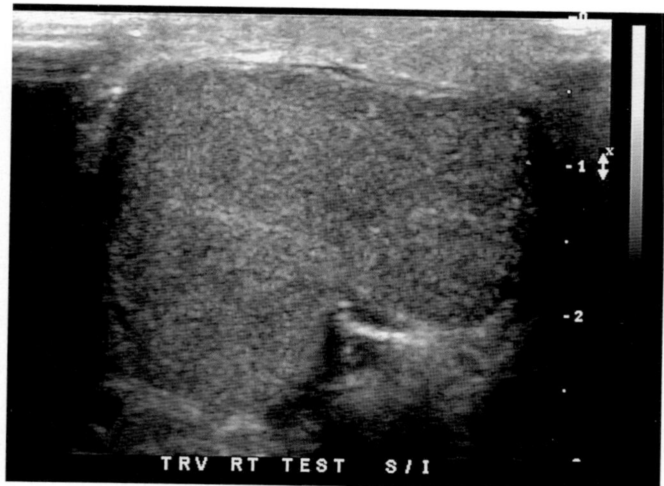

Figure 12-38 Testicular Deformity Post Orchiopexy Grayscale image shows a deformed-appearing right testicle, which demonstrated normal blood flow. The other testicle had a similar appearance. In this asymptomatic patient with history of orchiopexy, the deformity is consistent with postsurgical change.

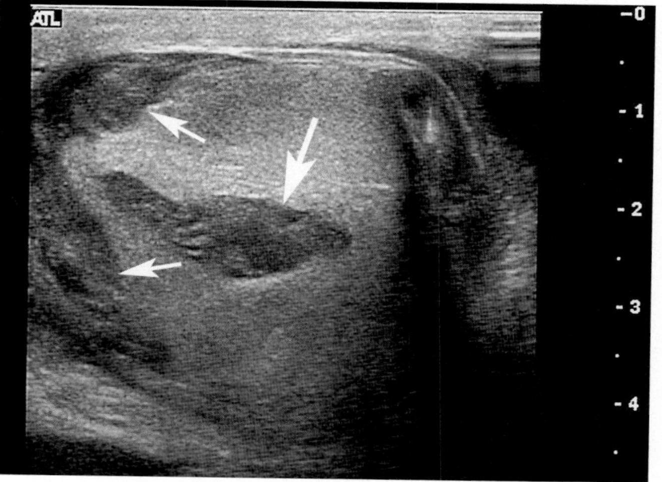

Figure 12-39 Testicular Fracture and Hematoma Grayscale image in a patient with blunt trauma shows a linear area (*large arrow*) representing a fracture as well as multiple areas of testicular hematoma (*small arrows*).

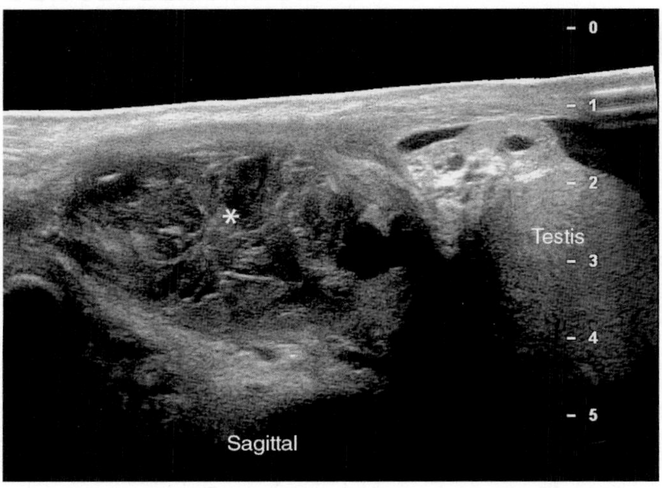

Figure 12-40 Inguinal Hematoma
This patient had experienced trauma to the scrotum. Grayscale image shows a heterogenous mass (*asterisk*) in the inguinal region superior to the testis due to a hematoma. It is important to asses for normal flow in the spermatic cord and testis to exclude vascular compromise either due to compression of the spermatic cord, or due to direct spermatic cord injury.

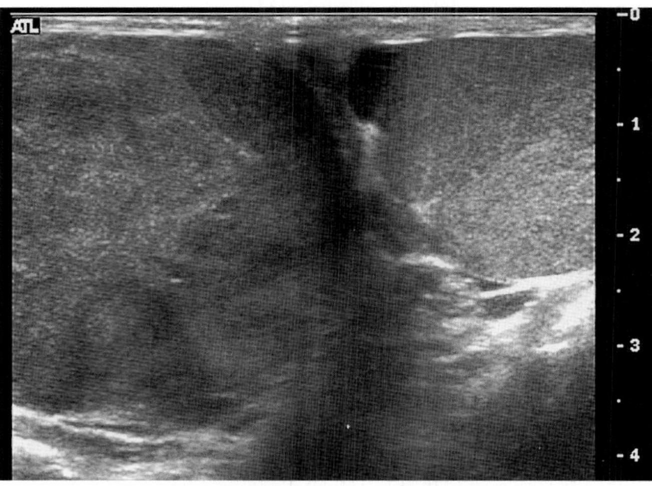

Figure 12-41 Seminoma
Grayscale image demonstrates mildly heterogenous hypoechoic enlargement of the right testicle. There is loss of normal testicular architecture and contour deformity, which is indicative of a mass (as opposed to inflammatory etiology). Right orchiectomy revealed a 6-cm seminoma.

Although clinical history usually points to the diagnosis of trauma, 10% to 15% of tumors first manifest after an episode of trauma.[1] Therefore, intratesticular abnormalities should be followed to resolution if they do not warrant immediate surgical treatment.

Neoplasms causing diffuse testicular abnormality

Several tumors can present with diffuse involvement of the testis, most commonly seminoma and lymphoma/leukemia. Seminoma completely replaces the testis in up to 50% of cases.[1] Diffuse infiltration of the testis is reported to be the most prevalent pattern of leukemia and is a frequent pattern of lymphoma. Compared with seminoma, leukemia and lymphoma are more commonly bilateral.[57] In most cases, tumor infiltration results in diffusely decreased echogenicity, heterogeneity, mass effect, and disruption of the testicular architecture as well as abnormal increased vascularity, which are clues to the presence of neoplasm, along with nonacute presentation, and failure to resolve on short term (weeks) follow-up (see Figure 12-41).

Testicular fibrosis/atrophy

The term *testicular atrophy* or *fibrosis* corresponds to seminiferous tubule sclerosis and interstitial fibrosis. Causes and predisposing conditions include cryptorchidism, gonadotropin deficiency, Klinefelter syndrome, cirrhosis, malnutrition, chemoradiation, trauma, infection such as mumps, ischemia, and hormonal causes such as estrogen therapy, hypothyroidism, hypogonadism, or idiopathic (Table 12-7).[19] Testicular atrophy has been reported in 14% of men older than age 50 years in 1 autopsy series.[58] It often appears as patchy-geographic ill-defined areas of altered echogenicity. It can also appear as a pattern of multiple hypoechogenic bands radiating from the mediastinum testis, which has been referred to as the "striated

Table 12-7. Causes of Testicular Fibrosis and Atrophy

1. Idiopathic
2. Infection (mumps)
3. Trauma
4. Ischemia
5. Hormonal
   a. Estrogen therapy
   b. Hypothyroidism
   c. Hypogonadism
      i. Cryptorchidism
      ii. Gonadotropin deficiency
      iii. Klinefelter syndrome
6. Cirrhosis
7. Malnutrition
8. Chemoradiation

Imaging Notes 12-11. The "Striated" Testicle

- A pattern of multiple hypoechogenic bands radiating from the mediastinum testis
- Caused by
  1. Testicular fibrosis[a]
  2. Ischemia
  3. Orchitis
  4. Lymphoma[b]

[a]Most likely etiology in an older asymptomatic male.
[b]Rare, usually associated with testicular enlargement.

Imaging Notes 12-12. Differentiating Features of Diffuse Testicular Abnormality

Diffusely Abnormal Testis	Helpful Features
Torsion	Abnormally decreased flow on color and spectral Doppler in testis, decreased flow in the epididymis unless late, "cord knot," "whirlpool," acute presentation
Trauma	Traumatic history, tunical disruption, hematocele
Severe epididymo-orchitis	Hyperemic testis unless severe and complicated by testicular infarction; hyperemic epididymis; clinical findings of infection
Atrophy	Normal vascularity, "striated pattern," stable on follow-up, the presence of predisposing factors (eg, history of cryptorchidism, mumps or hernia repair); normal epididymis
Tumor infiltration	Enlarged and hypervascular testis; typically normal epididymis; history of lymphoma/leukemia
Testicular prosthesis	Anechoic ovoid structure in the hemiscrotum, history

testicle" or septal pattern (see Figure 12-42). Ischemia, orchitis, and lymphoma may also give rise to a "striated testicle."[59] However, features favoring testicular atrophy as the etiology of "striation" include normal blood flow, lack of mass effect, lack of symptoms, and normal to small testicular size. In some cases, capsular retraction can be present in a region of chronic atrophy. On MRI, areas of fibrosis usually appear as low-signal areas on T2-weighted images that are hypoenhancing; however the appearance is variable (see Figure 12-42). If atrophy is suspected, follow-up is usually the most appropriate management option.[59]

Testicular prosthesis

Silicone prosthesis has a characteristic sonographic appearance as an anechoic oval structure in the hemiscrotum. Silicone prostheses cause moderate sound enhancement and reverberation artifacts (see Figure 12-43).[1] History and appearance are diagnostic.

Diffusely Hyperemic Testicle

In some conditions, the most striking finding is the presence of markedly increased testicular vascularity. This is most often a result of orchitis or intermittent torsion but can occasionally be due to neoplasms (Table 12-8).

Orchitis

In up to 40% of cases of orchitis, the grayscale appearance of the testicle is normal, and the only imaging finding is increased vascularity.[1] Most of the time, the typical findings of epididymitis are also present. However, viral orchitis, most commonly due to mumps, often occurs without epididymitis. The testicular hyperemia should resolve with appropriate treatment.

Torsion-detorsion (Intermittent torsion)

A transient increase in testicular blood flow occurs following the untwisting of the spermatic cord (detorsion), and can be associated with hyperemia of the paratesticular tissues (see Figure 12-44). This increased vascularity may mimic epididymo-orchitis. Features suggestive of torsion-detorsion include a history of acute sharp transient pain with spontaneous relief, horizontal testicular axis, as well as lack of marked tenderness at the time of the examination.[53] Another finding that should raise suspicion for torsion-detorsion is the presence of an unexplained testicular infarct.[32] By contrast, orchitis/epididymo-orchitis usually presents with clinical or laboratory evidence of infection, continuous (not intermittent) pain, and an exquisitely tender hemiscrotum at the time of examination.[60] If these differentiating features are not present, close follow-up is required.

Neoplasms

Increased vascularity may be seen in the setting of diffuse infiltration with tumor such as lymphoma, leukemia,

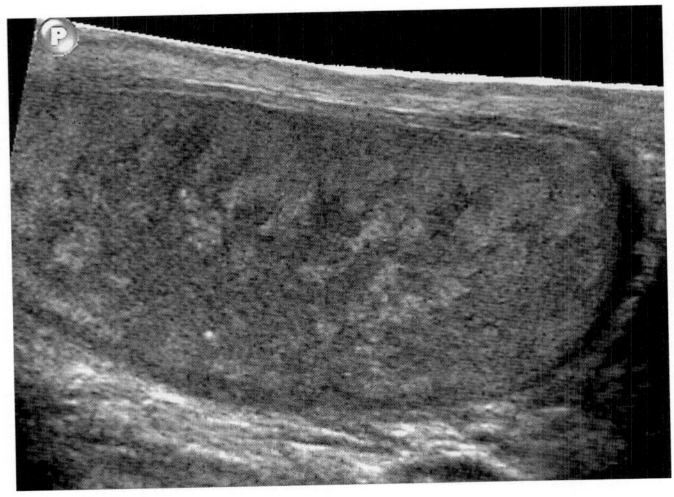

A

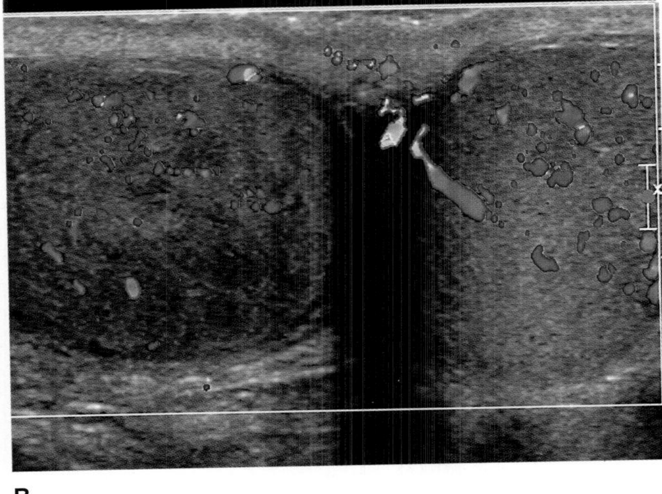

B

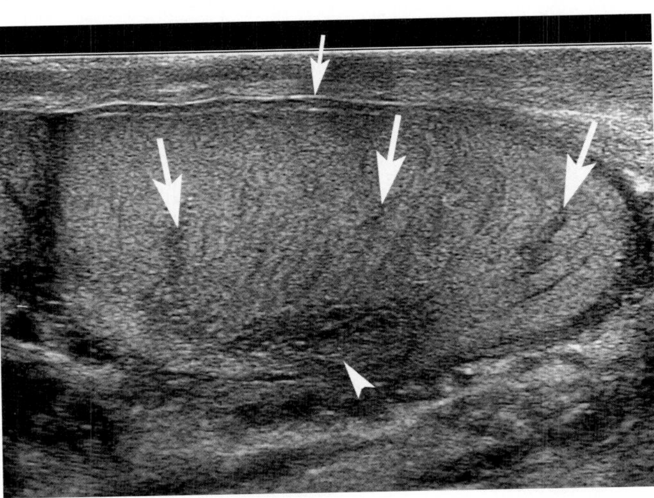

C

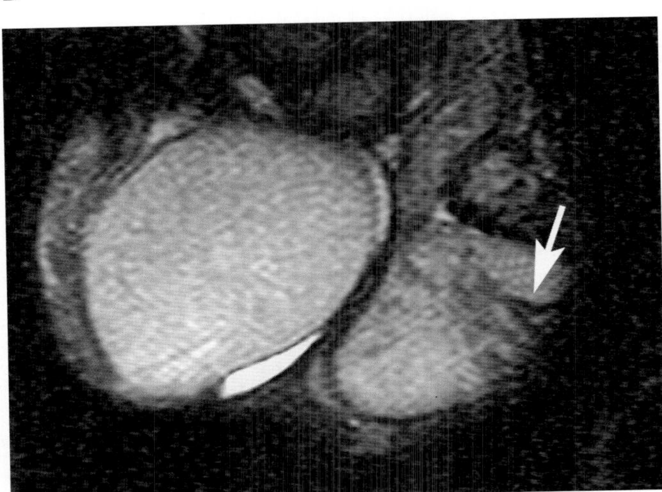

D

Figure 12-42 Testicular Atrophy in 3 Patients
The patient in **A** and **B** had a history of a palpable abnormality and a remote history of orchitis. (A) Grayscale and (B) color Doppler images demonstrate a diffusely heterogeneous normal-sized testicle with normal blood flow. Given the absence of pain and the presence of normal blood flow, this most likely indicates testicular atrophy due to prior orchitis. **C**. Grayscale image in a patient with a history of prior episodes of epididymitis shows prominence of the lobular septa ("striated testicle" *arrows*), reflecting testicular atrophy. Edema related to detorsion or acute orchitis could have a similar appearance but would be associated with pain and abnormal blood flow. Note also mild tubular ectasia of the rete testis (*arrowhead*) and the tunica albuginea (*small arrow*). **D**. This patient reported testicular pain and decrease in testicular size after hernia repair. Coronal T2-weighted image showing a small heterogeneous testicle with linear hypoenhancing areas of decreased T2 signal, typical of fibrosis.

or seminoma and can mimic orchitis (see Figure 12-45).[9] Findings suggestive of tumor include marked testicular enlargement and heterogeneity, persistence with time, as well as absence of paratesticular abnormalities. In equivocal cases, MRI and/or short-term follow-up following therapy may be helpful.

Other

Secondary testicular hyperemia may occur in the setting of inflamed paratesticular tissues including patients with hernia, torsed epididymis, and torsed appendage.

EXTRATESTICULAR DISORDERS

Disorders of the paratesticular tissues can be seen as a variety of extratesticular abnormalities on US and MRI examinations. These can broadly be divided into epididymal and nonepididymal abnormalities.

Focal Epididymal Disorders

As with most organ systems, focal lesions of the epididymis can be subdivided into neoplastic, inflammatory, posttraumatic, and other conditions (Table 12-9).

Imaging Notes 12-13. Differentiating Features of Diffuse Testicular Hyperemia

Entity	Features
Orchitis	Acute presentation, associated epididymitis, resolution with time, history of HIV, mumps, prior trauma
Infiltration with tumor	Subacute presentation, enlarged testicle with disorganized flow, + tumor markers or history of lymphoma/leukemia, normal epididymis
Torsion-detorsion	History of intermittent pain, hyperemia without mass or scrotal tenderness, and without findings of infection; upper pole infarct
Reactive	Secondary hyperemia due to other intrascrotal inflammatory process

Epididymal neoplasms

Epididymal tumors account for approximately 5% of scrotal masses, most of which are benign. Benign tumors tend to be smaller and less vascular than inflammatory processes. In 1 report, benign tumors tended to have a hypoechogenic or hyperechogenic rim more often than focal epididymitis.

Adenomatoid tumors: Adenomatoid tumor represents 32% of all paratesticular tumors, second only to lipoma of the spermatic cord.[4,14] It is most commonly located in the epididymis, involving the tail more frequently than the head by 4:1. Adenomatoid tumors are usually unilateral and more commonly occur on the left. Less common sites include the tunica albuginea (accounting for up to 14%)[61] and rarely the spermatic cord and testis.[14] Adenomatoid tumors are usually incidentally detected during physical examination, but in up to 30% present with pain.[62] On US, they appear as a well-circumscribed isoechogenic (to epididymis) solid mass ranging in size from 1 to 5 cm, usually diagnosed in patients aged 20 to 50 years (see Figure 12-46). Rarely adenomatoid tumors can be cystic. On MRI, these tend to be mildly T2 hypointense relative to the testis in the few available case reports, and enhance postcontrast.[4,61]

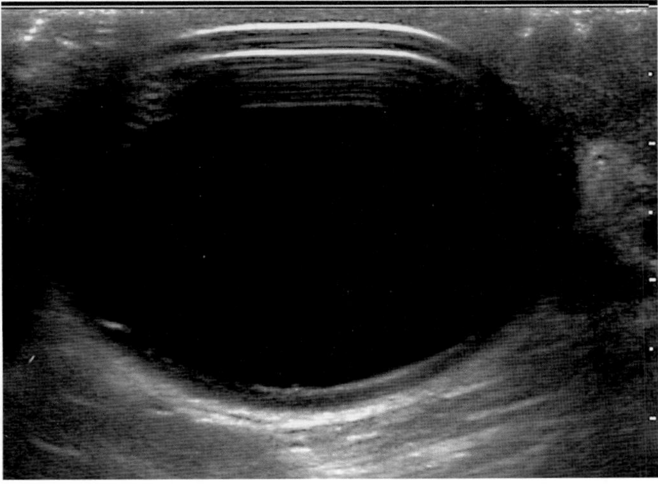

Figure 12-43 Testicular Prosthesis
Grayscale image shows the characteristic appearance of silicone prosthesis.

Table 12-8. Causes of Diffusely Hyperemic Testicle

1. Orchitis
2. Torsion-detorsion (intermittent torsion)
3. Neoplasms
4. Other

Leiomyoma: Leiomyoma is the second most common tumor of the epididymis after adenomatoid tumor, and is also usually incidentally detected as a slow-growing nontender palpable mass in the fifth decade of life.[14] It typically appears as a well circumscribed mass measuring between 1 and 4 cm. The US appearance is variable. The mass can be solid, partially cystic, and can contain calcifications or produce areas of refractory shadowing. The most common location is the epididymal head. Hydrocele is reportedly present in up to 50%. The MRI appearance has not been reported.

Papillary cystadenoma: Papillary cystadenoma is a benign epithelial tumor of mesonephric origin that has a strong association with von Hippel-Lindau syndrome (VHL). Up to 60% of those with VHL have papillary cystadenoma of the epididymis.[63] Approximately 40% of lesions are bilateral, which is thought to be almost pathognomonic for VHL.[44] Lesions associated with VHL are usually found at a younger age than sporadic lesions, which occur in middle-aged men.[62] Pathologically, papillary cystadenoma appears similar to renal cell carcinoma and therefore metastatic renal carcinoma to the epididymis should be ruled out before a diagnosis of papillary cystadenoma is made.[44] Accepted US criteria for diagnosis of papillary cystadenoma include a predominately solid epididymal mass larger than 14 × 10 mm, occurrence in a male with VHL, and demonstration of slow growth.[62] However, papillary cystadenoma is variable in appearance. The most common US appearance is as a predominately solid 1- to 2-cm mass with small cystic spaces in the head of the epididymis,[63] but papillary cystadenoma can be predominately cystic with solid components.

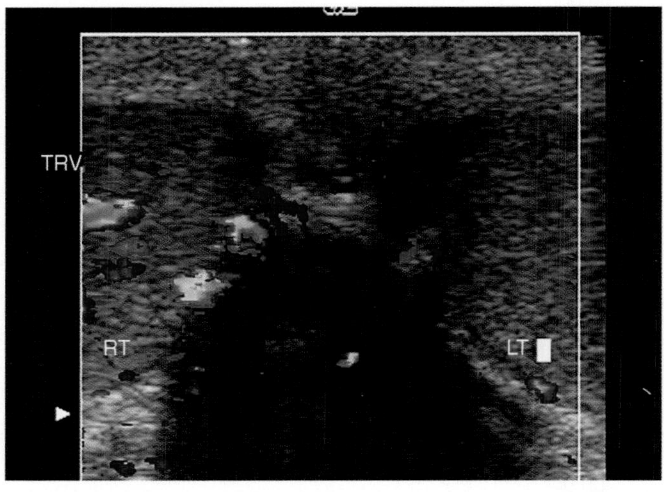

A

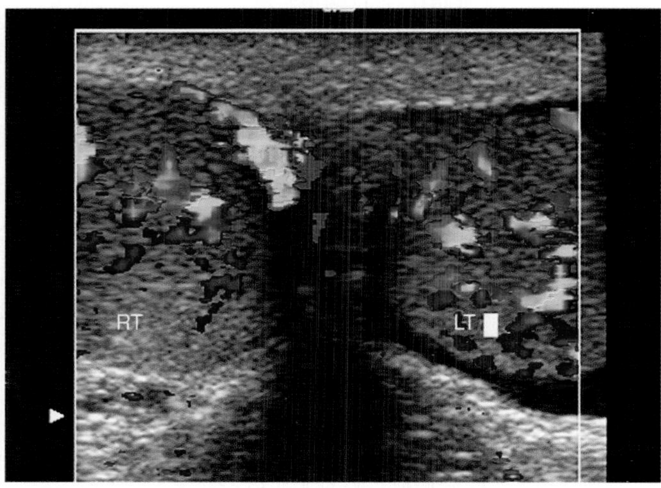

B

Figure 12-44 Torsion-detorsion
A. Color Doppler image through both testicles in a patient with left testicular pain shows markedly decreased flow in the left testicle in keeping with torsion. **B.** Color Doppler images through both testicles, obtained 10 minutes after the first image showing rebound hyperemia with low-resistance arterial flow in the left testicle. Hyperemia related to torsion-detorsion can be difficult to differentiate from orchitis.

Additionally, it can occasionally occur in the spermatic cord or close to the rete testis. Tumors in the region of the rete testis can result in obstruction and dilation of the intratesticular ductules.[64] At first glance, this may mimic tubular ectasia of the rete testis or a cystic testicular neoplasm; however, a dominant extratesticular component with or without a history of VHL should indicate extratesticular origin. MRI of papillary cystadenoma has not been studied beyond case reports.

Other benign epididymal neoplasms: Other rare benign epididymal tumors include fibroma, hemangioma, lipoma, rhabdomyoma, lymphangioma. Hemangioma of the scrotum is rare, usually occurs in children or young adults, and can mimic a varicocele.

Malignant tumors of the epididymis: Only about 5% of solid epididymal lesions are malignant;[65] however, up to 25% of the solid **tumors** of the epididymis have been

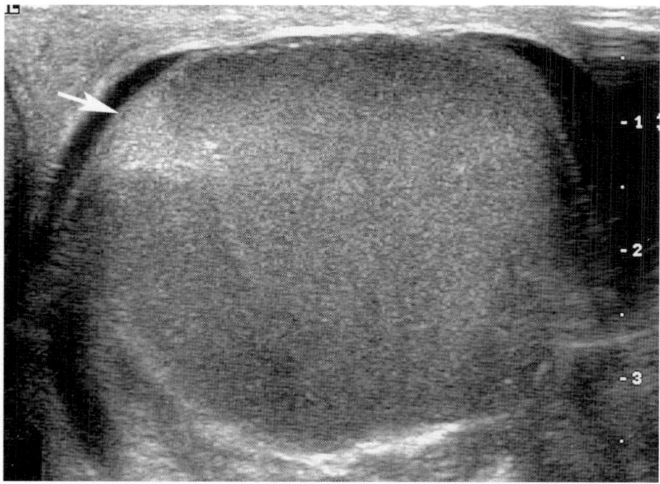

A

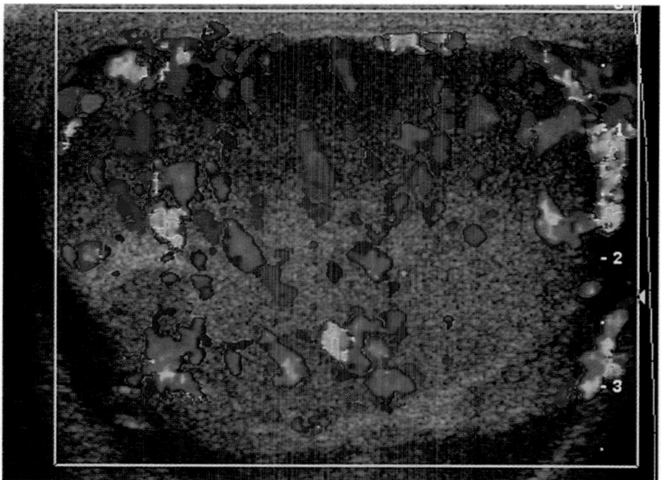

B

Figure 12-45 Hyperemia Due to Leukemic Infiltration
A. Grayscale and (**B**) color Doppler images of the left testicle in a patient with leukemia demonstrates hyperemic enlargement of the testicle due to diffuse tumor infiltration with sparing of a small amount of parenchyma (*arrow*). Orchitis can produce a similar appearance, but usually involves the epididymis whereas tumor infiltration does not.

Table 12-9. Causes of Epididymal Mass

1. Epididymal neoplasms a. Benign i. Adenomatoid tumors ii. Leiomyoma iii. Papillary cystadenoma b. Malignant i. Metastasis (testicular, prostate, kidney, GI tract) ii. Lymphoma iii. Epididymal adenocarcinoma iv. Epididymal sarcoma
2. Inflammatory disorders a. Epididymitis/abscess b. Chronic granulomatous disease i. Sarcoidosis ii. Tuberculosis c. Fibrous (inflammatory) pseudotumor d. Sperm granuloma
3. Trauma—Hematoma
4. Knot associated with torsion

reported to be malignant.[1] The most common malignant epididymal mass is a metastasis. Epididymal metastases tend to be from testicular carcinoma or prostatic carcinoma and less frequently from renal and gastrointestinal (GI) malignancies.[62] The epididymis can also be invaded directly by an adjacent testicular malignancy.

Primary epididymal malignancies include a variety of lesions such as adenocarcinomas and sarcomas, but are very rare. On US, malignant epididymal masses are difficult to distinguish from each other and can even be difficult to distinguish from benign chronic inflammatory lesions. However, in 1 report studying sonographic features of epididymal masses, a size >1.5 cm and increased vascularity were found to favor malignancy.[65] Also in that study, calcifications were found less commonly in malignant lesions but this did not reach statistical significance as many benign lesions were also noncalcified. Since the imaging features of epididymal malignancy are relatively nonspecific, consideration of clinical factors (eg, rapid growth, history of lymphoma, history of other primary tumor, systemic metastases, concurrent presence of testicular tumor, positive tumor markers), is usually necessary to suggest a correct diagnosis.

Inflammatory masses of the epididymis

The most common inflammatory masses of the epididymis are focal bacterial epididymitis and epididymal abscess. Less common inflammatory lesions include abnormalities due to sarcoidosis or due to a granulomatous infection such as tuberculosis, as well as fibrous pseudotumor and sperm granuloma.

Epididymitis/abscess: Acute pyogenic epididymitis usually results in diffuse enlargement of the epididymis and is discussed in greatest detail in the section **Diffusely Enlarged Epididymis.** However, occasionally acute epididymitis may appear as a focal area of increased vascularity, usually associated with epididymal thickening and heterogeneity (see Figure 12-47). In most cases, when pyogenic epididymitis is focal, it involves the tail of the epididymis. This is hypothesized to be due to the mechanism of infection,

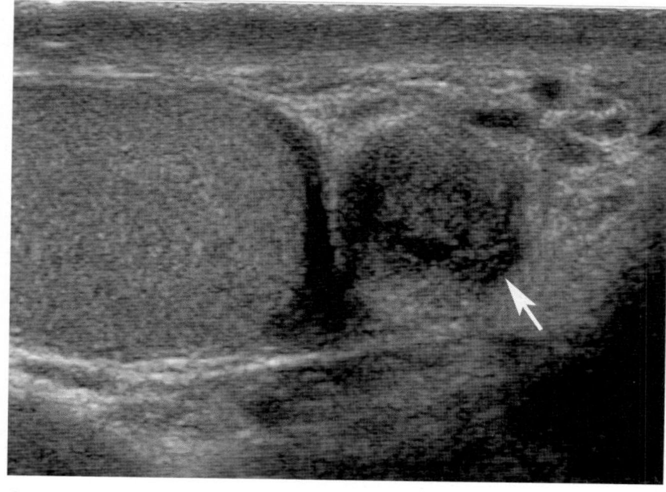

A

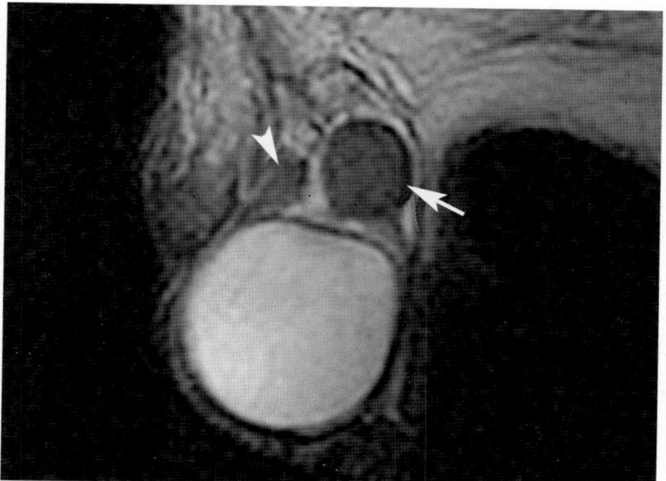

B

Figure 12-46 Adenomatoid Tumor
A. Grayscale US demonstrates a well-circumscribed mass (*arrow*) adjacent to the lower pole of the testis in the region of the epididymal tail. Surgical biopsy was diagnostic of an adenomatoid tumor of the epididymis. **B.** Sagittal T2 MRI image in a second patient demonstrates a well-circumscribed mass (*arrow*) separate from the epididymis (*arrowhead*), which on excision was a 1.5-cm adenomatoid tumor.

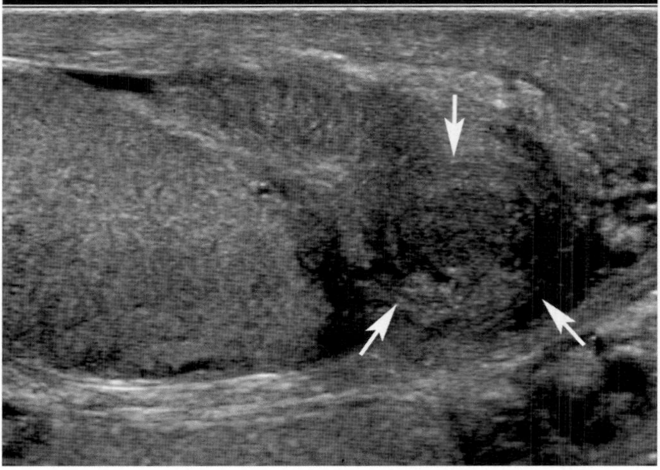

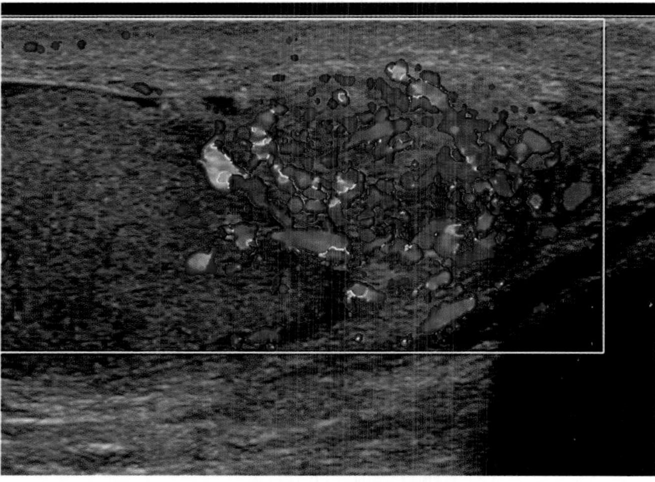

A B

Figure 12-47 Focal Acute Epididymitis
This patient presented with fever and acute scrotal pain. A. Sagittal grayscale and (B) color Doppler images of the epididymal tail show focal mass like expansion and heterogeneity (*arrows* in A) of the epididymis. This is associated with marked hypervascularity, typical of acute epididymitis.

in which bacteria ascend the vas deferens to reach the tail of the epididymis first, before spreading to the rest of the epididymis. Acute epididymitis can also produce abscesses, resulting in a focal mass (see Figure 12-48). Ultrasonographic features of a epididymal abscess are similar to an abscess located anywhere in the body and include shaggy irregular walls, low-level internal echoes, through transmission, peripheral hypervascularity, and occasionally intralesional gas.[2] The diagnosis of epididymitis is usually suggested clinically by symptoms of infection, including scrotal pain and fever, and may be confirmed by improvement/resolution following antibiotic treatment.

Chronic granulomatous epididymitis: Focal hypoechoic epididymal lesions can be due to chronic granulomatous inflammation from infection, such as tuberculosis (TB) or Bacille Calmette–Guérin (BCG), or other inflammatory conditions, such as sarcoid (see Figure 12-49). In most cases, granulomatous epididymitis can be differentiated from acute bacterial epididymitis by the lack of

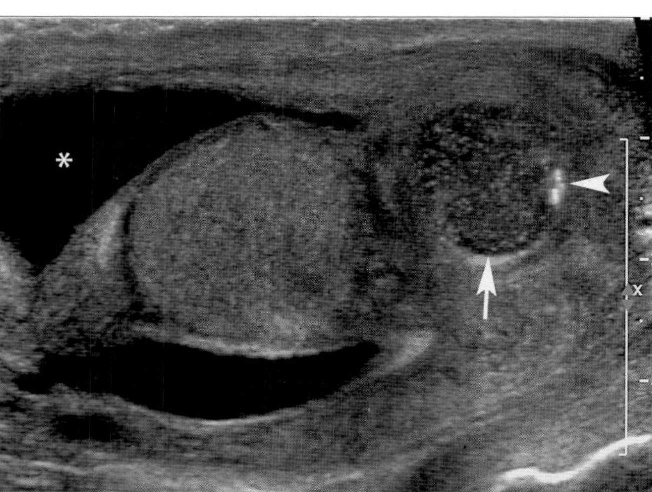

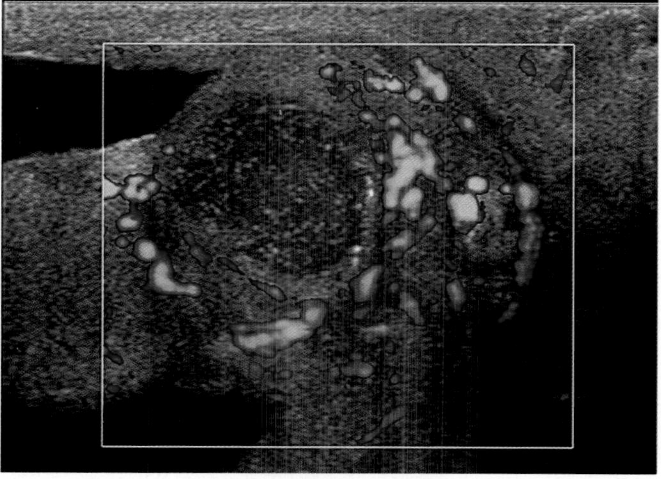

A B

Figure 12-48 Epididymal Abscess
This patient presented with fever and acute scrotal pain. A. Sagittal grayscale and (B) color Doppler images of the epididymal tail demonstrate a rounded mass (*arrow*) with through transmission. There are several internal echogenic foci (*arrowhead*) most likely reflecting gas, and peripheral hyperemia (B). This appearance is most consistent with an epididymal abscess. Note the hydrocele (*asterisk*) and scrotal wall thickening. Orchitis was also present (not shown).

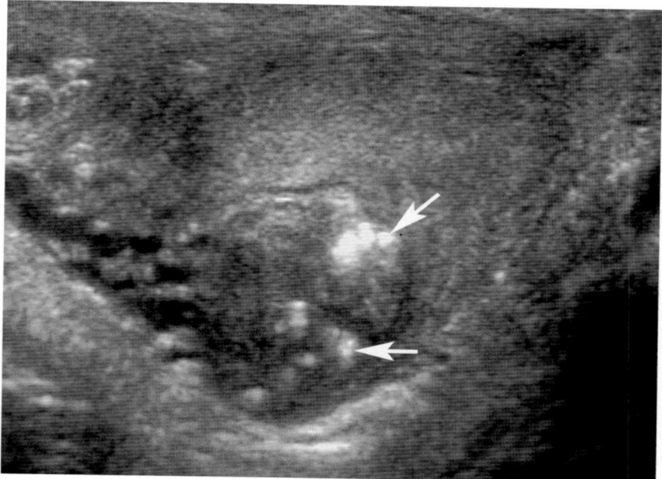

A

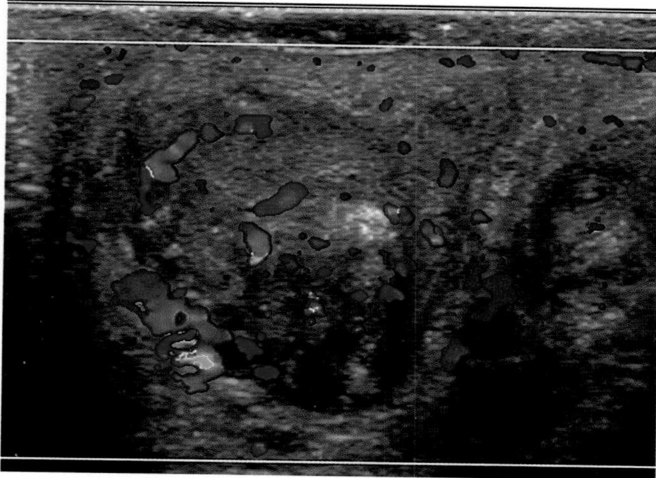

B

Figure 12-49 Chronic Epididymitis
This patient presented with history of a single episode of scrotal pain, which subsequently mostly resolved. Transverse grayscale (**A**) and color Doppler (**B**) images show enlargement and heterogeneity of the epididymal tail with punctate echogenic foci (*arrows*, A) representing calcifications. Mildly increased vascularity is present suggesting ongoing inflammation. However, the absence of acute scrotal pain and the presence of calcification suggest the process is subacute or chronic.

scrotal tenderness and indolent course. Furthermore, the epididymal lesions associated with tuberculosis tend to be larger and less vascular than those of pyogenic bacterial epididymitis.[66] When the granulomatous lesions are masslike, differentiation from epididymal neoplasms can be problematic. However, it has been reported that benign epididymal neoplasms are more likely than inflammatory lesions to have a hypoechogenic or hyperechogenic rim on US.[66] Additionally, systemic evidence of granulomatous disease can also provide a clue to the diagnosis of chronic granulomatous epididymitis.

Fibrous pseudotumor (inflammatory pseudotumor): This benign fibroinflammatory condition usually involves the tunica vaginalis or tunica albuginea but has been reported in the epididymis in approximately 10% of cases,[2] where it appears as a nonspecific solid mass with shadowing on US. The shadowing may either be due to calcification or due to the fibrous component. MRI can help to establish the diagnosis by demonstrating a low-T2-signal mass with little if any enhancement.[67]

Imaging Notes 12-14. Epididymal and Testicular Involvement-Tumor Versus Inflammation

Granulomatous epididymitis and lymphoma can both involve the testicle and epididymis. Inflammatory etiology typically involves the epididymis to a greater degree than the testis, whereas tumor (lymphoma) usually involves the testis to a greater degree.

Sperm granuloma: Sperm granuloma is a foreign body giant cell reaction to extravasated sperm cells that is seen in 2.5% of the general population and in up to 40% of patients postvasectomy.[14] About 3% of patients experience testicular pain. On US, sperm granulomas usually measure less than 1 cm and are variable in echogenicity but most often appear as hypoechoic solid lesions (see Figure 12-50). They may be

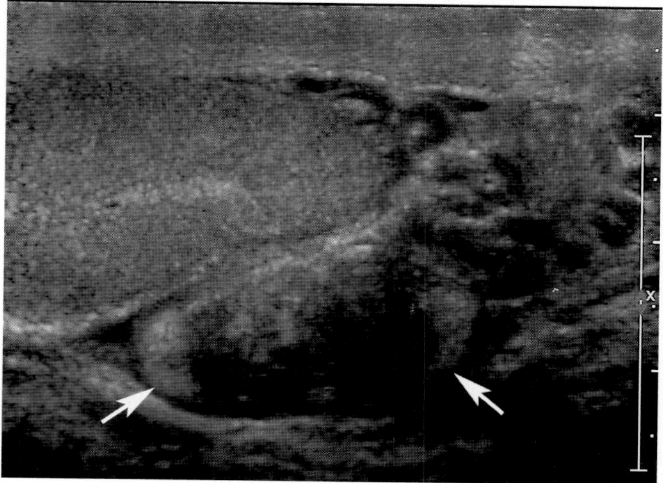

Figure 12-50 Sperm Granuloma
This patient had previously undergone vasectomy. Sagittal grayscale image of the region of the lower pole of the testis demonstrates a heterogenous extratesticular mass (*arrows*) in the region of the epididymal tail that demonstrated little vascularity on color Doppler (not shown). Excision revealed sperm granuloma.

located anywhere along the ductal system (epididymis and ductus deferens) but most commonly are found near the cut ends of the vas deferens.[14] Calcifications, seen as echogenic shadowing areas, are variably present. Chronic granulomatous inflammation due to other conditions such as TB, brucellosis, or fungal infections can have a similar imaging appearance. Clues to the diagnosis include a history of vasectomy and other postvasectomy imaging findings such as spermatoceles, tubular ectasia of the epididymis, and echogenic mobile foci in the epididymis representing clumps of nonmotile sperm and macrophages called "dancing megasperm."[29,83]

Traumatic mass—hematoma

Epididymal hematoma will appear as a focal mass within the epididymis, with the US appearance of a hematoma anywhere else, appearing hyperechoic in the acute phase and becoming more hypoechoic as the hemorrhage ages. In most cases, the diagnosis of epididymal hematoma can be made on the basis of a history of scrotal trauma and other imaging findings of scrotal trauma.

Complex epididymal cyst

Proteinaceous cysts can be difficult to differentiate from a hypovascular solid mass (see Figure 12-51) on US. Well-circumscribed border and through transmission can point to cystic nature, but if uncertainty remains, MRI can be obtained for clarification.

Other Paratesticular Masses

Nontesticular, nonepididymal intrascrotal masses include neoplasms of the spermatic cord, tunica vaginalis, tunica albuginea, and other paratesticular tissues, as well as a variety of nonneoplastic masses (Table 12-10).

Neoplasms of the spermatic cord and extratesticular tissues

A variety of soft-tissue neoplasms can arise from the paratesticular tissues, most of which are from the spermatic cord.

Spermatic cord lipoma: Seventy percent of extratesticular neoplasms are found in the spermatic cord. The most common extratesticular neoplasm is a spermatic cord lipoma, accounting for 45% of all paratesticular masses, with adenomatoid tumor of the epididymis second in frequency. On US, lipomas are variable in appearance depending on their composition but most commonly appear as an echogenic mass with little internal vascularity (see Figure 12-52). This US appearance is suggestive of fat but is not specific and, therefore, additional imaging with MRI or computed tomography (CT) scan may be indicated to confirm the presence of macroscopic fat. Aside from lipoma, the differential diagnosis for a fatty spermatic cord mass includes omentum containing inguinal hernia (see section on inguinal hernia), fibrolipoma, and liposarcoma.

Imaging Notes 12-15. Differentiating Features of Epididymal Masses

Epididymal Mass	Helpful Features
Acute epididymitis/abscess	Pain, hyperemia, secondary findings of inflammation (hydrocele, wall thickening), resolution with time
Granulomatous epididymitis	Less tender, less hyperemic, often larger than acute epididymitis
Adenomatoid tumor	Well-circumscribed solid mass, epididymal tail
Leiomyoma	Well-circumscribed solid mass, epididymal head
Papillary cystadenoma	Variable appearance, history of VHL, bilateral
Secondary malignancy	History of other malignancy, especially lymphoma, prostate, testis; lymphoma typically involves testis > epididymis compared with inflammatory lesions; usually larger and more vascular than benign tumors
Fibrous pseudotumor	Nonspecific, may show Ca^{2+}; MRI may show signal consistent with fibrous tissue
Torsion knot	Acute scrotum; decreased or absent ipsilateral testicular vascularity
Sperm granuloma	History of vasectomy, other postvasectomy changes including tubular ectasia epididymis
Hematoma	History of trauma, resolution with time

Fibrolipoma and/or liposarcoma should be suspected if there is a significant, nonfatty, soft-tissue component.

Other benign spermatic cord neoplasms: Other benign neoplasms of the spermatic cord include adenomatoid tumor, leiomyoma, fibroma, neurofibroma, lymphangioma, and dermoid, all very rare.

Imaging Notes 12-16. Most Common Extratesticular Masses

The spermatic cord lipoma and epididymal adenomatoid tumor are the most common benign extratesticular neoplasms. The primary differential consideration for spermatic cord lipoma is fat-containing inguinal hernia.

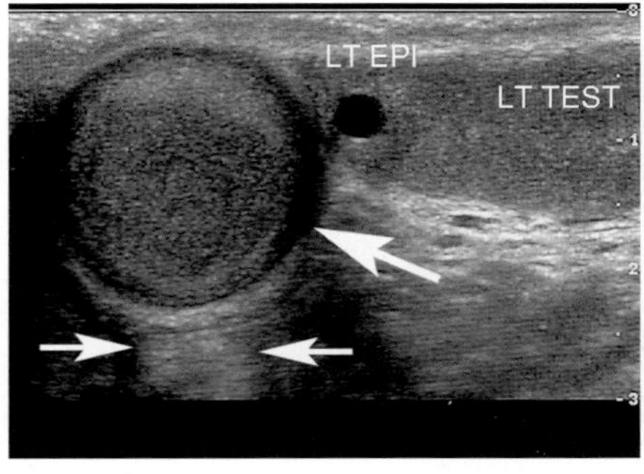

A

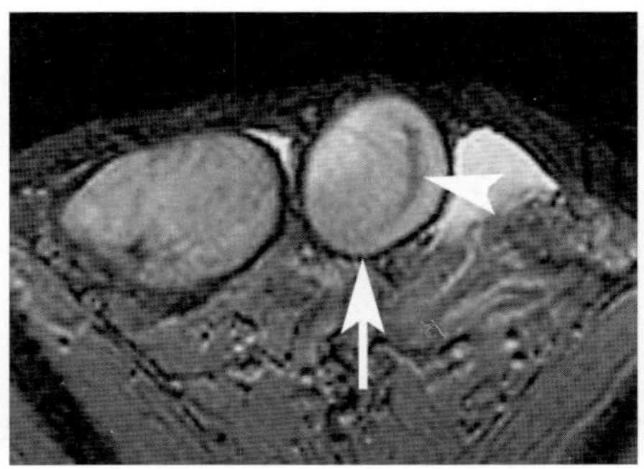

B

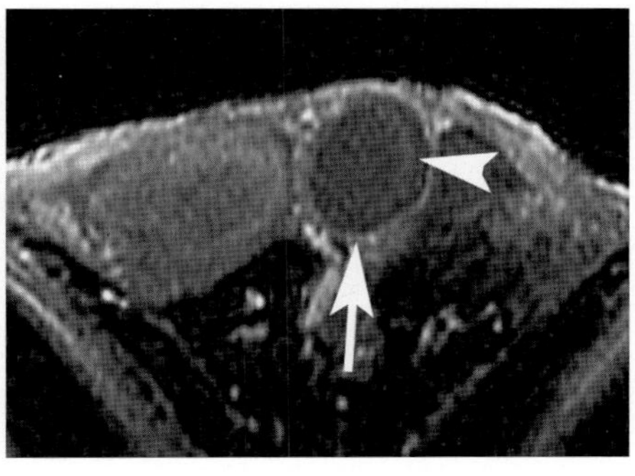

C

Figure 12-51 Complex Cyst
A. Sagittal grayscale image demonstrates an solid appearing hypoechoic extratesticular mass (*long arrow*) with through transmission (*short arrows*). It is unclear by US whether this is a complex cyst or a uniform solid mass. **B.** Axial T2-weighted and (**C**) axial postgadolinium fat-saturated T1-weighted MRI images demonstrate no enhancement of the mass (*arrows*) in keeping with a complex cyst. Note the presence of nonenhancing material (*arrowheads*) with in the cyst, reflecting debris/proteinaceous content.

Malignant spermatic cord tumors: Extratesticular, intrascrotal neoplasms are reported to have a 3% rate of malignancy in 1 larger urology series[68] and a 16% rate in a study with possible selection bias.[69] Furthermore, if lipomas are excluded, up to 56% of the neoplasms of the spermatic cord are reported to be malignant.[68] Most of these malignant tumors are sarcomas, which develop caudal to the external inguinal ring, thereby appearing as a scrotal mass rather than as an inguinal mass. Rhabdomyosarcoma is the most common sarcoma, accounting for 40% of malignant paratesticular neoplasms.[62] It usually occurs in children. The second most common sarcoma is liposarcoma, which occurs primarily in adults with a mean age of 56 years (see Figure 12-53).[14] Less common primary malignant tumors include leiomyosarcoma, fibrosarcoma, and malignant fibrous histiocytoma, which tend to occur in older adults. Other than liposarcoma, which is characterized by fat, these masses have no reliable differentiating imaging features and appear as nondescript large scrotal masses. However, malignancy may be suspected based on large size of the mass (greater than 5 cm), rapid growth, and evidence of metastases. Lymphoma and metastases from other primaries may also rarely involve the spermatic cord.

Table 12-10. Paratesticular Masses Unrelated to the Epididymis

Paratesticular Masses Unrelated to the Epididymis
1. Neoplasms a. Lipoma of the spermatic cord b. Liposarcoma and rhabdomyosarcoma of the spermatic cord c. Other benign and malignant tumors of the paratesticular tissues
2. Fibrous (inflammatory) pseudotumor
3. Sperm granuloma
4. Varicocele
5. Hemangioma
6. Splenogonadal fusion
7. Polyorchism
8. Inguinal hernia
9. Knot associated with testicular torsion
10. Torsion of the appendix testis
11. Hematoma

Nonneoplastic masses

Nonneoplastic masses include a variety of entities: inflammatory lesions (such as fibrous pseudotumor, and sperm granuloma), developmental lesions (splenogonadal fusion, polyorchidism, inguinal hernia), vascular lesions (varicocele and hemangioma), and masses seen in the setting of an acute scrotal pain.

Fibrous pseudotumor: Fibrous pseudotumor is the next most common mass in the testicular adnexa after adenomatoid tumors.[14,44] It is a benign inflammatory reaction of uncertain etiology that results in 1 or more nodules most commonly involving the tunica vaginalis or the testicular tunica albuginea, and rarely the spermatic cord or epididymis. Sonographic evaluation generally shows one or more solid masses attached to or closely associated with the capsule of the testis (see Figure 12-54). The echogenicity of the masses is variable, but if they contain substantial calcification, posterior acoustic shadowing can be present.[14] In some cases, the nodules detach from the tunical surface and give rise to small, free-floating bodies known as "scrotal pearls," which usually are calcified (see Figure 12-54).

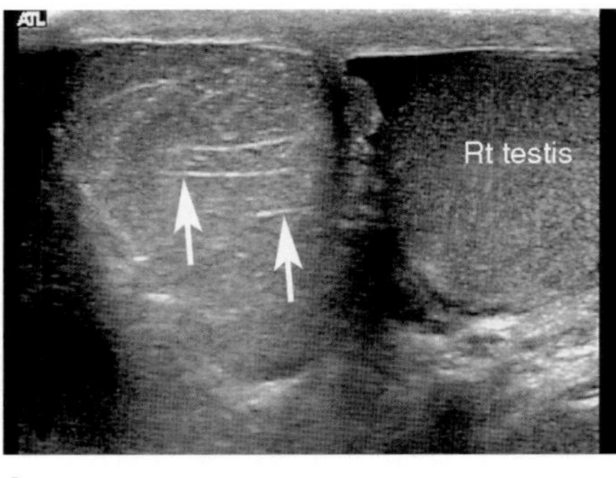

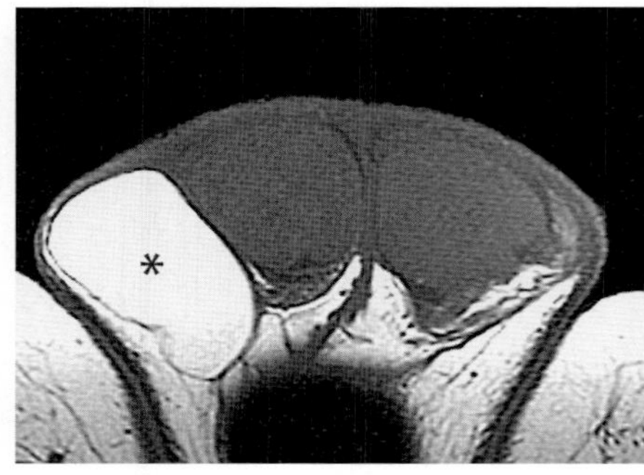
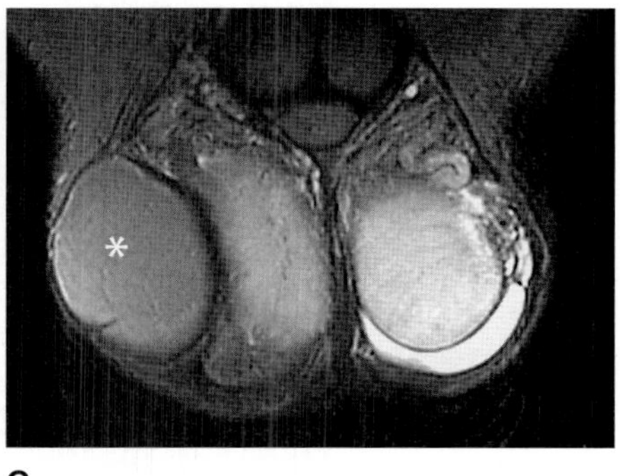

A B C

Figure 12-52 Testicular Lipoma
A. Transverse grayscale image of the right scrotum demonstrates a well-circumscribed mass isoechoic to subcutaneous fat and with echogenic lines parallel to the skin surface (*arrows*). These characteristics suggest a lipoma. **B.** Axial T1-weighted image and (**C**) coronal fat saturated T2-weighted image show a uniform mass (*asterisk*), which follows fat on all sequences, in keeping with a lipoma. By contrast to herniated fat, the mass is circumscribed and does not extend into the region of the inguinal canal.

Masslike inflammatory pseudotumors can occasionally be large (several centimeters)[62] and mimic a neoplasm. In such cases, MRI can be helpful by demonstrating low T1/low T2 signal typical of fibrous tissue, as well as showing a paucity of enhancement.[44]

Sperm granuloma: Sperm granulomas may occur in the region of the ductus deferens (which is separate from the epididymis). These are more completely discussed under the heading **Focal Epididymal Lesions**.

Varicocele: A varicocele is abnormal dilation of the veins of the pampiniform plexus and is present in 15% to 20% of the male population and 20% to 40% of men attending infertility clinics.[5] Complications of varicoceles include subfertility, testicular atrophy, and pain.

Varicoceles can be subdivided into primary and secondary types. Primary varicoceles are usually caused by incompetent valves in the gonadal vein. In 98% of cases, primary varicocele will be on the left; however, primary varicocele is bilateral 70% of the time.[23] Isolated right varicocele is uncommon. This left-sided predilection is hypothesized to be due to the longer course and more perpendicular insertion of the left testicular (a.k.a gonadal) vein into the left renal vein as well as compression of the left renal vein by the superior mesenteric artery (nutcracker effect),[44] or compression of the left testicular vein by the stool-filled descending colon.[1]

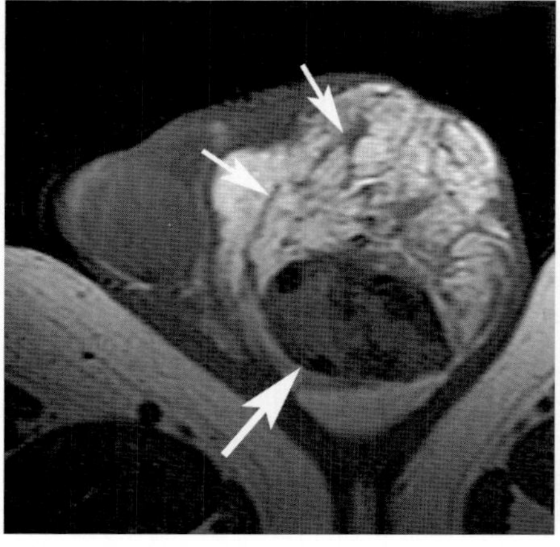
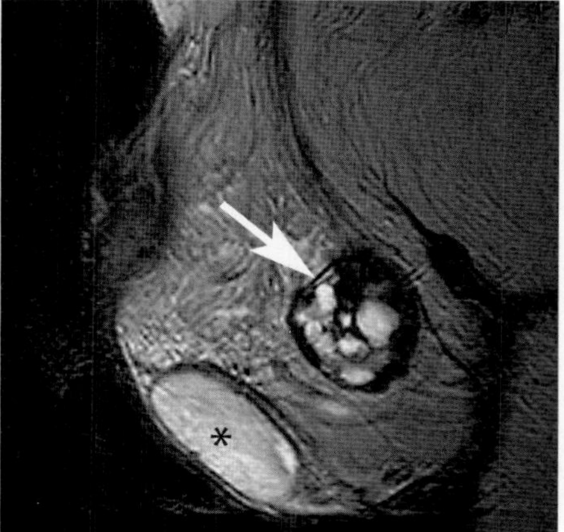
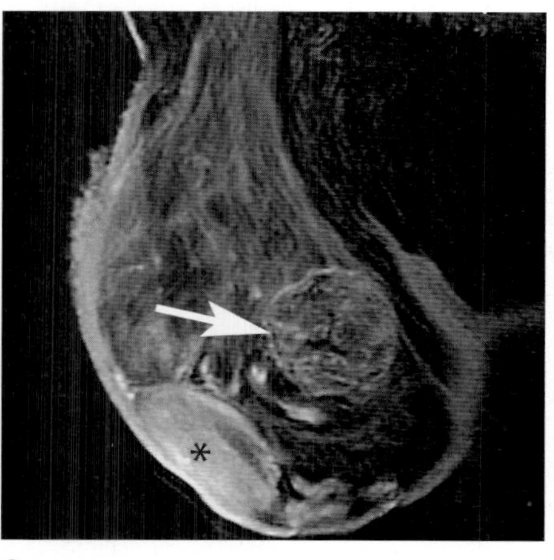

A B C

Figure 12-53 Spermatic Cord Liposarcoma
A. Axial T1-weighted, (**B**) sagittal T2-weighted, and (**C**) sagittal fat-saturated postgadolinium T1-weighted images demonstrate the presence of a spermatic cord mass. The mass is composed predominately of macroscopic fat but demonstrates moderately extensive low-level enhancing septa (*small arrows* in A), as well as a cystic and solid area (*larger arrows*) with low-signal areas likely representing calcifications. This mass is too complex to represent a lipoma and was suspected to represent a liposarcoma, which was proven at surgical excision. Testis is indicated by *asterisk* in B and C.

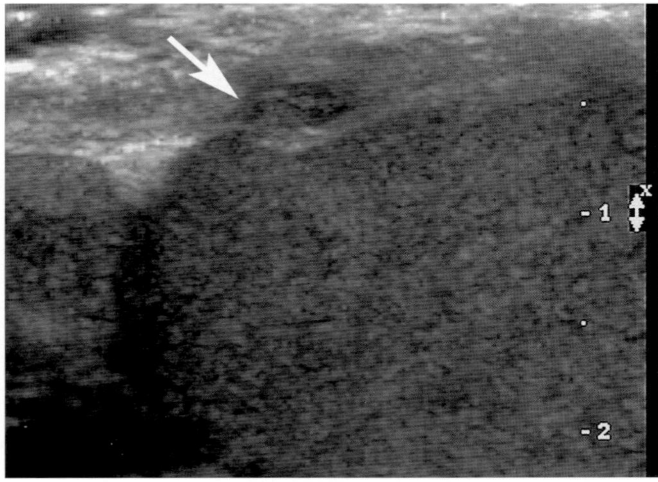

A

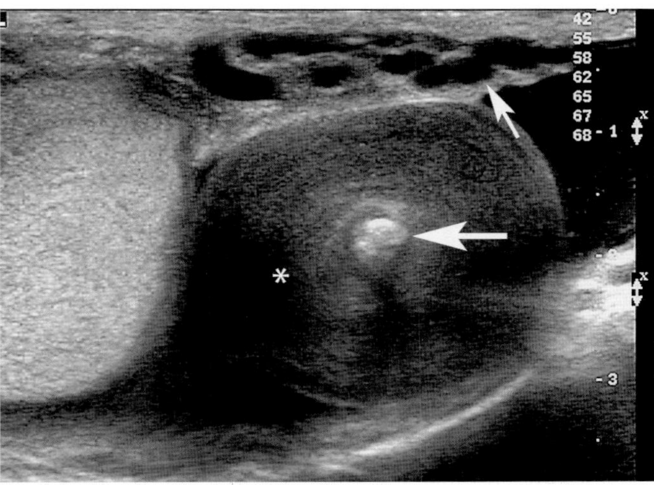

B

Figure 12-54 Fibrous Pseudotumor
A. Grayscale US image shows a hypoechoic elliptical mass (*arrow*) along the tunica albuginea which showed no appreciable internal blood flow on color Doppler. In this location, fibrous pseudotumor is the most likely diagnosis. **B.** Grayscale image in a second patient demonstrates an extratesticular mass (*asterisk*) with central calcification (*large arrow*) typical of a scrotal pearl, which was mobile during the examination. Some scrotal pearls are hypothesized to form from detached fibrous pseudotumors or detached testicular appendages. Note small varicocele (*small arrow*).

Most incidentally discovered varicoceles will be of the primary type.

Secondary varicoceles result from increased pressure within the paratesticular veins caused by extrinsic compression of the gonadal vein, or by thrombosis of the gonadal vein, IVC, or left renal vein. Compression most commonly is due to a retroperitoneal mass such as lymphadenopathy, but has also been reported due to hydronephrosis and hepatomegaly. Regarding thrombus, it is important to consider tumor thrombus, due to venous invasion by certain malignancies, such as renal cell carcinoma or adrenal cortical carcinoma. Secondary varicoceles have also been associated with cirrhosis. Secondary varicocele should be suspected if the varicocele is found only on the right side, is nondecompressible (not affected by patient position), and/or is newly discovered in a patient older than age 40.[23] It is important to recognize secondary varicoceles in order to search for a potential cause.

Sonographically, a varicocele consists of multiple serpiginous anechoic paratesticular structures that measure larger than 2 to 3 mm in diameter (see Figure 12-55). They are typically located superior and/or lateral to the testis but when large, will extend posteriorly and inferiorly. Color Doppler shows retrograde filling during Valsalva maneuver lasting greater than 1 second. Transient "flash" retrograde filling can occur in normal individuals.[70] On MRI, varicoceles have the same serpiginous appearance as on US scans, and enhance post contrast. The signal intensity on noncontrast sequences varies depending on the velocity of flow, with slow flow manifested as intermediate signal on T1-weighted images and high signal on T2-weighted images, and high-velocity flow manifesting flow voids (dark on T1 and T2-weighted images).

Scrotal hemangioma: Scrotal hemangiomas are very rare, accounting for <1% of all hemangiomas. Pathologically, hemangiomas are composed of numerous epithelial-lined vascular channels. On imaging, scrotal hemangioma may appear as a cluster of vessels resembling a varicocele on both MRI and US. However, unlike a varicocele, a scrotal hemangioma can occur in many locations in the scrotum and can involve the scrotal wall. On MRI, hemangiomas can demonstrate focal zones of decreased signal that are thought to be due to either fibrous, fatty, or smooth muscle components, relatively fast flow within portions of the hemangioma, or organized thrombus-containing calcification. These are not usually present in varicoceles. Additionally, scrotal hemangiomas tend to occur in infants and children as opposed to adults and may be associated with a history of Klippel-Trenaunay syndrome (cutaneous hemangiomas, varicose veins, and ipsilateral soft-tissue and bony hypertrophy) or with a family history of hemangiomas.[71]

Splenogonadal fusion: Splenogonadal fusion is a rare congenital malformation where an accessory spleen exists within the scrotum fused to either the testis, the epididymis, or the vas deferens.[29,44,62] In the majority of cases, this occurs in the left hemiscrotum. Splenogonadal fusion is subdivided into continuous and discontinuous types. In the continuous type, a cord of tissue, usually with a transperitoneal course, connects the ectopic and normal spleen. In the discontinuous type, no cord is present. On US, splenogonadal fusion typically appears as a homogeneous mass hypoechoic relative to the testicle. On color Doppler, a central vascular pattern with peripheral branching is often present as opposed to the disorganized flow seen in testicular neoplasms. Diagnosis of splenogonadal fusion can be

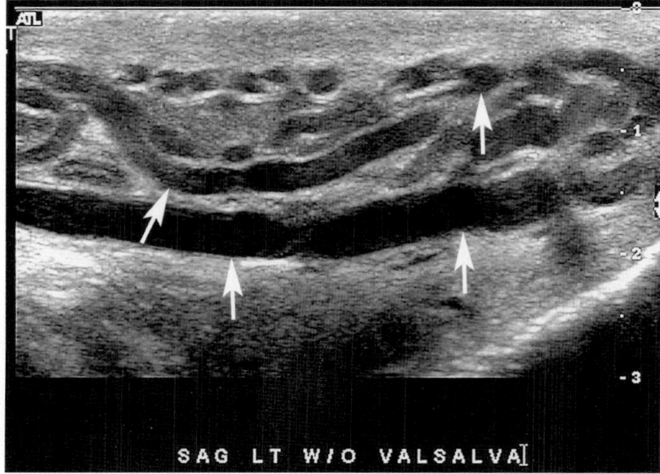

A

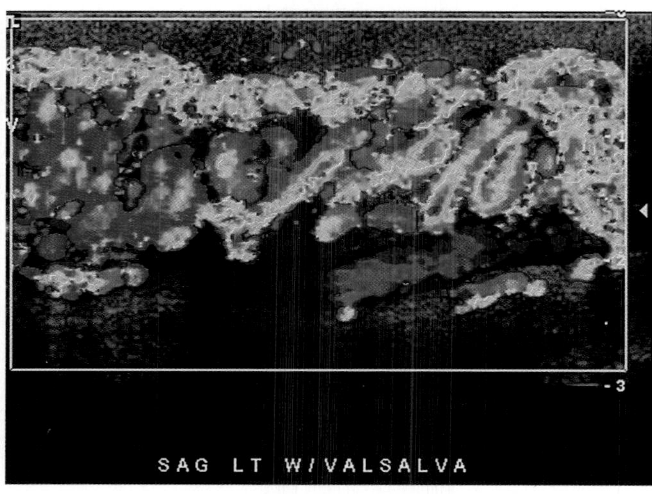

B

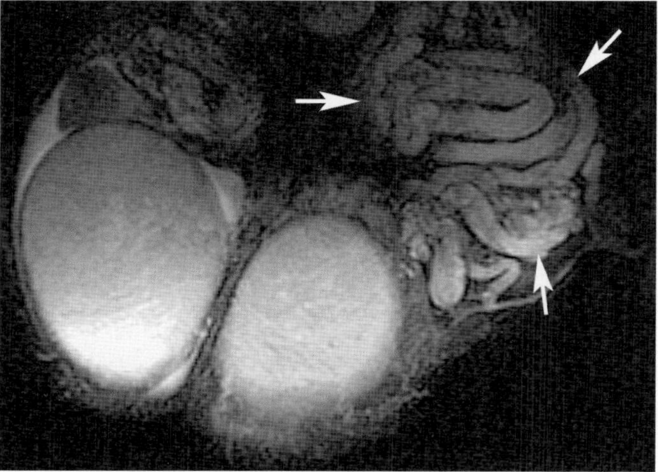

C

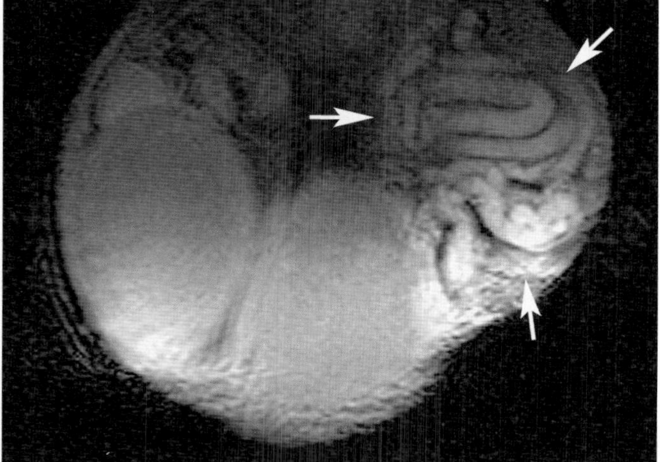

D

Figure 12-55 Varicocele
A. Grayscale and (**B**) color Doppler images during Valsalva maneuver demonstrate multiple veins (*arrows* in A) measuring greater than 2 to 3 mm, which show retrograde filling with Valsalva maneuver, diagnostic of a varicocele. **C**. Coronal T2-weighted and (**D**) coronal postgadolinium fat-saturated T1-weighted images in a different patient demonstrate multiple dilated veins along the superior aspect of the testis (*arrows*) typical of a varicocele.

problematic when the mass is inseparable from the testis. In this case, the accessory splenic tissue often mimics a testicular neoplasm and can lead to unnecessary orchiectomy. The presence of other congenital abnormalities, including cryptorchidism, inguinal hernia, peromelia, and micrognathia can be a clue to the diagnosis of splenogonadal fusion. These associated congenital anomalies occur more commonly with the continuous subtype. If the diagnosis is considered preoperatively, a 99mTc-sulphur colloid scan showing radiotracer uptake in the scrotum is diagnostic of splenogonadal fusion.

Polyorchidism: Polyorchidism, also called a supernumerary testis, is a rare congenital anomaly of the genitourinary tract thought to be due to a developmental accident in the union and division of the genital ridge with the mesonephric ducts, resulting in 3 or more testes.[72] Duplication of other scrotal structures such as the epididymis and vas deferens can occur simultaneously with duplication of the testis; however, in most cases, only the testis is duplicated. The supernumerary testis is intrascrotal in 75% of cases, inguinal in 20% of cases, and retroperitoneal in 5% of cases and is more common on the left.[14] Abnormal fixation of the supernumerary testis predisposes to torsion, which has been reported in up to 13% of cases.[72] An increased prevalence of testicular carcinoma has also been reported. In uncomplicated cases, US demonstrates an extratesticular mass similar in echogenicity to testis, which can be attached or separate from the ipsilateral testicle (see Figure 12-56). The sum of the lengths of the ipsilateral testicle and the

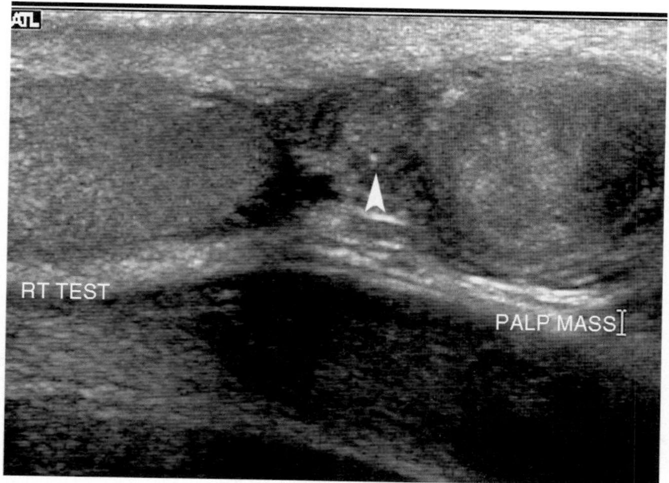

A

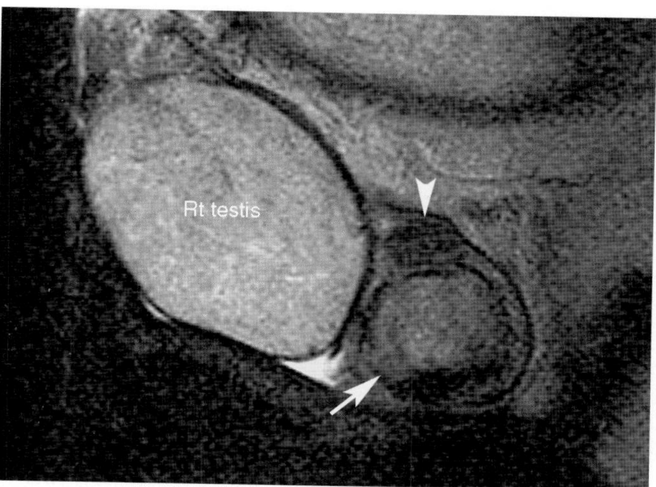

B

Figure 12-56 Supernumerary Testis
A. Sagittal grayscale image of the right scrotum in a patient with a palpable nodule demonstrates a well circumscribed mass that is similar in echogenicity and vascularity (not shown) to the ipsilateral testicle. In addition, an extratesticular structure adjacent to the mass (*arrowhead*) has an appearance suggestive of an epididymis. **B.** Sagittal T2-weighted image in the same patient demonstrates the mass (*arrow*) inferior to the right testis with its own epididymis (*arrowhead*) in keeping with a supernumerary testis. The signal intensity of the supernumerary testis is less than that of normal testis, likely reflecting atrophy.

supernumerary testis may approximate the length of the contralateral testicle. Bridging centripetal arterial vessels may be visualized between the ipsilateral testicles.[73] MRI demonstrates a well-circumscribed homogeneous mass with imaging signal similar to normal testicle. On both MRI and US, identification of a tunica albuginea surrounding the mass, a mediastinum testis or an associated epididymis may increase diagnostic confidence.[62]

Inguinal hernia: Inguinal hernia is a common paratesticular mass. Hernias are subdivided into indirect or direct types, based on the location of the orifice of the hernia lateral or medial to the inferior epigastric vessels, respectively.[74] Most hernias contain omentum and bowel, but sometimes ascites, urinary bladder, ureter, appendix, and Meckel diverticulum can be present in the hernia sac. The specific US appearance depends on the herniated contents. Hernias containing bowel can be identified based on (1) peristalsis in the scrotal sac or (2) the presence of paratesticular tubular structures containing gas and fluid that demonstrate a wall composed of alternating hyperechoic and hypoechoic layers corresponding to the histologic layers of bowel ("bowel signature") (see Figure 12-57). Importantly, herniated bowel can strangulate. Imaging findings suggesting strangulation include akinesia of the loop of bowel, bowel wall thickening, and/or hyperemia of the scrotal soft-tissues, as well as acute scrotal pain. By contrast to bowel, herniated omentum appears uniformly echogenic and can mimic spermatic cord lipoma (see Figure 12-58).[14] However, fat-containing hernia can be distinguished from spermatic cord lipoma by identification of the communication of the herniated fatty omentum with the pelvic cavity. Recognition of the communication with the pelvic cavity can be facilitated by the Valsalva maneuver or standing the patient upright. Such provocative maneuvers can be helpful in eliciting an otherwise occult inguinal hernia in a patient with a history of scrotal bulge.

Knot associated with testicular torsion: The spermatic cord knot sometimes visualized in the setting of torsion may be mistaken for an extratesticular or epididymal mass, or for focal epididymitis (see Figure 12-59). Clues include apparent spiraling of vessels in the torsion mass, paucity of ipsilateral testicular flow, and clinical presentation of acute testicular pain not relieved by elevating the hemiscrotum and an absent cremaster reflex. Details about testicular torsion can be found under the heading **Diffuse Testicular Disorders**.

Torsion of the appendix testis: Torsion of the appendix testis occurs mainly in prepubertal boys, typically aged 7 to 14 years. In that age group, it accounts for 20% to 40% of cases of acute scrotal pain and occurs more frequently on the left. The diagnosis may be suspected on physical examination if there is a palpable abnormality at the superior aspect of the scrotum associated with discoloration of the overlying skin, called the "blue dot sign."[28] On US, the torsed appendix appears as a variable echogenicity extratesticular mass located adjacent to the epididymal head that demonstrates peripheral but no internal blood flow. Secondary findings often include hydrocele, skin thickening, reactive enlargement of the epididymal head, and

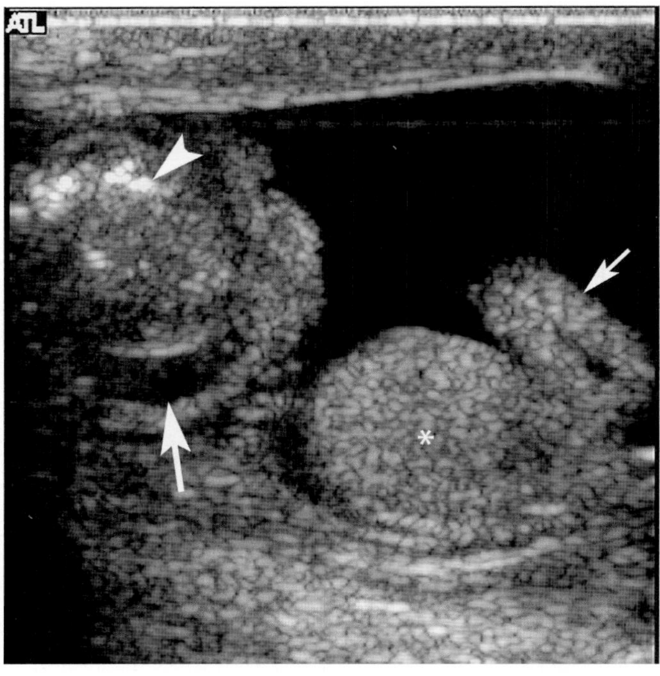

A

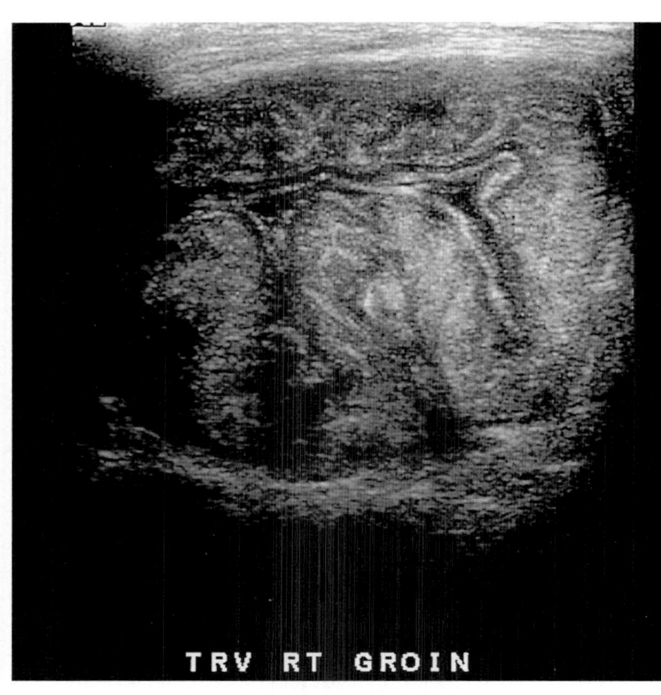

B

Figure 12-57 Bowel containing Hernia
This neonate presented with history of "scrotal swelling." **A.** Sagittal grayscale image of the scrotum shows a hernia containing gas-filled cecum (*large arrow* points to cecum, *arrowhead* to echogenic intraluminal gas) and appendix (*small arrow*). Testis is indicated by *asterisk*. **B.** Transverse image through the inguinal region of another patient with scrotal swelling demonstrates a hernia containing fluid and multiple loops of bowel. Note that the bowel is composed of hyperechoic and hypoechoic layers.

hyperemia of the periappendiceal tissues, including testicle, scrotum, and tunica vaginalis.[28,75] Within days, the twisted appendix can calcify and become detached from the epididymis, leaving a scrotal calcification, known as a scrotolith (or scrotal pearl).

Trauma: scrotal hematoma: Hematoma usually may be diagnosed on the basis of history and the presence of other findings of scrotal trauma. The appearance of hematoma varies, but typically appears as a complex cystic mass with variable echogenicity, as previously described.

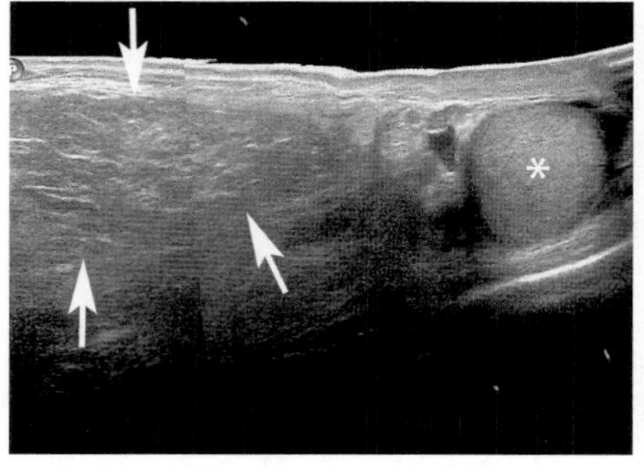

A

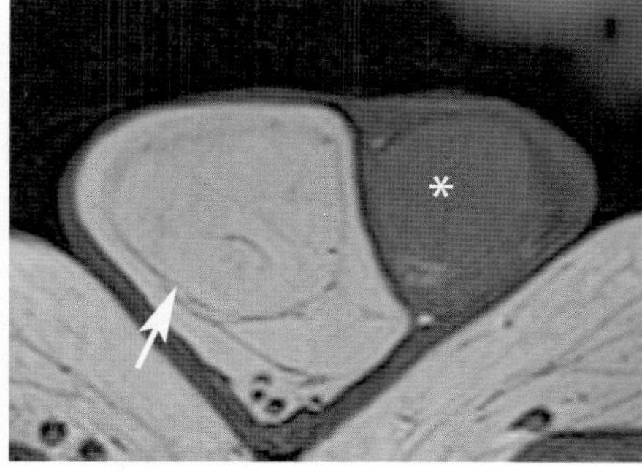

B

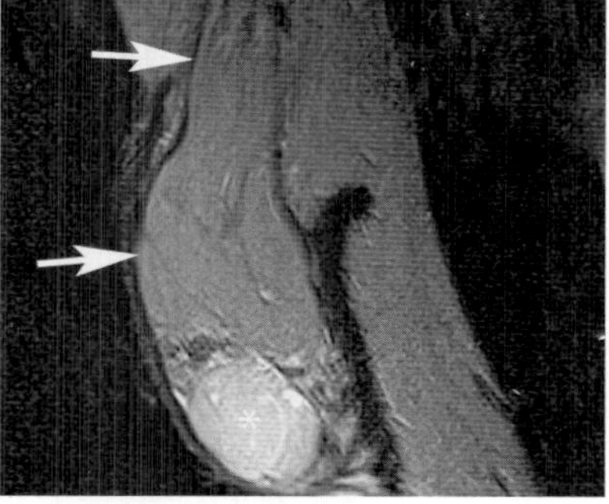

C

Figure 12-58 Fat-Containing Inguinal Hernia
A. Sagittal grayscale image of the scrotum and inguinal region shows a mass (*arrows*) in the scrotum superior to the testis (*asterisk*). The mass is isoechoic to subcutaneous fat with internal striations and extends into the inguinal region. The mass moved with Valsalva maneuver. These findings are all typical of herniated fat. **B.** Axial T1-weighted and (**C**) sagittal T2-weighted images in a different patient than A show a hyperintense mass (*arrow*) in the superior right scrotum that loses signal with fat saturation (not shown) in keeping with the presence of macroscopic fat. The sagittal image shows extension of the fatty mass (*arrows*) into the inguinal region, in keeping with herniated intra-abdominal fat.

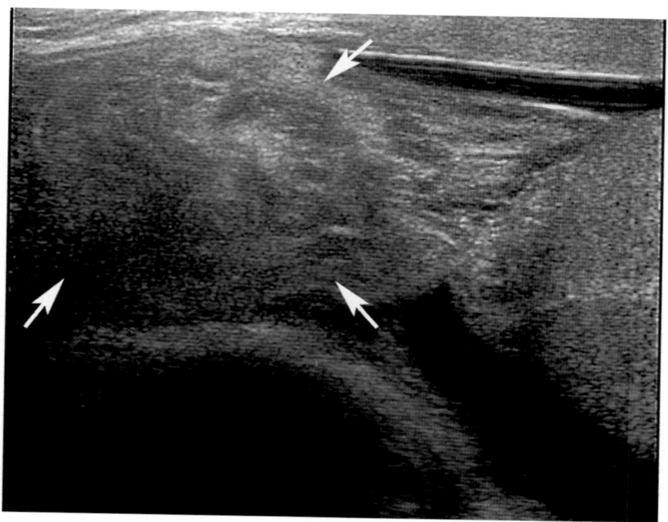

Figure 12-59 Spermatic Cord Torsion
This patient presented with acute-onset scrotal pain. Sagittal grayscale image shows a mass like area superior to the testis (*arrows*) reflecting torsed spermatic cord (same patient as in Figure 12-31). Clues to the diagnosis include the acute presentation and lack of flow in the testis.

Testicular hematomas are discussed under the heading **Solid-Appearing Intratesticular Nodule or Mass.** Follow-up US to confirm resolution can establish the diagnosis with more certainty.

Diffusely Enlarged Epididymis

By far, the most common cause of a diffusely thickened epididymis is acute epididymitis, which usually can be differentiated from less common causes based on hyperemia and acute clinical presentation. Less common causes include chronic inflammatory disorders (chronic epididymitis, sarcoidosis), tubular ectasia of the epididymis, torsion of the epididymis, and epididymal neoplasms (Table 12-11).

Epididymitis and epididymo-orchitis

Epididymitis is the most common cause of diffuse epididymal thickening. There are a variety of inciting conditions that can produce epididymitis, but in most cases the cause is ascending bacterial infection.

Acute epididymitis and epididymo-orchitis: Epididymitis and epididymo-orchitis are among the most common

Imaging Notes 12-17. Differentiating Features of Paratesticular Masses

Entity	Helpful Features
Inguinal hernia	Bowel containing—peristalsis, change with Valsalva maneuver, connection of herniated structure with pelvic cavity via inguinal canal (differentiates fat-containing hernia from spermatic cord lipoma)
Varicocele	Dilated veins >2-3 mm with reversal of flow >1 s on Valsalva maneuver, location near superior pole; left > right, remember to consider secondary varicocele
Torsion of appendix testis	Clinically, prepubertal males with "blue dot sign," avascular mass with peripheral flow along superior pole testis
Splenogonadal fusion	Homogeneous mass with organized branching flow, associated congenital abnormalities, confirm with Tc99 sulfur colloid scan
Polyorchidism	Left > right, homogeneous circumscribed mass similar in appearance to testis, ± associated epididymis; visualization of mediastinum or tunica makes the diagnosis; sometimes bridging flow to ipsilateral testis
Fibrous pseudotumor	May be masslike or present as tunical thickening; on US, can mimic tumor. MRI showing avascular low-T2-signal mass may be helpful
Hematoma	History, other findings of trauma, resolution with time
Spermatic cord lipoma	Echogenic extratesticular mass; main differential is herniated omental fat, and rarely liposarcoma if soft-tissue is present
Malignant spermatic cord tumor	Usually sarcomas, often large and complex, findings of metastatic disease or rapid interval growth
Scrotal metastases	Rare, history of primary malignancy; can either be hematogenous or lymphatic or due to extension of carcinomatosis through patent processes vaginalis
Benign tumors and nonneoplastic masses	Adenomatoid, leiomyoma, hemangioma, lymphangioma, noncalcified scrotal pearls, sperm granuloma (when in the region of the vas deferens)

Table 12-11. Causes of a Diffusely Thickened Epididymis

1. Epididymitis a. Acute bacterial b. Chronic epididymitis c. Granulomatous inflammation i. Tuberculous epididymitis ii. Sarcoidosis
2. Tubular ectasia of the epididymis
3. Epididymal torsion
4. Spermatic cord torsion
5. Tumor a. Leukemia and lymphoma

causes of acute scrotal pain. The scrotal pain is characteristically relieved when the testis is elevated over the symphysis pubis, called the Prehn sign, a finding that may help to clinically differentiate epididymitis from torsion. Epididymitis usually is due to an ascending infection, with inflammation initially involving the tail and progressing to involve the rest of the epididymis. In 20% to 40% of cases, the infection will progress to involve the testis.[1] In adolescents, the most commonly responsible organisms are *Chlamydia trachomatis* and *Neisseria gonorrhoeae,* with *Treponema pallidum* and other sexually transmitted diseases less likely, whereas in men older than age 45 and prepubertal males, the most common organisms are urinary coliform bacteria such as *E coli* and *P mirabilis.*[2] Other uncommon infectious causes of epididymitis include granulomatous organisms such as tuberculosis (discussed in the next heading), as well as opportunistic infections in patients who are immunocompromised, including cryptococcus, candida, brucellosis, other fungi, and cytomegalovirus. Viral causes in the immunocompetent patient include mumps, coxsackie virus A, and varicella and echovirus. Viral infections can be suspected based on the absence of pyuria.[2] In Asia, Africa, and the Western Pacific, *Wucheria bancrofti,* a filarial parasite, can be a cause of granulomatous epididymo-orchitis. Noninfectious causes of epididymitis include vasculitis (Behçet and Henoch-Schönlein purpura), trauma, amiodarone, and chemical epididymitis due to sterile reflux of urine through the vas deferens or due to a congenital anomaly. Epididymitis occurring before the age of 2 should prompt evaluation for predisposing factors, such as ectopic insertion of the ureter into the seminal vesicle, posterior urethral valves, voiding dysfunction, or bladder extrophy.[75]

Acute complications of epididymitis include epididymal or testicular abscess, pyocele, and testicular infarction or ischemia. Chronic complications include infertility, chronic pain, and testicular atrophy.

Sonographically, in acute epididymitis, the epididymis is usually diffusely enlarged and demonstrates variable echogenicity from normal to hypoechoic as a result of edema, to hyperechoic because of the presence of hemorrhage (see Figure 12-60). Occasionally, epididymitis can appear focal, as was discussed previously. Since reflux of urine via the vas deferens reaches the tail of the epididymis first, focal epididymitis involves the tail more commonly than the head of the epididymis. On color and spectral Doppler, the presence of increased blood flow has sensitivity for acute epididymitis approaching 100%. This is one of the most important imaging manifestation of acute epididymitis because 20% of cases of epididymitis and 40% of cases of orchitis demonstrate normal grayscale findings.[1] Associated findings include skin thickening, hydrocele, and echogenic paratesticular fat. MRI is not typically obtained during epididymitis. However, on MRI, acute epididymitis usually appears as epididymal enlargement and hyperenhancement; in some case, epididymal signal may be heterogeneous because of hemorrhage or edema.[76]

Chronic epididymitis: Chronic epididymitis is characterized by scrotal pain lasting greater than 3 months. It most commonly is a result of granulomatous infection (discussed further below) but can be due to persistent inflammation after an episode of acute bacterial epididymitis. Other causes include drug-induced epididymitis, proximal obstruction following vasectomy, other obstructive phenomena, Behçet vasculitis, and idiopathic.[2] The grayscale appearance of the epididymis in chronic epididymitis is similar to that seen in acute ependymitis, with diffuse thickening that may be associated with heterogeneity (see Figure 12-61). However, skin thickening is usually absent and hyperemia is often mild, reflecting the chronic nature of the disorder. The presence of calcifications also is suggestive of prior or chronic inflammation (see Figure 12-49).

Tuberculous epididymitis: Genitourinary tuberculosis is the most common location of extrapulmonary tuberculosis. When the genital organs are involved, the epididymis is the most common site of involvement and has been reported in 7% of those with tuberculosis in autopsy series. Epididymal tuberculosis can be due to spread of infection from the prostate or the kidney, or can be due to

Imaging Notes 12-18. Sonographic Findings of Epididymitis

1. Increased Doppler blood flow. Nearly 100% sensitivity
2. Usually diffuse involvement of epididymis. When focal, tail is the most common location.
3. Grayscale appearance of epididymis is variable, and may be NORMAL in 20%
4. Skin thickening
5. Hydrocele
6. Echogenic paratesticular fat

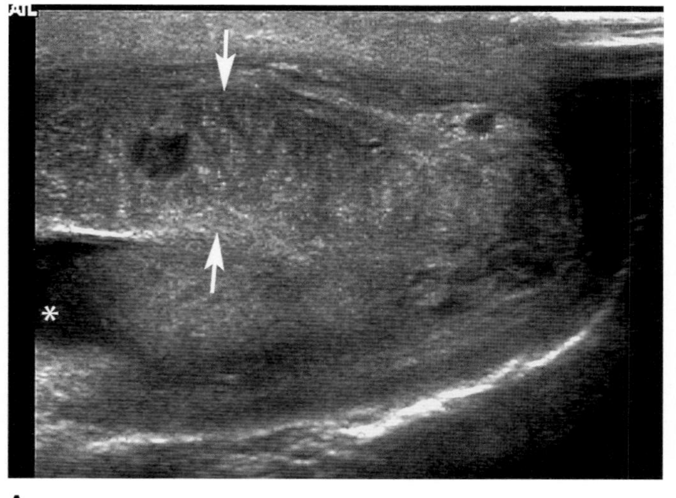

A

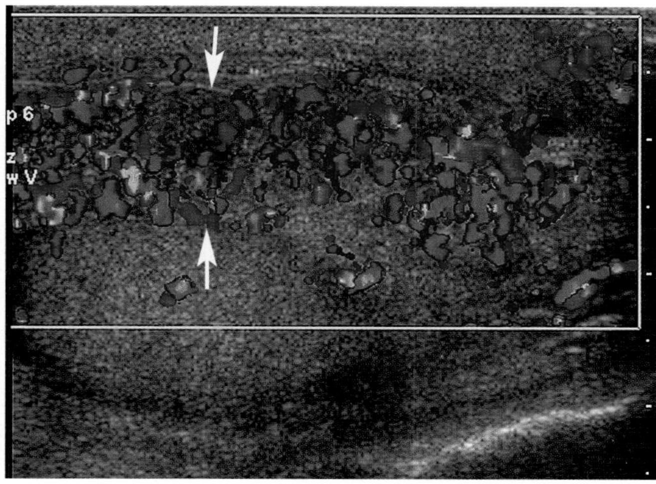

B

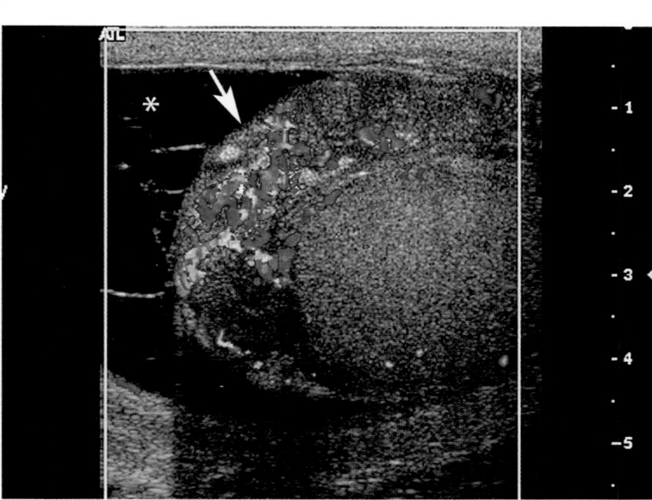

C

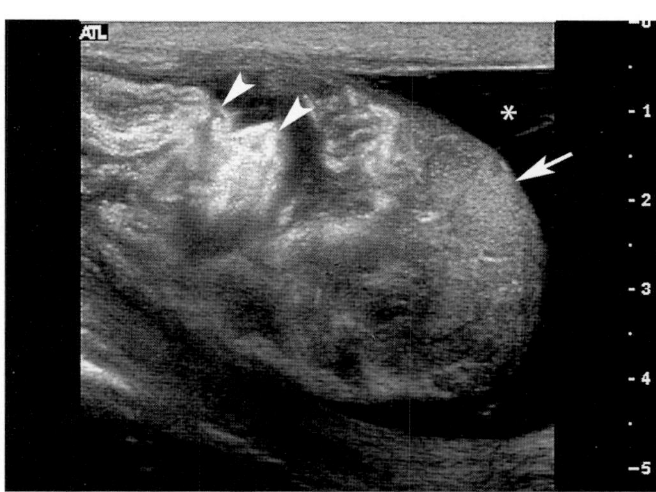

D

Figure 12-60 Epididymitis
This patient presented with acute scrotal pain. **A.** Sagittal grayscale and (**B**) color Doppler images demonstrate marked thickening, heterogeneity, and increased blood flow of the epididymal body and tail (*arrows* in A and B). Note small hydrocele (*asterisk*). **C.** Sagittal color Doppler and (**D**) transverse grayscale images of the region of the epididymal head demonstrate a thickened hypervascular epididymis (*arrow*), complex hydrocele with septations (*asterisk*), and increased echogenicity of the paratesticular tissue (*arrowheads* in **D**). These findings are in keeping with acute epididymitis with an probable associated pyocele.

hematogenous spread. Rarely, epididymal tuberculosis can result from sexual transmission or acquired from intravesical BCG therapy for bladder cancer. In patients with genital tuberculosis, pulmonary disease can be documented in 50% of patients, and renal tuberculosis can be documented in 80% to 85% of patients.[77] Tuberculous epididymitis can be either painless or cause scrotal pain.

Tuberculous involvement usually results in diffuse enlargement of the epididymis. This enlargement can be uniformly hypoechogenic, heterogeneously hypoechogenic, or with multiple hypoechogenic lesions.[26] The heterogeneously hypoechoic patterns of epididymal enlargement are believed to reflect various stages of fibrosis, necrosis, and granulomas and calcifications (see Figure 12-62).[85] The heterogeneously hypoechoic pattern of epididymal enlargement favors a diagnosis of tuberculous over bacterial epididymitis. Diffusely increased blood flow throughout the epididymis is seen in subjects with bacterial epididymitis, whereas focal linear or spotty blood flow within the periphery of the affected epididymis is typical of subjects with tuberculous epididymitis.[24] Additionally, tuberculous epididymal abscesses are reported to demonstrate a milder degree of peripheral hypervascularity compared with bacterial abscesses.[24] Other features that favor a diagnosis of tuberculous over bacterial epididymitis include sinus tracts, a miliary pattern of testicular orchitis, and a history/diagnosis of tuberculosis at other sites in the body.

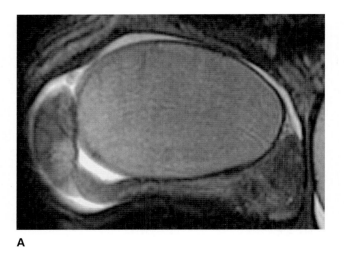

A

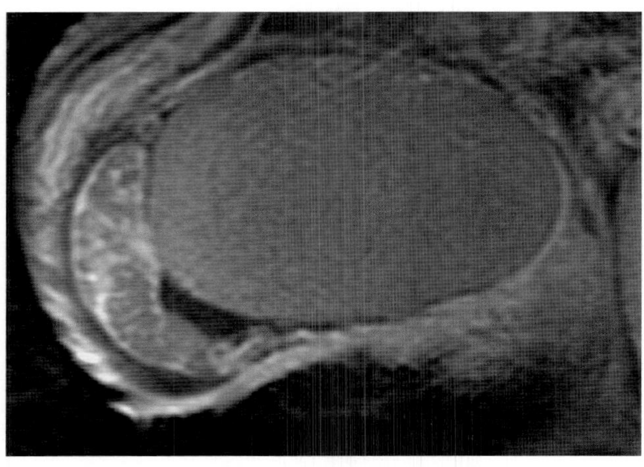

B

Figure 12-61 Chronic Epididymitis
This patient presented with a palpable abnormality of the testis. A. Coronal T2-weighted and (B) postgadolinium fat-saturated T1-weighted images show a diffusely heterogenous epididymis, in keeping with chronic inflammation.

Sarcoidosis

Sarcoidosis is a systemic disease characterized by formation of noncaseating granulomas in multiple origins. The prevalence of genital involvement on postmortem series in 5%; however, clinically diagnosed disease is present in less than 0.5%.[1,79] Of the reported cases of genitourinary sarcoid, 75% involve the epididymis and 50% involve the testis.[80] The epididymal involvement can be bilateral in up to one-third of cases.[81] The patients can present with systemic symptoms related to sarcoidosis, or with findings referable to the scrotum, including pain and palpable abnormality. On imaging, the epididymis usually is enlarged and heterogeneous with hypoechogenic nodules. Hypoechogenic nodules can also be present in the testis, where involvement is reportedly more commonly bilateral than in the epididymis. Combined testicular and epididymal nodules may be produced by other processes, including granulomatous infection and certain neoplasms, such as lymphoma (see **Tuberculous Orchitis and Other Granulomatous Orchitis** under **Focal Testicular Disorders**). Potential clues include African American race, history of sarcoid and elevated serum ACE levels, and in some cases response to steroids.[2,14]

Tubular ectasia of the epididymis

Tubular ectasia of the epididymis is believed to be due to upstream obstruction. It most commonly occurs as a sequela of vasectomy, where it is reported to occur in

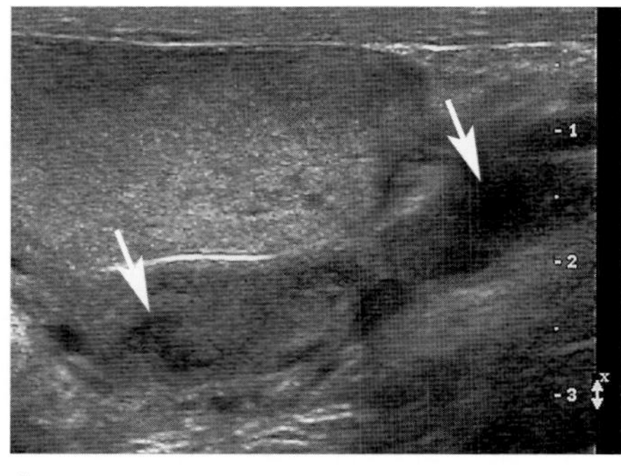

A

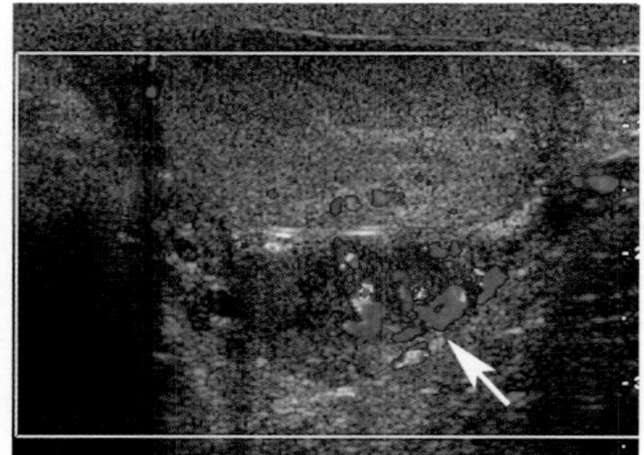

B

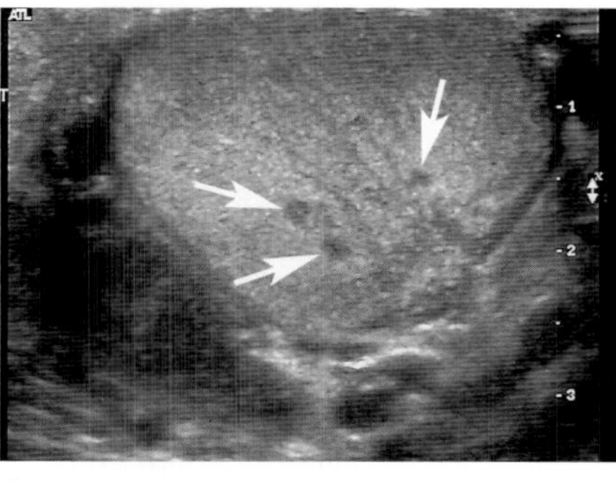

C

Figure 12-62 BCG Epididymitis
This patient had received BCG therapy for bladder cancer and presented with a palpable abnormality in the scrotum. A. Sagittal grayscale and (B) color Doppler images of the epididymal body and tail and (C) grayscale image of the testis demonstrate irregular thickening of the epididymal body and tail with focal areas of decreased echogenicity (*arrows* in A) and increased vascularity (*arrow* in B). There are tiny hypoechoic lesions (*arrows* in C) in the testis. This appearance, in combination with the lack of acute symptoms and history of BCG treatment, is most consistent with chronic granulomatous epididymal and testicular inflammation due to BCG therapy.

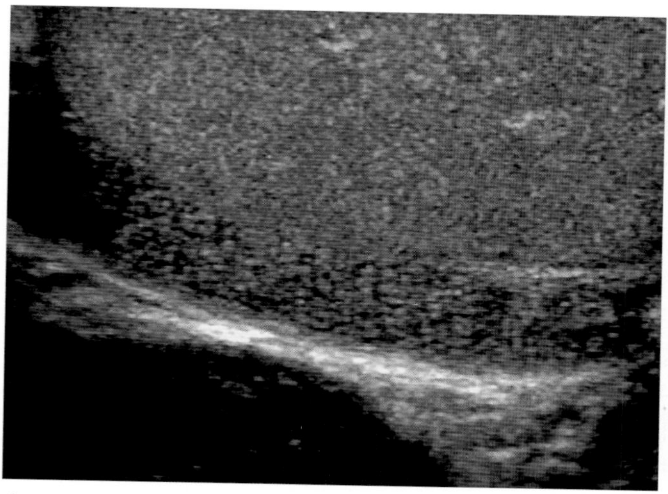

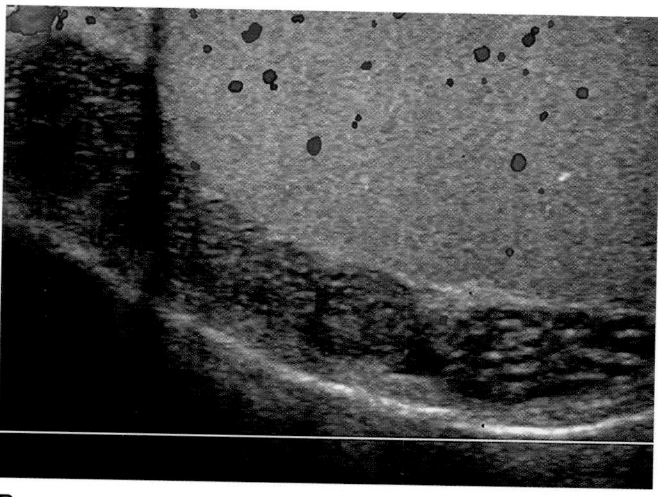

Figure 12-63 Tubular Ectasia of the Epididymis
This patient had undergone previous vasectomy. (**A**) Grayscale and (**B**) color Doppler images demonstrate a thickened epididymal body and tail which have a somewhat spongiform appearance. This appearance is typical of tubular ectasia, a finding that can be seen postvasectomy. This phenomenon can be differentiated from other causes of diffuse epididymal thickening by the lack of acute symptoms, spongiform appearance, and lack of increased blood flow.

43%.[82] Tubular ectasia results in an enlarged epididymis that can be differentiated from other causes of epididymal enlargement by (1) spongiform appearance due to visualization of the dilated epididymal tubules, (2) lack of increased vascularity, and (3) history of vasectomy (see Figure 12-63). Other findings commonly found postvasectomy include sperm granuloma (discussed previously under the heading **Focal Epididymal Disorders**), spermatocele, dilation of the vas deferens, and tubular ectasia of the rete testis, in addition to tubular ectasia of the epididymis.[83] Sometimes, the vasectomy clip may be identified by US.

Torsion of epididymis

Isolated epididymal torsion, without associated testicular torsion, is rare. Causes include an anomalous attachment of the epididymis to the testis or a long epididymis with a long meso-orchium.[2] Such anomalies are more common in patients who have undescended testes. Isolated torsion of the epididymis can be suspected if (1) the body and tail of the epididymis are markedly enlarged and heterogeneous with little or no blood flow detected by Doppler imaging, (2) the head of the epididymis is hypervascular, with a whorled appearance of the vessels indicating the site of torsion, (3) the testicle is normal in vascularity, and (4) the patient has acute scrotal pain.

Spermatic cord torsion

Spermatic cord torsion can result in an enlarged epididymis, but by contrast to epididymitis the vascularity is decreased (see Figure 12-64). See also section **Torsion of the Epididymis**.

Diffuse epididymal neoplasm: leukemia and lymphoma

Leukemia and lymphoma usually produce focal lesions, but can rarely result in a diffusely enlarged, hypoechogenic, hypervascular epididymis. However, isolated involvement of the epididymis by lymphoma and leukemia is rare, and in most cases the ipsilateral testicle will also be extensively involved by lymphoma.

UNIQUE SCROTAL LESIONS

Unique scrotal lesions include cystic lesions of the scrotum, causes of scrotal calcifications, and scrotal gas.

Cystic Lesions in the Scrotal Sac

Fluid within the scrotum will most often be due to a hydrocele or an epdidymal cyst but can occasionally be a result of herniation of fluid or fluid containing structures, and rarely can be caused by mesothelioma of the tunica vaginalis (Table 12-12).

Simple and complicated hydroceles

Serous fluid, blood, pus, lymphatic fluid, or urine can accumulate between the layers of the tunica vaginalis resulting in a hydrocele, hematocele, pyocele, and rarely lymphocele or urinoma, respectively.

Simple hydrocele is the most common cause of asymptomatic scrotal swelling and can be a congenital or acquired abnormality. Congenital hydroceles are usually seen in infants and are due to a patent processus vaginalis

Imaging Notes 12-19. Differentiating Features of Diffuse Epididymal Enlargement

Diffusely thickened epididymis

Entity	Helpful Differentiating Features
Acute epididymo-orchitis	Pain, hyperemia, hydrocele, scrotal wall thickening, associated increased testicular vascularity, resolution with treatment
Chronic epididymo-orchitis	Chronic pain, thickening without hyperemia, diagnosis of exclusion
Tuberculous epididymo-orchitis	Systemic findings of TB, heterogeneous hypoechoic enlargement with only mildly increased vascularity, calcification, sinus tracts, miliary involvement of testicle
Tubular ectasia	History of vasectomy, spongiform appearance without internal vascularity; other postvasectomy findings
Torsion of the epididymis (rare)	Acute scrotum with enlarged but hypovascular epididymis, normal testis, whorled vessels near enlarged epididymal head
Secondary involvement with tumor	For lymphoma, epididymal involvement is usually due to infiltration from testis
Sarcoid	Systemic findings of sarcoid, heterogeneous hypoechogenic enlargement, elevated ACE, ± testicular involvement

resulting in collection of peritoneal fluid in the scrotal sac. Most cases of congenital hydrocele will resolve by 18 months of age, but in about 15% a patent processes vaginalis may persist into adulthood.[14] The presence of calcifications complicating a congenital hydrocele should suggest the diagnosis of meconium periorchitis. This is a sequela of meconium peritonitis, which is a chemical peritonitis due to intrauterine bowel perforation. In adults, most simple hydroceles are acquired, occurring as a reaction to intrascrotal pathology such as tumors or infections. However, in some cases no cause for the acquired hydroceles can be identified. For both acquired and congenital hydroceles, when the hydrocele is small, the fluid tends to be located anterolateral to the testis. When large, intravaginal fluid collections can compress the testis, resulting in vascular compromise, which is manifested as diminished flow on color Doppler US or abnormal spectral Doppler waveforms.

On US, a hydrocele is usually anechoic but may contain a few low-level echoes due to a small amount of protein

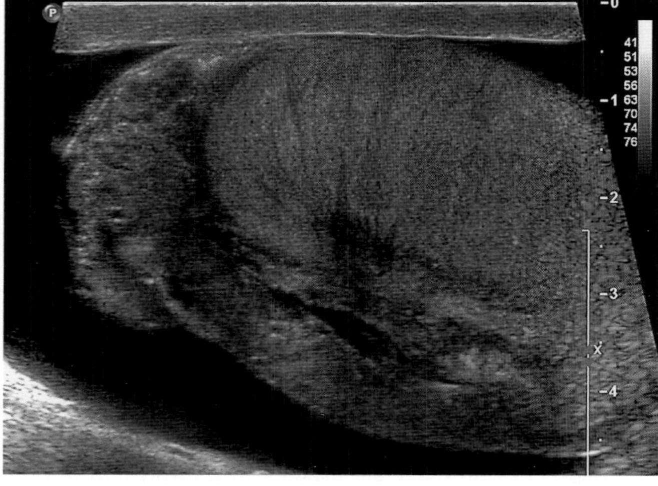

A

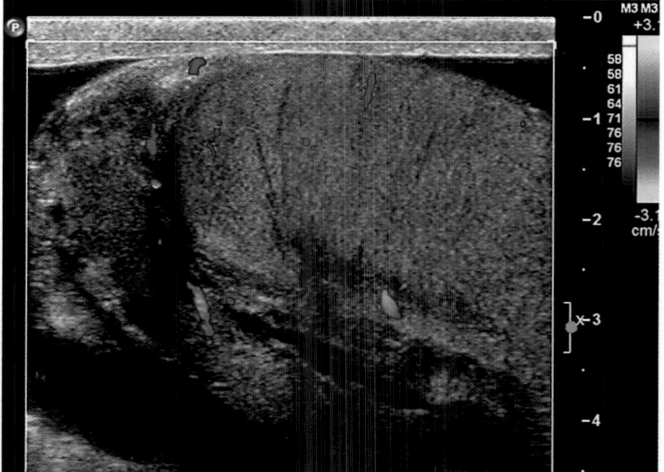

B

Figure 12-64 Epididymal Thickening Due to Spermatic Cord Torsion
A. Grayscale and (**B**) color Doppler images in a patient with acute scrotal pain demonstrate an enlarged epididymis and a hydrocele. However, the testicle and the epididymis demonstrate decreased blood flow. These findings should prompt consideration of spermatic cord torsion as the etiology, rather than epididymo-orchitis, which would have increased blood flow.

Table 12-12. Large Cystic Lesions in the Scrotal Sac

1. Fluid in the sac of the tunica vaginalis a. Hydrocele b. Hematocele c. Pyocele d. Lymphocele e. Scrotal urinoma
2. Epididymal cyst and spermatocele
3. Inguinal hernia a. Ascitic fluid b. Herniated fluid-filled bowel c. Herniated bladder
4. Mesothelioma of the tunica vaginalis

or cholesterol content (see Figure 12-65).[1] On MRI examinations, a simple hydrocele appears as simple fluid surrounding the testis. On both imaging studies, congenital hydrocele can be differentiated from acquired hydrocele by demonstrating a patent processus vaginalis, seen as fluid tracking from the peritoneal cavity through the inguinal region into the sac of the tunica vaginalis.

A hydrocele can appear complex because of a variety of reasons, including (1) chronic or prior inflammation, (2) the presence of blood (hematocele), (3) the presence of pus and infectious debris (pyocele), (4) rarely due to complex peritoneal fluid extending through a patent processes vaginalis into the scrotal sac, or primary malignancy of the tunica vaginalis (see **Mesothelioma of the tunica vaginalis** below). Complex hydroceles from all of these of causes have a similar sonographic appearance, demonstrating variable amounts of internal echoes, fluid-debris levels, septations, and loculations (see Figure 12-65). However, different etiologies can sometimes be distinguished based on other factors, as follows. Hematoceles are usually associated with a history of recent trauma and other imaging findings of scrotal injury. Pyoceles typically present with fever and leucocytosis, and are associated with other imaging findings of infection, such as epididymo-orchitis. Pyoceles occasionally can contain gas, suggesting infectious nature of the collection. On the other hand, complex hydrocele in an asymptomatic patient most likely represents sequela of prior inflammation. Rarely, a rapidly enlarging complex hydrocele can reflect extension of carcinomatosis into the scrotal sac through a patent processus vaginalis or a mesothelioma of the tunica vaginalis, in which case peripheral nodularity may be present. MRI can also occasionally add specificity by demonstrating T1 hyperintense fluid representing blood products in the case of a hematocele or by revealing the presence of enhancing nodules lining the scrotal sac in the case of malignancy (see Figures 12-66 and 12-67).

Intravaginal collections of lymphatic fluid can be due to congenital lymphedema or can be due to prior surgery. History is key to the diagnosis in this situation as the imaging appearance is not specific. Likewise, urinoma is indistinguishable based on imaging from a simple hydrocele, but might be suspected if there is new scrotal swelling in the setting of urinary tract injury.

Epididymal cyst and spermatocele

Epididymal cysts and spermatoceles are both believed to result from dilation of the epididymal tubules. Epididymal

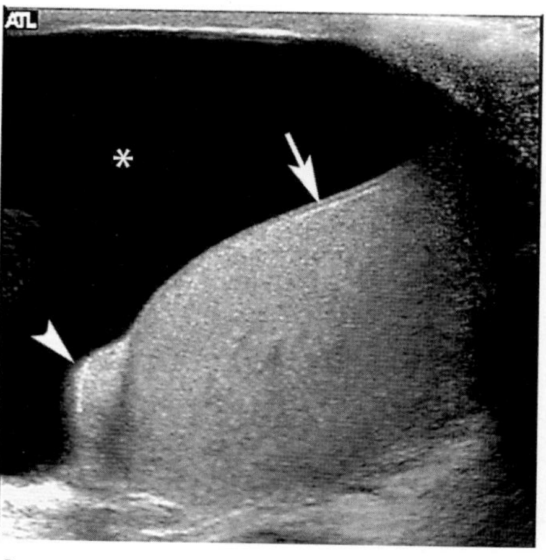

A

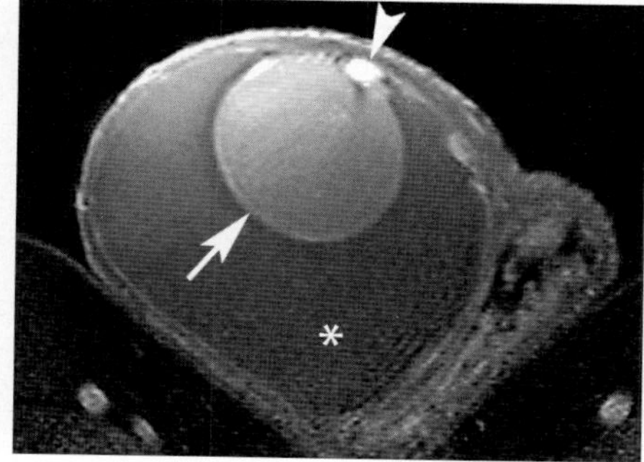

B

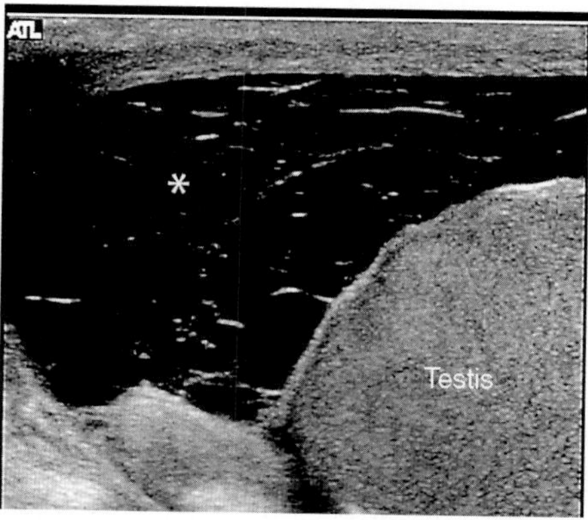

C

Figure 12-65 Hydrocele and Pyocele, in Different Patients
A. Grayscale US image demonstrating simple fluid (*asterisk*) surrounding and compressing the epididymis (*arrowhead*) and testis (*arrow*) characteristic of a large hydrocele. **B.** Enhanced post contrast fat-saturated T1-weighted MRI image in a different patient demonstrates fluid (*asterisk*) surrounding the testis (*arrow*) and epididymis (*arrowhead*) typical of a simple hydrocele. **C.** Grayscale image in a third patient with epididymo-orchitis demonstrates a scrotal fluid collection (*asterisk*) containing multiple lacy septations, suggestive of a pyocele.

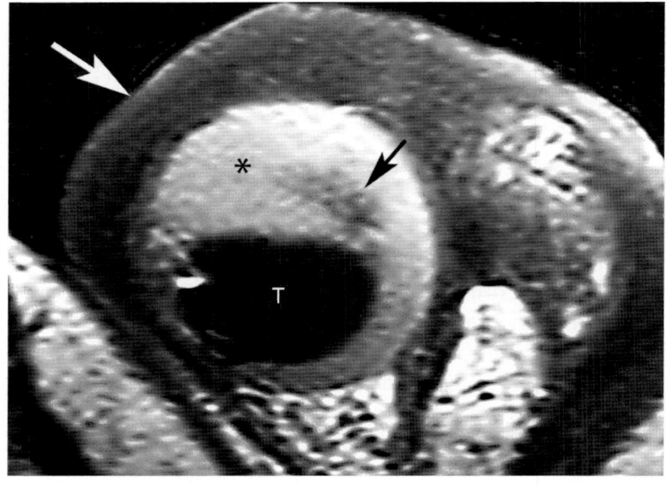

A

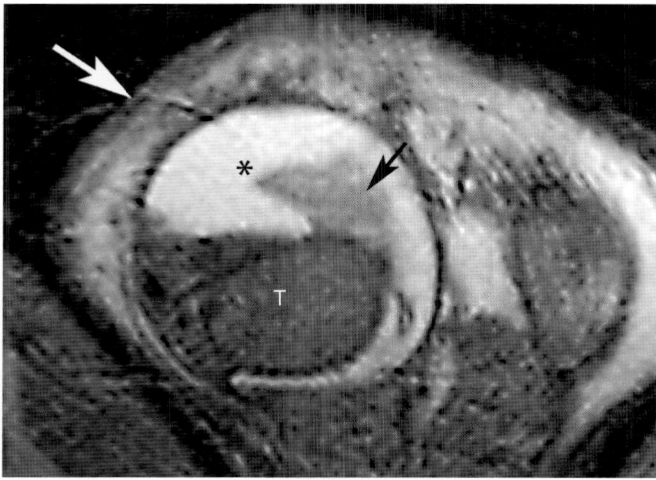

B

Figure 12-66 Hematocele
This patient presented with a history of testicular trauma. **A.** Axial T1 and (**B**) T2-weighted images demonstrate T1 hyperintense fluid (*asterisk*) in keeping with hemorrhage with associated blood clot (*small black arrow*) surrounding the testis (T), in keeping with hematocele. *White arrows* point to scrotal edema.

cysts and spermatoceles are differentiated on the basis of the presence of sperm in a spermatocele. Together, these lesions are reported to occur in 29% of asymptomatic men.[84] Epididymal cysts and spermatoceles have been reported more frequently in men who have undergone vasectomy or have had intrauterine exposure to diethylstilbestrol, or who demonstrate dilation of the rete testis. Spermatoceles are only found in the epididymal head whereas epididymal cysts can be found throughout the epididymis. Epididymal cysts and spermatoceles are otherwise indistinguishable by US, and in general, the distinction is not clinically important. Both lesions appear on US as cystic masses within the epididymis (see Figure 12-68). These can appear simple or can contain loculations, septations, and/or internal echoes. When large, they can be difficult to distinguish from a large hydrocele. However, epididymal cysts and spermatoceles tend to displace the testis, by contrast to hydroceles, which envelop the testis. This feature may suggest the correct diagnosis.[14]

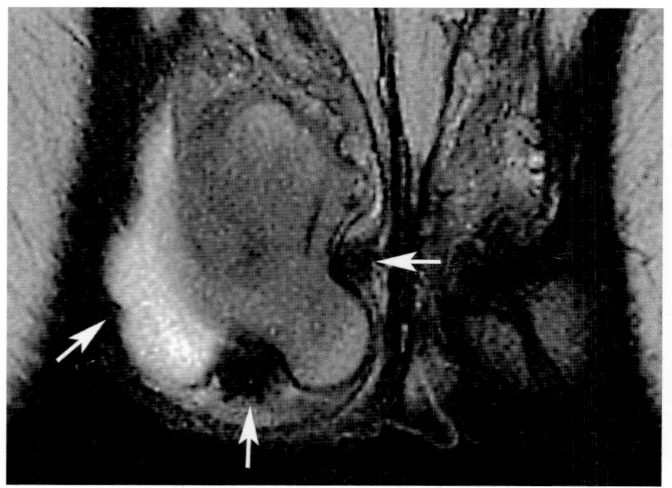

A

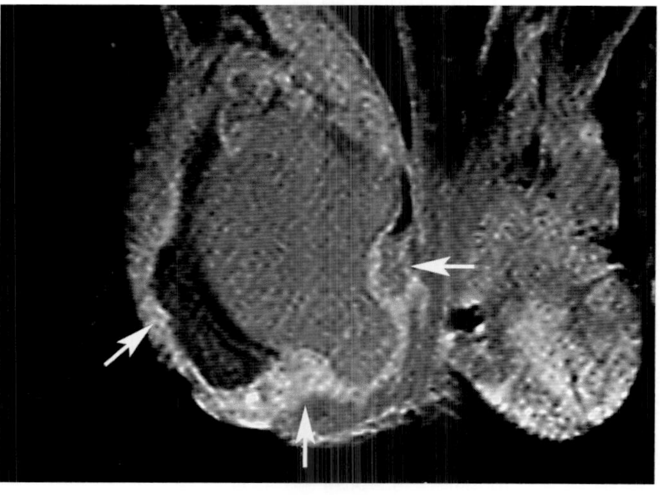

B

Figure 12-67 Scrotal Metastases
This patient had known peritoneal carcinomatosis from gallbladder carcinoma. **A.** Coronal T2-weighted and (**B**) coronal fat-saturated T1-weighted postgadolinium sequences reveal multiple small enhancing nodules along the tunica vaginalis (*arrows*) as well as a small hydrocele reflecting scrotal involvement by peritoneal spread through a patent process vaginalis.

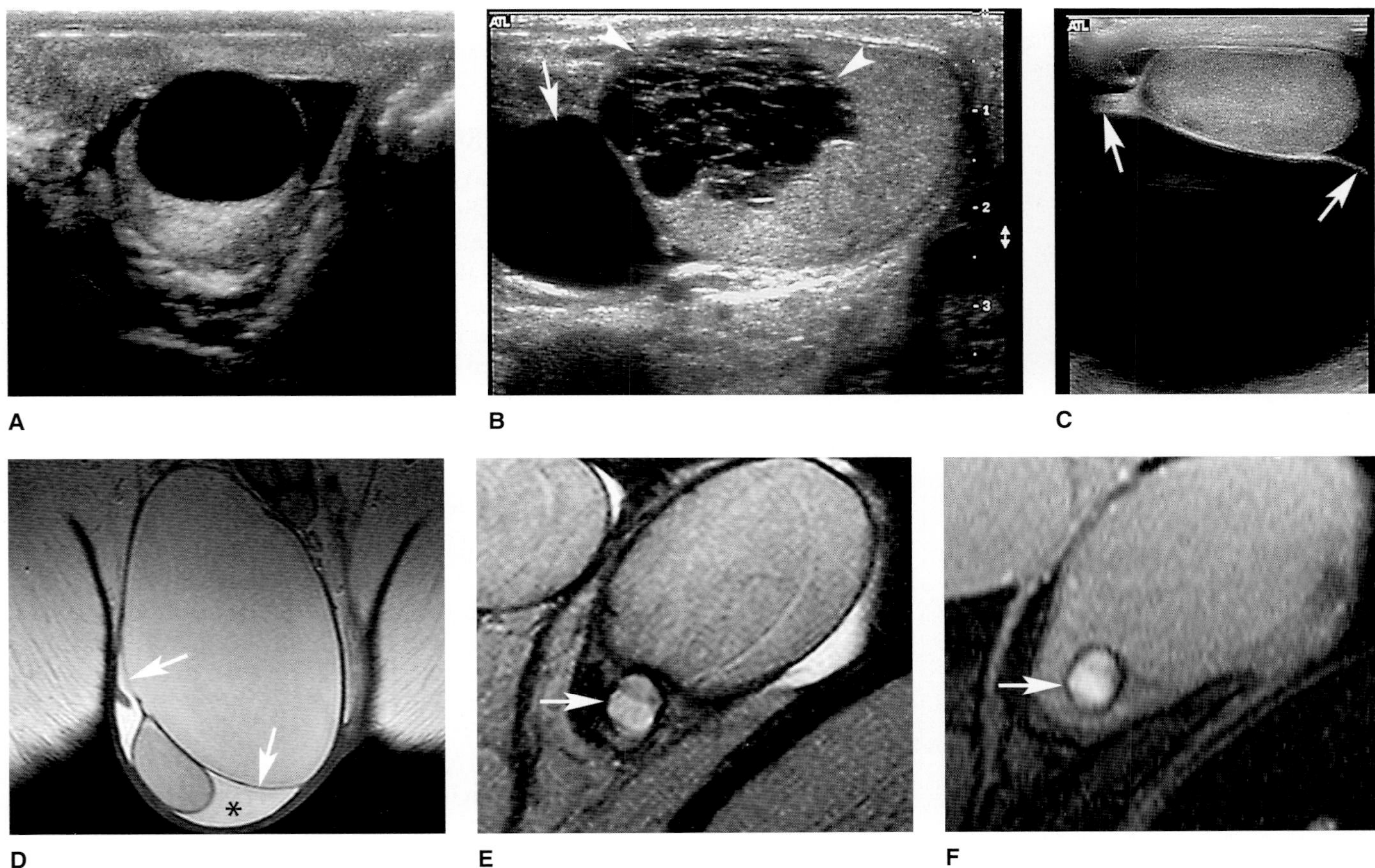

Figure 12-68 Epididymal Cysts in 4 Patients
A. Sagittal grayscale image through the epididymal head demonstrates an anechoic mass with a well-defined wall and through transmission characteristic of a simple epididymal cyst. A spermatocele can have an identical appearance. **B.** Transverse grayscale image demonstrates tubular ectasia of the rete testis (*arrowhead*), which is commonly associated with epididymal cysts (*arrow*). **C.** Grayscale image shows a large fluid collection in the scrotum. This appears to have a wall (*arrows*) and the testis is located in a nondependent location, features that are suggestive of a large epididymal cyst as opposed to hydrocele. **D.** Coronal T2-weighted image of the same patient as in C more clearly shows the cyst (*arrows*) as well as a small hydrocele (*asterisk*). The testis is displaced inferiorly to the left of the image. **E.** Axial T2-weighted and (**F**) axial T1-weighted images in a patient referred for evaluation of a solid-appearing epididymal mass demonstrates a mass with T1 hyperintensity (*arrows*) in the region of the epididymal head. This did not enhance postcontrast (not shown), indicative of an epididymal cyst complicated by protein or hemorrhage. This illustrates how MRI may be useful in cases where US is unable to determine if a mass is cystic or solid.

Inguinal hernia

Inguinal hernias may be classified as direct or indirect inguinal hernias. Both types of inguinal hernias can contain fluid-filled bowel or urinary bladder, each of which can be seen as an intrascrotal fluid collection (see Figure 12-57). The diagnosis of a hernia is made by examination of the inguinal region, which demonstrates communication of the herniated contents through the inguinal canal into the pelvic cavity. Valsalva maneuver can be helpful in eliciting an otherwise occult hernia.

Most inguinal hernias are asymptomatic and discovered as a groin bulge on physical examination. However, inguinal hernias can present with acute scrotal pain if bowel is incarcerated and strangulated, which occurs more frequently with the indirect type. A diagnosis of strangulation should be suspected on US if (1) the herniated bowel is akinetic and hyperemic or demonstrates wall thickening, (2) the scrotal wall is hyperemic, (3) the loop of bowel is not reducible, or (4) there is acute scrotal pain.[1]

Mesothelioma of the tunica vaginalis

Mesothelioma of the tunica vaginalis is a rare etiology of recurrent or enlarging hydrocele, with fewer than 100 cases reported in the literature (see Figure 12-69).[85] Scrotal mesothelioma arises from the tunica vaginalis and accounts for 0.2% to 5% of cases of mesothelioma. Asbestos exposure is a risk factor, but reported in less than 50% of cases.[14] Prospective diagnosis of scrotal

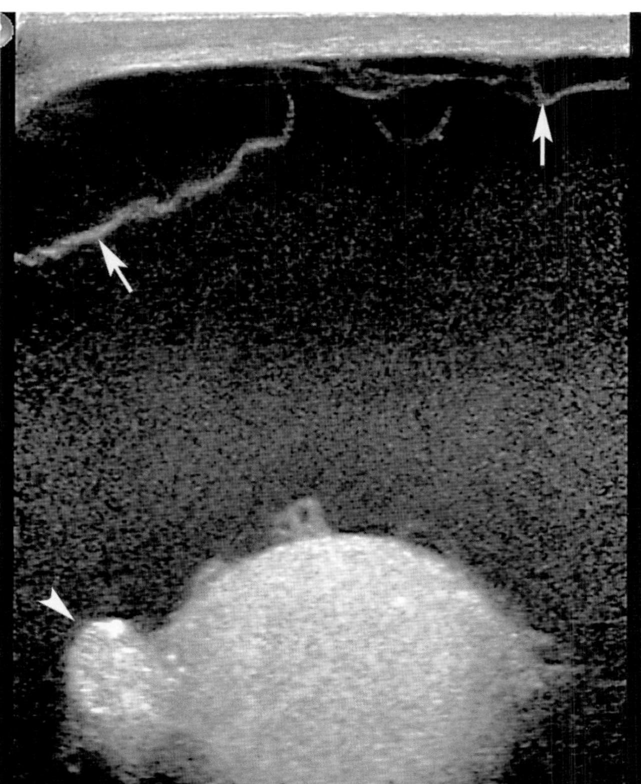

Figure 12-69 Scrotal Mesothelioma
Grayscale image reveals a large complex hydrocele with fine internal echoes and internal strands (*arrows*), without solid components or internal vascularity. This was thought to represent a hematocele or pyocele but found to represent scrotal mesothelioma. Epididymal head indicated by *arrowhead*.

mesothelioma is difficult. However, the diagnosis can be suspected in the setting of a recurrent or enlarging hydrocele associated with soft-tissue nodules along the tunica vaginalis. Mesothelioma is an aggressive tumor with metastatic disease found in 15% of patients at presentation, most commonly in retroperitoneal lymph nodes.[85]

A patent process vaginalis containing ascites and tumor nodules related to peritoneal carcinomatosis can produce a similar appearance (see Figure 12-67).

Scrotal Echogenic Foci

In most cases, echogenic foci within the testis will be a result of dystrophic calcifications but can occasionally be a result of intratesticular gas or foreign material like sutures or surgical clips deposited in the scrotum during surgery. Rarely, echogenic foci within testicular neoplasms can be due to focal areas of hemorrhage or fibrosis.[1] Calcifications can be associated with both malignant and benign conditions (Table 12-13).

Calcifications and other echogenic foci associated with testicular neoplasms

Viable neoplasms: A variety of testicular neoplasms can contain echogenic foci, the most common of which are NSGCT, which contain echogenic foci in 35% of cases. Echogenic foci in NSGCT can be due to hemorrhage, fibrosis, or dystrophic calcification and in tumors containing teratomatous elements can also be due to the presence of bone or cartilage (see Figure 12-70).[1] Other rare neoplasms with intralesional calcifications include large-cell calcifying Sertoli tumor, carcinoid tumor, osteosarcoma, epidermoid, and hemangioma of the testis.

Burned-out germ cell tumor: Rarely, a small fibrotic mass, without evidence of malignant cells, will be discovered within the testicle of a patient with evidence of metastatic germ cell tumor. It is believed that this fibrotic mass represents the primary testicular malignancy that has autoinfarcted as a result of such rapid growth that the malignancy outstripped its blood supply. This phenomenon has been termed *burned-out germ cell tumor* and occurs most commonly with teratocarcinoma or choriocarcinoma. The US appearance of burned-out germ cell tumor is variable, ranging from a single area of macroscopic calcification to a small hypoechogenic mass.[86]

Imaging Notes 12-20. Differentiating Features of Fluid in the Scrotal Sac

Large amount of fluid in the scrotal sac

Fluid in Scrotal Sac	Differentiating Features
Hydrocele, hematocele, pyocele	Surrounds and envelops the testis and epididymis, often anterolateral in location, can compress the testis
Epididymal cyst/spermatocele	Displaces, as opposed to envelops the testis (compared to hydrocele)
Hernia sac with ascites or bowel	Communication with pelvic cavity via inguinal canal; peristalsis
Mesothelioma	Recurrent or enlarging complex hydrocele with nodules along the tunica vaginalis
Scrotal metastases	Mixed cystic and solid masses associated with the hydrocele

Table 12-13. Causes of Scrotal Echogenic Foci

A. Calcifications 1. Associated with neoplasms a. More common i. Nonseminomatous germ cell tumor (most common) ii. Burnt-out germ cell tumor iii. Epidermoid b. Very rare i. Large-cell calcifying Sertoli tumor ii. Hemangioma iii. Carcinoid tumor iv. Osteosarcoma
2. Calcifications associated with benign conditions a. Dystrophic calcifications i. Prior infarction ii. Prior trauma iii. Prior abscess iv. Granulomatous diseases (tuberculosis, sarcoidosis) b. Testicular microlithiasis (benign, but associated with ITGCN)
B. Intratesticular gas (postoperative)
C. Iatrogenic material (sutures, surgical clips)

Calcifications associated with benign conditions

Calcifications associated with benign conditions can be macroscopic, typically due to prior insult, or tiny punctate calcifications representing microlithiasis.

Dystrophic macrocalcifications: Benign causes of coarse testicular calcifications include prior infarction, trauma, or abscess and previous granulomatous disease, including sarcoidosis and granulomatous infections. (see Figure 12-71). One unusual posttraumatic cause of dystrophic calcifications is chronic repetitive trauma in equestrians and mountain bikers.[87,88] This usually results in bilateral testicular calcifications measuring a few millimeters in size. Although relatively small, they are larger in size than the calcifications of microlithiasis. Rimlike testicular calcification can be seen in the setting of prenatal torsion. This rim calcification is associated with testicular atrophy and thickening of the tunica albuginea.[89] Vascular calcifications may also occasionally be identified as a cluster of tiny calcifications.[90]

Testicular microlithiasis: Testicular microliths are laminated calcium deposits within the lumen of the seminiferous tubules, which on US appear as nonshadowing echogenic foci measuring less than 2 to 3 mm.[91] These are differentiated from macrocalcifications by their small size. The presence of 5 or more microliths per transducer field has come to be accepted as the definition for classic testicular microlithiasis (CTM), with fewer microliths representing limited testicular microlithiasis (LTM) (see Figure 12-72).[92] Management of microlithiasis remains controversial because of the uncertain causal relationship between CTM and germ cell neoplasia. Early retrospective studies reported a low prevalence of CTM (0.6% of the general population), associated with a fairly high prevalence of GCT (40% in patients with CTM),[94] with a relative risk of testicular GCT of up to 21.6 comparing those with CTM with the general population,[95] suggesting a strong relationship between CTM and GCN. However,

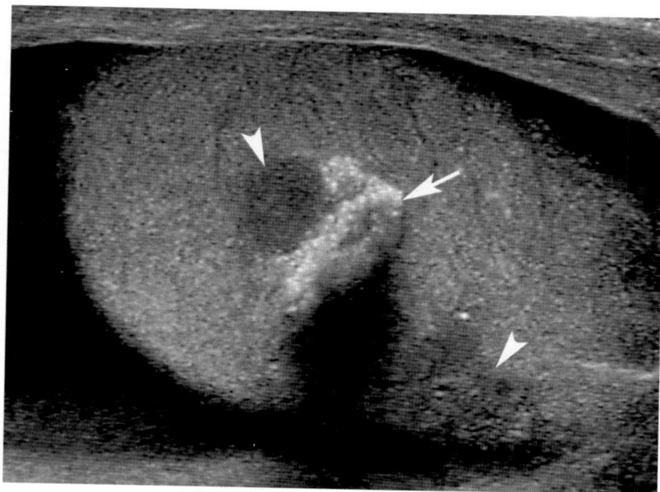
A

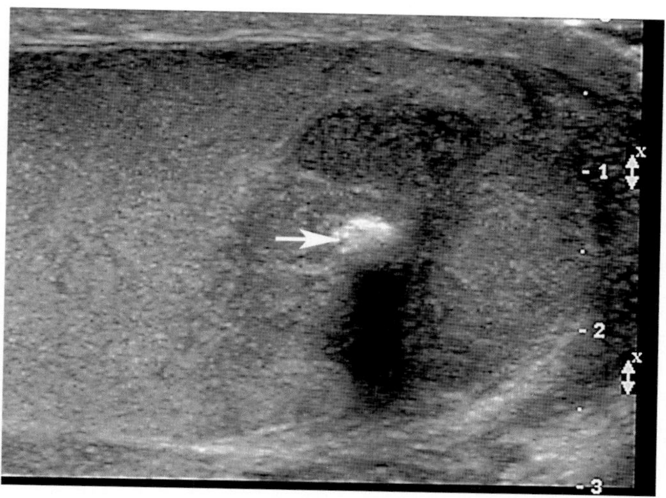

B

Figure 12-70 Calcifications in Nonseminomatous Germ Cell Tumors
A. Grayscale sonographic image demonstrates a coarse shadowing calcification (*arrow*) associated with a hypoechoic mass (*arrowheads*). Orchiectomy revealed a mixed germ cell tumor composed of seminoma and yolk sac components. **B.** Grayscale sonographic image in a different patient shows a hypoechoic mass with a coarse calcification (*arrow*). Orchiectomy revealed mixed germ cell tumor composed of mostly seminoma with a small component of embryonal cell carcinoma.

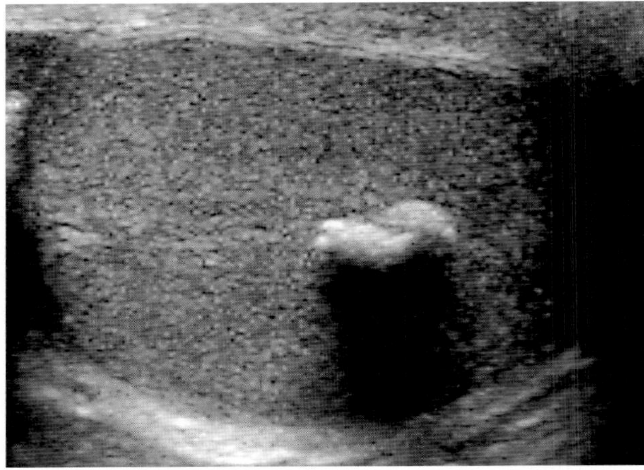

Figure 12-71 Dystrophic Calcifications
This patient was asymptomatic. Sonogram shows a coarse echogenic focus with shadowing indicating dystrophic calcification without known cause. Note the absence of associated mass or adjacent testicular abnormality.

later studies reported a higher prevalence of CTM of 1.7% in an asymptomatic population and 3.7% to 9% in a referred population and also reported a lower prevalence of testicular neoplasia of between 5.8% and 18% for CTM and between 0% and 5.8 % for LTM when compared with 0.3% to 0.7% in the control population.[92,98-101] The data from these newer studies indicates that the association of testicular microlithiasis with malignancy is likely not as strong as originally thought. Furthermore, while there have been case reports of testicular carcinoma developing in the setting of microlithiasis,[91,102] other studies with short-term follow-up have shown no tumor development.[92] Long-term large prospective studies have not yet been performed. At this time, it seems reasonable to consider patients with testicular microlithiasis as having an increased risk of developing a primary testicular tumor and to offer some kind of surveillance.[96,102] A combination of annual US and periodic self-examination has been suggested for patients at increased risk, such as men with testicular microlithiasis who are subfertile or have a history of prior GCT or who have cryptorchidism.[96] There is no consensus regarding management of patients with no risk factors other than testicular microlithiasis, and the decision regarding the type of surveillance, either self-examination or annual US, should be decided on an individual basis.[96]

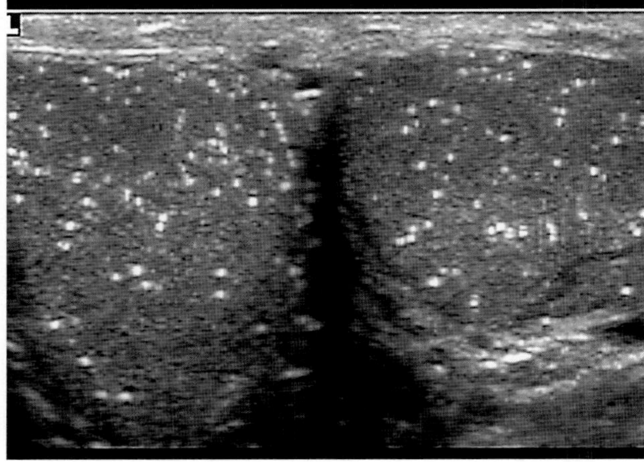

Figure 12-72 Microlithiasis
Ultrasonographic examination demonstrates innumerable tiny bilateral nonshadowing echogenic intratesticular foci characteristic of microlithiasis. These are not visible by MRI.

Intratesticular gas

Intratesticular gas can be due to iatrogenic intervention, penetrating trauma, or due to a gas-forming infection. Features suggestive of gas on US examinations include ring-down artifact, dirty shadowing, nondependent location, and mobility (see Figure 12-73).

Iatrogenic material

Regularly spaced nonshadowing echogenic foci can represent suture material, usually in the setting sperm harvesting procedure (see Figure 12-74).

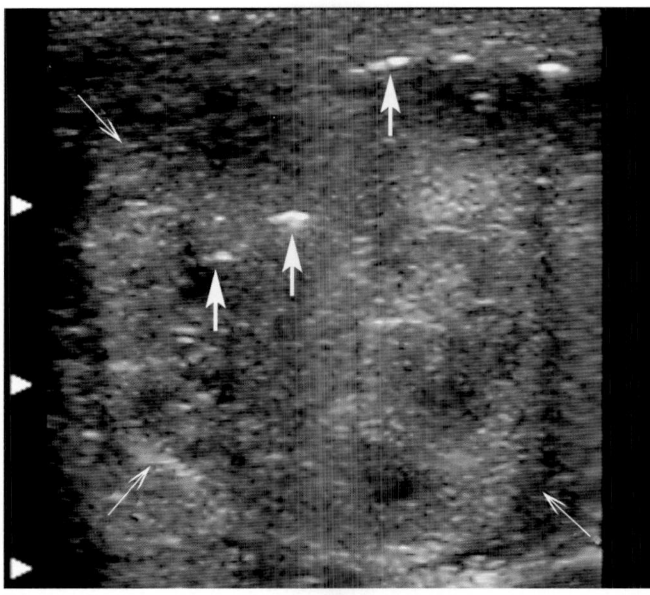

Figure 12-73 Intratesticular Gas
This grayscale US image shows multiple echogenic foci (*arrows*) in a diffusely heterogeneous testicle (*outlined by thin arrows*). On grayscale imaging, this could mimic a mass with calcifications; however, the patient had a history of gunshot to the scrotum and the testicle was avascular with tunica disruption (not shown), and therefore the echogenic foci represent gas due to the penetrating injury.

Imaging Notes 12-21. Differentiating Features of Intratesticular Echogenic Foci

Intratesticular Echogenic Foci

Entity	Differentiating Features
Burnt-out germ cell neoplasm	History of germ cell neoplasm/retroperitoneal LAN, +tumor markers
NSGCT	Soft-tissue component, +tumor markers, retroperitoneal LAN
Calcifying Sertoli cell tumor	May present as bilateral calcified masses, pediatric age group, ass with Peutz-Jaeger and Carney syndrome
Other rare calcifying tumors (carcinoid, osteosarcoma)	Rare, would be difficult to diagnose prospectively
Macrocalcifications (chronic trauma, hematoma, abscess, granulomatous disease, infarct)	Negative tumor markers, no soft-tissue component, history of repetitive trauma
Intrauterine spermatic cord torsion	Rim calcified atrophic testicle in a neonate
Microlithiasis	Tiny punctate calcifications, nonshadowing; association with testicular cancer
Intratesticular gas	History of surgery, instrumentation, infection, dirty shadowing, ring down, mobility of echogenic foci
Iatrogenic	Regularly spaced, history of testicular biopsy or sperm harvesting

Extratesticular Echogenic Foci

Extratesticular echogenic foci can be due to calcifications, gas, or foreign material (Table 12-14).

Extratesticular calcification

Most extratesticular calcifications are benign findings due to chronic or prior inflammation, and include scrotal pearls, and calcification of the tunica vaginalis, appendix testis, and epididymis. These are differentiated by location of the calcification.

The most common type of extratesticular calcification is a "scrotolith" or "scrotal pearl," which is a calcified

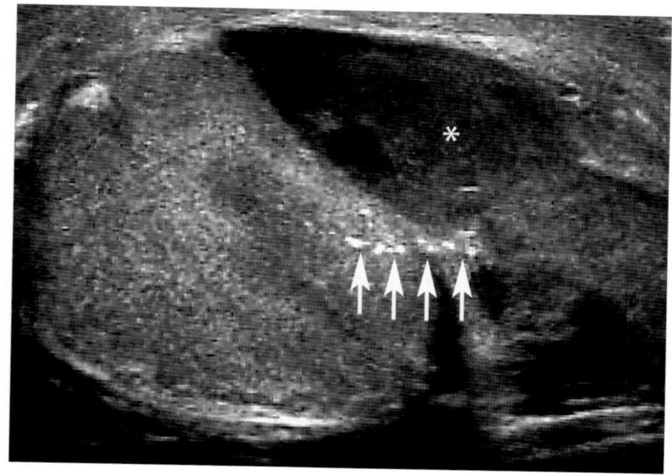

Figure 12-74 Suture Material
Grayscale image shows regularly spaced echogenic foci in a linear distribution (*arrows*) typical of sutures related to a recent sperm harvest. Note the large complex hydrocele (*asterisk*) with dependent debris representing a postoperative hematocele.

Table 12-14. Extratesticular Echogenic Foci

1. Extratesticular calcification
   a. Scrotolith ("scrotal pearl")
   b. Prior infarction of the appendix testis
   c. Calcification of the tunica vaginalis or tunica albuginea
   d. Epididymal calcifications
      i. Chronic epididymitis
      ii. Sperm granuloma
2. Gas
   a. Forniers gangrene
   b. Bowel containing hernia; gas may be extraluminal if perforation has occurred
   c. Prior recent surgery
   d. Scrotal abscess
   e. Fistula from the genitourinary or gastrointestinal tracts
   f. Dissection of subcutaneous gas from the thorax
3. Foreign bodies
   a. Prior penetrating trauma
   b. Prior surgery

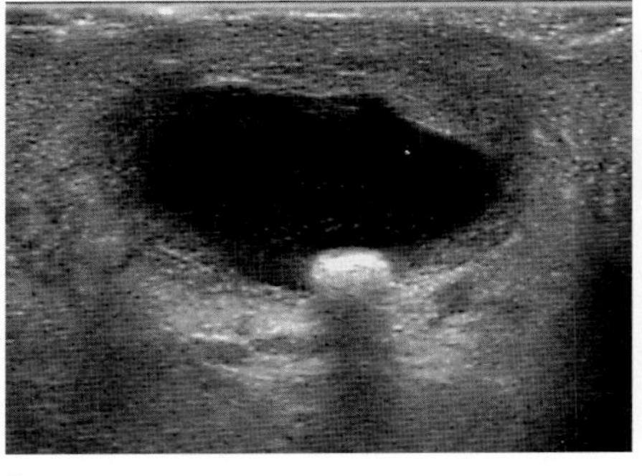
A

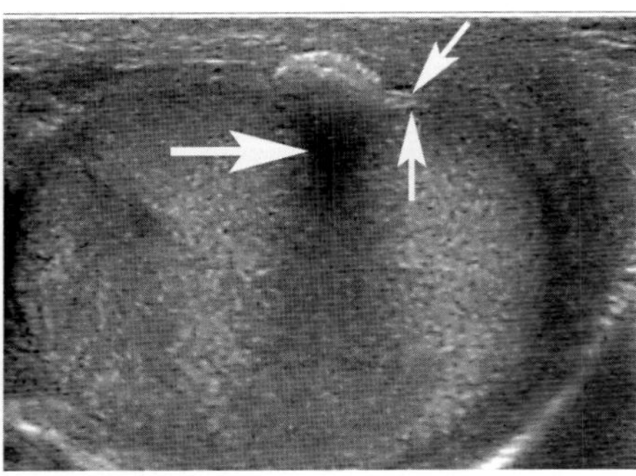
B

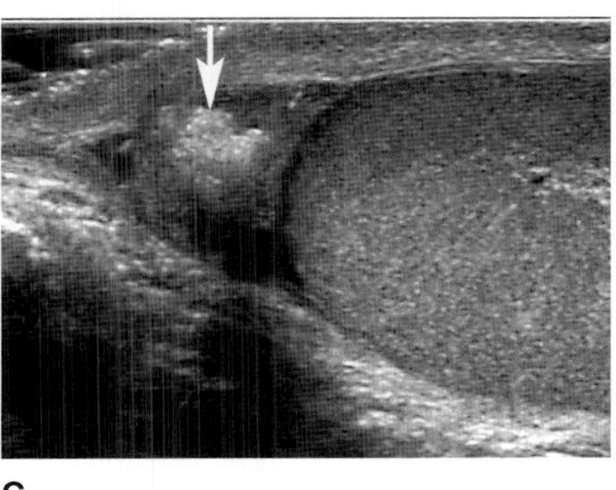
C

Figure 12-75 Extratesticular Calcifications
A. Grayscale US image demonstrating a coarse shadowing calcification in the dependent scrotal sac, which was mobile during real-time examination typical of a scrotolith (a.k.a scrotal pearl) **B.** Grayscale US image in a different patient demonstrating a nonmobile, linear calcification with posterior acoustic shadowing (*arrow*) in a nondependent location intimately associated with the tunica (*small arrows*) characteristic of a tunica albuginea calcification. **C.** Grayscale US image from a patient with history of prior vasectomy, demonstrating echogenic foci in the epididymal head (*arrow*) with shadowing, indicating dystrophic calcification related to the prior surgery.

loose body lying between the membranes of the tunica vaginalis. It is believed to originate from either a fibrinous deposit in the tunica vaginalis or as a remnant of a detached torsed appendix testis or appendix epididymis. Scrotoliths can occasionally be detected by physical examination but in most cases are not palpable because of an associated hydrocele. On US examinations, a scrotolith appears as a dependently located mobile small round or oval mass external to the testis, which can be completely calcified or may contain central calcifications (see Figure 12-75). In most cases, there will be an associated hydrocele.

Calcification of the appendix testis can be recognized by its characteristic position near the superior pole of the testis, and is often secondary to prior appendiceal torsion. Dystrophic calcification of the tunica albuginea or tunica vaginalis can be recognized on the basis of a linear or plaquelike configuration along the surface of the testis or along the scrotal wall, respectively and is usually from prior inflammation (see Figure 12-75). Calcification within the epididymis can be on the basis of prior inflammation in an asymptomatic patient, but can in some cases reflect chronic/granulomatous epididymitis and sperm granuloma (see Figure 12-75). (See **Chronic epididymitis** and **Tuberculous epididymitis** under **Diffusely Thickened Epididymis** and **Sperm Granuloma** under **Focal Epididymal Disorder**.)

Phleboliths can occur within intrascrotal, extratesticular hemangiomas and are one additional very rare cause of paratesticular echogenic foci.

Gas

Causes of extratesticular scrotal gas include Fournier gangrene, inguinal hernia, gas dissection from an air leak in the thorax, abscess, fistula, and recent prior surgery. Features suggesting gas include mobility as indicated by a change with position, "ring-down" artifact, and "dirty-shadowing." Gas can be confirmed by CT or plain-film radiography. The patient's clinical history and the location of the gas within the scrotum can aid in differentiating among different etiologies of scrotal gas.

Necrotizing gangrene of the perineum and genitalia, called Fournier's gangrene, is a severe infection of the perineum that is associated with underlying illnesses, including diabetes, renal failure, alcohol abuse, and perirectal disease. It is usually a result of polymicrobial infection and is most commonly caused by anaerobic cocci. The mortality rate is high. Patients will typically have fever, leucocytosis, and perineal pain and will frequently have crepitus on physical examination. Imaging examinations will demonstrate diffuse gas within the scrotal wall and surrounding perineum (see Figure 12-76).[97]

Inguinal hernia can also present with acute scrotum and extratesticular gas; however, unlike in Fournier gangrene, the gas is localized within bowel loops in the hernia sac, unless perforation has occured.

Rarely, gas within the skin of the scrotum can be due to extensive subcutaneous gas dissecting from an air leak in the thorax or due to dissection of gas due to a perforated abdominal viscus. Other etiologies of scrotal gas include organized abscess, fistula from the bowel in the abdomen or pelvis, fistula from the urethra, and gas introduced by surgery or trauma.

Foreign bodies

Shrapnel from penetrating injury or surgical clips appear as highly echogenic foci with shadowing and ring-down artifact. In most cases, this appearance plus a clinical history of penetrating trauma or prior surgery will identify the cause of the echogenic foci. If necessary, radiography can be performed to confirm the metallic composition of the echogenic focus.

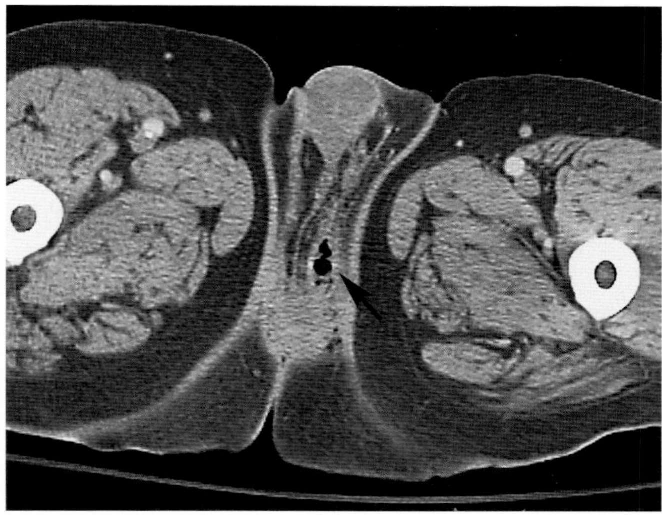

Figure 12-76 Fournier Gangrene
This 76-year-old man complained of increasing scrotal pain for 3 days. Images show thickening of the perineum with associated stranding and foci of gas (*arrow*), suspect for Fournier gangrene.

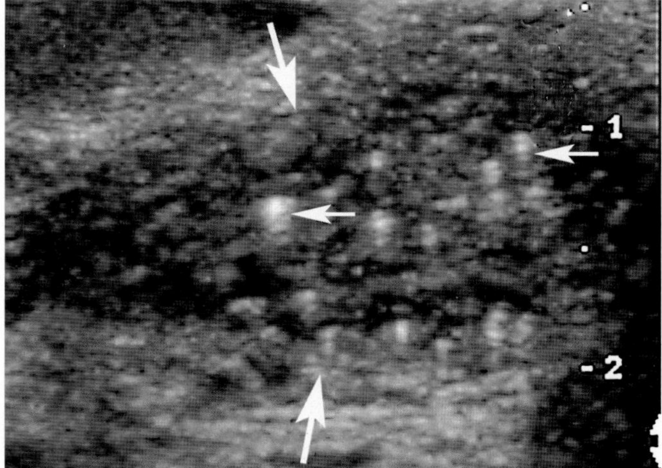

Figure 12-77 Dancing Megasperm
This grayscale image demonstrates marked thickening and tubular ectasia of the epididymal tail (*between large arrows*) with several echogenic foci (*small arrows*) that were seen to move in the dilated tubules in real time; this has been referred to as "dancing megasperm."

Other

Echogenic foci are commonly present in the epididymis postvasectomy, representing either fibrosis, calcification, or clumps of sperm. Occasionally, the clumps of sperm may be seen to move in real time in the tubules, which has been termed "dancing megasperm" (see Figure 12-77).[29]

Nonpalpable Testis

A testis can be nonpalpable due to resection, congenital absence, atrophy, retractile location or cryptorchidism, or dislocation due to trauma. The testis descends from the abdomen into the scrotum at 36 weeks' gestation. Cryptorchidism is defined as complete or partial failure of the testis to descend into the scrotal sac, which is found in 3.5% of newborns, decreasing to 1% at 1 year of age.[19] Complications associated with cryptorchidism include infertility and increased risk of testicular cancer, usually seminoma. The estimated rate of testicular cancer was initially reported to be as much as 50 times greater than the general population; however, more recent studies indicate a risk of 2.5- to 8-fold. Orchiopexy is usually performed between ages 1 and 10 and does not change the risk of malignant degeneration but does facilitate surveillance.

US is useful for identifying ectopic testicles located in the inguinal canal (72%) or in a prescrotal location, just distal to the external inguinal ring, but US is usually unable to detect intraabdominal testicles (8%) due to overlying bowel gas (see Figure 12-78).[1] In cases where the testicle is not identified sonographically, MRI should be obtained. On US, the cryptorchid testis is usually small and hypoechogenic and can be difficult to differentiate from a lymph node or from the distal bulbous portion of the gubernaculum testis.[23] Identification of the echogenic mediastinum testis is helpful in confirming that a structure represents the testis.[1,23]

Imaging Notes 12-22. Differentiating Features of Extratesticular Echogenic Foci

Extratesticular Echogenic Foci	Differentiating Features
Scrotal pearls	Mobile masses in the scrotal sac
Other extratesticular calcifications	Location (most commonly along the tunica albuginea or in the epididymis), usually due to chronic or prior inflammation
Gas in the setting of fistula, surgery/trauma, trauma or infection/abscess	Dirty shadowing, mobility, ring-down artifact, nondependent location
Gas within a bowel containing hernia	peristalsis
Iatrogenic	Shrapnel, staples—ring-down artifact, confirm with radiographs and history

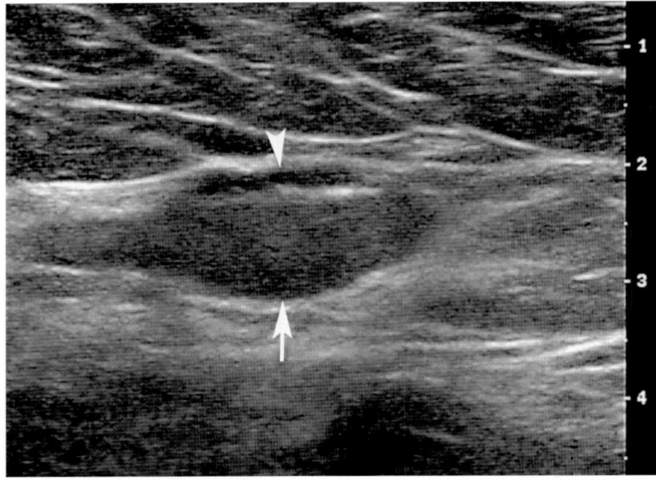

A

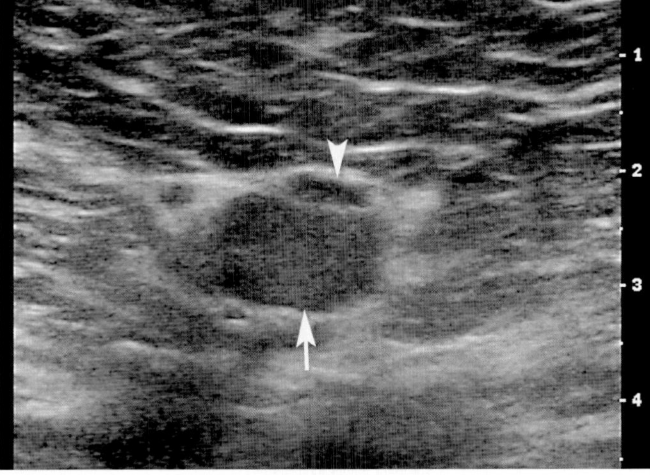

B

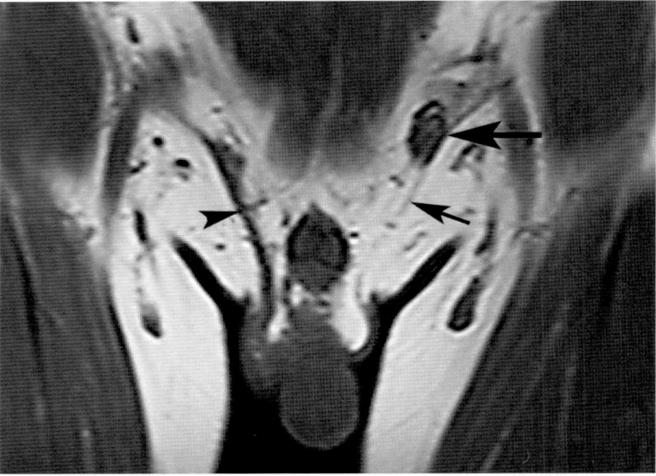
C

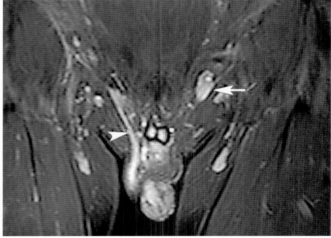

D

Figure 12-78 Cryptorchidism
A. Sagittal and (**B**) transverse US images through the left inguinal region reveal a small hypoechoic cryptorchid testis (*arrows*). Note the adjacent epididymis (*arrowheads*). **C.** Coronal T1-weighted and (**D**) fat saturated T2-weighted images in a different patient show a cryptorchid testis (*long arrows*) in the left inguinal region. Note the absence of the left spermatic cord in the scrotum when compared with the normal right spermatic cord (*arrowheads*) and the gubernaculum (*short arrow*, A).

ANATOMY OF THE PENIS

The penis is composed of three cylindrical bodies of endothelium-lined vascular spaces: the paired dorsolateral corpora cavernosa and a single ventral corpus spongiosum. The corpora cavernosa are in close apposition in the penile shaft and diverge at the base of the penis to become the crura, which are attached to the ischial tuberosities. The bulbar and pendulous portions of the male urethra are contained within the corpus spongiosum, which forms the penile bulb posteriorly and glans penis anteriorly. A fibrous sheath known as the tunica albuginea surrounds the corpus spongiosum and both corpora cavernosa.[103,104] External to this is another fascial layer (Buck's fascia).

The root is the proximal portion of the penis containing the crus of the paired corpora cavernosa and the bulb of the corpus spongiosum. The body of the penis extends from the root to the distal ends of the corpora cavernosa and is surrounded by the deep fascial layers. The distal portion of the penis consists of the expanded anterior end of the corpus spongiosum known as the glans penis.[103,105,106]

Numerous trabeculae extend across the corpora cavernosa, forming sinusoids or cavernous spaces that become engorged during erection. The cavernosal arteries are located slightly medially within the corpora cavernosa and feed capillary networks via helicine branches that open directly into the vascular sinusoids. Drainage of the corporal bodies is through emissary veins within the wall of the tunica albuginea into the deep dorsal vein of the penis, which courses within the shallow groove between the corpora cavernosa, deep to Buck's fascia. The superficial dorsal vein, which is superficial to Buck's fascia, drains blood from the pendulous penile skin and glans and communicates with the deep dorsal vein. During erection, engorgement of the corpora cavernosa causes compression of the draining veins, trapping blood within the corporal bodies. Branches from the paired dorsal arteries of the penis, which run adjacent to the deep dorsal vein, supply the glans penis, distal corpus spongiosum and penile skin, whereas the bulbar artery supplies the urethra, proximal corpus spongiosum, and bulbospongiosus muscle.[103,105,106]

IMAGING OF THE PENIS

US is the primary imaging modality to evaluate patients with penile disease. Clinical indications for penile US are palpable abnormality, penile fracture, erectile dysfunction, and priapism. MRI is generally reserved for cases where the ultrasound findings are not diagnostic, or for staging of known penile malignancies.[107,108]

For most indications, ultrasound of the penis is performed in the flaccid state, and consists primarily of grayscale axial and longitudinal images obtained with a high-frequency linear transducer (>12 megaHz). However, for evaluation of erectile dysfunction, a penile vascular flow study is also usually performed (described in more detail later), in which the penile vessels (cavernosal and dorsal arteries, deep dorsal vein) are evaluated by spectral and color Doppler, in both the flaccid state and the erect state. For these studies, erection is induced by intracavernosal injection of a vasoactive agent (most commonly Prostoglandin E1), if injection is not contraindicated by a condition predisposing to priapism, such as sickle cell disease, multiple myeloma, leukemia, tumors that invade the cavernosa, and partial cavernosal thromosis.[156,157]

In general, MRI is the preferred imaging modality for the evaluation and staging of penile malignancy due to superior soft-tissue contrast and multiplanar capabilities. The scrotum and penis are elevated by placing a folded towel between the patient's legs. The penis is subsequently dorsiflexed against the lower abdomen and taped in position to reduce motion during examination. A surface coil is employed to maximize signal-to-noise ratio at small fields of view. A pelvic coil is used when imaging the entire pelvis in staging penile malignancy. In general, both T1- and T2-weighted sequences are obtained in axial, sagittal, and coronal planes. Fat-saturated T1-weighted images are obtained before and after administration of gadolinium contrast agent. As with US, imaging of the erect penis can be performed after the intracavernosal injection of vasoactive drugs.[104,107]

NORMAL IMAGING APPEARANCE OF THE MALE URETHRA AND PENIS

Both sonography and MRI examinations can provide important information regarding diseases of the penis.

Ultrasonography

In the flaccid penis, the corpus spongiosum and corpora cavernosa appear as homogeneous cylindrical structures. The urethra can sometimes be seen as a slitlike structure in the corpora spongiosum, but is typically difficult to appreciate when not distended by retrograde injection of fluid. The combination of the tunica albuginea and Buck's fascia usually appear as a single thin echogenic line surrounding the corpora (see Figure 12-79). The cavernosal arteries appear as narrow tubular structures within the corpora cavernosa on longitudinal scans, measuring 0.3 to 1 mm (mean 0.3-0.5 mm) in the flaccid state. The dorsal vessels appear as anechoic structures along the dorsal aspect of the penile shaft, with the deep dorsal vein and dorsal arteries located deep to Buck's fascia and the superficial dorsal vein outside Buck's fascia (see Figure 12-80). In the flaccid state, peak systolic velocities in the cavernosal and dorsal arteries are similiar, in the range from 11 to 20 cm/s. At rest, flow within the cavernosal arteries demonstrates a high resistance pattern with no diastolic flow. During erection, flow within the cavernosal arteries undergoes a series of characteristic changes. Initially there is increased systolic flow with increased diastolic flow, followed by progressive decrease in diastolic flow due to venous occlusion, eventually resulting in reversal of diastolic flow. By contrast, the dorsal arteries normally maintain diastolic flow during erection (see Figure 12-80), although the peak systolic velocity increases.[156,157]

Magnetic Resonance Imaging

The paired corpora cavernosa and single corpora spongiosum are usually intermediate signal intensity on T1-weighted sequences and high signal intensity on T2-weighted sequences. The corpora cavernosa are typically isointense to each other as fenestrations in the membranous intercavernosal septum allows communication of blood within the cavernosal sinuses. The corpora spongiosum may have a slightly different signal intensity from the corpora cavernosa because of different rates of blood flow within the vascular sinusoids. Fluid levels can be present in the cavernosal bodies as a normal finding because of layering of blood in the cavernosal spaces. Both the tunica albuginea and Buck's fascia appear as low T1-weighted and low T2-weighted signal-intensity bands that surround the corporal bodies, the individual layers of which may not be distinguishable. The cavernosal arteries appear as hypointense foci within the corpora cavernosa on axial T2-weighted sequences (see Figure 12-81).[104]

The urethra is a low-signal-intensity tubular structure coursing within the midline corpus spongiosum in the root of the penis. Midline sagittal T2-weighted sequences in some cases will show the course of the male urethra extending from the bladder neck to the distal penile urethra. However, the proximal portion of the prostatic urethra and distal penile urethra are rarely seen on MRI in the absence of a Foley catheter.[111]

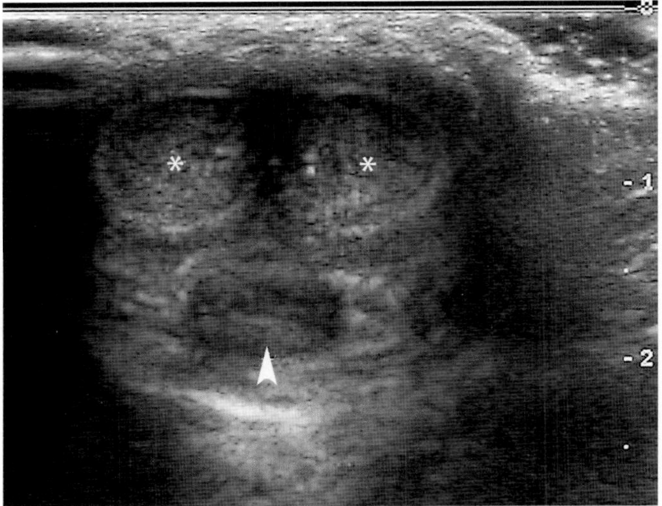

A

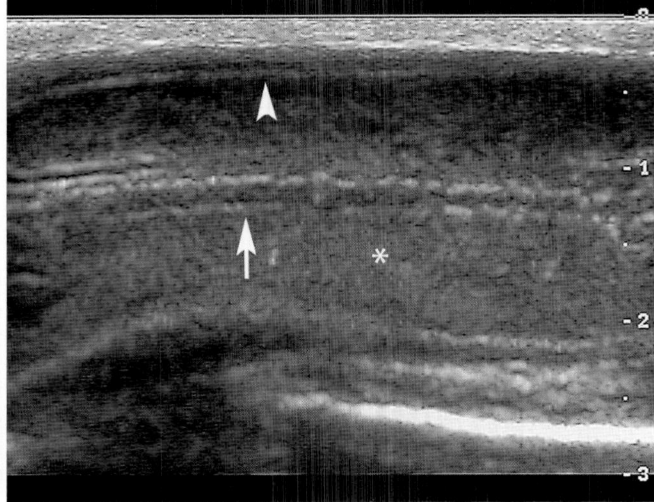

B

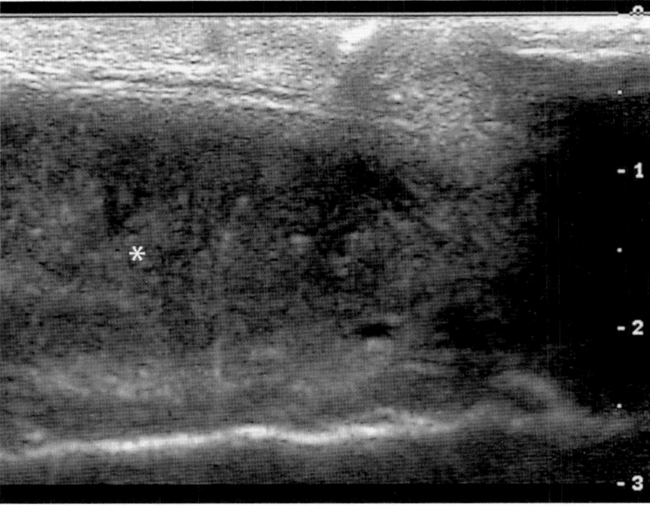

C

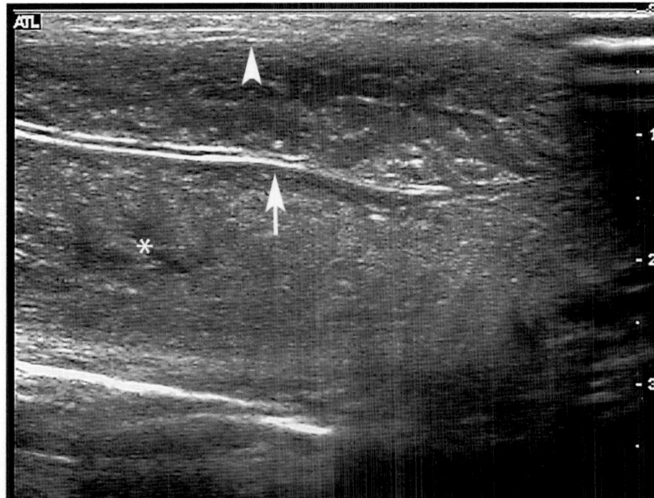

D

Figure 12-79 Normal US Appearance of the Penis
A. Grayscale transverse image at the mid-shaft penis demonstrating the paired corpora cavernosa (*asterisks*) and corpora spongiosum (*arrowhead*). **B.** Grayscale longitudinal image of the flaccid penis demonstrating the tunica albuginea (*arrowhead*) surrounding the corpora cavernosa (*asterisk*). The cavernosal artery (*arrow*) appears as a narrow tubular structure located centrally within the cavernosal body. **C.** Grayscale sagittal image of the flaccid penis demonstrating homogeneous echogenicity of the corpora spongiosum (*asterisk*). **D.** Grayscale sagittal image of the erect penis (following injection of prostaglandin E-1) demonstrating the engorged corpora cavernosum (*asterisk*) and cavernosal artery (*arrow*). The tunica albuginea is again visualized as a thin echogenic line (*arrowhead*) surrounding the corpora.

DISEASES OF THE PENIS

Penile pathology can be subdivided into solid lesions of the penis, cystic lesions of the penis, and some unique disorders of the penis.

Solid Lesions of the Penis

Solid lesions of the penis include benign and malignant neoplasms, fibrous plaques, and partial thrombosis of the corpora cavernosa (Table 12-15).

Primary malignancies of the penis

Primary malignant neoplasms of the penis are rare in Western countries, affecting an estimated 1000 to 1500 men per year, with approximately 300 deaths per year. By contrast, in some parts of Africa and South America, penile cancer may account for 10% to 20% of all male cancers.

Squamous cell carcinoma

Squamous cell carcinoma (SCC) accounts for 95% of penile cancers and usually occurs in the sixth to seventh

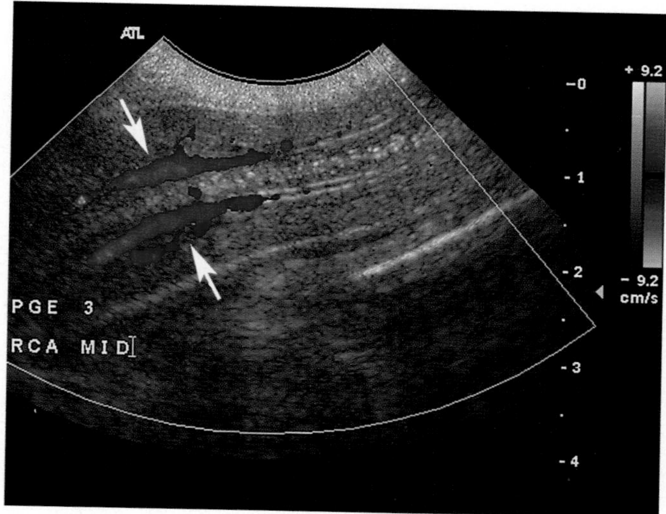

A

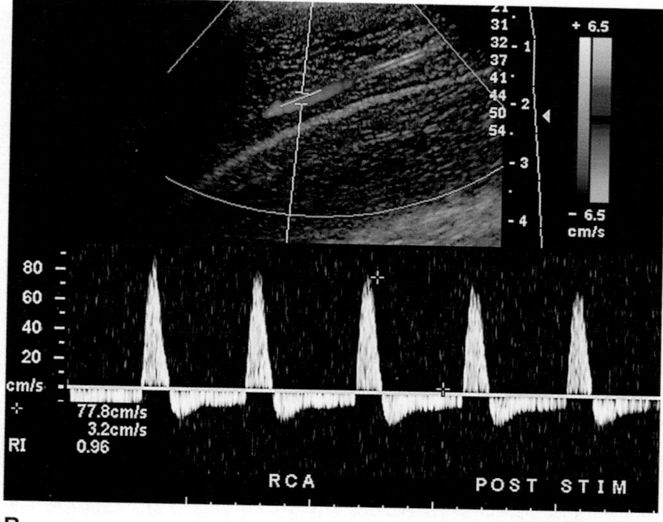

B

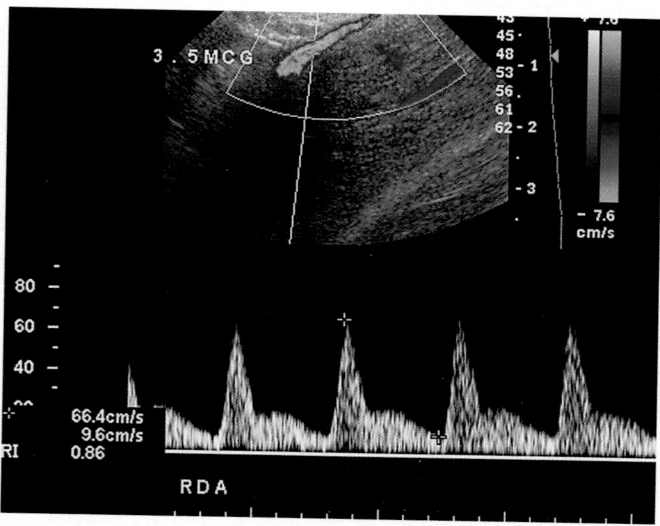

C

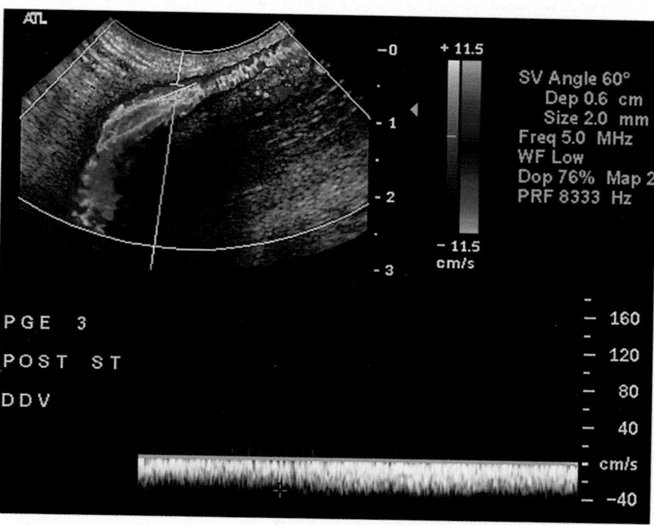

D

Figure 12-80 Normal US Appearance of the Penile Vessels
A. Coronal color Doppler image of the paired cavernosal arteries (*arrows*) demonstrating normal flow. **B.** Spectral Doppler tracing obtained from the right cavernosal artery 20 minutes following stimulation (injection of 3.5 µg of prostaglandin E-1) shows expected reversal of diastolic flow and a peak systolic velocity of >25 cm/s. **C.** Spectral Doppler tracing during erection obtained from a dorsal artery shows measurable diastolic flow, which is normal in the dorsal arteries, by contrast to the cavernosal arteries (B). **D.** Spectral Doppler tracing obtained following stimulation from the deep dorsal vein demonstrating a venous waveform, which may be present early post-stimulation, but should disappear as erection progresses.

decades of life, most commonly arising from the skin of the glans penis in 48% of patients. SCC is far more common in uncircumcised men, presumably as a result of chronic irritation from smegma. Therefore, circumcision in the neonatal period is considered a well-established prophylactic measure for penile carcinoma. Infection with human papilloma viruses 16 and 18 is an additional risk factor for the development of penile cancer.[104,107,111-119]

Sonographically, on grayscale imaging, SCC usually appears as a hypoechoic heterogeneous mass that may invade into the adjacent cavernosal bodies. In the region of the glans, invasion of subepithelial tissue is difficult to differentiate from invasion of the corpus spongiosum. However, elsewhere, deep invasion of the corpora cavernosa appears as interruption of the tunica albuginea, and early invasion may demonstrate focal thickening and decreased

---

Imaging Notes 12-23. Differentiating Features of Scrotal Wall Thickening

Squamous cell carcinoma is the most common malignancy of the penis typically arising from the skin of the glans penis and seen on the sixth and seventh decades of life.

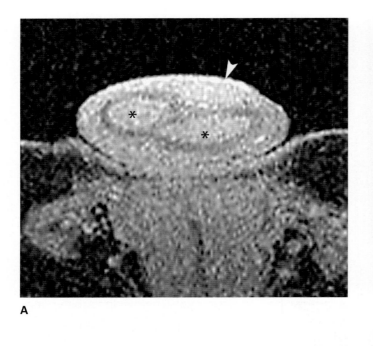

A

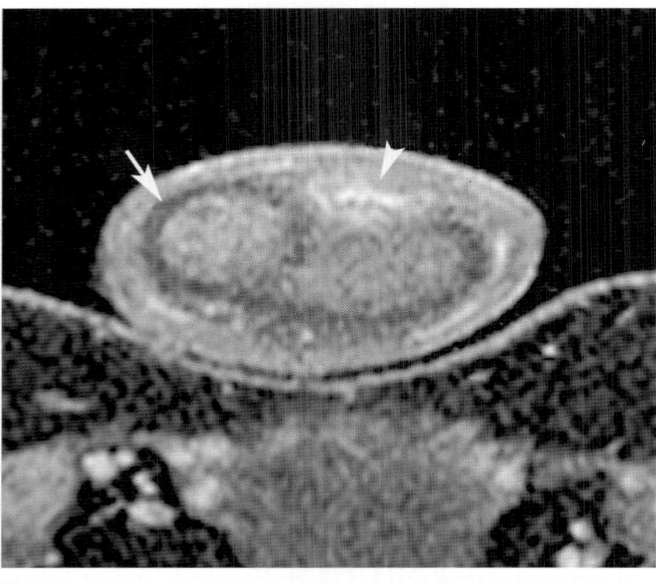

B

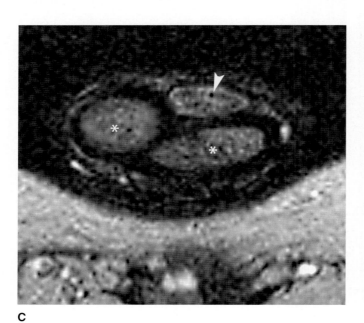

C

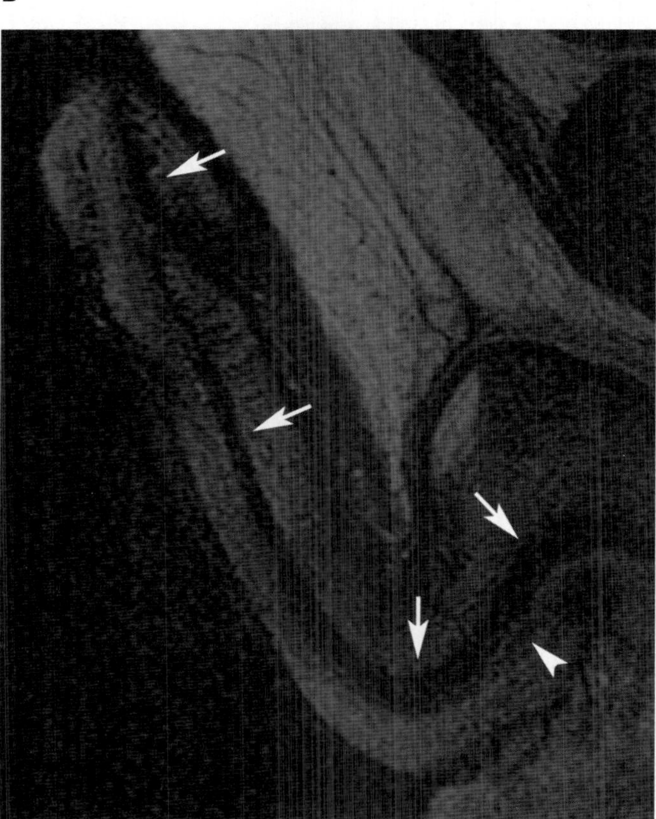

D

Figure 12-81 Normal MRI appearance of the Penis
A. Axial T1-weighted MRI of the penis with fat suppression demonstrating the intermediate-signal-intensity corpora cavernosa (*asterisks*) and corpus spongiosum (*arrowhead*). The thin, hypointense line surrounding the corpora cavernosa represents the tunica albuginea. **B.** Axial T1-weighted MRI of the penis with fat suppression obtained after the administration of gadolinium-containing contrast material demonstrating enhancement of the paired corpora cavernosa and corpora spongiosum. The tunica albuginea (*white arrow*) is thickened around the corpora cavernosa where it joins with Buck's fascia. The flattened urethra (*arrowhead*) is located centrally within the corpora spongiosum. **C.** Transverse T2-weighted MRI of the penis more clearly demonstrates the hypointense tunica albuginea surrounding the corpora cavernosa (*asterisks*) and corpus spongiosum (*arrowhead*). **D.** Sagittal T2-weighted MRI of the penis demonstrates the low signal tunica albuginea (*arrows*). The urethra is visible in the proximal corpora spongiosum (*arrowhead*).

Table 12-15. Causes of Solid Lesions of the Penis

1. Malignant neoplasms a. Penile shaft i. Squamous cell carcinoma ii. Melanoma iii. Epithelioid sarcoma iv. Leiomyosarcoma v. Rhabdosarcoma vi. Kaposi sarcoma b. Urethra i. Squamous cell carcinoma ii. Transitional cell carcinoma iii. Adenocarcinoma c. Metastasis
2. Benign neoplasms a. Penile shaft i. Hemangioma ii. Neurofibroma b. Urethra i. Fibrovascular polyp ii. Hemangioma
3. Fibrous plaques a. Peyronie disease b. Trauma (accidental and iatrogenic) c. Injection of intracavernosal drugs
4. Partial cavernosal thrombosis.

echogenicity of an intact tunica at the point of contact with the adjacent lesion. Color Doppler evaluation generally does not provide much additional information, other than to confirm that a penile lesion is solid. Nonetheless, it has been reported that SCC typically demonstrates poor vascularization, although associated inflammation may result in increased vascularity.[120-123]

On MRI, SCC of the penis is typically hypointense on both T1- and T2-weighted sequences with poor enhancement after the administration of gadolinium contrast material compared to the corpora. However, associated inflammation can result in areas of increased signal intensity on T2-weighted sequences with marked enhancement. Both T2-weighted and gadolinium-enhanced images can be used to determine the presence and extent of invasion of the corpora. Lymphatic drainage of SCC is via pelvic lymph node chains. The location of the primary lesion determines whether spread is via superficial inguinal nodes (shaft), deep inguinal nodes (glans and shaft), external iliac nodes (glans), or internal iliac nodes (urethra). Because there is significant communication between the lymphatic channels, bilateral lymphadenopathy can be seen with a unilateral tumor.[124]

There is no universally accepted staging system for primary penile carcinoma, and both the TNM and Jackson systems are used (Table 12-16). Tumors involving the glans and distal shaft are typically managed with partial penectomy to preserve a cosmetically acceptable and functional penis. Proximal tumors involving the base of the penis can require total penectomy. Surgical margins of 1 to 2 cm have been advocated to reduce the rate of local recurrence. Radiation therapy can be used as an alternative to surgery in young men with small (<3 cm), superficial, exophytic lesions or noninvasive cancers on the glans or distal shaft. Bilateral pelvic lymphadenectomy is necessary when nodes are palpable or appear abnormal or enlarged on CT or MRI. Patients with superficial tumors (not invasive of corpora) have a 95% 3-year survival rate following

Table 12-16. Staging System for Penile Cancer

TNM system of staging penile cancer	
TX	Primary tumor cannot be assessed
T0	No evidence of primary tumor
Ta	Noninvasive verrucous carcinoma
Tis	Carcinoma in situ
T1	Tumor invades subepithelial connective tissue
T2	Tumor invades corpora cavernosa or spongiosum
T3	Tumor invades the urethra or prostate
T4	Tumor invades other adjacent structures
NX	Regional lymph nodes cannot be assessed
N0	No regional lymph node metastases
N1	Metastasis in a single superficial inguinal lymph node
N2	Metastasis in multiple or bilateral superficial inguinal lymph nodes
MX	Presence of distant metastases cannot be assessed
N3	Extranodal extension of lymph node metastasis or pelvic lymph node(s) unilateral or bilateral
M0	No distant metastases
M1	Distant metastases
Jackson classification for staging penile cancer	
Stage I	Tumor is confined to the glans, prepuce, or both
Stage II	Tumor extends onto the shaft of the penis
Stage III	Tumor has inguinal metastasis that is operable
Stage IV	Tumor involves adjacent structures and is associated with inoperable inguinal metastasis or distant metastasis

Adapted from references 104 and 158.

penectomy. Survival decreases markedly with cavernosal invasion or with spread to regional lymph node chains.[125-131]

Nonsquamous penile malignancies

The remaining 5% of nonsquamous primary carcinomas of the penis are penile melanomas and sarcomas, which include epithelioid sarcoma, Kaposi sarcoma, leiomyosarcoma, and rhabdomyosarcoma in children.

Clinically, the diagnosis of primary penile melanoma is usually clear. Nonetheless, melanoma may sometimes be differentiated from SCC by MRI as it can appear hyperintense to skin on T1-weighted sequences because of the high melanin content of the lesion, and the tumor is usually avidly enhancing.

Rhabdomyosarcomas are aggressive tumors that primarily occur in the pediatric population. On MRI, these lesions generally appear isointense on T1-weighted sequences and hyperintense on T2-weighted sequences compared to skeletal muscle, with heterogeneous enhancement after administration of gadolinium contrast material.

Primary Kaposi sarcoma of the penis is extremely rare and usually seen with other synchronous cutaneous, mucosal, and visceral lesions in the setting of a history of HIV. The appearance has not been described on MRI.

Leiomyosarcomas arise from smooth muscle, either in the glans or in the corpora cavernosa, with the latter metastasizing early due to their proximity to the vasculature of the penis (see Figure 12-82).

Epithelioid sarcomas are rare malignant soft-tissue neoplasms with only about 15 cases reported in the literature. Patients present with a slowly growing palpable plaque or nodule that may or may not have caused penile deviation and can be associated with erectile dysfunction, which can therefore be clinically confused with Peyronie disease. The MRI and US features are not specific; however, a clue to the diagnosis of epithelioid sarcoma is the presence of multiple satellite nodules in the penile shaft between the primary lesion and local lymph nodes. Additionally, the plaques of Peyronie disease are always connected to the tunica albuginea and never completely intracavernosal.[114,119]

Penile Metastasis

Metastases to the penis are uncommon and indicate poor prognosis by virtue of the fact that they represent distant organ spread. Genitourinary tumors such as prostate and bladder cancer are the most common primary malignancies to metastasize to the penis, although metastases from the colon, stomach, esophagus, and pancreas have been reported. Metastases to the penile shaft can appear as circumscribed tumor nodules within the corpora cavernosa, diffuse infiltration, or both. In most cases, 1 or more discrete enhancing masses are seen in the corpora cavernosa. Metastatic infiltration of the normal venous drainage pathways can cause venous stasis and thrombosis, resulting in *malignant priapism*. Concomitant imaging of the pelvis in some cases will reveal a genitourinary or rectosigmoid primary tumor or adenopathy, or may reveal direct tumor invasion of the penis by prostate and bladder cancer (see Figure 12-83).[104,107]

Benign neoplasms of the penis

Benign neoplasms of the penis are very rare, and include mostly tumors of the subcutaneous tissues, including lipomas, hemangiomas, and nerve sheath tumors, among other rare things. Penile lipomas appear as a fat signal lesion in the subcutaneous tissues of the penis on MRI. A penile hemangioma appears as a focal hypoechoic mass on

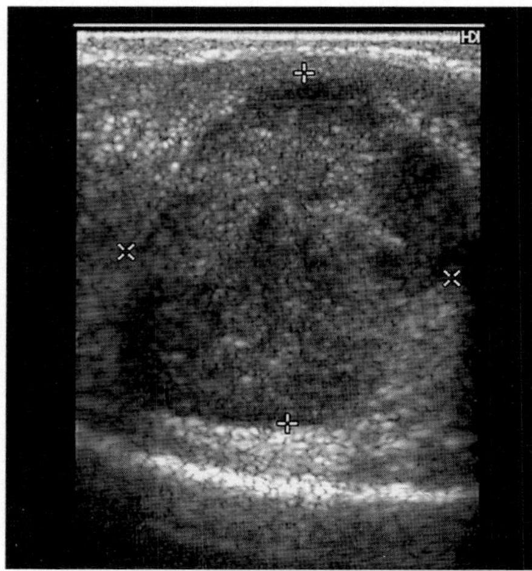

A

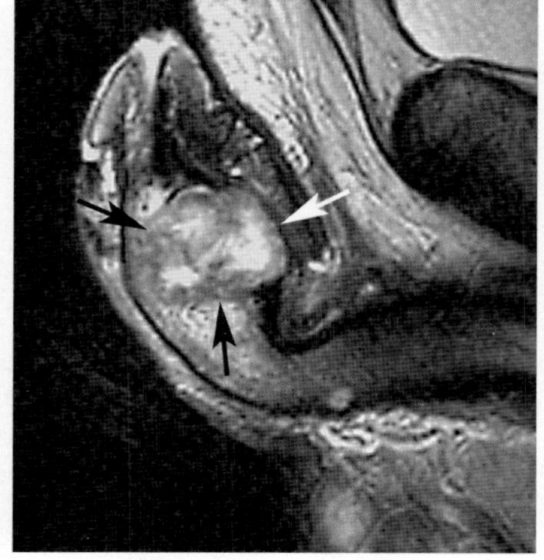

B

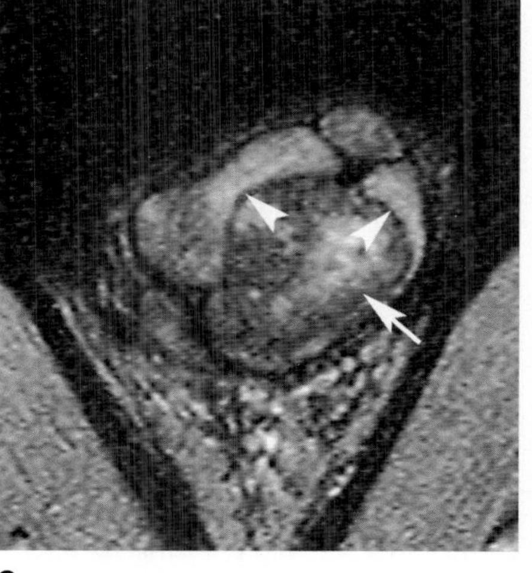

C

Figure 12-82 Penile Sarcoma
A. Sagittal grayscale image demonstrating a hypoechoic mass centered on the corpora cavernosa. **B.** Sagittal T2-weighted image showing a heterogeneous mass (*white and black arrows*) invading the corpora cavernosa. **C.** Axial T2-weighted MRI image demonstrating a heterogeneous mass (*arrow*) centered in the region of the corpora cavernosa (*arrowheads*). Surgically proven to represent a penile leiomyosarcoma.

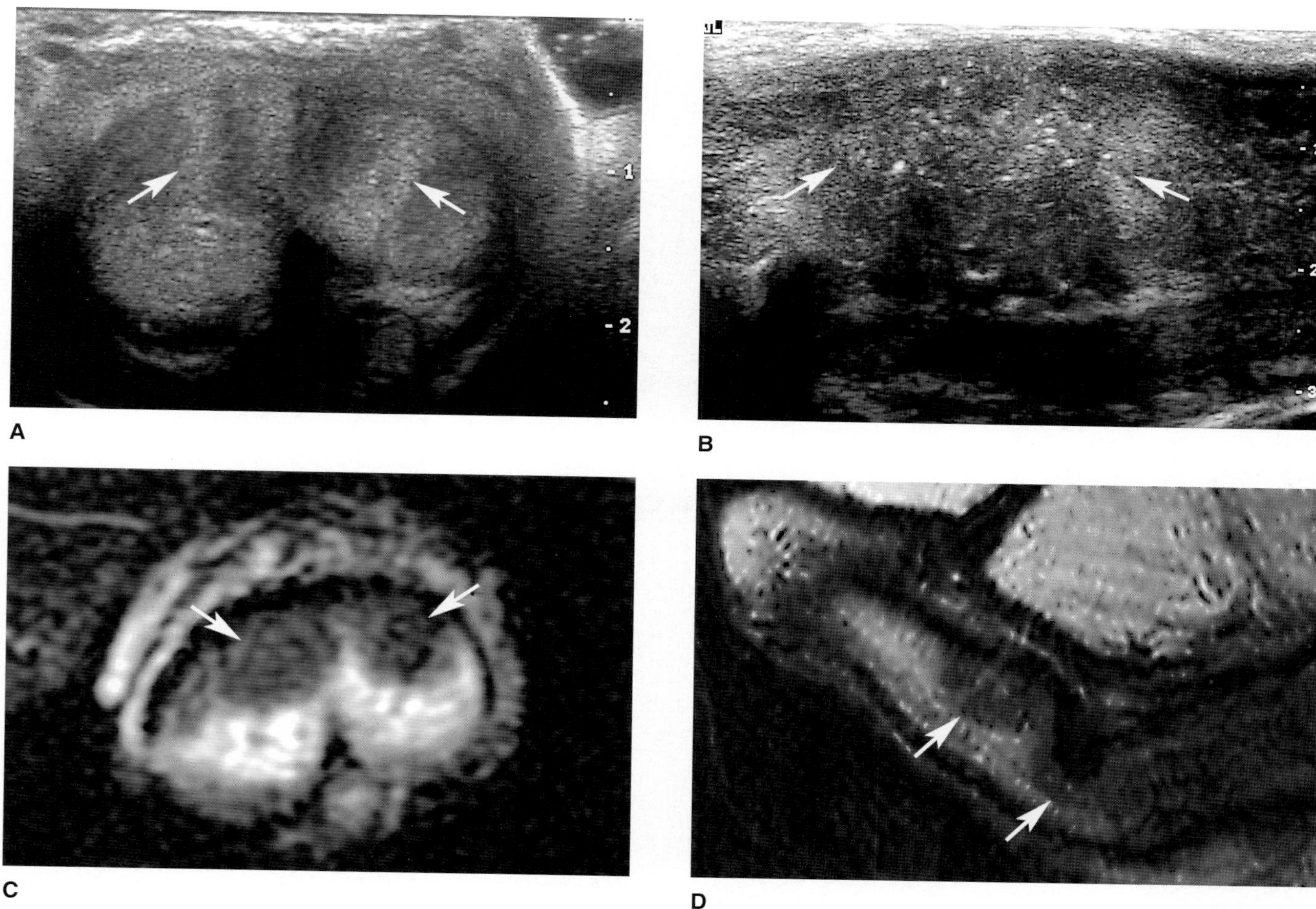

Figure 12-83 Penile Metastasis
A. Transverse and (B) sagittal grayscale images of the penis show masses (*arrows*) within both corpora cavernosa resulting in distortion of normal echotexture. C. Axial T2-weighted MRI demonstrates low-signal-intensity masses (*arrows*) in the corpora cavernosa, representing colon cancer metastasis. D. Sagittal T2-weighted image demonstrating low-signal-intensity colon cancer metastases (*arrows*) in the corpus cavernosa.

US (which sometimes is compressible) and demonstrates high signal intensity on T2-weighted sequences. A penile nerve sheath tumor is similar in appearance on MRI to nerve sheath tumors elsewhere in the body, demonstrating low signal intensity on T1-weighted sequences and high signal intensity on T2-weighted sequences. On ultrasound, nerve sheath tumors typically appear as hypoechoic masses, which may sometimes have thorough transmission (see Figure 12-84).[132-134]

Urethral neoplasms

Benign and malignant neoplasms of the urethra can appear as a penile mass centered on the urethra on US and MRI examinations of the penis. These include squamous cell carcinoma, transitional cell carcinoma, metastases, adenocarcinoma, fibroepithelial polyps, and extension of cancers of adjacent organs including the prostate, penis, and bladder. These disorders are discussed in Chapter 7: **Imaging of the Urinary System** (see Figure 12-85).

Peyronie's disease and other causes of penile fibrosis

Peyronie's disease is characterized by the formation of fibrous plaques within the tunica albuginea and adjacent corpus cavernosum from chronic inflammation, causing varying degrees of penile deformity and pain. The fibrin-containing plaques can be the result of aberrant healing

Imaging Notes 12-24. Peyronie's disease

Peyronie's disease, abnormal curvature of the erect penis, is caused by fibrous plaques of the tunica albuginea that are seen as echogenic thickening or calcified foci of the tunica albuginea on US exams and as focal hypointense thickening of the tunica albuginea on MRI exams.

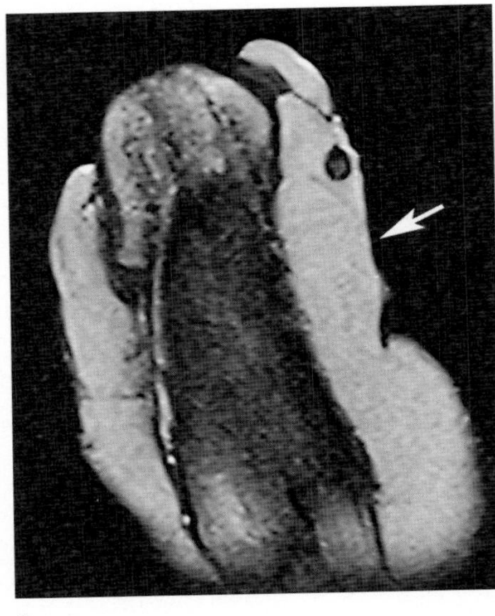

A

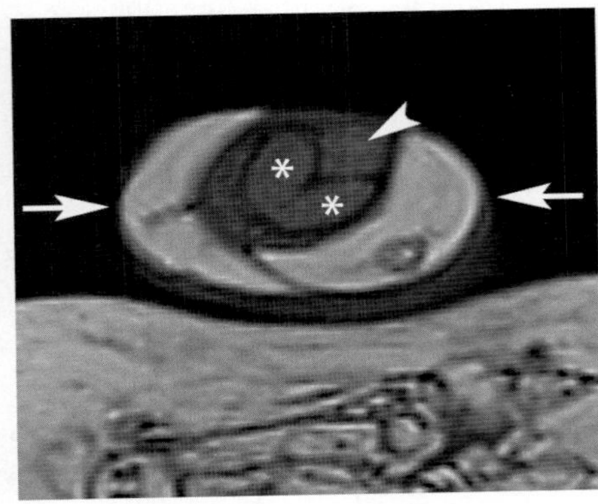

B

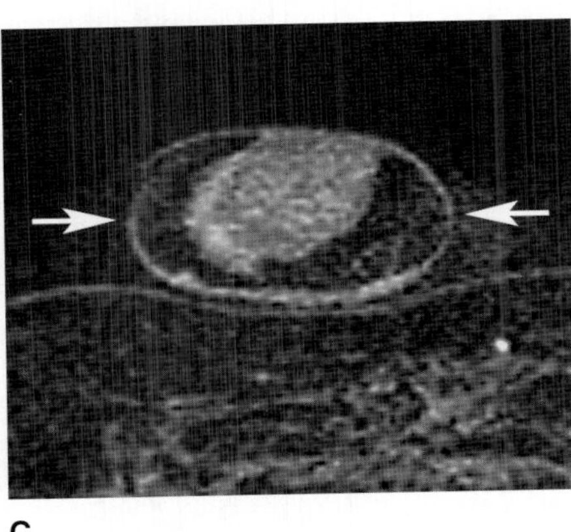

C

Figure 12-84 Penile Lipoma
Coronal T2-weighted image (**A**) demonstrates expansion of the tissues (*arrow*) surrounding the penile shaft. Axial T1-weighted images without (**B**) and with (**C**) fat saturation demonstrate that the expanded tissues (*arrows*) lose signal with fat saturation (C) in keeping with fatty composition, typical of a lipoma. Note the corpora cavernosa (*asterisks* in B) and corpora spongiosum (*arrowhead*, B).

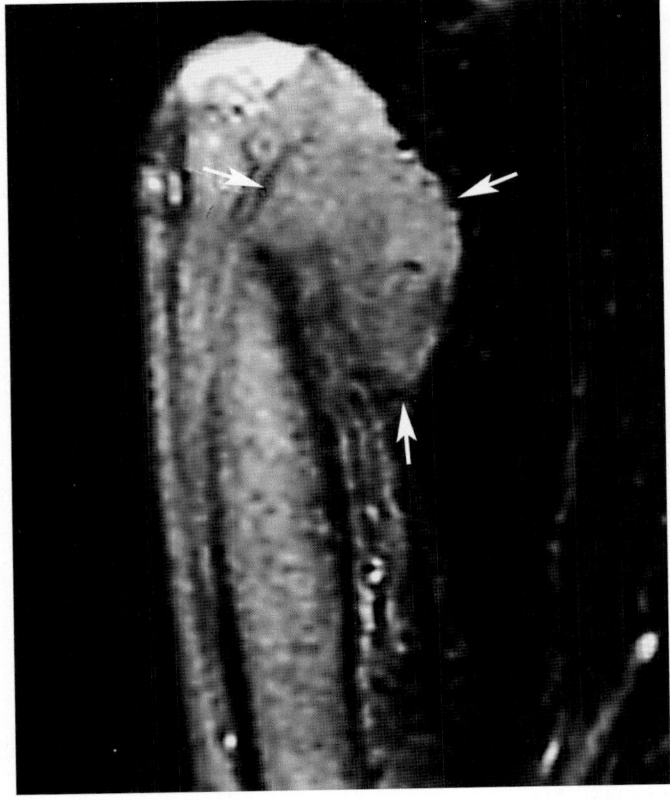

A

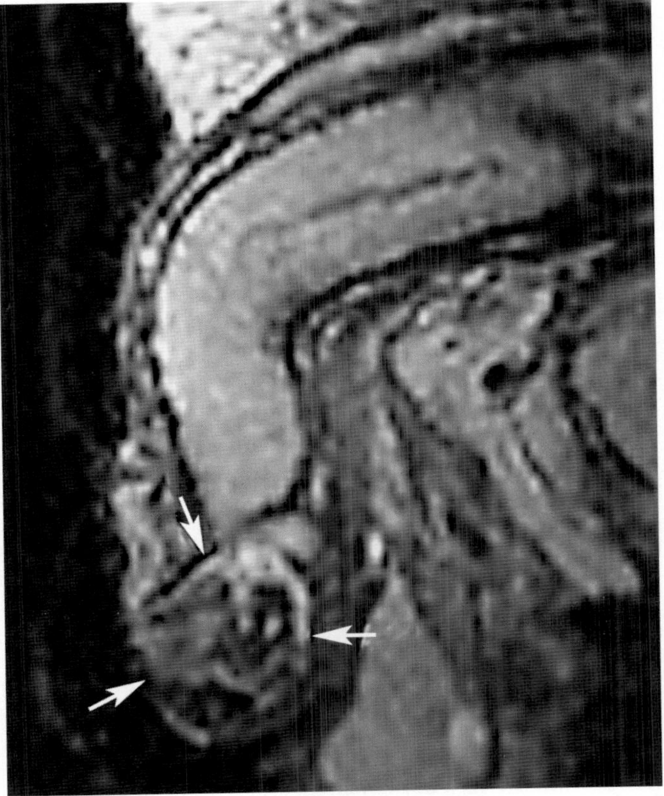

B

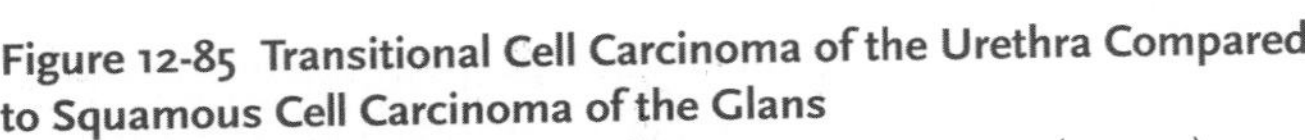

Figure 12-85 Transitional Cell Carcinoma of the Urethra Compared to Squamous Cell Carcinoma of the Glans
A. Sagittal T2-weighted image demonstrates a mass (*arrows*) involving the glans, pathologically proven to represent squamous cell carcinoma (SCC) of the penis. **B.** Sagittal T2-weighted image in a different patient demonstrates a similar-appearing mass (*arrows*, compare to A) located in the region of the glans, but pathology revealed transitional cell carcinoma (TCC) of the urethra, not SCC.

in response to minor penile trauma. Clinical features of Peyronie's disease include painful erection, penile deviation, and erectile dysfunction. The acute phase typically lasts for 6 to 18 months and is usually characterized by pain during erection. This is followed by the chronic phase with mature scar formation, resulting in painless penile deformity.

US and MRI are similar in their ability to demonstrate Peyronie's plaques, as well as the relationship of the plaques to adjacent structures such as the cavernosal and dorsal arteries. Plaques are more commonly located on the dorsal aspect of the penis but can be found on the ventral or lateral aspect. They can extend into the intercavernosal septum, or even into cavernosal sinusoids. Fibrous plaques appear as focal areas of thickening in the tunica albuginea that are usually hyperechoic on sonograms and are typically low in signal intensity on both T1- and T2-weighted sequences on MRI.[104,105,107,135,136] Fibrous plaques may eventually calcify, in which case they may also be visible on radiography or CT scan (see Figure 12-86).

Although the most common cause of penile fibrosis is Peyronie's disease, fibrosis can also occur with prolonged priapism, after trauma, after the removal of a penile prosthesis and with the use of intracavernosal drugs for erectile dysfunction (see Figure 12-87).[137]

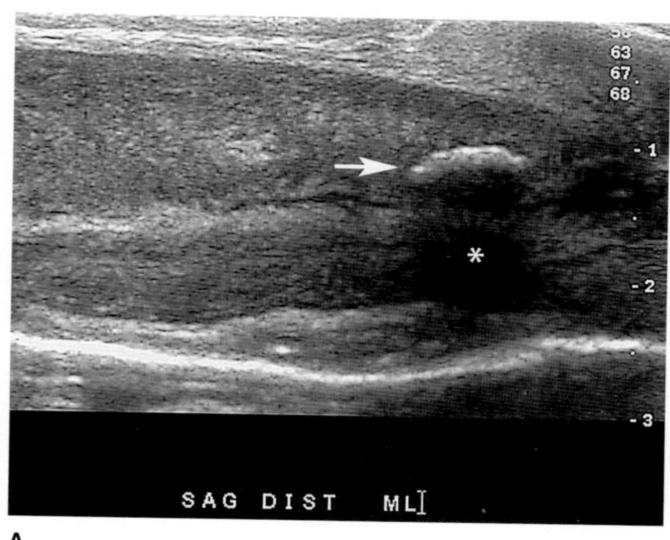

A

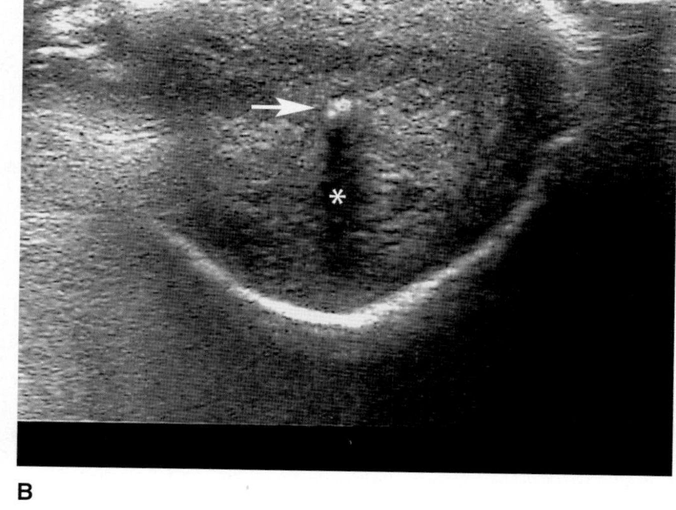

B

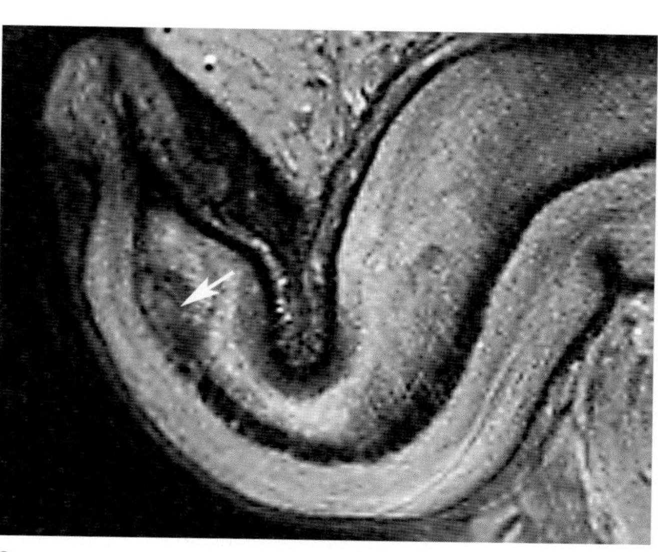

C

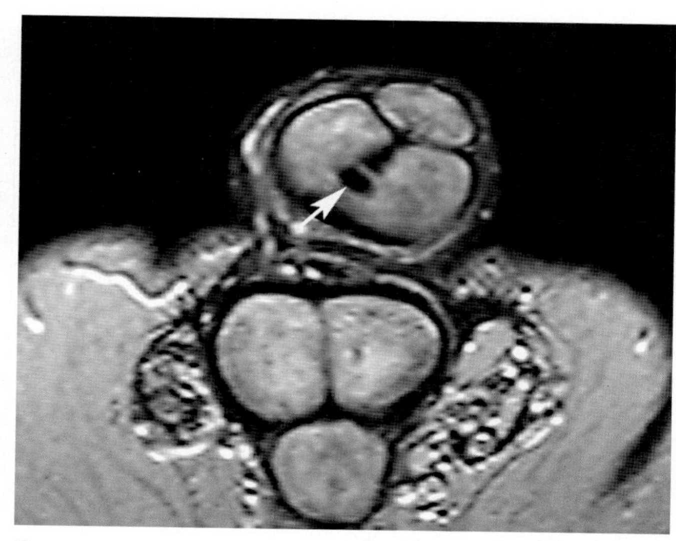

D

Figure 12-86 Peyronie Disease
A. Sagittal and (B) transverse grayscale images demonstrate a calcified plaque (*arrow*) with posterior acoustic shadowing (*asterisk*) representing a Peyronie's plaque in a 30-year-old male with painful erections. C. Sagittal T2-weighted and (D) axial T2-weighted MRI images demonstrate low-signal-intensity thickening of the tunica albuginea (*arrow*) between the corpora cavernosa, representing a Peyronie plaque.

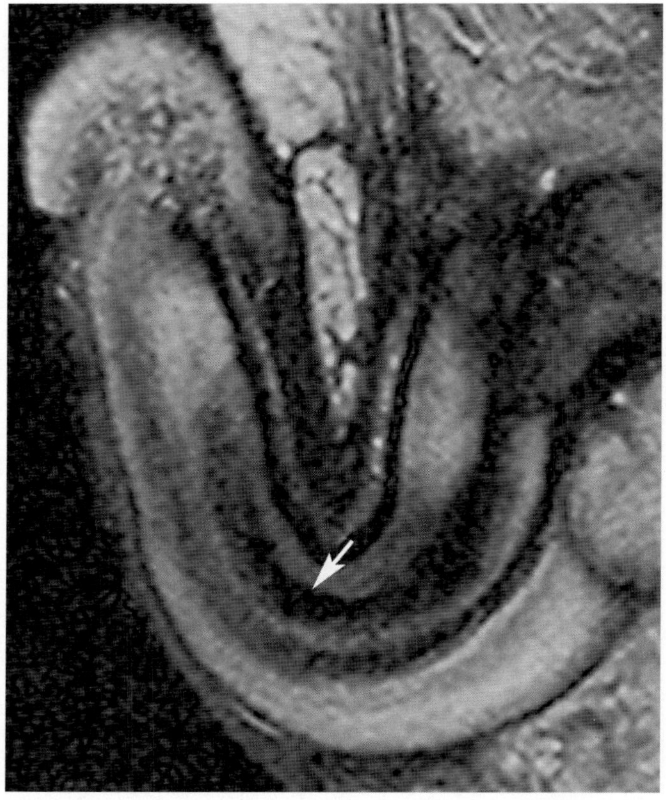

A

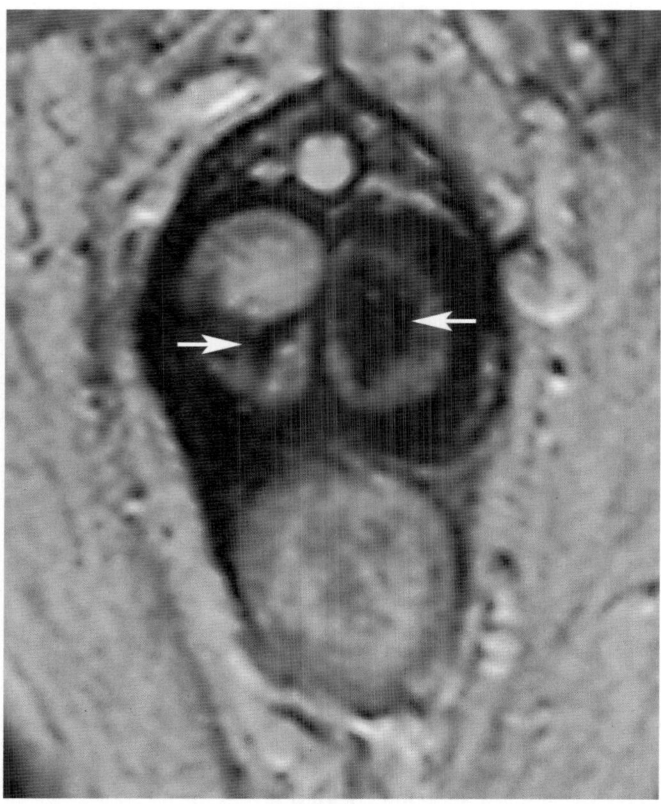

B

Figure 12-87 Fibrosis from Penile Implant
Seven months after removal of a penile prosthesis this patient noted deformity of his penis. **A**. Sagittal and (**B**) coronal T2-weighted MRI images demonstrate linear low-signal-intensity within the corpora cavernosa (*arrows*), representing fibrosis from the corporal cylinders of the prior penile prosthesis.

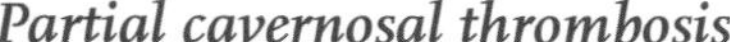

Partial cavernosal thrombosis

Partial cavernosal thrombosis can appear as a focal lesion within the penile shaft. Causes include trauma, not uncommonly related to cycling, hypercoagulable states, and vigorous intercourse. In some cases, no cause is identified. Patients will typically present with partial priapism, pain, palpable lump, or induration of the penile shaft. Sonographic evaluation demonstrates expansion and heterogeneity of the involved segment of the corpora cavernosa without detectable flow on color Doppler. At MRI, the signal intensity of the affected corpora is generally hyperintense on T1-weighted sequences and hypointense on T2-weighted sequences relative to the normal cavernosum, although the signal intensity is dependent on the age of the thrombus. Thrombosed blood in the affected corpora can cause distension and compression of the adjacent contralateral corpora cavernosa. Administration of gadolinium contrast material reveals the absence of enhancement in the affected segment. Conservative management is generally advocated because complete resolution of symptoms and return of normal erectile function are reported in most cases (see Figure 12-88).[103-105,107,138-140]

Cystic-Appearing Periurethral Lesions

There are a variety of cystic lesions of the penis, including Cowper duct syringocele, urethral diverticula, periurethral abscess, fistulas, and urethral duplications. These disorders are all related to the urethra and are discussed in Chapter 7: **Imaging of the Urinary System**.

UNIQUE PENILE DISORDERS

Unique disorders of the penis include penile fracture, dorsal vein thrombosis, priapism, and Peyronie disease.

Penile Trauma

Trauma to the **flaccid** penis usually results in extratunical or cavernosal hematoma, without fracture. Penile fracture is an uncommon urologic emergency caused by the exertion of axial forces on the **erect** penis, tearing the tunica albuginea and resulting in rupture of the corpus cavernosum. Penile fracture most often occurs during sexual intercourse, but can sometimes occur during masturbation or

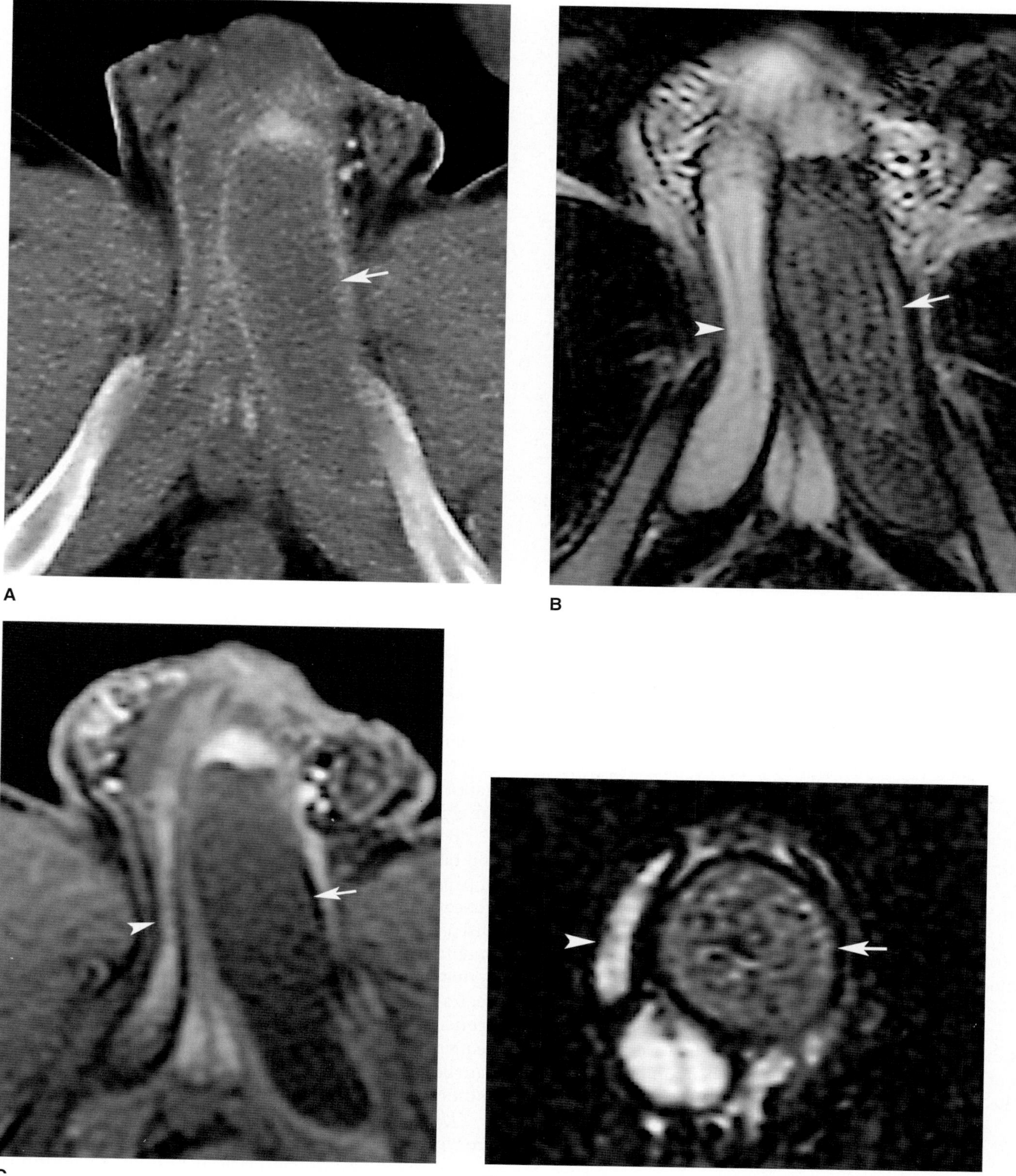

Figure 12-88 Partial Cavernosal Thrombosis
A. Axial contrast-enhanced CT image from a patient with a perineal mass demonstrating partial thrombosis of the left corpora cavernosum (*arrow*). **B.** Axial T2-weighted MRI image demonstrating low-signal-intensity distension (*arrow*) of the left corpus cavernosum, representing partial cavernosal thrombosis. Note compression of the contralateral corpora cavernosa (*arrowhead*). **C.** Axial T1-weighted MRI image obtained after intravenous administration of gadolinium demonstrates lack of enhancement of the partially thrombosed left corpus cavernosum (*arrow*). Note normal enhancement of the compressed contralateral corpus cavernosum (*arrowhead*). **D.** Coronal T2-weighted MRI image with fat suppression demonstrates expansion of the partially thrombosed corpus cavernosum (*arrow*) and compression of the contralateral cavernosum (*arrowhead*).

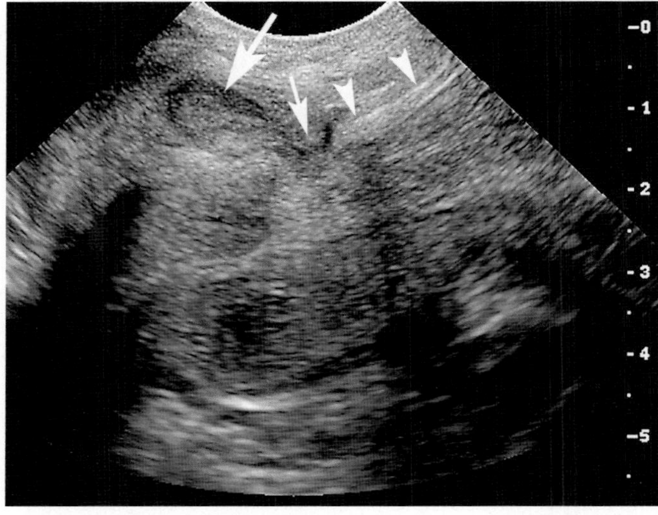

A

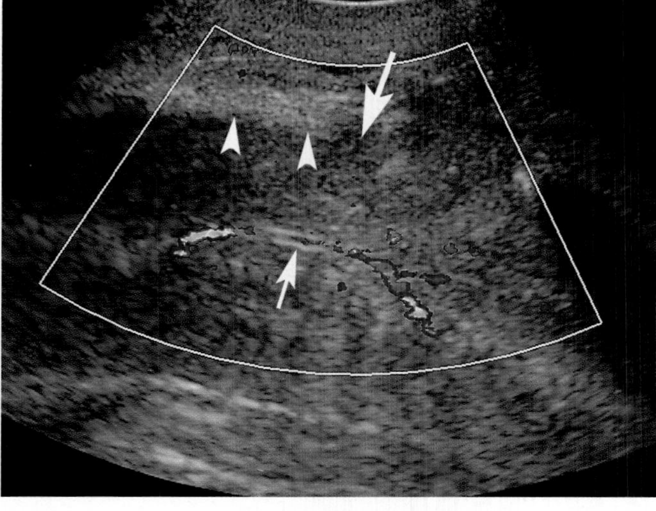

B

Figure 12-89 Penile Fracture
This 29-year-old patient suffered acute pain during intercourse. **A.** Coronal grayscale image demonstrates disruption (*thin arrow*) of the tunica albuginea (*arrowheads*) with hematoma (*thick arrow*). **B.** Coronal color Doppler image shows disruption (*thick arrow*) of the tunica albuginea (*arrowheads*) with an intact cavernosal artery (*thin arrow*).

even after rolling over in bed with an erect penis. Patients with penile fractures often describe a popping or cracking sensation with sharp pain followed by immediate detumescence, swelling, and discoloration, resulting in the so-called eggplant deformity. Penile fractures generally occur in the proximal or midshaft penis. Typically only 1 of the paired corpora cavernosa is injured, although bilateral involvement can also occur.[105,141-148] Additionally, urethral injury is associated with penile fracture in 10% to 20% of cases and can present with inability to urinate or urethrorrhagia.

The integrity of the tunica albuginea is the most important factor in determining the need for surgical intervention, as surgical repair is generally recommended if there is a tear of the tunica or if there is a urethral injury. The use of sonography may be limited because of severe pain and swelling at the site of injury; however, the exact site of the tear may be visualized on US as an interruption of the thin echogenic line of the tunica albuginea. This is usually associated with an irregular hypoechoic or hyperechoic mass, reflecting hematoma and cavernosal rupture, by which penile fracture can be suspected even if the tunical defect is not directly seen. Routine sonography does not directly demonstrate urethral defects; however, urethral trauma should be suspected if there is hematoma or gas in the corpora spongiosum (see Figure 12-89).

Because of multiplanar capabilities and excellent tissue contrast, MRI is more accurate than US in the identification of penile fractures and tears of the tunica albuginea, but is not commonly used due to expense and lack of availability. Discontinuity of the low-signal-intensity tunica albuginea on either T1- or T2-weighted sequences with interspersed hematoma indicates tear and is typically identified in the ventral portion of the corpus cavernosum. T1-weighted sequences are in some cases preferable to T2-weighted sequences to evaluate for tunical tear because hematomas can be low signal intensity on T2-weighted sequences, mimicking an intact tunica albuginea.

Unlike penile fractures, intracavernosal hematomas are typically bilateral and occur when the base of the penis is compacted against the pelvic bones. On US examinations, penile hematomas appear as hyperechoic or complex masses in the acute phase, and become cystic with septations as the hematoma evolves. On MRI examinations, acute intracavernosal hematomas may be isointense to the corpora cavernosa but can be identified as enhancement defects after the administration of contrast agent, although contrast is not routinely indicated. Associated anterior urethral tear can also be identified at MRI (see Figure 12-90).[104,105,110,144,146-152]

Imaging Notes 12-25. Imaging Features of Penile Fracture

1. Disruption or discontinuity of the tunica albuginea (diagnostic of penile fracture)
2. Irregular heterogeneous mass adjacent to the corpora cavernosa (suggestive of penile fracture)

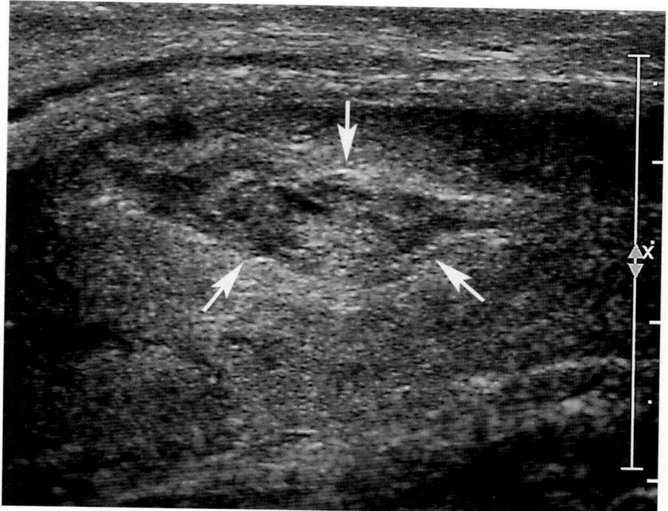

A

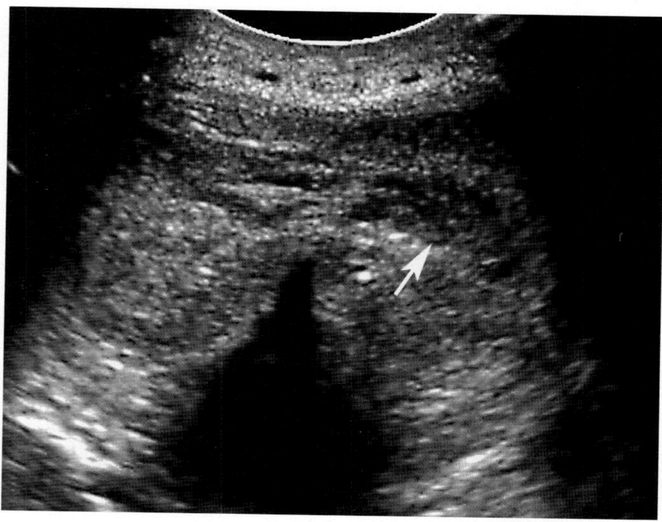

B

Figure 12-90 Intracavernosal Hematoma
This 26-year-old male had direct perineal trauma. **A.** Sagittal and (**B**) transverse grayscale images demonstrate a heterogeneous, hypoechoic mass (*arrows*) of the corpora cavernosa consistent with an intracavernosal hematoma.

Dorsal Vein Thrombosis

Dorsal vein thrombosis usually involves the superficial dorsal vein (Mondor's disease). It can be associated with trauma, hypercoagulable states, or vigorous intercourse, but in some cases occurs without known cause. Patients typically present with painful induration in the dorsal aspect of the penile shaft. US is indicated to exclude other lesions and confirm the clinical diagnosis. On color and spectral Doppler evaluation, no flow is detectable in the vein if the clot is occlusive. On grayscale imaging, the presence of thrombus makes the normally compressible dorsal vein enlarged and noncompressible. MRI is not typically performed. Spontaneous resolution can occur in 6 to 8 weeks, with treatment consisting of fibrinolytics, anticoagulation, and discontinuance of sexual activity.[104,107,153,154]

Priapism

Priapism is a defined by abnormal persistent, often painful, erection of the penis. High-flow priapism is characterized by the presence of forward flow in the cavernosal arteries of >25 cm/s and is usually due to the presence of a fistula between the cavernosal artery and the vascular spaces of the corpus cavernosum, known as an arterial-lacunar fistula. Patients usually present days or weeks after an injury with a painless nonrigid erection due to unregulated arterial inflow into the sinusoidal spaces. Grayscale US may reveal an irregular hypoechogenic region in the corpus cavernosum due to enlarged vascular spaces or tissue injury. Color Doppler shows a blush of turbulent flow extending from a feeding artery into the cavernosal tissues, with increased low-resistance flow in the cavernosal artery on spectral Doppler. High-flow priapism is generally not a surgical emergency (see Figure 12-91).[155]

Low-flow (ischemic) priapism results from sinusoidal thrombosis and veno-occlusion and manifests as a painful, rigid erection. Doppler sonography reveals high-resistance, low-velocity flow in the cavernosal arteries as well as little or no detectable flow in the deep dorsal vein. On grayscale imaging, the sinusoids will be engorged and of low or mixed echogenicity and can demonstrate lack of compressibility depending on the completeness of sinusoidal thrombosis. Low-flow priapism represents a urologic emergency, as severe cellular damage and long-term erectile dysfunction due to cavernosal fibrosis will result if it left untreated (see Figure 12-92).[156]

Imaging Notes 12-26. Clinical and Imaging Features of Priapism

High Flow:	1. Fistula between the cavernosal artery and the corpus cavernosum 2. Painless, nonrigid erection 3. Cavernosal artery flow >25 cm/s
Low Flow:	1. Sinusoidal thrombosis and venous occlusion 2. Painful, rigid erection 3. Cavernosal artery flow: high resistance, low velocity 4. Venous flow: Minimal or absent

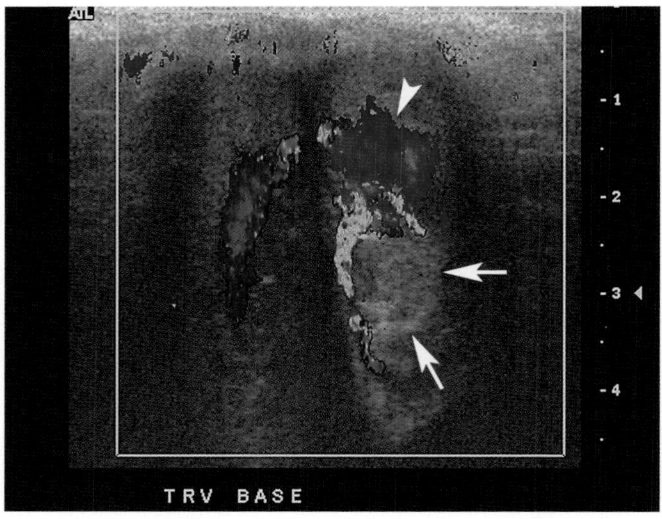

A

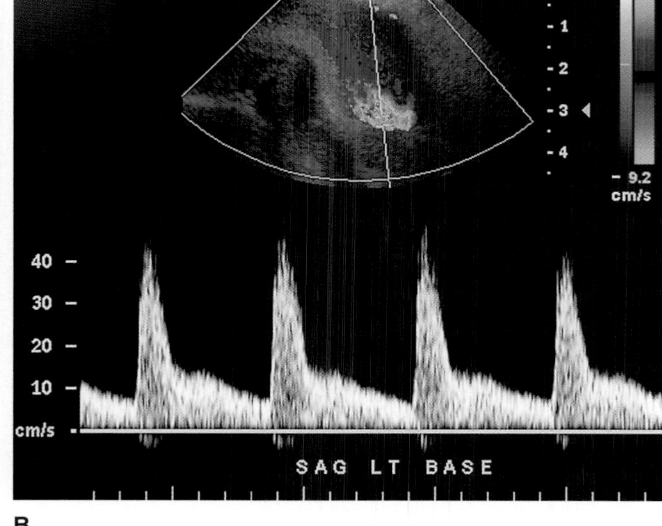

B

Figure 12-91 Arterial-lacunar Fistula
A. Color Doppler transverse image in a patient with partial priapism a few days following straddle injury demonstrates a hyperechogenic hematoma in the left corpora cavernosa (*arrows*) adjacent to an area of disorganized flow (*arrowhead*) which shows low resistance on spectral Doppler (**B**), in keeping with a cavernosal-lacunar fistula in the setting of high-flow priapism.

Peyronie's Disease

Peyronie's disease is a common disorder of the penis that typically results in a characteristic curved deformity of the penile shaft when erect. This disorder is caused by fibrous plaques within the tunica albuginea that appear as a focal lesion. This is discussed previously under the heading: **Solid Lesions of the Penis.**

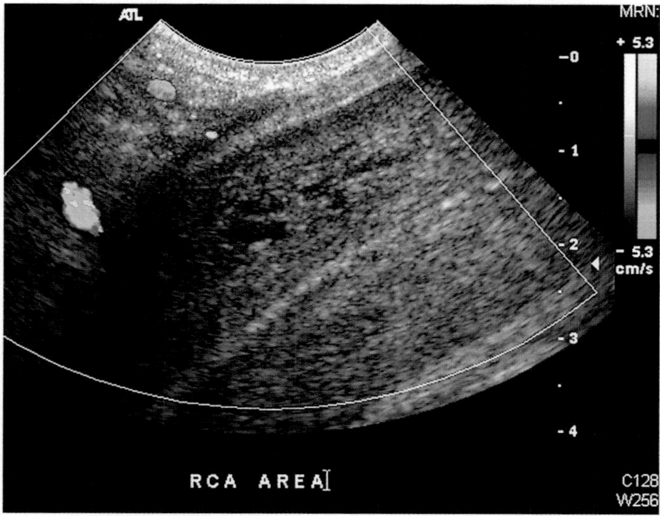

Figure 12-92 Low Flow Priapism
Sagittal color Doppler image obtained of one of the cavernosal bodies in a patient with priapism lasting >30 hours, showing no detectable flow in the cavernosal artery, in keeping with low flow priapism.

Imaging Evaluation of Erectile Dysfunction

Erectile dysfunction is defined as the persistent or repeated inability to attain or maintain an erection sufficient for satisfactory sexual performance, with a duration of at least 6 months. The pathophysiology of erectile dysfunction is complex with many potential contributing organic and psychogenic factors, a discussion of which is beyond the scope of this review. Sonographic penile flow evaluation is just one component of the evaluation of erectile dysfunction, which must encompass the complete sequence of male sexual function. US is used to evaluate the arterial and venous flow patterns within the erect penis to distinguish between arterial and venous causes of erectile dysfunction.

In a penile flow study, grayscale, color Doppler and spectral Doppler evaluation of penis are performed in the flaccid state. A vasoactive agent is then injected into the penis to stimulate penile erection and the peak systolic velocities in the cavernosal arteries (as well as the arterial diameter) are recorded every 5 minutes. The dorsal penile arteries and deep dorsal vein are also assessed on spectral Doppler.

The average peak systolic velocity (PSV) in the cavernosal arteries after cavernosal injection of vasoactive substances is approximately 30 to 40 cm/s. A PSV of less than 25 cm/s with a dampened waveform in the cavernosal artery is the standard criterion for a diagnosis of arterial insufficiency. Other findings of arterial insufficiency include (1) dilation of the cavernosal artery by less than 75%, (2) asymmetry of cavernosal peak systolic velocities by >10 cm/s, (3) focal stenosis or retrograde flow in a cavernosal artery (CA), (4) acceleration time of >100

Imaging Notes 12-27. Sonographic Evaluation of Erectile Dysfunction

Arterial Insufficiency

Primary criteria:	1. Peak **systolic** velocity in the cavernosal artery <25 cm/s following cavernosal injection of vasoactive substance with a dampened waveform
Secondary criteria:	1. Less than 75% dilation of the cavernosal artery 2. >10 cm/s difference in cavernosal peak systolic velocities 3. Focal stenosis/retrograde flow in cavernosal artery 4. Acceleration time >100 ms in the cavernosal artery 5. Peak systolic velocity <10 cm/s in the cavernosal arteries in flaccid state

Venous Insufficiency:

Primary criteria:	1. Arterial **diastolic** velocity >5 cm/s throughout all phases of erection (cavernosal arteries)
Secondary criteria:	1. Persistent flow in the deep dorsal vein 2. Resistive index in the cavernosal arteries less than 0.75 measured 20 min after cavernosal injection of vasoactive substance

Note: Venous insufficiency cannot be accurately diagnosed by US in the setting of arterial insufficiency.

ms, and (5) a PSV of less than 10 cm/s in the cavernosal artery in the flaccid state. The peak systolic velocities in the dorsal arteries are also measured for comparison and usually are similar to those in the cavernosal arteries. Normal PSV in the dorsal arteries with low cavernosal artery velocities suggests intrapenile arteriogenic disease whereas low velocities in the both the dorsal and cavernosal arteries suggests more proximal arterial disease (see Figure 12-93).

Normally, there is no diastolic flow in the cavernosal arteries during the tumescent phase of erection. An arterial diastolic velocity of >5 cm/s throughout all phases of erection is abnormal and indicates persistent arterial diastolic flow, a finding that suggests venous leak if the patient has normal arterial function. Venous leak/insufficiency can also be suggested by persistent flow in the deep dorsal vein. Note that in the setting of arterial insufficiency, the cavernosal sinusoids may never fill to the point of occluding the veins, resulting in persistent venous flow even in the setting of normal veins, and therefore venous insufficiency cannot be accurately diagnosed by US in the setting of arterial insufficiency (see Figure 12-94).[157]

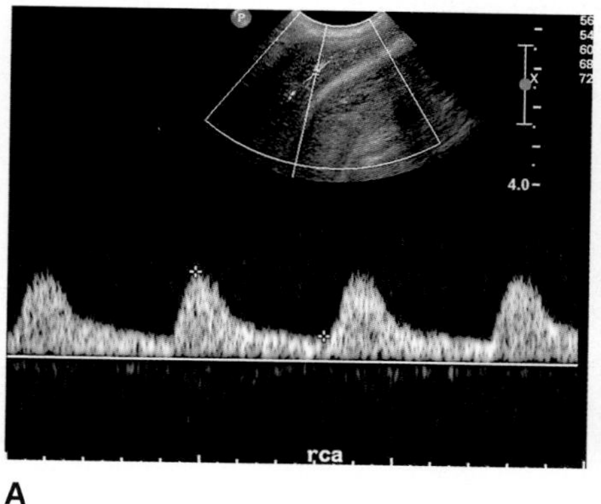

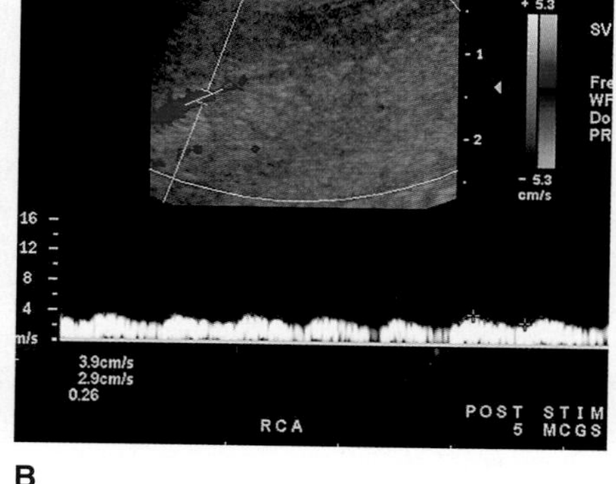

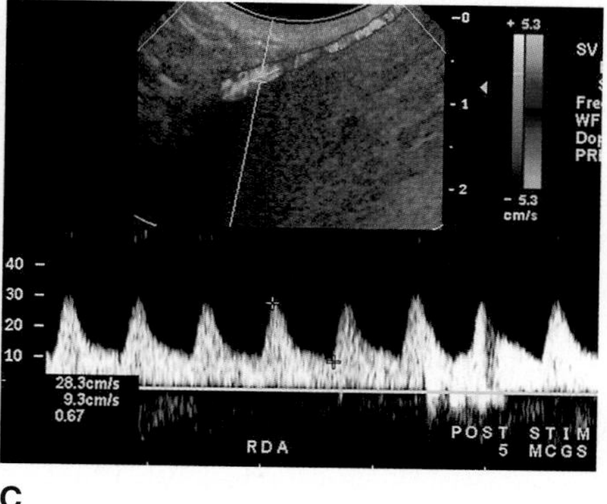

Figure 12-93 Penile Arterial Insufficiency in 2 Patients
A. Spectral Doppler waveform obtained from sampling the right cavernosal artery following stimulation demonstrates a tardus parvus appearance with abnormally low peak systolic velocity of 12.1 cm/s (normal > 25 cm/s). Similar waveforms were obtained from the left cavernosal artery and from the dorsal arteries, indicative of arterial insufficiency proximal to the penis. **B.** Spectral Doppler waveform obtained from the right cavernosal artery in a different patient following stimulation shows a parvus tardus appearance with very low peak systolic velocity, in keeping with arterial insufficiency. However, the spectral Doppler wave from the right dorsal artery is normal (**C**), suggesting intrapenile arterial disease.

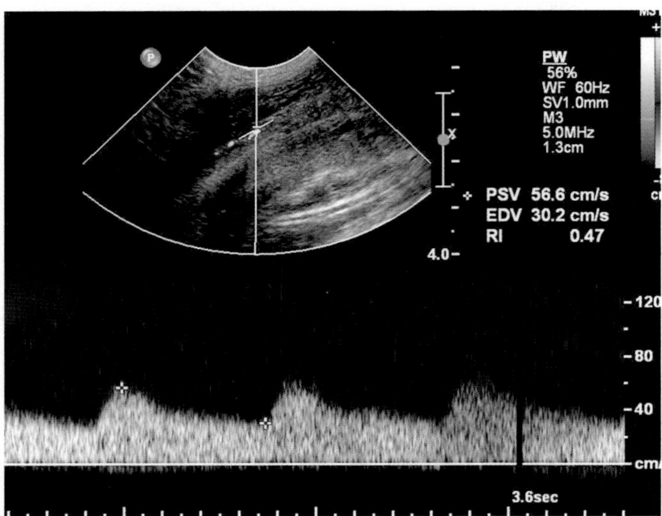

Figure 12-94 Penile Venous Insufficiency
Spectral Doppler waveform obtained from the cavernosal artery following stimulation demonstrates persistent elevated diastolic flow, a finding of venous leak/insufficiency, assuming normal arterial inflow.

REFERENCES

1. Dogra VS, Gottlieb RH, Oka M, Rubens DJ. Sonography of the scrotum. *Radiology.* 2003;227:18-36.
2. Lee JC, Bhatt S, Dogra VS. Imaging of the epididymis. *Ultrasound Q.* 2008;24:3-16.
3. Gerscovich EO. Scrotal Ultrasound Measurements. In: Goldberg BB, McGahan JP, eds. *Atlas of Ultrasound Measurements.* 2nd ed. Philadelphia, PA: Mosby Elsevier; 2006:375-381.
4. Kim W, Rosen MA, Langer JE, Banner MP, Siegelman ES, Ramchandani P. US MR imaging correlation in pathologic conditions of the scrotum. *Radiographics.* 2007;27:1239-1253.
5. Langer JE. Ultrasound of the scrotum. *Semin Roentgenol.* 1993;28:5-18.
6. Epstein JI. Chapter 21—the lower urinary tract and male genital system. In: Kumar V, Abbas AK, Fausto N, eds. *Kumar: Robbins and Cotran: Pathologic Basis of Disease.* 7th ed. Philadelphia, PA: Elsevier Saunders; 2005.
7. Woodward PJ, Sohaey R, O'Donoghue MJ, Green DE. From the archives of the AFIP: tumors and tumorlike lesions of the testis: radiologic-pathologic correlation. *Radiographics.* 2002;22:189-216.
8. Sohaib SA, Koh D-M, Husband JE. The role of imaging in the diagnosis, staging, and management of testicular cancer. *Am J Roentgenol.* 2008;191:387-395.
9. Kocakoc E, Bhatt S, Dogra VS. Ultrasound evaluation of testicular neoplasms. *Ultrasound Clin.* 2007;2:27-44.
10. Ryan CJ, Small EJ, Torti FM. Chapter 90—testicular cancer. In: Abeloff MB, Armitage MD, Niederhuber JO, Kastan JE, eds. *Abeloff's Clinical Oncology.* 4th ed. Philadelphia, PA: Churchill Livingstone Elsevier; 2008.
11. Tsili AC, Tsampoulas C, Giannakopoulos X, et al. MRI in the histologic characterization of testicular neoplasms. *Am J Roentgenol.* 2007;189:W331-W337.
12. Lorigan JG, Eftekhari F, David CL, Shirkhoda A. The growing teratoma syndrome: an unusual manifestation of treated, nonseminomatous germ cell tumors of the testis. *Am J Roentgenol.* 1988;151:325-329.
13. Aide N, Comoz F, Sevin E. Enlarging residual mass after treatment of a nonseminomatous germ cell tumor: growing teratoma syndrome or cancer recurrence? *J Clin Oncol.* 2007;25:4494-4496.
14. Woodward PJ, Schwab CM, Sesterhenn IA. From the archives of the AFIP: extratesticular scrotal masses: radiologic-pathologic correlation. *Radiographics.* 2003; 23:215-240.
15. Maizlin ZV, Belenky A, Kunichezky M, Sandbank J, Strauss S. Leydig cell tumors of the testis: grayscale and color Doppler sonographic appearance. *J Ultrasound Med.* 2004;23:959-964.
16. Fernandez GC, Tardaguila F, Rivas C, et al. MRI in the diagnosis of testicular Leydig cell tumour. *Br J Radiol.* 2004;77:521-524.
17. Maizlin ZV, Belenky A, Baniel J, Gottlieb P, Sandbank J, Strauss S. Epidermoid cyst and teratoma of the testis: sonographic and histologic similarities. *J Ultrasound Med.* 2005;24:1403-1409.
18. Mazzu D, Jeffrey RB Jr, Ralls PW. Lymphoma and leukemia involving the testicles: findings on gray-scale and color Doppler sonography. *Am J Roentgenol.* 1995;164:645-647.
19. Akin EA, Khati NJ, Hill MC. Ultrasound of the scrotum. *Ultrasound Q.* 2004;20:181-199.
20. Zicherman JM, Weissman D, Gribbin C, Epstein R. Best cases from the AFIP: primary diffuse large B-cell lymphoma of the epididymis and testis. *Radiographics.* 2005;25:243-248.
21. Stoffel TJ, Nesbit ME, Levitt SH. Extramedullary involvement of the testes in childhood leukemia. *Cancer.* 1975;35:1203-1211.
22. Lupetin AR, King W 3rd, Rich P, Lederman RB. Ultrasound diagnosis of testicular leukemia. *Radiology.* 1983;146:171-172.
23. Dambro TJ, Stewart RR, Carroll BA. Chapter 24: the scrotum. In: Rumack CM, Wilson SR, Charboneau JW, eds. *Diagnostic Ultrasound.* St Louis, MO: Mosby; 1998:791-821.
24. Muttarak M, Peh WCG. Case 91: tuberculous epididymo-orchitis. *Radiology.* 2006;238:748-751.
25. Drudi FM, Laghi A, Iannicelli E, et al. Tubercular epididymitis and orchitis: US patterns. *Eur Radiol.* 1997;7:1076-1078.
26. Muttarak M, Peh WCG, Lojanapiwat B, Chaiwun B. Tuberculous epididymitis and epididymo-orchitis: sonographic appearances. *Am J Roentgenol.* 2001;176:1459-1466.
27. Dogra VS, Gottlieb RH, Rubens DJ, Liao L. Benign intratesticular cystic lesions: US features. *Radiographics.* 2001;21:S273-S281.
28. Turgut AT, Bhatt S, Dogra VS. Acute painful scrotum. *Ultrasound Clin.* 2008;3:93-107.
29. Stewart VR, Sidhu PS. The testis: the unusual, the rare and the bizarre. *Clin Radiol.* 2007;62:289-302.
30. Gerscovich EO, Bateni CP, Kazemaini MR, Gillen MA, Visis T. Reversal of diastolic blood flow in the testis of a patient with impending infarction due to epididymitis. *J Ultrasound Med.* 2008;27:1643-1646.
31. Holloway BJ, Belcher HE, Letourneau JG, Kunberger LE. Scrotal sonography: a valuable tool in the evaluation of complications following inguinal hernia repair. *J Clin Ultrasound.* 1998;26:341-344.

32. Fernandez-Perez GC, Tardaguila FM, Velasco M, et al. Radiologic findings of segmental testicular infarction. *Am J Roentgenol.* 2005;184:1587-1593.
33. Ulbright TM, Young RH. Metastatic carcinoma to the testis: a clinicopathologic analysis of 26 nonincidental cases with emphasis on deceptive features. *Am J Surg Pathol.* 2008;32:1683-1693.
34. Dieckmann KP, Boeckmann W, Brosig W, Jonas D, Bauer HW. Bilateral testicular germ cell tumors. Report of nine cases and review of the literature. *Cancer.* 1986;57:1254-1258.
35. Adham WK, Raval BK, Uzquiano MC, Lemos LB. Best cases from the AFIP: bilateral testicular tumors: seminoma and mixed germ cell tumor. *Radiographics.* 2005;25:835-839.
36. Winter TC 3rd, Keener TS, Mack LA. Sonographic appearance of testicular sarcoid. *J Ultrasound Med.* 1995;14:153-156.
37. Carucci LR, Tirkes AT, Pretorius ES, Genega EM, Weinstein SP. Testicular Leydig's cell hyperplasia: MR imaging and sonographic findings. *Am J Roentgenol.* 2003; 180:501-503.
38. Dogra V, Nathan J, Bhatt S. Sonographic appearance of testicular adrenal rest tissue in congenital adrenal hyperplasia. *J Ultrasound Med.* 2004;23:979-981.
39. Avila NA, Premkumar A, Shawker TH, Jones JV, Laue L, Cutler GB Jr. Testicular adrenal rest tissue in congenital adrenal hyperplasia: findings at Gray-scale and color Doppler US. *Radiology.* 1996;198:99-104.
40. Nagamine WH, Mehta SV, Vade A. Testicular adrenal rest tumors in a patient with congenital adrenal hyperplasia: sonographic and magnetic resonance imaging findings. *J Ultrasound Med.* 2005;24:1717-1720.
41. Ors F, Lev-Toaff A, O'Kane P, Qazi N, Bergin D. Paraovarian adrenal rest with MRI features characteristic of an adrenal adenoma. *Br J Radiol.* 2007;80:e205-e208.
42. Hamm B, Fobbe F, Loy V. Testicular cysts: differentiation with US and clinical findings. *Radiology.* 1988;168:19-23.
43. Chen SS, Chou YH, Hsu CC, Tiu CM, Chang TE. Simple testicular cyst [in Chinese]. *Zhonghua Yi Xue Za Zhi.* (Taipei) 1990;46:285-288.
44. Rubenstein RA, Dogra VS, Seftel AD, Resnick MI. Benign intrascrotal lesions. *J Urol.* 2004;171:1765-1772.
45. Brown DL, Benson CB, Doherty FJ, et al. Cystic testicular mass caused by dilated rete testis: sonographic findings in 31 cases. *Am J Roentgenol.* 1992;158:1257-1259.
46. Smith SJ, Vogelzang RL, Smith WM, Moran MJ. Papillary adenocarcinoma of the rete testis: sonographic findings. *Am J Roentgenol.* 1987;148:1147-1148.
47. Gabriel H, Marko J, Nikolaidis P. Cystadenoma of the rete testis: sonographic appearance. *Am J Roentgenol.* 2007;189:W67-W69.
48. Cho CS, Kosek J. Cystic dysplasia of the testis: sonographic and pathologic findings. *Radiology.* 1985;156:777-778.
49. Das KM, Prasad K, Szmigielski W, Noorani N. Intratesticular varicocele: evaluation using conventional and Doppler sonography. *Am J Roentgenol.* 1999;173:1079-1083.
50. Kessler A, Meirsdorf S, Graif M, Gottlieb P, Strauss S. Intratesticular varicocele: grayscale and color Doppler sonographic appearance. *J Ultrasound Med.* 2005;24: 1711-1716.
51. Caesar RE, Kaplan GW. Incidence of the bell-clapper deformity in an autopsy series. *Urology.* 1994;44:114-116.
52. Middleton WD, Middleton MA, Dierks M, Keetch D, Dierks S. Sonographic prediction of viability in testicular torsion: preliminary observations. *J Ultrasound Med.* 1997;16:23-27; quiz 29-30.
53. Vijayaraghavan SB. Sonographic differential diagnosis of acute scrotum: real-time whirlpool sign, a key sign of torsion. *J Ultrasound Med.* 2006;25:563-574.
54. Horstman WG, Middleton WD, Melson GL, Siegel BA. Color Doppler US of the scrotum. *Radiographics.* 1991;11: 941-957.
55. Burks DD, Markey BJ, Burkhard TK, Balsara ZN, Haluszka MM, Canning DA. Suspected testicular torsion and ischemia: evaluation with color Doppler sonography. *Radiology.* 1990;175:815-821.
56. Deurdulian C, Mittelstaedt CA, Chong WK, Fielding JR. US of acute scrotal trauma: optimal technique, imaging findings, and management. *Radiographics.* 2007;27:357-369.
57. Phillips G, Kumari-Subaiya S, Sawitsky A. Ultrasonic evaluation of the scrotum in lymphoproliferative disease. *J Ultrasound Med.* 1987;6:169-175.
58. Harris RD, Chouteau C, Partrick M, Schned A. Prevalence and significance of heterogeneous testes revealed on sonography: ex vivo sonographic–pathologic correlation. *Am J Roentgenol.* 2000;175:347-352.
59. Casalino DD, Kim R. Clinical importance of a unilateral striated pattern seen on sonography of the testicle. *Am J Roentgenol.* 2002;178:927-930.
60. Dogra VS, Rubens DJ, Gottlieb RH, Bhatt S. Torsion and beyond: new twists in spectral Doppler evaluation of the scrotum. *J Ultrasound Med.* 2004;23:1077-1085.
61. Patel MD, Silva AC. MRI of an adenomatoid tumor of the tunica albuginea. *AJR Am J Roentgenol.* 2004;182:415-417.
62. Akbar SA, Sayyed TA, Jafri SZH, Hasteh F, Neill JSA. Multimodality imaging of paratesticular neoplasms and their rare mimics. *Radiographics.* 2003;23:1461-1476.
63. Choyke PL, Glenn GM, Wagner JP, et al. Epididymal cystadenomas in von Hippel-Lindau disease. *Urology.* 1997;49:926-931.
64. Uppuluri S, Bhatt S, Tang P, Dogra VS. Clear cell papillary cystadenoma with sonographic and histopathologic correlation. *J Ultrasound Med.* 2006;25:1451-1453.
65. Alleman WG, Gorman B, King BF, Larson DR, Cheville JC, Nehra A. Benign and malignant epididymal masses evaluated with scrotal sonography: clinical and pathologic review of 85 patients. *J Ultrasound Med.* 2008;27:1195-1202.
66. Yang DM, Kim SH, Kim HN, et al. Differential diagnosis of focal epididymal lesions with grayscale sonographic, color Doppler sonographic, and clinical features. *J Ultrasound Med.* 2003;22:135-142.
67. Saginoya T, Yamaguchi K, Toda T, Kiyuna M. Fibrous pseudotumor of the scrotum: MR imaging findings. *AJR Am J Roentgenol.* 1996;167:285-286.
68. Beccia DJ, Krane RJ, Olsson CA. Clinical management of non-testicular intrascrotal tumors. *J Urol.* 1976; 116:476-479.
69. Frates MC, Benson CB, DiSalvo DN, Brown DL, Laing FC, Doubilet PM. Solid extratesticular masses evaluated with sonography: pathologic correlation. *Radiology.* 1997;204:43-46.
70. Cornud F, Belin X, Amar E, Delafontaine D, Helenon O, Moreau JF. Varicocele: strategies in diagnosis and treatment. *Eur Radiol.* 1999;9:536-545.

71. Aizenstein RI, Wilbur AC, O'Neil HK, Gerber B. Clinical image. MRI of scrotal hemangioma. *J Comput Assist Tomogr.* 1996;20:888-889.
72. Hwang S, Aronoff DR, Leonidas JC. Case 82: polyorchidism with torsion. *Radiology.* 2005;235:433-435.
73. Amodio JB, Maybody M, Slowotsky C, Fried K, Foresto C. Polyorchidism: report of 3 cases and review of the literature. *J Ultrasound Med.* 2004;23:951-957.
74. Bhosale PR, Patnana M, Viswanathan C, Szklaruk J. The inguinal canal: anatomy and imaging features of common and uncommon masses. *Radiographics.* 2008;28:819-835.
75. Aso C, Enriquez G, Fite M, et al. Gray-scale and color Doppler sonography of scrotal disorders in children: an update. *Radiographics.* 2005;25:1197-1214.
76. Schnall M. Magnetic resonance imaging of the scrotum. *Semin Roentgenol.* 1993;XXVIII:19-30.
77. Turkvatan A, Kelahmet E, Yazgan C, Olcer T. Sonographic findings in tuberculous epididymo-orchitis. *J Clin Ultrasound.* 2004;32:302-305.
78. Kim SH, Pollack HM, Cho KS, Pollack MS, Han MC. Tuberculous epididymitis and epididymo-orchitis: sonographic findings. *J Urol.* 1993;150:81-84.
79. Eraso CE, Vrachliotis TG, Cunningham JJ. Sonographic findings in testicular sarcoidosis simulating malignant nodule. *J Clin Ultrasound.* 1999;27:81-83.
80. Reinecks EZ, MacLennan GT. Sarcoidosis of the testis and epididymis. *J Urol.* 2008;179:1147.
81. Koyama T, Ueda H, Togashi K, Umeoka S, Kataoka M, Nagai S. Radiologic manifestations of sarcoidosis in various organs. *Radiographics.* 2004;24:87-104.
82. Reddy NM, Gerscovich EO, Jain KA, Le-Petross HT, Brock JM. Vasectomy-related changes on sonographic examination of the scrotum. *J Clin Ultrasound.* 2004;32:394-398.
83. Kousei Ishigami MMA-YYE-Z. Tubular ectasia of the epididymis: a sign of postvasectomy status. *J Clin Ultrasound.* 2005;33:447-451.
84. Leung ML, Gooding GA, Williams RD. High-resolution sonography of scrotal contents in asymptomatic subjects. *AJR Am J Roentgenol.* 1984;143:161-164.
85. Boyum J, Wasserman NF. Malignant mesothelioma of the tunica vaginalis testis: a case illustrating Doppler color flow imaging and its potential for preoperative diagnosis. *J Ultrasound Med.* 2008;27:1249-1255.
86. Tasu J-P, Faye N, Eschwege P, Rocher L, Blery M. Imaging of burned-out testis tumor: five new cases and review of the literature. *J Ultrasound Med.* 2003;22:515-521.
87. Frauscher F, Klauser A, Stenzl A, Helweg G, Amort B, zur Nedden D. US findings in the scrotum of extreme mountain bikers. *Radiology.* 2001;219:427-431.
88. Turgut AT, Kosar U, Kosar P, Karabulut A. Scrotal sonographic findings in equestrians. *J Ultrasound Med.* 2005;24:911-917.
89. van der Sluijs JW, den Hollander JC, Lequin MH, Nijman RM, Robben SG. Prenatal testicular torsion: diagnosis and natural course. An ultrasonographic study. *Eur Radiol.* 2004;14:250-255.
90. Bushby LH, Miller FN, Rosairo S, Clarke JL, Sidhu PS. Scrotal calcification: ultrasound appearances, distribution and aetiology. *Br J Radiol.* 2002;75:283-288.
91. Miller FN, Sidhu PS. Does testicular microlithiasis matter? A review. *Clin Radiol.* 2002;57:883-890.
92. Bennett HF, Middleton WD, Bullock AD, Teefey SA. Testicular microlithiasis: US follow-up. *Radiology.* 2001;218:359-363.
93. Kim B, Winter TC 3rd, Ryu JA. Testicular microlithiasis: clinical significance and review of the literature. *Eur Radiol.* 2003;13:2567-2576.
94. Backus ML, Mack LA, Middleton WD, King BF, Winter TC 3rd, True LD. Testicular microlithiasis: imaging appearances and pathologic correlation. *Radiology.* 1994;192:781-785.
95. Cast JEI, Nelson WM, Early AS, et al. Testicular Microlithiasis: Prevalence and tumor risk in a population referred for scrotal sonography. *Am J Roentgenol.* 2000;175:1703-1706.
96. Teefey SA. Ask the Expert: Microlithiasis to follow or not to follow. *Soc Radiol Ultrasound Newslett.* 2007;17:12.
97. Kane CJ, Nash P, McAninch JW. Ultrasonographic appearance of necrotizing gangrene: aid in early diagnosis. *Urology.* 1996;48:142-144.
98. Peterson AC, Bauman JM, Light DE, McMann LP, Costabile RA. The prevalence of testicular microlithiasis in an asymptomatic population of men 18 to 35 years old. *J Urol.* 2001;166:2061-2064.
99. Middleton WD, Teefey SA, Santillan CS. Testicular microlithiasis: prospective analysis of prevalence and associated tumor. *Radiology.* 2002;224:425-428.
100. Bach AM, Hann LE, Hadar O, et al. Testicular microlithiasis: what is its association with testicular cancer? *Radiology.* 2001;220:70-75.
101. Lam DL, Gerscovich EO, Kuo MC, McGahan JP. Testicular microlithiasis: our experience of 10 years. *J Ultrasound Med.* 2007;26:867-873.
102. DeCastro BJ, Peterson AC, Costabile RA. A 5-year followup study of asymptomatic men with testicular microlithiasis. *J Urol.* 2008;179:1420-1423; discussion 1423.
103. Siegelman ES. Body MRI. Philadelphia, PA: Elsevier; 2004.
104. Pretorius ES, Siegelman ES, Ramchandani P, Banner MP. MR imaging of the penis. *Radiographics.* 2001;21 Spec No: S283-298; discussion S298-S299.
105. Kirkham AP, Illing RO, Minhas S, Minhas S, Allen C. MR imaging of nonmalignant penile lesions. *Radiographics.* 2008. 28(3):837-853.
106. Dunnick NR, Sandler CM, Newhouse JH, Amis ES. *Textbook of Uroradiology.* 2007.
107. Bertolotto M, Pavlica P, Serafini G, Quaia E, Zappetti R. Painful penile induration: imaging findings and management. *Radiographics.* 2009;29:477-493.
108. Middleton WD, Kurtz AB. *Ultrasound: The Requisites. 2nd ed.* 2003.
109. Pavlica P, Barozzi L, Menchi I. Imaging of male urethra. *Eur Radiol.* 2003:13(7): 1583-1596.
110. Bhatt S, Kocakoc E, Rubens DJ, Seftel AD, Dogra VS. Sonographic evaluation of penile trauma. *J Ultrasound Med.* 2005;24(7):993-1000; quiz 1001.
111. Ryu J, Kim B. MR imaging of the male and female urethra. *Radiographics.* 2001;21:1169-1185.
112. Sica GT, Teeger S. MR imaging of scrotal, testicular, and penile diseases. *Magn Reson Imaging Clin N Am.* 1996;4(3): 545-563.

113. McCance DJ, Kalache A, Ashdown K, et al. Human papillomavirus types 16 and 18 in carcinomas of the penis from Brazil. *Int J Cancer.* 1986;37(1):55-59.

114. Mostofi FK, Davis CJ Jr, Sesterhenn IA. Carcinoma of the male and female urethra. *Urol Clin North Am.* 1992;19(2):347-358.

115. Lucia MS, Miller GJ. Histopathology of malignant lesions of the penis. *Urol Clin North Am.* 1992;19(2):227-246.

116. Oto A, Meyer J. MR appearance of penile epithelioid sarcoma. *AJR Am J Roentgenol.* 1999;172(2):555-556.

117. Isa SS, Almaraz R, Magovern J. Leiomyosarcoma of the penis. Case report and review of the literature. *Cancer.* 1984;54(5): 939-942.

118. Agrons GA, Wagner BJ, Lonergan GJ, Dickey GE, Kaufman MS. From the archives of the AFIP. Genitourinary rhabdomyosarcoma in children: radiologic-pathologic correlation. *Radiographics.* 1997;17(4):919-937.

119. Barnholtz-Sloan JS, Maldonado JL, Pow-sang J, Giuliano AR. Incidence trends in primary malignant penile cancer. *Urol Oncol.* 2007;25(5):361-367.

120. Agrawal A, Pai D, Ananthakrishnan N, Smile SR, Ratnakar C. Clinical and sonographic findings in carcinoma of the penis. *J Clin Ultrasound.* 2000;28(8):399-406.

121. Lont AP, Besnard AP, Gallee MP, van Tinteren H, Horenblas S. A comparison of physical examination and imaging in determining the extent of primary penile carcinoma. *BJU Int.* 2003;91(6):493-495.

122. Horenblas S, Kröger R, Gallee MP, Newling DW, van Tinteren H. Ultrasound in squamous cell carcinoma of the penis; a useful addition to clinical staging? A comparison of ultrasound with histopathology. *Urology.* 1994;43(5):702-707.

123. Bertolotto M, Serafini G, Dogliotti L, et al. Primary and secondary malignancies of the penis: ultrasound features. *Abdom Imaging.* 2005;30(1):108-112.

124. Vossough A, Pretorius ES, Siegelman ES, Ramchandani P, Banner MP. Magnetic resonance imaging of the penis. *Abdom Imaging.* 2002;27:640-659.

125. Bermejo C, Busby JE, Spiess PE, Heller L, Pagliaro LC, Pettaway CA. Neoadjuvant chemotherapy followed by aggressive surgical consolidation for metastatic penile squamous cell carcinoma. *J Urol.* 2007;177(4):1335-1338.

126. Ozsahin M, Jichlinski P, Weber DC, et al. Treatment of penile carcinoma: to cut or not to cut? *Int J Radiat Oncol Biol Phys.* 2006;66(3):674-679.

127. Bouchot O, Rigaud J, Maillet F, Hetet JF, Karam G. Morbidity of inguinal lymphadenectomy for invasive penile carcinoma. *Eur Urol.* 2004;45(6):761-765; discussion 765-766.

128. d'Ancona CA, de Lucena RG, Querne FA, Martins MH, Denardi F, Netto NR Jr. Long-term followup of penile carcinoma treated with penectomy and bilateral modified inguinal lymphadenectomy. *J Urol.* 2004;172(2):498-501; discussion 501.

129. Brown CT, Minhas S, Ralph DJ. Conservative surgery for penile cancer: subtotal glans excision without grafting. *BJU Int.* 2005;96(6)911-912.

130. Burgers JK, Badalament RA, Drago JR. Penile cancer. Clinical presentation, diagnosis, and staging. *Urol Clin North Am.* 1992;19(2):247-256.

131. Busby JE, Pettaway CA. What's new in the management of penile cancer? *Curr Opin Urol.* 2005;15(5):350-357.

132. Forstner R, Hricak H, Kalbhen CL, Kogan BA, McAninch JW. Magnetic resonance imaging of vascular lesions of the scrotum and penis. *Urology.* 1995;46(4):581-583.

133. Kim SH, Lee SE, Han MC. Penile hemangioma: US and MR imaging demonstration. *Urol Radiol.* 1991;13(2):126-128.

134. Niku SD, Mattrey RF, Kalota SJ, Schmidt JD. MRI of pelvic neurofibromatosis. *Abdom Imaging.* 1995;20(2):176-178.

135. Jalkut M, Gonzalez-Cadavid N, Rajfer J. Peyronie's Disease: A Review. *Rev Urol.* 2003;5(3):142-148.

136. Hauck EW, Hackstein N, Vosshenrich R, et al. Diagnostic value of magnetic resonance imaging in Peyronie's disease—a comparison both with palpation and ultrasound in the evaluation of plaque formation. *Eur Urol.* 2003;43(3):293-299; discussion 299-300.

137. Moemen MN, Hamed HA, Kamel II, Shamloul RM, Ghanem HM. Clinical and sonographic assessment of the side effects of intracavernous injection of vasoactive substances. *Int J Impot Res.* 2004;16:143-145.

138. Horger DC, Wingo MS, Keane TE. Partial segmental thrombosis of corpus cavernosum: case report and review of world literature. *Urology.* 2005;66(1):194.

139. Zandrino F, Musante F, Mariani N, Derchi LE. Partial unilateral intracavernosal hematoma in a long-distance mountain biker: a case report. *Acta Radiol.* 2004;45(5): 580-583.

140. Ptak T, Larsen CR, Beckmann CF, Boyle DE Jr. Idiopathic segmental thrombosis of the corpus cavernosum as a cause of partial priapism. *Abdom Imaging.* 1994;19(6):564-566.

141. Al Saleh BM, Ansari ER, Al Ali IH, Tell JY, Saheb A. Fractures of the penis seen in Abu Dhabi. *J Urol.* 1985; 134(2):274-275.

142. Mydlo JH, Harris CF, Brown JG. Blunt, penetrating and ischemic injuries to the penis. *J Urol.* 2002;168(4 Pt 1): 1433-1435.

143. Bertolotto M, Neumaier CE. Penile sonography. *Eur Radiol.* 1999;9 Suppl 3:S407-S412.

144. Choi MH, Kim B, Ryu JA, Lee SW, Lee KS. MR imaging of acute penile fracture. *Radiographics.* 2000;20(5):1397-1405.

145. Beysel M, Tekin A, Gürdal M, Yücebaş E, Sengör F. Evaluation and treatment of penile fractures: accuracy of clinical diagnosis and the value of corpus cavernosography. *Urology.* 2002;60(3):492-496.

146. Bertolotto M, Mucelli RP. Nonpenetrating penile traumas: sonographic and Doppler features. *AJR Am J Roentgenol.* 2004;183(4):1085-1089.

147. Kervancioglu S, Ozkur A, Bayram MM. Color Doppler sonographic findings in penile fracture. *J Clin Ultrasound.* 2005;33(1):38-42.

148. El-Bahnasawy MS, Gomha MA. Penile fractures: the successful outcome of immediate surgical intervention. *Int J Impot Res.* 2000;12(5):273-277.

149. Fedel M, Venz S, Andreessen R, Sudhoff F, Loening SA. The value of magnetic resonance imaging in the diagnosis of suspected penile fracture with atypical clinical findings. *J Urol.* 1996;155(6):1924-1927.

150. Maubon AJ, Roux JO, Faix A, Segui B, Ferru JM, Rouanet JP. Penile fracture: MRI demonstration of a urethral tear associated with a rupture of the corpus cavernosum. *Eur Radiol.* 1998;8(3):469-470.

151. Uder M, Gohl D, Takahashi M, et al. MRI of penile fracture: diagnosis and therapeutic follow-up. *Eur Radiol.* 2002;12(1): 113-120.
152. Forman HP, Rosenberg HK, Snyder HM 3rd. Fractured penis: sonographic aid to diagnosis. *AJR Am J Roentgenol.* 1989;153(5):1009-1010.
153. Schmidt BA, Schwarz T, Schellong SM. Spontaneous thrombosis of the deep dorsal penile vein in a patient with thrombophilia. *J Urol.* 2000;164(5):1649.
154. Shapiro RS. Superficial dorsal penile vein thrombosis (penile Mondor's phlebitis): ultrasound diagnosis. *J Clin Ultrasound.* 1996;24(5):272-274.
155. Shweta Bhatt HG, Vikram Dogra. Sonographic evaluation of scrotal and penile trauma. *Ultrasound Clin.* 2007;2:45-56.
156. James Halls GB, Uday Patel. Erectile dysfunction: the role of penile Doppler ultrasound in diagnosis. *Abdom Imaging.* 2009;34:712-725.
157. Hossein Sadeghi-Nejad DB, Vikram Dogra. Male erectile dysfunction. *Ultrasound Clin.* 2007;2:57-71.
158. Greene FL, Page, DL, Felming ID, Fritz, AG, Balch, CM, Haller DG, Morrow M, eds. *AJCC Cancer Staging Handbook.* 6th ed. New York: Springer-Verlag; 2002;331-335 [chapter 33].

CHAPTER 13

Imaging of the Lymph Nodes and Lymphatic Ducts

Naraindеr K. Gupta, MD, DRM, MSc, FRCR
Wallace T. Miller Jr., MD

NORMAL LYMPH NODES ANATOMY AND DRAINAGE PATTERNS

Lymph nodes can be found throughout the body and normal lymph nodes may be identified noninvasively. Abnormal lymph nodes are found in many disease processes, including but not limited to malignancy, inflammation, and infection. Abnormalities of lymph node size, numbers, distribution, and imaging characteristics can be an important indicator of disease in the region of the abnormality. Careful review of the presence of lymph nodes is an important part of the evaluation of abdominal disease. Many inexperienced readers overemphasize the mere presence of lymph nodes. Small lymph nodes between 2 and 10 mm in short axis are normally observed in the abdomen. Faster scanning and thin collimation helps one distinguish between lymph nodes and vessels, which previously was more challenging. Scrolling through images also greatly aids the ability to distinguish lymph nodes from vessels. Lymph nodes appear as round or oval soft-tissue masses that appear and disappear over several images. These can be found in a variety of locations including behind the diaphragmatic crura (retrocrural lymph nodes); adjacent to the aorta; inferior vena cava; common, internal, and external iliac arteries and veins (retroperitoneal and pelvic lymph nodes); adjacent to the celiac axis (celiac axis lymph nodes); along the course of the portal vein (periportal lymph nodes); in the small bowel mesentery (mesenteric lymph nodes); and in the inguinal region.

In the majority of cases, lymph node abnormalities are secondary to diseases in the organs that the lymph nodes drain and therefore, discovery of enlarged or otherwise abnormal lymph node should lead to a search for pathology in the drainage distribution of the abnormal lymph nodes. Although the arrangement of abdomen and pelvic lymphatics and draining lymph nodes is complicated, there is a common principle of drainage, which will be explained in the text below.

Abdominal lymphatics are divided into parietal and visceral lymphatic vessels and nodes and drain the abdominal wall and abdominal viscera, respectively (see Figure 13-1). These lymphatics and lymph nodes follow the course of parietal and visceral branches of abdominal aorta and drain into venous blood via thoracic duct. Some of the lymphatics from liver drain via alternate routes.[1,2] Before draining into the thoracic duct, most of the lymphatics of the abdominal cavity are interrupted by retroperitoneal nodes called terminal lumbo-aortic nodes around the inferior vena cava and abdominal aorta.[3,4]

Parietal Abdominal Lymphatics

The superficial parietal lymphatics from the anterior and posterior abdominal skin and subcutaneous tissues drain cranially into the pectoral and subscapular axillary nodes.

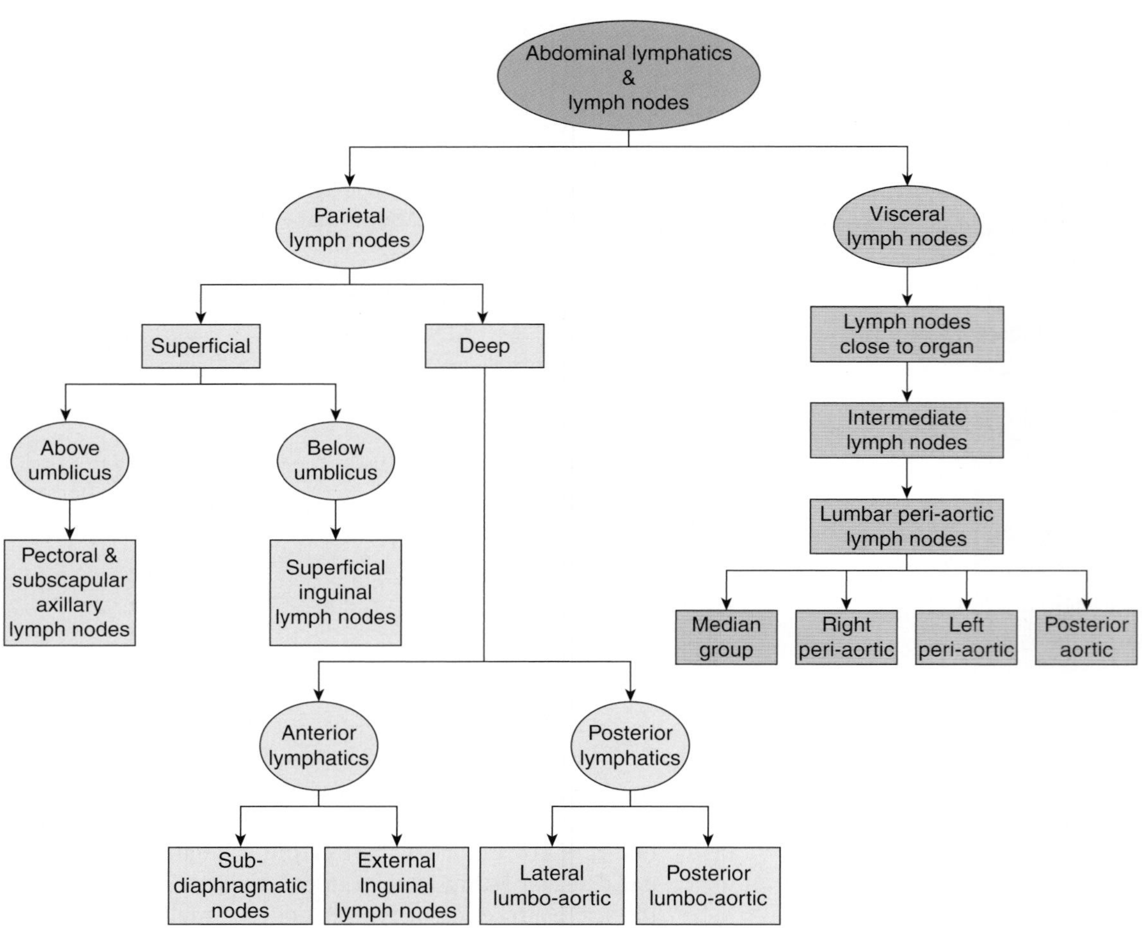

Figure 13-1 Patterns of Abdominal Lymphatic Drainage
Basic scheme and principle of abdominal lymphatic drainage is illustrated in this diagram. Note that the drainage of the superficial parietal abdominal tissues above the umbilicus is superior to the diaphragm. *Green* = drainage from the viscera; *gray* = drainage from the parietes.

However, below the umbilicus, the parietal drainage is to superficial inguinal lymph nodes (see Figure 13-2).[5]

The deep lymphatic vessels from the muscles and fasciae of abdomen run in the subperitoneal adipose tissue and superiorly drain into subdiaphragmatic nodes and inferiorly follow deep inferior epigastric vessels to drain into external iliac lymph nodes. From the posterior abdominal wall, the lymphatics drain into lateral or posterior lumbo-aortic lymph nodes.[1]

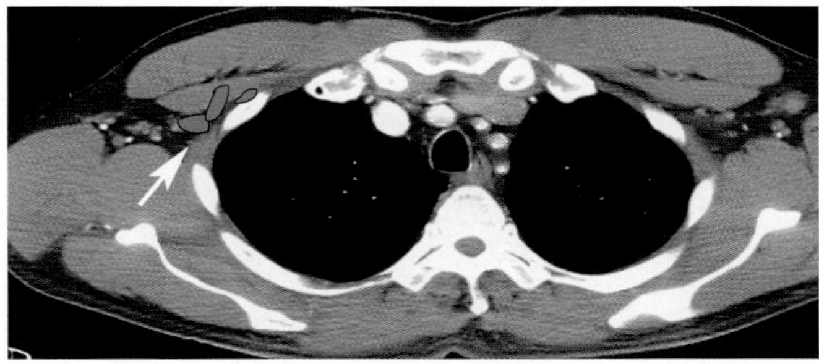
A

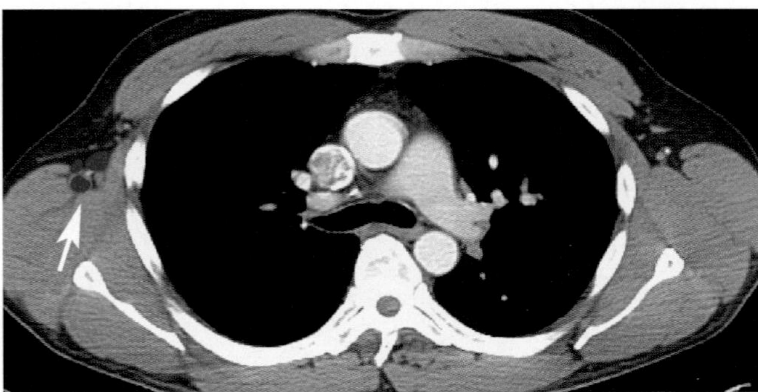
B

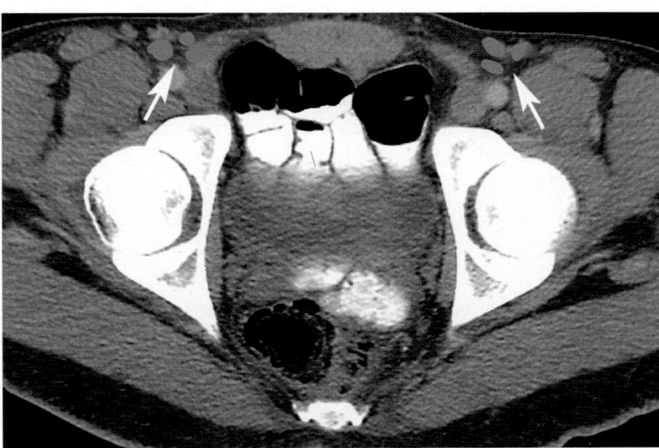
C

Figure 13-2 Lymphatic Drainage of the Skin and Subcutaneous Tissues of the Trunk
The CT sections illustrating the draining lymph nodes from the anterior and posterior abdomen skin and subcutaneous tissue above the umbilicus. **A** and **B.** Above the umbilicus, the drainage is into subpectoral and subscapular nodes. **C.** Below the umbilicus, the drainage is into superficial inguinal lymph nodes. *Green* = pectoral lymph nodes; *red* = subscapular lymph nodes; *blue* = inguinal lymph nodes

Visceral Abdominal Lymphatics

Figure 13-3 shows the normal distribution of abdominal lymph nodes. Lymphatic drainage from various abdominal viscera drain firstly to lymph nodes close to particular viscera, then to lymph nodes of peritoneal ligaments and mesentery and drain into the lymph nodes of paired or unpaired branches of the abdominal aorta, which finally drain to periaortic nodes in the lumbar area (see Figure 13-3). The lumbar periaortic lymph nodes are divided into preaortic, postaortic, and left and right lateral aortic lymph nodes.[4] The median preaortic lymph nodes drain the lymphatics of the gastrointestinal (GI) tract that are supplied by the ventral branches of the abdominal aorta. These drain into the cisterna chyli.[1]

The left and right lateral aortic lymph nodes receive lymphatics from the common iliac lymph nodes and lymphatics running along the lateral branches of the aorta, from the kidneys and adrenal glands, as well as male and female gonads. Hence, these lateral aortic nodes are main groups of drainage from the urogenital viscera in abdominopelvic cavity. These lateral aortic nodes drain into the cisterna chyli via paired left and right lumbar lymphatic trunks.[1,5] The posterior aortic lymph nodes do not directly drain any viscera and usually serve as communications between left and right lateral aortic lymph nodes along with draining posterior deep parietes and then drain into the thoracic duct.[2,3]

Preaortic lymph nodes

The preaortic groups of lymph nodes is located anterior to the aorta and are named after 3 unpaired vessels originating from the abdominal aorta named celiac, superior mesenteric, and inferior mesenteric nodes (see Figures 13-3 and 13-4).[3]

Celiac lymph nodes

The celiac lymph nodes drain lymphatics from the stomach, duodenum, most of the liver, gallbladder, spleen, and pancreas. The intermediate nodes for these organs are lined close to their supplying arteries and are called gastric, hepatic, and pancreaticosplenic nodes.[5,6]

Gastric nodes are found along the arterial vessels along the lesser and greater curvature of the stomach and are called right and left gastric nodes. On the lesser curvature side of the stomach, the lymph nodes lie in the lesser omentum, as right and left gastroepiploic nodes lying in the greater omentum in the lower portion of the greater curvature of the stomach. Cranial lymph nodes of the left gastric chain lie near the cardia and receive drainage from the abdominal portion of the esophagus. These predominantly drain into the celiac lymph nodes; however part of them is drained into the posterior lower mediastinal lymph nodes. A group of pyloric nodes 4 to 5 in number and lying close to the division of gastroduodenal artery receive

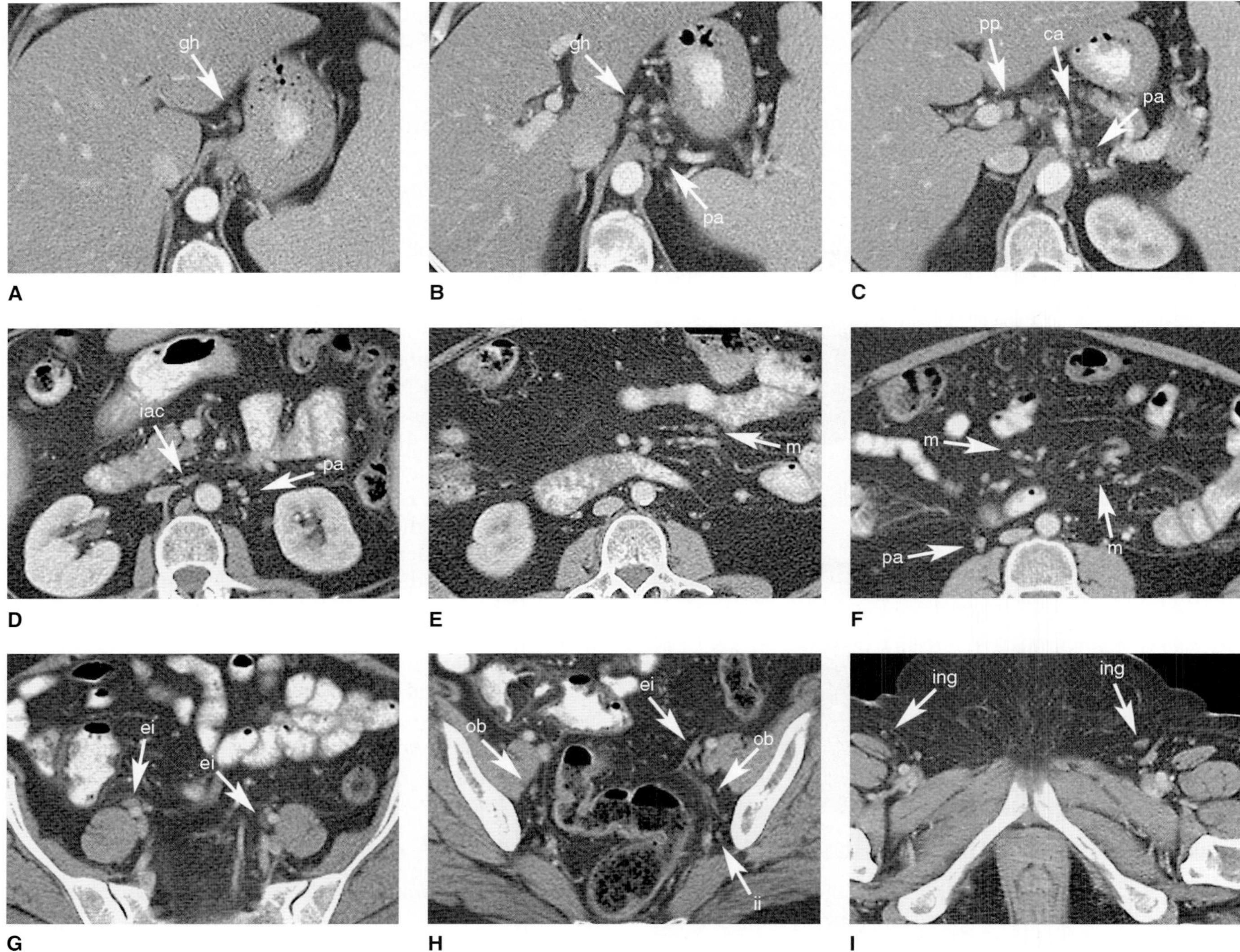

Figure 13-3 Normal Lymph Nodes of the Abdomen and Pelvis A-I. Axial CT of the abdomen demonstrates multiple small normal lymph nodes in the abdomen and pelvis. The celiac axis lymph nodes represent a type of preaortic lymph node; the para-aortic and interaortocaval lymph nodes are types of right and left lateral aortic lymph nodes. gh = gastrohepatic; ca = celiac axis; pp = periportal, iac = interaortocaval; pa = para-aortic; m = mesenteric; ei = external iliac; ob = obturator; ii = internal iliac; ing = inguinal.

afferent lymphatics from the pylorus, first part of the duodenum and pancreatic head and receive efferents from the right gastroepiploic nodes. These pyloric nodes usually drain into the celiac group of lymph nodes. Alternatively, these can drain into the superior mesenteric group of lymph nodes.

Hepatic nodes not only drain liver, bile ducts, and gallbladder but also receive efferents from stomach, duodenum, and pancreas. These nodes, 3 to 6 in number, are situated along the hepatic artery. The first hepatic nodes are situated at the origin of the hepatic artery and correspond to the superior border of the pancreas. Middle hepatic nodes are located along the anterior surface of the portal vein. The superior hepatic nodes are situated in the hepatic hilum and randomly distributed along left and right hepatic arteries. One of these hepatic nodes is constant in location at the junction of cystic and common bile duct and called the Quénu cystic node.

Splenic lymph nodes associated with the splenic artery are called pancreaticosplenic nodes and therefore situated along the superior and posterior part of the pancreas. The largest of these nodes lie behind the body of the pancreas. Lateral smaller pancreaticosplenic nodes lie near the hilum in the pancreaticosplenic ligament. These nodes receive lymphatics from the spleen, body, and tail of the pancreas and gastric fundus. The efferent drainage from the pancreaticosplenic nodes is into the celiac group.[7]

Superior mesenteric nodes

This group of lymph nodes surrounds the origin of the superior mesenteric artery, anterior to the aorta. They are

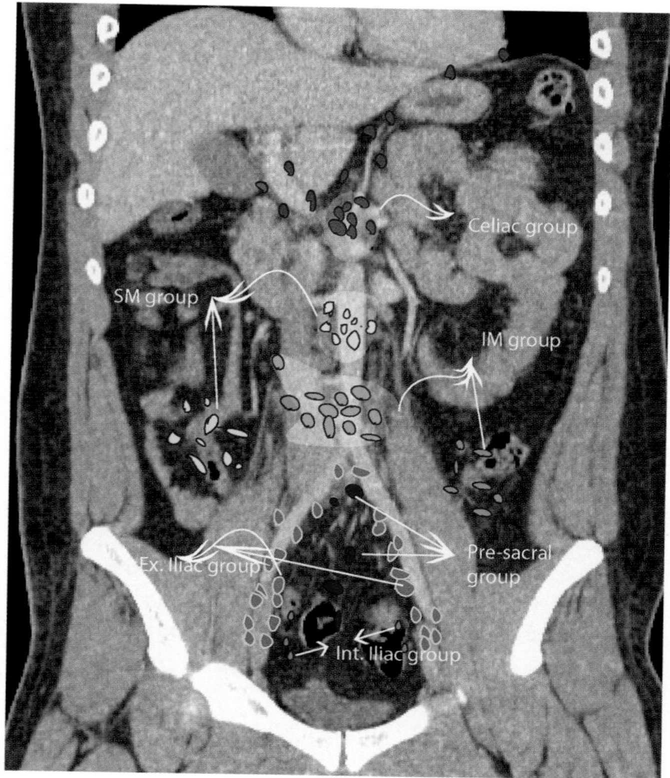

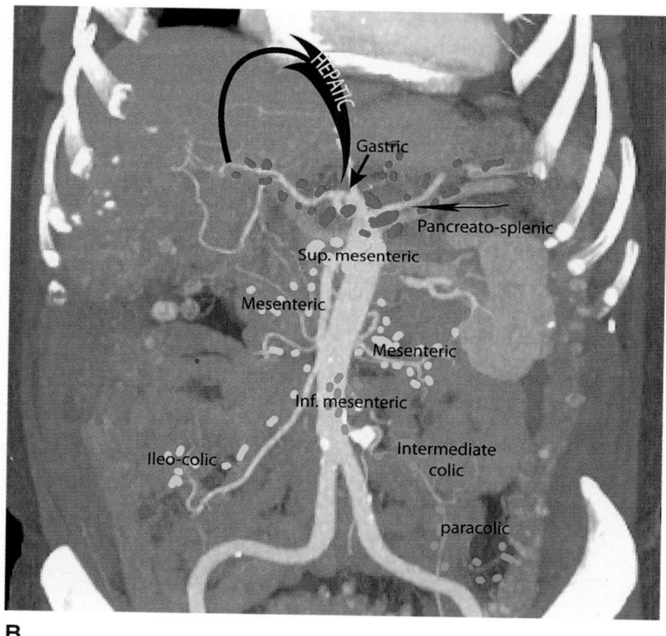

Figure 13-4 Preaortic and Mesenteric Lymph Nodes
A. Labeled illustration shows preaortic lymph nodes named after unpaired branches of abdominal aorta. Posterior aortic, left lateral aortic, and right lateral aortic lymph nodes are not shown in this picture. Major pelvic lymph node groups are shown. *Purple* = common and external iliac lymph nodes; *blue* = presacral lymph nodes; *yellow* = superior mesenteric (SM) artery lymph nodes; *green* = inferior mesenteric (IM) artery lymph nodes; *pink* = internal iliac lymph nodes; red= celiac axis lymph nodes. **B.** Coronal maximum-intensity projection showing group of celiac, superior mesenteric, and inferior mesenteric lymph nodes shown in *red*, *yellow*, and *green*, respectively. Different subtle shades of the same color represent the drainage territory and lymph nodes.

situated behind the pancreas and anterior to the aorta at the level of L1 lumbar vertebra. These lymph nodes are almost contiguous with the mesenteric lymph nodes at the root of mesentery. These lymph nodes drain the mesenteric and ileocolic lymph nodes, thus draining the distal duodenum, small intestine, and right-sided colon.[4,5]

Mesenteric lymph nodes approximately 100 to 150 in numbers are located in the mesenteric fat. Most peripheral of mesenteric nodes are located close to the intestinal wall between the terminal jejunal and ileal arteries and these are called juxtaintestinal mesenteric nodes. The intermediate or second group of mesenteric lymph nodes lie within the mesentery between the primary and secondary loops of the superior mesenteric artery and the last central mesenteric nodal group or the third group, which are slightly larger than the other 2 groups of mesenteric lymph nodes, lie along the main stem of superior mesenteric artery near the mesenteric root where these are indistinguishable from superior mesenteric lymph nodes.[1]

Ileocolic nodes are situated around the ileocolic artery and there are approximately 20 in number; 1 of these nodes is usually found in the mesoappendix (see Figures 13-3 and 13-4).[1]

Inferior mesenteric nodes

Inferior mesenteric nodes are usually a group of 2 lymph nodes situated on either side of origin of inferior mesenteric artery. These are usually at the level of L3 lumbar vertebra and drain the lymphatics from the upper rectum and left side of colon via epicolic, paracolic, and intermediate colic nodes. The epicolic nodes are situated in the walls of colon itself, paracolic nodes are located along the mesenteric borders of the colon and intermediate colic nodes are located along the middle and left colic arteries. Similarly, the ascending colon and part of transverse colon have similar arrangement of drainage but end in superior mesenteric nodes instead of inferior mesenteric nodes.[1,2,5]

Lateral aortic lymph nodes

Lateral aortic lymph nodes on the left are a continuous vertical chain of lymph nodes along the left side of abdominal aorta. These lymph nodes lie on vertebral attachments of the psoas muscle and left crus of diaphragm. Left renal vessels and sympathetic nervous trunks cross this chain anteriorly.[1] Right lateral aortic lymph nodes are located in the front of the inferior vena cava or behind it. Few of these can be lateral to the inferior vena cava or lie between the aorta and inferior vena cava. According to their relationship with the inferior vena cava, these are named as precaval, laterocaval, or postcaval lymph nodes. Their relationship otherwise is similar as the left counterpart.[2,5] The lateral aortic lymph nodes through tortuous networks not only receive lymphatic drainage from the structures supplied by the posterior and lateral paired branches of the abdominal aorta but also drain pelvic lymphatics through the common iliac nodes. These also drain adrenal glands and lymphatics running along the renal, suprarenal, and diaphragmatic vessels. Lateral aortic lymph nodes also drain lymph from the kidneys, perirenal fat, renal capsule, and abdominal ureter. Gonadal lymphatics from the ovaries and testes as well as the fallopian tubes lymphatics drain in these lymph nodes.[8]

Functionally, the proximal lymphatics from the digestive tract cannot be easily demarcated because of complex 3-dimensional drainage; however, distally the lymphatics drain into preaortic pathways of celiac, superior, and inferior mesenteric lymph nodes. However, drainage from genitourinary lymphatic pathways is more precise to the lateral aortic ascending chains.

Pelvic Lymphatics and Lymph Nodes

Similar to the abdominal lymphatics and lymph nodes, the pelvic lymphatics and lymph nodes are also divided into parietal and visceral networks. All lymphatics drain in the successive group of lymph nodes located at the level of pelvic inlet along the arcuate line of pelvis and L5 lumbar vertebra. These are mostly associated with iliac vessels and their branches and combine to form the ascending chains and then drain on the lateral aortic chains on the respective sides. Ascending chains are named after their location and called external iliac, internal iliac, common iliac, and sacral groups of lymph nodes (see Figures 13-3 and 13-5).[9]

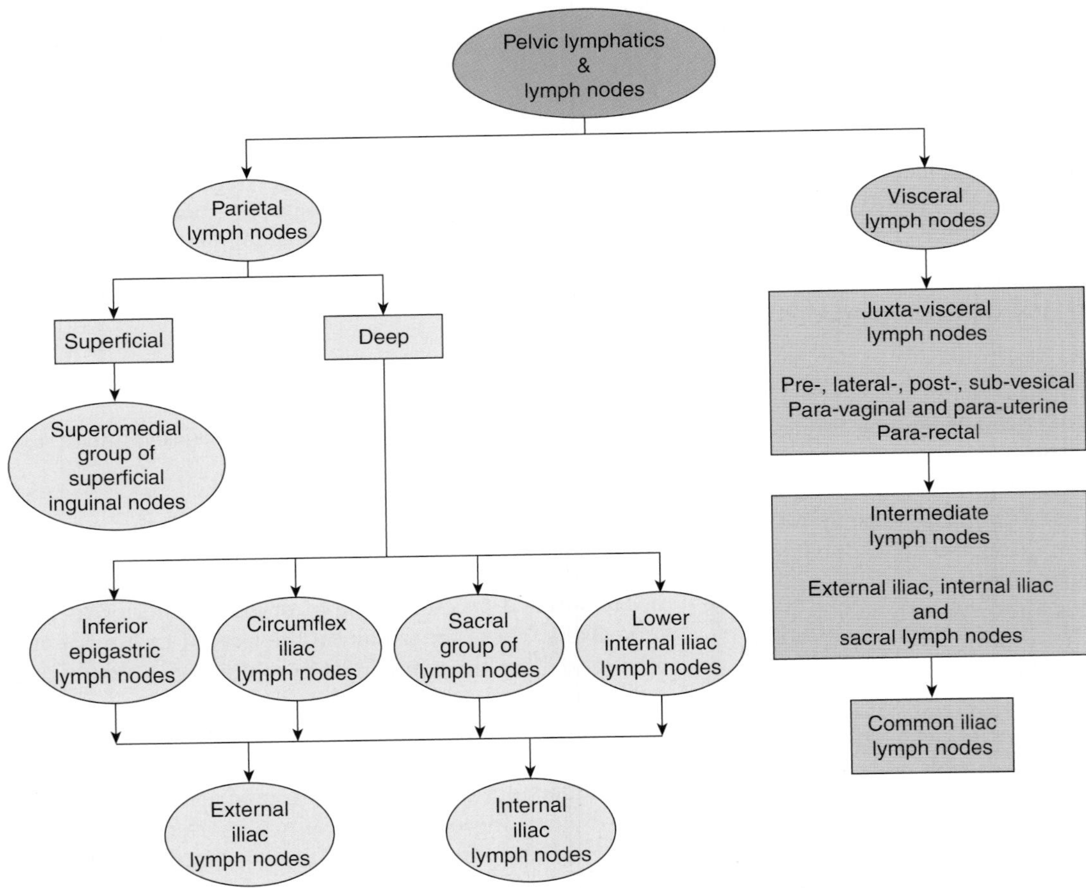

Figure 13-5 Patterns of Pelvic Lymphatic Drainage
Basic scheme and principle of pelvic lymphatic drainage is illustrated in this diagram. Note that the drainage principle is similar to the abdominal drainage principle and lymph nodes groups follow the names of accompanying blood vessels.

Parietal Pelvic Lymphatics

Parietal lymph vessels and nodes drain the lymph from all the pelvic walls and are arranged in superficial and deep lymphatic network that drain the superficial soft-tissue of perineum and the muscles covering the pelvis respectively.[2,3,9]

Superficial network on the pelvic floor runs from the coccyx region to pubic region to drain in the superomedial group of superficial inguinal nodes. Functionally, these drain all soft-tissues of perineum below the external fascial sheath of urogenital diaphragm, distal vagina below the hymen, and the inferior part of the anal canal below the anocutaneous line.[1]

Deep parietal lymphatics follow the parietal branches of the external and internal iliac vessels and first drain into the inferior epigastric, circumflex iliac, and sacral nodal groups. Deep inferior nodes drain the lower anterior abdominal wall and retropubic region of the anterior pelvic wall. Up the hierarchy, these drain into lateral groups of external iliac nodes. The deep circumflex iliac nodes are located around the deep circumflex iliac artery and receive afferent vessels arising from the iliac muscle and the parietal peritoneal lining of the iliac fossa and then drain into external iliac nodes. The sacral groups of lymph nodes are situated around the lateral and median sacral arteries and constitute 3 ascending lymph chains running, respectively, one each along the lateral borders of the sacrum and third in front of its anterior aspect on the midline. The sacral group of lymph nodes drain the presacral space between the fascia recti anteriorly and the sacrum posteriorly. The largest of the median sacral nodes is known as the promontorial node as it sits anterior to disc space at L5/S1.[8] Lateral pelvic wall lymphatics run on endopelvic fascia and drain to external and internal iliac nodes above the plane of levator ani and coccygeal muscles. Below the plane of the levator ani, the lymphatic vessels, which follow the internal pudendal artery along the surface of the obturator internus, drain the muscles and fasciae. These deep lymphatics originating in the prevesical space also collect the lymph vessels from the ischiorectal fossa, and then drain into the internal iliac chain.[9]

Visceral Pelvic Lymphatics

Similar to the abdominal viscera, the pelvic viscera first drain to closely located juxtavisceral lymph nodes, then along the vascular pedicles of each organ, and finally along the iliac vessels. At iliac levels, rich and extensively developed lymphatic plexus form ascending pathways draining toward the lateral aortic chains.

The juxtavisceral nodes are named in relation to the organ being drained.[4] For the urinary bladder, these are called prevesical, lateral vesical, posterior vesical, and subvesical corresponding to the respective bladder surfaces. Pararectal lymph nodes are named left and right and situated in the pararectal fat of posterior digestive pelvic compartment. Paravaginal and parauterine nodes correspond to the lymph nodes found on the lateral edges of vagina and cervix and situated in the parametrial fibrous tissue of the female pelvis. After receiving drainage from the neighboring organs, these nodes drain to the external iliac, internal iliac, or presacral chain of lymph nodes.[9]

External iliac lymphatics and lymph nodes

External iliac lymph nodes are a group of approximately 10 lymph nodes arranged around the external iliac vessels. These lymph nodes form 3 distinct groups called the lateral, medial, and middle group of external iliac lymph nodes. The lowest lymph node of the lateral group is located under the inguinal ligament. This group drains from the deep inferior epigastric and deep circumflex iliac lymph nodes situated along corresponding arteries. The medial group of the external iliac lymph nodes are situated medially to external iliac vessels, predominantly drain the lower limb, and there are very few draining lymphatics from the pelvis itself. This group is also called obturator nodes and should not be confused with the isolated small obturator nodes that sit in the obturator foramen of the obturator canal in the obturator fossa. These small lymph nodes are linked to the internal iliac lymph nodes rather than the external iliac group.[2,5,9] The external iliac lymph nodes group receives lymph from the lower limb through the superficial and deep inguinal lymph nodes. These also drain the subumbilical part of the abdominal wall, glans penis or clitoris, muscles of the medial compartment of the thigh, lateral lobes of the prostate, vesical fundus, cervix uteri, and upper vagina.[3,9]

Because of fetal positioning of prostate, vagina, and cervix uteri at the level of pelvic inlet, these organs develop drainage into nearby medial nodes of the external iliac chain rather than primarily draining in the internal iliac group of nodes. Similarly, this process explains the lymphatics of ovaries and testes, which drain in the lower lateral aortic nodes because of their lumbar origin fetally.[5] The lymphatic efferents from the external iliac chain drain to corresponding lower lymph nodes of the common iliac chain (see Figures 13-3 and 13-6).

Internal iliac lymphatic and lymph nodes

These lymph channels and lymph nodes are also called hypogastric lymphatics and lymph nodes. These surround the internal iliac artery and their corresponding branches. These are named superior-gluteal lymph nodes, uterine, internal pudendal, inferior gluteal, and middle rectal arteries.[1,4] The internal iliac lymph nodes drain lymph from all the pelvic organs including the posterior prostate, lateral and lower part of the bladder, membranous and prostatic urethra, seminal vesicles, lower two-thirds of the vagina, the uterine body, and midrectum.[4,6,10] Superior gluteal lymph nodes also draining the deep gluteal regions including glutei muscles. Internal pudendal lymph nodes drain to the internal iliac after receiving lymph from the deep

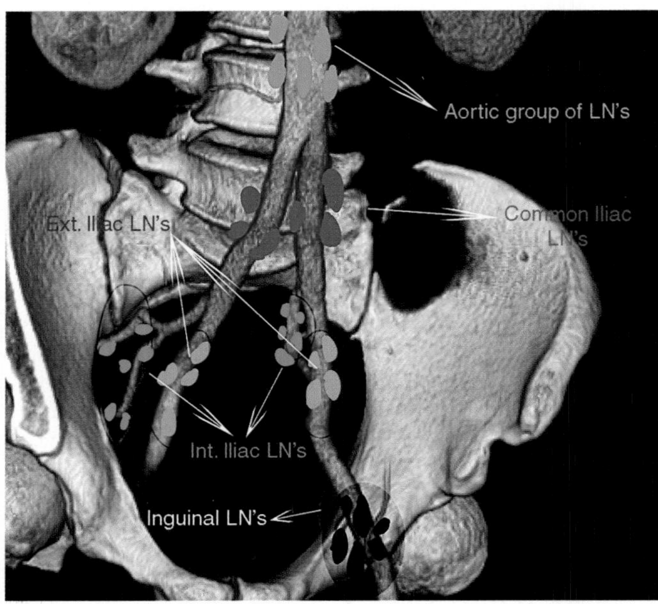

Figure 13-6 Pelvic Lymph Node Chains
Volume-rendered image of the pelvis illustrates the major groups of pelvic lymph nodes and named after the vessels adjacent to which these lie.

perineum, ischioanal fossa, and lower parts of the vagina, prostrate, and rectum.[5,7] Internal iliac lymphatics then travel upwards and drain into the intermediate group of common iliac lymph nodes.

Common iliac lymphatics and lymph nodes

Four to 7 in numbers, these nodes depending on their location are divided into medial, lateral, and intermediate groups.[4] Lateral common iliac lymph nodes lie between the medial border of psoas and lateral to the common iliac artery, and merges with the lateral aortic lymph nodes without clear demarcation. The middle or intermediate common iliac lymph nodes lie posteromedial to artery. The medial chain lies inner to the common iliac artery and travels upwards to meet its counterpart from the other side to form an uneven group just below the aortic bifurcation at the level of the L5 vertebra. The lateral and intermediate common iliac chains do not receive any direct lymphatics from the pelvic viscera. However, some lymphatics originating from the bladder neck, cervix uteri, and posterior rectum drains directly into the median subaortic group of lymph nodes.

Drainage Patterns of the Abdominal Organs

Importance of proper evaluation of lymph nodes cannot be stressed enough and, therefore, it is crucial that an inexperienced reader acquires a feel for the normal variation in the distribution, number, and size of lymph nodes in the abdomen in order to prevent overcalling the presence of disease. It is also important for the reader to be aware of the normal lymphatic drainage patterns for the organs of the abdomen. Malignancies and inflammatory conditions of each organ will commonly result in mild or moderate lymphadenopathy in the drainage distribution of the organ. These drainage distributions should be inspected for the presence of disease when an abnormality within the organ is discovered or vice versa to look for a diseased organ when lymphadenopathy is found. A list of the drainage distributions for many of the organs in the abdomen is shown (Table 13-1).

Table 13-1. Common Lymphatic Drainage Patterns

Organ	Drainage
Liver	Periportal – upper para-aortic[a] Right paracardiac
Stomach	Celiac axis – upper para-aortic Gastrohepatic Perigastric
Pancreas Duodenum	Celiac axis – upper para-aortic
Right kidney Right adrenal Right ovary Right testicle	Right mid para-aortic
Left kidney Left adrenal Left ovary Left testicle	Left mid para-aortic[b]
Jejunum Ileum	Small bowel mesentery – upper para-aortic
Cecum Ascending colon	Pericecal – small bowel mesentery – upper para-aortic
Transverse colon	Transverse mesocolon – upper para-aortic
Descending colon Sigmoid colon	Pericolonic fat LN – inferior para-aortic[c]
Rectum Prostate Uterus Cervix	Retroperitoneal fat LN – internal iliac/obturator – inferior para-aortic
Anus Perineum Skin of scrotum	Inguinal

[a]Upper para-aortic = from diaphragm to renal arteries
[b]Mid para-aortic = 1-2 cm above and below the origins of the renal arteries
[c]Lower para-aortic = from renal arteries to the iliac bifurcation
Note: Dashes between lymph node groups indicate sequential spread from first to last groups listed.

LYMPH NODE CHARACTERISTICS INDICATING DISEASE

Lymph node characteristics that can indicate disease include increased size, increased number, increased metabolic activity, increased or decreased attenuation, hyperenhancement, and decreased magnetic resonance imaging (MRI) signal.

Increased Size and/or Increased Number

The 2 most important characteristics of lymph nodes indicating the presence of disease is an increase in size or number of lymph nodes. Enlarged lymph nodes can be reactive, because of benign or malignant infiltration or lymphoproliferative disorders (Table 13-2). Many radiologists rely on the "1-cm" rule, a short axis diameter of greater than 1 cm, as a marker for "pathologic" enlargement of lymph nodes. The attraction of this rule is its simplicity of use. Unfortunately, numerous studies of a wide range of diseases throughout the body have shown the 1-cm rule to be seriously flawed. When used as a marker for lymphatic spread of cancer, wide ranges in sensitivity and specificity have been reported for the variety of cancers.[11-30] The poor sensitivity of the 1-cm rule is not surprising because

Imaging Notes 13-1. The One-Centimeter Rule

> Use of a short axis diameter of 1 cm as cutoff to distinguish normal lymph nodes from diseased lymph nodes results in very poor clinical accuracy and should be avoided.

Table 13-2. Causes of Lymphadenopathy

Reactive lymphadenopathy	***Infectious causes***	
	Viral	Inf. Mononucleosis, Rubella
	Bacterial	Pyogenic, cat-scratch disease
	Mycobacterial	Tuberculosis and atypical mycobacterium
	Spirochetal	*Treponema pallidum*, leptospirosis
	Chlamydial	Lymphogranuloma venereum
	Parasitic	Toxoplasmosis
	Fungal	Coccidioidomycosis
	Noninfectious causes	
	Sarcoidosis Connective tissue disorders [Systemic lupus erythematosus (SLE), RA, mixed connective tissue disease] Kawasaki disease Rosai-Dorfman disease Kikuchi disease Castleman disease Drug reaction/hypersensitivity (phenytoin)	
Infiltrative diseases	***Malignant***	***Nonmalignant***
	Metastatic carcinoma	Lipid storage disease eg, Gaucher disease
	Metastatic melanoma	
	Leukemia	Amyloidosis
	Germ cell tumor	
Primary lymphoproliferative diseases	Lymphomas - Hodgkin, Non-Hodgkin	
	Lymphomatoid granulomatosis	
	Angioimmunoblastic lymphadenopathy	
	Malignant histiocytosis	

microscopic spread of tumor will not change lymph node size. Some normal lymph nodes can be larger than 1 cm and the presence of inflammation in the drainage distribution of the lymph node can also result in an increase in diameter. Consequently, the specificity of the 1-cm rule for malignant spread is also relatively poor. Some researchers have attempted to increase sensitivity for spread by lowering the "pathologic cut-off" to a variety of subcentimeter values. This approach consistently increases sensitivity by reducing specificity and rarely results in a clinically useful accuracy in the diagnosis of lymph node metastasis. With the widespread availability of positron emission tomography (PET)–computed tomography (CT), there is a paradigm shift in how the lymph nodes are evaluated at present. It has been documented that PET is generally more sensitive and specific than CT, MRI, or other imaging methods for the detection of cancer.[31-34]

In this text, we would like to offer a new paradigm in the prediction of lymph node pathology that relies on a combination of lymph node size and the clinical pretest probability of disease in any lymph node distribution. The 1-cm rule as a gross rule of thumb is the starting point. The majority of **small lymph nodes**, those with a short axis less than 10 mm, will be normal and the majority of lymph nodes with a short axis greater than or equal to 10 mm will indicate the presence of pathology either in the drainage distribution of the lymph node or systemically within the lymph nodes and the majority of lymph nodes. However, there are important caveats: (1) When there is a known malignancy in the drainage distribution of a lymph node, any size lymph node can potentially harbor malignancy, and any small changes in lymph node number, location, or appearance should be viewed with suspicion. (2) One or 2 **intermediate lymph nodes**, those with a short axis between 10 and 20 mm, are indeterminate in significance. In the absence of a known disease in the drainage distribution of the lymph node. These intermediate lymph nodes will most often represent a normal variant. (3) **Large lymph nodes**, those with a short axis of greater than 20 mm, will virtually always indicate an underlying disease, most often a malignancy.

Lymph nodes with short axis less than or equal to 10 mm we will call "small lymph nodes" and will usually represent a normal variant. However, any lymph node found in a location where lymph nodes are not normally present should we evaluated for possible disease. For example, small lymph nodes in the perirectal fat are not seen in normal individuals and will usually indicate a malignancy of the nearby tissues such as the rectum, cervix, or prostate (see Figure 13-7). Therefore, it is imperative for the reader to become familiar with the normal distribution of abdominal and pelvic lymph nodes.

Furthermore, all lymph nodes, regardless of size, are potentially significant when they are found in the drainage distribution of a known cancer. In the setting of a cancer, any small variation from normal should be suspected to harbor metastasis. This includes an increase in number of small lymph nodes or lymph nodes in a location where they are not normally encountered.

Large lymph nodes, those greater than 20 mm in diameter, will in the majority of cases indicate the presence of malignancy in the drainage distribution of the lymph node or a lymphoproliferative malignancy such as Hodgkin lymphoma (HL), non-Hodgkin lymphoma (NHL), and chronic lymphocytic leukemia (CLL) (see Figure 13-8). The inflammatory disorders that can also result in lymph nodes with short axis greater than 20 mm are sarcoidosis; granulomatous infections with tuberculous or nontuberculous organisms and endemic fungi such as histoplasma, coccidioides, and cryptococcal species; and connective tissue disorders, especially systemic lupus erythematosus and rheumatoid arthritis (Table 13-3).

Lymph nodes with short axis between 11 and 20 mm we will call "intermediate lymph nodes." The significance of intermediate lymph nodes is dependent on the patient's clinical history and other characteristics of the lymph nodes, most importantly the number of intermediate lymph nodes. If the patient has a malignancy or inflammatory condition in the drainage distribution of the intermediate lymph nodes, then this mild lymph node enlargement will often be a result of the disorder. For example, it is common for patients with cirrhosis to have mildly enlarged, that is, intermediate, lymph nodes in the porta hepatis (see Figure 13-9). Similarly, intermediate lymph nodes in the celiac axis distribution of a patient with gastric carcinoma will have a high probability of harboring metastasis. On the other hand, 1 or 2 intermediate lymph nodes are commonly found in normal individuals and in the absence of a known disorder in the drainage distribution of the lymph node will usually represent a normal variant (see Figure 13-10).

The number of intermediate lymph nodes is also an important characteristic in identifying the clinical

Imaging Notes 13-2. New Paradigm for the Determination of Lymph Node Pathology

Short axis ≤10 mm	
No cancer in drainage distribution	Usually normal
Cancer in drainage distribution	Indeterminate significance Use other imaging criteria to determine significance
Short axis 11-20 mm	Indeterminate significance Use clinical history and other imaging criteria to determine significance
Short axis >20 mm	Nearly always indicated disease Usually lymphoma, CLL, or metastasis

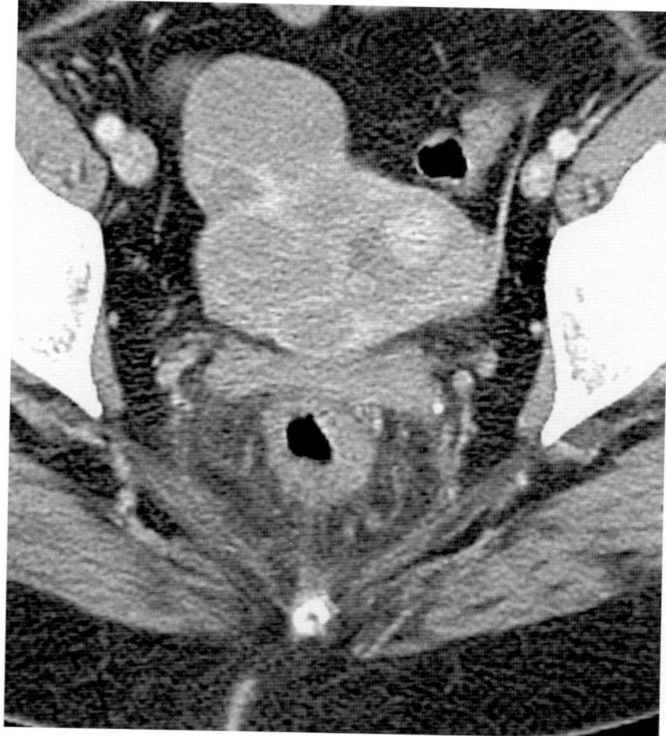

A

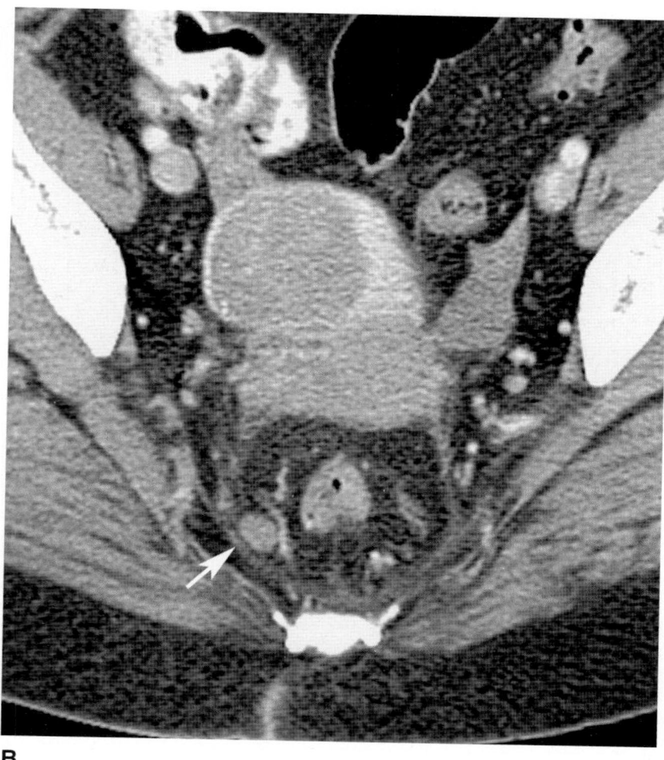

B

Figure 13-7 Perirectal Lymph Node Metastasis in Rectal Cancer This 55-year-old woman had blood in her stool. **A.** Enhanced CT of the pelvis shows asymmetric thickening of the rectal wall indicating the presence of a rectal carcinoma. Note the streaking of the perirectal fat, a finding suggesting local soft-tissue invasion. **B.** CT images 1 cm higher than in **A** shows 5 mm × 9 mm lymph node (*arrow*) in the perirectal fat. Although this lymph node has a short axis less than 10 mm, lymph nodes are not normally seen in this location. The presence of any perirectal lymph nodes will usually indicate the presence of disease in the region.

significance of intermediate lymph nodes. More than a few intermediate lymph nodes in any nodal group is usually abnormal and will indicate pathology in the drainage distribution of the nodes or a systemic disorder of lymph nodes (see Figure 13-11). There are also some locations where intermediate lymph nodes are a relatively common normal variant. This is especially true of inguinal lymph nodes and para-aortic lymph nodes between the celiac axis and the the inferior vena cava at the level of the kidneys. Lymph nodes of this size, even if few in number, will nearly always indicate malignancy. This is the characteristic location for lymphatic metastasis from testicular cancer because the lymphatic drainage travels with the venous supply to the gonads.

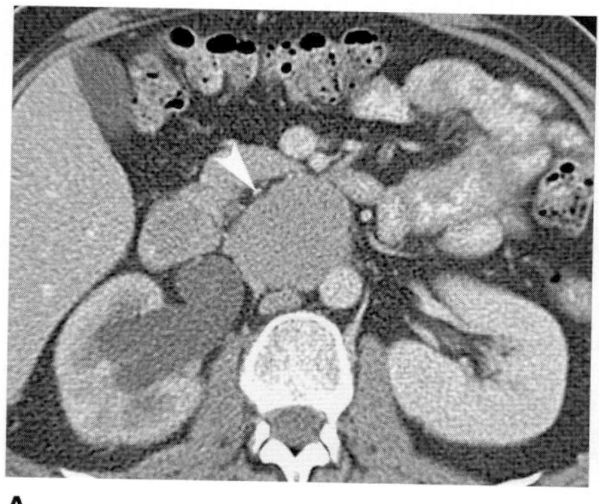

A

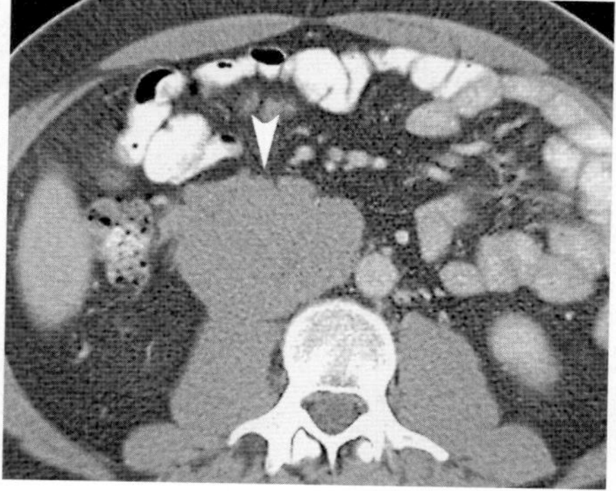

B

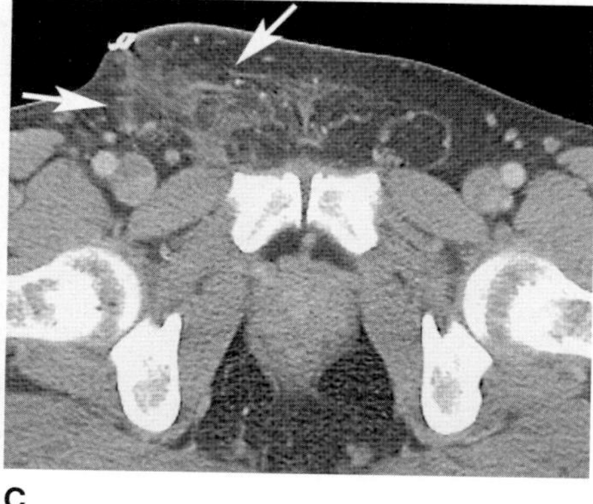

C

Figure 13-8 Lymph Node Metastasis From Testicular Carcinoma This 35-year-old man had testicular carcinoma. **A-C.** Contrast-enhanced CT shows infiltration of the fat of the right inguinal region typical of a previous right orchiectomy (*arrows*) and two markedly enlarged retroperitoneal lymph nodes (*arrowheads*) measuring 31 mm × 35 mm and 36 mm × 48 mm anterior to

Imaging Notes 13-3. Clinical Significance of Intermediate Lymph Nodes (Long axis 11 mm-20 mm)

1-2 intermediate lymph nodes + No clinical disease in drainage distribution	Usually normal variant
1-2 intermediate lymph nodes + Known disease in drainage distribution	Lymph nodes usually a result of known disease
>2 intermediate lymph nodes	Usually indicates disease Disease should be determined

Table 13-3. Disorders Commonly Causing Large Lymph Nodes (Short Axis >20 mm)

1. Metastatic tumor
2. Lymphoma
3. Chronic lymphocytic leukemia
4. Sarcoidosis
5. Granulomatous infections a. Tuberculosis b. Nontuberculous mycobacterial infection c. Histoplasmosis d. Coccidioidomycosis e. Cryptococcosis

renal hilum, and therefore intermediate lymph nodes in these locations are often clinically not significant.

In addition to increase in lymph node diameter, increased numbers of lymph nodes, more than is usually seen, can be a sign of disease. Increased numbers of large and intermediate-sized lymph nodes will usually indicate the presence of lymphoma or metastatic tumor but can occasionally be due to inflammatory diseases. Increased numbers of small lymph nodes that involve multiple nodal groups is usually a sign of an inflammatory disorder but can also be a manifestation of malignancy (see Figures 13-12 and 13-13).

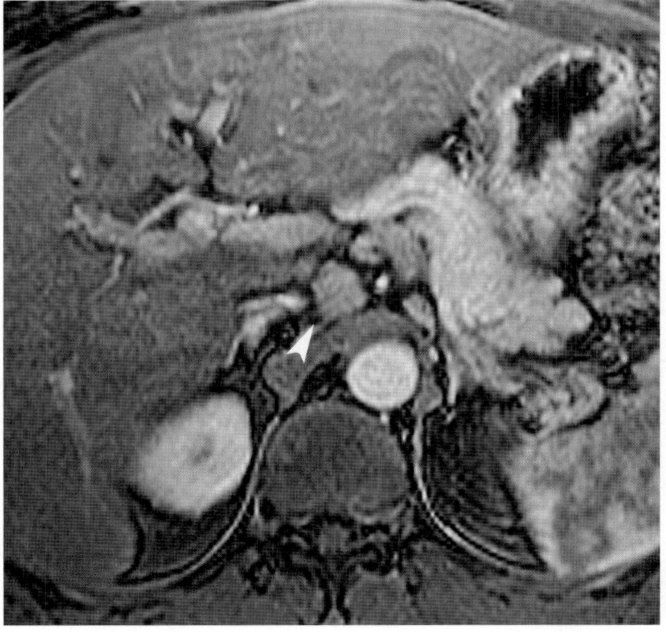

A

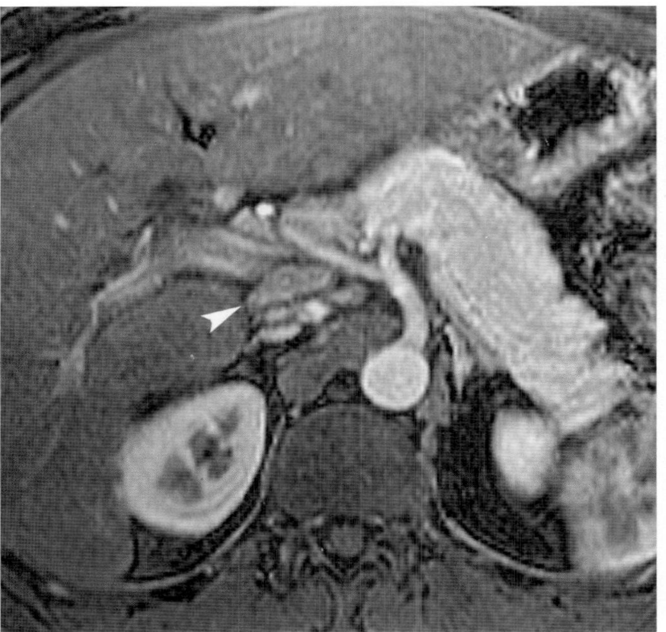

B

Figure 13-9 Periportal Lymphadenopathy due to Hepatitis This 51-year-old man with hepatitis C was being evaluated for the risk of hepatocellular carcinoma. **A** and **B**. Gadolinium-enhanced T1-weighted MRI sequences through the porta hepatis shows enlarged periportal lymph nodes (*arrowheads*) measuring 14 mm × 15 mm and 11 mm × 26 mm. No mass was found in the liver. Inflammatory diseases of the liver such as hepatitis and cirrhosis will commonly cause mild adenopathy in the periportal and celiac axis regions.

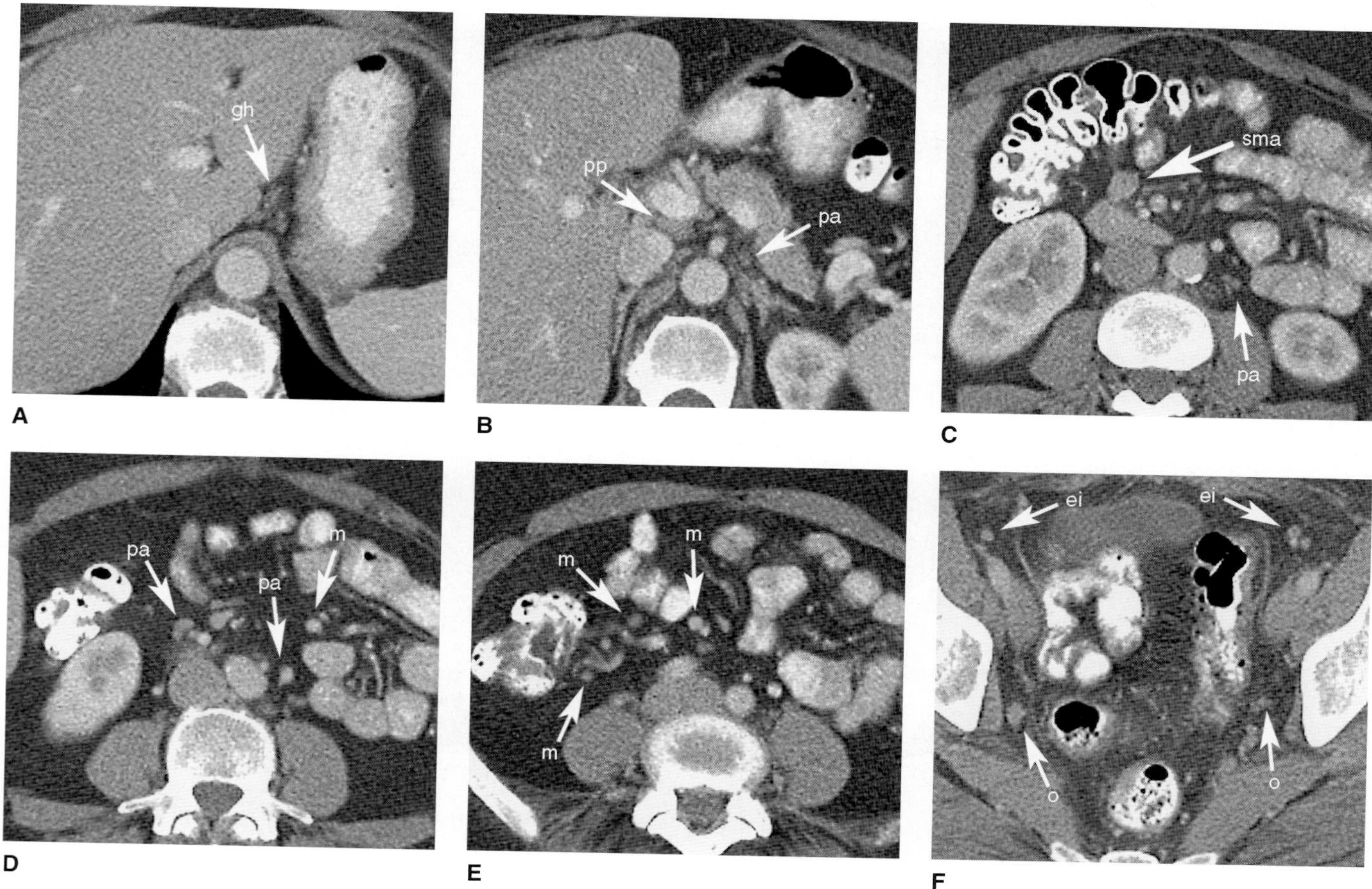

Figure 13-10 Normal Variant Intermediate Lymph Node This 49-year-old woman complained of abdominal pain. **A-F.** Contrast-enhanced axial CT images show multiple normal-sized lymph nodes in the gastrohepatic (gh), periportal (pp), para-aortic (pa), mesenteric (m), external iliac (ei), and obturator (o) locations. However, there is also an intermediate-sized superior mesenteric artery (SMA) lymph node (*large arrow*) in (C), measuring 12 mm × 15 mm. This was unchanged in size from a study 2 years previously. No other pathology was noted in the abdomen. This intermediate lymph node is likely to represent a normal variant.

Increased Metabolic Activity

Metabolic activity, as measured by PET scan, is increasingly being used as a measure of lymph node disease. Numerous studies have demonstrated increased sensitivity of PET scan or PET-CT over CT scans in the detection of both neoplastic and inflammatory disorders.[35] This is because PET scans have the opportunity to detect lymph node involvement by disease prior to enlargement of the lymph node (see Figure 13-14). Many studies have also suggested that PET scans have a higher specificity than CT scans.[35] Causes of false-positive PET scans include muscular activity, brown fat, peristalsis of bowel, and synchronous inflammatory conditions (see Figure 13-15). With more prevalent use of PET-CT hybrid scanners, the false-positive rate has decreased.[35]

When using PET and PET-CT scans to diagnose diseases, it is important to understand that the imaging agent, fluorodeoxyglucose (FDG), is a glucose analogue and measures metabolic activity. This is a nonspecific measure of disease and does not indicate the cause of the increased metabolic activity. In most cases, PET and PET-CT is used in the evaluation of the spread of malignancy and many individuals make the incorrect assumption that all increased metabolic activity indicates the spread of malignancy. Patients with a malignancy can have an unrelated inflammatory condition that results in the uptake of FDG. Similar to the interpretation of lymph node size, the significance of increased activity should be interpreted in the light of the patient's clinical history. False-positive nonmalignant FDG uptake is common in patients with malignancy who have undergone surgery or received radiotherapy or a combination of the 2. Lymph node activity in the expected distribution of disease will have a high positive predictive value for the spread of malignancy. However, increased activities in areas of unexpected spread of disease have an indeterminate significance and warrants further workup or accelerated follow-up.

Unique Lymph Node Characteristics

Most normal and abnormal lymph nodes will have imaging characteristics similar to skeletal muscle with x-ray

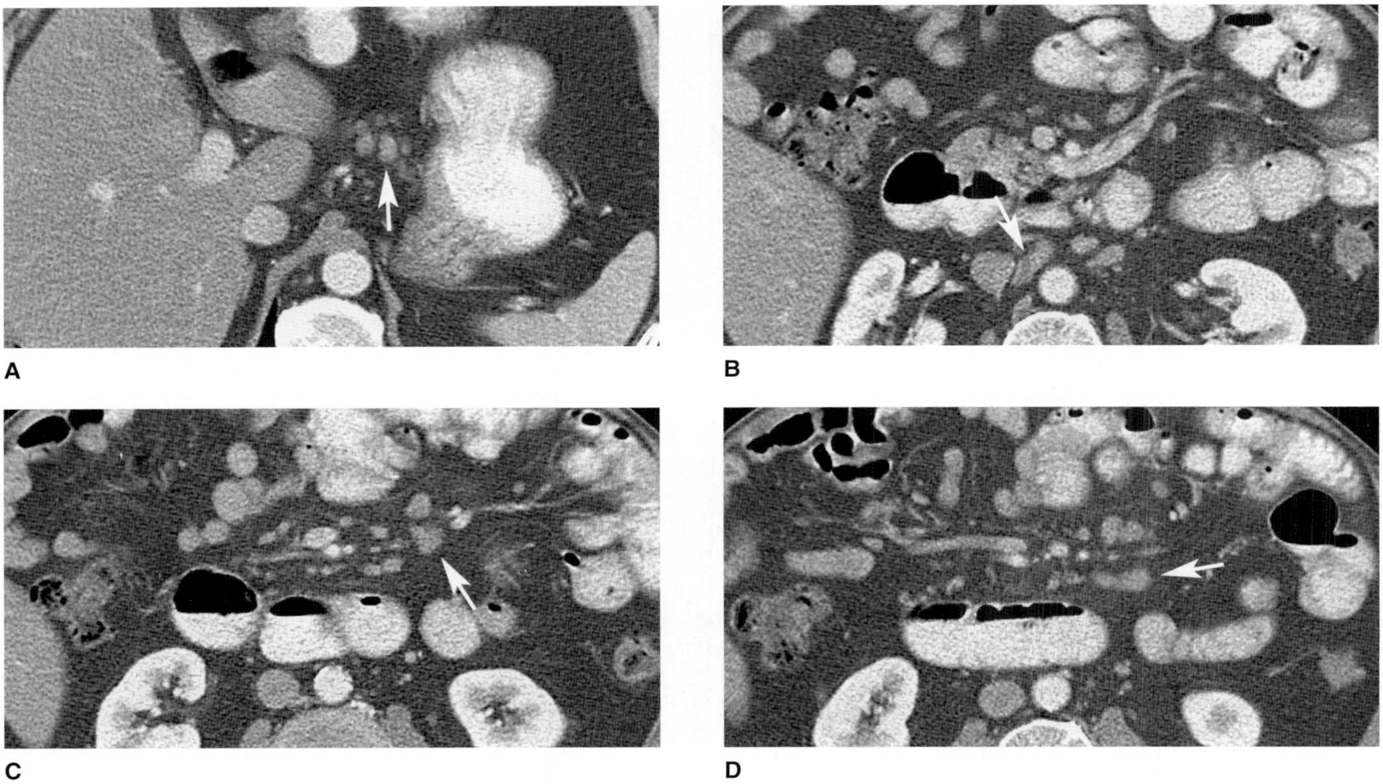

A

B

C

D

Figure 13-11 Follicular Lymphoma
This 54-year-old man presented with weight loss and diarrhea. **A-D.** Contrast-enhanced axial CT demonstrates multiple small and intermediate lymph nodes in the gastrohepatic (*arrow* in A, 7 mm × 12 mm), right para-aortic (*arrow* in B, 10 mm × 24 mm), and mesenteric (*arrow* in C, 13 mm × 17 mm and *arrow* in D) 10 mm × 17 mm). Any one of these intermediate lymph nodes could be a normal variant; however, this many intermediate lymph nodes will usually signal disease. Lymph node biopsy was diagnostic of low-grade, follicular lymphoma.

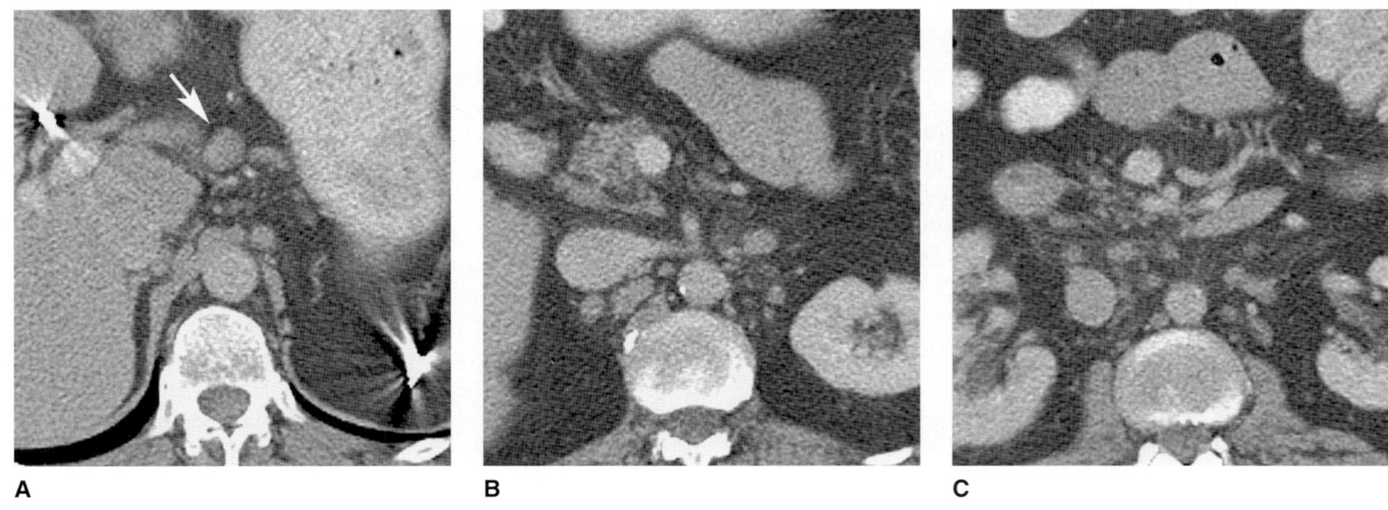

A

B

C

Figure 13-12 Multiple Small Lymph Nodes due to Chronic Lymphocytic Leukemia (CLL)
This 58-year-old woman had chronic lymphocytic leukemia. **A-C.** Contrast-enhanced axial images demonstrate 1 intermediate-sized gastrohepatic lymph node (14 mm × 16 mm) (*arrow*) and many small para-aortic lymph nodes. This is an abnormal pattern of lymph node distribution and will usually be a manifestation of inflammatory disease but can occasionally be due to a malignancy such as CLL as in this case.

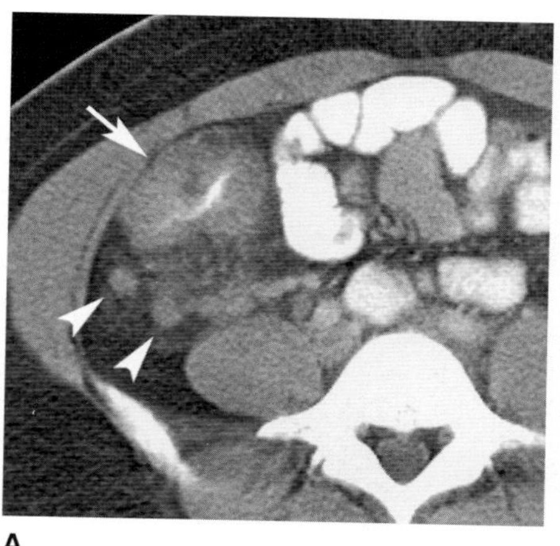
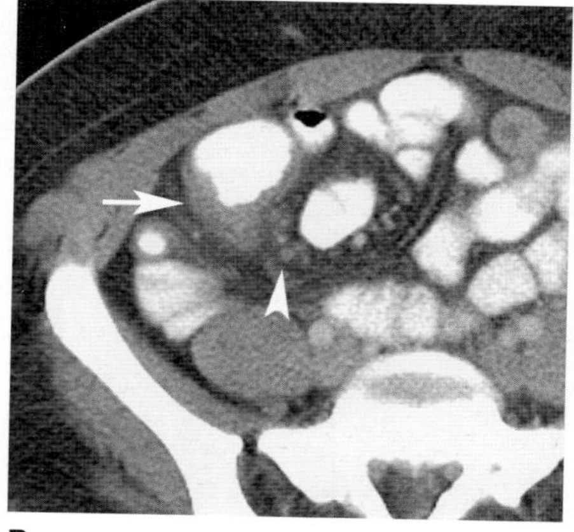
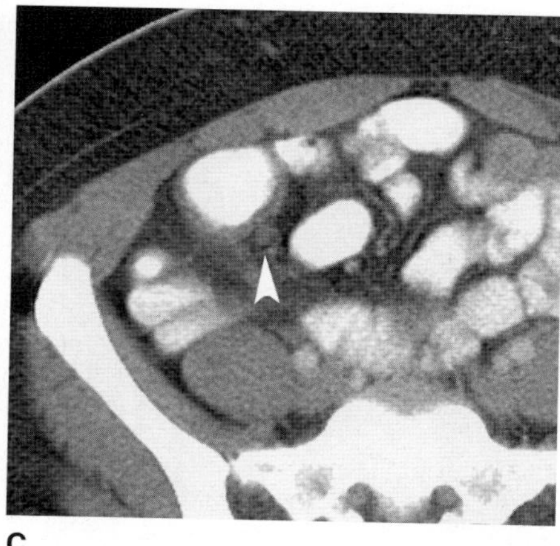

Figure 13-13 Pericecal Adenopathy Due to Crohn Ileitis-Colitis This 31-year-old woman presented with nausea, vomiting, and diarrhea. **A-C.** Contrast-enhanced CT through the right lower quadrant demonstrates a thickened cecal wall (*arrows*) and increase in number and size of pericecal lymph nodes (*arrowheads*). There is also streaking of the perirectal and mesenteric fat. Colonoscopic biopsy was diagnostic of Crohn disease.

attenuations similar to skeletal muscle on both enhanced and unenhanced CT and with T1-weighted, T2-weighted, and gradient echo signal characteristics similar to skeletal muscle. However, rarely lymph node pathology can be identified because of the presence of altered x-ray attenuation or signal intensity.

Occasionally special techniques in MRI can be employed to characterize the tissues involved with malignancy and to measure response to therapy. These techniques include MR spectroscopy to detect altered metabolism, diffusion MRI to detect cell proliferation, and dynamic MRI to detect angiogenesis and to identify hypoxia.[36,37] Detailed description of these techniques is beyond the scope of this chapter.

Lymph node calcification

High attenuation within lymph nodes will usually be a result of dystrophic calcification within the lymph node. Dystrophic calcification, calcification of tissues due to cell death, is most

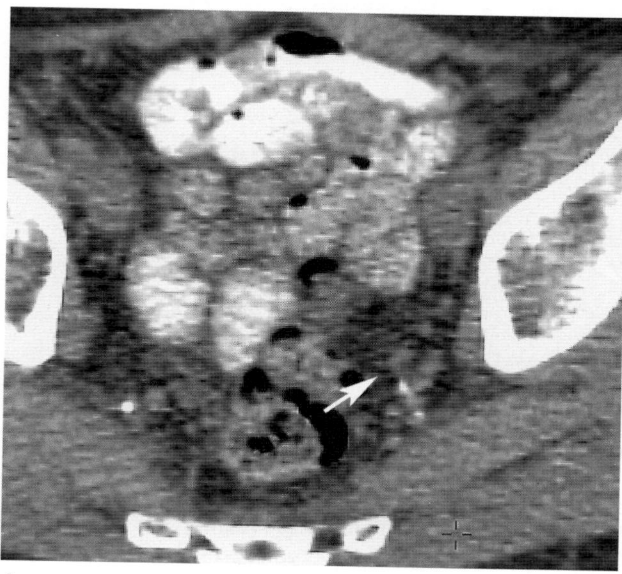
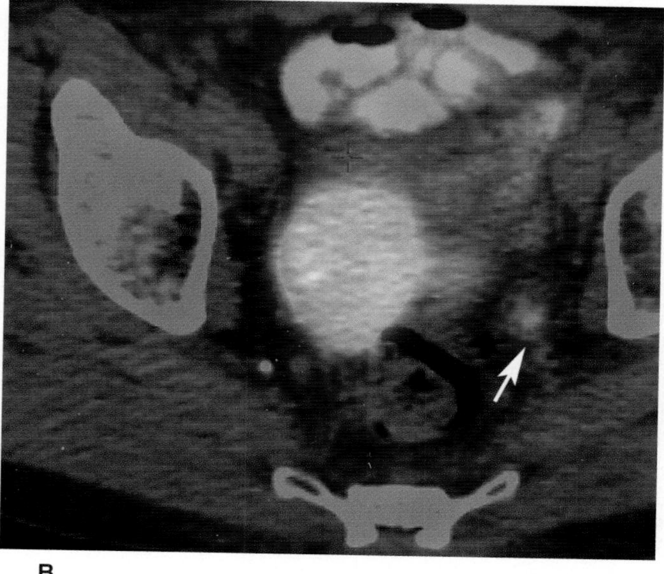

Figure 13-14 Perirectal Small Lymph Node Metastasis **A.** Unenhanced CT from a PET-CT shows a tiny perirectal lymph node (*arrow*). In most cases this will represent a normal variant. **B.** However, PET-CT fused image shows this lymph node to be FDG positive. In this 67-year-old patient with a known rectal carcinoma, this is highly likely to represent microscopic lymph node metastasis.

A

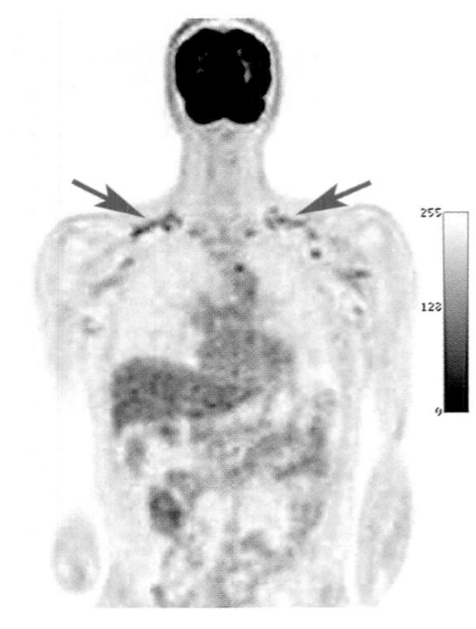

B

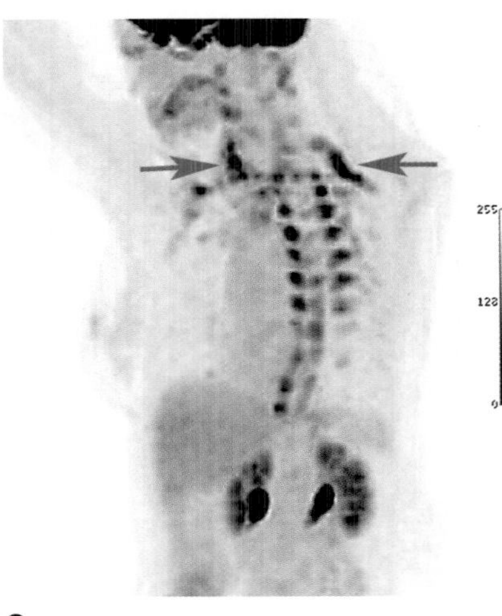

C

Figure 13-15 PET Activity Due to Brown Fat in 3 Patients
A. PET-CT and (**B** and **C**) PET images demonstrate increased activity in the soft-tissues of the neck and in the paraspinal location (*arrows*). This is the typical appearance of brown fat and should not be confused with metabolically abnormal tissues.

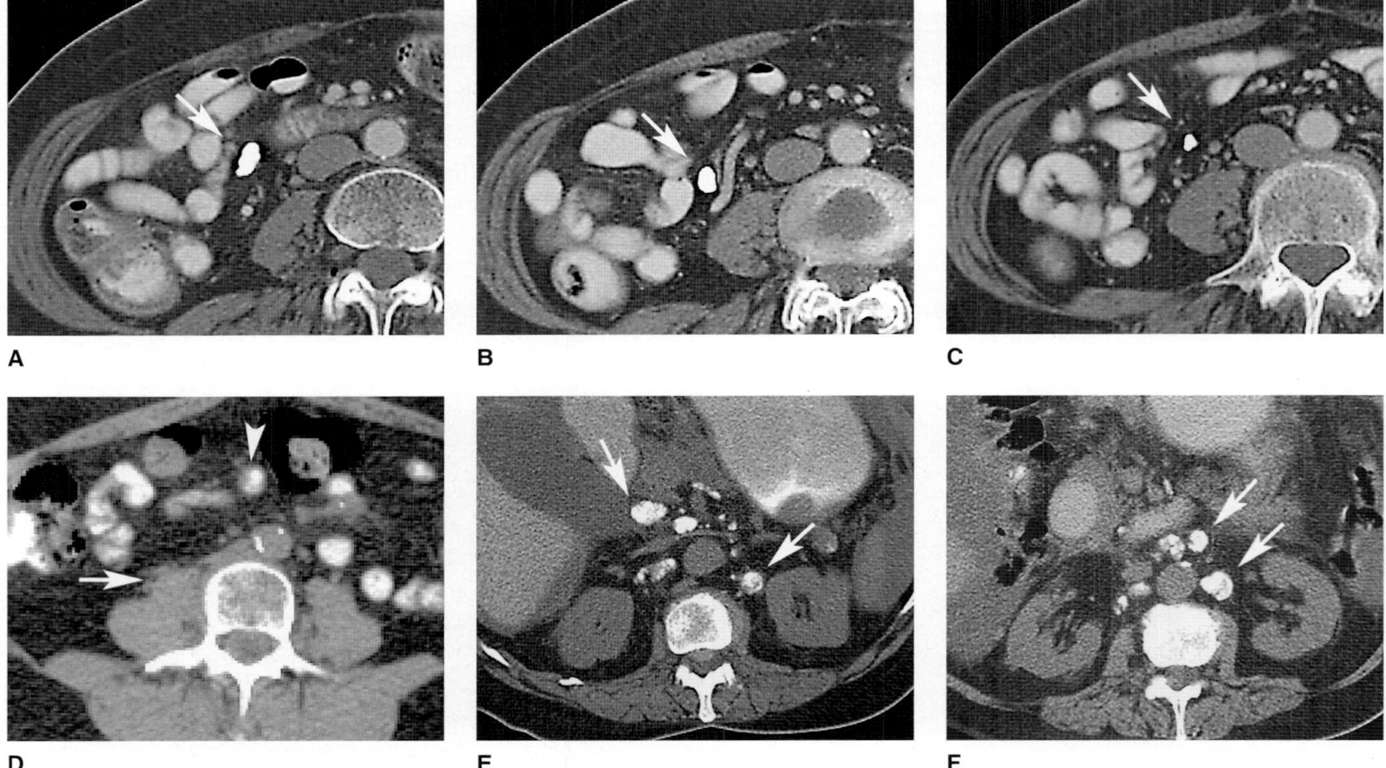

Figure 13-16 Lymph Node Calcification in 3 Patients
A-C. This 70-year-old woman was being evaluated for breast carcinoma. Contrast-enhanced CT demonstrates multiple calcified right lower quadrant mesenteric lymph nodes (*arrows*). Most lymph node calcifications will be secondary to prior granulomatous infection. The exact cause for these lymph nodes is not known but they have remained stable for many years. **D.** This 46-year-old woman is a known case of lymphoma and previously treated with chemotherapy. Calcified mesenteric (*arrowhead*) and noncalcified right psoas (*arrow*) lymph nodes are seen. **E** and **F.** This 54-year-old woman had mucinous cystadenoarcinoma of the ovary. Contrast-enhanced CT demonstrates multiple calcified lymph nodes (*arrow*) in the upper retroperitoneum. These will most often be due to prior granulomatous disease. However, this patient's primary tumor demonstrated coarse regions of calcification and these lymph nodes have slowly enlarged over 5 years, indicating widespread calcified lymph node metastasis.

Table 13-4. Causes of Hyperattenuating Lymph Nodes

A. Calcification 1. Granulomatous infection 2. Sarcoidosis 3. Treated lymphoma 4. Metastasis from calcified neoplasms
B. Hyperenhancement 1. Hypervascular metastasis 2. Castleman disease
C. Lymphangiographic contrast

often a result of prior granulomatous infection, prior sarcoidosis, or treated lymphoma and will typically appear as flocculent areas within the lymph node with very high attenuation similar to cortical bone (see Figure 13-16).

Rarely lymph nodes can be high attenuation due to calcified metastasis. Very few tumors exhibit macroscopic calcification; however, notable exceptions include some tumors of bone and cartilage such as osteosarcomas and chondrosarcomas and some mucinous adenocarcinomas (Table 13-4) see Figure 13-16.

Hyperenhancing lymph nodes

High attenuation within lymph nodes on CT can also be due to hyperenhancement of the lymph node following injection of intravenous contrast or the accumulation of lymphangiographic contrast. Hyperenhancing lymph nodes will most often be seen in lymph node metastasis from hypervascular tumors such as neuroendocrine tumors, melanoma, renal cell carcinoma, papillary thyroid carcinoma, and Kaposi sarcoma (see Figure 13-17).[38] Rarely, hyperenhancing lymph nodes will be due to Castleman disease (see Figure 13-18).[39-41]

Lymphangiographic contrast is a lipid based iodinated compound injected into the lymphatics of the feet and which accumulates in the lymph nodes. This has a characteristic attenuation and imaging appearance on plain films and CT scans. On plain films, the lymph nodes appear hyperdense. On CT scans lymphangiographic contrast is more attenuating than calcium and resemble the attenuation of metallic structures (see Figure 13-19).

Low-attenuation lymph nodes

Attenuation of lymph nodes less than the normal attenuation of skeletal muscle is an uncommon finding that can be due to the presence of fluid or lipid material within the lymph node. Causes of low-attenuation lymph nodes include necrotic metastasis, lymphoma, granulomatous infections, and several other unusual disorders (Table 13-5).

Recognition of low attenuation of lymph nodes will most often indicate central necrosis of the lymph node as a result of necrotic metastasis (see Figure 13-20). Neoplasms reported to cause low-attenuation lymph nodes include metastatic carcinoma from lung, germ cell tumors, ovary, and lymphoma.[42]

Granulomatous infections including tuberculosis, nontuberculous mycobacterial infection, and histoplasmosis can also cause low-attenuation lymph nodes.[42] This

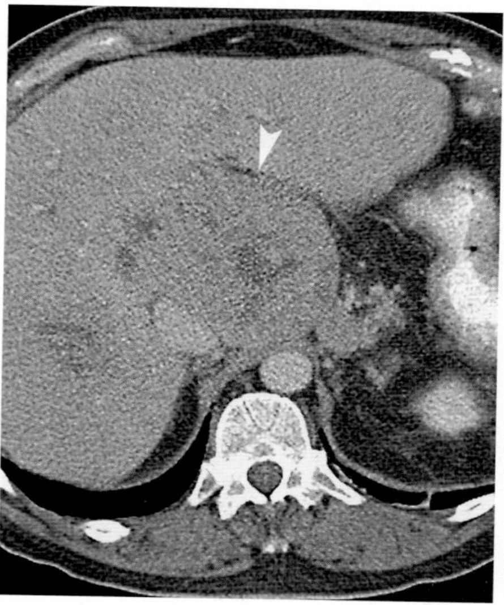
A

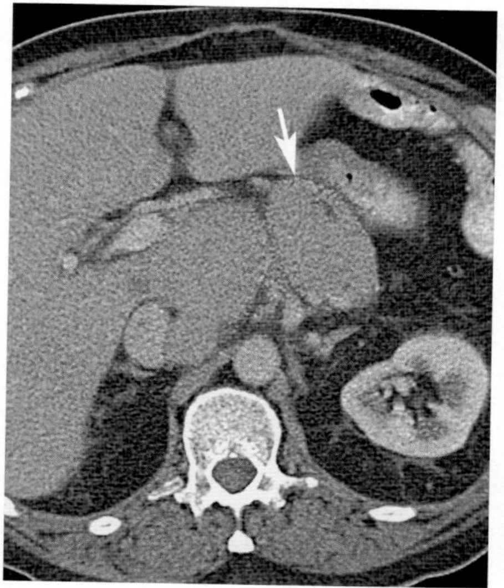
B

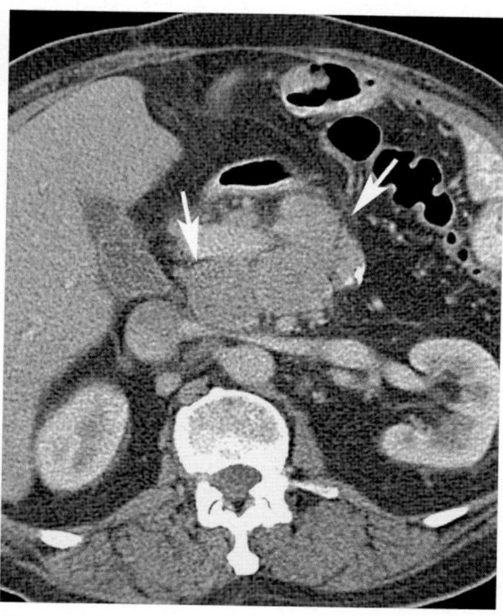
C

Figure 13-17 Hypervascular Lymph Node Metastasis This 69-year-old man had a pancreatic neuroendocrine carcinoma. **A-C.** Contrast-enhanced axial CT images show a large hypervascular liver metastasis (*arrowhead*) and multiple markedly enlarged hyperenhancing celiac axis lymph node metastasis (*arrows*). Note how the lymph nodes enhance as much as the normal liver parenchyma and more than the parasonal muscles. This indicates the presence of hypervascular disease, in this case metastasis.

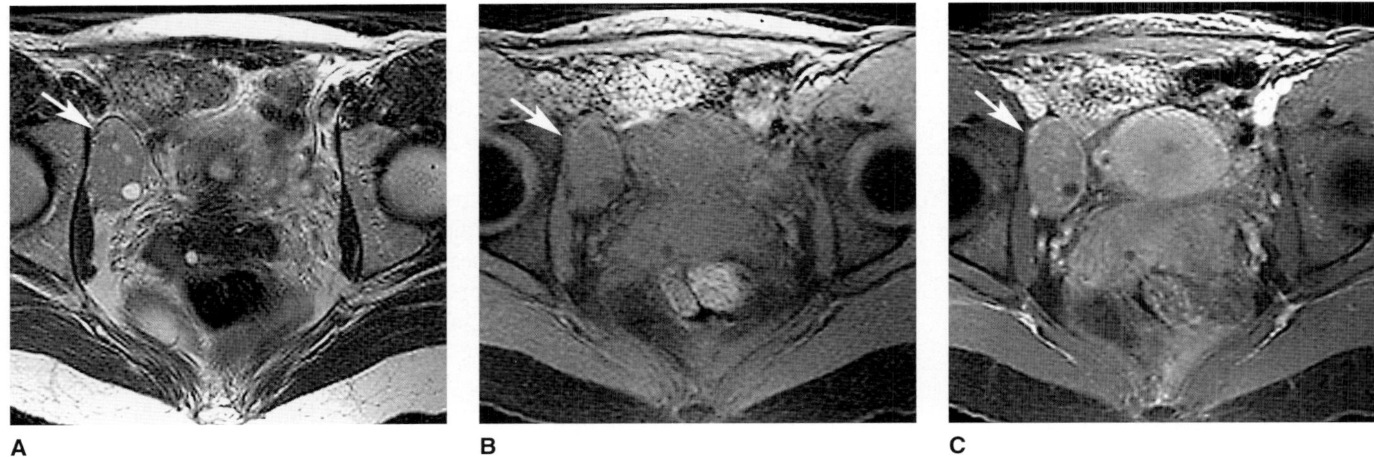

Figure 13-18 Castleman Disease
This 40-year-old woman had a palpebal pelvic abnormality. **A.** T2-weighted, (**B**) T1-weighted pregadolinium, and (**C**) T1-weighted postgadolinium axial MRI images of the pelvis show an enlarged right obturator lymph node (*arrows*). This node enhances (C) more brightly than the gluteus muscles following gadolinium enhancement. Surgical biopsy was diagnostic of Castleman disease.

finding was especially common in HIV-positive patients prior to highly active antiretroviral therapy (HAART). However, since HAART therapy has become the standard of care for HIV-infected individuals, recognition of low-attenuation lymph nodes due to granulomatous infections has become rare in industrialized countries. However, in developing countries, tuberculosis remains an important cause of low-attenuation lymph nodes (see Figure 13-21).

Whipple disease, a rare enteric infection caused by the bacterium *Tropheryma whippelii* causing bowel wall

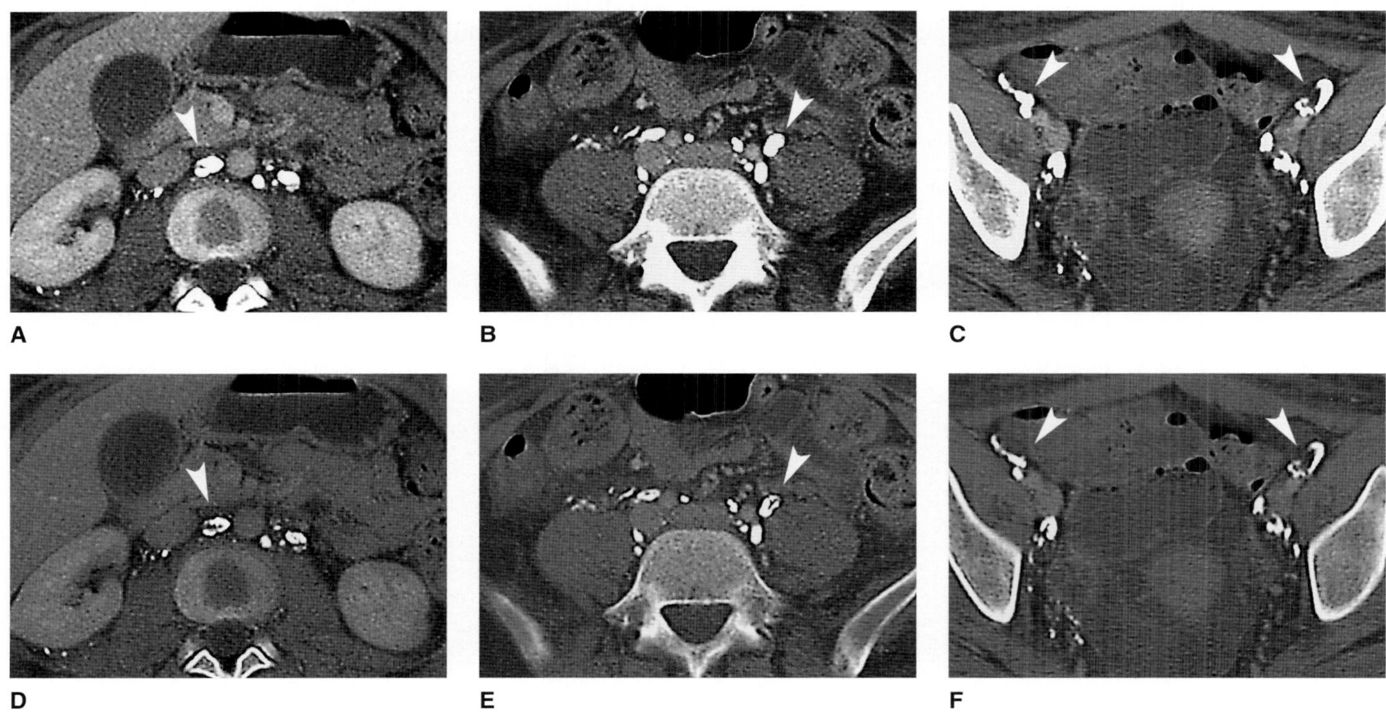

Figure 13-19 Lymphangiographic Contrast on CT Exams
A-C. Soft-tissue windows from an axial contrast-enhanced CT show multiple hyperattenuating lesions (*arrowheads*) in the distribution of abdominal and pelvic lymph nodes. Note these appear brighter than cortical bone. **D-F.** Bone windows show these to have fine curvilinear shapes outlining the cortex and hilum of individual lymph nodes. This appearance is characteristic of lymphangiographic contrast.

Table 13-5. Causes of Low-Attenuation Cystic Lymph Nodes

A. Necrotic metastasis
B. Whipple disease
C. Infections (primarily in HIV-positive patients) 1. Tuberculosis 2. *Mycobacterium avium-intracellulare* 3. *Histoplasma capsulatum*

thickening is also a rare cause of low-attenuation lymph nodes. This disorder is a cause for malabsorption and can present with weight loss, diarrhea, joint pain, and arthritis and is described in greater detail in Chapter 2. However, in this case, the low attenuation is not due to lymph node necrosis but is due to lipid accumulation in the lymph nodes related to accumulation of the Whipple organism within the lymph nodes.[42]

Patients with celiac disease can rarely present with low-attenuation lymph nodes, a phenomenon that has been called "cavitating mesenteric lymph node syndrome."[43,44] Histologic evaluation of the lymph nodes demonstrates a rim of atrophic lymphocytes with central cavitation containing milky fluid and lipid droplets. It is believed that cavitation is a result of mesenteric lymphoid depletion and the crossing of antigenic material over abnormal intestinal mucosa. Imaging examinations demonstrate enlarged low-attenuation lymph nodes with either fluid or fat attenuation (see Figure 2-53). Only Whipple disease and celiac disease are known to cause fat attenuation lymph nodes. Rarely, lymph nodes in celiac disease will contain fat-fluid levels, a finding that appears to be unique to celiac disease.[43]

Lymphangioleiomyomatosis (LAM) is a rare idiopathic disorder resulting in cystic interstitial lung disease. Although the clinically significant manifestations of LAM are primarily in the thorax, there are a variety of abdominal manifestations of LAM including angiomyolipomas of the kidney, LAM of the lymphatic ducts, chylous ascites, and abdominal lymphadenopathy.[45] Some studies suggest that lymphadenopathy can be found in up to 40% of cases and can be as large as 4 cm in diameter. Lymph nodes can contain water-attenuation regions because of the accumulation of lymph fluid.

Lymph nodes with decreased MRI signal

As a result of the paramagnetic effects of iron, iron deposition within lymph nodes will result in loss of signal on virtually all imaging sequences but is most pronounced on gradient echo sequences. Excessive iron deposition within lymph nodes is virtually diagnostic of hemosiderosis and will usually cause loss of signal in the liver and spleen because of similar iron deposition in those organs. These organs are part of the reticuloendothelial system that phagocytizes damaged red blood cells. Excessive red cell

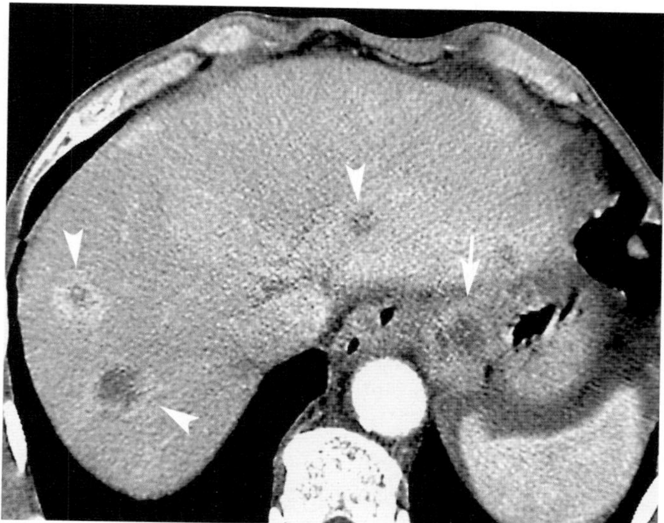
A

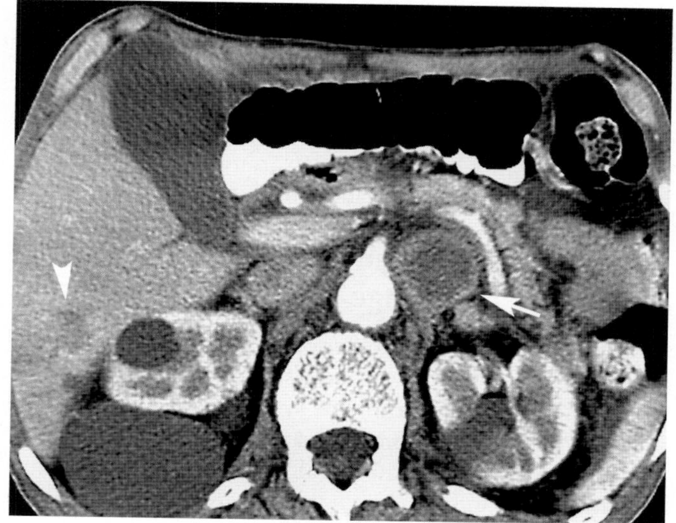
B

Figure 13-20 Necrotic Lymph Node Metastasis
This 83-year-old man with prostate cancer presented with right upper quadrant pain, anorexia, and weight loss. **A** and **B.** Contrast-enhanced axial CT images show multiple rim-enhancing, centrally low-attenuation liver lesions (*arrowheads*) typical of liver metastasis. There are also low-attenuation gastrohepatic (*arrow* in A) and celiac axis (*arrow* in B) lymph nodes. The central low attenuation of the liver metastasis and lymph nodes represents central necrosis of lymph node metastasis. This distribution and appearance of metastatic disease is unusual for prostate cancer. Further evaluation revealed an occult poorly differentiated esophageal adenocarcinoma.

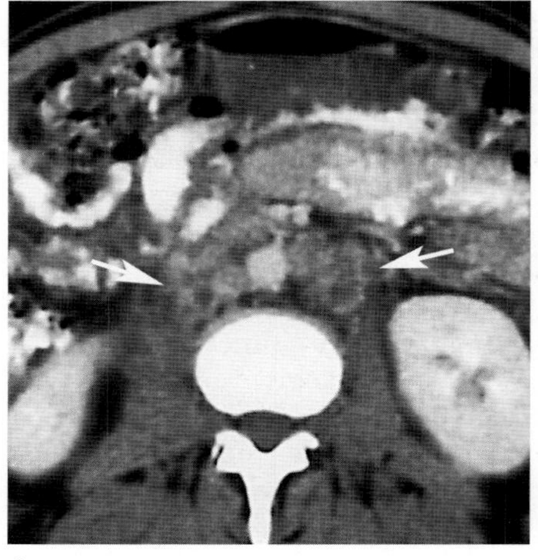

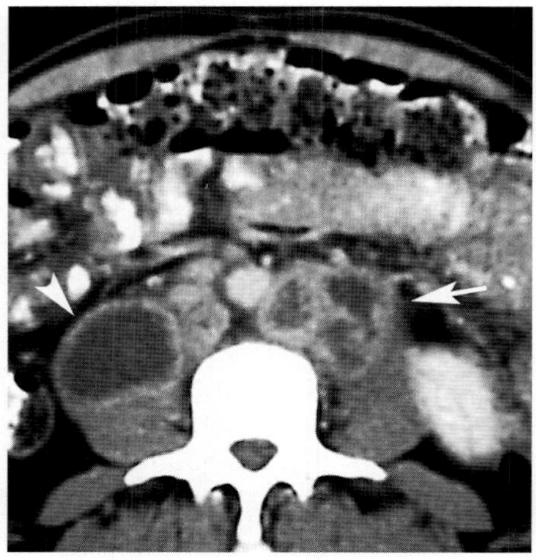

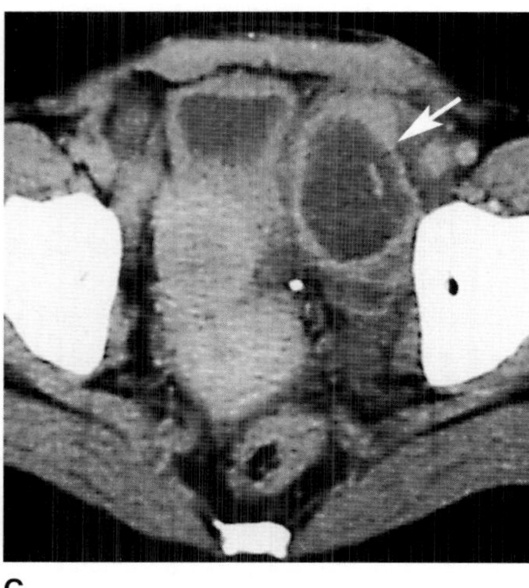

Figure 13-21 Disseminated Tuberculosis
This 37-year-old woman presented with fever, chills, and a 10-pound weight loss. **A-C.** Contrast enhanced axial CT images show centrally low attenuation, rim enhancing lymph nodes in the para-aortic (*arrows* in A and B) and external iliac (*arrow* in C) chains. There is also a low attenuation lesion in the right retroperitoneum that either represents a necrotic lymph node or psoas abscess. Thoracic imaging (not shown) demonstrated innumerable micronodules. This patient was ultimately diagnosed with disseminated tuberculosis.

destruction as seen in hemoglobinopathies and related to blood transfusions can lead to the deposition of iron in the tissues of the reticuloendothelial system. Deposition in the lymph nodes is much less common than that seen in the liver and spleen.

DISEASES AFFECTING LYMPH NODES

Metastatic tumor and lymphoma are the most common diseases to cause imaging-identifiable lymph node abnormalities. Hepatitis, infectious colitis, inflammatory bowel disease, and sarcoidosis are the most common infectious or inflammatory conditions to cause imaging identifiable lymphadenopathy but there are a variety of other causes of imaging identifiable lymphadenopathy.

Causes of Lymphadenopathy Affecting More Than 1 Drainage Distribution

Lymphadenopathy affecting more than 1 drainage distribution will usually indicate a systemic disorder that has manifestations in the lymphatic system. This is most often due to lymphoma or CLL but can occasionally be due to disseminated granulomatous infections or some systemic inflammatory conditions such as systemic lupus erythematosus and rheumatoid arthritis (Table 13-6).

Lymphoma

Lymphoma is cancer of lymphatic system and the most fifth most common malignancy in adults, the most common malignancy among teenagers and young adults and is the third most common neoplasm among children.[46] Lymphoma is typically divided into HL and NHL. In year 2010, a total of 74,030 cases of lymphoma were diagnosed in the United States, approximately 8490 of which were HL.[46]

Further, HL and NHL are among the most common causes of abdominopelvic lymphadenopathy. Para-aortic lymphadenopathy is one of the most common findings in HL

Table 13-6. Causes of Lymphadenopathy Affecting More Than 1 Drainage Distribution

A. Neoplasms
1. **Non-Hodgkin lymphoma**[a]
2. **Hodgkin disease**
3. **Chronic lymphocytic leukemia**
4. Systemic mastocytosis
5. Metastatic tumor

B. Infectious diseases (usually in HIV patients)
1. Tuberculosis
2. *Mycobacterium avium-intracellulare*
3. Histoplasmosis

C. Inflammatory disorders
1. Connective tissue disorders
    a. Systemic lupus erythematosus
    b. Rheumatoid arthritis
2. Henoch-Schönlein purpura
3. Sarcoidosis
4. Kikuchi disease

D. Other causes
1. Amyloidosis

[a]Items in bold are most common.

and NHL. Moreover, HL and NHL can present as lymphadenopathy of 1 or more groups of lymph nodes or often involving isolated organ or can present as widely disseminated disease. Lymph node involvement due to lymphoma usually causes displacement of structures without their invasion. This is an important finding on imaging that distinguishes lymphomas from the carcinomas. HL and NHL usually present with similar radiological features; however, there are some significant differences in their radiographic presentations.

Non-Hodgkin lymphoma: Non-Hodgkin lymphomas (NHLs) are a diverse set of diseases with varying histology, natural histories, and responses to therapy. At least 15 types of NHLs are recognized as distinct clinical entities.[47,48] About 85% of NHLs are B-cells. The others have T cell–type or NK cell–type histology. In general, NHL can be clinically subdivided into low-grade, intermediate-grade, and high-grade lymphomas, with survival without therapy measured in, respectively, years, months, and weeks.[47-49] As a group, they are the fifth most common malignancy in the United States in men and women.[46] The incidence of NHL progressively increases with age from childhood through advanced old age (see Figure 13-22).[50] The cause of NHL remains unknown but roles for infections, autoimmune disorders, ionizing radiation, and generalized immunodeficiency have been proposed. Epstein-Barr virus (EBV) infection has been associated with Burkitt and other lymphomas.[51] *Helicobacter pylori* infection has been associated with GI maltomas.[52,53] Therapeutic irradiation in patients with HL has been associated with an increase in the incidence of secondary NHL.[54-56] Patients with HIV/AIDS, organ transplantation, autoimmune diseases, and some congenital immunodeficiencies have also been associated with increased incidence of NHL.[57-59] The incidence of NHL has doubled in the United States from the 1980s to 2000, largely as a result of HIV/AIDS and the increasing use of immunosuppressive therapies in organ transplants and other chronic illnesses. However, incidence of NHL and Kaposi sarcoma have declined markedly in recent years, likely because of HAART-related improvements in immunity.

Patients with lymphoma will usually present with either (1) a variety of systemic symptoms such as weight loss, fever, malaise, fatigue, night sweats, and pruritis; (2) painless lymphadenopathy; or (3) a combination of both.[60]

Hodgkin lymphoma: HL has a bimodal incidence, with peaks occurring between 15 and 35 years and after age 50 (see Figure 13-23).[60] Further, HL accounts for approximately 10% of lymphomas and will most often present in the neck and thorax.[60] The histologic diagnosis of HL is dependent on demonstration of large, bilobed or double-nuclei cells with prominent inclusion-like nucleoli giving an "owl's-eye" appearance. These are known as Reed-Sternberg cells and with their mononuclear variants are thought to be the malignant cell in HL.[61] The many other cells that surround the Reed-Sternberg cells in HL are believed to be reactive populations of nonneoplastic lymphocytes, histiocytes, fibroblasts, eosinophils, and plasma cells.

HL can be subdivided into 4 histological subtypes. The nodular sclerosing subtype accounts for approximately 40% to 60% of cases.[62,63] The remainder represent lymphocyte-depleted, lymphocyte-predominant, and mixed-cellularity subtypes. Patients with mixed cellularity and lymphocyte depletion histology have a poorer prognosis than those with other histological subtypes.[64] Seroepidemiologic studies and localization of EBV DNA in Reed-Sternberg cells suggests a role of EBV infection in HL. Up to 40% of HL cases in developed countries can be associated with EBV infection.[65]

In most cases, HL will spread contiguously from 1 lymph node region to adjacent lymph node regions.[66,67] This contiguous pattern of spread makes staging prognostically and therapeutically important, with clinical stage being the most important determinant of prognosis in HL. Further, HL is commonly staged using the Ann Arbor classification system (Table 13-7). Most patients with Stage I or Stage II disease will be cured of their disease with appropriate radiation

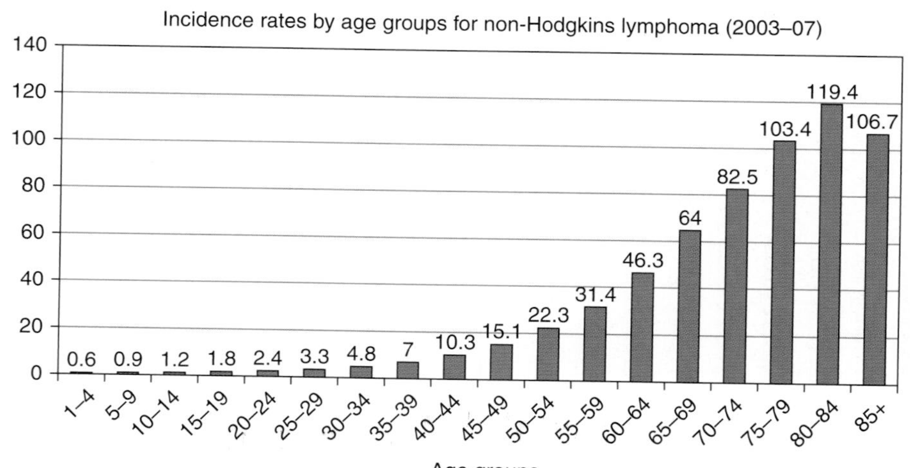

Figure 13-22 Age-Specific Incidence Rates for NHL (2003-2007)
Bar chart showing age-specific incidence rates for NHL (2003-07). On the *x*-axis, the incidence rates are shown per 100 000 population.
Data from Altekruse SF, Kosary CL, Krapcho M, et al, eds. *SEER Cancer Statistics Review, 1975-2007*, National Cancer Institute. Bethesda, MD.

Imaging Notes 13-4. Spread of Hodgkins Disease

Hodgkin lymphoma typically spreads in a contiguous fashion along lymph node chains.

therapy and/or chemotherapy.[64] Factors associated with poorer outcome include the presence of "B" symptoms, older age, bulky disease, and mixed cellularity and lymphocyte depletion histologies of the tumor.[64]

HL will typically present with asymptomatic enlargement of lymph nodes, especially of the cervical and axillary chains. Patients with symptoms will most often complain of dry cough or chest discomfort.[60] Approximately one-third of patients will complain of systemic or "B" symptoms, including fever, night sweats, and weight loss. Weight loss and loss of appetite, and dragging pain due to splenomegaly are the usual abdominal symptoms. Bone pain, especially that which is worsened by alcohol consumption, is an unusual but interesting symptom associated with HL.

HL is a chemotherapy-sensitive malignancy with an excellent response and cure rate. Five-year survival rates are approximately 80% to 85% for all races in the United States, and relapse will usually occur within the first 2 years following completion of therapy.[54,60,64] Development of lymphadenopathy or masses within organs more than a few years following completion of therapy should raise the suspicion of a second malignancy, a phenomenon that will occur in approximately 13% of patients.[54-56,68] Secondary malignancies are most frequently breast cancer, lung cancer, leukemia, and NHL.[54,68] Increased risk of a second malignancy is associated with combined chemotherapy-radiation therapy and is correlated with the size of the radiation portal. Breast cancer is at especially increased incidence when women are treated with radiotherapy at a young age.[54,68]

The majority of patients with HL will have presentations in the cervical, axillary, and thoracic lymph node chains.[69,70] Abdominal involvement was found in approximately 15% and 27% of patients in 2 series.[70,71] Lymph node involvement was found most often in retroperitoneal lymph nodes, followed by intraperitoneal and pelvic locations. In most cases, the PET and CT imaging will be concordant in their detection of specific disease loci. However, most studies have indicated that PET scans have greater sensitivity and specificity than CT scans in the staging of HL.[72-74] The combination of PET imaging and CT scanning has been shown to be complementary because in some instances disease will only be detected by one or the other of the imaging studies.[29] Further, PET-CT delivers the advantages of both examinations and is now an integral part of the staging and follow-up of HL.

Table 13-7. Ann Arbor Staging System of Hodgkin and Non-Hodgkin Lymphoma

Stage I	Involvement of a single lymph node region (I) or a single extralymphatic organ or site (IE).
Stage II	Involvement of 2 or more lymph node regions on the same side of the diaphragm (II) alone or with localized involvement of an extralymphatic organ or site (IIE).
Stage III	Involvement of lymph node regions on both sides of the diaphragm (III) alone or with localized involvement of an extralymphatic organ or site (IIIE) or spleen (IIIS) or both (IIISE).
Stage IV	Diffuse or disseminated involvement of 1 or more extralymphatic organs with or without associated lymph node involvement.
All patients are subclassified A or B to indicate the absence or presence, respectively, of unexplained weight loss of more than 10% body weight, unexplained fever with temperatures more than 38°C, and night sweats.	

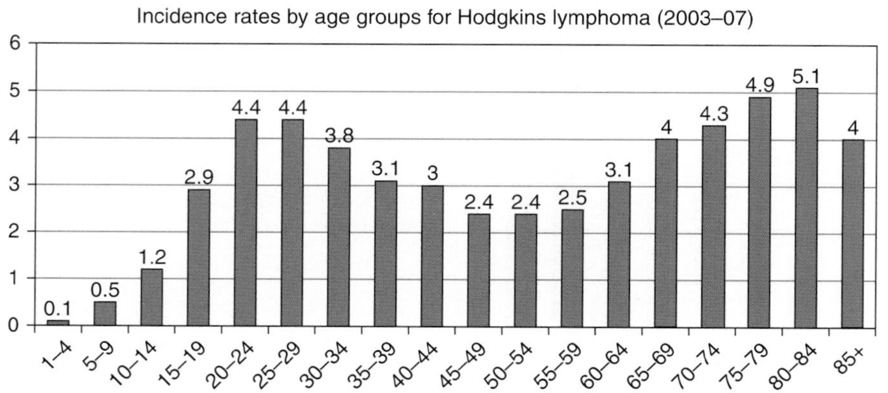

Figure 13-23 Age-Specific Incidence of Hodgkin Lymphoma (2003-2007)
Bar chart showing age-specific incidence rates for Hodgkin Lymphoma (2003-2007). On *x*-axis, the incidence rates are shown per 100 000 population.
Data from Altekruse SF, Kosary CL, Krapcho M, et al, eds. *SEER Cancer Statistics Review, 1975-2007*, National Cancer Institute. Bethesda, MD.

Older studies have suggested that approximately 60% to 75% of cases of HL will leave residual fibrotic soft-tissue masses following completion of chemotherapy and/or irradiation.[75-77] Some studies have suggested that patients with residual masses are twice as likely to have recurrence than those without residual masses, especially those who were treated with chemotherapy without radiation therapy.[75,77] However, other studies have failed to show this association.[76] It is the author's belief that residual masses are now much less common than previously reported. When found, residual masses typically appear as a non-descript soft-tissue mass at the sites of original disease. When noncalcified, these masses are indistinguishable from residual tumor on CT and MRI exams. However, cross-sectional imaging will show them to remains stable on serial follow-up exams and they will be cold on PET scans. A PET-CT study is very useful in the assessment of therapeutic response because of its discriminating power between benign fibrosis presenting as absent or low-grade FDG uptake and residual active lymphoma presenting as elevated FDG uptake. Persistent FDG activity in posttreatment scans is associated with early relapse and poor clinical outcome.[78,79] The larger the initial tumor, the greater the likelihood of a residual mass on CT scans. Most residual fibrotic masses will slowly decrease in volume over many years and often subsequently calcify.[80] In past decades, it was common to see dystrophic calcification developing in lymph nodes of previously treated HL.[75-77,80] However, this is now a relatively uncommon phenomenon.

Imaging features of Hodgkin lymphoma and non-Hodgkin lymphoma: The imaging characteristics of HL and NHL are similar and cannot be reliably distinguished. One of the distinguishing features between NHL and HL is that HL spreads in a contiguous fashion along the lymph node chains. Very large lymph nodes, greater than 4 cm in diameter, are uncommon in HL but are not infrequent in NHL. Also extranodal involvement in HL is much less common than NHL.

Imaging Notes 13-5. Lymph Node Size and Lymphoma

> Lymph nodes larger than 4 cm in diameter are uncommon in Hodgkin lymphoma but are not infrequent in non-Hodgkins lymphomas.

The imaging role of CT scans in the evaluation of lymphoma is multifold. It not only defines the full extent of disease for accurate staging but also assists in treatment planning, to evaluate response to therapy, to monitor progression of disease, and to detect possible relapse. Care should be made in attributing small changes in lymph node size with treatment response. Studies of interobserver variability in the measurement of lymph node diameters have suggested that observers will have an average of 3-mm difference in measurements of lymph node diameters.[81] CT has traditionally been the imaging modality of choice in the evaluation of lymphomas; however, it is limited in its accuracy because small lymph nodes can harbor lymphoma and large lymph nodes can be benign.[82] Increasingly, PET-CT is being employed in the surveillance of lymphoma because of its greater accuracy in identifying the sites of active disease.

Lymphoma can present as unifocal adenopathy, multifocal adenopathy, or as a diffusely infiltrating mass involving multiple lymph node sites (see Figures 13-11, 13-24, and 13-25). Any nodal chain within the abdomen and pelvis can

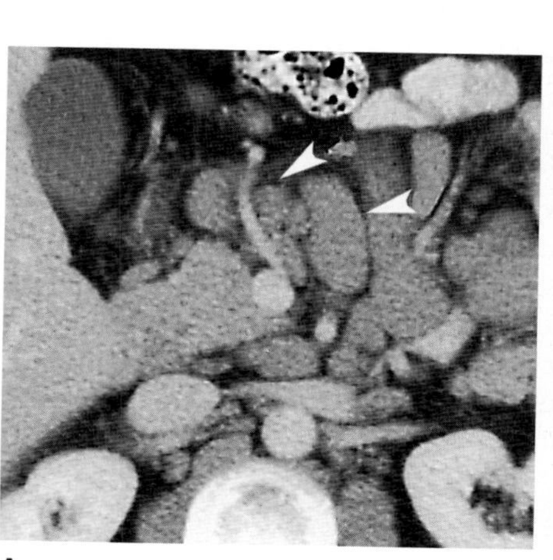
A

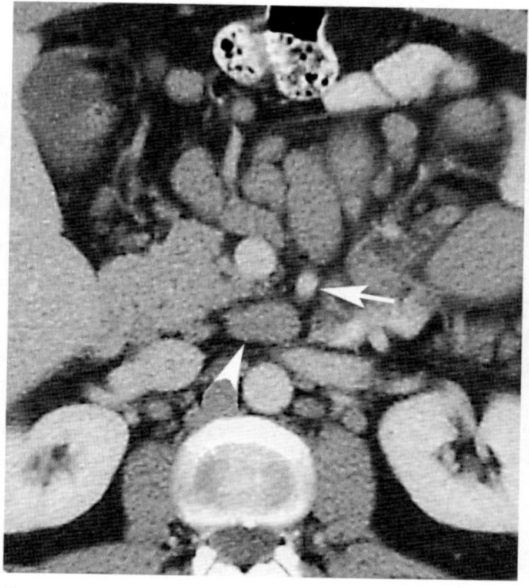
B

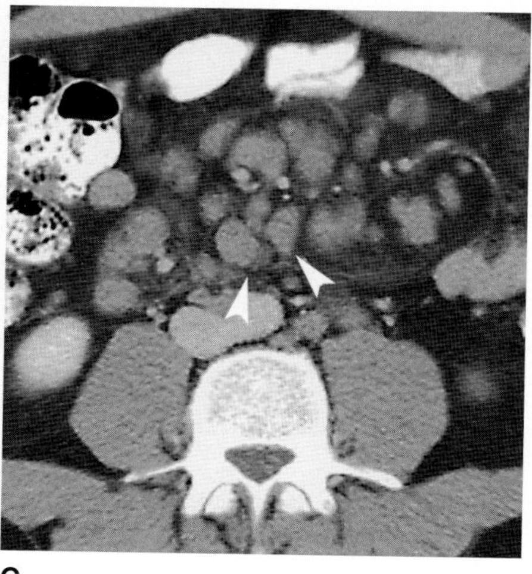
C

Figure 13-24 Non-Hodgkin Lymphoma
This 57-year-old man presented with fevers and weight loss. **A-C.** Contrast-enhanced axial CT images demonstrate enlarged para-aortic and mesenteric lymph nodes (*arrowheads*). Extensive multichain adenopathy like this will most often be due to lymphoma. The *arrow* in (B) points to the superior mesenteric artery. Node biopsy was diagnostic of non-Hodgkin lymphoma.

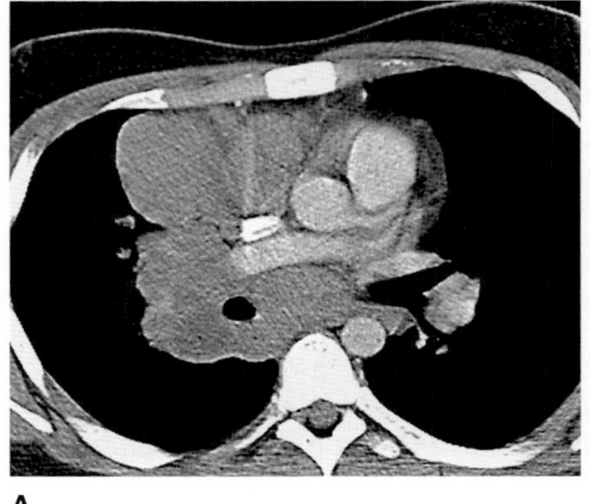

A

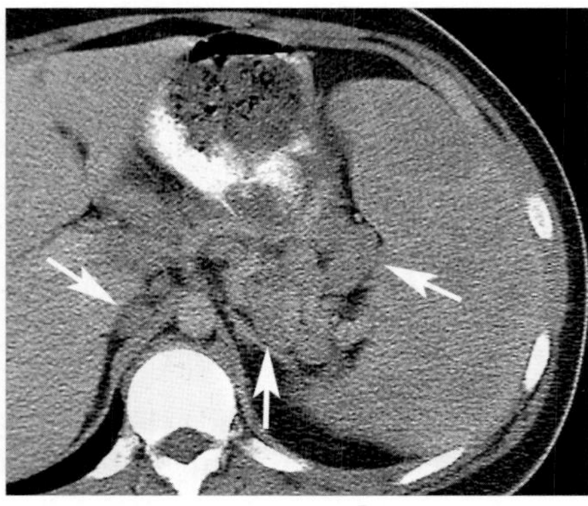

B

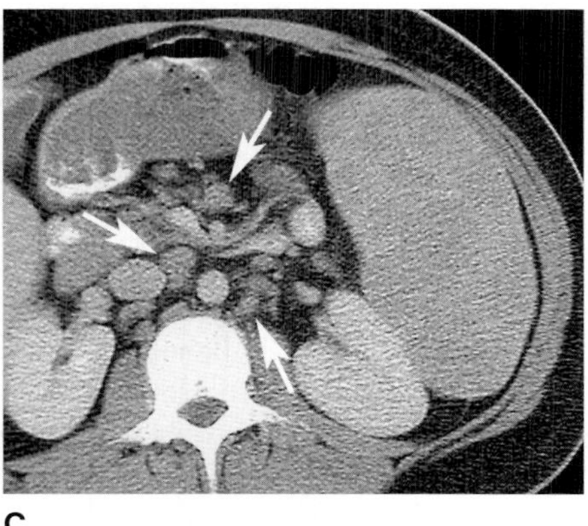

C

Figure 13-25 Hodgkin Lymphoma
This 19-year-old man presented with weight loss. **A-C.** Contrast-enhanced axial CT images demonstrate markedly enlarged mediastinal lymph nodes in (A) and increased numbers of small- and medium-sized lymph nodes (*arrows*) in the upper abdomen. The spleen is moderately enlarged and contains multiple hypoattenuating lesions. This constellation of finding is highly suggestive of lymphoma. Lymph node biopsy was diagnostic of Hodgkin disease.

be involved, but para-aortic and iliac chains are the most frequently involved. Mesenteric involvement is the predominant finding in 4% to 5% cases of HL and 30% to 50% cases of NHL. Mesenteric lymphoma can present as round, oval, or irregular masses within the fat of the mesentery. In some cases, the lymph nodes will form 2 conglomerate homogeneous masses on either side of the mesenteric arteries and veins. In cross section, the flat conglomerate masses resemble the bread and the mesenteric vessels the filling of a sandwich, a phenomenon called the "sandwich sign" (see Figure 13-26).[83]

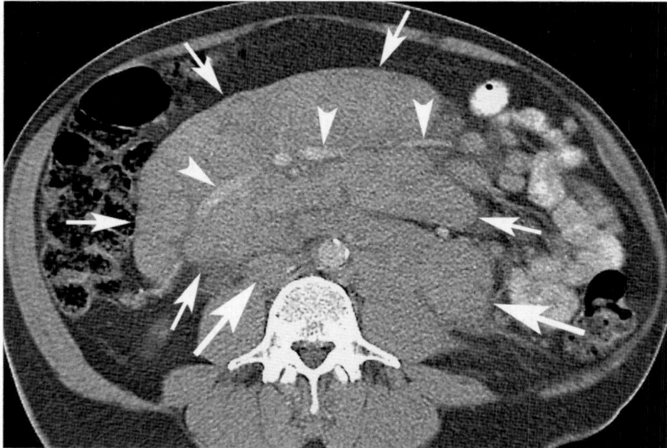

Figure 13-26 The Sandwich Sign
This 61-year-old man had a non-Hodgkin Lymphoma. Contrast-enhanced CT image shows massive mesenteric lymphadenopathy (*small arrows*) surrounding the mesenteric vessels (*arrowheads*). With the lymph nodes serving as the bun and the vessels serving as the filling, the combination resembles a sandwich. There are also multiple enlarged retroperitoneal lymph nodes (*large arrows*).

Lymphoma is a hypercellular malignancy and therefore can be mildly hyperattenuating on unenhanced CT scans. After contrast enhancement, lymphomatous lymph nodes will usually show homogenous low-level enhancement. If there is involvement of the extranodal organs of the abdomen, the organ involved typically shows greater enhancement than the lymphoma. Larger nodal masses can develop central necrosis. Calcification in lymphomas is nearly always a response to treatment and is uncommon as a primary manifestation of the malignancy.

Accuracy of MR in detection of lymph node and organ involvement due to lymphoma is similar to that of CT exams. Lymphomas are usually isointense to skeletal muscle on T1-weighted imaging. On T2-weighted imaging, lymphomas have a moderately high signal intensity because of increased water content in untreated lymphomas.[84,85] In general MRI is significantly more sensitive than CT for detecting bone marrow involvement. Nakayama et al recently showed that the lymphomas' diffusion coefficient of retroperitoneal lymphoma is significantly lower than those of the malignant and benign mesenchymal tumors of the retroperitoneum.[86] This principle can be exploited to distinguish between retroperitoneal lymphoma and nonlymphomatous involvement of the retroperitoneal structures.

Further, PET scanning has become an essential tool in the imaging evaluation of patients with both Hodgkin and NHLs. In general, PET scans will often identify a higher stage than CT scans, in the initial staging of HL.[72-74] Nearly one-third of patients with HL will be upstaged by PET over CT staging.[72] Foci of increased activity will usually indicate the presence of lymphoma (see Figure 13-27). However, low-grade lymphomas and foci of disease less than 1 cm in diameter can result in false-negative examinations.[74] False-positive foci of activity are frequently found in the neck and paraspinal locations because muscular activity, as a result of anxiety, can lead to metabolic activity at these

Imaging Notes 13-6. PET scanning and Hodgkins Disease

> PET or PET-CT is the preferred modality for staging Hodgkin lymphoma because nearly one-third of patients with Hodgkin lymphoma will be upstaged by PET over CT staging.

sites. This has been especially recognized in children and adolescents.[87] Increased metabolic activity can also be seen in the soft-tissues of the sites of brown fat. Uptake in the brown fat in the head and neck areas can result in false-positive results in 2.3% to 4% patients.[88,89] In the fetal life and neonates, brown adipose tissue is in abundance and plays an important role in thermoregulation. This is found usually in the cervical, axillary, paravertebral, mediastinal, and abdominal areas (see Figure 13-15).[90] Most experienced readers are aware of these phenomena and discount activity at these locations. False-positive activity can also occur as a result of unrelated inflammatory conditions. These are the most likely areas of increased activity to be a cause of a false-positive interpretation. Further, PET-CT is not only useful in the initial assessment of lymphoma but is now being extensively used in the treatment follow-up of PET-avid lymphoma.[82]

US has little role in the evaluation of the lymphomas and is predominantly used in real-time biopsies of the focal lesions of the liver and some other approachable lesions in lymphoma.

Involvement of abdominal organs other than the spleen is uncommon in patients with HL and NHL. Details of lymphomatous involvement of extranodal sites in the abdomen are detailed in the chapters dedicated to each organ.

Leukemia

Leukemia is a malignant disease of the bone marrow and blood characterized by uncontrolled accumulation and proliferation of blood cells. Two major categories of leukemia are myelogenous or lymphocytic and each can be subdivided into acute and chronic types. Acute leukemias can present with tiredness, shortness of breath on exertion, fever, night sweat, jaundice, excessive bleeding, slow healing, ecchymosis, and joint pains. Most leukemias have no or few abnormalities detected by imaging exams, with the exception of CLL that commonly causes widespread lymphadenopathy and splenomegaly. Chronic myeloid leukemia can show enlarged spleen on plain abdominal radiograph or CT of abdomen.

Chronic lymphocytic leukemia: CLL occurs as a result of a mutation to the DNA of lymphocytes. In 95% of the cases of CLL, the changes involve B-lymphocytes, but in 5% it can involve T-lymphocytes or natural killer (NK) cells. With time, the CLL cells replace normal lymphocytes in

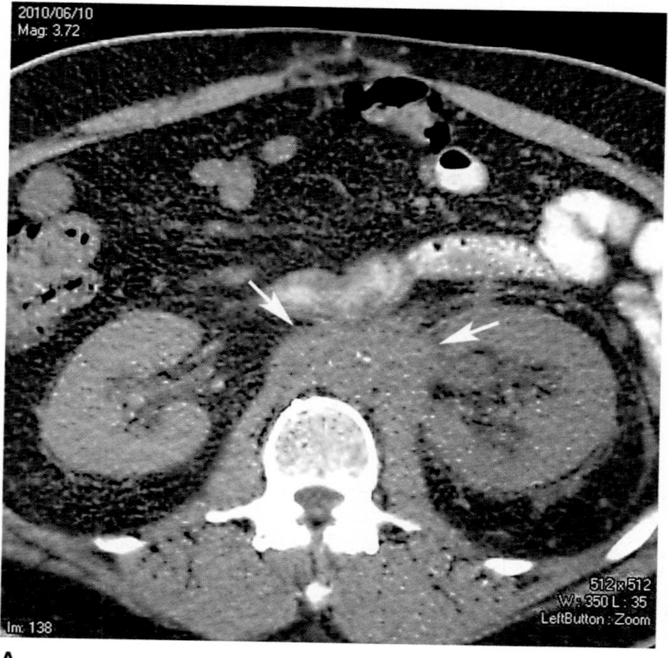

A

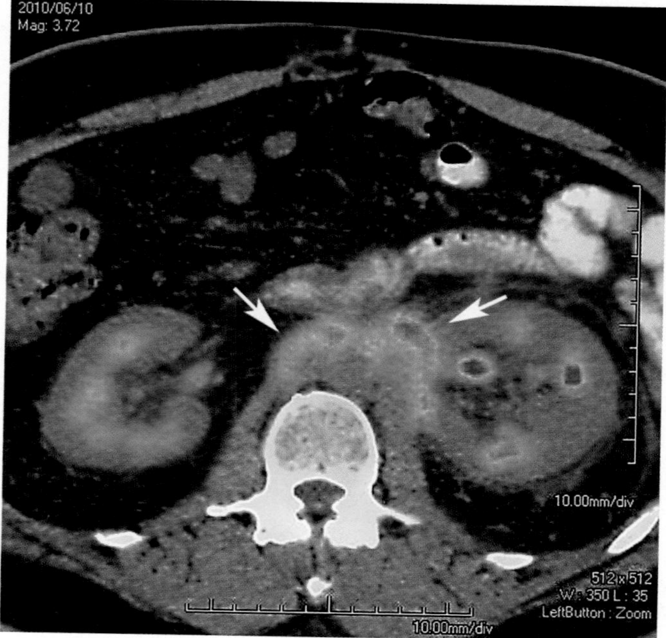

B

Figure 13-27 PET-CT of Non-Hodgkin Lymphoma
This 50-year-old woman presented for staging with known non-Hodgkin lymphoma before treatment. **A** and **B.** Low-dose CT portion of PET-CT examination showed a subtle mantle of retroperitoneal soft-tissue (*arrows*) (A) that showed moderately increased FDG activity on the combined PET-CT image (*arrows*) (B) consistent with active non-Hodgkin lymphoma.

the bone marrow and lymph nodes, thereby causing lower immunity and inability to fight infection. CLL is typically seen in patients older than age 60 years. The etiology of CLL is unknown but U.S. Department of Veterans Affairs has associated use of herbicides with CLL.

Many CLL patients will be asymptomatic and are identified as a result of incidentally discovered lymphadenopathy. Those with symptoms will typically present with tiredness, shortness of breath during exertion, lymphadenopathy, splenomegaly, weight loss, and/or infections. Faster-growing CLL is the type that can present with lymphadenopathy, and this lymphadenopathy can compress the neighboring structures, causing GI and urinary symptoms in the abdomen. As with other leukemias, the diagnostic tests for CLL primarily includes blood examination, bone marrow examination, immunophenotyping, and immunoglobulin-level measurements. Incidental lymphadenopathy and splenomegaly can be found on CT scans being performed for other reasons than CLL. It has been suggested that CT scans are not necessary to routinely evaluate disease extension in the CLL.[91] However, CT scans are being used increasingly in CLL to assess disease extension and treatment response. Recently, it has been shown that CT was a strong predictor of progression in patients with early-stage CLL.[92] In general, CT and MRI examinations will demonstrate innumerable small to moderate lymph nodes, widely distributed throughout the body. These are especially prevalent in the thorax but can also be seen in the abdomen (see Figures 13-12 and 13-28).

Systemic mastocytosis

Systemic mastocytosis is a rare lymphoproliferative disease, characterized by monoclonal proliferation of mast

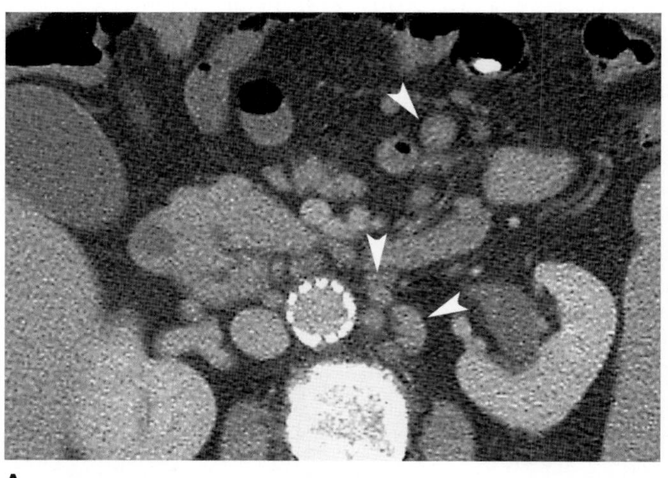

A

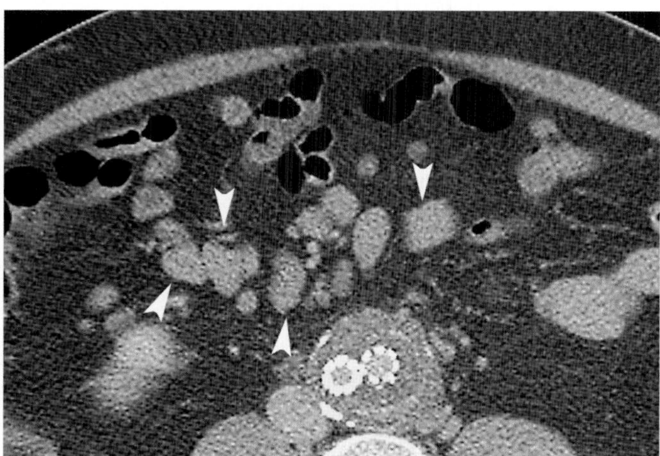

B

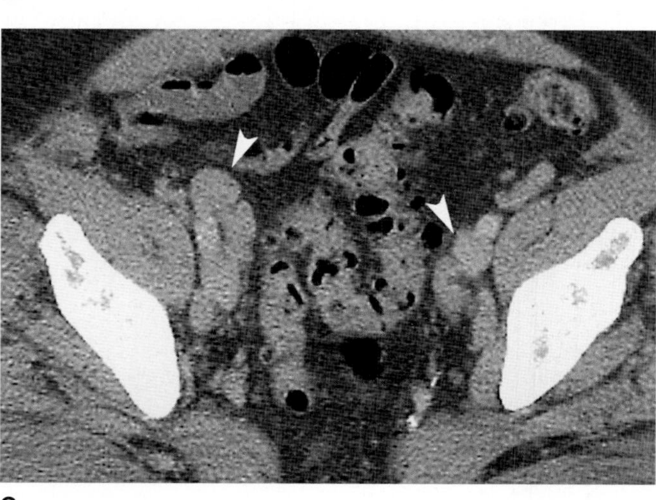

C

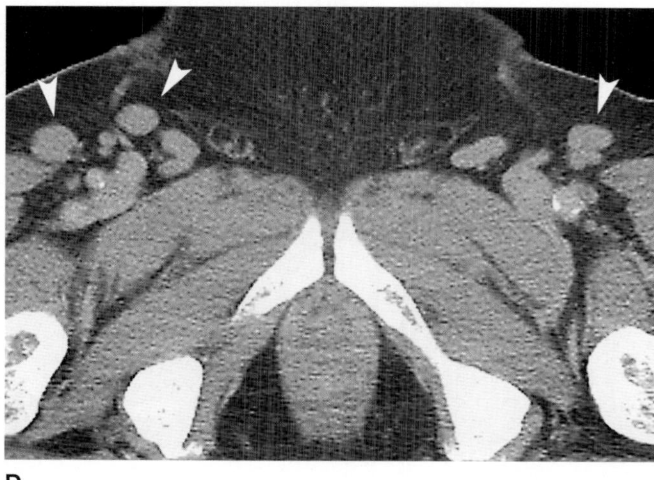

D

Figure 13-28 Chronic Lymphocytic Leukemia
This 68-year-old man had an abdominal aortic aneurysm for which he had received a stent graft. He was otherwise asymptomatic. **A-D.** Contrast-enhanced axial CT images demonstrate many intermediate and a few large lymph nodes (*arrowheads*) in the para-aortic, mesenteric, external iliac, internal iliac, and inguinal chains. Multidistribution moderate lymphadenopathy will usually indicate a lymphoprolipherative malignancy. This patient had chronic lymphocytic leukemia.

cells in organs throughout the body.[93] Systemic mastocytosis is almost always associated with KIT D816V mutation resulting in this unusual lymphoproliferative neoplasm. GI symptoms are common and include abdominal pain, diarrhea, nausea, and vomiting and can infiltrate any of the GI organs from the esophagus to the rectum. In a report by Barete et al, 74% (43/57) of the patients of systemic mastocytosis presented with abdominal symptoms. Lymphadenopathy and splenomegaly are common physical findings in systemic mastocytosis.[94] Abdominal lymphadenopathy has been found in 12 of 18 patients with systemic mastocytosis.[95] Hepatomegaly and/or splenomegaly has been found in approximately one half of patients with systemic mastocytosis.

Metastatic Carcinoma and Sarcoma

In the vast majority of cases, malignancies will metastasize in an orderly distribution along the lymphatic drainage path of the organ involved. However, rarely malignancies will cause widespread adenopathy across multiple drainage distributions.

Inflammatory Diseases Causing Adenopathy in More than 1 Drainage Distribution

Focal inflammatory diseases will typically cause lymphadenopathy in the drainage distribution of the affected organ. However, there are some systemic inflammatory conditions that can cause widespread lymphadenopathy across many drainage systems.

Disseminated granulomatous infections

Abdominal tuberculosis is the most common abdominal granulomatous infection. It typically involves the terminal ileum and cecum and gives rise to localized adenopathy in the drainage distribution of the terminal ileum and cecum. However, immunocompromised patients can develop disseminated granulomatous infections that can cause widespread adenopathy throughout the body (see Figure 13-21). Prior to HAART therapy, this was most often seen in HIV-positive patients infected with tuberculosis, *mycobacterium avium* complex (MAC), or histoplasmosis.

Although HIV is a relatively common cause of peripheral lymphadenopathy, it virtually never gives intrathoracic or abdominal adenopathy. Therefore, discovery of abdominal lymphadenopathy in an HIV-positive patient will usually indicate a superimposed disease, usually lymphoma or a disseminated granulomatous infection. The granulomatous infections most common to cause abdominal adenopathy are tuberculosis and MAC but less commonly histoplasmosis.[96]

Disseminated infection due to MAC usually presents with night sweats, abdominal pain, diarrhea, and weight loss. The most common CT findings are enlarged retroperitoneal and mesenteric lymph nodes in 42% of cases.[96] Other findings include hepatomegaly in 50%, splenomegaly in 46%, and small bowel thickening in 14% of patients.[96] Abdominal CT in more than 80% patients shows large, bulky, retroperitoneal, and mesenteric lymphadenopathy which can be soft-tissue or have low attenuation (see Figure 13-29).[97] The lymph nodes due to MAC are typically smaller and of uniform attenuation in comparison

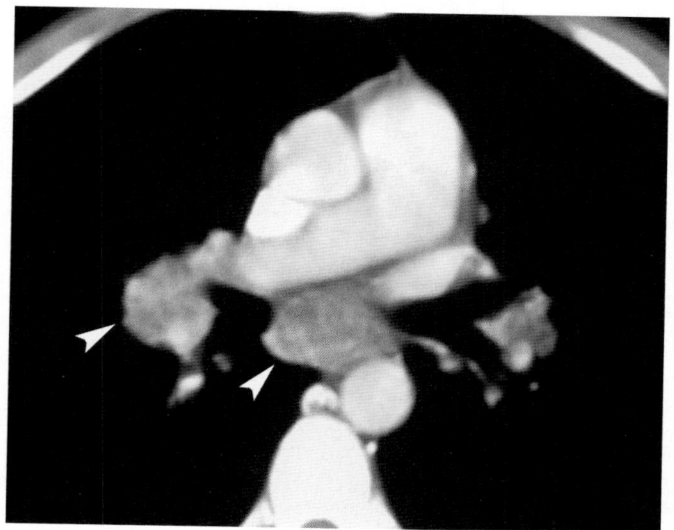
A

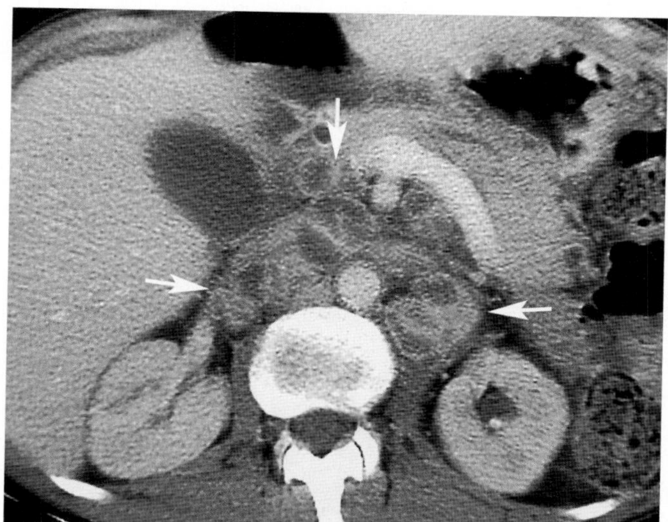
B

Figure 13-29 Lymphadenopathy Due to *Mycobacterium avium intracellulare* Infection
This 42-year-old HIV-positive man complained of abdominal pain, malaise, and weakness. **A** and **B**. Contrast-enhanced axial CT images show extensive low-attenuation lymph nodes in the subcarinal and right hilar locations in the thorax (*arrowheads*) and the anterior and lateral para-aortic locations (*arrows*) in the abdomen. Cultures of lymph node biopsies grew *Mycobacterium avium intracellulare.*

to the tuberculosis where the lymph nodes are typically larger and have low central attenuation. However, there is considerable overlap in the appearance of the 2 disseminated infections.

In 1993, tuberculosis was listed as AIDS-defining disease by the centers for disease control (CDC).[98] Necrotic lymph nodes showing low attenuation centers can be seen associated with tuberculosis.[99] Koh et al showed that lymph nodes with low attenuation are more common and lymph nodes are usually larger.[100] In non-HIV patients, abdominal tuberculosis will most frequently involve the ascending colon and terminal ileum.[101-103] Characteristics of tuberculous colitis are detailed in Chapter 2. In tuberculous colitis, there is usually an increased number of small, focal mesenteric lymphadenopathy, especially in the pericecal regions.

In acute progressive histoplasmosis, hepatosplenomegaly and lymphadenopathy may be seen. Progressive disseminated histoplasmosis occurs mostly in immunocompromised individuals, especially in AIDS patients with CD4 counts of less than 150 cells/μL. GI dissemination may produce diarrhea and abdominal pain. Abdominal CT findings in the disseminated histoplasmosis included abdominal homogenous lymphadenopathy in 44% patients, lymphadenopathy with diffuse or low central density in 13%, or both in 19% patients.[104]

Systemic inflammatory disorders

There are a variety of systemic inflammatory disorders that can result in lymphadenopathy that affects more than 1 drainage distribution. These include some connective tissue disorders, vasculitis, and sarcoidosis.

Connective tissue disorders: Connective tissue disorders including progressive systemic sclerosis, systemic lupus erythematosus, or rheumatoid arthritis can give rise to lymphadenopathy.[105] The overall incidence of lymphadenopathy in active rheumatoid arthritis was 82%, and axillary lymph nodes were involved more than cervical, supraclavicular, and inguinal lymph nodes.[106] In the active systemic lupus erythematosus, 69% patients showed lymphadenopathy, and similar to rheumatoid arthritis, there was more involvement of axillary lymph nodes than inguinal lymph nodes. With the exception of inguinal lymphadenopathy, abdominal and pelvic lymphadenopathy is rare in patients with connective tissue disorders (see Figure 13-30). These lymph nodes do not cavitate and are rarely larger than 2 cm. Lymphadenopathy will typically regress with the corticosteroid therapy.

Henoch-Schönlein purpura: Henoch-Schönlein purpura (HSP) is a systemic, generalized vasculitis and is a rare but reported cause of abdominal lymphadenopathy. Abdominal symptoms are common and sometimes precede the other manifestations of HSP. Disease predominantly involves the second part of duodenum but can also frequently involve other portions of the small intestine. Further, CT scans characteristically show multifocal bowel wall thickening with intervening normal segments.[107]

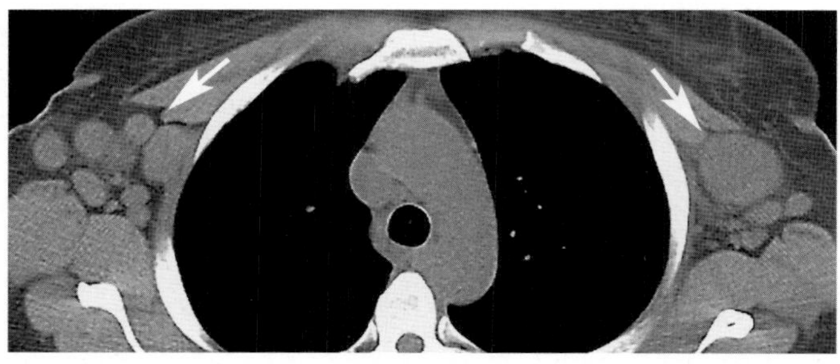

A

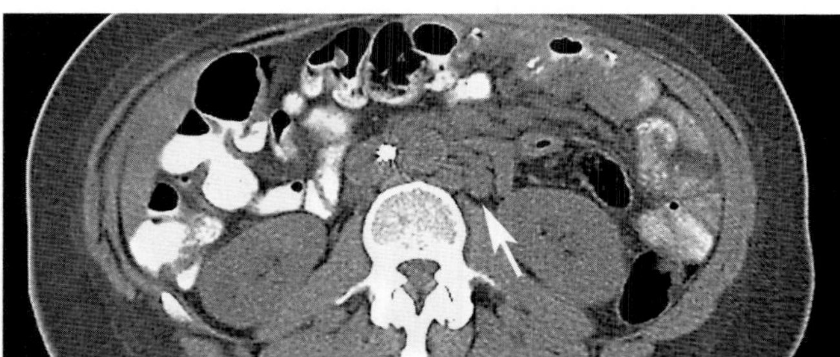

B

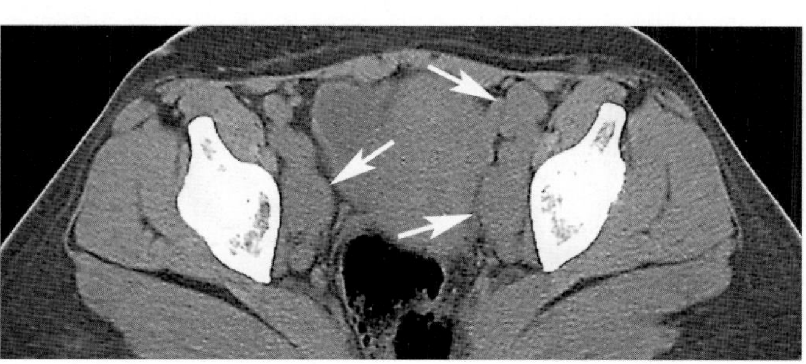

C

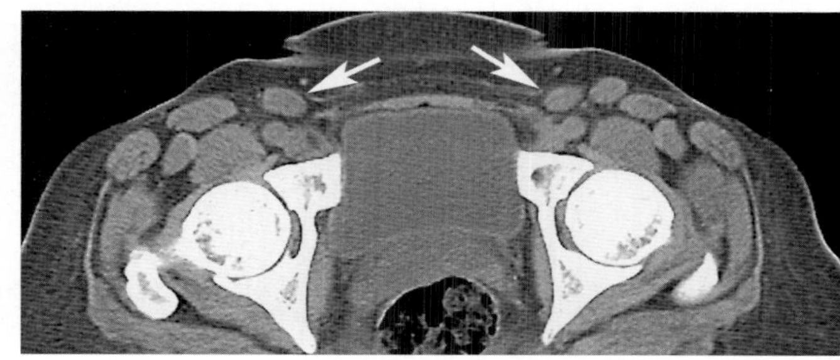

D

Figure 13-30 Systemic Lupus Erythematosis
This 46-year-old woman had persistent fevers and rash. **A-D.** Unenhanced axial CT images demonstrate multiple large axillary (*arrows* in A), obturator and external iliac (*arrows* in C) lymph nodes, and multiple moderate para-aortic (*arrow* in B) and inguinal (*arrow* in D) lymph nodes. Extensive adenopathy like this will usually indicate lymphoma but in this case was due to the patient's SLE.

Associated findings include mesenteric lymphadenopathy, mesenteric vascular engorgement, mesenteric fat stranding, ascites, pleural effusions, renal infarcts, and splenic infarcts.[107] Jeong et al showed mesenteric lymphadenopathy of less than 1.5 cm on CT in 6 of 7 patients.[107,108]

Sarcoidosis: Sarcoidosis is a multisystem disorder primarily involving the lungs and lymphoid system. In the majority of cases, adenopathy due to sarcoidosis will be confined to the thorax. However, occasionally abdominal involvement can be seen with or without intrathoracic sarcoidosis and include disease of the lymph nodes, liver, spleen, and gut.[109] In patients with hepatosplenic sarcoidosis, there is concomitant abdominal lymphadenopathy in 76%.[110] Lymph node enlargement can be seen without imaging evidence of disease in other abdominal organs. In most cases, lymphadenopathy will be confined to the upper abdominal chains above the level of the renal arteries. Retrocrural lymph nodes were seen in approximately 30% of patients.[110] In most cases, the lymph nodes will only be moderately enlarged between 10 and 20 mm in the short axis diameter. However, rarely sarcoidosis can cause bulky lymphadenopathy that can be confused with lymphoma (see Figure 13-31).[111] In 10% of patients, there was involvement of 4 or more sites with lymph node size greater than 2 cm.[110]

Kikuchi disease: Kikuchi disease is a rare, self-limited inflammatory condition that can cause lymphadenopathy.[112] Kikuchi disease can be misdiagnosed as malignant lymphoma or some other inflammatory diseases because of similar clinical and radiological findings.[113-115] Patients typically present with fever and painless lymphadenopathy. Rarely patients will complain of weight loss, diarrhea, chills, and/or sweats. Histology of the excised lymphadenopathy demonstrates geographic foci of central necrosis with extensive karyorrhectic debris surrounded by immunoblasts, histiocytes, and plasmacytoid monocytes. Necrosis is not very extensive. Unilocation lymphadenopathy in Kikuchi disease has been reported in 83% of cases.[116] Cervical lymphadenopathy is the commonest site but can involve any lymph node chains. Isolated intra-abdominal lymphadenopathy has been reported rarely.[116] A larger than normal number of small or mildly enlarged lymph nodes was observed by 1 of the authors.[112] The size of the affected lymph nodes is typically less than 4 cm (see Figure 13-32).

Amyloidosis

Amyloidosis is an uncommon systemic disorder that can involve a wide variety of organs giving diverse clinical features at presentation.[117] The most common presenting symptoms are weakness, fatigue, and weight loss. Other symptoms include pedal edema, paraesthesias, abdominal pain, periorbital, facial purpura, syncope, and orthostatic hypotension. In the abdomen, hepatosplenomegaly is often present. Lymph node enlargement is a less common manifestation and can be isolated or part of multisystem disease.[118-120] Generalized lymphadenopathy occurs in 8% of patients with systemic amyloidosis.[121] Hilar, mediastinal,

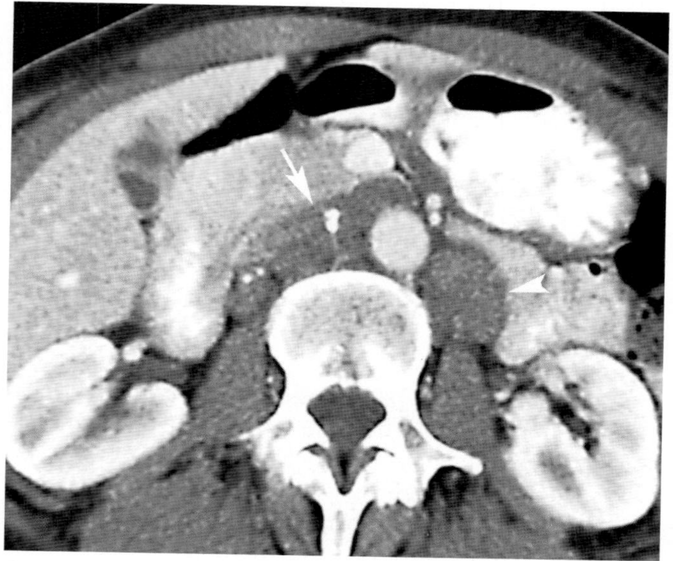

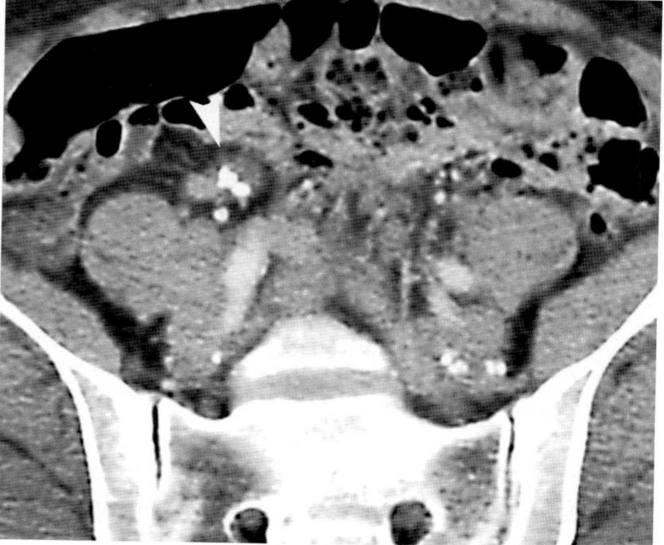

Figure 13-31 Abdominal Adenopathy Due to Sarcoidosis This 52-year-old woman had a long history of thoracic sarcoidosis. **A** and **B.** Contrast-enhanced CT of the abdomen and pelvis demonstrates enlarged left para-aortic (*small arrowhead*), inter-aortocaval (*arrow*), and right common iliac adenopathy (*large arrowhead*). Note that several of the lymph nodes have focal areas of calcification typical of chronic granulomatous diseases. These lymph nodes have remained stable for 8 years and are presumed to be secondary to sarcoidosis.

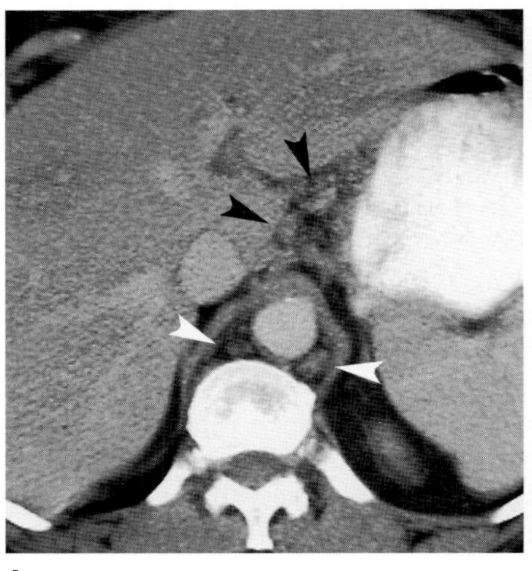
A

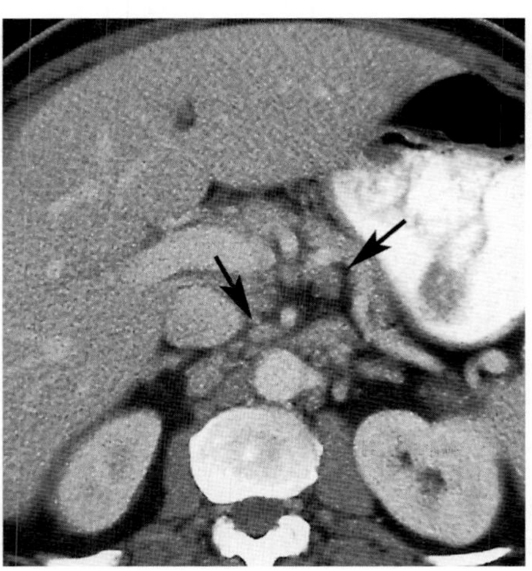
B

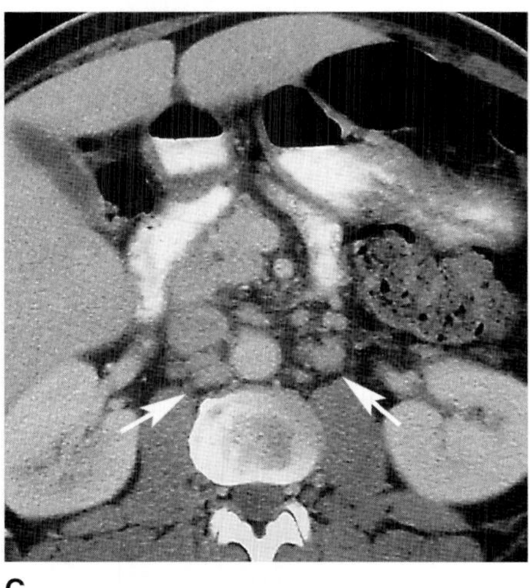
C

Figure 13-32 Kikuchi Disease
This 63-year-old man with diabetes mellitus presented with 3-week history of fatigue, myalgias, fever, and rigors. **A-C.** Contrast-enhanced axial CT images demonstrate increased numbers and slight increase in size of retrocrural (*white arrowhead*), gastrohepatic (*black arrowheads*), celiac axis (*black arrows*), and para-aortic (*white arrows*) lymph nodes. Lymph node biopsy was diagnostic of Kikuchi disease.

and/or para-aortic lymph nodes are the most common sites of involvement; however, abdominal lymphadenopathy has also been reported.[122]

Causes of Lymphadenopathy Affecting a Single Drainage Distribution

Adenopathy in a single drainage distribution will usually be due to diseases of the organs that drain into that distribution, and recognition of focal adenopathy should lead to an evaluation of the organ that supplies that distribution. In many cases, focal adenopathy will indicate lymph node metastasis from a cancer in the organ in question. However, infectious and inflammatory diseases of the organ can also cause lymphadenopathy in the drainage distribution of the organ.

Lymphoma

In most cases, lymphoma will cause lymph node abnormalities that involve multiple lymph node drainage distributions. However, occasionally, imaging abnormalities will be limited to a single drainage distribution.

Metastatic tumor

Lymphatic metastases from abdominal malignancies are a common mode of cancer spread. In the majority of cases, the distribution of lymphatic metastasis will follow the typical drainage pattern of the organ of origin. In most cases, the typical lymphatic distribution will parallel the vascular drainage of the organ (Table 13-1). Details of the lymphatic drainage and nodal staging for each organ will be reviewed in the chapters detailing diseases of that organ; however, these will be briefly mentioned individually for major abdominal-pelvic organs.

Gastrointestinal malignancies: Distal esophageal carcinoma will typically involve small periesophageal nodes first and then spread to the larger celiac axis lymph nodes.[123] Gastric carcinoma will initially involve small lymph nodes in the gastrohepatic ligament and perigastric fat and then also spread to the celiac axis lymph nodes (see Figure 13-33). Tumors of the small bowel and colon will initially involve small lymph nodes in the fat surrounding the primary tumor and then spread to lymph nodes in the small bowel or colonic mesentery. Tumors of the small bowel and proximal colon to the level of the sigmoid flexure will then spread to the periaortic lymph nodes adjacent to the origin of the superior mesenteric artery (see Figure 13-33). Tumors of the descending and sigmoid colons and proximal rectum will involve the para-aortic lymph nodes at the level of the inferior mesenteric lymph nodes, and distal rectal cancers will spread to the internal iliac chains.

Hepatobiliary and pancreatic malignancies: Nodal drainage of malignancy from the liver, gallbladder, and bile ducts is usually to hepatoduodenal, peripancreatic and aortocaval nodes (see Figure 13-34).[124] Pancreatic carcinoma frequently results in local lymph node spread in the retroperitoneum and peripancreatic distribution, but mesenteric lymph nodes involvement is not infrequent.

Prostate, cervix, uterine, and bladder malignancies: Tumors of the prostate, cervix, and uterus will typically first involve the pelvic fat surrounding each of the organs, followed by the internal iliac, obturator, and external iliac

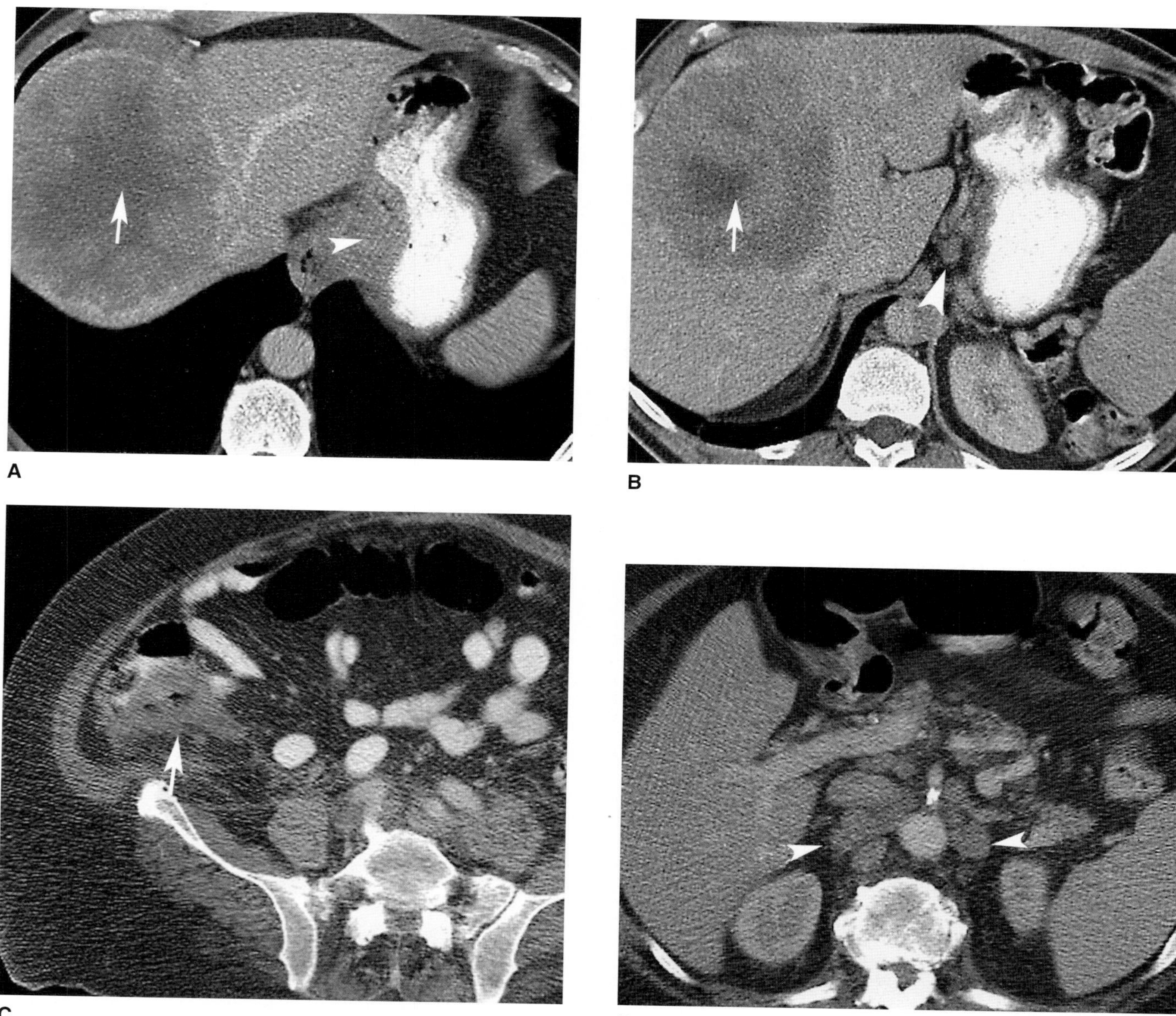

Figure 13-33 Gastrointestinal Malignancy Lymph Node Metastasis **A** and **B**. This 47-year-old man with gastric carcinoma (*small arrowhead*) has a large hepatic metastasis (*white arrow*) and gastrohepatic ligament lymph node metastasis (*large arrowhead*). The gastrohepatic ligament nodes and celiac axis nodes are the typical sites of lymph node metastasis from gastric malignancies. **C** and **D**. This 64-year-old woman with cecal carcinoma (*arrow*) has multiple enlarged para-aortic and SMA lymph nodes (*arrowheads*) typical of lymph node metastasis from a malignancy of the colon proximal to the splenic flexure.

nodes. Further spread is to the common iliac and retroperitoneal lymph nodes. Adenopathy outside of this distribution, for example, in the mesenteric lymph nodes of the pelvis, is rare and should prompt a search for another cause of lymph node enlargement (see Figure 13-35).[125] In most cases, the relative likelihood of lymphatic metastasis increases as the tumor invades into the muscles and soft-tissues of the cervix, uterus, and bladder and the surrounding pelvic fat.[126] For example, lymph node involvement has been seen in approximately 30% of the cases where bladder carcinoma has invaded beyond the muscle of the bladder wall (see Figure 13-35).[127]

Ovarian cancer: Ovarian cancer has 3 routes of lymphatic spread: (1) via lymphatics that ascend with the ovarian vessels to the retroperitoneal nodes of the upper abdomen; (2) via lymphatics draining laterally in the broad ligament to reach the internal iliac and obturator nodes in the pelvic sidewall; (3) via lymphatics in the round ligament to external iliacs and inguinal lymph nodes.

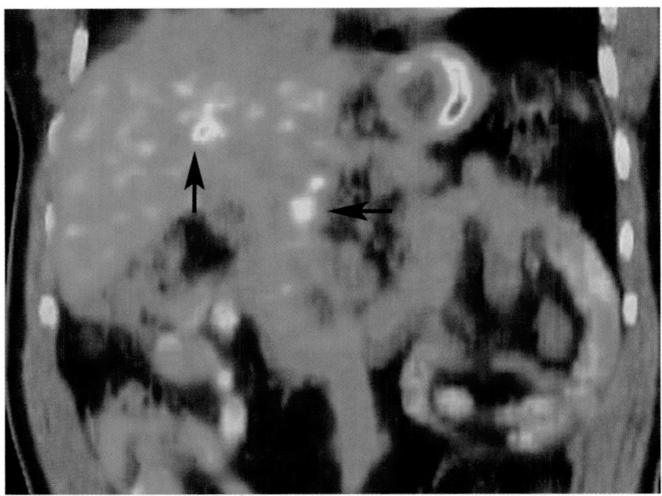

Figure 13-34 Cholangiocarcinoma and Metastatic Portocaval Lymph Nodes
A coronal fused PET-CT scan shows FDG-avid cholangiocarcinoma marked with the *vertical arrow* and metastatic portocaval lymph nodes marked with the *horizontal arrow*.

Testicular cancer: Nodal metastases are seen mostly in the para-aortic nodes between the renal and inferior mesentery arteries and are ipsilateral to the primary tumor (see Figure 13-8). Because of abundant collaterals, the contralateral para-aortic and aortocaval lymph nodes can be affected. Testicular cancer should always be considered in the differential diagnosis for the para-aortic lymphadenopathy of unknown etiology. Residual masses following chemotherapy are a relatively common phenomenon with nonseminomatous germ cell tumors. Further, PET-CT has been reported to show a higher accuracy for evaluating the residual tumor compared with CT.[128] In the American College of Radiology (ACR) appropriateness criteria, use of FDG-PET-CT is mentioned as appropriate and possibly indicated for the follow-up of residual or recurrent disease. It has been said that whole body FDG-PET has no clear benefit in initial staging over CT.

Vaginal carcinoma: Vaginal carcinomas spread to obturator and internal iliac nodes. Tumors from the posterior wall tend to spread to the superior and inferior gluteal nodes. Carcinomas from the lower third of the vagina usually spread to the pelvic and/or inguinofemoral nodes.

Penis, vulva, and anus: The lymph node drainage from these organs is typically to the superficial inguinal lymph nodes (see Figure 13-36). Subsequent spread to the deep pelvic lymph nodes is less common.

Accuracy of abdominal lymph node staging for abdominal malignancies: None of the imaging modalities has been shown to be highly accurate in the diagnosis of metastatic adenopathy from intra-abdominal

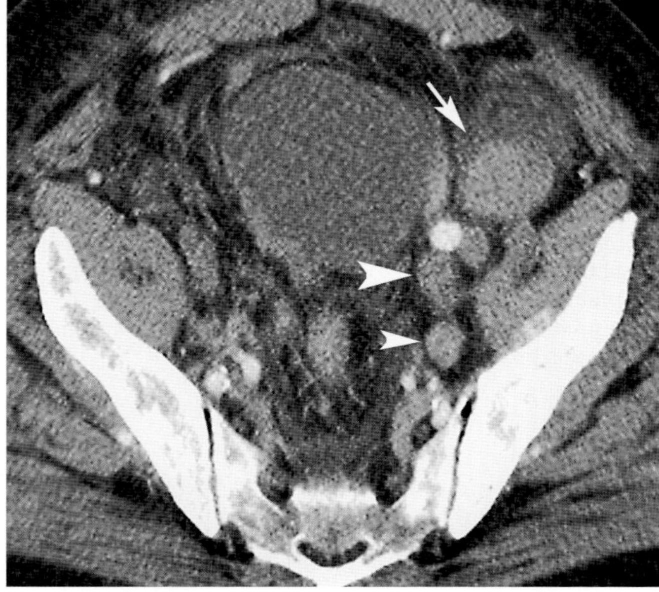

A

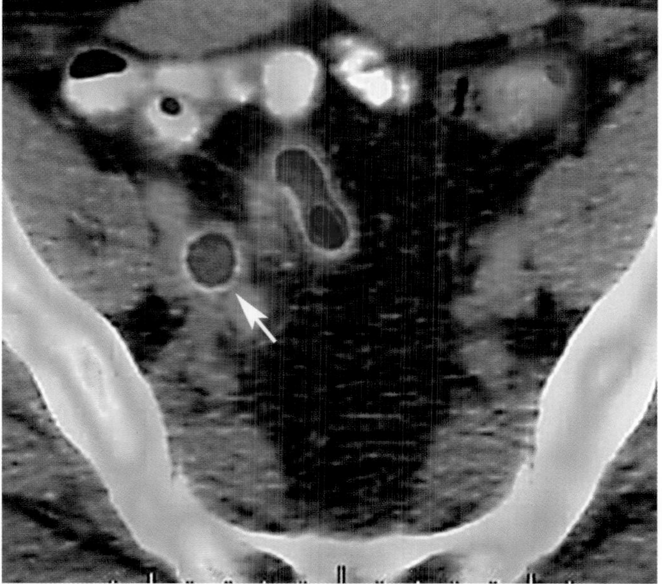

B

Figure 13-35 Pelvic Lymph Node Metastasis from Prostate Carcinoma and Bladder Cancer in 2 Patients
A. This 66-year-old man had prostate carcinoma. Contrast-enhanced CT through the pelvis shows enlarged obturator (*small arrowhead*), external iliac (*large arrowhead*), and external iliac (*arrow*) lymph nodes. This is the typical lymphatic drainage distribution for a pelvic malignancy including prostate cancer.
B. This 89-year-old had bladder carcinoma. Fused PET-CT image shows an enlarged FDG-positive right internal iliac lymph node (*arrow*) which likely represents lymphatic metastasis.

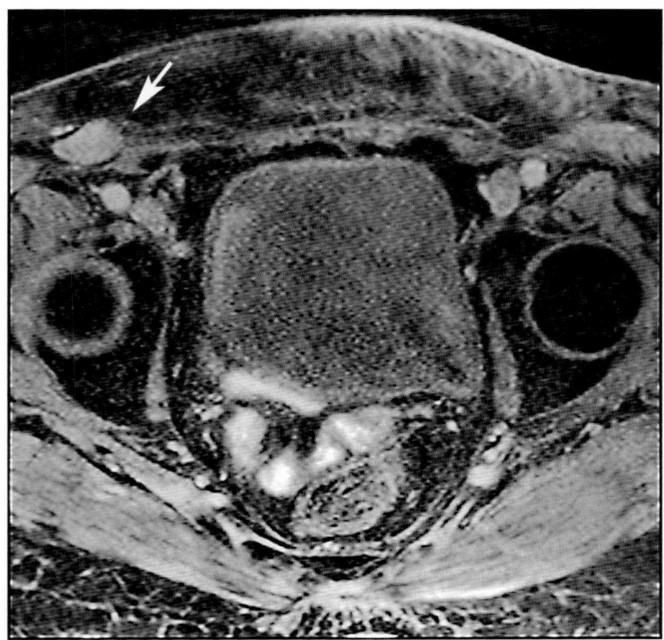

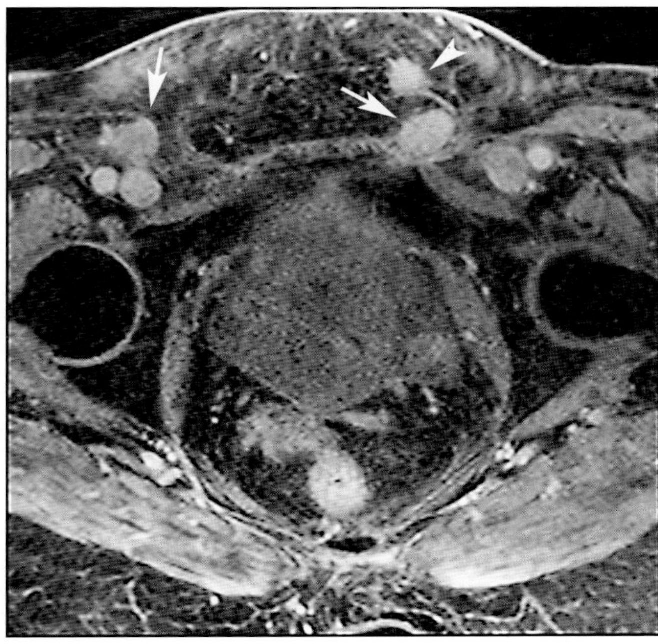

Figure 13-36 Inguinal Lymph Node Metastasis from Vulvar Cancer This 52-year-old woman had surgical resection of a vulvar carcinoma. **A** and **B.** Gadolinium-enhanced, fat-saturated T1-weighted MRI images of the inguinal regions demonstrate enlarged bilateral inguinal lymph nodes (*arrows*). There is also a subcutaneous metastasis to the anterior abdominal wall (*arrowhead*). These findings were not present on an MRI examination 6 months previously and are the typical lymphatic drainage for a perineal malignancy. Lymph node biopsy confirmed a diagnosis of metastatic vulvar carcinoma.

malignancies. For example, studies of colorectal carcinoma have shown accuracies of CT and MRI of between 66% and 83% in the diagnosis of lymphatic metastasis.[11,129,130] Studies of pancreatic, renal, prostate, bladder, endometrial, cervical, and ovarian malignancies have demonstrated similarly intermediate accuracies.[12-30]

In general, when using the 1-cm rule, anatomic imaging has had moderately high specificity in the range of 75% to 95%, with lower sensitivity for metastasis in the range of 50% to 75%.[11-30] Therefore, the presence of enlarged lymph nodes will in most cases indicate the presence of metastasis. However, microscopic metastases occur with moderate frequency and lower the sensitivity of anatomic imaging for metastatic lymphadenopathy. Addition of functional imaging with FDG-PET has only slightly increased the sensitivity for lymph node metastasis for GI malignancies but has been shown to increase sensitivities in the range of 80% to 90% and specificities at levels greater than 90% for other neoplasms such as endometrial carcinoma and cervical cancer.[131-137]

Researchers have attempted to increase accuracy in lymph node staging with a variety of novel MR and nuclear medicine contrast agents. It has been shown that using lymphotropic super-paramagnetic nanoparticles results in higher sensitivity in lymph node involvement with prostate carcinoma. A sensitivity of 82% to 100%, a specificity of 93% to 96%, and a negative predictive value of 96% to 100% has been reported.[138,139] Capromab pendetide scintigraphy is useful in prostate carcinoma staging and provides a sensitivity of 67% to 94% and a specificity of 42% to 80% in the detection of lymph node metastasis.[140-142] However, the reported accuracies for these newer agents are still not sufficiently high to obviate the need for histologic staging of lymph node metastasis.

Regional lymphadenopathy due to inflammatory conditions

Besides malignancy, lymph nodes respond to a wide variety of internal and external stimuli, including infectious, noninfectious inflammatory, systemic, and immunologic

Imaging Notes 13-7. Causes of Lymphadenopathy Affecting a Single Drainage Distribution

Lymphadenopathy in a single drainage distribution will usually indicate a disease in the organ drained by the abnormal lymph nodes. Although this is often attributed to malignancies, inflammatory conditions, especially those of the bowel and liver, are also frequent causes of lymphadenopathy in a single drainage distribution.

disorders. In general, an inflammatory condition within a given organ will cause mild lymphadenopathy in the drainage distribution of the organ. This can be seen as mild enlargement of 1 to 2cm or as increases in numbers of lymph nodes in the drainage distribution of the organ. Therefore, recognition of a focal or regional lymphadenopathy should engender a search of the organs in that drainage distribution for a malignant or inflammatory cause of the lymphadenopathy. Size, location, contour, density, relationship to aorta/vena cava, and presence of mass effect are of no value in distinguishing the malignant from benign causes of lymphadenopathy.[143,144] The significance of lymphadenopathy is therefore based on recognition of the primary lesion causing the lymphadenopathy. When no cause can be identified, either short-term clinical and CT follow-up or percutaneous or other biopsies may be necessary.

Appendicitis, diverticulitis, other causes of intra-abdominal abscess, and perforation of any abdominal viscera can give rise to mesenteric lymphadenopathy. In most cases, the adenopathy will be present in the mesenteric nodes that drain the region of affected bowel and in each of these disorders, and the mesenteric lymphadenopathy will be associated with the characteristic features of the primary bowel disorder. Many causes of bowel wall thickening will also be associated with mesenteric lymphadenopathy (see Figure 13-37). These include (1) inflammatory bowel diseases: Crohn disease and ulcerative colitis; (2) bowel infections: tuberculosis, *Yersinia enterocolitica*, *Campylobacter* species, *Giardia lamblia*; and (3) autoimmune disorders: celiac disease (see Figure 13-13).[145-147]

Abdominal tuberculosis is an important infection in developing countries. In most cases, the disease will involve the cecum and terminal ileum, causing thickening of the walls of the cecum and terminal ileum. Pericecal and mesenteric adenopathy is a common associated finding (see Figure 13-38). Multiple reports have suggested that these lymph nodes often have low attenuation centers and enhance peripherally with the administration of intravenous contrast.[148]

Biliary diseases and hepatitis of any cause, infectious, autoimmune, alcoholic, drug-induced, and others, will commonly give rise to mild periportal and celiac

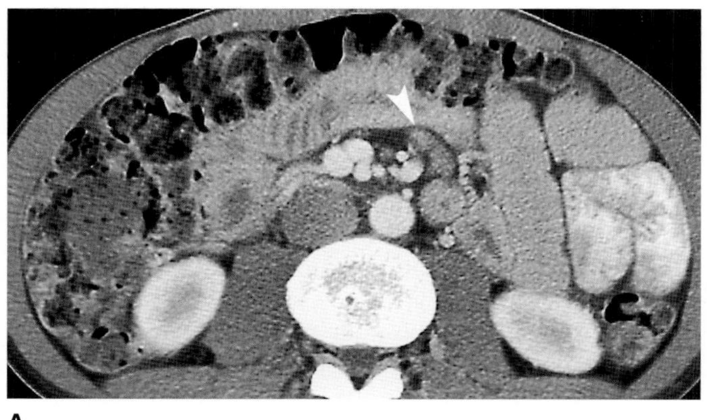

A

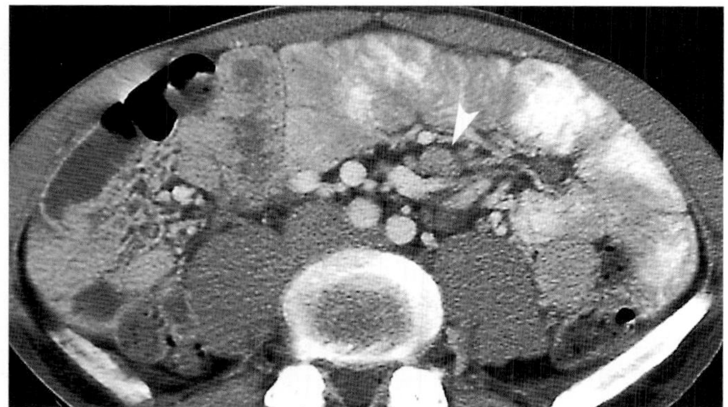

B

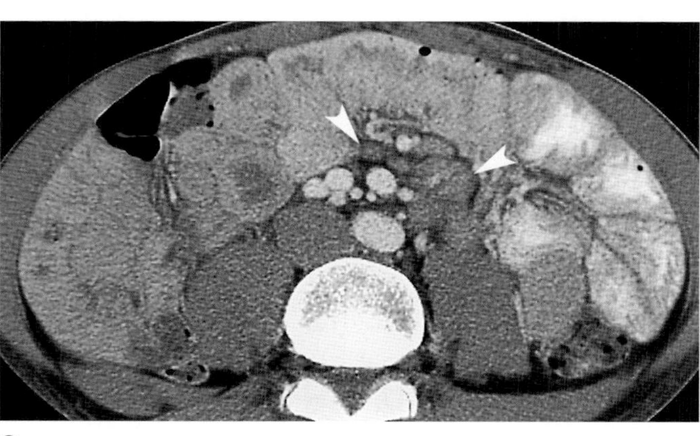

C

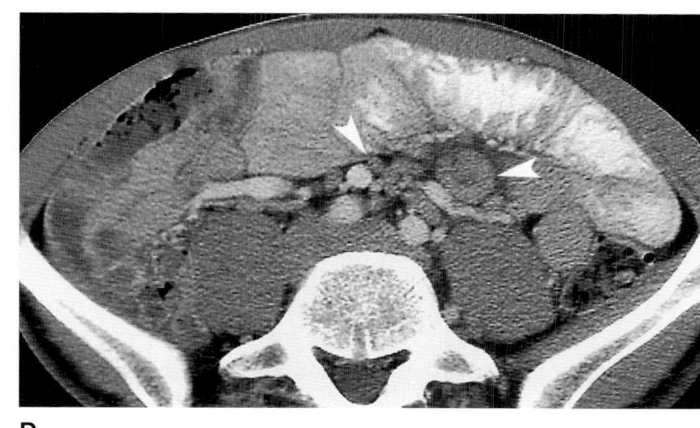

D

Figure 13-37 Mesenteric Adenopathy Due to Celiac Disease This 37-year-old man had testicular carcinoma. **A-D.** Contrast-enhanced CT demonstrates an increased number and size of mesenteric lymph nodes (*arrowheads*). With the history of testicular carcinoma, it might be tempting to attribute these nodes to metastatic cancer. However, this is the wrong drainage pattern for metastatic testicular carcinoma. Furthermore, the wall of the small bowel appears much thickened, suggesting diffuse edema due to inflammation. Further evaluation lead to a diagnosis of celiac sprue, which had not been known before this CT examination.

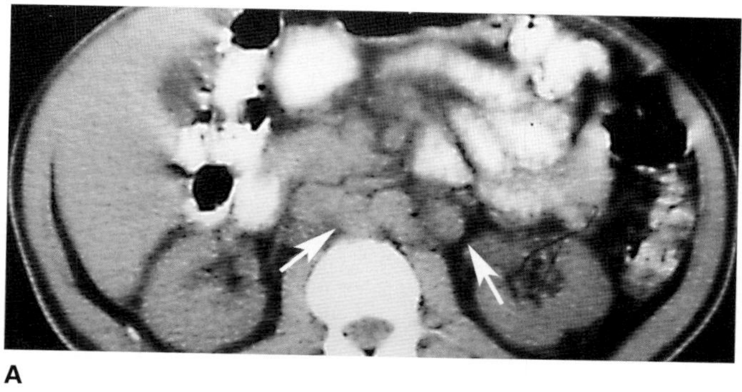
A

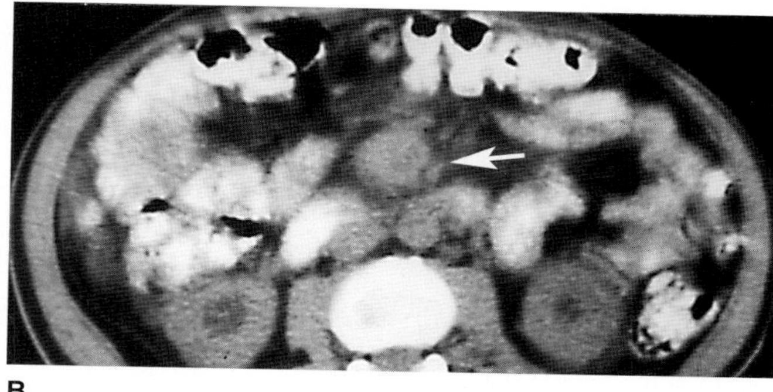
B

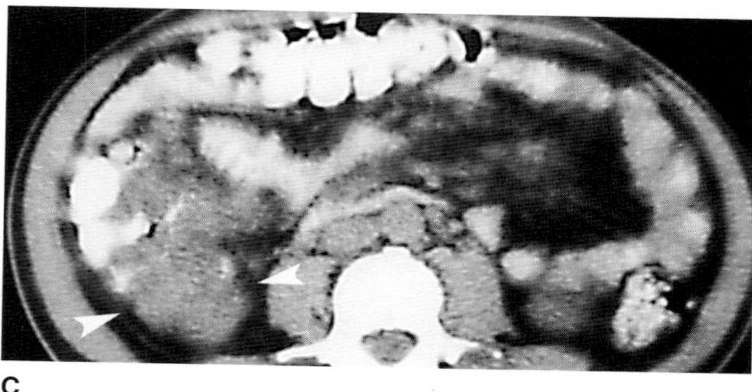
C

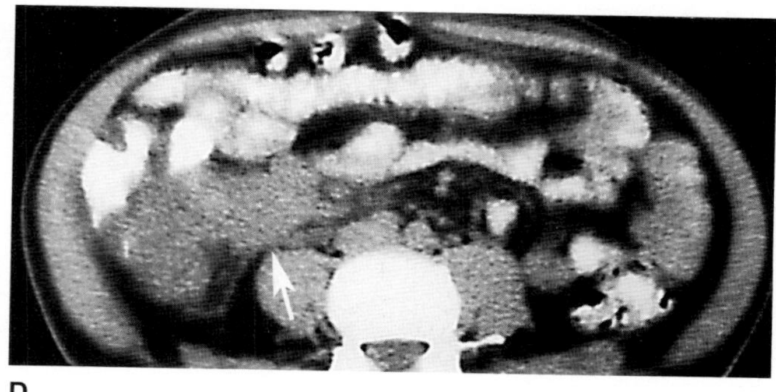
D

Figure 13-38 Abdominal Tuberculosis
This 43-year-old man presented with abdominal pain and hiccoughs. **A-D.** Unenhanced, axial CT images show thickening of the wall of the cecum (*arrowheads*) with a large matted area of pericecal adenopathy (*arrow* in D) and mesenteric (*arrow* in B) and para-aortic (*arrows* in A) adenopathy. This might have represented a colonic lymphoma or carcinoma; however, cultures were positive for *Mycobacterium tuberculosis*.

axis lymphadenopathy (see Figure 13-9). For example, lymphadenopathy, typically involving portohepatic and/or portocaval nodes, is seen in 80% cases of primary biliary cirrhosis (PBC).[149] The liver also drains to the cardiophrenic lymph nodes in the thorax and so hepatitis can also lead to adenopathy in that distribution. Other causes of cirrhosis have been shown to cause lymphadenopathy in 37% to 49% patients, ranging from approximately 50% in cases of hepatitis C–related hepatitis to less than 10% in cases of alcoholic cirrhosis and hepatitis B–related liver diseases.[149,150]

Interestingly, inflammatory diseases of the genitourinary tract such as pyelonephritis, prostatitis, and pelvic inflammatory disease do not usually cause abdominal or pelvic lymphadenopathy.

Sclerosing mesenteritis (panniculitis): Sclerosing mesenteritis is a nonspecific, idiopathic inflammatory condition affecting the fatty tissue of the mesentery.[151,152] The disorder is often associated with other idiopathic inflammatory disorders such as retroperitoneal fibrosis, sclerosing cholangitis, Riedel thyroiditis, and orbital pseudotumor. These associations suggest that sclerosing mesenteritis could be an autoimmune phenomenon, but infection, trauma, and ischemia have also been suggested as potential etiologies. Histologically, varying degrees of inflammation, fat necrosis, and fibrosis are found within the fat of the small bowel mesentery.[151,152] It is found more commonly in men than women and can be seen at any age but with an average age of 60 years. Some patients are discovered as an incidental asymptomatic finding on abdominal imaging exam. Symptoms are variable and include abdominal pain, fever, nausea, vomiting, and weight loss.[151,152] The appearance of the lesion can range from a well-defined soft-tissue mass to ill-defined areas of higher attenuation in the mesenteric fat.[151,152] There may be preservation of fat around the mesenteric vessels, a phenomenon that is referred to as the "fat ring sign," which can be an important distinguishing feature from other mesenteric processes such as lymphoma and carcinoid tumor.[151,152] Local mesenteric lymphadenopathy is also often present in cases of mesenteric panniculitis (see Figure 13-39).[151,152]

Focal Abdominopelvic Lymphadenopathy Without Other Abdominal Findings

There are a few rare causes of focal lymphadenopathy that do hot have associated intra-abdominal findings. These include mesenteric lymphadenitis, Castleman disease, and familial Mediterranean fever.

Mesenteric lymphadenitis: Mesenteric lymphadenitis is a well-established clinical entity and was first reported

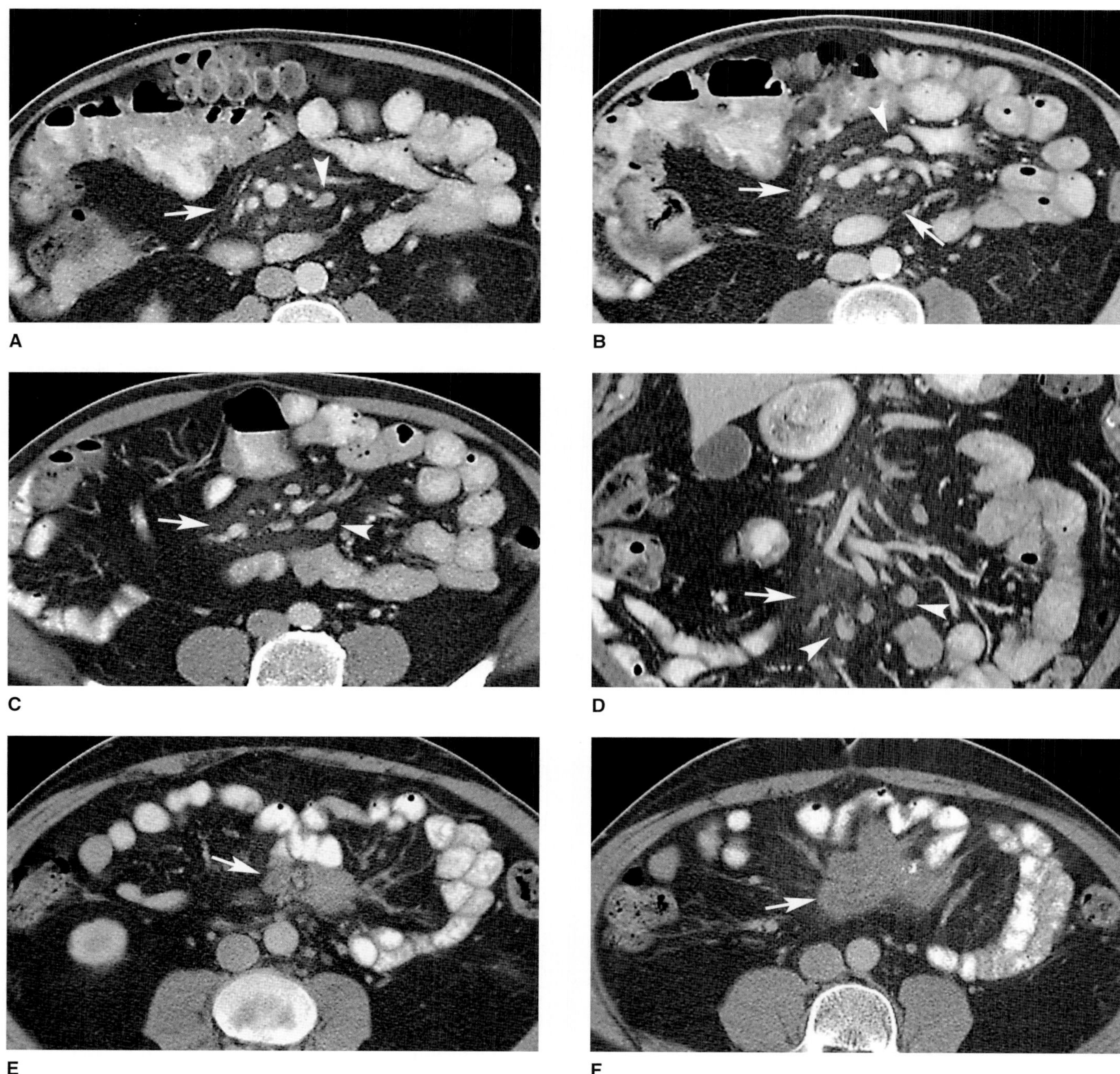

Figure 13-39 Sclerosing Mesenteritis (Paniculitis) in 2 Patients This 61-year-old man complained of dyspepsia. **A-C.** Contrast-enhanced axial CT images show a faint area of increased attenuation (*arrows* in A-C) within the central mesenteric fat. There are also mildly enlarged mesenteric lymph nodes (*arrowheads* in A-C). **D.** Coronal reconstruction also shows increased fat attenuation (*arrow*) and enlarged lymph nodes (*arrowheads*). This is a typical appearance of sclerosing mesenteritis. **E** and **F.** This 59-year-old man was being evaluated for a renal mass (not shown). Axial CT images demonstrate a spiculated, infiltrating mass (*arrows*) within the small bowel mesentery (*arrows* in E and F). Differential diagnosis would include a mesenteric sarcoma, desmoid tumor, fibrosis associated with carcinoid tumor, and sclerosing mesenteritis. Biopsy was diagnostic of sclerosing mesenteritis.

in 1913 and can occur at any age but is primarily reported in children.[153,154] Its clinical presentation mimics acute appendicitis without perforation, with symptoms of abdominal pain, fever being most prominent but also including nausea, vomiting, diarrhea, and malaise. Mesenteric lymphadenitis represents inflammation of the mesenteric lymph nodes, usually as a result of infection. Organisms that have been cultured include *Escherichia coli*, Bacteroides, Clostridia, Enterococci, β-hemolytic streptococcus, Staphylococcus, and Yersinia.[155,156] Viruses, including coxsackie viruses (A and B), rubeola virus, and adenovirus are also believed to be causes of mesenteric lymphadenitis. These organisms originate in the bowel and in many cases the primary bowel source can be identified. However, in some patients, 30% in 1 series, no bowel abnormality is identified and the only imaging abnormality is lymph node enlargement.[157] This latter group is called "primary mesenteric lymphadenitis" and may account for 7% to 14% of patients who are evaluated for suspected appendicitis.[158,159] Surgical evaluations usually show intense inflammatory reaction in the ileocecal region with omental adhesions and periappendicitis. Cross-sectional imaging can play an important role in the diagnosis of mesenteric lymphadenitis and can help avoid unnecessary surgery since the disorder can be confused with acute appendicitis, lymphoma, and regional enteritis as well as other entities. Diagnostic features of mesenteric lymphadenitis include enlarged mesenteric lymph nodes with or without associated ileocecal or ileal wall thickening, in the setting of normal appendix.[160] Rao et al showed that using their criteria of 3 or more nodes with a short axis diameter of at least 5 mm allowed a correct diagnosis of mesenteric adenitis in all patients.[158] Both US and CT have been used to diagnose this disorder (see Figure 13-40).[157,159]

Castleman Disease

Castleman disease, also known as giant lymph node hyperplasia and angiofollicular lymph node hyperplasia, is a rare disorder affecting the lymph nodes with noncancerous growths and is typically divided into unifocal and multifocal forms of disease. The cause is unknown but probably represents either a response to chronic inflammation or a hamartoma of the lymphatic system.[161,162] Pathologically, this disease is classified as hyaline, vascular, plasmacytic, or mixed-cellularity types. Castleman disease of the abdomen will typically present as abdominal pain, trouble eating, or abdominal fullness. Multicentric disease will also frequently have systemic symptoms such as fever, weakness, night sweats, weight loss, loss of appetite, nausea, vomiting, and neuropathy, whereas unicentric disease rarely presents with systemic symptoms.

Imaging exams will most often demonstrate a solitary, enhancing mass in the retroperitoneum, porta hepatis, mesentery, or pancreas.[39-41] Lesions less than 5 cm in diameter will usually appear as a uniformly enhancing mass; however, lesions greater than 5 cm in diameter will often display inhomogeneous enhancement with low-attenuation areas consistent with necrosis. Calcification can be seen in some cases (see Figures 13-18 and 13-41).[163]

Familial mediterranean fever: Familial Mediterranean fever is a recessive genetic disease also known as recurrent polyserositis.[164] It usually occurs in families and is more common in individuals of Mediterranean descent. It usually presents as fever with brief recurrent episodes of peritonitis, pleuritis, and arthritis.[165] The disease is commonly confused with appendicitis and cholecystitis often leading to unnecessary surgery. Pleural and pericardial effusions are common. Arthritis can last longer than abdominal symptoms and in between attacks, joints are normal, with permanent damage rare. Rash and muscle pain can be other symptoms.

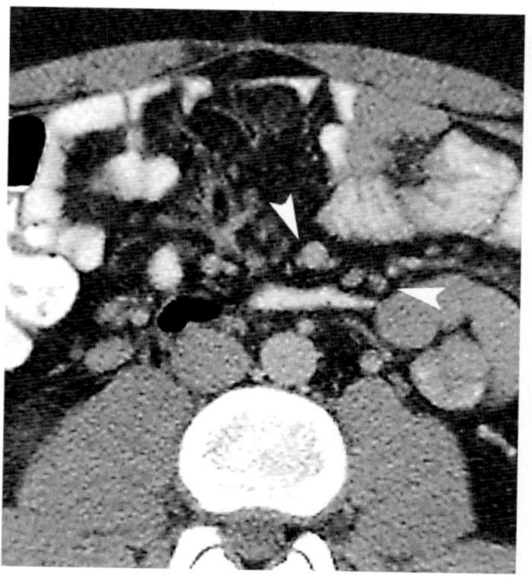
A

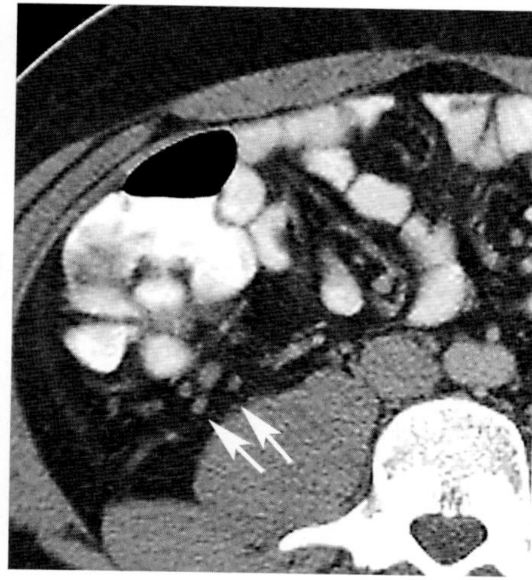
B

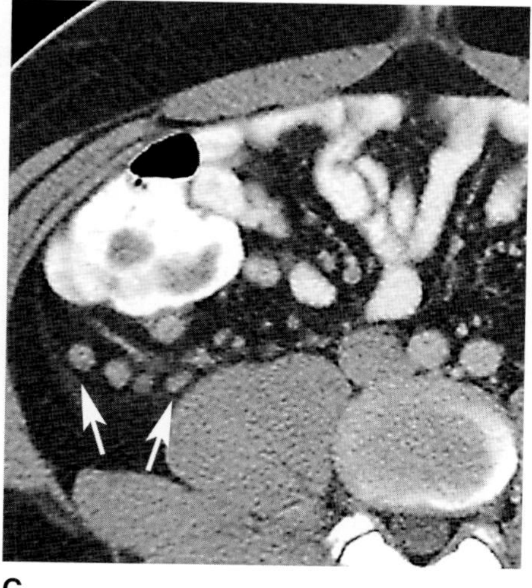
C

Figure 13-40 Mesenteric Lymphadenitis
This 19-year-old man presented with right lower quadrant pain and fever. **A-C.** Contrast-enhanced axial CT shows an increased number of small pericecal lymph nodes (*arrows*), with normal or minimally increased number of lymph nodes in the mesentery (*arrowheads*). The appendix (not shown) appeared normal. This appearance was presumed to represent mesenteric lymphadenitis, and the patient was observed with serial clinical exams. The patient's symptoms resolved 2 days later without therapy.

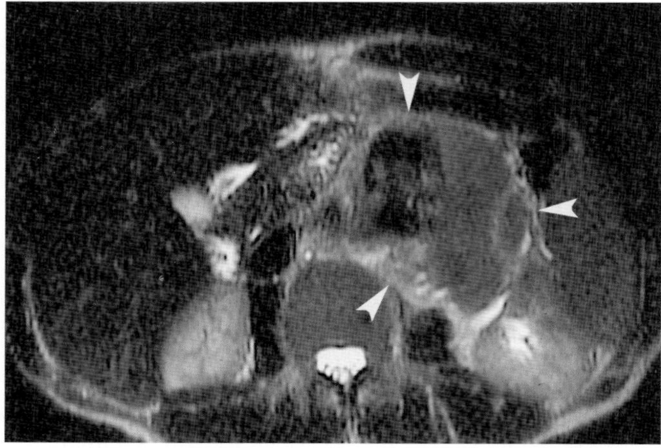

A

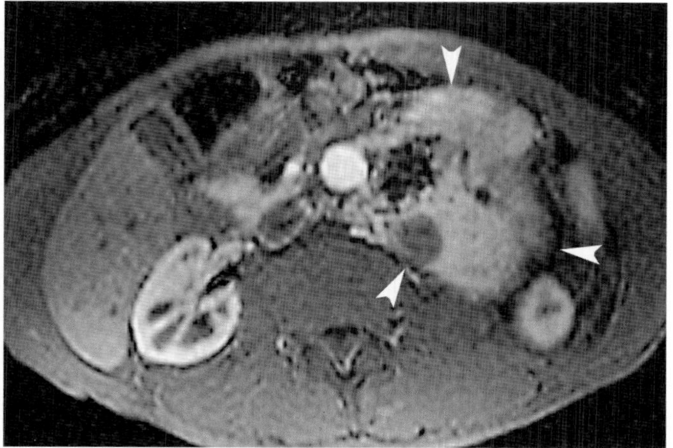

B

Figure 13-41 Castleman Disease Appearing as a Retroperitoneal Mass
This 51-year-old man complained of dyspepsia. **A.** T2-weighted and (**B**) T1-weighted postgadolinium axial MRI images show a heterogenous mass in the left retroperitoneum that has regions that densely enhance. This appearance would be consistent with a soft-tissue sarcoma, but biopsy was diagnostic of Castleman disease.

Imaging studies have shown that mesenteric lymphadenopathy is the predominant finding, present in 86% of patients as with familial Mediterranean fever.[166] Other findings include engorged mesenteric vessels, thickened mesenteric folds, ascites, focal peritonitis, splenomegaly, dilated small bowel loops, and mural thickening of the ascending colon. CT can be an important tool in the evaluation of patients with familial Mediterranean fever because of its ability to exclude other causes of abdominal pain, including acute appendicitis and bowel obstruction.[167-169]

ANATOMY AND IMAGING OF THE LYMPHATIC DUCTS

Anatomy

Interstitial lymph is drained via afferent lymphatics, which converge toward the outer nodal surfaces of lymph nodes before exiting via efferents at centrally located medullary sinuses. Numerous small lymph channels join to form a small tubular structure in the superior retroperitoneum called the cisterna chyli. This is the only lymphatic duct structure that can be seen by conventional cross-sectional imaging. On transaxial images, it appears as a small, round or oval fluid-filled structure anterior to the vertebral bodies at the level of the diaphragmatic crux (see Figure 13-42). The cisterna chyli then empties into 1 or several lymphatic channels that run anterior to the thoracic vertebra and collectively are called the thoracic duct. At the level of the thoracic inlet, if multiple, these channels rejoin to form a single duct that drains lymph in the venous circulation by opening usually at the angle between the left jugular vein and the left subclavian vein.

Imaging Studies

Very few tools are available at present for imaging the lymphatics. There are 2 primary techniques to evaluate the lymphatic channels, lymphography that utilized radiopaque contrast to anatomically define the lymphatics and functionally define the transport of lipid materials and lymphoscintigraphy, which utilizes a radioactive agent to functionally evaluate the lymph flow. In the past few years, new macromolecular agents, gadolinium-labeled dendrimers, fluorescent quantum dots, fluorescent labeled immunoglobulins have been used to image lymphatics and sentinel lymph node with MRI and optical imaging.[170] With the exception of the cisterna chyli, the lymph channels cannot be seen with conventional cross-sectional imaging.

Lymphography

Lymphographic studies are useful in the detection of lymphatic fistulas or lymphatic leakage. Lymphography is diagnostically more accurate than CT in normal-sized lymph nodes or small lymph nodes by CT criteria, as this demonstrates internal architecture. Since the advent of cross-sectional imaging, especially CT, the use of lymphographic studies has significantly decreased because of the difficulty in performing the procedure and its moderately invasive nature. First, methylene blue is injected into the soft-tissues between the toes. Then an incision is made into the dorsum of the foot, allowing for direct visualization and cannulation of the methylene blue–filled lymphatic ducts. Fatty (Lipiodol, Ethiodol) or water-soluble contrast is injected into the lymphatics and radiographs of the pelvis, abdomen, and thorax demonstrate the contrast-filled

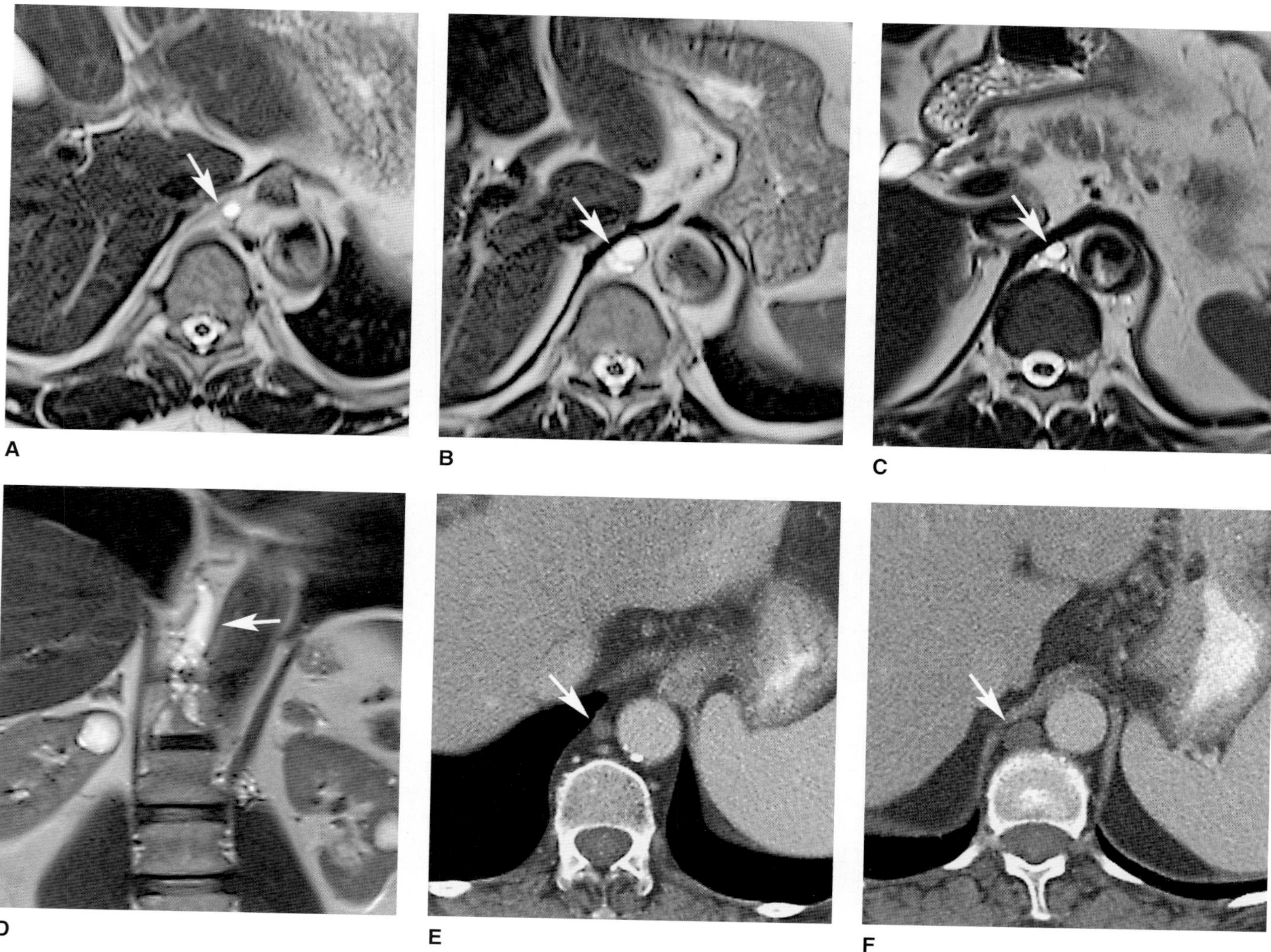

Figure 13-42 Cisterna Chyli in 2 Patients
A-C. Axial T2-weighted MRI images show a bright oval structure (*arrows*) behind the crux of the diaphragm. Note how this is narrow at the top and bottom and wider in the middle image, indicating a tubular structure. This is the typical axial appearance of the cisterna chyli, a small reservoir of lymph fluid as the lymph passes from the lower extremities and trunk into the thorax. **D.** The tubular character of the cisterna chyli (*arrow*) is seen better on this longitudinal T2-weighted MRI sequence. **E** and **F.** Contrast-enhanced axial CT images show an oval low-attenuation structure (*arrows*) behind the crux of the diaphragm, typical of the CT appearance of the cisterna chyli. This can be confused with a retroperitoneal lymph node. However, note how the cisterna chyli is lower attenuation than the crux of the diaphragm. A lymph node would have similar attenuation to the diaphragm crux.

lymphatic ducts and lymph nodes (see Figure 13-43). Oily lymphatic contrast will remain in lymph nodes for years and will be seen on all subsequent x-ray and CT examinations of the pelvis, abdomen, thorax, and neck. The contrast is very strongly attenuating and appears nearly metallic on CT scans of the pelvis, abdomen, and thorax (see Figure 13-19).

Complications of the procedure are not rare and most often consist of pulmonary oil embolization but also include pulmonary infarction, allergy to methylene blue and Ethiodol, intra-alveolar hemorrhage, systemic embolization, and hypothyroidism.[171-176] Lymphography is still an important part of the diagnosis of chylous ascites, chylothorax, chyluria, external genital lymphedema, and preplanning for thoracic duct embolization. In spite of the decline of lymphography worldwide, its role in diagnosis and localization of damage in lymph vessel is indisputable.[177]

Lymphoscintigraphy

Lymphoscintigraphy has recently replaced the lymphography for the assessment of lymphedema. Lymphoscintigraphy is done by injecting the 99-m-Tc-rhenium sulfide nanocolloids (50-100 nm is average diameter) in a subcutaneous space of the toes and follow its progression with the help of

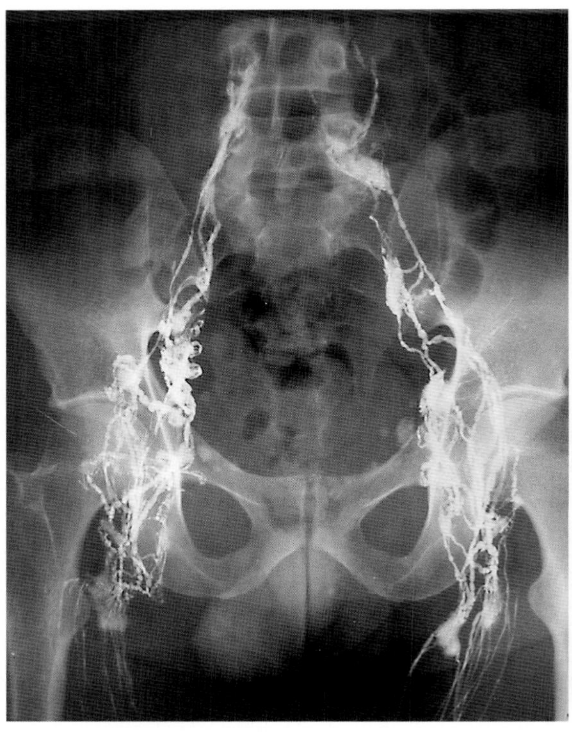

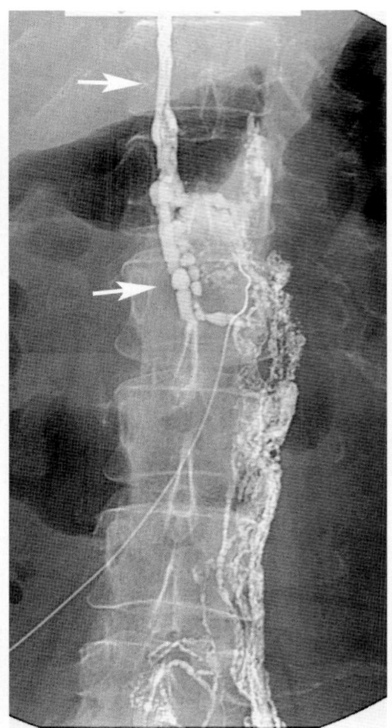

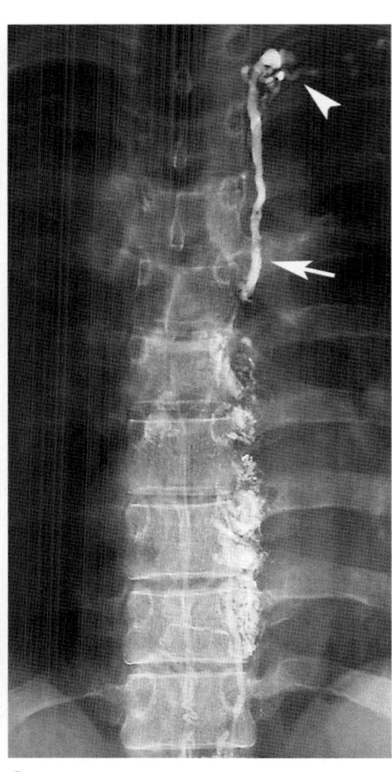

Figure 13-43 Lymphangiogram in Two Patients
A. Image of the pelvis following injection of lymphangiographic contrast show innumerable, fine parallel channels extending along the iliac lymph node chains bilaterally. **B.** Image of the abdomen in a second patient shows lymphangiographic contrast in fine parallel lymphatics in the left para-aortic chain. The larger tubular structure (*arrow*) in the superior abdomen represents the cisterna chyli and beginnings of the thoracic duct. **C.** Image of the thorax in the same patient as (A) shows continuation of fine lymphatic channels until a single large thoracic duct (*arrow*) forms in the superior thorax and then empties into the left subclavian vein.

a gamma camera, including static images. In the last 5 to 10 years, renewed interest in the use of lymphoscintigraphy for sentinel node mapping has been seen. The sentinel node is defined as the first lymphatic relay in the drainage territory of a primary tumor and is thought to be the first site of metastasis. This technique is well established for melanoma and breast carcinoma sentinel node mapping (see Figure 13-44).[178]

Disorders of the Lymphatic System

Disruption or obstruction of the lymphatic system can lead to lymphedema and or lymphatic fistulas and chylous collections in the thorax or abdomen.

Lymphedema

Lymphedema also known as lymphatic insufficiency is characterized by the accumulation of lymphatic fluid in the interstitium causing soft-tissue swelling, primarily of the legs or arms, but occasionally involving other parts of the body. Skin affected by chronic lymphedema can become fibrotic with a loss of the normal skin architecture, function, and mobility and can lead to life-threatening infection.

Lymphedema can be inherited (primary) or result from injury to the lymphatic vessels (secondary). Primary lymphedema is an inherited disease with incidence of less than 1% of live births. Lymphatic vessels are missing or maldeveloped and will typically present as swelling of 1 limb or several limbs and/or internal organs. Secondary causes are most often a result of prior surgical lymphadenectomy or irradiation for cancer, especially breast cancer, but can also be seen with accidental trauma and neoplastic obstruction of the lymph channels. In tropical climates, lymphatic filariasis, 90% of which is caused by the organism *Wucheria bancrofti*, is an important cause of lymphedema.

Lymphatic trauma

The lymphatic system has a remarkable regenerating ability, and very rarely does injury cause significant morbidity. However, surgical or accidental traumatic injury to lymphatics or obstructing neoplasms can cause lymphatic fistula/lymphocele, or chylous ascites.[179] Lymphatic fistula can be diagnosed by lymphangiography or lymphoscintigraphy, showing that the abnormal drainage or fluid collection contains lymph fluid.

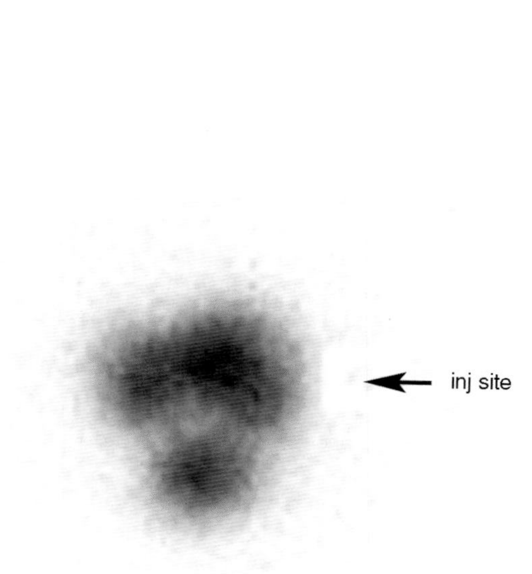

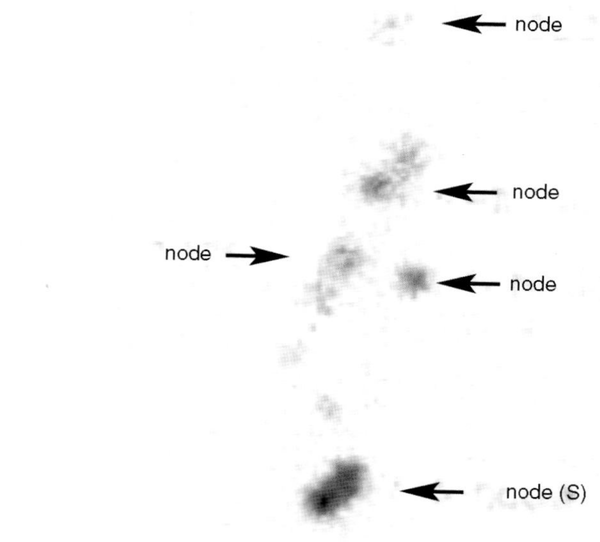

Figure 13-44 Sentinel Node Mapping in Melanoma
This 47-year-old male is a known patient of melanoma of the left knee. **A.** After the injection of 99-m-Tc-sulfur nanocolloid subcutaneously at the left knee, (**B**) the draining nodes were mapped, and a sentinel node is highlighted by "(S)."

SUMMARY

A wide array of imaging techniques is available for imaging of the lymph nodes and lymphatic ducts. Differentiation of normal and abnormal lymph nodes on cross-sectional imaging has become progressively better, but further refinements in the techniques, especially use of molecular imaging, is necessary so that pathologically small lymph nodes can be detected more accurately. Fundamental knowledge of anatomy of lymphatic drainage pathways is crucial for the staging of abdominopelvic malignancies as prognosis is linked to the initial staging in every malignancy. There is a wide differential diagnosis for lymphadenopathy; however, disease-specific clues can be demonstrated on imaging to reach the diagnosis or at least for narrowing the differential diagnosis.

REFERENCES

1. Poirier P, CuneoB, Delamere G. *The Lymphatics*. Westminster: Archibald Constable & Co, Ltd; 1903.
2. Sappey P. *Des vaisseaux lymphatiques*. Paris: Delahaye A, Lecrosnier E; 1888:731-842.
3. Warwick R, Williams P. Topography of the lymph nodes and vessels. In: *Gray's Anatomy*. Edinburgh: Longman; 1973: 727-744.
4. Whitmore I. Lymphoid system. In: *Federative Committee on Anatomical Terminology – Terminologica Anatomica*. Stuttgart: Thieme Verlag; 1998:100-103.
5. Testut L. Des lymphatiques. In: Testut L, ed. *Traite´ d'anatomie humaine*. Paris: Doin; 1893:267-308.
6. Lengele B. The lymphatic system. In: Gregoire V, Scalliet P, Ang K, eds. *Clinical Target Volume in Conformal and Intensity Modulated Radiotherapy A Clinical Guide to Cancer Treatment*. Berlin: Springer Verlag; 2004:1-36.
7. Rouviere H, Tobias M. *Anatomy of the Human Lymphatic System*. Ann Arbor: Edwards; 1938.
8. Plentl A, Friedman E. *Lymphatic System of the Female Genitalia. The Morphologic Basis of Oncologic Diagnosis and Therapy*. Philadelphia, PA: WB Saunders; 1971.
9. Lengelé B, Nyssen-Behets C, Scalliet P. Anatomical bases for the radiological delineation of lymph node areas. Part II: upper limbs chest and abdomen. *Radiother Oncol*. 2007;84: 335-347.
10. Henrikson E. The lymphatic spread of carcinoma of the cervix and of the body of the uterus. A study of 420 necropsies. *Am J Obstet Gynec*. 1949;58:924.
11. Kwok H, Bissett I, Hill G. Preoperative staging of rectal cancer. *Int J Colorectal Dis*. 2000;15:9-20.
12. Bluemke D, Cameron J, Hruban R, et al. Potentially resectable pancreatic adenocarcinoma: spiral CT assessment with surgical and pathologic correlation. *Radiology*. 19956;197:381-385.
13. Diehl S, Lehmann K, Sadick M, Lackmann R, Georgi M. Pancreatic cancer: value of dual-phase helical CT in assessing resectability. *Radiology*. 1998;206:373-378.
14. Gmeinwieser J, Feuerbach S, Hohenberger W, et al. Spiral CT in diagnosis of vascular involvement of pancreatic cancer. *Hepatogastroenterology*. 1995;42:418-422.
15. Studer U, Scherz S, Scheidegger J, et al. Enlargement of regional lymph nodes in renal cell carcinoma is often not due to metastases. *J Urol*. 1990;144(2 pt 1):243-245.

16. Perrotti M, Kaufman RJ, Jennings T, et al. Endo-rectal coil magnetic resonance imaging in clinically localized prostate cancer: is it accurate? *J Urol.* 1996;156:106-109.
17. Bezzi M, Kressel H, Allen K, et al. Prostatic carcinoma: staging with MR imaging at 1.5 T. *Radiology.* 1988;169:339-346.
18. Jager G, Barentsz J, Oosterhof G, et al. Pelvic adenopathy in prostatic and urinary bladder carcinoma: MR imaging with a three-dimensional TI-weighted magnetization-prepared-rapid gradient- echo sequence. *AJR Am J Roentgenol.* 1996;167:1503-1507.
19. Kier R, Wain S, Troiano R. Fast spin-echo MR images of the pelvis obtained with a phased-array coil: value in localizing and staging prostatic carcinoma. *AJR Am J Roentgenol.* 1993;161: 601-606.
20. Tuzel E, Sevinc M, Obuz F, et al. Is magnetic resonance imaging necessary in the staging of prostate cancer? *Urol Int.* 1998;61:227-231.
21. Hall T, MacVicar A. Imaging of bladder cancer. *Imaging.* 2001;13:1-10.
22. Barentsz J, Jager G, van Vierzen P, et al. Staging urinary bladder cancer after transurethral biopsy: value of fast dynamic contrast-enhanced MR imaging. *Radiology.* 1996;20:185-193.
23. Barentsz J, Ruijs S, Strijk S. The role of MR imaging in carcinoma of the urinary bladder. *AJR Am J Roentgenol.* 1993;160:937-947.
24. Tavares N, Demas B, Hricak H. MR imaging of bladder neoplasms: correlation with pathologic staging. *Urol Radiol.* 1990;12:27-33.
25. Creasman W, Morrow C, Bundy B, et al. Surgical pathologic spread patterns of endometrial cancer: a Gynecologic Oncology Group study. *Cancer.* 1987;60:2035-2041.
26. Manfredi R, Mirk P, Maresca G, et al. Local-regional staging of endometrial carcinoma: role of MR imaging in surgical planning. *Radiology.* 2004;231:372-378.
27. Kim S, Choi B, Kim J, et al. Preoperative staging of uterine cervical carcinoma: comparison of CT and MRI in 99 patients. *J Comput Assist Tomogr.* 1993;17:633-640.
28. Yang W, Lam W, Yu M, et al. Comparison of dynamic helical CT and dynamic MR imaging in the evaluation of pelvic lymph nodes in cervical carcinoma. *AJR Am J Roentgenol.* 2000;175:759-766.
29. Tempany C, Zou K, Silverman, et al. Staging of advanced ovarian cancer: comparison of imaging modalities—report from the Radiology Oncology Group. *Radiology.* 2000;215: 761-767.
30. Ricke J, Sehouli J, Hach C, et al. Prospective evaluation of contrast-enhanced MRI in the depiction of peritoneal spread in primary or recurrent ovarian cancer. *Eur Radiol.* 2003;13: 943-949.
31. Antoch G, Saoudi N, Kuehl H, et al. Accuracy of whole-body dual-modality fluorine-18-2-fluoro-2-deoxy-D-glucose positron emission tomography and computed tomography (FDG-PET/ CT) for tumor staging in solid tumors: comparison with CT and PET. *J Clin Oncol.* 2004;22:4357-4368.
32. von Schulthess G, Steinert H, Hany T. Integrated PET/CT: current applications and future directions. *Radiology.* 2006; 238:405-422.
33. Gambhir S, Czernin J, Schwimmer J, Silverman D, Coleman R, Phelps M. A tabulated summary of the FDG PET literature. *J Nucl Med.* 2001;42(5 suppl):1S-93S.
34. Bar-Shalom R, Yefremov N, Guralnik L, et al. Clinical performance of PET/CT in evaluation of cancer: additional value for diagnostic imaging and patient management. *J Nucl Med.* 2003;44:1200-1209.
35. Mikosch P, Gallowitsch HJ, Zinke-Cerwenka W, et al. Accuracy of whole-body ^{18}F-FDP-PET for restaging malignant lymphoma. *Acta Med Austriaca.* 2003;30:41-47.
36. Al-Hallaq H, River J, Zamora M, Oikawa H, Karczma G. Correlation of magnetic resonance and oxygen microelectrode measurements of carbogen induced changes in tumor oxygenation. *Int J Radiat Oncol Biol Phys.* 1998;41:151-159.
37. Rosen M, Schnall M. Dynamic contrast-enhanced magnetic resonance imaging for assessing tumor vascularity and vascular effects of targeted therapies in renal cell carcinoma. *Clin Cancer Res.* 2007;13(2 pt 2):770s-776s.
38. Herts B, Megibow A, Birnbaum B, Kanzer G, Noz M. High-attenuation lymphadenopathy in AIDS patients: significance of findings at CT. *Radiology.* 1992;185:777-781.
39. Rahmouni A, Golli M, Mathieu D, Anglade M-C, Charlotte F, Vasile N. Castleman disease mimicking liver tumor: CT and MR features. *J Comput Assist Tomogr.* 1992;16:699-703.
40. Lepke R, Pagani J. Pancreatic Castleman disease simulating pancreatic carcinoma on computed tomography. *J Comput Assist Tomogr.* 1982;6:1193-1195.
41. Garber S, Shaw D. Case report: the ultrasound and computed tomography appearance of mesenteric Castleman disease. *Clin Radiol.* 1991;43:429-430.
42. Glazer H, Semenkovich J, Gutierrez F. Mediastinum. In: Lee J, Sagel S, Stanley R, Heiken J, eds. *Computed Body Tomography With MRI Correlation.* 3rd ed. Philadelphia, PA: Lippincott-Raven Publishers; 1998:261-349.
43. Reddy D, Salomon C, Demos TC, Cosar. E. Mesenteric lymph node cavitation in celiac disease. *AJR Am J Roentgenol.* 2002;178:247.
44. Huppert B, Farrell M. Case 60: cavitating mesenteric lymph node syndrome. *Radiology.* 2003;228:180-184.
45. Pallisa E, Sanz P, Roman A, Majó J, Andreu J, Cáceres J. Lymphangioleiomyomatosis: pulmonary and abdominal findings with pathologic correlation. *RadioGraphics.* 2002;22:S185-S198.
46. *Facts 2009-2010.* White Plains: The Leukemia and Lymphoma Society; 2010.
47. Skarin A, Dorfman D. Non-Hodgkin's lymphomas: current classification and management. *CA Cancer J Clin.* 1997;47: 351-372.
48. Harris N, Jaffe ES, Stein H, et al. A revised European-American classification of lymphoid neoplasms: a proposal from the International Lymphoma Study Group. *Blood.* 1994;84: 1361-1392.
49. NCI Non-Hodgkin's Classification Project Writing Committee: National Cancer Institute sponsored study of classification of non-Hodgkin's lymphomas: summary and description of a Working Formulation for Clinical Usage. *Cancer.* 1982;49: 2112-2135.
50. Altekruse S, Kosary C, Krapcho M, et al. *SEER Cancer Statistics Review, 1975-2007.* Bethesda: National Cancer Institute; 2010.
51. Stewart S, King JB, Thompson TD, Friedman C, Wingo PA. Cancer mortality surveillance—United States, 1990-2000. *MMWR Surveill Summ.* 2004;53:1-108.

52. Bouzourene H, Haefliger T, Delacretaz F, Saraga E. The role of *Helicobacter pylori* in primary gastric MALT lymphoma. *Histopathology.* 1999;34:118-123.
53. Ratner L. Adult T cell leukemia lymphoma. *Front Biosci.* 2004;1:2852-2859.
54. Wooldridge J, Link B. Post-treatment surveillance of patients with lymphoma treated with curative intent. *Semin Oncol.* 2003;30:375-381.
55. Coleman C, Williams C, Flint A, Glatstein E, Rosenberg S, Kaplan H. Hematologic neoplasia in patients treated for Hodgkin's disease. *N Engl J Med.* 1977;297:1249-1252.
56. Canellos G, Arseneau J, DeVita V, Whang-Peng J, Johnson R. Second malignancies complicating Hodgkin's disease in remission. *Lancet.* 1975;26:947-949.
57. Killebrew D, Shiramizu B. Pathogenesis of HIV-associated non-Hodgkin lymphoma. *Curr HIV Res.* 2004;2:215-221.
58. Adami J, Gabel H, Lindelof B, et al. Cancer risk following organ transplantation: a nationwide cohort study in Sweden. *Br J Cancer.* 2003;89:1221-1227.
59. Fisher S, Fisher R. The epidemiology of non-Hodgkin's lymphoma. *Oncogene.* 2004;232:6524-6534.
60. *Facts 2008-2009.* White Plains: The Leukemia and Lymphoma Society, 2009:1-21.
61. Banks P. The pathology of Hodgkin's disease. *Semin Oncol.* 1990;17:683.
62. Colby T, Hoppe R, Warnke R. Hodgkin's disease: a clinicopathologic study of 659 cases. *Cancer.* 1982;49:1848-1858.
63. Shankar A, Ashley S, Radford M, Barrett A, Wright D, Pinkerton C. Does histology influence outcome in childhood Hodgkin's disease? Results from the United Kingdom Children's Cancer Study Group. *J Clin Oncol.* 1997;15:2622-2630.
64. Smolewski P, Robak T, Krykowski E, et al. Prognostic factors in Hodgkin's disease: multivariate analysis of 327 patients from a single institution. *Clin Cancer Res.* 2000;6:1150-1160.
65. Alexander F, Jarrett R, Cartwright R, et al. Epstein-Barr virus and HLA-DPB1-*0301 in young adult Hodgkin's disease: evidence for inherited susceptibility to Epstein-Barr virus in cases that are EBV(+ve). *Cancer Epidemiol Biomarkers Prev.* 2001;110:705-709.
66. Cobby M, Whipp E, Bullimore J, et al. CT appearances of relapse of lymphoma in the lung. *Clin Radiol.* 1990;41:232-238.
67. Rosenberg S, Kaplan J. Evidence for an orderly progression in the spread of Hodgkin's disease. *Cancer Res.* 1966;26:1225-1231.
68. Tucker M, Coleman C, Cox R, Varghese A, Rosenberg S. Risk of second cancers after treatment for Hodgkin's disease. *N Engl J Med.* 1988;318:76-81.
69. Bangerter M, Moog F, Buchmann I, et al. Whole-body 2-^{18}F-fluoro-2-deoxy-D-glucose positron emission tomography (FDG-PET) for accurate staging of Hodgkin's disease. *Ann Oncol.* 1998;9:1117-1122.
70. Jerusalem G, Beguin Y, Fassotte MF, et al. Whole-body positron emission tomography using ^{18}F-fluorodeoxyglucose compared to standard procedures for staging patients with Hodgkin's disease. *Haematologica.* 2001;86:266-273.
71. Kabickova E, Sumerauer D, Cumlivska E, et al. Comparison of ^{18}F-FDG-PET and standard procedures for the pretreatment staging of children and adolescents with Hodgkin's disease. *Eur J Nucl Med Mol Imaging.* 2006;33:1025-1031.
72. Munker R, Glass J, Griffeth L, et al. Contribution of PET imaging to the initial staging and prognosis of patients with Hodgkin's disease. *Ann Oncol.* 2004;15:1699-1704.
73. Kumar R, Maillard I, Schuster S, Alavi A. Utility of fluorodeoxyglucose-PET imaging in the management of patients with Hodgkin's and non-Hodgkin's lymphomas. *Radiol Clin North Am.* 2004;42:1083-1100.
74. Jerusalem G, Beguin Y, Najjar F, et al. Positron emission tomography (PET) with ^{18}F-fluorodeoxyglucose (^{18}F-FDG) for the staging of low-grade non-Hodgkin's lymphoma (NHL). *Ann Oncol.* 2001;12:825-830.
75. Radford J, Cowan R, Flanagan M, et al. The significance of residual mediastinal abnormality on the chest radiograph following treatment for Hodgkin's disease. *J Clin Oncol.* 1988;6:940-946.
76. Jochelson M, Mauch P, Balikian J, Rosenthal D, Canellos G. The significance of the residual mediastinal mass in treated Hodgkin's disease. *J Clin Oncol.* 1985;3:637-640.
77. Orlandi E, Lazzarino M, Brusamolino E, et al. Residual mediastinal widening following therapy in Hodgkin's disease. *Hematol Oncol.* 1990;8:125-131.
78. Jerusalem G, Beguin Y, Fassotte M, et al. Whole-body positron emission tomography using ^{18}F-fluorodeoxyglucose for posttreatment evaluation in Hodgkin's disease and non-Hodgkin's lymphoma has higher diagnostic and prognostic value than classical computed tomography scan imaging. *Blood.* 1999;94:429-433.
79. Zijlstra J, van der Werf G, Hoekstra O, et al. ^{18}F-fluoro-deoxyglucose positron emission tomography for post-treatment evaluation of malignant lymphoma: a systematic review. *Haematologica.* 2006;91:522-552.
80. Nyman R, Forsgren G, Glimelius B. Long-term follow-up of residual mediastinal masses in treated Hodgkin's disease using MR imaging. *Acta Radiol.* 1996;37:323-326.
81. Buerke B, Puesken M, Muter S, et al. Measurement accuracy and reproducibility of semiautomated metric and volumetric lymph node analysis in MDCT. *AJR Am J Roentgenol.* 2010;195:979-985.
82. Rademaker J. Diagnostic imaging modalities for the assessment of lymphoma with special emphasis on CT, MRI and US. *PET Clin.* 2006;1:219-230.
83. Mueller P, Ferrucci JJ, Harbin W, et al. Appearance of lymphomatous involvement of the mesentery by ultrasound and body computed tomography: the sandwich sign. *Radiology.* 1980;134:467-473.
84. Moog F, Bangerter M, Diederchs C, et al. Lymphoma: role of whole-body 2-deoxy-2-{F-18} fluoro-D-glucose (FDG) PET in nodal staging. *Radiology.* 1997;203:795-800.
85. Rahmouni A, Divine M, Lepage E, et al. Mediastinal lymphoma: quantitative changes in gadolinium enhancement at MR imaging after treatment. *Radiology.* 2001;219:621-628.
86. Nakayama T, Yoshimitsu K, Irie J. Usefulness of the calculated apparent diffusion coefficient value in the differential diagnosis of retroperitoneal masses. *Magn Reson Imaging.* 2004;20:735-742.
87. Dobert N, Menzel C, Hamscho N, Wordehoff W, Kranert W, Grunwald F. Atypical thoracic and supraclavicular FDG-uptake in patients with Hodgkin's and non-Hodgkin's lymphoma. *Q J Nucl Med Mol Imaging.* 2004;48:33-38.

88. Cohade C, Osman M, Pannu H, Wahl R. Uptake in supraclavicular area fat ("USA-Fat"): description on 18F-FDG PET/CT. *J Nucl Med.* 2003;44:170-176.

89. Yeung H, Grewal R, Gonen M, Schoder H, Larson S. Patterns of ^{18}F-FDG uptake in adipose tissue and muscle: a potential source of false-positives for PET. *J Nucl Med.* 2003;44: 1789-1796.

90. Johansson B. Brown fat: a review. *Metabolism.* 1959;8:221-240.

91. Cheson B, Bennett J, Grever M, et al. National Cancer Institute-sponsored Working Group guidelines for chronic lymphocytic leukemia: revised guidelines for diagnosis and treatment. *Blood.* 1996;87:4990-4997.

92. Muntañola A, Bosch F, Arguis P, et al. Abdominal computed tomography predicts progression in patients with Rai stage 0 chronic lymphocytic leukemia. *J Clin Oncol.* 2007;25:1576-1580.

93. Vardiman J, Thiele J, Arber D, Brunning R, Borowitz M, Porwit A. The 2008 revision of the World Health Organization (WHO) classification of myeloid neoplasms and acute leukemia: rationale and important changes. *Blood.* 2009;114:937-951.

94. Ben Romdhane K, Ben Romdhane N, Ben Younes M, Ayadi S, Ben Ayed M. Systemic mastocytosis: a case report. *Arch Anat Cytol Pathol.* 1990;38:100-103.

95. Avila NA, Ling A, Worobec AS, Mican JM, Metcalfe DD. Systemic mastocytosis: CT and US features of abdominal manifestations. *Radiology.* 1997 Feb;202(2):367-372.

96. Pantongrag-Brown L, Krebs T, Daly B, et al. Frequency of abdominal CT findings in AIDS patients with M. avium complex bacteraemia. *Clin Radiol.* 1988;53:816-819.

97. Nyberg D, Federle M, Jeffrey R, Bottles K, Wofsy C. Abdominal CT findings of disseminated *Mycobacterium avium-intracellulare* in AIDS. *AJR Am J Roentgenol.* 1985;145:297-299.

98. 1993 Revised classification system for HIV infection and expanded surveillance case definition for AIDS among adolescents and adults. *MMWR Recomm Rep.* 1992;41(RR-17):1-19.

99. Yee J, Wall S. Gastrointestinal manifestations of AIDS. *Gastroenterol Clin North Am.* 1995;24:413-434.

100. Koh D, Burn P, Mathews G, Nelson M, Healy J. Abdominal computed tomographic findings of Mycobacterium tuberculosis and Mycobacterium avium intracellulare infection in HIV seropositive patients. *Can Assoc Radiol J.* 2003;54:45-50.

101. Bhargava D, Tandon H, Chawla T, Shriniwas, Tandon B, Kapur B. Diagnosis of ileocecal and colonic tuberculosis by colonoscopy. *Gastrointest Endosc.* 1985;31:68-70.

102. Shah S, Thomas V, Mathan M, et al. Colonoscopic study of 50 patients with colonic tuberculosis. *Gut.* 1992;33:347-351.

103. Singh V, Kumar P, Kamal J, Prakash V, Vaiphei K, Singh K. Clinicocolonoscopic profile of colonic tuberculosis. *Am J Gastroenterol.* 1996;91:565-568.

104. Radin D. Disseminated histoplasmosis: abdominal CT findings in 16 patients. *AJR Am J Roentgenol.* 1991;157:955-958.

105. Kitsanou M, Andreopoulou E, Bai M, Elisaf M, Drosos A. Extensive lymphadenopathy as the first clinical manifestation in systemic lupus erythematosus. *Lupus.* 2000;9:140-143.

106. Calguneri M, Ozturk M, Ozbalkan Z, et al. Frequency of lymphadenopathy in rheumatoid arthritis and systemic lupus erythematosus. *J Int Med Res.* 2003;31:345-349.

107. Jeong Y, Ha H, Yoon C, et al. Gastrointestinal involvement in Henoch-Schönlein syndrome: CT findings. *Am J Roentgenol.* 1997;168:965-968.

108. Siskind B, Burrell M, Pun H, Russo RJ, Levin W. CT demonstration of gastrointestinal involvement in Henoch-Schönlein syndrome. *Gastrointest Radiol.* 1985;10:352-354.

109. Akinyemi E, Rohewal U, Tangorra M, et al. Gastric sarcoidosis. *J Natl Med Assoc.* 2006;98:948.

110. Warshauer D, Molina P, Hamman S, et al. Nodular sarcoidosis of the liver and spleen: analysis of 32 cases. *Radiology* 1995; 195:757-762.

111. Fazzi P, Solfanelli S, Morelli G, et al. Sarcoidosis: single bulky mesenteric lymph node mimicking a lymphoma. *Sarcoidosis.* 1995;12:75-77.

112. Miller WTJ, Perez-Jaffe LA. Cross-sectional imaging of Kikuchi disease. *J Comp Assist Tomogr Issue.* 1999;23:548-551.

113. Kim C, Hyun O, Yoo I, Kim S, Sohn H, Chung S. Kikuchi disease mimicking malignant lymphoma on FDG PET/CT. *Clin Nucl Med.* 2007;32:711-712.

114. Chamulak G, Brynes R, Nathwani B. Kikuchi-Fujimoto disease mimicking malignant lymphoma. *Am J Surg Pathol.* 1990;14:514-523.

115. Jayaraj S, Lloyd J, Frosh A, Patel K. Kikuchi-Fujimoto's syndrome masquerading as tuberculosis. *J Laryngol Otol.* 1999;113:82-84.

116. Dorfman R, Berry G. Kikuchi's histiocytic necrotizing lymphadenitis: an analysis of 108 cases with emphasis on differential diagnosis. *Semin Diagn Pathol.* 1988;5: 329-345.

117. Falk R, Comenzo R, Skinner M. The Systemic Amyloidoses. *N Engl J Med.* 1997;337:898-909.

118. Kyle R, Gertz M. Primary systemic amyloidosis: clinical and laboratory features in 474 cases. *Semin Hematol.* 1995;32:45-59.

119. Spitale L, Jimenez D, Montenegro R. Localised primary amyloidosis of inguinal lymph node with superimposed bone metaplasia. *Pathology.* 1998;30:321-322.

120. Kahn H, Strauchen J, Gilbert H, Fuchs A. Immunoglobulin-relate d amyloidosis presenting as recurrent isolated lymph node involvement. *Arch Pathol Lab Med.* 1991;115:948-950.

121. Kyle R, Bayrd E. Amyloidosis: review of 236 cases. *Medicine.* 1975;54:271-299.

122. Takebayashi S, Ono Y, Sasaki F, et al. Computed tomography of amyloidosis involving retroperitoneal lymph nodes mimicking lymphoma. *J Comput Assist Tomogr.* 1984;8:1025-1027.

123. Suga K, Shimizu K, Kawakami Y, et al. Lymphatic drainage from esophagogastric tract: feasibility of endoscopic CT lymphography for direct visualization of pathways. *Radiology.* 2005;237:952-960.

124. Efremidis S, Vougiouklis N, Zafiriadou E, et al. Pathways of lymph node involvement in upper abdominal malignancies: evaluation with high-resolution CT. *Eur Radiol.* 1999;9: 868-874.

125. Coakley F, Lin R, Schwartz L, Panicek D. Mesenteric adenopathy in patients with prostate cancer: frequency and etiology. *AJR Am J Roentgenol.* 2002;178:125-127.

126. Creasman W, Morrow C, Bundy B, et al. Surgical pathologic spread patterns of endometrial cancer: a Gynecologic Oncology Group study. *Cancer.* 1987;60:2035-2041.

127. MacVicar A. Bladder cancer staging. *BJU Int.* 2000;86(suppl 1): 111-122.

128. Kumar R, Zhuang H, Alavi A. PET in the management of urologic malignancies. *Radiol Clin North Am.* 2004;42:1141-1153.

129. Low RN, McCue M, Barone R, Saleh F, Song T. MR staging of primary colorectal carcinoma: comparison with surgical and histopathologic findings. *Abdom Imaging.* 2003;28:784-793.

130. Brown g, Richards C, Bourne M, et al. Morphologic predictors of lymph node status in rectal cancer with use of high-spatial-resolution MR imaging with histopathologic comparison. *Radiology.* 2003;227:371-377.

131. Lowe V, Booya F, Fletcher J, et al. Comparison of positron emission tomography, computed tomography, and endoscopic ultrasound in the initial staging of patients with esophageal cancer. *Mol Imaging Biol.* 2005;7:422-430.

132. Pfau P, Perlman S, Stanko P, et al. The role and clinical value of EUS in a multimodality esophageal carcinoma staging program with CT and positron emission tomography. *Gastrointest Endosc.* 2007;65:377-384.

133. McAteer D, Wallis F, Couper G, et al. Evaluation of ^{18}F-FDG positron emission tomography in gastric and oesophageal carcinoma. *Br J Radiol.* 1999;72:525-529.

134. Yun M, Lim J, Noh S, et al. Lymph node staging of gastric cancer using (18)F-FDG PET: a comparison study with CT. *J Nucl Med* 2005;46:1582-1588.

135. Tian J, Chen L, Wei B, et al. The value of vesicant ^{18}F-fluorodeoxyglucose positron emission tomography (18F-FDG PET) in gastric malignancies. *Nucl Med Commun.* 2004;25:825-831.

136. Chen J, Cheong J, Yun M, et al. Improvement in preoperative staging of gastric adenocarcinoma with positron emission tomography. *Cancer.* 2005;103:2383-2390.

137. Saga T, Higashi T, Ishimori T, et al. Clinical value of FDG-PET in the follow up of post-operative patients with endometrial cancer. *Ann Nucl Med.* 2003;17:197-203.

138. Heesakkers RAM, Hövels AM, Jager GJ, et al. MRI with a lymph-node-specific contrast agent as an alternative to CT scan and lymph-node dissection in patients with prostate cancer: a prospective multicohort study. *Lancet Oncol.* 2008;9:850-856.

139. Harisinghani M, Barentsz J, Hahn P, et al. Noninvasive detection of clinically occult lymph-node metastases in prostate cancer. *N Engl J Med.* 2003;348:2491-2499.

140. Lange P. ProstaScint scan for staging prostate cancer. *Urology.* 2001;57:402-406.

141. Bermejo C, Coursey J, Basler J, et al. Histological confirmation of lesions identified by ProstaScint scan following definitive treatment. *Urol Oncol.* 2003;21:349-352.

142. Polascik T, Manyak M, Haseman M, et al. Comparison of clinical staging algorithms and ^{111}Indium-capromab pendetide immunoscintigraphy in the prediction of lymph node involvement in high risk prostate carcinoma patients. *Cancer.* 1999;85:1586-1592.

143. Harris R. Computerized tomography of retroperitoneal lymphadenopathy: benign or malignant? *Comput Tomogr.* 1979;3:73-80.

144. Subramanyam B, Balthazar E, Homii S, Hilton S. Abdominal lymphadenopathy in intravenous drug addicts: sonographic features and clinical significance. *AJR Am J Roentgenol.* 1985; 144:917-920.

145. Goldberg H, Gore R, Margulis A, Moss A, Baker E. Computed tomography in the evaluation of Crohn disease. *AJR Am J Roentgenol.* 1983;140:277-282.

146. Nagamata H, Inadama E, Arihiro S, Matsuoka M, Torii A, Fukuda K. The usefulness of MDCT in Crohn's disease. *Nippon Shokakibyo Gakkai Zasshi.* 2002;99:1317-1325.

147. Trommer G, Bewer A, Kosling A. Mesenteric lymphadenopathy in *Yersinia enterocolitica* infection. *Radiologe.* 1998;38:37-40.

148. Yang Z, Min P, Sone S, et al. Tuberculosis versus lymphomas in the abdominal lymph nodes: evaluation with contrast-enhanced CT. *AJR Am J Roentgenol.* 1999;172:619-623.

149. Blachar A, Federle M, Brancatelli G. Primary biliary cirrhosis: clinical, pathologic, and helical CT findings in 53 patients. *Radiology.* 2001;220:329-336.

150. del Olmo J, Esteban J, Maldonado L, et al. Clinical significance of abdominal lymphadenopathy in chronic liver disease. *Ultrasound Med Biol.* 2002;28:297-301.

151. Horton KM, Lawler LP, Fishman EK. CT findings in sclerosing mesenteritis (panniculitis): spectrum of disease. *Radiographics.* 2003;23:1561-1567.

152. Sabate JM, Torrubia S, Maideu J, Franquet T, Monill JM, Perez C. Sclerosing mesenteritis: imaging findings in 17 patients. *AJR Am J Roentgenol.* 1999;172:625-629.

153. Mitchell OWH. Acute suppurative lymphadenitis abdominal due to diplostreptococcus; autopsy. *Am J Med Sci.* 1913;145:721-723.

154. Asch MJ, Amoury RA, Toulukian RJ, Santulli TV. Suppurative mesenteric lymphadenitis. *Am J Surg.* 1968;115:570-573.

155. Collins DG. Mesenteric lymphadenitis in adolescents simulating appendicitis. *Can Med Assoc J.* 1936;34:402-405.

156. Domingo T, Alvear T, Kain M. Suppurative mesenteric lymphadenitis, a forgotten clinical entity: report of two cases. *J Pediatr Surg.* 1975;19:969-970.

157. Macari M, Hines J, Balthazar E, Megibow A. Mesenteric adenitis: CT diagnosis of primary versus secondary causes, incidence, and clinical significance in pediatric and adult patients. *Am J Roentgenol.* 2002;178:853-858.

158. Rao P, Rhea J, Novelline R. CT diagnosis of mesenteric adenitis. *Radiology.* 1997;202:145-149.

159. Puylaert J. Mesenteric adenitis and acute terminal ileitis: US evaluation using graded compression. *Radiology.* 1986;161: 691-695.

160. Borgia G, Ciampi R, Nappa S, et al. Tuberculous mesenteric lymphadenitis clinically presenting as abdominal mass: CT and sonographic findings. *J Clin Ultrasound.* 1985;13:491-493.

161. Abell M. Lymphoid hamartoma. *Radiol Clin North Am.* 1868; 6:15-24.

162. Gloviczki P, Lowell R. Lymphatic complications of vascular surgery. In: Rutherford R, ed. *Vascular Surgery.* Philadelphia, PA: WB Saunders; 2001:781-789.

163. Meador TL, McLarney JK. CT features of Castleman disease of the abdomen and pelvis. *AJR Am J Roentgenol.* 2000;175:115-118.

164. Gershoni-Baruch R, Brik R, Shinawi M, Livneh A. The differential contribution of MEFV mutant alleles to the clinical profile of familial Mediterranean fever. *Eur J Hum Genet.* 2002; 10:145-149.

165. Ben-Chetrit E, Levy M. Familial Mediterranean fever. *Lancet.* 1998;351:659-664.

166. Zissin R, Rathaus V, Gayer G, Shapiro-Feinberg M, Hertz M. CT findings in patients with familial Mediterranean fever during an acute abdominal attack. *Br J Radiol.* 2003;76:22-25.

167. Rao P, Rhea J, Novelline R, Mostafavi A, McCabe C. Effect of computed tomography of the appendix on treatment of patients and use of hospital resources. *N Engl J Med.* 1998;15: 141-146.

168. Burkill G, Bell J, Healy J. The utility of computed tomography in acute small bowel obstruction. *Clin Radiol.* 2001;56: 350-359.

169. Boudiaf M, Soyer P, Terem C, Pelage J, Maissiat E, Rymer R. CT evaluation of small bowel obstruction. *Radiographics.* 2001;21:613-624.

170. Lucarelli R, Ogawa M, Kosaka N, Turkbey B, Kobayashi H, Choyke P. New approaches to lymphatic imaging. *Lymphat Res Biol.* 2009;7:205-214.

171. Vogl T, Bartjes M, Marzec K. Contrast-enhanced lymphography: CT or MR imaging? *Acta Radiol Suppl* 1997;412:47-50.

172. Mortazavi S, Burrows B. Allergic reaction to patent blue dye in lymphangiography. *Clin Radiol.* 1971;22:389-390.

173. Dupont H, Timsit J, Souweine B, Gachot B, Bedos J, Wolff M. Intra-alveolar hemorrhage following bipedal lymphography. *Intensive Care Med.* 1996;22:614-615.

174. Fein D, Hanlon A, Corn B, Curran WJ, Coia L. The influence of lymphangiography on the development of hypothyroidism in patients irradiated for Hodgkin's disease. *Int J Radiat Oncol Biol Phys.* 1996;36:13-18.

175. Kusumoto S, Imamura A, Watanabe K. Case report: the incidental lipid embolization to the brain and kidney after lymphography in a patient with malignant lymphoma—CT findings. *Clin Radiol.* 1991;44:279-280.

176. Winterer J, Blum U, Boos S, Konstantinides S, Langer M. Cerebral and renal embolization after lymphography in a patient with non-Hodgkin lymphoma: case report. *Radiology.* 1999;210:381-383.

177. Guermazi A, Brice P, C H, Sarfati E. Lymphography: an old technique retains its usefulness. *Radiographics.* 2003;23: 1541-1558.

178. Morton D, Wen D, Wong J, et al. Technical details of intraoperative lymphatic mapping for early stage melanoma. *Arch Surg.* 1992;127:392-399.

179. Gloviczki P, Lowell R. Lymphatic complications of vascular surgery. In: Rutherford R, ed. *Vascular Surgery.* Philadelphia, PA: WB Saunders; 2001:781-789.

CHAPTER

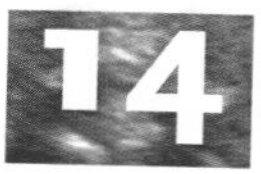

Imaging of the Spleen

Lauren Ehrlich, MD
Wallace T. Miller Jr., MD

ANATOMY OF THE SPLEEN

The spleen is a functionally diverse organ with active roles in immunosurveillance, red blood cell breakdown, splenic contraction for blood volume augmentation during hemorrhage, and hematopoiesis.

The spleen lies within the left upper quadrant of the peritoneal cavity and abuts ribs 9 to 12, the fundus of the stomach, the upper pole of the left kidney, the splenic flexure of the colon, and the tail of the pancreas. During childhood, the size of the spleen is based on age and weight, and tables of normal splenic size are available in the literature.[1] A normal adult spleen weighs approximately 150 g and is approximately 11 cm in craniocaudal length. A craniocaudal measurement of 11 to 13 cm is frequently used as the upper limit of normal for splenic size in imaging studies. The spleen is composed of lymphatic follicles and reticuloendothelial cells ("white pulp") and vascular sinusoids ("red pulp"). The relative percentage of white pulp increases with age because of accumulated antigenic exposure. The spleen has a lenticular shape, convex superolateral, and concave inferomedial.

Clefts and lobules are common. Accessory spleens, also known as supernumerary spleens or splenules, are the most common congenital anomalies of the spleen, detected in 10% to 30% of patients at autopsy, and in approximately 16% of CT studies.[2] Their location is variable, but most often are near the hilum and tail of the pancreas.[3] The vast majority of accessory spleens are asymptomatic and discovered incidentally. However, recognizing them is important in order not to misdiagnose an accessory spleen for lymphadenopathy or for a tumor arising from adjacent organs. Also, before splenectomy in a patient with a hematologic or autoimmune disorder, the presence of an accessory spleen must be known in order to remove all functional splenic tissue. Accessory spleens are usually less than 4 cm in diameter, are round or ovoid, have well-demarcated margins, and are characterized by their similar imaging characteristics to normal splenic parenchyma (see Figure 14-1). These characteristics should enable the reader to distinguish splenules from other causes of left upper quadrant masses.

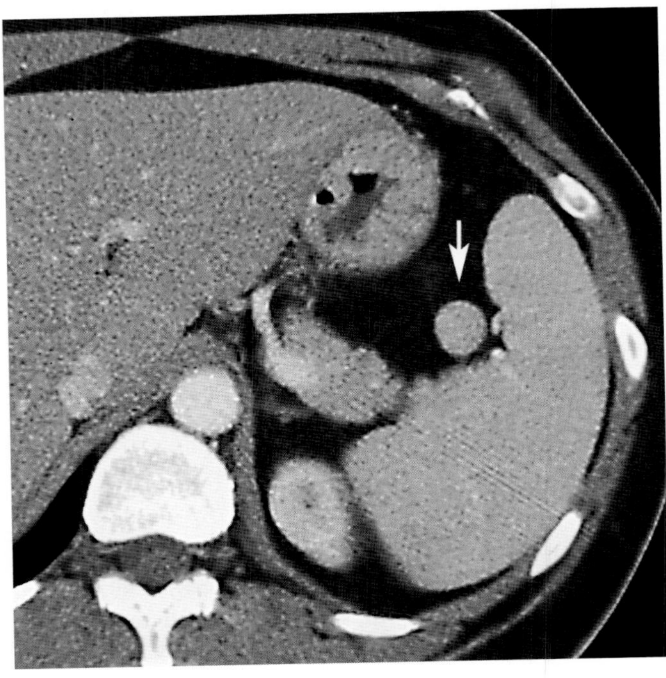

Figure 14-1 Splenule
Contrast-enhanced CT shows a small uniformly enhancing nodule (*arrow*) medial to the body of the spleen. This is a typical appearance of a splenule or small accessory spleen, a common normal variant. Splenules will have imaging characteristics that match the main body of the spleen on all imaging modalities.

IMAGING OF THE SPLEEN

On abdominal and chest radiographs, the spleen will appear as a lenticular-shaped opacity in the left upper quadrant of the abdomen beneath the diaphragm. In some individuals, the medial edge of the spleen will be sharply defined because of the different attenuation of adjacent abdominal fat (see Figure 14-2). In other individuals, the size and location of the spleen can only be inferred by the displacement of adjacent gas-containing intestines. Splenomegaly is 1 of the few abnormalities of the solid abdominal viscera that can be reliably demonstrated on abdominal x-rays. In addition, calcified splenic abnormalities may be detected by plain film, including splenic artery aneurysms, calcified cysts, calcified granulomas, and calcified hematomas.

Sonography is frequently the first imaging modality employed to evaluate the spleen, because it is noninvasive and relatively inexpensive. Ultrasonography (US) of the spleen is performed with the patient in the supine or right lateral decubitus position, with the spleen visualized beneath the left costal margin or between rib interspaces. A 3.0- to 5.0-MHz transducer is generally used. On US, the spleen is homogeneous, slightly more echogenic than normal kidney, and isoechoic or slightly greater in echogenicity than liver. The spleen is relatively hypervascular on Doppler interrogation (see Figure 14-3).

On unenhanced CT, the spleen is homogeneous, with attenuation typically measuring 40 to 60 Hounsfield units (HUs). Unenhanced splenic attenuation is normally 5 to 10 HU less than that of liver. With contrast, spleen enhancement is initially heterogeneous, likely reflecting variation in the flow rate through red pulp in the spleen.[4] Bizarre enhancement patterns are the norm, particularly during the arterial and early venous phases of enhancement. Later venous-phase images or delayed images

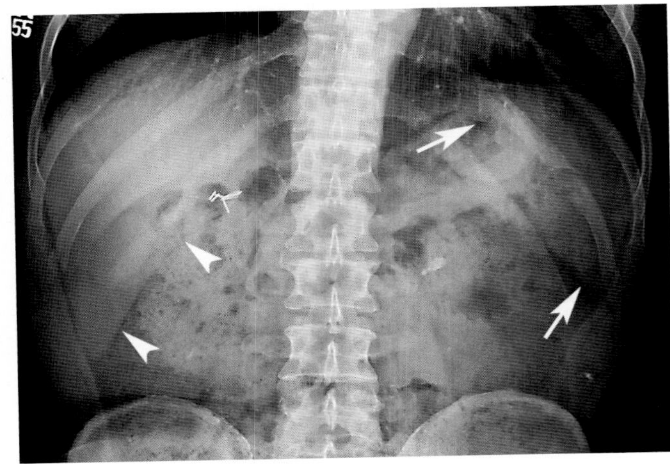

Figure 14-2 Spleen on Abdominal X-ray
This 57-year-old man was being evaluated for nephrolithiasis. The presence of abdominal fat makes the outline of the spleen (*arrows*) and liver (*arrowheads*) visible on this abdominal x-ray.

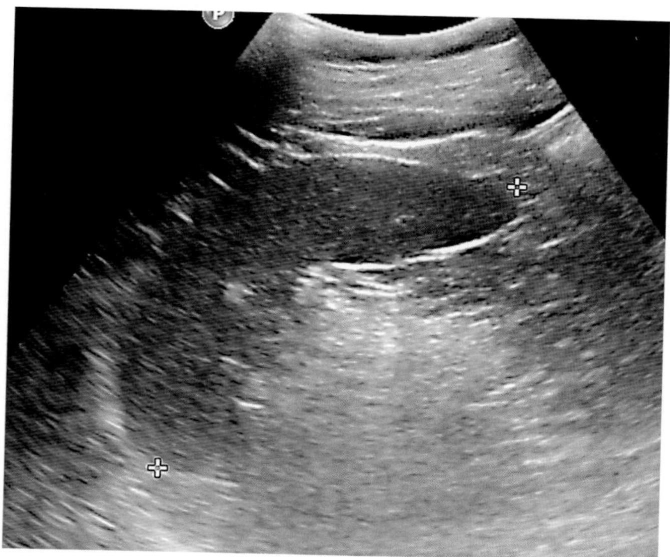

Figure 14-3 Normal Splenic Ultrasonography
US image of the normal spleen shows the normal crescentic shape and uniform echogenicity.

greater than 70 seconds after the initiation of contrast injection will show homogeneous enhancement of the normal spleen (see Figure 14-4). Normally, the liver and spleen densities are within 25 HU on dynamic contrast-enhanced CT scan images.

On MR, the spleen is usually evaluated with both T1- and T2-weighted spin-echo sequences. On T1-weighted imaging, the spleen is hypointense to hepatic tissue and slightly greater than that of skeletal muscle. The spleen appears high signal on T2-weighted imaging, greater than the liver. Inhomogeneous and bizarre enhancement patterns of gadolinium enhancement of the spleen are similar to those seen with iodinated contrast on CT (see Figure 14-5).[5]

^{104m}Tc-sulfur colloid is now only occasionally used to clarify splenic anatomy. ^{104m}Tc-labeled heat-damaged red cells can be used to assess splenic function and anatomy. The advantage of this technique is uptake only by the spleen, not the liver as also occurs with sulfur colloid. ^{18}F-FDG-PET/CT is now used as a noninvasive imaging modality, predominantly in assessing solid splenic masses. Physiologic uptake of ^{18}F-FDG by normal splenic tissue is generally uniformly low.[6]

UNIFOCAL SPLENIC LESIONS

Unifocal splenic lesions can be cystic or solid appearing and spherical or nonspherical in shape. Our differential diagnosis of solitary splenic lesions will revolve around these imaging characteristics.

Cystic-Appearing Nodules and Masses of the Spleen

A solitary cystic-appearing nodule is the most common imaging abnormality identified on routine cross-sectional imaging. Hemangiomas before contrast enhancement are the most common cause, with other causes including lymphangiomas, splenic abscesses, and posttraumatic or infarction cysts (Table 14-1).

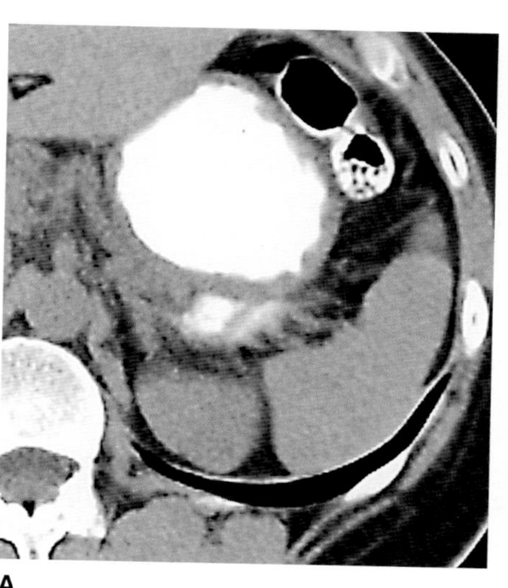

A

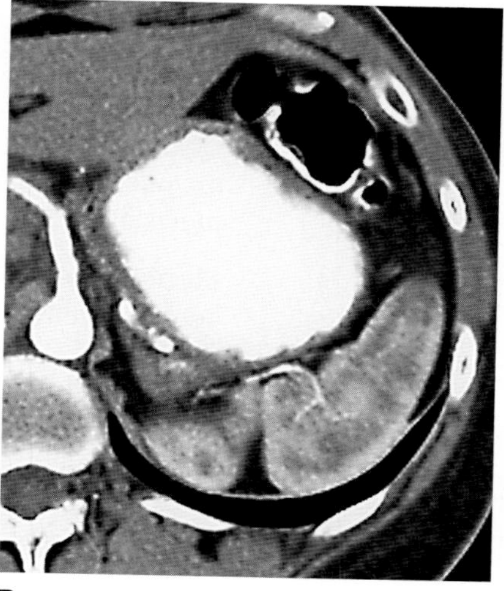

B

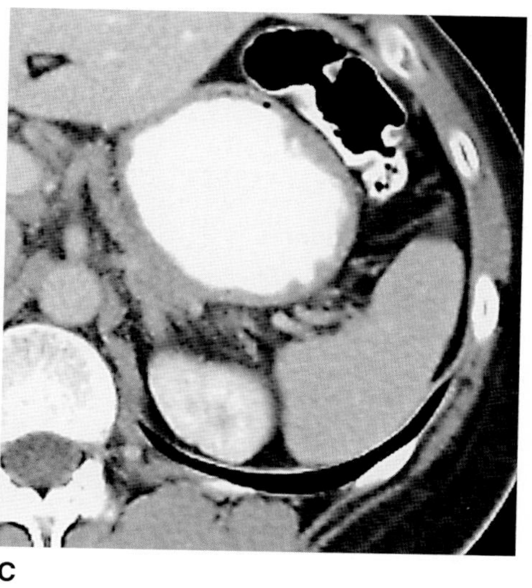

C

Figure 14-4 CT of the Spleen
A. Unenhanced image of the spleen shows the typical crescent-shaped spleen with attenuation similar to the kidney, liver, and other soft-tissue organs. **B.** Arterial-phase image shows the normal inhomogeneous enhancement of the spleen. **C.** Late venous-phase image now shows uniform enhancement of the spleen similar to liver and hyperattenuating relative to paraspinal muscle.

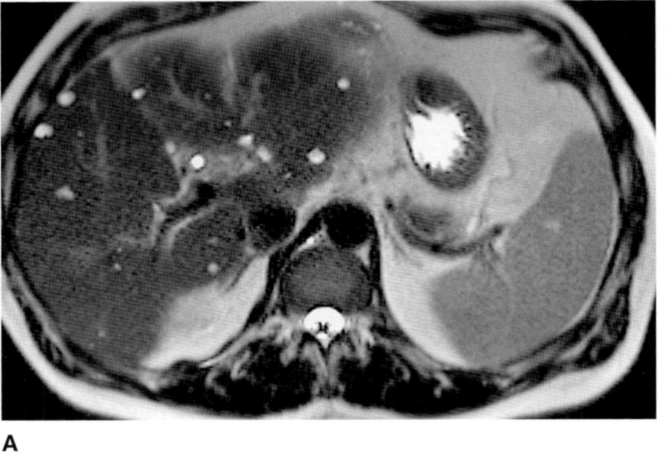

A

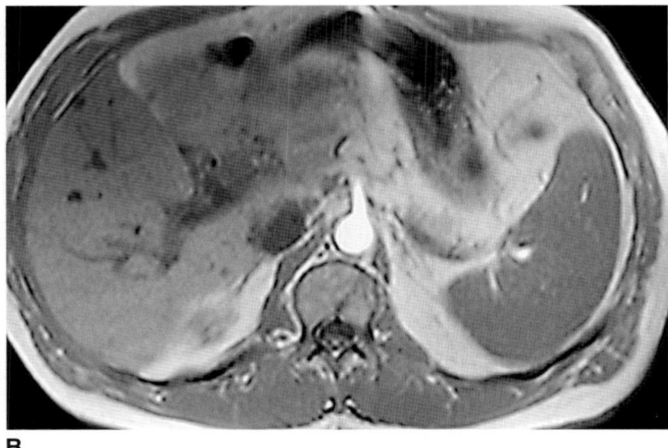

B

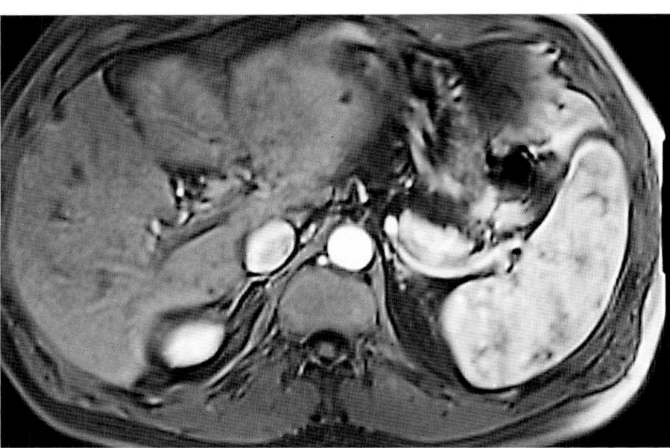

C

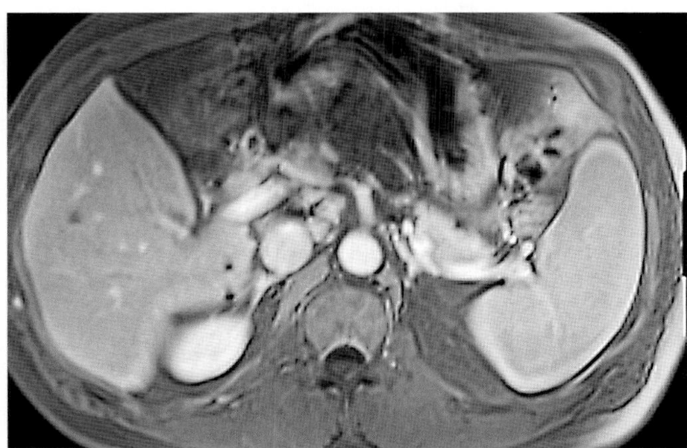

D

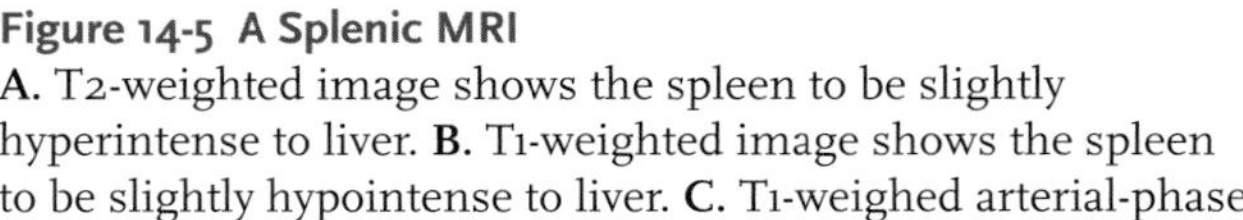

Figure 14-5 A Splenic MRI
A. T2-weighted image shows the spleen to be slightly hyperintense to liver. **B.** T1-weighted image shows the spleen to be slightly hypointense to liver. **C.** T1-weighed arterial-phase image shows the typical inhomogeneous enhancement of the spleen. **D.** T1-weighted venous-phase image shows the typical uniform enhancement of the spleen on late-phase images.

Table 14-1. Solitary Cystic Appearing Splenic Nodules or Masses

A. Neoplasms 1. **Hemangioma**[a] 2. Lymphangioma 3. Cystic metastasis
B. Infections 1. Pyogenic abscess 2. Amebic abscess 3. Echinococcus
C. Hematoma
D. **Posttraumatic and postinfarction cysts**
E. Epidermoid cysts
F. Pancreatic pseudocyst

[a]Disorders in bold are most common.

Neoplasms

Cystic-appearing neoplasms of the spleen are common and include hemangiomas, lymphangiomas, and rarely cystic metastasis.

Hemangioma: Hemangiomas are the most common benign splenic neoplasm and can occur as either solitary, multiple, or diffuse lesions.[7] They have a prevalence at autopsy ranging from 0.3% to 14%.[8] Histologically, they are composed of endothelial-lined blood-filled spaces of varying size and can be characterized by the size of these spaces as capillary or cavernous lesions. The latter are more common. Infrequent associations include Kasabach-Merritt syndrome (anemia, thrombocytopenia, and consumptive coagulopathy) and Klippel-Trénaunay-Weber syndrome (cutaneous hemangiomas, venous varicosities, and soft-tissue and bony hypertrophy of an extremity). In most cases, hemangiomas of the spleen are small asymptomatic lesions that are discovered accidentally.

Imaging Notes 14-1. Hemangioma

Hemangioma is the most common cause of an incidentally detected focal lesion of the spleen.

Splenic hemangiomas have a variety of imaging appearances depending on the proportion of cavernous and capillary features. They are the most common incidentally discovered focal lesion in the spleen. Calcification can occur as either scattered, punctuate, curvilinear, or radiating densities but is unusual. US may show both hypoechoic and hyperechoic regions.[9]

Focal hemangiomas typically appear as well-defined hypoattenuating lesions on noncontrast CT, resembling small cysts but can be isoattenuating to the spleen and be missed entirely (see Figure 14-6).[8] On US examinations, the multiple vascular walls of hemangiomas will usually make them uniformly echogenic and are, therefore, rarely confused with cystic lesions (see Figure 14-7). Although, occasionally they will appear as a complex cystic and solid mass where the larger cavernous channels appear as cystic regions.[10] On MRI, hemangiomas typically appear hypointense or isointense with the remainder of the spleen on T1-weighted images. They are usually hyperintense relative

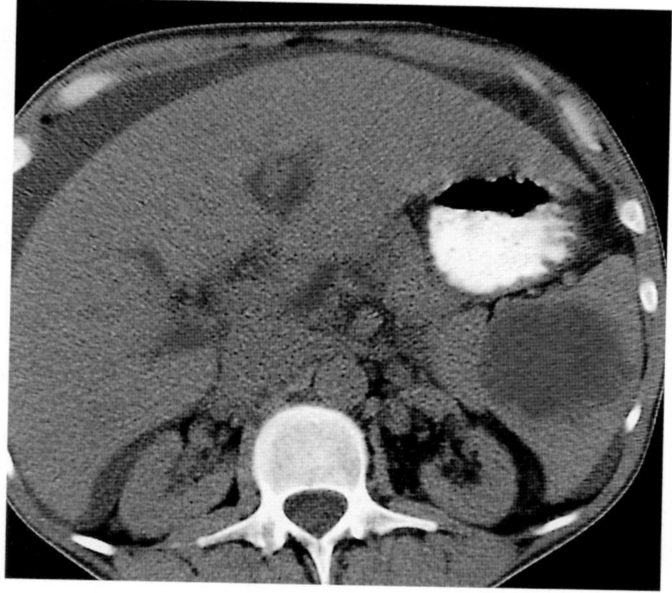

Figure 14-6 Hemangioma on Unenhanced CT
This 38-year-old man had end-stage renal disease. Unenhanced CT shows a large hypoechoic mass in the spleen that is slightly more hyperattenuating than the ascites surrounding the liver. This is a nonspecific mass but is statistically most likely to represent a hemangioma. US examination (not shown) had the typical appearance of a hemangioma.

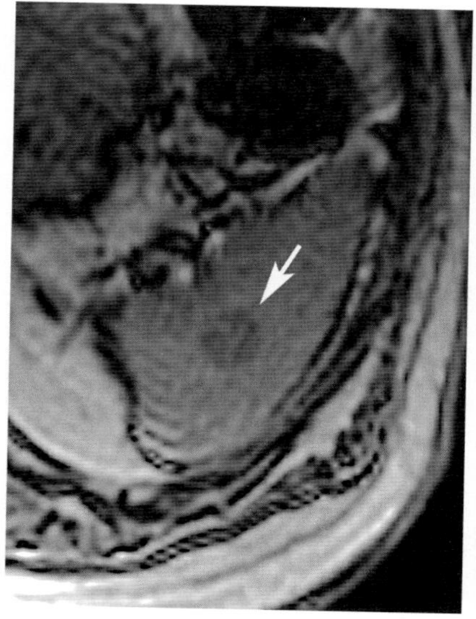

A

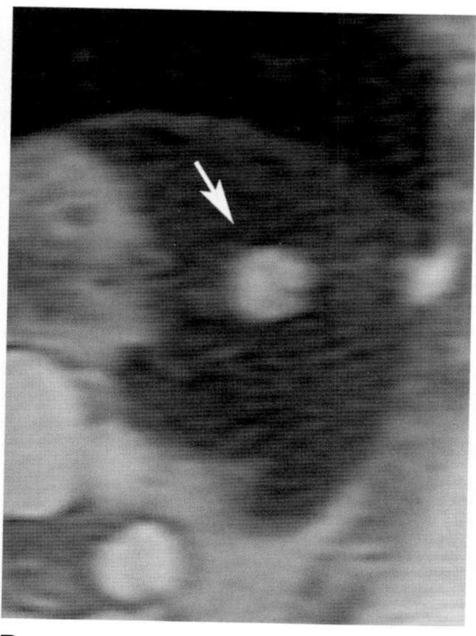

B

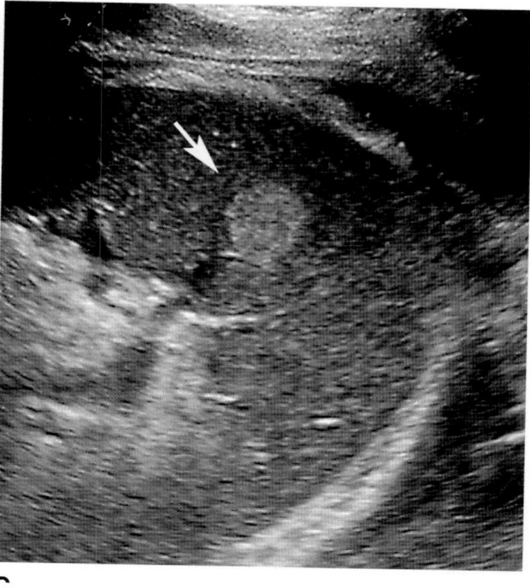

C

Figure 14-7 Splenic Hemangioma
This 85-year-old man had chronic renal disease. **A.** Axial T1-weighted MRI sequence demonstrates a faintly hypointense 1.8-cm nodule (*arrow*) in the spleen. **B.** The nodule (*arrow*) is very intense on this coronal T2-weighted MRI sequence. This is most likely to represent a hemangioma but could indicate a small lymphangioma. **C.** Longitudinal US of the spleen shows the nodule (*arrow*) to be very echogenic, a feature characteristic of hemangioma but would be atypical for a lymphangioma.

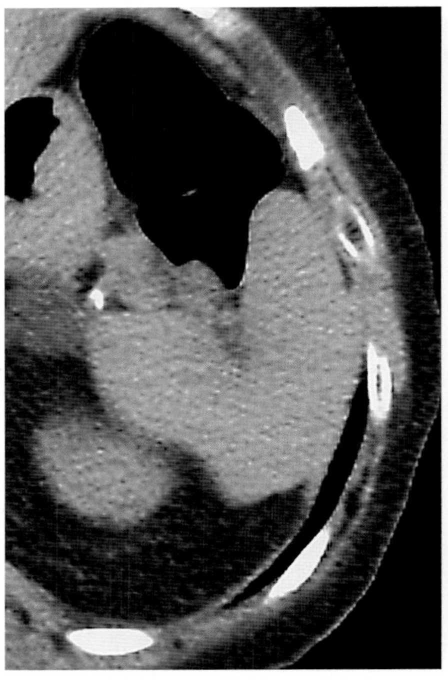
A

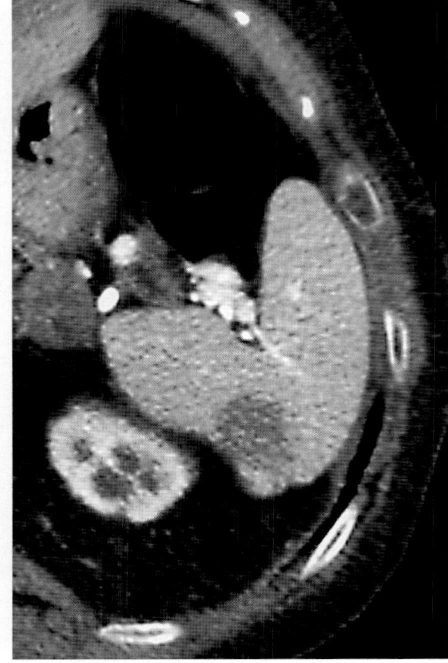
B

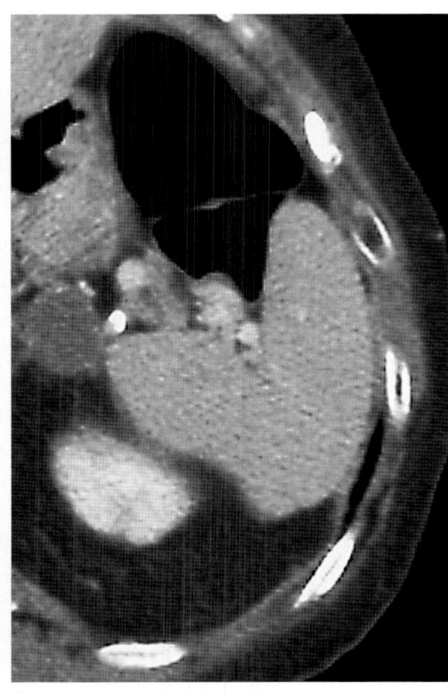
C

Figure 14-8 CT of Splenic Hemangioma
This 75-year-old woman was being evaluated for an abdominal aortic stent graft. **A.** Unenhanced CT shows a normal-appearing spleen. **B.** Arterial-phase image taken at 35 s after injection shows a small focal low-attenuation lesion. **C.** Late venous-phase image taken at 2 min after injection shows the lesion to be isoattenuating with the spleen. Most standard enhanced CT scans are taken between 35 and 60 s after injection, and therefore hemangiomas of the spleen will typically appear as a hypoattenuating mass. Note the incidental left adrenal adenoma.

to normal spleen on T2-weighted images, although slight heterogeneity is sometimes seen, reflecting the variation in the size of blood-filled spaces and the varying amounts of internal fibrosis and hemorrhage (see Figure 14-7).[8]

Following intravenous (IV) contrast administration, the appearance of hemangiomas also shows considerable variation. In the arterial phase and of enhancement, approximately 35 seconds after contrast administration, they will appear as hypoattenuating/hypointense nodules relative to the enhancing spleen and can resemble a cyst (see Figure 14-8). During the early venous phase, at approximately 60 seconds after contrast administration, the lesions will demonstrate centripetal enhancement from the periphery with persistence on delayed images. Unlike the classic peripheral nodular discontinuous enhancement characteristic of hepatic hemangiomas, this pattern of enhancement is rare in splenic hemangiomas, with most lesions showing a continuous peripheral rim of enhancement of variable thickness with an irregular inner margin (see Figure 14-9).[8] Others can show immediate homogeneous enhancement (see Figure 14-10). Mottled enhancement has also been described, with areas remaining hypoattenuating relative to normal spleen, particularly in hemangiomas containing fibrotic components. In the late venous phase, 90 to 120 seconds after contrast administration, the mass will typically become isoattenuating to the spleen.

When the appearance is atypical, Tc-99m-labeled RBC scintigraphy can be utilized to confirm a diagnosis by demonstrating increased activity within the lesion on delayed images.[11] With Tc-99m radiocolloid scanning, both photopenic areas and areas of increased activity have been reported with splenic hemangiomas.[12]

Lymphangioma: Splenic lymphangioma is a rare benign lesion usually diagnosed in childhood.[13] It can occur as solitary or multiple splenic lesions, or as diffuse involvement replacing most of the splenic parenchyma, called lymphangiomatosis.[14] An association with lymphangiomas in other sites (most commonly mediastinum, axilla, and neck) has also been noted.[15] Although typically asymptomatic, lymphangiomas can grow quite large, causing splenomegaly and pain, or compressing adjacent structures. Lesions can be characterized as capillary, cavernous, or cystic depending on the size of the lymphatic channels.

On imaging, the typical cystic lymphangioma is a well-defined, multilocular cystic lesion with thin septations. Cross sectional imaging typically reveals cysts of various sizes, ranging from a few millimeters to several centimeters in diameter.[8] They are often found in a subcapsular location or around larger trabeculae.[16] Lesions are anechoic or hypoechoic on US, and hypoattenuating on CT.[17]

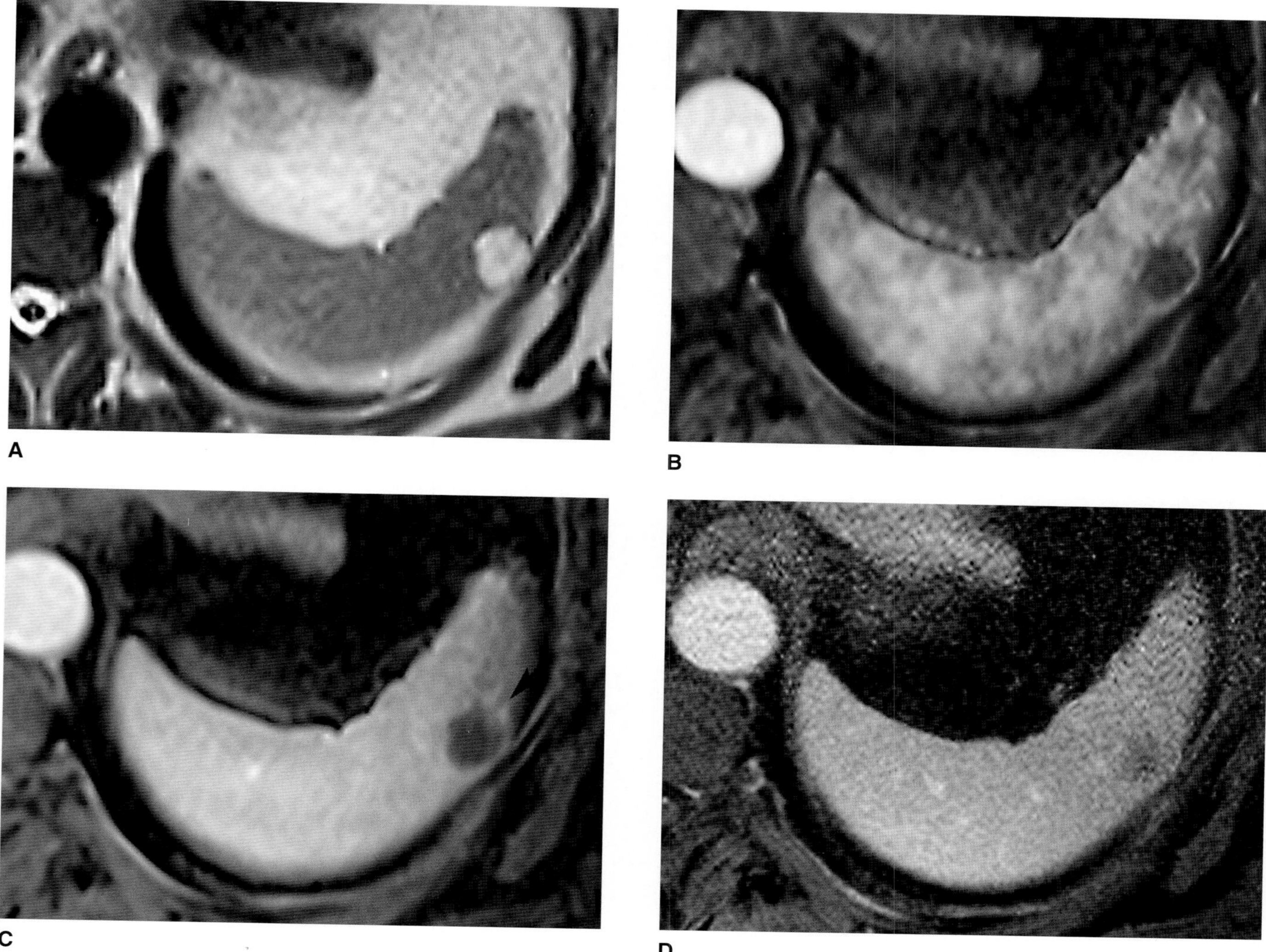

Figure 14-9 Centripetal Enhancement of Splenic Hemangioma This 55-year-old man had colon cancer. **A.** T2-weighted MRI sequence demonstrates a 2-cm lobulated nodule in the spleen that most likely represents a hemangioma or lymphangioma. Contrast-enhanced T1-weighted sequences in the (**B**) arterial phase, (**C**) early portal phase, and (**D**) late portal phase of enhancement show the nodule to progressively decrease in size, typical of centripetal enhancement seen in hemangiomas. Note the faint nodular enhancement (*arrow*) in the periphery of the nodule in (C).

Smaller lymphatic spaces, as can occur in capillary or cavernous lesions, can appear solid on CT and hyperechoic on US.[18] Calcification is occasionally noted. No enhancement of the cystic spaces is noted following IV contrast administration, but moderate enhancement of the septa can be seen. On MRI, the lesions show typical hyperintense signal on T2-weighted images and are usually hypointense on T1-weighted images.[19] The presence of proteinaceous fluid or hemorrhage may result in increased T1 signal (see Figure 14-11).

Cystic metastasis: The majority of metastasis will appear as solid nodules or masses within the spleen. Some will demonstrate central cavitation but will still show solid elements in the periphery of the nodule. In very rare instances, a metastasis could appear as a thin-walled cyst within the substance of the spleen.

Focal infections and abscesses of the spleen

Focal infections of the spleen are rare and include bacterial, mycobacterial, fungal, and protozoal causes. Bacterial and echinococcal infections are typically solitary and will be discussed here; however, mycobacterial and fungal abscesses typically cause multiple small cystic lesions and will be discussed in the subsequent section called **Multifocal Splenic Lesions**.

Pyogenic abscesses of the spleen: Pyogenic or bacterial abscesses involving the spleen are rare. In 1 study of hospitalizations in Denmark, only 20 splenic abscesses were

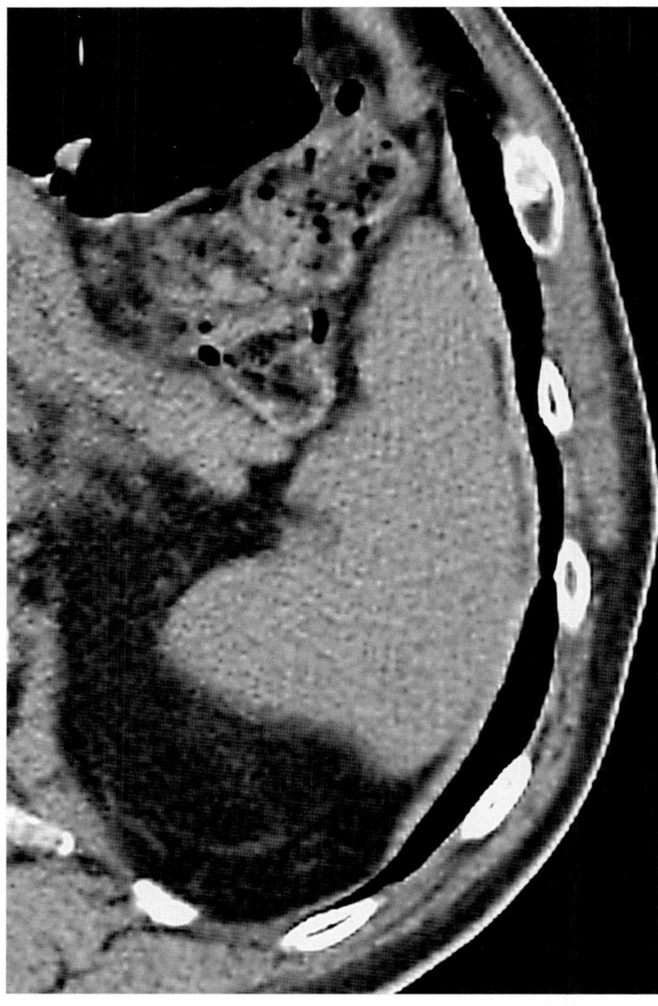

A

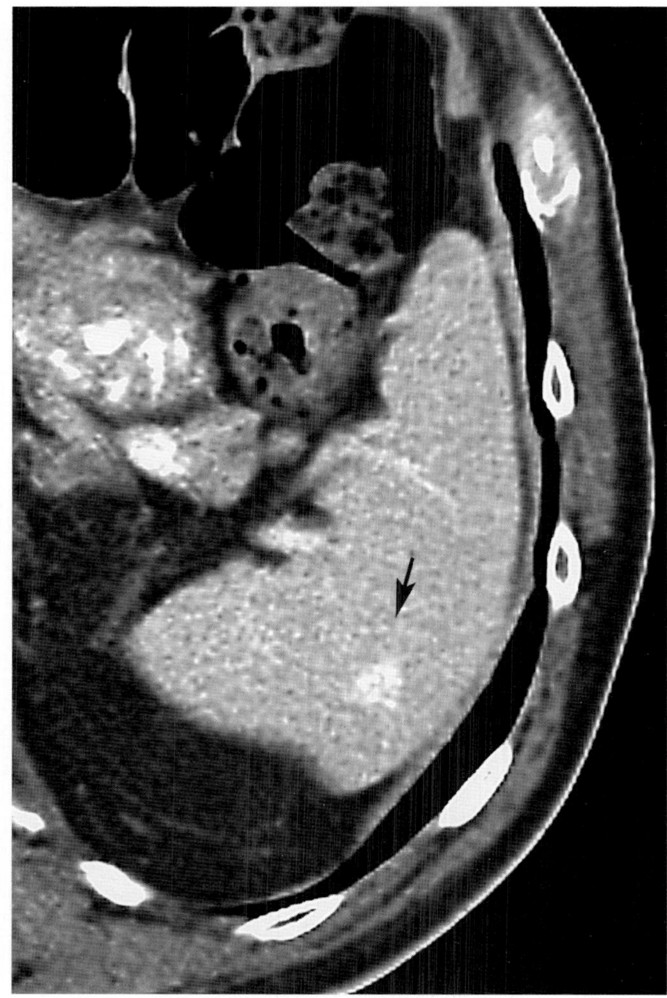

B

Figure 14-10 Uniformly Enhancing Splenic Hemangioma This 72-year-old man had bladder cancer. **A.** Unenhanced CT shows no splenic abnormality. **B.** Contrast-enhanced CT image shows a focal hyperenhancing lesion (*arrow*) in the posterior aspect of the spleen. Although most hemangiomas will have slow-flowing blood and will appear as a hypointense nodule resembling a cyst on early-phase images and will fill in slowly over time, occasionally, some flash-filling hemangiomas will appear uniformly hyperattenuating on early-phase images, like this example.

seen over a 5-year period, accounting for 0.05% of hospitalizations and 0.005% of hospital deaths.[20] The most common mechanism of splenic abscess is via hematogenous dissemination of organisms from another site of infection. This is most often a result of endocarditis but can be due to a wide variety of sites, including urinary tract infections, gastrointestinal infections, pneumonia, mycotic aneurysms, and osteomyelitis.[21-23] Superinfection of necrotic tissue following splenic infarction or splenic trauma is also a well recognized cause for splenic abscess.[23-28] Direct extension of infection from an adjacent organ can also occasionally occur from diverticulitis, subphrenic abscesses, pancreatic abscess, and other retroperitoneal infections.

A variety of conditions have been associated with splenic abscesses, including, trauma, malignancies, corticosteroid use, AIDS, IV drug abuse, cirrhosis, alcoholism and diabetes mellitus.[28-31] Immunocompromised patients account for an increasing proportion of patients with splenic abscess, between one-fourth and one-third of patients.[30,31] Patients typically present with fever, left upper quadrant pain, splenomegaly, and a left pleural effusion.[22,28,32] Most will have a leukocytosis and approximately 2/3rds of patients will have positive blood cultures.[23] Imaging, primarily CT and to a lesser extent US and MRI, is the primary diagnostic method for diagnosing splenic abscesses. CT has been shown to have a 92% to 98% sensitivity and US has been shown to have an approximately 87% sensitivity for splenic abscess.[28,30,31] Splenic abscess carries a 15% to 35% mortality rate.[20,28,32] Standard therapy, as with most abdominal abscesses, is systemic antibiotics and percutaneous or surgical abscess drainage or splenectomy.[20,22,28,33]

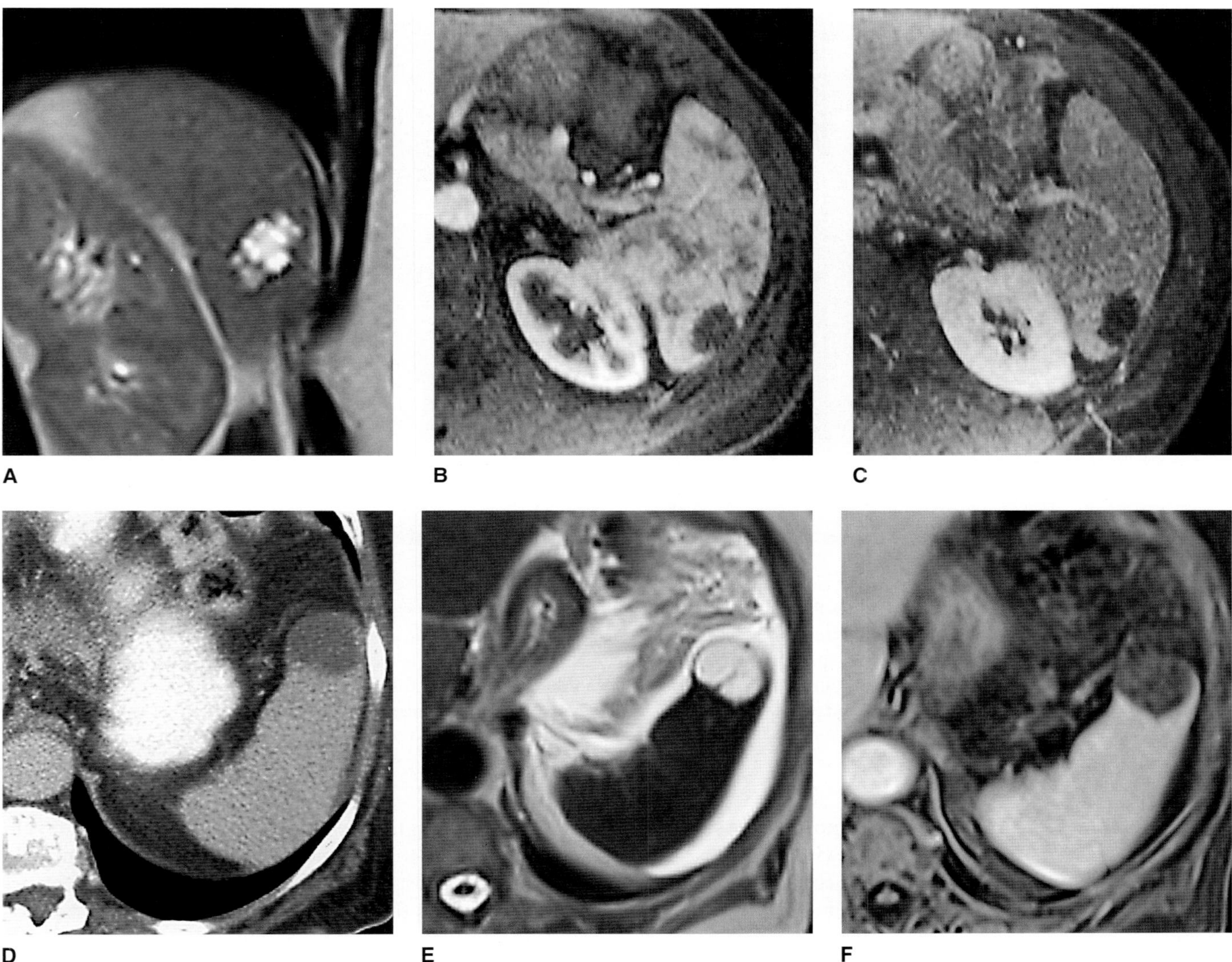

Figure 14-11 Two Splenic Lymphangiomas
A-C. This 65-year-old woman had small cell lymphoma. (A) Coronal T2-weighted MRI sequence demonstrates a lobulated hyperintense mass in the spleen. (B) Arterial-phase and (C) venous-phase T1-weighted MRI images show the nodule to remain low attenuation without enhancement. This could represent a hemangioma with very slow flow but probably represents a small lymphangioma. **D-F.** The second patient was an 83-year-old woman with breast cancer. (D) Venous-phase (60 s post injection) contrast-enhanced CT shows a hypoattenuating mass. (E) T2-weighted MRI image shows a septated high-signal mass indicating a complex cyst. (F) Late venous phase (90 s post injection) gadolinium-enhanced MRI shows a nonenhancing mass. These findings are most consistent with a diagnosis of a splenic lymphangioma.

Bacterial infections are the most common cause of splenic abscesses, accounting for between 56% and 80% of abscesses in 4 large series.[28-31,34] No organisms are discovered in 11%-29% of cases. A wide variety of bacteria have been cultured from splenic abscess including gram negative and gram positive, aerobic and anaerobic organisms.[22,28] A metaanalysis of reported cases from 1987 to 1995 showed Staphylococcus, Salmonella, and Escherichia coli to be the most common organisms cultured.[31] The majority, approximately 70%, of bacterial abscesses will appear as a solitary fluid filled mass.[28,35] Patients with multiple abscesses will often have underlying immunosuppression as a result of malignancies, corticosteroid use, AIDS, cirrhosis, alcoholism, or diabetes mellitus.[28] Most fungal and mycobacterial abscesses will appear as multiple abscesses and so the majority of unilocular abscesses will be bacterial in origin.[36]

On US, lesions are typically internally avascular and may show either low echogenicity or complex internal echoes from debris.[37] A solitary splenic abscess appears as a hypodense (20-40 HU) area on CT with low signal on T1-weighted MR images and intermediate or increased

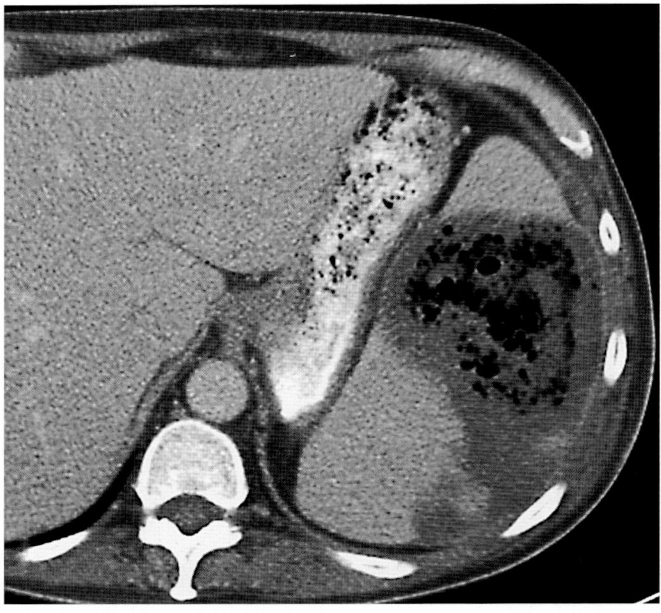

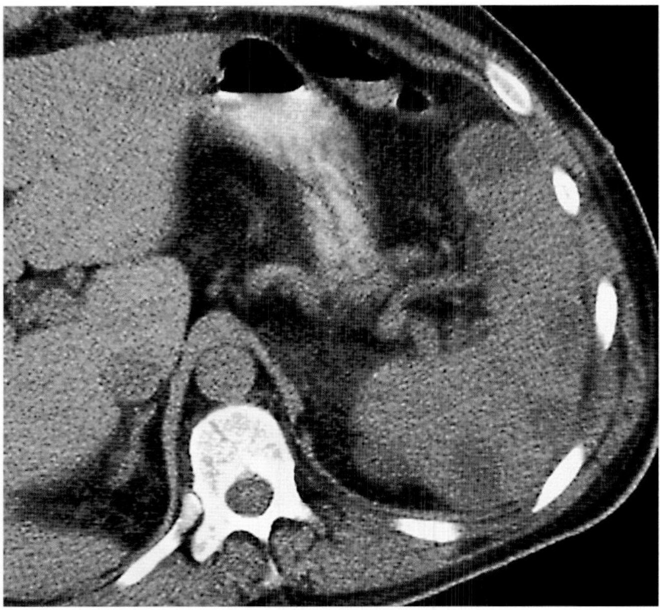

Figure 14-12 Pyogenic Splenic Abscesses in 2 Patients
A. This 63-year-old man with non-Hodgkin lymphoma developed splenic infarctions (not shown) as a result of splenomegaly. One month later, he developed fevers and *Clostridium septicum* septicemia. Contrast-enhanced CT shows a large low-attenuation mass with multiple small bubbles of gas indicating development of a pyogenic splenic abscess complicating splenic infarction. **B.** The second patient is a 42-year-old man with *Staphylococcus aureus* endocarditis. CT of the spleen without contrasts shows multiple hypoattenuating masses in the spleen indicating septic emboli.

signal on T2-weighted images. The margins may be smooth or irregular.[37] Gas is infrequently seen within the abscess. Following IV contrast administration, peripheral enhancement may be seen (see Figure 14-12).[36]

Amebic abscess: Amebic abscesses of the spleen are rare but have been reported to represent between 0% and 12% of splenic abscesses.[28-31,34] Their appearance is indistinguishable from the more common bacterial abscess.

Echinococcal infection of the spleen: Although rare in the United States, echinococcal cysts historically have been the most common non-neoplastic cause worldwide for a cystic lesion in spleen.[38] *Echinococcus* has a complex life cycle that requires development within both a canine animal, usually the dog, and a herd animal, usually a sheep. Humans are accidental hosts and become infected with the organism through contact with canine feces, usually in the form of contaminated, raw vegetables.

Echinococcal infection results in the formation of complex cysts in a variety of organs, most commonly the liver and lung. Splenic involvement with *Echinococcus granulosa* is unusual, occurring in only between 1% and 3% of echinococcal infections.[39] Isolated splenic involvement is very uncommon.[40]

Echinococcal cysts have 3 layers: an outer layer, or pericyst; a middle laminated membrane; and an inner germinal membrane.[41] The pericyst represents the response of the host to the parasite and consists of modified host cells, fibroblasts, giant cells, and eosinophils, which create a few-millimeter-thick, rigid protective layer. The middle laminated membrane is a fibrous 2-mm, acellular structure that permits the passage of nutrients but is impervious to bacteria. Disruption of the laminated membrane predisposes to dissemination of the infection within the host. Outpouchings of the thin translucent inner germinal membrane, also called the brood capsule, produce scolices, the infectious embryonic tapeworms. Freed scolices together with brood capsules form a granular, sometimes calcified, material called hydatid sand that settles in the dependent part of the cyst. The clear cyst fluid is a transudate of serum, containing echinococcal proteins. This fluid is highly antigenic and, if released into the circulation of the host, can cause eosinophilia or anaphylaxis.[41]

Hydatid cysts are usually solitary. The cysts can be unilocular, in which case they are indistinguishable from other cysts, or they can contain multiple internal "daughter cysts," a finding that is pathognomonic for echinococcal infection.[41] Many cysts will demonstrate partial or complete rim calcification. Some cysts will develop fine psammomatous calcifications within the fluid of the cyst, a finding that represents hydatid sand. In some cases, the membranes of the cyst can collapse and float centrally within the fluid-filled exocyst. This appearance is essentially diagnostic of echinococcal cysts. Most of the various findings of echinococcal cysts can be demonstrated by US, CT, and MRI.

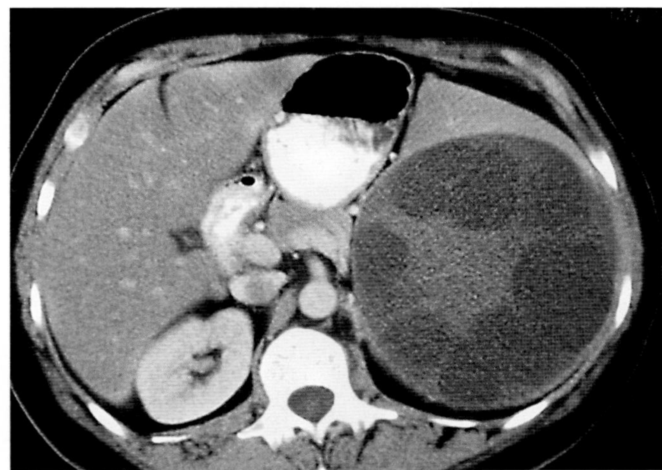

Figure 14-13 Echinococcal Cyst of the Spleen
This 38-year-old woman had emigrated from Uzbekistan. She had a family history of polycystic kidney disease. Contrast-enhanced CT scan shows the characteristic cyst within cyst appearance of echinococcal infection.

In most cases, plain films of the abdomen and chest will fail to detect echinococcal cysts of the spleen. In some cases, radiographs of the abdomen will show a soft-tissue mass in the left upper quadrant of the abdomen displacing the stomach, left kidney, and/or splenic flexure of the colon. Rarely, rim calcification of the cyst will indicate the cystic nature of the left upper quadrant mass. Chest radiograph can demonstrate an elevated left hemidiaphragm or pleural effusion in some cases.[42]

Various sonographic patterns of hydatid cysts have been described. A simple anechoic cyst is observed most often—a nonspecific finding with the differential diagnosis of all causes of splenic cysts.[43] Presence of collapsed membranes within a cystic lesion is pathognomonic for hydatid disease.[44] Demonstration of daughter cysts is also diagnostic of echinococcal infection.

Echinococcal cysts appear as well-circumscribed, low-density lesions on CT.[41] Lesions are often large and can be unilocular or contain daughter cysts distributed either peripherally or throughout the lesion (see Figure 14-13).[41] The multiple cysts within larger cysts are diagnostic of hydatid disease and in most cases are easily distinguished from loculated cysts. The daughter cysts appear as perfect spheres within the larger cyst, rather than multiple septations as are seen in multiloculated cysts. In most cases, the daughter cysts are slightly less dense on CT relative to fluid in the parent cyst.[41] A "serpent" or "snake" sign is occasionally noted, representing collapsed parasitic membranes within the cyst.[41] Cyst wall calcification is noted commonly, and when extensive, suggests that the cyst is dead. Rarely, small calcified granules can be found in the dependent portions of the cysts and represent hydatid sand. Typically, no enhancement is noted following IV contrast administration.

MRI is capable of adequately demonstrating all features of hydatid disease with the exception of calcifications. On MRI, the cysts are hyperintense on T2-weighted images and hypointense on T1-weighted images.[45] Daughter cysts are typically hypointense on T1-weighted images relative to fluid in the parent cyst.[45] A continuous low-intensity rim surrounding the cyst corresponding to the dense fibrous capsule encasing the parasitic membranes is frequently seen.[46]

Splenic trauma

Splenic trauma can result in a variety of focal lesions, including lacerations, hematomas, and vascular injuries resulting in pseudoaneurysms or active bleeding. Splenic trauma is discussed in detail under the heading **Nonspherical Focal Lesions of the Spleen.** However, splenic hematomas can appear as a cystic mass in the spleen and, in some cases, will leave a posttraumatic cyst and will be discussed briefly here.

Hematoma: Hematomas are among the most common causes of a cystic mass in the spleen. Subcapsular hematomas are more common than intraparenchymal hematomas and will appear lenticular or crescentic shaped adjacent to the capsule of the spleen. These are discussed in detail in a subsequent section of this chapter titled: **Nonspherical Focal Lesions of the Spleen**.

Intraparenchymal hematomas will appear as round, oval, or irregularly shaped lesions within the substance of the spleen. In the early phases, the margins will often be indistinct and the contents of the hematoma will appear hyperattenuating to nonenhanced spleen on CT, will have multiple internal echoes on US, and will appear hyperintense on T1- and T2-weighted MRI sequences. As the hematoma ages, it will become progressively more sharply marginated with the splenic parenchyma and the contents will become progressively more simple-appearing: water attenuation on CT, anechoic on US, and hypointense on T1 to hyperintense on T2 MRI sequences (see Figure 14-14).

Posttraumatic and postinfarction cysts: Traumatic and ischemic damage to the spleen can evolve into a cyst that will remain for the lifetime of the individual. These posttraumatic and postinfarction cysts are the most common cyst of the spleen accounting for approximately 80% of splenic cysts.[47,48] In some cases, the wall of these cysts will become calcified (see Figure 14-15).

Other causes of cystic nodules and masses

The remaining causes of solitary cystic lesions of the spleen are epidermoid cysts and pancreatic pseudocysts.

Epidermoid cysts: Epidermoid or mesothelial cysts are uncommon congenital lesions of the spleen. They constitute less than 10% of nonparasitic splenic cysts and were incidentally found in 32 of 42 327 autopsies at 1 institution.[49]

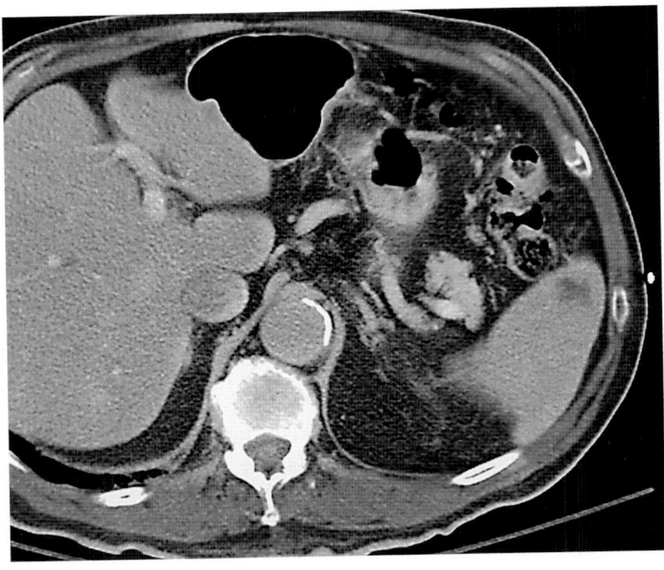

A

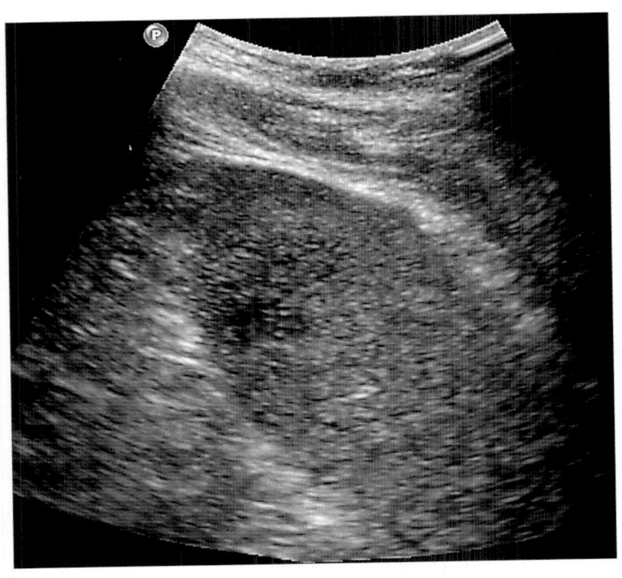

B

Figure 14-14 Small Intrasplenic Hematoma
This 86-year-old woman was in a motor vehicle accident. **A.** Enhanced CT scan demonstrates an irregularly shaped hypoechoic mass in the spleen. This could represent a small intrasplenic hematoma or an incidentally discovered hemangioma. **B.** US examination shows the lesion to be hypoechoic, a finding consistent with a small hematoma and not a hemangioma that would be echogenic.

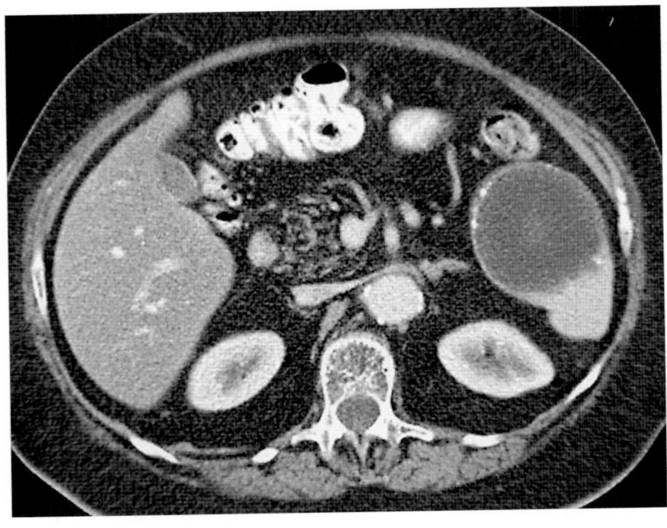

A

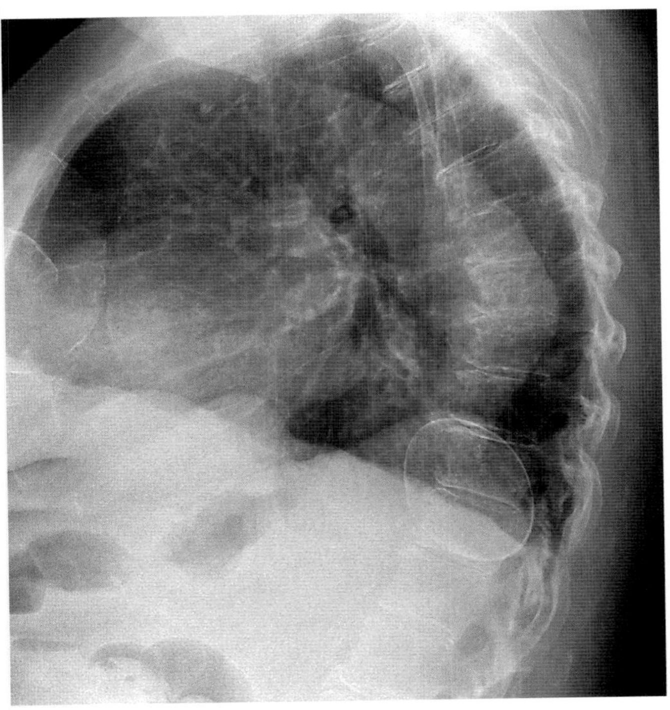

B

Figure 14-15 Postinfarction Splenic Cyst
This 74-year-old woman had a history of non-Hodgkin lymphoma many years previously. **A.** The current examination shows a 3.5-cm cystic mass in the anterior aspect of the spleen with multiple small punctate rim calcifications seen as high attenuation foci in the rim of the cyst. It is likely that this woman had lymphoma-related splenomegaly and this cyst formed from a splenic hematoma caused by infarction or trauma to the enlarged spleen. **B.** As a result of the rim calcification, the cyst could be seen on the lateral view of this patient's chest radiograph.

These are true cysts with a fibrous wall and stratified squamous epithelium filled with serous fluid.[50] They appear as simple cysts on all cross-sectional imaging.

Pancreatic pseudocyst: Rarely, pancreatic pseudocysts can dissect along the splenorenal ligament into the splenic parenchyma resulting in an intrasplenic pseudocyst.[51] This will appear as a simple or complex cyst within the substance of the spleen. In most cases, there will be other imaging findings of pancreatitis evident in the pancreas and peripancreatic tissues.

Solid-Appearing Nodules and Masses of the Spleen

All solitary solid-appearing nodules and masses of the spleen are neoplasms. They are most often due to lymphoma or metastasis but can occasionally be due to several other benign or malignant neoplasms of the spleen (Table 14-2).

Lymphoma

The combination of Hodgkin disease and non-Hodgkin lymphoma is the most common malignancy affecting the spleen.[52] Isolated or primary splenic involvement occurs in 1% to 2% of all lymphomas, the majority of which will represent Hodgkin disease.[53] Lymphoma of the spleen can have a variety of imaging appearances, most commonly as splenomegaly. However, lymphoma can also appear as solitary or multiple round or oval lesions in the spleen. These lesions can have a miliary appearance or appear as larger nodular lesions (see Figure 14-16).

Metastasis

Although metastases to the spleen are uncommon, they represent 1 of the most common causes of solitary and multiple solid nodules in the spleen. When splenic metastases are present, multiple other metastatic sites such as lymph nodes, liver, and lungs are usually present.[54] Common primary cancers that metastasize to the spleen include breast, lung, melanoma, ovary, stomach, pancreas, liver, and colon cancer. Splenic metastatic lesions may be solitary or multiple in number and can range from a few millimeters to several centimeters in diameter (see Figure 14-17). Splenic metastases are discussed most completely under the heading **Multifocal Splenic Lesions** later in this text.

Table 14-2. Solitary Solid-Appearing Splenic Nodules or Masses

1. **Lymphoma**[a]
2. **Metastasis**
3. **Hemangioma**
4. Angiosarcoma
5. Hamartoma
6. Inflammatory pseudotumor

[a]Disorders in bold are most common.

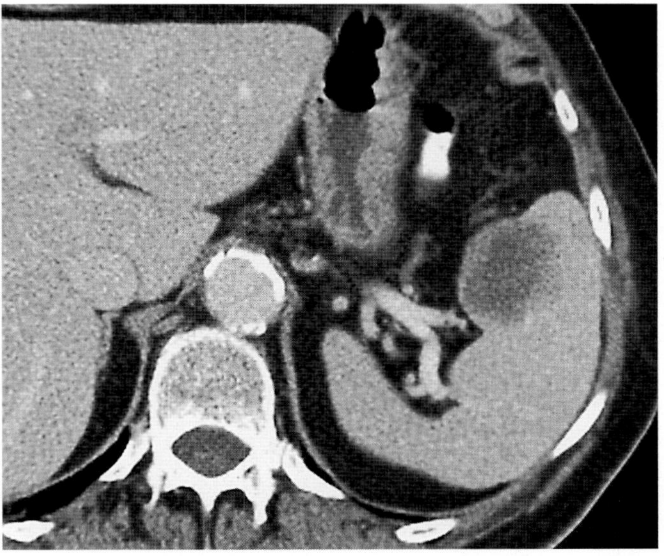

Figure 14-16 Lymphoma Appearing as a Solitary Splenic Mass This 73-year-old woman had right upper quadrant pain when this unsuspected mass in the spleen was discovered. Follow-up examinations showed progression of the mass and development of new abdominal adenopathy. Lymph node biopsy was diagnostic of non-Hodgkin lymphoma.

Hemangioma

Hemangiomas are composed of tangles of blood vessels ranging from small capillaries to large venules. Because the majority of the mass of a hemangioma represents blood coursing through the lesion, most hemangiomas will appear as a small round or oval lesion mimicking a simple cyst on MRI and CT examinations, appearing low attenuation on CT and low signal on T1-weighted sequences and very high signal on T2-weighted MRI sequences. However, some hemangiomas can have a solid appearance on CT, US, and MRI imaging because they will show homogenous or heterogenous enhancement on CT and MRI examinations (see Figure 14-10). On US examinations, the multiple vascular walls of the hemangioma make them uniformly echogenic and are therefore rarely confused with cystic lesions (see Figure 14-7). Hemangiomas are discussed in detail in the previous section titled: **Cystic-Appearing Nodules and Masses of the Spleen**.

Angiosarcoma

Splenic angiosarcomas are rare highly aggressive lesions with nearly 80% of patients dead at a median interval of 6 months following diagnosis.[55] Metastases are frequently present at diagnosis. The most common symptoms of

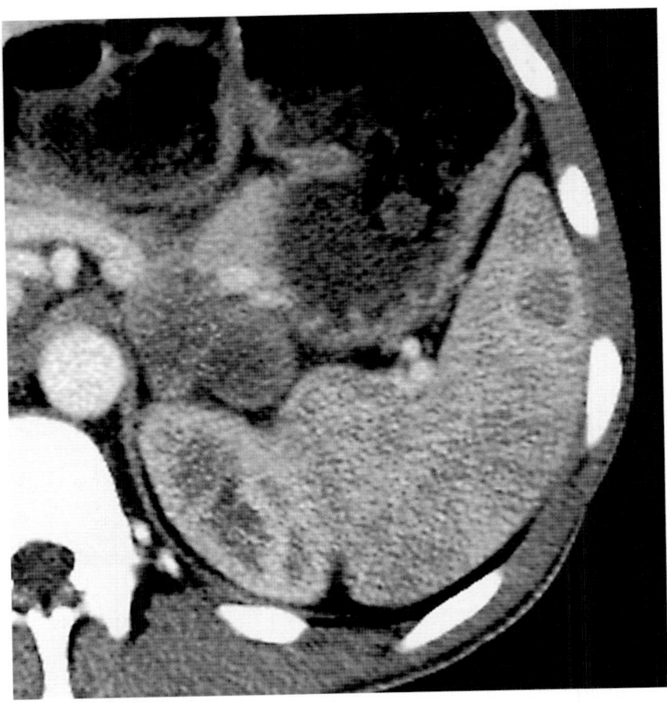

A

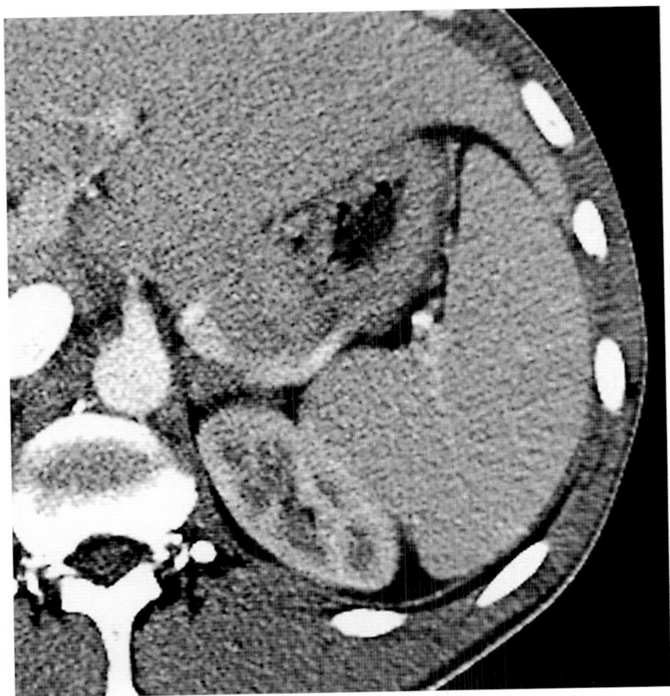

B

Figure 14-17 Solitary Splenic Metastasis from Lung Cancer This 49-year-old man had lung cancer. **A.** Image from a contrast-enhanced CT shows a solitary focal low-attenuation mass in the anterior aspect of the spleen. There is also vague heterogeneity of the remainder of the spleen typical of the early phase of contrast enhancement of the spleen. **B.** CT image from 2 years prior shows no evidence of the mass. These findings are indicative of a splenic metastasis from lung cancer. Also note the enlarged left adrenal gland in (A) indicating an adrenal metastasis.

angiosarcoma are abdominal pain and weight loss. Splenomegaly is common, with splenic rupture also noted.

Splenic angiosarcoma has a heterogeneous appearance on imaging. US may show a large mass with areas of both increased and decreased echogenicity. CT, most commonly, demonstrates an enlarged spleen in which the normal parenchyma is almost entirely replaced by a heterogeneously attenuating mass or masses. Less common is a discrete solitary mass. Lesions range in size considerably and may show areas of necrosis. Areas of increased density may be noted from acute hemorrhage, hemosiderin deposits, or calcification.

At MRI, lesions are heterogeneously hypointense on T1-weighted images and hyperintense on T2-weighted images. Areas of increased T1 signal can also be noted and may correspond to regions of hemorrhage. Enhancement with IV contrast is variable, with lesions showing both hypo- and hyperenhancement relative to normal spleen.[56]

Hamartoma

Splenic hamartomas are rare benign lesions composed of an anomalous mixture of normal splenic red pulp elements and have an incidence at autopsy of 0.024% to 0.13%.[8] They are, in part, distinguished from normal splenic tissue by the absence of organized lymphoid follicles. Splenic hamartomas are usually solitary lesions and can range in size up to 20 cm in diameter.[57] They are discovered incidentally or due to mass-related symptoms.

Typically, a splenic hamartoma appears as a well-circumscribed mass. On US, lesions typically are uniform solid masses, however, rarely they can have a heterogeneous echotexture from cystic regions.[8] Calcification is occasionally noted. On noncontrast CT, the lesions are usually iso- or hypodense relative to spleen and can be missed entirely or only recognized by the contour abnormality produced by the mass (see Figure 14-18).[8] As a consequence, both US and MRI are more sensitive for their detection.[8] On MRI, hamartomas are usually isointense on T1-weighted images and heterogeneously hyperintense on T2-weighted images. A mildly hypointense appearance on T2-weighted imaging has also been reported and may reflect an increased fibrous component.[58]

After IV contrast administration, there is usually diffuse heterogeneous enhancement on both CT and MRI.[9] The diffuse nature of early enhancement may be useful in distinguishing this lesion from the typical peripheral enhancement noted with hemangiomas. On delayed images, persistent hyperenhancement has been noted and may help distinguish hamartoma from lymphoma. Persistent areas of hypodensity or hypointensity may be seen and correspond to areas of necrosis within the lesion.

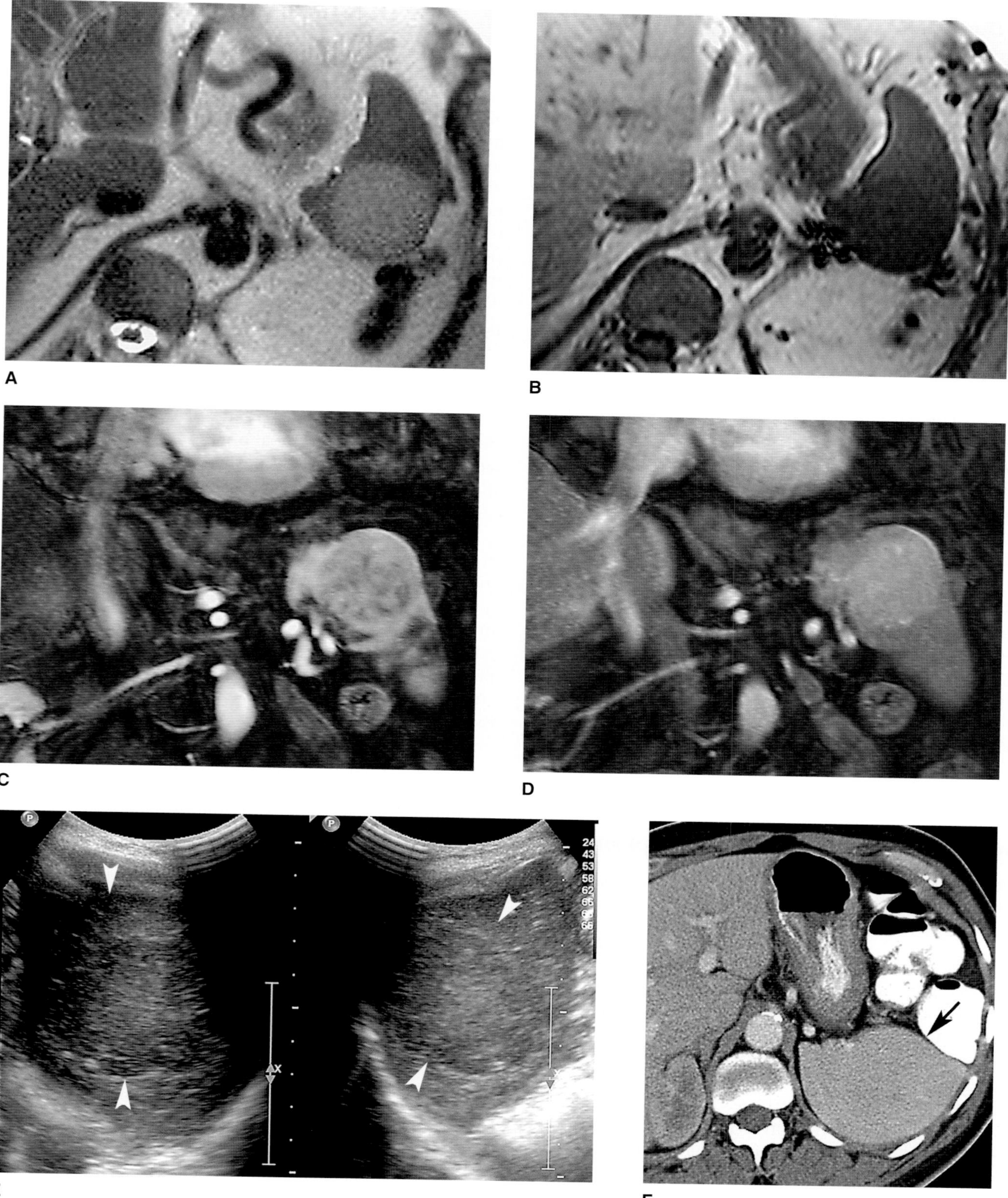

Figure 14-18 Splenic Hamartomas in 2 Patients

A-D. This 69-year-old man had a renal cell carcinoma of the kidney. Contrast-enhanced CT (not shown) of the spleen appeared normal. (A) T2-weighted MRI examination shows a faintly hyperintense smoothly marginated mass in the spleen. (B) T1-weighted image shows the mass to be nearly isointense with spleen. Coronal T1-weighted images in (C) arterial phase and (D) portal venous phase of enhancement shows initial heterogenous enhancement followed by uniform enhancement. These features are essentially diagnostic of a splenic hamartoma. **E** and **F.** Patient 2 is an 80-year-old man who had right upper quadrant pain. (E) US of the spleen in the longitudinal and transverse plane demonstrates a large solid, homogenous mass (*arrowheads*) that is slightly hypoechoic relative to the spleen. (F) On CT scan, the mass is isoattenuating to the spleen and is only recognizable because it deforms the surface of the spleen (*arrow*). MRI showed similar findings to the first patient.

Reticuloendothelial activity, either increased or somewhat decreased relative to normal spleen, has been noted on scintigraphy with either Tc-99m stannous phytate or sulfur colloid or with heat-treated Cr-51-labeled RBCs but is not invariably present. Such activity has also been noted with hemangioma, but when present may help distinguish hamartoma from lymphoma or metastasis where it is generally absent.[59]

Inflammatory pseudotumor

Inflammatory pseudotumor consists of a polymorphous population of inflammatory and spindle cells with varying amounts of granulomatous reaction, fibrosis, and necrosis.[60] Inflammatory pseudotumors are rare, benign, and of uncertain etiology. Patients can be asymptomatic or present with a mass and vague systemic symptoms of fever and malaise. These lesions are more common in adults than children.

Inflammatory pseudotumor typically appears as a well-circumscribed solitary mass that ranges in size from a few centimeters to greater than 12 cm.[61] On noncontrast CT, the lesions are generally heterogeneously hypodense. Peripheral and stippled calcification has been noted.[62] Lesions have been reported as hypoechoic on US.

On T1- and T2-weighted MRI, the lesions have been described as both slightly hypo- as well as slightly hyperintense relative to background spleen. Following IV contrast, mild-to-moderate enhancement has been noted with the lesion remaining hypo- or isodense and intense relative to normal spleen.[63]

Nonspherical Focal Lesions of the Spleen

Posttraumatic lesions and infarction are the 2 most common nonspherical lesions of the spleen.

Trauma

The spleen is the intra-abdominal organ most often injured as a result of blunt trauma, and is the second most commonly injured solid organ in penetrating trauma. The spleen is the most vascular organ in the body, and therefore bleeding from splenic injury is potentially life-threatening. Furthermore, delayed hemorrhage days and weeks after splenic injury is a known complication of splenic injury. When other abdominal injuries are excluded from analysis, the mortality rate for isolated splenic injury is still substantial at approximately 8.3% of patients, and the most severe splenic injury, a completely shattered spleen or one with a hilar vascular injury has a mortality of approximately 17.4%.[64] Since the 1970s, management of splenic injuries has progressively moved from operative to nonoperative management. Between 53% and 77% of patients with blunt splenic injury meet currently accepted criteria for selective nonoperative management.[65-69] Of those managed nonoperatively, 2% to 11% will require subsequent surgical intervention. Management decisions are based on the clinical presentation, especially hemodynamic stability and on the cross-sectional imaging appearance of the splenic injury. Therefore, imaging plays a critical role in management decisions of splenic injuries. Splenic injuries include intraparenchymal and subcapsular hematomas, lacerations, acute bleeding, and vascular injuries.

Focused assessment with sonography for trauma (FAST) is a quick and noninvasive method used by the majority of level 1 trauma centers in the United States for detecting intraperitoneal blood as a marker of blunt intraperitoneal injury.[70] Four areas are surveyed for the presence of blood: the pericardial cavity, right upper quadrant, left upper quadrant, and pelvis. Studies have shown that US can detect as little as 100 mL of fluid in the most dependent areas of the peritoneal cavity.[71] However, a high number of significant abdominal organ injuries occur without associated hemoperitoneum, and US detection of these injuries has been inconsistent such that other diagnostic tests are often necessary.[72-74]

The availability of multidetector-row CT (MDCT) at most trauma centers in the United States has led to increased detection and diagnostic accuracy in splenic injury. In general, MDCT is the imaging modality of choice in the patient who is hemodynamically stable. It is important to image for splenic injury during the portal venous phase of enhancement.[75] Theoretically, MRI would have similar diagnostic accuracy; however, its use is impractical in most settings.

Since the early 1980s, angiography with splenic artery embolization has been used as an adjunct to increase the number of patients managed nonoperatively.[76] Multiple techniques can be used, including proximal main splenic artery embolization, selective distal embolization, and a combination of these techniques.[76] No significant differences in outcomes or complication rates have been reported between proximal and distal splenic artery embolization.[77] Indications for splenic arteriography reported in the literature include CT evidence of active bleeding, vascular injury, high-grade injury, and large-volume hemoperitoneum.[78] However, 1 cohort study of 154 patients comparing splenic artery embolization with splenectomy demonstrated a significantly higher incidence of ARDS in the embolization group and demonstrated a 22% failure rate of nonoperative management requiring subsequent surgery and questioned the use of splenic artery embolization.[17]

Grading system for splenic trauma: The American Association for the Surgery of Trauma has developed a detailed organ injury scaling (OIS) system for the evaluation of blunt organ injuries (Table 14-3). This is based on the most accurate assessment of the injury at imaging examinations, laparotomy, or autopsy. Grade I injuries are small subcapsular hematomas or small lacerations. Grade II lesions represent intermediate subcapsular and small intraparenchymal hematomas and intermediate lacerations. Grade III lesions are large subcapsular

Table 14-3. American Association for the Surgery of Trauma Splenic Injury Scale

Grade	Injury Type	Description of Injury
I	Hematoma subcapsular Laceration	Surface area < 10% < 1 cm
II	Hematoma subcapsular Hematoma intraparenchymal Laceration	Surface area 10% to 50% ≤5 cm 1-3 cm, trabecular vessel not involved
III	Hematoma subcapsular Hematoma intraparenchymal Hematoma ruptured Laceration	Surface area > 50% or expanding > 5 cm or expanding Either subcapsular or intraparenchymal Depth > 3 or involving trabecular vessels
IV	Laceration	Involving segmental or hilar vessels or producing devascularization > 25% of spleen
V	Hematoma Laceration	Completely shattered spleen Hilar vascular injury devascularizes spleen

Note: Organ injury scale (OIS) for the spleen, based on the most accurate assessment at autopsy, laparotomy, or radiologic study (1994 revision)[198]
Source: American Heart Association.

or intraparenchymal hematomas or large lacerations. Grade IV lesions are lacerations that produce infarction of greater than 25% of the spleen. Grade V lesions represent either a completely shattered spleen or one that is completely infarcted. In a review of 1 130 093 patients, there was a statistically significant increase in mortality between grade II-III and grade IV-V injuries of 14.1% and 29.3%.[64] Mortality rates for patients with isolated splenic injury are listed in Table 14-4. Thus, the primary determinant of mortality is related to significant vascular injury to the spleen. This vascular injury is predicted by 3 imaging findings: (1) evidence of active extravasation of contrast on venous phase imaging, (2) laceration involving the splenic hilum and causing significant infarction of the spleen, and (3) evidence of hemoperitoneum.[79]

Laceration: A laceration represents a focal linear defect in the surface of the spleen. The OIS grading system differentiates between small (<1 cm), intermediate (1-3 cm), and large (>3 cm) lacerations and whether the laceration involves the trabecular vessels in the splenic hilum. Of these features, only vascular involvement has been shown to be a significant predictor of increased risk of mortality.[64] In particular, vascular injuries that lead to infarction of greater than 25% of the spleen have an increased risk of mortality. Therefore, evaluation for the presence of associated infarction is an important feature that should be evaluated by imaging (see Figure 14-19).

Lacerations of the spleen can be difficult to identify on unenhanced CT scans but can appear as linear or branching areas of low attenuation with sharply defined margins. Following contrast enhancement, the nonenhancing laceration will typically become more distinct from the enhancing splenic parenchyma (see Figure 14-20). With time, lacerations decrease in size and number, margins become less well defined, and the area becomes isodense to normal splenic parenchyma. On US examinations, a laceration will appear as a linear or branching hypoechoic defect in the splenic parenchyma.

Imaging Notes 14-2. Imaging Features That Predict Need for Surgical or Angiographic Intervention in Splenic Trauma

1. Active extravasation of contrast
2. Splenic laceration causing infarction of >25% to 50% of the spleen
3. Shattered spleen
4. Hemorrhagic acites associated with splenic injury

Table 14-4. Mortality Rates for Splenic Injury by Grade[a]

Grade	Mortality with Other Injuries	Mortality Isolated Injury
I-II	9.9%	6.9%
III	10.4%	7.1%
IV	14.1%	9.4%
V	29.8%	22.7%

[a]Data from Tinkoff G, Esposito TJ, Reed J, et al. American Association for the Surgery of Trauma Organ Injury Scale I: Spleen, Liver, and Kidney, validation based on the National Trauma Data Bank. *J Am Coll Surg* 2008;207(5):646-655.

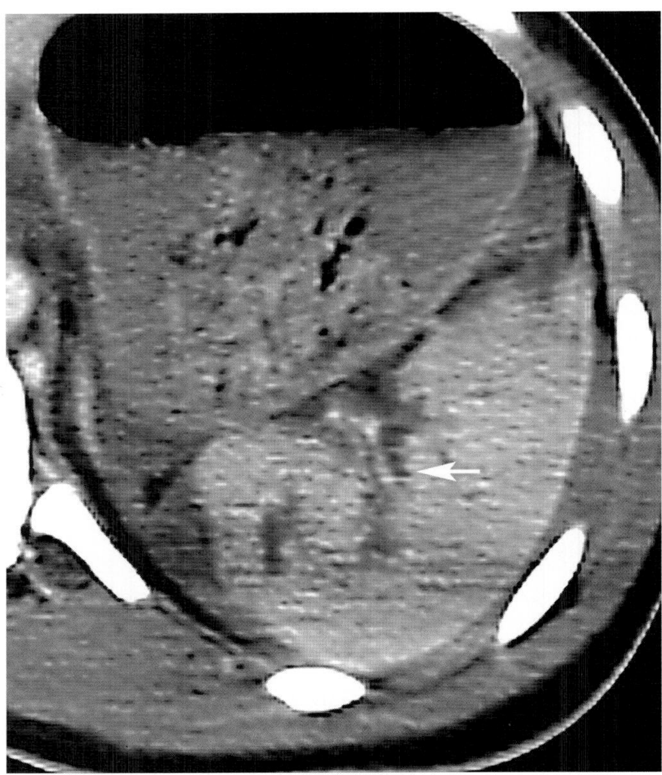

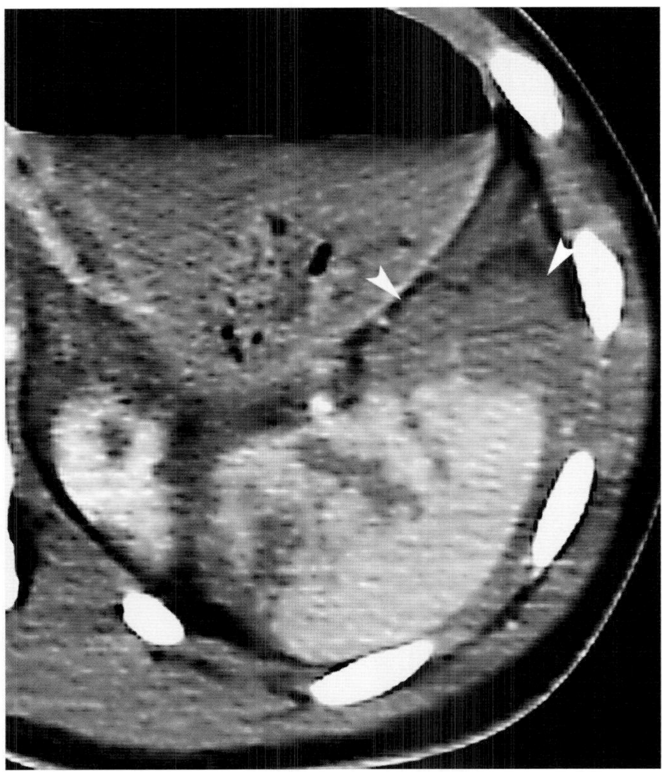

Figure 14-19 Splenic Laceration with Associated Infarction This 17-year-old woman was an unrestrained passenger in an automobile accident. **A** and **B.** Contrast-enhanced CT shows multiple linear and branching defects (*arrow*) in the spleen typical of lacerations. These extend into the hilum of the spleen and cause infarction of the anterior portion (*arrowheads*) of the spleen in (B). Involvement of hilar vessels and infarction of greater than 25% of the spleen are both associated with increased mortality.

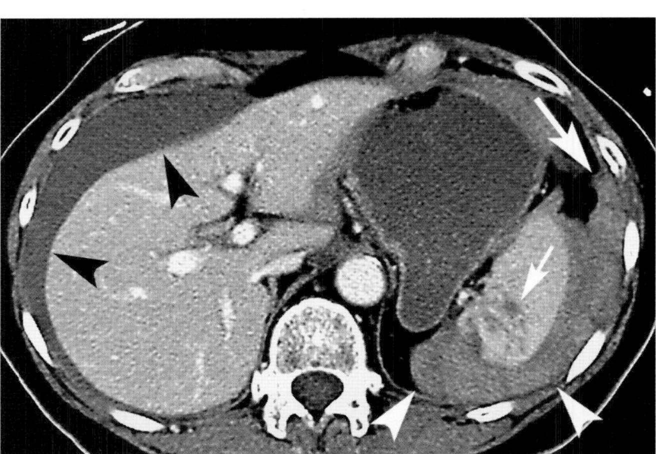

Figure 14-20 Splenic Laceration with Subcapsular Hematoma This 67-year-old woman was in an automobile accident. Contrast-enhanced CT shows multiple linear defects (*small arrow*) in the spleen characteristic of lacerations. There is also a crescentic hypoattenuating region surrounding the spleen (*white arrowheads*) typical of a subcapsular hematoma. Compare the attenuation of the subcapsular hematoma with the ascites surrounding the liver (*black arrowheads*). Note that the acute hematoma has a higher attenuation than the simple fluid surrounding the liver.

Intraparenchymal and subcapsular hematoma: Splenic hematoma represents a focal collection of blood within the spleen. These are most often subcapsular in location but can less commonly be found within the spleen parenchyma. Although the OIS grading system distinguishes among small, medium, and large subcapsular hematomas and small and large intraparenchymal hematomas, the presence of a hematoma of any size or location without active extravasation of contrast will not alter the management of the patient with the exception of a completely shattered spleen (see Figure 14-21).[64]

On unenhanced CT, acute subcapsular hematomas are typically hyperdense compared with adjacent normal parenchyma (see Figure 14-20). After contrast administration, subcapsular hematomas are seen as low-attenuation collections between the splenic capsule and enhancing splenic parenchyma. The subcapsular hematoma will compress the underlying splenic parenchyma. With time, the attenuation of the hematoma will decrease and will appear hypoattenuating relative to unenhanced spleen. Intraparenchymal hematomas appear as irregular high- or low-attenuation areas within the spleen parenchyma. In some individuals, a splenic hematoma will persist as a simple cyst for years later. How commonly this occurs is not known.

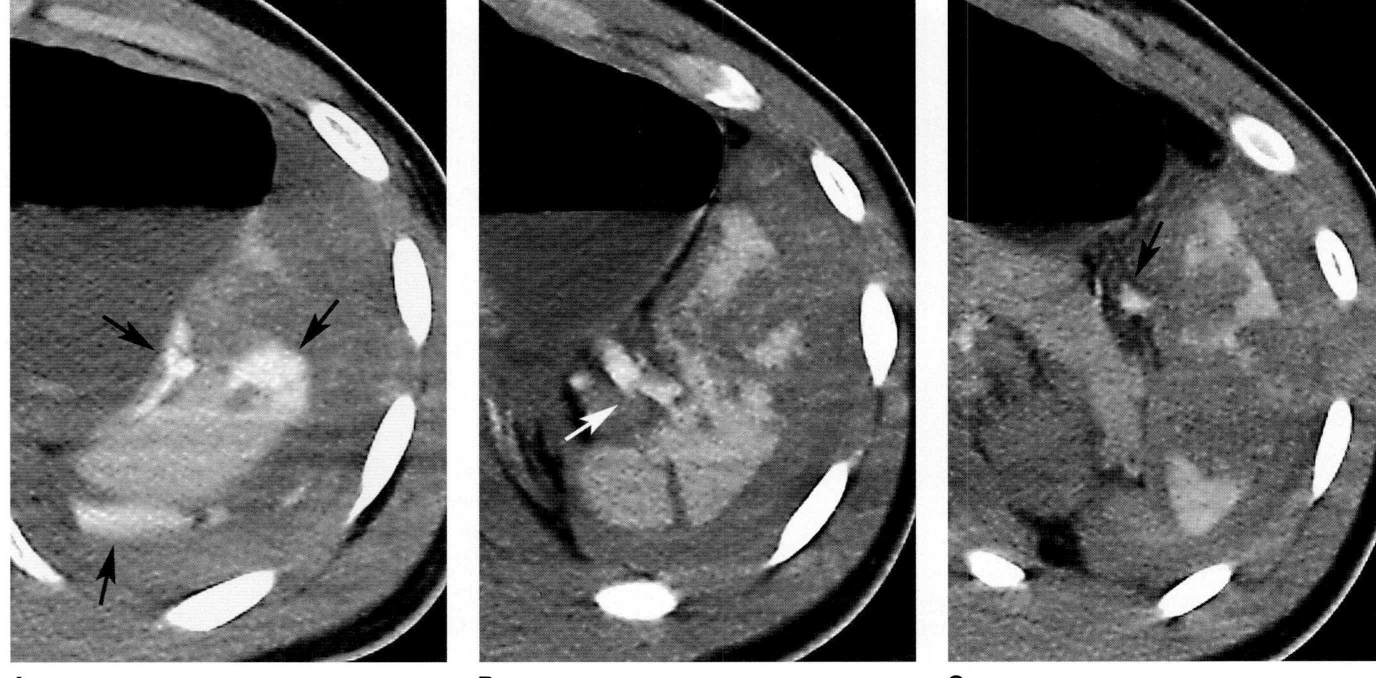

Figure 14-21 Shattered Spleen
This 23-year-old man was involved in a motor vehicle accident. **A-C.** Contrast-enhanced CT demonstrates a fragmented spleen with disruption of a major vessel in the hilum (*white arrow*) and active extravasation of contrast (*black arrows*). There is also extensive subcapsular and retroperitoneal hematoma surrounding the spleen. Active extravasation is a surgical emergency to prevent exsanguination.

Subcapsular hematomas on US examinations will typically appear as a crescentic hypoechoic structure with through transmission, adjacent to the surface of the spleen. In most cases, the hematoma will contain the low-level echoes typical of hematomas in any location (see Figure 14-20). Intraparenchymal hematomas will typically appear as complex irregularly shaped cystic lesions within the spleen parenchyma. Internal echoes due to blood products will usually be present.

Vascular injuries: Posttraumatic splenic vascular injuries include active bleeding, acute pseudoaneurysms, and arteriovenous fistulae. These, especially active bleeding, are the most clinically significant findings associated with splenic trauma. The hypotension and/or the presence of active bleeding as demonstrated by contrast-enhanced CT are the most common indications for surgical or angiographic intervention of patients with splenic injuries.[17,64-69]

Active bleeding: Active bleeding is the most significant imaging finding of splenic injury. This finding has been used as the primary feature identifying surgical or angiographic intervention of splenic injuries.[17,65-69] It is identified by the extravasation of IV contrast during enhanced CT scanning. This is seen as a nodular, irregular, or linear area of contrast material extravasation into the splenic parenchyma or perisplenic tissues (see Figure 14-21). The attenuation of the extravasated contrast material (85-350 HU) will be significantly higher than that of clotted blood (40-70 HU).[80] On delayed imaging, the area of active extravasation remains high in attenuation and increases in size.

Splenic pseudoaneurysm and arteriovenous fistula: These lesions have a similar appearance on CT examinations and can be differentiated only on splenic angiography. On enhanced CT examinations, both types of vascular lesions appear as well-circumscribed focal nodular areas of increased attenuation in the region of the splenic hilum. They are often surrounded by indistinctly marginated low-attenuation rims of inflammatory tissue (see Figure 14-22).

A pseudoaneurysm is formed by an incomplete tear of the arterial wall. The defect in the intima and possibly media results in a weakening of the tensile strength of the vascular wall. The vessel then dilates in response to the arterial pressure, resulting in a pseudoaneurysm. The weakened wall is predisposed to rupture of the wall and subsequent high-volume extravasation of blood that can lead to hypotension, hypovolemia, and shock.

Splenic arteriovenous fistulae develop as a result of injury to both the artery and the adjacent vein, resulting in a direct communication. On diagnostic angiography, arteriovenous fistulae can be differentiated from pseudoaneurysms by the characteristic early filling of veins.

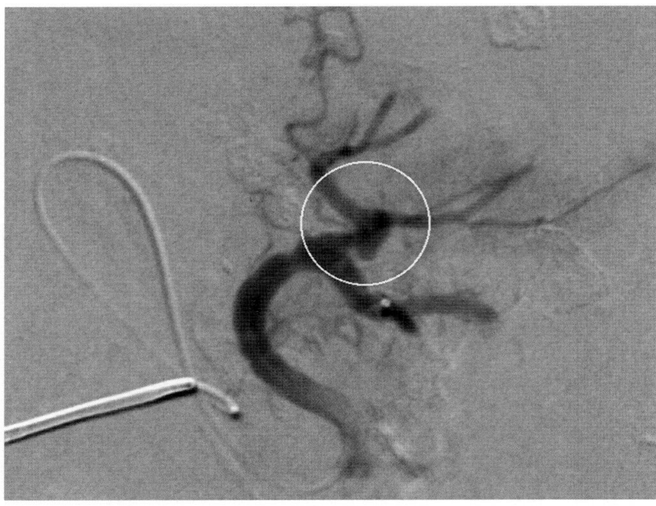

Figure 14-22 Splenic Artery Pseudoaneurysm
This 70-year-old woman was involved in a motor vehicle accident and had evidence of deep splenic lacerations on a CT scan (not shown). Selective digital subtraction angiogram of the splenic artery demonstrates a small focal nodular area of contrast (*circle*) typical of a posttraumatic pseudoaneurysm.

Infarction

Splenic infarction is caused by occlusion of the splenic artery (global) or one of its branches (segmental). Splenic-portal-mesenteric venous thrombosis may also cause splenic infarcts because of venous stasis and resultant ischemia. There are numerous causes of splenic infarcts, which are summarized in Table 14-5.[81] Generally, however, the etiology varies with age. In older patients, an embolic event is the most frequent cause, whereas in patients younger than age 40 years, the etiology is most often an underlying hematologic disorder.[82]

Table 14-5. Etiologies of Splenic Infarction

Etiologies
1. Hematological disorders
Sickle cell disease
Lymphoma
Leukemia
Myelofibrosis
Gaucher disease
2. Thromboembolic disorders
Embolism
Atherosclerosis
Pancreatic disease with vascular involvement
Splenic artery aneurysm
Vasculitis
Hypercoagulable state
3. Mechanical disorders
Splenic torsion
Wandering spleen
Portal hypertension

On US examinations, acute splenic infarcts classically appear as wedge-shaped, hypoechoic, and well-demarcated lesions, with absent flow in the infarcted area on color Doppler.[83] This appearance is diagnostic of a splenic infarction. However, the presence of coexisting edema, bleeding, or necrosis can lead to different sonographic appearances, including round or irregular-shaped lesions that can be confused with other focal lesions of the spleen. As they age, infarcts become progressively hyperechoic due to fibrosis and scarring (see Figure 14-23). If large areas of the spleen become infracted, the volume decreases, resulting in a small irregularly-surfaced spleen.

On noncontrast CT, infarcts can be poorly visualized because of the small attenuation difference between viable and infarcted spleen. Hemorrhagic infarcts can be more easily detected on unenhanced examinations because of the presence of scattered areas of increased attenuation representing acute blood.[84] After contrast administration, infarcted areas become more distinct, usually appearing as peripheral, wedge-shaped, sharply marginated defects (see Figures 14-23 and 14-24). This classic appearance, however, is present in less than half of all acute splenic segmental infarcts.[83] Many splenic infarctions will appear as round or irregular hypoattenuating regions within the spleen that can be difficult to differentiate from other splenic lesions such as tumors, hematomas, or abscesses.

Global splenic infarction will show complete nonenhancement of the spleen with or without a "cortical rim sign." The "cortical rim sign" consists of a thin layer of peripheral enhancement, representing residual capsular flow surrounding the nonenhancing splenic parenchyma (see Figure 14-25).

In the chronic phase, infarcts may disappear completely or, more commonly, will appear as small, peripheral, linear, or wedge-shaped areas of low attenuation in the splenic parenchyma. In many cases, there will also be a focal contour deformity of the peripheral surface of the spleen because of retraction of the fibrous tissue in the splenic scar (see Figure 14-26). When large regions of the spleen have been infarcted, the overall volume of the spleen will decrease. In some instances, there can be calcifications from repeated infarctions. This is especially common in infarctions related to hemoglobinopathies. The end-stage appearance of a globally infarcted spleen is a very small and calcified lenticular or sickle-shaped structure beneath the left hemidiaphragm. This phenomenon is often called an "autosplenectomy." Autosplenectomy is most commonly a manifestation of sickle cell disease (see Figure 14-27).

On MRI, the signal intensity of the infarct depends on its age, the degree of hemorrhagic necrosis, and the amount of different blood products within the infarcted area.[85] Recent hemorrhagic areas are increased in T1 signal intensity. Chronic infarcts are decreased in signal intensity on all pulse sequences. After gadolinium administration, most infarcts appear as wedge-shaped perfusion defects.[85]

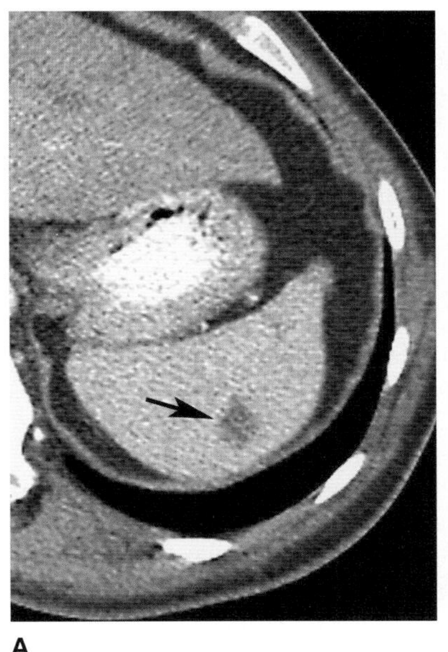

A

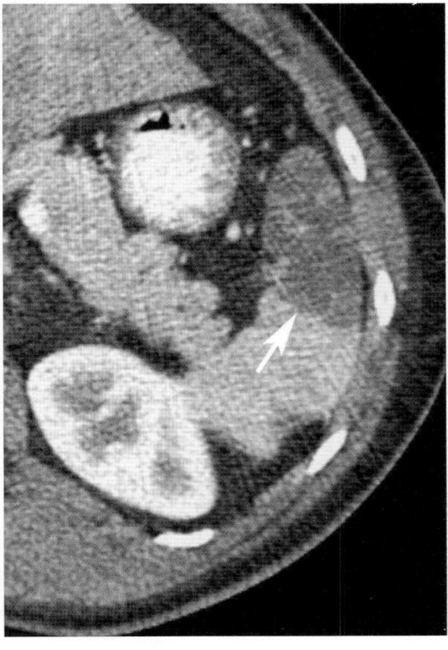

B

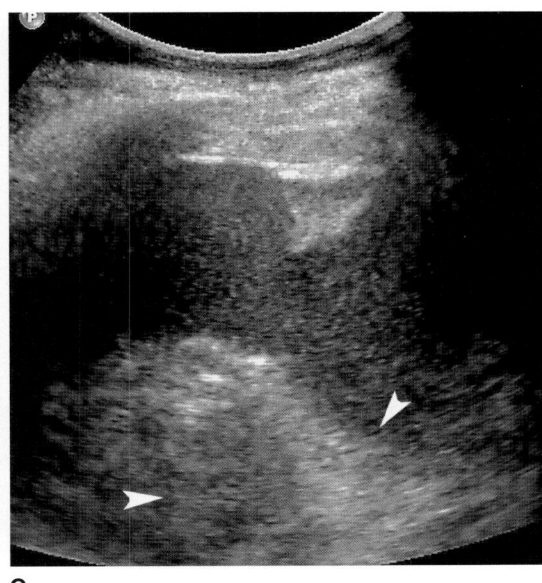

C

Figure 14-23 Splenic Infarction Due to Emboli
This 26-year-old man had a complex congenital heart disease. **A** and **B**. Contrast-enhanced CT of the spleen shows a focal wedge-shaped hypoattenuating region in the midspleen (*black arrow*) and a second larger infarction of the inferior aspect of the spleen (*white arrow*). These infarcts were a result of thromboemboli from intracardiac thrombi because of slow flow in a dilated chamber. **C**. Transverse US 1 year later shows a focal wedge-shaped hyperechoic lesion (*arrowheads*) in the midbody of the spleen, characteristic of a chronic infarct.

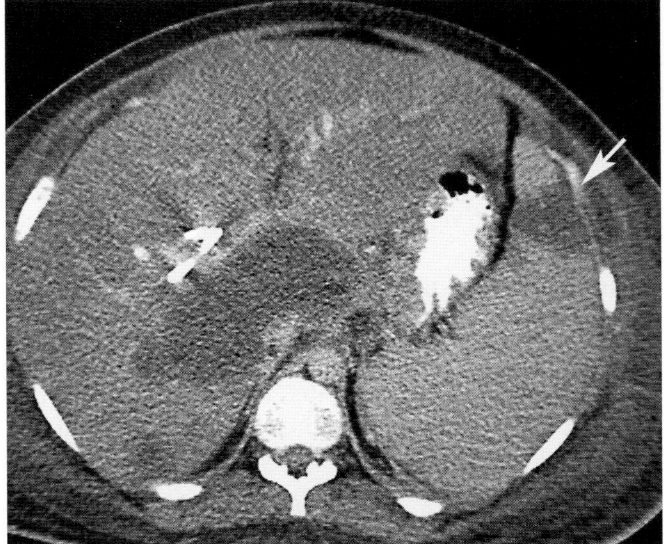

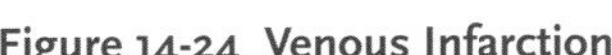

A

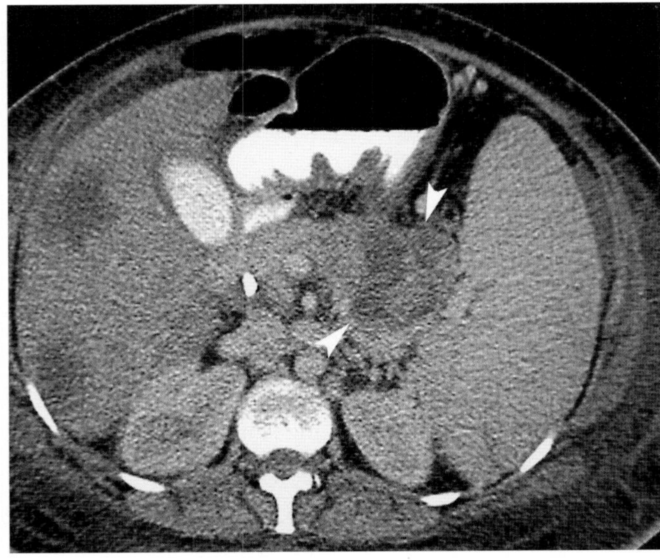

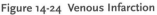

B

Figure 14-24 Venous Infarction
A and **B**. Enhanced CT images through the upper abdomen demonstrate a large mass in the tail of the pancreas (*arrowheads*) that causes occlusion of the splenic vein by direct invasion. The spleen is diffusely enlarged because of the venous obstruction and has a small wedge-shaped area of hypodensity (*arrow*), characteristic of an infarction. In this case, the infarction is probably a result of the venous hypertension. The examination also shows multiple irregularly marginated hepatic lesions representing liver metastasis.

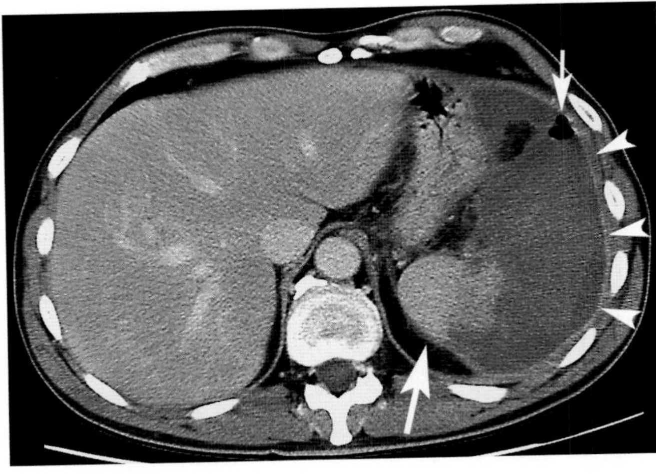

Figure 14-25 The Cortical Rim Sign of Infarction with Secondary Pyogenic Abscess
This 54-year-old man recently underwent a distal pancreatectomy and now has persistent fevers. Enhanced CT shows the majority of the spleen to be mixed fluid attenuation representing a large region of infarction with only a small amount of residual normal splenic tissue (*large arrow*). Note the enhancing splenic capsule (*arrowheads*) surrounding the infarcted spleen, the "cortical rim sign." There is also a small dot of gas (*small arrow*) indicating secondary bacterial abscess.

MULTIFOCAL SPLENIC LESIONS

Multifocal splenic lesions can be due to malignant and benign tumors, hematogenous infections, sarcoidosis, and the rare disorder peliosis (Table 14-6).

Multifocal Neoplasms

Multifocal splenic masses will most often be due to lymphoma or hematogenous metastasis to the spleen. However, rarely they can be due to multiple hemangiomas, lymphangiomas, or littoral angiomas.

Lymphoma

The combination of Hodgkin disease and non-Hodgkin lymphoma is the most common malignancy affecting the spleen.[52] Isolated or primary splenic involvement occurs in 1 to 2% of all lymphomas, the majority of which will represent Hodgkin disease.[53] Lymphoma of the spleen can have a variety of imaging appearances most commonly as splenomegaly. However, lymphoma can also appear as solitary or multiple round or oval lesions in the spleen. These lesions can have a miliary appearance or appear as larger nodular lesions (see Figure 14-28).

Metastasis

The spleen is an infrequent site of tumor metastasis despite its vascularity. When splenic metastases are present, multiple other metastatic sites such as lymph nodes, liver, and lungs are often seen, indicating a worse prognosis.[54] Common primary cancers that metastasize to the spleen include breast, lung, ovary, melanoma, stomach, pancreas, liver, and colon cancer. Calcification in splenic metastases is rare unless the primary tumor is a mucinous adenocarcinoma.[85] Melanoma can cause cystic metastases. Metastatic ovarian cancer produces cystic implants along the peritoneal surfaces of the spleen.

Splenic metastatic lesions may be solitary, multiple, or diffuse and vary in number and size from a few millimeters to several centimeters. On US, splenic metastases predominantly appear as small hypoechoic target lesions or may be well defined as either cystic or solid masses.

A cystic or solid mass may show contrast enhancement at the periphery and within the septa of the lesion on CT and MRI (see Figure 14-29). Because metastatic disease often follows the MR signal of normal spleen, nonhemorrhagic splenic metastases may be difficult to see or the size may be underestimated on noncontrast T1- or T2-weighted MR sequences.[86] Internal hemorrhage, necrosis, or contour deformity are often clues to the presence of splenic metastasis. In patients with transfusional iron overload, metastatic disease can be seen against a background of low T2 signal in surrounding abnormal spleen.

Multifocal vascular tumors

Vascular tumors are the most common nonhematolymphoid tumors of the spleen.[87] Several of these—hemangiomas, lymphangiomas, and littoral cell angiomas—can appear as multifocal masses within the spleen. Hemangiomatosis, multiple hemangiomas widely

Imaging Notes 14-3. Distinguishing Features of the Common Focal Lesions of the Spleen

Hemangioma	Small, round, or oval	Incidentally discovered
Infarction	Wedge shaped	
Hematoma	Features of blood products	History of trauma
Metastasis	Usually multiple	History of a malignancy
Lymphoma	Usually multiple	History of lymphoma

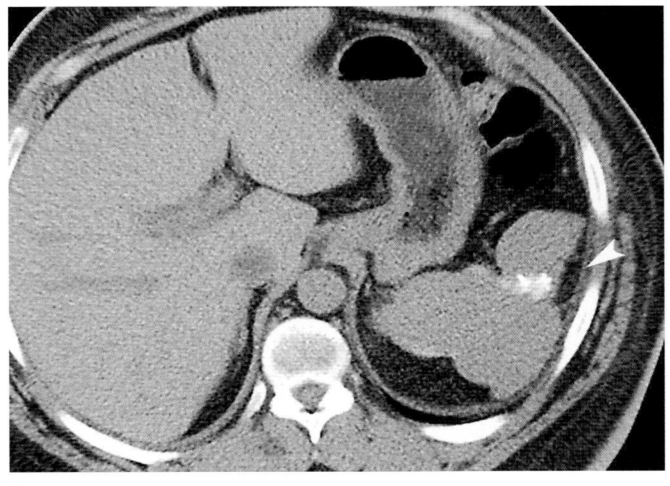

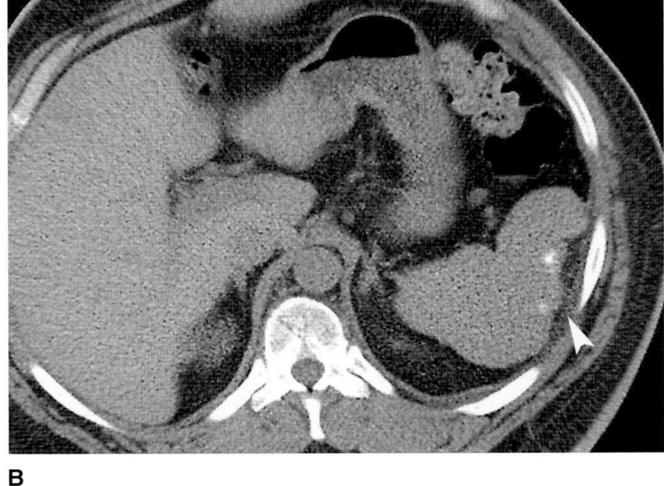

Figure 14-26 Focal Splenic Atrophy due to Prior Infarction or Trauma Unenhanced CT demonstrates a focal defect in the surface of the spleen (*arrowheads*) with associated dystrophic calcification. This is typical of focal scarring and atrophy due to prior infarction or trauma.

involving the spleen, is usually a manifestation of a generalized angiomatosis such as Klippel-Trénaunay syndrome.[87] Similarly, lymphangiomatosis, multiple lymphangiomas widely involving the spleen, is usually a manifestation of lymphangiomatosis, a syndrome where lymphangiomas involve multiple organs (see Figure 14-30). However, littoral cell angiomas are usually multiple in number and not associated with other syndromes.[87]

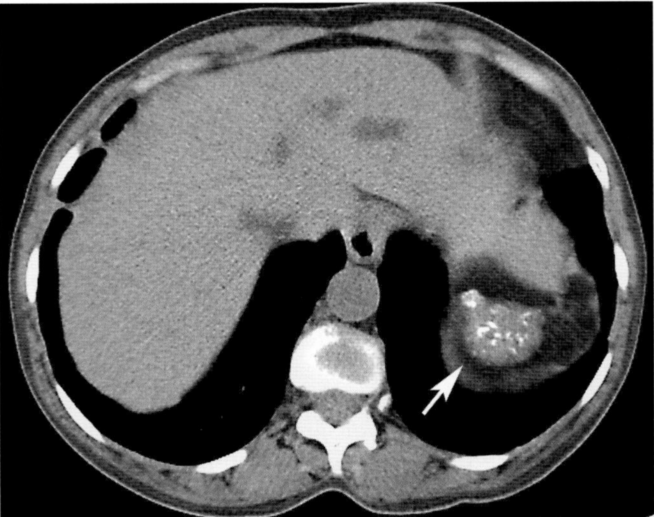

Figure 14-27 Autosplenectomy in Sickle Cell Disease This 51-year-old woman with sickle cell disease presented with chest pain. Axial CT image through the upper abdomen shows a diminutive spleen (*arrow*) with multiple punctate calcifications. This calcified atrophy is typical of the autosplenectomy of sickle cell disease caused by multiple infarcts of the spleen.

Littoral cell angioma: Littoral cell angioma is a rare tumor of the spleen that is derived from the littoral cells of the splenic red pulp sinuses and has features intermediate between those of endothelial cells and macrophages. These tumors can contain foci of extramedullary hematopoiesis, hemosiderin pigment, or calcification.[87] To date, many cases have been found because of anemia, thrombocytopenia, or during evaluations for abdominal malignancies. It is possible that this is a result of meaningful association between these symptoms and the presence of the tumor, or

Table 14-6. Causes of Multiple Splenic Nodules

A. Neoplasms
1. **Lymphoma**[a]
2. **Metastasis**
3. **Hemangioma**
4. Lymphangioma
5. Littoral cell angioma
B. Infections
1. Granulomatous infections
a. Tuberculosis
b. Histoplasmosis
c. Cryptococcosis
2. Disseminated candidiasis
3. *Pneumocystis jiroveci* (HIV only)
4. Hepatosplenic cat scratch disease (*Bartonella henselae*)
C. **Sarcoidosis**
D. Peliosis

[a]Disorders in bold are most common.

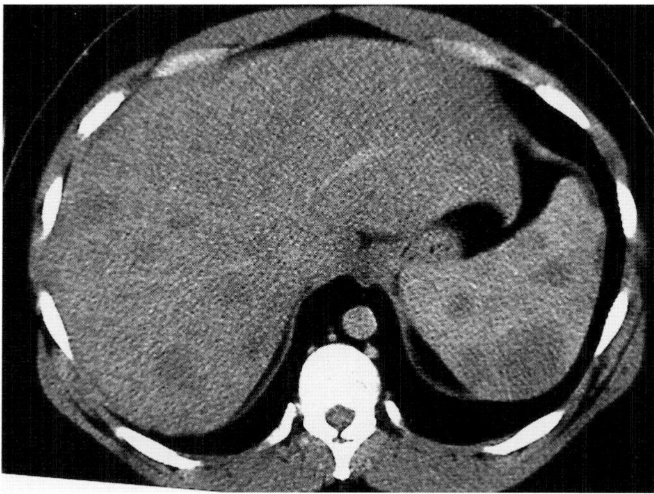

A

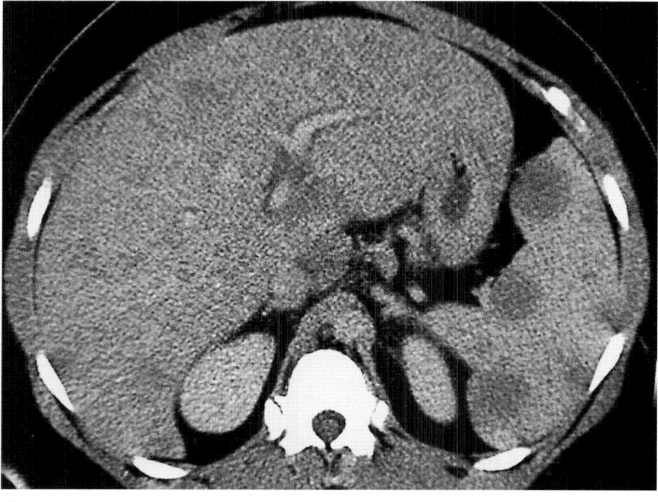

B

Figure 14-28 Multifocal Nodules Due to Lymphoma
This 38-year-old man presented with nausea, vomiting, and a 15-pound weight loss. **A** and **B.** Axial contrast-enhanced images demonstrate multiple large nodular masses in the spleen and innumerable small nodules in the liver. Images of the lower abdomen also demonstrated multiple retroperitoneal lymph nodes. Lymph node biopsy was diagnostic of a non-Hodgkin lymphoma.

it is possible that these tumors are accidentally discovered because of imaging related to these conditions.

Like hemangiomas, the US appearance of littoral cell angiomas has been reported to range from hypoechoic to isoechoic to hyperechoic, depending on the size of the vascular channels created by the tumor, but they are probably most commonly hyperechoic.[87] On unenhanced CT examinations, littoral cell angiomas will typically appear as multiple hypoechoic masses within the spleen. With contrast enhancement, the tumors will initially enhance in an inhomogeneous fashion and on delayed contrast-enhanced images, littoral cell angiomas homogeneously enhance and become isoattenuating relative to the remaining splenic parenchyma.[87] In most cases, both T1- and T2-weighted MRI sequences will have markedly low signal intensity. This reflects the presence of hemosiderin in the lesions, a finding that can be an important clue to the diagnosis (see Figure 14-31).[87]

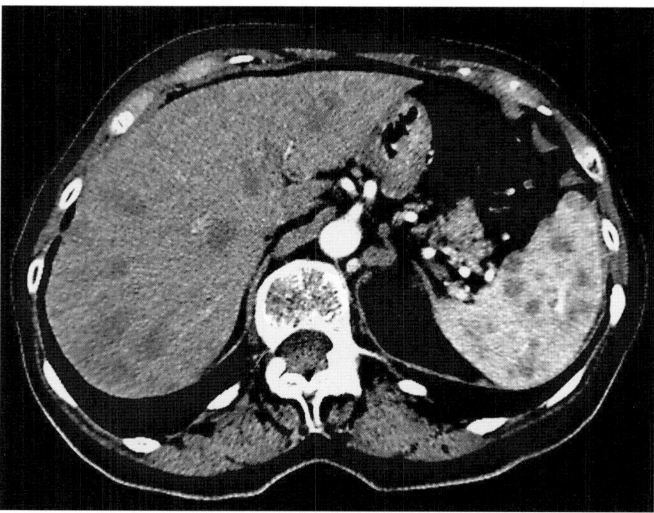

Figure 14-29 Splenic Metastasis from Breast Cancer
This 79-year-old woman had a history of breast cancer. Enhanced CT image through the upper abdomen demonstrates many small hypoattenuating nodules within the spleen and liver. In this clinical setting, this is most likely to represent multiple metastases from the patient's breast cancer.

Multifocal Infections

Multifocal infections of the spleen are usually a result of hematogenous dissemination of organisms. Intravascular foci of infection such as bacterial endocarditis can result in multiple septic emboli to the spleen and have been discussed previously under the heading **Cystic-Appearing Nodules and Masses of the Spleen** (see Figure 14-12). However, granulomatous infections of the spleen and fungal abscesses typically appear as multiple small nodular lesions of the spleen and are discussed here. Rarely, infections with *Pneumocystis jiroveci* and hepatosplenic cat scratch disease can also produce multiple small splenic lesions.

Granulomatous infections of the spleen

Granulomatous infections, including tuberculosis, nontuberculous mycobacteria, and histoplasmosis are uncommon causes of splenic infection and have been reported to account for 0% to 5% of splenic abscesses.[88-92] In the majority of cases, the splenic aspect of these infections will

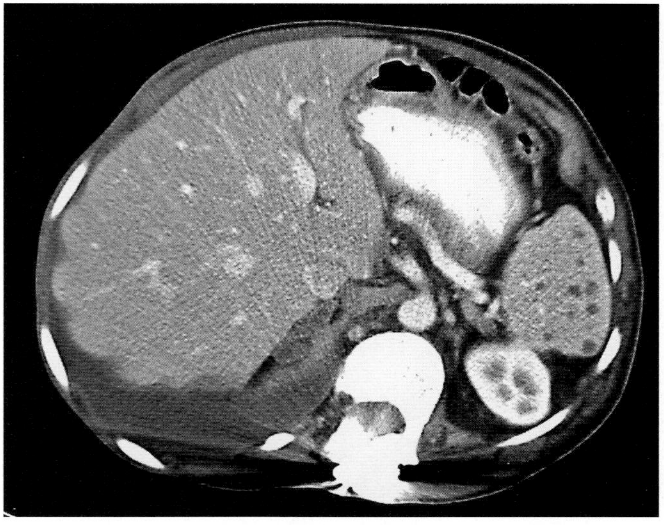

A

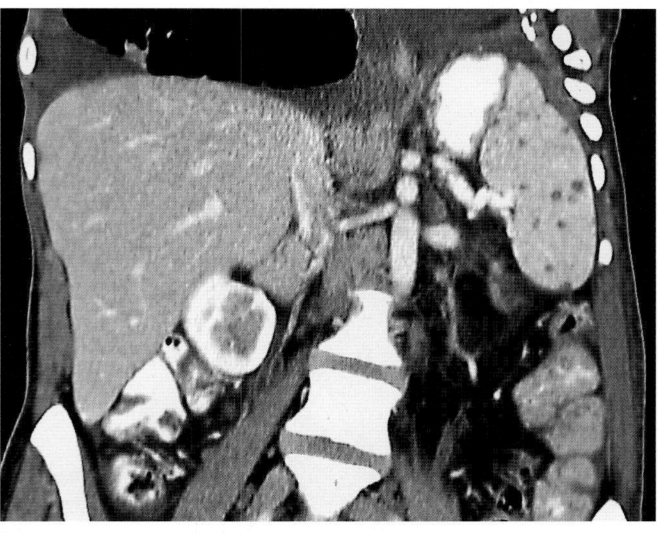

B

Figure 14-30 Splenic Lymphangiomas in Lymphangiectasia This 32-year-old woman had congenital lymphangiectasia. **A.** Axial and (**B**) coronal contrast-enhanced CT images of the spleen demonstrate multiple small splenic lesions with an attenuation similar to the right pleural effusion. Although unproven, these likely represent multiple splenic lymphangiomas.

be clinically silent and require no specific therapy other than general systemic antituberculous or antifungal medications when indicated.

In one study of 57 patients with clinically diagnosed abdominal tuberculosis, splenic involvement was detected in 7 (12%).[93] Most patients who have clinically detected splenic tuberculosis will have severe disseminated disease elsewhere and will often be immunocompromised.[94,95] Focal splenic lesions have been detected in 30% of patients with tuberculosis and AIDS.[96] In the active phase of disease, TB will most often appear as multiple small, few-millimeter to few-centimeter, lesions in the spleen that appear hypoechoic on US and hypoattenuating on CT examinations (see Figure 14-32).[94,95,97,98] These are thought to represent small granulomas because of hematogenous dissemination of the infection.[99] CT is more sensitive than US for the presence of these small lesions.[95] In up to one-third of cases, tubercular infection will appear as a large unilocular fluid collection with or without rim enhancement and mimic the more common bacterial abscess.[95,100] Tubercular abscesses may be more common in HIV-infected patients.[95,101] In some cases, the spleen will appear enlarged with or without the presence of cystic lesions in the spleen. Once the infection is controlled, the small hypoechoic nodules will frequently leave multiple small splenic calcifications that persist for the lifetime of the patient.[95]

Histoplasmosis is the most common granulomatous fungal infection to involve the spleen. In most cases, the infection is clinically silent and so multiple small punctate calcified granulomas is the most common imaging manifestation of splenic histoplasmosis.[98] Like tuberculosis, during the acute infection, cross-sectional imaging will, in some cases, demonstrate multiple small nodular lesions that appear hypoechoic on US studies, hypoattenuating on CT scans, and hyperintense on T2 MR sequences.[96,98] Splenomegaly, with or without the small nodular lesions, can also be seen in some patients.[98,102] One study noted diffuse splenic hypoattenuation in 2 of 6 HIV-positive patients with histoplasmosis.[102] This may be a rare but specific manifestation of histoplasmosis in this population.

Splenic involvement with nontuberculous mycobacteria, *Coccidioides* and *Cryptococcus*, only occurs in HIV-positive individuals who remain severely immunosuppressed with diminished CD4 counts. Imaging manifestations mimic those of tuberculosis and include small nodular lesions that appear low attenuation on CT scans and splenomegaly.[98] Small low attenuation nodular lesions have been detected in 7% and splenomegaly in 20% of patients with MAI and AIDS.[96,103]

Fungal microabscesses

Fungal infection in the spleen is uncommon and accounts for between 1% and 25% of all splenic abscesses.[28-31,34,96] Splenic fungal abscess most often occurs as a result of hematogenous dissemination in an immunocompromised patient.[30,96,104] Patients at risk include those with hematologic malignancies, those that have received organ or bone marrow transplants, and those with cell-mediated immunodeficiencies, including AIDS.[30,98,104] The typical patient presents with fevers, malaise, and weight loss and laboratory evaluations show neutropenia. The large majority of cases will be caused by *Candida* species; however,

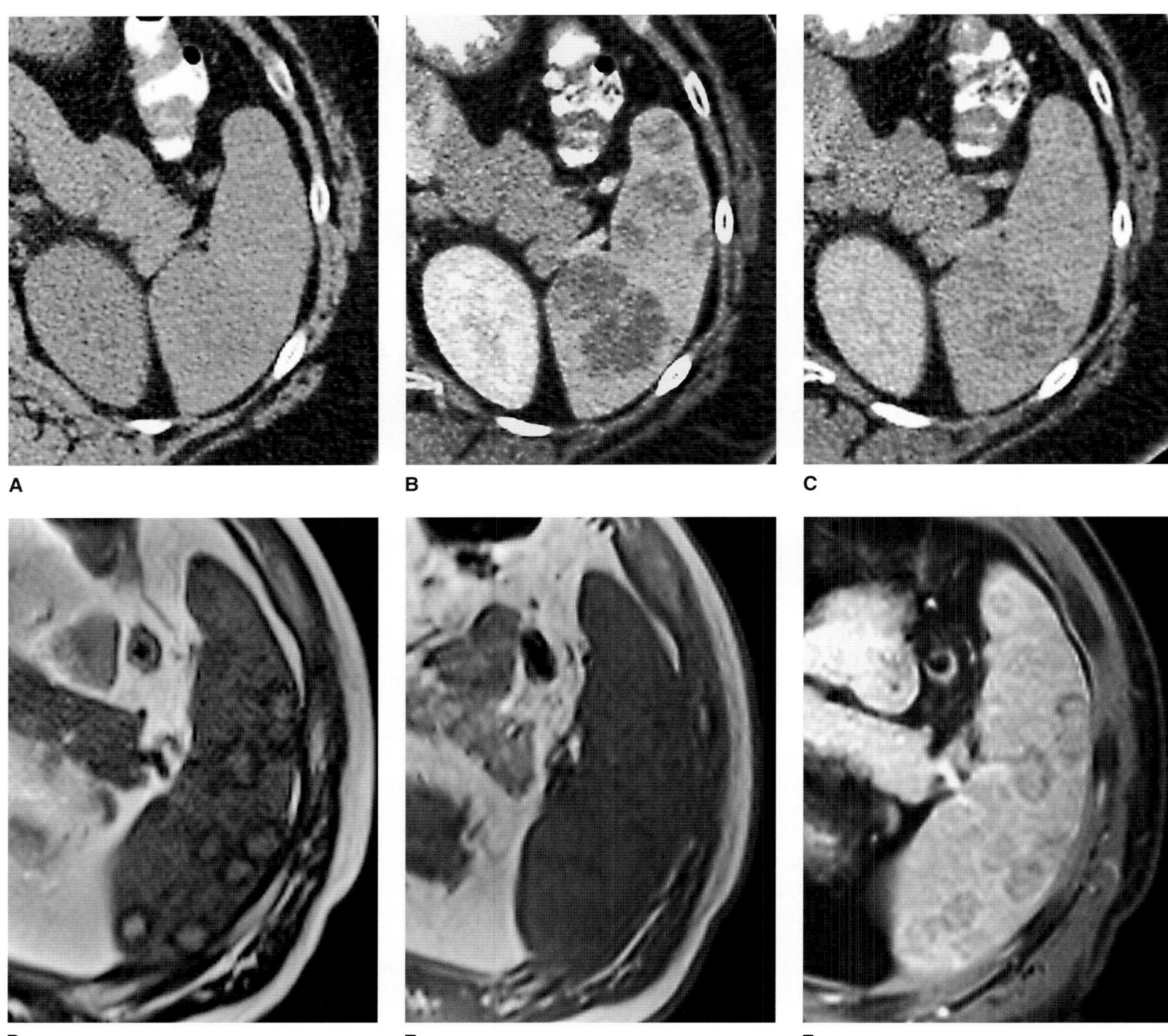

Figure 14-31 Littoral Cell Angiomas of the Spleen in 2 Patients
A-C. This 65-year-old woman had a renal cell carcinoma of the left kidney. (A) Unenhanced, (B) arterial-, and (C) venous-phase CT images demonstrate multiple irregularly marginated masses in the spleen. They demonstrate irregular predominantly peripheral enhancement on arterial-phase images and nearly completely fill in with contrast on the venous-phase images. These lesions remained stable over multiple years. This combination of findings indicates that these represent primary vascular tumors of the spleen, either multiple splenic hemangiomas or littoral cell angiomas. **D.** T2-weighted, (**E**) T1-weighted, and (**F**) T1-weighted postgadolinium images in a 56-year-old man with prostate carcinoma demonstrate multiple irregularly shaped lesions distributed throughout the spleen. These are poorly seen on the T1-weighted sequence and filled in with contrast on delayed images. They have a remarkably similar appearance to those of first patient and likely represent multiple littoral cell angiomas of the spleen. These have remained stable on MRI examinations for several years.

occasionally *Aspergillus* or *Cryptococcus* organisms are discovered.[96,105] Patients at risk include those that have received organ transplants or bone marrow transplants and patients with cell-mediated immunodeficiencies, including AIDS.[30,98]

Fungal infections of the spleen can only be seen on cross-sectional imaging studies. This hematologically disseminated infection causes multiple small splenic and hepatic abscesses that are sometimes imperceptible by imaging examinations.[96,106] When detectable, US, CT,

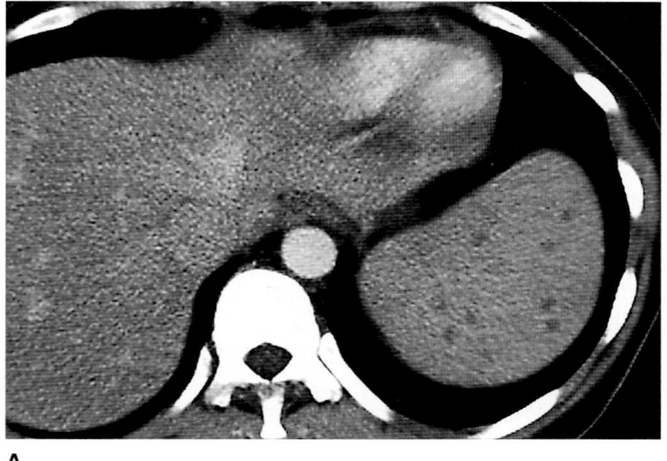

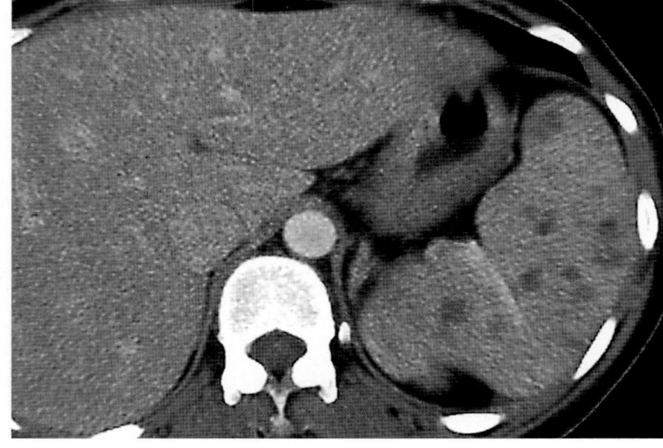

A B

Figure 14-32 Splenic Tuberculosis
This 33-year-old African man was HIV-positive and febrile with cough and hemoptysis. Chest CT (not shown) demonstrated multiple low attenuation lymph nodes. **A, B.** Contrast enhanced CT exam demonstrates multiple small hypoattenuating lesions of the spleen. Subsequent lymph node biopsy was diagnostic of tuberculosis."

and/or MRI will typically demonstrate innumerable small, 5- to 10-mm, cysts widely distributed across the spleen.[96,98,105,107,108] Occasionally, the cyst can be as large as 20 mm in diameter. In most cases, similar microabscesses will be seen in the liver. In many cases, these individuals will have a recent CT of the abdomen in which these small lesions were absent. The acute presentation of many tiny cysts in the liver and spleen of an immunocompromised patient is virtually diagnostic of disseminated fungal infection, usually with *Candida* species (see Figure 14-33). Occasionally, US examinations will demonstrate a central focus of higher echogenicity, or a wheel-within-a-wheel pattern can be seen within the small cystic lesions.[106]

Pneumocystis infection

Extrapulmonary *P jiroveci* infection is a rare phenomenon that has primarily been detected in patients who are severely immunocompromised by HIV infection. With the

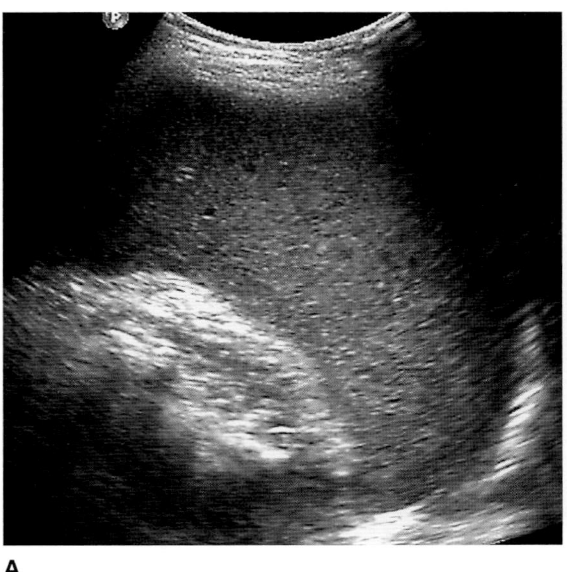

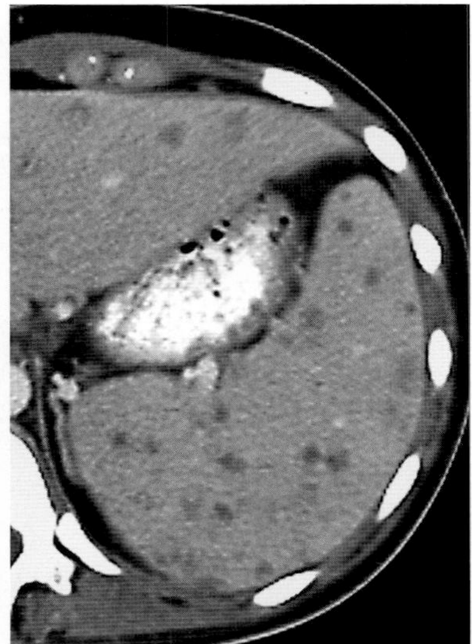

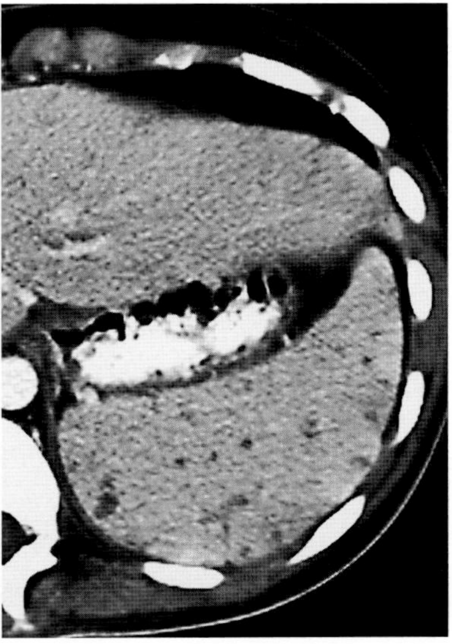

A B C

Figure 14-33 Candida Microabscesses
This 22-year-old woman with AML was neutropenic and febrile. **A.** US of the spleen shows multiple tiny hypoechoic lesions scattered throughout the spleen. **B.** Enhanced CT image confirms the presence of multiple low-attenuation lesions. Note the similar lesions in the left lobe of the liver. In this clinical setting, these findings are highly likely to represent multiple candidal abscesses. Blood cultures confirmed the presence of disseminated candidiasis.

advent of HAART therapy, fewer and fewer HIV-positive individuals remain immunocompromised and so splenic infection with *Pneumocystis* rarely occurs. Splenic involvement by *Pneumocystis* is typically asymptomatic and discovered incidentally on imaging examinations. In the acute phase of the infection, the spleen will be enlarged and contain multiple small nodular lesions that resemble fungal microabscesses on imaging examinations.[96,109,110] With time, these lesions will become diffusely calcified and resemble multiple calcified granulomas within the spleen.[111]

Hepatosplenic cat scratch disease

Cat scratch disease is an unusual lymphoreticular infection due to *Bartonella henselae* primarily seen in patients with T-cell immunodeficiency, such as AIDS.[112] Imaging findings include splenomegaly with or without multiple nodular lesions that appear hypoechoic on US examinations and hypoattenuating on CT scans.[112-114]

Infiltrative Diseases

Less commonly mulitiple splenic lesions can be due to the infiltrative diseases: sarcoidosis, Gaucher disease and peliosis.

Sarcoidosis

Splenic involvement occurs in approximately 7% of patients with sarcoidosis and is usually asymptomatic.[115,116] On imaging, there may be splenomegaly or the presence of multiple splenic nodules. Splenomegaly is the most common finding, occurring in approximately one-third of patients with splenic sarcoidosis.[117] Nodules occur more often when the spleen is enlarged.

On US, splenic nodules are hypoechoic relative to background splenic parenchyma.[118] They may also produce a diffuse heterogeneous pattern. Splenic nodules are visible on CT in approximately 6% to 33% of sarcoid patients.[119] With contrast-enhanced CT, nodules appear hypodense relative to normal background spleen, are diffusely distributed through the spleen, and range in size from 1 mm to 2 cm in diameter.[120] With increasing size, nodules tend to become confluent (see Figure 14-34). With MRI, splenic nodules associated with sarcoidosis are hypointense relative to background spleen on T1- and T2-weighted sequences. Following IV gadolinium administration, nodules show no substantial enhancement.[121]

Gaucher disease

Gaucher disease is an autosomal recessive lysosomal disorder in which lack of an enzyme results in accumulation of glucocerebrosides in the cells of the reticuloendothelial system, causing hepatosplenomegaly. On T1-weighted MR images, signal intensity is low relative to normal spleen secondary to glucocerebroside. On T2-weighted images, signal intensity is indeterminate except for nodal clusters of Gaucher cells, which appear hypointense to spleen (see Figure 14-35).[122]

Peliosis

Splenic peliosis is a rare condition of unknown cause, characterized by multiple, variously sized, blood-filled cysts distributed throughout the spleen. The liver is more often involved than the spleen. Its clinical significance lies in the

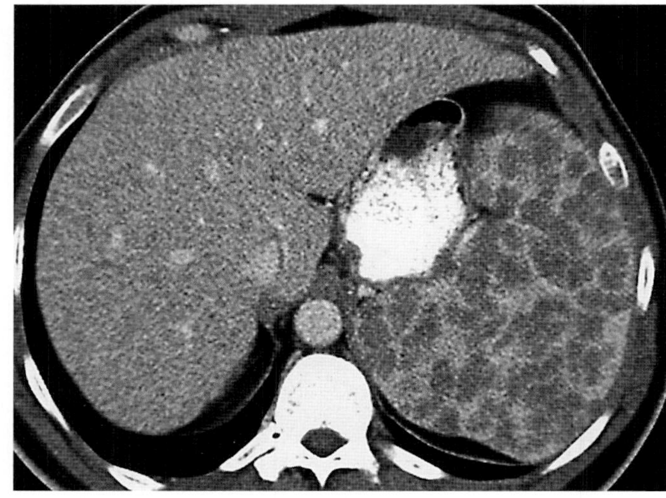

A

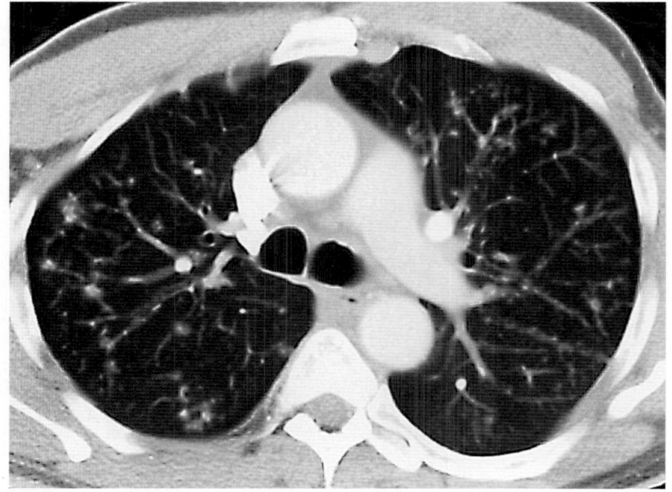

B

Figure 14-34 Multifocal Nodules Due to Sarcoidosis
This 44-year-old man had unexplained weight loss. **A.** Contrast-enhanced CT demonstrates multiple low-attenuation nodules in the spleen and more subtle, smaller nodules in the liver. There is also moderate splenomegaly. **B.** CT image of the lungs shows small nodules in a bronchovascular pattern. Lung biopsy was diagnostic of sarcoidosis.

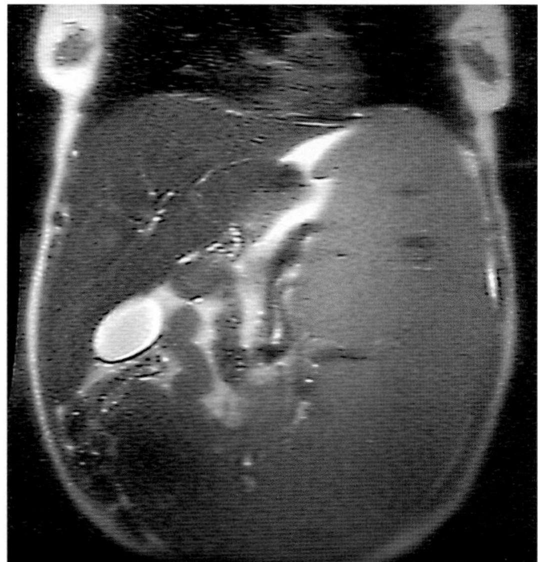

A

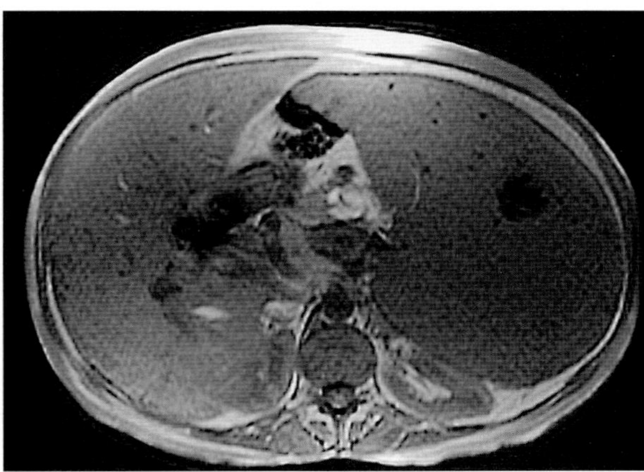

B

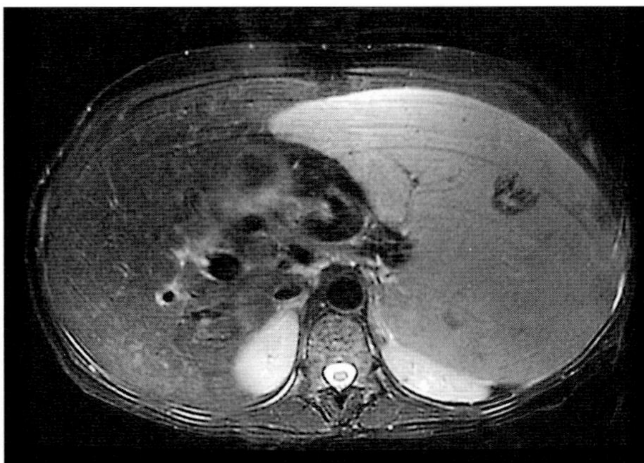

C

Figure 14-35 MRI of Gaucher Disease
This 58-year-old woman had a history of Gaucher disease. **A.** Coronal T1-weighted sequence demonstrates massive splenomegaly that fills the left upper quadrant of the abdomen and pelvis. **B.** Axial T1- and (**C**) T2-weighted sequences show splenomegaly and multiple small, low-signal lesions distributed throughout the spleen. These are nodal clusters of Gaucher cells.

potential of peliotic lesions on the splenic surface to rupture and cause intraperitoneal hemorrhage.[87]

Hepatosplenomegaly and multiple small hepatosplenic lesions are seen on all imaging modalities. On US, these lesions are hypoechoic. On unenhanced CT, lesions are hypodense but may contain fluid-fluid levels reflecting hematocrit effect.[87] Following administration of IV contrast, lesions may not enhance if thrombosed or may demonstrate central enhancing foci if the thrombus becomes recanalized. On MRI, signal intensity within lesions varies depending on the stage of intralesional blood products.

SPLENOMEGALY AND OTHER DIFFUSE DISORDERS

Diffuse abnormalities of the spleen are characterized by diffuse enlargement (splenomegaly) and diminished sized (atrophy, autosplenectomy).

Splenomegaly

There is no universally accepted definition of splenomegaly. Furthermore, several studies have shown that splenic size is directly correlated with the size of the individual and is inversely correlated with age.[123-126] The most accurate means of identifying splenic size is to determine splenic volume by measuring the cross-sectional area of the spleen on individual CT or MRI slices, multiplying by the thickness of the slice and then summing the total number of slices. Using this method, 2 studies of 140 and 149 consecutive adult patients who underwent abdominal CT for indications not related to splenic disease identified the 95% confidence limit of the upper limit of normal splenic volume of 314.5 to 378 cm^3.[127,128] This method of determining splenic size is not generally practical, and fortunately studies have shown that measurement of the maximal length of the spleen is strongly correlated with splenic volume ($r = 0.81$ to 0.86).[129,130] A study of 783 Chinese patients not known to have any condition likely to be associated with splenic enlargement recommended a length of 12 cm as the upper limits of normal.[126] However, 2 studies of college athletes of 631 subjects and 129 subjects demonstrated mean splenic length of 10.65 ± 1.55 cm and 11.4 ± 1.7 cm.[123] Therefore, 75% of normal young adult spleens will be less than 12.2 to 13.1 cm and 95% of normal young adult spleens will be less than 13.75 to 14.8 cm. This study corroborates

Imaging Notes 14-4. Splenomegaly

Splenic length of <12 cm is within the range of normal variation
Splenic length of >15 cm indicates splenomegaly
Splenic length of 12-15 cm is a gray zone between normal and mild splenomegaly

the generally accepted criteria that a spleen with a maximal length of less than 12 cm is within the range of normal variation, that a spleen of greater than 15 cm maximal length is indicative of splenomegaly, and a spleen between 12 and 15 cm in length is within a gray zone between normal and mild splenomegaly.

On physical examination and abdominal plain films, some large focal splenic lesions can be confused with splenomegaly. However, cross-sectional imaging can distinguish uniform splenic enlargement from enlargement of a focal portion of the spleen. We will reserve the term *splenomegaly* for uniform splenic enlargement without focal abnormality.

Plain-film findings suggestive of splenomegaly are mass effect in the left upper quadrant of the abdomen, elevation of the left hemidiaphragm, medial and anterior displacement of the stomach, and inferomedial displacement of bowel (see Figure 14-36). In addition to length and volume measurements, cross-sectional imaging findings suggestive of splenomegaly include extension beyond the lower pole of the left kidney, extension medial to the aorta, and loss of inferomedial concavity.

Splenomegaly can result from several pathophysiologies: (1) venous congestion, (2) infiltrative diseases, and (3) increased splenic function. Infiltrative diseases can be subdivided into neoplastic and nonneoplastic conditions. Increased splenic function can be due to infections, noninfectious inflammatory diseases (autoimmune disorders), removal of defective red cells (hemoglobinopathies), and extramedullary hematopoiesis (Table 14-7). Occasionally, the etiology for splenomegaly can be suggested based on other nonsplenic imaging findings such as liver cirrhosis, occlusion of the splenic vein, and retroperitoneal lymphadenopathy (usually indicating lymphoma), but often the cause of splenomegaly cannot be determined by imaging.

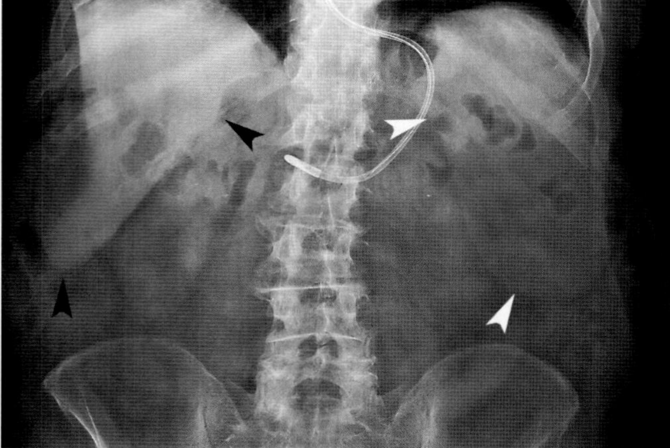

Figure 14-36 Splenomegaly due to Portal Hypertension
This 77-year-old man with a history of cirrhosis had abdominal pain. Abdominal plain film demonstrates a small liver shadow (*black arrowheads*) and an enlarged spleen (*white arrowheads*), which measured 18 cm in craniocaudad length. These findings are typical of cirrhosis and splenomegaly due to portal hypertension.

Table 14-7. Causes of Splenomegaly

A. Splenic congestion
1. **Cirrhosis**[a]
2. Splenic vein obstruction
a. Pancreatic carcinoma
b. Pancreatitis
3. Portal or hepatic vein obstruction
4. Right heart failure
B. Infiltrative diseases
1. Neoplasms
a. **Leukemia**
b. **Lymphoma**
c. Malignant histiocytosis
2. Nonneoplastic
a. Gaucher disease
b. Niemann-Pick disease
c. Alpha-mannosidosis
d. Hurler syndrome
e. Other mucopolysaccharidoses
f. Amyloidosis
g. Histiocytosis
C. Increased splenic function
1. Infections
a. **Infectious mononucleosis**
b. **Malaria**
c. Leishmaniasis (Kala Azar)
d. Other infections
2. Noninfectious inflammatory conditions
a. Rheumatoid arthritis
b. Systemic lupus erythematosus
c. Autoimmune hemolytic anemia
d. **Sarcoidosis**
3. Hematologic disorders
a. Thalassemia
b. Hereditary spherocytosis
c. Early sickle cell disease
d. Autoimmune hemolytic anemia
e. Other causes of anemia
f. Polycythemia vera
4. Extramedullary hematopoiesis
a. **Myelofibrosis**
b. Marrow infiltration by neoplasms

[a]Disorders in bold are most common.

Venous congestion

Occlusion or hypertension of the splenic vein leads to edema of the spleen and splenomegaly. In many cases, cross-sectional imaging will also reveal secondary findings of portal hypertension such as perisplenic varices and dilation of the splenic vein.

Cirrhosis: Cirrhosis with portal hypertension is the most common cause of splenomegaly in the United States. Although the splenic enlargement is nonspecific,

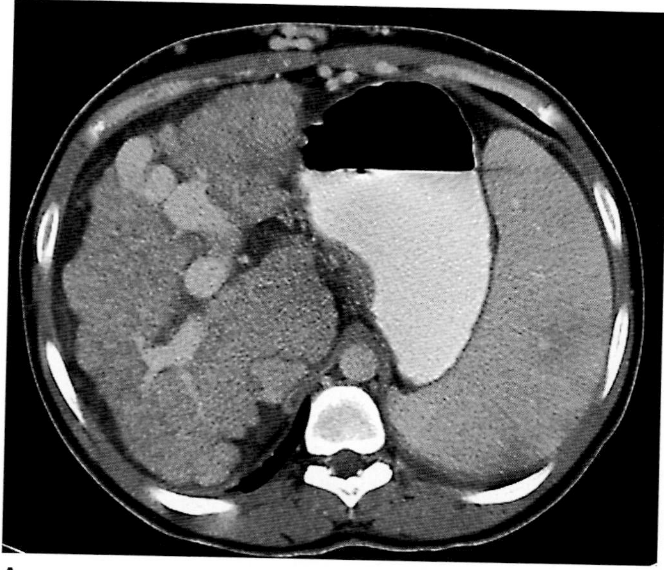

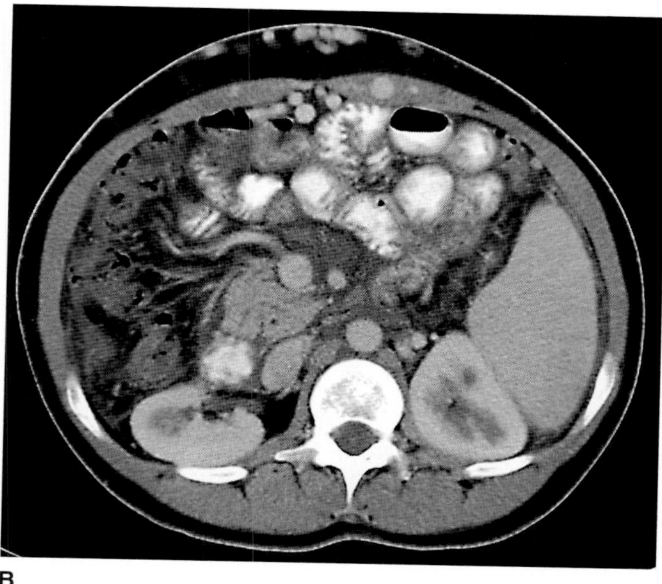

Figure 14-37 Splenomegaly due to Cirrhosis
This 22-year-old woman had cirrhosis due to autoimmune hepatitis. **A** and **B**. The liver is small and nodular in appearance, typical of cirrhosis. There are multiple abdominal wall varices due to a recanalized umbilical vein indicating portal hypertension. Contrast-enhanced axial CT images demonstrate an enlarged spleen that extends into the lower abdomen and displaces the left kidney.

imaging will usually demonstrate findings of cirrhosis, including hepatic nodularity and relative caudate and left hepatic lobe hypertrophy (see Figure 14-37). On MRI, splenic foci of hemosiderin deposition are seen in 9% to 12% of patients with portal hypertension. These foci are called Gamna-Gandy bodies and are due to small areas of intrasplenic hemorrhage. They appear as multiple tiny foci of decreased signal intensity with all pulse sequences, and exhibit "blooming" on gradient echo sequences secondary to iron deposition.[82] Gamna-Gandy bodies are discussed in greater detail under the heading: **Many Small Splenic Calcifications or Hemosiderin Foci.**

Venous obstruction: Obstruction of the splenic, portal, or hepatic vein can also result in splenomegaly. Causes of portal and hepatic vein obstruction are discussed in Chapter 3.

Splenomegaly due to splenic vein obstruction is uncommon and can be due to surrounding inflammation, compression, or invasion by an adjacent mass or by in situ thrombosis of the splenic vein. The most common causes are acute and chronic pancreatitis and pancreatic cancer (see Figure 14-24).[131,132] However, rarely mass effect or invasion from a renal cyst or cancer, direct injury from trauma, or thrombosis from blood dyscrasia can cause splenic vein occlusion.

Infiltrative malignancies

Many forms of lymphoma and leukemia can cause splenomegaly. Malignant histocytosis is another rare infiltrative malignancy of the spleen.

Lymphoma: Lymphoma is the most common malignancy affecting the spleen, most often, secondary involvement by disseminated disease but occasionally as the primary focus.[52] Splenic involvement is common in both Hodgkin disease and non-Hodgkin lymphoma. Although splenic involvement in disseminated Hodgkin disease and non-Hodgkin lymphoma is common, isolated or primary splenic involvement is rare, occurring in approximately 1% to 2% of all lymphomas at presentation.[53] The vast majority of primary splenic lymphomas are non-Hodgkin type. Patients with AIDS have an increased risk of splenic involvement in lymphoma, in addition to a more aggressive course of disease.

The imaging features of splenic lymphoma include (1) a normal-appearing spleen in which the involvement is only microscopic, (2) splenomegaly in which the spleen is diffusely infiltrated without focal mass lesion, and (3) focal lesions of the spleen in which there are solitary or multiple discrete regions of lymphoma within the splenic parenchyma (see Figure 14-38). Focal and multifocal lymphomatous lesions will typically appear as round or oval nodules or masses within the normal spleen (see Figure 14-16). Multifocal involvement can be further subdivided into miliary/micronodular configuration, with nodules less than 1 cm in diameter or large masses between 1 and 10 cm (see Figure 14-28).[53] Focal involvement can occur in both normal and enlarged spleens.

Splenic size alone is an unreliable predictor of lymphomatous involvement. Although massive splenomegaly, in the setting of a patient with known lymphoma, is invariably indicative of splenic involvement by lymphoma, mild-moderate splenomegaly without lymphomatous

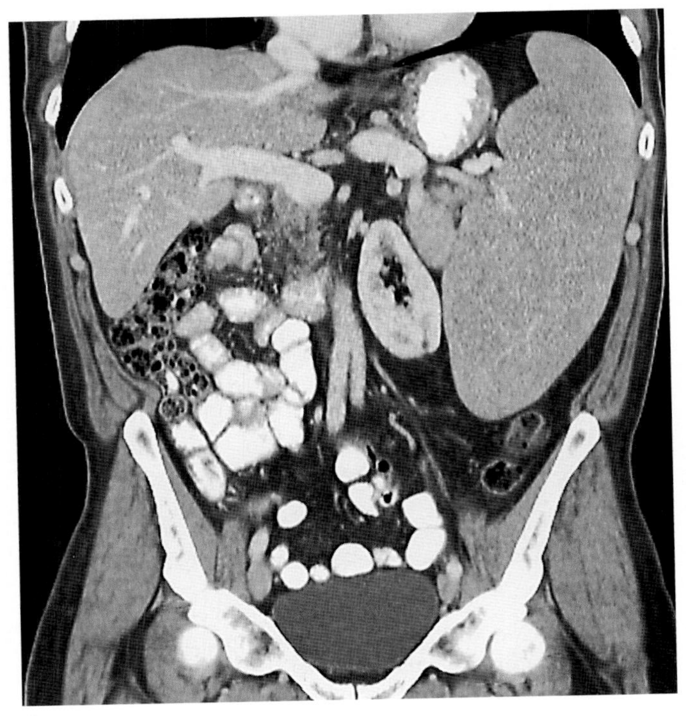

A

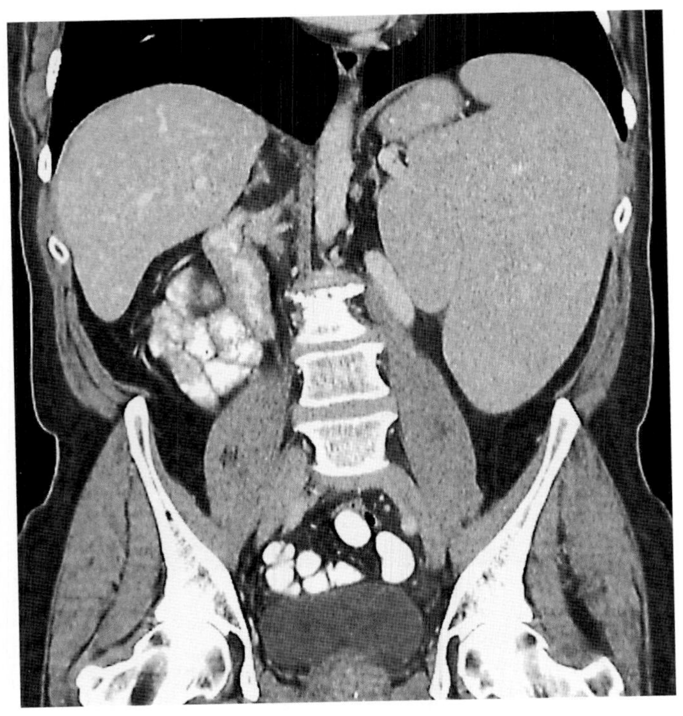

B

Figure 14-38 Splenomegaly due to Lymphoma
This 65-year-old man had a low-grade B-cell lymphoma. **A** and **B.** Coronal reconstruction from an enhanced CT demonstrates massive enlargement of the spleen, the most common splenic manifestation of lymphoma.

infiltration occurs in approximately 30% of patients with Hodgkin lymphoma and 70% of patients with non-Hodgkin lymphoma.[133] Accepting these limitations, it has been shown that alterations in serial splenic volume on CT correlate with changes in disease. Consequently, alterations in serial CT measurements may be used to assess treatment response or disease progression.[134]

CT is the most widely used imaging modality for lymphoma assessment. However, it has a low accuracy for detecting splenic involvement. Quoted sensitivities vary between 22% and 65%, but have increased with advances in multidetector imaging.[135] This low sensitivity is primarily due to poor lesion-to-spleen contrast for lymphomatous deposits on CT. Consequently, even gross infiltrates that are clearly evident on US can be missed on CT. When focal splenic involvement is detected, deposits are of lower attenuation than adjacent normal splenic parenchyma on unenhanced CT and demonstrate little or no enhancement on enhanced images. Deposits may be markedly hypodense, of near water density, which can represent areas of liquefactive necrosis or hypovascular solid tumor. Rim enhancement has also been documented.[136]

US has limited accuracy in detecting splenic involvement in lymphoma. Sensitivities vary widely but have also improved over time, likely reflecting technical advances. US is more sensitive than CT for detecting splenic involvement, approaching 63% as compared to 37% for CT in 1 study, with US preferentially demonstrating inhomogeneities as well as small nodular infiltrates.[137,138] On US, the majority of detectable foci are hypoechoic relative to normal splenic tissue and have scattered and penetrating vascularity on color Doppler. Focal deposits may have smooth or indistinct margins. Solid lymphoma deposits can appear deceptively cystic on B-mode US, although color Doppler can be used to confirm internal vascularity. Hypoechoic splenic deposits may become isoechoic as they regress with treatment or become hyperechoic secondary to fibrosis.

Conventional T1- and T2-weighted MR sequences have poor sensitivity for splenic involvement in lymphoma, because of similar relaxation times of lymphoma and normal splenic tissue using these sequences.[16] Identifiable splenic deposits are hypointense on T1-weighted images and hyperintense on T2-weighted images. Improvements in MRI have improved lesion detection. In 1 study using gradient echo sequences resulting in predominantly T2* and proton density-weighted images, MRI demonstrated splenic lymphoma with greater lesion-to-spleen contrast than US or CT.[139] Gadolinium-enhanced MRI further increases conspicuity of lymphoma deposits as a consequence of their relatively poor enhancement compared to normal splenic parenchyma, although this is dependent on the timing of acquisition. Studies using dynamic-enhanced MR suggest that the optimal timing to demonstrate splenic lesions is between 20 seconds and 1 minute from commencement of bolus injection.[5]

In general, CT, US, and MRI have similar limited specificity, with difficulty differentiating lymphomatous involvement from leukemic infiltrates, sarcoid deposits, healed infarcts, and secondary infection.

Although currently limited in its availability, FDG-PET imaging has established a definite role in imaging of patients with lymphoma at all stages in management. It is the radionuclide of choice for the evaluation of lymphoma. In terms of splenic assessment, benign and malignant splenic pathologies may be separated in patients with or without known malignancy based on their differing metabolic activities, which can be described quantitatively by standardized uptake values. Recent reports have documented greater accuracy of PET compared to CT for detecting splenic involvement in lymphoma.[140] Inherent limitations of PET include false positives produced by other processes with high metabolic activity such as infection and false negatives that are a recognized feature of indolent, low-grade lymphomas.[141]

Leukemia: Both acute and chronic forms of leukemia are common causes of splenomegaly. They typically result in uniform enlargement of the spleen without focal defect. Some leukemias, specifically, chronic lymphocytic, acute myelocytic, and hairy cell leukemia are predisposed to massive splenomegaly (Table 14-8). Massive splenomegaly is traditionally defined as a weight greater than 1000 g (pathologic definition) or a spleen palpable more than 8 cm below the costal margin (clinical definition). The imaging criterion for massive splenomegaly is typically a maximal length of greater than 20 cm.

Malignant histiocytosis: Malignant histiocytosis is a rare neoplastic transformation of macrophages characterized by a syndrome of systemic symptoms such as fever wasting and malaise, pancytopenia, adenopathy, and hepatosplenomegaly.[142] Splenomegaly without systemic symptoms has been rarely reported.[143]

Table 14-8. Causes of Massive Splenomegaly

1. Leukemia (CLL, CML, hairy cell)
2. Lymphoma
3. Myelofibrosis
4. Sarcoidosis
5. Malaria
6. Thalassemia
7. Polycythemia vera
8. Autoimmune hemolytic anemia
9. Schistosomiasis
10. Visceral leishmaniasis (Kala Azar)

Nonneoplastic infiltrative diseases

There are a variety of rare metabolic disorders that can cause infiltration of the spleen and resultant splenomegaly. These include Gaucher disease, Niemann-Pick disease, α-mannosidosis, Hurler syndrome and other mucopolysaccharidoses, amyloidosis, and Tangier disease. Discussion of these entities is beyond the scope of this text. We have briefly discussed Gaucher disease under the heading **MULTIFOCAL SPLENIC LESIONS** because it can sometimes be differentiated from the other etiologies of splenomegaly because of multiple, small low-signal lesions seen on MRI examinations (see Figure 14-35).

Infectious causes of splenomegaly

Increased functioning of the spleen as a response to systemic infection can result in splenic enlargement. Infections that have been reported to cause splenomegaly include Epstein-Barr virus (mononucleosis), cytomegalovirus, HIV, viral hepatitis, malaria, typhoid fever, brucellosis, leptospirosis, tuberculosis, histoplasmosis, leishmaniasis, trypanosomiasis, *Bartonella henselae* (hepatosplenic cat scratch disease), and ehrlichiosis (see Figure 14-39). The most common of these are Epstein-Barr virus and malaria and will be discussed briefly.

Infectious mononucleosis: Infectious mononucleosis is a common clinical syndrome of pharyngitis, fever, and lymphadenopathy that can occur at any age; it is most frequently encountered in adolescents and young adults.[144,145] Infectious mononucleosis is most often due to primary infection with Epstein-Barr virus but is occasionally a result of primary infection with cytomegalovirus. These organisms are transmitted through bodily secretions, primarily saliva in the case of Epstein-Barr virus and primarily via semen or vaginal secretions in the case of cytomegalovirus (CMV). Transmission can be subclinical in many cases, but can also cause the syndrome of infectious mononucleosis in other individuals. Epstein-Barr virus remains latent in human lymphocytes and CMV remains latent in human bone marrow–derived myeloid progenitors. The infection remains suppressed by the activity of human T cells and, therefore, T-cell immunosuppression, as seen in AIDS and organ transplantation, can result in reactivation of

Imaging Notes 14-5. Causes of Splenomegaly

In the industrialized nations, the most common causes of splenomegaly are cirrhosis, leukemia, and lymphoma followed by sarcoidosis and myelofibrosis. In developing countries, the most common causes of splenomegaly are malaria and anemia[144,150]

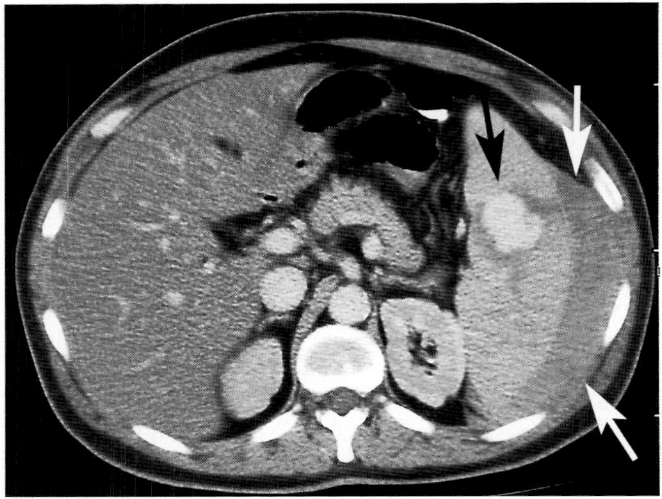

A

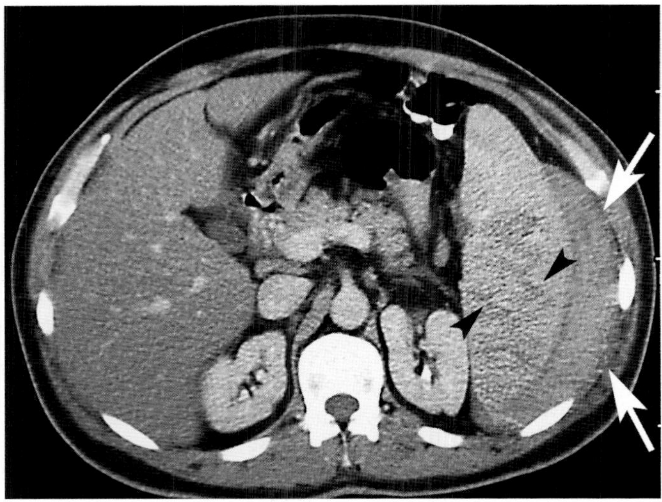

B

Figure 14-39 Splenomegaly and Rupture in Cat Scratch Disease This 37-year-old man was HIV-positive and had bilateral lower quadrant pain and a falling serum hematocrit. **A** and **B.** Contrast-enhanced CT images demonstrate moderate splenomegaly with multiple splenic fractures (*small black arrowheads*), acute contrast extravasation (*black arrow*), and a large subcapsular hematoma (*white arrows*). Patients with splenomegaly have an increased incidence of rupture probably due to minor trauma. The surgical specimen was diagnostic of bacillary angiomatosis or cat scratch disease.

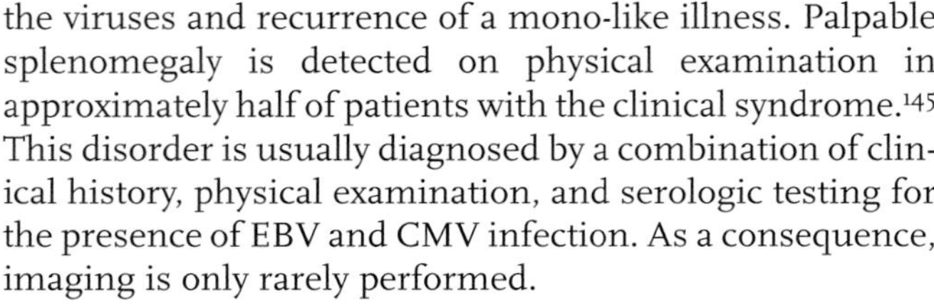

the viruses and recurrence of a mono-like illness. Palpable splenomegaly is detected on physical examination in approximately half of patients with the clinical syndrome.[145] This disorder is usually diagnosed by a combination of clinical history, physical examination, and serologic testing for the presence of EBV and CMV infection. As a consequence, imaging is only rarely performed.

Malaria: Malaria is among the most common infectious diseases in tropical and subtropical regions of the world, including Asia, Africa, and the Americas. It is caused by the protozoa of the genus *Plasmodium* of which 5 species, *falciparum, vivax, ovale, malariae,* and *knowlesi,* can cause human illness.[146] There are approximately 350 to 500 million cases of malaria annually, causing the death of 1 to 3 million people, the majority of whom are young children in sub-Saharan Africa.[147,148] Mosquito bites act as the vector from an infected individual to a new uninfected host. After a short incubation period in the liver, the parasite infects circulating red blood cells. Symptoms typically include fever and headache but can also include anemia, arthralgias, vomiting, anemia, and coma.

In the developing world, malaria is among the most common causes of splenomegaly and accounted for 25% of cases in a study of 1400 patients in Pakistan and for 53% of cases of children in the Ivory Coast.[149,150] In most cases, this is a direct result of the infection and the clearance of infected red blood cells. However, tropical splenomegaly syndrome, a rare complication of recurrent malarial infection thought to be secondary to an abnormal immunologic response to repeated infection, can also be a cause for splenomegaly.[151]

Noninfectious inflammatory conditions causing splenomegaly

The autoimmune disorders rheumatoid arthritis, systemic lupus erythematosus, and autoimmune hemolytic anemia are all associated with splenomegaly as is the idiopathic granulomatous condition sarcoidosis. In these conditions, the splenomegaly is thought to be a result of increased lymphoreticular splenic function and subsequent hypertrophy of these splenic elements.

Sarcoidosis: Asymptomatic splenic involvement occurs in approximately 7% of patients with sarcoidosis.[115,116] On imaging, there may be splenomegaly or the presence of multiple splenic nodules. Splenomegaly is the most common finding, occurring in approximately one-third of patients, but is a nonspecific finding (see Figure 14-40).[117]

Hemoglobinopathies and splenomegaly

As a response to excessive hemolysis of red blood cells, the spleen can hypertrophy in order to process the extra damaged red cells. As a consequence, hemoglobinopathies, including thalassemia, hereditary spherocytosis, sickle cell disease, autoimmune hemolytic anemia, and some other causes of anemia can be a cause of splenomegaly. In patients with homozygous sickle cell disease, splenomegaly is seen only early in childhood because of the propensity for autoinfarction of the spleen in patients with sickle cell disease. However, patients with heterozygous sickle cell disease will commonly have splenomegaly.[152]

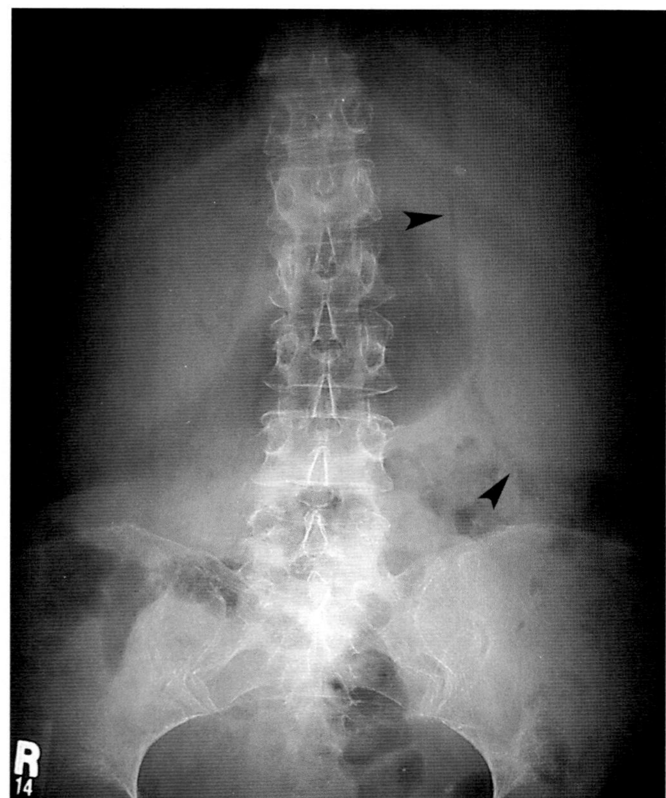

Figure 14-40 Splenomegaly due to Sarcoidosis
This 38-year-old man with a history of sarcoidosis had abdominal pain. Abdominal x-ray reveals a massively enlarged spleen (*arrowheads*) due to sarcoidosis.

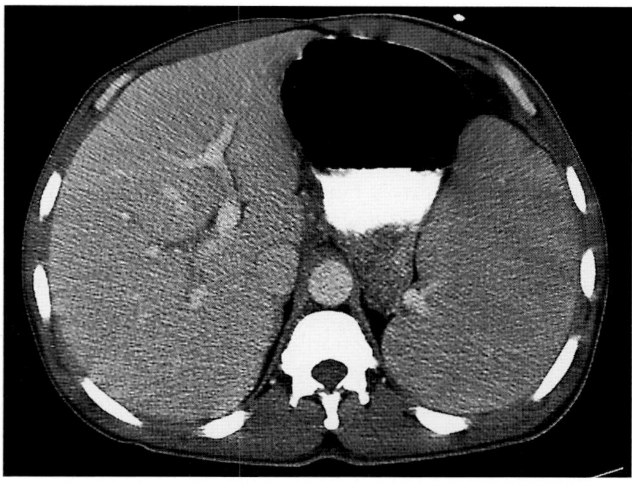

A

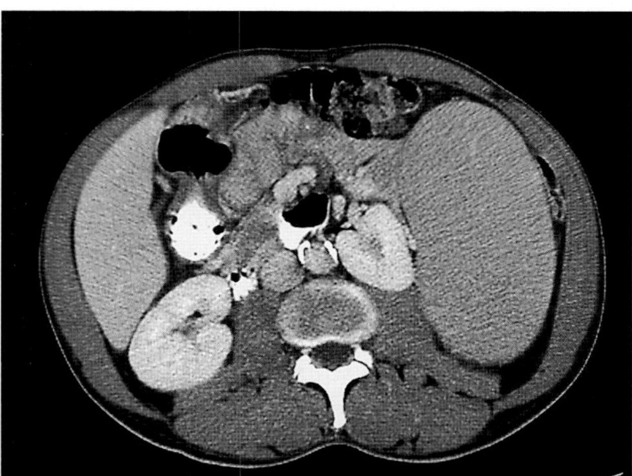

B

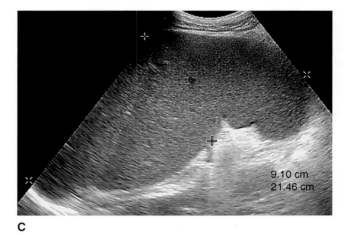

9.10 cm
21.46 cm

C

Figure 14-41 Splenomegaly in Myelofibrosis
This 50-year-old man had a history of myelofibrosis. **A** and **B.** Contrast-enhanced axial CT shows a spleen that has a rounded bulbous appearance, extends inferior to the liver tip, and displaces the left kidney medially. These are all transaxial imaging features indicating splenomegaly, in this case as a result of the myelofibrosis. **C.** US of the spleen also shows the bulbous nature of the spleen and confirms the increased length of nearly 22 cm.

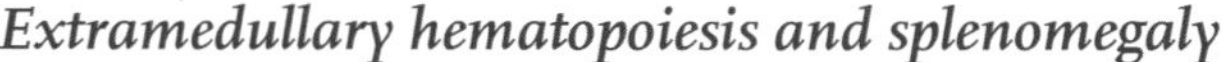

Extramedullary hematopoiesis and splenomegaly

Disorders that lead to the destruction of the normal functioning of the bone marrow can result in extramedullary hematopoiesis in the spleen and other sites around the body. This activity in the spleen can be a cause for splenomegaly. Conditions causing this phenomenon include myelofibrosis, marrow infiltration by leukemia and lymphoma and marrow destruction by irradiation, medications, and other toxins.

Myelofibrosis: Myelofibrosis is a disorder of the bone marrow, in which the marrow is replaced by fibrous (scar) tissue resulting in anemia. Symptoms include fatigue, bruising, easy bleeding, bone pain, and increased susceptibility to infections. The cause of myelofibrosis is unknown and there are no known risk factors. Myelofibrosis typically develops after the age of 50 but can occur at any age. Splenomegaly due to extramedullary hematopoiesis is a characteristic finding on physical examination and in imaging of patients with myelofibrosis (see Figure 14-41).

Splenic Atrophy: Autosplenectomy

The term *autosplenectomy* is used to denote the atrophy of the spleen secondary to spontaneous widespread infarction, leading to loss of splenic function. In the vast majority of cases, this is a complication of homozygous sickle cell disease but has rarely been reported as a complication of pneumococcal septicemia and SLE.[153,154] The spleen is prone to infarction in sickle cell disease because the slow flow and relative hypoxemia of the spleen results in sickling of red cells leading to microvascular occlusion and infarction. Complete infarction of the spleen has typically occurred by the age of 8.[155] In most cases, patients are asymptomatic but are predisposed to bacterial infections with encapsulated organisms because of the loss of splenic function. Repeated episodes of infarction result in atrophy of the spleen. Chronically, the spleen can become diffusely calcified.

Imaging examinations demonstrate diminished size of the spleen in all cases and will often demonstrate diffuse calcifications as increased opacity on plain films, increased attenuation on CT, and shadowing on US.[152,156,157] Calcification can diffusely involve the spleen, be seen as multiple punctate foci or as curvilinear calcification (see Figures 14-27 and 14-42). Calcifications are common, demonstrated on plain films in 31% of 182 subjects, with an increasing prevalence with increasing age of the subject.[156] On MRI examinations, the spleens of patients with sickle cell disease are typically decreased in signal intensity on both T1- and T2-weighted sequences because of the iron deposition in the spleen.[158]

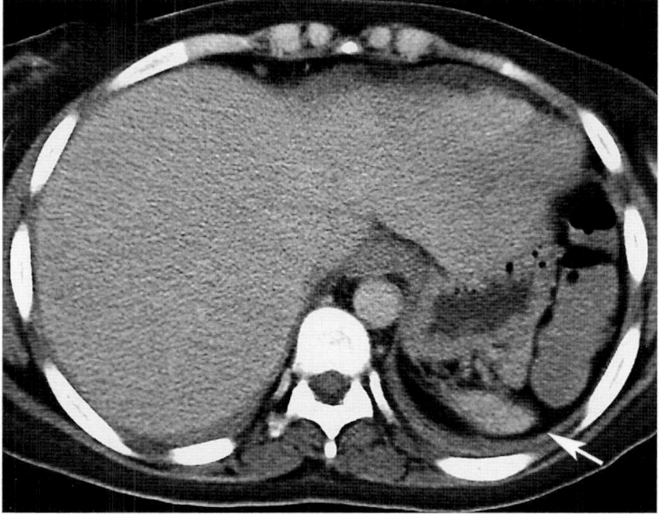

Figure 14-42 Sickle Cell Autosplenectomy
This 21-year-old woman with sickle cell disease presented with fever and jaundice. The spleen (*arrow*) is diminutive and minimally increased in attenuation. This splenic atrophy is a result of repeated splenic infarction.

Unique Anomalies of the Spleen

There are several congenital anomalies of the spleen that can result in an abnormal appearance, location, or number of splenic tissue.

Wandering spleen

Wandering or ectopic spleen refers to migration of the spleen from its normal site in the left upper quadrant to a more caudal location in the abdomen as a result of laxity or maldevelopment of the supporting splenic ligaments.[159] It is a rare entity, found incidentally in less than 0.2% of patients undergoing splenectomy.[160]

The long pedicle renders the spleen hypermobile, predisposing it to torsion. Patients can be asymptomatic; present with a mobile mass in the abdomen; or present with acute, chronic, or intermittent abdominal pain due to torsion of the wandering spleen.[161]

The most characteristic imaging finding is absence of the spleen in its normal position and a soft-tissue mass resembling the spleen located somewhere else in the abdomen or pelvis.[159] The most common location of the spleen is in the left midabdomen.

The whirl sign of the splenic pedicle, representing the twisted splenic vessels and surrounding fat, is reported to be specific for splenic torsion.[160] Twisting of the tail of the pancreas along with torsion of the splenic pedicle has been reported in cases with acute splenic torsion and can cause clinical signs of acute pancreatitis.[162,163] An additional finding in acute torsion is total or partial splenic infarction, the imaging findings of which are described in detail earlier in this chapter.

Heterotaxy syndromes

Heterotaxy is defined as the abnormal placement of organs. There are 2 defined heterotaxy syndromes, polysplenia and asplenia, that are due to failure to establish the normal left-right patterning during embryonic development. Although abnormalities of the spleen are some of the most recognizable features of these syndromes, clinical outcomes of these patients are primarily related to the severity of congenital heart disease.

Polysplenia syndrome: Polysplenia syndrome is a complex congenital anomaly characterized by partial visceral heterotaxia (situs ambiguous) and concomitant levo isomerism (bilateral left-sidedness). It is usually diagnosed in childhood because of the various and often severe cardiac anomalies that are a part of the syndrome.[164] Most patients with polysplenia syndrome die by the age of 5 years due to severe cardiac anomalies.[165] Five percent to 10% of patients with polysplenia syndrome have a normal heart or only minor cardiac defects and reach adulthood without symptoms, and the syndrome may then be incidentally discovered by US, CT, or MRI of the abdomen.[164]

As the name of the syndrome implies, multiple discrete spleens are considered the hallmark of the syndrome.

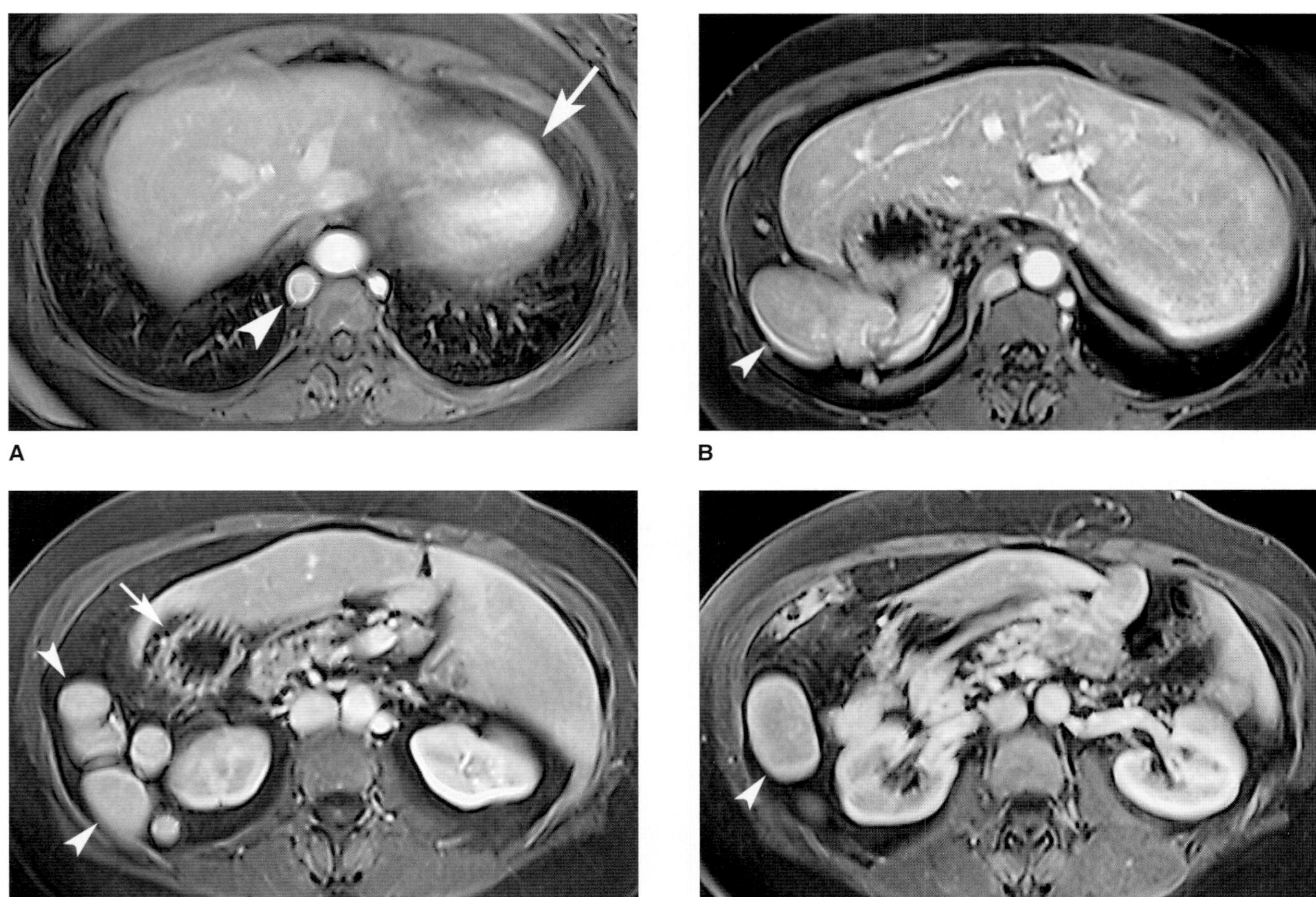

Figure 14-43 Polysplenia
This 52-year-old woman had congenital heart disease. **A-D.** Axial T1-weighted contrast-enhanced images show a left-sided heart (*large arrow*), right-sided stomach (*small arrow*), and multiple splenules (*small arrowheads*) and a large midline liver. Features are characteristic of polysplenia. Note the dilated hemiazygous vein (*large arrowhead* in A) indicating interruption of the IVC and azygous continuation.

However, there is a wide variation ranging from many very small spleens to a multilobular spleen with tiny accessory spleens and even an undivided spleen.[164] The spleens may be left-sided or right-sided and are always on the same side as the stomach and almost always along the greater curvature (see Figure 14-43).[166]

The liver is most often located in the midline extending symmetrically to both sides of the upper abdomen. The gallbladder is usually in a central location, and anomalies may also affect the branching pattern of the biliary tree. A shortened pancreas, consisting only of the pancreatic head, may be associated with polysplenia syndrome.[167] Mirror image location of the bowel and mesenteric vessels is frequently seen in polysplenia.[168]

The most common venous anomaly associated with polysplenia syndrome is interruption of the inferior vena cava with azygos or hemiazygos continuation, occurring in 65% to 80% of individuals with polysplenia.[169] Caudal to the caval interruption, the inferior vena cava may lie to the right or the left of the midline, or may be duplicated. The hepatic segment of the inferior vena cava is often absent, and the hepatic veins drain directly into the right atrium.[170]

Asplenia syndrome: Asplenia is generally characterized by an abnormal arrangement of the abdominal organs and absence of the spleen. As in polysplenia, there is partial visceral heterotaxia (situs ambiguous) but in this case there is generally dextro isomerism (bilateral right-sidedness). Congenital heart disease complicates this anomaly in up to 99% to 100% of patients, accounting for a very high mortality rate of up to 95% of patients in the first year of life.[168]

As the name implies, the spleen is absent or rudimentary. The liver and gallbladder are often midline in location.[169] The pancreas can be shortened, consisting only of the pancreatic head.[168] Venous anomalies can include bilateral inferior vena cava (see Figure 14-44).

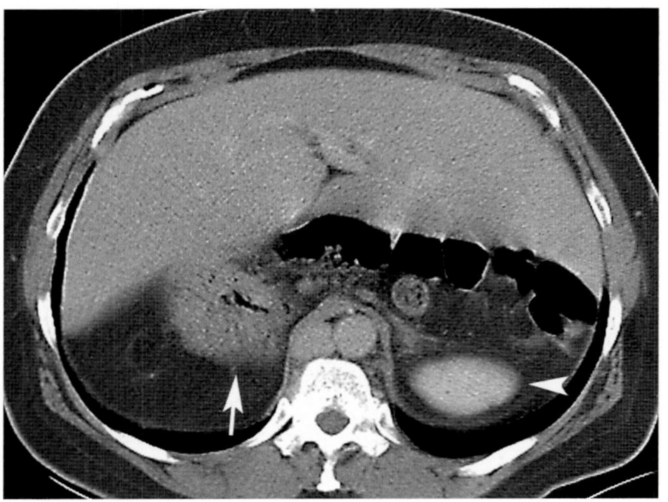

Figure 14-44 Asplenia
This 50-year-old woman was being evaluated for a neck mass. Contrast-enhanced CT shows a large midline liver with the stomach (*arrow*) in the right upper quadrant and absence of all splenic tissue. The oval structure in the left upper quadrant is the top of the left kidney (*arrowhead*). This patient had situs inversus of the thorax but had no congenital heart disease and is one of a tiny minority of patients with tiny minority of patients with asplenia to survive to adulthood.

Table 14-9. Causes of Multiple Calcified Splenic Nodules

1. Granulomatous infection a. **Histoplasmosis**[a] b. **Tuberculosis**
2. Other infections a. *Pneumocystis jiroveci* b. Schistosomiasis
3. Amyloidosis
4. Sarcoidosis
5. Anthrasilicosis
6. Gamna-Gandy bodies (cirrhosis)

[a]Disorders in bold are most common.

Splenic calcifications

Calcifications will appear as increased opacity on plain films, increased attenuation on CT scans, and as echogenic structures on US examinations. Diffuse calcification is usually seen with splenic atrophy and is a manifestation of sickle cell disease and has been discussed previously under the heading: **Splenic Atrophy: Autosplenectomy**. Small punctate calcifications are most often due to granulomatous infections but can be a result of a variety of other disorders (Table 14-9).

Splenic granulomas: One or many small spherical calcifications in the spleen will most often be a manifestation of granulomatous disease, most often tuberculosis or histoplasmosis.[171,172] These are a common incidental finding on imaging examinations and have no clinical significance other than as a marker for previous granulomatous infection (see Figure 14-45). The presence of more than a few calcified nodules will usually indicate histoplasmosis as the cause, whereas smaller numbers of granulomas will often be due to tuberculosis.[173,174] In areas where histoplasmosis is endemic, the majority of splenic

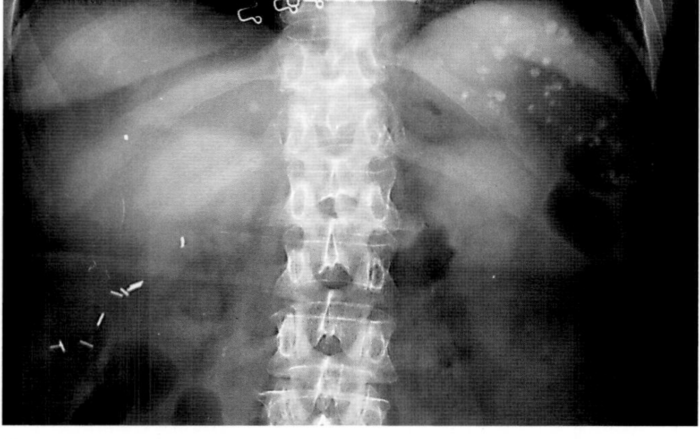

A

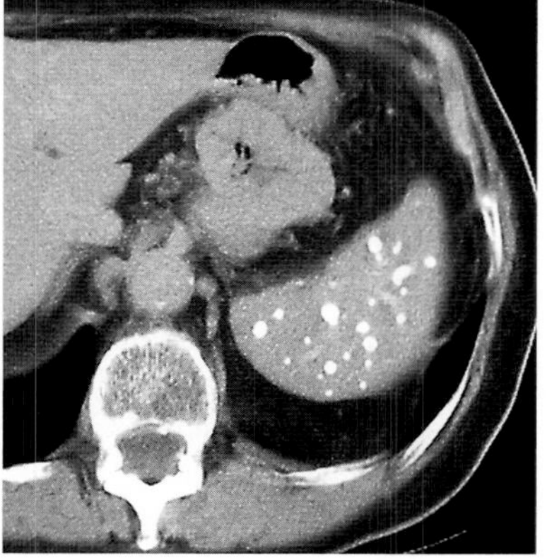

B

Figure 14-45 Calcified Granulomas of the Spleen
A. Abdominal x-ray and (**B**) CT scan both demonstrate multiple oval calcifications in the spleen, typical of splenic granulomas probably secondary to histoplasmosis.

calcifications will be secondary to histoplasmosis. In regions of the world where histoplasmosis is uncommon, tuberculosis will be the most common cause of small focal splenic calcifications.

Rare causes of multiple small splenic calcifications: Rarely primary and secondary amyloidosis, sarcoidosis, anthrasilicosis, *Pneumocystis jiroveci* infection, and schistosomiasis can result in multiple small calcifications in the spleen and liver.[111,175-178] Gamna-Gandy bodies due to liver cirrhosis will occasionally calcify and appear as multiple punctate calcifications in the spleen on CT and US examinations; however, their primary manifestation is signal loss on MRI and will be discussed in detail under the subsequent heading: **Iron deposition.**

Iron deposition in the spleen

Hemosiderin deposits in the spleen in most cases do not cause abnormalities detectable by plain films, CT, or US. However, the paramagnetic properties of hemosiderin result in T1 and T2 shortening and cause loss of signal of the spleen on both T1- and T2-weighted images. In hemosiderosis, this results in diffuse signal loss of the spleen; however, in the case of cirrhosis, small petechial hemorrhages called Gamna-Gandy bodies result in characteristic multiple small foci of signal loss.

Hemosiderosis: Iron overload can be due to 1 of 2 underlying causes: (1) multiple transfusions or (2) increased gut resorption of iron.[179] Excess iron from blood transfusions is deposited in the reticuloendothelial system and in the parenchymal cells of the liver, spleen, and other organs, including the heart and lymph nodes and is known as hemosiderosis.[180] Hemosiderosis can be distinguished from hemochromatosis, the other primary cause of iron overload, by the presence of iron overload in the spleen. Iron deposition in hemochromatosis will spare the spleen and bone marrow but involve the liver and pancreas, whereas hemosiderosis will involve all 4 organs. The amount of iron overload can be quantified by MRI examinations when necessary (see Figure 14-46).[181]

Gamna-gandy bodies: Gamna-Gandy bodies, also called siderotic nodules, are small fibrotic nodules that occur within the spleen as a result of small petechial hemorrhages. These will contain hemosiderin, the chronic byproduct of hemorrhage and can also contain small areas of dystrophic calcification.[182-185] These small lesions are typically a result of portal hypertension but can rarely be due to hemolytic anemia and leukemia.

Gamna-Gandy bodies can be detected on cross-sectional imaging because of the imaging characteristics of hemosiderin and calcium. In general, MRI examinations are the most sensitive study for the detection of Gamna-Gandy bodies which can be seen in 10% to 15% of patients with portal hypertension and approximately 6% of patients with chronic liver disease.[182] The ferritin in hemosiderin causes susceptibility artifact, leading to loss of signal in the surrounding tissues. This appears as multiple small low-signal foci within the spleen. Gradient echo sequences are more sensitive to susceptibility artifact and therefore the lesions will appear larger on gradient echo sequences.[182] Further, US and CT examinations can detect Gamna-Gandy bodies through the presence of small dystrophic calcifications that appear as small echogenic foci on US examinations and as punctate hyperattenuating dots on CT examinations.[182-185] The small areas of fibrosis can also appear as tiny hypoattenuating nodules on contrast-enhanced CT (see Figure 14-47).

POSTOPERATIVE FINDINGS RELATED TO SPLENIC SURGERY

There are various normal and abnormal imaging findings related to splenectomy that can be detected by abdominal imaging, including long-term regeneration of small residual amounts of splenic tissue, called splenosis.

Normal Postoperative Findings

Accumulation of a small amount of sterile, reactive peritoneal effusion of water density is a common normal finding in the immediate postoperative period. Most of these collections are not encapsulated, are confined to the surgical bed, and resolve on follow-up studies. A small amount of left-sided pleural effusion and posterior displacement of the stomach into the subphrenic space is also expected.[186]

Pneumoperitoneum is another common finding following recent intra-abdominal surgery, which usually disappears within days. A persistent or increasing amount of free air in the peritoneum beyond the first postoperative week in the absence of an abdominal drain or dehiscent incision is suggestive of perforation of the gastrointestinal tract.[187]

Splenosis

Splenosis is defined as autotransplantation of splenic tissue in various abnormal sites after splenic injury that can be either traumatic or iatrogenic during surgery. Iatrogenic splenosis occurs more often during laparoscopic splenectomy. Abdominal splenosis is the most common form, and although it usually has no clinical significance, may cause relapse of hematologic disorders.[188] Thoracic splenosis is less common, usually occurring following combined diaphragmatic and splenic injury, leading to the formation of left-sided, pleural-based pulmonary nodules or masses.[189]

Residual splenic function following splenectomy may occur due to an unidentified accessory spleen in

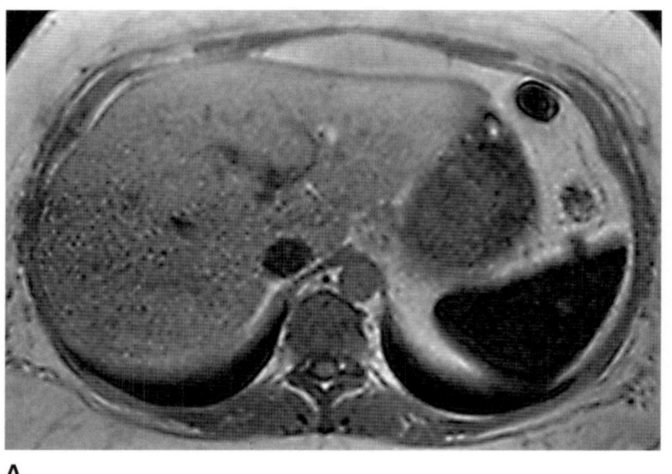
A

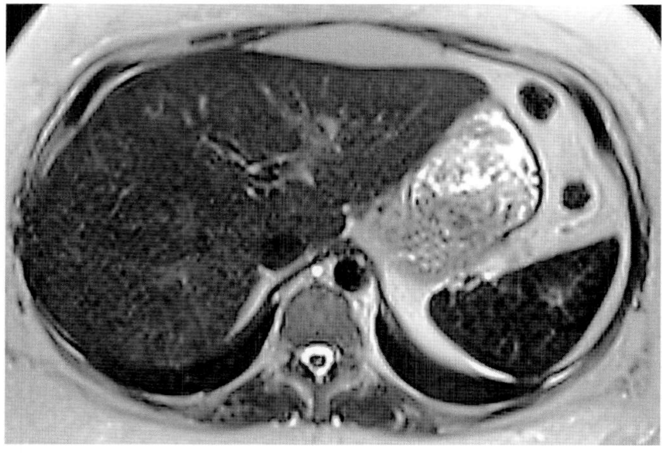
B

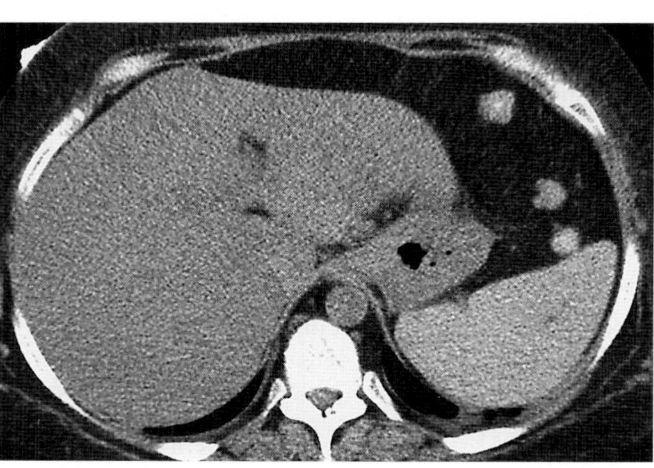
C

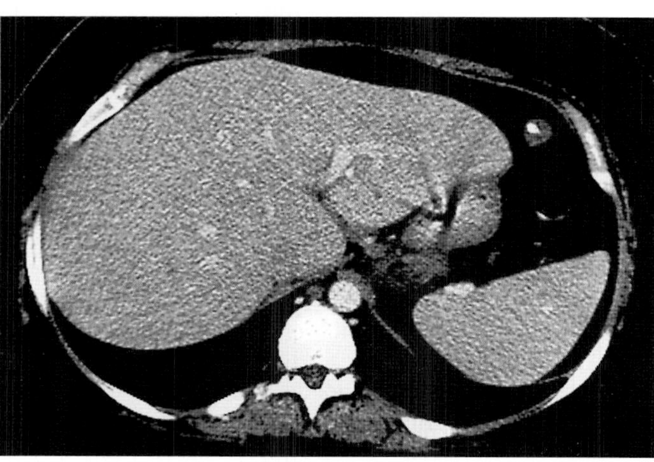
D

Figure 14-46 Hemosiderosis of the Spleen
This 33-year-old woman had undergone stem cell transplant for Hodgkin lymphoma. **A.** T1-weighted and (**B**) T2-weighted MRI sequences show the spleen to be diffusely low signal. The liver is also lower signal than normal, although to a lesser degree than the spleen. This is the typical finding of hemosiderosis. **C.** Unenhanced CT shows the spleen to be slightly higher attenuation than the liver, also indicating the greater deposition of hemosiderin in the spleen. **D.** The difference in attenuation between liver and spleen is masked by the presence of IV contrast in this contrast-enhanced image.

the abdominal cavity that was left in situ or from aforementioned splenosis auto-transplants left behind (see Figure 14-48). Such residual functioning splenic tissue helps preserve the host defense mechanism. However, when splenectomy was performed for the management of hematologic disease, residual functioning splenic tissue may induce relapse and is considered failure of surgical management.

The diagnosis of splenosis or residual splenic tissue can be confirmed using nuclear scintigraphy with radiolabeled heat-damaged red blood cells or 99mTc-sulfur colloid, which detects functioning splenic tissue foci as small as 2 cm or smaller when using SPECT.[190] Further localization of functioning tissue can then be demonstrated with CT prior to repeat surgery.

Complications of Splenic Surgery

Complications of splenic surgery include intra-abdominal abscess, portal or splenic vein thrombosis, and injury to adjacent structures.

Intra-abdominal abscess

Intra-abdominal abscess remains the main cause of morbidity in the postsplenectomy patient. CT is highly accurate in diagnosing postoperative abscess and is the preferred imaging modality in assessing its presence, location, and size. The CT features of an abscess include a well-circumscribed fluid collection, occasionally with peripheral enhancing rim, which may contain gas bubbles or an air-fluid level. The abscess may, however, appear as a mass of

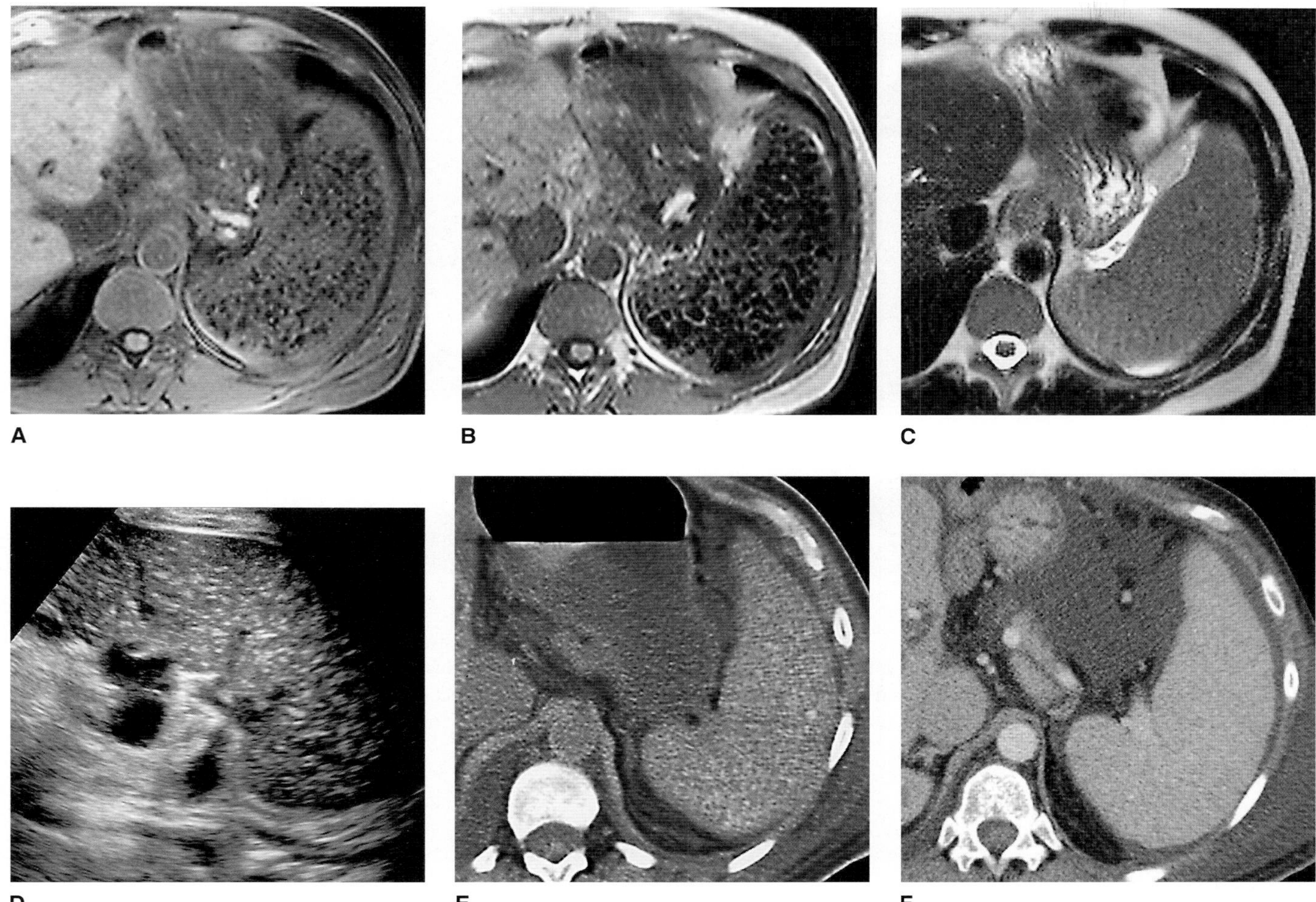

Figure 14-47 Gamna-Gandy Bodies
This 55-year-old woman had alcoholic cirrhosis. **A.** T1-weighted and (**B**) T1*- and T2-weighted MRI sequences show innumerable small low-signal lesions throughout the spleen. Note how the lesions appear larger on the T1* sequence. This is a susceptibility artifact and indicates the presence of a paramagnetic substance, most often hemosiderin. **C.** The low-attenuation regions are much less apparent on this T2-weighted sequence. **D.** US image shows innumerable small echogenic foci in the spleen, most likely due to many small splenic calcifications. **E.** Unenhanced and (**F**) contrast-enhanced CT images show a combination of multiple tiny hyperattenuating foci typical of calcifications, associated with multiple small hypoattenuating foci, in this case due to small foci of fibrosis. These are all imaging findings of Gamna-Gandy bodies due to small foci of hemorrhage in this patient with portal hypertension.

soft-tissue density within inflamed peritoneal planes. In addition, CT plays a therapeutic role by guiding percutaneous drainage of an abscess.

Portal or splenic vein thrombosis

Thrombosis of the portal venous system is an infrequent complication after splenectomy, but occurs more often following laparoscopic than open splenectomy.[191] On contrast-enhanced CT, a filling defect within the portomesenteric vein is diagnostic of venous thrombosis. If unrecognized and left untreated, this may appear later as cavernous transformation of the portal vein.

Injuries to adjacent structures

Intraoperative manipulation or improper use of electrocautery during splenectomy may lead to direct pancreatic injury and postoperative pancreatitis that may become complicated with pseudocyst formation.[10] Gastric injury, including perforation and mural necrosis, may be caused during dissection and ligation of the short gastric vessels in the splenogastric ligament.[192] On CT, gastric wall injury and perforation present as a localized fluid collection with gas bubbles and/or ingested oral contrast in the splenic bed, or with large-volume hydropneumoperitoneum. Injury to adjacent colon is a rare additional possible complication.

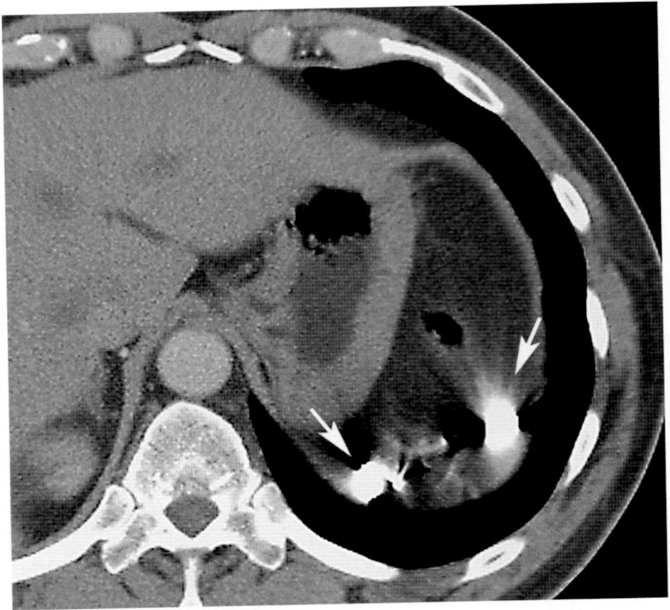

A

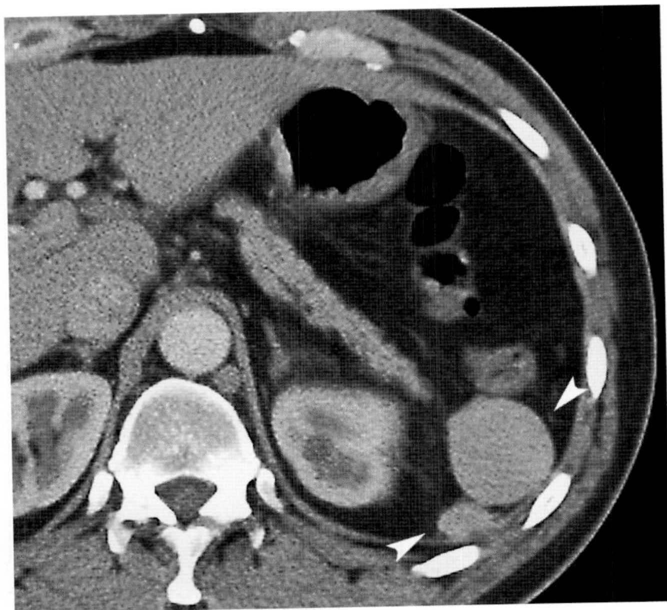

B

Figure 14-48 Splenosis
This 53-year-old man had a splenectomy for splenic trauma several years previously. **A.** Contrast-enhanced CT of the left upper quadrant shows several surgical clips (*arrows*) and absence of the spleen consistent with the prior splenectomy. **B.** Image a few centimeters lower shows 2 rounded masses (*arrowheads*) in the inferior aspect of the surgical bed. These represent regenerated splenic nodules: splenosis.

REFERENCES

1. Megremis S, Vlachonikolis I, Tsilimigaki A. Spleen length in childhood with US: normal values based on age, sex, and somatometric parameters. *Radiology.* 2004;231:129-134.
2. Dodds W, Taylor A, Erickson S, et al. Radiologic imaging of splenic anomalies. *AJR Am J Roentgenol.* 1990;155: 805-810.
3. Paterson A, Frush D, Donnelly L, et al. A pattern-oriented approach to splenic imaging in infants and children. *Radiographics.* 1999;19:1465-1485.
4. Donnelly L, Foss J, Frush D, et al. Heterogeneous splenic enhancement patterns on spiral CT images in children: minimizing misinterpretation. *Radiology.* 1999;210: 493-497.
5. Mirowitz S, Brown J, Lee J, et al. Dynamic gadolinium-enhanced MR imaging of the spleen: normal enhancement patterns and evaluation of splenic lesions. *Radiology.* 1991;179:681-686.
6. Gallagher B, Ansari A, Atkins H, et al. Radiopharmaceuticals XXVII: ^{18}F-labeled 2-deoxy-2-fluoro-D-glucose as a radiopharmaceutical for measuring regional myocardial glucose metabolism in vivo—tissue distribution and imaging studies in animals. *J Nucl Med.* 1977;18:990-996.
7. Abbott R, Angela D, Aguilera N, et al. Primary vascular neoplasms of the spleen: radiologic-pathologic correlation. *Radiographics.* 2004;24:1137-1163.
8. Abbott R, Angela D, Aguilera N, et al. Primary vascular neoplasms of the spleen: radiologic-pathologic correlation. *Radiographics.* 2004;24:1137-1163.
9. Ramani M, Reinhold C, Semelka R, et al. Splenic hemangiomas and hamartomas: MR imaging characteristics of 28 lesions. *Radiology.* 1997;202:166-172.
10. Targarona E, Espert J, Bombuy E, et al. Complications of laparoscopic splenectomy. *Arch Surg.* 2000;135:1137-1140.
11. Wijaya J, Kapoor R, Roach P. Tc-99m-labeled RBC scintigraphy and splenic hemangioma. *Clin Nucl Med.* 2001; 26:1022-1023.
12. Gulenchyn K, Dover M, Kelly S. Splenic hemangioma presenting as a hot spot on radiocolloid scintigraphy. *J Nucl Med.* 1986;27:804-806.
13. Solomou E, Patriarheas G, Mpadra F, et al. Asymptomatic adult cystic lymphangioma of the spleen: case report and review of the literature. *Magn Reson Imaging.* 2003;21:81-84.
14. Morgenstern L, Bello J, Fisher B, et al. The clinical spectrum of lymphangiomas and lymphangiomatosis of the spleen. *Am Surg.* 1992;58:599-604.
15. Wadsworth D, Newman B, Abramson S, et al. Splenic lymphangiomatosis in children. *Radiology.* 1997;202:173-176.
16. Warnke R, Weiss L, Chan J, et al. *Tumors of the lymph nodes and spleen.* 3rd series ed. Washington, DC: Armed Forces Institute of Pathology; 1995.
17. Duchesne JC, Simmons JD, Schmieg RE Jr, McSwain NE Jr, Bellows CF. Proximal splenic angioembolization does not improve outcomes in treating blunt splenic injuries compared with splenectomy: a cohort analysis. *J Trauma.* 2008;65:1346-51.
18. Bader T, Ranner G, Kimpfinger M. Case report: CT appearance of capillary and cavernous lymphangiomatosis of the spleen in an adult. *Clin Radiol.* 1998;53:379-387.

19. Bezzi M, Spinelli A, Pierleoni M, et al. Cystic lymphangioma of the spleen: US-CT-MRI correlation. *Eur Radiol.* 2001;11: 1187-1190.

20. Westh H, Reines E, Skibsted L. Splenic abscesses: a review of 20 cases. *Scand J Infect Dis.* 1990;22:569-573.

21. Fotiadis C, Lavranos G, Patapis P, et al. Abscesses of the spleen: report of three cases. *World J Gastroenterol.* 2008;14: 3088-3091.

22. Losanoff J, Basson M. Splenic abscess. emedicine.medscape. com/article/194655-overview.

23. Lee C, Leu H, Hum T, Liu J. Splenic abscess in southern Taiwan. *J Microbiol Immunol Infect.* 2004;37:39-44.

24. Tung C, Chen F, Lo C. Splenic abscess: an easily overlooked disease? *Am Surg.* 2006;72:322-325.

25. Ulhaci N, Meteoglu I, Kacar F, Ozbas S. Abscess of the spleen. *Pathol Oncol Res.* 2004;10(4):234-236.

26. Villamil-Cajoto I, Lado F, Van den Eynde-Collado A, Díaz-Peromingo J. Splenic abscess: presentation of nine cases. *Rev Chilena Infectol.* 2006;23:150-154.

27. Al-Salem A, Qaisaruddin S, Al Jam'a A, Al-Kalaf J, El-Bashier A. Splenic abscess and sickle cell disease. *Am J Hematol.* 1998;58:100-104.

28. Chang K, Chuah S, Changchien C, et al. Clinical characteristics and prognostic factors of splenic abscess: a review of 67 cases in a single medical center of Taiwan. *World J Gastroenterol.* 2006;12:460-464.

29. Chun C, Raff M, et al. Splenic Abscess. *Medicine (Baltimore).* 1990;59:50-65.

30. Nelken N, Ignatius J, Skinner M, Christensen N. Changing clinical spectrum of splenic abscess. *Am J Surg.* 1987;154:27-34.

31. Ooi L, Leong S. Splenic abscess from 1987-1995. *Am J Surg.* 1997;174:87-93.

32. Alvi A, Kulsoom S, Shamsi G. Splenic abscess: outcome and prognostic factors. *J Coll Physicians Surg Pak.* 2008;18:740-743.

33. Zerem E, Bergsland J. Ultrasound guided percutaneous treatment for splenic abscesses: the significance in treatment of critically ill patients. *World J Gastroenterol.* 2006;12: 7341-7345.

34. Ferraioli G, Brunetti E, Gulizia R, Mariani G, Marone P, Filice C. Management of splenic abscess: report on 16 cases from a single center. *Int J Infect Dis.* 2009;13:524-530.

35. Chiang I, Lin T, Chiang I, Tsai M. Splenic abscesses: review of 29 cases. *Kaohsiung J Med Sci.* 2003;19:510-515.

36. Urrutia M, Mergo P, Ros L, et al. Cystic masses of the spleen: radiologic-pathologic correlation. *Radiographics.* 1996;16: 107-129.

37. Ng K, Lee T, Wan Y, et al. Splenic abscess: diagnosis and management. *Hepatogastroenterology.* 2002; 49:567-571.

38. Fowler R. Hydatid cysts of spleen. *Int Abstr Surg.* 1953;96:105-116.

39. Manterola C, Vial M, Losada H, et al. Uncommon locations of abdominal hydatid disease. *Trop Doct.* 2003;33:179-180.

40. Durgun V, Kapan S, Kapan M, et al. Primary splenic hydatidosis. *Dig Surg.* 2003; 20:38-41.

41. Polat P, Kantarci M, Alper F, et al. Hydatid disease from head to toe. *Radiographics.* 2003;23:475-494; quiz 536-537.

42. Atmatzidis K, Papaziogas B, Mirelis C, et al. Splenectomy versus spleen-preserving surgery for splenic echinococcus. *Dig Surg.* 2003;20:527-531.

43. Franquet T, Montes M, Lecumberri F, et al. Hydatid disease of the spleen: imaging findings in 9 patients. *AJR Am J Roentgenol.* 1990;154:525-528.

44. von Sinner W, Stnidbeck H. Hydatid disease of the spleen: ultrasonography, CT, and MR imaging. *Acta Radiol.* 1992;33:459-461.

45. von Sinner W, te Strake L, Clark D, et al. MR imaging in hydatid disease. *AJR Am J Roentgenol.* 1991;157:741-745.

46. Marani S, Canossi G, Nicoli F, et al. Hydatid disease: MR imaging study. *Radiology.* 1990;175:701-706.

47. Ito K, Mitchell K, Honjo K, et al. MR imaging of acquired abnormalities of the spleen. *AJR Am J Roentgenol.* 1997;168: 697-702.

48. Garvin D, King F. Cysts and nonlymphomatous tumors of the spleen. *Pathol Annu.* 1981;16:61-80.

49. Robbins F, Yellin A, Lingua R, Craig J, Turrill F, Mikkelsen W. Splenic epidermoid cysts. *Ann Surg.* 1978;187:231-235.

50. Maskey P, Rupakheti S, Regmi R, Adhikary S, Agrawal C. Splenic epidermoid cyst. *Kathmandu Univ Med J.* 2007;5: 250-252.

51. Heider R, Behrns K. Pancreatic pseudocysts complicated by splenic parenchymal involvement: results of operative and percutaneous management. *Pancreas.* 2001;23:20-25.

52. Georg C, Schwerk W, Georg K, et al. Sonographic patterns of the affected spleen in malignant lymphoma. *J Clin Ultrasound.* 1990;18:569-574.

53. Ahmann D, Kiely J, Harrison EG Jr, Payne WS. Malignant lymphoma of the spleen. A review of 49 cases in which the diagnosis was made at splenectomy. *Cancer.* 1966;19:461-469.

54. Schon C, Gorg C, Ramaswamy A, et al. Splenic metastases in a large unselected autopsy series. *Pathol Res Pract.* 2006;202: 351-356.

55. Falk S, Krishnan J, Meis J. Primary angiosarcoma of the spleen. *Am J Surg Pathol.* 1993;17:959-970.

56. Thompson W, Levy A, Aguilera N, et al. Angiosarcoma of the spleen: imaging characteristics in 12 patients. *Radiology.* 2005; 235:106-115.

57. Krishnan J, Frizzera G. Two splenic lesions in need of clarification: hamartoma and inflammatory pseudotumor. *Semin Diagn Pathol.* 2003;20:94-104.

58. Ohtomo K, Fukuda H, Mori K, et al. CT and MR appearances of splenic hamartoma. *J Comput Assist Tomogr.* 1992;16:425-428.

59. Gulenchyn K, Dover M, Kelly S. Splenic hemangioma presenting as a hot spot on radiocolloid scintigraphy. *J Nucl Med.* 1986;27:804-806.

60. Safran D, Welch J, Requke W. Inflammatory pseudotumor of the spleen. *Arch Surg.* 1991;126:904-908.

61. Monforte-Mujnoz H, Ro J, Manning J. Inflammatory pseudotumor of the spleen: report of two cases with a review of the literature. *Am J Clin Pathol.* 1991;96:491-495.

62. Franquet T, Montes M, Aizcorbe M, et al. Inflammatory pseudotumor of the spleen: ultrasound and computed tomographic findings. *Gastrointest Radiol.* 1989;14:181-183.

63. Glazer M, Lally J, Kanzer M. Inflammatory pseudotumor of the spleen: MR findings. *J Comput Assist Tomogr.* 1992;16:980-983.

64. Tinkoff G, Esposito T, Reed J, et al. American Association for the Surgery of Trauma Organ Injury Scale I: Spleen, Liver, and Kidney, Validation Based on the National Trauma Data Bank. *J Am Coll Surg.* 2008;207:646-655.

65. Peitzman A, Heil B, Rivera L, et al. Blunt splenic injury in adults: multiinstitutional study of the Eastern Association for the Surgery of Trauma. *J Trauma.* 2000;49:177-189.

66. Haan J, Scott J, Boyd-Kranis R, Ho S, Kramer M, Scalea T. Admission angiography for blunt splenic injury: advantages and pitfalls. *J Trauma.* 2001;51:1161-1165.

67. Pachter H, Guth A, Hofstetter S, Spencer F. Changing patterns in the management of splenic trauma: the impact of nonoperative management. *Ann Surg.* 1998;227:708-719.

68. Bee T, Croce M, Miller P, et al. Failures of splenic nonoperative management: is the glass half empty or half full? *J Trauma.* 2001;50:230-236.

69. Velmahos G, Chan L, Kamel E, et al. Nonoperative management of splenic injuries: have we gone too far? *Arch Surg.* 2000;135:674-681.

70. Boulanger B, Kearney P, Brenneman F, et al. Utilization of FAST (Focused Assessment with Sonography for Trauma) in 1999: results of a survey of North American trauma centers. *Am Surg.* 2000;66:1049-1055.

71. Goldberg B, Goodman G, Clearfield H. Evaluation of ascites by ultrasound. *Radiology.* 1970;96:15-22.

72. Shanmuganathan K, Mirvis S, Sherbourne C, et al. Hemoperitoneum as the sole indicator of abdominal visceral injuries: a potential limitation of screening abdominal US for trauma. *Radiology.* 1999;212:423-430.

73. Röthlin M, Näf R, Amgwerd M, Candinas D, Frick T, Trentz O. Ultrasound in blunt abdominal and thoracic trauma. *J Trauma.* 1993;34:488-495.

74. Goletti O, Ghiselli G, Lippolis P, et al. The role of ultrasonography in blunt abdominal trauma: results in 250 consecutive cases. *J Trauma.* 1994;36:178-181.

75. Becker D, Metha G, Terrier F. Blunt abdominal trauma in adults: role of CT in the diagnosis and management of visceral injuries Part 1: liver and spleen. *Eur Radiol.* 1998;8:553-562.

76. Sclafani S. The use of angiographic hemostasis in salvage of the injured spleen. *Radiology.* 1981;141:645-650.

77. Haan J, Biffl W, Knudson MM, et al. Splenic embolization revisited: a multicenter review. *J Trauma.* 2004;56:542-547.

78. Shanmugnathan K, Mirvis S, Boyd-Kranis R, et al. Nonsurgical management of blunt splenic injury: use of CT criteria to select patients for splenic arteriography and potential endovascular therapy. *Radiology.* 2000;217:75-82.

79. Thompson B, Munera F, Cohn S, et al. Computed tomography scan scoring system predicts the need for intervention after splenic injury. *Trauma.* 2006;60:1083-1086.

80. Shanmuganathan K, Mirvis S, Sover E. Value of contrast-enhanced CT in detecting active hemorrhage in patients with blunt abdominal or pelvic trauma. *AJR Am J Roengenol.* 1993;161:65-69.

81. De Schepper A, Vanhoenacker F, de Beeck BO, et al. Vascular pathology of the spleen, part II. *Abdom Imaging.* 2005;30: 228-238.

82. Jaroch M, Broughan T, Hermann R. The natural history of splenic infarction. *Surgery.* 1986;100:743.

83. Goerg C, Schwerk W. Splenic infarction: sonographic patterns, diagnosis, follow-up, and complications. *Radiology.* 1990;174:803.

84. Robertson F, Leander P, Ekberg O. Radiology of the spleen. *Eur Radiol.* 2001;11:80-95.

85. Rabushka L, Kawashima A, Fishman E. Imaging of the spleen: CT with supplemental MR examination. *Radiographics.* 1994; 14:307-332.

86. Hahn P, Weissleder R, Stark D, et al. MR imaging of focal splenic tumors. *AJR Am J Roentgenol.* 1988;150:823-827.

87. Abbott R, Levy A, Aguilera N, Gorospe L, Thompson W. From the archives of the AFIP primary vascular neoplasms of the spleen: radiologic-pathologic correlation. *Radiographics.* 2004;24:1137-1163.

88. Chang KC, Chuah SK, Changchien CS, Tsai TL, Lu SN, Chiu YC, et al. Clinical characteristics and prognostic factors of splenic abscess: a review of 67 cases in a single medical center of Taiwan. *World J Gastroenterol.* Jan 2006;12(3):460–464.

89. Chun CH, Raff MJ, Contreras L, Varghese R, Waterman N, Daffner R, et al. Splenic abscess. *Medicine (Baltimore).* 1990;59:50–65.

90. Nelken N, Ignatius J, Skinner M, Christensen N. Changing clinical spectrum of splenic abscess. *Am J Surg.* 1987;154:27–34

91. Ooi LL, Leong SS. Splenic abscess from 1987-1995. *Am J Surg.* 1997;174:87–93.

92. Ferraioli G, Brunetti E, Gulizia R, Mariani G, Marone P, Filice C. Management of splenic abscess: report on 16 cases from a single center. *Int J Infect Dis.* Jul 2009;13(4):524–530

93. Tan K, Chen K, Sim R. The spectrum of abdominal tuberculosis in a developed country: a single institution's experience over 7 years. *J Gastrointest Surg.* 2009;13:142-147.

94. Topal U, Savci G, Yurtkuran Sadikoglu M, Parlak M, Tuncel E. Splenic involvement of tuberculosis: US and CT findings. *Eur Radiol.* 1994;4:577-579.

95. Sharma S, Smith-Rohrberg D, Tahir M, Mohan A, Seith A. Radiological manifestations of splenic tuberculosis: a 23-patient case series from India. *Indian J Med Res.* 2007;125:669-678.

96. Rabushka L, Kawashima A, Fishman E. Imaging of the spleen: CT with supplemental MR examination. *Radiographics.* 1994;14:307-332.

97. Malik A, Saxena N. Ultrasound in abdominal tuberculosis. *Abdom Imaging.* 2003;28:574-579.

98. Radin R. HIV infection: analysis in 259 consecutive patients with abnormal abdominal CT findings. *Radiology.* 1995;197: 712-722.

99. Kapoor R, Jain A, Chaturvedi U, Saha M. Ultrasound detection of tuberculomas of the spleen. *Clin Radiol.* 1991;43:128-129.

100. Hasan M, Sarwar J, Bhuiyan J, Islam S. Tubercular splenic abscess. *Mymensingh J Med.* 2008;17:67-69.

101. Reichel C, Theisen A, Rockstroh J, Muller-Miny H, Spengler U, Sauerbruch T. Splenic abscesses and abdominal tuberculosis in patients with AIDS. *Z Gastroenterol.* 1996;34:494-496.

102. Radin D. Disseminated histoplasmosis: abdominal CT findings in 16 patients. *AJR Am J Roentgenol.* 1991;157(5): 955-958.

103. Buckner C, Leithiser R, Walker C, et al. The changing epidemiology of tuberculosis and other mycobacterial infections in the United States: implications for the radiologist. *AJR Am J Roentgenol.* 1991;156:255-264.

104. von Eift M, Essink M, Roos N, Hiddemann W, Buchner T, van de Loo J. Hepatosplenic candidiasis, a late manifestation of Candida septicaemia in neutropenic patients with haematologic malignancies. *Blut.* 1990;60:242-248.

105. Cho J, Kim E, Varma D, et al. MR imaging of hepatosplenic candidiasis superimposed on hemochromatosis. *J Comput Assist Tomogr.* 1990;14:774-776.

106. Pastakia B, Shawker T, Thaler M, O'Leary T, Pisso P. Hepatosplenic candidiasis: wheels within wheels. *Radiology.* 1988;166:417-421.

107. Chew F, Smith P, Barboniak D. Candidal splenic abscesses. *AJR Am J Roentgenol.* 1991;156:474.

108. Semelka R, Shoenut J, Greenberg H, Bow E. Detection of acute and treated lesions of hepatosplenic candidiasis: comparison of dynamic contrast-enhanced CT and MR imaging. *J Magn Reson Imaging.* 1992;2:341-345.

109. Lubat E, Megibow A, Balthazar E, et al. Extrapulmonary Pneumocystis carinii infection in AIDS. *Radiology.* 1990;174:157-160.

1110. Fishman E, Magid D, Kuhimanj E. Pneumocystis carinii involvement of the liver and spleen: CT demonstration. *J Comput Assist Tomogr.* 1990;14:146-148.

1111. Radin DR, Baker EL, Klatt EC, et al. Visceral and nodal calcification in patients with AIDS-related Pneumocystis carinii infection. *AJR Am J Roentgenol.* 1990;154:27-31.

112. Kahr A, Kerbl R, Gschwandtner K, et al. Visceral manifestation of cat scratch disease in children. A consequence of altered immunological state? *Infection.* 2000;28:116-118.

113. Ishikawa T, Suzuki T, Shinoda M, et al. A case of hepatosplenic cat scratch disease [in Japanese]. *Nippon Shokakibyo Gakkai Zasshi.* 2006;103:1050-1054.

114. Luciano A, Rossi F, Bolognani M, Trabucchi C. Hepatic and splenic micro-abscess in cat scratch disease. Report of a case [in Italian]. *Pediatr Med Chir.* 1999;21:89-91.

115. Baughman R, Teirstein A, Judson M, et al.; Case Control Etiologic Study of Sarcoidosis (ACCESS) research group. Clinical characteristics of patients in a case control study of sarcoidosis. *Am J Respir Crit Care Med.* 2001;164:1885-1889.

116. Judson M. Hepatic, splenic, and gastrointestinal involvement with sarcoidosis. *Semin Respir Crit Care Med.* 2002;23:529-541.

117. Warshauer D, Dumbleton S, Molina P, et al. Abdominal CT findings in sarcoidosis: radiologic and clinical correlation. *Radiology.* 1994;192:93-98.

118. Kessler A, Mitchell D, Israel H, et al. Hepatic and splenic sarcoidosis: US and MR imaging. *Abdom Imaging.* 1993;18: 159-163.

119. Folz S, Johnson C, Swensen S. Abdominal manifestations of sarcoidosis in CT studies. *J Comput Assist Tomogr.* 1995;19: 573-579.

120. Warshauer DM, Molina PL, Hamman SM, et al. Nodular sarcoidosis of the liver and spleen: analysis of 32 cases. *Radiology.* 1995;195:757-762.

121. Warshauer D, Molina P, Hamman S, et al. Nodular sarcoidosis of the liver and spleen: analysis of 32 cases. *Radiology.* 1995; 195:757-762.

122. Poll L, Koch J, vom Dahl S, et al. Gaucher disease of the spleen: CT and MR findings. *Abdom Imaging.* 2000;25:286-289.

123. Hosey RG, Mattacola CG, Kriss V, Armsey T, Quarles JD, Jagger J. Ultrasound assessment of spleen size in collegiate athletes. *Br J Sports Med.* 2006;40:251-254.

124. Spielmann AL, DeLong DM, Kliewer MA. Sonographic evaluation of spleen size in tall healthy athletes. *AJR Am J Roentgenol.* 2005;184:45-49.

125. Kaneko J, Sugawara Y, Matsui Y, Makuuchi M. Spleen size of live donors for liver transplantation. *Surg Radiol Anat.* 2008;30:515-518.

126. Loftus WK, Metreweli C. Normal splenic size in a Chinese population. *J Ultrasound Med.* 1997;16:345-347.

127. Prassopoulos P, Daskalogiannaki M, Raissaki M, Hatjidakis A, Gourtsoyiannis N. Determination of normal splenic volume on computed tomography in relation to age, gender and body habitus. *Eur Radiol.* 1997;7:246-248.

128. Geraghty EM, Boone JM, McGahan JP, Jain K. Normal organ volume assessment from abdominal CT. *Abdom Imaging.* 2004;29:482-490.

129. Bezerra AS, D'Ippolito G, Faintuch S, Szejnfeld J, Ahmed M. Determination of splenomegaly by CT: is there a place for a single measurement? *AJR Am J Roentgenol.* 2005;184:1510-1513.

130. Lamb PM, Lund A, Kanagasabay RR, Martin A, Webb JAW, Reznek RH. Spleen size: how well do linear ultrasound measurements correlate with three-dimensional CT volume assessments? *Br J Radiol.* 2002;75:573-577.

131. Weber SM, Rikkers LF. Splenic vein thrombosis and gastrointestinal bleeding in chronic pancreatitis. *World J Surg.* 2003;27:1271-1274.

132. Koklu S, Koksal A, Yolcu O, et al. Isolated splenic vein thrombosis: an unusual cause and review of the literature. *Can J Gastroenterol.* 2004;13:173-174.

133. Castellino R. Hodgkin disease: practical concepts for the diagnostic radiologist. *Radiology.* 1986;159:305-310.

134. Rueffer U, Sieber M, Stemberg M, et al.; German Hodgkin's Lymphoma Study Group (GHSG). Spleen involvement in Hodgkin's lymphoma: assessment and risk profile. *Ann Hematol.* 2003;82:390-396.

135. Breiman R, Castellino R, Harrell G, et al. CT-pathologic correlations in Hodgkin's disease and non-Hodgkin's lymphoma. *Radiology.* 1978;126:159-166.

136. Dachman A, Buck J, Krishnan J, et al. Primary non-Hodgkin's splenic lymphoma. *Clin Radiol.* 1998;53:137-142.

137. Munker R, Stengel A, Stabler A, et al. Diagnostic accuracy of ultrasound and computed tomography in the staging of Hodgkin's disease. Verification by laparotomy in 100 cases. *Cancer.* 1995;76:1460-1466.

138. Siniluoto T, Tikkakoski T, Lahde S, et al. Ultrasound or CT in splenic diseases? *Acta Radiol.* 1994;35:597-605.

139. Hess C, Griebel J, Schmiedl U, et al. Focal lesions of the spleen: preliminary results with fast MR imaging at 1.5 T. *J Comput Assist Tomogr.* 1988;2:569-574.

140. Rini J, Leonidas J, Tomas M, et al. ^{18}F-FDG PET versus CT for evaluating the spleen during initial staging of lymphoma. *J Nucl Med.* 2003;44:1072-1074.

141. Hicks R, Mac Manus M, Seymour J. Initial staging of lymphoma with positron emission tomography and computed tomography. *Semin Nucl Med.* 2005;35:165-175.

142. Egeler RM, Laura S, Pieter S, Carlos M, Mark EN. Malignant histiocytosis: a reassessment of cases formerly classified as histiocytic neoplasms and review of the literature. *Med Pediatr Oncol.* 1995;25:1-7.

143. James WV, Gerald EB Jr, Henry R. Malignant histiocytosis with massive splenomegaly in asymptomatic patients. A possible chronic form of the disease. *Cancer.* 1975;36: 419-427.

144. Hirsch MS. Cytomegalovirus infection. In: Braunwald E, Isselbacher KJ, Petersdorf RG, Wilson JD, Martin JB, Fauci AS, eds. *Harrison's Principles of Internal Medicine.* New York: McGraw-Hill; 1987:697-699.
145. Schooley RT. Epstein-Barr virus infections, including infectious mononucleosis. In: Braunwald E, Isselbacher KJ, Petersdorf RG, Wilson JD, Martin JB, Fauci AS, eds. *Harrison's Principles of Internal Medicine.* New York: McGraw-Hill; 1987: 699-703.
146. Singh B, Kim Sung L, Matusop A, et al. A large focus of naturally acquired Plasmodium knowlesi infections in human beings. *Lancet.* 2004;363:1017-1024.
147. Snow R, Guerra C, Noor A, Myint H, Hay S. The global distribution of clinical episodes of Plasmodium falciparum malaria. *Nature.* 2005;434:214-217.
148. Malaria Facts. Centers for Disease Control and Prevention.
149. Nadeem A, Ali N, Hussain T, Anwar M. Frequency and etiology of splenomegaly in adults seeking medical advice in Combined Military Hospital Attock. *J Ayub Med Coll Abbottabad.* 2004;16:44-47.
150. Timite-Konan M, Kouame K, Konan A, et al. Etiology of splenomegaly in children in the tropics. 178 cases reviewed at the university hospital center of Abidjan-Cocody (Ivory Coast) [in French]. *Ann Pediatr (Paris).* 1992;39:136-141.
151. Betticher D, Nicole A, Pugin P, Regamey C. The hyperreactive malarial splenomegaly syndrome in a European: has the treatment of a modulatory effect on the immune system? *J Infect Dis.* 1990;161:157-159.
152. Magid D, Fishman EK, Siegelman SS. Computed tomography of the spleen and liver in sickle cell disease. *AJR Am J Roentgenol.* 1984;143:245-249.
153. Eshel Y, Sarova-Pinhas I, Lampl Y, Jedwab M. Autosplenectomy complicating pneumococcal meningitis in an adult. *Arch Intern Med.* 1991;151:998-999.
154. Leipe J, Hueber AJ, Kallert S, Rech J, Schulze-Koops H. Autosplenectomy: rare syndrome in autoimmunopathy. *Ann Rheum Dis.* 2007;66:566-567.
155. Claster S, Vichinsky EP. Managing sickle cell disease. *BMJ.* 2003;327:1151-1155.
156. McCall I, Vaidya S, Serjeant G. Splenic opacification in homozygous sickle cell disease. *Clin Radiol.* 1981;32: 611-615.
157. Walker T, Serjeant G. Focal echogenic lesions in the spleen in sickle cell disease. *Clin Radiol.* 1993;47:114-116.
158. Adler DD, Glazer GM, Aisen AM. MRI of the spleen: normal appearance and findings in sickle-cell anemia. *AJR Am J Roentgenol.* 1986;147:843-845.
159. Gayer G, Zissin R, Apter S, et al. CT findings in congenital anomalies of the spleen. *Br J Radiol.* 2001;74:767-772.
160. Raissaki M, Prassopoulos P, Daskalogiannaki M, et al. Acute abdomen due to torsion of wandering spleen: CT diagnosis. *Eur Radiol.* 1998;8:1409-1412.
161. Taori K, Ghonge N, Prakash A. Wandering spleen with torsion of vascular pedicle: early diagnosis with multiplaner reformation technique of multislice spiral CT. *Abdom Imaging.* 2004;29:479-481.
162. Desai D, Hebra A, Davidoff A, et al. Wandering spleen: a challenging diagnosis. *South Med J.* 1997;90:439-443.
163. Deux J, Salomon L, Barrier A, et al. Acute torsion of wandering spleen: MRI findings. *AJR Am J Roentgenol.* 2004;182:1607-1608.
164. Winer-Muram H, Tonkin I. The spectrum of heterotaxic syndromes. *Radiol Clin North Am.* 1989;27:1147-1170.
165. Peoples W, Moller J, Edwards J. Polysplenia: a review of 146 cases. *Pediatr Cardiol.* 1983;4:129-137.
166. Lee FT Jr, Pozniak M, Helgerson R. US case of the day. Polysplenia syndrome. *Radiographics.* 1993;13:1159-1162.
167. Soler R, Rodriguez E, Comesana M, et al. Agenesis of the dorsal pancreas with polysplenia syndrome: CT features. *J Comput Assist Tomogr.* 1992;16:921-923.
168. Fulcher A, Turner M. Abdominal manifestations of situs anomalies in adults. *Radiographics.* 2002;22:1439-1456.
169. Applegate K, Goske M, Pierce G, et al. Situs revisited: imaging of the heterotaxy syndrome. *Radiographics.* 1999;19:837-852; discussion 853-854.
170. Marx M, Van AR. SIR 2005 film panel case: heterotaxia with polysplenia. *J Vasc Interv Radiol.* 2005;16:1055-1059.
171. Serviansky B, Schwarz J. The incidence of splenic calcifications in positive reactors to histoplasmin and tuberculin. *Am J Roentgenol Radium Ther Nucl Med.* 1956;76:53-59.
172. Grey EF. Calcifications of the spleen. *AJR Am J Roentgenol.* 1944;51:336-351.
173. Topin J, Mutlu GM. Splenic and mediastinal calcifications in histoplasmosis. *N Engl J Med.* 2006;354:179.
174. Okudaira M, Straub M, Schwarz J. The etiology of discrete splenic and hepatic calcifications in an endemic area of histoplasmosis. *Am J Pathol.* 1961;39:599-611.
175. Jacobs JE, Birnbaum BA, Furth EE. Abdominal visceral calcification in primary amyloidosis: CT findings. *Abdom Imaging.* 1997;22:519-521.
176. Vanhoenacker F, Van den Brande P, De Schepper A. Hepatosplenic anthracosilicosis: a rare cause of splenic calcifications. *Eur Radiol.* 2001;11:1184-1186.
177. Radhakrishnan S, al Nakib B, Sivanandan R, Menon N. Hepatosplenic and small bowel calcification due to Schistosoma mansoni infection. *Dig Dis Sci.* 1988;33: 1637-1640.
178. Ishizaki T, Kuroda H, Kuroda T, Nakai T, Miyabo S. Sarcoidosis with multiple calcification. *Jpn J Med.* 1988;27:191-194.
179. Fischer R, Harmatz PR. Non-invasive assessment of tissue iron overload. *Hematology.* 2009;2009:215-221.
180. Salo S, Alanen A, Leino R, Bondestam S, Komu M. The effect of haemosiderosis and blood transfusions on the T2 relaxation time and 1/T2 relaxation rate of liver tissue. *Br J Radiol.* 2002;75:24-27.
181. Wood JC, Enriquez C, Ghugre N, et al. MRI R2 and R2* mapping accurately estimates hepatic iron concentration in transfusion-dependent thalassemia and sickle cell disease patients. *Blood.* 2005;106:1460-1465.
182. Sagoh T, Itoh K, Togashi K, et al. Gamna-Gandy bodies of the spleen: evaluation with MR imaging. *Radiology.* 1989;172: 685-687.
183. Bhatt S, Simon R, Dogra V. Gamna-Gandy bodies: sonographic features with histopathologic correlation. *J Ultrasound Med.* 2006;25:1625-1629.

184. Luo T, Itai Y, Yamaguchi M, Kurosaki Y, Saida Y. Gamna-Gandy bodies of the spleen depicted by unenhanced CT: report of two cases. *Radiat Med.* 1998;16:473-476.

185. Selçuk D, Demirel K, Kantarci F, Mihmanli I, Oğüt G. Gamna-Gandy bodies: a sign of portal hypertension. *Turk J Gastroenterol.* 2005;16:150-152.

186. Ghahremani G, Gore R. CT diagnosis of postoperative abdominal complications. *Radiol Clin North Am.* 1989;27: 787-804.

187. Gayer G, Hertz M, Zissin R. Postoperative pneumoperitoneum: prevalence, duration, and possible significance. *Semin Ultrasound CT MR.* 2004;25:286-289.

188. Khosravi M, Margulies D, Alsabeh R, et al. Consider the diagnosis of splenosis for soft tissue masses long after any splenic injury. *Am Surg.* 2004;70:967-970.

189. Osadchy A, Zissin R, Shapiro-Feinberg M. Thoracic splenosis. *Isr Med Assoc J.* 2001;3:547.

190. Sharma R, Mondal A, Kashyap R, et al. Radiolabeled denatured RBC scintigraphy in autologous splenic transplantation. *Clin Nucl Med.* 1996;21:534-536.

191. Winslow E, Brunt L. Perioperative outcomes of laparoscopic versus open splenectomy: a meta-analysis with an emphasis on complications. *Surgery.* 2003;134:647-653.

192. Martinez C, Waisberg J, Palma R, et al. Gastric necrosis and perforation as a complication of splenectomy. Case report and related references. *Arq Gastroenterol.* 2000;27:227-230.

193. Moore EE, Cogbill TH, Jurkovich GJ, Shackford SR, Malangoni MA, Champion HR. Organ injury scaling: spleen and liver (1994 revision). *J Trauma.* 1995;38(3):323-324.

CHAPTER 15

Imaging of the Arteries and Veins of the Abdomen and Pelvis

Saurabh Jha, MBBS, MRCS
Wallace T. Miller Jr., MD

Given that arteries and veins of a caliber detectable by modern-day imaging permeates virtually every organ system, imaging of any organ system can be considered imaging of the vascular tree. However, the vascular tree is an organ in its own right afflicted by a range of unique pathology and amenable to unique forms of treatment.

There are differences in principle between arterial pathology and its management and management of pathology in other organ systems. These differences must be appreciated by imagers in order to provide the most insightful and clinically useful reports.

Imaging of the arteries carries with it 2 major responsibilities. The first is to aid in the diagnosis of arterial disease, the predominant etiology of which is atherosclerosis. The second purpose of imaging is that it helps the clinician decide the best course of intervention which, broadly speaking, falls into 3 groups: (1) do nothing surgically, either because nothing needs to be done or because nothing can be done; (2) open surgical intervention; and (3) percutaneous surgical intervention. What distinguishes imaging of the arteries from other organs is that it is generally assumed that information for surgical planning will be needed.

There are a narrow range of morphologic end points that can result from a range of pathologic processes. However, both the morphology of the abnormality and the underlying pathology can affect the type of intervention. For example, there is no single management strategy for atherosclerosis. The management depends on what exactly atherosclerosis does to the artery and is a different strategy, if the result is occlusion of the artery from or if the result is an aneurysm of the artery. As a corollary, aneurysms caused by infection are managed differently to aneurysms caused by atherosclerosis in that the size threshold for surgical intervention is reduced, and aggressive medical management in the form of organism-specific antibiotics is also instituted.

The abdominal arteries, particularly the aorta, are seldom afflicted in isolation and the systemic nature of the arterial pathology obliges a search for disease in unsuspected arterial beds. Also, extrinsic pathology can involve the aorta or the arteries of the lower extremities, a finding that can affect the type of intervention.

IMAGING MODALITIES

The mainstay of imaging for arterial disease includes computed tomographic angiography (CTA) and magnetic resonance angiography (MRA), with ultrasonography (US) and conventional angiography (CA) having a less central role.

CT Angiography

The combination of helical CT technology and multiple detectors have enabled interrogation of a large field of view within an achievable breath hold. From the vantage point of arterial imaging, this combination has been revolutionary, and now high-quality arterial contrast is all but routinely assumed.

The typical vascular CT protocol is, of course, tailored to the clinical circumstance but generally comprises precontrast, arterial-phase and delayed (venous phase) imaging.

Precontrast images are not mandatory but are useful particularly in a patient post surgical intervention or with suspected acute rupture. This is to distinguish between in situ high-attenuating materials (calcium, graft, stent) from iodinated contrast, particularly if such distinction makes a difference to the interpretation. Similarly, a venous phase is valuable in certain situations such as the search for endoleaks post stent, but is not required routinely.

The timing of the acquisition is the key to a diagnostic arterial phase. To best synchronize the acquisition of the images with the peak maximal enhancement of iodinated contrast in the artery of interest, guesswork should be kept to a minimum. Two recognized methods of achieving this are the bolus tracking and the test bolus methods. The former relies on placing a tracker on a certain part of the arterial tree, for example the suprarenal aorta, and performing low-dose single-slice images until a certain attenuation threshold, typically on the order of 130 Hounsfield units (HUs), is attained; thereafter, the scan commences after a fixed delay, typically 6 seconds. The ease of the bolus tracking method accounts for its greater popularity than the test bolus in which a smaller volume of contrast, approximately 20 mL, is injected at the same injection rate as used in the subsequent diagnostic scan and the time at which peak maximal enhancement occurs for a particular section of the aorta is graphed. The time to peak maximal enhancement is noted to guide the main injection.

Nonionic low or iso-osmolar iodinated contrast agents are used for CT angiograms. The slices are reconstructed at a thickness between 0.6 to 3 mm to achieve near-isotropic resolution, in order that the images are processed with a variety of 3-dimensional (3D) rendering technologies (see Figure 15-1).

MR Angiography

Arterial contrast can be achieved without the administration of exogenous contrast using flow-dependent methods, although many are still evolving and have yet to make a widespread clinical impact. The main method of achieving arterial contrast is the administration of gadolinium chelates and subsequent exploitation of the T1 shortening properties of gadolinium. With current hardware and pulse sequence design, high-quality arterial-phase images can be achieved with near isotropic resolution within an achievable breath hold. The availability of step table and moving table technology means that multiple contiguous body parts can be imaged with a single injection of contrast (see Figure 15-2).

Advantages of MR over CT include (1) absence of ionizing radiation and (2) easier postprocessing because it is easier to remove nonarterial structures from MRI images than CT images. There are several disadvantages of MR relative to CT: (1) MR does not assess calcification—this is an important blind spot as the amount and location of calcification affects the suitability of the vessel for percutaneous interventions. (2) Stents cause a signal drop on MR due to the susceptibility artifact, making it impossible to measure stent stenosis and/or occlusion. (3) Finally, MR takes a longer time than CT to acquire images.

Ultrasonography

US has been proposed as a screening modality for asymptomatic abdominal aortic aneurysms (AAAs). Its role in

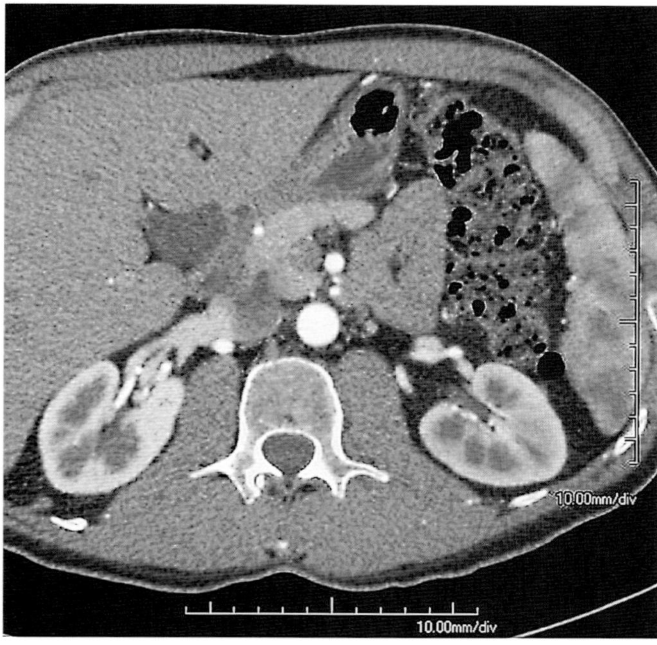

A

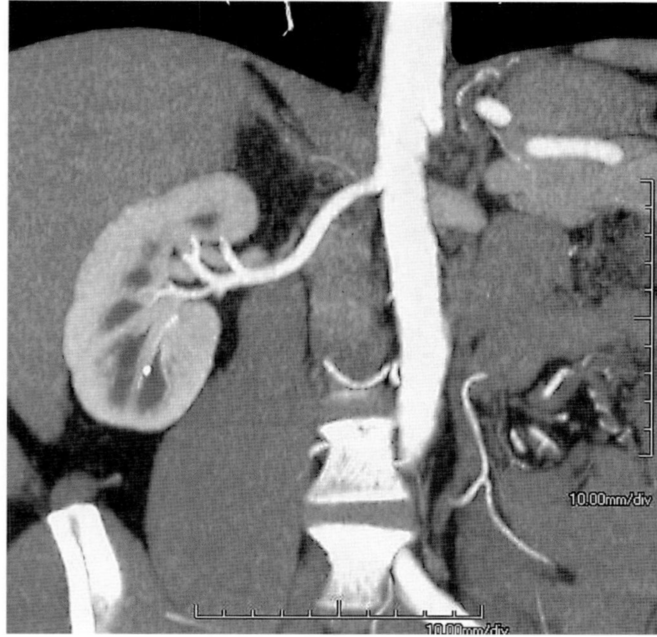

B

Figure 15-1 Normal CTA
A. Axial CTA shows intense opacification of the abdominal aorta. The 3 layers of the normal wall are imperceptible. **B.** Coronal-oblique MIP shows the right renal artery extending from the origin to the hilum. Note the smooth, tapered appearance with the absence of luminal irregularity, typical of normal vessels.

diagnosis is not surprising as it is relatively inexpensive, available, and free of ionizing radiation and the use of exogenous contrast agents. However, it is not comparable to CT and MR for definitive diagnosis or surgical planning because it is unable to interrogate the entire vascular tree with the same clarity, precision, and reproducibility (see Figure 15-3).

Ultrasound is not only operator-dependent but is also disadvantaged by nonoperator issues such as body habitus and the presence of bowel gas. It is for these reasons that barring the renal vasculature, US has not made any headway into the interrogation of vascular trees.

However, duplex US has certain advantages. It is better able to appreciate the hemodynamic significance of narrowing than a purely anatomical modality such as CT and MR. It does so by measuring velocities across stenosis, quantifying a gradient, and by measuring resistive indices of stenosis such as in the renal arteries.

Ultrasound has much to offer in certain clinical situations and in patients in whom it can be predicted a priori that the operator is less likely to be encumbered by technical challenges.

Catheter Angiography

Biplane 2-dimensional (2D) catheter angiograms were the initial imaging method to evaluated the vascular tree but have been sidelined by CTA and MRA for a variety of reasons. Catheter angiogram offers a luminogram but does not provide information about the arterial wall, including the presence of luminal thrombus or calcification, or extravascular structures. Catheter angiogram is less sensitive to contrast enhancement than CTA or MRA. Projectional images from catheter angiograms are less accurate at quantifying asymmetric stenosis than 3D images from CTA and MRA. Additionally, 3D images do not suffer from the problems due to overlap of vessels seen with projectional images. Catheter angiogram is invasive with puncture site complications, and it is more resource intensive than cross-sectional imaging.

Despite its limitations, catheter angiograms have some advantages over cross-sectional imaging. (1) The temporal resolution of catheter angiogram is very high and multiple frames can provide information about the directionality of blood flow and (2) catheter angiogram has a higher spatial resolution than cross-sectional imaging. (3) Catheter angiogram is not susceptible to metallic artifact and assessment of in-stent stenosis is superior to CTA and MRA. (4) Finally, catheter angiogram has a role during intraprocedural guidance of intravascular intervention.

ANATOMY OF THE ABDOMINAL ARTERIES

The aorta enters the abdominal cavity through an opening in the diaphragm opposite T12. The aorta bifurcates into the common iliac arteries opposite L4 into the right and left common iliac arteries.

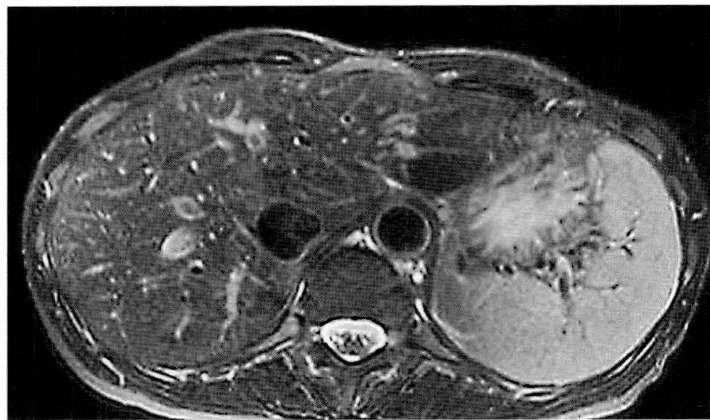

A

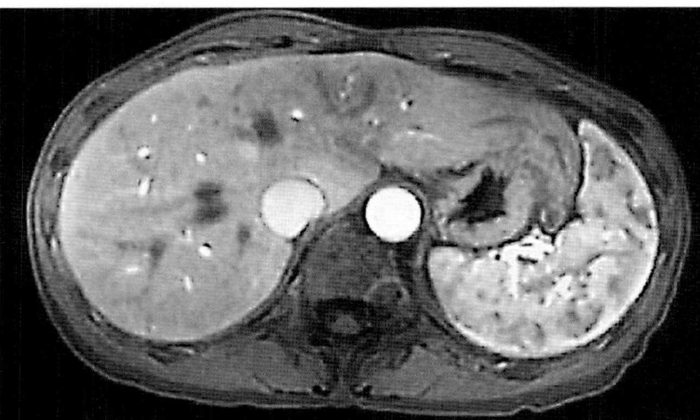

B

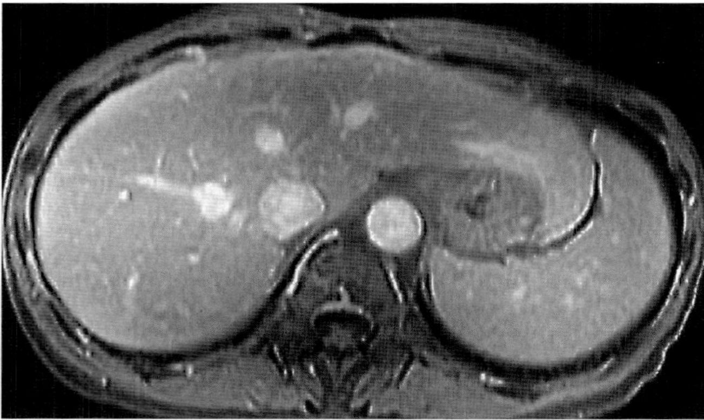

C

Figure 15-2 Normal MRA
A. Axial T2-weighted, (**B**) axial reformation from 3D postgadolinium MRA, and (**C**) axial 2D postgadolinium gradient echo shows the normal aorta. Note the imperceptible aortic wall, which is composed of the intima, media, and the adventitia. Note the absence of detectable mural enhancement on the delayed images.

The abdominal aorta provides blood supply to the viscera of the abdomen and pelvis. The major visceral arteries include the celiac trunk, the superior mesenteric artery (SMA), the inferior mesenteric artery (IMA), and the bilateral renal arteries. In addition, the aorta gives rise to the inferior phrenic artery, adrenal and lumbar arteries, the gonadal artery, and the median sacral artery.

The celiac divides into the left gastric, common hepatic, and splenic arteries. The celiac provides blood supply to the upper abdominal viscera, the descendants of the foregut. There is a rich anastomotic network about the stomach and pancreas from branches of the celiac trunk and between the celiac trunk and the SMA.

The common hepatic artery gives off the gastroduodenal artery (GDA) and right gastric artery and continues as the proper hepatic artery. The proper hepatic artery gives rise to the cystic artery and then divides into the right and left hepatic arteries. The GDA divides into the superior pancreaticoduodenal and right gastroepiploic artery. The superior pancreaticoduodenal artery then divides into an anterior and posterior branch that anastomoses with their counterparts from the inferior pancreaticoduodenal branch of the SMA. The right gastroepiploic artery anastomoses with the left gastroepiploic artery, which is a terminal branch of the splenic artery. The splenic artery, in addition, gives rise to several short gastric arteries and several branches to the pancreas including the dorsal pancreatic, transverse pancreatic, caudal pancreatic, and pancreatic magna arteries.

The SMA gives rise to the inferior pancreaticoduodenal artery, jejunal arteries, the ileocolic artery, ileal arteries, and the right and middle colic arteries. The SMA provides blood supply to the descendants of the midgut as far as the splenic flexure. There is a rich intramesenteric anastomotic network along the transverse colon between branches of the SMA and the IMA.

The IMA gives rise to the left colic artery, several sigmoid arteries, and terminates as the superior hemorrhoidal artery that anastomoses with the middle hemorrhoidal branch of the anterior division of the internal iliac artery.

Renal arteries divide at the renal hilum into anterior and posterior division. The anterior division supplies the apical, upper, middle, and lower segments of the kidney whereas the posterior division supplies the middle segment. Further subdivision into the lobar and thence interlobar arteries occurs. The interlobar arteries terminate at the corticomedullary junction into arcuate arteries. The arcuate arteries generally give rise to the interlobular artery, which becomes the afferent arteriole.

The common iliac artery bifurcates into the internal and external iliac arteries opposite the pelvic brim. The internal iliac artery divides into an anterior and posterior branch. The posterior branch of the internal iliac arteries gives rise to the lateral sacral, iliolumbar, and superior gluteal arteries. The anterior division gives off the inferior gluteal, obturator, vesicle, middle hemorrhoidal, internal pudendal, and in females the uterine and in males the deferential arteries. The external iliac artery becomes the common femoral artery below the inguinal ligament. Before that it gives rise to the circumflex iliac, external pudendal, and inferior epigastric arteries.

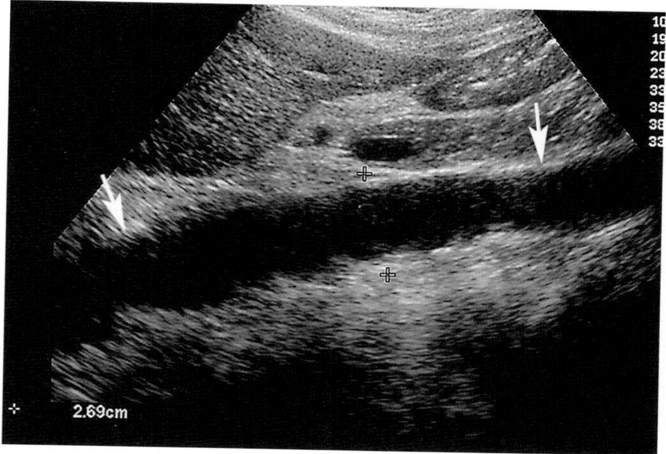

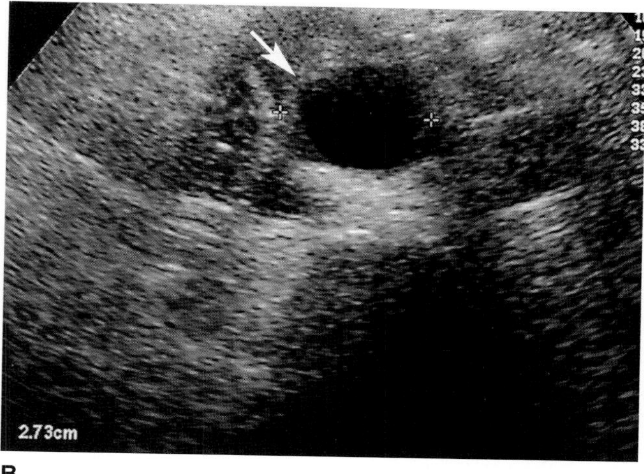

Figure 15-3 Normal US Abdominal Aorta
A. Longitudinal and (**B**) transaxial US images of the abdomen demonstrate a smooth, anechoic tubular structure (*arrows*), with increased through transmission, measuring approximately 2.7 cm in diameter typical of the normal abdominal aorta.

Branches of the external and internal iliac arteries become important pathways for collaterals during aortoiliac occlusion. For example, blood in the inferior epigastric artery flows retrograde to reconstitute the external iliac artery in upstream occlusion, through its anastomosis with the superior epigastric artery. Also, the middle hemorrhoidal branch of the anterior division of the internal iliac artery anastomoses with the superior hemorrhoidal branch of the IMA to provide blood to the distal left colon in IMA occlusion.

Noting the rich anastomotic network about the pelvic arteries, it is important for the imager to comment on the health of the parent arteries, so that a sense of potential for collateral recruitment may be gained, in the event of deliberate or accidental occlusion of the arteries during vascular intervention.

A major congenital variant to be aware of is the persistent sciatic artery. This artery normally regresses but when persistent is associated with diminutive or absent ipsilateral external iliac and femoral arteries. The classic presentation is that of patient with absent femoral pulses but palpable pedal pulses. The persistent sciatic artery travels with the sciatic nerve through the greater sciatic foramen into the posterior thigh.

DISEASES OF THE ABDOMINAL ARTERIES

Arterial disease can be classified according to etiology (eg, atherosclerosis) or morphological end point (eg, aneurysm). In the following section, grouping of disease will be made according to morphologic end points. This is because such classification is most favorable to an imager seeking pattern recognition and applying a differential diagnosis based on pattern.

The arteries in the abdomen and pelvis can be affected by a range of acute and chronic conditions. These disorders begin with an abnormality of the arterial wall that can be radiographically occult or result in wall thickening or calcification or both. Structural abnormalities in the aortic wall can further lead to vascular stenosis, dilation (aneurysm formation), disruption, and perivascular soft tissue abnormalities (Table 15-1). The imaging features, pattern of vascular involvement, and the age of the patient can often indicate the underlying cause of vascular diseases. Because the disease begins with structural abnormalities in the vessel wall, we will begin our discussion of vascular diseases with a discussion of causes of wall thickening and calcification and then continue on to the complications of vascular diseases: stenosis, aneurysm formation, wall disruption, and perivascular soft-tissue changes.

Table 15-1. Imaging Descriptors for Abdominal Arterial Pathology

1. Wall thickening
2. Wall calcification
3. Stenosis/occlusion
4. Aneurysm
5. Wall disruption
6. Perivascular abnormality
7. Intraluminal abnormalities a. Clot b. Gas

Table 15-2. Causes of Wall Thickening

Causes of Wall Thickening
A. Subintimal
1. Atherosclerotic plaque
2. Mural thrombus
B. Intramural and adventitial
1. Intramural hematoma
2. Vasculitis
3. Bacterial infection (mycotic aneurysm)
4. Aneurysm with a chronic leak
5. Graft repair of the aorta

Wall Thickening

The arterial wall is histologically composed of the intima, media, and adventitia. The arterial wall, although comprising 3 layers, is normally imperceptible on imaging examinations (see Figures 15-1 and 15-2). Pathologic conditions can occur in subintimal, intramural, and periadventitial locations (Table 15-2). Atherosclerotic plaque and mural thrombus are the principal causes of subintimal deposits and result in focal wall thickening. Calcification can be superimposed on either. Subintimal thickening tends to be irregular, noncircumferential, and discrete.

Intramural thickening is thickening of the medial layer of the aorta and can be a result of edema and inflammatory expansion of the tissues or due to bleeding within the wall of the vessel. Inflammatory thickening of the media can be a result of vasculitis and bacterial infection (mycotic aneurysm). Intramural thickening typically is uniform, circumferential, and diffuse or segmental.

Atherosclerotic plaque

Atherosclerosis is the leading cause of death in the western world. Atherosclerosis is a chronic inflammatory process and is responsible in the vast majority of systemic arterial disease. It results from the combination of vessel wall injury, angiogenesis, and inflammation, leading to the deposition of lipid, fibrous tissue, and calcification in varying amounts, which constitutes the atherosclerotic plaque. The plaque affects both the lumen and the arterial wall, leading to luminal narrowing, stenosis, and occlusion. In addition, plaque can undergo ulceration, which can progress beyond the plaque and disrupt the intimal layer of the aorta leading to a penetrating atherosclerotic ulcer (PAU).

Atherosclerosis is chronic and progressive although the rate of progression can be retarded by appropriate therapy, including lipid lowering and antiplatelet drugs and attention to certain risk factors. Atherosclerosis is a multifactorial phenomenon with a familial predisposition augmented by risk factors many of which are reversible or can be modified, such as smoking, hypertension, diabetes, serum lipid profile, obesity, and inactivity, and some which cannot be reversed such as male gender and age.

Focal wall thickening due to both calcified and noncalcified plaque are easily visualized on contrast-enhanced CT and MRI. Noncalcified plaque typically appears as soft-tissue attenuation, plateau-shaped protuberance into the lumen of the vessel in question, and can extend over a few millimeters to many centimeters in length (see Figure 15-4). The surface can be smooth or irregular. Some plaques will contain foci of lipid attenuation/signal within them. Occasionally, plaque can be polypoid in morphology and attached to the wall with a narrow neck. This morphologic

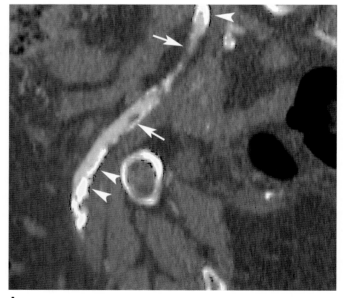

A

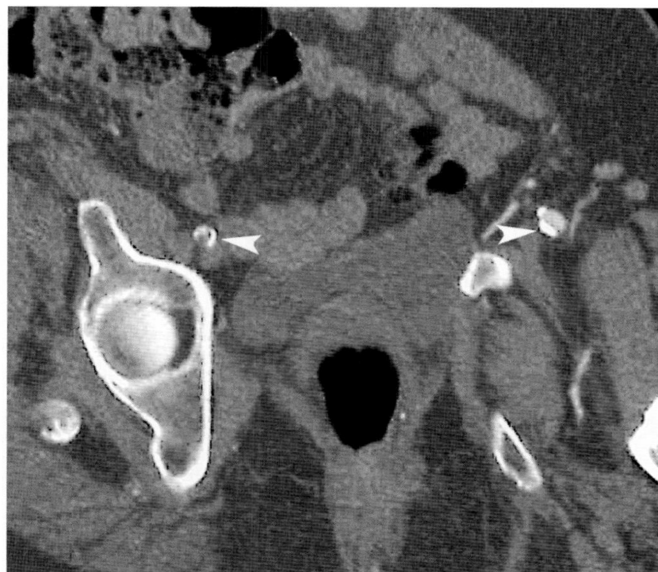

B

Figure 15-4 Atherosclerotic Plaque
A. Sagittal and (**B**) oblique-axial reformations show calcified and noncalcified plaque in the right external iliac artery in this 81-year-old female with rest pain. The plaques cause narrowing of the iliac vessels.

feature predisposes the plaque to becoming dislodged during catheter angiography, leading to distal emboli and the potential for distal ischemia. Therefore, it is important for these lesions to be specifically noted to alert physicians performing catheter angiography of the potential for emboli.

Much research has focused on detection of plaque vulnerability morphologically on CT and MR. Vulnerable plaque is plaque likely to rupture, leading to vessel thrombosis. Such plaques have a large amount of lipid core and a thin fibrous capsule. With improving spatial and low-contrast resolution, in vivo histological characterization of plaque is becoming increasingly possible.

As atherosclerotic plaque ages, it develops regions of dystrophic calcification. As a consequence, the extent of plaque calcification increases with the age of the individual. Calcification can be detected on abdominal radiographs, US, and CT (see Figure 15-4). Calcification is not reliably detected on MRI.

Mural thrombus

According to Virchow triad, thrombogenicity is increased when there is an abnormality of (1) the vessel wall, (2) blood flow, or (3) the nature of blood itself. Mural thrombus is the name given to the thrombus that forms in areas of arterial ectasia/aneurysm because of the altered flow patterns (see Figure 15-5). This thrombus is attached to the wall of the artery. Mural thrombus can also form in nondilated arterial

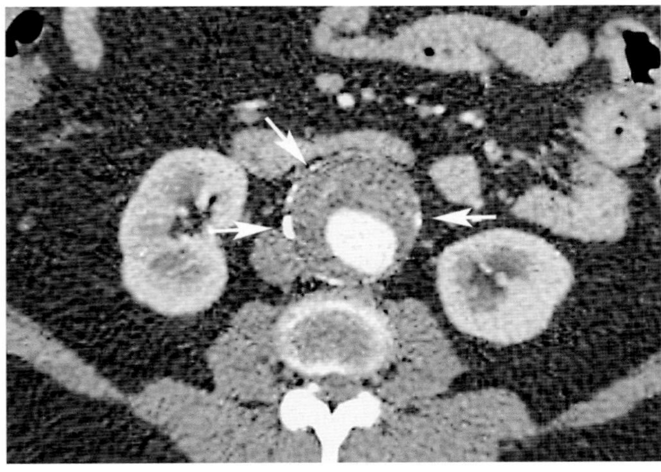

A

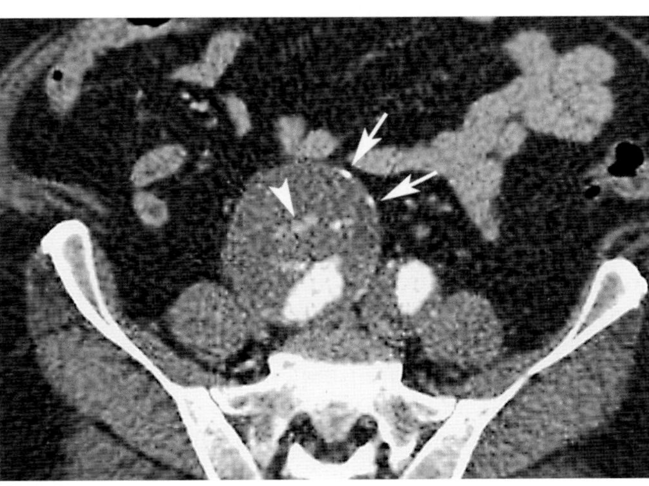

B

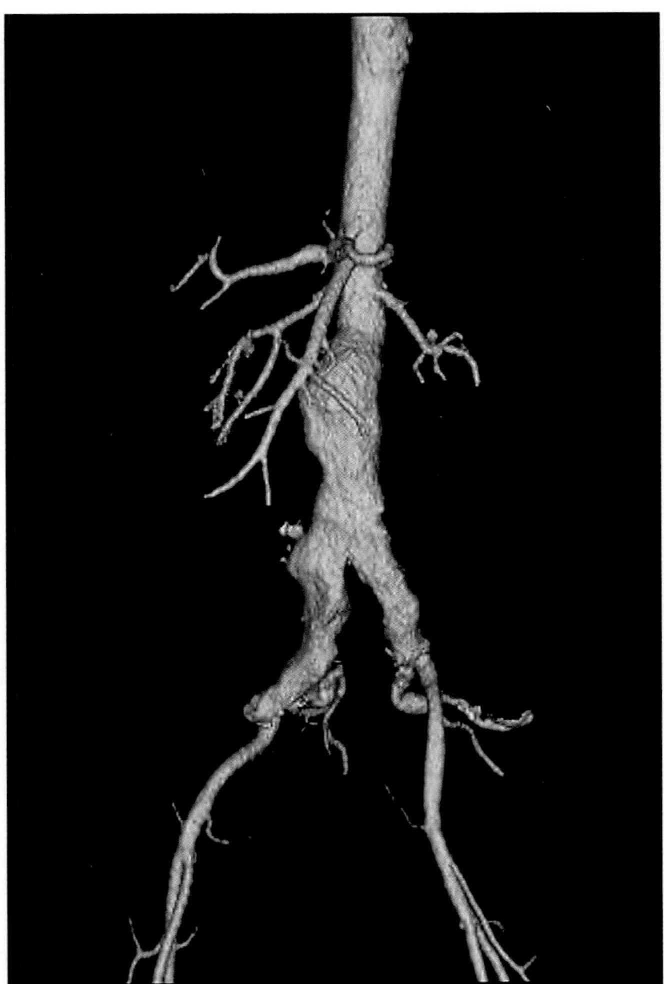

C

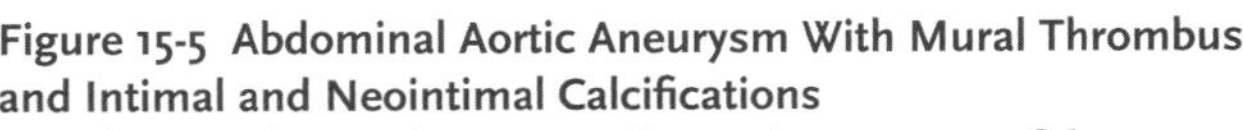

Figure 15-5 Abdominal Aortic Aneurysm With Mural Thrombus and Intimal and Neointimal Calcifications

A and **B.** Axial CTA shows an infrarenal aneurysm of the aorta (A) and right common iliac artery (B). The peripheral, curvilinear calcification (*arrows*) marks the intimal layer of the aorta and iliac arteries. The low-attenuation material between the aortic wall and the contrast-enhanced lumen represents mural thrombus that is subintimal in location. The medial and adventitial layers of the aorta remain imperceptible. Curvilinear calcification is a landmark for the intimal layer of the aorta in patients with atherosclerosis. However, chronic mural thrombus can also calcify, and this is known as neointimal calcifications, which is seen as small flecks of high attenuation within the mural thrombus (*arrowhead*).
C. Volume-rendered image shows the distribution of contrast and calcification. Note how this underestimates the diameter of the aneurysm because of the presence of mural thrombus.

segments if the flow dynamics are altered, such as in areas of atherosclerotic plaque. As a consequence, plaque and thrombus frequently coexist.

The imaging differentiation of plaque from thrombus can be difficult. Both mural thrombus and plaque tend to have an irregular surface. Thrombus tends to have a higher attenuation than plaque and will not have the areas of fat attenuation seen in plaque. As mentioned, plaque can ulcerate and the ulceration can form a fissure, which extends to the intimal layer, a feature that is not seen as frequently in mural thrombus but can happen. Like plaque, thrombus can occasionally have a polypoid morphology that is predisposed to dislodgement and distal embolization. As is evident from this discussion, the imaging distinction between plaque and mural thrombus is not always possible. Fortunately, the distinction between plaque and thrombus is usually clinically irrelevant.

Intramural hematoma

Rupture of the vaso vasorum of the aorta and other great vessels will result in an intramural hematoma.[1] Intramural hematomas most commonly occur spontaneously in association with systemic hypertension but can also be a result of penetrating atherosclerotic ulcers (PAUs).[2,3]

Spontaneous aortic intramural hematomas are typically discovered in elderly patients, with a mean age of presentation of 74 years and a range of 63 and 87 years.[1,4,5] Systemic hypertension is seen in the majority of patients and many will have a variety of comorbidities such as chronic obstructive pulmonary disease (COPD), heart disease, and chronic renal insufficiency.[1,5,6] Symptoms mimic an aortic dissection such as severe, midscapular, substernal, or anterior chest or back pain.[1,6]

On histologic examination, there is degeneration of the aortic media, and the hematoma will typically be present in the outer third of the media only a few cells from the adventitia.[1] This is in comparison with aortic dissections, which will normally involve the more central aspects of the media, closer to the intima.

The natural history of intramural hematomas is quite variable. Approximately one-half of medically treated intramural hematomas will regress within 6 months and will ultimately resolve within 1 year.[1,7,8] Twelve percent to 24% will evolve into dissections and 13% to 30% evolve into aneurysms or and will usually require surgical or endovascular intervention.[4,6,9] Some series have identified a 35% to 51% incidence of acute rupture of intramural hematomas either spontaneously or associated with progression to dissections or aneurysms.[1,6] Involvement of the ascending aorta increases the likelihood of rupture.[1,5,6,8,10-13] The majority of complications of intramural hematomas, approximately 90%, will happen within a few weeks of presentation but rarely, others will occur months to years later.[6]

The majority, approximately 70%, of intramural hematomas will occur in the descending thoracic aorta.[1] Intramural hematoma of the abdominal aorta is rare in isolation and is usually an extension of an intramural hematoma that originates in the thoracic aorta. On CT scans, intramural hematoma will appear as high attenuation thickening of the aortic wall on precontrast images.[14-16] MRI will most often reveal increased signal intensity on T1-weighted images, indicating subacute blood.[14,17] Following contrast injection, the attenuation of intramural hematoma will remain unchanged (see Figure 15-6).

Intramural hematoma must be distinguished from mural thrombus, which can also contain blood products. Intramural hematoma tends to be circumferential, smooth and continuous whereas mural thrombus is irregular and discrete. Intimal calcification, when present, can aid in distinguishing mural thrombus from intramural hematoma. Calcification generally tends to be intimal/ subintimal. The consequence of this is that intramural hematoma tends to surround the calcification whereas mural thrombus is on the luminal side of the calcification.

Vasculitis

Vasculitis is typically classified according to the size of vessel involved. Large vessel vasculitis, such as Takayasu and giant cell arteritis, affects the aorta and major branches. Medium vessel vasculitis, such as polyarteritis nodosa (PAN), affects the primary arteries to major organs such as the celiac artery and the SMA and their branches. Small vessel vasculitis, such as microscopic polyarteritis, Churg-Strauss vasculitis, and Wegener granulomatosis affects capillaries.

In addition to the primary vasculitides, vessel wall inflammation can also be secondary to medications, infection, and malignancy. From the perspective of imagers it is best to think of vasculitides as those that are occult on cross-sectional imaging (small vessel vasculitis) and those that are seen on imaging (large and medium vessel vasculitis). In a patient suspected of vasculitis, a negative CTA or MRA does not rule out small vessel vasculitis.

The primary imaging abnormality of medium and large vessel vasculitis is inflammatory thickening of the media.[18-27] On precontrast CT and MRI images, the thickened media have an attenuation and signal intensity similar to or less than that of muscle. This is an important distinguishing feature from intramural hematoma, which should be of higher attenuation than skeletal muscle on CT and high signal on T1-weighted MR sequences. Further, following contrast administration, the thickened vessel wall on both CT and MRI may enhance, whereas intramural hematoma will have an unchanged attenuation. In the acute phase of the vasculitis, wall thickening is a result of mural edema, which can be detected by T2-weighted MRI as increased signal of the vessel wall or as a hypoechoic halo on sonography.[26,28] As with intramural hematoma, the thickened vessel wall in vasculitis is smooth and the thickening is circumferential, features that help distinguish it from atherosclerotic plaque and most cases of mural thrombus. The thickening also tends to be more symmetrically circumferential in vasculitis than intramural

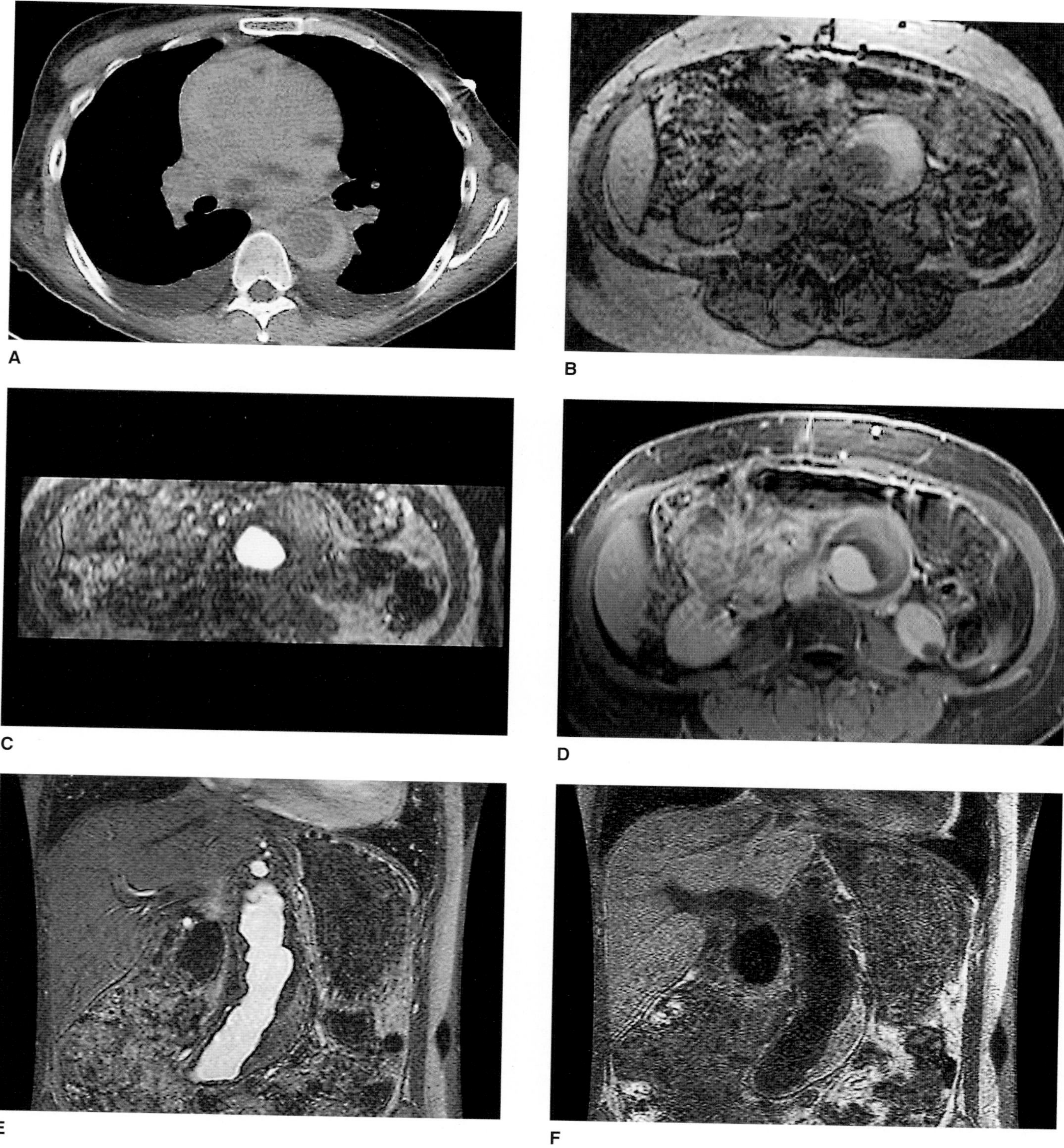

Figure 15-6 Intramural Hematoma in 2 Patients
A. A crescenteric area of high attenuation can be seen in the ascending and descending aorta. This is the typical appearance of an intramural hematoma on unenhanced CT. **B-F.** MRI exam in a second patient. (B) Axial T1 through the abdomen shows high-signal crescent along the levolateral wall of the abdominal aorta suggestive of IMH. (C) Axial reformation of 3D gadolinium MRA does not show any enhancement of the area of high signal. (D) Axial postgadolinium delayed image reveals 2 different signal intensities. The inner aspect of the crescent has a markedly low signal and is thought to represent calcified intima, which is displaced by an intramural hematoma. (E) Axial 3D pregadolinium and (F) postgadolinium shows high signal along the levolateral wall of the aorta, which does not enhance in keeping with an intramural hematoma.

hematoma. In comparison with intramural hematoma that is typically a single long focus of wall thickening adjacent to the site of primary injury, vasculitis tends to be uniformly diffuse across the entire extent of the involved vessel or multifocal with thickening of noncontiguous arterial segments/beds.[18-25,28] Vasculitis tends to have luminal narrowing associated with the wall thickening (see Figure 15-7).

In addition to the primary abnormality, wall thickening, vasculitis can lead to the gamut of other vascular morphologic disturbances including stenosis, occlusion, aneurysm formation, and arterial rupture, which will be discussed later in this chapter. Further, vasculitis, like other systemic vascular pathologies, can present on imaging with end organ stigmata of ischemia and hemorrhage. These

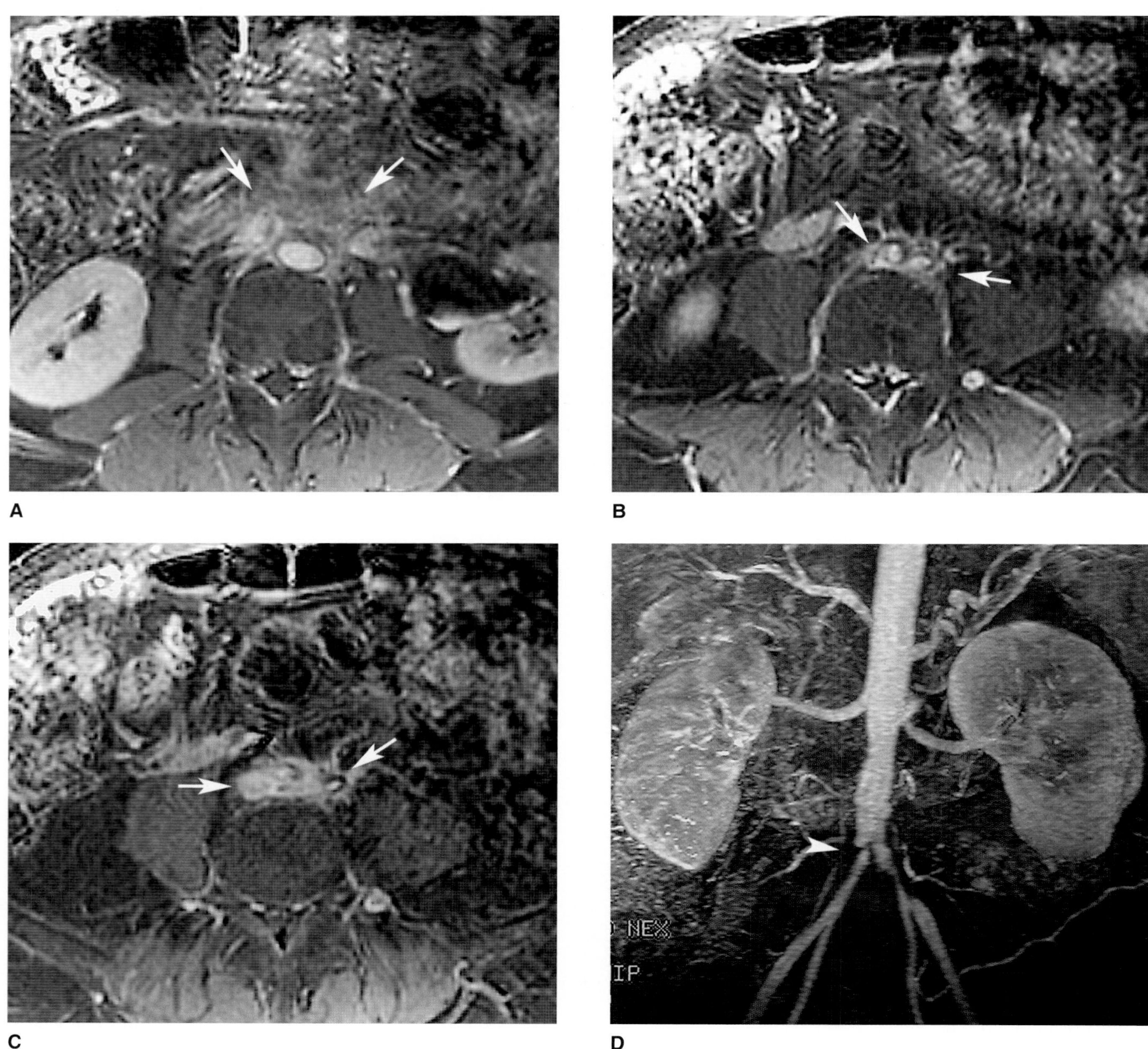

Figure 15-7 Wall Thickening due to Takayasu Arteritis
This 47-year-old man presented with lower extremity edema. **A-C.** Axial contrast-enhanced T1-weighted images through the abdomen demonstrate extensive periaortic soft-tissue enhancement (*arrows*). The caliber of the iliac arteries is small, and careful observation of the iliac arteries in (B and C) shows modest wall thickening. Note the low signal ring around the iliac arteries bilaterally, which is believed to represent nonenhanceing intima. These features suggest an inflammatory process involving the abdominal great arteries, probably a large vessel vasculitis. **D.** Coronal MIP shows tight stenosis (*arrowhead*) of the proximal iliac arteries bilaterally. Further evaluation lead to a diagnosis of Takayasu arteritis.

findings are discussed in many other chapters as imaging features of the affected organ.

Takayasu arteritis: Takayasu arteritis is a rare idiopathic inflammatory disorder of the large vessels primarily involving the aorta, the aortic branch vessels, and pulmonary arteries.[19,20,29] Takayasu arteritis has a worldwide distribution, but is seen most frequently in Asian populations.[19,20,29] It is primarily a disorder of young and middle-aged women, with median age of presentation of 36 years (range 19-57 y).[18] Chronic inflammation of the aortic wall can lead to arterial stenosis and occlusion or weakening of the wall and aneurysm formation.[19,20,29-31] Stenosis is the more common manifestation of Takayasu arteritis; however, aortic aneurysm and subsequent rupture is the most common fatal complication.[32,33]

Histologic examination of the acute phases of the disease will demonstrate extensive inflammation and thickening of the media and adventitia.[19,34] With disease progression, there is marked thinning of the media, disruption of elastic fibers and pronounced fibrotic thickening of the adventitia leading to vascular stenosis.[19,35] Aneurysms appear to be a result of degeneration and weakening of the media.[19,36] Some researchers suggest that the development of aortic aneurysms is most closely associated with elevations in blood pressure.[37]

Patients typically present with the insidious onset of vague systemic symptoms such as fever, malaise, and weakness. With progressive disease, arterial stenoses can result in diminished or absent peripheral pulses. It causes inflammation of the aortic wall, which can lead to stenosis, occlusion, and aneurysm formation.[19,20,29-31]

In general, CT and MRI examinations will demonstrate extensive wall thickening of 1-mm to 4-mm thickness in the acute phases of disease.[18-25] Arterial-phase imaging and delayed-phase imaging following intravenous contrast administration will demonstrate extensive wall enhancement, in patients with active arteritis.[18] In some patients, a thin low attenuation ring is seen between the enhancing lumen and the enhancing aortic wall and is thought to represent nonenhancing intima (see Figure 15-7).[18] Further, CT and MRI can be of value in monitoring for active disease. Studies have shown decreases in vascular wall thickening on CT and MRI examinations following administration of corticosteroids.[24,25] This is especially important because clinical markers of disease in some cases may fail to identify patients with histologically active disease.[38]

With progression of disease, regions of stenosis, aneurysm formation or both are common.[18-20] The presence of wall thickening is associated with greater likelihood of aneurysm progression and rupture.[37] In the late phases of disease, chronic inflammation can also lead to dystrophic calcification within the wall of the aorta. Vascular stenosis, aneurysm formation, and wall calcifications as a complication of Takayasu arteritis are discussed more completely in the subsequent section titled: **Aneurysms**.

Giant cell arteritis (temporal arteritis): Giant cell arteritis is a granulomatous arteritis of large vessels. It primarily involves the arteries of the head, especially the extracranial branches of the carotid artery, but can also involve the aorta and other aortic branch vessels.[39] Giant cell arteritis is also called "temporal arteritis" because of predisposition to involving the superficial temporal artery. Giant cell arteritis is an autoimmune disorder resulting in T-cell and macrophage-driven inflammation of the media of large arteries.[39] The triggers leading to development of giant cell arteritis are not certain but appear to include genetic factors (HLA–DRB1*04 alleles and others), infectious agents, and other environmental factors.[39] Giant cell arteritis is the most common arteritis in Europe and the United States and primarily affects the elderly, with an average age of onset of 70 years, and it rarely presents in patients younger than age 50 years.[39] It primarily affects individuals from northern European descent, especially those with Scandinavian heritage.[39] Patients often present cranial symptoms such as headache, scalp tenderness, jaw claudication, and visual disturbances (double vision, visual loss, blindness) or systemic symptoms such as fatigue, weight loss, and malaise.[40] Ocular ischemic complications are the primary source of chronic disability in patients with giant cell arteritis. There is an association with the rheumatologic condition polymyalgia rheumatica, and approximately 10% to 15% of patients with polymyalgia rheumatica will develop giant cell arteritis.[39,40]

The disease primarily causes wall thickening and occlusion of the branch arteries originating from the aortic arch but can occasionally involve any of the large vessels of the body. The superficial temporal, vertebral, ophthalmic, and posterior ciliary arteries are most commonly affected followed by the internal and external carotid arteries. The inflammation is typically not continuous and therefore regions of thickening can be interspersed with areas of normal wall thickness.[41] With active inflammation, US examinations show a hypoechoic halo of wall thickening due to edema of the arterial wall.[26] The sensitivity and specificity of this finding are not established. With fibrosis, the arterial wall becomes hyperechoic.[42,43] In general, MRI examinations will demonstrate increased thickness of the wall of the affected vessels and will also demonstrate wall enhancement following gadolinium administration.[27] In a study of 20 patients with suspected giant cell arteritis, MRI was able to identify 16 of 17 patients with disease.[27] One incidentally discovered case of giant cell arteritis was on ^{18}F fluorodeoxyglucose (FDG) positron emission tomography (PET)-CT imaging.[44] This finding may suggest that PET-CT could be used to identify patients with active inflammation due to giant cell arteritis.

The major features that distinguish giant cell arteritis from Takayasu arteritis are the age (elderly females), predisposition to involve the temporal arteries, dramatically elevated ESR (>100), and disease disproportionately centered on the branches of the aortic arch.

Imaging Notes 15-1. Differentiating Features of Arterial Wall Thickening

Cause	Distribution	Surface	BP[a]	Aneurysm	Stenosis
Atherosclerotic plaque	multifocal	irreg[b]	no	sometimes	sometimes
Mural thrombus	mutlifocal	irreg	yes	sometimes	sometimes
Intramural hematoma	diffuse	smooth	yes	rarely	rarely
Vasculitis	diffuse	smooth	no	often	often
Bacterial infection	diffuse	smooth	no	always	never
Inflammatory aneurysm	diffuse	smooth	no	always	never
Chronic leak	diffuse	smooth	no	always	never

[a]Blood products.
[b]Irregular.

Polyarteritis nodosa: PAN is a necrotizing, medium vessel vasculitis due to autoimmune-mediated vessel wall inflammation. Because the primary abnormality of PAN is inflammation of the arterial wall, it is expected that this disease would also cause thickening of the walls of the affected arteries. However, because of the small size of these vessels, vascular wall thickening is difficult to appreciate. Imaging examinations will most often identify multiple aneurysms of the medium arteries supplying the abdominal viscera, especially the kidneys, bowel, liver, and spleen. PAN is discussed most completely under the heading: **Aneurysm.**

Mycotic aneurysm

Infection of the wall of the great vessels will virtually always lead to inflammatory thickening of the vessel wall. However, vascular infections will virtually always result in an associated aneurysm of the vessel involved. Therefore, mycotic aneurysms will be discussed most completely in the subsequent section titled: **Aneurysms.**

Periadventitial Fat Stranding

Fat stranding in the soft tissues surrounding an artery will in most cases indicate inflammation of the periadventitial soft tissue. In many cases, the stranding will indicate the presence of an inflammatory process in the adjacent vessel. In most cases, the differential diagnosis for periadventitial fat stranding will be similar to the inflammatory causes of wall thickening such as vasculitis and mycotic aneurysm. Chronic leak of an aneurysm and a chronic reaction to graft repair of an aneurysm are other causes of soft tissue stranding. Rarely periadventitial thickening can be due to the condition retroperitoneal fibrosis (RPF) (Table 15-3).

Retroperitoneal fibrosis (Chronic periaortitis, inflammatory AAA, perianeurysmal retroperitoneal fibrosis)

The 3 rare retroperitoneal fibrosing conditions RPF, inflammatory AAA, and perianeurysmal RPF are now believed to be differing manifestations of the same disorder.[45] It has been suggested that these can be grouped under the umbrella term *chronic periaortitis*. All 3 conditions are characterized by advanced atherosclerosis, thinning of the media, and chronic inflammation and fibrosis of the adventitia of the abdominal aorta and periaortic soft tissues.[45] This inflammation and fibrosis can be associated with formation of an AAA or can strangle adjacent structures, most commonly the ureters. Inflammation and fibrosis in isolation has been called "retroperitoneal fibrosis," but when associated with aneurysm formation has been called "inflammatory abdominal aortic aneurysms" and when spreading to involve adjacent structures has been called "perianeurysmal retroperitoneal fibrosis."

The majority of cases are idiopathic; however, occasionally disease can be associated with a variety of factors,

Table 15-3. Causes of Periadventitial Inflammation

1. Vasculitis
2. Bacterial infection (mycotic aneurysm)
3. Aneurysm with a chronic leak
4. Graft repair of the aorta
5. Retroperitoneal fibrosis

including drugs (methysergide, bromocryptine, B-blockers, etc), malignancies (Hodgkin and non-Hodgkin lymphoma, cancer of the prostate breast and stomach), infections (tuberculosis, histoplasmosis, actinomycosis), prior surgery (lymphadenectomy, colectomy, hysterectomy, aortic aneurysmectomy), and miscellaneous other disorders (amyloidosis).[45] Most cases associated with malignancies and infections appear to be an exaggerated desmoplastic response to retroperitoneal lymph node involvement by the process.

Some data have suggested that idiopathic RPF is an inflammatory reaction to antigens from atherosclerotic plaques of the abdominal aorta.[46,47] However, more recent research has suggested that the idiopathic forms of chronic periaortitis are probably an autoimmune disorder. Findings suggesting an autoimmune etiology include frequent systemic symptomatology, frequent association with other autoimmune disorders, and preliminary evidence suggesting that autoantibodies to fibroblasts can be seen in up to one-third of patients with chronic periaortitis.[45,48,49]

Patients will most often complain of side, back, or abdominal pain and some will develop lower extremity edema because of compression of the vena cava.[45] Constitutional symptoms such as fatigue, fever, weight loss, nausea anorexia, and myalgias will often precede the localizing symptoms. Elevations in acute phase reactants (erythrocyte sedimentation rate, C-reactive protein) are commonly discovered.

It is seen more commonly in men with a frequency of 2:1 to 3:1.[45] The mean age of presentation is between 50 and 60 years but cases have been reported in children and the elderly. There are no standardized criteria for the diagnosis of chronic periaortitis but the diagnosis is typically based on a typical CT or MRI appearance associated with characteristic symptoms and elevated acute phase reactants or based on the histologic evaluation of tissues.[45]

On CT and MRI examinations, RPF appears as an infiltrative soft tissue mass, typically surrounding the infrarenal abdominal aorta and iliac arteries and occasionally enveloping the ureters and inferior vena cava.[45,50,51] Ureteral involvement can also result in ureteral obstruction. The ureters are typically drawn into the fibrotic mass and are, therefore, medially displaced, a finding that can be seen on intravenous urogram.[51] The aorta is variably dilated or narrowed. On CT scans, the mass is typically isoattenuating with skeletal muscle.[50,51] MRI examinations show the mass to be isointense to muscle on T1-weighted sequences. On T2-weighted sequences, the signal from the mass is variable depending on the stage of disease. In the early phases, the RPF will typically be hyperintense because of the presence of edema and inflammatory cells but late in disease will appear hypointense as a result of mature fibrosis.[50,51] Inhomogeneous T2 signal has been associated with RPF due to malignancies.[52] In comparison with lymphoma and other retroperitoneal neoplasms, RPF will usually not elevate the aorta away from the spine. In general, FDG-PET and PET-CT scans have been used to assess for disease activity (see Figure 15-8).[53]

Wall Calcification

Vascular calcification occurs at 2 distinct sites within the vessel wall: the intima and the media. Intimal calcification is a manifestation of atherosclerosis, whereas medial calcification can exist independently of atherosclerosis and is associated with aging, chronic renal failure, and diabetes mellitus.[54] Rarely, Takayasu arteritis and syphilitic aortitis will also be a cause of large vessel calcification.

Atherosclerosis and intimal calcification

Atherosclerosis results in focal calcification of the intima. Intimal calcification only occurs within atherosclerotic plaques and can be seen pathologically as early as the second decade of life but is typically first discovered on imaging examination of patients older than age 50 years.[54] Calcification appears to be a result of apoptotic cell death of intimal vascular smooth muscle cells, the presence of lipids and lipoproteins within the intima of the vessel, and mechanisms that increase calcium and phosphate extracellular concentrations.[54]

Calcified plaque typically appears as high-attenuation, plateau-shaped protuberance into the lumen of the vessel in question on CT scans and can extend over a few millimeters to many centimeters in length (see Figures 15-4, 15-9, and 15-10). Calcification typically occurs at the base of the plaque. Abdominal plain films can also demonstrate vascular calcifications as linear opacities in the distribution of the aorta and iliac vessels. On US examinations, atherosclerotic plaque calcifications will be seen as areas of shadowing along the surface of the aorta.

Aging, end-stage renal disease, diabetes mellitus, and medial calcification

Unlike atherosclerosis, aging, end-stage renal disease (ESRD), and diabetes mellitus cause calcification of the media of the vascular wall.[54,55] Medial calcification histologically appears as linear deposits along the elastic lamina and at its most severe can form dense circumferential calcification of the vessel wall. Atherosclerotic calcifications typically involve the large and medium arteries of the body such as the aorta and its main branch vessels. Whereas medial calcification will typically involve the small branch arteries of the periphery of the abdominal organs or lower extremities. This phenomenon is most commonly a complication of diabetes mellitus and chronic renal failure.[56] It also occurs in the small vessels of the foot and lower legs in otherwise healthy elderly patients, where it is called Mönckeberg sclerosis. Medial calcifications are associated with an increased incidence of neuropathy and

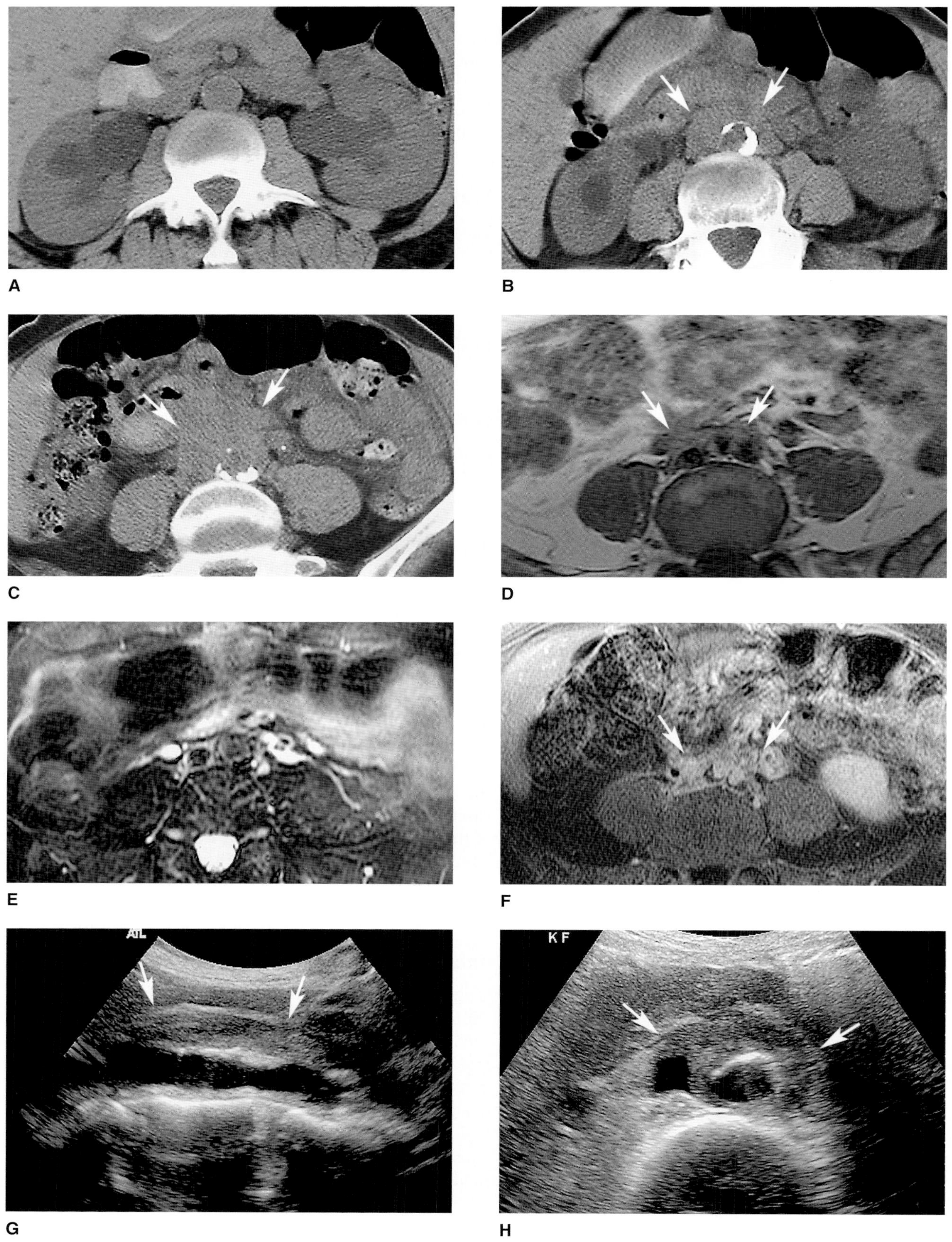

Figure 15-8 Retroperitoneal Fibrosis
This 52-year-old woman presented with renal insufficiency. **A-C.** Unenhanced CT shows bilateral hydroureteronephrosis and a poorly defined soft tissue mass (*arrows*) surrounding a heavily calcified aorta and iliac arteries. **D.** T1-weighted, (**E**) T2-weighted, and (**F**) postgadolinium MRI also shows a vague retroperitoneal soft-tissue mass, with intermediate T1, high T2 signal that moderately enhances. **G.** Longitudinal and (**H**) transaxial US also shows amorphous soft tissue surrounding the aorta and a diffusely thickened aortic wall. Biopsy was diagnostic of retroperitoneal fibrosis without evidence of malignancy.

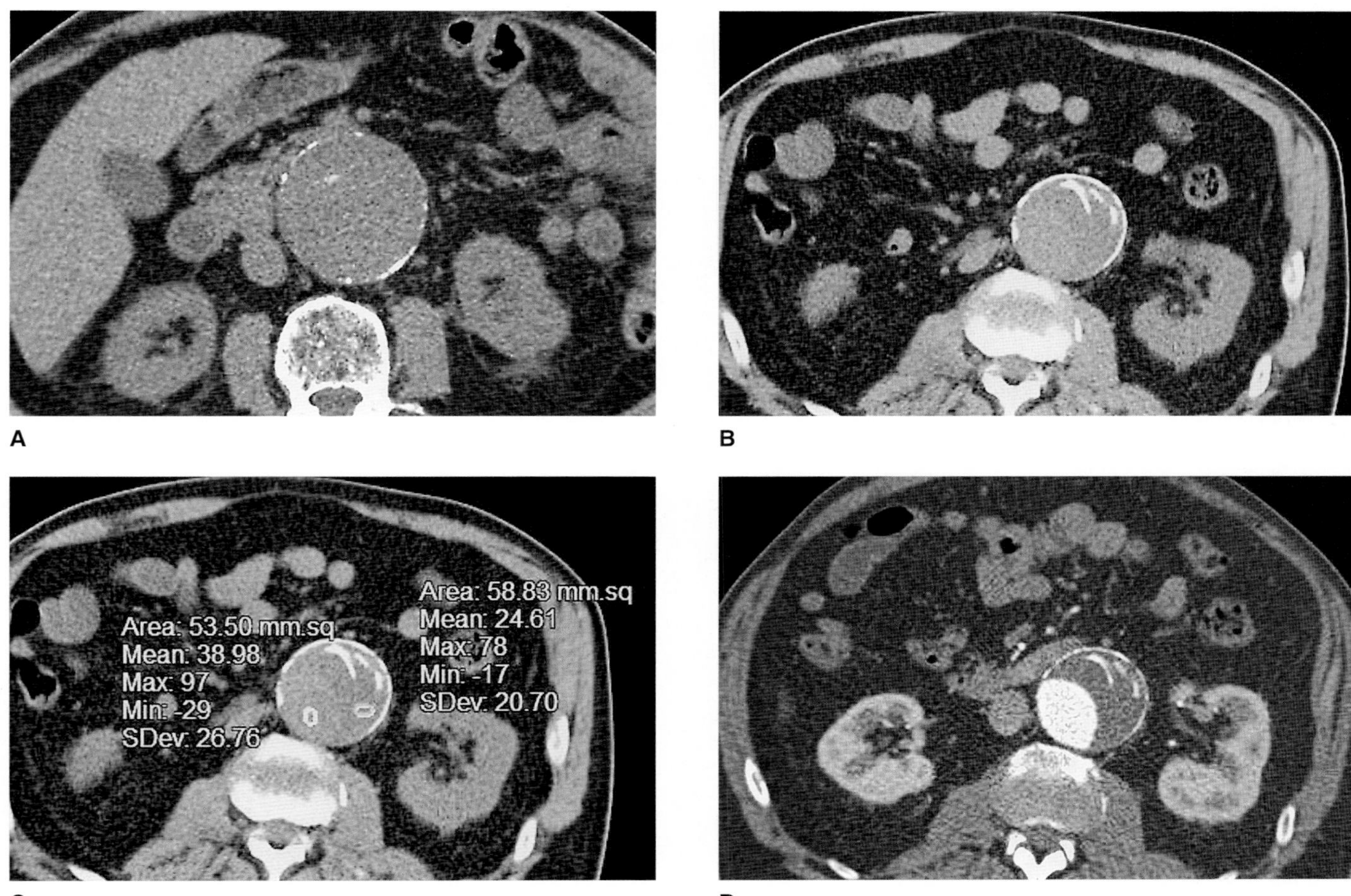

Figure 15-9 Intimal and Neointimal Calcifications in 2 Patients **A.** Axial unenhanced CT in the first patient shows an abdominal aortic aneurysm with both peripheral "rim" calcification and nonperipheral calcification. Rim calcification indicates intimal calcification. Nonperipheral calcification can represent displaced intimal calcifications or neointimal calcification, where neointimal calcification represents calcification of thrombus. **B-D.** CT images in a second patient with an abdominal aneurysm demonstrates similar peripheral and nonperipheral calcifications. The peripheral rim calcification are intimal calcification. In this case, we can prove that the nonperipheral calcifications are calcifications of thrombus, ie, neointimal calcification. Careful observation of (B) shows there to be a region of decreased attenuation surrounding the nonperipheral calcification, which is confirmed by the attenuation measurements in(C). Thrombus has a lower attenuation than blood in the lumen on unenhanced CT. Contrast-enhanced image (D) confirms the presence of thrombus within the lumen of the aneurysm with several areas of neointimal calcification.

are associated with increased cardiovascular mortality in patients with diabetes.[57,58]

Calcifications are typically identified in small and medium arteries throughout the body and can be seen in the extremities on x-rays of the hands, forearms, feet, and lower leg as paired linear opacities, which often demonstrate a branching pattern. Medial calcifications can also be seen in small vessels of the abdominal organs such as the kidneys, liver, and spleen on CT scans and appear as smooth, usually continuous, linear calcifications within the walls of small vessels with the involved organ (see Figures 15-11 and 15-12).[59] Small vessel calcification in most cases will indicate the presence of diabetes mellitus or chronic renal failure.

Vasculitis

Calcification as a manifestation of vasculitis is relatively uncommon, but is a known phenomenon in patients with Takayasu arteritis.

Takayasu arteritis: As noted previously, Takayasu arteritis is an uncommon idiopathic inflammatory condition of the large arteries of the body, seen predominantly in young and middle aged women. The most characteristic features of Takayasu arteritis are wall thickening, vascular stenosis, and aneurysm formation. However, as the disease becomes quiescent, the walls of involved vessels can develop extensive wall calcification.[18] Histologically, the calcification begins within the intima of the diseased vessel but can

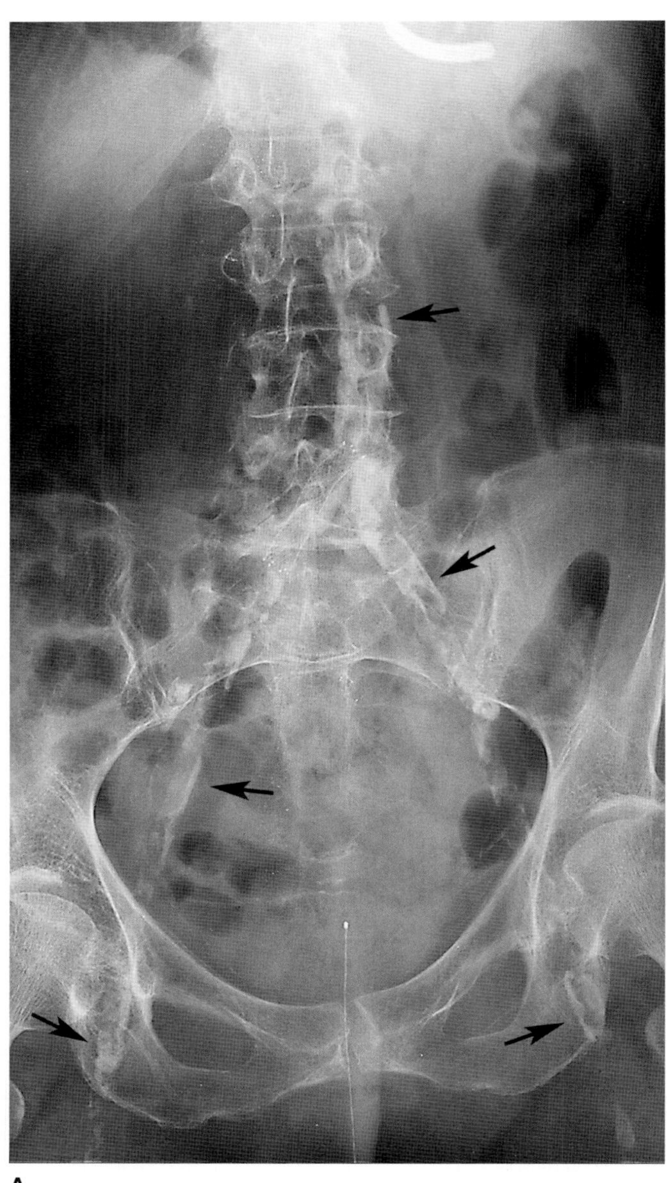

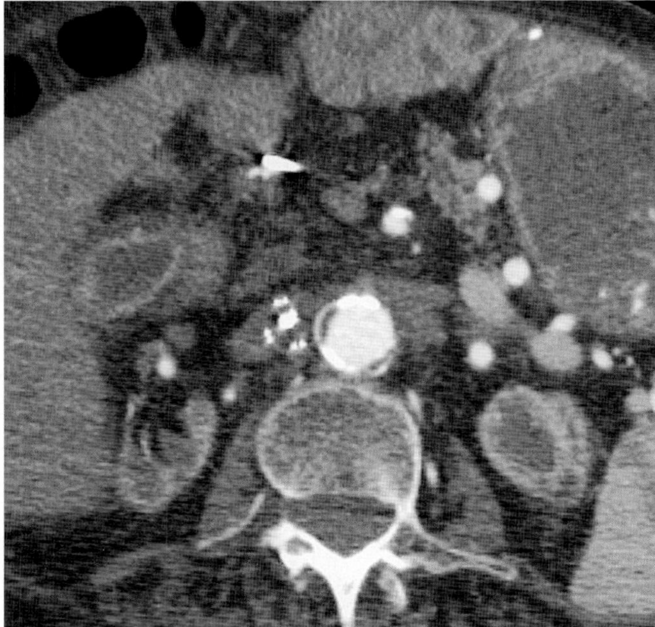

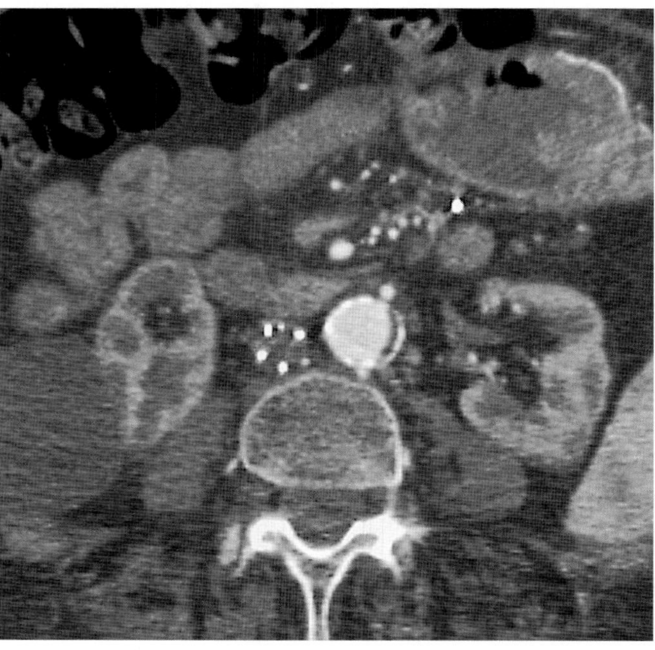

Figure 15-10 Calcified Atherosclerotic Plaque in 2 Patients
A. Abdominal radiograph shows tubular calcifications outlining the wall of the abdominal aorta, iliac arteries, and femoral arteries (*arrows*). In most cases, this will represent calcification of atherosclerotic plaque. **B** and **C.** Axial images of CTA through the abdominal aorta in a second patient shows calcification of the intima and noncalcified plaque deposited subintimally.

extend diffusely throughout the aortic wall. Diffuse calcification is not seen in patients with atherosclerosis and may be a specific finding of Takayasu arteritis.[18] Further, atherosclerosis is predominantly a disease of the elderly. The presence of extensive aortic calcification in a patient younger than age 40 years can suggest a diagnosis of Takayasu arteritis (see Figure 15-13). Some authors believe that the presence of mural calcification is protective against aneurysm formation.[37] They have found that most aneurysms form in regions of the aorta relatively devoid of wall calcification.

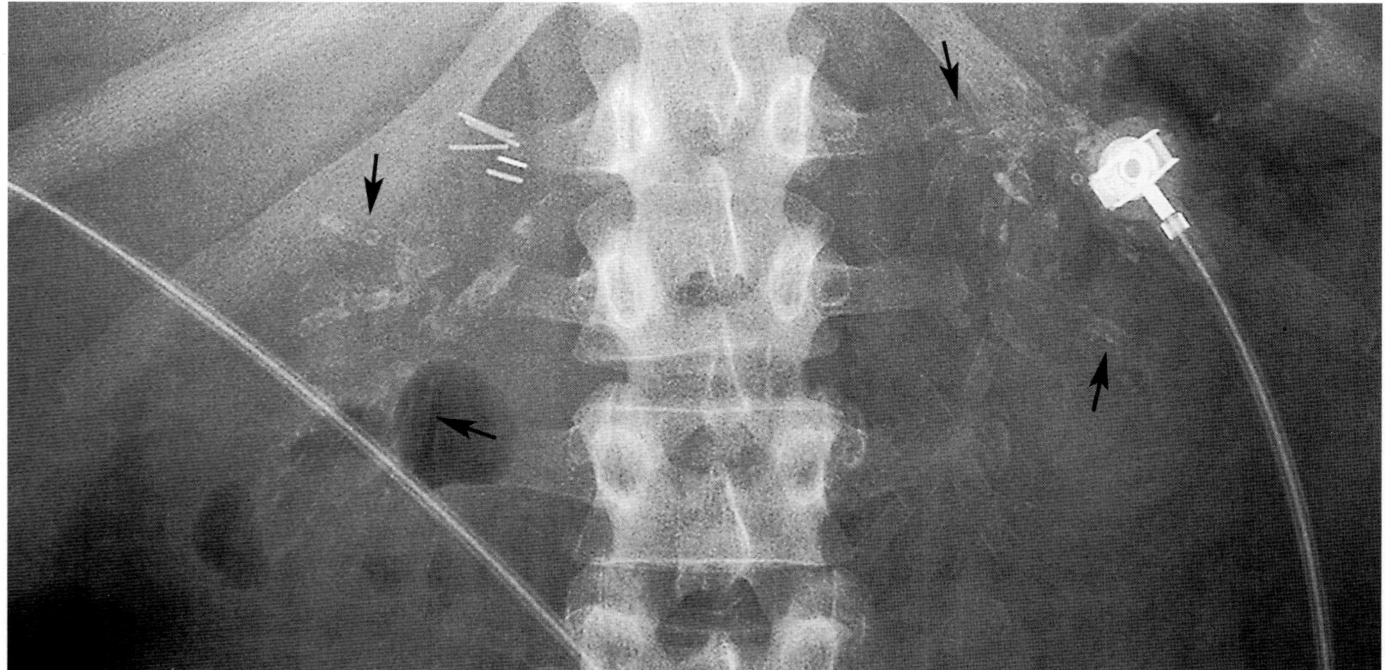

A

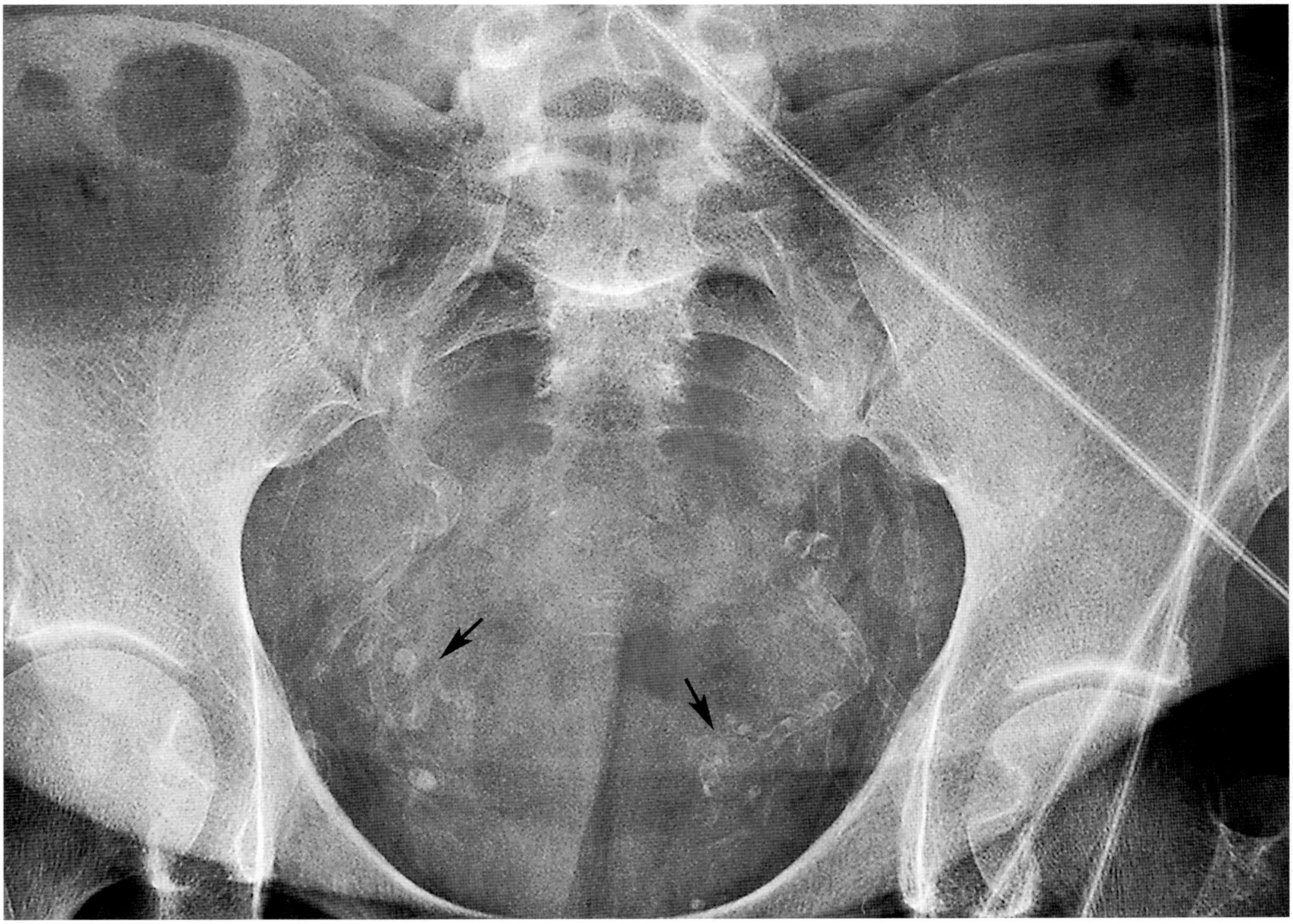

B

Figure 15-11 Small Vessel Calcifications on an Abdominal Radiograph This 36-year-old woman had childhood diabetes mellitus and chronic renal failure. Magnified views of the (**A**) upper abdomen and (**B**) pelvis from an abdominal radiograph demonstrate extensive vascular calcifications of the small arteries of the kidneys (*arrows* in A) and the branches of the internal iliac arteries (*arrows* in B).

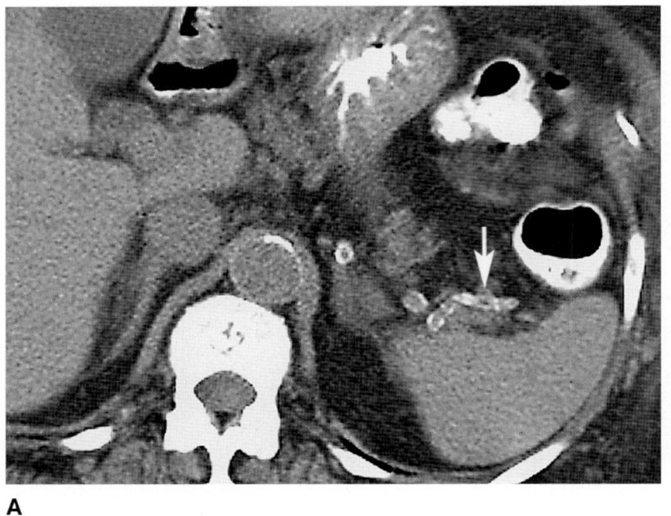
A

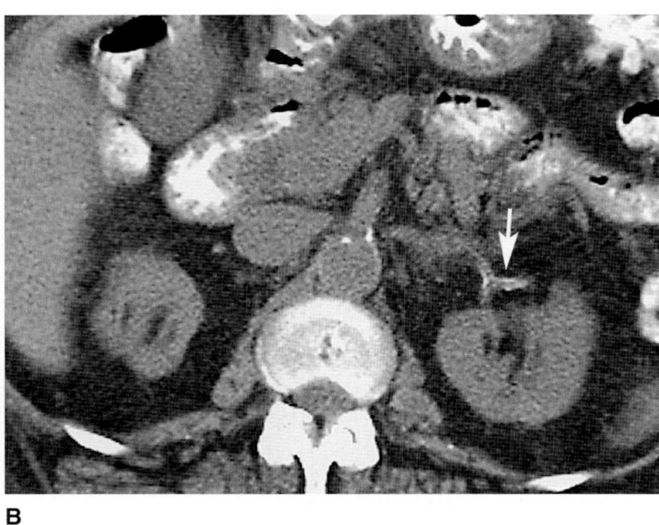
B

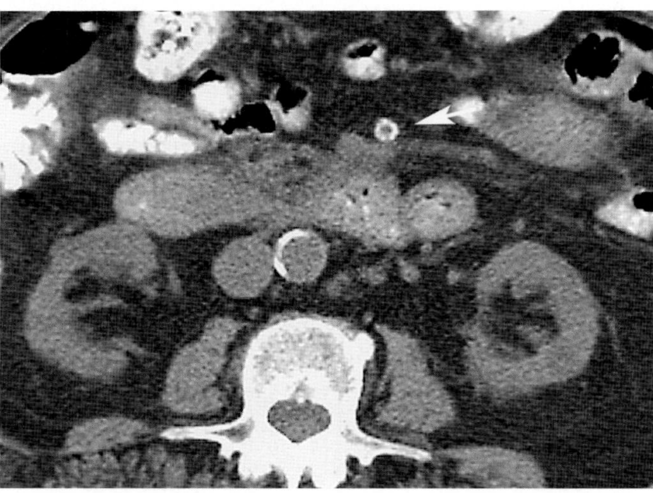
C

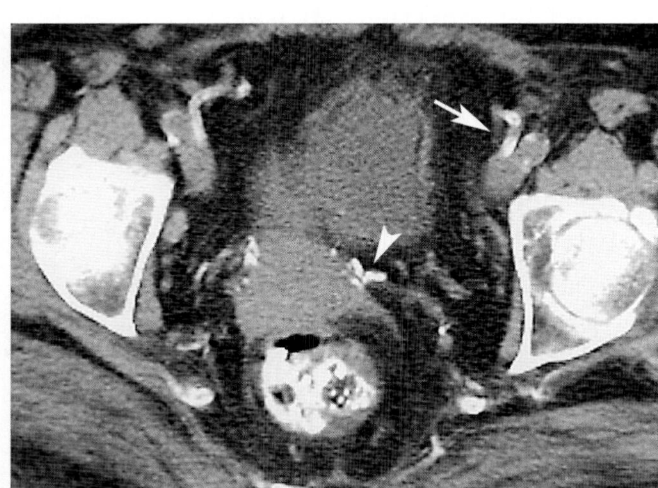
D

Figure 15-12 Small Vessel Calcification
This 77-year-old woman had both diabetes mellitus and chronic renal insufficiency. **A-D.** Axial CT images demonstrate multiple intermediate and small vessel calcifications of the splenic artery (*arrow* in A), the renal arteries (*arrow* in B), the SMA (*arrow* in C), and branches of the external iliac (*arrow* in D) and uterine arteries (*arrowhead* in D). Small vessel calcifications are often a manifestation of diabetes mellitus, renal dysfunction, or both.

Stenosis and Occlusion

The progressive narrowing of an arterial lumen produces end-organ ischemia. The most common cause of arterial narrowing is atherosclerosis. Nonatherosclerotic entities such as vasculitis and connective tissue disease should be considered in the younger individuals, in the absence of findings of atherosclerotic involvement, and with certain patterns of wall thickening or intimal disruption. Occasionally, vascular stenosis can be a result of external compression of an artery. This is best typified by the arcuate ligament syndrome.

Progressive narrowing will eventually occlude the artery. An artery can also be acutely occluded by an embolus or, more rarely, in situ thrombus. It is important to distinguish between an acute occlusion and chronic narrowing, as the former requires emergent intervention.

Patients will typically present with symptoms of end organ ischemia such as abdominal pain, renal insufficiency, and claudication.

In general, CTA and MRA will show narrowing of the involved vessel. Percentage of luminal narrowing is a predictor of end organ ischemia, with studies in some arterial beds suggesting that diameter narrowing greater than 70% is likely to be associated with hemodynamic compromise.[39] However, there is no universally accepted dividing line largely because each vascular bed is unique and there may be varying degrees of contribution from collateral vessels (Table 15-4).

An abrupt transition from enhanced vessel to unenhanced vessel, the meniscal sign, at the site of occlusion suggests the presence of acute thromboembolism whereas a smooth tapered narrowing will typically indicate stenosis

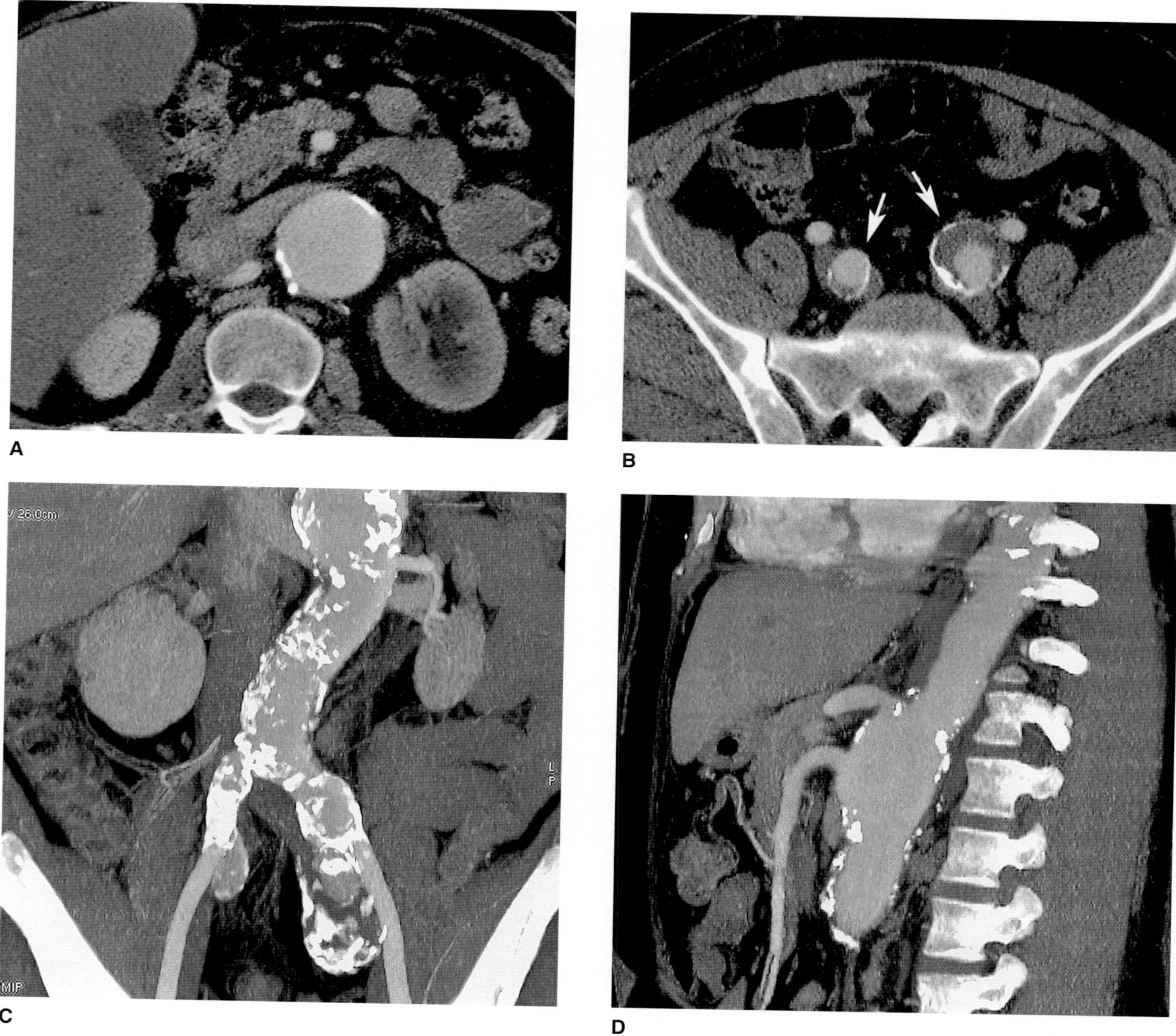

Figure 15-13 Abdominal Aneurysm due to Takayasu Arteritis This 34-year-old man had been diagnosed with Takayasu arteritis for several years. **A** and **B**. Contrast-enhanced axial CT images and MIP projection images in the (**C**) coronal and (**D**) sagittal planes show dilation of the infrarenal abdominal aorta and both internal iliac arteries (*arrows*). There are multiple plaquelike areas of calcification within the walls of the great vessels. In an elderly individual, this would most often be a result of degenerative aneurysms but in this young man are due to Takayasu arteritis.

(see Figures 15-14 and 15-15). The presence of enlarged collateral vessels will indicate a more long-standing stenosis. It can be difficult to distinguish between acute and chronic narrowing in cases of in situ thrombosis where there is a background of chronic narrowing with ischemia. In the presence of potential arterial compromise, the most important point to ascertain is the presence or risk of end-organ ischemia, in other words, whether the lesion is hemodynamically significant. Imaging features of end-organ ischemia on imaging ranges from asymmetry in the degree

Imaging Notes 15-2. Arterial Occlusion

- Where possible, a distinction between an acute occlusion and chronic occlusion of the arteries should be made
- The presence of collaterals suggests a chronic process
- The surrogate of the significance of arterial compromise is the organ itself

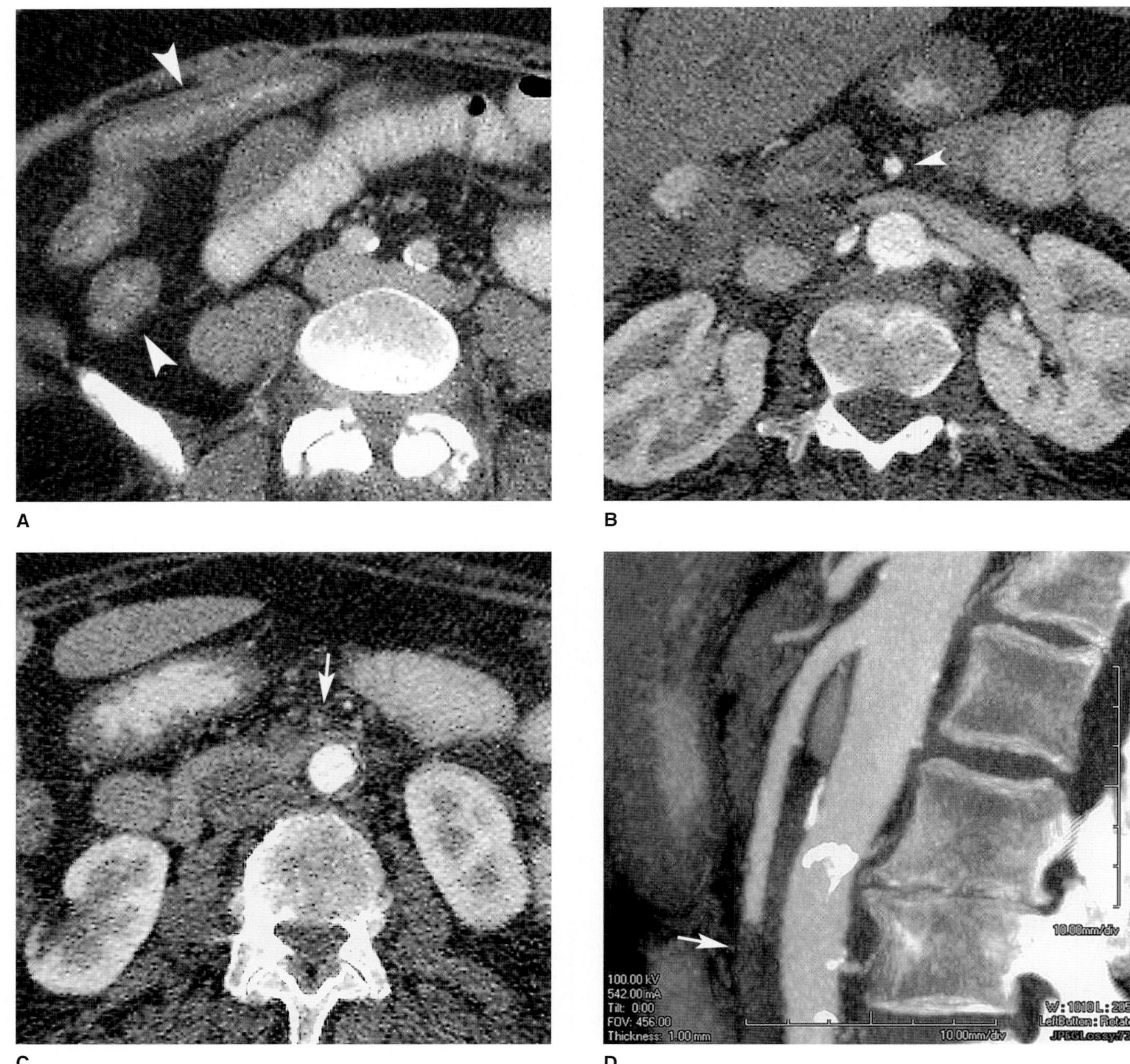

Figure 15-14 SMA Embolus
This 62-year-old woman with the recent onset of atrial fibrillation complained of 2 days of abdominal pain. **A.** Axial CT image through the midabdomen demonstrates thickening of the wall (*large arrowheads*) of the ascending and transverse colon. In this clinical setting, the possibility of ischemic colitis should be considered. **B** and **C.** Axial CTA confirms contrast in the proximal SMA (*small arrowhead*) but absence of contrast in the distal SMA (*arrow*). **D.** This abrupt transition between contrast-enhanced (*arrowhead*) and unenhanced (*arrow*) SMA is seen better on this sagical reconstruction and indicates the presence of an acute embolus (*arrow*) to the SMA causing colonic ischemia.

of vascular enhancement of the organ to an infarct whose morphology can take the classical wedge shape with the apex pointing centrally. The bowel shows some sign with ischemia/infarction with varying specificity. These include wall thickening with mural stratification, narrowing, pneumatosis coli, mesenteric venous air, and portal venous air. Although these findings are individually not specific for ischemia, the distribution, in particular of the wall thickening and location of the luminal narrowing, can be highly suggestive of an ischemic process if it conforms to

Table 15-4. Causes of Vascular Stenosis or Occlusion

1. Atherosclerosis
2. Emboli
3. Vasculitis
4. Connective tissue disease
5. Spontaneous thrombosis

a vascular territory. Features of end-organ ischemia have been discussed in detail in prior chapters under the organ of interest.

Atherosclerosis

Atherosclerosis is a chronic degenerative process causing the proliferation of smooth muscle cells that results in the production of fatty intimal lesions known as atherosclerotic plaques.[60] Plaques and plaque complications such as plaque rupture and associated arterial thrombosis can cause acute or chronic narrowing of arteries. As a result, many of the complications of atherosclerosis are a consequence of arterial stenosis and subsequent tissue ischemia and infarction. Both calcified and noncalcified plaque can lead to narrowing of an artery, creating flow-limiting stenosis and occlusion. The degree of atherosclerosis does not usually correlate with the degree of narrowing. This is because plaque can cause wall thickening without concomitant luminal narrowing, an observation known as the Glagov phenomenon.[61]

Stenosis due to atherosclerosis is identified by the presence of calcified and noncalcified plaque within the stenotic vessel. As noted previously, plaque typically appears as a calcified or noncalcified, plateau-shaped protuberance into the lumen of the vessel in question and can extend over a few millimeters to many centimeters in length (see Figure 15-16).

In addition to in situ narrowing and occlusion, atherosclerotic plaque can be a source of emboli. Friable plaque can be located in the descending aorta or the aortic arch. The presence of plaque ulceration is an important marker of an increased risk of embolization. Emboli as a cause for vascular occlusion are discussed later in this section.

Takayasu arteritis

One of the important complications of the large and medium vessel vasculitides is the development of vascular stenosis leading to end-organ stenosis.

Vascular stenosis is the most common complication of Takayasu arteritis. Histologically, the chronic inflammation of Takayasu arteritis leads to marked thinning of the media with disruption of elastic fibers and pronounced fibrotic thickening of the adventitia.[19,35] These changes result in

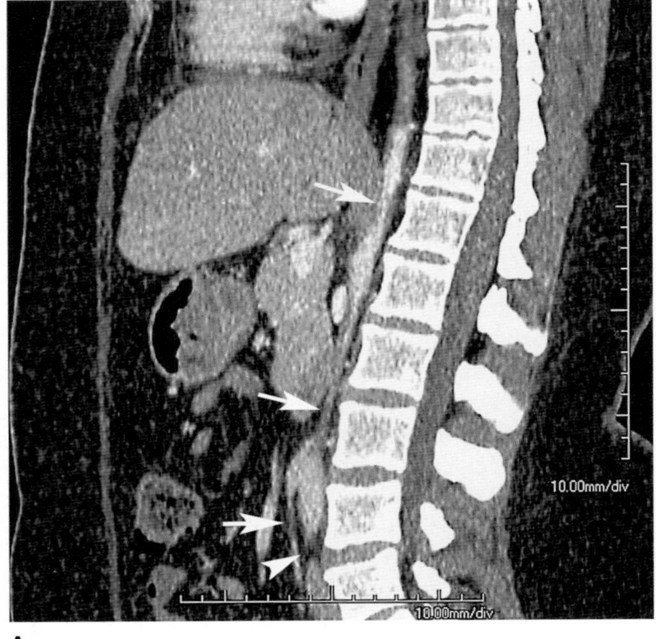

A

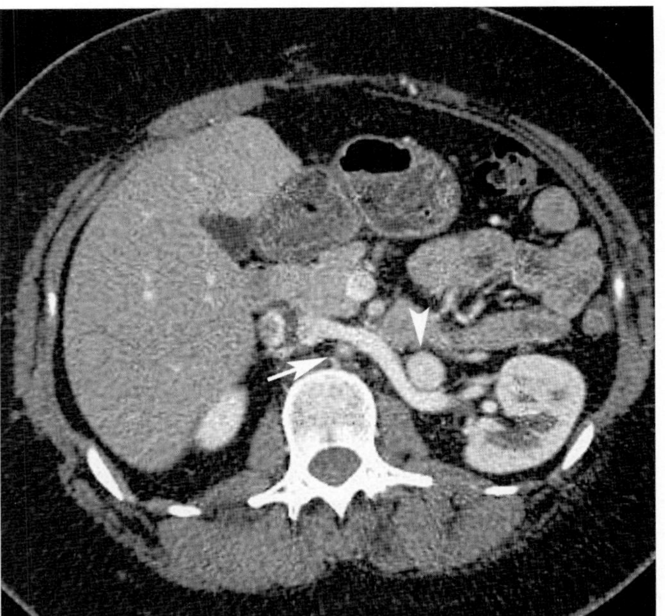

B

Figure 15-15 Stenosis due to Takayasu Arteritis
A. Sagittal MPR from CTA shows multisegment narrowing (*arrows*) of the abdominal aorta and branch vessels culminating in occlusion (*arrowhead*). **B.** Axial image at the level of the left renal vein shows an unidentifiable abdominal aorta (*arrow*) but a vascular structure anterior to the left renal vein (*arrowhead*) which is an extra-anatomical bypass graft connecting the proximal aorta to the prebifurcation abdominal aorta.

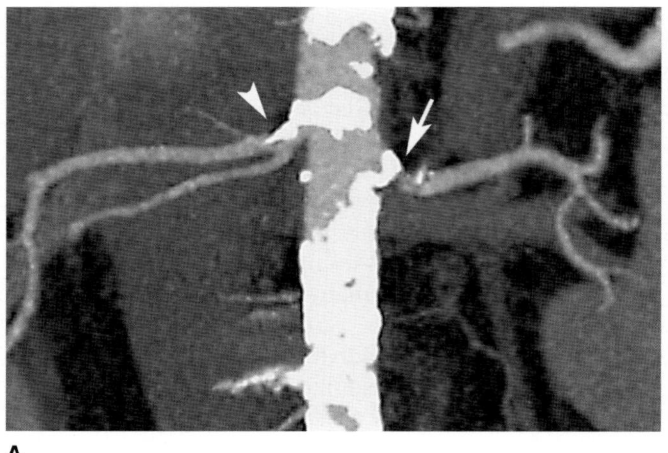

A

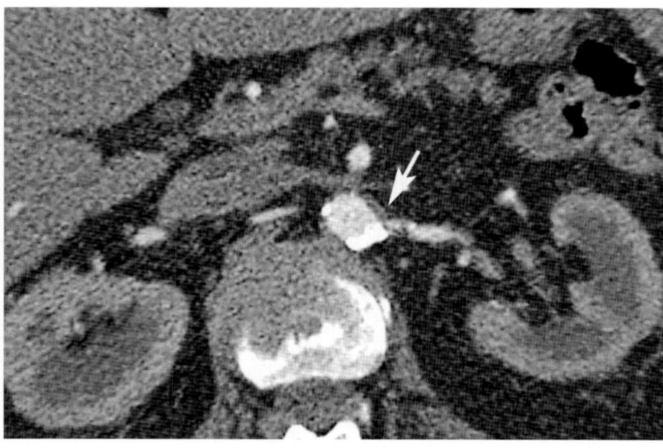

B

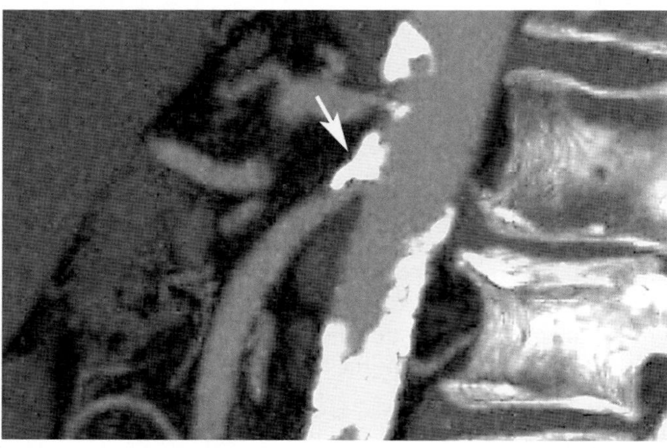

C

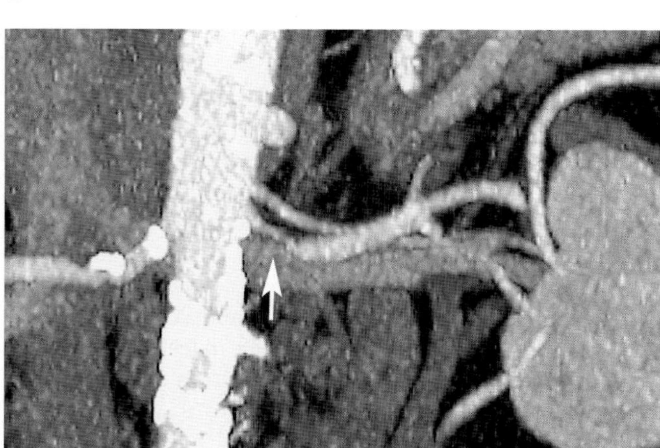

D

Figure 15-16 Stenosis due to Atherosclerosis in 2 Patients This 75-year-old woman had systemic hypertension. **A.** Maximum intensity projection (MIP) image from a CTA shows an approximately 50% ostial stenosis of the right renal artery (*arrowhead*) and what appears to be complete occlusion of the left renal artery (*arrow*) caused by large atherosclerotic plaques. **B.** Source axial image through the left renal artery shows a tight stenosis (*arrow*) but not occlusion due to aortic and renal artery plaque. **C.** Sagittal MIP through the SMA also shows plaque (*arrow*), causing an approximately 50% ostial stenosis. **D.** Coronal MIP in a 75-year-old man with claudication demonstrates a long noncalcified stricture of the left renal artery (*arrow*) due to atherosclerosis. He also had strictures of his femoral arteries (not shown), which were the cause of his claudication.

narrowing of the lumen of the vessel. The disease is seen primarily in young and middle-aged women, with median age of presentation of 36 years (range 19-57 y) and will usually present with systemic symptoms of fever, malaise, and weakness.[18] Arterial stenoses can also cause diminished or absent peripheral pulses and symptoms of ischemia in the affected territory (see Figures 15-7 and 15-16).

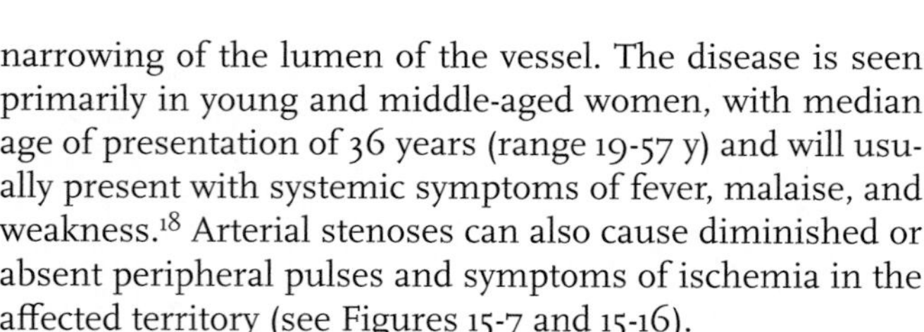

Connective tissue disease

A variety of connective tissue diseases can have vascular manifestations. The most common connective tissue disease that is associated with abdominal arterial stenosis is fibromuscular dysplasia.

Fibromuscular dysplasia: Fibromuscular dysplasia is a nonatherosclerotic, noninflammatory disorder of the arterial wall that most commonly affects the renal and common carotid arteries.[62] The etiology of fibromuscular dysplasia remains a mystery. However, the disease has an increased incidence in individuals who are current or former smokers and in those with systemic hypertension.[62] An increased incidence of fibromuscular dysplasia in first-degree relatives suggests that there are heritable factors in the development of disease.[62] Fibromuscular dysplasia has also been associated with Ehlers-Danlos syndrome type IV.

Fibromuscular dysplasia is subclassified depending on involvement of the layers of the vessel, the media, intima or adventitia.[62] **Medial fibromuscular dysplasia** is the most common type accounting for nearly 80% of all cases of fibromuscular dysplasia and is further subclassified into medial fibroplasia, perimedial fibroplasia, and medial hyperplasia. **Medial fibroplasia** is the most common subtype of medial fibromuscular dysplasia and is characterized by a hypertrophied media and a thin or absent internal elastic lamina. Weakening of the wall leads to multiple adjacent aneurysms in medium-sized arteries and causes the classic "string of pearl" appearance on imaging examinations.[62] In **perimedial fibroplasias**, the outer layer of the media undergoes fibrosis. This phenomenon primarily causes stenosis without aneurysm formation. The rarest subtype is the **medial hyperplasia** and appears as smooth concentric stenosis of the involved vessel.

Intimal fibroplasia accounts for <10% of all fibromuscular dysplasia and typically causes stenosis progressing to occlusion and end-organ ischemia.[62] The stenosis is smooth, mid vessel, and can be either an abrupt focal narrowing or a gradual elongated tubular narrowing.

Adventitial (periadventitial, periarterial) hyperplasia is the least common type of fibromuscular dysplasia. The fibrosis is centered in the adventitia and compresses the arterial lumen resulting in stenosis without aneurysm formation.[62]

Fibromuscular dysplasia is most commonly found in individuals from 15 to 50 years of age, although rarely it can be seen in patients older than 60 years.[62] It is more common in women and occasionally can be discovered incidentally during imaging performed for unrelated reasons. Clinical presentations are dependent on the vessels involved. Renal artery involvement is most common and typically presents as renovascular hypertension in a young individual, where it accounts for approximately 10% to 25% of cases of renovascular hypertension.[56,59,63] Renovascular hypertension accounts for approximately 5% of all cases of systemic hypertension.

Involvement of the carotid artery is the second most common site of disease and will typically present with nonspecific cranial symptoms such as headache, tinnitus, vertigo, lightheadedness, and syncope and occasionally with the more vascular specific symptoms such as transient ischemic attack, amaurosis fugax, stroke, Horner syndrome, and cranial-nerve palsies.[62] Fibromuscular dysplasia can also involve the iliac, hepatic, splenic, superior mesenteric, and inferior mesenteric arteries, causing symptoms of ischemia in the vascular territory involved.

Fibromuscular dysplasia most often appears as stenosis or aneurysm formation of the medium arteries of the abdomen on CTA, MRA, and angiographic examinations.[59,64-66] Conventional angiography remains the criterion standard for this diagnosis because of its greater spatial resolution. However both CTA and MRA have been shown to have high sensitivities and specificities for the diagnosis of fibromuscular dysplasia and are commonly used as screening studies because of their noninvasive nature.[59,64-66] Renal arteries are most commonly involved; however, hepatic, splenic, superior mesenteric, inferior mesenteric, and iliac arteries can also be diseased. In many subtypes, fibromuscular dysplasia will result in smooth stenosis of medium arteries of the abdomen and neck. Features that help distinguish fibromuscular dysplasia related stenosis from atherosclerotic stenoses include (1) nonostial location, (2) lack of atherosclerosis elsewhere, and (3) young age of the patient (see Figure 15-17).[62] Fibromuscular dysplasia will typically involve the distal two-thirds of the renal artery and its branch vessels, whereas atherosclerotic stenoses will characteristically involve the ostia of the renal arteries.[59]

Some patients will demonstrate combination of multiple sequential foci of narrowing and aneurysm resulting in the "string of beads" appearance (see Figure 15-17). This appearance is virtually diagnostic of a diagnosis of fibromuscular dysplasia and will usually indicate the medial fibroplasia subtype of disease.[62]

Angiographic studies have demonstrated progression of disease in up to 37% of patients with fibromuscular dysplasia, when progression is defined as the occurrence of a new focal lesion, worsening arterial stenosis, or the enlargement of an aneurysm.[64,67]

Thromboembolism

Whereas stenosis is typically a slow, progressive, chronic phenomenon that will result in nonemergent intervention, thromboembolism is typically an acute event that requires immediate medical response. Embolism to arterial branches leads to acute or acute on chronic ischemia and arise from thrombus in the upstream arterial tree. The most common sources of upstream thrombus are the left atrial appendage in a patient with atrial fibrillation, and the apex of the left ventricle post myocardial infarction or dilated cardiomyopathy. Occasionally, thrombus originating in the venous system can cross into the arterial system through a patent foramen ovale or septal defect [atrial septal defect (ASD) and ventricular septal defect (VSD)], a phenomenon known as a paradoxical embolus. Thrombus associated with atherosclerotic plaque and other vascular injury can also be a source of downstream embolism. This is especially problematic following vascular intervention.

An acute thromboembolism will typically take 1 of 2 appearances, depending on whether the thromboembolus completely or partially occludes the vessel in question. With partial occlusion, the thromboembolus will appear as an elongated linear filling defect within the lumen of the vessel in question. By "filling defect," we mean a linear region of nonenhancement surrounded by the enhanced blood within the lumen of the vessel. The emboli will often get caught at the branching of a vessel and so it is common for emboli to be centered at the bifurcation of a vessel, with one end of the thromboembolus causing a filling defect in one branch and the other end of the embolus causing a filling defect in the other branch. If the thromboembolus completely occludes the vessel, there will be an abrupt termination of the contrast filled vessel (see Figure 15-14).

Spontaneous thrombosis

Certain hypercoagulable states can lead to in situ thrombosis. Examples of such entities include deficiency of proteins C, S, and antithrombin 3, nephrotic syndrome, and

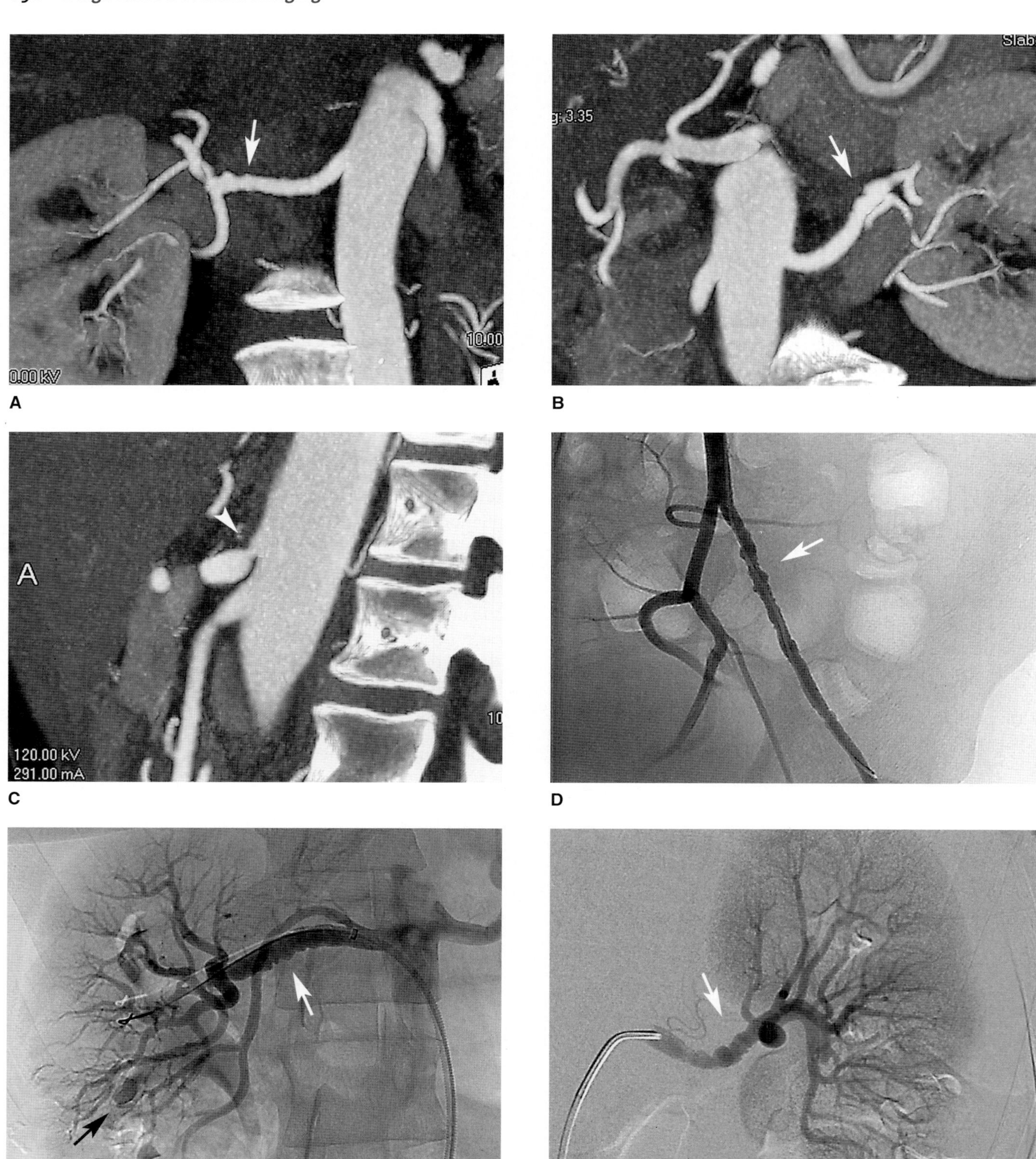

Figure 15-17 Fibromuscular Dysplasia in 2 Patients
Both of these patients presented with renovascular hypertension. **A-C.** Multiplanar reconstructions from a CTA in this 40-year-old woman demonstrate an undulating appearance of aneurysms and strictures (*white arrows*) of the (A) right and (B) left renal arteries characteristic of fibromuscular dysplasia. (C) There is also a smooth stricture of the celiac axis (*arrowhead*). This appearance is specific for fibromuscular dysplasia. **D-F.** This 37-year-old woman presented with hypertension. Selective angiograms of the (D) superior mesenteric artery, (E) right renal artery, and (F) left renal artery show the typical undulating narrowing and dilation of medium vessels (*white arrows*) characteristic of fibromuscular dysplasia. There are also several peripheral aneurysms (*black arrows*) in the lower pole of the right kidney.

paroxysmal nocturnal hemoglobinuria. Occasionally, treatment with heparin for thromboembolic disease can lead to a paradoxical hypercoagulable state called heparin-induced thrombocytopenic syndrome. Patients will typically present with symptoms of end-organ ischemia.

Median arcuate ligament syndrome

The median arcuate ligament is a fibrous arch that unites the diaphragmatic crura across the aortic hiatus. In the majority of patients, the ligament passes superior to the origin of the celiac axis; however, in 13% to 50% of people, the ligament crosses anterior to and can cause compression of the anterior wall of the celiac axis.[68-70] In most cases, this is a clinically insignificant finding without symptoms; however, in a minority of individuals, compression can compromise blood flow, causing symptoms of gut ischemia. Thus, the radiographic finding of celiac axis compression is usually not significant, unless it is associated with clinical symptoms.

Median arcuate ligament syndrome typically occurs in patients between 20 and 40 years of age and is more common in thin individuals and in women.[68,71] Symptoms include epigastric pain, which can be exacerbated by eating, and weight loss.[68,70] Physical examination in some cases will demonstrate an abdominal bruit in the midepigastric region.

In general, CT and MR angiograms demonstrate a characteristic focal narrowing in the proximal celiac axis. The focal narrowing is seen as depression of the anterior wall of the celiac artery on sagittal images or 3D reconstructions, giving the proximal celiac artery a "hooked" appearance (see Figure 15-18).[68] This appearance can also be demonstrated by Doppler US.[71] Axial images alone can miss the narrowing associated with arcuate ligament compression. Typically compression occurs at end expiration.[68] Some cases will demonstrate poststenotic dilation of the artery just distal to the compression.

Aneurysms

An aneurysm is dilation of the blood vessel usually to greater than 1.5 times the normal diameter. General agreement has defined the "normal" diameter of the suprarenal abdominal aorta to be 28 mm and the infrarenal abdominal aorta to be 20 mm.

Degenerative aneurysms associated with atherosclerosis and systemic hypertension are the most common cause of AAA. Other causes of abdominal aneurysms include connective tissue disorders such as Marfan syndrome, Ehlers-Danlos syndrome, mycotic aneurysms, large vessel vasculitis, such as Takayasu and giant cell arteritis, aortic dissections, intramural hematomas, PAUs, and trauma.[18,37,72-78]

Aneurysms represent a medically important condition because of the risk of rupture and sudden death. The risk of aneurysm rupture is proportional to the diameter of the aneurysm.[79-81] Various studies have shown a growth rate of aortic aneurysms between 0.22 and 0.57 cm per

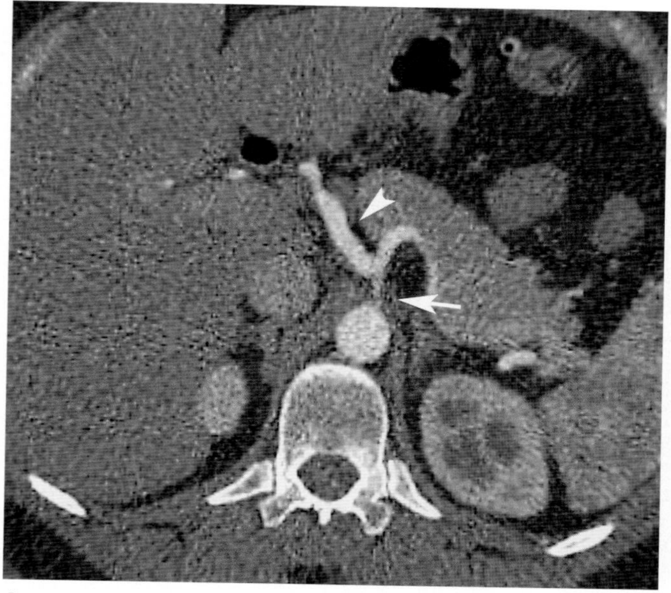

A

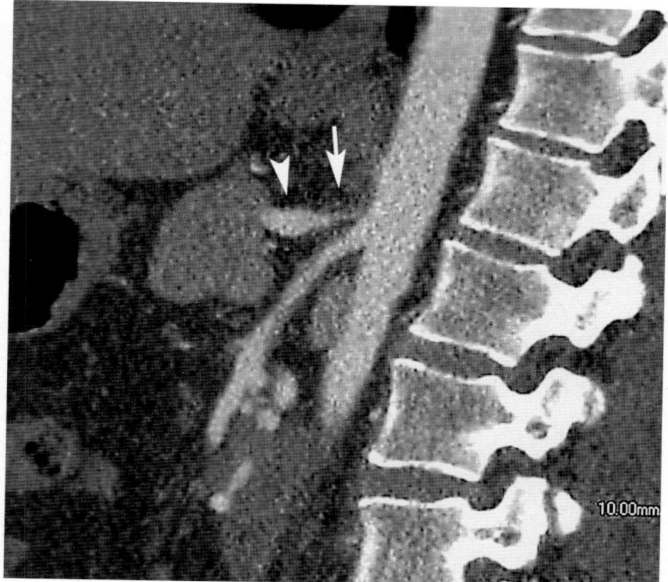

B

Figure 15-18 Median Arcuate Ligament Syndrome
A. Axial and (**B**) sagittal multiplanar reconstruction CTA shows compression of the celiac artery (*arrow*) by the arcuate ligament with poststenotic dilation (*arrowhead*). The compression leads to an imprint on the anterior wall, which is greater in expiration. Depending on the degree of compression there can be, as in this case, poststenotic dilation.

year.[82-91] The growth rate increases with increasing sized of the aneurysm.[79] Thoracic aortic aneurysms appear to have higher growth rates than AAAs, especially those involving the aortic arch.[79]

The majority of AAAs are clinically silent.[92] As a consequence, screening for abdominal aneurysms has been advocated by some physicians. Two studies have suggested that 1-time ultrasonographic screening of men, at the age of 65 years, is sufficient to identify nearly all those who are at risk.[92,94] Aneurysms are often found incidentally as a pulsatile mass on physical examination or as vascular dilation on imaging examinations performed for other indications (see Figure 15-19). When symptomatic, they will most often present with back pain and can present with signs of acute rupture that include back pain, severe hypotension, and sudden death. Many aneurysms will develop mural thrombus that can lead to vascular occlusion or distal emboli, either of which can cause signs and symptoms of ischemia.

Morphologically, aneurysms can take 1 of 2 shapes, fusiform or saccular. Fusiform aneurysms demonstrate uniform dilation of the blood vessel, characterized by smooth progressive dilation and then smooth resumption of normal size. Saccular aneurysms have nonuniform dilation of the wall, characterized by abrupt dilation of one side of the vessel that balloons out from the main vascular channel. Different etiologies of aneurysm are more likely to produce 1 of the 2 morphologies of aneurysm. In general, systemic diseases of the vasculature, such as atherosclerosis, vasculitis, and connective tissue disorders will produce fusiform aneurysms, whereas focal lesions of the vessel, such as trauma, infection, and PAUs, will cause saccular aneurysms.

Imaging Notes 15-3. Pathophysiology of Fusiform and Saccular Aneurysms

- Fusiform aneurysm will most often indicate the presence of a systemic disease of the vasculature such as atherosclerosis, vasculitis, or connective tissue disorder.
- Saccular aneurysms will usually indicate a focal lesion of the aorta such as infection, trauma, or penetrating atherosclerotic ulcer.

Because they are by large measure the most common, it is reasonable to assume that most AAAs are degenerative aneurysms associated with hypertension and atherosclerosis. Imaging features that should suggest that an aneurysm may not be degenerative in origin include (1) saccular morphology, (2) involvement of branch vessels while sparing the abdominal aorta, and (3) absence or limited extent of atherosclerotic plaque. Saccular aneurysms should raise the possibility of infection, PAU and trauma. Selective aneurysms of the branch arteries with sparing of the abdominal aorta in the absence of atherosclerosis in a young patient should raise the possibility of connective tissue disease and vasculitis. Isolated aneurysms of the branch artery in the absence of features of atherosclerosis can also be due

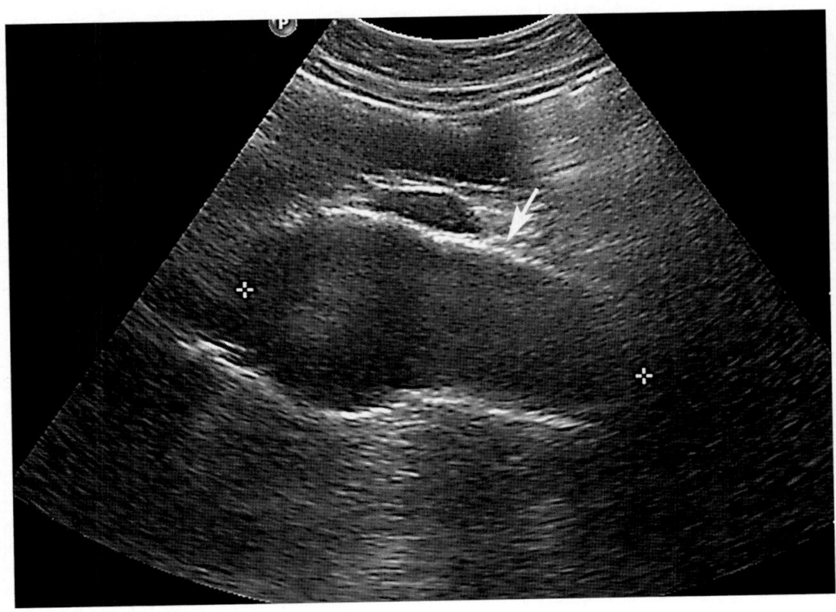

A

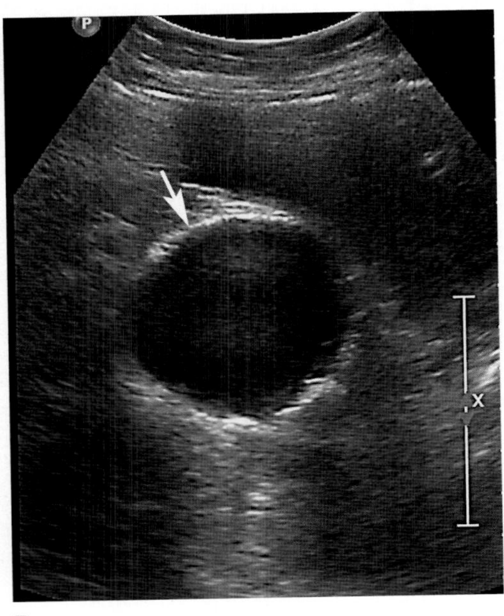

B

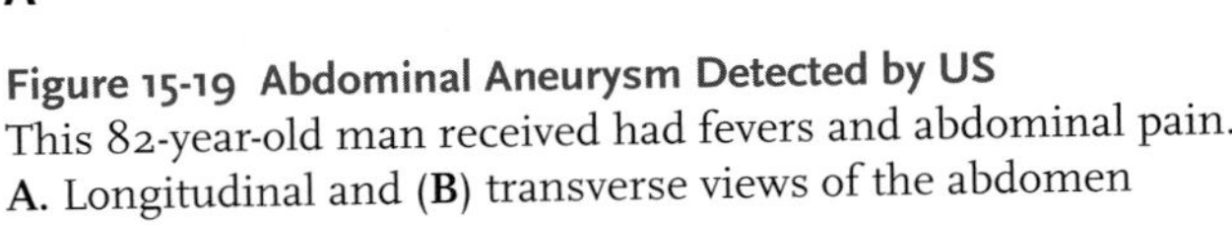

Figure 15-19 Abdominal Aneurysm Detected by US
This 82-year-old man received had fevers and abdominal pain. **A.** Longitudinal and (**B**) transverse views of the abdomen demonstrate a markedly dilated abdominal aorta (*arrows*), indicating the presence of a fusiform aneurysm. The maximum cross-sectional distance was 4.7 cm.

Table 15-5. Causes of Aneurysms in the Abdominal Aorta and Branches

1. Atherosclerosis
2. Intramural hematoma and dissection
3. Vasculitis and connective tissue disorders
4. Infection
5. Inflammatory aneurysms
6. Trauma/surgery
7. Pancreatitis
8. Compression

to local extravascular processes such as arcuate ligament compression of the celiac artery, pancreatitis, or surgery. Often isolated aneurysms will not have a specific etiology (Table 15-5).

It is important for radiologists to evaluate aortic aneurysms for signs of instability and/or rupture. Rapid growth of an aneurysm is a sign of aneurysm instability. The high attenuation crescent sign, the draped aorta sign, and discontinuity of intimal calcifications are signs associated with impending rupture.[95,96] The presence of a periaortic hematoma indicates rupture.[97-100]

A high-attenuation crescent within the mural thrombus on CT images is a sign of impending rupture and is a relative indication for emergent surgery. Twenty-one percent (11/52) of ruptured aneurysms and no unruptured aneurysms exhibited this sign in one study.[101] It is generally believed that the high attenuation crescent represents an area of acute hemorrhage into organized thrombus within the lumen of the aneurysm.[102] This high-attenuation crescent is seen best on unenhanced scans because of greater conspicuity of acute blood on unenhanced images. However, careful inspection can also reveal this sign on enhanced images (see Figure 15-20).

The "draped aorta" sign is an additional imaging finding associated with impending aortic rupture. In this sign, the wall of the aorta adjacent to the spine is indistinct (see Figure 15-20).

Focal discontinuity of intimal calcifications within the aortic wall also has been associated with rupture of aortic aneurysms in some series.[101] However, others have suggested that this is an unreliable finding of aortic rupture.[98,103,104]

Imaging Notes 15-4. The Crescent Sign

- High attenuation within the mural thrombus, the crescent sign, is an indicator of instability of the aneurysm

Degenerative AAAs (Atherosclerotic aneurysm, AAA)

Most AAAs are a result of chronic inflammation and degeneration of the aortic wall associated with aging, male sex, history of smoking, systemic hypertension, and hyperlipidemia.[92,105] The risk factors for AAAs are the same as those for atherosclerosis and in the past, this has been used to suggest that these aneurysms are caused by atherosclerosis. However, current thinking suggests that AAAs are associated with but have a separate pathophysiology to atherosclerosis.[97-109] This phenomenon lacks a specific name and is referred to as "abdominal aortic aneurysm" in the medical literature without distinguishing this disorder from other causes of AAAs such as vasculitis, connective tissue diseases, and infection. In this text, we use the term *degenerative abdominal aortic aneurysm* or *degenerative aneurysm* to identify this disorder from other causes of aneurysms.

Degenerative aneurysms are among the most common disease in the adult population. A population-based study of 6386 men and women aged 25 to 84 years in Tromsø, Norway, revealed a prevalence of degenerative aneurysms of 8.9% in men and 2.2% in women.[92] The primary pathologic mechanism for the formation of degenerative aneurysms is the degeneration of elastin, mediated by an increase in the presence of proteolytic enzymes, particularly matrix metalloproteinase.[107] This leads to the progressive atrophy of the musculolamellar units of the media of large arteries, which is replaced by fibrosis. This process reduces the elasticity of the arterial wall, causing dilation of systemic arteries in response to pulsations of systolic blood pressure. Laplace's law states that the wall tension of the wall of a spherical object (T) is directly proportional to product of the transmural pressure gradient and the diameter and inversely proportional to the radius. By Laplace's law, as the artery dilates, there is progressive increase in the force on the arterial wall, further increasing the tendency toward aneurysm formation.[110]

Imaging examinations will typically demonstrate fusiform dilation of the aortic wall (see Figures 15-5, 15-9, and 15-19).

Inflammatory aneurysms (chronic periaortitis, retroperitoneal fibrosis)

Inflammatory aneurysms of the aorta were at one time thought to be a variant of atherosclerotic aneurysms characterized by inflammation and/or fibrosis in the aortic wall or periaortic tissues and were thought to be an inflammatory reaction to atherosclerotic plaques.[111,112] However, inflammatory aneurysms are now believed to be part of the spectrum of RPF and are thought to be a result of an autoimmune disorder. Abnormal proteolysis of the media results in degeneration of the wall associated with deficiencies in collagen and elastin.[113-117] Loss of collagen and elastin

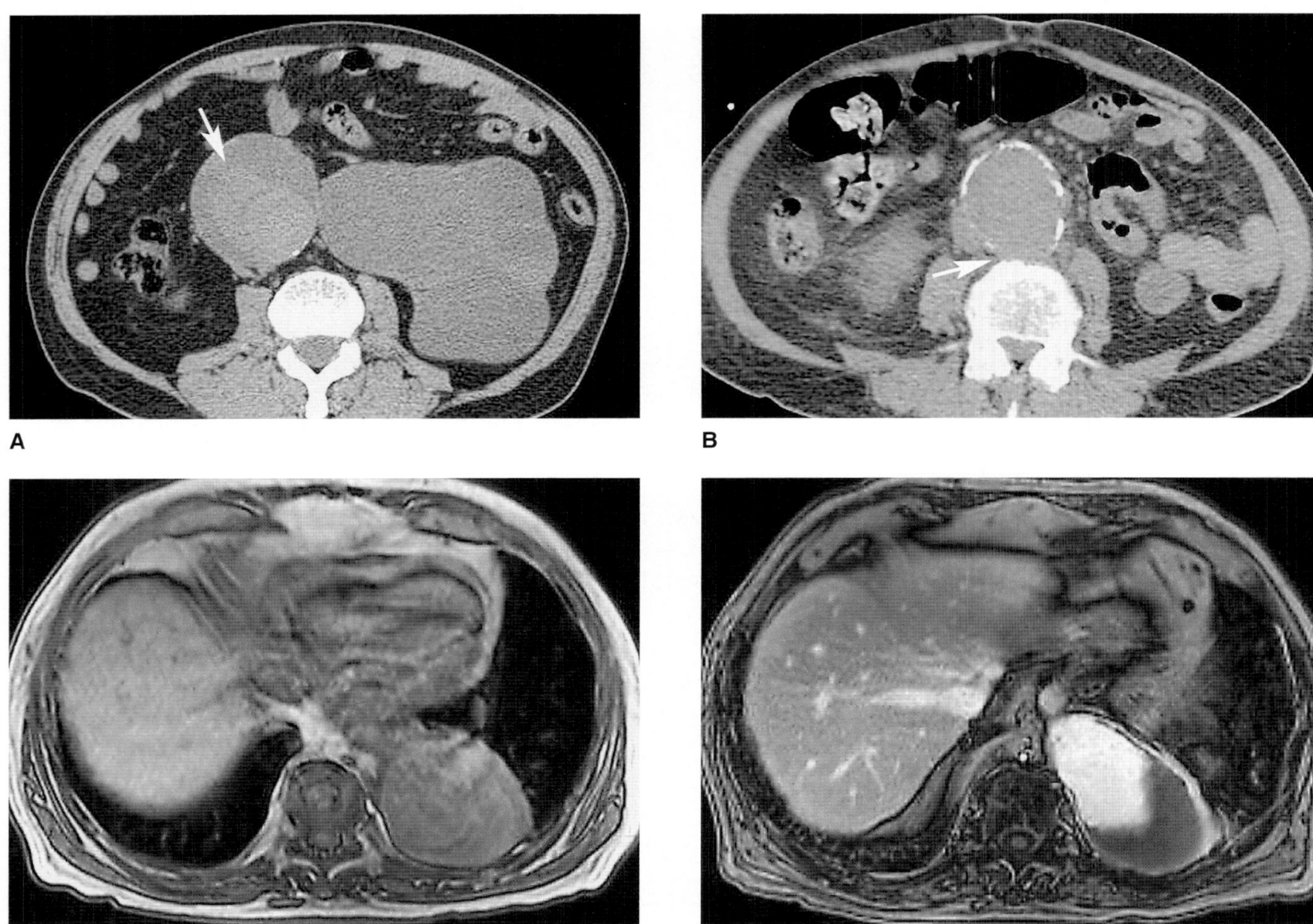

Figure 15-20 Signs of Aneurysm Instability in 3 Patients
A. This 74-year-old male with bladder cancer and severe hydronephrosis. Note the subtle high attenuation crescent (*arrow*) within the center of the mural thrombus in this patient with an AAA. This finding indicates acute hemorrhage into the thrombus and is a sign of instability. **B.** This 60-year-old male with AAA had abdominal pain. Note the loss of fat plane (*arrow*) between the aorta and the vertebral body with the appearance of the aorta actually sitting on the vertebral body is known as the "draped aorta" sign. This is a sign of instability of aneurysm and such aneurysms have a higher chance of rupturing. **C** and **D.** This 82-year-old man had back pain. (C) Axial T1-weighted sequences shows a large descending thoracic aortic aneurysm with high signal in the lateral aspect. (D) Postcontrast T1-weighted sequence shows this high signal to be within thrombus. This high signal indicates subacute hemorrhage into the clot and is a sign of instability.

reduces the elasticity and strength of the aortic wall and results in dilation.

Patients characteristically present with back or flank pain and tenderness. Laboratory tests, such as erythrocyte sedimentation rate or C-reactive protein, will be elevated in some patients, indicating the presence of indicate active inflammation.[118-120] Some patients will have constitutional symptoms such as weight loss.[120] Because of the extensive RPF associated with inflammatory aneurysms, surgical correction is often difficult with increased incidence of complications.[119,121]

Inflammatory aneurysms will usually take 1 of 2 appearances on CT scans. In some cases, it will resemble diffuse thickening of the aortic wall in addition to aortic dilation.[118-120,122] When taking this appearance, inflammatory aneurysms may be confused with a large vessel vasculitis, such as Takayasu arteritis or with mycotic aneurysms. In other instances, inflammatory aneurysms will appear as a soft-tissue mass surrounding and contiguous with the aortic wall, a finding that has been termed the "mantle core" sign.[118,122] In this situation, the disorder can be confused with lymphoma or a soft tissue neoplasm. In most cases, the perianeurysmal inflammation and/or fibrosis will spare the region of the aorta adjacent to the spine.[122-124] Following contrast administration, the reactive tissue will demonstrate variable enhancement.[122-124]

Penetrating atherosclerotic ulcer

Ulceration is an important complication of atherosclerotic plaque that can lead to the development of aortic aneurysms and aortic dissections. PAUs are seen primarily in the elderly and can present with symptoms of chest or abdominal pain similar to that seen with aortic dissection. In other situations, PAUs will be discovered incidentally during imaging for other purposes. Aneurysms represent one of the life-threatening complications of PAUs and will typically appear as saccular dilations of the thoracic or abdominal aorta. PAU is discussed most completely under the subsequent heading: **Wall Disruption** (see Figures 15-21 and 15-22).

Intramural hematoma and dissection

As noted previously, intramural hematoma in some patients leads to the development of an aneurysm. It is believed that intramural hematoma weakens the wall of the involved vessel, subjecting the wall to greater degrees of transmural pressure, leading to dilation of the vessel by Laplace law. Intramural hematoma can result in both saccular and fusiform aneurysms. Intramural hematoma is discussed most completely under the previous heading: **Wall Thickening.**

Similar to intramural hematoma, dissection can become aneurysmal over time. Dissection is discussed most completely under the subsequent heading: **Wall Disruption.**

Mycotic aneurysm

The term *mycotic* is a misnomer. Causative agents are most often bacteria and not fungal organisms, with *Staphylococcus aureus*, *Salmonella* species, and *Escherichia coli* the most commonly isolated organisms.[74,125-129] Bacterial infection of the vascular wall can occur via 1 of 4 routes: (1) implantation on the intimal surface, (2) seeding of bacterial via the vasa vasorum, (3) direct extension from a contiguous extravascular site, and (4) direct traumatic inoculation of a vessel with contaminated material.[74] Aneurysms will in most cases rapidly form over the course of a few days after the

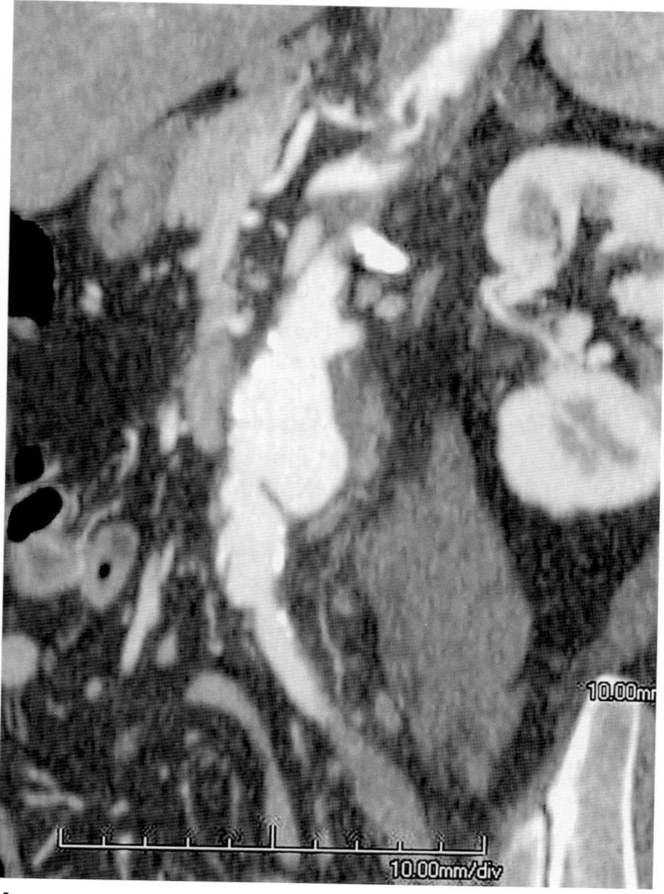

A

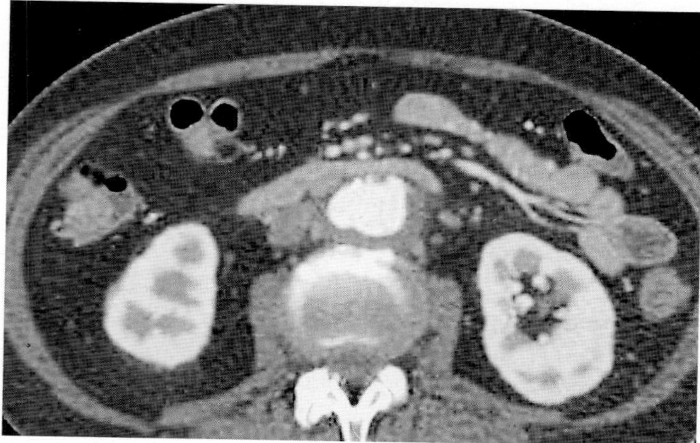

B

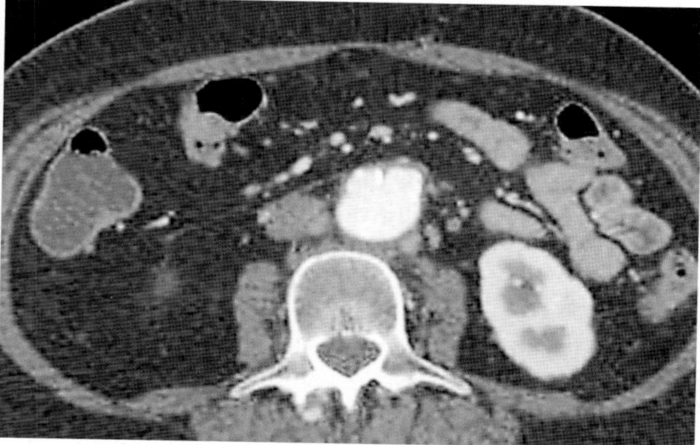

C

Figure 15-21 Aneurysm due to a Penetrating Atherosclerotic Ulcer **A.** Sagittal MPR and (**B** and **C**) axial source images show an irregularly shaped saccular aneurysm of the infrarenal abdominal aorta. Saccular aneurysms of the aorta are most often secondary to penetrating atherosclerotic ulcers or infection of the aortic wall. Note the multiple calcified atherosclerotic plaques and the absence of perianeurysm fat stranding, features indicating that this aneurysm is a result of a penetrating ulcer.

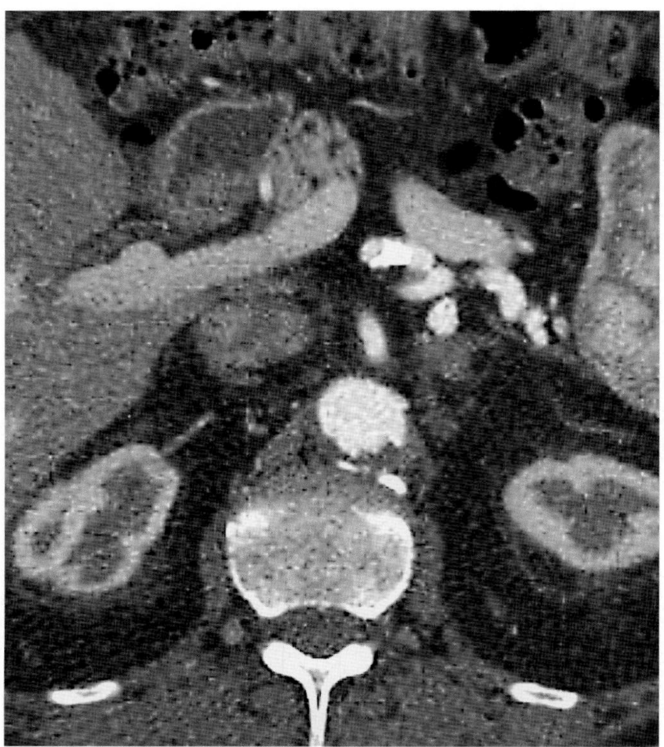

A

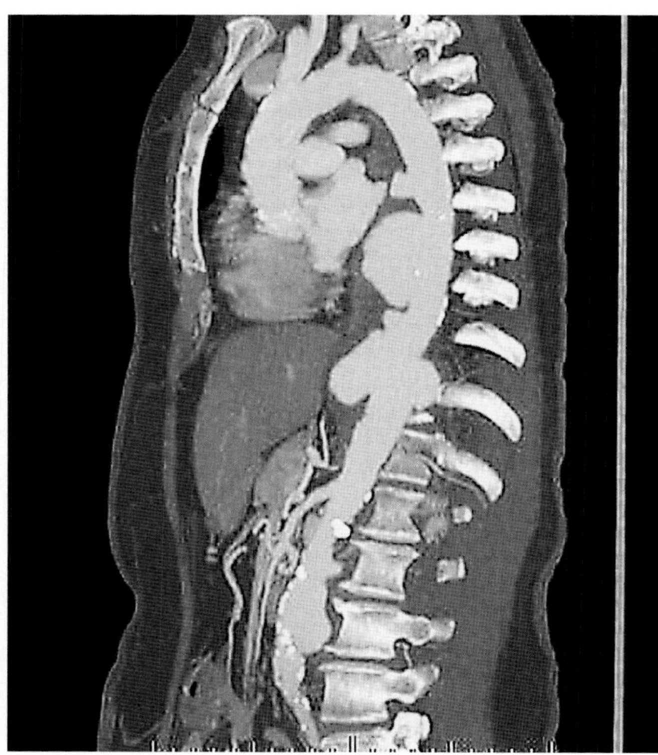

B

Figure 15-22 Penetrating Atherosclerotic Ulcer
A. Axial CTA shows a small irregular depression in the left lateral and posterior walls of the aorta, typical of an ulcerated atherosclerotic plaque. In plaque ulceration, the subintimal plaque is ulcerated but the intimal layer is not disrupted and the smooth aortic contour is maintained. Compare this to (**B**) the sagittal oblique MIP showing multiple penetrating ulcers leading to multiple saccular aneurysms.

initial inoculation.[126] Mycotic aneurysms will most commonly form in the femoral artery (56%) but will also occur in the abdominal aorta (18%) and thoracic aorta (15%).

Before the widespread availability of antibiotics, endocarditis was the most common cause of mycotic aneurysm.[130] However, currently intravenous drug use is the most common cause.[131] Immunosuppressed individuals such as those taking corticosteroids and those with malignancies are also at increased risk of mycotic aneurysms.[97,132] Up to 70% of individuals have been immunocompromised in some series of mycotic aneurysms.[133] The annual incidence of mycotic aneurysm is quite low. The Mayo Clinic identified only 43 cases of aortic mycotic aneurysms over a 25-year period.[133] Among intravenous drug users, it is estimated to be 0.03%.[134] Intravenous drug users are most likely to have mycotic aneurysms of the peripheral arteries but can occasionally have infections of the aorta or great vessels.[133,134] Aortic involvement is most common in the abdominal aorta but may rarely involve the thoracic aorta.[129,133,135] Patients typically present with fevers and leucocytosis and may complain of back or abdominal pain.[129,135] Blood cultures can fail to identify an infective organism in up to one-half of cases and, therefore, the absence of culture-proven bacteremia should not dissuade a diagnosis of a mycotic aneurysm.[136]

Imaging will typically demonstrate a saccular aneurysm with disproportionate wall thickening and periaortic stranding resulting in a soft-tissue rind.[130,131,137] Some cases will demonstrate an enhancing fluid collection, typical of an abscess, adjacent to the aneurysm (see Figure 15-23).[130,131,137] Gas within the aorta in the absence of recent surgical manipulation is suggestive of a mycotic aneurysm.[131] However, if there has been recent surgery, the gas can be a normal post operative phenomenon. The presence of foreign bodies such as stents or aortic grafts can predispose to the development of a vascular infection.

Aortoenteric fistula and osteomyelitis are potential complications or causes of aortic infection. An aortoenteric fistula typically involves the duodenum and can be a life threatening event. Aortoenteric fistula is discussed in greatest detail under the subsequent heading: **Gas in the Arterial Lumen or Wall of the Vessel.** Adjacent vertebral osteomyelitis can be due to spread of infection from the aorta to the adjacent vertebra or vice versa.

Trauma and surgery

Traumatic aortic rupture or aortic transection is a surgical emergency most commonly a result of blunt thoracic trauma such as a motor vehicle accident (MVA) or a fall

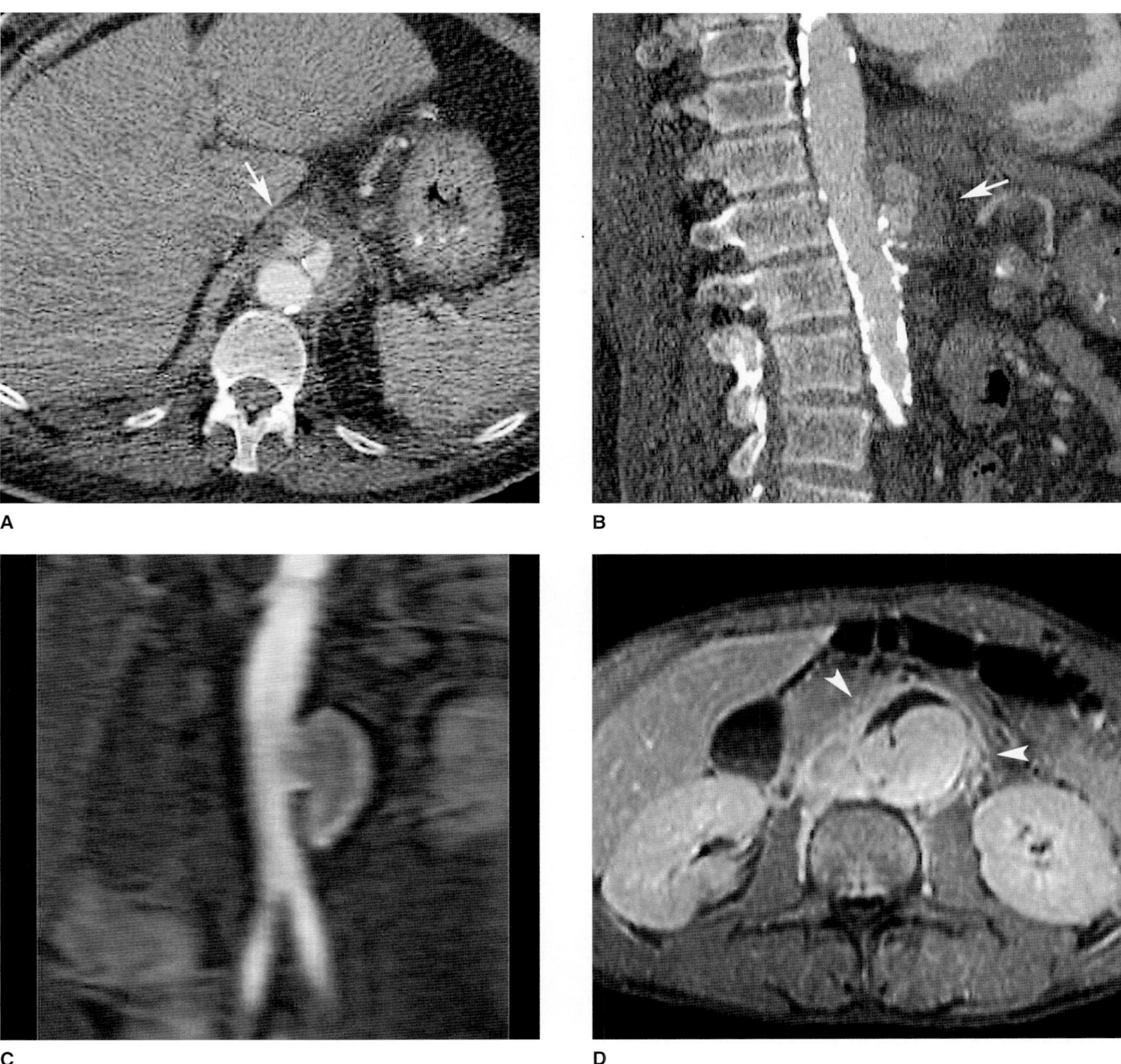

Figure 15-23 Mycotic Aneurysm in 2 Patients
A and **B.** This 67-year-old man presented with positive blood cultures and fever of unknown origin. (A) Axial CTA with (B) sagittal reformation shows a focal complex aneurysm (*arrows*) arising from the anterior wall of the abdominal aorta with considerable soft-tissue rind. The saccular character and the excessive soft-tissue rind are features suggesting an infected aortic aneurysm. These findings coupled with the clinical presentation are essentially diagnostic of a mycotic aneurysm.

C and **D.** This 41-year-old man presented with abdominal pain. (C) Sagittal contrast-enhanced MRA demonstrates a saccular aneurysm of the abdominal aorta. The remainder of the aorta appears relatively normal. Differential diagnosis would include saccular aneurysms from trauma and penetrating atherosclerotic ulcer. (D) Axial postgadolinium enhanced image also demonstrates extensive enhancement of the periaortic soft tissue (*arrowheads*), a finding that in conjunction with a mycotic aneurysm will most often indicate a mycotic aneurysm.

from a height.[138] Rapid deceleration results in shearing and bending forces across the aortic wall causing an intramural hematoma, less severe cases, and laceration of the intima and media, in more severe cases.[138,139] Extravasation is often prevented by an intact adventitia, however, pressures at the site of injury create a pseudoaneurysm.

Ninety percent of aortic transections occur just distal to the left subclavian artery near insertion of the ligamentum arteriosum. The ligamentum arteriosum inhibits the mobility of the aorta at this location, creating a point of maximum wall shear forces.[140-143] Other less common sites of aortic transection include the aortic root and the aorta at the diaphragmatic hiatus.[138,144] In these locations, the aorta is similarly constrained resulting in similar sheering forces and the risk of aortic tear. The thoracic aorta at the isthmus faces the brunt of blunt traumatic injuries and the aorta at the hiatus is the second most common site of injury.

The imaging hallmark of traumatic pseudoaneurysms is the presence of a pseudoaneurysm and short intimal flap.[145,146] A pseudoaneurysm will appear as a focal, saccular widening of a short segment of the aortic lumen. Since imaging does not identify the individual layers of vascular wall, a pseudoaneurysm is indistinguishable from other causes of a saccular aneurysm. However, in most cases, a small flap of intima will be seen as a linear filling defect within the aortic lumen, outlined by intravascular contrast, at the superior and inferior margins of the pseudoaneurysm. The combination of a saccular aneurysm with short proximal and distal intimal flaps at the aortic isthmus is the most common appearance of an acute aortic transection.

Injuries to the abdominal aorta can also occur in penetrating abdominal trauma. Isolated traumatic injuries to the abdominal aorta are rare in blunt trauma but can occur as part of the complex of retroperitoneal injury in association with a Chance fracture. Iatrogenic trauma can also lead to aneurysm formation. Iatrogenic causes of aneurysm include renal artery aneurysms from renal biopsy and aneurysms of the celiac branches from upper gastrointestinal surgery.

Vasculitis

Vasculitis is a great mimicker of atherosclerosis in terms of clinical features including the formation of aneurysms. Large vessel vasculitis can cause aortic aneurysms and aneurysms of major visceral arteries. Medium vessel vasculitis cause microaneurysms.

Takayasu arteritis: Takayasu arteritis, although rare, is the most common large vessel vasculitis. The primary lesion of Takayasu arteritis is inflammation of media and adventitia of the aorta and the large branch vessels of the aorta.[19,34] Vascular stenosis is the most common complication of Takayasu arteritis but aneurysm formation is also common. Studies of patients with Takayasu arteritis have identified aneurysms in 0% to 85% of individuals,[37,147,148] and aortic aneurysm with subsequent rupture is the most common fatal complication of Takayasu arteritis.[32,33]

Aneurysms appear to be a result of degeneration and weakening of the media.[19,36] Some researchers suggest that the development of aortic aneurysms is most closely associated with elevations in blood pressure.[37]

In patients with Takayasu arteritis, solitary aneurysms are uncommon and cross-sectional imaging will frequently show aneurysms at multiple locations.[18-20] There are, frequently, additional sites of vascular stenosis. In the active phases of inflammation, diffuse wall thickening and wall enhancement will also be present.[18-25] Clues to the diagnosis of Takayasu-related aortic aneurysm include young age of the patient, multifocality of the aneurysms, and the presence of associated vascular stenoses and wall thickening (see Figure 15-13). The major differential diagnosis for these findings is the other large vessel vasculitis: giant cell arteritis.

Polyarteritis nodosa: PAN is a necrotizing, medium vessel vasculitis due to autoimmune-mediated vessel wall inflammation. In most cases, the underlying cause is unknown. However, it is estimated that approximately 7% to 21% of cases of PAN will be associated with hepatitis B virus seropositivity.[149,150] A causal relationship is likely and patients develop PAN with a mean of 12 months after clinical evidence of infection.

PAN can involve multiple organ systems, most commonly the skin, joints, kidney, gastrointestinal tract, and nerves and occasionally involved the heart.[149] Patients can have a wide variety of presentations, depending on the organs involved. Systemic symptoms of fever, malaise, and weight loss are often present. Organ-specific symptoms include polyarthralgia due to joint disease, renal insufficiency, proteinuria and malignant hypertension due to renal involvement, abdominal pain due to bowel involvement, asthenia and neuropathy due to nerve involvement, and heart failure due to a nonobstructive cardiomyopathy with cardiac involvement.[149,151]

Cutaneous and muscular involvement is primarily identified by biopsy of the affected organ. However, deep tissue disease, primarily renal and gastrointestinal involvement, is often inferred based on abnormal imaging examinations and a set of positive and negative clinical criteria.[152] As such, imaging plays a crucial role in the diagnosis of this rare disorder.

Imaging examinations will typically demonstrate aneurysms occurring at branch points within the medium vessels of the abdominal viscera (see Figure 15-24). In one study of 7 patients with PAN, aneurysms of the major arteries to the kidney, bowel, liver, and spleen were the most common manifestation.[153] Aneurysms were most commonly found in the renal arteries (5), SMA (5), hepatic artery (4), splenic artery (2), and IMA (1). Multiple vessel involvement was the norm and evidence of end-organ ischemia, including bowel wall thickening and enhancement, renal infarctions, and splenic infarctions was common. Thrombotic occlusion of medium vessel arteries can also be demonstrated in some cases.[151]

The presence of multiple aneurysms involving the arteries of the abdominal viscera will most often suggest a diagnosis of PAN.

Connective tissue disorders

A variety of connective tissue diseases can have involvement of the large and medium vessels of the body (Table 15-6).

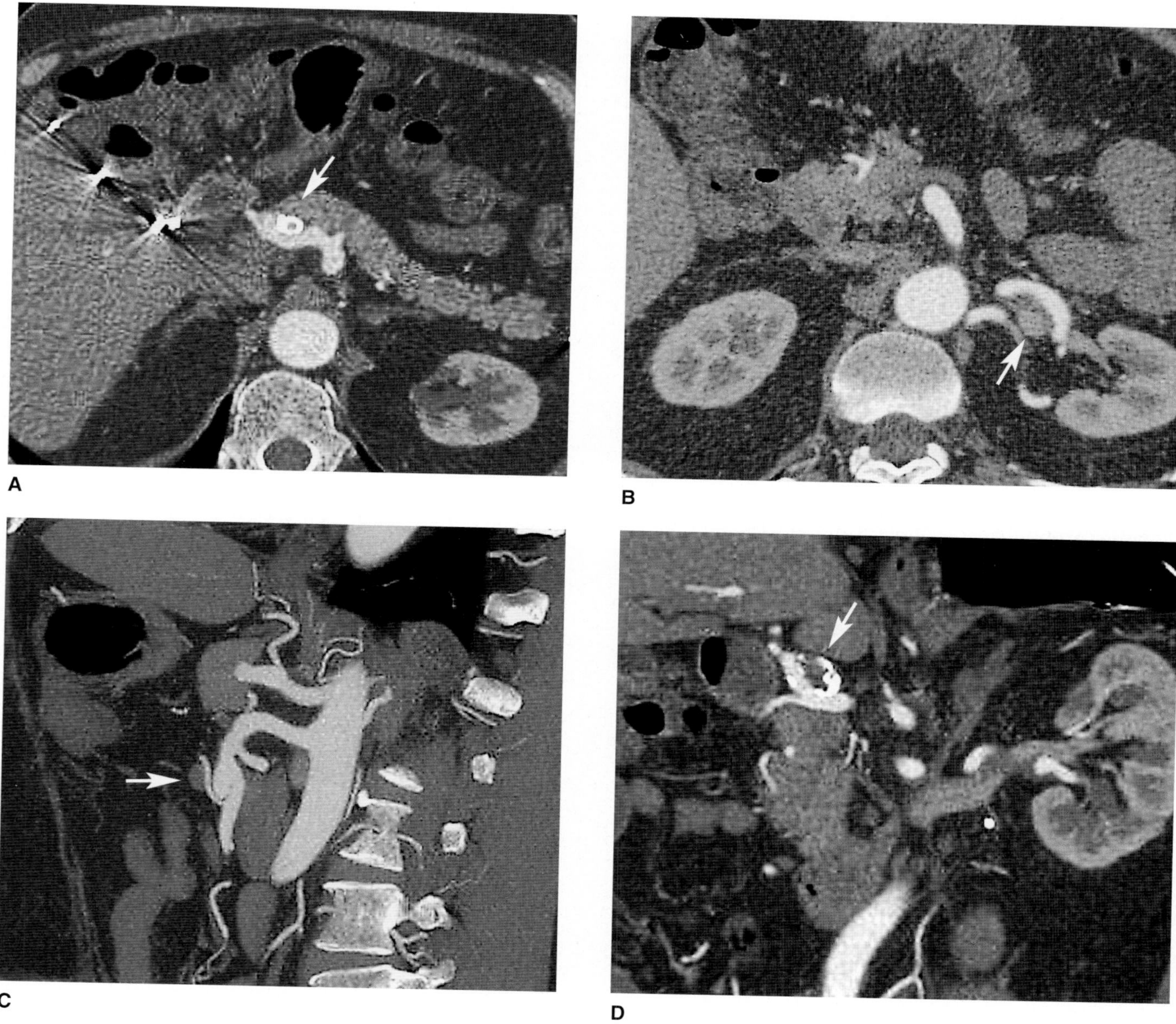

Figure 15-24 Polyarteritis Nodosa
This 57-year-old man had a clinical diagnosis of polyarteritis nodosa. **A** and **B**. Axial, (**C**) sagittal reconstruction, and (**D**) coronal oblique reconstructions from a CT angiogram show multiple visceral artery aneurysms (*arrows*) of the common hepatic (A), left renal (B), SMA (C), and proper hepatic (D) arteries. Note the absence of atherosclerosis. This appearance would be most commonly seen as a complication of medium vessel vasculitis or a connective tissue disorder.

Because these are systemic disorders, involvement tends to be multicompartmental and may or may not involve contiguous arterial segments.

Marfan syndrome: Marfan syndrome is a genetic disorder of fibrillin of varying phenotype characterized by skeletal, ocular and cardiovascular disorders, with an estimated prevalence is 1/4000.[40] It is an autosomal dominant disorder with high penetrance but with considerable variability of clinical expression.[72,154] There are a variety of defects on chromosome 15 that result in the abnormal production of fibrillin, an important element of elastic tissues and leads to weakening of the vascular wall.[155-160] As a consequence, the aorta and other capacitance arteries are predisposed to the development of aneurysms and dissections.[161-163] Histologically, patients have cystic medial necrosis that is characterized by loss of elastic fibers and smooth muscle cells with deposition of pools of collagen and glycosaminoglycan.[164]

Clinical features include tall stature and elongated limbs, including arachnodactyly, joint hypermobility,

Table 15-6. Aneurysms due to Connective Tissue Diseases

1. Marfan syndrome
2. Ehlers-Danlos syndrome
3. Loeys-Dietz syndrome
4. Fibromuscular dysplasia
5. Segmental arterial mediolysis
6. Neurofibromatosis
7. Pseudoxanthoma elasticum

myopia, retinal detachment, mitral valve prolapse and aneurysms, and dissection of the aorta. Aortic aneurysm represents the most serious and potentially lethal complications of Marfan syndrome.[75-77] The aortic root and ascending aorta are typically involved with aneurysms or dissections or both. Involvement of the abdominal aorta is usually through extension of a dissection that commences in the thoracic aorta.

Ehlers-Danlos syndrome: The vascular variant of Ehlers-Danlos syndrome (EDS) is an autosomal dominant disorder affecting the gene encoding procollagen type 3.[164] This disorder is thought to affect 1/100 000 people of which approximately 50% of the mutations are spontaneous. The disorder is clinically characterized by joint hypermobility, hyperextensibility of the skin, and fragile tissues that easily bruise and scar.[74] At least 9 distinct forms of Ehlers-Danlos syndrome have been identified with various clinical and pathologic overlap.[164] Aortic complications are only seen with type IV Ehlers-Danlos syndrome that is caused by a congenital defect in type III collagen. This subgroup can develop aneurysms without dissection, most commonly of the abdominal aorta and its branches but also the origins of the great vessels and the large arteries of the legs and arms.[78] The hallmark of this disorder is the propensity of the arterial system to rupture sometimes in the absence of aneurysms or dissection. Indeed, it is not only the arterial system that could rupture but the bowel, uterus, and pleura.[92] Noninvasive imaging is of particular importance in the diagnosis of vascular complications in these patients because invasive arteriography carries with it the risk of arterial laceration.

Ehlers-Danlos syndrome can result in aneurysms of both the abdominal aorta and its branch vessels. Aneurysms have been reported to involve the renal arteries, hepatic artery, and abdominal aorta and can potentially occur in any vessel (see Figure 15-25).[165-167]

Loeys-Dietz syndrome: Loeys-Dietz syndrome is a rare autosomal dominant inherited disorder first described in 2005. It involves a mutation in the gene encoding transforming growth factor–β.[168] Affected children can have a variety of morphologic abnormalities including hypertelorism, a bifid or broad uvula, and in a small percentage of patients, craniosynostosis, cleft palate, and club foot. The majority of children will also have skin abnormalities, including a translucent appearance with easy bruising and scarring.[168] Approximately 15% of individuals have cervical spine instability. This is an aggressive disorder causing vascular dissections and rupture with the rupture occurring at size thresholds lower than that for Marfan syndrome or other aneurysms without a history of connective tissue disease.[168] Aortic dissection with rupture is the most common cause of death with thoracic aortic dissections accounting for 67% and abdominal aortic dissections accounting for 22% of deaths in 1 series.[168]

Imaging examinations will typically demonstrate marked tortuosity of the vessels, especially, the larger vessels of the neck. Multiple large and medium vessel aneurysms are seen throughout the body but most commonly involve the thoracic aorta. Aneurysms of the abdominal aorta or abdominal branch vessels are found in approximately 10% of individuals.[168]

Fibromuscular dysplasia: Fibromuscular dysplasia is a moderately common connective tissue disorder of the arterial wall that primarily causes stenosis of arterioles, especially the renal arteries, and has been most completely reviewed under the previous heading: **Stenosis and Occlusion**. However, the **medial fibroplasia** subtype of fibromuscular dysplasia is characterized by multiple adjacent aneurysms and stenoses of arterioles that cause the classic string-of-pearl appearance on imaging examinations.[62,64-66] This appearance is virtually diagnostic of a diagnosis of fibromuscular dysplasia (see Figure 15-17).

Segmental arterial mediolysis: Segmental arterial mediolysis involves, as the nomenclature suggests, breakdown of the medial layer of the artery. This split in media leads to dissection. The dissection affects medium-sized arteries and, instead of maintaining a double lumen, the artery frequently thromboses with resulting ischemia in the supplied territory. Bowel and kidneys can be affected. The SMA is the most commonly affected artery. This entity can lead to multifocal aneurysms in a pattern not dissimilar to fibromuscular dysplasia (see Figure 15-26).

Neurofibromatosis: Neurofibromatosis type 1 (NF1), a genetic disorder of the neurologic and dermatologic systems, also affects the vascular system, causing aneurysms, stenosis, and mural weakening. Along with the abdominal aorta, NF1 affects the renal arteries and is an important cause of secondary hypertension in children.

Pseudoxanthoma elasticum: Pseudoxanthoma elasticum (PXE) is a rare genetic disorder, which affects the elastic media. The term *pseudoxanthoma* relates to the cutaneous lesions in this disorder, which are yellow papules resembling true xanthomas. On the vascular side, this

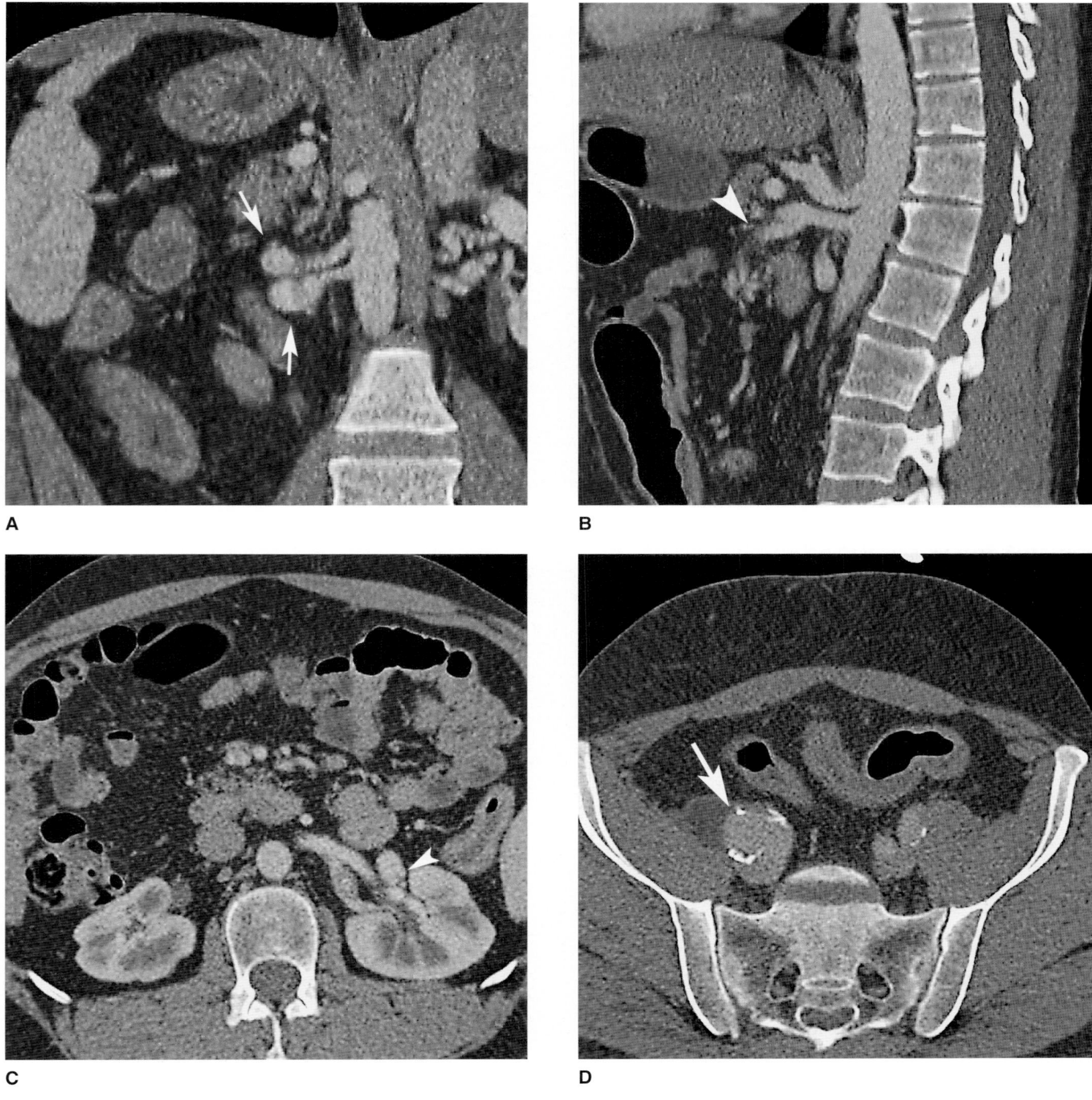

Figure 15-25 Aneurysms due to Ehlers-Danlos Syndrome This 33-year-old man has known Ehlers-Danlos type 4. **A.** Coronal reconstructions, (**B**) sagittal reconstructions and (**C** and **D**) axial images from a CTA shows 2 aneurysms of the duplicated right renal arteries (*small arrows*) and the right external iliac artery (*large arrow*). There is also a subtle intimal flap involving a branch of the left renal artery (*small arrowhead*) indicating a dissection and intimal disruption of the proximal SMA (*large arrowhead*). Patients with Ehlers-Danlos syndrome are predisposition to visceral artery aneurysms and dissection.

entity leads to aneurysm, stenosis, and bleeding due to arterial rupture of small and medium-sized arteries. The medial layer of the arteries typically calcifies in a manner similar to Mönckeberg arteriosclerosis.

External factors leading to abdominal aneurysms

Local inflammation originating in the tissues external to a blood vessel can lead to disruption of the connective tissues

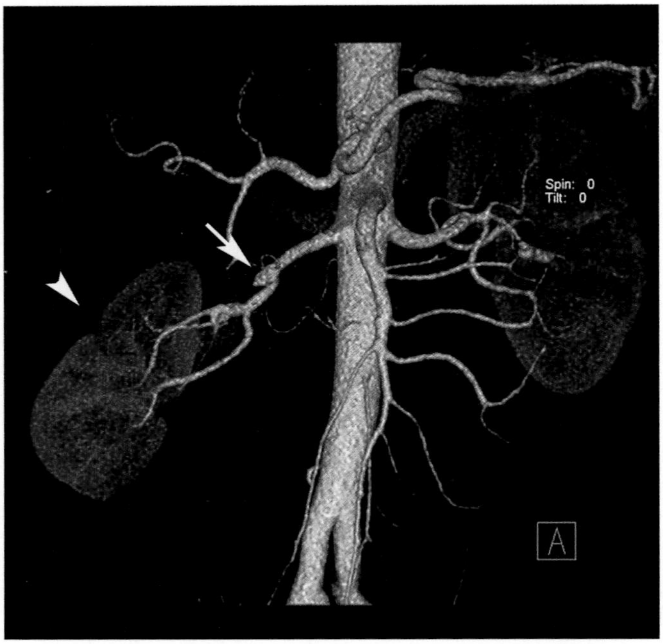

Figure 15-26 Systemic Arterial Mediolysis
Coronal volume rendered image from CTA shows an aneurysm (*arrow*) just before the bifurcation of the main right renal artery. In addition, there is a parenchymal defect (*arrowhead*) along the lateral aspect of the kidney from an infarct. These findings were shown to be due to systemic arterial mediolysis. This condition leads to spontaneous dissections and occlusions.

of the vascular wall and lead to the development of an aneurysm. In the abdomen, this is most often associated with pancreatitis. External compression of arteries can lead to poststenotic dilation that appears as a small aneurysm, distal to the narrowing. This phenomenon is associated with median arcuate ligament syndrome.

Pancreatitis: Pancreatitis generally affects arteries surrounding the pancreas including the splenic, gastroduodenal, and pancreaticoduodenal arteries. The inflammation and pancreatic enzymes can result in the development of a pseudoaneurysm. These aneurysms are at risk of rupture, and the rupture of a visceral artery aneurysm should be considered in the differential diagnosis of a patient with pancreatitis whose condition worsens with abdominal pain and shock. In general, CT is the best modality to assess the pancreas and the surrounding vessels for the presence and complications of pseudoaneurysm formation (see Figure 15-27).

Median arcuate ligament syndrome: Compression of the celiac artery by the arcuate ligament of the diaphragm can lead to focal narrowing and poststenotic dilation. This can appear as a small focal aneurysm of the proximal celiac artery (see Figure 15-18). Median arcuate ligament syndrome is discussed more completely under the previous heading: **Stenosis and Occlusion**.

Wall Disruption

The intima can be disrupted by a PAU, instrumentation, trauma, or infection. This is recognized as a break in the smooth contour of the arterial wall. Disruption of the medial layer of the artery with an exit and entry point and 2 lumina are features of a dissection. Disruption of all 3 layers of the aortic wall leads to aortic rupture or, if contained by adventitia, a pseudoaneurysm.

Penetrating atherosclerotic ulcer

PAU is a frequent sequelae of atherosclerosis.[1,169] In the mid-1980s, it was realized that atheromatous plaques can develop surface ulcerations that can propagate into the media.[1,7,169,170] Complications of PAUs include intramural hematoma, dissection, and aneurysm formation. In most cases, the intramural hematoma and dissection involve a relatively short segment of the aorta. They are prevented from extending further by surrounding transmural inflammation, which results in a relative fusion of the aortic wall layers.[3]

These ulcers typically form in regions of locally advanced atherosclerotic disease. Disruption of the intima and internal elastic lamina is the characteristic pathologic feature of PAUs.[1,171] Histologic examination will also demonstrate cholesterol clefts deep within the aortic media. Varying degrees of intramural hematoma and/or medial dissection can be seen histologically.

PAUs are typically found in patients in their 60s, 70s, and 80s.[1,169,172,173] The majority of patients will have systemic hypertension and many will have a variety of comorbidities such as COPD, heart disease, and chronic renal insufficiency.[1,169,172,173] In some cases, patients will be clinically asymptomatic and discovered on imaging examinations performed for other reasons. In other cases, they will present with back or chest pain similar to aortic dissection.[1,169,172,173]

The natural history of PAUs is quite variable. Some will persist unchanged and asymptomatic for years, others will result in aneurysmal dilation, dissection, or rupture of the aorta.[171,174] Rupture is believed to be more likely in patients with clinical symptoms and occurs in 16% and 42% of PAUs.[1,171,173]

Enhanced CT examinations or MRI sequences with lumen-to-wall contrast will demonstrate a focal area of ulceration within the aortic wall that resembles a gastric ulcer (see Figures 15-21 and 15-22).[1,17,169,174] Typically, CT will also demonstrate extensive aortic calcifications, indicating severe atherosclerosis nearby to the area of the ulceration.[1,169,171] Most ulcers will develop in the descending thoracic aorta but they can also be found in the ascending and abdominal aortas. Some ulcers will undermine the wall of the aorta, producing a small intimal flap. In most

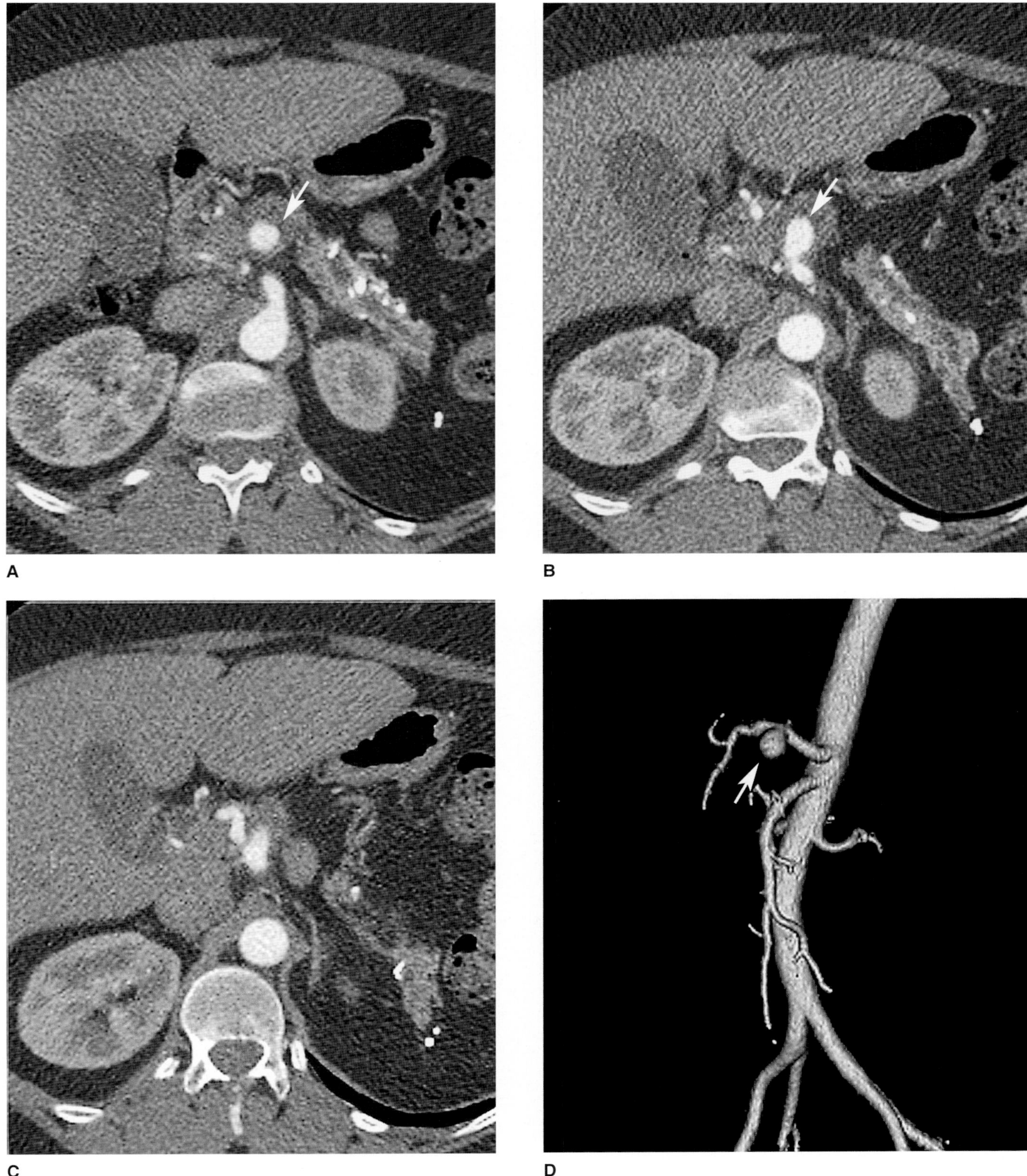

Figure 15-27 Pseudoaneurysm as a Complication of Pancreatitis This 46-year-old woman complained of chronic abdominal pain. **A-C.** Contrast-enhanced axial CT images shows focal dilation (*arrows*) of the origin of the splenic artery, with occlusion of the distal splenic artery, indicating the presence of an aneurysm or pseudoaneurysm. **D.** The small pseudoaneurysm (*arrow*) is seen to better advantage on the shaded surface display of the aorta and branch vessels. Images (**A** and **B**) also show multiple calcifications of the pancreas and dilation of the pancreatic duct, typical of chronic pancreatitis.

cases, the intimal flap is short in length, unlike the extensive intimal flap of an aortic dissection. The adjacent aortic wall will often demonstrate focal enhancement and/or thickening and the lumen.[169,171,174] Some penetrating ulcers will have an associated intramural hematoma.[17,169,171,174] The ulcer frequently weakens the aortic wall and long-term follow-up will often show development of saccular or fusiform aortic aneurysms or pseudoaneurysms (see Figure 15-21 and 15-22).[1,174] One study noted a mean diameter of 6.2 cm at the site of the ulcer.[1] Unfortunately, imaging findings were not predictive of the need for surgery in 2 series.[169]

Dissection

Aortic dissections are the most common medical emergency to involve the aorta, and occur 2 to 3 times more frequently than the second most common medical emergency involving the aorta: acute rupture of AAAs.[175] The dissection starts with a medial tear.[1,176-179] The combination of the tear and high pressure arterial pulsations force blood to dissect through the media of the aorta and allow propagation of the dissection over a variable distance. The dissection has an entrance and an exit tear and a variable number of fenestrations. Dissections can begin as an intramural hematoma.[180-183] Finally, dissections can be caused by PAU, either directly or through an intramural hematoma. If untreated, the false lumen of a dissection can progressively dilate leading to an aneurysm of the affected aorta. Dissection involving the abdominal aorta usually originates in the thoracic aorta and is a continuation of either a Stanford type A or type B dissection.

The primary risk factor for the development of an aortic dissection is systemic hypertension.[184,185] Other risk factors include Marfan syndrome, Ehlers-Danlos syndrome, Turners syndrome, and cystic medial necrosis, pregnancy, aortic stenosis, and coarctation of the aorta.[184,185]

The most accepted nomenclature for aortic dissection is the Stanford classification system. Type A dissections involve some portion of the ascending aorta and can be isolated to the proximal aorta or can progress to involve portions of the descending aorta including the abdominal aorta. Type B dissections involve the aorta distal to the left subclavian artery.[186]

Acute type A dissections represent a surgical emergency and require immediate surgical repair because of several life-threatening complications, including rupture, pericardial tamponade, acute aortic insufficiency, myocardial infarction, and stroke.[186-195] Acute type B dissections have a lower operative morbidity and mortality than type A dissections and are in most cases initially treated with antihypertensive therapy aimed to reduce blood pressure.[190,193-195] Surgical intervention is reserved for those individuals who fail medical therapy, including persistent symptoms, development of visceral, renal, or peripheral ischemia, and imaging evidence of progression of the dissection or creation of an aneurysm.[196]

The mean age of presentation of aortic dissection is in the sixth decade with ages ranging from the teens to the 80s.[192,193,197,198] Type A lesions on average present at a younger age, mean 52 years, than Type B lesions, mean age of 59.[192] Patients characteristically present with severe, tearing, chest or back pain.[198,199] Other symptoms include neck or epigastric pain and signs of shock. Up to one-quarter of patients will have no clinical symptoms referable to a dissection and are discovered incidentally on imaging studies.[199]

Prospective, direct comparison of the accuracy of CT, MRI, and transesophageal echocardiography in the evaluation of aortic dissection has shown that CT and MRI are very reliable in the diagnosis of this dissection with accuracies between 90% and 100%.[200-202] Transesophageal echocardiography has a lower sensitivity than the other techniques but has the advantage of being portable.

All 3 cross-sectional imaging techniques diagnose this disorder by demonstrating the presence of an intimal flap separating a true and false lumen producing a "double-barrel" appearance to the aorta (see Figure 15-28).[203-207] In most cases, the true lumen is smaller and better opacified with contrast than the false lumen.[196,203,208,209] Further, MRI can show slow flow of blood in the false lumen, relative to more rapid flow in the true lumen on flow-sensitive pulse sequences. The true lumen can be followed to the nondissected aorta. The false lumen can be recognized by the presence of incompletely sheared media, which appear as strands in the false lumen. If the flap is calcified, the lumen closest to the calcification is the true lumen (see Figure 15-29).

On noncontrast studies, displacement of intimal calcifications away from the periphery of the aorta suggests a dissection, with blood in the false lumen displacing the calcification from the external surface of the aorta. Unfortunately, occasionally chronic mural thrombus can calcify, known as "neointimal calcification," causing non-peripheral calcification that can mimic displacement of mural calcification in dissections (see Figure 15-30).

Aortic dissections, which cause branch vessel occlusions, that involve the brain, gastrointestinal tract, kidneys, and extremities, have up to 7 times increased mortality when compared with uncomplicated dissections.[210] Therefore, it is important to evaluate all branch vessels for involvement by the dissection (see Figure 15-31).

Imaging Notes 15-5. Dissection vs. Mural Thrombus

- Intravenous contrast is required for the detection of wall thickness and determination of its etiology.
- Displaced intimal calcifications on noncontrast scan should raise the possibility of wall disruption due to dissection, wall thickening from intramural hematoma, or calcification of mural thrombus.

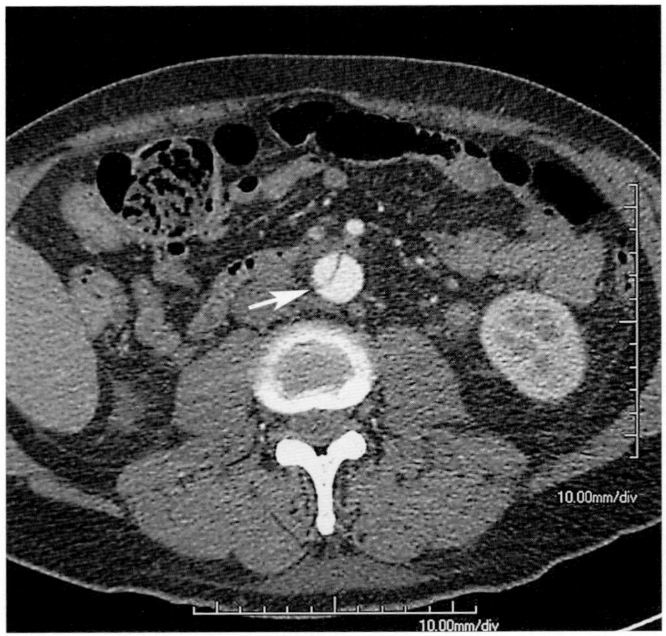

A

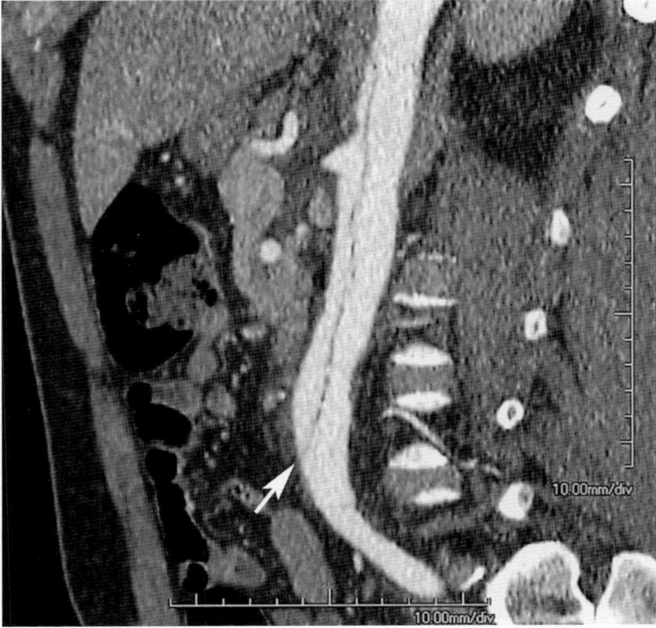

B

Figure 15-28 Dissection in the Abdominal Aorta
A. Axial CTA with (**B**) coronal multiplanar reconstruction shows a long intimal flap (*arrows*) indicating the presence of a dissection of the abdominal aorta. Dissection is a split in the media. The flap is composed of both the intima and media. The true lumen (anteriorly located in this case) is surrounded by intima, as is the case with the normal aorta. The false lumen is bounded by the intima-medial flap anteriorly and the media/adventitia posteriorly. Features of a dissection include dual lumen, flap, and an entry and exit point.

Follow-up cross-sectional imaging for all patients regardless of how they are managed is routinely performed.[211,212] The aorta is evaluated for progression of the dissection, new involvement of branch vessels, and the development of secondary aneurysms.

The imaging evaluation and report of a patient with and abdominal aortic dissection should evaluate a variety of features of the dissected aorta, including (1) the relationship of the major branch arteries to the true and false lumen, (2) extension of the dissection flap extending into the major branch arteries of the abdominal aorta, (3) relationship of the dissection flap to the origins of the major branch arteries, (4) the sites of re-entry points, (5) presence of false lumen thrombosis, (6) presence of true lumen collapse, and (7) signs of end-organ ischemia. All of these findings either identify the presence or predict the development of end-organ ischemia and the possible need for surgical intervention.

Rupture

Causes of abdominal vascular rupture include spontaneous rupture of AAAs and dissections and penetrating or blunt trauma.

Aortic aneurysm: An important cause of aortic rupture is an infrarenal AAA. For a given size threshold, mycotic aneurysms are more likely to rupture as are aneurysms due to connective tissue disease. The risk of rupture of aneurysm depends on the size of the aneurysm. For AAAs 4 to 5 cm, the risk is 0.5% to 3% per year and for aneurysms 6 to 7 cm, it is 20% to 40% per year. The mortality rate of those with treated rupture is 50%.[41]

Imaging Notes 15-6. Reporting and Evaluation of Aortic Dissection

The imaging evaluation and report of a patient with and abdominal aortic dissection should answer the following questions:

1. Do the major branch arteries arise from the true lumen, false lumen or both?
2. Does the dissection flap extend into the major branch arteries of the abdominal aorta?
3. Does the flap straddle the origin of the artery?
4. Where are the re-entry points?
5. Is the false lumen thrombosed?
6. Is the true lumen collapsed?
7. Are there any signs of end-organ ischemia?

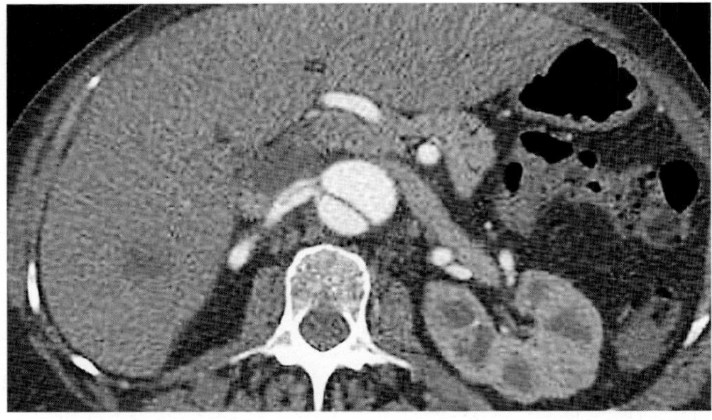

A

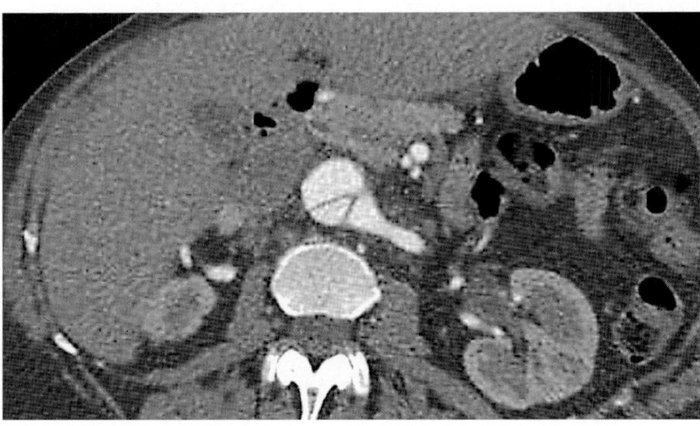

B

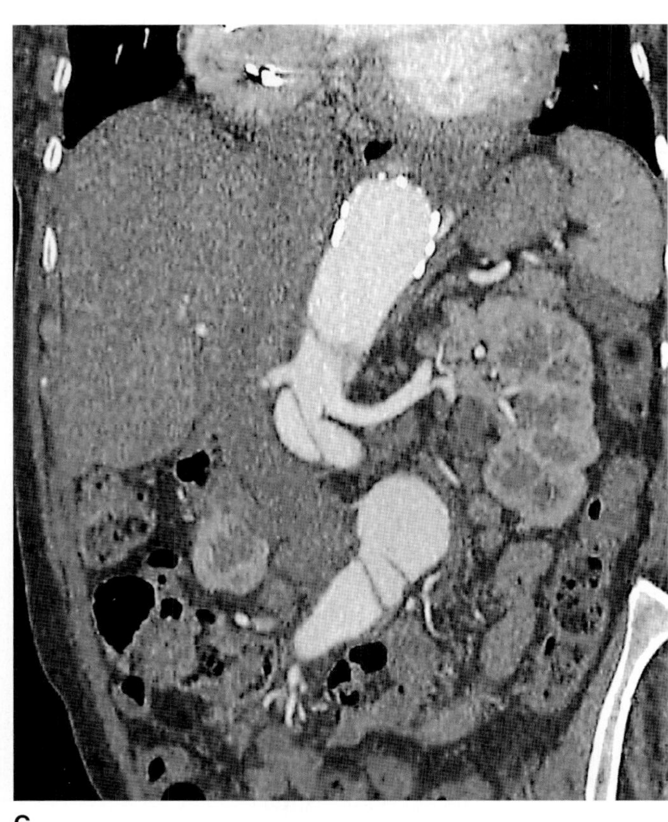

C

Figure 15-29 Dissection with Involvement of Branch Vessels
A and **B**. Axial and (**C**) Coronal reconstructions from a CTA show an intimal flap typical of a dissection. Visceral supply can be from the true lumen or false lumen or there can be extension of the flap into the artery. Note the flap extension into the right renal artery in (A). The left renal artery arises from the false lumen, which is placed more anteriorly (B and C). However, the flap straddles the origin of the right renal artery, predisposing to dynamic compression.

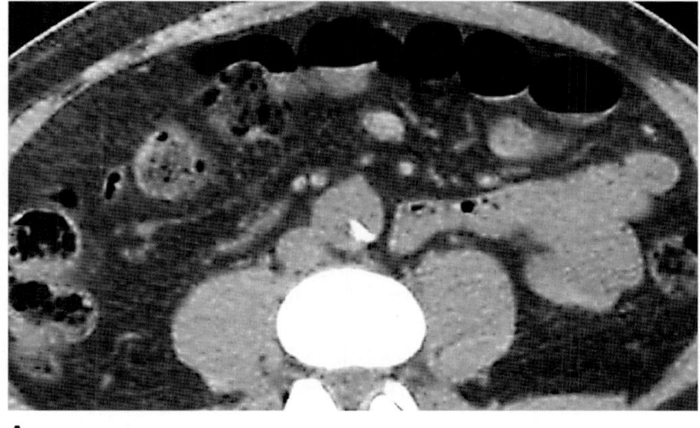

A

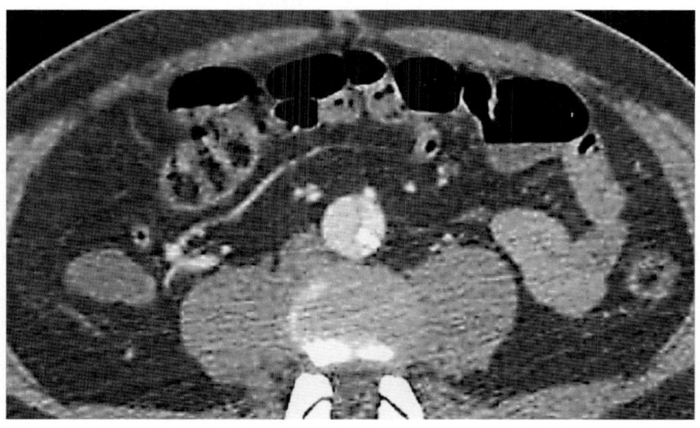

B

Figure 15-30 Displaced Intimal Calcification in 2 Patients
Nonperipheral intimal calcifications due to displaced intima indicate either dissection or intramural hematoma. **A.** Unenhanced CT in 1 patient shows a displaced calcification due to an intramural hematoma. **B.** Contrast-enhanced CT in a second patient shows an intramural flap and displaced intimal calcification indicating a dissection.

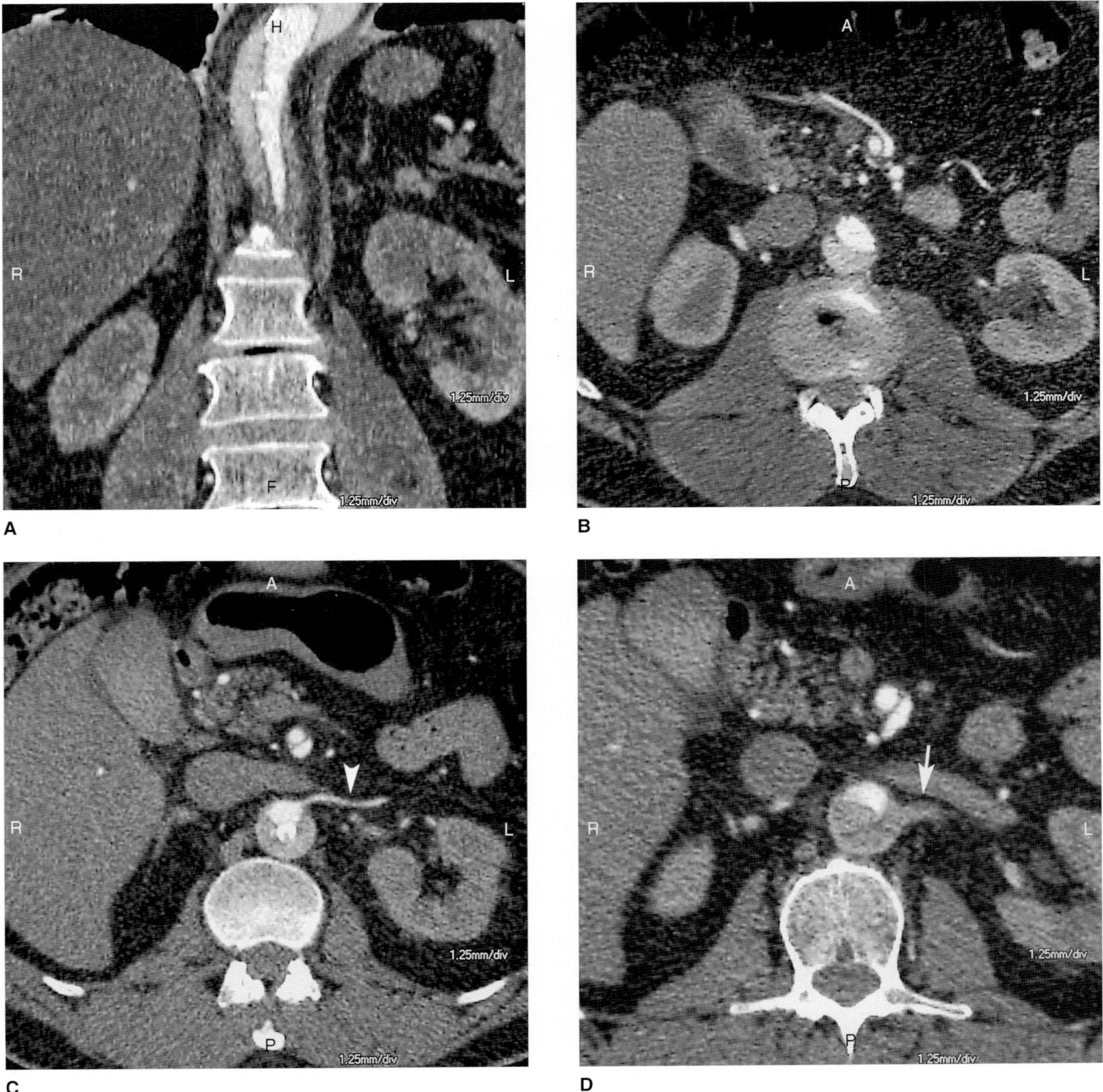

Figure 15-31 Dissection with Compromise of Renal Blood Flow A. Coronal reconstruction and (**B-D**) Axial CT images from a CTA demonstrates an intimal flap and a true and false lumen indicative of an aortic dissection. Note the subtle difference in perfusion between the anterior and posterior aspects of the lower pole of the left kidney in (A and B). This is because the accessory left renal artery arises from the true lumen (*arrowhead* in C), whereas the main left renal artery comes from the false lumen (*arrow* in D).

The presence of high-attenuation material in the periaortic space on the noncontrast study is a sign of aortic rupture (see Figure 15-32).[26] On MRI, such a hematoma is best revealed as areas of high signal on T1-weighted images. The hematoma frequently tracks to retroperitoneal compartments such as the perirenal and pararenal spaces and the psoas muscle. Periaortic hematoma can be accompanied by active extravasation of contrast, indicating active bleeding. However, the absence of extravasation does not exclude the diagnosis of rupture.[26]

There are certain imaging signs that have been associated with aneurysm rupture. These include the hyperattenuating crescent sign (hemorrhage into the mural thrombus), loss of a plane between the posterior wall of the aorta and the anterior aspect of the vertebral body (the draping aorta sign), reduction in the ratio of thrombus and lumen, and a break in the intimal calcification. These signs have been discussed in detail under the heading: **Aneurysm.** It is uncertain by what degree the risk of rupture of an AAA increases in the presence of these signs. If present, these merit emphasis in the impression of the report.

A chronic slow leak of the aorta may not be as clinically catastrophic as an acute rupture. One of the consequences of a slow leak is the formation of an aortocaval fistula. Like any other arteriovenous (AV)-fistulae, these patients can present with high-output cardiac failure and symptoms of distal ischemic steal. On imaging, there is opacification of the inferior vena cava (IVC) during the arterial phase of imaging and expansion of the IVC. Aortocaval fistula can also be a consequence of surgery such as discectomy and an infected aortic aneurysm.

Trauma: The majority of trauma-related abdominal arterial rupture is due to laceration of small arteries. This can be due to penetrating trauma or blunt trauma with laceration of the vessel by bone fragments. Vascular laceration is accompanied by hematoma in the respective compartment, be it intraperitoneal, retroperitoneal, or extraperitoneal.

The "sentinel clot sign" is an important sign of vascular laceration seen on unenhanced and enhanced CT examinations. It is seen as an area of high attenuation on CT adjacent to the site of injury and is helpful in locating the inured vessel or organ (see Figure 15-33).[213,214] Extravasation of contrast on contrast-enhanced examinations is seen as an amorphous pool of contrast that does not conform to a vascular structure in the tissues adjacent to the vascular injury. The contrast pool changes shape and dilutes in the venous phase of imaging (see Figure 15-34). Contrast extravasation indicates active bleeding requiring angiographic or surgical intervention.

Gas in the Arterial Lumen or Wall of the Vessel

In the vast majority of cases, gas in the lumen or wall of a vessel will be iatrogenic and related to recent instrumentation or surgery (see Figure 15-35). In this situation, the gas is usually of no consequence and will resolve spontaneously.

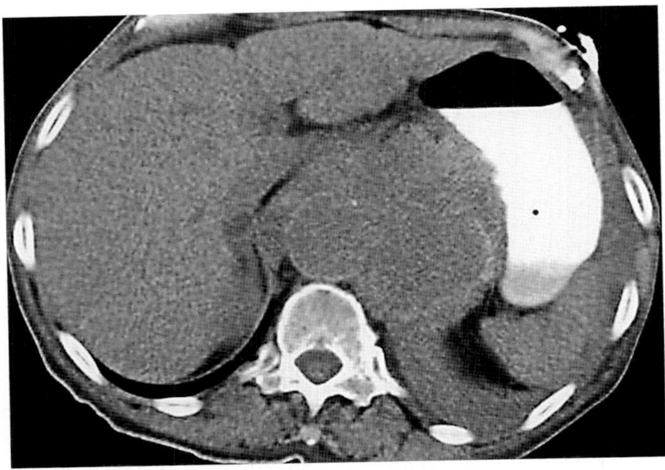

A

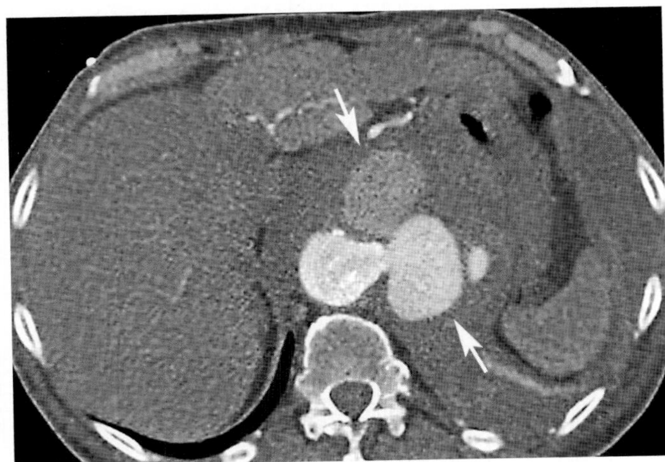

B

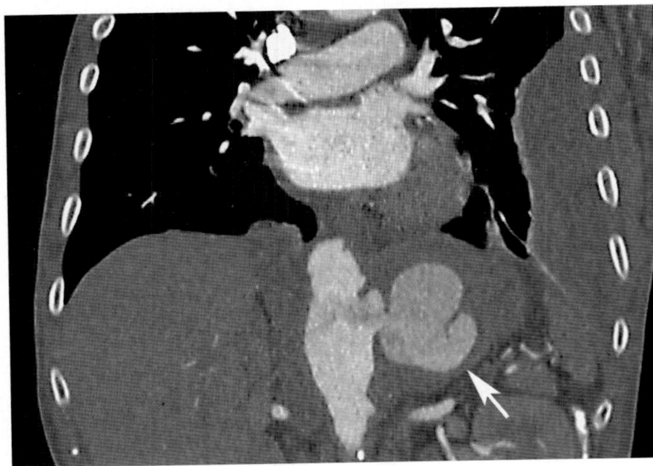

C

Figure 15-32 Contained Aortic Rupture
This 62-year-old man complained of back pain. **A.** Axial noncontrast CT shows an enlarged thoracic aorta at the diaphragmatic hiatus with expanded soft tissue. **B.** Axial and (**C**) coronal CTA show well-defined extraluminal contrast collection (*arrow*), indicating a contained aortic rupture, in this case due to a penetrating atherosclerotic aortic ulcer.

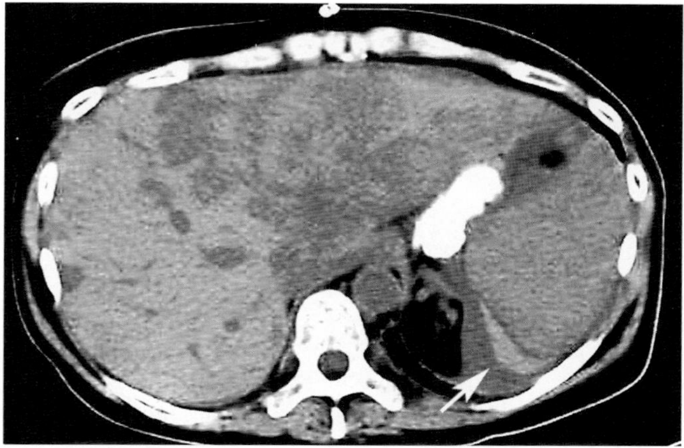

Figure 15-33 Sentinal Clot Sign
Axial noncontrast CT in this 42-year-old woman post hepatic transplant with left flank pain shows high attenuating fluid (*arrow*) posterior to the splenic tip indicating the presence of hemoperitoneum. This is an example of the sentinal clot sign and indicates the presence of significant bleeding. Note the extensive area of low attenuation in the liver indicating the presence of contusion.

However, in the absence of instrumentation gas can indicate an infection and/or fistula to the bowel.

Mycotic aneurysm and infected aortitis

Mycotic aneurysms are among the most common, nonoperative causes of gas in the arterial lumen or wall. They represent a infection of the vessel wall, most commonly the femoral artery (56%) followed by the abdominal aorta (18%) and the thoracic aorta (15%).[126] Aneurysms will in most cases rapidly form over the course of a few days after the initial inoculation; however, rarely the wall can be infected without development of an aneurysm.

Patients typically present with fevers and leucocytosis and may complain of back or abdominal pain.[129,135] Blood cultures are negative in up to one-half of cases.[136]

Imaging will typically demonstrate a saccular aneurysm with disproportionate wall thickening and periaortic stranding, resulting in a soft-tissue rind.[130,131,137] Some cases will demonstrate an enhancing fluid collection, typical of an abscess, adjacent to the aneurysm.[130,131,137] Gas within the wall of the aorta is in the absence of recent surgical manipulation is diagnostic of a mycotic aneurysm.[131] Patients with infected aortitis without aneurysm will have wall thickening with or without intramural gas.

Mycotic aneurysms are discussed most completely under the previous heading: **Aneurysm.**

Aortoenteric fistula

The most common site of aortoenteric fistula is the transverse duodenum.[42] The duodenum is retroperitoneal in

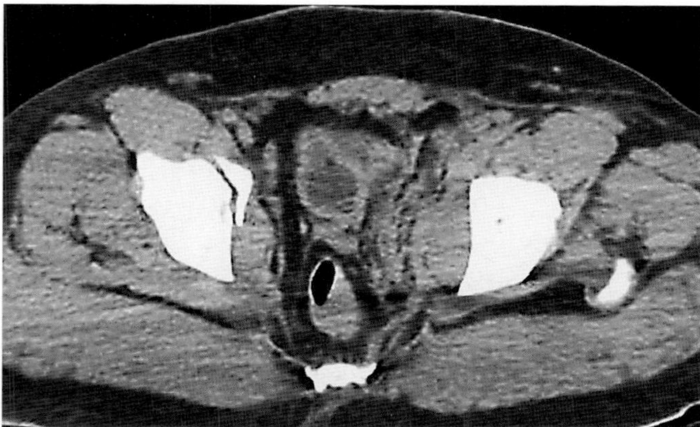

A

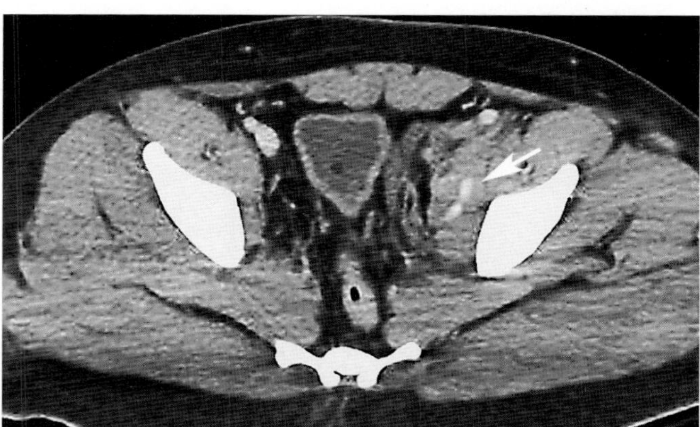

B

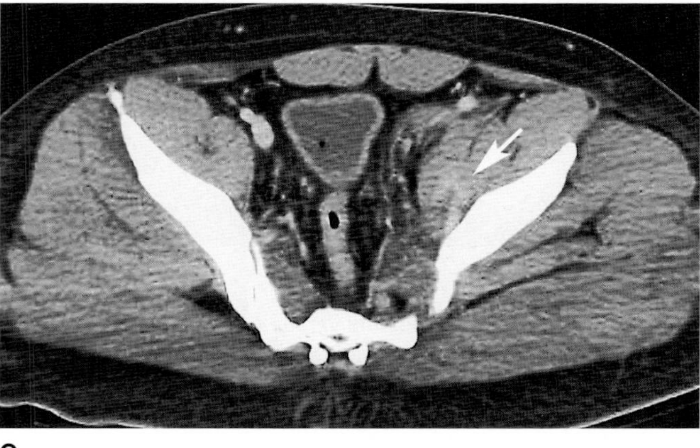

C

Figure 15-34 Extravasated Contrast due to an Arterial Injury
This 19-year-old man had a pelvic fracture. **A.** Noncontrast image through the pelvis shows expansion of the left sidewall muscle. **B.** CTA in the arterial phase and **(C)** venous phase shows an irregular area of contrast opacification (*arrows*) in the left hemipelvis that is asymmetric, does not conform to a vessel, and changes morphology between the arterial and venous phases, indicating active extravasation of contrast.

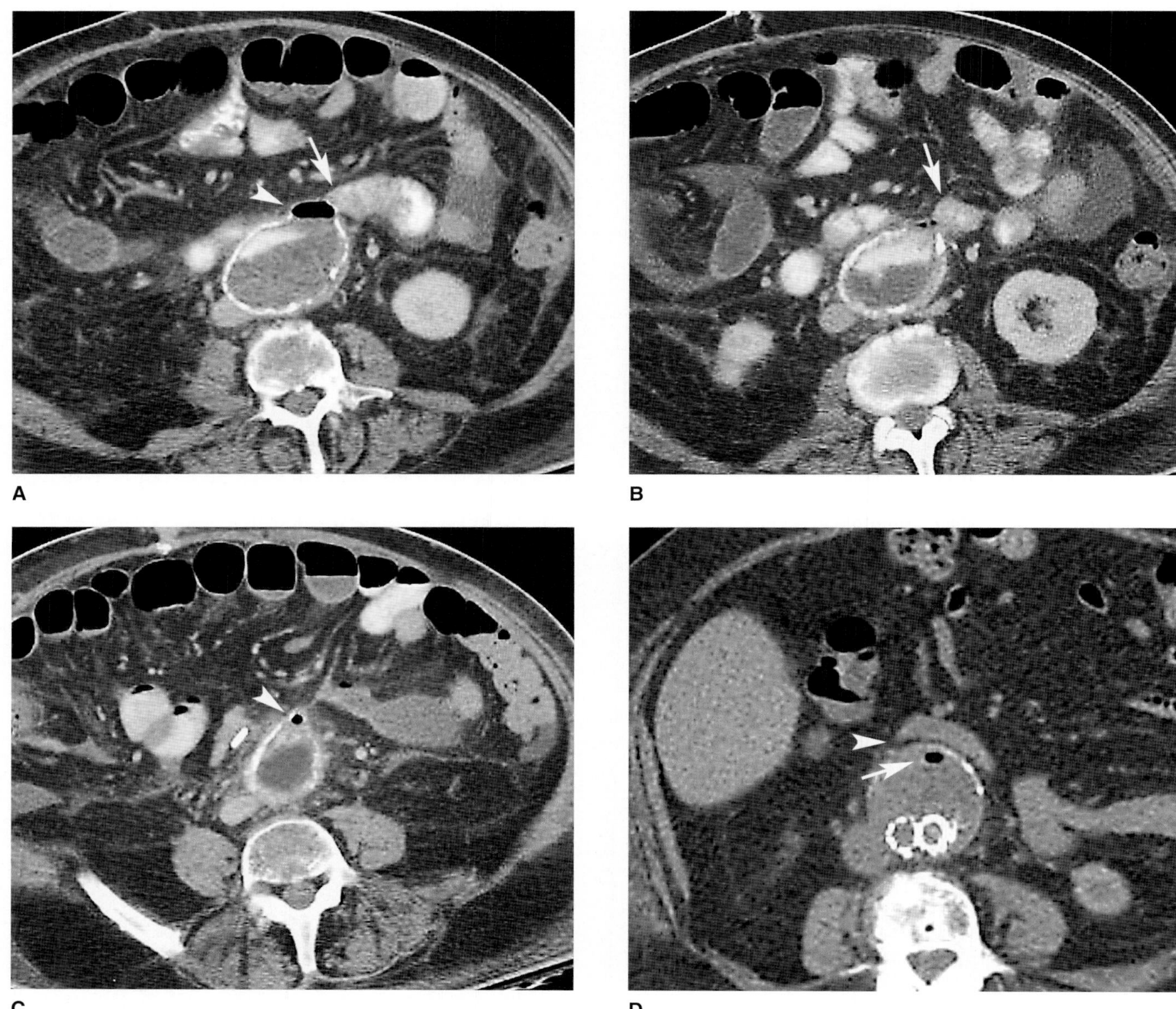

Figure 15-35 Aorto-Enteric Fistula versus Arterial Gas due to Recent Instrumentation in 2 Patients
A-C. This 67-year-old man complained of weakness. Axial CTA through the abdomen shows air (*arrowheads*) in the anterior aspect of the aorta with loss of the fat plane and tethering (*arrow*) of a small bowel loop anterior to the aorta. There is also mild haziness of the periaortic fat, suggesting surrounding inflammation and discontinuity of the intimal calcification along the anterior surface of the aorta. In the absence of recent instrumentation, this combination of findings is suspicious for infection and/or fistula with the bowel. **D.** This 78-year-old man had undergone recent placement of an aortic stent graft. There is air in the anterior aspect of the aorta (*arrow*), which was presumed to be due to the intervention. Note the maintained fat plane (*arrowhead*) between the aorta and transverse duodenum, which would normally be disrupted in an aorto-enteric fistula.

location and is directly adjacent to the abdominal aorta. Infection originating in the aorta has free passage via the retroperitoneal soft tissues into the adjacent structure.

Fistulization is most commonly seen in patients that have had surgical or endovascular repair of the aorta and is known as a secondary aortoenteric fistula. The annual incidence post graft repair is as high as 0.6% to 2%.[43] Primary aortoenteric fistula, fistula in the absence of aortic repair, is rare and almost invariably occurs in the presence of an aneurysm.[27] Primary aortoenteric fistula can also rarely be associated with conditions such as tuberculosis, syphilis, and infected aortitis.[44]

Aortoenteric fistula is nearly always accompanied by the presence of vascular infection, and the order of occurrence of these processes can be difficult to determine. Infection can lead to development of a fistula, and fistulas can lead to the development of vascular infection. If signs of abdominal aortic infection are identified on imaging, a concerted effort should be made to search for signs of aortoenteric fistula. Further, recognition of an aortoenteric fistula should lead to the suggestion of the possibility of coexisting infection.

The mortality of untreated aortoenteric fistula is 100%. The signs and symptoms are nonspecific and include hematemesis, melena, hematochezia, and abdominal pain.[149] Classically the patient has a seemingly insidious gastrointestinal bleed (herald bleed) that is followed by catastrophic hemorrhage. The suspicion of aortoenteric fistula must be especially elevated in a patient with gastrointestinal bleed and a history of aneurysm repair.

The definitive diagnosis of aortoenteric fistula is made by identification of the transmission of intravenous contrast from the aorta into the bowel lumen. If this diagnosis is suspected, oral contrast should be withheld to optimize the detection of intravenous contrast within the bowel lumen. Because bleeding can be intermittent, the absence of extravascular contrast in the bowel lumen does not exclude the presence of an aortoenteric fistula. Ancillary imaging signs of aortoenteric fistula include air in the anterior aspect of the aorta, loss of fat plane between the bowel and the aorta, tethering of the bowel, and bowel wall thickening.[152] Recognition of any of these findings should raise the suspicion of an aortoenteric fistula. In many cases, there will also be a nonspecific periaortic hematoma (see Figure 15-35).

DISEASES OF THE ABDOMINAL VEINS

Veins in the abdomen and pelvis include the systemic venous system comprising the inferior vena cava and its tributaries and the portal venous system comprising the portal vein, superior mesenteric vein, and inferior mesenteric vein.

Veins can have thrombi (bland or tumor), can be narrowed or dilated, and can have reversal of flow. The veins can be affected by local or systemic pathology.

Imaging Notes 15-7. Patterns of Venous Disease

1. Thrombus
2. Narrowing of vein
3. Dilation of vein
4. Reversal of flow

Thrombus

Thrombus can be acute or chronic, occlusive or nonocclusive, tumor or bland.

On imaging examinations, acute thrombus is characterized by central filling defect within the lumen of the vein, expansion of the vein, perivenular soft tissue stranding, and perivenular enhancement (see Figure 15-36).[153] Both US and MR examinations can visualize the thrombus directly. On CT, recognition of venous thrombosis will in most cases require the use of intravenous contrast to outline the filling defect. However, occasionally acute thrombus can be identified as hyperattenuated lumen of an expanded artery (see Figure 15-36).

Chronic thrombi tend to demonstrate eccentric and nonocclusive filling defects within the lumen of the vessel.[150] The vein is of smaller caliber than normal and in many cases, there will be collateral vessels carrying blood back to the heart (see Figure 15-37). Collateral vessels appear as contrast- or blood-filled tubular and/or serpentine structures in the soft tissues surrounding the venous obstruction. They represent dilation of normally small venous channels in the surrounding soft tissues.

Tumor thrombus can be distinguished from bland thrombus by the presence of contrast enhancement of the thrombus (see Figure 15-38).[151] Thus, a diagnosis of tumor thrombus requires both pre- and postcontrast enhanced CT or MRI images. In general, MRI is more sensitive for the presence of thrombus enhancement than CT. In most cases, tumor thrombus is a result of direct extension of tumor from a neoplasm arising within the abdomen. This is most commonly a complication of renal cell carcinoma, hepatocellular carcinoma, and adrenal carcinoma.[215] Rarely, tumor thrombus can be a result of hematogenous metastasis or a primary tumor of the vein.

Primary venous tumors include leiomyosarcoma, vascular leiomyomas, epithelioid hemangioendotheliomas, intravascular papillary endothelial hyperplasia (Masson tumor), and angiosarcoma, of which the former is most common. The tumor presents with signs of venous obstruction such as lower extremity swelling. Prognosis is dismal. On imaging, the slow growth of the tumor allows for ample collateral vessel formation.

Vascular leiomyomas are benign tumors of the smooth muscle. The Masson tumor is characterized by endothelial proliferation and overgrowth, and imaging cannot distinguish this from angiosarcoma with sufficient diagnostic certainty.

Narrowing of Veins

Narrowing of the large and medium veins of the abdomen is uncommon and can be subdivided into (1) focal, short-segment and (2) diffuse, long-segment narrowing. Diffuse, long-segment narrowing is caused by 2 processes: chronic thrombus and radiation therapy (see Figure 15-37). In the

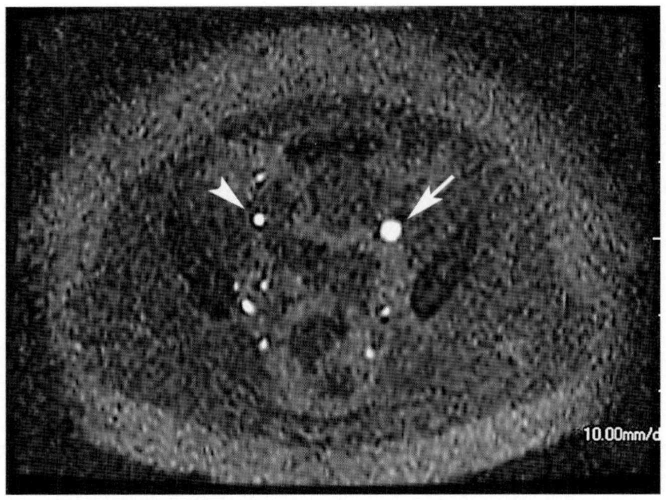

A

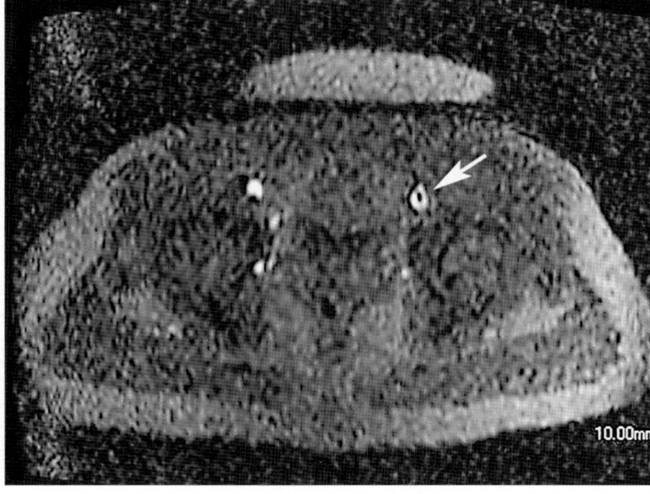

B

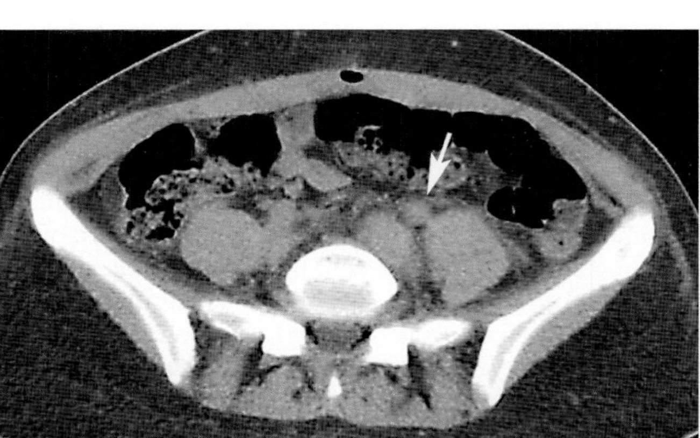

C

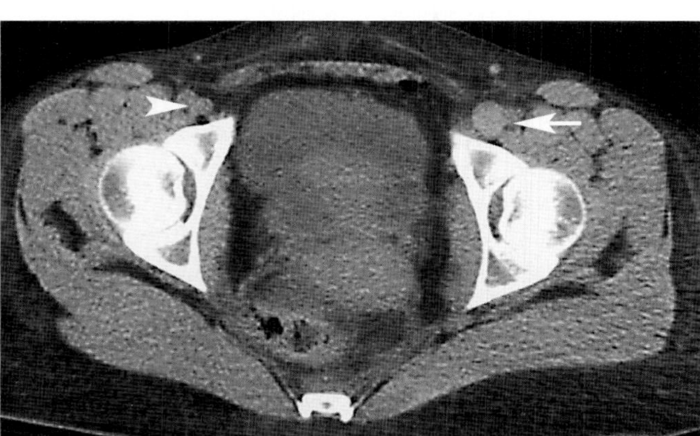

D

Figure 15-36 Imaging Manifestations of Venous Thrombosis in 2 Patients
A and **B**. Axial time-of-flight images through the pelvis of the first patient are obtained with placement of superior saturation bands to suppress signal from arteries. (A) The right external iliac vein (*arrowhead*) is smaller than the left iliac vein (*arrow*) because of chronic thromboembolic disease. (B) The left external iliac vein has a central filling defect that is nonocclusive thrombus (*arrow*). The second patient, a 20-year-old woman, complained of pelvic pain. **C** and **D**. Axial noncontrast CT through the pelvis shows 2 important features of acute thrombus (*arrows*) within the left common femoral vein to the left common iliac vein—high attenuation in the lumen representing the acute thrombus and expansion of the vein. Compare the diameter of the right (*arrowhead*) and left (*arrows*) common femoral veins. A third feature of acute thrombus is noted in (D), which is perivenular soft-tissue stranding. Although contrast should be given to assess thrombus in the venous system, occasionally features of acute thrombus may be evident on unenhanced CT and the reader should be cognizant of these features.

majority of cases, focal narrowing of the vein indicates the presence of external compression. This can be due to external mass lesions, bowel volvulus, and compression by the surrounding normal structures such as those seen in the nutcracker and May-Thurner syndromes.

Nutcracker syndrome

Nutcracker syndrome is an uncommon syndrome of left renal vein compression, which can be a cause of left-sided abdominal, flank, or testicular pain.[216] The left renal vein passes between the aorta and SMA as it travels from the inferior vena cava to the left kidney. In rare instances, the aorta and SMA (the 2 arms of the nutcracker) can compress the left renal vein (the nut) leading to partial obstruction of the left renal vein. Because the left gonadal vein empties into the left renal vein, there is also partial obstruction of venous outflow of the left testis or ovary. Symptoms are a result of venous obstruction of the left kidney and gonad.

Nutcracker syndrome can be found in individuals of any age but is most frequently discovered in teenage and young adult patients.[216] Some studies indicate a slight female predominance. Hematuria is the most commonly

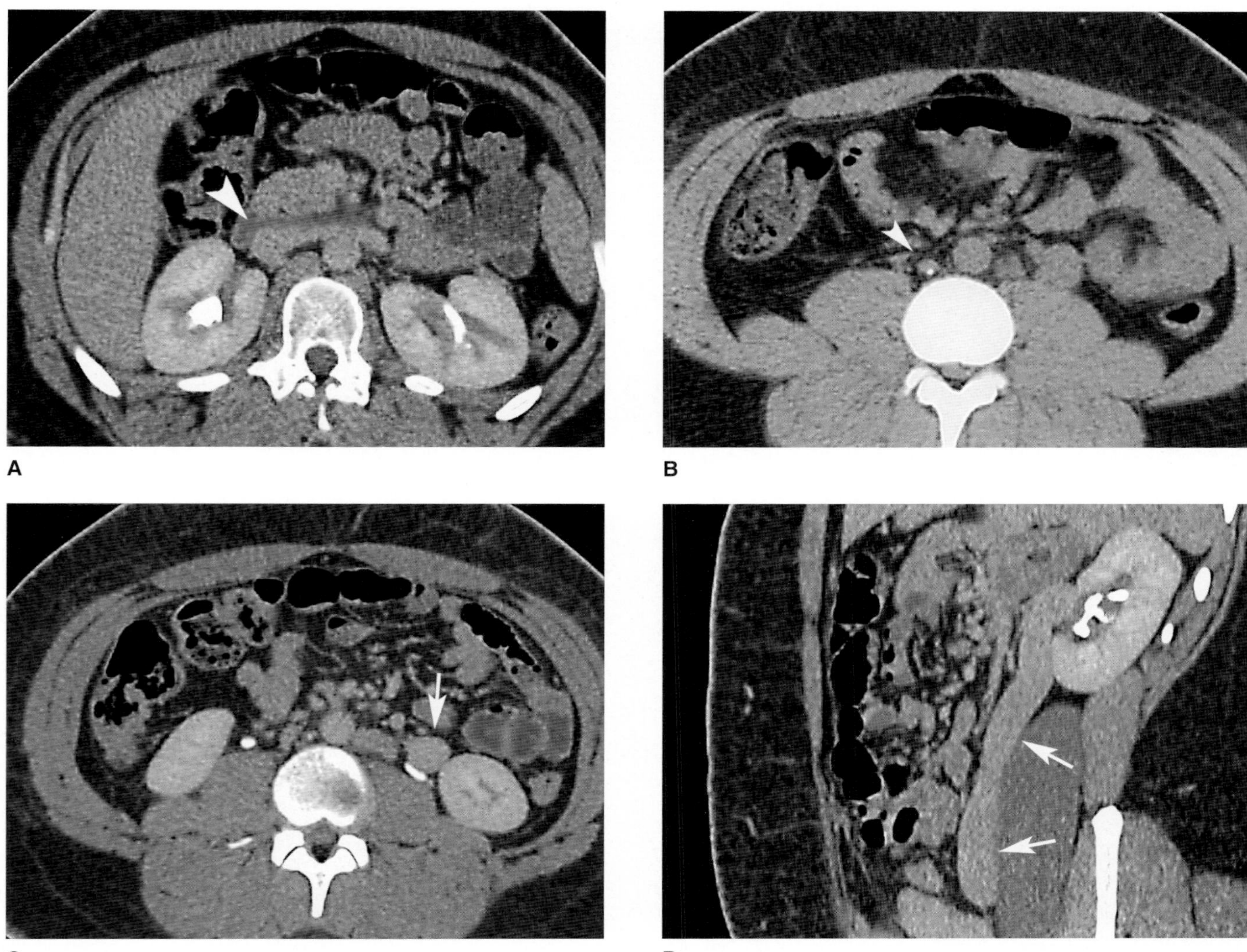

Figure 15-37 Chronic Venous Thrombosis
A-C. Axial contrast-enhanced CT venogram shows a narrow infrarenal IVC (*small arrowhead* in B) with a fleck of calcification on the posterior wall from chronic obstruction. Note that the caliber of the IVC (*large arrowhead* in A) is normal at the level of the left renal vein. An additional hallmark of the chronicity of the obstruction is the presence of extensive retroperitoneal collaterals, including an enlarged left gonadal vein (*arrows*) seen in the (C) axial images and (**D**) coronal oblique reconstruction.

reported symptom and is attributed to rupture of small intrarenal varices into the collecting system of the kidney. Pain—abdominal, flank, pelvic or testicular—is the second most common symptom. The pain is often exacerbated by sitting, standing, walking, or riding in a vehicle that shakes.[216] Nutcracker syndrome can also result in a left-sided varicocele and in one series was a common cause of left varicoceles.[217]

On cross-sectional imaging examinations, the left renal vein is narrowed in the anteroposterior dimension as it passes between the aorta and SMA. The proximal left renal vein is often mildly dilated as a result of the partial obstruction (see Figure 15-39). A retroaortic left renal vein can also be compressed between the aorta and lumbar spine—a phenomenon that is sometimes called the "posterior nutcracker."[216]

May-Thurner syndrome (iliocaval compression syndrome)

May-Thurner syndrome is a syndrome of left iliac vein compression leading to an increased incidence of deep venous thrombosis. Although first noted by Virchow, this syndrome was first substantially documented by May and Thurner who demonstrated that the right iliac artery compressed the left iliac vein against the fifth lumbar vertebra in 22% to 32% of 430 cadavers.[218] It has been suggested that from 18% to 49% of patients with left-sided lower

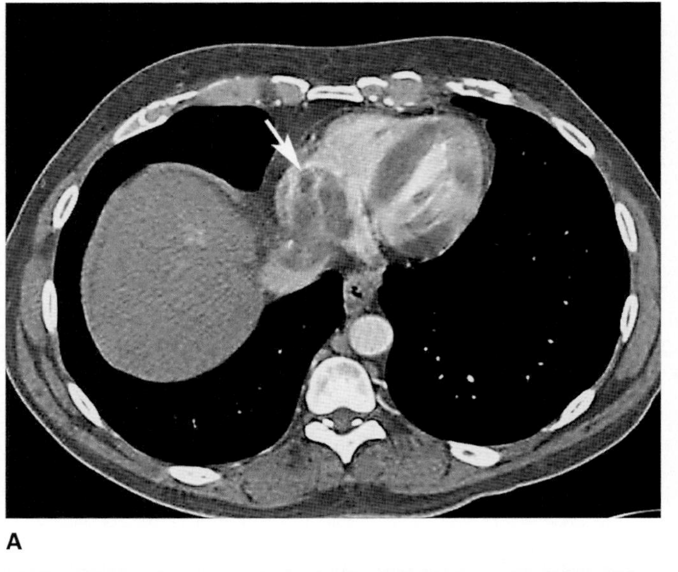

A

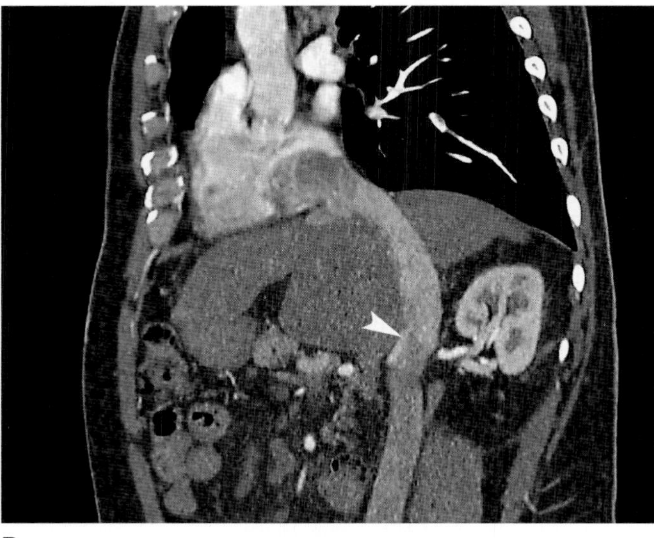

B

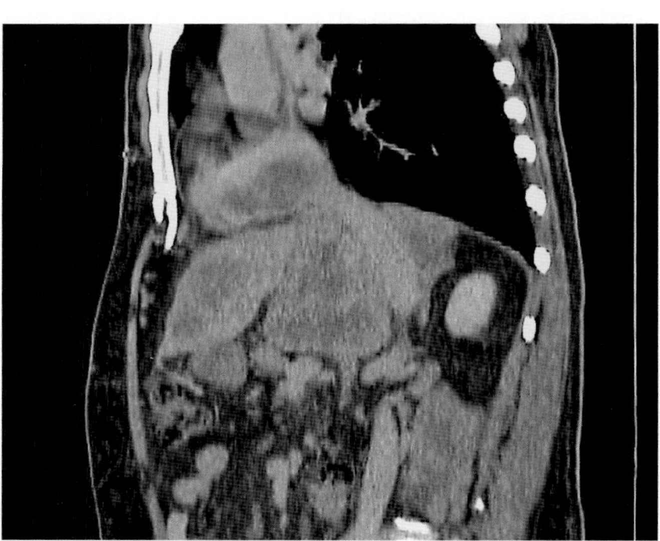

C

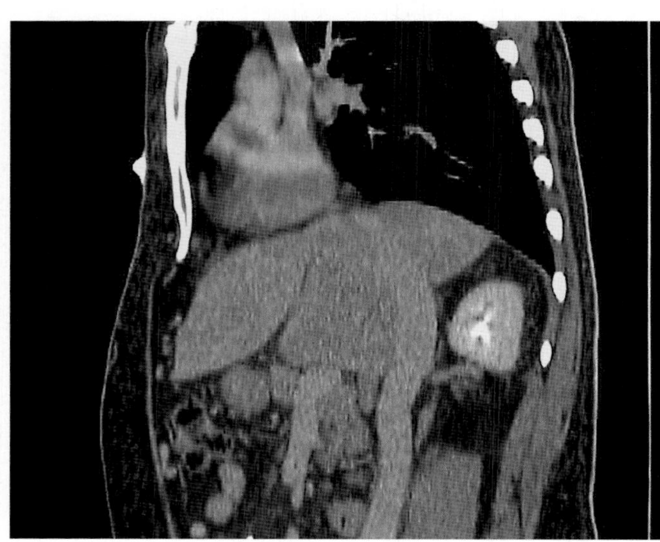

D

Figure 15-38 Tumor Thrombus
This 54-year-old man had hepatocellular carcinoma. Invading the IVC and extending into the right atrium. **A.** Axial and (**B**) sagittal CTA in the arterial phase through the liver shows expansion of the IVC by a mass that invades the RA (*arrow*). Note the high attenuation contrast in the hepatic segment of the IVC with abrupt cut-off at the level of the left renal vein (*arrowhead*). It is common for the hepatic IVC to opacify in the arterial phase because of transit of contrast through the renal veins. However, the infrarenal IVC is the last to opacify because it has to wait for the contrast to recirculate through the lower extremity veins. As a consequence, it is unclear whether this represents an enhancing IVC mass or return of contrast from the kidneys to the heart. **C** and **D**. Sagittal images through the liver in the venous phase show uniform opacification of the IVC with a persistent mass in the left atrium confirming the presence of IVC-LA tumor thrombus from the hepatocellular carcinoma.

extremity deep vein thrombosis (DVT) will have May-Thurner syndrome.[219] It is believed that a combination of external compression and irritation of the venous wall by pulsation of the artery can predispose these individuals to the development of DVT.

Patients typically present with symptoms of left DVT such as lower extremity edema and pain or symptoms of chronic venous stasis such as pigmentation changes, phlebitis, varicose veins, and skin ulceration.[220] It is most commonly discovered in women in the second to fourth decade of life after prolonged immobilization or pregnancy.

The diagnosis of May-Thurner syndrome is based on clinical symptoms of left iliac vein venous stasis and the demonstration of compression of the left iliac vein by the right iliac artery on US, CT, MRI, or conventional

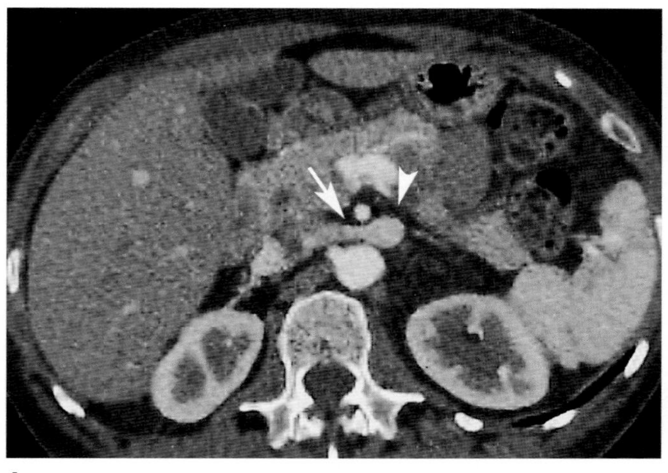

A

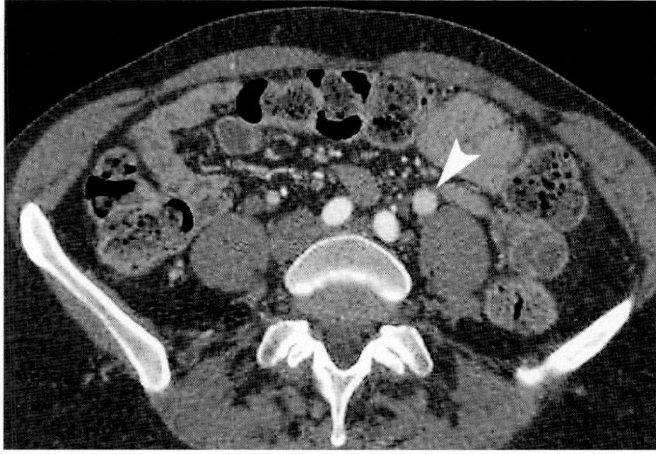

B

Figure 15-39 Nutcracker Syndrome
This 58-year-old woman complained of pelvic pain. **A** and **B**. Contrast-enhanced CT shows narrowing of the left renal vein as it crosses between the aorta and SMA (*arrow*) with dilation of the gonadal vein (*large arrowhead*) and renal vein (*small arrowhead*) proximal to the narrowing. This is an example of the Nutcracker syndrome and can be a cause of pelvic pain.

venography examinations.[221] Care must be taken in diagnosing May-Thurner syndrome in the absence of symptoms. One study of asymptomatic patients showed that two-thirds of all patients studied had at least 25% compression of the left iliac vein.[222]

Dilation of Veins

Vein dilation will usually reflect downstream compression or occlusion but in some cases is due to venous stasis because of incompetent valves. Rarely vein dilation can be a marker for an arteriovenous fistula or arteriovenous malformation.

Venous stenosis or occlusion

Venous stenosis/compression or occlusion will cause increased venous pressures downstream to the blockage. The elevated pressures will then result in dilation of the pressurized veins. Also, blood will search for alternative pathways to return to the heart. These alternative pathways will become dilated in order to carry the excess blood, a phenomenon called varices.

Portal hypertension resulting in varices or Budd-Chiari syndrome is among the most common causes of venous hypertension in the abdomen. Obstruction of the portal sinusoids as a result of fibrosis leads to elevated portal venous pressures and the development of enlarged veins throughout the upper abdomen, most commonly around the esophagus, stomach, and spleen (see Figure 3-39). Similarly, obstruction of the inferior vena cava will result in dilation of intra-abdominal and abdominal wall collateral veins. Discovery of varices should lead to a search for the site of obstruction, which is most often due to benign causes but can rarely be due to malignancy. In most cases, varices are of little clinical significance; however, occasionally they can result in clinically important complications, such as variceal bleeding in patients with cirrhosis and unsuspected passage for pulmonary emboli in patients with IVC occlusion following IVC filter placement.

One of the more commonly identified downstream compressive causes of venous dilation is dilation of the left gonadal vein from left renal vein compression. This is often due to the nutcracker syndrome, which has been discussed in the previous section of this chapter titled **Narrowing of Veins** (see Figure 15-39).

Pelvic congestion syndrome

Pelvic congestion syndrome is a common medical condition causing chronic pelvic pain in middle aged women. The disorder is due to stasis or retrograde flow of blood within dilated ovarian veins, which can be found in up to 10% of middle-aged women of whom 60% will develop pelvic congestion syndrome.[223] This syndrome is only seen in premenopausal women, suggesting that there are hormonal factors involved in the development of the syndrome. Ovarian varices have an increased incidence with increased parity and can also be associated with the nutcracker syndrome (discussed previously in this chapter).[223]

Patients typically complain of dull aching pelvic pain that is increased in severity, at the end of the day, just prior to menses and during pregnancy. Pain is often exacerbated by fatigue, standing, and coitus. Bladder irritability and increased urinary frequency can also be encountered.[223]

Imaging is an important tool in the evaluation of patients with pelvic congestion syndrome. US, CT, MRI, and pelvic venography will demonstrate multiple ovarian varices seen as numerous dilated veins in the adnexa on either side of the uterus.[223-225] The uterus is often enlarged and there are frequently polycystic changes in the ovaries on the side of the pelvic congestion.[12] There are 4 primary diagnostic criteria for pelvic congestion syndrome by US[226,227]: (1) tortuous pelvic veins with diameter greater than 6 mm, (2) slow blood flow (≤3 cm/s) or reversal of the normal caudal blood flow within the ovarian vein, (3) dilated arcuate veins of the uterus that communicate between the bilateral pelvic varices, and (4) polycystic changes in the ovaries. CT and MRI will show similar dilated tortuous pelvic veins on either side of the uterus and polycystic ovaries and MRI can demonstrate flow reversal within the ovarian vein (see Figure 15-40).

Arteriovenous fistula/malformation

Direct communication between arteries and veins without the intervening capillaries is an abnormal condition that can be a result of a congenital malformation or due to a pathologic condition that creates the abnormal communication. Arteriovenous malformations and fistulas can occur anywhere within the body but are most commonly recognized in the extremities.[228] In the abdomen, they can be found in the liver, kidney, alimentary tract, and between the aorta and inferior vena cava. Causes include penetrating trauma (accidental or iatrogenic), neoplasm, cirrhosis, erosions of aneurysms into adjacent veins, or can be congenital in origin, either sporadic or associated with hereditary hemorrhagic telangiectasia.[228] Aortocaval fistulas are typically a complication of AAAs and may be seen in up to 6% of ruptured AAA (see Figure 15-41).[228]

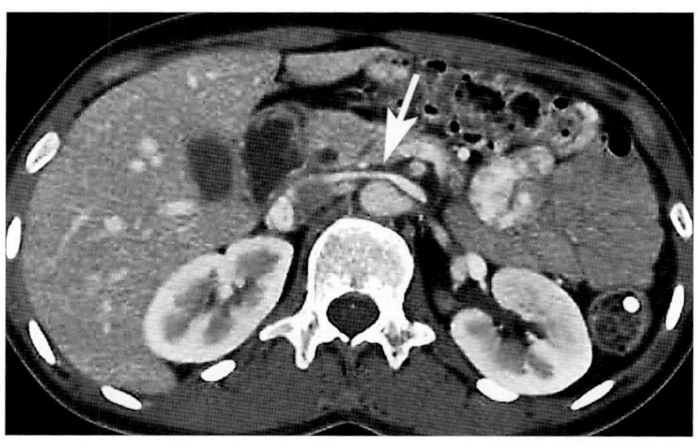

A

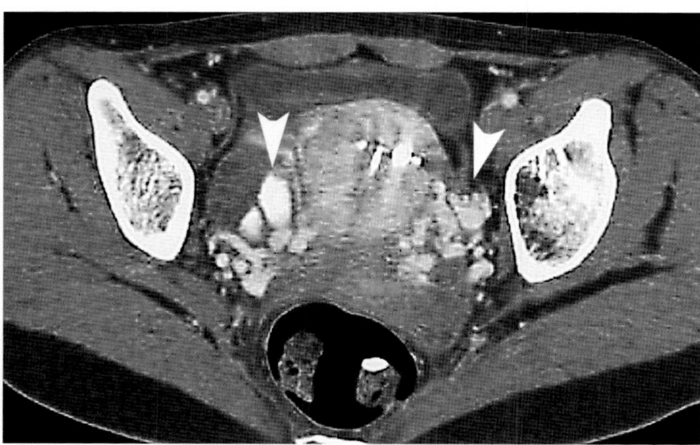

B

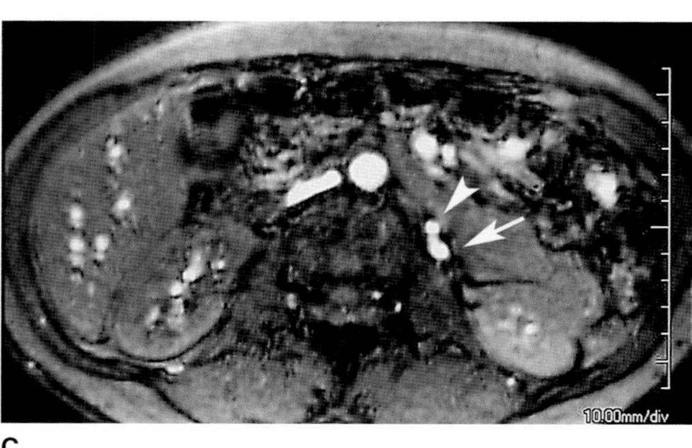

C

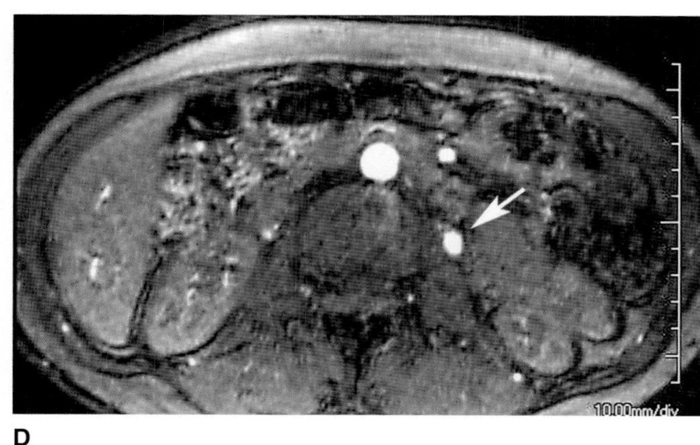

D

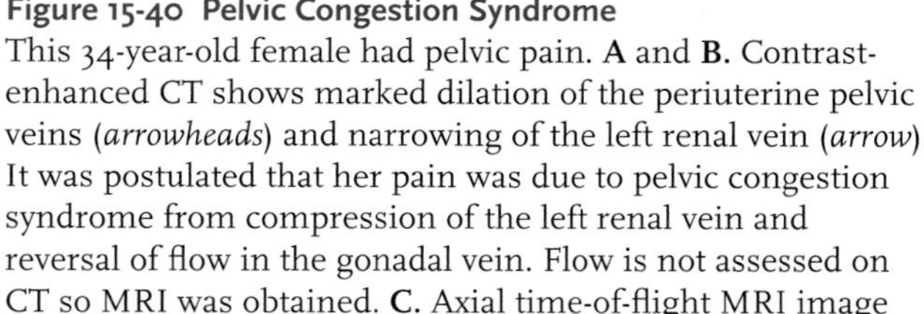

Figure 15-40 Pelvic Congestion Syndrome
This 34-year-old female had pelvic pain. **A** and **B.** Contrast-enhanced CT shows marked dilation of the periuterine pelvic veins (*arrowheads*) and narrowing of the left renal vein (*arrow*). It was postulated that her pain was due to pelvic congestion syndrome from compression of the left renal vein and reversal of flow in the gonadal vein. Flow is not assessed on CT so MRI was obtained. **C.** Axial time-of-flight MRI image with no saturation band shows signal in the IVC, aorta, IMV (*small arrowhead*), and left gonadal vein (*small arrow*). **D.** Axial time-of-flight MRI image shows an inferior saturation band suppresses the signal in the IVC and IMV but not the left gonadal vein (*arrow*), which has reversal of flow, proving that the dilated pelvic veins were due to reversal of flow. This phenomenon can be a cause of pelvic pain.

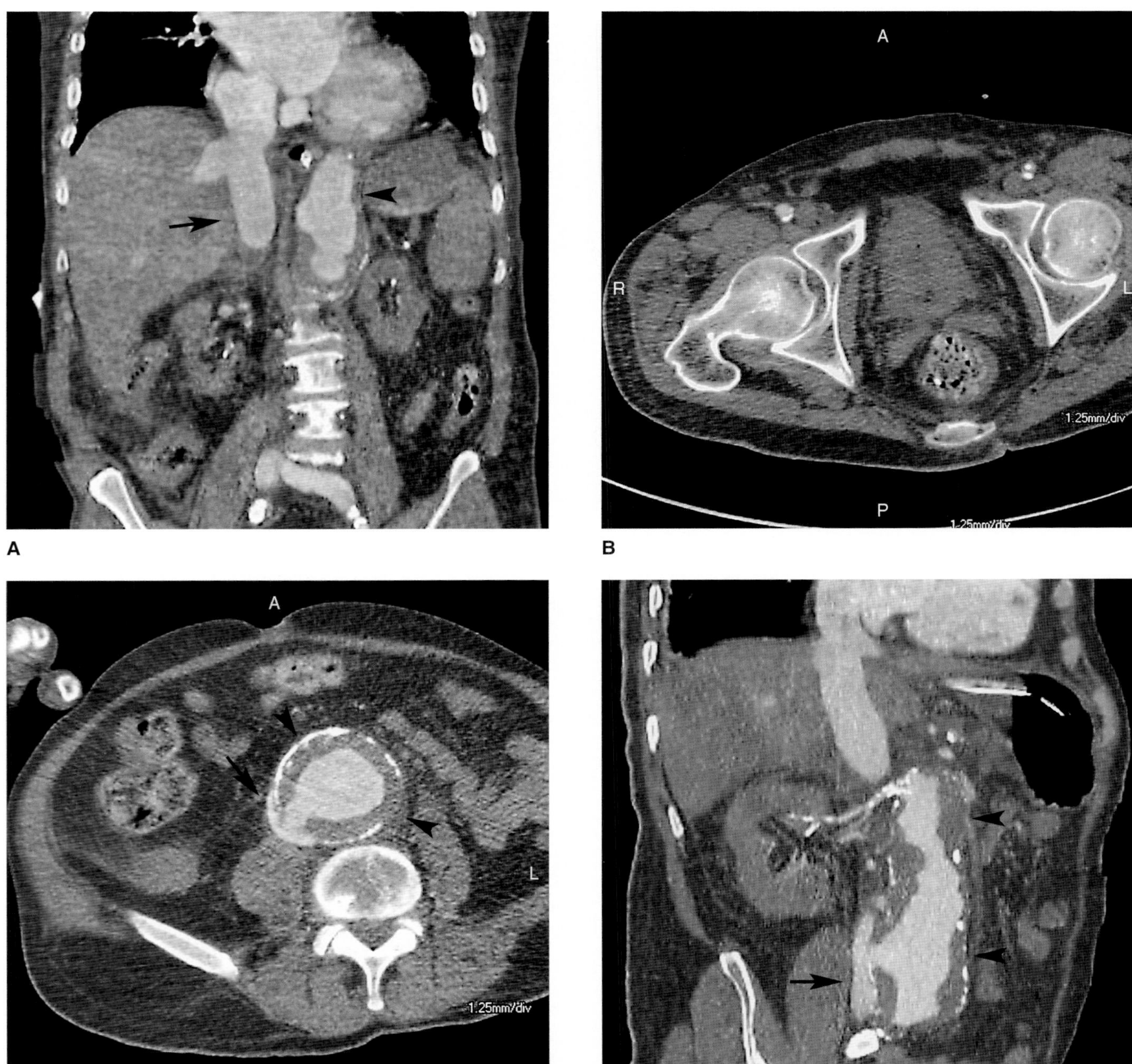

Figure 15-41 Aortocaval Fistula
This 61-year-old man presented with increasing lower extremity ischemia. **A.** Coronal CTA demonstrates early opacification of the IVC (*arrow*), which has a similar attenuation to the aorta (*arrowhead*), which is not due to reflux of contrast from the SVC. **B.** Axial CTA at the same time as (A) shows that the iliac veins are unopacified, indicating that the contrast in the IVC is not due to recirculation of contrast from the lower extremities and suggests an anomalous communication between the arterial and venous systems proximal to the legs. **C.** Axial CTA shows a dilated, thick-walled, calcified abdominal aortic aneurysm (*arrowheads*). The IVC is seen as a flattened curved structure (*arrow*) right lateral and posterior to the aorta. There is also direct communication between the aorta and the compressed IVC at approximately 7 o'clock on the aortic wall. **D.** The aortocaval fistula can also be seen on this coronal oblique image between the IVC (*arrow*) and the aorta (*arrowheads*).

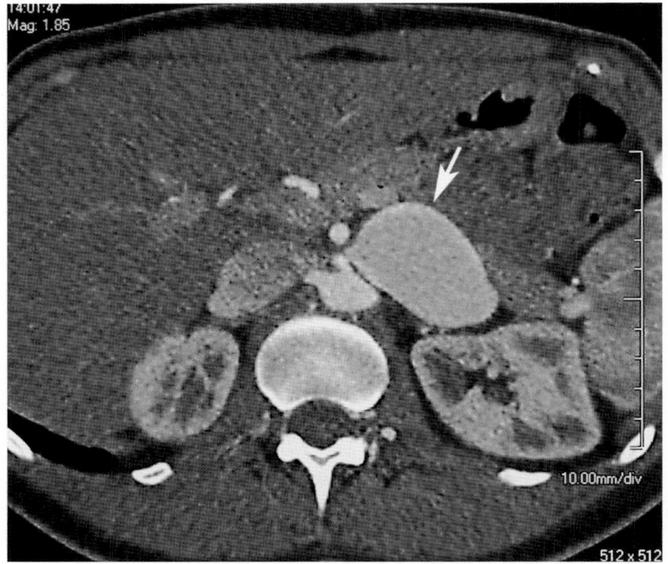

A

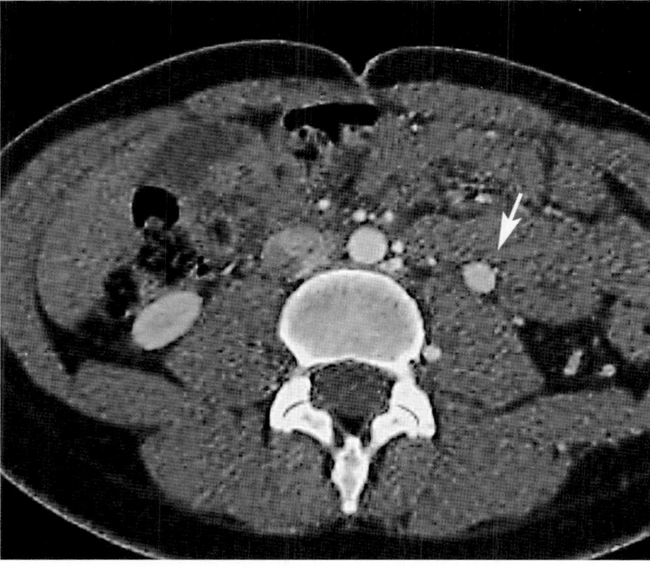

B

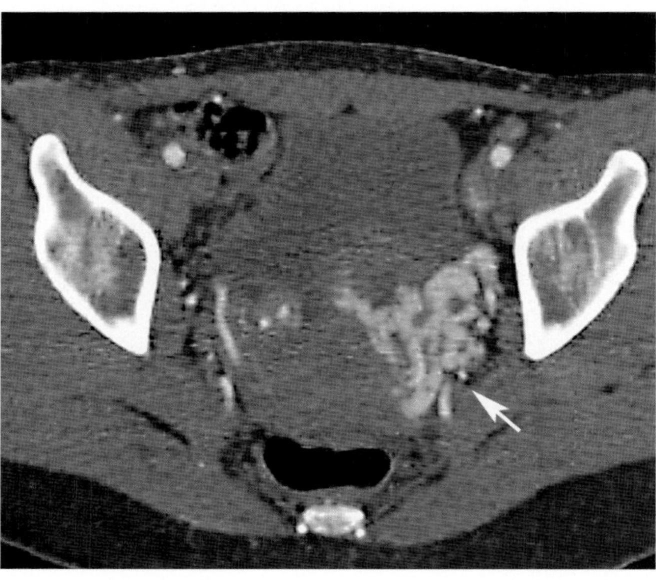

C

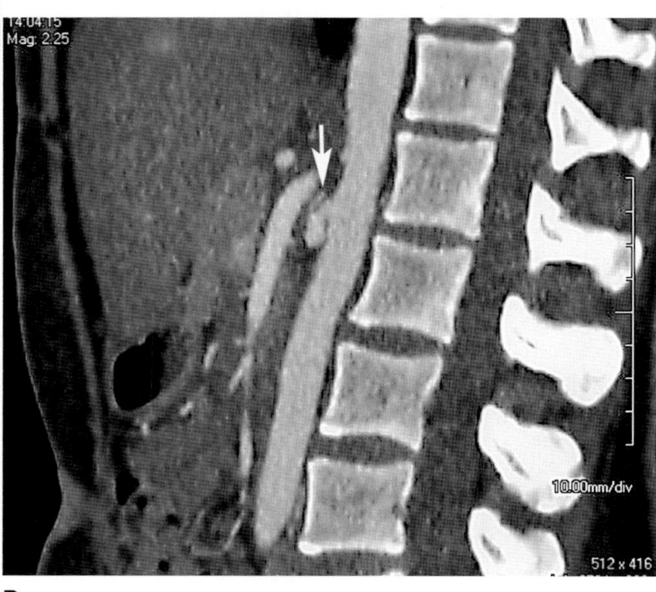

D

Figure 15-42 Arteriovenous Fistula
This 30-year-old female presented with abdominal pain and with dilated pelvic veins on US. **A-C.** Axial CTA shows a dilated left renal vein (*arrow* in A) that has the same opacification as the aorta. There is also dilation of the left gonadal vein (*arrow* in B) and there are left pelvic varices (*arrow* in C). These findings suggest an arteriovenous communication into the left renal vein system. **D.** Sagittal reconstruction from a CTA shows subtle communication between the left renal vein and the aorta (*arrow*).

Posttraumatic AV fistulas will typically demonstrate a single direct communication between an artery and vein, whereas AV malformations will typically be composed of multiple communicating channels. In both AV malformations the involved vein will become dilated as a result of the arterial-level pressures within the vein. On US, an AV fistula is characterized by pulsatile venous flow and low-resistance arterial flow.[228] On contrast-enhanced CT and MRI, an AV fistula is characterized by early venous opacification and dilated vein (see Figure 15-42).[228]

Reversal of Flow

Reversal of flow within veins is indicative of obstruction downstream from the flow reversal and is always associated with vein dilation. Examples of flow reversal include portal hypertension due to cirrhosis and compression of the left renal vein. The reversal of flow in the left gonadal vein can lead to engorgement of pelvic veins and, if associated with pelvic pain, is part of the pelvic congestion syndrome (see Figure 15-40).

Congenital abnormalities of the abdominal veins

The embryogenesis of the IVC is a complex process because of the formation of several anastomoses between 3 paired embryonic veins. Abnormalities in the creation of these anastomoses can result is numerous variations in the venous anatomy of the abdomen and pelvis.[229] The infrarenal IVC derives from the right supracardinal vein and the suprarenal IVC develops from the right subcardinal vein. The intervening segment of the IVC (renal segment) is formed from the anastomosis between the right subcardinal and right supracardinal veins. The hepatic segment of the IVC forms from the right vitelline vein. The iliac veins are persistent posterior cardinal veins. There is further anastomosis between the right subcardinal vein and the right vitelline vein and the right supracardinal vein and the posterior cardinal veins, all of which complete the formation of the IVC.

The left renal vein forms from an anastomosis between the right and left subcardinal veins (intersubcardinal anastomosis). This anastomosis courses anterior to the aorta.

A **double IVC** forms from persistence of bilateral supracardinal veins. The left-sided IVC drains into the left renal vein, which then empties into the right-sided IVC, which continues as the normal IVC into the right atrium. The prevalence of a double IVC is between 1% and 3% (see Figure 15-43).[229]

Left IVC is persistence of the left supracardinal vein and regression of the right supracardinal vein. The left IVC joins the left renal vein, which then empties into the suprarenal segment of a right-sided IVC that continues into the right atrium. The prevalence of left IVC is between 0.2% and 0.5% (see Figure 15-44).[229]

Azygous continuation of the IVC is due to both the failure of anastomosis between the right subcardinal vein and the right vitelline vein and atrophy of the right subcardinal vein. The infrarenal IVC continues as the azygous vein, which is typically dilated. The hepatic veins drain into a short nub, which connects to the right atrium. The prevalence of this abnormality is 0.6%.[229] However, azygous continuation of the IVC is associated with situs abnormalities, particularly polysplenia. Polysplenia is discussed in detail in Chapter 14: **Imaging of the Spleen**.

The **retroaortic left renal vein** occurs when there is persistence of anastomosis between the supracardinal veins and regression of the intersubcardinal veins. This occurs with a prevalence of 1.7% to 3.4%.[229] Persistence of both intersupracardinal and intersubcardinal veins results in a **circumaortic left renal vein** (see Figure 15-45). The preaortic component is located cranially and the retroaortic component is located caudally. The retroaortic component, which typically receives the gonadal vein, is predisposed to compression. This abnormality is seen in 2.4% to 8.4% of patients.[229] Acknowledgement of variants of renal vein anatomy is important in patients who will undergo laparoscopic nephrectomy for renal donation.

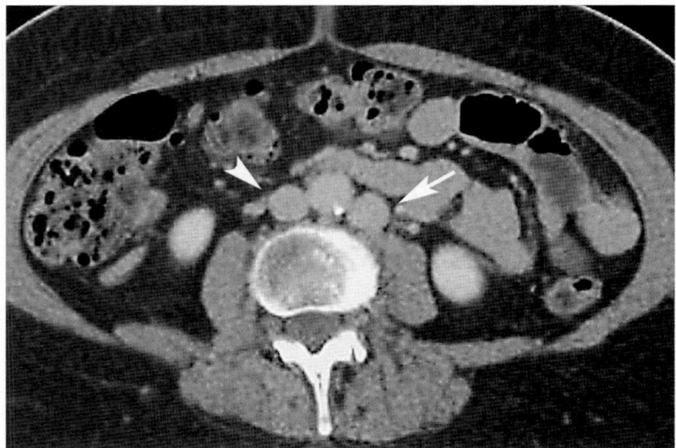

A

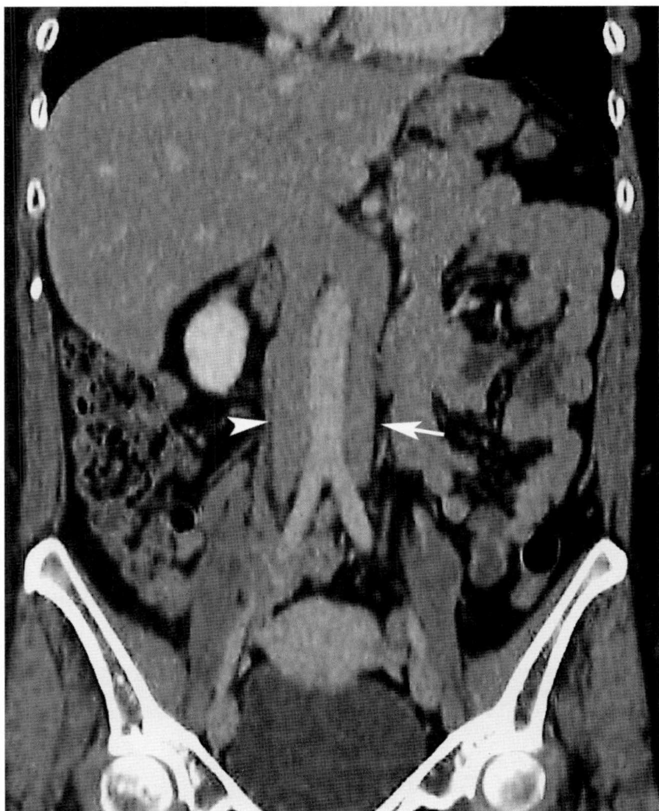

B

Figure 15-43 Double IVC
A. Axial CT demonstrates 3 oval structures anterior to the spine when there should only be 2. **B.** Coronal reconstruction shows these to represent a right IVC (*arrowheads* in A and B) and persistent left IVC (*arrows* in A and B) with a central normal aorta. Double IVC is composed of a left IVC, which is a continuation of the left iliac vein, and a right IVC, which is a continuation of the right iliac vein. The left IVC receives the left renal vein, and the right IVC receives the right renal vein and the left IVC before forming the common IVC just below the liver.

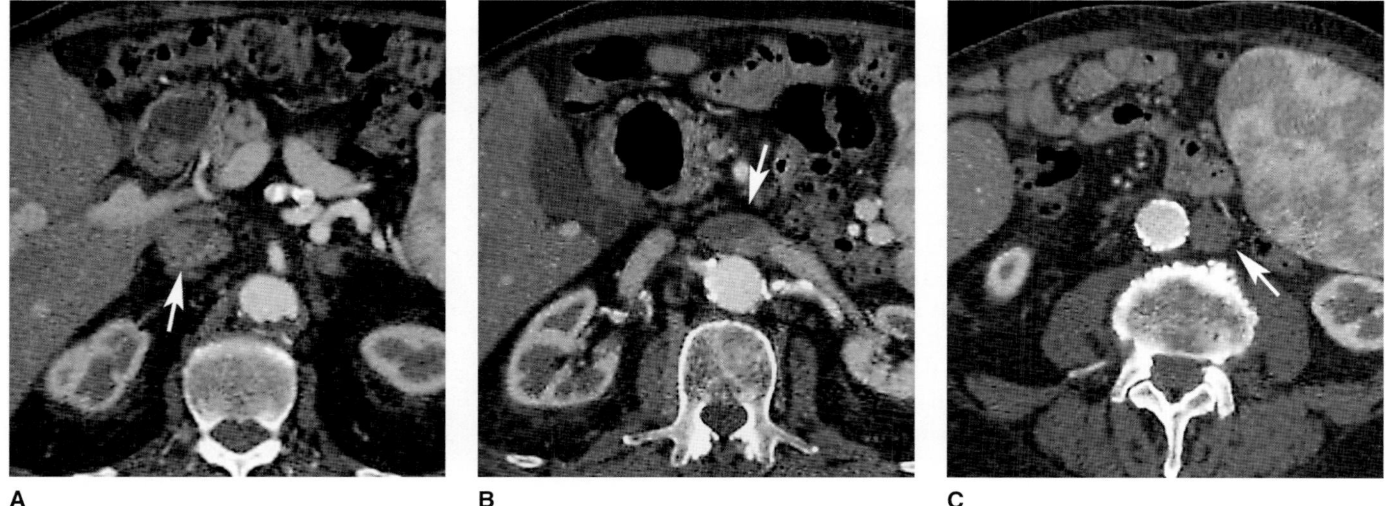

Figure 15-44 Left IVC
A-C. Axial CT images show no IVC to the right of the aorta but show it to the left of the aorta (*arrow* in C) at a level below the renal veins. The IVC then crosses from left to right (*arrow* in B) after it receives the left renal vein. Cephalad to the renal veins, the IVC course in the normal position (*arrow* in A) to the right of the aorta.

A

B

C

D

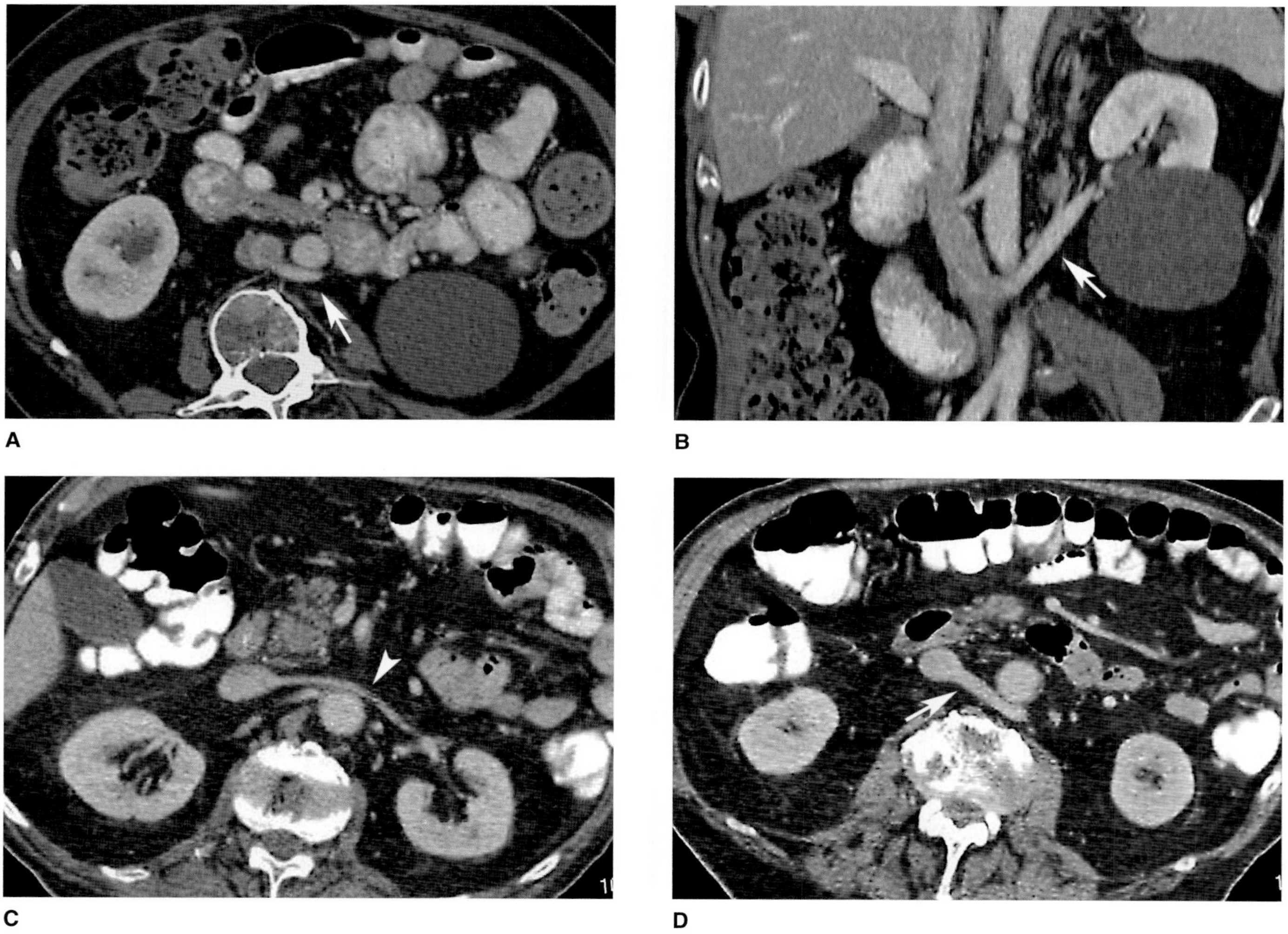

Figure 15-45 Congenital Anomalies of the Left Renal Vein in 2 Patients
A. Axial and (**B**) coronal reconstructions from an enhanced CT show the left renal vein (*arrows*) to course posterior to the aorta, a common congenital anomaly. **C** and **D.** Axial CT images in a second patient show 2 veins draining the left kidney, an anterior, preaortic vein (*arrowhead* in C) in the normal position and a retroaortic vein (*arrow* in D). This is called a "circumaortic" renal vein and typically the retroaortic component is inferior to the preaortic component.

REFERENCES

1. Coady, Rizzo JA, Elefteriades JA. Pathologic variants of thoracic aortic dissections. Penetrating atherosclerotic ulcers and intramural hematomas. *Cardiol Clin.* 1999;17:1-20.
2. Alfonso F, Goicolea J, Aragoncillo P, Hernandez R, Macaya C. Diagnosis of aortic intramural hematoma by intravascular ultrasound imaging (abstract). *Am J Cardiol.* 1995;76:735-738.
3. Roberts WC. Aortic dissection: anatomy, consequences, and causes. *Am Heart J.* 1981;101:195-214.
4. Song JK, Kim HS, Kang DH, et al. Different clinical features of aortic intramural hematoma versus dissection involving the ascending aorta. *J Am Coll Cardiol.* 2001;37:1604-1610.
5. Motoyoshi N, Moizumi Y, Komatsu T, Tabayashi K. Intramural hematoma and dissection involving ascending aorta: the clinical features and prognosis. *Eur J Cardiothorac Surg.* 2003;24: 237-242.
6. von Kodolitsch Y, Csösz SK, Koschyk DH, et al. Intramural hematoma of the aorta: predictors of progression to dissection and rupture. *Circulation.* 2003;107:1158-1163.
7. Yamada T, Takamiya M, Naito H, Kozuka T, Nakajima N. Diagnosis of aortic dissection without intimal rupture by x-ray computed tomography [in Japanese]. *Nippon Acta Radiol.* 1985;45:699-710.
8. Nishigami K, Tsuchiya T, Shono H, Horibata Y, Honda T. Disappearance of aortic intramural hematoma and its significance to the prognosis. *Circulation.* 2000;102:243-247.
9. Evangelista A, Dominguez R, Sebastia C, et al. Long-term follow-up of aortic intramural hematoma: predictors of outcome. *Circulation.* 2003;108:583-589.
10. Evangelista A, Dominguez R, Sebastia C, et al. Prognostic value of clinical and morphologic findings in short-term evolution of aortic intramural haematoma. Therapeutic implications. *Eur Heart J.* 2004;25:81-87.
11. Sueyoshi E, Imada T, Sakamoto I, Matsuoka Y, Hayashi K. Analysis of predictive factors for progression of type B aortic intramural hematoma with computed tomography. *J Vasc Surg.* 2002;35:1179-1183.
12. Kaji S, Nishigami K, Akasaka T, et al. Prediction of progression or regression of type A aortic intramural hematoma by computed tomography. *Circulation.* 1999;100:281-286.
13. Murray JG, Manisali M, Flamm SD, et al. Intramural hematoma of the thoracic aorta: MR image findings and their prognostic implications. *Radiology.* 1997;204:349-355.
14. Yamada T, Tada S, Harada J. Aortic dissection without intimal rupture: diagnosis with MR imaging and CT. *Radiology.* 1988;168:347-352.
15. Oliver TB, Murchison JT, Reid JH. Serial MRI in the management of intramural haemorrhage of the thoracic aorta. *Br J Radiol.* 1997;70:1288-1290.
16. Neinaber CA, von Kodolitsch Y, Petersen B, et al. Intramural hemorrhage of the aorta: diagnostic and therapeutic implications. *Circulation.* 1995;92:1465-1472.
17. Yucel EK, Steinberg FL, Egglin TK, Geller SC, Waltman AC, Athanasoulis CA. Penetrating aortic ulcers: diagnosis with MR imaging. *Radiology.* 1990;177:779-781.
18. Park JH, Chung JW, Im JG, Kim SK, Park YB, Han MC. Takayasu arteritis: evaluation of mural changes in the aorta and pulmonary artery with CT angiography. *Radiology.* 1995;196:89-93.
19. Matsuaga N, Hayashi K, Sakamoto I, Ogawa Y, Matsumoto T. Takayasu arteritis: protean radiologic manifestations and diagnosis. *Radiographics.* 1997;17:579-594.
20. Tanigawa K, Eguchi K, Kitamura Y, et al. Magnetic resonance imaging detection of aortic and pulmonary artery wall thickening in acute stage of Takayasu arteritis: improvement of clinical and radiologic findings after steroid therapy. *Arthritis Rheum.* 1992;35:476-480.
21. Link KM, Lesko NM. The role of MR imaging in the evaluation of acquired diseases of the thoracic aorta. *AJR Am J Roentgenol.* 1992;158:1115-1125.
22. Mandalam KR, Joseph S, Rao VR, et al. Aortoarteritis of abdominal aorta: an angiographic profile in 110 patients. *Clin Radiol.* 1993;48:29-34.
23. Yamada I, Numano F, Suzuki S. Takayasu arteritis: evaluation with MR imaging. *Radiology.* 1993;188:89-94.
24. Hayashi K, Fukushima T, Matsunaga N, Hombo Z. Takayasu's arteritis: decrease in aortic wall thickening following steroid therapy, documented by CT. *Br J Radiol.* 1986;59:281-283.
25. Tanikawa K, Eguchi K, Kitamura Y, et al. Magnetic resonance imaging detection of aortic and pulmonary artery wall thickening in the acute stage of Takayasu arteritis: improvement of clinical and radiologic findings after steroid therapy. *Arthritis Rheum.* 1992;35:476-480.
26. Rosen V, Korobkin M, Silverman PM, Moore AV Jr, Dunnick NR. CT diagnosis of ruptured abdominal aortic aneurysm. *AJR Am J Roentgenol.* 1984;143:265-268.
27. Voorhoeve R, Moll FL, de Letter JA, Bast TJ, Wester JP, Slee PH. Primary aortoenteric fistula: report of eight new cases and review of the literature. *Ann Vasc Surg.* 1996;10:40-48.
28. Jee KN, Ha HK, Lee IJ, et al. Radiologic findings of abdominal polyarteritis nodosa. *AJR Am J Roentgenol.* 2000;174:1675-1679.
29. Yamada I, Nakagawa T, Himeno Y, Numano F, Shibuya H. Takayasu arteritis: evaluation of the thoracic aorta with CT angiography. *Radiology.* 1998;209:103-109.
30. Yamato M, Lecky JW, Hiramatsu K, Kohda E. Takayasu arteritis: radiographic and angiographic findings in 59 patients. *Radiology.* 1986;161:329-334.
31. Lande A, Bard R, Rossi P, Passariello R, Castrucci A. Takayasu's arteritis. A world wide entity. *NY State J Med.* 1976;76:1477-1482.
32. The Aortitis Syndrome Research Committee of Japan organized by the Ministry of Health and Welfare. A report of the survey of aortitis syndrome in Japan (in Japanese) Tokyo. Ministry of Health and Welfare;1993:8-10.
33. Ishikawa K, Maetani S. Long-term outcome for 120 Japanese patients with Takayasu's disease: clinical and statistical analyses of related prognosis factors. *Circulation.* 1994;90: 1855-1860.
34. Virman R, Lande A, McAllister HA. Pathological aspects of Takayasu's arteritis. In: Lande A, Berkmen YM, McAllister HA, eds. *Aortitis: Clinical, Pathologic and Radiographic Aspects.* New York: Raven; 1986:55-79.
35. Nasu T. Pathology of pulseless disease: a systematic study and critical review of twenty-one autopsy cases reported in Japan. *Angiology.* 1963;14:225-235.
36. Kozuka T, Nosaki T, Sato K, Tachiiri H. Aneurysm associated with aortitis syndrome. *Acta Radiol.* 1968;7:314-320.
37. Sueyoshi E, Sakamoto I, Hayashi K. Aortic aneurysms in patients with Takayasu's arteritis: CT evaluation. *AJR Am J Roentgenol.* 2000;175:1727-1733.
38. Kerr GS, Hallahan CW, Giordano J, et al. Takayasu arteritis. *Ann Intern Med.* 1994;120:919-929.

39. Moneta GL, Edwards JM, Chitwood RW, et al. Correlation of North American Symptomatic Carotid Endarterectomy Trial (NASCET) angiographic definition of 70% to 99% internal carotid artery stenosis with duplex scanning. *J Vasc Surg.* 1993;17:152-157.
40. Wilcken DE. Overview of inherited metabolic disorders causing cardiovascular disease. *J Inherit Metab Dis.* 2003;26(2-3):245-257.
41. Hoornweg LL, Storm-Versloot MN, Ubbink DT, Koelemay MJ, Legemate DA, Balm R. Meta analysis on mortality of ruptured abdominal aortic aneurysms. *Eur J Vasc Endovasc Surg.* 2008;35(5):558-570.
42. Bernard VM, ed. *Aortoenteric Fistulas.* 3rd ed. Philadelphia, PA: WB Saunders; 1989:528-535.
43. O'Hara PJ, Hertzer NR, Beven EG, Krajewski LP. Surgical management of infected abdominal aortic grafts: review of a 25-year experience. *J Vasc Surg.* 1986;3:725-731.
44. Dossa CD, Pipinos II, Shepard AD, Ernst CB. Primary aortoenteric fistula: part I. *Ann Vasc Surg.* 1994;8:113-120.
45. Albert DM, Frederick A. Jakobiec, eds. *Principles and Practice of Ophthalmology.* Vol. 5. Philadelphia, PA: WB Saunders; 2000:4570-4576.
46. Gonzalez-Gay JA, Martin J, Liorca J. Epidemiology of giant cell arteritis and polymyalgia rheumatic. *Arthritis Rheum.* 2009;61:1454.
47. Salvarani C, Cantini F, Hunder GG. Polymyalgia rheumatica and giant cell arteritis. *Lancet.* 2008;372:234-245.
48. Francois M, Koussa D, Declerck D. Periarterial temporal halo in the ultrasonographic image of polyarteritis nodosa. *Presse Med.* 1999;28(3):133.
49. Aloisi D. Doppler color ultrasonography in the assessment of epiaortic vessels in giant-cell arteritis. *Minerva Cardioangiol.* 1999;47(12):645-646.
50. Ghanchi FD, Williamson TH, Lim CS, et al. Colour Doppler imaging in giant cell (temporal) arteritis: serial examination and comparison with non-arteritic anterior ischaemic optic neuropathy. *Eye.* 1999;10(4):459-464.
51. Bley TA, Wieben O, Uhl M, Thiel J, Schmidt D, Langer M. High-resolution MRI in giant cell arteritis: imaging of the wall of the superficial temporal artery. *AJR Am J Roentgenol.* 2005;184:283-287.
52. Henegar C, Pagnoux C, Puéchal X, et al.; French Vasculitis Study Group. A paradigm of diagnostic criteria for polyarteritis nodosa: Analysis of a series of 949 patients with vasculitides. *Arthritis Rheum.* 2008;58(5):1528-1538.
53. Guillevin L, Lhote F, Cohen P, et al. A prospective study with long-term observation of 41 patients. *Medicine.* 1995;74:238-253.
54. Vaglio A, Salvarani C, Buzio C. Retroperitoneal fibrosis. *Lancet.* 2006;367:241-251.
55. Ebert EC, Hagspiel KD, Nagar M, Schlesinger N. Gastrointestinal involvement in polyarteritis nodosa. *Clin Gastroenterol Hepatol.* 2008;6:960-966.
56. Proudfoot D, Shanahan CM. Biology of calcification in vascular cells: intima versus media. *Herz.* 2001;26(4):245-251.
57. Adaletli I, Ozpeynirci Y, Kurugoglu S, Sever L, Arisoy N. Abdominal manifestations of polyarteritis nodosa demonstrated with CT. *Pediatr Radiol.* 2010;40:766-769.
58. Parums DV. *The spectrum of chronic periaortitis. Histopathology.* 1990;16:423-431.
59. Capron L. Medial arterial calcification and diabetic neuropathy. *Br Med J (Clin Res Ed).* 1982;284(6320):1711-1712.
60. Gotlieb, et al. Atherosclerosis: pathology and pathogenesis. In: Silver MD, Gotlieb AI, Schoen FJ, eds. *Cardiovascular Pathology.* Chapter 4, 3rd ed. Philadelphia, PA: Churchill Livingstone; 2001:68-106.
61. Vaglio A, Buzio C. Chronic periaortitis: a spectrum of diseases. *Curr Opin Rheumatol.* 2005;17:34-40.
62. Vaglio A, Corradi D, Manenti L, Ferretti S, Garini G, Buzio C. Evidence of autoimmunity in chronic periaortitis: a prospective study. *Am J Med.* 2003;114:454-462.
63. Kottra JJ, Dunnick NR. Retroperitoneal fibrosis. *Radiol Clin North Am.* 1996;43:1259-1275.
64. Vivas I, Nicolás AI, Velázquez P, Elduayen B, Fernández-Villa T, Martínez-Cuesta A. Retroperitoneal fibrosis: typical and atypical manifestations. *Br J Radiol.* 2000;73:214-222.
65. Arrivé L, Hricak H, Tavares NJ, Miller TR. Malignant versus nonmalignant retroperitoneal fibrosis: differentiation with MR imaging. *Radiology.* 1989;172:139-143.
66. Nastri MV, Baptista LP, Baroni RH, et al. Gadolinium-enhanced. Three-dimensional MR Angiography of Takayasu Arteritis. *Radiographics.* 2004;24:773-786.
67. Vaglio A, Versari A, Fraternali A, Ferrozzi F, Salvarani C, Buzio C. 18F-fluorodeoxyglucose positron emission tomography in the diagnosis and follow-up of idiopathic retroperitoneal fibrosis. *Arthritis Rheum.* 2005;53:122-125.
68. Horton KM, Talamini MA, Fishman EK. Median arcuate ligament syndrome: evaluation with CT angiography1. *Radiographics.* 2005;25(5):1177-1182.
69. Lindner HH, Kemprud E. A clinicoanatomical study of the arcuate ligament of the diaphragm. *Arch Surg.* 1971;103(5): 600-605.
70. Dunbar JD, Molnar W, Beman FF, Marable SA. Compression of the celiac trunk and abdominal angina. *Am J Roentgenol Radium Ther Nucl Med.* 1965;95(3):731-744.
71. Sproat IA, Pozniak MA, Kennell TW. US case of the day. Median arcuate ligament syndrome (celiac artery compression syndrome). *Radiographics.* 1993;13(6):1400-1402.
72. Shores J, Berger KR, Murphy EA, Pyeritz RE. Progression of aortic dilatation and the benefit of long-term B-adrenergic blockade in Marfan's syndrome. *N Engl J Med.* 1994;330: 1335-1341.
73. Kawamoto S, Bluemke DA, Traill TA, Zerhouni EA. Thoracoabdominal aorta in Marfan syndrome: MR imaging findings of progression of vasculopathy after surgical repair. *Radiology.* 1997;203:727-732.
74. Virmani, et al. Nonatherosclerotic diseases of the aorta and miscellaneous diseases of the main pulmonary arteries and large veins. In: Silver MD, Gotlieb AI, Schoen FJ, eds. *Cardiovascular Pathology.* Chapter 5, 3rd ed. Philadelphia, PA: Churchill Livingstone; 2001:107-137.
75. Silverman DI, Burton KJ, Gray J, et al. Life expectancy in the Marfan syndrome. *Am J Cardiol.* 1995;75:157-160.
76. Pyeritz RE. Marfan syndrome: current and future clinical and genetic management of cardiovascular manifestations. *Semin Thorac Cardiovasc Surg.* 1993;5:11-16.
77. Pyeritz RE, McKusick VA. The Marfan syndrome: diagnosis and management. *N Engl J Med.* 1979;300:772-777.

78. Byers PH. Disorders of collage biosynthesis and structure. In: Scriver, et al., eds. *The Metabolic and Molecular Bases of Inherited Diseases.* New York: McGraw Hill; 1995:4029.
79. Hirose Y, Hamada S, Takamiya M, Imakita S, Naito H, Nishimura T. Aortic aneurysms: growth rates measured with CT. *Radiology.* 1992;185:249-252.
80. Dapunt OE, Galla JD, Sadeghi AM, et al. The natural history of thoracic aortic aneurysm. *J Thorac Cardiovasc Surg.* 1994;107:1323-1333.
81. Masuda Y, Takanashi K, Takasu J, Morooka N, Inagaki Y. Expansion rate of thoracic aortic aneurysm and influencing factors. *Chest.* 1992;102:461-466.
82. Guirguis EM, Barber GG. The natural history of abdominal aortic aneurysms. *Am J Surg.* 1991;162:481-483.
83. Bernstein EF, Chan EL. Abdominal aortic aneurysm in high-risk patients: outcome of selective management based on size and expansion rate. *Ann Surg.* 1984;200:255-263.
84. Bernstein EF, Dilley RB, Goldberger LE, Gosink BB, Leopold GR. Growth rates of small abdominal aortic aneurysms. *Surgery.* 1976;80:765-773.
85. Kremer H, Weigold B, Dobrinski W, Schreiber MA, Zöllner N. Sonographische verlaufsbeobachtungen von bauchaortenaneurysmen. *Klin Wochenschr.* 1984;62:1120-1125.
86. Stepetti AV, Schultz RD, Feldhaus RJ, Peetz DJ Jr, Fasciano AJ, McGill JE. Abdominal aortic aneurysm in elderly patients: selective management based on clinical status and aneurysmal expansion rate. *Am J Surg.* 1985;150:772-776.
87. Cronenwett JL, Murphy TF, Zelenock GB, et al. Actuarial analysis of variables associated with rupture of small abdominal aortic aneurysms. *Surgery.* 1985;98:472-483.
88. Sterpetti AV, Schultz RD, Feldhaus RJ, Cheng SE, Peetz DJ Jr. Factors influencing enlargement rate of small abdominal aortic aneurysms. *J Surg Res.* 1987;43:211-219.
89. Collin J, Araujo L, Walton J. How fast do very small abdominal aortic aneurysms grow? *Eur J Vasc Surg.* 1989;3:15-17.
90. Nevitt MP, Ballard DJ, Hallett JW Jr. Prognosis of abdominal aortic aneurysms: a population-based study. *N Engl J Med.* 1989;321:1009-1014.
91. Delin A, Ohlsén H, Swedenborg J. Growth rate of abdominal aortic aneurysms as measured by computed tomography. *Br J Surg.* 1985;72:530-532.
92. Lindbom A. Arteriosclerosis and arterial thrombosis in the lower limb; roentgenological study. *Acta Radiol Suppl.* 1950;80:1-80.
93. Beregi JP, Louvegny S, Gautier C, et al. Fibromuscular dysplasia of the renal arteries: comparison of helical CT angiography and arteriography. *AJR Am J Roentgenol.* 2006;172:27-34.
94. Sabharwal R, Vladica P, Coleman P. Multidetector spiral CT renal angiography in the diagnosis of renal artery fibromuscular dysplasia. *Eur J Radiol.* 2007;61(3):520-527.
95. Lindsay, et al. Disease of the aorta. In: Hurst, et al., eds. *The Heart.* 7th ed. New York: McGraw-Hill; 1990:1411-1414.
96. Louridas G, Reilly K, Perry MO. The role of the aortic aneurysm diameter aortic diameter ratio in predicting the risk of rupture. *S Afr Med J.* 1990;78:642-643.
97. Siegel CL, Cohan RH. CT of abdominal aortic aneurysms. *AJR Am J Roentgenol.* 1994;163:17-29.
98. Garb M. The CT appearances of ruptured abdominal aortic aneurysm. *Australas Radiol.* 1989;33:154-156.
99. Johnson WC, Gale ME, Gerzof SG, Robbin AH, Nabseth DC. The role of computed tomography in symptomatic aortic aneurysms. *Surg Gynecol Obstet.* 1986;162:49-53.
100. Kreel L. Leaking aortic aneurysm. *Postgrad Med J.* 1987;63:107-109.
101. Siegel CL, Cohan RH, Korobkin M, Alpern MB, Courneya DL, Leder RA. Abdominal aortic aneurysm morphology: CT features in patients with ruptured and nonruptured aneurysms. *AJR Am J Roentgenol.* 1994;163:1123-1129.
102. Arita T, Matsunaga N, Takano K, et al., Abdominal aortic aneurysm: rupture associated with the high-attenuating crescent sign. *Radiology.* 1997;204:765-768.
103. Morehouse HT, Hochstztein JG, Lonwie W, et al. Pitfalls in the CT diagnosis of ruptured abdominal aortic aneurysm (abstr). *Radiology.* 1992;185:181.
104. Marston WA, Ahlquist R, Johnson G Jr, Meyer AA. Misdiagnosis of ruptured abdominal aortic aneurysms. *J Vasc Surg.* 1992;16:17-22.
105. Slovut DP, Olin JW. Fibromuscular dysplasia. *N Engl J Med.* 2004;350:1862-1871.
106. Joyce JW, Fairbairn JF 2nd, Kincaid OW, Juergen JL. Aneurysms of the thoracic aorta: a clinical study with special reference to prognosis. *Circulation.* 1964;29:176-181.
107. Lehto S, Niskanen L, Suhonen M, Rönnemaa T, Laakso M. A neglected harbinger of cardiovascular complications in non-insulin- dependent diabetes mellitus. *Arterioscler Thromb Vasc Biol.* 1996;16:978-983.
108. Glagov S, Weisenberg E, Zarins CK, Stankunavicius R, Kolettis GJ. Compensatory enlargement of human atherosclerotic coronary arteries. *N Engl J Med.* 1987;316:1371-1375.
109. Safian RD, Textor SC. Renal-artery stenosis. *N Engl J Med.* 2001;344:431-442.
110. Tilson, et al. The abdominal aortic aneurysm. *Ann NY Acad Sci.* 1996;80:1-298.
111. Pennel RC, Hollier LH, Lie JT, et al. Inflammatory abdominal aortic aneurysms: a thirty year review. *J Vasc Surg.* 1985;2:859-869.
112. Leseche G, Schaetz A, Arrive L, Nussaume O, Andreassian B. Diagnosis and management of 17 consecutive patients with inflammatory abdominal aortic aneurysm. *Am J Surg.* 1992;164:39-44.
113. Busuttil RW, Rinderbriecht H, Flesher A, Carmack C. Elastase activity: the role of elastase in aortic aneurysm formation. *J Surg Res.* 1982;32:214-217.
114. Brown SL, Backstrom B, Busuttil RW. A new serum proteolytic enzyme in aneurysm pathogenesis. *J Vasc Surg.* 1985;2:393-399.
115. Cannon DJ, Read RC. Blood elastolytic activity in patients with aortic aneurysm. *Ann Thorac Surg.* 1982;34:10-15.
116. Nicod P, Bloor C. Collagen types and matrix protein content in human abdominal aortic aneurysm. *J Am Coll Cardiol.* 1989;13:811-819.
117. Rizzo RJ, McCarthy WJ, Dixit SN, et al. Collagen types and matrix protein content in human abdominal aortic aneurysms. *J Vasc Surg.* 1989;10:365-373.
118. Sasaki S, Yasuda K, Takigami K, Yamauchi H, Shiiya N, Sakuma M. Inflammatory abdominal aortic aneurysms and atherosclerotic abdominal aortic aneurysms—comparisons of clinical features and long-term results. *Jpn Circ J.* 1997;61(3):231-235.

119. Crawford JL, Stowe CL, Safi HJ, Hallman CH, Crawford ES. Inflammatory aneurysms of the aorta. *J Vasc Surg.* 1985;2:113-124.
120. Gans RO, Hoorntje SJ, Rauwerda JA, Luth WJ, van Hattum LA, Donker AJ. The inflammatory abdominal aortic aneurysm. Prevalence, clinical features and diagnostic evaluation. *Neth J Med.* 1993;43:105-115.
121. Seltzer SE, D'Orsi C, Kirshner R, DeWeese JA. Traumatic aortic rupture: plain radiographic findings. *AJR Am J Roentgenol.* 1981;137:1011-1014.
122. Arrive L, Corréas JM, Lesèche G, Ghebontni L, Tubiana JM. Inflammatory aneurysms of the abdominal aorta: CT findings. *AJR Am J Roentgenol.* 1995;165:1481-1484.
123. Cullenward MJ, Scanlan KA, Pozniak MA, Acher CA., Inflammatory aortic aneurysm (periaortic fibrosis): radiologic imaging. *Radiology.* 1986;159:75-82.
124. Baskerville PA, Blakeney CG, Young AE, Browse NL. The diagnosis and treatment of periaortic fibrosis ("inflmmatory" aneurysm). *AJR Am J Roentgenol.* 1983;70:381-385.
125. Worrell JT, Buja LM, Reynolds RC. Pneumococcal aortitis with rupture of the aorta. Report of a case and review of the literature. *Am J Clin Pathol.* 1988;89:565-568.
126. Carreras M, Larena JA, Tabernero G, Langara E, Pena JM. Evolution of salmonella aortitis towards the formation of abdominal aneurysm. *Eur Radiol.* 1997;7:54-56.
127. Huppertz HI, Sandhage K. Reactive arthritis due to Salmonella enteritidis complicated by carditis. *Acta Paediatr.,* 1994;83:1230-1231.
128. Oz MC, McNicholas KW, Serra AJ, Spagna PM, Lemole GM. Review of Salmonella mycotic aneurysms of the thoracic aorta. *J Cardiovasc Surg.* 1989;30:99-103.
129. Moneta GL, Taylor LM Jr, Yeager RA, et al. Surgical treatment of infected aortic aneurysm. *Am J Surg.* 1998;175(5):396-399.
130. Gonda RL Jr, Gutierrez OH, Azodo MV. Mycotic aneurysms of the aorta: radiologic features. *Radiology.* 1988;168:343-346.
131. Shetty PC, Krasicky GA, Sharma RP, Vemuri BR, Burke MM. Mycotic aneurysms in intravenous drug abusers: the utility of digital substraction angiography. *Radiology.* 1985;155:319-321.
132. Johansen K, Devin J. Mycotic aortic aneurysms: a reappraisal. *Arch Surg.* 1983;118:583-588.
133. Oderich GS, Panneton JM, Bower TC, et al. Infected aortic aneurysms: aggressive presentation, complicated early outcome, but durable results. *J Vasc Surg.* 2001;34(5):900-908.
134. Tsao JW, Marder SR, Goldstone J, Bloom AI. Presentation, diagnosis, and management of arterial mycotic pseudoaneurysms in injection drug users. *Ann Vasc Surg.* 2002;16(5):652-662.
135. Fillmore AJ, Valentine RJ. Surgical mortality in patients with infected aortic aneurysms. *J Am Coll Surg.* 2003;196(3):435-441.
136. Mendelowitz DS, Ramstedt R, Yao JS, Bergan JJ. Abdominal aortic salmonellosis. *Surgery.* 1979;85:514-519.
137. Parellada JA, Palmer J, Monill JM, Zidan A, Giménez AM, Moreno A. Mycotic aneurysm of the abdominal aorta: CT findings in three patients. *Abdom Imaging.* 1997;22(3):321-324.
138. Creasy JD, Chiles C, Routh WD, Dyer RB. Overview of traumatic injury of the thoracic aorta. *Radiographics.* 1997;17:27-45.
139. Parmley LF, Mattingly TW, Manion WC, Jahnke EJ Jr. Nonpenetrating traumatic injury of the aorta. *Circulation.* 1958;17:1086-1101.
140. Lundevall J. The mechanism of traumatic rupture of the aorta. *Acta Pathol Microbiol Scand.* 1964;62:34-46.
141. Clark DE, Zeiger MA, Wallace KL, Packard AB, Nowicki ER. Blunt aortic trauma: signs of high risk. *J Trauma.* 1990;30:701-705.
142. Crowley RA, Turney SZ, Hankins JR, Rodriguez A, Attar S, Shankar BS. Rupture of thoracic aorta caused by blunt trauma: a fifteen year experience. *J Thorac Cardiovasc Surg.* 1990;100:652-660.
143. Kirsh MM, Behrendt DM, Orringer MB, et al. The treatment of acute traumatic rupture of the aorta: a 10 year experience. *Ann Surg.* 1976;184:308-315.
144. Groskin SA. Selected topics in chest trauma. *Radiology.* 1992; 183:605-617.
145. Gavant ML, Flick P, Menke P, Gold RE. CT aortography of thoracic aortic rupture. *AJR Am J Roentgenol.* 1996;166:955-961.
146. Gavant ML, Menke PG, Fabian T, Flick PA, Graney MJ, Gold RE. Blunt traumatic aortic rupture: detection with helical CT of the chest. *Radiology.* 1995;197:125-133.
147. Sharma S, Rajani M, Kamalakar T, Kumar A, Talwar KK. The association between aneurysm formation and systemic hypertension in Takayasu's arteritis. *Clin Radiol.* 1990;42:182-187.
148. Kumar S, Subramanyan R, Mandalam KR, et al. Aneurysmal form of aortoarteritis (Takayasu's disease): analysis of thirty cases. *Clin Radiol.* 1990;42:342-347.
149. Pipinos II, Carr JA, Haithcock BE, et al. Secondary Aortoenteric Fistula. *Ann Vasc Surg.* 2000;14:688-696.
150. Castañer E, Gallardo X, Ballesteros E, et al. CT diagnosis of chronic pulmonary thromboembolism. *Radiographics.* 2009;29:31-50.
151. Glazer GM, Callen PW, Parker JJ. CT diagnosis of tumor thrombus in the inferior vena cava: avoiding the false-positive diagnosis. *AJR Am J Roentgenol.* 1981;137(6):1265-1267.
152. Vu QD, Menias CO, Bhalla S, Peterson C, Wang LL, Balfe DM. Aortoenteric fistulas: CT features and potential mimics. *Radiographics.* 2009;29:197-209.
153. Garg K, Mao J. Deep venous thrombosis: spectrum of findings and pitfalls in interpretation on CT venography. AJR *Am J Roentgenol.* 2001;177:319-323.
154. Godfrey M. The Marfan syndrome. In: Beighton P, ed. *McKusick's Heritable Disorders of Connective Tissue.* 5th ed. St. Louis, MO: Mosby-Year Book; 1993:51-135.
155. Lee B, Godfrey M, Vitale E, et al. Linkage of Marfan syndrome and a phenotypically related disorder to two different fibrillin genes. *Nature.* 1991;352:330-334.
156. Dietz HC, Cutting GR, Pyeritz RE, et al. Marfan syndrome caused by a recurrent de novo missense mutation in the fibrillin gene. *Nature.* 1991;352:337-339.
157. Milewicz DM, Pyeritz RE, Crawford ES, Byers PH. Marfan syndrome: defective synthesis, secretion and extracellular matrix formation of fibrillin by cultured dermal fibroblasts. *J Clin Invest.* 1992;89:79-86.
158. Tsipouras P, Del Mastro R, Sarfarazi M, et al. Genetic linkage of the Marfan syndrome, ectopia lentis and congenital contractural arachnodactyly to the fibrillin genes on chromosomes 15 and 5. *N Engl J Med.* 1992;326:905-909.
159. Dietz HC, Saraiva JM, Pyeritz RE, Cutting GR, Francomano CA. Clustering of fibrillin (FBN1) missense mutations in Marfan syndrome patients at cysteine residues in EGF like domains. *Hum Mutat.* 1992;1:366-374.

160. Dietz HC, McIntosh I, Sakai LY, et al. Four novel FBN1 mutations: significance for mutant transcript level and EGF like domain calcium binding in the pathogenesis of Marfan syndrome. *Genomics.* 1993;17:468-475.

161. Sakai LY, Keene DR, Engvall E. Fibrillin, a new 350-kD glycoprotein is a component of extracellular microfibrils. *J Cell Biol.* 1986;103:2499-2509.

162. Claeary EG. The microfibrillar component of the elastic fibers: morphology and biochemistry. In: Uitto, et al., eds. *Connective Tissue Disease: Molecular Pathology of the Extracellular Matrix.* New York: Dekker; 1987:55-81.

163. Godfrey M, Nejezchleb PA, Schaefer GB, Minion DJ, Wang Y, Baxter BT. Elastin and fibrillin mRNA and protein levels in the ontogeny of normal human aorta. *Connect Tissue Res.* 1993;29:61-69.

164. Lester, et al. Cardiovascular Effects of Systemic Diseases and Conditions, Chapter 16. In: *Cardiovascular Pathology, 3rd edition,* Silver MD, Gotlieb AI, Schoen FJ, eds. *Cardiovascular Pathology.* 3rd ed. Philadelphia, PA: Churchill Livingstone; 2001:493-540.

165. Kincaid OW, Davis GD, Hallermann FJ, Hunt JC. Fibromuscular dysplasia of the renal arteries: arteriographic features, classification, and observations on natural history of the disease. *Am J Roentgenol Radium Ther Nucl Med.* 1968;104:271-282.

166. Schreiber MJ, Pohl MA, Novick AC. The natural history of atherosclerotic and fibrous renal artery disease. *AJR Am J Roentgenol.* 1984;172:27-34.

167. Willoteaux S, Faivre-Pierret M, Moranne O, et al. Fibromuscular dysplasia of the main renal arteries: comparison of contrast-enhanced MR angiography with digital subtraction angiography. *Radiology.* 2006;241:922-929.

168. Loeys BL, Schwarze U, Holm T, et al. Aneurysm syndromes caused by mutations in the TGF-beta receptor. *N Engl J Med.* 2006;355(8):788-798.

169. Kazerooni EA, Bree RL, Williams DM. Penetrating atherosclerotic ulcers of the descending thoracic aorta: evaluation with CT and distinction from aortic dissection. *Radiology.* 1992;183:759-765.

170. Stanson AW, Kazmier FJ, Hollier LH, et al. Penetrating atherosclerotic ulcers of the thoracic aorta: natural history and clinicopathological correlations. *Ann Vas Surg.* 1986;1:15-23.

171. Hayashi H, Matsuoka Y, Sakamoto I, et al. Penetrating atherosclerotic ulcer of the aorta: imaging features and disease concept. *Radiographics.* 2000;20:995-1005.

172. Vilacosta I, San Román JA, Aragoncillo P, et al. Penetrating atherosclerotic ulcer: documentation by transesophageal echocardiography. *J Am Coll Cardiol.* 1998;32:83-89.

173. Coady MA, Rizzo JA, Hammond GL, Pierce JG, Kopf GS, Elefteriades JA. Penetrating ulcer of the thoracic aorta: what is it? How do we recognize it? How do we manage it? *J Vasc Surg.* 1998;27:1006-1015.

174. Harris JA, Bis KG, Glover JL. Penetrating atherosclerotic ulcers of the aorta. *J Vasc Surg.* 1994;19:90-98.

175. Sorensen HR, Olsen H. Ruptured and dissecting aneurysms of the aorta. *Acta Chir Scand.* 1964;128:644-650.

176. Larson EW, Edwards WD. Risk factors for aortic dissection: a necropsy study of 161 cases. *Am J Cardiol.* 1984;53:849-855.

177. Wheat MW. Pathogenesis of aortic dissection. In: Doroghazi, et al., eds. *Aortic dissection.* New York: McGraw-Hill; 1983:55-70.

178. Schlatmann TJ, Becker AE. Pathogenesis of dissecting aneurysm of aorta. *Am J Cardiol.* 1977;39:21-26.

179. Anagnostopoulos CE. *Acute aortic dissections.* Baltimore: University Press; 1975:76-100.

180. Wilson SK, Hutchins GM.et al. Aortic dissecting aneurysms: causative factors in 204 subjects. *Arch Pathol Lab Med.* 1982; 106:175-180.

181. Gore I, Hirst AE Jr. Dissecting aneurysm of the aorta. *Cardiovasc Cl.* 1973;2:103-111.

182. Gore I. Pathogenesis of dissecting aneurysm of the aorta. *Arch Pathol.* 1952;53:142-153.

183. Hirst AE Jr, Johns VJ Jr, Kime SW Jr. Dissecting aneurysm of the aorta: a review of 505 cases. *Medicine.* 1958;37:217-279.

184. Fisher ER, Stern EJ, Godwin JD 2nd, Otto CM, Johnson JA. Acute aortic dissection: typical and atypical imaging features. *Radiographics.* 1994;14:1263-1271.

185. Wolff KA, Herold CJ, Tempany CM, Parravano JG, Zerhouni EA. Aortic dissection: atypical patterns seen at MR imaging. *Radiology.* 1991;181:489-495.

186. Daily PO, Trueblood HW, Stinson EB, Wuerflein RD, Shumway NE. Management of acute aortic dissections. *Ann Thorac Surg.* 1970;10:237-247.

187. DeBakey ME, Cooley DA, Creech O Jr. Surgical considerations of dissecting aneurysm of the aorta. *Ann Surg.* 1955;142:586-610.

188. Miller DC. Surgical management of aortic dissections: indications, perioperative management and long-term results. In: Doroghazi, et al., eds. *Aortic Dissection.* New York: McGraw Hill; 1983:193-243.

189. Crawford ES, Svensson LG, Coselli JS, Safi HJ, Hess KR. Aortic dissection and dissecting aortic aneurysms. *Ann Surg.* 1988;208:254-273.

190. Wheat MW Jr. Acute dissection of the aorta. *Cardiovasc Clin.* 1987;17:241-262.

191. Reul GJ, Cooley DA, Hallman GL, Reddy SB, Kyger ER 3rd, Wukasch DC. Dissecting aneurysm of the descending aorta. *Arch Surg.* 1975;110:632-640.

192. Eagle KA, DeSanctis RW. Aortic dissection. *Curr Probl Cardiol.* 1989;14:225-278.

193. Crawford ES. The diagnosis and management of aortic dissection. *J Am Med Assoc.* 1990;264:2537-2541.

194. Wheat MW Jr. Acute dissecting aneurysms of the aorta: diagnosis and treatment—1979. *Am Heart J.* 1980;99:373-387.

195. DeSanctis RW, Doroghazi RM, Austen WG, Buckley MJ. Aortic dissection. *N Engl J Med.* 1987;317:1060-1067.

196. Petasnick JP. Radiologic Evaluation of Aortic Dissection. *Radiology.* 1991;180:297-305.

197. Stein HL, Steinberg I. Selective aortography, the definitive technique for diagnosis of dissecting aneurysm of the aorta. *AJR Am J Roentgenol Radium Ther Nucl Med.* 1968;102:333-348.

198. Dinsmore RE, Rourke JA, DeSanctis RD, Harthorne JW, Austen WG. Angiographic findings in dissecting aortic aneurysm. *N Engl J Med.* 1966;275:1152-1157.

199. Luker GD, Glazer HS, Eagar G, Gutierrez FR, Sagel SS. Aortic dissection: effect of prospective chest radiographic diagnosis on delay to definitive diagnosis. *Radiology.* 1994;193:813-819.

200. Nienaber CA, von Kodolitsch Y, Nicolas V, et al. The diagnosis of thoracic aortic dissection by noninvasive imaging procedures. *N Engl J Med.* 1993;328:1-10.

201. Sommer T, Fehske W, Holzknecht N, et al. Aortic dissection: a comparative study of diagnosis with spiral CT, multiplanar transesophageal echocardiography and MR imaging. *Radiology.* 1996;199:347-352.

202. Cigarroa JE, Isselbacher EM, DeSanctis RW, Eagle KA. Diagnostic imaging in the evaluation of suspected aortic dissection. *N Engl J Med.* 1993;328:35-43.

203. Gross SC, Barr I, Eyler WR, Khaja F, Goldstein S. Computed tomography in dissection of the thoracic aorta. *Radiology.* 1980; 136:135-139.

204. Egan TJ, Neiman HL, Herman RJ, Malave SR, Sanders JH. Computed tomography in the diagnosis of aortic aneurysm dissection or tramatic injury. *Radiology.* 1980;136:141-146.

205. Lardé D, Belloir C, Vasile N, Frija J, Ferrané J. Computed tomography of aortic dissection. *Radiology.* 1980;136:147-151.

206. Moncada R, Salinas M, Churchill R, et al. Diagnosis of dissecting aortic aneurysm by computed tomography. *Lancet.* 1981;1:238-241.

207. Thorsen MK, San Dretto MA, Lawson TL, Foley WD, Smith DF, Berland LL. Dissecting aortic aneurysms: accuracy of computed tomographic diagnosis. *Radiology.* 1983;148:773-777.

208. Godwin JD, Herfkens RL, Skiöldebrand CG, Federle MP, Lipton MJ. Evaluation of dissections and aneurysms of the thoracic aorta by conventional and dynamic CT scanning. *Radiology.* 1980;136:125-133.

209. Demos TC, Posniak HV, Marsan RE. CT of aortic dissection. *Semin Roentgenol.* 1989;24:22-37.

210. Cavaye DM, French WJ, White RA, et al. Intravascular ultrasound imaging of an acute dissecting aortic aneurysm: a case report. *J Vasc Surg.* 1991;13:510-512.

211. Deutsch HJ, Sechtem U, Meyer H, Theissen P, Schicha H, Erdmann E. Chronic aortic dissection: comparison of MR imaging and transesophageal echocardiography. *Radiology.* 1994;192:645-650.

212. Gauber JY, Moulin G, Mesana T, et al. Type A dissection of the thoracic aorta: use of MR imaging for long-term follow-up. *Radiology.* 1995;196:363-369.

213. Orwig D, Federle MP. Localized clotted blood as evidence of visceral trauma on CT: the sentinel clot sign. AJR *Am J Roentgenol.* 1989;153(4):747-749.

214. Hamilton JD, Kumaravel M, Censullo ML, Cohen AM, Kievlan DS, West OC. Multidetector CT evaluation of active extravasation in blunt abdominal and pelvic trauma patients. *Radiographics.* 2008;28:1603-1616.

215. Didier D, Racle A, Etievent JP, Weill F. Tumor thrombus of the inferior vena cava secondary to malignant abdominal neoplasms: US and CT evaluation. *Radiology.* 1987;162(1):83-89.

216. Youngberg SP, Sheps SG, Strong CG. Fibromuscular disease of the renal arteries. *Med Clin North Am.* 1977;61:623-641.

217. Singh K, Bønaa KH, Jacobsen BK, Bjørk L, Solberg S. Prevalence of and risk factors for abdominal aortic aneurysms in a population-based study. *Tromsø J Epidemiol.* 2001;154: 236-244.

218. Golledge J, Norman PE. Pathophysiology of abdominal aortic aneurysm relevant to improvements in patients' management. *Cardiology.* 2009;24:532-538.

219. Golledge J, Muller J, Daugherty A, Norman P. Abdominal aortic aneurysm: pathogenesis and implications for management. *Arterioscler Thromb Vasc Biol.* 2006;26:2605-2613.

220. Johnsen SH, Forsdahl SH, Singh K, Jacobsen BK. Atherosclerosis in abdominal aortic aneurysms: a causal event or a process running in parallel. *Arterioscler Thromb Vasc Biol.* 2010;30:1263-1268.

221. Lumsden AB, Salam TA, Walton KG. Renal artery aneurysm: a report of 28 cases. *Cardiovasc Surg.* 1996;4(2):185-189.

222. Golledge J, Norman PE. Atherosclerosis and abdominal aortic aneurysm cause, response, or common risk factors? *Arterioscler Thromb Vasc Biol.* 2010;30:1075-1077.

223. Nosher JL, Trooskin SZ, Amorosa JK. Occlusion of a hepatic arterial aneurysm with gianturco coils in a patient with the Ehlers-Danlos syndrome. *Am J Surg.* 1986;152(3):326-328.

224. Crow P, Shaw E, Earnshaw JJ, Poskitt KR, Whyman MR, Heather BP. A single normal ultrasonographic scan at age 65 years rules out significant aneurysm disease for life in men. *Br J Surg.* 2001;88:941-944.

225. Scott RA, Vardulaki KA, Walker NM, Day NE, Duffy SW, Ashton HA. The long-term benefits of a single scan for abdominal aortic aneurysm (AAA) at age 65. *Eur J Vasc Endovasc Surg.* 2001;21:535-540.

226. Bade MA, Queral LA, Mukherjee D, Kong LS. Endovascular abdominal aortic aneurysm repair in a patient with Ehlers-Danlos syndrome. *J Vasc Surg.* 2007;46(2):360-362.

227. Bloom SL, Uppot R, Roberts DJ. Case 32-2010: a pregnant woman with abdominal pain and fluid in the peritoneal cavity. *N Engl J Med.* 2010;363:1657-1665.

228. Mohammadi A, Ghasemi-Rad M, Mladkova N, Masudi S. Varicocele and nutcracker syndrome: sonographic findings. *J Ultrasound Med.* 2010;29:1153-1160.

229. May R, Thurner J. The cause of the predominately sinistral occurrence of thrombosis of the pelvic veins. *Angiology.* 1957;8: 419-427.

Index

Page references followed by *f* indicate figures; followed by *t* indicate tables and followed by *n* indicate notes.

B

D

H

M

S